REPTILE
Medicine
and Surgery

Second Edition

REPTILE
Medicine
and Surgery

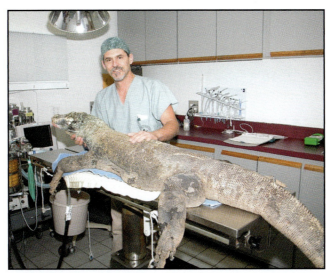

(Photograph courtesy of S. Monier, Miami Metro Zoo)

Douglas R. Mader, MS, DVM, DABVP
Diplomate, American Board of Veterinary
Practitioners (CA)
Fellow, Royal Society of Medicine
Marathon Veterinary Hospital
Marathon, Florida

With 72 Contributing Authors

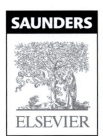

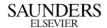

11830 Westline Industrial Drive
St. Louis, Missouri 63146

REPTILE MEDICINE AND SURGERY

ISBN-13: 978-0-7216-9327-9
ISBN-10: 0-7216-9327-X

Copyright © 2006, 1996 by Elsevier Inc.

All rights reserved. No part of this publication may be reproduced or transmitted in any form or by any means, electronic or mechanical, including photocopying, recording, or any information storage and retrieval system, without permission in writing from the publisher.

Permissions may be sought directly from Elsevier's Health Sciences Rights Department in Philadelphia, PA, USA: phone: (+1) 215 239 3804, fax: (+1) 215 239 3805, e-mail: healthpermissions@elsevier.com. You may also complete your request on-line via the Elsevier homepage (http://www.elsevier.com), by selecting 'Customer Support' and then 'Obtaining Permissions'.

Notice

Knowledge and best practice in this field are constantly changing. As new research and experience broaden our knowledge, changes in practice, treatment and drug therapy may become necessary or appropriate. Readers are advised to check the most current information provided (i) on procedures featured or (ii) by the manufacturer of each product to be administered, to verify the recommended dose or formula, the method and duration of administration, and contraindications. It is the responsibility of the practitioner, relying on their own experience and knowledge of the patient, to make diagnoses, to determine dosages and the best treatment for each individual patient, and to take all appropriate safety precautions. To the fullest extent of the law, neither the Publisher nor the Author assume any liability for any injury and/or damage to persons or property arising out or related to any use of the material contained in this book.

The Publisher

ISBN-13: 978-0-7216-9327-9
ISBN-10: 0-7216-9327-X

Publishing Director: Linda Duncan
Acquisitions Editor: Penny Rudolph
Developmental Editor: Shelly Stringer
Publishing Services Manager: Patricia Tannian
Project Manager: Sarah Wunderly
Cover Designer: Paula Ruckenbrod
Text Designer: Paula Ruckenbrod

Printed in Canada

Last digit is the print number: 9 8 7 6 5 4 3

Working together to grow libraries in developing countries

www.elsevier.com | www.bookaid.org | www.sabre.org

ELSEVIER | BOOK AID International | Sabre Foundation

*This book,
with all of the hours and effort that went into it,
is dedicated, with even more emotion,
to my wonderful wife, Gerry.
Ich liebe Dich*

CONTRIBUTORS

Stephen L. Barten, DVM
Vernon Hills Animal Hospital
Mundelein, Illinois
Reference Sources for Reptile Clinicians
Lizards (Biology)
Lizards (Differential Diagnoses by Symptoms)
Bites from Prey
Penile Prolapse
Shell Damage

R. Avery Bennett, DVM, MS, DACVS
Staff Surgeon
Bay Area Veterinary Specialists
San Leandro, California
Neurology
Surgery (Soft Tissue and Orthopedics)
Cloacal Prolapse
Upper Alimentary Tract Disease

Barbara Blanchard, M.Sc. (Zoology)
Animal Registrar/Librarian and Captive Management
Co-ordinator for Tuatara
Life Sciences
Wellington Zoo Trust
Wellington, New Zealand
Biology, Captive Management, and Medical Care of Tuatara

Wayne Boardman, B.Vet.Med., MRCVS., MACVSc
Associate Lecturer
Royal Veterinary College
London, United Kingdom
Head of Veterinary Services
Zoological Society of London
London, United Kingdom
Biology, Captive Management, and Medical Care of Tuatara

Donal M. Boyer
Curator of Herpetology
Reptile Department
San Diego Zoo
San Diego, California
Turtles, Tortoises, and Terrapins (Biology)

Thomas H. Boyer, DVM
Owner, Pet Hospital of Penasquitos
Editor-in-Chief, *Journal of Herpetological Medicine and Surgery*
San Diego, California
Turtles, Tortoise and Terrapins (Biology)
Turtles, Tortoise and Terrapins (Differential Diagnosis by Symptoms)
Hypovitaminosis A and Hypervitaminosis A

Ellen Bronson, Med.vet
Veterinary Resident
Department of Animal Health
Smithsonian National Zoological Park
Washington, District of Columbia
Paramyxovirus

Daniel R. Brown, B.S., M.S., PhD
Assistant Professor
Department of Pathobiology
College of Veterinary Medicine
University of Florida
Gainesville, Florida
Upper Respiratory Tract Disease (Mycoplasmosis) in Tortoises

Mary B. Brown, MS, PhD
Professor
Department of Pathobiology
College of Veterinary Medicine
University of Florida
Gainesville, Florida
Upper Respiratory Tract Disease (Mycoplasmosis) in Tortoises

Terry W. Campbell, MS, DVM, PhD
Associate Professor
Department of Clinical Sciences
College of Veterinary Medicine and Biomedical Sciences
Fort Collins, Colorado
Clinical Pathology of Reptiles
Hemoparasites

Professor John E. Cooper, DTVM, FRCPath, FIBiol, FRCVS, DECVP
Professor of Pathology
Veterinary Pathology
School of Veterinary Medicine
University of the West Indies (UWI)
St. Augustine, Trinidad and Tobago
Visiting Professor
Wild Animal and Resource Management
Faculty of Veterinary Medicine
Makerere University, Uganda, East Africa
Dermatology
Hepatic Lipidosis

Contributors

Margaret E. Cooper, LLB FLS
Guest Lecturer
University of the West Indies
St. Augustine, Trinidad and Tobago
Visiting Lecturer
Wild Animal and Resource Management
Makerere University
Kampala, Uganda, East Africa
Reptile Laws and Regulations: European

Michael R. Cranfield, DVM
Faculty
Comparative Department Medicine
Johns Hopkins School of Medicine
Baltimore, Maryland
Adjunct Assistant Professor
Maryland Regional Veterinary College
University of Maryland Medicine
College Park, Maryland
Adjunct Faculty
College of Forest Research
Mississippi State University
Starkville, Mississippi
Director of Animal Management and Research and Conservation
Medical Department
Maryland Zoo in Baltimore
Baltimore, Maryland
Director of the Mountain Gorilla Veterinary Project
Medical Department
Maryland Zoo in Baltimore
Baltimore, Maryland
Cryptosporidiosis
Paramyxovirus

Dale DeNardo, DVM, PhD
University Veterinarian and Assistant Professor
School of Life Sciences
Arizona State University
Tempe, Arizona
Stress in Captive Reptiles
Reproductive Biology
Dystocias

Lisa B. Done, DVM, MPVM
Veterinarian
California Wildlife Center
Calabasas, California
Oncology
Neurologic Disorders

Geraldine Diethelm, Dr.vet.med
Chief of Staff
Marathon Veterinary Hospital
Marathon, Florida
Digit Abnormalities
Hematologic and Blood Chemistry Values in Reptiles
Reptile Formulary

Orlando Diaz-Figueroa, DVM, MS
Affiliated Veterinary Specialists
Maitland, Florida
Gastrointestinal Anatomy and Physiology

Susan Donoghue, MS, DMD, DACVN
Owner
Nutrition Support Services, Inc.
Pembroke, Virgina
Nutrition

Bruce Ferguson, DVM, MS (Animal Behavior)
Instructor
TCVM Acupuncture, Herbal Medicine and Tui Na
Chi Institute of Chinese Medicine
Reddick, Florida
Alternative and Complementary Veterinary Therapies

Kevin T. Fitzgerald PhD, DVM, DABVP (Canine/Feline)
Staff Veterinarian
Alameda East Veterinary Hospital
Denver, Colorado
Surgery (Biotelemetry)
Acariasis
Dysecdysis
Spinal Osteopathy
Reported Toxicities in Reptiles

Richard S. Funk, MA, DVM
Mesa Veterinary Hospital
Mesa, Arizona
Snakes (Biology)
Surgery (Venemoid)
Snakes (Differential Diagnoses by Symptoms)
Anorexia
Diarrhea
Tail Damage
Vomiting and Regurgitation
Reptile Formulary

Michael M. Garner, DVM, DACVP
President
Northwest ZooPath
Monroe, Washington
Overview of Biopsy and Necropsy Techniques

William H. Gehrmann, PhD
Professor of Biology
Department of Biology
Texas Christian University
Forth Worth, Texas
Artificial Lighting

Donald Scott Gillespie, DVM
Staff Veterinarian
Animal Health
Montgomery Zoo
Montgomery, Alabama
Lizards (section on Komodo Dragons)
Large Collections: Special Considerations

Contributors

Barry S. Gold, MD, FACP
Assistant Professor, Division of Emergency Medicine
Department of Surgery
School of Medicine
University of Maryland
Baltimore, Maryland
Associate Professor
Department of Medicine
School of Medicine
Johns Hopkins University
Baltimore, Maryland
Working with Venomous Species: Emergency Protocols

Ellis C. Greiner, PhD
Professor
Department of Pathology
College of Veterinary Medicine
University of Florida
Gainesville, Florida
Parasitology

Thaddeus K. Graczyk, M.Sc., PhD
Associate Professor
Department of Environmental Health Sciences and
Department of Molecular Microbiology and Immunology
Johns Hopkins Bloomberg School of Public Health
Baltimore, Maryland
Cryptosporidiosis

Stephen J. Hernandez-Divers, BVetMed, CBiol MIBiol, DZooMed, MRCVS, DACZM, RCVS Recognized Specialist in Zoo and Wildlife Medicine
Associate Professor
Exotic Animal, Wildlife and Zoological Medicine
Department of Small Animal Medicine and Surgery
College of Veterinary Medicine
University of Georgia
Athens, Georgia
Associate Editor, *Journal of Zoo & Wildlife Medicine*
Associate Editor, *Journal of Herpetological Medicine & Surgery*
Co-Director of the Veterinary Endoscopy Training Symposia
Department of Small Animal Medicine and Surgery
College of Veterinary Medicine
University of Georgia
Athens, Georgia
Diagnostic Techniques
Surgery (Laser and Radiosurgery)
Hepatic Lipidosis
Renal Disease in Reptiles: Diagnosis and Clinical Management
Appendix A
Appendix B

Peter Holz
Associate Veterinarian
Healesville Sanctuary
Healesville, Victoria, Australia
Renal Anatomy and Physiology

Charles J. Innis, VMD
Adjuct Professor
Department of Conservation Medicine
Cummings School of Veterinary Medicine
Tufts University
North Grafton, Massachusetts
Associate Veterinarian
Animal Health Department
New England Aquarium
Boston, Massachusetts
Renal Disease in Reptiles: Diagnosis and Clinical Management

Cathy A. Johnson-Delaney, BS, DVM, DABVP (Avian)
Consultant
Bird and Exotic Clinic of Seattle
Seattle, Washington
Associate
Exotic Pet and Bird Clinic
Kirkland, Washington
Medical Director
Washington Ferret Rescue and Shelter
Bothell, Washington
Attending Veterinarian
NW Zoological Supply/Terantulas.com
Edmonds, Washington
Reptile Zoonoses and Threats to Public Health

Gretchen Kaufman, DVM
Assistant Professor
Department of Environment and Population Health
Cummings School of Veterinary Medicine
Tufts University
North Grafton, Massachusetts
Allometric Scaling

Paul A. Klein, PhD
Professor Emeritus
Department of Pathology, Immunology, and Laboratory Medicine
College of Medicine
University of Florida
Gainesville, Florida
Upper Respiratory Tract Disease (Mycoplasmosis) in Tortoises

Thomas Lane, BS, DVM
Professor Emeritus College of Veterinary Medicine
Large Animal Clinical Sciences
College of Veterinary Medicine
University of Florida
Gainesville, Florida
Program Director
Department of Equine Science
International Equine School
Ocala, Florida
Crocodilians (Biology)

Martin P.C. Lawton, BVetMed, CertVOphthal, CertLAS, DZooMed, MIBiol, FRCVS
RCVS Specialist in Exotic Animal Medicine
Exotic Animal and Ophthalmic Referral Centre
England

Daniel T. Lewbart, JD, MSEL
Partner
Litigation
Gerolamo McNutly Divis & Lewbart, PC
Philadelphia, Pennsylvania
Reptile Laws and Regulations: American

Gregory A. Lewbart, MS, VMD, DACZM
Professor of Aquatic Medicine
Department of Clinical Sciences
North Carolina State University
College of Veterinary Medicine
Raleigh, North Carolina
Reptile Laws and Regulations: American

Brad A. Lock, DVM, DACZM
Adjunct Professor
Small Animal Medicine and Surgery (Exotic Animal, Wildlife and Zoological Medicine Service)
University of Georgia
Athens, Georgia
Assistant Curator
Herpetology
Zoo Atlanta
Atlanta, Georgia
Behavioral and Morphologic Adaptations

Douglas Mader, MS, DVM, DABVP, Fellow, Royal Society of Medicine
Co-owner
Marathon Veterinary Hospital
Staff Veterinarian
Marathon Sea Turtle Hospital
Key West Aquarium
Monroe County Animal Farm
Theater of the Sea
Florida Keys (Conch Republic), Florida
Adjunct Professor
School of Veterinary Medicine
Western University of the Health Sciences
Pomona, California
Understanding the Human-Reptile Relationship
Microbiology: Fungal and Bacterial Diseases of Reptiles
Parasitology
Perinatology
Emergency and Critical Care
Euthanasia
Surgery
Abscesses
Cloacal Prolapse
Calculi: Urinary
Gout
Metabolic Bone Diseases
Thermal Burns
Medical Care of Seaturtles (Medicine and Surgery)
Radiographic Anatomy

Bonnie S. Mader-Weidner, MS (Marriage, Family, Child Counseling and School Counseling)
Founder, Coordinator
The Pet Loss Support Hotline
Center for Animals in Society
School of Veterinary Medicine
University of California, Davis
Davis, California
Understanding the Human-Reptile Relationship

G. Neal Mauldin, DVM, DACVIM (Internal Medicine and Oncology), DACVR (Radiation Oncology)
Associate Professor of Veterinary Oncology
Veterinary Clinical Sciences
Louisiana State University
Baton Rouge, Louisiana
Oncology

Joerg Mayer, Dr.med.vet., M.Sc
Clinical Assistant Professor, Head of Exotics Service
Department of Clinical Service
Cummings School of Veterinary Medicine
Tufts University
North Grafton, Massachusetts
Allometric Scaling

Stephen J. Mehler, DVM
Small Animal Surgery Resident
Department of Clinical Studies
Matthew J. Ryan Veterinary Hospital
University of Pennsylvania
Philadelphia, Pennsylvania
Neurology
Upper Alimentary Tract Disease

Constance Merigo
Director of the Marine Mammal and Sea Turtle Stranding Program
Marine Animal Rescue and Rehabilitation
New England Aquarium
Boston, Massachusetts
Medical Care of Seaturtles (Medical Management of Cold-Stunned Seaturtles)

Mark A. Mitchell, DVM, MS, PhD
Associate Professor
Veterinary Clinical Sciences
Louisiana State University
Baton Rouge, Louisiana
Gastrointestinal Anatomy and Physiology
Therapuetics
Salmonella: Diagnostic Methods for Reptiles

Michael J. Murray, DVM
Staff Veterinarian
Monterey Bay Aquarium
Monterey, California
Cardiopulmonary Anatomy and Physiology
Cardiology
Aural Abscesses
Pneumonia

Contributors

Javier Nevarez, BS, DVM
Clinical Instructor
Veterinary Clinical Sciences
School of Veterinary Medicine
Louisiana State University
Baton Rouge, Louisiana
Contract Veterinarian
Louisiana Alligator Industry
Louisiana Department of Wildlife and Fisheries
Baton Rouge, Louisiana
Crocodilian Differential Diagnosis

Nancy O'Leary, DVM, CVA
Tufts University School of Veterinary Medicine
Grafton, Massachusetts
Certified Veterinary Acupuncturist
Chi Institute
Reddick, Florida
China National Society of TCVM
Bejing China
Alternative and Complementary Veterinary Therapies

Francesco C. Origgi, DVM, PhD
Scientist
Immumology and Infectious Diseases
San Raffaele Scientific Institute
Milano, Italy
Herpesvirus in Tortoises

Jean A. Paré, DVM, DVSc, DACVM
Assistant Professor
Special Species Health
Department of Surgical Sciences
School of Veterinary Medicine
University of Wisconsin
Madison, Wisconsin
Fungal Diseases of Reptiles

Lonny B. Pace, DVM
Resident
Advanced Critical Care and Internal Medicine
Tustin, California
Glossary

Mark Pokras, BS, DVM
Associate Professor and Director
Wildlife Clinic
Department of Environmental and Population Health
Cummings School of Veterinary Medicine
Tufts University
N. Grafton, Massachusetts
Allometric Scaling

Bran Ritchie, DVM, MS, PhD, DABVP
Interim Department Head and Professor
Department of Small Animal Medicine and Surgery
College of Veterinary Medicine
University of Georgia
Athens, Georgia
Virology

Karen L. Rosenthal, MS, DVM, DABVP (Avian)
University of Pennsylvania
School of Veterinary Medicine
Veterinary Hospital
Philadelphia, PA
Microbiology: Fungal and Bacterial Diseases of Reptiles

John V. Rossi, DVM, MA
Small/Exotic Animal Practitioner
Riverside Animal Hospital
Jacksonville, Florida
General Husbandry and Management

Elke Rudloff, DVM, DACVESS
Director of Education
Animal Emergency Center
Glendale, Wisconsin
Emergency and Critical Care

Juergen Schumacher, Dr.med.vet., DACZM
Associate Professor of Avian and Zoological Medicine
Department of Small Animal Clinical Sciences
College of Veterinary Medicine
The University of Tennessee
Knoxville, Tennessee
Anesthesia and Analgesia
Inclusion Body Disease Virus

Sam Silverman, DVM, PhD, DACVR
Clinical Professor
Department of Surgical and Radiological Science
University of California, Davis
Davis, California
Radiologist
Private Practice
Sausalito, California
Diagnostic Imaging

Lynne Sigler, M.Sc.
Professor and Curator
University of Alberta Microfungus Collection
and Herbarium
Devonian Botanic Garden and Medical Microbiology
and Immunology
Edmonton, Alberta, Canada
Microbiology: Fungal and Bacterial Diseases of Reptiles

Eileen Slomka-McFarland, LVT
Marathon Veterinary Hospital
Marathon, Florida
Disinfectants for the Vivarium

Scott J. Stahl, DVM, DABVP (Avian)
Stahl Exotic Animal Veterinary Services
Vienna, Virginia
Hyperglycemia in Reptiles

Geoff Stein, DVM
Studio City Animal Hospital
Studio City, California
Hematologic and Blood Chemistry Values in Reptiles

Contributors

Mark D. Stetter, DVM, DACZM
Veterinary Services Director
Disney's Animal Programs
Walt Disney World
Lake Buena Vista, Florida
Ultrasonography

Gregory W. Stoutenburgh
Aliso Viejo, California
Building a Successful Reptile Practice

W. Michael Taylor, DVM
Service Chief
Avian and Exotic Medicine
Veterinary Teaching Hospital
Ontario Veterinary College
University of Guelph
Guelph, Ontario, Canada
Endoscopy

E. Scott Weber III, MSc Aquatic Veterinary Sciences, VMD
Head Veterinarian and Research Associate
Animal Health Department
New England Aquarium
Boston, Massachusetts
Medical Care of Seaturtles (Medical Management of Cold-Stunned Seaturtles)

Jim Wellehan, DVM, MS, Dipl ACZM
Resident, Zoological Medicine
Small Animal Clinical Sciences
University of Florida
Gainesville, Florida
Understanding Diagnostic Testing

Lori D. Wendland, DVM
Assistant Scientist
Department of Pathobiology
University of Florida
Gainesville, Florida
Associate Veterinarian
Micanopy Animal Hospital
Micanopy, Florida
Upper Respiratory Tract Disease (Mycoplasmosis) in Tortoises

Brent R. Whitaker, MS, DVM
Research Associate Professor
Center of Marine Biotechnology
Baltimore, Maryland
Deputy Executive Director for Biological Programs
Biological Programs
National Aquarium in Baltimore
Baltimore, Maryland
Working with Venomous Species: Emergency Protocols

Kevin M. Wright, DVM
Associate Veterinarian
University Animal Hospital
Tempe, Arizona
Conservation Associate
National Aquarium in Baltimore
Baltimore, Maryland
Overview of Amphibian Medicine
Amphibian Formulary

Jeanette Wyneken, PhD
Assistant Professor
Department of Biological Sciences
Florida Atlantic University
Boca Raton, Florida
Medical Care of Seaturtles (Species Identification and Biology)
Computed Tomography and Magnetic Resonance Imaging

Rebecca Vera, AAS, CVT
Veterinary Technician
Alameda East Veterinary Hospital
Denver, Colorado
Surgery (Biotelemetry)
Acariasis
Dysecdysis
Spinal Osteopathy
Reported Toxicities in Reptiles

Trisha Yelen, BS
College of Veterinary Medicine
The University of Tennessee
Knoxville, Tennessee
Anesthesia and Analgesia

FOREWORD

It is an honor and a pleasure to write this foreword to the second edition of *Reptile Medicine and Surgery*. Dr. Douglas Mader, an outstanding practitioner, lecturer, and author, has assembled authorities in every aspect of reptilian medicine to write this book.

Veterinary care of reptiles uses the same diagnostic and therapeutic modalities as those for domestic animals, but significant differences in detail make this specialty unique. Being ectothermic, reptiles are dependent on the environment for control of body temperature and regulation of metabolism. However, reptiles are found in climates ranging from arctic to tropical, in deserts, meadows, swamps, jungles, and oceans. Species have adapted to these environments, and it is reasonable to presume that optimal care for them in captivity should mimic their natural ecology as much as possible. Veterinarians need to add that information to their database.

It is part of the art of veterinary medicine to interact positively with clients and understand what motivates people to own reptiles. The reasons can be trivial (curiosity, seeking status symbols), psychologic (machismo, counter-phobic), practical (wants a pet, but is allergic to birds and mammals), academic (professional biologist) or economic (breeders, pet stores). Clients should be encouraged to develop interest in the more serious aspects of keeping reptiles because that will result in greater commitment to veterinary care and better health for the animal.

Unique aspects of veterinary ethics apply in reptilian medicine. Many species are in danger of extinction through habitat loss, environmental pollution, and deliberate killing and hunting or collecting for food, leather, trinkets, or the pet trade. Veterinarians should support conservation efforts through legislation, participation in organizations, and personal example. They should not condone or support the trade in endangered species. They should become familiar with and be compliant with federal, state, and local laws regarding ownership and care of reptiles and other exotic animals.

Some reptiles are extraordinarily dangerous. Veterinarians should not put themselves, their staff, owners, or others at risk by interacting with these animals without reasonable assurance of safety to all concerned.

When I first became interested in reptilian medicine almost 50 years ago, very little information was available in veterinary curricula, journals, or textbooks. The few practitioners in the field gained knowledge from biologic literature and by empirical experience. Since then several texts on the subject have been published, relevant articles frequently appear in veterinary journals, significant time is devoted to reptiles at veterinary meetings, and there is an Association of Reptilian and Amphibian Veterinarians that currently has almost 200 members from several countries.

This text is a significant addition to the specialty of reptilian medicine, covering technical, ethical, business, public health, and safety aspects of the field. To Dr. Mader and his coauthors, congratulations on a job well done!

Leonard Marcus VMD, MD

PREFACE

If you're gonna talk the talk, you have to walk the walk.
Anonymous

Walk before you run.
A Different Anonymous

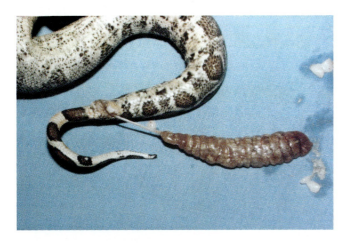

Boa constrictor with a prolapsed kidney.

According to me, Douglas Mader, MS, DVM, DABVP, snakes have the ability to "sense" when one of their kidneys is going bad, and, in a self-preserving purge, "spontaneously slough" the organ. Hence the phenomenon, "Spontaneous Kidney Sloughing."

Readers can readily confirm this by performing a quick Internet search using the term "Spontaneous Kidney Sloughing in Snakes."

It is amazing what knowledge we can gain by just a few simple keystrokes. It is also amazing what bad information is available to anyone, also with just a few simple keystrokes.

I think the biggest change that has occurred in the field of herpetologic medicine since the first edition of *Reptile Medicine and Surgery* is the advent of, and accessibility to, the Internet. No longer do you have to live near a big university to have access to a sophisticated library. Again, with just a few keystrokes, you can access journals, books, and other information and never leave your computer.

This edition of *Reptile Medicine and Surgery* refers to the Internet throughout. Readers are referred to many websites, portals to the world of herpetologic medicine through the guidance and direction of over 70 expert authors from around the globe. The Internet is constantly evolving, and keeping current on new websites will be a dynamic and worthwhile exercise. However, the information on each website should be scrutinized and carefully evaluated.

Having more than 70 authors contribute to a text is a wonderful thing. No one person can have the experience and knowledge to write a comprehensive book such as this. Putting together contributors from the best in the field creates pure synergy.

The reader of *Reptile Medicine and Surgery* will be able to look up information in this book and often find not one, but two or three viewpoints. As mentioned in the first edition, I don't necessarily agree with all the viewpoints—but that is what makes this text so great. One thing I have learned is that there is always someone out there who has more experience or knowledge than you do—all the more reason to have more than one opinion.

In some cases the reader may find the differences of opinion frustrating. I agree. As an editor, I did not always find clear-cut ways to handle this. Some contributors are adamant about using the term "Preferred Optimal Temperature Zone," and others find it scientifically unacceptable. Some like the term "Selected Temperature Zone" or "Preferred Optimal Temperature Range." I feel it is best to allow the contributors to use the terms with which they are most comfortable.

The Committee of Standard English and Scientific names has published new guidelines for the spelling and "naming" of all North American reptiles and amphibians. Effective in 2001, many of the old spellings have been changed; unfortunately, the publication has not been widely disseminated (Society for the Study of Amphibians and Reptiles [SAAR], Circular No. 29).

In some cases the name changes were subtle, such as capitalizing first and second common names (e.g., green iguana, became Green Iguana.) In other cases common names were both capitalized and combined; for instance garter snake became Gartersnake, corn snake became Cornsnake, loggerhead sea turtle became Loggerhead Seaturtle. In still other cases the change was slightly more complicated; for example, the hog nose snake became the Hog-nosed Snake.

For this textbook I made every effort to use these new spellings. Keep in mind that these recommended changes are for amphibians and reptiles in North America, not around the world. That posed two problems for me as an editor.

First, what do I do with the names of animals that are not North American in origin? I consulted several herpetologists and got many different opinions. Some thought it a travesty to change any of the names, some believed it would be appropriate to change only the North American names, and others felt it best to follow the guidelines as closely as possible and change them all in a similar fashion for the sake of consistency.

I followed the third approach. For instance, even though the bearded dragon is not a North American lizard, you will see that it is capitalized as Bearded Dragon in the text.

Now for the second problem. If I change the spelling and capitalization of the names in the text, what should I do with the names as they appear in the references? For instance, if Gartersnake is changed in the text of a chapter, how should it read in the reference—Gartersnake as written in the chapter, or garter snake as it appears in the title of the published document?

That was a tough call because it would appear inconsistent if I chose the latter option. However, I decided the proper thing to do was to leave the spelling as it originally stood in the published title in the references. If a person wanted to do a literature search, and the spelling of the subject was changed, the cybertrail would be lost.

I am sure there will be complaints about my decisions, but I believe we must make every effort to comply with scientific changes, whatever challenges they present. I take full responsibility for stretching the rules and applying them to species not included in the SSAR publication. As I said, I wanted to try and maintain some consistency in the written word.

Finally, and for the record, there is no such medical entity as Spontaneous Kidney Sloughing in Snakes. Many years ago I reported on a case of a neonatal Red Tailed Boa Constrictor that literally had its insides forced out by an overly aggressive pet store clerk whose diagnosis was that the animal had constipation. After the clerk squeezed and squeezed the snake's midsection, trying to get it to pass its fecal impaction, a funny tissue popped out of the cloaca, hanging tenuously by a tendril of tissue. In a flash of brilliance, although not exactly sure what he had done, the clerk recommended that the owner take the baby snake to a herp vet.

The tissue was the animal's kidney, and the tendril was its ureter. Hence the birth of Spontaneous Kidney Sloughing.

Douglas R. Mader, MS, DVM, DAVBP

ACKNOWLEDGMENTS

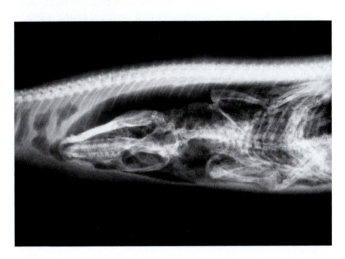

This is one of the few slides that survived Hurricane Georges. It is also one my all-time favorites. Animal Control brought a 12-foot-long Burmese Python to my hospital. It was found under a woman's house trailer—her cat was missing. Animal Control wanted me to check if the snake had eaten the woman's cat ....

On September 25, 1998, my life turned upside down. Hurricane Georges blew through the Conch Republic, blasting winds of 113 mph and pushing a tidal surge of 8 feet. Although the wind did little damage, the tides, the waves, and the surge washed away everything I owned, including approximately 20,000 slides and all of the teaching radiographs I had collected during my career.

But, you know what? It was just stuff. I was safe, thank God my wife was safe, and my pets were safe. That was really all I cared about.

Compared to the devastation along the Gulf Coast (after hurricanes Katrina and Rita) and the suffering in Indonesia and surrounding areas after the horrible tsunamis, I was blessed.

Even more so, I have the most wonderful colleagues, associates, friends, and family in the world.

Writing and editing a book like this does require resources, especially a comprehensive reference library and a plethora of photographic images. A picture is worth a thousand words, and this is especially true when you are trying to describe or teach a technique or illustrate a concept.

I cannot even begin to list all the people who have helped me out after the hurricane. However, those who directly aided in the production of this second edition of *Reptile Medicine and Surgery* warrant mention.

Always on top of my list is my colleague, mentor, and most important, friend, Dr. Fred Frye. Dr. Frye has unselfishly lent me image after image, helping support my personal slide library and augment many chapters in this book. Dr. Frye has an infectious enthusiasm for the profession, one that I hope will continue to spread in perpetuity.

This book really should be called *Reptile Medicine and Surgery* by Douglas Mader, with images by Dr. Steve Barten. I could not have produced such an attractive book without his constant help with images and text.

Another source of spectacular photographs had been Dr. Richard Funk, a consummate veterinary professional with a sharp eye for photography. Dr. Funk has been more than generous in sharing images and experience, as well as contributing to many fine chapters in the book.

Dr. Karen Rosenthal has long been my friend, colleague, and connection to the Ivory Tower. Over the years she has shared numerous references, images, and case studies with me. Also a splendid photographer and a computer genius, Dr. Rosenthal has been a source of information and support.

Dr. Mike Garner has been a wonderful asset in reviewing chapters and providing images and general guidance. It is a comfort to know that he is always there whenever I need him.

Dr. Jeanette Wyneken, my partner in Focus Groups and Seaturtles, has been a great source of support, information, and knowledge. Dr. Wyneken has been a fantastic resource for the Association of Reptilian and Amphibian Veterinarians (ARAV). I hope they realize how lucky they are to have her as part of their group.

Dr. Geoff Stein was the artist for the first edition of *Reptile Medicine and Surgery*. Many of his fine drawings are used again in this edition. I thank him for his work.

Ray Kersey, formerly of WB Saunders, was instrumental in the first and second editions of this book.

Over the past couple of years I have had the honor and privilege of hosting dozens of senior veterinary students at my hospital for their senior rotations. Several of these students have contributed to the development of this book. Most have since graduated and received their veterinary degree—they will all make excellent veterinarians: Chad Givens, Sophia Chiang, Jeana Knowling, Melissa Thomas, and Mariah Kochavi.

I am blessed with a terrific professional staff, many of whom have in one way or another contributed to this text. I thank them for going outside their normal job descriptions to help with production: Lindy Starliper, Teresa Spencer, Linda Dwyer, Debbie Turner, Sonya Whitt, Bret Newton, Eileen Slomka-McFarland, Kelly Martin, Dawn Sandoval, Joe Gessler, Liz Smith, Della Schular, Emily Witcher, Melissa Liakas, Celeste Weimer, and Julie Roth.

My associate veterinarians graciously helped out with collecting data, images, and cases. Drs. Lonny Pace, Kristin

Hall, Stephen Anderson, Alissa Raymond, and Nikki Johnson have all been generous with their time and experience.

"Badger," my client, colleague, friend, and herpetologist extraordinaire, has always been there with a "yes, whatever you need, Doc." It is the good people like Badger who motivate me to keep going when I feel like quitting.

Several organizations and attractions, such as the Key West Aquarium, the Monroe County Animal Farm, the Key West Butterfly Conservancy, and the Theater of the Sea, have given me many opportunities for which I am most grateful.

The Marathon Sea Turtle Hospital has been my second "hospital" for the past 11 years. I have watched it mature from a "turtle rehab" facility to a world-class seaturtle hospital and research center. My thanks to Richie Moretti, Sue Schaf, and Corinne Rose for all of their help with this book and much more.

The ARAV has grown and matured over the years. It is wonderful to see how the membership has increased and the quality of the journal and conferences has improved. It is a world-class organization with a world-class product. I am proud to be a member.

It is always important to recognize your roots. I have to thank the Eastern States Veterinary Association, the organizing force behind the North American Veterinary Conference, for giving me my first real opportunity to lecture on a professional level. In 1987, as the undercard for Dr. Fred Frye, I presented three lectures: Reptile Anatomy, The Effects of Temperature on the Reptilian Immune System, and Antibiotic Therapy in Reptiles. There were fewer than 20 people in the room—all of whom, I am positive, were there to see Dr. Frye. Regardless, I must have done something right, because I was invited back and have been on the program ever since. I thank the NAVC (and the 20 people in the room) for the opportunity.

My connection with the amateur and professional herpetologic community for the past 12 years has been *REPTILES* magazine. Educated herpers are the best clients and take the best care of their charges. *REPTILES,* thanks for giving me that opportunity.

I wish to thank the wonderful editorial staff at Elsevier. In particular, Shelly Stringer and Sarah Wunderly have been a constant source of encouragement and nudging when I needed it. They have been most patient and tolerant of my work schedule, family crises, and other excuses (stranded whales, dolphins, and loss of power from hurricanes). They are all professionals and it is their efforts that will make this book shine.

This book would not be successful without the help of my pets—Bailey, Stanley, Puck, Pixel, and Simon. Of the tortoises, Stella, Tracy, and Dewe, the latter two were here for the first edition and will likely be around for the 75th as well.

Last, and most important, I need to express heartfelt thanks and love to Geraldine, my partner in business and in life. She has been most supportive and understanding over the last 3 years—with manuscript issues and otherwise.

DRM

CONTENTS

Section I Introduction
1 Building a Successful Reptile Practice, 1
2 Reference Sources for Reptile Clinicians, 9
3 Understanding the Human-Reptile Relationship, 14

Section II Biology and Husbandry
4 General Husbandry and Management, 25
5 Snakes, 42
6 Lizards, 59
7 Turtles, Tortoises, and Terrapins, 78
8 Crocodilians, 100

Section III Anatomy, Physiology, and Behavior
9 Stress in Captive Reptiles, 119
10 Cardiopulmonary Anatomy and Physiology, 124
11 Renal Anatomy and Physiology, 135
12 Gastrointestinal Anatomy and Physiology, 145
13 Behavioral and Morphologic Adaptations, 163

Section IV Medicine
14 Cardiology, 181
15 Dermatology, 196
16 Microbiology: Fungal and Bacterial Diseases of Reptiles, 217
17 Neurology, 239
18 Nutrition, 251
19 Oncology, 299
20 Reptilian Ophthalmology, 323
21 Parasitology, 343
22 Perinatology, 365
23 Reproductive Biology, 376
24 Virology, 391

Section V Clinical Techniques/Procedures
25 Allometric Scaling, 419
26 Alternative and Complementary Veterinary Therapies, 428
27 Anesthesia and Analgesia, 442
28 Clinical Pathology of Reptiles, 453
29 Diagnostic Imaging, 471
30 Diagnostic Techniques, 490
31 Emergency and Critical Care, 533
32 Endoscopy, 549
33 Euthanasia, 564
34 Overview of Biopsy and Necropsy Techniques, 569
35 Surgery, 581
36 Therapeutics, 631
37 Ultrasonography, 665

Section VI Differential Diagnoses by Symptoms
38 Snakes, 675
39 Lizards, 683
40 Turtles, Tortoises, and Terrapins, 696
41 Crocodilian Differential Diagnosis, 705

Section VII Specific Diseases and Clinical Conditions
42 Abscesses, 715
43 Acariasis, 720
44 Anorexia, 739
45 Aural Abscesses, 742
46 Bites from Prey, 747
47 Cloacal Prolapse, 751
48 Cryptosporidiosis, 756
49 Calculi: Urinary, 763
50 Diarrhea, 772
51 Digit Abnormalities, 774
52 Dysecdysis, 778
53 Dystocias, 787
54 Gout, 793
55 Hemoparasites, 801
56 Hepatic Lipidosis, 806
57 Herpesvirus in Tortoises, 814
58 Hyperglycemia in Reptiles, 822
59 Hypovitaminosis A and Hypervitaminosis A, 831
60 Inclusion Body Disease Virus, 836
61 Metabolic Bone Diseases, 841
62 Neurologic Disorders, 852
63 Paramyxovirus, 858
64 Penile Prolapse, 862
65 Pneumonia and Lower Respiratory Tract Disease, 865
66 Renal Disease in Reptiles: Diagnosis and Clinical Management, 878
67 Shell Damage, 893
68 *Salmonella:* Diagnostic Methods for Reptiles, 900
69 Spinal Osteopathy, 906
70 Tail Damage, 913
71 Thermal Burns, 916
72 Upper Alimentary Tract Disease, 924
73 Upper Respiratory Tract Disease (Mycoplasmosis) in Tortoises, 931
74 Vomiting and Regurgitation, 939

Section VIII Special Topics
75 Overview of Amphibian Medicine, 941
76 Medical Care of Seaturtles, 972

77 Biology, Captive Management, and Medical Care of Tuatara, 1008
78 Large Collections: Special Considerations, 1013
79 Reptile Zoonoses and Threats to Public Health, 1017
80 Laws and Regulations: European and American, 1031
81 Working with Venomous Species: Emergency Protocols, 1051
82 Understanding Diagnostic Testing, 1062
83 Reported Toxicities in Reptiles, 1068
84 Artificial Lighting, 1081
85 Disinfectants for the Vivarium, 1085
86 Computed Tomography and Magnetic Resonance Imaging Anatomy of Reptiles, 1088
87 Radiographic Anatomy, 1097
88 Hematologic and Blood Chemistry Values in Reptiles, 1103
89 Reptilian Formulary, 1119
90 Amphibian Formulary, 1140

Appendixes

A. Reptile Viral Diseases—Summary Table, 1147
B. Reptile Parasites—Summary Table, 1159
C. Environmental, Dietary, and Reproductive Characteristics Reptiles, 1171
D. Selected Sources of Reptilian Products, 1173
E. United States Commercial Analytical Laboratories, 1174
F. Weights and Measures Conversions, 1176
G. Fahrenheit versus Centigrade Conversion, 1177
H. US-IU (Blood Values) Conversion, 1178
I. Pharmacology Abbreviations, 1179

Glossary, 1181

Index, 1189

Section I
INTRODUCTION

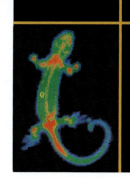

1
BUILDING A SUCCESSFUL REPTILE PRACTICE

GREGORY W. STOUTENBURGH

The dynamic field of reptile medicine tends to foster innovation of many sorts. Most reptile veterinarians work with reptiles because of a love and fascination developed in their formative years. This devotion, although healthy to the practice of medicine, can tend to buffer the business aspects of reptile medicine from scrutiny within practices. Consequently, an equivalent level of business optimization is rarely seen in reptile practice compared with other aspects of the practice. Equally unfortunate is that subpar business success in reptile medicine is a clear indication that the medicine was subdued, usually because of the [perceived] financial concerns of the owner. Reptile medicine can and should be profitable and beneficial to the practice as a whole. Although reptile medicine may act synergistically with other types of medicine within a given practice, it possesses its own unique benefits, pitfalls, economy, challenges, and clientele.

This chapter focuses on the unique challenges that face the business of reptile medicine. Concentration is on understanding and meeting these challenges to optimize the success and profitability of reptile medicine either in an exclusively exotics practice or in a mixed practice. Readers of this text are assumed to be already committed to the practice of reptile medicine; therefore, this discussion focuses on a realistic, pragmatic, and holistic approach to making reptile medicine profitable and successful rather than on an attempt to convert veterinarians with no interest in treating exotics.

THE INTEGRATED PRACTICE

In an integrated practice, reptiles and other exotic pets are seen and treated along with companion animals. Reptile medicine can be a worthwhile and profitable venture in most practices. A synergy may occur, on many fronts, that improves financial, staffing, medical, and marketing results of the practice.

Beyond the obvious benefit when reptiles are seen of an increased gross from a larger client base, many clients who were attracted for a clinic's capabilities with reptiles also bring their other pets, which may be more economically significant than the reptile patient. In addition, the staff at veterinary practices with regular treatment of exotics frequently have higher levels of loyalty and pride because of the unique capabilities of the practice and the added variety in work. The presence of exotic animals in the lobby generates interest and conversation for clients without exotics, which can foster client loyalty and increase referrals because clients commonly equate the variety of patients a veterinarian sees with the veterinarian's skill as a practitioner.

Achievement of financial success is often easier in an integrated practice than in reptile or general exotic animal medicine alone because of the relative market sizes of domestic companion animals compared with that of exotic pets and because of the willingness of pet owners to spend money on these pets. Further, with no conflicting factors for a given service, a wise practice is consolidation of a wide range of services under a single roof that results in a larger potential client base without significant increase in overhead costs.

EQUIPMENT AND FACILITIES

Because of the nature of the reptile-owning client (discussed subsequently), the degree of medical success achieved with reptiles is more critical to the long-term financial health of the venture than with domestic companion animals. Whether reptiles are wild caught, farm bred, or captive bred, all have specific habitat and dietary requirements that are necessary for survival and even more specific requirements that are necessary if they are to thrive. Just as a dog with pneumonia is not expected to recover well if kept outside in a Minnesota winter, less than healthy reptiles are certainly not expected to improve if kept outside of optimal conditions. Morphologic, behavioral, and physiologic characteristics of reptiles must be understood and accounted for in equipment and in methods.

The diversity of reptiles seen by veterinarians greatly exceeds the diversity in any other group of pets. Unfortunately, this point is poorly recognized, and the result is a mindset of "one size fits all husbandry" for reptiles as people attempt to make these animals conform to a household environment. **That reptile veterinarians understand the needs and biology of the animals that they treat is essential for medical and marketing success.**

Although a veterinarian's ability to remember the natural history and habitat requirements of every potential patient is unreasonable, knowledge of the basics for the most commonly kept captive reptiles is quite reasonable. For the rest, a comprehensive reference library should be readily available. For proper treatment, correct husbandry advice, and adequate respect of often skeptical reptile owners, a reference library for natural history, dietary, and behavioral information is essential.

For hospitalization of reptiles, adequate caging facilities must be available as they are not only ethically necessary but also essential to success (Figure 1-1). The methods and costs involved can vary greatly according to how elaborate the setup is and what materials and methods are used to provide the facilities. Although caging may be discussed elsewhere in this text, it is of significant importance to this discussion for capital concerns and for overall success and gaining the confidence of reptile-owning clients. The following criteria should be considered in cage design:

Cages should be designed for temperature and humidity control (different species have different requirements).
The cages or environments should be disposable or capable of complete and easy disinfection.
The cages must be escape proof.
The environments must mimic natural conditions as well as reasonable to minimize stress of the patients (e.g., chameleons in screen cages with trees; all animals with hiding places, appropriate water sources, appropriate type of heat for active versus passive thermoregulators, appropriate lighting on timers).

Some important medical and surgical equipment may be used for exotics exclusively. This equipment includes a gram scale, a microliter syringe, sexing probes, metal feeding tubes with ball tips, small endotracheal tubes, and safe-handling equipment. All of these items should have a total cost of less than $500.00.

CLIENT SERVICES

From the business perspective, the base unit for assessment of the success of a veterinary facility is the interaction between the client and the hospital staff. Every interaction should end with:

The client feeling that they have friends at the hospital.
The client feeling that the hospital staff is competent and is giving the best possible care.
The client understanding the care given and content with the value for the money spent.
The client having had a positive experience they would want to have again.

Staff

Essential to the success of client interactions is that the lay staff of a hospital be up to the task of service with compassion. The staff must understand the needs and anxieties of the client if the client is to be satisfied. Service is entirely about respect and problem solving. Use of this notion to its fullest extent is important so that the staff members understand and respond to the client's emotional state and needs. Through this understanding, the staff gains the client's loyalty and trust.

With the hiring of staff, one should know upfront exactly what to look for. A receptionist should be engaging, warm, intelligent, and well spoken with good people skills. An exotics practice must have staff members interested in and knowledgeable about exotic pets.

Most interactions with clients actually do not involve doctors. A huge mistake is for a veterinarian to be the sole repository of the ability to impress clients with herpetological expertise or to charm clients with service-oriented warmth. The utmost care and effort should be placed in the hiring and training of lay staff.

Establishing Value

To state the obvious, gross revenue is a result of the number of clients seen multiplied by the per-client charge. The per-client charge is far more influential in profitability than is the client volume because increased client volume results in more costs to the practice than does a rise in per-client charge. Unfortunately, **minimization of care and costs to save the client money and reduce the risk of rejection of services is common, especially among reptile veterinarians.** A veterinarian should never minimize the care recommended because of a perception of the client's financial wherewithal or any rationalization that takes cost into consideration. Clients visit veterinarians to receive the best possible care and recommendations. Neither the client nor the veterinarian is served when cost plays a part in the development of the medical recommendations.

Clients have the right and responsibility to take care of their own finances. A client may refuse any services that are

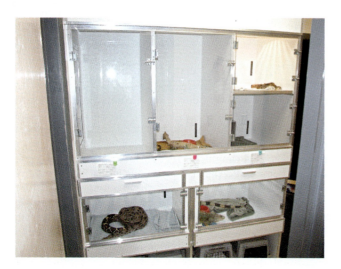

FIGURE 1-1 Proper reptile caging is mandatory for hospitals that offer services to exotic clientele.

unwanted after the value of said services has been established. A veterinarian should consider only the best quality care in development of a medical plan. Cost is irrelevant.

Clearly, however, for a veterinarian to practice the best medicine possible and make the reptile practice profitable, the client must be willing to pay for the care. As with any type of veterinary medicine, understanding the client's perspective, including motivations and valuations, is critical. Again, the overriding goal in the examination room is to get the client to accept, in full, an estimate of charges to provide the animal with the best possible care. All that is necessary to obtain this result is to cause the client to feel that the service is worth the cost. In other words, value needs to be established. A specific method can be used to do this with all veterinary patients. Value establishment is most difficult and the technique most critical with animals the client may value least, emotionally and financially.

A basic method for value establishment is as follows:

- A knowledgeable lay staff member speaks with the client and forms a relationship before the doctor enters the room.
- The doctor performs an examination and discusses what care the patient needs and how that care benefits the patient. The doctor does not discuss money because this wastes a client's time and clouds the client's mind about the purity of the doctor's motivation.
- The doctor writes the chart and gives the staff enough information to construct an estimate of charges.
- While a staff member constructs an estimate, the original lay staff member discusses with the client what the doctor recommends and how that care benefits the patient. Options for lesser care are not given. The relationship previously established fostered trust for this exchange, and the repetition of the doctor's recommendations provides greater understanding and an increased perception of the correctness of the plan.
- After the client has agreed to the treatment plan in principle, the estimate, complete with costs, is presented to the client in a matter-of-fact way.

Note that the most important element of this procedure is the client's agreement to the medical plan in principle, on the basis of a solid understanding of the importance of each item on the estimate, before the cost of the services is shown. When a client says, "I cannot afford that," they are often saying, "My money is worth more to me than what you are selling," usually because the client does not understand the product and the estimate may as well be written in Greek. **Services that a client does not understand have no value.** Only services that directly help the pet have value.

If the client receives an estimate without a prior thorough understanding of the value of the services on the estimate, no value exists. From this position, convincing the client of the value is an uphill battle. Or the quality of care is simply reduced to reduce the price and placate the client. However, now the client may believe unnecessary items were added to the estimate. This client from then on will not trust the estimates until they are reduced and will not be terribly loyal. If the previously described methodology is followed with adherence to all the principles from which it was constructed, many clients when presented with the price say, "Oh, that's all? I thought it would be more."

For this system to work best, the system of charges should display only charges for services or items that give the client/patient clear and direct benefit and, thus, value. Charges such as blood draw fees and waste disposal fees are valueless to a client and commonly lead to uneasiness and a lack of perceived value. However, if these costs are added into items that do provide value, such as a radiograph, blood panel, or injection, the client perceives greater value and overall satisfaction.

A client does not know whether a blood panel should cost $55, $85, or $100. The client can be educated to understand that the blood panel is essential to the diagnosis and treatment of the pet, and then the client will pay the cost of the test. When charges that do not have such value appear, a client feels "nickeled-and-dimed" and is more skeptical of the entire estimate or invoice. Line items for services that are actually steps of other services can be beneficial provided zeros accompany these items and only the main value carrying service carries charges. With this method, the invoice/estimate can actually total more while providing greater value. For example, consider the following two estimates for the same services:

Estimate of Charges
Physical Examination	$ 39.00
CBC & Biochemistry Panel	$ 65.00
Blood Draw	$ 15.00
Injectable Anesthetic	$ 20.00
Intubation	$ 10.00
Isoflurine Anesthesia	$ 55.00
Technician Time	$ 55.00
Coeliotomy (bladder stone removal)	$175.00
Hospitalization × 3	$ 90.00
Injections × 9	$ 54.00
Waste disposal/OSHA	$ 2.50

Estimate of Charges
Physical Examination	$ 39.00
CBC & Biochemistry Panel	$ 98.00
Ceoliotomy (bladder stone removal)	$365.00
Anesthetic Induction/Intubation	$ 0.00
Isoflurine Anesthesia	$ 0.00
Pulmonary Assistance	$ 0.00
Anesthetic Monitoring	$ 0.00
Hospitalization × 3	$120.00
Injections × 9	$ 54.00

Clients tend to respond far better to the second estimate even though the total cost is $95.50 greater. With a set of estimates similar to the previous example, 40 veterinary clients from three veterinary hospitals of various demographic areas in Southern California were asked which estimate they would rather be given. Of the 40, 36 chose the estimate that was higher but contained zeros. The four clients who chose the other estimate all took the time to add the items and realized that the cost was lower. **The point that should be clear is that an estimate of the second style provides clients with a greater feeling of value and satisfaction.** This system allows for charging higher prices while improving estimate acceptance, thus increasing per-client charge significantly. In addition, clients leave the facility with greater satisfaction, which improves client loyalty and referrals.

Diagnosis and the Client

With companion animals, clients more often then not consider their pets part of the family. The replacement cost of the animal is irrelevant in consideration of the value of the services. In addition, veterinarians have a long-standing and solid reputation of good care to companion animals. Value is easy to establish with these clients.

On the other hand, reptile owners can be divided into three groups:

- The first is pet owners who are very attached to the reptile as though it were a companion animal. This group establishes value most easily because the clients are motivated by emotion and devotion to the pet.
- The second group is composed of clients who keep reptiles as a novelty or to "be cool." This group is the least savvy and generally waits until the animal is seriously ill before consulting a veterinarian. This group is the one from whom the line is heard "I could get a new iguana for a lot less than that!" Some individuals from this group may be fostered, by the veterinary staff, into the first group.
- The third group consists of clients who breed reptiles or keep rare animals. This group is generally more knowledgeable and more skeptical of veterinary expertise than the other groups. This group also tends to lack an emotional attachment to the pet, and value decisions are made on the basis of economics, time invested, and difficulty of replacement.

In the assessment of the success of client-handling methodologies within any clinic, the category of client should be noted. The general methodology for estimate presentation described previously optimizes success for each of these groups. The discussions of care and husbandry, however, should be modified to appeal best to the individual at hand and should always take place before any financial discussion, and usually before the examination.

For clients in the first group, a dog and cat approach with some added technical details and a discussion of how the pet is an important family member is effective. For the second group, husbandry should be a basic and pragmatic discussion. If client interest is exceeded or the clients are intimidated, they are likely to give up the endeavor or just ignore the advice altogether. Every effort should be made to excite this group and encourage evolution toward the first group. Discussion with the third group should be precise and technically oriented. A solid understanding of the natural history of the patient is necessary before discussion with a third-group client.

MARKETING

As with any type of marketing, identification of a target client and establishment of a goal for that client is essential to success. Put simply, the marketing plan should be aimed at reptile owners from group one and at having them as loyal clients of $200 to $300 per year. Several methods can be used for marketing, and a multipoint approach is usually most effective. Methods of marketing vary greatly in cost and efficacy among both methods and geographic regions. Referral sources must be recorded from new clients so that methods can be refined over time. Equally important is keeping track of costs for each method so that a cost per client can be assessed for each method. When budgets are established, the cost/client numbers should be taken into account so that resources can be equitably distributed. Keep in mind that the cost/client number is not linear and a point of optimization exists above which returns diminish. Further, some synergy probably will occur among methods; therefore, marketing efforts should remain diverse, but adjustments in emphasis may pay dividends.

Establish a Practice Identity

An appropriate name and logo are essential to successful marketing. Clients today choose a veterinarian on the basis of quality above all else. Name and logo should express quality and any other feelings or philosophies that are part of the practice. The logo should make the practice stand out from the crowd and be clearly and easily identifiable. Most veterinary practices use generic pictures of cute animals for a logo. If the logo does not stand out from this group, it is not effective. The purpose of a logo is not to tell a client what services a business offers. A logo's purpose is served if it is recognizable and noticeable. Well constructed advertising lets the client know about services much more effectively than a logo and can be customized to the media. The logo also must work in grayscale even if the standard is color. The following examples show two types of logos that meet all criteria effective for establishing practice identity:

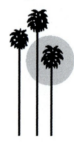

An exotics-only practice may be served well by a logo that depicts an exotic animal, but for practices that derive most income from mammals, creation of a logo that is effective and uses animals is difficult. With this understanding, an effective logo can take virtually any form as long as it is unique and consistently used.

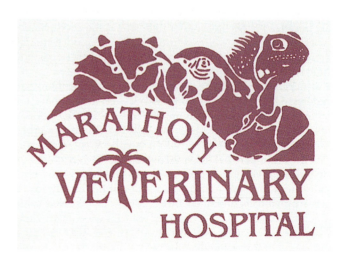

Hiring a professional to help create a logo and, if needed, even change the hospital name is worthwhile. Colors and paper choices should also be part of this process. The name and logo of the practice should then appear in the same form everywhere possible.

Print/Yellow Pages

Print and telephone book advertisements can be effective but also expensive. A poorly done ad is a waste of money, but a well-done ad can be a windfall. Again, hiring a professional (who does not work for the phone book company) to help create a cost-effective ad is a good idea. The cost of hiring is recovered in response if professionals hired are worth their salt. A few characteristics of a good ad are:

- Eye catching (this does not require color)
- Professional look and quality oriented
- Low prices are not advertised
- Name and logo are clear and obvious
- Clutter and too much copy are avoided
- Phone number is large and easy to read
- All unique and special characteristics are listed (e.g., open 7 days/evenings; reptiles; birds; luxury boarding)

Once a good ad is created, it should be presented digitally (on disk) and as a photo-ready print so that it can be used over and over. A consideration in hiring a professional is that the ad belongs to the veterinarian and is not just licensed for use.

Pet Stores

A wonderful idea is the establishment and maintenance of a relationship with pet stores and reptile dealers in the area. Treatment at a reduced cost of animals that belong to these vendors and even regular on-site visits to evaluate animals and maintain a relationship is worthwhile. These dealers then should be expected to refer clients to the practice. Experience shows that offers of free examinations for new pet purchases are not workable. These offers tend to clog the practice with the least desirable and least loyal clients who take more than they give. A discounted examination may be workable if done properly because this eliminates the thriftiest of clients. Note that if a policy is not worked out with the store, a bad situation frequently occurs when a client must be told that the animal they got from a referring store is ill.

Establishment as a Member of the Community

Various herpetile organizations exist virtually anywhere people keep herpetiles as pets (Table 1-1). Establishment as a member of these organizations, attendance at functions, and even the presentation of lectures is well worth the time. Word of mouth is the best referral source, and these are great ways to develop it quickly. A list of organizations is provided at the end of this chapter.

Internet

Although the Internet has become a huge part of our culture, it is not currently a significant source of new client referrals. A well-done web site may be an increasingly worthwhile venture if it acts synergistically with other aspects of a marketing strategy.

The Internet may serve as a conduit to the herpetological community at large. A simple Internet search with a word such as "reptile" or "herpetology" can yield a plethora of information and opportunities to engage with individuals and organizations that may be of benefit to the practice.

Television, Radio, Newspapers

Commercials and ads may be successful, but they tend to be costly and whether they are worthwhile is questionable. A wonderful irony is that free media are almost always successful. Free media can come from a weekly column in the local newspaper or a short spot on a radio or television show. If effort is put into arranging such a situation, the payoff can be substantial.

Promotional Items

Promotional items, such as t-shirts and refrigerator magnets with the practice name and logo, can be effective marketing tools. T-shirts encourage recognition of the practice, and magnets on refrigerators are in easy reach when the time comes to call a veterinarian. The design of such items should be kept clear and simple but eye catching to achieve the best results.

When an advertising campaign is put together, the psychology of the optimal client should always be kept in mind. A well-conceived effort convinces potential clients that the practice is the highest quality option and makes contacting the practice easy for the client. The value of any particular type of advertising may vary by region and demographic. The key to success in marketing lies in understanding the client.

REVENUE

Revenue generated by the reptile portion of a practice varies too widely among practices for comparisons to be of much use. Monitoring the profitability of the reptile portion of the practice is important so that it may be optimized.

The reptile portion of the practice likely has higher estimate rejection and lower charge per client than do domestic companion animals in the same practice. This difference is the result of the difficulties and limitations of the clients as discussed previously. A mixed practice that is new to reptile medicine or only generates a small portion of the revenue from reptiles may find reptiles extremely profitable because they do not add significantly to the overhead and may fill in otherwise vacant appointment slots with paying clients. A practice that deals exclusively or mostly with reptiles may have a more difficult time finding strong profitability because of the lower per-client charge.

Costs for outside laboratory tests, medical supplies, and lay staff time are comparable with reptiles and domestic pets. A relative savings may be experienced with drugs because smaller amounts are generally given with reptiles. Prices should therefore be equivalent to a successful scale for dogs and cats. If money is lost on a case, the case was not worth doing because that loss just compromised the quality given to

Table 1-1 Herpetological Societies

Alabama

West Alabama Herpetological Society
4404 Alabama Avenue NE
Tuscaloosa, AL 35404

Arizona

Arizona Herpetological Association
PO Box 64531
Phoenix, AZ 85082-4531

Arkansas

Arkansas Herpetological Association
C/O Perk Floyd
Route 2
Box 16
16 Lakeside
Hensley, AK 72065

California

BAARS
Palo Alto Museum
1451 Middlefield Road
Palo Alto, CA 94301

The Bridge
160 N Fairview Avenue #D231
Goleta, CA 93177

California Turtle & Tortoise Club
PO Box 7300
Van Nuys, CA 91409-7300

Chameleon Information Network
13419 Appalachian Way
San Diego, CA 92129

Island Empire Herpetological Society
2024 Orange Tree Lane
Redlands, CA 92373

North Bay Herpetological Society
PO Box 1117
Santa Rosa, CA 95402

Northern CA Herpetological Society
PO Box 661738
Sacramento, CA 95866

Sacramento Turtle & Tortoise Club
25 Starlit Circle
Sacramento, CA 95831

San Diego Herpetological Society
PO Box 4036
San Diego, CA 92164-4036

San Diego Herpetological Society
PO Box 4439
San Diego, CA 92104-0439

San Diego Turtle Society
PO Box 519
Imperial Beach, CA 91933-0519

Southern CA Herpetological Association
PO Box 90083
Long Beach, CA 90809-0083

Southwestern Herpetological Society
PO Box 7469
Van Nuys, CA 91409

Turtle & Tortoise Education Media
3245 Military Avenue
Los Angeles, CA 90034

Connecticut

Connecticut Herpetological League
CT State Agriculture Research Station
New Haven, CT 06430

Southern New England Herpetological
Society
2325 Burr Street
Fairfield, CT 06430-1806

Delaware

Delaware Herpetological Society
Ashland Nature Center
Brackenville & Barley Mill Road
Hockessin, DE 19707

Florida

American Society of Herpetologists
Florida St. Museum
University of Florida
Gainesville, FL 32611

Bay County Reptile Society
10531 Nona Wood Road
Fountain, FL 32438

Calusa Herpetological Society
11600 Gladiolus Drive #312
Fort Meyers, FL 33908

Caribbean Conservation Group
PO Box 2866
Gainesville, FL 32602-2866

Central Florida Herpetological Society
PO Box 3277
Winter Haven, FL 33885

Everglades Herpetological Society
PO Box 431242
Miami, FL 33243-242

Florida Panhandle Herpetological Society
5801 Gulf Breeze Parkway
Gulf Breeze, FL 32561

Florida West Herpetological Society
1312 S. Evergreen Avenue
Clearwater, FL 33516

Florida West Coast Herpetological Society
PO Box 2725
Dunedin, FL 34697

Gainesville Herpetological Society
PO Box 14353
Gainesville, FL 32614-0353

Gopher Tortoise Council
University of Florida
Department of Biology
4000 Central Park Boulevard
Orlando, FL 32816

League of Florida Herpetological Society
PO Box 3277
Winter Haven, FL 33881

Manasota Herpetological Society
PO Box 20381
Bradenton, FL 34203-0381

Palm Beach County Herpetological Society
13837 54th Lane North
Royal Palm Beach, FL 33411

Sawgrass Herpetological Society
PO Box 4852
Margate, FL 33063

South Marion Herpetological Society
PO Box 1817
Belleview, FL 32620

Suncoast Herpetological Society
PO Box 2725
Dunedin, FL 34697

Tallahassee Herpetological Society
PO Box 931
Crawfordville, FL 32327

Treasure Coast Herpetological Society
PO Box 650654
Vero Beach, FL 32965

Volusia County Herpetological
Society
PO Box 250553
Holly Hill, FL 32125

Georgia

Georgia Herpetological Society
PO Box 464778
Lawrenceville, GA 30246

Idaho

Idaho Herpetological Society
PO Box 44484
Boise, ID 83711-0484

Illinois

Central Illinois Herpetological
Society
PO Box 6413
Peoria, IL 61601-6413

Chicago Herpetological Society
2060 N Clark Street
Chicago, IL 60614

Chicago Turtle Club
1393 W Lunt
Chicago, IL 60626

Indiana

Hoosier Herpetological Society
PO Box 40544
Indianapolis, IN 46240-0544

Iowa

Iowa Herpetological Society
PO Box 250
Huxley, IA 50124

Kansas

Kansas Herpetological Society
327 West 24th Street
Hays, KS 67601-3007

Louisiana

Louisiana Gulf Coast Herpetological
Society
6713 Wilty Street
Metairie, LA 70004

Louisiana Herpetological Society
5025 Tulane Drive
Baton Rouge, LA 70808

Maine

Maine Herpetological Society
99 Water Street
Millinocket, ME 04462

Maryland

Maryland Herpetological Association
Department of Herpetology
2643 N Charles Street
Baltimore, MD 21218

Massachusetts

New England Herpetological Society
PO Box 1082
Boston, MA 02103

Table 1-1 Herpetological Societies—cont'd

Michigan
Great Lakes Herpetological Society
4308 N Woodward Avenue
Royal Oak, MI 48072

Michigan Society of Herpetologists
321 Oakland Street
Lansing, MI 48906

Minnesota
Minnesota Herpetological Society
10 Church Street SE
Minneapolis, MN 55455-1014

Mississippi
Southern Mississippi Herpetological Association
PO Box 10047
Gulfport, MS 39505

Missouri
Mid-Missouri Herpetological Society
4054 Victoria Court
Columbia, MO 65201

Mid-Missouri Herpetological Society
7501 N Highway VV
Columbia, MO 65202

St. Louis Herpetological Society
PO Box 410346
St. Louis, MO 63141-0346

Nebraska
Nebraska Herpetological Society
Biology Department
University of Nebraska, Omaha
Omaha, NE 68182-0040

Nevada
Northern Nevada Herpetological Society
PO Box 5812
Reno, NV 89513-5812

New Hampshire
New Hampshire Herpetological Society
PO Box 4020
Concord, NH 03302

New Jersey
NY Turtle Society
PO Box 878
Orange, NJ 07051

New York
Long Island Herpetological Society
476 N. Ontario Avenue
Lindenhurst, NY 11757

New York Herpetological Society
PO Box 1245 Grand Central Station
New York, NY 10163-1245

Reptile Adoption & Rescue
60 Bright Street
Buffalo, NY 14206

SNEHA
16 Roaring Brook Road
Chappaqua, NY 10514

Upstate Herpetological Association
HCR 68 Box 30 B
Springfield Center, NY 13468

Western New York Herpetological Society
686 Taunton Place
Buffalo, NY 14214

Ohio
Greater Cincinnati Herpetological Society
1720 Gilbert Avenue
Cincinnati, OH 45202

Greater Dayton Herpetological Society
2600 DeWeese Parkway
Dayton, OH 45414

Mid-Ohio Herpetological Society
PO Box 6
Powell, OH 43065

Northern Ohio Association of Herpetologists
Department of Biology
Case Western Reserve University
Cleveland, OH 44106

Toledo Herpetological Society
1587 Jermain Drive
Toledo, OH 43606

Oklahoma
Oklahoma Herpetological Society
5812 Coleman Avenue
Oklahoma City, OK 73179

Pennsylvania
Lehigh Valley Herpetological Society
PO Box 9171
Allentown, PA 18105-9171

Philadelphia Herpetological Society
PO Box 52261
Philadelphia, PA 19115-7261

Susquehanna Herpetological Society
211 South Market Street
Muncy, PA 17756

Rhode Island
William Hynes
Rhode Island Herpetological Society
547 Pleasant Valley Parkway
Providence, RI 02908

Tennessee
Clarksville Area Herpetological Society
PO Box 30852
Clarksville, TN 37040

Texas
Central Texas Herpetological Society
1405 Rabb Road
Austin, TX 78704

Dallas-Fort Worth Herpetological Society
7111 Layla Road
Arlington, TX 76016

East Texas Herpetological Society
8 Leisure Lane
Houston, TX 77024-5123

East Texas Regional Herpetological Society
703 Southoak Drive
Athens, TX 75751

Greater San Antonio Herpetological Society
134 Aldrich Street
San Antonio, TX 78227

Horned Lizard Conservation Society
PO Box 122
Austin, TX 78767

North Texas Herpetological Society
Attn: Mark Pyle
3744 Waxwing Circle
Fort Worth, TX 76137

North Texas Herpetological Society
PO Box 1043
Euless, TX 76039-1043

South Texas Herpetological Association
1405 Rabb Road
Austin, TX 78704

South Texas Herpetological Society
PO Box 780073
San Antonio, TX 78278-0073

Texas Herpetological Society
535 Guerin Drive
Arlington, TX 76012

Texas Herpetological Society
1810 W Mulberry
San Antonio, TX 78730

West Texas Herpetological Society
PO Box 60844
San Angelo, TX 76906

Utah
Utah Herpetological Society
PO Box 9361
Salt Lake City, UT 84109

Virginia
Blue Ridge Herpetological Society
PO Box 727
Brookneal, VA 25428

Wisconsin
Wisconsin Herpetological Society
PO Vox 366
Germantown, WI 53022

Wyoming
Wahsatch Alliance of Herpetoculturists
TAH
PO Box 1907
Casper, WY 82602

every other case. If value is established with the clients and good medicine is practiced without compromise, per-client charge is optimized and reptile medicine can be significantly profitable even with little volume if done in a mixed practice.

CONCLUSION

Reptile medicine can be a rewarding pursuit financially and personally. An understanding of the psychology of the reptile client is always important so that the situation may be optimized toward success. This understanding leads to success in marketing, estimate acceptance, client loyalty and referrals, and profitability.

If an understanding and proper handling of the client is put together in a situation with adequate facilities, good medicine, understanding of differences between species, and a good pricing structure, reptile medicine is successful.

2
REFERENCE SOURCES FOR REPTILE CLINICIANS

STEPHEN L. BARTEN

Two main bodies of literature serve herpetological medicine: traditional veterinary medical literature and herpetological literature. Unfortunately, veterinarians often overlook the latter. Nevertheless, herpetological literature contains a wealth of information, as academic herpetologists have been studying reptile biology, natural history, anatomy, physiology, nutrition, behavior, taxonomy, and so on literally for centuries. Moreover, as the popularity of captive reptiles soared in the nineties, so did the demand by veterinarians for books, journals, articles, and lectures on herpetological medicine. Publishers and conference organizers met the demand faster than colleges of veterinary medicine could supply it, resulting in the unique situation of a specialty where most of the so-called experts were private practitioners with heavy case loads but little formal academic experience or training. Most professionals did an admirable job, but much of the information was anecdotal and based on few cases. Some irrational and inaccurate information was published and presented, and unfortunately, these so-called data are still passed down in more recent papers that cite older literature. Herpetological medicine had to start somewhere, but references always should be critically evaluated and not accepted at face value. Papers reviewed by knowledgeable academic peers may carry more weight than those reviewed by private practitioners, but even those may be more accurate than some unreviewed papers. Of course, conference presentations usually are not edited or reviewed so the quality varies substantially. Although attractive to busy practitioners, simplistic answers to complex situations should be avoided. Rather, all veterinarians should strive to understand the basic principles of anatomy, physiology, pathophysiology, and natural history of their herpetologic patients.

Since the first edition of this textbook was published, the addresses for virtually every society and journal listed have changed. A significant number of journals and societies mentioned in the first edition no longer exist, and other new ones have cropped up. Although the following information was accurate at the time of writing, information sources change rapidly and current information at the time of reading should be verified. Almost every journal and society maintains a web page, and any standard search engine on the Internet, such as www.yahoo.com or www.google.com, makes finding the location and verification of current information easy. Subscriptions and memberships often can be ordered directly from these web pages.

ASSOCIATIONS AND SOCIETIES

Besides the usual veterinary associations, two associations regularly deal with reptilian medicine: the Association of Reptilian and Amphibian Veterinarians (ARAV; PO Box 1897, Lawrence, KS 66044-8897, www.arav.org) and the American Association of Zoo Veterinarians (AAZV; Attn: Tracy Candelaria, PO Box 7065, Lawrence, KS 66044, www.aazv.org). Each publishes a journal and hosts an annual conference with proceedings. Membership in the ARAV is recommended highly for all veterinarians who treat reptiles. The AAZV regularly publishes papers on reptiles.

Professional herpetological societies have publications that often benefit the reptile practitioner, and they host annual conferences as well. National societies include the following organizations:

- The Society for the Study of Amphibians and Reptiles (SSAR), PO Box 253, Marceline, MO 64658-0253, www.ssarherps.org. Of all the national herpetological societies, the SSAR is the most useful for veterinarians. The SSAR publishes *Herpetological Review*, which contains legislative updates; husbandry, field, and laboratory techniques; captive reproduction data; and book reviews. The SSAR also publishes the *Journal of Herpetology*, which is more scientific and contains articles on biology and natural history, and occasional pamphlets that cover topics such as longevity in captivity and standard common and scientific names.
- The Herpetologists League, c/o Dr Lora Smith, PO Box 519, Bainbridge, GA 39818, www.inhs.uiuc.edu/cbd/HL/HL.htm. This organization publishes *Herpetologica*.
- The American Society of Ichthyologists and Herpetologists, ASIH Business Office, PO Box 1897, Lawrence, KS 66044-8897, www.asih.org. This society publishes *Copeia*.

These three societies produce the most respected scientific herpetological journals.

Regional herpetological societies publish various newsletters that often contain useful husbandry and breeding techniques. Some are more professional than others, but few are peer reviewed. Some of the most well-known include:

- California Turtle and Tortoise Club, with over a dozen chapters, www.tortoise.org for addresses.
- Chicago Herpetological Society, 2060 N Clark Street, Chicago, IL 60614, www.chicagoherp.org.
- League of Florida Herpetological Societies, Jacqueline Sheehan, editor, PO Box 3277, Winter Haven, FL 33885, http://jaxherp.tripod.com/league.htm.
- New York Herpetological Society, PO Box 1245, New York, NY 10163-1245, www.nyhs.org/index1.html.

Northern California Herpetological Society, PO Box 661738, Sacramento, CA 95866-1738, www.norcalherp.com.

Northern Ohio Association of Herpetologists, Department of Biology, Case Western Reserve University, Cleveland, OH 44106-7080, www.noahonline.net.

Virtually every large city has a regional herpetological society. Local zoos, museums, and pet stores may have the names and addresses of regional herpetological societies in the area. Numerous web sites, such as www.kingsnake.com and www.anapsid.org, also have links to regional herpetological society web pages.

JOURNALS

Veterinary Journals

Standard veterinary journals, including the *Journal of the American Veterinary Medical Association (JAVMA)* and the *Compendium on Continuing Education for the Practicing Veterinarian*, occasionally carry papers on reptilian medicine. *Seminars in Avian and Exotic Pet Medicine* and *The Veterinary Clinics of North America: Exotic Animal Practice* are available from Elsevier, Inc., Periodicals Department, 6277 Sea Harbor Drive, Orlando, FL 32887-4800, elspcs@elsevier.com. Individual issues of both are dedicated to a single topic, such as soft tissue surgery or respiratory medicine. Each article is a thorough review of the given topic, and articles are scientific and of excellent quality. One or more herpetological papers are presented per issue. Both periodicals are highly recommended.

Exotic DVM veterinary magazine, PO Box 541749, Lake Worth, FL 33454-1749, www.exoticdvm.com, also caters to the veterinary care of exotic pets. This journal, contains large numbers of high-quality color photographs and photo essays, and articles tend to address more specific topics rather than general ones or reviews.

Herpetological Journals

Again, the Internet should be used to verify current addresses and information for the following journals. Most have web pages. Often subscriptions may be ordered online.

Amphibian-Reptilia, www.gli.cas.cz/SEH/, the journal of the Societas Europaea Herpetologica.

The Chameleon Information Network, c/o Andi Abate II, 13419 Appalachian Way, San Diego, CA 92129, www.animalarkshelter.org/cin/. The newsletters contain specialized information about chameleons not available elsewhere and names and phone numbers of dozens of experienced chameleon keepers for networking.

Herpetological Natural History, Editorial Office, Herpetological Natural History, Department of Biology, La Sierra University, Riverside, CA 92515-8247, www.hnh.no-frills.net/about.html. This is a peer-reviewed publication covering behavior, ecology, and life history.

Iguana: Conservation, Natural History and Husbandry of Reptiles, The International Reptile Conservation Foundation, 3010 Magnum Drive, San Jose, CA 95135, http://www.ircf.org/. The IRCF evolved from the International Iguana Society to cover a wider spectrum of reptilian species than iguanas and include more husbandry topics. The journal and website are both high quality.

Reptiles, PO Box 58700, Boulder, CO 80322-8700, http://www.reptilesmagazine.com/reptiles/home.aspx. A popular, slick, color magazine that caters to the reptile keeper. This is an important reference, and clients enjoy it in the reception area.

World Chelonian Trust Newsletter, World Chelonian Trust, 685 Bridge Street Plaza PMB #292, Owatonna, MN 55060, www.chelonia.org. The website and newsletter cover husbandry and natural history of turtles and tortoises. The website has many care sheets and images to facilitate species identification.

REFERENCE SOURCES AND TEXTBOOKS

Many standard veterinary textbooks have exotic animal chapters with excellent herpetological references. *Current Veterinary Therapy*, Elsevier, Inc, Periodicals Department, 6277 Sea Harbor Drive, Orlando, FL 32887-4800, is among the best of these, and veterinarians who treat reptiles should familiarize themselves with current and back editions. *The Merck Veterinary Manual*, Merck & Co, Inc, Rahway, NJ 07067, also has a surprisingly complete reptile section.

Biology of the Reptilia, a massive, multivolume work edited by Carl Gans and others, is the definitive herpetological text. Volumes 1 through 13 were published from 1969 to 1982 by Academic Press, London, UK. Three different publishers issued volumes 14 through 18, and the most recent volume 19 was published by the SSAR in 1998. Titles of individual volumes include morphology, physiology, ecology and behavior, neurology, and development. Each chapter is a comprehensive review of its topic and includes an exhaustive reference list. For instance, volume 19 contains, among others, three chapters titled "Lungs: Comparative Anatomy, Functional Morphology, and Evolution," "The Lungs of Snakes," and "Pulmonary Function in Reptiles," for a total of 374 pages, of which 85 pages are reference lists. Any serious literature search begins here.

Krieger Publishing (www.krieger-publishing.com) offers a long list of books devoted to herpetological subjects. Zoo Book Sales (www.zoobooksales.com) stocks virtually every book on herpetology and reptiles currently in print.

Additional important herpetological texts include:

Ashley LM: *Laboratory anatomy of the turtle*, Dubuque, Iowa, 1962, Wm C Brown. 48 pp. The title is out of print and hard to find but is an excellent reference.

Bartlett PP, Griswold B, Bartlett RD: *Reptiles, amphibians and invertebrates: an identification and care guide*, Hauppauge, NY, 2001, Barron's Educational Series. 279 pp. This is a wonderful, inexpensive book that illustrates a couple hundred of the most commonly kept species of reptiles and amphibians. It is a good reference for identification of patients and husbandry advice and is especially useful to veterinarians new to reptile practice.

Boyer TH: *Essentials of reptiles: a guide for practitioners,* Lakewood, Colo, 1998, AAHA Press. 252 pp. Basic advice for practitioners new to treating reptiles, with lots of husbandry information.

Carpenter JW editor: *Exotic animal formulary,* ed 3, Philadelphia, 2005, Elsevier, 564 pp. A terrific, up-to-date formulary of published drug dosages for reptiles that also has charts of normal blood values and more.

Conant R, Collins JT: *A field guide to reptiles and amphibians, Eastern and Central North America,* ed 3, Boston, 1991, Houghton Mifflin. 450 pp. Identification of reptiles and amphibians, including those from other areas of the country, is an important part of reptile practice.

Cooper JE, Jackson OF, editors: *Diseases of the reptilia,* vol 2, San Diego, 1981, Academic Press. 584 pp. By now somewhat dated, this text is still a valuable and scientific overview of herpetological medicine.

De Vosjoli P, et al: *The herpetocultural library,* Lakeside, Calif, Advanced Vivarium Systems, PO Box 40833, Lakeside, CA 92040, www.avsbooks.com. These short, paperback booklets on commonly kept species have thorough and accurate husbandry advice for the veterinarian and pet owner alike.

Dodd CK Jr: *North American box turtles; a natural history,* Norman, 2001, University of Oklahoma Press. 231 pp. Natural history translates to husbandry information; reptiles in captivity need the same diet and conditions that they do in the wild.

Duellman WE, Trueb L: *Biology of amphibians,* New York, 1986, McGraw-Hill Book Co. 670 pp.

Ernst CH, Barbour RW: *Turtles of the world,* Washington, DC, 1989, Smithsonian Institution Press. 313 pp. The text contains natural history information for all turtle species known at the time of publication and is useful when unusual species of chelonians are presented for treatment.

Ernst CH, Ernst EM: *Snakes of the United States and Canada,* Washington, DC, 2003, Smithsonian Books. 668 pp. This detailed natural history on all North American snakes is very well done.

Ernst CH, Lovich JE, Barbour RW: *Turtles of the United States and Canada,* ed 2, Washington, DC, 2000, Smithsonian Books. 682 pp. The text is a detailed natural history on all North American chelonians and is very well done.

Fowler ME, editor: *Zoo and wild animal medicine: current therapy,* ed 3, Philadelphia, 1993, WB Saunders. 617 pp. The book includes a good amphibian chapter. The first two editions (1978 and 1986) also contain reptile sections.

Fowler ME, editor: *Zoo and wild animal medicine: current therapy,* ed 4, Philadelphia, 1999, WB Saunders. 747 pp. The book includes several chapters on reptiles, including crocodilians and factors to consider when releasing turtles to the wild.

Frye FL: *Biomedical and surgical aspects of captive reptile husbandry,* ed 2, vol 2, Melbourne, Fla, 1991, Krieger Publishing. By now this title is somewhat dated, but it is still a standard reference. This huge two-volume set contains a wealth of information found nowhere else and has literally hundreds of color images.

Frye FL: *A practical guide to feeding reptiles,* Melbourne, Fla, 1991, Krieger Publishing. 171 pp. Aimed more at keepers than veterinarians, the title is self-descriptive.

Frye FL, Townsend W: *Iguanas: a guide to their biology and captive care,* Melbourne, Fla, 1993, Krieger Publishing. 145 pp. This text contains useful information, especially on iguana behavior in captivity.

Fudge AM: *Laboratory medicine: avian and exotic pets,* Philadelphia, 2000, WB Saunders. 486 pp. Several chapters discuss clinical pathology of reptiles.

Girling S, Raiti P, editors: *BSAVA manual of reptiles,* Ames, Iowa, 2004, Blackwell Publishing. 383 pp. Thorough and concise, this multiauthored text has contributors from both sides of the Atlantic.

Greene HW: 1997. *Snakes: the evolution of mystery in nature.* University of California Press, Berkeley, CA, 351 pp. A terrific summary of snake biology, lavishly illustrated with color images.

Grzimek HCB (ed): *Grzimek's animal life encyclopedia, volume 5: fishes II and amphibia,* and *volume 6: reptiles,* New York, 1972, Van Nostrand Reinhold. These large volumes are loaded with natural history on virtually every species known at the time of publication and include many illustrations. This is a useful reference for obscure species.

Gurley R: *Keeping and breeding freshwater turtles,* Ada, Okla, 2003, Living Art Publishing. 297 pp. This terrific summary of modern aquatic turtle husbandry has reference to many individual species and is a must-have for turtle keepers.

Hawkey CM, Dennett TB: *Color atlas of comparative veterinary hematology,* Ames, Iowa, 1989, Iowa State University Press. 192 pp. This older text covers mainly avian hematology but is one of the few that also mentions reptiles. It includes many photomicrographs.

Heatwole HF, Taylor, J: *Ecology of reptiles,* Chipping Norton, NSW, Australia, 1987, Surrey Beatty & Sons Pty Ltd. 325 pp. This is a terrific summary of how reptiles live in the wild, with detailed information on topics such as heat exchange and water relations.

Heatwole HF, Barthalmus GT: *Amphibian biology, volume 1: the integument,* Chipping Norton, NSW, Australia, 1994, Surrey Beatty & Sons Pty Ltd. 1-418 pp.

Heatwole HF, Sullivan BK: *Amphibian biology, volume 2: social behaviour,* Chipping Norton, NSW, Australia, 1995, Surrey Beatty & Sons Pty Ltd. 419-710 pp.

Heatwole HF, Dawley EM: *Amphibian biology, volume 3: sensory perception,* Chipping Norton, NSW, Australia, 1998, Surrey Beatty & Sons Pty Ltd. 711-972 pp.

Jacobson ER, editor: *Biology, husbandry and medicine of the green iguana,* Malabar, Fla, 2003, Krieger Publishing. 188 pp. This succinct, multiauthored book is limited to the green iguana. Half of the chapters cover biology and husbandry, and the other half discuss veterinary medicine. The book is short but packed with practical and important information.

Jacobson ER, Kollias GV, editors: *Contemporary issues in small animal practice, volume 9: exotic animals,* New York, 1988, Churchill Livingstone. pp 1-74. This text is now somewhat dated, but in its time, it was complete, accurate, and concise. Like an abridged version of Frye, the reptile section succinctly covers a scientific approach to reptile medicine.

Kaplan M: *Iguanas for dummies,* Foster City, Calif, 2000, IDG Books Worldwide, Inc. 353 pp. The title may be off-putting, but this is one of the best iguana husbandry books ever written. Kaplan is a well-known and respected expert on iguanas in captivity.

Marcus LC: *Veterinary biology and medicine of captive amphibians and reptiles,* Philadelphia, 1981, Lea and Febiger. 239 pp. Although this is one of the first texts on reptile medicine, it still has value and a strong parasitology section.

Mattison C: *The care of reptiles and amphibians in captivity,* ed 2, New York, 1987, Sterling Publishing. 304 pp. This book contains sound husbandry advice.

McArthur S, Wilkinson R, Meyer J: *Medicine and surgery of tortoises and turtles,* Ames, Iowa, 2004, Blackwell Publishing. 579 pp. This is a huge book that resembles Frye's text with detailed, experience-based information and lavish illustrations.

Oldham JC, Smith HM: *Laboratory anatomy of the iguana,* Dubuque, Iowa, 1975, Wm C Brown. 106 pp. This reference is old but excellent.

Pianka ER, Vitt LJ: *Lizards: windows to the evolution of diversity,* Berkeley, 2003, University of California Press, 333 pp. A companion to Harry Greene's book listed previously, this one offers a terrific summary of lizard biology and is full of exceptional color images.

Pough FH, Andrews RM, Cadle JE, et al: *Herpetology,* ed 3, Upper Saddle River, NJ, 2004, Pearson Prentice Hall. 726 pp. This is one of two modern herpetology texts.

Ross RA, Marzec G: *The reproductive husbandry of pythons and boas,* Stanford, Calif, 1990, Institute for Herpetological Research. 270 pp. PO Box 2227, Stanford, CA 94305. This older book covers boid reproduction thoroughly, with specific data and advice on each species.

Rossi JV, Rossi R: *Snakes of the United States and Canada; natural history and care in captivity,* Melbourne, Fla, 2003, Krieger Publishing. 520 pp. The book is somewhat pricey, but this is the only book that offers husbandry advice on every North American snake species on the basis of personal experience.

Rubel GA, Isenbugel E, Wolvekamp P, editors: *Atlas of diagnostic radiology of exotic pets,* Philadelphia, 1991, WB Saunders. 224 pp. This text is a good complement to radiology chapters in herpetological medical texts.

Shine R: *Australian snakes, a natural history,* Ithaca, NY, 1991, Cornell University Press. 223 pp. This excellent work covers basic natural history. Although Australian species are featured, the information can be extrapolated to the snakes kept as pets in the United States.

Stebbins RC: *A field guide to Western reptiles and amphibians,* ed 2, Boston, 1998, Houghton Mifflin. 336 pp. Identification of patients is important.

Warwick C, Frye FL, Murphy JB, editors: *Health and welfare of captive reptiles,* London, 1995, Chapman & Hall. 299 pp. Health and welfare issues are ignored in virtually every other herpetological and care-in-captivity reference. The chapter on stress in captivity is a topic that is crucial to reptile practice.

Wright KM, Whitaker BR, editors: *Amphibian medicine and captive husbandry,* Malabar, Fla, 2001, Krieger Publishing. 499 pp. This huge, multiauthored book covers this topic for the first time. Previous papers on amphibian medicine were limited to single chapters. Extensive husbandry information is included.

Zug GR, Vitt LJ, Caldwell JP: *Herpetology: an introductory biology of amphibians and reptiles,* ed 2, San Diego, 2001, Academic Press. 630 pp. This book is one of two modern herpetology texts.

This list is far from comprehensive. A number of textbooks cover various aspects of herpetology, and more are published all the time. Several of the journals listed regularly run book reviews of new releases in the herpetological field. Many dealers in used, out-of-print, and hard-to-find natural history books advertise in herpetological journals and are excellent sources for textbooks.

HERPETOLOGY ONLINE

The Internet is an essential tool in any search for information. A textbook is probably not the best place to list web sites because information and addresses change with astonishing speed. As already mentioned, a user must be familiar with at least one good search engine, of which many exist, such as www.google.com or www.yahoo.com. If the listed web sites are no longer valid, appropriate key words should be used to search for the current information.

Two information networks exist for veterinarians. The Veterinary Information Network (VIN) offers services for a fee. Subscribers have access to interactive message boards, a reference center, Occupational Safety and Health Administration (OSHA) center, continuing education classes, and free classified ads. One message board is dedicated to reptile medicine and is monitored by a number of nationally renowned experts. Contact www.vin.com. The American Veterinary Medical Association (AVMA) Network Of Animal Health (NOAH) is similar to VIN and offers discussion groups, a resource center, AVMA literature database, AVMA membership list, and helpful topics like product information, material safety data sheets (MSDS), legal briefs, zoonoses updates, and the like. Access is available free to AVMA members with their membership identification number and for a fee to nonmembers. Contact www.avma.org/noah/noahlog.asp.

Tufts University, in their Wildlife Rehabilitation Database (www.wpi.edu/Projects/Tufts/amphibian.html), lists normal blood values for some species of reptiles and amphibians.

The International Species Information System (ISIS) Reference Ranges for Physiological Values in Captive Wildlife is available on CD-ROM. Orders may be placed at http://www.isis.org/products/physref/physreforder2002.rtf. Other useful web sites include:

> www.kingsnake.com. This site is a good jumping off page for anything herpetological. It contains several hundred links, including breeders, dealers, stores,

classified ads, forums specific to various species, organizations, events, care sheets, frequently asked questions (FAQs), and products.

www.anapsid.org. The Melissa Kaplan Herp Care Collection web site is one of the finest web sites on herpetological care because it is comprehensive, current, accurate, well referenced, and frequently updated. The site contains hundreds of articles on the care of most herpetological species seen in the pet trade with an exhaustive section on Green Iguanas. It also lists information on herpetological societies and veterinarians, literature, supplies, and links to other important sites.

www.ncbi.nih.gov/entrez/query.fcgi?db=PubMed. The PubMed site is a searchable database of more than 4300 health journals; abstracts are available at no charge, and full text can be ordered.

www.medvet.umontreal.ca/biblio/vetjr.html. MedVet is a searchable database of veterinary journals that do not appear in PubMed. Some abstracts are available, but full text articles are not.

www.nal.usda.gov/ag98/ag98.html. APT Online is a searchable database of abstracts from zoological and wildlife journals, including the major herpetological journals.

www.herplit.com. This is the web site of Bibliomania, a group that offers out-of-print and hard-to-find herpetological literature for sale. Other important resources on this site include the current contents of more than 80 herpetological journals and newsletters and a herpetological literature database with more than 50,000 citations that range from the year 1586 to the present.

www.pondturtle.com/longev.html. Frank and Kate Slavens' web page lists longevity records collected from surveys of public and private reptile collections and is updated annually. Data for an amazing number of species are presented here.

www.embl-heidelberg.de/~uetz/LivingReptiles.html. The EMBL database covers current reptile classification and taxonomy. It has information and links to online photographs of virtually every species of reptile. However, the species are organized by scientific name, so searching photos to find a match is not practical.

For specific husbandry advice, the name of the target species followed by the word "care" should be entered into the search engine (e.g., "Leopard Gecko care" or "Jungle Carpet Python care"). This process leads to numerous sites that post specific care sheets for various species.

CONFERENCES

The Association of Reptilian and Amphibian Veterinarians and the American Association of Zoo Veterinarians both host annual conferences. They can be contacted at the previously mentioned addresses for times, locations, and program lists for upcoming conferences.

The North American Veterinary Conference in Orlando, Fla, held in January, has one of the most comprehensive reptilian medicine programs of any national meeting. The annual program has 3 days of lectures on reptile medicine, including both basic and advanced sessions, plus a variety of reptile techniques wet laboratory studies. Contact Eastern States Veterinary Association, 2614 SW 34th Street, Suite 4, Gainesville, FL 32608, http://gainesville.tnavc.org/portal/.

The Western Veterinary Conference has a large exotic animal program, which often includes reptilian medicine. The conference takes place in Las Vegas in February. Contact 2425 East Oquendo Road, Las Vegas, NV 89120, www.wvc.org.

The International Conference on Exotics is held in Florida each May by the publishers of *Exotic DVM* magazine. Contact PO Box 541749, Lake Worth, FL 33454-1749, www.exoticdvm.com.

The International Herpetological Symposium, PO Box 16444, Salt Lake City, UT 84116-0444, www.kingsnake.com/ihs/, is a large annual conference of herpetologists and herpetoculturists. Topics include biology, natural history, captive care, breeding techniques, and some veterinary topics. The conference is held in a different city every year.

3
UNDERSTANDING THE HUMAN-REPTILE RELATIONSHIP

DOUGLAS R. MADER and
BONNIE S. MADER-WEIDNER

Reptile ownership represents the fastest growing population of pets in the United States. At one time, the adage was "a sick reptile is a dead reptile," or in simple financial terms, buying a new reptile was cheaper than taking an ill reptile to the veterinarian. This is simply no longer the case.

With the rapid advance in veterinary medical knowledge in exotic pets and the strengthening of the human-animal bond, reptile owners are now seeking health care which once was not even considered an option. Services that were only seen in dog and cat patients are now offered on a routine basis to reptile patients.

Common knowledge is that a person does not enter the veterinary profession to avoid working with people; in most cases, the "people part" is the biggest part of the job. Veterinarians who are weak in the bedside manner aspect of their training lose out on both the financial and personal satisfaction aspects of this wonderful profession.

Preparation for work with owners and caretakers of non-traditional pets takes extra training—training that generally does not come from a classroom. The veterinarian learns this extra knowledge either in the field through trial and error (at the expense of the owner and often the pet) or from an experienced mentor. This chapter offers the serious veterinary clinician and technician a scaffold for building a better understanding of the concerns of clients and non-traditional patients.

THE HUMAN-ANIMAL BOND

Who gets attached to a pet and why? The many answers to this question probably equal the number of clients in a practice. In general, people are attracted to pets for companionship, for the sense of security they provide, and for the unconditional love that is free of criticism and judgment (Figure 3-1). For many people, experiencing consistent positive feelings with animals is easier than it is with people (Figure 3-2). Relationships with animals do not take as much emotional work to maintain.

Much truth can be found in the previous statements, even with reptiles (and amphibians) as pets. Depending on the reptile in consideration, many owners claim that their pets show reciprocal affection (Figure 3-3). That affection is a matter of interpretation, and one person's definition likely differs from the next. Regardless of how the veterinarian rationalizes a particular animal's ability to relate, the owner's emotional interplay is what matters.

Three general categories of the human-reptile bond are considered in this chapter: the "pet" reptile, the "commercial" reptile, and the "large collection" group.

THE PET REPTILE

The pet reptile usually has the most emotional significance. To take the position of "pet," the animal must assume and fill some niche in a person's life. The relationship may be as simple as the owner dropping some crickets in the animal's cage every morning, or it may be as complex as the owner

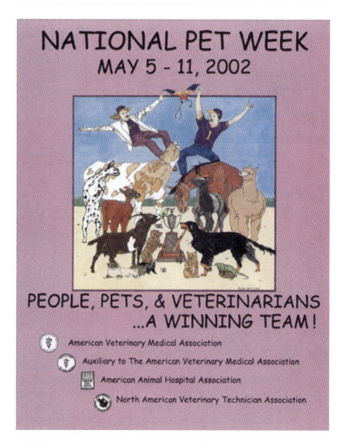

FIGURE 3-1 American Veterinary Medical Association (AVMA) has historically not recognized reptiles as companion animals. However, a recent "National Pet Week" poster sponsored by the AVMA featured a lizard as one of many pets.

Understanding the Human-Reptile Relationship

considering the animal a true part of the family, with conversations had with the pet and Christmas presents bought in the animal's name.

Some pets have a more ornamental or decorative value. Reptiles are often used to enhance an image, such as the outlaw biker with the pet rattlesnake, the dancer with the python, or the surfer kid with the pet iguana at the beach. These animals, although important facets in the lives of these individuals, likely do not take on the same significance as the reptile pet considered to be a part of the family.

Reptiles and amphibians can be anywhere from mundane, bland creatures to exquisite, colorful reflections of nature's art. Terraria can be simple plastic boxes or elaborate pieces of furniture. Some clients collect reptiles and amphibians for display in their terraria, as part of the decorum or art in their homes. Again, these animals are an important part of their lives but may take on more of an emotional resemblance to fish in a tank rather than the family dog or cat that sleeps on the couch.

The pet reptile has an intrinsic value as a pet. That intrinsic value is the value seen with any pet, be it a dog, a cat, or otherwise. Examples of this value are seen when the existence of the reptile somehow influences the decision making and daily lives of the owners.

People have been known to decline lucrative job offers because they were not allowed to bring their pet reptiles with them (import/export restrictions in overseas locations). Relationships have ended because one of the pair objected to the other having reptiles in the house (or feeding live prey, etc).

Pet reptiles can be a significant part of a client's life, and every consideration must be given to this relationship.

THE COMMERCIAL ANIMAL

The commercial animal refers to a reptile that is part of a breeding collection and is essentially a farm animal (Figure 3-4). Some professional herpetoculturists have thousands of breeders. The loss of a single animal may not take on much significance unless it happens to have significant financial value. For instance, some animals carry unique recessive genes (color patterns, albinism) that are worth thousands of dollars. These deaths also may take on significance if the loss of the individual animal may indicate a potential risk to the rest of the colony. The financial investment generally far outweighs the emotional attachment.

LARGE COLLECTIONS

The last general category in the human-reptile bond group is the large collection. Examples include animals on display, such as zoo animals, or animals in a research colony.

In this last category, the bond between caretaker (note: not an owner but someone assigned to provide daily care for the animals) and the animal often may be just as strong as that between an owner and the pet reptile (Figure 3-5). Caretakers may be asked to spend a significant part of their lives attending

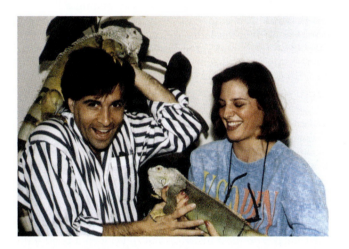

FIGURE 3-2 Reptiles have replaced more common dog and cat pets in some "childless" families.

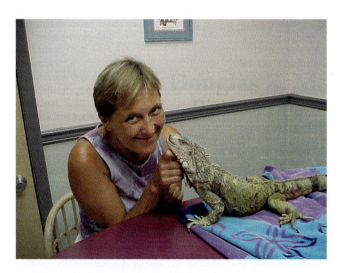

FIGURE 3-3 Some owners report that their pet reptiles have complex personalities and show affection.

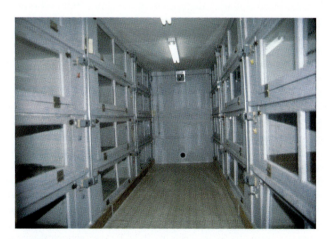

FIGURE 3-4 Even caretakers with large collections take interest in their charges. This feeling may be based on emotion or finance or a combination of the two. Oftentimes when finances come into consideration, feelings of guilt may be associated with decisions that may affect health of animals.

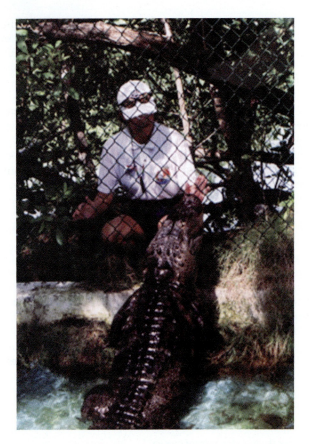

FIGURE 3-5 Curators and caretakers develop strong bonds with animals in their care.

to these captive animals. Emotional attachment is not uncommon when one of the animals becomes ill or has to be killed, in the case of a research setting.

The first-step approach to take with a client and animal, in any situation, is to assume that some degree of emotional investment exists. This emotional investment could be in the form of "my lizard Iggy is deathly ill, and I may lose him" or "my lizard breeder number 14 is sick, and I could be out several hundred dollars." Regardless of the connection, whether an obvious true emotional dependence or a financial dependence, some type of emotion is almost always playing a part in the decision making.

EUTHANASIA

For the emotionally attached client, regardless of the category, the decision of euthanasia for a cherished animal is agonizing and heart wrenching. Some people withdraw into a state of denial that gives relief from the psychological pain of a beloved animal in declining health. Caretakers in large collections have quit their jobs over the loss of some of their charges or the perceived handling of the terminal health care of the animals they keep.

Many different conflicts and questions must be addressed in each category. An experienced veterinarian (and staff) is a great help to the client in making these difficult decisions.

With pets, regardless of the type of animal, the dilemma is always "treat or don't treat" or "euthanize and replace."

A consideration with reptile pets, one that is not seen with dog and cats, is the potential longevity of the animal in question.

Some reptile pets have extended life expectancies. Some of the smaller lizards may only live a few years, but some of the larger snakes may live much longer and certainly the tortoises may live more than 100 years.

Longevity has an obvious impact on the decision for treatment or euthanasia. Although an owner's treatment of a 15-year-old German Shepherd may not seem appropriate because the life expectancy is nearly complete, treatment of a 30-year-old tortoise that may be expected to live another 70 or more years may be totally appropriate.

In a commercial situation, the decision to treat an animal may not be financially wise unless the patient in question has great financial value (i.e., if the cost of treatment can be recuperated with production profits). The decision for euthanasia may not be emotional but intellectual and financial.

An effete breeder with no productive value may well be better off with euthanasia. However, as an option to the owner, "retirement" for the animal (i.e., finding a home as a pet) rather than euthanasia may be wise to recommend. Many people find this latter option more appealing.

In some cases, euthanasia may be a scientific/diagnostic recommendation rather than a medical one. In large collections, all members of the colony are at a potential risk. If an animal is ill and a risk of infectious disease (or other colony danger) exists, then sacrifice of an ill or dying individual for the benefit of the colony is often wise.

Even in this situation, a veterinarian is wise to be cognizant of the owner's emotions because the inherent loss of any animal, commercial or not, may have an emotional impact.

The animals in the large collection category present their own concerns regarding the human-reptile bond. An obvious connection exists with the display animals, such as in a zoo. The caretaker in most instances has developed a bond with the animals. In addition, in many instances, the general public may also develop bonds with certain display animals (although this bond may not be the same as that with the caretaker). The public watches an animal grow, reproduce, and exist. Often some zoo specimens live for many years. Parents take their children to see the same animals that they themselves saw as children. When one of these special animals die, the event often makes the newspapers.

In a research setting, the value of an animal to a caretaker/scientist takes on different meanings. Again, caretakers commonly form bonds, even with caged research specimens, especially with animals on a long-term project. The animals in the cages take on personalities, and many astute technicians can tell apart seemingly identical animals just by their behavior.

When one of these animals die or are sacrificed, an emotional toll may result on the caretaker. From a more objective perspective, if a colony animal is ill and is in imminent danger of dying or may have to be sacrificed, the associated loss of scientific worth (i.e., lost data and future potential data) also brings some consternation.

The caretakers in these situations (i.e., large collections) may find themselves stuck in the middle of a euthanasia situation. In many cases, the decision for euthanasia or treatment may be a financial one and completely out of their control.

For instance, a zoo caretaker has a sick green iguana. The animal has been part of the petting zoo for 10 years and quite a bond has developed over that time. The animal falls ill, and the estimated cost of treatment far exceeds the minimal cost of replacement. Because of financial constraints of the zoo's budget, euthanasia may be the chosen option.

The loss of control can have a serious effect on the caretaker. Feelings of guilt ("If I had only taken better care of the lizard, it may not have had to undergo euthanasia.") and feelings of estrangement ("I have taken care of the lizard for 10 years, why don't I get any say in his treatment?") can have a heavy toll on a person's emotions.

The client who wants heroic efforts made at all costs to keep the terminal animal alive can create resentment in some veterinarians and staff who would like that client to end the animal's suffering with euthanasia. Practitioners also may disagree with clients who, in their opinion, prematurely or inappropriately choose euthanasia rather than attempt to treat an apparently correctable health problem.

With current law as it applies to veterinary medicine, animals are property of the owner. The owner has the right to make the decision to euthanize a pet. Owners who feel they are discouraged from or coerced into a euthanasia decision may leave the office feeling misunderstood and manipulated. They may also feel angry enough to seek legal action.

Euthanasia of a beloved pet can be the single event by which a pet owner judges the veterinary service. People saying good-bye to a deeply valued relationship with a precious animal forever remember the final moments of that animal's life.

See Chapter 33 for a technical discussion of euthanasia.

COMMON REACTIONS TO LOSS

Loss is an individual emotion, and whether it concerns a person, dog, cat, or reptile, it is just as real. Regardless of the species involved, when the lost loved one is not a person, the reaction by others is often seemingly callous. "For heaven's sake, it is just a dog, cat, horse, etc." And reptile owners often suffer the additional stigma attached to the concept of "It is just a reptile." Many question whether or not reptiles even show affection or exhibit a personality.

This chapter is not the place for discussion of those questions but rather for acknowledgement of the existence of the bond between the owner and the pet.

People dealing with the loss of a treasured relationship grieve for what they cannot have again and for what will never be. Feelings of grief can be had before a loss (anticipatory grief) just as they can after a loss. These feelings encompass all of one's being: feelings, thoughts, and behavior. Grief can leave a feeling of abandonment by a faith thought to give protection from such pain. It affects a person spiritually and can take a physical toll. A person who is grieving may commonly feel "out of control" or "crazy."

Feelings of helplessness, fear, emptiness, despair, pessimism, irritability, anger, guilt, and restlessness are all considered normal reactions. People can also have hallucinations, imagining that they see, hear, or smell the animal that has died. Not uncommonly, people awaken at night with the sensation of weight next to them on the bed where a pet used to sleep.

Losses of concentration, hope, motivation, and energy are also common. Changes in appetite, sleep patterns, or sexual drive may occur. More fatigued and error-prone behavior is also seen. During the normal grief process, a person can be sad and crying one day and smiling the next. People can feel tremendous guilt if they catch themselves laughing spontaneously or feeling happy because they interpret any positive feelings as disrespectful to the animal being mourned.

Elisabeth Kübler-Ross, MD, was a pioneer in helping the medical profession better care for dying patients and their families. In her extensive work, she learned the common patterns of reactions as people dealt with their own issues of mortality, dying, and death. She referred to these common reactions as the stages of grief. Although these stages are well documented in her work, no two people experience the awareness of mortality or loss exactly the same way and people often do not experience these stages in a linear fashion. Also, the many other aspects of grief include mind, body, spirit, and soul, which may seem to be overlooked with this model of grief. Regardless, Dr Kübler-Ross's paradigm for grief is made on the basis of solid work and can help people in the veterinary profession better understand what clients face with loss of a beloved animal. The following section includes concepts based on Dr. Kübler-Ross's work (*The Five Stages of Grief: Shock/Denial, Anger, Bargaining, Depression and Acceptance/Resolution*) and includes adaptations from *Pet Loss and Bereavement* by Sandra Barker.

Shock/Denial

Disbelief, shock, and numbness characterize this stage.
Denial of the reality of death, real or impending, is a protective defense.
Time is needed to comprehend the severity of the situation.
Hasty decisions during this time can result in regrets and added suffering.
Time is needed to accept the finality of the pet's situation before euthanasia decisions.

How to Help

Shock is a common reaction to overwhelming news, bad or good. It is a temporary state of mind characterized by emotional numbness. When the reality of the situation begins to be understood, then a person's coping style takes over.

Denial is one of the many different types of defense mechanisms used when reality becomes too overwhelming and coping skills can not keep up. In the context of veterinary medicine, dealing with someone in a perceived state of denial is one of the most challenging aspects of the profession—particularly when the veterinary professional's idea of proper care for the animal patient clashes vehemently with that of the pet owner's. Sometimes veterinary professionals believe that an animal is being kept alive for the selfish reasons of the pet's owner. "Can't she see how much that animal is suffering? How selfish to keep it alive when she knows we can do nothing more!" Those thoughts and feelings are common for people who accept euthanasia as a humane act and want to intervene on behalf of a pet they believe is needlessly suffering because of a selfish owner.

People have a number of reasons to not choose euthanasia, and many of the reasons have nothing to do with being selfish. Some people have strong religious values that prohibit euthanasia as an option. Some truly believe that death needs to happen "naturally." Others simply need more time to psychologically come to terms with saying goodbye and do not morally disagree with the act of euthanasia.

A few clients truly are in a state of denial about the animal's condition. People who are clinically in denial need compassion rather than judgment. Compassion provides patience to a person struggling with reality. For people who can not cope with the reality of losing a pet, hospice care is a most humane option. Home hospice care gives the person in denial more time to come to terms with the impending loss of their precious animal. The hospice approach allows the animal to be kept under the watchful eye of a veterinarian skilled at palliative care. This type of an arrangement can help clients accept the fate of their mortal pet. Although hospice is not a common practice in reptile-amphibian medicine at present, the door must be left open for the future.

With interaction with a person perceived as in denial, one should keep in mind that emotional distance from the situation makes it easier to be objective, unlike the client who probably has a strong emotional dependency. The veterinarian and the client should explore how the client would like the situation with the pet to be (ideal fantasy). Options should be identified and suggestions made, if possible. If offering hope to the client is based in reality, then hope should be offered. Hope can help with coping. This may require a judgment call because the interpretation of reality may at times be more subjective than objective. If the client may benefit from another medical opinion, then this should be offered as a suggestion.

In the gentlest way, comments can be made about how frightening thinking about life without this beloved pet can be. Fear of being left alone keeps many people from facing the reality that someday, and perhaps soon, they will be permanently without the animal that is such a major part of their daily routine and emotional life. During this time, patience, support, and respect for a client's tremendous fear about losing their beloved animal is most needed. **Use of logic to sway a client's decisions or to get them to understand is usually not productive.** If a clinician is feeling short on patience and easily irritated with such clients, the best interests of everyone (the clinician, staff, and client) might be served by referring the client to a different veterinarian.

Anger

A fearful or threatened feeling, common when facing a loss, is often expressed as anger.

Blaming, accusing, or desperately trying to find precisely why death occurred allows the client to focus on something other than the death of the pet and the resulting deeply painful feelings of grief.

How to Help

Anger needs to be accepted and understood. Refrain from becoming defensive and hostile in return. Sympathetic responses help to defuse anger. Acknowledge the client's feelings with a phrase like, "I know you are worried about Iggy right now. We are keeping a close eye on him and will do everything we can to help him. I will keep you informed of any changes."

If clients are abusive with anger expression, then one may need to say, "I know you are worried about Iggy. I assure you we are keeping a close eye on him and are doing everything we can. If you have decided you do not like the care we are giving him, you are welcome to take him to a different doctor. If you want us to continue treating him, we will, but you will need to control your anger and your behavior." If a client remains obnoxious and difficult, in spite of requests to change the inappropriate behavior, a clinician has the right to ask that client to stop coming to the practice.

Before a client is "fired," some allowances should be made for bad behavior if they are struggling to take care of an ill, beloved animal. **Remember, anger is a normal emotional component of grief.** Everyone can behave badly when frazzled with stress, so be patient. **Abusive anger is never appropriate, and it does not need to be accommodated.**

Guilt/Bargaining

Guilt can stem from regret for things that should have been done or should not have been done. Some tragedies are realistically preventable. People can feel guilty looking back at a euthanasia decision; perhaps in hindsight, they decided their pet was given euthanasia too soon or they feel they waited too long. People can feel guilty if they blame their pet for dying and have thoughts of "why did you leave me?" As they remember their pet, they can feel guilty if they decide the pet gave them more love and affection than they gave the pet.

Guilt may be unrealistic, taking responsibility for something out of one's control.

Guilt may be realistic, an act of real negligence.

People may make bargains to influence the outcome of a dying individual (e.g., "I will play with Iggy every day and clean her cage and give her fresh water if she doesn't die").

How to Help

Let clients know that it is common for an owner to want to do anything possible to prevent the loss of a pet. Doubting choices made is typical. When we believe we are solely responsible for the welfare of our animal and we have the need to be in control of what happens, becoming overwhelmed with feelings of inadequacy, frustration, and guilt for not being able to keep our pet from suffering or dying is easy.

If guilt is unrealistic, help the client to understand that it was a situation that was beyond anyone's control. Give reassurances that the client did everything possible.

If guilt is realistic, gently acknowledge the client's part in the injury or demise of their pet. "We all make mistakes. Unfortunately, this mistake had tragic consequences." Assure the client that what happened was unintentional. If what happened was truly an act of negligence, support clients if they express regrets. To honor their pet, they can prevent something similar from happening again by learning from this terrible experience.

A classic example of this with pet reptiles is the owner that forgets to turn the heat lamp off and accidentally bakes their pet. They know they made a terrible mistake, and furthermore, they know that they caused their pet tremendous pain and suffering.

Depression

True sadness about the loss is felt.
Depression can be a normal reaction that lasts from a few days to a few weeks. If a person's depression does not seem to diminish even after many weeks and it seriously interferes with normal daily functioning, than a physician or therapist should be consulted about appropriate medical or therapeutic interventions.

How to Help

People need to talk about their loss. Offer to listen, and/or refer the client to a specific resource that provides support for grief and bereavement. Hearing that they did all they could for their pet and were good caretakers is helpful to clients. Sympathy cards or letters can be comforting and appreciated at this time. Some people ignore their own needs in the face of depression. Encourage them to take care of themselves.

Acceptance/Resolution

Death has been accepted (more or less), and the person is able to think of the pet with fond memories and less pain.
Adjustment occurs to the environment that no longer includes the pet.
A desire may exist to reinvest the emotional energy that previously went to the pet into other relationships.
Healthy grief allows people to recognize through thoughts, actions, and feelings, the meaningfulness of a lost relationship. When people work through the painful feelings of loss, acceptance of that loss can occur. Acceptance of a loss does not mean that the animal, or person, is forgotten. On the contrary, healthy resolution includes fond memories that can be valued for a lifetime. Healthy resolution of a loss allows people to move on in their lives and become emotionally available to love again.
Complicated bereavement means that something has blocked the normal expression of grief and may interfere with normal grief resolution. The length of normal bereavement varies from person to person. As impossible as it may seem to someone in deep pain, people can start to feel emotionally able to experience joy again within a year or so after a loss. A more normal participation in life happens somewhere from 1 to 3 years after a profound loss.

COMPASSIONATE EUTHANASIA GUIDELINES

Reptilian euthanasia can be a technically difficult procedure and should not be learned by trial an error in front of a client. See Chapter 33 for procedures to follow. Learn the techniques on either non–client owned animals or on patients with clients who do not want to be present.

> From beginning to end, all cases of euthanasia should be handled with the utmost sensitivity and compassion.

Acknowledge to the client the difficulty of saying goodbye. If possible, reminisce with the client about the animal.
Offer at-home euthanasia, particularly for special clients.
Give the client the option to be with the animal during the procedure. Many people need to feel that they were at the animal's side, particularly at this time of saying the last goodbye. If a practice is not comfortable with this, a referral should be made to a practice where clients can be present during the pet's euthanasia. Many clients appreciate honoring their feelings about being present and remain loyal to the practice in the future.
Take time to educate the client. Talk about the process of euthanasia: the solutions that are used and how they work on the body; the length of time for an animal to die; that twitching, writhing, and elimination can occur; and that animals may die with their eyes open.
Let the client know about options for handling the animal's remains. Give names of pet cemeteries that offer cremation or burial services. If a client wants specific information on how animal remains are handled, be honest about rendering. Uninformed clients can become horrified when they find out what really happened (as with rendering) after they left their pet's body with their veterinarian.
If possible, handle financial matters beforehand. If the client is billed, consider a phrase like "special services" rather than "euthanasia" on the billing statement.
Schedule euthanasia when people are not feeling rushed between other client appointments (e.g., during lunchtime or after hours).
Once the animal is deceased, allow the client to see the veterinarian check for a heartbeat with a stethoscope, Doppler scan, or electrocardiogram. The client can even be allowed to listen for the pet's heartbeat through a stethoscope. This can be reassuring to some clients who may not be convinced that their animal has actually died (a common concern, particularly if the animal's eyes remain open after death).
Keep facial tissue within reach.
Some clients might appreciate a private moment to say goodbye to their pet. Ask clients who are upset to have someone drive them home, or keep them at your practice until they seem calm enough to drive.
Handle the body of a deceased animal with respect and gentleness.
A condolence or sympathy card signed by the veterinarian and the staff is an appreciated thoughtful gesture. Some practices send flower arrangements for extra-special clients. A follow-up call a few days or so after an animal's death is also considerate.
Acknowledge that this is a difficult time. **Show support by making a referral to a local pet loss support group or hotline even before the death of a pet has occurred.** This does not have to be awkward. Simply hand them a brochure telling them that they might be interested in attending a support group or calling a hotline because other clients have found these resources to be quite helpful. In this way, clients are

informed but still make their own decisions. If a group in the area is not known, the client should be given a number for one of the many Pet Loss Support Hotlines. The volunteers who respond to calls provide an understanding ear and use a national referral directory to let callers know about available local support. The practitioner should have compassion for this difficult time, but the primary support should come from an outside source.

- Update the client's records to reflect the death of the animal so reminders of future examinations, parasite checks, etc, are not sent. If applicable, note what examination room was used for the euthanasia and then refrain from using that room for that client who may bring other pets. Clients commonly avoid returning to the site of their goodbye to their beloved animal. A client can be retained by assurances of understanding they may feel sad on returning to the practice. Providing a photo of the pet to add to a memorial board in the waiting room or web page may give them the courage to return to the practice's compassionate care.

COMMON CONCERNS FOR THE CLINICIAN AND THE CLIENT REGARDING ANIMAL LOSS

Delivering Bad News

As a health care provider, delivering unpleasant news is part of the job. No one relishes sharing bad news. The skills needed to do so are straightforward and become second nature as experience broadens and interactions with clients remain thoughtful.

Keep in mind that every meeting with a client can result in the client's education about the animal's state of health. The initial bad news is softer for the client when a gentle voice and demeanor is used and the conversation is started with something like "We got the blood results back, and I'm afraid that there are some values indicating that Iggy's kidneys are starting to fail." When an animal is aged or has a life-threatening illness, chronic bad news is continually shared as the animal's health declines. With simple honest communication to the client about the ongoing health status of the animal, over time the client is gently prepared for the animal's eventual death.

In some cases, the bad news cannot be broken in stages but needs to be done all at once. **With an unexpected death, the clinician needs to prepare before delivering such serious and sudden bad news to the client.** Collect your thoughts and ready yourself for your client's reaction, which can be extreme shock or anger or both. Be sure to remain calm and pace the message so it is not blurted out.

One can start by saying, "I have some bad news to tell you." Then the client is given a brief moment to adjust to hearing even that much. Then one continues gently, "Iggy went into cardiac arrest during his surgery. In spite of our best efforts, we were not able to revive him. I am terribly sorry."

Your client may become upset and might even yell. One should be reminded that this is a normal reaction to such news, as unpleasant as it is for the clinician and perhaps the staff. Work at containing feelings of defensiveness; rather, express understanding at the shock. The clinician can express shock as well. Once the clients are over the initial shock (which may take days or a few weeks), many can rationally understand that some things happen in life that cannot be prevented and do not hold the clinician responsible.

Depending on the circumstances, the clinician may deal with an irate client for a time. Be empathetic and truthful about what happened. Continue to contain any defensive feelings—and hang in there. Remind yourself that you are a good doctor and that your client is understandably upset because of suffering from an unexpected loss. With certain clients anything you do will not be good enough. In these situations, it is always better to listen and document all conversations.

Answering the Question, "What Would You Do If You Were Me?"

The decision for euthanasia of a beloved animal leaves many people struggling with the feeling that they must "play God." Commonly, the pet owner turns to the veterinary professional for advice and guidance, often pleading, "What would you do if you were me?" No one perfect answer exists for this situation. If the client is well known, clear communications are likely maintained about the state of health of the animal with every visit for medical care. The client comes to trust the clincian's judgment.

As seriously ailing or aged pets are cared for, clients can be gently prepared in advance for thinking about the mortality of the pet. One may say something such as, "Right now, we have different options to try to keep his quality of life good, but eventually, our options will decrease and he will start to deteriorate in a serious way." End-of-life decisions (whether euthanasia, body care, or memorialization options) certainly do not need to be decided prematurely.

When a client looks to the clinician for the answer to the question of whether euthanasia is right for their animal, the clinician can respond as if the pet were the clinicians, but one should be very careful about this. Review everything that has been done for the animal and if anything can yet be done. Consider all variables, particularly financial constraints. **Acknowledge that this is a most difficult time and that making the decision to say goodbye is perhaps the hardest ever to make for a person who loves their pet.**

The client is in the best position to judge whether the animal is no longer enjoying a quality of life, for the client, not the veterinarian, knows the animal's normal personality. Some examples: "You know your pet better than anyone does, and as difficult as it is, you can judge your animal's quality of life today compared with how your pet used to be. You know your pet's normal personality better than I do. Does he seem to be himself? Do you think he's enjoying life as he used to?" One can also ask in a gentle way, "Do you think you might be keeping your pet alive more for yourself than for him?"

One should remember that the clinician has more of an objective relationship with the animal, unlike the client who is emotionally attached and shares an intimate history with the animal. The clinician therefore can probably see reality more clearly and easily than the client. The person faced with a euthanasia decision should rightly be given the truth about the state of the animal's health, including an honest prognosis.

Telling people what they "should" do can be dangerous. Owners may feel resentment because after the animal is dead, they may feel that they were not ready to say goodbye and that they were pressured. Some people can be so bitter that they pursue legal action. From a more philosophical perspective, telling people what to do denies them the experience of taking responsibility for their own tough decisions.

An option for people who are not able to make a euthanasia decision is to suggest hospice care for the animal that needs intensive care. In this way, the owner keeps the animal at home, with the more technologic treatment administered or supervised by a veterinary professional. This allows the owner to feel less pressure about euthanasia, and any staff members who feel resentment can have some relief from a client they feel is selfish.

Why Do People Often Feel Guilty about the Death of a Pet?

Guilty feelings having to do with a pet's loss often involve the questions, "Did I wait too long to put my animal to sleep, causing my pet to suffer?" and "Maybe I acted in haste and put my animal to sleep too soon." A reassuring and truthful response to both these concerns is that in making such a hard decision, a perfect answer usually does not exist. All we can do when faced with tough choices is to make decisions on the basis of the information we have at the time. Maybe after the irreversible decision is made, we wish we had chosen something different. This is useless because we did the best we could at the time we felt we had to act. Beating ourselves up over our "wrong choice" keeps us from moving on with our lives.

Sometimes a real act of negligence leads to a traumatic incident that results in a pet's injury or death. Most people feel acute guilt and perhaps shame when they realize they should have acted sooner or taken measures to prevent the situation from happening in the first place. We are all vulnerable to errors in judgment and making mistakes. From a veterinary point of view, educate, gently when possible, to help prevent a repeat occurrence of negligent care. For the rare client who may have a truly apathetic attitude about animal care, a more direct approach may be necessary.

What about a Pet's Remains?

Many people never think to ask their veterinarian about their pet's remains. They just assume that the veterinarian handles this and that other considerations do not exist. People need to be educated about the different options available for handling their pet's remains. If a pet's death is anticipated, the client may benefit from thinking about the available options, such as burial, cremation, and freeze-drying. For clinicians who live in a state that supplies rendering services, one would be wise to let the client know what that means.

How Can a Pet be Memorialized?

A big fear for many people is that they will someday *forget* about their pet. They think that if they ever recover from their painful feelings, they will have forgotten about everything they loved about this special animal. Suggestions for keeping memories alive can be reassuring. Ways in which to memorialize a pet are as many as a person's creativity. Making a donation in the pet's name to a charitable organization that benefits animals, collecting a collage of favorite pictures, or planting a tree can memorialize a pet. Some people find that writing down a detailed description of favorite behaviors or personality traits assures them that those special memories are always preserved.

How Does One Talk with Children about the Loss of a Family Pet?

Never lie to children about what happened or is happening to a pet. If a client asks you to collude with them into telling their child (or children) something other than the truth about their animal, refrain from doing so. Understand that when parents want to hide the truth from their children, their motivation mostly comes from not wanting their children to suffer. They may also feel unsure about how to talk to their children about such sad things. If you are comfortable and confident about these situations, then coach parents about how to talk to their kids. You can also suggest a book on the topic of children and pet loss (there are many) that they can use.

Young children can be told about death, although before the age of 7 years or so, they do not have the cognitive ability to understand the finality of death. An older child is more able to mentally comprehend the meaning of death and can have an emotional reaction to the reality of the situation. In all cases, the best way to support children is to be truthful with answers that do not over explain. Give children your undivided attention when they ask questions. This is an opportunity to teach children about regarding death with respect and dignity and that losing a special being, animal or person, can be a sad thing because that animal or person was unique and can never been replaced. Holding a memorial service that everyone helped create is a nice way to say goodbye to a dear animal family member. Children can also benefit from memorializing a beloved pet in their own personal way, such as drawing pictures of their pet, putting together a scrapbook, or establishing a special spot in a garden.

How Does One Address the Fears of Older Persons about Caring for Pets Later in Life?

"What will happen to my pet if I go to the hospital or I die before my pet does?" For older persons or persons with failing health, these are the most common, unspoken concerns about having a pet. Considering that some reptile pets long outlive their owners, this is a real concern.

After losing a special animal, many older people feel too many risks are involved in bringing another pet into their lives, even though the companionship of a pet would be a most healthful relationship for them. Taking a solution-oriented approach is most helpful in dealing with these concerns. Explore all the available resources the older person has. Think about all the people (friends, relatives, their veterinarian) who would be willing to adopt the animal in case of the owner's death or at least provide short-term care if the owner needs to be in the hospital for a time. Other possibilities include an animal sanctuary or an arrangement with an informed attorney who can help a person provide ongoing care for a pet should the person die. Some veterinary schools have programs that provide arrangements for the lifetime care of pets of deceased owners. This may include providing loving homes and medical care for the lifetime of the pet. Owners should contact their regional veterinary universities to enquire about the availability of these options.

Should a Veterinary Professional Encourage Clients Who Have Lost Special Animals to Get Another One?

This dilemma is similar to that of euthanasia. Because all people have unique reactions to the loss of a pet, following their lead when suggesting that they get another pet is respectful. Some people need time to mourn their loss. Others cannot imagine their home without an animal, so they might bring in a new pet before they lose the other one. People know when they are ready. Also, giving animals as gifts is often a bad idea. Depending on the type of animal, a person could be sharing a significant number of years with this pet. For a close relationship to develop, a certain amount of chemistry is essential and can only be felt by the person who will be caring for the animal.

Is It Okay to Cry in Front of a Client?

Although you are a veterinary professional, you are first a human being. Undoubtedly, at times, you will be moved emotionally and will feel like crying. If you are a sensitive person, you are susceptible to this. Getting teary-eyed on occasion is normal. Keep in mind, though, that you have a job to do, so tell yourself that you will take some private time to feel and express emotion after you are done with the job at hand. Clients appreciate sensitivity and can feel especially supported when the veterinary staff shares in the emotional climate of a particular event or experience.

CONCLUSION

The profession of veterinary medicine is full of trials, tribulations, and triumphs. It can be demanding when, within the same day, you find yourself sharing the excitement of a client's new puppy or kitten only to enter the next examination room to deliver bad news about the beloved pet of a familiar client. Euthanasia of animals you have come to know and like also takes its toll on your emotional well being. Given the emotional challenges you face as a veterinary professional, you need to keep yourself "tuned-up" so that you can maintain patience and a sense of compassion for your clients. Keeping tuned-up means staying current with your medical skills and having confidence with your interpersonal skills. You also need to take good care of yourself physically and emotionally.

If you find that you are feeling impatient or you are reacting to people in a cold fashion, you could be experiencing some symptoms of burnout. Instead of focusing on the complaints you have about work, think about some possible solutions to what you have identified as problems. Then, take action. Do what you can to make some constructive changes and accept the aspects of your job you feel you cannot change. If you definitely cannot accept certain things, maybe a different strategy will help. Of course, you can always quit that job and find something you think will suit you better. If you are discovering a pattern of discontent in your work history, you may have to take a serious look at your work choices, habits, and expectations.

Working in the veterinary field, especially in a unique discipline such as reptile medicine, can be a most rewarding experience. Because of the compassion you show, the job is one in which you can truly make a difference in the lives of many animals and the people who love them. You will be intimately involved in creating final, permanent memories for many people who must say goodbye to animals they hold so dear in their hearts. Through your actions and words, you can bring grace to these memories. Take good care of yourself so you can keep compassion in all the wonderful work you do.

Animals are family!
Keep up with your own grief work.
You cannot do others' emotional work for them.
You do not have to like all clients.
Give clients a break when they are stressed, allowing for bad behavior. *You never have to tolerate* abusive *behavior*.
Maintain respectful interactions with clients.
A real limit exists as to what you can provide your clients—know this!
Be aware of what stresses you and learn effective strategies to cope.
A client's denial is almost impenetrable in the context of your relationship.
Denial does not respond easily (if at all) to logic.
Be kind and patient. People need time to let reality sink in that their pet is absolutely mortal and will die someday, perhaps very soon.
Be honest about the animal's health.
Be careful not to give false hope, but be sure to give hope when realistically possible.
Offer hospice care (comfort care, pain management) as a way to keep a pet comfortable while a client struggles with decision making.
Honor the client's right to make decisions about when and where they want to say goodbye to their beloved animal, even if it means you need to refer them to a different veterinarian who accommodates them if you cannot.

SUGGESTED READING

Mader B, Binder M: *Attitudes of people about their pets; unpublished survey*, Davis, 1998, Program for Veterinary Family Practice, School of Veterinary Medicine, University of California.

Catanzaro TE: A survey on the question of how well veterinarians are prepared to predict their client's human-animal bond, *JAVMA* 192:1707-1711, 1988.

Lee M, Lee L: *Absent friend, coping with the loss of a treasured pet*, High Wycombe, Bucks, England, 1992, Henston Ltd.

Kubler-Ross E: *On death and dying*, New York, 1969, Macmillan Publishing.

Barker S: Pet loss and bereavement, *Veterinary Practice Staff* 1(1):1989.

Harris J, Hancock G, Mader B: Animal hospice, Portland, Oregon, 1991, *Abstracts of Presentations of the Delta Society Tenth Annual Conference*.

Randolf M: *Dog law*, Berkeley, Calif, 1989, Nolo Press.

Hart L, Hart B, Mader B: Humane euthanasia and companion-animal death: caring for the animal, the client, and the veterinarian, *JAVMA* 197(10):1292-1299, 1990.

Lagoni L, Butler C, Hetts S: *The human-animal bond and grief*, Philadelphia, 1994, WB Saunders.

Milani M: *The art of veterinary practice; a guide to client communication*, Philadelphia, 1995, University of Pennsylvania Press.

RESOURCES AND ADDITIONAL INFORMATION

Delta Society
PO Box 1080
Renton, WA 98057-9906
(206) 226-7357
Ask for the "Pet Loss and Bereavement Packet."

The American Veterinary Medical Association (AVMA)
 Committee on the Human-Animal Bond
AVMA
1931 N Meacham Road, Suite 100
Schaumburg, IL 60173-4360
(800) 248-2862

Printed Material

"Death of the Family Pet: Losing a Family Friend" pamphlet
The ALPO Center
PO Box 4000
Lehigh Valey, PA 18001-4000
(215) 395-3301
Free to veterinarians.

"Pet Loss and Human Emotion: When the Question is Euthanasia" pamphlet
AVMA
1931 N Meacham Road, Suite 100
Schaumburg, IL 60173-4360
(800) 248-2862
First pamphlet free; small cost for additional pamphlets.

"The Loss of Your Pet" pamphlet
The American Animal Hospital Association's Member Service Center
PO Box 150899
Denver, CO 80215-0899
(800) 252-2242 or (303) 986-2800
Fax (303) 986-1700
A fee is charged for the brochures; call for prices.

Pet-Loss Support Groups and Web Sites

Many support groups are available. Some are private, and many are nonprofit and supported by veterinary associations and veterinary schools. Contact the local or state Veterinary Medical Association for referrals, or enter a keyword search "Pet Loss" on the Internet. Amazon.com also offers many excellent resources on pets and pet loss.

Section II
BIOLOGY AND HUSBANDRY

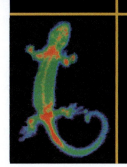

4
GENERAL HUSBANDRY AND MANAGEMENT

JOHN V. ROSSI

In the last 10 years, major advances have been made in the captive maintenance of reptiles. Yet the basics are still the same. Certain procedures must be carried out and certain requirements must be met if reptiles are to remain healthy in captivity. Clinicians need to be aware of basic reptile biology and husbandry to properly diagnose and treat this group of animals. Procedures of critical importance include quarantine, disinfection, regular examination, fecal examinations, and deworming if necessary. In collections of reptiles, disease transmission must be prevented. With increasing regularity, reptile keepers create multiindividual or multispecies enclosures, which complicate the issue even further. Also, a shift has been seen away from simple enclosures to those that are more environmentally enriched. More complex environments had traditionally been considered more difficult to maintain and were not being used for many reptiles. The benefits of such enriched enclosures have become increasingly obvious in the last several years (Figure 4-1). These benefits appear to be both behavioral and physiological. Increased environmental complexity leads to increased activity, which appears to result in leaner, more reproductively active animals. The physiological benefits of microclimates within the enclosure include enabling the reptile to regulate body temperature and cutaneous water losses accurately. These benefits are believed to be extremely important in allowing the reptile to function normally and live to an age approximating genetic potential and are also critical for disease prevention. Another recent advance in herpetoculture involves the use of bioactive substrates in reptile enclosures. Bioactive substrates are believed to encourage the growth of bacteria and fungi that compete with pathogenic bacteria and fungi, thereby protecting the captive reptile from infection.

BASIC BIOLOGY

More than 7000 species of reptiles have been divided into three major orders and one minor order. The species vary widely in terms of size, shape, physiology, and diet. Their captive requirements may vary just as widely. Providing every detail for each of these species is beyond the scope of

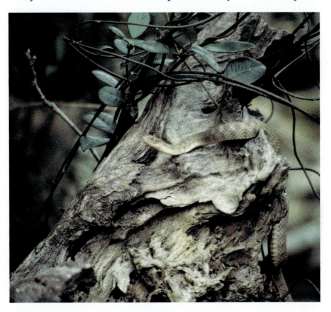

FIGURE 4-1 A Brazos Watersnake *(Nerodia harteri)* in a natural enclosure is more wary and maintains a leaner appearance than those housed in a typical aquarium-style cage. This snake also grows at rate more similar to those found in wild.

this chapter. However, basic important similarities in the biology of reptiles must be considered in designing an enclosure or attempting to treat a captive reptile. The most important factor is that reptiles are ectothermic, which means they derive the vast majority of their body heat from outside heat sources. Some reptiles are considered stenothermal, accurately controlling body temperature within a narrow range, and others are eurythermal, allowing body temperature to vary widely according to external temperatures. In general, terrestrial reptiles are more stenothermal than arboreal or aquatic reptiles. However, all reptiles are believed to thermoregulate to some extent, making use of thermal gradients within their environment. Most aspects of their physiology are intimately tied to body temperatures, and hence, so is their behavior and ultimately their health. The preferred body temperature range of reptiles is referred to as the preferred optimum temperature range (POTR); this range is known for most wild reptiles (Table 4-1; Figure 4-2).

Table 4-1 Preferred Optimum Temperature Ranges for Commonly Housed Captive Reptiles

Common Name	Scientific Name	Preferred Optimum Temperature Range (°F)			Buried Hot Rock or Under Enclosure with Heat Tape Necessary	50-Watt to 75-Watt Sun Spotlight Bulb Necessary	Natural Spectrum Lighting Necessary
		Day	*Night*	*Winter Cool Down**			
Snakes							
Boa Constrictor	*Boa constrictor*	Mid-80s	70-80	60-70	Yes	Optional	No
Rosy Boa	*Lichanura trivirgata*	80-85	70-75	58-60	Yes	No	No
Ball Python	*Python reguis*	Mid-80s	70-80	60-70	Yes	Optional	No
Burmese Python	*Python molurus*	Mid-80s	70-80	60-70	Yes	Optional	No
Green Tree Python	*Morelia viridis*	75-82	70-75	60-64	Yes	Optional	Optional
Carpet Python	*Morelia spilota*	80-85	70-75	60-64	Yes	Optional	Optional
Cornsnake	*Elaphe guttata*	77-84	67-75	55-60	Yes	Optional	No
Yellow Ratsnake	*Elaphe obsoleta*	77-84	67-75	55-60	Yes	Optional	No
Gopher/Bullsnake	*Pituophis melanoleucus*	77-84	67-74	50-60	Yes	Optional	No
Common Kingsnake	*Lampropeltis getula*	78-84	68-74	55-60	Yes	Optional	No
Mountain Kingsnake	*Lampropeltis zonata*	78-84	66-74	55-60	Yes	Optional	No
Gray-banded Kingsnake	*Lampropeltis alterna*	79-84	70-75	58-60	Yes	Optional	No
Gartersnakes	*Thamnophis sp.*	75-80	65-72	54-59	Yes	Optional	No
Lizards							
Green Iguana	*Iguana iguana*	84-90	67-77	64-69	Optional	Yes	Yes
Basilisks	*Basiliscus sp.*	82-87	75-77	68-70	No	Yes	Yes
Leopard Gecko	*Eublepharis macularius*	77-85	65-75	None	Yes	No	No
African Fat-tailed Gecko	*Hemitheconyx caudicinctus*	78-85	67-75	None	Yes	No	No
Day Geckos	*Phelsuma sp.*	85	75	None	No	Yes	Yes
Madagascar Leaf-tailed Gecko	*Uroplatus sp.*	81-84	72-78	None	No	No	Optional
Chameleons (montane)	*Chamaeleo sp.*	77-84	55-67	None	No	Yes	Yes
Chameleons (lowland)	*Chamaeleo sp.*	80-84	70	None	No	Yes	Yes
Bearded Dragons	*Pogona sp.*	84-88	68-74	62-69	Optional	Yes	Yes
Blue-tongued Skinks	*Tiliqua sp.*	80-85	67-75	60-65	Optional	Yes	Optional
Monitor Lizards	*Varanus sp.*	84-88	74-78	66-70	No	Yes	Optional
Tegus	*Tupinambis sp.*	80-86	70-78	60-70	No	Yes	Optional
Turtles							
Semiaquatic turtles	Most species	80-84	65-70	Optional	No	Yes	Optional
Tropical turtles	Most species	82-86	74-80	None	Optional	Yes	Yes
Box Turtles	*Terrapene sp.*	Outdoors in backyard for late spring, summer, early fall					
		78-89	70	50-65	No	Yes	Yes
Tortoises	Most species	Outdoors in backyard for late spring, summer, early fall					
		82-88	70-76	Temperate climate species only	No	Yes	Yes

*(with no food in gut).

General Husbandry and Management

Another factor that is important for the health and reproduction of reptiles is photoperiod. Seasonal reproduction is often strongly influenced by the amount of light and darkness per day. Some reptiles (e.g., many iguanid lizards and the Tuatara) actually have a light receptor on top of the head called the pineal eye.

Water regulation of reptiles also varies dramatically from one group of reptiles to another and even considerably from species to species that are considered closely related. Once again, emphasis is placed on researching the natural history of each animal if one is contemplating captive maintenance or advising a client of such. Generally speaking, reptiles from dry environments are uricotelic, essentially producing the large, relatively insoluble molecules of uric acid in an effort to conserve water at the renal tubule level. Those reptiles from aquatic environments generally produce the smaller, more soluble urea, or in some cases ammonia, to eliminate nitrogenous wastes (Figure 4-3). Many use various combinations. All reptiles have insensitive cutaneous and respiratory water loss, however, which may be minimized with microhabitat selection; that is, seeking an environment with a higher humidity. This is properly termed **hydroregulation**, and all reptiles appear to engage in microhabitat selection and possibly hydroregulation to some extent. The ability to reduce these minute water losses is now considered important for long-term health and possibly for reduction of the likelihood for kidney disease. These microenvironments may also harbor beneficial bacteria and fungi that compete with pathogenic bacteria and fungi, thereby providing other benefits to the reptile. See the subsequent discussion on bioactive substrates.

The immune response of reptiles appears to vary dramatically on a seasonal basis and is also intricately tied to the temperature range available to the reptile in question. Maximum immune response appears to occur in most reptiles when they are held in or near their POTR, or preferred optimum temperature range. This range needs to be researched for the species in question. Both the humoral and cellular immune responses appear to be measurably lower in winter months, and thus, reptiles may be more vulnerable to infection during this time. Certainly, the subject of stress and its relationship to disease in captive reptiles has been discussed in detail by a number of authors. Perhaps the most interesting and detailed discussion on the subject is that of Cowan.[1]

For the sake of discussion, the amount of stress may be directly related to differences between the captive environment and the wild environment. Therefore, those captive environments that lack suitable temperature and humidity clines and secure hiding places or have inappropriate photoperiods are more likely to result in diseased reptiles than those that have these key factors addressed (Figure 4-4). Thus, the clinician must strive to recommend the proper temperature and humidity gradients and hiding areas in new reptile enclosures. For those established reptiles undergoing treatment, captive environments must be reevaluated whenever a disease outbreak occurs. Basic requirements and husbandry techniques are discussed herein. The subject of stress is also discussed in more detail in Chapter 9.

BASIC HUSBANDRY REQUIREMENTS

The basic requirements for captive reptiles are based on their basic needs in nature as discussed previously. These requirements are summarized in the following sections.

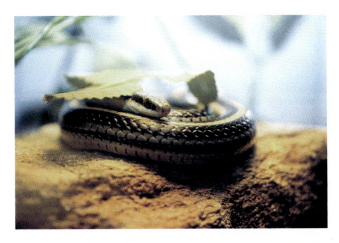

FIGURE 4-2 Texas Patch-nosed Snake *(Salvadora grahamiae)* basks on a rock in its cage. Ability to thermoregulate is absolutely critical for long-term successful maintenance and reproduction of captive reptiles.

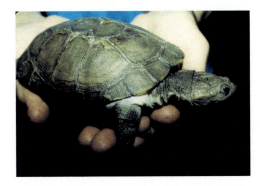

FIGURE 4-3 Side-necked Turtle *(Pelomedusa* sp.*)* is a highly aquatic turtle that is more likely to produce urea as a primary nitrogenous waste product; many tortoises and desert lizards produce primarily uric acid.

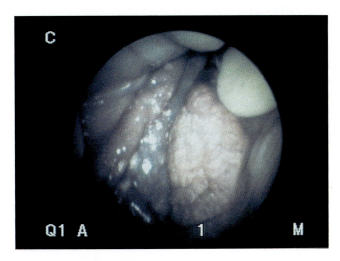

FIGURE 4-4 Visceral gout in Blue-tailed Monitor *(Varanus doreanus)*. Many diseases of captive reptiles are related to inadequate captive environment or diet. A causal relationship is often difficult to prove, however.

Unlike domestic animals, these animals have not been bred for generations to survive in "human habitations." In combination with their unique dietary requirements, their ectothermic nature must be understood and addressed by keepers and clinicians alike or their efforts to maintain or heal these creatures will meet with failure. Photoperiod is also important for reptiles. Thus, a thermal gradient and proper photoperiod should be maintained for all captive reptiles. Humidity is also important and needs to be addressed as well.

Long-term hospitalization of these animals with their unique requirements is often extremely difficult, and clinicians may be forced to provide these animals with the bare necessities of a thermal gradient and a clean cage (Figure 4-5). Thus, for many reptiles, diagnosing and beginning treatment for release to the owner as soon as possible for return into the new and improved cage is often beneficial. In many cases, environmental corrections may be instituted by the owner while the reptile is hospitalized, which of course requires that the owner is reeducated to correct the environment and can medicate the reptile at home. Some animals must be hospitalized for longer periods of time, however, which requires daily maintenance by the staff, such as cleaning the cages and soaking or spraying some of the patients.

The staff needs extra training to care for reptiles during their stay in the hospital. They should be made aware of handling techniques to prevent injury to themselves or clients and the reptiles in question (Figure 4-6). Many reptiles may be easily injured if dropped, and many technicians may be bitten or scratched if they handle reptiles carelessly. In addition, cage security is critical. Snakes and lizards are especially good at escaping, and this is unacceptable in a veterinary hospital. In addition to surprised clients being informed about the absence of the animals left in the hospital's care, a risk also exists that a large boa or python may ingest an endothermic patient or frighten clients at the time of its sudden reappearance. The clinician's responsibility is to take every precaution needed to secure reptile patients in proper cages, even if it means keeping snakes overnight inside of a secured cloth bag. Larger snakes, lizards, and tortoises may be secured inside of plastic containers with locking lids and then placed inside of standard stainless steel cages with the doors closed and locked. This provides an extra measure of security. Clinics that hospitalize many reptiles should invest in a rack style system, where small to medium reptiles may be housed in plastic drawers in a rack (Figure 4-7). These racks are often on wheels and can be conveniently moved from place to place with some degree of ease. Unfortunately, this style of cage makes providing a light source difficult, but most reptiles seem to tolerate this for the short periods of time that they are hospitalized, just as they tolerate the absence of the usual environmental enrichment they have in their regular home cage.

Ideally, one should have separate rooms or at least separate racks for long-term healthy reptiles and those that have been recently captured or been in another collection. This allows a limited hospital quarantine, which is extremely important for reptiles. A more complete discussion of quarantine and disinfection follows. Remember that wild reptiles often show no outward signs of infection or parasitism at the

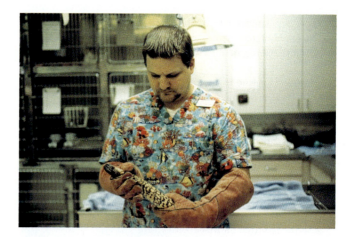

FIGURE 4-6 Training technicians to handle reptiles and provide for their daily needs is critical to successful treatment. This experienced technician is handling a venomous Gila Monster (*Heloderma suspectum*) for treatment.

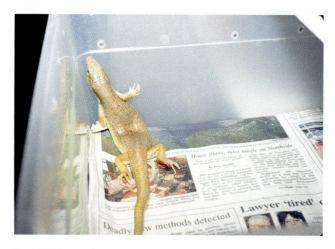

FIGURE 4-5 A hospital cage often provides only bare necessities. These include cleanliness, warmth, and security. A high-humidity retreat can be provided for some. The most commonly used substrate in a hospital setting is newspaper, which can be quickly changed.

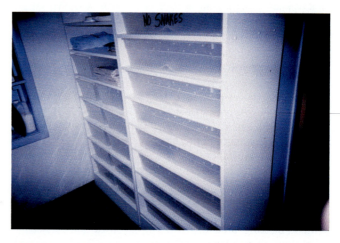

FIGURE 4-7 Reptile rack. These mobile units house light, easily cleaned, and heated drawers that can house many reptiles in a relatively small space. A separate rack may be used for quarantine purposes, but ideally this should be in a separate room.

time they are captured. In some cases, reptiles may not show signs of a virus they contracted for up to 6 months.[2,3] Therefore, precautions must be taken when handling reptiles of unknown origin (all reptiles). With large numbers of hospitalized reptiles, wearing gloves to handle or examine new reptiles may be beneficial.

The following sections outline some of the requirements of reptiles that a clinician should understand and be able to share with reptile clients.

Temperature

A useable thermal gradient should be provided to every captive reptile. In addition, daily temperature fluctuations and seasonal temperature fluctuations should be provided. Heating pads and heat tapes usually provide a useable thermal gradient for most terrestrial reptiles. These same devices, however, do not provide a useable thermal gradient for aquatic or arboreal reptiles. For aquatic reptiles, a submersible water heater may be necessary, and for arboreal reptiles, a radiant heat source is often necessary to create a hot spot somewhere among the branches in which they reside. Basking areas are considered important for most reptiles, which includes many aquatic reptiles. The preferred temperature ranges of many commonly kept reptiles are listed in Table 4-1. **A simple rule of thumb is to maintain a hot spot in the cage that is near the upper end of the POTR**. Then reptiles can achieve the highest temperatures that they would normally seek in nature but also can choose lower temperatures, including those that may be outside the POTR. McKeown[4] defines a *primary* heat source as that which is used to maintain an appropriate background temperature in the enclosure. For most people, this is the central heating unit in their house. *Secondary* heat sources are those used to create additional heat in some areas of the enclosure to provide a thermal gradient.[4] If either is insufficient or unusable to the reptile, disease is a likely occurrence for that reptile.

Hot rocks, a source of artificial heat, are commonly used by reptile keepers. These generally provide very focal heat, directed from the ground upwards, and generally are not useable by all but the smallest reptiles. They often become progressively hotter with age, and larger reptiles frequently burn themselves, presumably trying to stay warm. Better heat sources include adjustable heating pads placed under the cage and incandescent bulbs placed at various heights above the cage. Ceramic heaters have recently become more popular because they produce radiant heat with no light emission. One must remember, however, that sick reptiles often do not thermoregulate properly, so the background heat must be controlled carefully for these animals. Another group of reptiles at risk are male snakes during breeding season. Male boas and pythons commonly seek out the coolest area of the cage at this time, only to become too cold and have a bacterial infection develop. Once again, this may be avoided with careful control of the background temperature.

A general guideline for daytime air temperatures to provide for most diurnal reptiles is 80°F to 95°F (27°C to 35°C), with a basking area of 120°F to 130°F (49°C to 54.5°C). Nocturnal or montane reptiles often do well with daytime air temperatures of 70°F to 80°F (21°C to 27°C) but still seem to benefit by having a warmer area of 90°F to 95°F (32°C to 35°C) present in the enclosure (Figure 4-8). Nighttime air temperatures for most reptiles should not drop below 70°F during the active season, although temperate zone reptiles can usually tolerate temperatures lower than this for short periods with access to a heat source. Experience shows that maintaining most reptiles for prolonged periods at temperatures ranging from 60°F to 70°F (15°C to 21°C) is potentially harmful. This temperature range appears to be too cold to allow normal digestion or immune system response and too warm to allow for normal brumation (hibernation). Without any supplemental heat or the absence of a daytime temperature that rises sharply into the 90°F to 95°F (32°C to 35°C) range, many reptiles kept consistently in this 60°F to 70°F temperature range often become ill (Figure 4-9).

Brumation (hibernation) temperatures for temperate zone reptiles generally may be maintained between 35°F to 59°F (3.8°C to 15°C) for a minimum of 10 weeks. Montane reptiles or those from cold climates may need brumation (hibernation) temperatures at the lower end of this range and possibly for a longer period of time. Of course, no feeding should occur at this time (Figure 4-10). Subtropical reptiles can be brumated (hibernated) at similar temperatures but should have access to some heat source at all times. Tropical reptiles should not be brumated (hibernated) but instead may be exposed to nighttime lows that are lower than those to which they are exposed to in the summer, and daytime highs remain similar to that which are provided during the summer. Typically, nighttime low temperatures for tropical reptiles should not drop below 70°F (21°C). Python and boa breeders often

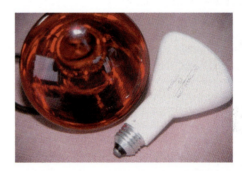

FIGURE 4-8 Heat sources commonly used for captive reptiles include heat lamps and heating pads. The heating pad should be kept in low position and monitored frequently to ensure it does not overheat or short out. Heat lamps are also commonly incriminated in reptile burns because people tend to underestimate the amount of heat they produce and fail to provide reptiles with suitable escape. *(Photograph courtesy D. Mader.)*

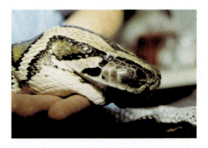

FIGURE 4-9 Python with cellulitis. This snake was maintained at room temperature with little or no access to a useable primary heat source. Constant exposure to these "middle temperatures" often results in various manifestations of the disease.

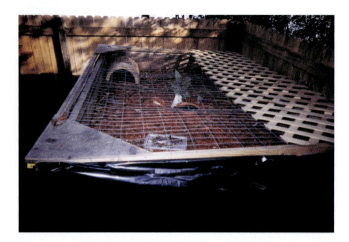

FIGURE 4-10 This turtle table has thick mulch and a plastic barrier as insulation against cold for turtles overwintering here. They may not eat for up to 6 months during brumation (hibernation).

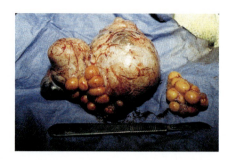

FIGURE 4-11 Fist-sized ovarian teratoma from a Green Iguana (*Iguana iguana*). These tumors appear common in long-term captive reptiles that are not being cycled and bred regularly.

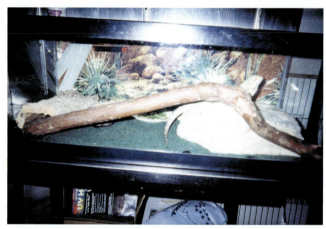

FIGURE 4-12 Natural light is powerful medicine for captive reptiles and should be provided whenever possible.

attempt to cycle their snakes by dropping the temperatures below this level at night during the late fall and winter to induce breeding behavior and ovulation. This is not necessary for most snakes and is also potentially dangerous, often resulting in respiratory infections. The photoperiod can safely be shortened during this time, however (see subsequent discussion).

Photoperiod and Light Quality

The amount of light received per day, or photoperiod, is important to reptiles. In general, day length and temperature should be decreased during the winter months. Failure to do so often results in reproductive failure or disease in many reptiles. Present hypothesis shows that inappropriate photoperiod and temperature fluctuations result in repeated reproductive failure as a result of abnormal vitellogenesis, with chronic resorption of yolk and ultimately ovarian granulomas or tumors (Figure 4-11). Obesity is another possible sequelae to abnormal photoperiod; those animals that are normally inactive and anorectic during the winter months may continue eating when exposed to the same photoperiod, even though their metabolism is lower because of ambient temperature reduction. In most cases with temperate zone or subtropical zone reptiles, the artificial photoperiod may mimic that which is naturally occurring outside. Modifications may be made depending on the latitude of the reptile's origin and the latitude where the reptile is being housed (i.e., increase the day length slightly for tropical reptiles housed at a subtropical area and more if housed in a temperate zone, even though still following seasonal changes; decrease the day length if housing a northern temperate zone reptile in a subtropical area, even though still following seasonal changes).

Electric timers are inexpensive and widely available, and lights may be set to mimic the naturally occurring photoperiod or to adjust it in either direction. Not surprisingly, reptiles housed with access to the natural light cycle (i.e., a window or skylight) respond more strongly to the natural light than to an artificial light source. This must be taken into consideration when cycling reptiles for breeding purposes. A general guideline relating to photoperiod is to provide about 14 hours of light in the summer and 12 hours of light in the winter. Another author suggested that temperate zone reptiles be exposed to 15 hours of light during the summer, 12 hours during spring and fall, and 9 hours during the winter, with tropical reptiles exposed to 13 hours of light during the summer and 11 hours of light during the winter.[5]

The quality of light is also important. Some ultraviolet (UV) light is necessary for most reptiles to manufacture vitamin D_3 within their skin. Vitamin D_3 is necessary for the absorption of calcium from the intestinal tract. A deficiency of UV light, particularly UVB, or light in the 290 to 320 nm range often results in metabolic bone disease of nutritional origin (NMBD). UVA light, or light in the 320 to 400 nm range does not assist in converting vitamin D into an active molecule in the skin but may have some beneficial effects in terms of behavior (i.e., improved visualization of prey or mates). Types of lights are discussed subsequently under lighting. Most curators and experienced herpetoculturists believe that natural lighting is the best light and may even be a requirement for some of the more demanding captive reptiles (Figure 4-12). See Chapter 84 for a discussion of artificial lighting.

Humidity

Providing a high humidity retreat or a humidity gradient may be slightly more difficult. In doing so, one must remember that the higher humidity areas in the cage must not be created

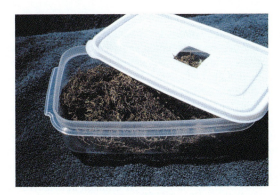

FIGURE 4-13 A humidity box is a plastic box containing substrate that holds some moisture. The most commonly used substrate for this purpose at this time is sphagnum moss.

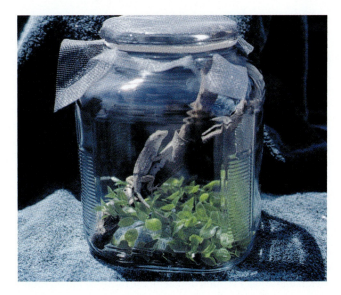

FIGURE 4-14 A small open-topped plastic container is ideal for many species of arboreal reptiles. Baby chameleons and Emerald Tree Boas (*Corrallus caninus*) are often housed in this manner.

at the expense of total cage ventilation. If ventilation is severely restricted, stagnant air often contributes to the growth of bacterial or fungal pathogens. Instead, high humidity zones within otherwise well-ventilated cages should be created. This may be done in confined areas, such as plastic boxes of varying sizes, or with moisture-containing substrates in different parts of the cage. The most commonly used method of providing a high humidity retreat for some reptiles is the use of the aforementioned humidity box, in which a plastic box is filled with a moisture-containing substrate, such as sphagnum moss or peat moss (Figure 4-13). A small hole is created in the cover of such a box to allow the reptile to enter or exit the structure. These boxes often show visible condensation within and provide the moisture needed to aid in ecdysis, or egg deposition, and to prevent chronic dehydration via cutaneous and respiratory water loss.

Many reptile keepers use vaporizers or humidifiers to humidify the enclosure directly or indirectly. This is acceptable because it does not interfere with ventilation. Chameleon keepers have been known to place intravenous (IV) drip–type systems or ice above a screen lid to allow water to drip into the environment. A number of keepers of both lizards and snakes simply maintain moistened sphagnum moss at the bottom of the cage. For some strictly arboreal reptiles, the bottom of the cage may filled with several inches of water. In a well-ventilated cage, this maintains a high and constant humidity. Small chameleons and arboreal snakes, such as Emerald Tree Boas (*Corallus caninus*) and Green Tree Pythons (*Morelia viridis*) have been successfully maintained in gallon jars with water on the bottom, a branch to perch on, and a screen top (Figure 4-14).

Substrate

Perhaps the next most important factor in determining the success or failure of a captive reptile is the substrate used. Both artificial and natural substrates may be used to achieve a level of humidity, physical support, and psychological security. Shredded newspaper, butcher's paper, and artificial turf have been popular with many herpetoculturists because of their availability and low price. However, although these materials are satisfactory and readily cleanable substrates for many reptiles, they are not aesthetically pleasing and do not appear to provide microenvironments similar to those which are found in nature. Certain kinds of wood chips, such as cypress chips, appear to provide a substrate with all of the features previously listed and an aesthetic appearance. Large, smooth stones have been successfully used as a substrate for many lizards and snakes; small stones and gravel, however, may be ingested. One of the more recent substrates that appears to have a great deal of promise is shredded coconut shells. Many species of snakes, lizards, and tortoises can be maintained on a variety of substrates; however, refer to herpetocultural sources for specific recommendations on the species in question. Substrates that are too basic, too acidic, too dry, too moist, or dirty contribute to dermatological or respiratory conditions in captive reptiles. Substrates that contain irritating aromatic compounds, such as cedar shavings, may also result in skin or respiratory irritation with secondary infection possible. Natural substrates that absorb moisture, such as wood chips of any kind, are likely to harbor heavy growth of potentially pathogenic bacteria or fungi if they are placed in a poorly ventilated cage. Thus, wood chip substrates should not be used in plastic shoe box or drawer style cages, unless good ventilation is present.

In general, tortoises do well on a substrate of rabbit pellets, but occasionally loose footing may lead to splay leg in young tortoises. Also, tortoises, such as Burmese Mountain Tortoises (*Manourid emys*), that need higher moisture substrates do not do well on this substrate. Semi-moist cypress mulch works better for these species. In addition, rabbit pellets may also contribute to respiratory disease if the pellets get wet and moldy. Most of the larger snakes commonly kept as pets do well on shredded newspaper, indoor/outdoor carpet, and wood chips, such as cypress or aspen. Smaller species of snakes generally do not do well on newspaper but may thrive when cypress mulch is used. Lizards often do well on dry, loose sand or indoor/outdoor carpet. Crushed pecan or walnut shells have been associated with many intestinal impactions in smaller lizards and are best avoided. However, crushed pecan or walnut shells have been used successfully with many snakes. Sand may also be ingested and has been associated with impactions in smaller lizards, so it must be used with care. In addition, sand in poorly ventilated cages may retain a large amount of water, which may lead to contact dermatitis. However, loose, dry sand as a substrate in a well-ventilated cage is frequently successfully used. One must often provide some sand-free areas, such as large flat rocks, on which to feed.

Water itself may be considered as a specialized substrate for some reptiles. However, tap water is often a poor substitute for the naturally occurring acidic bacteria-laden water from which many of our freshwater reptiles are derived. Tap water is also not useable for brackish or saltwater reptiles. Aquatic reptiles placed in cages where water is available frequently spend a great deal of time in that medium, which is to be expected. However, these reptiles often have skin lesions develop under these circumstances, most likely because the neutral tap water contaminated with reptile feces forms a suitable medium for many of the bacteria and fungi that may be opportunistic pathogens. Combined with the fact that the water is often devoid of the bacterial milieu found in the reptile's natural habitat, and often not in the appropriate temperature range, these animals succumb to superficial infections, which ultimately may result in sepsis. The warm acidic bacteria-laden water found in many natural situations is believed to form a bioactive substrate, which interferes with the growth of pathogens on many of those animals that have evolved to live there (see the discussion on bioactive substrates in this chapter). Thus, attempting to recreate this bioactive milieu by acidifying the water and providing organic material that maintain acid-loving bacteria may be indicated. Some authors have used dilute mixtures of tea; others have added peat to filters, and some have just used swamp mud and live plants.[5-7] Interestingly, an alternative that seems to help fresh water reptiles avoid skin lesions is the addition of some salt to the water. The addition of 1 cup of table salt per 20 gallons (approximately 80 L) of water often provides a brackish water solution that reduces the likelihood of infection but does not result in dehydration. This is particularly true if the temperature is maintained at a minimum of 82°F to 85°F (28°C to 29.5°C) with drying/basking areas available in which the reptile can raise its body temperature to more than 90°F (32°C) during the daytime. In some cases, merely a diurnal rise in the water temperature is suitable, and this can be achieved with incandescent lights placed over the water during the daytime. Full-strength seawater may be created by purchasing one of the commercially available seawater mixes (e.g., Instant Ocean, www.aquariumsystems.com) and following the directions. However, this is only necessary for marine reptiles.

Keep in mind that many reptiles do not follow these general guidelines, and the reader is referred to one of the many references listed for specific information on the species in question.[6-26]

Cage Size and Construction

In general, the larger the enclosure for any captive reptile, the better the reptile fares. Larger cages are associated with less self-inflicted injuries and better body condition. Captive reproduction is also more likely to occur when larger cages or enclosures are used. Refer to specific references for cage sizes for various reptiles, but some cages sizes are listed in Table 4-2.

The material from which cages are constructed is also important. Cages should be made of smooth, nonabrasive, and nonabsorbent materials. Examples of such materials are glass, plastic, plexiglass, and stainless steel. These materials are not as likely to cause rostral abrasions as are rough materials, and they are easily cleaned and disinfected. Bare wood is the most notorious problem material used in the construction of large reptile cages. Not only is it abrasive, but it is difficult to clean and nearly impossible to disinfect. Furthermore, eliminating mites from such a cage is difficult once they are introduced. Eliminating mites from wooden cages often requires that the cage be repainted. Otherwise, such infected cages may need to be destroyed.

The most common cage shape used in herpetoculture is the rectangle. These cages are structurally sound, and readily available, and they minimize the angles into which a reptile might collide. Unusual shapes such as pentagons, hexagons, octagons, and others often provide less useable space and are associated with more injuries than the simple rectangular cages. The height of a cage is also an important parameter of that cage. For terrestrial reptiles, the "foot space" is more important than the vertical height of the enclosure; however, the top of the cage must not be so low as to allow the reptile to reach it easily and traumatize itself or facilitate an easy escape. For arboreal reptiles, the opposite is true; a cage with

Table 4-2 Minimum Cage Sizes for Adults of Various Commonly Kept Reptiles

		Size of Cage
Snakes		
Gartersnakes	*Thamnophis* sp.	10 G
Ball (Royal) Python	*Python regius*	20 GL
Kingsnake	*Lampropeltis getula*	20 GL
Ratsnake and Cornsnake	*Elaphe* sp.	20 GL
Indigo Snake	*Drymarchon corais*	40 GL
Boa Constrictor	*Boa constrictor*	75 GL
Burmese Python	*Python molurus*	8 (L) × 4 (W) × 2 (H) ft
Lizards		
Bearded Dragon	*Pogona vitticeps*	40 GL or 4 (L) × 2 (W) × 2 (H) ft
Fence Lizard	*Sceloporus* sp.	20 GL
Water Dragon	*Physignathus* spp.	40 GL
Savannah Monitor	*Varanus exanthematicus*	40 GL
Green Iguana (juvenile)	*Iguana iguana*	30 GL
Green Iguana (adult)		8 (L) × 2 (W) × 6 (H) ft
Chameleons (juvenile)		20 GL
Chameleons (most adults)		2 (L) × 2 (W) × 3 (H) ft
Chelonians		
Musk, Mud, Sideneck		20 GL
Spotted, Bog, Box		40 GL
Sliders, Painted Turtle, Sawbacks		40 GL
Snapping Turtle	*Chelydra serpentina*	75 GL
Alligator Snapper	*Macrochelys temminckii*	100 GL

L, Long; *H*, high; *W*, wide; *G*, gallon; *GL*, gallon-long aquarium.

increased height provides more useable habitat than a cage with increased foot space. Mass-produced aquariums, which are commonly converted in reptile terrariums, use terminology that may be helpful to the herpetoculturist and veterinarian. Aquariums with the maximum floor space are referred to as "long" aquariums, and those of the same volume with a smaller foot space are referred to as "high" aquariums. High aquariums are more suitable for arboreal reptiles because they can use this vertical space.

Hospitalization

Hospitalizing a sick or debilitated reptile requires some of the same basic requirements as listed previously. However, temporary housing may be somewhat stark and sterile compared with permanent housing. Perhaps the most important physical requirement of sick reptiles is heat. These animals should be housed at or near the upper end of their preferred optimum temperature range (see Table 4-1).

The author's clinic maintains both heated and unheated racks, where plastic boxes may be slid into their respective slots. These cages are easily disinfected between patients and are space efficient. In addition, many of these racks are mobile (see Figure 4-7). They may be easily rolled from one area to another for a variety of reasons. Many veterinarians use incubators because they may precisely regulate a reptile's temperature.

Regular dog and cat cages may be used to house many large lizards and tortoises and small crocodilians. Supplemental heat may be provided via heat lamps or heating pads, which can be attached to or placed in the cage, respectively (Figure 4-15).

The substrate of choice for most hospitalized reptiles appears to be newspaper or some other nontoxic absorbent paper material. It should be checked daily and changed as necessary. As a general rule, these substrates should be completely dry. Those reptiles that have special high-humidity requirements may need humidity boxes in their cages; these were discussed previously under basic husbandry. All small reptiles, particularly neonates and juveniles, may benefit from access to these high-humidity retreats. For short periods of time, high-humidity microenvironments may be created by adding water-soaked paper or clean cotton towels to an enclosure. Snakes that need assistance in shedding their skin may often be soaked in moistened pillowcases placed within the confines of their hospital cage for 6 to 24 hours. When the snake is removed after the prescribed period, the skin is usually sufficiently moistened to facilitate its manual removal. High humidity provided for long periods of time can be detrimental, however, if the temperature and ventilation in the hospital cage are not adequate. This is especially true for plastic box–style cages.

Another cage accessory of importance for a hospitalized reptile is a place to hide. Hide boxes should be placed in the cage of hospitalized reptiles if the cages have clear sides and no secure hiding areas are within. A number of commercially manufactured plastic boxes are produced, but any plastic box may be modified for this purpose. Sometimes water bowls have a hollow space under them that provides a suitable retreat.

Branches of the correct size also provide some security and an opportunity for a reptile to exercise. These branches should be stable, however, because collapsing branches are potentially harmful to cage occupants. As with birds, branches must be of an appropriate diameter to be fully used by the species in question. Another consideration is the positioning of the branch. Some species, such as certain geckos, prefer vertical branches, and others, such as large lizards, prefer horizontal perches.

One of the most important aspects of hospitalizing reptiles is identification. In a busy exotic practice, numerous iguanas, tortoises, and bearded dragons may be in the hospital at the same time. If the cages are well marked with cards, errors in treatment are unlikely. Tortoises may also be easily marked with a strip of masking tape or white tape on the carapace. Most lizards may be marked with a small strip of white tape or self-adhesive bandage material wrapped around a lower limb. More permanent methods of identification include microchipping, tattooing, toe clipping, scale clipping, and notching marginal scales of a chelonian's shell, but these are generally reserved for study animals and not pet reptiles. The cage card mentioned previously should also have spaces for observations and daily treatments, in addition to the patient's name and owner's name.

Quarantine

Isolating reptiles from each other during their initial maintenance in a collection is critical. All too often parasitic or infectious diseases have been introduced into a collection because of a lack of any quarantine period. A recommended period of 3 months is advisable for most reptiles. Some experts have suggested that snakes be quarantined for up to 6 months because of the risk of paramyxovirus or other viruses that may devastate a collection.[2,3] Isolation should theoretically be accomplished in separate rooms that do not exchange air with each other. However, this is not often practical or possible with hospitalized reptiles. Under these circumstances, prevention of direct contact is often all that can be achieved. Animals that enter a hospital reptile kennel or bank of cages should be carefully examined first for any evidence of external parasitism. Snake mites and lizard mites may rapidly travel from cage to cage in a rack-style arrangement.

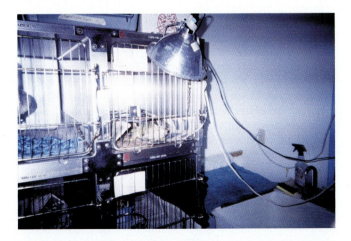

FIGURE 4-15 Regular stainless steel dog and cat cages can be modified to house larger reptiles by adding a heat source. Here a heat lamp is hung on the outside of the bars for this Green Iguana (*Iguana iguana*).

Snakes with mites are not housed in the same room as other reptiles. After the newly arrived reptile has been placed in its new enclosure, the bag or box used to transport that reptile should either be disinfected or discarded.

Also, remember that reptiles from different areas of the world should never be housed together because organisms that may be commensals for reptiles from one area may be pathogens for reptiles from other areas. Healthy animals, or long-term hospital patients, should be treated first, and new arrivals, or quarantined animals, should be taken care of last. In some cases, reptiles of the same species, captured in the same area and shipped at the same time, can be quarantined in a communal cage. However, this should only be attempted if the species in question is not cannibalistic and all of the previous conditions are met. Reptiles housed together may compete with each other for food and basking sites, so care should be exercised when housing communally. See Chapter 78 for a thorough discussion of quarantine procedures.

Disinfection

Use of disposable paper towels instead of a single cleaning rag is imperative when going from cage to cage. Keep in mind that no disinfectant is 100% effective against all pathogens, and therefore, one should dispose of towels after use in a single cage. Only clean paper towels are dipped into the chosen disinfectant bucket. In this manner, the disinfectant solution itself does not become contaminated. Hands should also be washed between cages with a suitable antibacterial soap or perhaps some of the disinfectant solution in a separate container from that used to disinfect the cages. For more information on disinfectants see Chapter 85. A common, inexpensive, and effective disinfectant is household bleach (sodium hypochlorite), which can be diluted to a concentration of one part bleach to 30 parts water (30 mL per liter of water or $1/2$ cup per gallon). Full strength bleach is not necessary and has been associated with the destruction of respiratory epithelium and death of birds and reptiles when used in their cages. A 5% ammonia solution is effective against coccidia and *Crytosporidia*, but remember that bleach and ammonia cannot be mixed.

Another commonly used and effective disinfectant is Roccal-D. This is a quaternary ammonium compound that has a broad spectrum of activity against common reptile pathogens. McKeown[4] recommends a diltution with water of 1:200 to 1:400 for reptile cages and bowls.

Remembering that disinfection cannot occur without first physically removing the organic debris is imperative. Thus, the clinician should advise herpetoculturists, zookeepers, and technicians to thoroughly clean a cage first and then disinfect it. Cleaning should occur daily unless a bioactive substrate is being used, in which case, nonpathogenic bacteria breaks down the fecal matter. See the discussion on bioactive substrates.

Ideally, hospitals that treat reptiles benefit by having foot pump water faucets and soap dispensers. This helps prevent cross contamination of hands and cages and cage accessories at the sink/faucet level. An important point to remember about cleaning these cage accessories, including water bowls, hide boxes, and artificial plants, is to avoid placing them together in the same water-filled sink. Even when soap and a disinfectant are added, certain infectious agents may not be eliminated and instead spread from dish to dish within the ineffective soapy solution. For example, if one placed a water bowl contaminated with coccidia in a sink filled with bleach water, all other dishes in that sink may be contaminated with coccidia because sodium hypochlorite is an ineffective disinfectant against coccidia.

Examinations

Careful examination of reptiles entering a facility where other reptiles are housed is critically important in protecting that collection. Any signs of illness, including nasal or ocular discharges; excessive sneezing or wheezing; loose, mucous, or bloody stools; neurological signs; or skin lesions, should alert the clinician to isolate such an animal immediately. Far too many stories exist of large stable collections with huge losses after a new "unquarantined" animal is admitted. A collection of reptiles that does not admit new animals is referred to as a closed collection.

A physical examination should be both thorough and systematic. Start at one end and work to the other in every animal. Look in the mouth, nares, eyes, and ears, where present. Palpate musculature, and examine the skin carefully. Closely examine folds of skin for ticks or mites, and watch for soft subcutaneous swellings, which could be indicative of pathology. Check the abdomen by palpation, and carefully examine the cloaca, looking for swelling or an abnormal discharge. Some urates in the cloaca are acceptable, but if they are excessive or if a mucous or abnormally colored discharge (e.g., florescent green) is found, a potential problem exists.

A fecal examination is advisable for all reptiles immediately after acquisition and again 3 months later. Annual or semiannual fecal examinations are advisable after that. See the subsequent discussion.

Hematology and blood chemistry may also be extremely helpful in determining the apparent health of a reptile. All too often, a reptile appears healthy outwardly but has a disorder that is only revealed with a complete blood cell count (CBC) or chemistry. A blood smear evaluation may reveal parasites in many imports. Normal blood values for numerous species of reptiles have now been published and are readily accessible (see Chapter 88).[27,28]

Parasite Control

All recently captured reptiles or any reptiles that are new to a collection should be suspected of parasites. Repeated fecal examinations should be performed during the first several months in captivity and then regularly thereafter. The eggs of many parasites may not appear immediately in the first fecal examination performed on a recently captured reptile; they often appear on fecal examinations performed 3 to 6 months later. The cause of this is not known. Presumably, the parasite infections are present at the time of capture, but either they are not yet reproductive and need time to mature and produce ova or else the stress of captivity may suppress the immune response of the captive reptile and allow the parasites to increase in numbers. Thus, fecal examinations performed right after the time of capture should be considered as necessary screens for animals with heavy parasite loads but not as definitive tests to rule out parasitism. Fecal analyses should be performed both at the beginning and the end of the quarantine period.

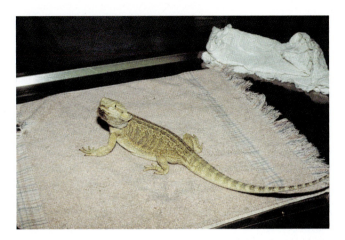

FIGURE 4-16 Bearded Dragons (*Pogona vitticeps*) are commonly parasitized with coccidia. These parasites can be difficult to eliminate.

Once parasitism is diagnosed, appropriate parasiticides should be administered at the doses recommended elsewhere in this book. Some authors recommend a routine deworming be performed even in the absence of positive fecal examination results. Furthermore, those parasites with direct life cycles are particularly difficult to eliminate, even in a single animal enclosure, so a regular deworming schedule may be indicated even for some long-term captives. An example of a parasite that is extremely difficult to eliminate is coccidia in bearded dragons (Figure 4-16).

Parasites and other infectious agents may be brought into a collection by wild rodents, birds, insects, and other arthropods. Mosquitos are well-known vectors for certain blood parasites, and flies can serve as mechanical vectors for many pathogenic bacteria. Thus, a simple but extremely effective method of disease control is to maintain insect screens over and between all cages. Flies, mosquitos, and roaches are not able to move easily from cage to cage with this manner of protection. Unfortunately, most insect screens do not stop fruit flies, gnats, or mites, and other methods are necessary for the control of these pests.

Snake mites and lizard mites are the bane of many herpetoculturists. Once in a collection, they are extremely difficult to eliminate, so major efforts should be made to prevent their entrance into a collection. Usually all new reptiles should be quarantined for at least 1 month, and probably longer to visualize a potential infection. If the newly acquired animal is found to have these ectoparasites, treating this individual is far easier than treating an entire collection. Food items and other individuals may also serve as vectors for mites.

The author once had a young volunteer come to his house to help clean up some snake cages. A week later, a major outbreak of mites occurred in the bank of cages cleaned by that volunteer. Nothing else had changed in the husbandry of that group of snakes, and no mite outbreaks in that group of snakes had occurred in the previous 2 years. Questioning of the individual revealed that he had just been to a pet shop and had handled some of the animals there.

Food items such as live mice have also been incriminated in transferring snake mites into collections. Pet shops all too commonly maintain rodent cages near snake cages, and when the snakes have mites, they often get into the rodent cages. Thus, an unsuspecting owner may carry home mites with a live prey item. The clinician should warn owners of this potential risk. This problem may be eliminated by purchasing rodents from clean reputable sources where reptiles are not housed near rodents or by purchasing frozen rodents. Freezing prekilled rodents appears to kill all of the snake mites on those animals. The same cannot be said for pathogenic bacteria or protozoans. If one must use live rodents from a potentially parasitized source, one may place the rodents in question in a cage with a Sevin-impregnated substrate for 48 hours before attempting to feed. One may simply sprinkle liberal amounts of 5% Sevin dust over the substrate before adding the rodents. Such rodents are best removed from this substrate 24 hours before feeding them to a reptile. This usually allows them to clean themselves and pass most of the Sevin before ingestion by the reptile.

Other techniques for controlling mites on reptiles include sprinkling 5% Sevin dust directly on the reptile in question and leaving it on for at least several hours and then rinsing it off or using a pyrethrin spray. A product named Provent-a-Mite was recently tested and appeared both safe and effective in all reptiles tested.[29] See Chapter 43 for more details.

As mentioned previously, insects, including prey insects, may also serve as vectors for the transmission of parasites or other pathogenic organisms. Prey insects arriving with flies, maggots, or the larvae of other insects should be suspect, and one might want to consider recommending a different supplier if these are observed in an insect shipment.

Control of Disease Transmission in Closed Collections

A closed collection is a group of reptiles to which new specimens are prevented from entering. This arrangement has tremendous advantages in the prevention of disease. The only reason to allow a new animal into a closed breeding colony is to add more genetic diversity to the group. This reduces the likelihood of inbreeding and associated diseases.

Multiindividual and Multispecies Enclosures

Recently, herpetoculturists have made efforts to house reptiles in naturalistic enclosures that mimic not only the naturally occurring physical environment but also the biological environment of the animals in question. Numerous species of plants and animals that coexist with the species in question may be considered for the captive environment, if the cage is suitably sized and complex enough to provide the proper habitat for all species considered. However, if two or more species are to be considered for cohabitation, their relationship to each other must be determined. Will they compete with each other for food and habitat? Will they prey on each other? Do they carry any diseases or parasites that may negatively affect the other species? What is a suitable population density for the species in question? These and other questions need to be answered to safely house reptiles together. For many years, we have correctly advised clients to house reptiles alone when they are using small cages. Only in this way can feeding be monitored and competition for food reduced. Larger more complex cages may house more than one individual of the same species, but one must watch them carefully. Tortoise keepers have been known to create a feeding stall arrangement so that tortoises in the same enclosure can eat without disturbance from other tortoises yet gain the benefit of social contact.

Generally speaking, **reptiles from different geographic areas should not be maintained together because of the risk of introducing a disease into a susceptible (immunologically naive) population**. If reptiles from different geographic areas are to be mixed, one should avoid mixing those which occupy the same ecological niche (i.e., those that eat the same food, occupy the same microhabitat, or are active at the same time of the day). Two individual rodent-eating snakes maintained in a small enclosure or two groups of rodent-eating snakes in a large enclosure may not be compatible. Similarly, two species of tortoises that feed on the same food at the same time of the day may compete directly or indirectly. Also, chelonians and crocodilians appear to naturally carry a number of commensal protozoans that may be pathogenic for some snakes and lizards. Thus, chelonians and terrestrial snakes should not be housed together in small enclosures. Crocodilians, of course, are likely to eat snakes, thereby making their cohabitation doubtful in a small enclosure.

In a large, outdoor enclosure maintained by the author, six species of snakes were maintained. These included Watersnakes (*Nerodia harteri harteri*), Queen Snakes (*Regina septemvittata*), Hog-nosed Snakes (*Heterodon simus*), Rough Greensnakes (*Opheodrys aestivus*), Foxsnakes (*Elaphe vulpina*), and Ribbonsnakes (*Thamnophis proximus*) (Figure 4-17). Theoretically, these snakes should have been able to cohabitate on the basis of their differing food preferences. Their preferred foods included, respectively, fish, crayfish, toads, insects, rodents, and small amphibians. However, the Ribbonsnakes also preyed on small fish, effectively competing with young Watersnakes. The Foxsnakes and Greensnakes contracted amoebiasis, presumably from drinking water contaminated by the heavy population of Watersnakes and Queen Snakes, for which the amoeba appeared to be nonpathogenic commensals. The Hog-nosed Snakes were preyed on by large local birds. Thus, one can see just how complicated these enclosures can become. Even when predation was controlled, the Watersnakes increased rapidly to such a number that parasitism, fungal disease, and even cannibalism became significant factors for these snakes housed outdoors.[30,31] See the discussion on outdoor enclosures to follow.

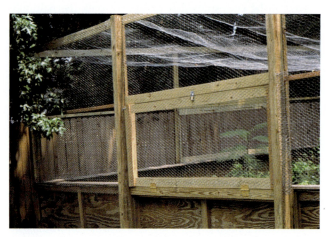

FIGURE 4-17 A large outdoor enclosure allows reptiles to establish territories, forage, and avoid confrontations with cage mates. These behaviors are not often observed in those reptiles housed in indoor aquarium-style cages.

Environmental Enhancement and Outdoor Enclosures

As a small boy visiting the large cat enclosure at the Bronx Zoo (now called the New York Zoological Garden) in the early 1960s, I was struck by the constant activity level of the caged cats. In small concrete-bottomed bare cages, they appeared to pace back and forth incessantly. In short, they were probably bored. Reptiles caged in similarly stark cages appear to show similar behavior, and, generally speaking, reptiles that pace are much more likely to have health problems in captivity. A direct observation that may be associated with pacing is rostral abrasion, which often leads to stomatitis, anorexia, and a rapid decline. However, a constantly pacing reptile likely has stress and all the sequelae of that stress, including immune system suppression and ultimately disease. Ideally, one should observe that a captive reptile finds certain areas within its enclosure and stays in one of those areas for periods of time, rather than constantly wandering.

Numerous hiding, resting, and activity areas should be provided. Activities might include foraging for food or water, seeking mates, thermoregulating, or seeking more suitable shelter. Admittedly, some energy may be directed towards escaping from an enclosure, but in a large well-designed enclosure, this activity should be minimized. In open outdoor enclosures, some reptiles establish territories and defend them. They may exhibit normal escape reactions when approached and normal defensive actions when approached closely or picked up (e.g., they may bite, flail wildly, or defecate on the keeper). In short, they may live like and behave much more like wild reptiles than captive ones.[30] All of those factors that affect them in nature may affect them in a large outdoor enclosure (i.e., competition, predation, parasitism, disease, starvation, dehydration, cold exposure). However, these animals are not wild but rather captive reptiles in fancy cages. They may become more heavily parasitized than their wild counterparts because they are confined to much smaller areas, thereby increasing exposure to parasite ova in the environment. They may become much heavier than their wild counterparts because of reduced activity associated with confinement. And they may exhibit unusual behaviors not seen in wild reptiles of the same species. Large outdoor enclosures have been used successfully for years with crocodilians and tortoises; only recently have they become more popular for lizards and snakes.

Bioactive Substrates

Recent advances in herpetoculture may revolutionize the way we keep reptiles in captivity and think about their captive requirements. DeVosjoli[32] discusses in detail the use of bioactive substrate systems (BSS). The basic theory behind these substrates is that they provide an environment where beneficial bacteria compete with pathogenic bacteria and fungi to support a healthy microhabitat for the captive. Stirring the substrate is apparently the key. Stirring mixes the competitive bacteria in lower layers with fecal bacteria and others at the surface, thereby inhibiting their growth. Successful creation of the bioactive substrate, according to DeVosjoli, requires that the substrate is at least 6.5 cm (2.5 in) deep and that it allows for good oxygenation and moisture retention. If the substrate dries out, it does not work. This system has been tested primarily on snakes, but theoretically it is useful for many captive reptiles.

The moisture-containing substrate mentioned previously probably has other benefits as well. Lillywhite[33] and others have recently commented on cutaneous water loss that captive snakes endure when they are placed in completely dry cages. This chronic water loss is suspected of being a major factor leading to the premature demise of these captive snakes; it may result in kidney damage. Thus, a moist substrate may create a microhabitat that protects a captive reptile from both dehydration and infection. Indeed, the author has seen many small species of snakes do well in moist substrates or where moist substrates are offered as one of the choices available to these reptiles.

Lighting

As mentioned previously, the provision of proper lighting for captive reptiles is necessary to successfully maintain them for long periods of time. The act of basking is thought to be a behavior that maximizes the use of not only the heat but also the light available. Both natural and artificial lighting may be beneficial for these animals. Natural lighting that is unfiltered by glass has the advantage that it has a spectrum that can be used for the production of vitamin D in the skin of many reptiles. It also has the advantage of providing some heat. However, two kinds of artificial lights are commonly used. Incandescent bulbs, which are generally bulb like, provide both heat and light. Florescent bulbs, which are generally tubular, provide a wider spectrum of light but little heat. Popular florescent bulbs that produce light in the proper spectrum discussed previously are ZooMed's Reptisun lights (www.zoomed.com). Diurnal lizards, diurnal snakes, small crocodilians, and basking species of turtles and tortoises do well with the Reptisun 5.0 or 7.0, and amphibians and many temperate zone snakes do well with the Reptisun 2.0. Providing both kinds of light for most reptiles is advisable, unless a combination light is used. See Chapter 84 on lighting for more details. Generally speaking, however, no substitute exists for natural light for many reptiles. It is perhaps one of the most powerful medicines known in captive reptile management. It is also a potent appetite stimulant for many reptiles and may have many other unknown beneficial effects.

Water

That water should be available at all times for most reptiles is generally believed. However, exceptions do exist. The constant presence of water in poorly ventilated cages often becomes a health hazard for many reptiles. Unable to escape the excessively humid air in such a cage, these animals become susceptible to dermatitis or respiratory disease. The situation may be aggravated by excessive substrate moisture, leaving the reptile no escape. However, with suitable conditions in a well-ventilated cage, the presence of a clean reliable source of water is extremely important to most captive reptiles. As mentioned previously, definite cutaneous and respiratory water losses must be compensated for or the captive reptile suffers either acute or chronic dehydration. This concept of chronic dehydration, and possibly associated kidney disease, has captured the interest of some physiologists and zookeepers recently. Some have suggested that merely providing sufficient drinking water cannot prevent chronic dehydration and kidney disease if the reptile is not placed in a suitable microenvironment that reduces cutaneous and respiratory water loss. See the discussion on basic husbandry requirements.

How water is provided is also important. An arboreal reptile, such as a vine snake, a tree boa, or a chameleon, may rarely come to the ground level. Therefore, a water bowl on the floor of the cage may be futile as a method of providing drinking water. However, misting the branches on a regular basis or providing a tree mounted water bowl may be effective. Desert reptiles may also benefit tremendously from a misting of the rocks in their enclosure on a regular basis, as they often lap water from these rocks but may not always use a water bowl. Conversely, some may sit in their water bowls for excessively long periods of time if these are provided, which may lead to dermatitis. Many tortoises seem to need a daily rain to thrive, but the substrate should not stay excessively moist on a continual basis.

The size and shape of a container is another factor that should be considered. Steep-sided water containers may prevent easy entry or exit by many chelonians, resulting in dehydration or drowning. Terrestrial chelonians and even some aquatic species are not strong swimmers and may easily drown if the water is deeper than their legs are long. As a general rule, no chelonian should be put in water deeper than this unless one is familiar with the habits of the species and the health of the individual in question. Even the most aquatic of reptiles, including crocodilians and certain snakes, need a resting area or "haul out" where they can climb out to bask or rest.

Be aware that daily soakings are an important maintenance requirement for many terrestrial chelonians. We soak every hospitalized tortoise for at least one half hour daily in shallow water. The tortoises may drink at this time, but often the soaking merely facilitates defecation and appears to encourage activity and alertness (Figure 4-18).

Additives to reptile water have been the subject of many discussions during the last 10 years. Several commercial vitamin and mineral formulations are presently available, but the values of these products are largely unknown. The dosing of

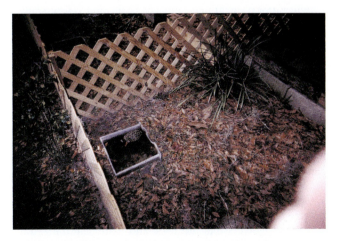

FIGURE 4-18 Hospitalized tortoises should be soaked in shallow water at least every other day. Some hospitals recommend soaking for at least a half hour per day.

such products is purely empirical. Some authors have recommended the use of dilute bleach in the drinking water to control bacteria. At 1 to 5 mL per gallon (4 L), this addition is both safe for the reptile and efficacious against some bacteria. This addition is probably unnecessary for most captive reptiles, however, but may be helpful in cases where a particular bacterial disease is spreading rapidly through a group of reptiles in the same cage.

Feeding

Inadequate nutrition of captive reptiles rivals inadequate environment in terms of being a leading cause of disease (see Chapter 18). Together, these factors are believed to be responsible directly or indirectly for more than 90% of illness in captive reptiles. Both the quantity and quality of the food are important. Feed reptiles the highest quality food items possible. Fresh food items are ideal. "Old" food items or those that have been stored improperly may be contaminated with various fungi or bacteria.

Items that have been frozen for more than 6 months may have the loss of some nutrients. Nevertheless, short-term freezing of most food items is an economical and convenient way to store food. Freezing may actually increase the digestibility of certain plant materials by rupturing the cell wall and thereby making the cell contents more accessible at an earlier stage of the digestive process. Unfortunately, the freezing process has also been associated with a reduced thiamin content in certain species of fish (see Chapter 18 for more details on the effects of storing food items).

Cooking some vegetables accomplishes the same function of breaking down cell walls but does not reduce the thiamin content, and this process may be helpful in softening some very hard vegetables, such as sweet potatoes, for reptile consumption. Under normal circumstances, however, most herbivorous reptiles should be fed uncooked green leafy vegetables. Mustard greens, collard greens, turnip greens, dandelion greens, escarole, endive, and water cress are all excellent foods. Other vegetables are also well accepted and nutritious. These include squash, snap peas, and carrot tops. Vegetables to avoid in large quantities include cabbage, brussels sprouts, cauliflower, broccoli, kale, bok choi, and radish because they contain goiterogenic substances (i.e., iodine-binding agents). Another group, including spinach, beets, and celery stalks, contains oxalic acid in a sufficient quantity to interfere with normal calcium uptake and metabolism but can be fed in moderation. Many fruits are nutritious but are low in calcium or have a poor calcium to phosphorus ratio or both. Bananas and grapes also contain tannins, which can interfere with protein metabolism in reptiles. As with birds, avocados are generally considered toxic to reptiles, although it is not uncommon to see wild iguanas eating avocados that have fallen from trees. Rhubarb and eggplant are also believed by some to be toxic for reptiles. It is always best to be safe; if concern exists over the safety of a food item, it is best left out of the captive diet.

Some flowers are considered safe and nutritious. The most notable and common among these are dandelions, hibiscus, and roses. Flowers that are toxic and extremely dangerous are azaleas, daffodils, and tulips. Marijuana is also toxic to reptiles (see Chapter 83 for more information).

The use of live prey food has been delegated to the realm of the last resort method of feeding over the last several years by a number of experts. The reasons for this include everything from increased risk of injury to the captive reptile to the inhumanity of placing a frightened prey in with one of its predators. The latter observation notwithstanding, some benefits may exist to feeding live prey over dead prey. First, the energy spent hunting and subduing food represents a significant percentage of the total energy expenditure of some reptiles. Second, the act of hunting may represent a series of necessary intellectual stimuli for the maintenance of normal behavior. Certainly, it is a survival skill that is needed if a reptile is to be released back into the wild. The combination of physical activity and intellectual stimulation helps to maintain a predatory reptile in much better condition than a stationary, stagnant, and stimulus-free environment. The same may be said for herbivorous reptiles, although the hunting behavior is limited to finding suitable forage.

Food may serve as a vector for a parasite, bacteria, fungus, or virus, so every effort must be made to advise clients to avoid wild caught food and the transfer of food items from one cage to another.

The nutritional requirements of different groups of reptiles are discussed elsewhere in this book and are not discussed in detail here. The preferred foods of many reptiles are discussed in the nutrition chapter in this book and discussed in detail in many references.[9,16,27,28,34] Generally, however, all snakes are carnivores, with foods ranging in size from insects, slugs, and earthworms to mammals the size of capybaras, deer, and antelope. Most of the snakes likely to be seen by clinicians are rodent or rabbit eaters, but a small percentage eat birds, fish, or other vertebrates. Many lizards and turtles are also carnivorous, with foods ranging from insects to large rodents, birds, fish, and small deer. The entire family Varanidae (Monitors), with a few rare exceptions, is carnivorous, with the most commonly seen captive species (e.g., Savannah, Water, and Nile Monitors) all being primarily small vertebrate eaters. The family Teiidae, commonly known as Whiptails and Tegus, occupy the same niche in the Western hemisphere as the Monitors do in the Eastern hemisphere and eat primarily insects and small vertebrates. Certainly most members of five other huge lizard families are insectivorous, namely the Scincidae (Skinks), Chamaeleonidae (Chameleons), Iguanidae (New World Anoles, Fence Lizards, Swifts, Chuckwallas, and Iguanas), Agamidae (Old World lizards occupying the same niche as the New World iguanids [e.g., Agamas, Water Dragons]), and Gekkonidae (Geckoes). Other species of lizards are herbivorous, including many of the species commonly kept as pets (e.g., Green Iguanas [*Iguana iguana*] and Bearded Dragons [*Pogona vitticeps*]).

Most tortoises and turtles are herbivorous, but many are omnivorous and a few are primarily carnivorous. Box Turtles (*Terrapene* sp. and *Cuora* sp.) and Hingeback Tortoises (*Kinyxis* sp.) are examples of chelonians that are primarily carnivorous. Among aquatic turtles, carnivorous or scavenging species include Mud Turtles family Kinosternidae, Chicken Turtles (*Deirochelys reticularia*), and Snapping Turtles (*Chelydra serpentina* and *Macroclemmys temminicki*).

Crocodilians are all carnivorous, with the preferred prey of adults varying from fish in some species to mammals and birds in others. The young of all species of crocodilians may consume some insects but rapidly switch to vertebrate prey, which has a higher calcium content.

Knowledge of the basic diets always is helpful in establishing guidelines for a captive or hospitalized patient. Typically, in an emergency situation, leafy greens or a high-quality pelletized rodent food may be used for a herbivorous reptile, a (quality) canned dog food may be used for an omnivous reptile, and a (quality) canned cat food may be used for a carnivorous reptile. The latter two options, however, may be too high in protein for long-term use in many reptiles. Gout or renal disease can result from such diets.

Fruits may have limited nutritional value but are often added to diets to stimulate consumption for herbivorous reptiles. Reptiles are capable of seeing color. Brightly colored fruits such as strawberries, tomatoes, bananas, and melons often attract the attention of many herbivorous lizards and tortoises and invite consumption. These are particularly valuable in many cases to entice recently captured or ill animals to eat, and they contain large quantities of water. Yellow (summer) squash and cooked sweet potato are also brightly colored valuable additions to the diet of many herbivorous reptiles. Some lizards, such as the Uromastyx, consume significant quantities of seeds in the wild, so a variety of seeds should be included as part of the captive diet.

Insects raised in captivity are also often of questionable value as a balanced diet. Captive raised crickets and mealworms often have a low calcium content and must be treated in such a manner as to increase this nutrient. Perhaps the most widely accepted method of raising the calcium content is to "dust" these food items with calcium powder; however, feeding the insects a high calcium diet for 24 hours or more before feeding them to a reptile has been shown to be much more efficient at providing the needed calcium to the reptile.[35] This is referred to as "gut loading" in the herpetological vernacular.

Mice and rats raised in captivity are usually considered to be a good quality food. However, those rodents and the reptiles that eat them are ultimately affected by what those rodents have been fed. Rodents fed a diet of exclusively dog food have a tendency to be fat and "greasy," and snakes and monitors that have eaten rodents fed this way also have a tendency to become obese. In fact, many of the rat snakes that have had lipomas develop have a common item in their history, the consumption of ex-breeder mice or those fed largely a dog food diet. Feeding young lean mice that have been fed a high-quality plant-based rodent chow is considered to be much healthier for those reptiles that consume them. Furthermore, this food should be available to the rodents right up until the time they are fed to the reptile. These gut contents probably contain valuable nutrients and roughage for the reptilian predator, and thus, multivitamin and mineral supplementation for rodent eaters is usually not considered necessary. In fact, one study showed no significant difference in size, weight, or bone density in two groups of hatchling cornsnakes fed supplemented and nonsupplemented mice.[36]

Herbivorous reptiles need a quality vitamin and mineral supplement. However, the vitamin and mineral requirements for most reptiles have not been determined, and most recommendations are anecdotal. Oversupplementation has occurred when vitamins are administered too frequently or in large quantities. Also, be aware that oversupplementation does not always balance an otherwise deficient diet (i.e., appropriate vitamin and mineral intake in the absence of sufficient roughage may still result in an unhealthy reptile). As in mammals, sometimes oversupplementation of one nutrient may result in a deficiency of another. In most cases, multivitamin and mineral supplementation once or twice weekly are sufficient.

Stress

Stress is a significant factor for captive reptiles (see Chapter 9). Stress is difficult to define but may be thought of as the increased energy required by a reptile to maintain itself when compared with that which is required in the normal habitat (Figure 4-19). Reptiles generally survive for prolonged periods and may reproduce if they are maintained in low-stress environments. Clean adequately sized cages with the proper substrate, thermal gradients, light quality and photoperiod, good ventilation, and the proper humidity are considered to be the physical requirements of the captive environment that reduce stress. Predators, competitors, parasites, and pathogens are the biological factors that must be controlled to reduce stress, but these factors act independently to increase the morbidity and mortality of captive reptiles in high-stress environments.

Constantly changing cages, substrates, cage accessories, or cage mates also adds stress to the life of a captive reptile. Even a change of keepers may be devastating. However, many reptiles can adapt to the captive environment and the routine provided. Indeed, reptiles appear to thrive once they adjust to a certain routine and any changes in a routine may be stressful. To put it another way, reptiles seem to be creatures of habit; once they have adapted to a routine, they may stay healthy for many years in captivity.

Other factors that may contribute to stress include handling, prodding, or poking. In addition, placing a cage in a high traffic area where there are many vibrations is also likely to be stressful. We often advise our clients not to handle any anorexic reptile until those animals have adapted and begun feeding again.

CONCLUSION

Reptile clinicians should be aware that reptiles are not domestic pets. Even though some species are bred extensively in

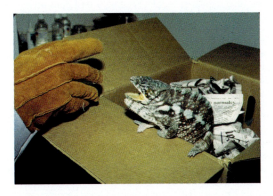

FIGURE 4-19 Measuring stress in a captive reptile is difficult but a major factor affecting survival, longevity, and reproduction.

captivity, millions of years of evolution cannot be erased in a few generations of captive propagation. As wild animals in captivity, they need a recreation of many of the physical and biological features of their natural habitat. Successful management of reptiles in a contrived environment, therefore, requires that veterinarians become familiar with the habitat, diet, and preferred temperature range of the species in question, and they should approximate those parameters as much as possible in the captive setting.

Some reptile species appear to be more adaptable than others. Many of these adaptable species have the ability to tolerate a wide range of captive habitats, but as clinicians we need to be aware of what the ideal temperature and humidity range is for our patients so that we can guide our clients in improving the captive environment. Reptiles that are housed in a different environment from what they should be housed in may survive but not thrive. This difference between ideal and realized captive environment is what leads to stress, and chronic stress leads to reproductive failure, disease, and death. As discussed previously, the first step in successfully treating reptiles is often examination of the captive environment and correction of it. The second step is educating the client.

The following practical guidelines may be given to reptile clients:

1. Maintain cage cleanliness. A clean cage looks and smells good not only to people but also probably to a captive reptile. This may result in a better appetite and an overall sense of well being. Cleaning and disinfection reduces the number of potentially pathogenic bacteria and breaks the life cycle of those parasites that have direct life cycles (e.g., oxyurids).
2. Provide clean water (and good ventilation). Even though some reptiles may not drink from a bowl, many species must have the option available. Many desert reptiles consume water from a bowl if given a choice. If not, water may be provided by frequent misting of the cage. Remember that the water must be changed frequently and that the water bowl must be scrubbed and disinfected regularly. Many professional snake breeders only provide water once weekly. Tortoises do best with daily soakings. Chameleons often need misting once or twice daily. One must remember that the presence of water in the cage at all times requires good ventilation. If the cage is poorly ventilated, the humidity in the cage may reach unhealthy levels, predisposing the occupant to disease.
3. Feed on a regular schedule. Feeding is best done on a routine schedule, with the same kind of food (same texture, size, dead versus alive, etc). So feed at the same time of the day or at the same intervals during the day. An observant keeper should learn the idiosyncrasies of a particular animal's food preferences. Captive reptiles often become accustomed to one particular keeper, and changes may be stressful.
4. Provide a regular light cycle. Timers are necessary for keeping light cycles regular. Estimating their value in terms of stress reduction, successful thermoregulation, and breeding is impossible, but the repeatable and controllable cycles that they maintain are likely healthful.
5. Keep specimen handling to a minimum. In nature, when something picks up a reptile, the reptile is about to be eaten. Thus, handling may be stressful for many reptiles and should be restricted. A well-adapted good-feeding reptile that has been raised in captivity may accommodate human intervention and in fact may even appear to enjoy being touched, but excessive handling should be avoided. Remember that handling also increases the risk of exposure to pathogenic organisms, especially if the handler has recently handled other reptiles. Accidental trauma is also more likely with frequent handling.
6. Never keep reptiles from different geographic regions together. Remember that organisms that may be normal in a reptile from one locale area (or a collection) may cause disease in a reptile from another area (or collection).
7. Avoid transferring anything from one cage to another. It is better to clean each cage with disposable paper towels and thereby avoid spreading potentially dangerous microorganisms from one cage to another on a cleansing towel. Along the same lines, do not wash cage accessories from different cages in the same soapy water.
8. Fecal examinations should be performed on a regular schedule. Even animals treated previously may not have had parasites entirely eliminated. Fecal examinations should be performed at the time of capture/purchase and then 3 months later and annually thereafter.
9. If only two words were chosen for successful reptile maintenance, they would be **clean** and **routine.**

ACKNOWLEDGMENTS

I would like to thank Sean McKeown for setting the standard for this chapter in the first edition and all of his guidance in so many areas of herpetoculture. Dr Alicia Esser and Dr Kim Niessen reviewed the manuscript for this chapter and made helpful suggestions. In addition, I would like to extend thanks to the staff of Riverside Animal Hospital in Jacksonville, Fla, for their suggestions on practical solutions to common reptile problems.

REFERENCES

1. Cowan D: Adaptation, maladaptation and disease. In Murphy JB, Collins JT, editors: *SSAR contributions to herpetology, number 1, reproductive biology and diseases of captive reptiles,* 1980.
2. Funk R: Quarantine procedures and protocol for reptiles. In *Proceedings of the North American Veterinary Conference 2002,* Gainesville, Fla, 2002, Eastern States Veterinary Association.
3. Jacobson E, Morris P, Norton T, Wright K: Quarantine, *J Herp Med Surg* 11(4):24-30, 2002.
4. McKeown S: General husbandry and management. In Mader DR, editor: *Reptile medicine and surgery,* Philadelphia, 1996, WB Saunders.
5. DeVosjoli P: Designing environments for captive amphibians and reptiles. In Jeffrey Jenkins J, editor: *The Veterinary Clinics of North America: exotic animal practice,* January 1999, Husbandry and Nutrition, 1999.
6. Rossi J: *Snakes of the United States and Canada: keeping them healthy in captivity,* vol 1, eastern area, Malabar, Fla, 1992, Krieger Publishing.
7. Rossi J: *Snakes of the United States and Canada: keeping them healthy in captivity,* vol 2, western area, Malabar, Fla, 1995, Krieger Publishing.
8. Alderton D: *Turtles and tortoises of the world,* New York, 1988, Facts on File, Inc.
9. Behler J: *The Audubon Society field guide to North American reptiles and amphibians,* New York, 1979, Alfred E. Knopf Publishers.

10. Bennet D: *A little book of monitor lizards*, Aberdeen, Great Britain, 1995, Viper Press.
11. Conant R: *A field guide to reptiles and amphibians of eastern and central North America*, Boston, 1975, Houghton Mifflin.
12. Delisle H: *The natural history of monitor lizards*, Malabar, Fla, 1996, Krieger Publishing.
13. Ernst C, Barbour R: *Turtles of the world*, Washington, DC, 1989, Smithsonian Institute Press.
14. Ernst C, Lovich J, Barbour R: *Turtles of the United States and Canada*, Washington, DC, 1994, The Smithsonian Press.
15. Grenard S: *Handbook of alligators and crocodiles*, Malabar, Fla, 1991, Krieger Publishing.
16. Highfield A: *The Tortoise Trust guide to tortoises and turtles*, London, 1994, Carapace Press/Tortoise Trust.
17. Mattison C: *Keeping and breeding snakes*, London, 1988, Blandford Press.
18. McKeown S: *The general care and maintenance of day geckos*, Santee, Calif, 1993, Advanced Vivarium Systems.
19. Obst F, Klaus R, Udo J: *Completely illustrated atlas of reptiles and amphibians for the terrarium*, Neptune City, NJ, 1988, TFH Publications.
20. Palika L: *The complete idiot's guide to turtles and tortoises*, New York, 1998, Alpha Books, Simon & Schuster.
21. Pritchard P: *Encyclopedia of turtles*, Neptune, NJ, 1979, TFH Publications.
22. Rogner M: *Lizards*, vols 1, 2, Malabar, Fla, 1997, Krieger Publishing.
23. Ross R, Marzec G: *The reproductive husbandry of pythons and boas*, Stanford, Calif, 1990, Institute for Herpetological Research.
24. Stebbins R: *A field guide to western reptiles and amphibians*, Boston, 1985, Houghton Mifflin.
25. Tyning T: *A guide to amphibians and reptiles; Stokes nature guide*, Boston, 1990, Little, Brown.
26. Wilke H: *Turtles: a complete owner's manual*, Woodbury, NY, 1983, Barron's.
27. Carpenter J, Mashima T, Rupiper D: *Exotic animal formulary*, Philadelphia, 2001, WB Saunders.
28. Harrison L, editor: *Exotic companion medicine handbook for veterinarians*, Lake Worth, Fla, 1998, Zoological Education Network.
29. Burridge M, Simmons L-A: *Control and eradication of exotic tick infestations on reptiles*, 2001, Proceedings of the ARAV Eighth Annual Conference.
30. Rossi J: *Use of outdoor snake enclosures for maintenance and breeding of difficult snakes, rehabilitation of injured wild snakes, and the medical problems of snakes kept in this manner*, Cincinnati, 1999, Proceedings of the 6th Annual Meeting of the ARAV.
31. Rossi J: *Fungal dermatitis in a large collection of Brazos water snakes housed in an outdoor enclosure*, 2000, Reno, Nev, Proceeding of the 7th Annual Meeting of the ARAV.
32. DeVosjoli P: *The art of keeping snakes* (in press).
33. Lillywhite H: *Physiology of captive snakes*, Cincinnati, 1997, Proceedings of the International Herpetological Symposium.
34. Donoghue S, McKeown S: Nutrition of captive reptiles. In: Jenkins J, editor: *The veterinary clinics of North America exotic animal practice, Husbandry and Nutrition*, 1999.
35. Allen M: From blackbirds and thrushes ... to the gut loaded cricket; a new approach to zoo animal nutrition, *Br J Nutr* 78: 8135-8143, 1997.
36. Backner B: *The effects of calcium phosphate and vitamin D_3 supplementation on the growth rates in hatchling rat snakes*, 1991, 14th International Symposium on Captive Propagation of Reptiles.

5
SNAKES

RICHARD S. FUNK

Of all the reptiles, few evoke such positive and negative reactions from people as do snakes. Snakes have figured in folklore, mythology, religion, and medicine and now figure more prominently in the pet trade than ever before. Of the approximately 2500 species of living snakes, few are well known in nature and some are threatened with extinction. Snake species seen by the practicing veterinarian are mainly from two diverse groups, the colubrids and the boids (boas and pythons) (Figure 5-1, *A, B*). We cannot assume that the physiology or medication dosages are identical for all these species, and yet we are asked to extrapolate from research on a handful of species and treat most any snake.

Snakes and lizards are related and classified together in the order Squamata. Snakes are placed in the suborder Serpentes. Among the more than 70 anatomic features shared by lizards and snakes are the paired hemipenes in the base of the tail. Limb reduction has occurred with evolution in at least 62 lineages among the Squamata.[1] In pythons, with more than 300 precloacal vertebrae, limb loss, body elongation, and loss of axial regionalization are the result of the expression of Hox (homeobox) genes; the Hox genes for the thoracic development are expressed, but those programming for forelimb development are not.[2,3]

Snakes are essentially limbless with a rigid brain case that has the frontal and parietal bones articulating with the sphenoid bones and a kinetic skull with a joint between the frontals and the nasal region. They lack external ear openings. The ophthalmic branch of the trigeminal nerve enters the orbit via the optic foramen, whereas in other squamates it enters the orbit posteriorly. They have a large number of precloacal vertebrae, which can exceed 400. Snakes have no scleral ossicles and no muscle in the ciliary body, and the eye is covered with a transparent spectacle or reduced and covered with a scale. They have no dermal osteoderms.[3-5]

This discussion of snake biology focuses on the clinically significant aspects of their lives for an appreciation of their uniqueness and diversity. Few disease conditions are mentioned in this discussion because these are more fully covered elsewhere in this text.

SNAKE TAXONOMY

Snake systematics is constantly changing. Difficulties occur when trying to arrange the snakes into a meaningful higher classification because of a poor fossil record; and because most snakes, in evolving an elongated body adapted for a crawling mode of existence, have relatively few external features, systematists rely heavily on features of internal morphology and, more recently, molecular data. As yet, no universal agreement exists on the phylogeny of snakes. For example, about 70% of the living snakes are currently placed in the family Colubridae, which has not been shown to be monophyletic.

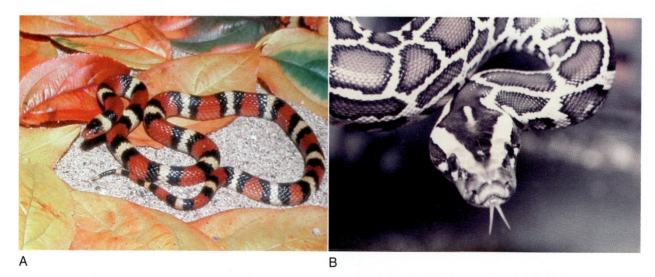

FIGURE 5-1 The two most common groups of snakes seen by veterinarians in clinical practice are colubrids, such as **(A)** the Scarlet Kingsnake *(Lampropeltis triangulum elapsoides)*, and boids, such as **(B)** the Burmese Python *(Python molurus bivittatus)*. (Photographs by R. Funk and D. Mader, respectively.)

Snakes are characterized by features that are shared with some of the lizards. Recent trends in phylogenetics, considering both molecular and morphological data, place the lizards, snakes, and the Tuatara in the clade Lepidosauria, as a sister taxon to the Archosauria, which includes the crocodilians and birds.[3]

The classification listed here is taken from a number of sources,[3,5-12] is based on a recent herpetology text[3] that attempts to synthesize the recent literature, and is quite different from classifications used only 10 to 15 years ago. Many of the details of this taxonomic arrangement are based on features not clinically important to the veterinary practitioner and so are not detailed (e.g., nerve foramina, bony processes of skull bones, insertions of jaw and other muscles). Table 5-1 summarizes this classification.

A brief listing of the content and some characteristics of the higher snake taxa may be useful in appreciation of the diversity of living species. Brief listings are also given of the geographic distribution of the various taxa. The * indicates families most often seen in herpetoculture (Figures 5-2 to 5-14).

Table 5-1 Higher Classification of Snakes

Infraorder Cholophidia (three extinct families)
Infraorder Scolecophidia: Blind Snakes
    Family Anomalepididae
    Family Typhlopidae: Blind Snakes
    Family Leptotyphlopidae: Slender Blind Snakes
Infraorder Alethinophidia
    Family Anomochilidae: Dwarf Pipe Snakes
    Family Cylindrophidae: Asian Pipe Snakes
    Family Uropeltidae: Shield-tail Snakes
    Family Aniliidae: Red Pipe Snakes
    *Family Xenopeltidae: Asian Sunbeam Snakes
    *Family Loxocemidae: Neotropical Sunbeam Snakes
    *Family Boidae: Boas and Pythons
    Family Bolyeriidae: Round Island Boas
    Family Xenophidiidae
    *Family Tropidophiidae: Caribbean Wood Snakes
Infraorder Caenophidia
    *Family Acrochordidae: File Snakes
    *Family Viperidae: Vipers and Pit Vipers
    *Family Colubridae: the colubrid snakes
    *Family Elapidae: cobras, kraits, sea snakes
    Family Atractaspidae: Stiletto snakes

*Indicates families most often seen in herpetoculture.

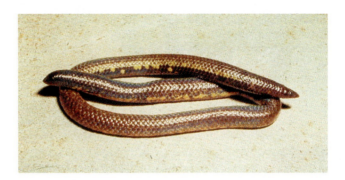

FIGURE 5-3 Sri Lankin Shield-tailed Snake *(Uropeltis phillipsi)* of family Uropeltidae. The head is the small pointed end. The soil adheres to the robust tail and helps block the burrow from behind.

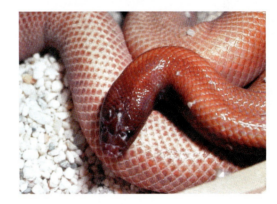

FIGURE 5-4 Neotropical Sunbeam Snake *(Loxocemes bicolor)* was formerly called the "New World Python." This oviparous and fossorial snake feeds on lizards, reptile eggs, and rodents.

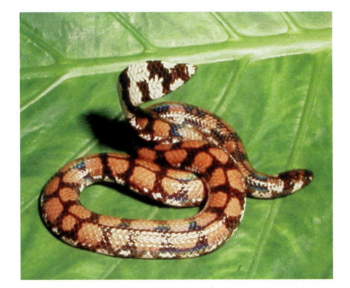

FIGURE 5-2 This adult Sri Lankin Pipe Snake *(Cylindrophis maculatus)* of the family Cylindrophidae exhibits automimicry with a flattened, elevated tail that is slowly moved in a side-to-side fashion. These viviparous snakes eat relatively large, elongated prey.

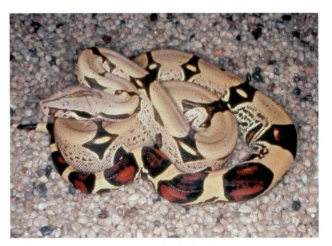

FIGURE 5-5 Boa Constrictor *(Boa constrictor)*, a common pet snake, is generally considered docile. It is now available in a number of colors and patterns. Although these snakes can attain lengths of more than 3 m (10 ft), most do not grow that large.

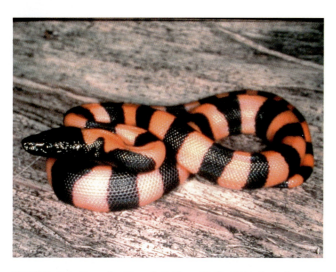

FIGURE 5-6 Juvenile Ringed Python (*Bothrochilus boa*) from the Bismark Archipelago. An active species in which adults are brown ringed with black or uniformly brown, with high iridescence.

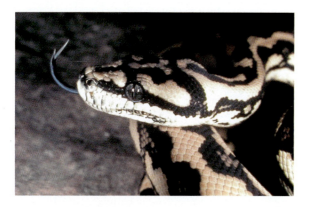

FIGURE 5-7 The popular Carpet Python (*Morelia spilotus variegatus*) is from Australia. This photo shows the typical forked tongue and also, in this case, the labial heat pits. This python typically reaches lengths of 2 m (6 to 7 ft).

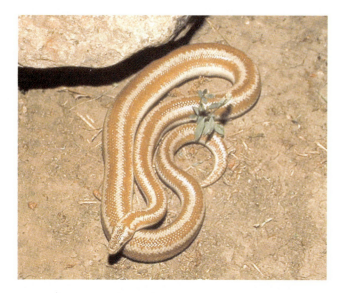

FIGURE 5-8 One of the North American Boas, the Rosy Boa (*Charina trivirgata*) is a quiet snake that is seen in different colors. These small boas are popular and easily kept. (*Photograph courtesy D. Mader.*)

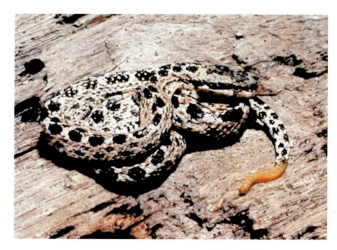

FIGURE 5-9 The Dwarf Boa (*Tropidophis canus curtus*) of the family Tropidophiidae is a live-bearing snake. Species in this genus have a defensive behavior involving flushing blood across the subspectacular space and out of the mouth onto a predator (or human handler). This species possesses a yellowish tail tip that functions as a caudal lure for its prey of frogs and lizards.

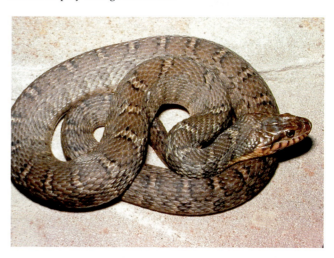

FIGURE 5-10 The Yellow-bellied Water Snake (*Nerodia erythrogaster flavigaster*) is representative of a group of colubrids called Natricines, which are mostly associated with aquatic habitats. North American Natricines are viviparous, but most Old World species are oviparous.

Infraorder Scolecophidia: The Blind Snakes

These snakes have blunt heads, short tails, vestigial eyes with only rods in the retina, and a multilobed liver. They are oviparous and fossorial, have smooth scales with no enlarged ventral scales, and feed on small prey, usually ants and termites.

- Family Anomalepididae: Four genera, Central and South America.
- Family Typhlopidae: Blind Snakes; six genera; Central and South America, West Indies, southern Africa, Eurasia, Australasia, Australia; one species parthenogenetic.
- Family Leptotyphlopidae: Slender Blind Snakes (or Thread Snakes); two genera; Southwest United States to northern South America, Middle East, Africa;

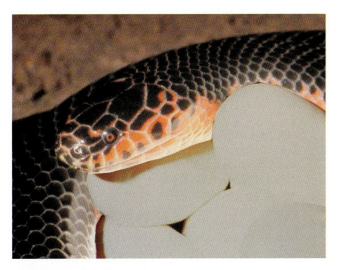

FIGURE 5-11 This adult Mud Snake (*Farancia abacura reinwardti*) is exhibiting parental care, coiling around her clutch of eggs until they hatch. This type of parental care is also seen in some pit vipers and notoriously among pythons, the latter of which thermoregulate to control their clutch's incubation temperature.

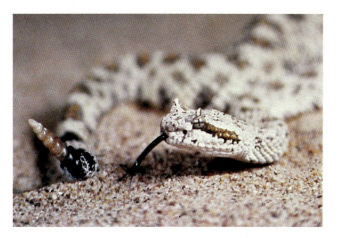

FIGURE 5-13 The Sidewinder (*Crotalus cerastes laterorepens*) is a species of rattlesnake from the deserts of the southwestern United States. Shown are the rattle on the tail tip, facial heat pit, forked tongue, and supraocular horns that may function to keep blowing sand off the eyes or shade the eyes. Rattlesnakes occur only in the New World, and all species are viviparous. A new rattle segment is added with each shed, and rattles may break off. Certain African vipers that sidewind also have supraocular horns.

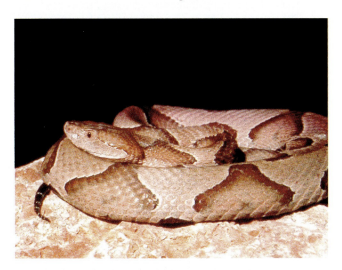

FIGURE 5-12 The Copperhead (*Agkistrodon c. contortrix*) is a terrestrial pit viper from the eastern United States with a pattern that is cryptic among leaves on the ground.

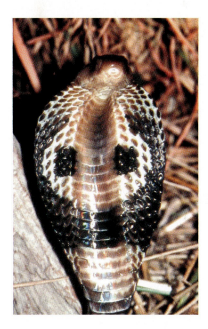

FIGURE 5-14 This Spectacled Cobra (*Naja naja*) is showing the "hood," an expanded portion of the neck that can be spread by expanding the neck ribs laterally. Cobras are highly venomous elapids, and some species can even spit venom at a predator's (or human's) face or eyes. Cobras account for many human deaths and also figure widely in religious and folk tales.

unique among vertebrates in having a mandibular feeding mechanism used to rake food into the mouth.

Infraorder Alethinophidia

The infraorder includes all living snakes except the blind snakes. Features these snakes share include a kinetic skull and details of palatine, laterosphenoid, and other osteologic traits.

- Family Anomochilidae: Dwarf Pipe Snakes; two small species, known from three specimens each; Sumatra, Borneo, Malaysia.
- Family Cylindrophidae: Asian Pipe Snakes; one genus, eight species; closely related to (and sometimes placed with) the Uropeltidae; Sri Lanka, Southeast Asia, Indoaustralian Archipelago.
- Family Uropeltidae: Shield-tail Snakes; specialized burrowers with blunt tails and a unique locomotion with skin purchasing holds on the burrows and the inner body moving along relative to the skin; 45 species; India and Sri Lanka.
- Family Aniliidae: Red Pipe Snakes; one fossorial red and black species; northern South America.
- *Family Xenopeltidae: Asian Sunbeam Snakes; iridescent fossorial and terrestrial constrictors, no pelvic

vestiges, oviparous; hinged teeth that change ontogenetically reflecting dietary shifts, hinged and bicuspid in juveniles; two species; India and Southeast Asia.

*Family Loxocemidae: Neotropical Sunbeam Snakes (called "New World Pythons" in older literature); also iridescent fossorial and terrestrial constrictors, no pelvic vestiges, oviparous; one species; Mexico to Costa Rica.

*Family Boidae: Boas and pythons; family includes the largest of the living snakes; however, many of the Boidae are small; all are constrictors, and many have facial infrared-receptive pits (heat pits or facial pits); they are from a wide variety of habitats and body forms; three subfamilies.

Subfamily Boinae: Boas; viviparous; with the pythons, include the longest living snakes; eight genera and about 40 species; New World plus Madagascar, New Guinea, the Solomon Islands.

Subfamily Pythoninae: Pythons; oviparous with maternal care of the eggs; include the longest living snakes; eight genera, 25 species; Africa, Indoaustralia, Australia.

Subfamily Erycinae: Rosy, Rubber, and Sand Boas; viviparous; three to four genera, 15 species; West North America, North Africa, South Europe, Southwest Asia.

Family Bolyeriidae: Round Island Boas; two unusual genera from Round Island in the Indian Ocean; *Bolyeria* probably went extinct about 1975; unique among tetrapod vertebrates in having divided (hinged) maxillary bones; *Casarea* is oviparous, endangered; formerly placed with the Boidae.

Family Xenophidiidae: Two species known from one specimen each; hinged teeth; Borneo and Malaysia.

*Family Tropidophiidae: Caribbean Wood Snakes (also called Dwarf Ground Boas); viviparous small constrictors with a well-developed tracheal lung and the left lung reduced or absent; most with pelvic vestiges; a unique defensive mechanism starts with ocular (subspectacular) hemorrhage that progresses to oral hemorrhage, the function of which is conjectural; two genera, 30 species; West Indies and South America to Panama.

Infraorder Caenophidia

Includes all of the families listed subsequently, the more "advanced" snakes, based mainly on features of internal anatomy such as lacking coronoid bones and having hemipenes with spines.

*Family Acrochordidae: File Snakes, Wart Snakes (or Elephant Trunk Snakes); aquatic, including marine and brackish habitats; scales small and strongly keeled giving them a sandpaper-like feeling, with a loose skin; can catch fish with body folds and skin; viviparous, one species at least occasionally parthenogenetic; one genus, three species; India to Northern Australia and Solomon Islands.

Superfamily Colubroidea (not recognized by all authorities): a grouping of the four most "advanced" families, sharing, among other things, the lack of a right common carotid artery.

*Family Viperidae: the Vipers and pit vipers; solenoglyph dentition, all venomous; fang erection in a posterior-anterior direction; includes the true vipers, the pit vipers, rattlesnakes, moccasins, and their allies; many habitats and life styles, both oviparous and viviparous, some with parental care; largest venomous snakes are the Bushmasters (three species of *Lachesis*) in Central and South America, which may reach 3 m in length; about 25 genera, 230 species; North, Central, and South America; Africa; Eurasia, Asia; Indonesia; Japan.

*Family Colubridae: the colubrid snakes; a huge family, difficult to characterize except to say these genera have not been placed in other families; this family is probably polyphyletic, and we expect future changes in the taxonomy of this group; worldwide, with more than 70% of living snakes comprising probably 325 genera and more than 1700 species; many habits and habitats; oviparous and viviparous, some species venomous; some are constrictors; colubrids, boas, and pythons comprise the majority of pet snakes; familiar species include the kingsnakes and milksnakes, ratsnakes, racers, watersnakes, gartersnakes, bullsnakes, and gophersnakes.

*Family Elapidae: the elapids; proteroglyph dentition and all venomous; some not dangerous to humans, with others are among the deadliest; mostly oviparous; North, Central, and South America; Africa; South Asia; Indoaustralia, Australia, and (Sea snakes) Indian and Pacific Oceans; familiar species include the cobras, mambas, coralsnakes, sea snakes, kraits, death adders, and taipans.

Family Atractaspidae: Stiletto Snakes; small African snakes; one genus with less than 20 species; affinities in dispute—formerly placed as a subfamily of the Colubridae and called mole vipers; they have a large maxillary fang and are able to retract this fang laterally, biting with one erect fang at a time with lateral-posterior head motion, biting the prey with the fang tip scarcely protruding from the mouth; humans who try to hold these snakes as they would other snakes are generally bitten. These animals are oviparous.

ANATOMY

The following sections refer to Figure 5-15.

Cardiovascular System

Snakes have a three-chambered heart with a complete atrial septum and an interventricular canal (see Chapter 10). Although this communication exists between the ventricular

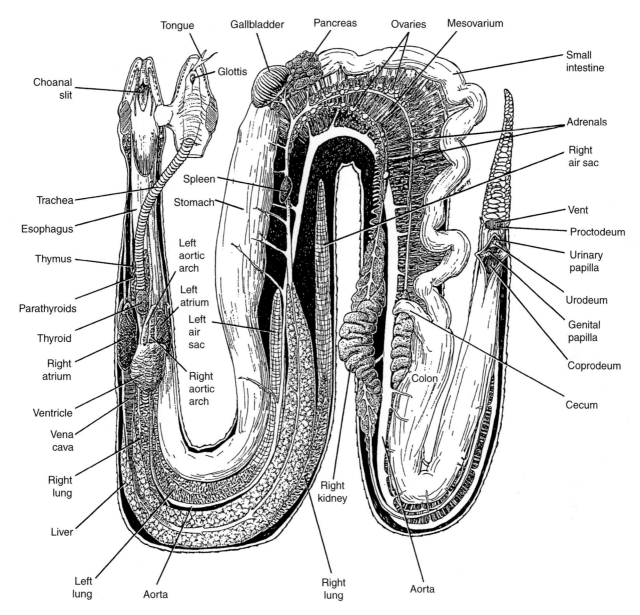

FIGURE 5-15 Gross anatomy of the snake, ventral view.

halves, considerable functional separation exists between the oxygenated and unoxygenated circuits leaving the heart. The heart becomes functionally five chambered, with the two systemic arches and a pulmonary artery all exiting the ventricle. Further, right-to-left and left-to-right shunting is also possible between the oxygen-rich and the oxygen-poor circuits, under control of several mechanisms.[3,13] Details of this are complex and beyond the scope of this brief introduction (see Chapter 10). Two aortae are present, with the right aorta exiting the left side of the ventricle and the left aorta exiting the right side; they fuse caudal to the heart and form the abdominal aorta. The left systemic arch is larger than the right, opposite most tetrapods.

Paired carotid arteries and jugular veins are located anterior to the heart near the trachea. The jugulars may be easily cannulated via a simple cutdown for placement of an intravenous (IV) catheter for obtaining samples or administering fluids and medications.

The position of the heart within the snake's body varies somewhat with its ecologic niche and phylogenetic position; but with no diaphragm, the heart is mobile within the rib cage, perhaps facilitating passage of relatively large prey. Snakes have been found to be able to control arterial pressure reflexly, but this control is reduced when the snake's body temperature is higher or lower than preferred.[14] Oxygen dissociation curves of snake blood are also influenced by temperature.[14] Snakes have both renal and hepatic portal circulations. For this reason, it may be necessary to administer parenteral medications that are eliminated from the body renally in the front portion of the body to avoid potential nephrotoxicity or first pass effects; however, future work may prove this to be unnecessary (see Chapter 11 for a thorough discussion of the renal portal system).[15] A ventral abdominal vein courses through much of the abdomen, and it should be avoided when making a surgical approach to the abdominal cavity by entering at the edge of the rib cage at about the level of the second and third dorsal scale rows.

The sites for obtaining blood samples in snakes include a ventral tail vein and cannulated jugular vein and via cardiocentesis. Venipuncture of the dorsal palatine vein is frequently referenced but, in reality, is difficult to use and fraught with complications. These sites are discussed in greater detail in Chapter 30.

The normal hematocrit (packed cell volume) of a snake is about 20% to 30%. On the basis of a study in the Black Ratsnake (*Elaphe* sp.), the blood volume is equivalent to approximately 6% of the animal's body weight.[16] All of the circulating cells are nucleated, and a finding of occasional mitotic figures in the peripheral blood is normal. Azurophils are present as in other reptiles, but snakes lack eosinophils (see Chapter 28).

Respiratory System

Although lizards have two lungs, in most snakes, the left lung is either reduced, never more than 85% the length of the right lung, or absent.[5] The right lung generally courses from near the heart to just cranial to the right kidney. The anterior part of the lung is vascularized, functioning in gas exchange, and the posterior portion of the lung is nonrespiratory and mainly functions as an air sac (see Chapter 10).

The trachea has incomplete cartilaginous rings, the ventral portion being rigid cartilage and the dorsal fourth being membranous. In many snakes, the vascular portion of the lung extends anteriorly dorsally into the dorsal trachea forming a "tracheal lung"; in extreme cases, the functional portion of the lung is tracheal.[5] The Acrochordidae have tracheal air sacs; and in some aquatic snakes, the lung extends posteriorly nearly to the cloaca as a hydrostatic adaptation. Variations in lung and tracheal morphology are useful taxonomic characteristics.

The glottis opens in the floor of the mouth posterior to the tongue and is generally easily visualized, making intubation for anesthesia easy. When feeding, the glottis may be moved laterally to facilitate breathing during the long process of ingesting large prey. The epiglottal cartilage may be greatly enlarged and modified to facilitate defensive hissing in such snakes as gophersnakes (*Pituophis* spp.).

Digestive System

The digestive tract is essentially a linear duct from the oral cavity to the cloaca, which also receives products from the urinary and reproductive systems (see Chapter 12). The following sets of mucus-secreting glands in the oral cavity moisten the mouth and lubricate prey: palatine, lingual, sublingual, and labial groups. Venom glands are modified labial glands and have evolved independently in several snake lineages. Snake venoms are mainly used for obtaining prey, and the venoms are extremely complex.

The tongue lies in a sheath beneath the epiglottis and glottis and functions in olfaction; snakes that lose their tongues through trauma or infection may not feed. The epiglottis fits into a recess in the upper jaw when the mouth is closed, and the openings of the vomeronasal or Jacobson's organs are in the cranial aspect of this groove within reach of the tongue tips.

The esophagus is usually quite distensible, and about half its length is largely amuscular. Snakes generally use their axial musculature and skeleton to help transport food from the mouth to the stomach. Snakes do not masticate food items; rather, they swallow food whole. They have no well-defined cardiac (gastroesophageal) sphincter.

The stomach is muscular and distensible. The process of prey digestion begins in the stomach. The small intestines are relatively uncoiled (compared with mammals and birds). The pancreas is generally located in a triad together with the spleen and gallbladder, the latter being distal to the caudal tip of the elongated, spindle-shaped liver. Some species have a combined organ, called the splenopancreas.

The small intestine empties into the colon, which may store feces for a time. In boas and pythons, a small cecum is located at the proximal colon. Urates may be retained in the distal colon until passed with the feces. The cloaca receives the products of the urinary, digestive, and reproductive systems. The intestines and cloaca have important roles in water conservation.

Dentition and Venom

Six rows of teeth are generally present in snakes found in the pet trade, with one row on each of the lower jaws and two rows on each side of the upper jaw. Teeth are generally not regionally differentiated except for modified fangs in some species or in species with specialized feeding habits (none have molars, incisors, etc). The dentigerous bones include the mandibles, maxillae, palatines, pterygoids, and sometimes the premaxillae. The teeth, including fangs, continue to be replaced throughout life. Usually a membranous flap covers the fangs when not in use. In vipers and pit vipers, the fangs fold caudodorsally and lie sheathed when the mouth is closed; but in elapids and colubrids with fangs, the fangs remain erect and cannot fold.

Snake teeth are basically elongated, slender, and slightly curved posteriorly. Snake teeth are modified pleurodont teeth with a rudimentary socket and are attached to the side of the jaw.[3,17] More primitive snakes have all the teeth about the same (homodont), whereas in the more advance snakes, some teeth may be modified into grooved and hollow fangs. Historically, variations in the maxillary teeth have been classified as follows[18]:

Aglyphous: having homodont maxillary teeth.
Opisthoglyphous: "rear-fanged" with enlarged teeth on the rear of the maxilla.
Proteroglyphous: a solitary enlarged fang on the long maxillary bone that does not allow for erection of the fang (elapid type).
Solenoglyphous: only tooth is a hollow fang on the short maxilla that can be erected by maxillary rotation on the prefrontal bone (viper type).

Many variations occur among these types.

In elapids and vipers, the anterior fangs are hollow with a distinctive venom canal. These fangs are shed periodically, and commonly, examination of a snake leads to observation of a functional fang and an adjacent replacement fang destined to replace the functional one. The fangs may be lost as prey is bitten and may pass through the snake relatively undigested and appear in the feces.

Snake venom glands are located in the upper jaw below the orbit. In contrast, the only venomous lizards, *Heloderma* spp., have venom glands in the lower jaw. The size and shape of the glands vary with the species. Rarely the venom glands extend far caudally into the body perhaps to the level of the heart (*Maticoura*, Elapidae; *Atractaspis*, Atractaspidae; *Causus*, Viperidae).

Snake venoms are quite complex and contain toxins that are proteins varying from a few amino acids to high molecular weight. These toxins have been characterized by their activities: neurotoxins act at neuromusclar junctions and synapses; hemorrhagins act to destroy blood vessels; and myotoxins act on skeletal muscle. Among the venom toxins are RNAses, DNAses, phospholipases, proteolytic enzymes, thrombin-like enzymes, hyaluronidases, lactate dehydrogenases, acetylcholinerases, nucleotidases, and l-amino acid oxidases and others.[19]

At least 10 enzymes are found in nearly all snake venoms, and a particular venom may contain more than two dozen different proteins. Any particular venom may have a number of receptor sites, and venoms also have digestive functions. In fact, these snake venoms are theorized to have evolved from digestive enzymes.[20] Older classifications of snake venoms as hemotoxic and neurotoxic are oversimplifications and inaccurate, and some venoms have mixtures of both. The relative abundance of venom components in a particular species can vary geographically, seasonally, or with age.

Recently, a number of colubrid snakes have been reported to have elicited toxic reactions in humans. These reports need to be evaluated further and with caution; some species, lacking discrete venom glands, apparently have other oral secretions with some toxic properties. But some colubrids are venomous and capable of serious human envenomation. Two renowned herpetologists were killed by colubrid snake bite: Karl P. Schmidt by a Boomslang (*Dispholidus typus*) and Robert Mertens by an African Twig Snake (*Thelotornis capensis*).[4,21] A number of colubrids have venoms that are toxic to their prey but not to humans. Individual human reactions to any snake bite can vary with the person, the general health status of the person, the nature of the bite, the species that bit the person, the amount of venom injected, the site of the bite, the depth of the bite, the activity of the venom, and so on.

A full discussion of human snakebites is beyond the scope of this chapter. If you choose to treat venomous reptiles, you should understand the risks involved to yourself, your staff, and your clients. Many jurisdictions have restrictions regarding the possession of venomous reptiles, and you must abide by these laws. Not all local hospitals have the appropriate antivenom on hand to treat bites from exotic species, nor are all hospitals experienced at treating snakebites. Proper identification of an exotic venomous snake may be difficult. Prevention of snakebites is superior to a cure (see Chapter 81).

Reproductive and Urinary Systems

The paired kidneys are located in the dorsal caudal abdomen, with the right kidney situated cranial to the left, far forward from the cloaca (see Chapter 11). The kidneys are lobulated and elongated and arranged in an anteroposterior orientation. The ureters empty into the urodeum portion of the cloaca; no urinary bladder is found in snakes. Male snakes have a so-called sexual segment, consisting of the posterior renal segments, that enlarges during the reproductive season to produce a contribution to the seminal fluid (Figure 5-16). When this happens, the kidneys appear abnormal because their size and color change dramatically. To the untrained eye, these kidneys may appear diseased.

The Blind Snake *Rhamphotyphlops braminus* is parthenogenetic (no males) and has been transported by man to various ports and around the tropics mainly by "hitching" rides in potted plants; it now occurs in Africa, Southeast Asia, the Philippines, Hawaii, Mexico, Arizona, and Florida and has been called the Flowerpot Snake (Figure 5-17). Parthenogenesis has also recently been reported in one file snake (*Acrochordus arafurae*) and a couple of North American snakes; further investigation will prove interesting.

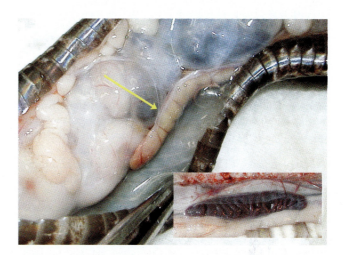

FIGURE 5-16 Male snakes have a so-called "sexual segment" in their kidneys *(yellow arrow)*, consisting of the posterior renal segments, that enlarge during reproductive season to produce a contribution to the seminal fluid. When this happens, the kidneys appear abnormal because their size and color change dramatically. To the untrained eye, these kidneys may appear diseased. Inset shows a normal kidney during nonreproductive season. *(Photograph courtesy D. Mader.)*

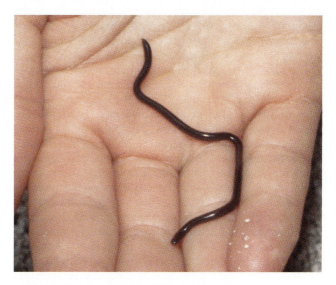

FIGURE 5-17 Blind Snake *(Rhamphotyphlops braminus)* is parthenogenetic (no males exist). *(Photograph courtesy D. Mader.)*

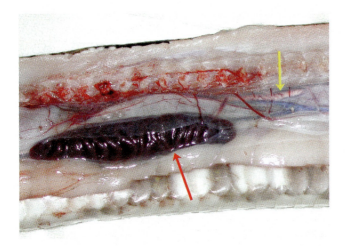

FIGURE 5-18 Fusiform testes *(yellow arrow)* are seen cranial to the kidneys *(red arrow)*, the right being more cranial than the left. During the breeding season, testes undergo recrudescence, often doubling in size. *(Photograph courtesy D. Mader.)*

All male snakes have two paired intromittent organs that lie invaginated in pouches in the ventral tail base. Each is called a hemipenis (plural, hemipenes). Hemipenial morphology has proven to be a valuable taxonomic character. During copulation, a hemipenis evaginates into the cloaca of the receptive female. The functional surface of the hemipenis facing her cloacal wall, when not in use, lines the lumen of a cavity in the tail.

Because of the presence of these hemipenes, a smooth blunt-tipped probe may be inserted into the hemipenial lumen to probe the snake as a male; the male probes relatively deeply compared with a conspecific female because she lacks the hemipenes (see Figure 23-6, *A, B*). In many snakes, the tail base is relatively wider and straighter in males than in females owing to the presence of these hemipenes. With practice, probing is safe and easy, and the author recommends sexing most snakes that come to the clinic as part of the physical examination.

In males and females, the gonads are situated with the right more anterior than the left. The ovaries are located nearer the pancreas. A few fossorial species have lost one ovary and oviduct. In females, the developing embryos or eggs in the right uterus are carried anterior to those on the left.

The fusiform testes are intracoelomic, situated between the pancreatic triad and the kidneys, and enlarge and regress in size as the season changes (Figure 5-18). Sperm is carried in the Wolffian ducts to the base of the hemipenis during copulation and travels up the sulcus spermaticus on the outside of the hemipenes into the female.

Some snakes are oviparous (egg-laying), and some are viviparous (live-bearing). Some snakes build nests (King Cobra) for egg incubation, and egg-brooding behavior by females has evolved in several lineages (pythons, *Farancia* in the Colubridae, and some *Trimeresurus* in the Viperidae). These females coil around their eggs until they hatch (see Figures 5-11 and 23-3).

No temperature-dependent sex determination has yet been documented in snakes, although it has in chelonians, crocodilians, and lizards. Where studied, snakes have genetic sex determination and the female is heterogametic. Sexual dimorphism

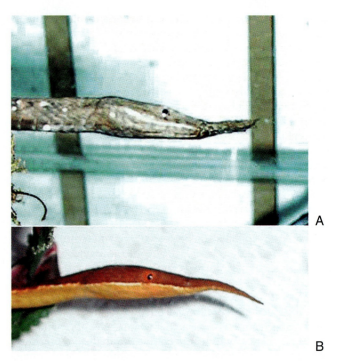

FIGURE 5-19 Sexual dimorphism in coloration or external morphology is rare in snakes. *Langaha* sp., Leaf-nosed snakes of Madagascar, exhibit dimorphism in nasal protuberances. The female **(A)** has a larger, more elaborate appendage compared with the male **(B)**. *(Photograph courtesy D. Mader.)*

in coloration or external morphology is rare. *Langaha sp.*, the Leaf-nosed Snakes of Madagascar, exhibit dimorphism in nasal protuberances (Figure 5-19, *A, B*). In general, female snakes attain larger sizes than males but not in all species. Reproductive cycles of males and females may not coincide because, in some species, females may store sperm.

Nervous System and Special Senses

Snakes have a typical reptilian brain with 12 pairs of cranial nerves.

The snake ear has no tympanic membrane or middle ear cavity. For years, snakes were presumed to be unable to hear airborne sounds, merely substrate vibrations. However, snakes have been shown electrophysiologically to hear airborne sound in a low frequency range of 150 to 600 Hz.[22]

The eyes of snakes are unique among vertebrates in lacking ciliary bodies, so that accommodation occurs by moving the lens toward or away from the retina by means of iris muscle movements, whereas in other vertebrates movements of the ciliary body muscles change the shape of the lens.[3,5,18] The eyelids fuse embryologically to form a spectacle that is keratinized and covers the eye and is continuous with the epidermis. The outer portion of the spectacle is shed during ecdysis along with the remainder of the snake's skin. When a snake nears shedding, the eye may look cloudy or "blue" like the rest of the skin. Lacrimal secretions flow through the subspectacular space between the spectacle and the cornea and drain into the roof of the mouth. The shape of the pupil varies with habitat and activity (see Figures 5-3, 5-7, 5-9, 5-13, and 5-22 for examples). Some fossorial snakes have the eyes reduced and covered by a head scale without a separate spectacle. Additional details of eye anatomy, clinical examination, and disease conditions are discussed in Chapter 20.

Independent evolution of specialized infrared receptors has occurred in the heat pits of pit vipers and the labial pits of different groups of boas and pythons[10,23]; they do not appear to be homologous.[24] In pit vipers, one organ occurs on each side of the head, slightly ventral to a line drawn between the nostril and the orbit. In the boas and pythons, these organs occur in labial or rostral scales or both, but the location, arrangement, and number vary with the species. Innervation is via the trigeminal nerve but with different branches.

Pit viper pits have a thin membrane stretched over an air-filled inner cavity. The pit organs are extremely sensitive to infrared radiation changes as small as 0.002°C.[24] These pits provide not only infrared information but also direction and distance, and because these pits are integrated in the brain with the optic region, they provide the snake with both infrared and visual imaging apparently superimposed.[25] Research shows that many pitless snakes also have the ability to detect infrared radiation with other nerve endings in the head, and some (many?) snakes may be able to "see" their environment nearly as well with this infrared system as they can optically.[3,23-26] Snake keepers are commonly bitten when feeding cool (e.g., frozen and thawed to room temperature) rodents to snakes because the snakes may smell prey and "aim" for the heat source (the keeper's hand).

Ticks and mites may use these pits as shelter.

Central nervous system diseases are poorly understood in snakes (see Chapters 17 and 62).

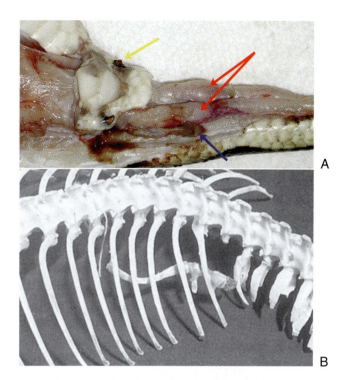

FIGURE 5-20 **A,** Male boids have vestigial pelvic appendages. The *yellow arrow* points to the "spurs," *red arrows* highlight paired hemipenes, and *blue arrow* points to the scent gland. **B,** Skeleton shows relationship of the "spur" to the vestigial pelvis. The tail is to the right in both **A** and **B**. *(Photographs by D. Mader and R. Funk, respectively.)*

Musculoskeletal System

Snakes show great modifications in their skeletal system from their lizard-like ancestry. Snakes do not have thoracic limbs, but a few have pelvic vestiges, including external spurs, that may be used during courtship, particularly in the boas and pythons (Figure 5-20, *A, B*). The diversity of snake locomotory types has been classified as follows[4,18]:

Lateral undulation: involves bending the vertebral column, where contractions occur on opposite sides of the body; this is characteristic of most tetrapods. The fastest terrestrial snakes use this method.

Rectilinear locomotion: a "caterpillar crawling" in which muscle contractions are bilaterally symmetrical in waves, with the body contacting the substrate at intervals and the progression occurring essentially in a straight line. Common in boas, pythons, and stocky vipers.

Concertina locomotion: the body moves forward by making a purchase and moving a portion of the body to gain a new purchase. Common in arboreal and fossorial snakes; the most energy-expensive method of locomotion.

Sidewinding: a difficult mode to describe, much more easily understood when observed; used by snakes on smooth surfaces such as sand or mud; the body essentially contacts the substrate at two points and creates a series of separate parallel straight lines as it progresses.

A snake can switch from one form of locomotion to another as it changes habitat, substrate, or activity.

Locomotion centers around a skeletal system of precloacal vertebrae, which may exceed 400 in number, most of which have ribs, and large axial skeletal muscles with multiple attachments. The ribs and vertebrae have only minor regional differentiation. Snake locomotion has been found to be relatively low in energy expenditure. A gartersnake expends only about 31% as much energy in locomotion as does a lizard of comparable body size.[14]

The brain case is solid. However, the skull is kinetic, with the quadrate bones articulating with the lower jaw and the palatomaxillary arch to facilitate, along with the elasticity in lacking a mandibular symphysis, the ingestion of prey items that are much larger than the head or the diameter of the body. Caudal autotomy, widespread in lizards, is known in only a few colubrid snakes (such as Neotropical *Pliocercus* spp. and *Scaphiodontophis* spp.) and in none of the species commonly kept in captivity. In these snakes, no autotomy plane or regeneration is present, the separation occurring between the vertebrae.[3,4,27]

Integument

Snake scales are essentially made of folds of the epidermis and dermis, but the scales themselves are epidermal in origin. Except for the head, they typically overlap each other. A variety of pits, ridges, keels, and tubercules of unknown function are present on snake scales. Regional differences are seen, with enlarged head shields, a series of rows of small dorsal scales covering the body and tail dorsally and laterally, and larger and wider ventral scales that provide support and

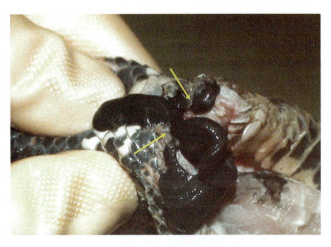

FIGURE 5-21 Almost no skin glands occur in snakes, but cloacal scent glands (anal glands) are characteristic *(yellow arrows)*. Note the thick, tar-like secretions. These foul-smelling sticky substances are used for marking territories, scenting the environment, and repelling predators. See also Figure 5-20, *A*. *(Photograph courtesy D. Mader.)*

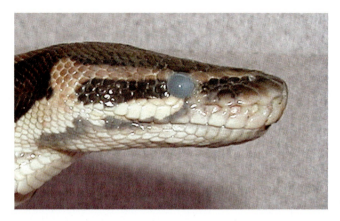

FIGURE 5-22 A shedding snake has a dull blue look to it as fluid forms between old and new layers of skin. Herpetoculturists call their snakes blue or opaque at this time. A snake "goes blue" for several days, then clears up, and then sheds. *(Photograph courtesy D. Mader.)*

protection ventrally. (Scolecophidia spp. and some Sea Snakes lack enlarged ventral scales.) Most snakes have an enlarged scale that covers the cloacal opening. Dorsal scales are usually in odd numbers of rows, with a maximum number near midbody and fewer rows near the neck and cloaca. The keratinized scales protect the snake from abrasion and dehydration.

Almost no skin glands occur in snakes, but cloacal scent glands (anal glands) are characteristic (Figure 5-21). These glands are a pair of organs in the base of the tail, dorsal to the hemipenes in a male, and they open into the posterior margin of the cloaca. Their unpleasant odor plays a role in defense and may also carry social signals. In captivity, they can become enlarged, impacted, or abscessed.

Shedding or ecdysis is a complex event histologically (see Chapter 15).[3,4,28,29] During shedding, a synchronous proliferation of the epithelial cells from the stratum germinativum occurs. This forms a new epidermal generation between the stratum germinativum and the older outer epidermal layer; this inner (younger) epidermal layer keratinizes and comes to resemble the (older) outer layer. During separation of these two generations of epithelium, anerobic glycolysis assists in separating the outer layer and acid phosphatase helps break down the cementing material.

The snake has a dull "blue" look to it as a fluid forms between the two layers. Herpetoculturists call their snakes "blue" or "opaque" at this time (Figure 5-22). A snake goes blue for several days, then clears up, and then sheds. Healthy snakes shed the entire outer layer as one event, but the older outer skin may tear in shedding especially in larger snakes. The epithelium over the spectacles (the eyecap) is also normally shed. While getting ready to shed, many snakes become inactive and seek shelter, often in a moist or humid site. Snakes often do not feed while they are in the blue or opaque but often eat immediately after shedding.

Dysecdysis is improper or incomplete shedding that may occur because of mites, incorrect humidity, lack of a proper substrate, improper handling, malnutrition, dermatitis, or trauma (see Chapters 15 and 52).

Most snakes have pigments that create the skin coloration, but microscopic surface structures can yield an iridescence. Ontogenetic color changes occur in some species. Some species, especially in juveniles, have brighter colored (usually yellow) tail tips that are used as caudal lures to attract prey. Coloration may also vary geographically. Polymorphism is unusual, but the California Kingsnake (*Lampropeltis getula californiae*) and the Turk's Island Boa (*Epicrates chrysogaster*), for example, have both striped and blotched individuals in the same populations. Many boas are darker during the day and paler at night.

In recent years, the captive propagation of a variety of genetic mutations, including partial albinos and leucistic individuals and a number of pattern types, has contributed to the marketing of "designer snakes" or "cultivars" (Figure 5-23, *A, B*). For example, at this writing, more than three dozen varieties are available of the Cornsnake (*Elaphe guttata*), including "morphs," as termed in the commercial trade, with names such as: Oketee, reverse Oketee, Miami, Zigzag, Aztec, Motley, Butter, Amber, Mocha, Sunglow, Fluorescent orange, Blood red, "Jungle" (hybridized with the California Kingsnake), Caramel, Creamsicle, Lavender, Striped, Crimson, Ghost, Pewter, and on and on; and some of these morphs are, or can be, combined with the traits for amelanistic partial albinisim or anerythristic partial albinism, and there are even Snow and Blizzard Cornsnakes that combine the genes for both amelanism and anerythrism.[30,31] Of course, prices vary with pattern and color.

Endocrine System

The single or paired thyroid glands lie just anterior to the heart (Figure 5-24). Thyroid function is involved in the shedding cycle and growth. The thymus does not involute in adult snakes as it does in mammals and is easily lost in the adipose tissue cranial to the thyroid gland. Parathyroid tissue is paired and often imbedded in the thymus tissue cranial to the heart and thyroid and plays a roll in calcium metabolism. The adrenal glands are usually located between the kidneys and the gonads (Figure 5-25). The pituitary seems to function as a master gland just as it does in mammals. The clinical significance of endocrine function is poorly understood in snakes.

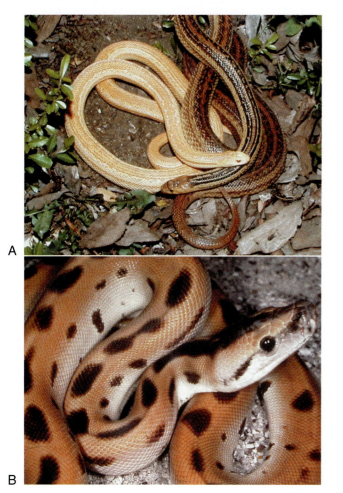

A

B

FIGURE 5-23 Captive propagation has produced a variety of genetic mutations, including partial albinos and leucistic individuals, and a number of pattern types, and has contributed to marketing of designer snakes or cultivars. **A,** Albino Gophersnake (*Pituophis catenifer*). **B,** Green phase Burmese Python (*Python molurus bivitattus*). (*Photographs by D. Mader and R. Funk, respectively.*)

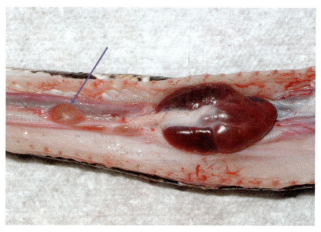

FIGURE 5-24 Single or paired thyroid gland (*blue arrow*) is found just cranial to the heart. (*Photograph courtesy J. Wyneken.*)

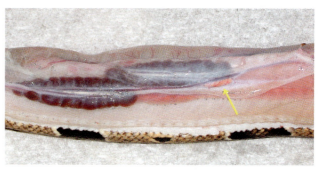

FIGURE 5-25 Pink adrenal glands are located just cranial and medial to the kidneys. (*Photograph courtesy J. Wyneken.*)

ENVIRONMENT AND MAINTENANCE

Thermoregulation

Snakes, like other reptiles, are ectotherms. In a captive setting, thermal regimens should closely resemble temperatures in the wild. A variety of commercially available products exist to give the herpetoculturist an opportunity to provide such a regimen. Heat tapes are popular and may be used with thermostats. Light bulbs are inefficient sources of heat and may lead to thermal burns, as may hot rocks, which the author never recommends. A readable discussion of thermoregulation in Diamond Pythons (*Morelia spilotes spilotes*) in nature is provided by Shine,[32] including changes with the seasons and differences in the genders.

Both the clinician and the client must understand the thermal physiology of reptiles. Each species needs to reach its selected (or preferred) body temperature (T_s or T_p), which occurs within the range of physiologically tolerated temperatures or the thermal neutral zone (TNZ).[33] Snakes that are ill, gravid, or digesting food often seek out situations that allow attainment of slightly elevated body temperatures.

Herpetoculturists find that their captives thrive better when provided with a thermal gradient that incorporates the T_s for species being housed. Summary discussions of research on thermoregulation are available.[33,34]

Feeding and Nutrition

No vegetarian snakes exist; all species are carnivorous. But among the snakes are species that eat mainly warm-blooded prey, only invertebrates, specialized diets (e.g., slugs, eggs, frogs, fish eggs, termites), or a wide variety of prey items (see Figure 44-2). Therefore, critical to the care of a captive animal is that both the clinican and the client understand what the normal diet is for the snake (Table 5-2). One of the most common reasons for a snake to fail to feed is that the type of food offered is incorrect. Species with specialized diets are difficult to maintain unless the owner is painstakingly dedicated.

Most of the snake species in the pet trade feed on captive-reared rodents, and because they eat whole animals, nutritional problems are infrequently seen among feeding snakes. Rodents must be fed a suitable diet so that they become a suitable diet for the snakes. No excuse exists for feeding dog food or swine food to rats and mice when so many nutritionally complete rodent diets are available. Similarly, if a client is

Table 5-2 Suggested Diets for Snakes

Snake Group	Example	Primary Food Preferences Adults	Young
Scolecophidia	Blind Snakes	A	
Acrochordidae	Elephant Trunk Snake	F	
Uropeltidae	Shield-tail Snakes	A	
Xenopeltidae	Asian Sunbeam Snakes	M	L
Loxocemidae	Neotropical Sunbeam Snakes	M	
Boas	Anaconda	F, M, B	
	Boa Constrictor, Dumeril's, Tree	M, B	
	Pacific/Solomon Island	L, M, B	
	Rubber	L, M	
	Amazon, Emerald, Annulated	M, B	L, M
	Rainbow/Caribbean	M, B	L, Am, M
	Sand Boas	M	L, M
	Rosy Boas	M	
Pythons	Burmese, Black-Headed African Burrowing, Carpet, Diamond, Reticulated, Indian, Ball	M, B	
	Rock, Short-tailed (blood), Green Tree	M, B	L, M
	Indoaustralian	M, B	L, M
Tropidophiidae	Wood Snakes	Am, L, M	
Viperidae	Copperheads and Asian relatives	M	Am, L, M
	Cottonmouth	F, M, B	Am, F, M
	Rattlesnakes	M, B	L, M
	Most other Pit Vipers (*Calloselasma, Bothriechis, Bothriopis, Bothrops*, etc.)	M, B	Am, L, M
	Sawscale Vipers	A, M	
	Horned, Sand Vipers	L, M	
	Most other Vipers (*Atheris, Bitis, Vipera*)	M, B	L, M
Colubridae	Brown, Red-bellied	OI	
	Garter and Ribbon	F, Am, M	
	Glossy	L, M	
	Gopher, Bull, Pine	M, B	
	Green	A, L	
	Hog-nosed	Am, M	
	House	M	
	Indigo, Cribo	F, M, B	Am, L, M
	Kingsnake	M	L, M
	Long-nosed	L, M	
	Madagascan Hog-nosed	M, B	
	Milksnake	M	L, M
	Patchnosed	L, M	
	Racers	M, B	L, M
	Ratsnakes	M, B	Am, L, M
	Ringneck	OI, Am, S	
Elapidae	King Cobra	S, M	
	Most other Cobras	M, B	
	Kraits	M, B	
	Coralsnakes	(F), S, M	

A, Arthropods; *OI*, other invertebrates; *F*, fish; *Am*, amphibians; *L*, lizards; *S*, snakes; *M*, mammals; *B*, birds.

feeding crickets or fish to a snake, the crickets and fish should be fed well to make better meals nutritionally for the snake. The author recommends feeding dead rodents to those animals eating rodents to avoid bite wounds and trauma to the snake; the rodents can be offered fresh-killed or purchased frozen and thawed (see Chapter 46). If the snake does not feed, review the husbandry requirements and check the identification and temperature (see Chapter 44).

Frequency of meals varies with the age and species of snake. Many juvenile and adult rodent-feeding species thrive and grow on once a week feedings, but a baby may need two or more feedings per week to do well. Active snakes may need more frequent feedings; for example, gartersnakes fed goldfish do poorly with only weekly meals. Most herpetoculturists increase the feedings to a female as the breeding season approaches. Many gravid female snakes go off feed during gestation. The best method is to feed snakes one at a time in isolation to avoid the possibility of inadvertent cannibalism.

ENVIRONMENTAL CAPTIVITY REQUIREMENTS

Cages may be plastic shoe boxes; modified aquaria; homemade from wood; or expensive, commercially manufactured, and made of fiberglass or acrylonitrate-butadiene-styrene (ABS) plastic.

Table 5-3 lists the minimum standards for caging (see also Chapter 4). Lighting requirements for captive snakes are less

Table 5-3	Minimal Requirements for Snake Caging

Escape proof with latch or lock.
Easy access for cleaning, feeding, and monitoring occupant.
Few places for ectoparasites, baby snakes, or uneaten prey items to hide.
Easy to clean and disinfect.
An appropriate substrate both for snake's needs and for serviceability.
Hiding box or shelter, perhaps multiple shelters.
Constructed so that water or feces is not absorbed.
Appropriate lighting, ventilation, and humidity for snake's needs.
Large enough to accommodate snake and allow some activity.
With number of animals, uniform or modular cages are conducive to good husbandry.

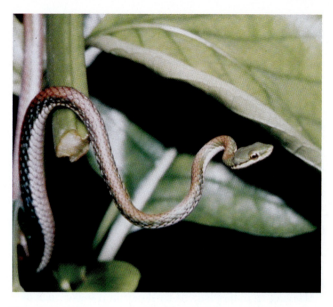

FIGURE 5-26 Snakes maintained in plastic boxes without environmental enrichment undoubtedly experience immeasurable stress. Attempts should be made toward offering a more naturalistic environment. (*Photograph courtesy D. Mader.*)

well understood than for lizards. Many successful breeders, for example, provide dim artificial lighting for their snakes and have excellent results, including breeding. However, attention to the photoperiod is believed to promote good health and successful reproduction.

Cages kept in dim light generally do not get cleaned well enough because filth may not be properly observed. Fresh water should always be available in the cage and should be cleaned frequently if the snake soaks in the water bowl. Arboreal species may do better with the bowl placed higher in the cage. Replacement water bowls should be available to clean and disinfect at least weekly.

Humidity varies geographically and seasonally. During the winter, when forced air heat is on in the home, the temperature may be maintained, but a drying effect may cause problems, such as dysecdysis. Too much humidity, as in Florida in the summer, may be harmful to a desert-adapted species. Many snakes do well if the humidity is between 50% and 70%, but without adequate ventilation, the humidity inside a cage could rise dramatically. Desert or xeric-adapted species may obviously fare better with less humidity than riparian or semiaquatic species.

Snakes kept in aquaria or plastic sweater boxes, with only a water bowl and a hide box, always look like prisoners rather than pets. A recent trend is to use larger cages (*vivaria* is perhaps a better term) with cage furnishings such as plants, rocks, and tree branches. Most clients feel that their snakes are "happier" in these environments, even though maintenance may involve a little more work (Figure 5-26). This type of cage projects a caring image.

For basic caging, the author prefers a newspaper substrate for hospitalized patients unless their needs dictate otherwise (such as fossorial or aquatic species). For clients, simple (spartan or barren) cages may also work well. But many species, especially fossorial or more secretive species, need more attention to cage setup, including some attempt to duplicate the conditions under which the captives are found in nature. Woodland burrowers cannot be expected to survive in dry sand, and vice versa for desert burrowers. Briefly we can provide several different styles of caging for captive snakes as follows[35]:

Basic enclosure setup. One type of substrate, with a water bowl, a hide box, and perhaps with a plant or a tree branch added.
Wet-dry enclosure setup. Similar to the basic, but this type has two (maybe one) type of substrate, with a moist area and a dry area, providing a horizontal moisture gradient.
Three-layer enclosure setup. As implied by the name, three layers of substrate are used: from bottom upward they are gravel, sand, and then mulch. The gravel can be moistened, and a vertical moisture gradient achieved.
Desert enclosure setup. Basically a thick layer of sand for the substrate. Small water bowl, good ventilation, perhaps some (or occasional) moisture in one small area.
Swamp tea setup. Rarely used, for swamp snakes, with a dilute solution of tea for the water environment.
Natural setups and outdoor enclosures. Indoor vivaria can be fascinating and functional, and esthetically pleasing, but the difficulty in maintaining them increases with the complexity of the enclosure. Outdoor enclosures must be escape proof, vermin proof, disaster proof, and vandal proof, which makes them difficult but at the same time rewarding.

BEHAVIOR

If the cage is opened mainly for feeding, the snake is likely to begin exhibiting a feeding response every time the cage is opened. If the snake is large and potentially dangerous, feeding it outside the cage is safer.

Social behavior in snakes usually involves reproductive activities. Observation of the interactions between individual snakes at this time is fascinating. Visual and tactile cues, and probably pheromones, may be involved in these complex behaviors, which tend to vary among the species. During the mating season, the behavior of some snakes is completely different, and courtship/mating/combat can occasionally result in injuries to participating snakes. Most clients can watch the behavior of their animals change as the mating season arrives, and they can also learn when a female is ready to oviposit or give birth.

In most circumstances, housing captive snakes singly is preferable. If housed in groups, close attention must be paid during feeding times and during the breeding season to avoid injuries or even cannibalism. For example, if two snakes both attempt to swallow the same prey item, a larger snake may be able to keep going and ingest both the prey and the other (attached) snake.

Hands should be washed after handling prey species, such as rats, mice, hamsters, and birds, or after handling predator species, such as cats, ferrets, or kingsnakes, and before handling a snake, so as not to present the snake with mixed signals and perhaps get bitten as either a feeding response or a defensive behavior.

Having an ophiophagous (snake-eating) snake, such as a Kingsnake *(Lampropeltis getula)*, housed in an adjacent cage, or having just treated one on the same examination table, can change the behavior of another snake.

BRUMATION

Brumation is the term now used for winter dormancy in reptiles (as opposed to a true hibernation).[36-38] Many temperate zone snakes must be brumated to induce successful reproduction. The snakes are well fed during the summer and fall; then feeding is stopped, and the snakes are allowed to pass stools. The cage temperature is slowly dropped over a period of several weeks. Dropping the temperature 2.8°C (5°F) per day or every few days for a total drop of 10°C to 14°C (20°F to 25°F) "conditions" the snakes to enter the brumation period. They are maintained with water available but no food for about 3 months, then slowly warmed up.

Feeding may begin 2 to 3 weeks later. Most tropical boas and pythons, when cooled for breeding situation, do not need as drastic a temperature drop (sometimes 5°C [10°F] suffices) as brumated colubrids and if cooled too low can have neurological or respiratory signs develop.

Some neonate temperate zone snakes that are not yet feeding, if in good physical condition, can be brumated, and this may induce them to feed after the brumation period. No snake, regardless of age, should be brumated if it is not in excellent condition or if it is showing signs of illness.

LONGEVITY

Clients frequently ask about the life expectancy of their snake. A Ball Python *(Python regius)* set the longevity record at 47.5 years in the Philadelphia Zoo.[14] Table 5-4 lists longevity records for a number of commonly kept snakes, showing that the potential exists to keep many for quite some time. Little available evidence of longevity exists in nature, but experts doubt that many snakes reach these ages in the wild. Many herpetoculturists believe that at least female snakes, bred repeatedly for high production, may have their lives shortened by this process.

Table 5-4 Longevity of Some Selected Snakes in Captivity, in Years[40]

	Longevity (y)
Xenopeltidae	
Asian Sunbeam Snake, *Xenopeltis unicolor*	12
Loxocemidae	
Neotropical Sunbeam Snake, *Loxocemus bicolor*	32
Boidae	
Dumeril's Ground Boa, *Acrantophis dumerili*	26
Children's Python, *Antaresia childreni*	24
Woma, *Asidites ramsayi*	16
Black-headed Python, *Aspidites melanocephalus*	22
Boa Constrictor, *Boa c. constrictor*	40
Solomon Island Ground Boa, *Candoia carinata*	16
Rubber Boa, *Charina bottae*	26
Coastal Rosy Boa, *Charina trivirgata*	31
Emerald Tree Boa, *Corallus caninus*	19
Columbian Rainbow Boa, *Epicrates cenchria maurus*	31
Smooth Sand Boa, *Eryx johni*	31
Anaconda, *Eunectes murinus*	31
Brown Water Python, *Liasis mackloti fuscus*	26
Carpet Python, *Morelia spilota variegata*	19
Green Tree Python, *Morelia viridis*	20
Short-tailed Python, *Python. curtus*	27
Burmese Python, *Python molurus bivittatus*	28
Indian Python, *Python m. molurus*	34
Ball Python, *Python regius**	47
Reticulated Python, *Python reticulatus*	29
African Rock Python, *Python sebae*	27
Viperidae, Crotalinae	
Northern Copperhead, *Agkistrodon contortrix mokeson*	29
Western Cottonmouth, *Agkistrodon piscivorus leucostoma*	26
Jumping Pit Viper, *Atropoides nummifer*	19
Eyelash Palm Pit Viper, *Bothriechis schlegeli*	19
Terciopelo, *Bothrops asper*	20
Eastern Diamondback Rattlesnake, *Crotalus adamanteus*	22
Western Diamondback Rattlesnake, *Crotalus atrox*	27
South American Rattlesnake, *Crotalus durissus terrificus*	17
Timber Rattlesnake, *Crotalus h. horridus*	30
Banded Rock Rattlesnake, *Crotalus lepidus klauberi*	33
Southern Pacific Rattlesnake, *Cortalus viridis herlleri*	24
Central American Bushmaster, *Lachesis stenophrys*	24
Western Massasauga, *Sistrurus catenatus tergeminus*	20
Pope's Pit Viper, *Trimeresurus popeorum*	13
Viperidae, Viperinae	
Puff Adder, *Bitis arietans*	15
Gaboon Viper, *Bitis gabonica*	18
Russell's Viper, *Daboia russelli*	15
Horned Sand Viper, *Cerastes cerastes*	18
Carpet Viper, *Echis coloratus*	28
Common Adder, *Vipera berus* spp.	19
Colubridae	
Trans-Pecos Ratsnake, *Bogertophis subocularis*	23
Eastern Indigo Snake, *Drymarchon corais couperi*	25
Cornsnake, *Elaphe g. guttata*	32

Table 5-4	Longevity of Some Selected Snakes in Captivity, in Years[40]—cont'd	
		Longevity (y)
Black Ratsnake, *Elaphe o. obsoleta*		22
Western Mud Snake, *Farancia abacura reinwardti*		18
Plains Hog-nosed Snake, *Heterodon n. nasicus*		19
False Water Cobra, *Hydrodynastes gigas*		16
Grey-banded Kingsnake, *Lampropeltis alterna*		19
Prairie Kingsnake, *Lampropeltis c. calligaster*		23
California Kingsnake, *Lampropeltis getula californiae*		44
Arizona Mountain Kingsnake, *Lampropeltis p. pyromelana*		22
Scarlet Kingsnake, *Lampropeltis triangulum elapsoides*		23
Coastal Mountain Kingsnake, *Lampropeltis zonata multicincta*		28
Grass Snake, *Natrix natrix*		20
Blotched Watersnake, *Nerodia erythrogaster transversa*		14
Great Basin Gophersnake, *Pituophis catenifer deserticola*		33
Northern Pinesnake, *Pituophis m. melanoleucus*		20
Queen Snake, *Regina septemvittata*		10
Northwestern Gartersnake, *Thamnophis ordinoides*		15
Elapidae		
Black Mamba, *Dendroaspis polylepis*		21
Texas Coralsnake, *Micrurus fulvius tenere*		19
Monocled Cobra, *Naja kaouthia*		32
Black Forest Cobra, *Naja melanoleuca*		29
Cape Cobra, *Naja nivea*		26
King Cobra, *Ophiophagus hannah*		22
Taipan, *Oxyuranus scutellatus*		15

*Reference 41.

GIANT SNAKES

Among the snakes are species that mature at less than 10 cm (4 inches) in total length and those that reach huge proportions and consume large prey. Much discussion centers around the so-called giant snakes. Many of the records of truly huge snakes remain dubious and unsubstantiated because they are poorly documented. A recent review[39] of the literature on giant snakes lists four species that probably exceed 6 m (20 ft) in length: the Anaconda (*Eunectes murinus*) of South America, the Burmese Python (*Python molurus bivittatus*) of Southeast Asia, the Reticulated Python (*Python reticulatus*) of Southeast Asia, and the African Rock Python (*Python sebae*) of Africa. The two largest species are the Anaconda and the Reticulated Python, which approach 9 m (30 ft), but no valid records are seen of either over 9 m (30 ft) in length. An Anaconda has a greater girth and weight than a Reticulated Python of the same length.

REFERENCES

1. Greer AE: Limb reduction in squamates: identification of the lineages and discussion of the trends, *J Herpetol* 25:166-173, 1991.
2. Cohn MJ, Tickle C: Developmental basis of limblessness and axial patterning in snakes, *Nature* 399:474-479, 1999.
3. Pough FH, Andrews RM, Cadle JE, Crump ML, Savitxky AH, Wells KD: *Herpetology*, ed 3, Upper Saddle River, NJ, 2004, Prentice Hall.
4. Greene HW: *Snakes: the evolution of mystery in nature*, Berkeley, 1997, University of California Press.
5. Underwood G: *A contribution to the classification of snakes*, London, 1967, British Museum (Natural History).
6. Cadle JE: Phylogenetic relationships among advanced snakes, snakes: a molecular perspective, *Univ Calif Publ Zool* 119:1-70, 1988.
7. Heise PJ, Maxson LR, Dowling HG, Hedges SB: Higher-level snake phylogeny inferred from mitochondrial DNA sequences of 12S rRNA and 16s rRNA genes, *Mol Biol Evol* 12:259-265, 1995.
8. Groombridge BC: Variations in morphology of the superficial palate of henophidian snakes and some possible systematic implications, *J Nat Hist* 13:447-475, 1979.
9. Kluge AG: Boine snake phylogeny and research cycles, *Misc Publ Mus Zool Univ Mich* 178:1-58, 1991.
10. Kluge AG: Aspidites and the phylogeny of pythonine snakes, *Rec Aust Mus Suppl* 19:1-77, 1993.
11. McDowell SB: Systematics. In Seigel RA, Collins JT, Novak SS, editors: *Snakes: ecology and evolutionary biology*, New York, 1987, MacMillan.
12. Rieppel O: A review of the origin of snakes, *Evol Biol* 22: 37-130, 1988.
13. Hicks J: Cardiac shunting in reptiles: mechanisms, regulation, and physiological functions. In Gans C, Gaunt AS, editors: *Biology of the Reptilia, vol 19, morphology C*, Ithaca, NY, 1998, Society for the Study of Amphibians and Reptiles.
14. Lillywhite HB: Temperature, energetics, and physiological ecology. In Seigel RA, Collins JT, Novak SS, editors: *Snakes: ecology and evolutionary biology*, New York, 1987, MacMillan.
15. Holz PH: The reptilian renal-portal system: influence on therapy. In Fowler ME, Miller RE, editors: *Zoo & wild animal medicine, current therapy 4*, Philadelphia, 1999, WB Saunders.
16. Lillywhite H, Smith LH: Haemodynamic responses to haemorrhage in the snake, *Elaphe obsoleta obsoleta*, *J Exp Biol* 94:275, 1981.
17. Zaher H, Rieppel O: Tooth implantation and replacement in squamates, with special reference to mosasaur lizards and snakes, *Am Museum Novitates* 3271:1-19, 1999.
18. Bellairs Ad'A: *The life of reptiles*, vol 2, London, 1969, Weidenfeld & Nicholson.
19. Russell FE: *Snake venom poisoning*, Great Neck, NY, 1983, Scholium International, Inc.
20. Strydom DH: The evolution of toxins found in snake venoms. In Lee C-Y, editor: *Snake venoms*, Berlin, 1979, Springer-Verlag.
21. Pope CH: Fatal bite of captive African rear-fanged snake (Dispholidus), *Copeia* 280-282, 1958.
22. Wever EG: *The reptile ear: its structure and function*, Princeton, NJ, 1978, Princeton University Press.
23. de Cock Buning TJ: Qualitative and quantitative explanation of the forms of heat sensitive organs in snakes, *Acta Biotheoretica* 34:193-206, 1985.
24. Molenaar GJ: Anatomy and physiology of infrared sensitivity of snakes. In Gans C, Ulinski PS, editors: *Biology of the Reptilia, vol 17, neurology C, sensorimotor integration*, Chicago, 1992, University of Chicago Press.
25. Hartline PH, Kass L, Loop MS: Merging of modalities in the optic tectum: infrared and visual integration in rattlesnakes, *Science* 199:1225-1229, 1978.
26. Newman EA, Hartline PH: The infrared "vision" of snakes, *Sci Am* 246:116-127, 1982.
27. Bellairs Ad'A, Bryant SV: Autotomy and regeneration in reptiles. In Gans C, Billett F, editors: *Biology of the Reptilia. development B*, vol 15, New York, 1985, John Wiley & Sons.

28. Alibardi L: Presence of acid phosphatase in the epidermis of the regenerating tail of the lizard *(Podarcis muralis)* and its possible role in the process of shedding and keratinization, *J Zool London* 246:379-390, 1998.
29. Maderson PFA: The structure and development of the squamate epidermis. In Lyne AG, Short BF, editors: *Biology of skin and hair growth*, Sydney, 1965, Angus & Robertson.
30. Bechtel HB: *Reptile and amphibian variants—colors, patterns, and scales*, Malabar, Fla, 1995, Krieger Publishing.
31. Love B, Love K: *The corn snake manual*, Escondido, Calif, 2000, Advanced Vivarium Systems.
32. Shine R: *Australian snakes: a natural history*, Ithaca, NY, 1991, Cornell University Press.
33. DeNardo DF: Reptile thermal biology: a veterinary prespective, *Proc Bull Assoc Reptile Amphibian Vet* 2002.
34. Avery RA: Field studies of body temperatures and thermoregulation. In Gans C, Pough FH, editors: *Biology of the Reptilia, vol 12, physiology C*, New York, 1982, Academic Press.
35. Rossi JV, Rossi R: *Snakes of the United States and Canada; keeping them healthy in captivity*, vol 2, western area, Malabar, Fla, 1995, Krieger Publishing.
36. Heatwole H: *Reptile ecology*, 1976, University Queensland Press.
37. Mayhew WW: Hibernation in the horned lizard, Phrynosoma m'calli, *Comp Biochem Physiol* 16:103-119, 1965.
38. Mayhew WW: Biology of desert amphibians and reptiles. In Brown GW, editor: *Desert biology*, vol I, New York, 1968, Academic Press.
39. Murphy JC, Henderson RW: *Tales of giant snakes: a historical natural history of anacondas and pythons*, Malabar, Fla, 1997, Krieger Publishing.
40. Slavens FL, Slavens K: *Reptiles and amphibians in captivity; breeding-longevity and inventory*, Seattle, WA, 1999, Slaveware.
41. Conant R: The oldest snake, *Bull Chicago Herp Soc* 28(4):77, 1993.

6
LIZARDS

STEPHEN L. BARTEN

EVOLUTION AND CLASSIFICATION

Systematics has undergone a shift from the traditional, morphology-based system of Carolus Linnaeus to the evolution-based system called cladistics. The Linnaean system assigns each animal a unique binomial genus and species name, then groups these into morphologically related families, orders, and classes. Cladistics describes evolutionary relationships and places organisms into monophyletic groups called *clades*, each consisting of a single ancestor and all its descendants.[1] Relationships between clades are shown in a diagram called a cladogram, which consists of a series of bipolar branching lines. A discussion of cladistics in detail is beyond the scope of this chapter, but veterinarians and herpetologists alike should become familiar with current concepts in systematics.

Living reptiles are divided into three clades. The first reptilian clade is the chelonians (turtles and tortoises), and the second is the archosaurs, which contains the crocodilians and the birds (one example of how cladistics is based on evolutionary relationships rather than morphology: crocodilians and birds share a common ancestor). The third clade is the lepidosaurs, which consists of tuataras, snakes, and lizards.[1] Snakes and lizards are grouped together in the Squamata, a monophyletic taxon that shares more than 50 derived features. Thus, snakes are not considered a sister group (sharing a common ancestor) to all lizards but rather are a subgroup of lizards; snakes are simply lizards with absent or reduced limbs. So, squamates have a precise definition, but a group consisting of lizards without snakes does not.[1] Nevertheless, that is exactly the group this chapter discusses. Current squamate relationship hypotheses do not enjoy universal acceptance at this writing, and the relationships between groups or families may change as more data come to light.

Squamates are the most successful group of living reptiles with about 7200 species. The traditional lizards, as opposed to snakes, comprise about 4450 of these.[1] The first branch of the squamate cladogram divides them into the Iguania and all the others, which collectively are called the Scleroglossa.

The Iguania contains three groups: the Iguanidae, the Agamidae, and the Chamaeleonidae. The family Iguanidae is the dominant group of lizards in the New World and differs from the other two by having pleurodont dentition (teeth attached to the medial side of the jaws without sockets that are regularly shed and replaced) and fracture planes in the caudal vertebrae. Examples of this family include the Green Iguana *(Iguana iguana;* Figure 6-1), Green Anole *(Anolis carolinensis)*, Basilisks *(Basiliscus* spp.), Horned Lizards *(Phrynosoma* spp.), Spiny Lizards *(Sceloporus* spp.), and West Indian Rock Iguanas *(Cyclura* spp.).

Together the Agamidae and Chamaeleonidae make up the Acrodonta because of their acrodont dentition (teeth attached to the biting edge of the jaw without sockets that are not shed and replaced). This group also lacks caudal vertebral fracture planes, except some *Uromastyx*. The family Agamidae is the dominant family of lizards in the Old World. Members include the Bearded Dragon *(Pogona vitticeps)*, Agama *(Agama agama)*, Frilled Lizard *(Chlamydosaurus kingii)*, Water Dragon *(Physignathus cocincinus)*, Egyptian Spiny-tailed Lizard *(Uromastyx aegyptius)*, and Sail-fin Lizard *(Hydrosaurus pustulatus)*. The family Chamaeleonidae consists of the Old World, or True, Chameleons. Examples include the Veiled Chameleon *(Chamaeleo calyptratus)*, the Panther Chameleon *(Furcifer pardalis)*, and the dwarf *Brookesia* spp.

The relationships between the remaining squamate groups in the Scleroglossa are less certain, and multiple hypotheses have been proposed. The first main group, the Nyctisaura, contains a number of families. The Gekkonidae include the geckos and pygopods. Geckos are primarily nocturnal insectivores, and the pygopods are snakelike without forelimbs, their hindlimbs reduced to flaps of skin containing a few phalanges. Examples of the former are the Leopard Gecko *(Eublepharis macularius)*, Crested Geckos *(Rhacodactylus* spp.), Leaf-tailed Geckos *(Uroplatus* spp.), and Day Geckos *(Phelsuma* spp.). Examples of the latter are the Snake Lizards *(Lialis* spp.) and the Scalyfoot *(Pygopus* spp.). The Dibamidae, or Blind Lizards *(Dibamus* and *Anelytropsis* spp.), also are snakelike lizards with no forelimbs and flaplike hindlimbs. The Amphisbaenidae, or Worm Lizards, are legless, covered with wormlike annular rings made of scales, and all species are fossorial. The Xantusiidae contain the desert Night Lizards *(Xantusia* spp.).

The remaining squamates, the Antarchoglossa, contain a number of diverse groups. The subgroup Lacertoiformes includes the family Lacertidae, or Wall and Sand Lizards. Some examples are the Oscellated Green Lizard *(Lacerta lepida)*, Rock Lizard *(Lacerta saxicola)*, and Viviparous Lizard

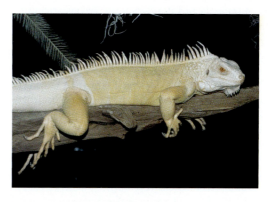

FIGURE 6-1 Amelanistic Green Iguana *(Iguana iguana)*. The skin is dull white with yellow highlights, and the irises are pink. Concern exists that such an animal could be prone to sunburn if exposed to unfiltered sunlight.

(*Lacerta vivipara*). The Teiidae are the New World equivalent of the Lacertidae and include the Whiptails and Racerunners (*Aspidoscelis* [*Cnemidophorus*] spp.), Jungle Runners (*Ameiva* spp.), and Tegus (*Tupinambis* spp.). The second subgroup is the Diploglossa, which contains the remaining lizard groups. One is the family Scincidae or true Skinks, familiar species of which include the Blue-tongued Skink (*Tiliqua* spp.), Prehensile-tailed Skink (*Corucia zebrata*), Five-lined Skink (*Eumeces fasciatus*), and the Casqueheads (*Tribolonotus* spp.). Two others are the Cordylidae or Girdle-tailed Lizards (*Cordylus* spp. and others) and Gerrhosauridae or Plated Lizards (*Gerrhosaurus* spp. and others). The Diploglossid group also incorporates a lesser subgroup, Anguimorpha, which contains several families. The Xenosauridae includes the New World viviparous Xenosaurs (*Xenosaurus* spp.) and the Shinisauridae contains only the Chinese Crocodile-tailed Lizard (*Shinisaurus crocodilurus*). The family Anguidae are long and snake-like in form. They include the Alligator Lizards (*Elgaria* spp.), Glass Lizards (*Ophisaurus* spp.), Legless Lizards (*Anniella* spp.), and the Sheltopusik (*Ophisaurus apodus*). The final families in the Anguimorpha are members of the Varanoidea group. The Helodermatidae contain only two species, but these are the only venomous lizards: the Gila Monster (*Heloderma suspectum*) and the Mexican Beaded Lizard (*Heloderma horridum*). The family Varanidae consists of the Monitor Lizards and Goannas. Familiar examples include the Savannah Monitor (*Varanus exanthematicus*), the Nile Monitor (*Varanus niloticus*), and the Komodo Dragon (*Varanus komodoensis*). Lanthanotidae has a single species, the Bornean Earless Lizard (*Lanthanotus borneensis*).[1-5]

ANATOMY

The following sections refer extensively to Figures 6-2 to 6-5.

Cardiovascular System

In lizards, the heart is three chambered with left and right atria and a single ventricle. The ventricle is divided into three chambers: the cavum arteriosum, cavum venosum, and cavum pulmonale. The cavum venosum receives unoxygenated venous blood from the right atrium, and the cavum arteriosum receives oxygenated blood from the left atrium. Blood leaves the heart through the pulmonary artery arising from the cavum pulmonale and the two aortic arches arising from the cavum venosum. All three cava communicate, but a muscular flap and two-stage ventricular contraction minimizes mixing among the three cava. Unoxygenated blood flows from the cavum venosum into the cavum pulmonale. An atrioventricular valve prevents mixing of this blood with the oxygen-rich blood in the cavum arteriosum. Next the ventricle contracts, forcing the unoxygenated blood in the cavum pulmonale into the pulmonary artery. The atrioventricular valve then closes, allowing oxygenated blood to flow from the cavum arteriosum into the cavum venosum and out the aortic arches. Thus the three-chambered squamate heart function is similar to that of a four-chambered heart.[1,4]

Paired left and right aortic arches fuse caudal to the heart to form the dorsal aorta.

The renal portal system of reptiles is well documented in the literature for its parenteral therapeutic implications.[6-10] Although the anatomy of the blood vessels varies somewhat from group to group, venous circulation from the tail, and little from the hind limbs, routes directly to the kidneys via the renal portal system. The injection of drugs that are cleared via tubular secretion into the caudal half of the body could result in lower than anticipated serum concentrations because of their excretion in the urine before entering the systemic circulation. This practice also could result in increased renal toxicity in the case of nephrotoxic drugs, such as aminoglycosides. Only limited pharmacokinetic studies on the effect of the renal portal system on serum drug concentrations have been done, but the results suggest that the renal portal system has less effect on drug uptake and distribution than was once

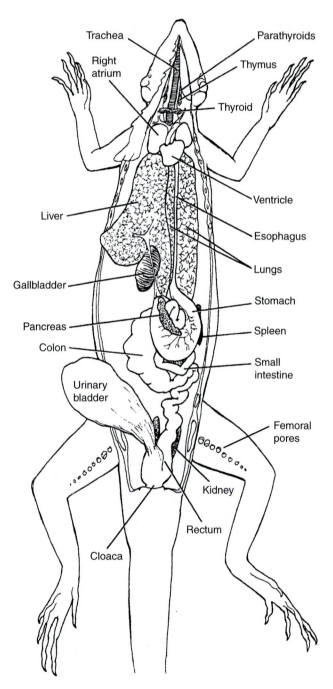

FIGURE 6-2 Ventral view of a Green Iguana (*Iguana iguana*). Note the relatively anterior location of the heart between the shoulder joints. Also, note the relatively caudal position of the kidneys within the pelvic canal.

thought.[10] Moreover, shunts exist that carry blood directly from the renal portal system to the postcava, bypassing the renal parenchyma.[5]

Lizards have a large ventral abdominal vein that lies along the inner surface of the abdominal wall on the midline (Figure 6-6).[6,11-13] This vein must be avoided in a celiotomy incision. One way to avoid and preserve the vein is with a paramedian incision. Alternatively, a ventral midline incision may be used if the linea is incised with caution, as the ventral abdominal vein is suspended in a broad ligament and is a few millimeters away from the linea alba.[14] The vein should be protected with saline solution–moistened gauze during the remainder of the procedure. With the surgical approach, the benefit of incising between muscles rather than through them must be weighed against the risk of damaging this large vein. Reports have shown that this vein can be ligated without clinical effect.[15]

Venipuncture may be done with the ventral caudal vein in species that do not undergo tail autotomy, with the axillary venous plexus or with the jugular vein (Figure 6-7). In large

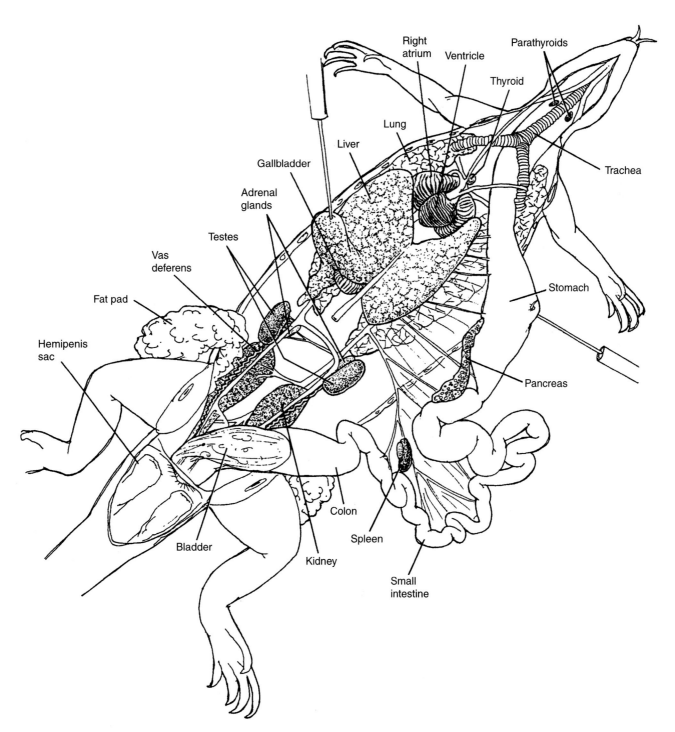

FIGURE 6-3 Ventral view of a Savannah Monitor Lizard *(Varanus exanthematicus)*. Note a more typical location of the heart compared with the Green Iguana *(Iguana iguana)*. Likewise, although the caudal portions of the kidneys extend into the pelvic canal, the cranial portions are within the coelomic cavity, unlike the Green Iguana.

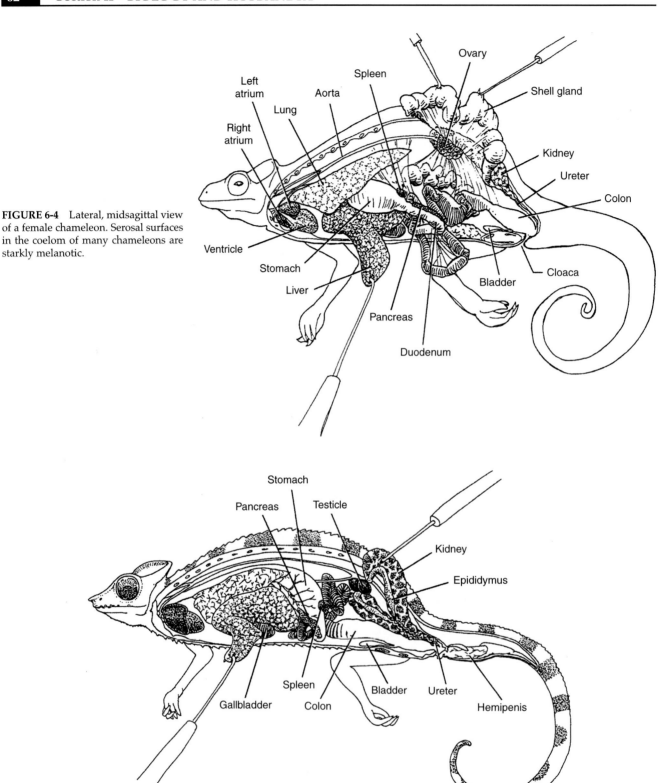

FIGURE 6-4 Lateral, midsagittal view of a female chameleon. Serosal surfaces in the coelom of many chameleons are starkly melanotic.

FIGURE 6-5 Lateral, midsagittal view of a male chameleon.

specimens intravenous (IV) catheters may be placed in the cephalic vein or jugular vein (in species with long necks) with a cutdown technique, or in the ventral caudal vein using a lateral approach aiming craniad.[16,17] IV fluids may be given by this route or through an intraosseous catheter placed in the femur or tibia. The curve of the femur in most species allows placement of a catheter into the distal end without invasion of the stifle joint.

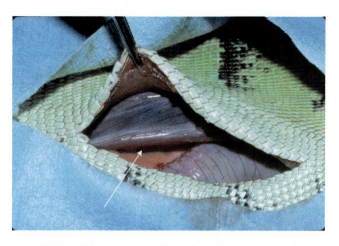

FIGURE 6-6 Paramedian celiotomy incision in a Green Iguana (*Iguana iguana*). The medial body wall has been elevated to show the large ventral abdominal vein as it hangs in its suspensory ligament (mesovasorum) from the medial aspect of the linea alba. This vessel must be avoided during celiotomy incisions. This may be accomplished with a careful midline incision, as the vein hangs several millimeters from the linea, or with a paramedian incision.

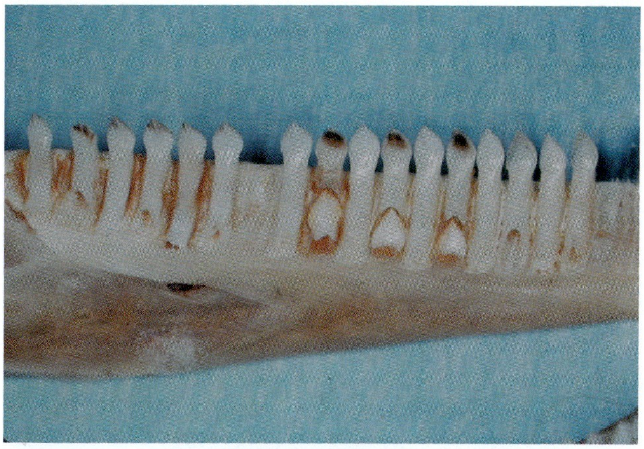

FIGURE 6-8 Mandible of a Green Iguana (*Iguana iguana*) showing pleurodont dentition. Teeth are attached to the medial side of the jaw without sockets. Note that alternate teeth have shortened roots with buds of new teeth below them. Teeth are shed and replaced throughout life. Rostral is to the right.

Digestive System

The lips of lizards are flexible skin but are not moveable. The teeth are generally pleurodont (attached to sides of mandible without sockets), but in some families, such as the Agamidae and Chamaeleonidae, they are acrodont (attached to the biting edges of the jaws without sockets). Pleurodont teeth are regularly shed and replaced (Figure 6-8). Acrodont teeth are not replaced except in very young specimens, although new teeth may be added to the posterior end of the tooth row as the lizard grows. Some agamids have a few canine tooth–like pleurodont teeth on the anterior jaws along with the normal acrodont teeth (Figure 6-9). Care should be taken to avoid damaging the irreplaceable acrodont teeth in agamids and chameleons when opening the mouth with a rigid speculum during physical examination. Likewise, periodontal disease has been reported in species with acrodont dentition but not pleurodont dentition.[18] Lizard teeth generally grasp, pierce, or break up food. In many monitors, the teeth slice and cut. Mollusk-eating Caiman Lizards (*Dracaena guianensis*) and adult Nile Monitors (*Varanus niloticus*) have broad rounded cheek teeth for crushing shells (Figure 6-10).

The only venomous species of lizards are the Gila Monster and the Mexican Beaded Lizard. These species have grooved rather than hollow teeth, which have no direct connection to the venom glands. The venom glands are sublingual rather than temporal as seen in snakes. Venom flows from the glands along the dental grooves and is injected with chewing action. Symptoms of envenomation include pain, hypotension, tachycardia, nausea, and vomiting. Commercial antivenin is not available for these species.[19]

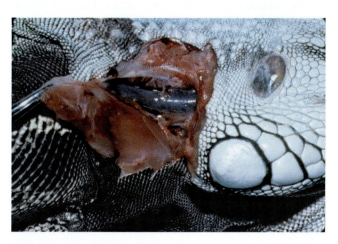

FIGURE 6-7 Necropsy specimen of a Green Iguana (*Iguana iguana*) to show the large jugular vein on the lateral neck caudal to and slightly below the tympanum. The depressor mandibularis muscle has been reflected to expose the jugular deep to it. The lizard's head is to the right. This site can be located by drawing an imaginary line from the ear to the point of the shoulder and used for venipuncture or intravenous catheters.

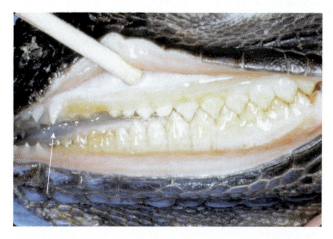

FIGURE 6-9 Teeth of a live Soa-soa Sailfin Lizard (*Hydrosaurus amboinensis*) showing acrodont dentition. The teeth rest on the occlusal surface of the jaw bones without sockets and are neither shed nor replaced if damaged. Most agamid lizards also have a few sharp pleurodont teeth on the anterior jaws that function like canine teeth (*arrow*); these are regularly shed and replaced. Rostral is to the left.

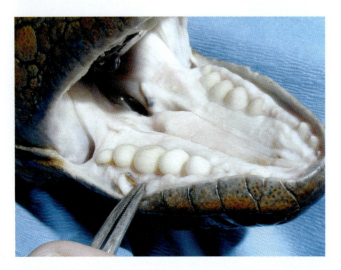

FIGURE 6-10 Cheek teeth of this Caiman Lizard (*Dracaena guianensis*), restrained in dorsal recumbency, are broad and rounded for crushing shells of snails on which it feeds exclusively.

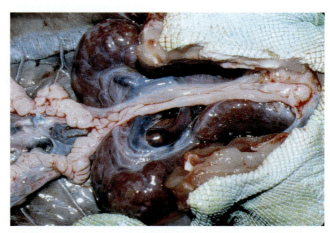

FIGURE 6-11 Granulomatous nephromegaly in a Green Iguana (*Iguana iguana*). The skin and body wall have been removed to the level of the pelvis, the symphysis of which has been split to reveal the bodies of kidneys within the pelvic canal. Note how these massively enlarged organs extend anterior to the pelvic brim, which was detected with antemortem palpation. Likewise, enlarged kidneys were shown to fill the pelvic canal on digital cloacal palpation before death. The colon and bladder have been removed to allow the kidneys to be seen. Cranial is to the left.

The tongue of the lizard varies with the species. In general, it is mobile and protrusible. Taste buds are abundant in species with fleshy tongues and reduced in those with keratinized tongues, like monitors. Taste buds also are found in the lining of the pharynx. Lizards with deeply forked tongues, such as monitors and tegus, protrude the tongue to bring scent particles to the vomeronasal (Jacobson's) organ for olfaction. The tongue is projectile for food gathering in Chameleons (*Chamaeleo* spp.). In Green Iguanas, the tip of the tongue is darker than the rest and should not be mistaken for a lesion. The paired vomeronasal (Jacobson's) organs have tiny openings in the anterior roof of the mouth, and the paired internal nares open just caudal to those.

The stomach of lizards is simple, J-shaped, and not gizzard-like. Swallowing stones to aid digestion is not a normal behavior.

A cecum is present in many species.[5] The large intestine is thin-walled and not as muscular as the stomach or small intestines.

A number of vegetarian species have a colon that is divided into sacculations to facilitate hindgut fermentation for more complete digestion. These types have relatively high optimal body temperatures (T_o) zones to enhance microbial fermentation. Lizards in this group include the Green Iguana, Prehensile-tailed Skink, Egyptian Spiny-tailed Lizard, and Chuckwalla (*Sauromalus obesus*).[20]

A cloaca is present and is divided into three parts: the coprodeum, which collects feces; the urodeum, which collects urinary waste and receives the sexual structures (vas deferens/oviducts); and the proctodeum, which is the final chamber before elimination.[5,21] The cloacal slit is transverse in lizards.

Reproductive-Urinary System

The kidneys are metanephric and are located in the caudal coelom or deep within the pelvic canal, depending on the species. In the latter, nephromegaly from any cause can result in obstruction of the colon as it passes between the kidneys within the pelvic canal. Granulomatous nephritis causing colonic obstruction or dystocia is relatively common in the Green Iguana (Figure 6-11).

The posterior segment of the kidney in some male geckos, skinks, and members of the iguana family is sexually dimorphic. This area is called the sexual segment. It becomes swollen during the breeding season and contributes to the seminal fluid. The color of the sexual segment may change dramatically during the breeding season and may be misinterpreted as pathology by the untrained eye (see Figure 5-16).

Nitrogenous waste is excreted as uric acid, urea, or ammonia. Reptile kidneys have relatively few nephrons, lack a renal pelvis, and also lack the loop of Henle and thus are unable to concentrate urine. However, water may be resorbed from the bladder, resulting in the postrenal concentration of urine. The excretion of ammonia or urea results in significant water loss, and the excretion of insoluble uric acid allows water conservation. Thus, ammonia and urea are excreted in significant amounts only in aquatic and semiaquatic species.[5]

A thin-walled bladder is present in most species of lizard. When absent, urine is stored in the distal colon. Because urinary waste flows from the kidney through the ureter into the urodeum of the cloaca before entering the bladder (or colon in species that lack a bladder), it is not sterile as in mammals. Urine may change within the bladder, so urinalysis results may not indicate renal function as in mammals.[22] Cystic calculi occur and may be caused in part by water deprivation and diets containing excessive levels of protein.[6] The calculi tend to be singular, smooth-surfaced, layered, and quite large when discovered (see Chapter 49).

Lizards have breeding seasons determined by cycles of photoperiod, temperature, rainfall, and availability of food. In males, a corresponding fluctuation is seen in testicular size. Male iguanas and other lizards are often noted to be more territorial and aggressive during their breeding season.

Fertilization is internal. Male lizards have paired hemipenes that are sac-like and lack erectile tissue. They are stored in an inverted position in the base of the tail and may produce noticeable bulges in the ventral proximal tail. Only one

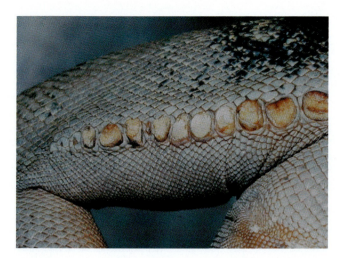

FIGURE 6-12 The large femoral pores on the ventral aspect of the thighs of this Green Iguana *(Iguana iguana)* indicate that it is male. Femoral pores of adult male iguanas are larger than those of females, although this specimen has unusually large pores. Femoral pores of juvenile iguanas resemble those of females.

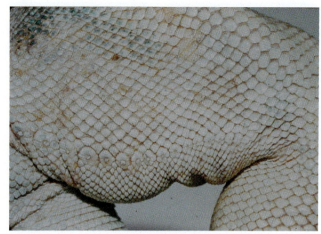

FIGURE 6-13 Small femoral pores of this Green Iguana *(Iguana iguana)* indicate that it is female.

hemipenis is used at a time during copulation. The hemipenes are not involved in urination.

Female lizards have paired ovaries and oviducts, which enter into the urodeum of the cloaca. Egg retention may be preovulatory, where ovulation does not occur and the mature follicles remain within the ovaries, and postovulatory, with the shelled or nonshelled ova within the oviducts. Preovulatory and postovulatory egg retention also have been referred to as follicular stasis and egg binding, respectively.

Gender identification is difficult in juvenile specimens, but most adult lizards are sexually dimorphic. Mature male iguanas have taller dorsal spines, larger dewlaps, and larger operculum scales than do females and have bilateral hemipenis bulges at the base of the tail. Male chameleons often have elaborate head ornamentation in the form of horns, crests, and plates that are lacking in females. Many other male lizards have larger heads, bigger crests, brighter colors, or erectable dewlaps or are larger than females.

Femoral and precloacal pores, when present, are larger in adult males than females (Figures 6-12 and 6-13). These are probably the most reliable means of determining the gender of adult lizards. Sexing probes may be used in iguanas and monitors but with less consistent accuracy than in snakes. A technique of injection of saline solution into the base of the tail to evert the hemipenis has been described, but care must be taken to prevent trauma to the exposed hemipenis before it is withdrawn.[6,23] Pressure necrosis also may result from this technique. This method might be considered in species that are otherwise difficult to sex, such as monitors, Tegus, large skinks, Beaded Lizards, and Gila Monsters. Hemipenes may be temporarily everted in anesthetized males with application of gentle pressure to the base of the tail, just caudal to the cloaca. The hemipenes of mature male monitor lizards of many species calcify and are demonstrable on radiographs.[6,23] Endoscopy to visualize the gonads may be used to identify gender.[22] Ultrasonic evaluation of the gonads in the coelom or the presence or absence of hemipenes in the proximal tail also may be used to identify the gender of a lizard[24] (see Chapter 23 for more information).

Lizard reproductive strategies vary and may be oviparous, ovoviviparous (the eggs are retained within the female until birth), viviparous (with a placental type of circulatory connection), or parthenogenic. Several populations of certain *Lacerta* spp. and *Aspidocelis (Cnemidophorus)* spp. consist entirely of females and reproduce via parthenogenesis[5] (see Chapter 23 for more information).

Nervous System

The reptile brain is more advanced with a larger cerebrum and cerebellum than that of amphibians or fishes. Still, the brain is small, not exceeding 1% of the body mass. Reptiles are the earliest group of vertebrates with 12 pairs of cranial nerves. The spinal cord differs from that of mammals in that it extends to the tail tip.

Neurologic disorders are poorly understood and documented in reptiles, but basic neurologic reflexes should be examined during any evaluation. Nutritional requirements and history must also be evaluated because unbalanced diets may result in neurologic symptoms, such as hypocalcemic tetany.[25]

Special Senses

The Ear

The ear has both auditory and vestibular functions. The tympanic membrane is generally visible within a shallow depression on the side of the head. It is covered with thin transparent skin, the outer layer of which is shed during ecdysis (Figure 6-14). In some lizards, such as the Earless Lizard *(Holbrookia maculata)* and Horned Lizards, the tympanic membrane is covered with scaly skin. Although mammals have three auditory ossicles, lizards only have two: the slender columnar stapes and its cartilagenous tip, the extracolumella. The eustachian tubes connect the middle ear cavities to the dorsolateral pharynx.

The Eye

The structure of the reptile eye is similar to that of other vertebrates. The iris contains striated, not smooth, musculature,

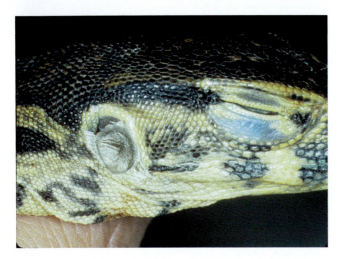

FIGURE 6-14 A monitor lizard (*Varanus* spp.) undergoing ecdysis here sheds the outer layer of transparent skin that covers the tympanic membrane.

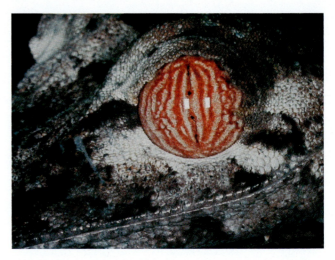

FIGURE 6-15 Madagascar Leaf-tailed Gecko (*Uroplatus fimbriatus*). The serrated vertical pupil is completely closed in the bright light used for photography, resulting in a series of pinholes (seen as a vertical line of tiny black dots in the center of the highly ornamented iris). These allow acute vision.

and common mydriatics have no effect. General anesthesia or d-tubocurare injected into the anterior chamber with a fine needle may be used for mydriasis,[26] although this technique is not recommended for the inexperienced practitioner.

The pupil is usually round and relatively immobile in diurnal species and is usually vertically slit-like in nocturnal species. Many geckos have a serrated pupillary opening that results in a series of small holes when the pupil is completely closed. The images that pass through these holes are superimposed on the retina, resulting in acute vision even in dim light (Figure 6-15). The lens does not move for accommodation, but rather muscles in the ciliary body change the lens shape for this purpose.

Consensual pupillary light reflex is absent. The cornea does not contain Descemet's membrane. A ring of bony scleral ossicles is present in most species.

Eyelids are usually present, except for some geckos and the Oscellated Skink (*Ablepharus* sp.), which have snake-like spectacles. The lower lid is more movable and moves upward to close the eye. In some lizards, the lower lid may be transparent, allowing vision when the lids are closed and the eyes protected. The nictitating membrane is usually present.

The retina is relatively avascular but contains a conus papillaris, a large vascular body that protrudes into the vitreous. The fovea centralis, a depression in the retina responsible for acute vision, is often present in diurnal species.

Certain Horned Lizards (*Phrynosoma cornutum*, *P. coronatum*, and *P. solare*) can squirt an alarming amount of blood from their eyes in response to threats from predators. They rarely do this in response to humans but do so when molested by dogs, coyotes, and foxes. If the blood spray enters their mouth, canines shake their heads and salivate as if it were distasteful. The lizards accomplish this by means of a pair of muscles that constrict the venous outflow from the head, causing an increase in blood pressure and leakage from the ocular venous sinuses. When threatened, the Horned Lizard arches its back and closes its eyes, which become swollen. A fine stream of blood then shoots out from the margins of the eyelids of one or both eyes for a distance of up to 4 feet. The hemorrhage lasts 1 or 2 seconds and may be repeated two or three times. The lizard may repeat this performance after a brief rest if another predator threatens. The amount of blood lost appears considerable, but the lizards recover rapidly with no visible signs of harm.[27,28]

A well-developed parietal eye is found on the dorsal midline of the head in some lizards, such as the Green Iguana. It is a degenerate eye that contains a lens and retina and connects neurologically to the pineal body. It plays a role in hormone (especially reproductive) production, thermoregulation, and regulation of the amount of time a lizard basks in sunlight. It does not form images.[5,26]

Respiratory System

Nasal salt glands are present in herbivorous iguanid lizards such as the Green Iguana. When the plasma osmotic concentration is high, excessive sodium and potassium is excreted by these glands. The lizards sneeze and expel a clear fluid that dries to a fine white powder consisting of sodium and potassium salts (Figure 6-16). This mechanism allows water conservation and may be mistaken for an upper respiratory infection. The paired internal nares are anterior in the roof of the mouth and are a common site for discharges to accumulate and a good site for bacteriologic sampling when respiratory infection is present.

In primitive lizards, the lungs are hollow sacs lined with faveoli (small sacs) that are more sponge-like than sac-like to increase surface area for gas exchange. In more advanced lizards, the lungs are further divided into interconnected chambers by few large septae.[5] Monitors have multichambered lungs with bronchioles that each end in a faveolus.[1] Chameleons have hollow, smooth-sided finger-like projections on the margins of their lungs that must be identified and avoided during coelomic surgery. These are not used in gas exchange but rather to inflate the body and intimidate would-be predators.[1] Some chameleons also have an accessory lung lobe that projects from the anterior trachea cranial

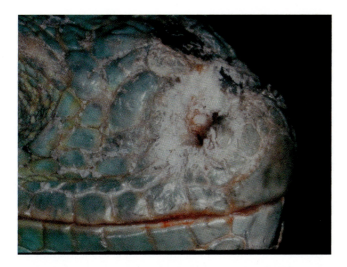

FIGURE 6-16 The nostril of this Green Iguana (*Iguana iguana*) is enlarged from chronic sinusitis. It also has a layer of fine white sodium chloride crystals around it. This is a product of the nasal salt-excreting gland and is a normal physiologic process but may be mistaken for an upper respiratory infection.

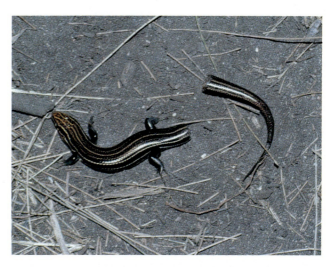

FIGURE 6-17 Tail autotomy in a Five-lined Skink (*Eumeces fasciatus*). The tail has fracture planes of cartilage through the vertebral bodies, allowing it to break off easily when grabbed by a predator. The detached tail writhes violently, allowing the lizard a chance to escape.

to their forelimbs. This may fill with secretions when infected, resulting in swelling of the ventral neck (see Figure 6-17).

Vocal cords are occasionally present, notably in some geckos, that can produce loud vocalizations.[5]

Lizards lack a diaphragm and move tidal volume with expansion and contraction of the ribs. The monitors and Gila Monsters have an incomplete postpulmonary fascia-like septum that divides the thoracic cavity from the abdominal cavity but does not aid respiratory movements.[29] The glottis is normally closed except during inspiration or expiration. The fluttering of the ventral throat does not result in significant respiration but probably ventilates the oropharynx for olfaction.[5] Lizards often inflate their lungs to maximum capacity to appear larger when threatened.

Some lizards can revert to anaerobic metabolism during prolonged periods of apnea.

Skeletal System

Many lizards are capable of tail autotomy, or loss of the tail (Figure 6-17). The advantage of autotomy is to escape from or distract predators when grabbed by the tail. Tails are often brightly colored to attract the attention of predators and wiggle extensively for a few minutes when they detach. Those species that undergo autotomy possess a vertical fracture plane through the body and part of the neural arch of each caudal vertebra. This is a plate of cartilage or connective tissue that develops after ossification.[5] Fracture planes are absent in the cranial part of the tail to protect the hemipenes, fat deposits, and other structures. In iguanas, the fracture plane is replaced by bone during maturation, resulting in a more stable tail in adults. The lost tail is regenerated with a cartilaginous rod for support. It generally has smaller darker scales in a more irregular pattern than the original tail and may be shorter and blunter.

Most iguanid lizards undergo autotomy, and most agamids, their Old World counterparts, do not. Likewise, the Monitors and True Chameleons (*Chamaeleo* spp.) do not have fragile tails. Those species with strong tails usually cannot regenerate a complete tail if the original is lost (see Chapter 70).

Ribs are usually present on all vertebrae except in the tail. Vertebral number is highly variable between species.

The forefeet and hindfeet are usually pentadactyl. The typical phalangeal formula is 2-3-4-5-3 in the forefoot and 2-3-4-5-4 in the hindfoot.[1] Bipedal locomotion is seen in some lizards, such as the Basilisk and the Collared Lizard (*Crotaphytus collaris*) and results in great speed.

Integument

Lizards have relatively thick skin with ectodermal scales formed by folding of the epidermis and outer dermal layers. Epidermal growth is cyclic, and lizards undergo regular periods of shedding or ecdysis, during which the skin comes off in large pieces in most lizards rather than in one piece as seen in snakes. Some species eat their sloughed skin. Normal shedding is one indication of good health. The frequency of ecdysis varies with species, temperature, humidity, state of nutrition, and rate of growth. Rapidly growing juveniles may shed every 2 weeks.[30] Wounds and skin infections cause more frequent shed cycles.

The skin contains few glands. Many lizards, notably iguanas, have femoral pores in a single row on the ventral aspect of the thigh (see Figures 6-12 and 6-13), and many geckos have both femoral and precloacal pores, the latter in a V-shaped row anterior to the cloaca. These tend to be larger in mature males.

Chromatophores are abundant in species that have rapid color changes, such as *Chamaeleo* spp. and *Anolis* spp. Control of the chromatophores may be hormonal, neurologic, or both. Chromatophores may react to stimulation from light or changes in temperature.[5]

Osteoderms, or dermal bony plates, are present in Gila Monsters, Beaded Lizards, some skinks, legless lizards, and

Girdle-tailed Lizards. These are usually confined to the back and sides.

Dewlaps, spines, crests, and horns may be present and often are secondary sex characteristics, more prominent in males. Spines serve a protective function in Bearded Dragons, Horned Lizards and the Moloch *(Moloch horridus).*

A lateral skin fold is usually present between front and hind legs. This is a convenient site for the injection of subcutaneous fluids.

Claws in large species like iguanas and monitors are large and well developed with sharp points. These must be trimmed at regular intervals to prevent deep scratches that would occur inadvertently even with casual handling. The nails should be trimmed before a physical examination.

Endocrine System

Reproductive hormone levels are influenced by photoperiod, temperature, and seasonal cycles.

The thyroid gland varies with the species and may be single, bilobed, or paired. The thyroid controls normal ecdysis. Lizards have paired parathyroid glands that control plasma calcium and phosphorus levels. Nutritional and renal secondary hyperparathyroidism are among the most commonly diagnosed diseases in captive reptiles.

Adrenal glands are suspended in the mesorchium or mesovarium and must be avoided during surgery for neutering.

The reptile pancreas has both exocrine and endocrine functions. The beta cells produce insulin, but diabetic changes are rare and often associated with widespread disease. Insulin and glucagon have the same functions in controlling blood sugar levels as they do in other vertebrates (see Chapter 58).

Endocrine disorders are poorly documented in reptiles and are probably underdiagnosed.

ENVIRONMENTAL CAPTIVITY REQUIREMENTS

Philosophy

Captive reptile husbandry has two main schools. Traditionally, spartan, easily cleaned cages were recommended and popular. Bare cages with newspaper substrate and a single branch and water bowl were considered adequate. The advantage was ease of maintenance at the cost of stimulation and enrichment for the cage inhabitants. More recently, lush complex naturalistic vivaria have become quite popular. Although these vivaria are more aesthetically pleasing for both the owner and the pet, they do not come without cost. Such cages are labor intensive to maintain, and if inadequately done, bacteria and fungi build up to levels that result in illness for the cage inhabitants. Few but the most dedicated and experienced hobbyists do an adequate job of maintaining hygiene in such complex cages. If a keeper cannot properly maintain a complex vivarium, then a simpler setup is a better choice. Likewise, ingestion of substrate is common when sand, gravel, or bark is used, especially if the diet is unbalanced or inadequate in amount. In spite of the potential problems, cages should be enriched to reduce stress and allow normal behaviors among the inhabitants.

Caging

Lizards need large cages to accommodate their active behavior, and most keepers provide cages that are too small for the lizards they keep. De Vosjoli[31] recommends that the cage length equal 1.5 to 2 times the total length of the lizard housed within and the cage width at least half that length (Figure 6-18). Divers[32] suggests even more space, quantifying requirements as 0.2 m² cage space per 0.1 m total length for terrestrial lizards and 0.4 m³ cage space per 0.1 m total length for arboreal lizards. That equals a cage two times as long and one time as wide as a terrestrial lizard is long or two times as long, two times as high, and one time as wide as an arboreal lizard is long. Thus, a 1 m–long iguana should have a cage measuring 2 m long, 2 m high, and 0.5 to 1 m wide, and a 2 m–long one needs a huge cage measuring 4 m long, 2 m high, and 1 m wide, almost the size of a whole room. Few commercial cages exceed 1.2 m long, so once a lizard reaches a length of 0.8 m, it needs a custom-built or room-sized cage. Aquariums sold for juvenile iguanas and monitors rarely are adequate for more than a year. Chameleons need proportionately more space than even this, and cages varying from $1 \times 0.5 \times 0.6$ m high for dwarf species to $1.3 \times 0.6 \times 1.3$ m high for large species are minimum standards.[33]

Many reptiles are escape artists and can squeeze through narrow cracks. Therefore, cages should be secure with tightly fitting lids. The sides should be smooth to prevent rostral abrasions. Metal screening should be used with caution because this screening does not retain heat and can result in foot and rostral trauma. Plastic mesh, polyethylene hardware cloth, or plastic-coated wire mesh is less abrasive. Cages made of wood must be sealed with polyurethane or a similar waterproofing agent and the joints caulked to allow cleaning and disinfection. Fresh polyurethane must be allowed to cure for several days, and the cage should be thoroughly aired out before placing a reptile in the cage or toxicity may result. Ventilation is crucial because ample air exchange is necessary to prevent the harmful buildup of bacteria and fungi.

Lizards allowed to roam free in the house are subject to chilling (lack of access to a heat source, too much access to cold outside walls and windows, and drafty floors), trauma (being stepped on, closed in doors, falling from high shelves or curtains, and attacked by dogs and cats), and escape.

Arboreal species need vertical space and climbing branches. Dry climbing branches of appropriate diameter may be used to make a three-dimensional pathway for them. Certain species have specific requirements; for instance, Frilled Lizards and *Corytophanes cristatus* need vertical or strongly inclined branches on which to perch and become anorectic if these are not available (Figure 6-19).[34] Likewise, geckos with adhesive lamellae on their feet prefer solid surfaces to screening. Live nontoxic plants that lack spines and slippery surfaces and are big enough to bear the weight of the lizard are recommended. These act as cage furniture and add humidity, shelter, egg-laying sites, and visual enhancement. They should be potted to facilitate cleaning.[33] Silk plants may be coated with toxic water-soluble stiffeners and should not be used.[33]

Substrate

Many different types of substrate are available. Each has advantages and disadvantages. Selection can be tailored to

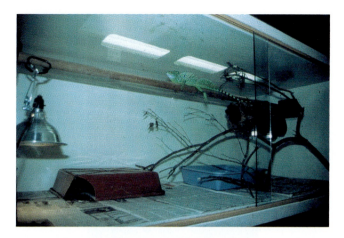

FIGURE 6-18 Lizards are active and need relatively large cages. Cages are recommended to be twice as long and one time as wide as the length of the lizard housed within. Nevertheless, this Basilisk (*Basilicus plumifrons*) is housed in a spacious cage at least three times its length, yet it has chronic rostral abrasion from repeatedly running into the glass.

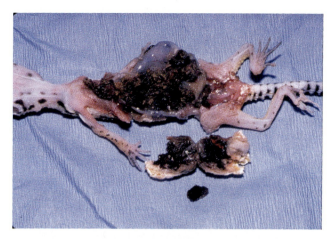

FIGURE 6-20 Gastrointestinal impaction in a Leopard Gecko (*Eublepharis macularius*) with fine-grade bark sold as substrate especially for reptiles. Cloaca, shown here in front of the body, was impacted, swollen, and abscessed. The entire gastrointestinal tract was distended with bark chips.

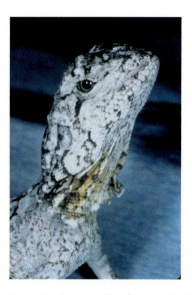

FIGURE 6-19 Some lizard species like this juvenile Frilled Dragon (*Chlamydosaurus kingii*) need vertical branches on which to perch or they fail to thrive.

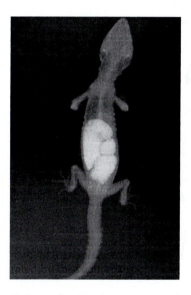

FIGURE 6-21 Radiograph of fatal gastrointestinal impaction in a Leopard Gecko (*Eublepharis macularius*) with so-called "digestible sand" sold as reptile bedding.

the particular needs of the client and species being housed. An ideal substrate is one that is inexpensive, aesthetically pleasing, easily cleaned, absorbent, and digestible if swallowed. Substrate can be flat newspaper, indoor-outdoor carpet, orchid or so-called "reptile" bark chips, cyprus mulch, potting soil, or commercial animal bedding made from recycled paper or wood pulp.[6,11,31,33,35,36] Newspaper is inexpensive and clean and easy to use but not aesthetically pleasing. Carpet is labor intensive and requires washing. Orchid bark products made from fir may be used but never redwood or cedar. If bark chips are excessively dusty, they could be rinsed and dried before use. Coarse-grade bark is too large to accidentally be swallowed by most lizards but can irritate the feet of lizards that dig repeatedly, such as monitors. Fine-grade bark can cause fatal gastrointestinal impaction if swallowed by a lizard (Figure 6-20). A shallow feeding dish can be used to minimize the risk of accidental substrate ingestion, but the bark should be removed if a keeper sees the lizard eat some or finds it in the droppings. Potting soil for lizard bedding should not contain perlite, pesticides, or fertilizers. It is basically harmless if swallowed but can become muddy or dusty if too wet or too dry. Recycled paper animal bedding currently is a popular bedding to use because it is more absorbent and less dusty than alfalfa pellets, it can be changed less frequently, it is more or less digestible if swallowed, and it is compostable.

Sand or a mixture of soil and sand may be used for desert species. Calcium carbonate marketed as digestible sand can be useful, but fatal gastrointestinal impactions in geckos have been reported (Figure 6-21).[37] Offering a powdered calcium supplement in a dish may minimize this risk. Silica sand is not recommended because it is abrasive and generates silica dust.

Cedar shavings contain aromatic resins that may be toxic to small reptiles.[6,38] Other substrates to *avoid* include alfalfa pellets, gravel, crushed corn cob, clay kitty litter, and miscellaneous wood shavings.[6,11,38] Alfalfa pellets are digestible if ingested and look nice but are dusty and odiferous when wet. Particulate substrates are difficult to clean, so many keepers fail to clean the cages thoroughly or with regular frequency. These substrates also retain moisture from animal waste and spilled water, which in the warm environment of the cage can promote microbial growth and infections in the animal. Reptiles may ingest these substrates, which results in gastrointestinal impaction (Figure 6-22). Fine bark chips and sand, except for desert species, used to be recommended against for these same reasons but are beginning to gain favor because of the current popularity of naturalistic vivaria. Now many keepers believe the risks of bark and sand are minimal and that the advantages outweigh these risks. Species that burrow are the exception and must be provided with sand or other suitable material in which to burrow.

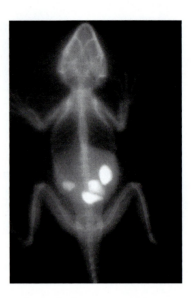

FIGURE 6-22 Radiograph of gastrointestinal impaction in a Collared Lizard *(Crotaphytus collaris)* with pea gravel sold as "too large to swallow."

Thermoregulation

Reptiles are ectothermic and need supplemental heat in captivity. The preferred body temperature (T_p) is a behavioral choice and is the temperature range a reptile selects when placed in a thermal gradient. The optimal body temperature (T_o) is a physiologic constant that represents the temperature at which performance is maximized. T_o is necessary to optimize metabolic processes including digestion, growth, healing, reproduction, and immune system function. T_p and T_o usually overlap.

One commonly used heat source for captive lizards is the hot rock, which is an artificial rock that contains an electric heating element. This rock is inappropriate in many cases because most lizard species derive external heat from basking in the sun (radiant heating) and not from lying on rocks heated by the sun (conductive heating). Hot rocks also do not heat the air adequately. Hot rocks also can be dangerous because they allow direct contact with the heat source, which may result in dehydration and severe burns. Substrate heat supplied by a thermal pad outside of the cage bottom is a safer alternative. A radiant heat source is better for most lizards, and keepers should be aware of the difference between overhead and substrate heat sources. Radiant heat sources include spot and flood lamps, ceramic heaters, and radiant heat panels. When radiant heat sources are used, direct contact must be prevented to avoid burns.

Heat sources should be used in conjunction with a thermostat so that the temperature in the cage can be precisely controlled. A number of models designed for use with reptile heating systems are commercially available. Temperatures within the cage must be monitored with a thermometer. It is important to know and adjust the temperature where the reptile rests and in the hottest and coolest parts of the enclosure. Remote infrared thermometers or "temp guns" are useful for this, but thermometers attached to the back of the cage provide little useful information.

Heating supplies for reptiles, including heat sources, thermostats, and infrared thermometers are widely available from various Internet-based reptile supply dealers who advertise in herpetological magazines and websites.

Thermal gradients must be provided. In nature, the environment consists of multiple microenvironments with varying temperatures and humidity levels. Reptiles in the wild control their core body temperature to within a few degrees of their T_o via thermoregulation—they move all or parts of their bodies into or out of direct sunlight. A thermally complex environment is recommended for captive reptiles to allow them to adjust their body temperature behaviorally as they would in the wild. A thermal gradient on both a horizontal and vertical axis is ideal. This can be created by providing a focal hot spot on one side of the cage with a combination of substrate and radiant heat. This area should reach the T_o for the species being housed. A captive can heat up in the morning by sitting in the focal hot spot and move out of the hot spot when it exceeds its T_o. Having the entire cage maintained at a uniform temperature is unnatural.

Diurnal temperature fluctuations occur between day and night in the wild, so heat sources should not be left on 24 hours a day. Daily fluctuations in temperature seem to be important for lizards.[33] The best method of supplying supplemental heat is to use a substrate heater under, rather than within, the cage in combination with a radiant heat source. Substrate heat can be provided with various commercially available reptilian heating pads or heat tape set to keep the floor of the cage at the low end of the T_p for the species being kept. The substrate heat source should be left on 24 hours a day. Radiant heat sources can then be used to raise the focal hot spot by 10 or 15 degrees during the day reaching the T_o. Timers can be used to turn the heaters off at night. Red or amber lamps may be used at night to maintain cage temperatures in colder climates.

Diurnal cage temperatures should range from 26.5°C to 37°C (80°F to 98.5°F) and 24.0°C to 29.5°C (75°F to 85°F) for tropical and temperate species, respectively. The particular needs of a given species should be researched because some require hotter or cooler temperatures than these (see Table 4-1).

Stressed, sick, or injured reptiles need to reach their T_o to optimize immune system function. Drug uptake and distribution is influenced by temperature, and reptiles should maintained at their T_o when receiving medications or anesthetics.

Osmoregulation

Pseudomonas spp. bacteria grow rapidly in water bowls, so bowls should be changed and disinfected or washed in hot soapy water daily.[39]

Arboreal species, such as Old World Chameleons, geckos, and anoles, only lap dew from leaves. These species need a daily misting of the cage or a drip system. A simple drip system can be made with old IV tubing pushed through the bottom of a water-filled plastic milk bottle. The IV set is adjusted to allow a steady drip over broad leaves in the cage, and a bowl is placed on the cage floor to catch the excess. A single pinhole in the bottom of a milk jug provides a simpler but less adjustable drip system. Alternatively, an aquarium pump may be connected to a large pan of water so that water is pumped up through tubing and allowed to drip over leaves and then flow back into the pan. Commercial misters and drip systems are available from reptile suppliers.

Tap water usually is adequate, but bottled water might be used where the tap water quality is in question. Aging the water or dechlorination is not necessary.

Humidity is an important but often overlooked factor.[38,40] In general, jungle species need higher humidity and desert species lower humidity. Most species do well at humidity levels of 50% to 70%.[38] High humidity and temperature can result in rapid growth of bacteria and mold in the cage, but this can be prevented with adequate ventilation.

Correct ambient humidity is necessary to ensure proper ecdysis in winter when humidity in the average home can get as low as 10%. Low humidity can be corrected by placing damp sponges in the hide boxes or by using a so-called humidity box. This is made by cutting an access hole in the side or top of a plastic storage container and partially filling it with damp but not soaked sphagnum moss. Frequent spraying with a plant mister is also effective but is more labor intensive. Commercial misting machines for reptile cages are available. Room humidifiers or vaporizers may be more efficient for controlling humidity in collections with numerous cages.

Feeding and Nutrition

Herbivores

Green Iguanas are herbivorous and in the wild feed almost entirely on leaves of trees and vines.[20,41,42] They do not have gizzard-like stomachs and do not need grit or gravel to help digest their food. In fact, intestinal obstruction with gravel is a common problem when iguanas are kept on this substrate.[6,11,12] Likewise, they are not insectivorous as juveniles that gradually transform to herbivores as they mature; they are herbivorous from birth (although an insect occasionally might be taken opportunistically).[20,42] This misinformation was in the literature in the 1960s and has been perpetuated in many poorly researched pet store "how to" books. They do use microbial fermentation in the hindgut to digest high-fiber diets as efficiently as ruminants. However, this requires high environmental temperatures. Newly hatched iguanas lack the microbes necessary for hindgut fermentation and obtain them in the wild by eating the feces from adult iguanas.[43,44] Whether the oral inoculation of captive hatched iguanas with the parasite-free feces of adult captive iguanas is beneficial for digestion is unknown, but the captive diet is relatively more digestible than the leaves that make up the bulk of their diet in the wild. However, this practice can be a useful part of the treatment of diarrhea in this species.[43]

Other species of herbivorous lizards, such as the Caicos Rock Iguana (*Cyclura carinata*) and Gray's Monitor Lizard (*Varanus olivaceous*), do undergo an ontogenetic change from a carnivorous diet as juveniles to an hebivorous one as adults. These two species use very different feeding strategies. The Rock Iguana is a generalist, feeding on 80% of the local plant species and using many parts of the plants but focusing on leaves. Adult Gray's Monitors are specialists that restrict their diet to ripe fruit of only a dozen or so of the thousands of local plant species.[45]

Ground Iguanas (*Cyclura* spp.), the Prehensile-tailed Skink, Spiny-tailed Iguanas (*Ctenosaura* spp.), Spiny-tailed Lizards (*Uromastyx* spp.), and the Chuckwalla are herbivores with hindgut fermentation like Green Iguanas and in general do well with iguana husbandry techniques.[20]

In captivity, herbivorous lizard diets should be based on a variety of chopped, dark green, leafy vegetables. Greens that contain oxalates, like spinach, or goitrogens, like kale, should be used sparingly. Fruit should be minimized, not because it is toxic but because it dilutes the beneficial nutrients of the other ingredients. In one study, adding 1 cup of strawberries to 1 cup of romaine reduced the protein and calcium concentrations by two thirds compared with romaine alone.[46] Recommended diets, including ingredients, amounts, and schedules and vitamin and mineral supplementation, are listed in Table 6-1. Commercial iguana diets are available but vary in quality and palatability. Their use should be limited to less than half of the total diet (see Chapter 18).

Wild Green Iguanas are specialized folivores and eat primarily leaves from trees. Captive iguanas are exposed to a number of food items they would never see in the wild. The owner must patiently work with the pet iguana and train it to eat a balanced diet. The lizard should never be allowed to choose what it eats because taste and palatability do not necessarily equate to nutritional value.

No captive iguana diet can be accurately described as proper. Precise nutritional requirements for this species are not known, and wild iguanas eat leaves from trees that are not available in captivity. We can approximate a nutritious diet, but most formulations are based on anecdote, experience, and speculation rather than scientific feeding trials.

Hatchling Green Iguanas in retail outlets are often anorectic, underweight, and weak. They may weigh less than 10 g and have a sunken abdomen and bony pelvic girdle. These lizards should be assist fed an appropriate vegetarian diet, such as a commercial tube feed mixture for rabbits or a gruel of rabbit pellets, as opposed to a liquid diet for carnivorous dogs and cats, at 1% to 3% of their body weight every 2 days. At the same time, the juvenile lizards should be offered a finely chopped diet, as described in Table 6-1, until they are eating on their own.[13,47]

Insectivores

Crickets, readily available in pet stores, are overused in lizard diets. Crickets by themselves are low in protein

Table 6-1	Recommended Diet for Captive Green Iguanas[58,59]

All plant material must be **washed, chopped** (a food processor is recommended), and **thoroughly mixed** to ensure a balanced diet in which **all** food items are eaten rather than just the favorite or tasty ones. Prepare enough for 4 to 7 days, store it in the refrigerator between feedings, and serve it at room temperature or slightly warmer. Offer food after the iguana has had several hours to bask under its heat source in the morning, leave it in all day, and remove uneaten food in the evening.

Hatchlings up to 14 inches in length:
Feed twice a day or provide continuous availability
Plant matter **finely chopped** or shredded
Juveniles up to 2.5 years or 3 ft in length:
Feed once a day
Plant matter **fine to medium chopped** or shredded
Adults over 2.5 years and 3 ft in length:
Feed daily or every other day; overfeeding an iguana is impossible with the high-fiber vegetarian diet recommended here
Plant matter **coarsely chopped**

Ingredients: **EACH MEAL** contains ingredients from **ALL FIVE** of the following categories:

1. Calcium-rich leafy greens, 40% to 45% of the diet or more, three or more items per feeding: turnip greens, mustard greens, collards, pesticide-free dandelion greens and flowers, clover, escarole, carrot tops, parsley, nasturtium leaves and flowers, and hibiscus leaves and flowers. Also offer endive, romaine, mint, and cilantro.
   Spinach, chard, and beet greens have high levels of oxalates that can tie up calcium; and kale, bok choy, and broccoli leaves have high levels of goitrogens. Both groups can be used but in moderation.
   Iceberg, Boston, butter, and head lettuces have little nutritional value compared with the dark leafy greens. Romaine is intermediate in value and should only be used in combination with the dark leafy green mentioned previously.
2. Other vegetables, 40% to 45% of the diet, a variety weekly: raw green beans, snow and snap peas, squash, sweet potato, okra, bell pepper, mushrooms, and yams. Thawed frozen mixed vegetables can be used occasionally. Grated carrot should be used occasionally only because it also contains high levels of oxalates.
   Vegetables with low nutritional value include cucumbers, tomatoes, onions, olives, zucchini, and radishes.
3. Alfalfa is a good source of fiber and protein. Alfalfa is available as minibales or pellets for small mammals from pet and feed stores. Read pellet ingredient labels to ensure alfalfa is the first ingredient listed. Do not use mixes that contain seeds and other ingredients. Alfalfa also is available as powder, tablets, or capsules from health food stores. Pellets and powder should be softened by soaking them in water before feeding. Be sure to use mature leaves and stems rather than sprouts. If an iguana refuses to eat alfalfa as offered, powder or crushed tablets can be added at low levels to the salad, with a gradual increase in the amount over several weeks.
4. Fruits, occasional treat or supplement. Fruits are low in most nutrients, including protein and calcium, and have high levels of phosphorus. They should not make up a large portion of the diet. Fruits dilute the good nutrients found in the leafy greens and vegetables. The following may be offered: figs, papaya, melon, apple, peaches, plums, strawberries, banana (with skin), and kiwi. Grapes and raisins have caused toxicities in dogs; use with caution, if at all.
5. Vitamin/mineral supplementation: supplementation is advised because vitamin and mineral deficiencies are common in iguanas. However, calcium and the fat-soluble vitamins (A, D, E, and K) can be both oversupplemented and undersupplemented. To avoid oversupplementation, natural sources from a varied diet are the best choice, with moderate vitamin/mineral use to balance the diet. To date, no documented studies exist on specific requirements for any lizard species.

Many **commercial products** are available for reptiles, but no manufacturers are required to prove potency or safety of their products. Products vary widely in levels of ingredients. Look for a ratio of roughly 100 parts vitamin A to 10 parts vitamin D_3 to 1 part vitamin E. Human products with vitamin D_3 rather than D_2 may also be used.

Minerals: Use powdered calcium carbonate (cuttlebone shavings is one source) or calcium gluconate.
Hatchlings and juveniles: 1 small pinch per feeding. Give vitamins 4 to 5 days a week and calcium 7 days a week.
Adults: 1 full pinch per 2 lbs body weight. Give vitamins two to three times a week and calcium four to five times a week (unless gravid or sick, then five to six times a week).
Vitamin powder on top of the salad may make it unpalatable. It should be mixed in thoroughly. If you can see the powder, you probably used too much.

A word about grains: grains such as bread, crackers, pasta, and seed are recommended in some iguana diet recipes. This food group is low in the nutrients that iguanas need, especially fiber, protein, and calcium. Grains should be limited to occasional treats if used at all.

A comment about animal protein sources: Traditionally, animal protein sources have been recommended in the diets of iguanas. However, in the wild, they are folivores, a type of vegetarian that eats primarily leaves. Some iguana books falsely claim that Green Iguanas eat insects until they mature then switch to a vegetarian diet as adults. This is not the case. They are vegetarians from birth, although they may occasionally accept unnatural foods, such as crickets or even mice in captivity. Although animal protein sources traditionally have been recommended for iguanas, their necessity has not been scientifically documented. Protein should be supplied as a plant-based source.

Little nutritional value: crickets, mealworms, king mealworms
  Too much protein or calcium: small prekilled mice, primate diets, trout chow, dog and cat food

A comment about commercial iguana diets: The advantage of these products is that they are easier to use than preparing a balanced salad several times a week. The disadvantage is that **in spite of claims that the commercial diets are complete and balanced, they may not be so.** The exact nutritional requirements for Green Iguanas have never been scientifically determined. Commercial diets that have high levels of protein (sometimes derived from animal sources rather than plant sources), fat, corn, soy, wheat, grains, goitrogenic vegetables, fruits, or flowers should be avoided. The main ingredient, which is always mentioned first on the ingredient list, should be alfalfa. Pelleted or powdered diets must be moistened with water before feeding. Frozen diets can be deficient in thiamine.

Commercial iguana diets may have a role in iguana nutrition but should only be part of the diet until more is known.

Captive Diet References:
Kaplan M: *Iguanas for Dummies.* Foster City, CA, 94404, IDG Books Worldwide, Inc., 2000.
Hatfield JW: *Green Iguana: the Ultimate Owner's Manual.* Portland, OR, Dunthorpe Press, 1996.

and calcium.[33,43,48,49] Many pet stores do not feed the crickets before sale for less mess to clean, but this practice results in less nutritional value.[48,49] Commercial cricket foods are available and should be fed to the crickets for at least 48 hours before their use as prey items, a practice called gut loading. Nevertheless, crickets should not be more than 50% of the diet.[32,47,48] The remainder of the diet can consist of a variety of wild-caught and captive-raised insects and other prey items, including but not limited to mealworms, king mealworms, wax worms, earthworms, cockroaches, giant cockroaches, flies, cicadas, grasshoppers, field crickets, caterpillars, silk worms, and newborn pinkie mice.[43,48,49] One should note that fireflies can be potentially toxic and lizard deaths have resulted from the ingestion of a single firefly (see Chapter 83).[50] "Sweepings" are obtained by sweeping a butterfly net through a grassy field and provide a variety of insect life.[48,49] Porch lights attract a variety of nocturnal insects. Hard-shelled beetles make up most of the diet of many lizards in the wild, such as Bengal (*Varanus bengalensis*) and Savannah Monitors (*V. exanthematicus*).[51]

Vitamins and minerals of the types listed in Table 6-1 are recommended. These may be applied to the insect prey with a salt shaker or by shaking the insects in a plastic bag with a small amount of supplement powder.[48,49] Insects groom themselves and remove this powder, so they should be offered immediately to the lizard. Young growing lizards should receive vitamin supplements once or twice a week and calcium supplements daily, and adults should receive vitamins every other week and calcium three to four times a week. Insects should be presented in a controlled manner so that the appetite can be monitored.[33] No more insects than would be eaten at once should be placed in the cage.

For chameleons, the best method is to hand feed. The insect may be held in front of the chameleon or may be placed in a smooth-sided bowl suspended in the climbing branches.[33] Juvenile chameleons must be fed several times a day, and a single daily feeding suffices for adults.[33]

Carnivores

Carnivorous lizards should be fed prekilled whole prey.[6,43] Rodents are preferable to chicks, and chicks are preferable to fish. Live rodents should never be offered as a food source. Not only does this prevent rodent bites to the lizard, but it is also more humane for the prey.[6,43] Appropriate-sized prey should be offered to prevent undue stress in swallowing. Juveniles should be fed once or twice a week, and adults every week or two. Obesity is common in adults, and these animals should be fed smaller amounts or less frequently.

If whole rodents and chicks make up the bulk of the diet, vitamin and mineral supplementation is not necessary.[6,43] Newborn pinkie mice have less total calcium than do adult mice, and calcium should be supplemented if these are used.[6,43]

Other items may be offered to help reduce feeding costs, but these are less optimal than whole prey items and should always be less than 50% of the diet. Chicken parts may be offered but should be washed and cooked to lessen the risk of harboring *Salmonella* bacteria. Bones are digested. Ground beef is high in fat and low in calcium and is nutritionally inadequate. Dog food, cat food, and trout pellets are not designed or formulated for reptiles and only should be used as supplements if at all.[6,35,43]

Ultraviolet Light Requirements

The full spectrum of natural light, specifically the ultraviolet wavelengths (UV), is important for vitamin D synthesis and calcium metabolism in diurnal lizards that do not eat vertebrate prey.[6,11,33,35,36,38,52] UV-A (nearwave, 320 to 400 nm) produces beneficial behavioral and psychologic effects but does not activate vitamin D precursors in the skin. UV-B (middle-wave, 290 to 320 nm) is necessary for vitamin D activation. Reptiles benefit from *both* UV-A and UV-B light.[33,35] Nevertheless, scientific studies into the specific requirement for UV light in captive lizards are lacking, and specific requirements for UV wavelength, intensity, and length of exposure are largely unknown (see Chapter 84).[38]

No artificial UV source matches the sun, but certain precautions must be taken before exposing captive lizards to direct sunlight. First, window glass filters out UV rays, so sunlight through a window is of no benefit. A reptile in a glass cage should never be placed in direct sunlight or overheating and death may occur.[6,36] Reptiles should be in a screen or mesh cage to allow sunlight to enter but at the same time prevent the escape of the lizard. Part of this enclosure must be shaded with an overhang or plants to allow the animal to get out of the sun. Another advantage of a screen or wire cage over hand holding a lizard or using a leash is that direct sunlight can result in temporary changes in personality, and normally tame lizards can become agitated and aggressive.[6] These changes reverse readily when the lizard is brought back inside. Lizards basking in sunlight should be monitored to prevent overheating, exposure to predators or theft, or any problem that might arise. Basking outside should not be allowed if the ambient temperature is excessively high. Even 15 to 30 minutes of direct sunlight a week can be quite beneficial.

A number of artificial UV-B light sources for reptiles are commercially available.[33,35,36,38,40,52] Obviously, a bulb producing 5.0% of its emitted light as UV-B is more efficient than one producing 2.0% UV-B. Moreover, a 48-inch tube produces more light than an 18-inch tube, and two tubes produce twice as much light as a single tube. Traditionally, fluorescent tubes have been considered better UV-B sources than incandescent bulbs, but mercury vapor bulbs that provide UV-B and heat in a single bulb are now available. These lamps get very hot and must be used with caution and only with larger lizards. New UV light sources are becoming available on a regular basis, and each should be evaluated on the basis of the wavelengths of UV produced.

There should never be glass or plastic between a UV light source and the reptile, as it will filter out the beneficial UV rays. Follow manufacturer recommendations for distance between the lamp and the reptile, and how frequently to replace the bulb.

Caution should be taken to avoid human exposure or eye contact with the UV rays because these have been associated with skin cancer and cataract formation.[33,35] Artificial UV light sources should mimic natural photoperiods and be turned off at night.

Artificial light sources cannot replace natural sunlight, and those reptiles with access to the sun in outdoor enclosures, even on a screen porch or patio, invariably have better growth, health, behavior, reproduction, and longevity than those kept indoors.[33,35,36]

Visual Security

Visual security is beneficial, especially for nervous species.[6,30,32,37] A hide box, which is a place where the caged reptile can retreat for some privacy, should be provided for all cage inhabitants. Hide boxes can be made from a cardboard box, terra cotta pottery, cardboard tubes, PVC tubes, corrugated black plastic drainage tubes, sheets of cork bark, or the saucer that fits under a flowerpot. The latter is inverted and a hole is cut through the top or side to allow access. Arboreal species should be provided with real or artificial plants in which to hide.[31,33] Many animals refuse to eat and may become stressed if they lack a secure hiding place. If the lizard does not use the hiding place, something is wrong with it and a different size or shape should be tried.

Disinfection

Cages and food and water bowls must be cleaned frequently. A solution of 3% sodium hypochlorite is an effective and economical disinfectant.[38,40] The cage and its furniture must be rinsed thoroughly before returning a lizard to the cage. Keepers must wash their hands thoroughly after cleaning each cage and not transfer water bowls, uneaten food, or climbing branches between cages without disinfecting them first (see Chapter 85).

Quarantine

New reptiles to a collection must be kept in a separate area from the main collection for a minimum of 3 months (see Chapter 4).[39,53] New arrivals should have physical examinations, recorded body weights, fecal examinations, parasite treatment, and monitoring for appetite, normal behavior, and symptoms of illness. At the very least, the owner should inspect new arrivals. The main collection should be fed and cleaned first and the quarantined animals second, with no transfer of animals, cages, food and water bowls, uneaten food items, or cage furniture between the two. Keepers must wash their hands and consider clothing changes after working with either collection to prevent the inadvertent transfer of pathogens. Ideally, different keepers should care for the two collections. The farther apart the two collections are physically, the less likely an epizootic will occur. No transfer of air should occur between the two groups. When multiple animals are quarantined, they should enter and leave the quarantine area as a group.

Communal Housing/Handling

Pet stores often display lizards for sale in crowded community tanks, suggesting that these are social animals. However, lizards are highly territorial and are stressed by the presence of conspecifics.[11,36,40] Male lizards are more territorial than females and react more violently to other males than to females. Hormone fluctuations, and thus territoriality, are seasonal and are manifested most acutely during the breeding season.[54] Chameleons are especially territorial.[33] When two or more lizards are kept together, the larger or more aggressive individual may physically attack the subordinate one, sometimes inflicting serious wounds (Figure 6-23). More often, it dominates in more subtle ways by keeping the subordinate lizard away from the food and heat sources. This allows the dominant one to digest its food more efficiently, grow faster, and have a more effective immune system than the subordinate lizard. The subordinate lizard in a pair invariably has chronic stress and thus fails to thrive. Symptoms include slow growth, emaciation, poor muscle tone, poor color, lethargy, and susceptibility to infections and parasites. The treatment is to separate the lizards. Reflective surfaces and mirrors should be avoided, especially for male lizards that attack their own reflection.

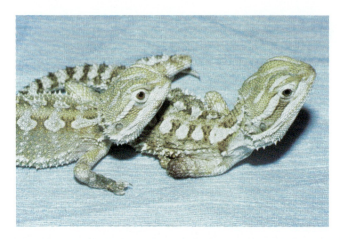

FIGURE 6-23 Large groups of juvenile Bearded Dragons (*Pogona vitticeps*) were housed together by a breeder for lack of cage space. They commonly bit each other, resulting in infection, abscessation, and avascular necrosis necessitating amputation of limbs and tails.

Keepers might occasionally observe two lizards in a cage to lay in the same spot and overinterpret that they have a relationship. However, stress is still present. If providing each lizard with its own cage is impossible, only same-sized members of the same species should be kept together and placing two males together should be avoided. A large cage is necessary, with enough spatial complexity so that the lizards are able to stay out of sight of one another while maintaining separate access to heat, UV light, water, and food.

Human nature is to be enthused about pet lizards, especially newly acquired ones, and to want to handle them frequently. However, unless a pet lizard is tame and acclimated to captivity, this practice causes stress and leads to anorexia.[11,36,40,49] In general, the relatively large species, such as iguanas and monitors, are less prone to panic and flight behavior and tolerate handling better than small species. Bearded Dragons (*Pogona* spp.) and Plated Lizards (*Gerrhosaurus* spp.) are especially docile and easily handled. Small high-strung species and juveniles or hatchlings of any species are easily startled and try to escape frantically, leaping from the keeper's grasp and scurrying frantically for cover across the room. Many Day Geckos (*Phelsuma* spp.) have fragile skin that is easily torn. None of these should be handled. Excessive handling of all lizards should be avoided. Handling, when done, should be in a closed room with little furniture for escaped lizards to hide behind or inside. Holding lizards over a table or in a lap lessens the distance they fall if they should try to escape.[49] Clients and employees who handle reptiles should be encouraged to wash their hands thoroughly when finished.

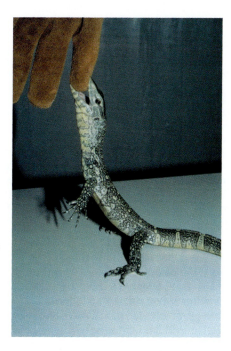

FIGURE 6-24 Some species of lizards, like this juvenile Nile Monitor (*Varanus nioloticus*), are naturally aggressive and do not make suitable pets. Only the most experienced herpetoculturists should attempt to keep them.

Table 6-2	Longevity Records for Some Notably Long-Lived Lizards[60,61,62]
Lizard	**Longevity**
Green Iguana (*Iguana iguana*)	19 y, 10 mo[62]*
	"Nearly 28 years" (purchased early 1968; died January 14, 1996)[61]
Cayman Island Ground Iguana (*Cyclura nubila lewisi*)	47 y, 7 mo[62]*
Spiny-tailed Iguana (*Ctenosaura similis*)	22 y, 5 mo[62]*
Prehensile-tailed Skink (*Corucia zebrata*)	16 y, 8 mo[60]*
	24 y, 4 mo[60]*
Green Water Dragon (*Physignathus cocincinus*)	11 y, 5 mo[60]*
	15 y, 4 mo[62]
Bearded Dragon (*Pogona vitticeps*)	10 y, 1 mo[62]
Jackson's Chameleon (*Chamaeleo jacksoni*)	8 y, 2 mo[62]
Panther Chameleon (*Furcifer pardalis*)	5 y, 2 mo[62]
Parson's Chameleon (*Chamaeleo parsoni*)	4 y, 0 mo[62]
Tokay Gecko (*Gekko gecko*)	23 y, 6 mo[62]
Leopard Gecko (*Eublepharis macularius*)	21 y, 1 mo[60]
	28 y, 6 mo[62]*
Mexican Beaded Lizard (*Heloderma horridum*)	34 y, 5 mo[62]*
Green Anole (*Anolis carolinensis*)	7 y, 2 mo[62]
Common or Black Tegu (*Tupinambis teguixin*)	13 y, 7 mo[60]
	16 y, 1 mo[62]
Savannah Monitor Lizard (*Varanus exanthematicus*)	12 y, 8 mo[62]

*Still alive at time of survey.

BEHAVIOR

Lizards tend to be alert and responsive, almost inquisitive. Captive-born lizards tend to be tame and docile. They tolerate handling and seem to relax when lightly stroked. Wild-caught lizards tend to be shy and wary. They frantically try to escape at the slightest disturbance.

Iguanas, monitors, and other lizards may exhibit defensive aggression when threatened. They stand sideways to the threat, swallow air to increase their size, stand high off the ground to look bigger, and lash at the threat with their tails. Some may gape and threaten to bite if provoked (Figure 6-24).

Offensive aggression is rare and usually involves sexually mature iguana males during the breeding season from December to March. They may attack anyone entering their territory and attempt to bite. These lizards must be confined to their cage during these times. A series of unprovoked attacks by adult male iguanas on their female human owners that occurred during the owner's menstrual period has been noted. Pheromones were postulated to have played a role in the aggressive behavior.[55]

Many lizards exhibit head bobbing and push-ups when another lizard or human invades their territory.

Iguanas, some geckos, and others frequently defecate in the same spot. If papers are put in that spot, the lizard may be more or less paper-trained and housebroken. Iguanas loose in the house frequently defecate in the bathtub, which is easy to clean.

RESTRAINT

Lizards are best restrained with a light touch. The more pressure that is exerted, the more a lizard struggles. Care must be taken to prevent tail autotomy. A lizard must never be grasped by the tail. Small geckos have delicate skin that can tear during handling. These may be confined in a plastic tube or anesthetized with isoflurane or sevoflurane for examination.

A large lizard may be enveloped in a towel to protect the handler from teeth, claws, and tail. If the nails are long and sharp, they should be clipped before the examination to prevent the handler from being scratched. One hand may grasp the forequarters around the neck and shoulders. The thumb and index finger should be just caudal to the head to prevent bites. The second hand grasps the hindquarters over the dorsal pelvis. The tail may be tucked under one arm during transport. Gauze or cotton placed over the eyes and held in place with self-adherent bandage material is a useful way to calm large, hyperactive, or aggressive lizards for handling.

Reptiles must be kept warm during transport in cold weather. Small reptiles may be carried in a jar with air holes punched in the lid, a cardboard box, or cloth bag under the owner's coat for warmth. Large ones should be placed in an insulated picnic cooler with a warm water bottle wrapped in towels to prevent it from crushing the lizards.

Lizards do not tolerate leashes well. They do not walk to follow an owner. When the leash is tugged, the lizards usually spin and end up tangled in the leash.

LONGEVITY

Lizards are relatively long-lived animals. A list of longevity records for captive reptiles in North American collections has been published.[56] These records reflect respondents to a national survey and primarily involve zoological institutions. Another publication documents inventory, breeding, and longevity based on surveys of public and private reptile collections.[57] Current information updated annually from surveys of 661 public and private collections by the same authors is available at the website Reptiles and Amphibians in Captivity—Longevity—Home Page, www.pondturtle.com/longev.html. Additional unreported records from private collectors may exceed some of those listed by these sources. Records for some of the more common pet lizards and some of the most long-lived species are shown in Table 6-2. As husbandry and veterinary techniques improve, many of these records will be eclipsed. A big difference does exist between the record lifespan for a given species of lizard and the average lifespan that owners might expect to observe in their own collection.

REFERENCES

1. Zug GR, Vitt LJ, Caldwell JP: *Herpetology: an introductory biology of amphibians and reptiles*, ed 2, San Diego, 2001, Academic Press.
2. Cooper JE, Lawton MPC: Introduction. In Beynon PH, Lawton MPC, Cooper JE, editors: *Manual of reptiles*, Gloucestershire, England, 1992, British Small Animal Veterinary Association.
3. Grzimek B, Hediger H, Klemmer K, et al, editors: *Grzimek's animal life encyclopedia, vol 6, reptiles*, New York, 1972, Van Nostrand Reinhold.
4. Halliday TR, Adler K, editors: *The encyclopedia of reptiles and amphibians*, New York, 1986, Facts on File.
5. Porter KR: *Herpetology*, Philadelphia, 1972, WB Saunders.
6. Frye FL: *Biomedical and surgical aspects of captive reptile husbandry*, ed 2, Malabar, Fla, 1991, Krieger Publishing.
7. Jacobson ER: Use of chemotherapeutics in reptile medicine. In Jacobson ER, Kollias GV, editors: *Contemporary issues in small animal practice: exotic animals*, New York, 1988, Churchill Livingstone.
8. Mader DR: Antibiotic therapy in reptile medicine. In Frye FL, editor: *Biomedical and surgical aspects of captive reptile husbandry*, ed 2, Malabar, Fla, 1991, Krieger Publishing.
9. Williams DL: Cardiovascular system. In Beynon PH, Lawton MPC, Cooper JE, editor: *Manual of reptiles*, Gloucestershire, England, 1992, British Small Animal Veterinary Association.
10. Holz PH: The reptilian renal portal system: a review, *Bull Assoc Rept Amphib Vet* 9:4-9, 1999.
11. Anderson NL: Husbandry and clinical evaluation of *Iguana iguana*, *Compend Cont Ed Pract Vet* 13:1265-1269, 1991.
12. Bennett RA: Reptilian surgery, part I: basic principles, *Compend Cont Ed Pract Vet* 11:10-20, 1989.
13. Boyer TH: Common problems and treatment of the green iguana, *Iguana iguana*, *Bull Assoc Rept Amphib Vet* 1:8, 1991.
14. Millichamp NJ: Surgical techniques in reptiles. In Jacobson ER, Kollias GV, editors: *Contemporary issues in small animal practice: exotic animals*, New York, 1988, Churchill Livingstone.
15. Mader DR, Wyneken J: The anatomy and clinical application of the renal portal system and the ventral abdominal vein, *Proc ARAV* 183-186, 2002.
16. Mader DR: *Intravenous catheters*, vol 6, Orlando, Fla, 1992, North American Veterinary Conference Proceedings Manual.
17. Wellehan JFX, Lafortune M: Coccygeal vascular catheterization in lizards and crocodilians, *J Herpe Med Surg* 14:26-28, 2004.
18. McCracken H, Birch CA: Periodontal disease in lizards—a review of numerous cases, *Proc Assoc Rept Amphib Vet* 108-114, 1994.
19. Boyer DM: *Venomous reptiles: an overview of families, handling, restraint techniques, and emergency protocol*, 1995, Proceedings of the Association of Reptilian and Amphibian Veterinarians.
20. Iverson JB: Adaptions to herbivory in iguanine lizards. In Burghardt GM, Rand AS, editors: *Iguanas of the world: their behavior, ecology, and conservation*, Park Ridge, NJ, 1982, Noyes Publications.
21. Bone RD: Gastrointestinal system. In Beynon PH, Lawton MPC, Cooper JE, editors: *Manual of reptiles*, Gloucestershire, England, 1992, British Small Animal Veterinary Association.
22. Zwart P: Urogenital system. In Beynon PH, Lawton MPC, Cooper JE, editors: Manual of reptiles, Gloucestershire, England, 1992, British Small Animal Veterinary Association.
23. Frye FL: Sexual dimorphism and identification in reptiles. In Kirk RW, editor: *Current veterinary therapy 10: small animal practice*, Philadelphia, 1989, WB Saunders.
24. Morris PJ, Henderson C: Gender determination in mature Gila monsters, *Heloderma suspectum*, and Mexican beaded lizards, *Heloderma horridum*, by ultrasound imaging of the ventral tail, *Bull Assoc Rept Amphib Vet* 8:4, 1998.
25. Lawton MPC: Neurological diseases. In Beynon PH, Lawton MPC, Cooper JE, editors: Manual of reptiles, Gloucestershire, England, 1992, British Small Animal Veterinary Association.
26. Lawton MPC: Ophthalmology. In Beynon PH, Lawton MPC, Cooper JE, editors: *Manual of reptiles*, Gloucestershire, England, 1992, British Small Animal Veterinary Association.
27. Sherbrooke WC: *Horned lizards: unique reptiles of Western North America*, Phoenix, 1981, Southwest Parks and Monuments Association.
28. Schmidt KP, Inger RF: *Living reptiles of the world*, Garden City, NY, 1957, Doubleday.
29. Coke RL: Respiratory biology and diseases of captive lizards (Sauria), *Vet Clin North Am Exotic Anim Pract* 3:531, 2000.
30. Cooper JE: Integument. In Beynon PH, Lawton MPC, Cooper JE, editors: *Manual of reptiles*, Gloucestershire, England, 1992, British Small Animal Veterinary Association.
31. de Vosjoli P: Designing environments for captive amphibians and reptiles, *Vet Clin North Am Exotic Anim Pract* 2: 43, 1999.
32. Divers SJ: Clinical evaluation of reptiles, *Vet Clin North Am Exotic Anim Pract* 2:291, 1999.
33. de Vosjoli P: *The general care and maintenance of true chameleons, parts I and II*, Lakeside, Calif, 1990, Advanced Vivarium Systems.
34. Barnett SL: Think "up": meeting the needs of arboreal lizards, *Proc Assoc Rept Amphib Vet* 41-56, 1997.
35. de Vosjoli P: *The green iguana manual*, Lakeside, Calif, 1992, Advanced Vivarium Systems.
36. Boyer TH: Green iguana care, *Bull Assoc Rept Amphib Vet* 1:12, 1991.
37. Bradley T: Coelomitis secondary to intestinal impaction of Calcisand in a leopard gecko, *Eublepharis macularius*, *Proc Assoc Rept Amphib Vet* 27-28, 2000.
38. Jacobson ER: Evaluation of the reptile patient. In Jacobson ER, Kollias GV, editors: *Contemporary issues in small animal practice: exotic animals*, New York, 1988, Churchill Livingstone.
39. Jacobson ER: Snakes, *Vet Clin North Am Small Anim Pract* 23:1179-1212, 1993.
40. Jarchow JL: Hospital care of the reptile patient. In Jacobson ER, Kollias GV, editors: *Contemporary issues in small animal practice: exotic animals*, New York, 1988, Churchill Livingstone.
41. McBee RH, McBee VH: The hindgut fermentation in the green iguana, *Iguana iguana*. In Burghardt GM, Rand AS, editors: *Iguanas of the world: their behavior, ecology, and conservation*, Park Ridge, NJ, 1982, Noyes Publications.

42. Rand AS, Degan BA, Monteza H, et al: The diet of a generalized folivore: *iguana iguana* in Panama, *J Herpetol* 24:211, 1990.
43. Frye FL: *A practical guide to feeding reptiles*, Malabar, Fla, 1991, Kreiger Publishing.
44. Troyer K: Transfer of fermentative microbes between generations in a herbivorous lizard, *Science* 216:540, 1982.
45. Auffenberg W: Herbivory in lizards: a comparison of feeding strategies. *Proc Assoc Rept Amphib Vet* 38-39, 1995.
46. Donoghue S: Nutrition of the green iguana (*iguana iguana*), *Proc Assoc Rept Amphib Vet* 99-106, 1996.
47. Anderson NL: Diseases of *Iguana iguana*, *Compend Cont Ed Pract Vet* 14:1335, 1992.
48. de Vosjoli P: *The right way to feed insect eating lizards*, Lakeside, Calif, 1989, Advanced Vivarium Systems.
49. de Vosjoli P: *The lizard keeper's guide*, Lakeside, Calif, 1994, Advanced Vivarium Systems.
50. Glor R, Means C, Weintraub MJH, Knight M, Adler K: Two cases of firefly toxicosis in bearded dragons, *Pogona vitticeps*, *Proc Assoc Rept Amphib Vet* 27-30, 1999.
51. Auffenberg W: The Bengal monitor (*Varanus bengalensis*): a model for insectivorous feeding strategies, *Proc Assoc Rept Amphib Vet* 1-2, 1995.
52. Gehrmann WH: Spectral characteristics of lamps commonly used in herpetoculture, *The Vivarium* 5(5):16, 1994.
53. Barten SL: The medical care of iguanas and other common pet lizards, *Vet Clin North Am Small Anim Pract* 23:1213, 1993.
54. Dugan B: The mating behavior of the green iguana, *Iguana iguana*. In Burghardt GM, Rand AS, editors: *Iguanas of the world: their behavior, ecology, and conservation*, Park Ridge, NJ, 1982, Noyes Publications.
55. Frye FL, Mader DR, Centofanti BV: Interspecific (lizard:human) sexual aggression in captive iguanas *(Iguana iguana)*: a preliminary compilation of eighteen cases, *Bull Assoc Rept Amphib Vet* 1:4, 1991.
56. Snider AT, Bowler JK: *Longevity of reptiles and amphibians in North American collections*, ed 2, 1992, Herpetological Circular No. 21. Society for the Study of Amphibians and Reptiles.
57. Slavens FL, Slavens K: *Reptiles and amphibians in captivity: breeding, longevity and inventory*, Seattle, 1992, Slaveware.
58. Kaplan M: *Iguanas for dummies*, Foster City, Calif, 2000, IDG Books Worldwide, Inc.
59. Hatfield JW: *Green iguana: the ultimate owner's manual*, Portland, Ore, 1996, Dunthorpe Press.
60. Snider AT, Bowler JK: *Longevity of reptiles and amphibians in North American collections*, ed 2, 1992, Herpetological Circular No. 21. Society for the Study of Amphibians and Reptiles.
61. Rogers KL: Iguana iguana (green iguana), longevity, *Herpetol Rev* 28:203, 1997.
62. Slavens FL, Slavens K: *Reptiles and amphibians in captivity: longevity home page*, 2001, www.pondturtle.com/longev.html

7
TURTLES, TORTOISES, AND TERRAPINS

THOMAS H. BOYER and DONAL M. BOYER

Turtles, tortoises, and terrapins are not as well represented in zoological institutions and private reptile collections as the squamate herpetofauna (lizards and snakes), perhaps in part because they often need more space and time to care for properly. Nonetheless, chelonians are brought to veterinarians on a regular basis and remain a challenge both in husbandry and medicine.

Chelonians face many threats on a worldwide basis. They are exploited primarily for food and traditional medicine; however, the international animal trade also takes its toll. The role of human consumption dramatically took a turn for the worse in recent years and has decimated Asian species. Once common species have become so scarce as to be considered commercially extinct. Of the 90 Asian species, 75% are currently threatened with extinction. These factors, compounded by ever-increasing habitat loss and degradation from expanding human population, have endangered many species. Disease is increasingly observed in wild populations. Population levels for many species remain unknown but are believed to be declining. A global conservation plan for chelonians has been developed by private individuals, government agencies, and conservation groups. For more information, contact the Turtle Conservation Fund (Kurt Buhlmann, Executive Director, Turtle Conservation Fund, 1919 M Street NW, Suite 600, Washington, DC 20036, k.buhlmann@conservation.org, 803-725-5293). For information on opportunities for veterinary involvement with the Turtle Survival Alliance, contact Charles Innis, VMD, Westboro VCA Animal Hospital, 155 Turnpike Road, Westboro, MA 01581, clemmys@aol.com.

Anyone who obtains chelonians is encouraged to act responsibly and observe all regulations set forth by the Convention on the International Trade in Endangered Species (CITES) in addition to other applicable wildlife laws. Asking questions about chelonian origin and verification of legal importation are important. Whenever possible, one should seek captive-born animals.

Gibbon[1] states that, among vertebrates, turtles are near the top in the number and proportion of species that have been known to live more than 50 years in captivity. He cites several examples of longevity—a Greek Tortoise *(Testudo graeca)* living 57 years and an Aldabra Tortoise *(Dipsochelys gigantea)* living 63 years. However, in captivity, inadequate care is more likely to result in mortality than old age.

Unfortunately, many veterinarians and turtle owners are not aware of what constitutes proper care for these animals. Accordingly, this chapter reviews basic chelonian taxonomy, anatomy, physiology, and husbandry in the hope that veterinarians will be better informed and use this information to improve veterinary care of this rapidly fading group. Keep in mind that for such a diverse group an overview of captive husbandry can only be that.

TAXONOMY

Within the Reptilia is a fundamental split that gives rise to two clades, the Anapsida (which includes the chelonia [Testudines]) and the Diapsida (which includes all other reptiles). Anapsid reptiles are characterized by a primitive skull with no temporal openings.[2] Turtles are the only living representatives of this clade and belong to one order variously referred to as Testudines, Testudinata, or Chelonia. Thus, when we refer to chelonians, we refer to turtles, tortoises, and terrapins as a group. Currently, approximately 12 families, 90 genera, and 250 species are within this order.[3] Taxonomy is a dynamic science; therefore, expect changes in chelonian nomenclature in the future.

The common names of chelonians vary throughout the world and change from language to language.[4] Tortoise usually refers to terrestrial turtles, such as members of the family Testudinidae. Australians, however, refer to all but one of their turtles as tortoises, despite the fact that no true tortoises exist there and all of their chelonians are aquatic. In the United Kingdom, terrapin refers to freshwater chelonians, turtle refers to marine chelonians, and tortoise refers to terrestrial chelonians. To North Americans, turtle refers to both aquatic and terrestrial chelonians and terrapins can be freshwater or marine. One can begin to appreciate the value of scientific names that are the same from language to language. Iverson[5] attempted to standardize English common names with generic names by compiling a checklist of turtles of the world.

The two suborders of chelonians are the Cryptodira (Hidden-neck Turtles) (Figure 7-1) and the Pleurodira (Side-neck Turtles) (Figure 7-2). A number of anatomic differences exist between these groups, the most recognizable of which is the mode of head retraction. Cryptodiran turtles are able to retract the neck straight back into the shell, thereby hiding the neck. Pleurodirans are not able to retract the neck and must fold it up sideways; hence, the common name of Side-necks. Unfortunately for veterinarians, cryptodirans are the turtles most commonly seen. Veterinarians who have struggled to get a cryptodiran's head out of its shell may not realize what a cruel twist of fate evolution has produced for us.

Pleurodirans are the smaller suborder and are composed of two aquatic to semiaquatic families. The Pelomedusidae include five genera and 25 species[2] distributed in tropical Africa, South America, and some Indian Ocean islands. The Chelidae consist of 14 genera and 49 species found in Australia, New Guinea, and South America. Food preference varies from carnivory to herbivory.

The cryptodirans were apparently more successful evolutionarily because they include the majority of extant chelonians. Of the seaturtles, the Cheloniidae include five genera and six species, and the Dermochelyidae contain only a single species, the Leatherback Seaturtle *(Dermochelys coriacea)*. Seaturtles inhabit all tropical oceans, with several species ranging into temperate water (Figure 7-3). Only one species, the Green Seaturtle *(Chelonia mydas)*, is largely herbivorous and grazes on sea grasses. The remaining species of seaturtles are mainly carnivorous and feed on jellyfish, molluscs, crustaceans, fish, sponges, and other marine creatures (see Chapter 76).

Kinosternidae, the Mud and Musk Turtles, are a family of small-sized to medium-sized, semiaquatic carnivorous species found from North to South America (Figure 7-4). They feed on a variety of invertebrate and vertebrate prey and can be quite aggressive; some species even feed on other kinosternid species.

Dermatemydidae are represented by a large, totally aquatic, freshwater herbivore called the Central American River Turtle *(Dermatemys mawii)*. This turtle is from Mexico, Guatemala, and Belize and is rare in captivity. Another monotypic family, Carettochelyidae, is represented by the Pig-nosed or Fly River Turtle from New Guinea and Australia (Figure 7-5). This omnivore has a skin-covered shell and front flippers reminiscent of seaturtles.

Trionychidae, the Softshell Turtles, are found in North America, Africa, and through Asia and the Indo-Australian archipelago (Figure 7-6). They vary in size from 28 to 95 cm,[2] and they have a soft, flattened, oval-shaped carapace and a long proboscis on the snout. Both the carapace and plastron are covered by a leathery skin. These turtles are aquatic specialists; their paddle-like feet make them excellent swimmers. Several taxa, such as Chitra and Pelochelys, are known to enter saltwater environs. They are mainly carnivorous.

The Emydidae are the largest group of turtles and are composed of two subfamilies, the Batagurinae (Old World Pond Turtles) and Emydinae (New World Pond Turtles; Figure 7-7). Within these groups are 35 genera and 97 species.[2] They are found on all continents except Australia and Antarctica. Emydid turtles vary in habitat from terrestrial to semiaquatic and are often omnivorous. This family is well represented in both public and private collections. Natural history information is abundant for some species and nonexistent for others.

Chelydridae, the Snapping Turtles, are composed of two genera, the Common Snapping Turtle *(Chelydra serpentina)* and the Alligator Snapping Turtle *(Macrochelys temminckii;* Figure 7-8). The family ranges from Canada to South America. These are large, semiaquatic turtles with an aggressive disposition when disturbed. Macrochelys is restricted to

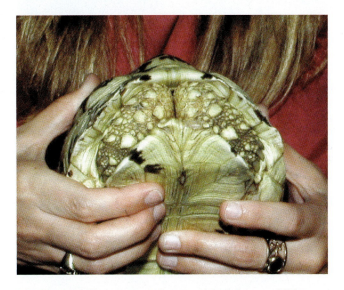

FIGURE 7-1 This Leopard Tortoise *(Geochelone pardalis)* is an example of the Hidden-neck Turtles in the suborder Cryptodira. *(Photograph courtesy D. Mader.)*

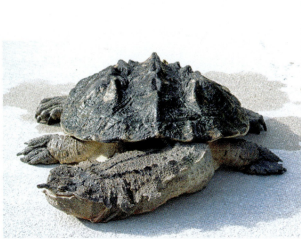

A

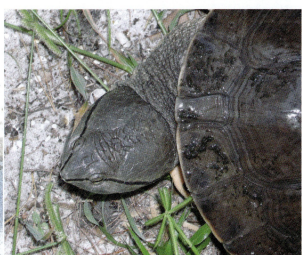

B

FIGURE 7-2 **A,** This Mata Mata *(Chelus fimbriatus)* is a bizarre-looking member of the side-neck turtles, suborder Pleurodira. **B,** Members of the genus *Phrynops*, including this Hilaire's Side-neck, are from South America. *(**A,** Photograph courtesy S. Monier; **B,** Photograph courtesy J. Wyneken.)*

the southeastern United States. This species is unique among the chelonians because of a worm-like fleshy appendage on its tongue used to lure fish within striking range. Overexploitation for food has decimated wild populations. It is protected in some portions of its range. Both species eat a wide variety of invertebrate and vertebrate species, including other reptiles.

The true tortoises, Testudinidae, consist of 12 genera with 46 living species found throughout the tropic, subtropic, and temperate zones of the world. These are all terrestrial species. Many species are successfully maintained and reproduced in captivity (Figure 7-9). Many are critically endangered or threatened.

The last family, Platysternidae, is monotypic and represented by the Big-headed Turtle (*Platysternon megacephalum*) (Figure 7-10). The Big-headed Turtle is found in small rocky mountain streams in Southeast Asia. This species is one of

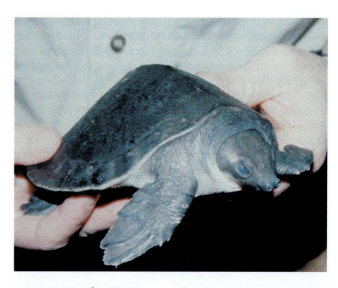

FIGURE 7-5 The Fly River or Pig-nosed Turtle (*Carettochelys insculpta*) is an excellent swimmer because of its broad flipper-like feet. (*Photograph courtesy D. Mader.*)

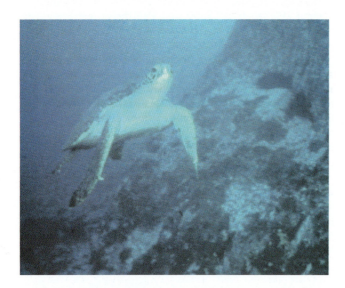

FIGURE 7-3 Free-swimming Green Seaturtle (*Chelonia mydas*). (*Photograph courtesy D. Mader.*)

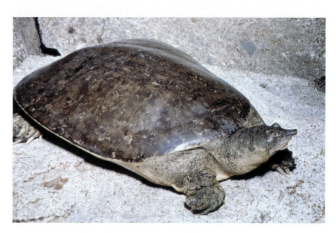

FIGURE 7-6 Spiny Softshell (*Apalone spinifera*). Softshells are a widely distributed group of North American turtles with eight subspecies. (*Photograph courtesy J. Tashjian.*)

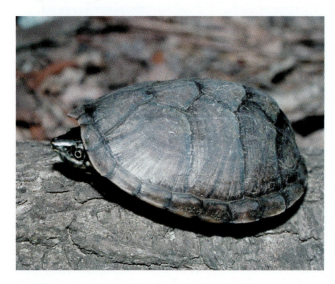

FIGURE 7-4 This Stinkpot (*Sternotherus odoratus*) shows typical morphologic appearance of Musk Turtles in the family Kinosternidae. (*Photograph courtesy S. Barten.*)

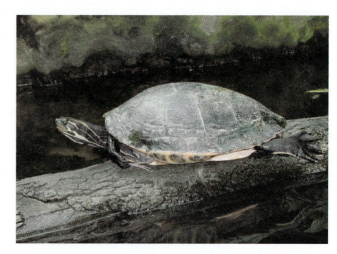

FIGURE 7-7 The Southern Painted Turtle (*Chrysemys picta dorsalis*) is representative of the largest group of turtles in the family Emydidae. (*Photograph courtesy D. Mader.*)

Turtles, Tortoises, and Terrapins

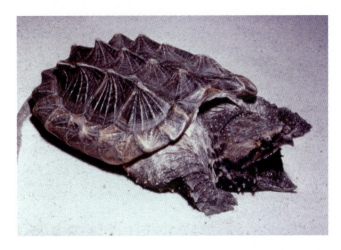

FIGURE 7-8 The Alligator Snapping Turtle (*Macrochelys temminckii*) is capable of inflicting a severe bite if handled carelessly. (*Photograph courtesy J. Tashjian.*)

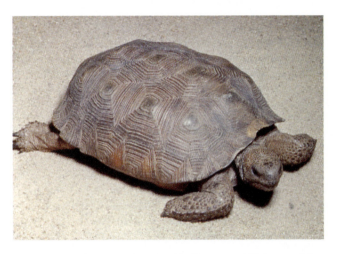

FIGURE 7-9 The Desert Tortoise (*Gopherus agassizii*) is one of four North American species of true tortoise. (*Photograph courtesy J. Tashjian.*)

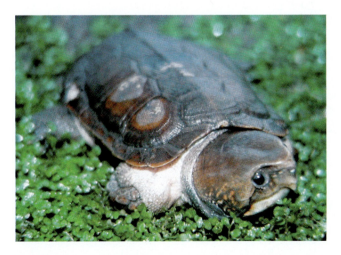

FIGURE 7-10 The Big-headed Turtle (*Platysternon megacephalum*) is an agile species known for its climbing abilities. (*Photograph courtesy D. Mader.*)

the best climbers of the order. It prefers cooler temperatures, 12°C to 17°C (54°F to 63°F), than most turtles and is carnivorous.[2]

CLINICAL ANATOMY AND PHYSIOLOGY

Chelonians are vertebrates, but because they are significantly different from other vertebrates, a brief review of their anatomy and physiology is in order. Figures 7-11 and 7-12 illustrate the gross anatomy of the tortoise.

Musculoskeletal System

Turtles are immediately recognizable because of their shell. The shell consists of an upper carapace and lower plastron connected laterally by bony bridges. The carapace consists of some 50 bones derived from ribs, vertebrae, and dermal elements of the skin. The plastron evolved from the clavicles, interclavicles, and gastralia (abdominal ribs).

The bony shell is covered by a superficial layer of keratin shields called scutes. Scutes do not precisely overlap the underlying bones of the shell. Instead they are staggered so that the seams between scutes are not directly over bone sutures. Both scutes and underlying bone are capable of regeneration. Turtles produce new scutes with each major growth period and retain or shed the scutes from the preceding growth period.[6] In some species, scute growth zones or rings can be used to estimate age. This technique requires considerable expertise and is reliable only when a distinct growth period is present, as in wild temperate turtles.[6] The difficulty of estimating age from scute growth zones is further appreciated when one considers that some species shed scutes (particularly temperate aquatic turtles) and that multiple growth zones can be produced per year. Continuous growth is common in captivity, and growth zones can smooth with age and wear. Therefore, contrary to popular belief, the age of most turtles cannot be determined accurately by counting so-called growth rings on the scutes.[7]

Scute terminology is useful to veterinarians to describe shell lesions and surgical sites and to identify species.[6] Nomenclature is easy to remember because scutes are named for their adjacent body portion (Figure 7-13).

Shell modifications are numerous. The bones in the shells of Leatherback Seaturtles, Softshells, and Fly River Turtles have been reduced and the scutes replaced with tough leathery skin; hence, the common names of the first two.[2] Most hatchling tortoises have fenestrae (openings) between carapacial bones that fuse as the tortoise ages (provided bone growth is normal). Some species, such as Pancake Tortoises, *Malacochersus tornieri*, female and immature male giant Asian River Turtles (*Batagur baska*, *Kachuga kachuga*, and *K. dhongoka*),[8] and Softshell Turtles (Trionychidae) retain these fenestrae (Figure 7-14).[2]

Many chelonians have hinges in their shell. These include plastronal hinges in Box Turtles (*Terrapene* spp., *Cuora* spp.), Spider Tortoises (*Pyxis* spp.), and Mud Turtles (*Kinosternon* spp.), a caudal carapacial hinge in Hinged-back Tortoises (*Kinixys* spp.), and slight caudal plastron mobility in female Mediterranean Tortoises (*Testudo* spp.).

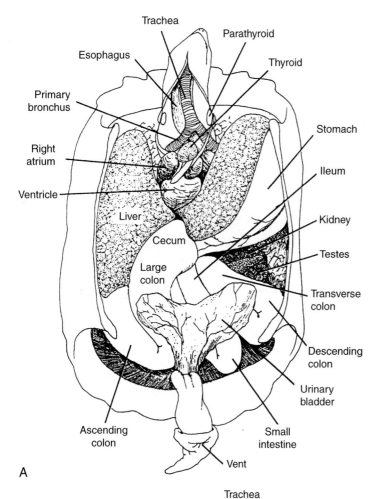
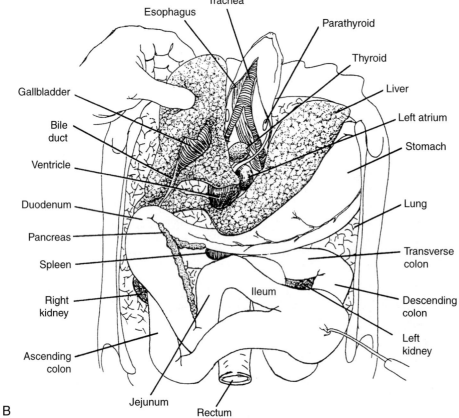

FIGURE 7-11 A, Gross anatomy of the tortoise. Ventral view. The plastron has been removed. **B,** Ventral view. The bladder has been removed to permit visualization of the intestinal tract. The right lobe of the liver is reflected to expose the gallbladder.

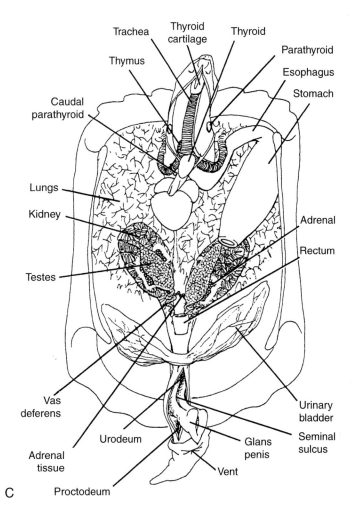

FIGURE 7-11, cont'd C, Ventral view. The liver and intestinal tract have been removed. In this male, the testicles are attached to the ventral aspect of the kidneys.

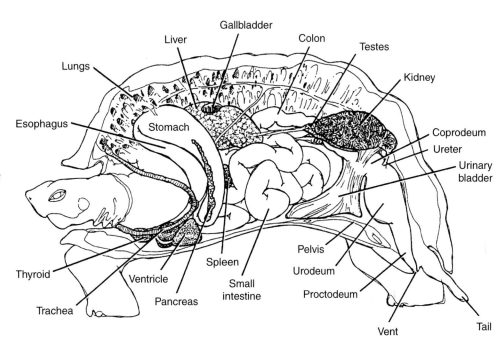

FIGURE 7-12 Midsagittal view of the gross anatomy of the tortoise.

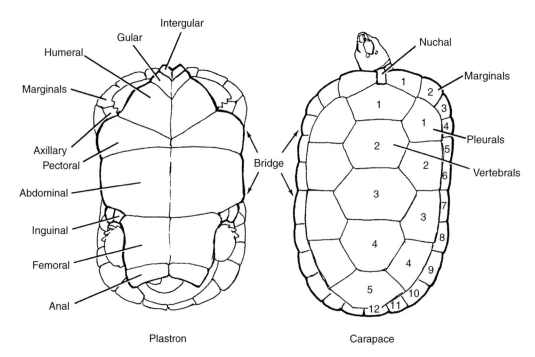

FIGURE 7-13 Nomenclature of plastron and carapace scutes.

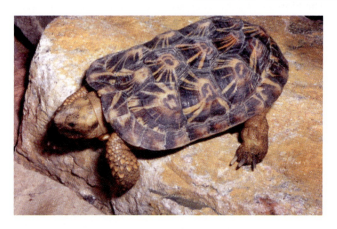

FIGURE 7-14 The Pancake Tortoise (*Malacochersus tornieri*) has a flattened shell that allows it to escape predators and heat by retreating into rock crevices. *(Photograph courtesy J. Tashjian.)*

In calculation of drug dosages, some practitioners subtract 33% to 66% of the body weight to compensate for shell weight. **Because bone is metabolically active, calculation of doses on the basis of total body weight is more logical and practical.**

Another remarkable feature of chelonians is that their pectoral and pelvic girdles are within the rib cage. The vertical orientation of the pectoral and pelvic girdles buttresses the shell and provides strong ventral anchors for the humerus and femur.

With few exceptions, the appendicular bones are typical of other vertebrates. Marine species and one freshwater species, the Fly River Turtle, have increased the digits to form elaborate forelimb flippers so that they can "fly" through water.

A large mass of muscles is associated with retraction of the head and neck.[9] Large masses also run from the pectoral and pelvic bones to the plastron and are visible radiographically. Appreciating the plastronal boundaries of these muscles is important when celiotomy is contemplated.

Integumentary System

The skin of chelonians varies from smooth and scaleless to thickly scaled. A tendency toward thicker scales is seen among the Testudinidae. Injections should be given through finely scaled areas, with avoidance of areas with larger, thicker scales that are difficult to penetrate. As with all reptiles, skin is shed periodically, although in a much more piecemeal fashion than in squamates. This is particularly noticeable in aquatic turtles.

Respiratory System

The rigid shell makes respiration much different for chelonians compared with other vertebrates with expandable chests. Chelonians breathe in and out through the nares. Mouth breathing is abnormal. The glottis is located at the base of the tongue. In cryptodiran turtles, the trachea is relatively short and quickly bifurcates into two main-stem bronchi that open directly into the surface of the paired lungs. The cranial bifurcation of the trachea enables chelonians to breath unimpeded when the neck is withdrawn.[10] The lungs attach dorsally to the ventral surface of the carapace and ventrally to a membrane that is weighted by attachments to the liver, stomach, and intestinal tract. No true diaphragm separates the lungs from other internal organs. Grossly, the lungs are large, partitioned, saccular structures reminiscent of hollow porous sponges. The lung surface is reticular and interspersed with bands of smooth muscle and connective tissue. Although lung volume is large, respiratory surface area is much less than that of mammals but adequate for animals with a lower metabolic rate.[11] Large lung volume provides an obvious advantage as a buoyant organ for aquatic turtles.

Respiration involves many structures. Antagonistic pairs of muscles essentially decrease or increase visceral volume and thus lung volume.[11] This action is supplemented with limb and head movements. Amphibians breathe in, in part, through positive pressure gular pumping. Turtles are capable of gular pumping, but this assists olfaction, not ventilation.[11]

In the submerged snapping turtle, inspiration is active and expiration passive because of hydrostatic pressure that affects visceral volume. On land, the opposite is true; inspiration is passive, and expiration is active.[11] Chelonians do not rely on negative thoracic pressure for respiration. Thus, open fractures of the shell, exposing lung, do not result in obvious respiratory distress. Many factors make removing secretions or foreign bodies from the lungs difficult for chelonians. These include termination of the mucociliary elevator outside the glottis, poor drainage through the bronchi, compartmentalization of the lungs, large potential space within the lungs, and lack of a complete muscular diaphragm to initiate coughing.[12] Consequently, pneumonia is often disastrous in chelonians. During brumation (hibernation), cloacal bursae are used for underwater respiration in pond, snapping, and side-necked turtles.[13] One study found that a quiet submerged Nile Softshell (*Trionyx triunguis*) received 30% of its oxygen through vascularized papillae in the pharnyx and the remainder through the skin.[14]

Many Australian species are capable of oxygen absorption through cloacal bursae, which allows for periods of longer submersion, particularly in the winter. The champion of cloacal respiration is the Fitzroy River Turtle, *Rheodytes leukops*, which can pump water in and out of its cloaca 15 to 60 times per minute.[15] Underwater respiration may sustain aquatic turtles during periods of low activity, but when they are active, they still need to surface for air.[7] Turtles are capable of long periods of apnea that makes induction of gas anesthesia difficult without injectable preanesthetics or intubation coupled with positive pressure ventilation.

Gastrointestinal System

Chelonians have large, fleshy tongues that are not able to distend from the mouth as in squamates. As a general rule, most terrestrial species are herbivores, whereas aquatic species are carnivorous or omnivorous; however, numerous exceptions exist.[7]

Chelonians lack teeth and depend on the scissor-like actions of their horny beak, or rhamphotheca, for biting off pieces of food that are swallowed whole. In captivity, periodic rhamphothecal trimming may be needed. Underlying calcium deficiency may produce deformity of the rhamphotheca. Salivary glands produce mucus to enable swallowing of bite-sized pieces,[16] but no digestive enzymes are used. Aquatic turtles eat under water. The esophagus courses along the neck. Passing a stomach tube with the neck extended rather than retracted is easier except in very large tortoises. However, the mouth is much easier to open with the head retracted than if extended. Thus, passing a rigid or flexible stomach tube without extending the head and neck is possible (Figure 7-15).

The stomach lies along the ventral left side and has gastroesophageal and pyloric valves. The small intestine is relatively short (compared with mammals) and mildly convoluted and absorbs nutrients and water.[13] The stomach, small intestine, pancreas, liver, and gallbladder produce digestive enzymes. The pancreas empties into the duodenum via a short duct and has exocrine and endocrine functions similar to other vertebrates. The pancreas is pale orange-pink in color and may be in direct contact with the spleen or separate in the mesentery along the duodenum.

The liver is a large, ventral, saddle-shaped organ that spreads from side to side under the lungs. It has two major lobes, envelops the gallbladder, and has indentations for the heart and stomach. The liver is dark red; some species may be normally pigmented with melanin.[10] Pale yellow to tan color is abnormal. The small intestine joins the large intestine at the ileocolic valve. The cecum is not well developed. The large intestine is the primary site of microbial fermentation in herbivorous tortoises. The colon terminates in the complex cloaca.

Gastrointestinal (GI) transit time is affected by many factors including temperature, feeding frequency, and water or fiber content of food. Captive diets generally move faster through the GI tract than natural diets, especially in tortoises. For example, GI transit times for Spur-thighed Tortoises (*Testudo graeca*) kept at 28°C varied from 3 to 8 days when fed *ad libitum* lettuce but increased to 16 to 28 days when fed thistles, grasses, and dog food.[17] Metoclopramide, cisapride, and erythromycin did not significantly reduce GI transit time compared with water in Desert Tortoises (*Gopherus agassizii*).[18]

Genitourinary Systems

The kidneys of chelonians are located on the ventral caudal carapace and posterior to the acetabulum, except in marine turtles in which they are usually anterior to the acetabulum.[10] The kidneys are metanephric.

Reptiles cannot concentrate urine, presumably because of the absence of the loop of Henle.[13] Soluble urinary nitrogenous

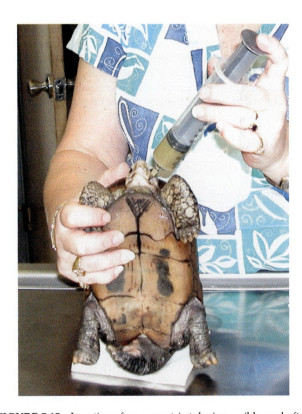

FIGURE 7-15 Insertion of an orogastric tube is possible, and often easier and less stressful, with the animal's head and neck withdrawn into the shell rather than with an extended neck of an unwilling patient. (*Photograph courtesy D. Mader.*)

wastes, such as ammonia and urea, require relatively large amounts of water for excretion. This is only practical for aquatic and semiaquatic chelonians. Terrestrial chelonians cannot afford to produce as much soluble nitrogenous wastes. To conserve water, they produce more insoluble urinary wastes, such as uric acid and urate salts, that can be passed from the body in a semisolid state, requiring much less water.[13] These differences make detection of kidney disease on the basis of mammalian markers of blood urea nitrogen and creatinine difficult. Serum uric acid levels are sometimes, but not consistently, increased with kidney disease.

Chelonians are different from other reptiles in that the urogenital ducts empty into the neck of the bladder instead of into the wall of the urodeum. The bladder is bilobed with a thin, membranous, distensible wall.[10] Terrestrial chelonians often use the urinary bladder for water storage. The cloaca, colon, and urinary bladder can reabsorb urinary water,[13] which can have interesting effects on pharmacokinetics of drugs excreted through the urinary system.

The paired gonads are located anterior to the kidney. Fertilization is internal in chelonians. The upper part of the oviduct secretes albumin for the passing ovum, and the lower portion produces the shell. Male chelonians possess a single, large, dark-colored, smooth, expansible penis. When not erect, it lies in the ventromedial floor of the proctodeum and is not used for urine transport. When engorged, the muscular penis extends from the cloaca with a seminal groove for transport of sperm (Figure 7-16). No inversion of the penis occurs as it does in squamates.[13]

Sexual Dimorphism

Sexual dimorphism is known to occur in many chelonians. Where present, differences can be seen in coloration, tail or claw length, size, and shell shape.

Sexual dichromatism is especially common among the Emydid and Geomydid turtles. Males and females may differ in coloration of the head, iris, chin, or markings on the head. A well-known example in the Eastern Box Turtle *(Terrapene carolina carolina)* is the bright-red iris of males compared with the yellow to reddish brown iris of females (Figure 7-17). Some of these differences are observable only in males during the breeding season. For example, during breeding season, the head of the male Painted Terrapin, *Callugar borneoensis*, changes from charcoal gray to white with a vivid red stripe between the eyes.[2]

Many male aquatic turtles have elongated foreclaws that they use to court females. Claw length is dimorphic in *Trachemys, Pseudemys, Chrysemys,* and *Graptemys*.[2] Male Box Turtles have a thickened, curved inner rear claw to assist in mating. Sexually mature female Leopard Tortoises, *Geochelone pardalis*, have elongated rear claws, perhaps as an aid to nest digging.

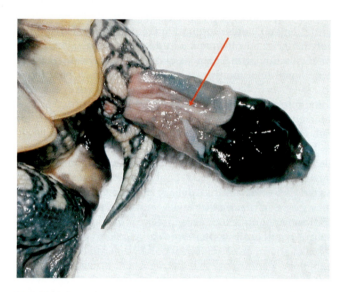

FIGURE 7-16 The muscular penis extends from the cranial base of the cloaca. The seminal groove *(red arrow)* transports sperm during copulation. *(Photograph courtesy S. Barten.)*

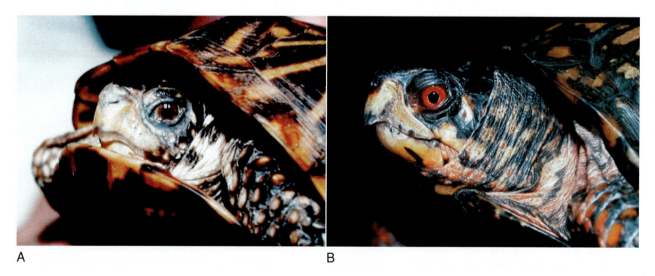

FIGURE 7-17 A, Note the brown iris color of the female Eastern Box Turtle *(Terrapene carolina carolina)*. **B,** The male Eastern Box Turtle *(Terrapene carolina carolina)* has a bright-red iris. *(A, Photograph courtesy D. Mader; B, Photograph courtesy S. Barten.)*

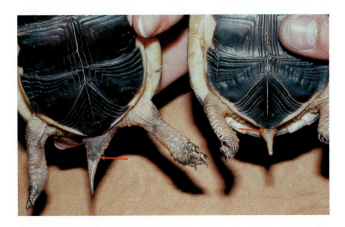

FIGURE 7-18 One of the most consistent, distinguishing characteristics between male and female turtles and tortoises is the length of the tail. In the male, not only is the tail longer and broader but the cloacal opening is beyond the margin of the carapace; in the female, the cloacal opening is between the margins of the plastron and carapace (*see red arrows*). (*Photograph courtesy D. Mader.*)

Perhaps the most obvious form of sexual dimorphism is tail length and shell shape (Figure 7-18). In many species, to facilitate intromission, mature males have longer, thicker tails, a more distal vent, a concave plastron, and, if present, an anal notch on the plastron that is narrower and deeper than that of the female. In contrast, females have shorter tails that abruptly taper posterior to the vent. The female vent tends to be proximal to the carapace margin. The plastron in females is usually flat, and the anal notch wider and shallower, perhaps as an aid to oviposition. With the onset of sexual maturity, these differences may allow for easy sex determination. Often, however, these differences are subtle and sex determination is more difficult. By far the most reliable difference is that the cloacal opening in males lies beyond the carapace. Males sometimes evert their penis during defecation or caudal manipulation. Little difference is seen in tail length between the sexes in the Chaco Tortoise, *Geochelone chilensis*.[8]

A difference in size between the sexes is common among cryptodiran turtles. In 70% of 50 taxa examined by Fitch,[19] females were larger, especially in highly aquatic turtles. Males were larger in 22% of the taxa, and in the remaining 8%, the sexes were equal in size. In taxa with larger males, the size difference was less pronounced and generally involved terrestrial forms. Males are larger than females in the following taxa: Galapagos Tortoise, *Geochelone nigra*; Bowsprit Tortoise, *Chersina angulata*; Desert Tortoise; Box Turtle, *Terrapene carolina*; Bog Turtle, *Clemmys muhlenbergii*; Blanding's Turtle, *Emydoidea blandingii*; Snapping Turtle; and Yellow Mud Turtle, *Kinostemon flavescens*.

Circulatory System

Chelonians have typical reptilian three-chambered hearts (see Chapter 10).

Renal portal systems (RPS) exist in chelonians, as in other reptiles. The significance of this is debatable; however, drugs may be given in the front half of the body to avoid the potential for renal toxicity or clearance if there are any questions (see Chapter 11 for a detailed discussion of the RPS).

CAPTIVE CARE

General Considerations

Lighting

Sunlight is by far the best source of ultraviolet (UV) light and should be provided for chelonians whenever practical. Unfortunately, indoors, UV light in the 290 to 320 nm wavelength is almost completely filtered by normal glass or plastics. This can be avoided through open windows or with UV transmissible windows or skylights (Acrylite OP-4 Acrylic Sheet, CYRO Industries, Rockaway, NJ; Starphire, PPG Industries Inc, Pittsburgh, Pa; or Polycast Solacyrl SUVT, Spartech Polycast, Stanford, Conn). UV transmissible glass or plastics allow for 60% to 75% UV transmission and are expensive. Another option for animals housed indoors long term is special broad-spectrum lights with some UV output between 290 and 320 nm (see Chapter 84). UV meters (UVX Radiometer, UVP Inc., Upland, Calif) can be used to measure UV output.

Behavioral Thermoregulation

Chelonians are heliotherms, which means they seek sunlight for heat. In captivity, a temperature gradient within the preferred optimal temperature zone (POTZ) is best so that the chelonian can regulate its own body temperature.

For tortoises, the POTZ is 26°C to 38°C (79°F to 100°F) and 25°C to 35°C (77°F to 95°F) for aquatic and semiaquatic turtles. Basking areas can be created with various incandescent light bulbs with reflector hoods shining into the cage. In addition, one can place a heating pad underneath the cage in the basking area. Incandescent 50-watt to 100-watt light bulbs, 250-watt infrared bulbs, or porcelain heating elements work well. Chelonians should not be within the 18-inch focal heating range of infrared fixtures or severe burns occur.

Water for aquatic turtles can be heated with submersible aquarium heaters. Provide barriers around submersible heaters to prevent contact burns on the turtle. In larger setups, an in-line heater can be plumbed to the filtration system. Room temperature can be thermostatically controlled with heating or cooling systems. Ambient temperatures should be regularly monitored with minimum-maximum thermometers. Indoor-outdoor varieties allow ambient and basking temperature monitoring. Noncontact temperature measurement guns (Raytek Ranger ST, Total Temperature Instrumentation Inc, Williston, Vt) are also useful to spot check temperatures throughout enclosures.

Predators

Predators, especially dogs, are fond of chewing on chelonians' shells and appendages and can wreak havoc in a short time (Figure 7-19). Small chelonians can be devoured without a trace. Raccoons and opossums enter yards at night to prey on turtles. Rats can chew on the limbs and heads of turtles even indoors. Other mammals and birds, and even crocodilians, are also potential predators. Smaller terrestrial and aquatic chelonians should always have screened outdoor cages.[20] In the southern United States, fire ants, *Solenopsis*, and in southern California, Argentine ants, *Linepithema*, can attack and kill small tortoises. Certain species, such as Snapping Turtles, large Softshells, and Big-headed Turtles, may be quite aggressive to other turtles, including conspecifics. Some male tortoises, such as Bowsprits, Desert, and Spurred Tortoises can also be aggressive to other males.

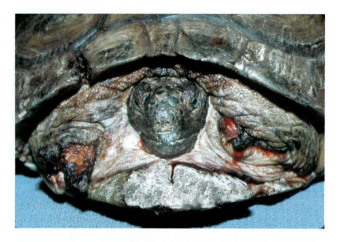

FIGURE 7-19 Severe dog-gnawing trauma is common in turtles. *(Photograph courtesy D. Mader.)*

Brumation (Hibernation)

Brumation (hibernation) is recommended for temperate terrestrial species, such as northerly distributed Box Turtles (*Terrapene carolina carolina, Terrapene c. triunguis, Terrapene ornata ornata*), several tortoise species (*Testudo marginata, T. hermanni*, most *T. graeca, T. horsfieldi, Gopherus agassizii, G. polyphemus*, and *G. berlandieri*), and many aquatic turtles. *Terrapene bauri* and *Terrapene c. major* do not brumate (hibernate). Keep in mind that within a given species animals from warmer microclimates may not brumate (hibernate) at all. Some temperate species may skip brumation (hibernation) in captivity, especially if the conditions stay warm and the day length remains artificially long. Others, particularly Box Turtles, stop eating in the early fall regardless of artificial conditions. Brumation (hibernation) is recommended for healthy specimens in good body weight.

To survive brumation (hibernation), the turtle must be in good body weight and health. A physical examination several weeks before brumation (hibernation) is advisable. Sick, convalescing, or underweight turtles should not brumate (hibernate). Weight gain over the summer is a prerequisite for brumation (hibernation). Prebrumation (prehibernation) weight and fecal checks are a good idea. Jackson's ratio[21] compares body weight with carapace length and is a simple and accurate method of determination of normal or healthy body weight for *Testudo graeca* and *T. hermanni*. Sick tortoises are often below this weight, and obese tortoises are above this weight. Mader and Stroutenburgh[22] charted maximum carapace length, width, and height against weight (compared with volume), which is an excellent means of assessing the health status of California Desert Tortoises (see discussion in nutrition, Chapter 18) (Figure 7-20). More charts need to be produced for other species of chelonians. Keep in mind that such charts are not foolproof because some diseases can increase the weight of a patient.

Frye[10] recommends preconditioning tortoises with carbohydrate-rich foods, such as steamed winter squashes, sprouts, alfalfa pellets, and mixed fruits (figs, melons, apples, etc.), 6 weeks before the onset of brumation (hibernation). Carrots and winter squashes are important to provide an adequate supply of vitamin A during brumation (hibernation).

Most chelonians that brumate (hibernate) noticeably decrease their food intake as brumation (hibernation) approaches. Water should be constantly available before brumation (hibernation); soaking encourages drinking. In early October, or as soon as the turtle's appetite noticeably decreases in early fall, withhold food (but not water) for 1 to 2 weeks for smaller turtles and up to 3 weeks for larger tortoises but keep the turtle between 21°C to 27°C (70°F to 80°F). This gives the turtle time to clear its GI tract of potentially fermentable ingesta. After this, remove external heat sources and allow the turtle to acclimate to room temperature of 16°C to 21°C (60°F to 70°F). After a week at room temperature, the turtle should be ready to enter the hibernaculum.

Chelonians can brumate (hibernate) indoors or outdoors. Outdoor brumation (hibernation) is potentially more dangerous because one has less control over environmental conditions. For indoor brumation (hibernation), select an area that can be kept between 2°C and 10°C (35°F and 50°F)[23] for the winter, such as a basement, garage, back porch, crawl space, wine cellar, or north-facing or east-facing closet, window, or wall. Use a minimum-maximum thermometer to check temperatures several weeks before brumation (hibernation). Persistent temperatures above 16°C (60°F) are not cool enough for brumation (hibernation), and the turtle's metabolism will be high enough that it will slowly starve. Prolonged temperatures below 2°C (35°F) are too cold; temperatures below freezing should be avoided. The ideal target temperature is 5°C (41°F).[23]

An indoor hibernaculum can be set up with a large box, crate, cooler, or aquarium with a foot of slightly humid peat-based potting soil and a 3-inch to 6-inch layer of shredded newspaper, shredded recycled cardboard, or dried leaves on top. Make sure the hibernaculum is not resting directly on cold cement. The turtle should burrow into the soil and remain inactive. The soil should be humid enough that the turtle does not dehydrate but is not wet.

If low humidity is a problem indoors, consider monitoring body weight and periodic soaking to prevent dehydration. Chelonians can be awakened every 2 to 4 weeks and allowed to drink or soak in shallow 24°C (75°F) water for 2 hours.[24] During soaking, the turtle's eyes should reopen. If the turtle appears healthy, let it dry off and then return it to the hibernaculum. If any signs of illness are present, warm the turtle up to 27°C (80°F) and begin antibiotic treatment immediately. Contrary to popular belief, disturbing turtles during brumation (hibernation) is not harmful.[23]

Species that naturally brumate (hibernate) in a given geographic area can brumate (hibernate) outdoors. Outdoor brumation (hibernation) is not advisable in areas with severe winters. For Box Turtles select an area sheltered from the wind with 2 to 3 feet of loosened soil; loose soil near a foundation works well. Spread a foot or two of loose leaves or hay over the soil. Compost piles are not suitable for brumation (hibernation). Be sure the area drains well and is not prone to flooding.

Tortoises can brumate (hibernate) outdoors in milder climates in artificial burrows or doghouses. A burrow can be constructed with partially or fully buried concrete blocks along the sides and ¾-inch plywood on the top. Cover a southern exposure entrance with a heavy tarp or opaque plastic and place hay or straw inside. A simpler alternative is a well-insulated dog house filled with a thick layer of leaves or soil. Place a tarp or plastic over the entrance. Outdoor hibernacula should be protected against freezing and flooding. Low humidity is generally not a problem outdoors, but turtles should still be encouraged to drink if active on warmer days.

Typically, chelonians brumate (hibernate) outdoors for 5 to 6 months from mid-October until early April. Indoor brumation (hibernation) can be shorter, from early November to late

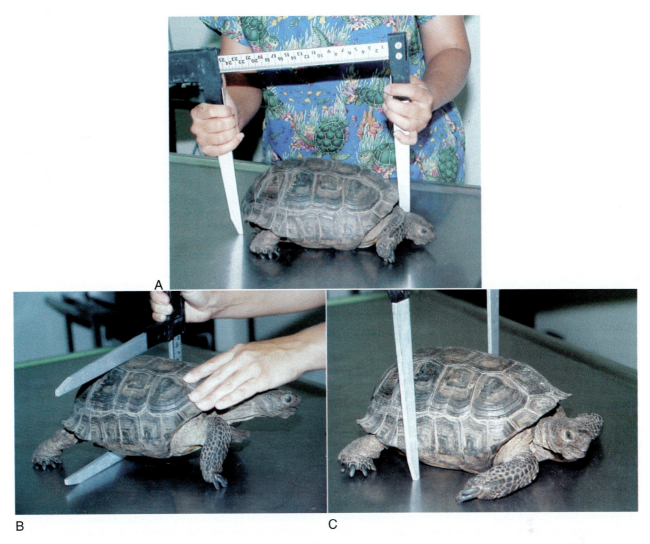

FIGURE 7-20 **A, B,** and **C,** Measurements of length, height, and width in the California Desert Tortoise (*Gopherus agassizii*) have proven to be an excellent means of assessing the animal's overall health status. (See Chapter 18 for a discussion on evaluating body condition.) *(Photograph courtesy D. Mader.)*

February or early March. Highfield[23] recommends 8 to 10 weeks for small specimens and no longer than 12 to 14 weeks for large specimens. Once the turtle becomes active in the spring, it should be soaked in lukewarm water and start eating well within a week or two. Healthy tortoises should lose less than 6% to 7% of their body weight over the winter brumation (hibernation).[24] A loss of greater than 7% body weight is indicative of disease.[25]

Brumation (hibernation) of juveniles is controversial.[23] Some experts believe that turtles less than 3 to 4 years of age should not brumate (hibernate). Much depends on the experience of the keeper and the stability of hibernaculum temperatures. When in doubt, skipping brumation (hibernation) for the first few years does no harm.

Box Turtles

Box Turtles[26-28] are one of the most common reptile pets in the United States (Figure 7-21). With proper care, they are long-lived, with life spans of 30 to 40 years and perhaps much longer. Unfortunately, they are among the most neglected reptiles in captivity because most people just do not appreciate how to care for them properly.

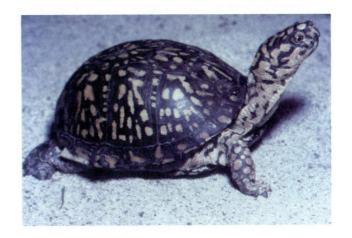

FIGURE 7-21 Box Turtles, such as this Eastern Box Turtle (*Terrapene carolina*), are one of the most common reptilian pets in the United States. *(Photograph courtesy J. Tashjian.)*

Several subspecies of Box Turtles are common in the pet trade, including the Eastern Box Turtle, *Terrapene carolina carolina*; Gulf Coast Box Turtle, *Terrapene c. major*; Three-toed Box Turtle, *Terrapene c. triungius*; the Ornate Box Turtle, *Terrapene ornata ornata*; and the Desert Box Turtle, *Terrapene o. luteola*.

Reproduction

Most species lay two to eight (normally four to six) eggs from May through July. Multiple clutches are possible. Females can store sperm and lay fertile eggs for up to 4 years after fertilization. Eggs hatch in 2 to 3 months if fertile.

Outdoor Housing

During the late spring, summer, and early fall months, turtles do best outdoors in a back yard or fenced enclosure. Provide shade with dense shrubbery, dry leaves, or a wooden shelter so the turtles can escape the hot sun when needed. Box Turtles are good at digging under fences and escaping. Often this explains the observation of so many proud novice Box Turtle owners that "it just wandered into our yard." The yard perimeter should be carefully sealed with bricks, rocks, boards, or buried fencing and periodically patrolled for developing breaks. Box Turtles can also climb over fencing less than 12 inches high.[29] Bring turtles indoors whenever the temperature drops into the low 60°F range (15°C to 18°C) unless brumation (hibernation) is anticipated.

Indoor Housing

Twenty-gallon aquaria are the minimum size for Box Turtles. Consider larger aquaria or make larger cages out of plywood (see tortoise care) or use concrete mixing containers available in most hardware stores. Larger enclosures are always better. The bottom of the cage should be filled with humid substrates such as medium-to-large wood chips mixed with peat moss, cypress mulch, or a sand and soil mixture. Drier substrates promote skin cracking and poor health. Avoid sand, gravel, clay cat litter, and crushed corn cob or walnut shells because they can cause GI impaction. Substrates need to be completely changed every few months, and feces need to be scooped out weekly. A hide box that the turtle can get under and out of sight is important. Many turtles prefer to sleep in them. Loose-leaf litter can be spread in the cage.

Temperature

The indoor cage should get no colder than 15°C (60°F) at night and gradually warm to 21°C to 27°C (70°F to 80°F) during the day. A 75-watt to 100-watt incandescent bulb with a reflector can provide a warm basking area at one end of the cage between 27°C to 32°C (80°F to 90°F). Lights should be turned off during the night, so supplemental heat from heat tape or heating pads also should be provided under one half of the cage if temperatures drop below 15°C (60°F). Hot rocks do not work well for turtles because the rigid shell inhibits conductive heat transfer.

Water

An easy-to-clean shallow water dish, big enough for the turtle to get into, should always be available (Figure 7-22). Water depth should be no deeper than the turtle's chin when its head is partially retracted. Turtles prefer to defecate in their water bowl, so it should be cleaned several times per week. Juvenile Box Turtles are often much more aquatic than adults.

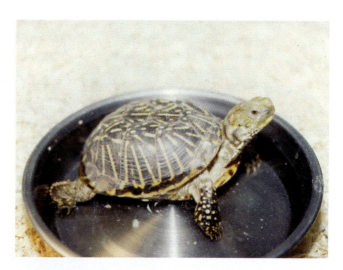

FIGURE 7-22 Chelonians should have access to water at all times.

Box Turtles drown in deep water, such as in a swimming pool. Highfield[23] notes that *Terrapene c. bauri* and *Terrapene c. triunguis* are better swimmers than other Box Turtles and even forage underwater.

Feeding

Box Turtles are much more carnivorous than most people realize. Adult Eastern Box Turtles are opportunistic omnivores that consume beetles, grasshoppers, millipedes, centipedes, land snails, slugs, earthworms, spiders, sowbugs or pillbugs, crayfish, carrion, fish, frogs, tadpoles, toads, small mammals, birds, salamanders, lizards, snakes, smaller turtles, and plant material such as mushrooms, strawberries, raspberries, blackberries, blueberries, mulberries, tomatoes, and grasses. Youngsters are primarily carnivorous. Ornate Box Turtles are mainly insectivorous and consume dung beetles, caterpillars, cicadas, and grasshoppers, but they also eat mulberries, leaves, tender shoots, and carrion. Unlike other Box Turtles, Ornates frequently use burrows and prefer more arid habitat such as open prairie.

In captivity chronic nutritional problems are typical for most Box Turtles yet difficult to appreciate. Nutritional diseases can be avoided with a well-balanced diet that is continually varied (see Table 7-1 and carnivore-omnivore diet in Tables 7-2 and 7-3). Interpret these guidelines liberally. Different species have different dietary preferences. For instance, some species, such as Ornate and Gulf Coast Box Turtles, are not fond of vegetables. Wash fruits and vegetables, and chop all items into bite-sized pieces.

Box Turtles have a continuous need for vitamin A–rich foods. Liver (in whole mice or fish) is an excellent source of vitamin A, as are rich yellow or dark orange–colored vegetables (carrots, sweet potatoes, butternut and winter squashes) and dark leafy greens (dandelion greens and flowers, spinach, turnip and mustard greens). Steaming (not boiling) hard squashes makes them much more palatable and easier to chop.

Acclimatization

Most pet Box Turtles are wild-caught adults and may adapt poorly to captivity, although some do well from the start. Fall and winter are particularly difficult times to establish brumating (hibernating) species because they are not

Table 7-1	Box Turtle Diet[26-28,33,36,38,39]

Items listed in italics often entice anorexic animals to eat. Adults should be fed three or more times per week in the morning, and juveniles fed daily. Juveniles tend to be much more carnivorous than adults.[8] For every feeding, lightly dust food with calcium lactate, carbonate, citrate, or gluconate. Every 2 to 4 weeks, lightly dust food with multivitamins (if vitamin-fortified foods are not available). Limit vitamin D–fortified foods to less than 5% of the total diet.

50% Animal or High-Protein Foods. *Earthworms, crickets, grasshoppers, slugs, snails, pill bugs, cicadas, whole skinned chopped mice, baby mice (pinkies),* goldfish, waxworms, mealworms, silk moth larvae, other insects, low fat, adult, soaked, dry dog chow, trout, or box turtle chow.

50% Plants (25% Fruits and 75% Vegetables)

25% Fruits. Tomatoes, strawberries, raspberries, blackberries, mulberries, blueberries, apples, grapes, cherries, oranges, peaches, pears, plums, nectarines, figs, *melons* (remove seeds), bananas, mangos, and grapefruit.

75% Vegetables. Dark leafy greens (mustard, collard, radish, beet and turnip greens or tops, kale, cabbage, *dandelion leaves, stems or flowers,* spinach, bok-choy, pak-choi, broccoli rape), red leaf or romaine lettuce (be careful not to overfeed lettuces), Swiss chard, steamed chopped squashes, sweet potatoes, shredded (not chopped) carrots, thawed frozen mixed vegetables (peas, corn, carrots, green beans, lima beans); alfalfa, radish, clover, or bean sprouts; soaked alfalfa pellets, *mushrooms,* bell peppers, broccoli, green beans, peas in the pod, okra, and prickly pear (*Opuntia* spp.) cactus pads (shave off spines).

Table 7-2	Herbivore and Carnivore-Omnivore Gel Diets Used for Chelonians at the Zoological Society of San Diego

Dr Mark Edwards formulated these diets from information provided by the Tennessee Aquarium.

Components:

Turtle Brittle, Nasco International, Inc, 901 Janesville Avenue, PO Box 902, Fort Atkinson, WI 53538; (920) 568-5565.
Leafeater Diet, Marion Zoological, Inc, 13803 Industrial Park Boulevard, Plymouth, MN 55441.
Gelatin (dry, unsweetened).
Carrots, raw.
Greens, raw (kale, collard, dandelion, mustard).

Preparation (1 kg gel):

Carnivore-Omnivore Gel

200 g Nasco turtle brittle (ground)
45 g Knox gelatin
90 g chopped leafy greens
90 g chopped/grated carrot
575 g hot water

Herbivore Gel

65 g Nasco turtle brittle (ground)
110 g Leafeater (ground)
45 g Knox gelatin
90 g chopped leafy greens
90 g chopped/grated carrot
600 g hot water

1. Add prepared greens and carrots to high-power blender, followed by all dry ingredients.
2. Add hot water to blender; immediately homogenize all ingredients for 3 minutes. Mixture should be a thick liquid.
3. Pour into a shallow pan and allow gel to set up in refrigerator. Cut gel with a knife or food processor to obtain appropriately sized pieces. Feed free choice as the primary diet; consumption varies by species. Remove uneaten gel on a daily basis.
4. Additional items can be added to gels: mealworms, extra chopped fruits or vegetables, crushed limestone, or oyster shell for mollusc eaters. Gels can also be used as a vehicle for medications.

Keep gels refrigerated and use within 7 days. Gels can be frozen and stored in an airtight container for up to 3 months.

---

normally eating. If healthy, brumation (hibernation) is one option; artificially increasing the photoperiod is another. If healthy, new arrivals should be set up in as large a cage as possible or placed outdoors if the weather is favorable. Box Turtles are naturally secretive animals, and frequent handling or watching deters them from settling into captivity. For finicky eaters, try some of their favorite foods (listed in italics) and keep in mind that Box Turtles are particularly attracted to red, yellow, and orange-colored foods. Live moving food often stimulates feeding; pinkies and earthworms often entice the most recalcitrant specimens to feed. Box Turtles are most active in early morning, or late afternoon, when it is not too hot, so these are good times to try and feed them. Rainstorms often increase activity; thus, spraying the cage can stimulate appetite. Mix favored food items into salads heavily at first then gradually decrease over a period of weeks. Bad dietary habits can be difficult to overcome and often require months to correct. Continue to offer foods even if they are not eaten initially; as the turtle adjusts to a varied salad, it gradually increases dietary diversity.

Tortoises

The true tortoises[20,27,28] are all members of the family Testudinidae. Testudinidae encompass 12 genera with 46 living species found throughout much of the tropic, subtropic, and temperate world. Many of these species are commonly found in the pet trade.

The genus *Gopherus* includes four North American tortoises: Desert Tortoise, *G. agassizii*; Texas Tortoise, *G. berlandieri*; Bolson Tortoise, *G. flavomarginatus*; and Gopher Tortoise, *G. polyphemus*. None are sold in the pet trade, but they are still common pets (except Bolsons). Chronic upper respiratory tract disease is a common problem in Desert and Gopher Tortoises. One must be aware of introducing this to other turtles (see Chapter 73).

The genus *Testudo* consists of five species native to Mediterranean Europe, Africa, and parts of the Middle East. These include Hermann's Tortoise, *T. hermanni*; Marginated Tortoise, *T. marginata*; Russian, Afghan, or Steppe Tortoise, *T. horsfieldi*; Greek Tortoise, *T. graeca*; and Egyptian Tortoise, *T. kleinmanni*. All Testudo tortoises (especially Russians) are potential carriers of herpesvirus, so quarantine these carefully before introducing them to other chelonians (see Chapter 57).

Most species of the genera *Gopherus* and *Testudo* are temperate tortoises that brumate (hibernate). In contrast, the genus *Geochelone* is pantropic and has the largest number of species, and the largest tortoises, but they do not brumate (hibernate). No adults are less than 25 cm in carapace length.[2]

Table 7-3 Selected Nutrient Analysis (Dry Matter Basis, Except Moisture)

Nutrient	Herbivore Gel	Carnivore-Omnivore Gel
Moisture (%)	77.5	75.4
Crude protein (%)	43.7	53.7
Crude fat (%)	4.5	5.2
Ash (%)	7.2	10.0
Crude fiber (%)	5.6	2.6
Calcium (%)	1.1	1.7
Phosphorus (%)	0.8	1.3
Sodium (%)	0.5	1.0
Magnesium (%)	0.1	0.2
Iron (ppm)	192.9	251.6
Zinc (ppm)	85.6	83.5
Manganese (ppm)	37.0	10.7
Thiamin (ppm)	4.4	4.0
Riboflavin (ppm)	6.1	8.0
Vitamin B_{12} (ppb)	23.7	32.5
Niacin (ppm)	47	56
Vitamin A (IU/kg)	7941	11356
Vitamin D (IU/kg)	2317	4059
Vitamin E (IU/kg)	155.6	76.0

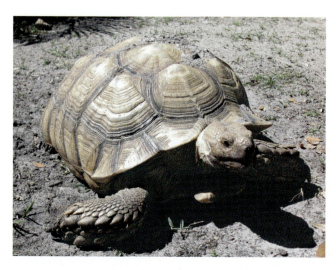

FIGURE 7-24 African Spurred Tortoises (*Geochelone sulcatta*) are rapidly becoming one of the most popular tortoise pets. They are fast growing and reproduce well in captivity. (*Photograph courtesy D. Mader.*)

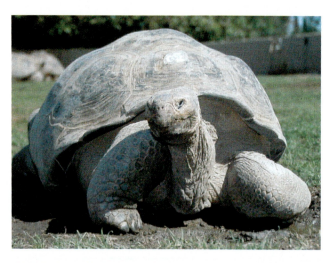

FIGURE 7-23 The Galapagos Tortoise (*Geochelone nigra*) is a common display animal in zoos and is also occasionally seen in private collections. (*Photograph courtesy D. Mader.*)

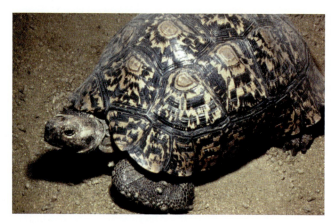

FIGURE 7-25 Leopard Tortoises (*Geochelone pardalis*) are hardy, prolific pets. (*Photograph courtesy J. Tashjian.*)

South American *Geochelone* include the Red-footed Tortoise, *G. carbonaria*; the larger Yellow-footed or Forest Tortoise, *G. denticulata*; and the Chaco or Argentine Tortoise, *G. chilensis*.

The Galapagos Islands are home to a single giant species, the Galapagos Tortoise with 12 subspecies. This is the largest living species of tortoise; large specimens can weigh up to 263 kg.[30] Captive-born specimens are now available in the reptile trade, although they are listed in Appendix 1 of the CITES and are subject to permit requirements (Figure 7-23).

Another island species, the Aldabran Giant Tortoise, *G. gigantea*, has been split into three species of *Dipsochelys*. *Dipsochelys* is the second largest species of tortoise and weighs up to 120 kg. They live on the Aldabra Atoll and have been introduced on other islands in the Indian Ocean. Aldabrans can be easily distinguished from Galapagos tortoises by the more wedge-shaped head, a thicker more domed carapace, and the presence of a single nuchal scute.

African *Geochelone* include two other large species, the Spurred Tortoise, *G. sulcata*, and the Leopard Tortoise, *G. pardalis* (Figures 7-24 and 7-25). Spurred Tortoises are the largest mainland tortoises and can grow to 84 kg.[7] Given their potential size and proclivity for burrowing, they are not a good choice for suburban living. Spurred Tortoises are generally erroneously referred to as Spur-thighed Tortoises, which refers to *Testudo graeca iberia*.

Leopard tortoises are a handsomely marked species with a high-domed shell; some specimens exceed 40 kg in weight.[4] Both Spurred and Leopards are fairly hardy and among the most prolific of tortoises in captivity. In 2000, the United States Department of Agriculture banned importation of Spurred, Leopard, and Hingeback Tortoises into the United States because they can carry ticks capable of introducing heartwater disease and cowdriosis to ruminants.

Other *Geochelone* include the Indian Star Tortoise, *G. elegans* (Figure 7-26), and a closely related species, the Asian Star

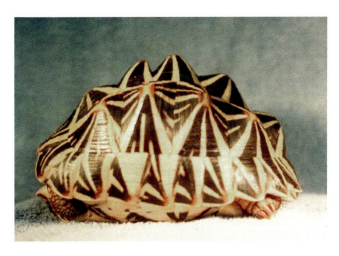

FIGURE 7-26 The Indian Star Tortoise (*Geochelone elegans*) is a beautifully marked species. *(Photograph courtesy C. Innis.)*

Tortoise, *G. platynota*. Several other species of *Geochelone* are not commonly found in the pet trade.

The Burmese Brown Tortoise, *Manouria emys*, can also be hardy and possibly one of the most prolific species. However, wild imports are difficult to establish because they often arrive in poor condition and heavily parasitized. Browns favor moist tropical temperatures. Browns are the only chelonians to construct mounds of vegetation to incubate their eggs.

Outdoor Housing

Whenever possible, tortoises should be kept outdoors, even if only for a small portion of the day or year. This allows tortoises space to exercise, graze, and bask in the sun, which is important for vitamin D synthesis. Well-acclimated adult tropical tortoises can be housed outdoors when morning temperatures are above 18°C (65°F) and midday temperatures exceed 24°C (75°F). The tortoises should be brought in at night when temperatures are below 18°C (65°F). Adult temperate species tolerate temperatures 3°C (5°F) less than those listed for tropical species. For small juveniles, temperatures should always be above 24°C (75°F; see neonatal care).

Tethering a tortoise by a leg or through a hole in the shell is not acceptable and is potentially harmful. Leg tethers can cut into flesh and result in severe infection. Drilling a hole through the shell should be considered inhumane.

When planning outdoor enclosures, several factors should be considered. Desert species can tolerate higher temperatures and drier enclosures than can tropical rainforest species. Outdoor enclosures can be modified to suit the needs of species. For tropical forest forms, such as *Geochelone carbonaria*, *G. denticulata*, *Manouria emys*, *Kinixys*, and *Indotestudo*, densely planted enclosures are ideal. For grassland or desert species, such as *Gopherus* and *Testudo*, *Geochelone sulcata*, *G. pardalis*, and *G. elegans*, enclosures can be more sparsely planted with shrubs and grasses. In either type of enclosure, shelters should be provided for shade and retreat from the elements. In areas with cool nights and warm days, insulated shelters with supplemental heat can be used. Plywood shelters can be insulated and heated with a fiberglass heating pad or other heat source. The door can be weatherproofed with overlying strips of thick clear vinyl.

Outdoor enclosures should have secure perimeters. Tortoises generally pace at the perimeters and constantly try to get through perimeters they can see through. Therefore, solid barriers, such as wooden fencing or smooth concrete, at tortoise eye level are preferable to open fencing. Chicken wire can entrap and cut tortoise legs or necks and is not advisable. If open fencing is used, 1/2-inch by 3-inch, medium gauge, welded wire (used for aviary construction) works well and is rat proof. Ideally, one should bury 6 to 12 inches of perimeter fencing to prevent underground escape.

Outdoor Hazards

See the predator section for more information. A potential hazard is pesticide spraying. Do not spray tortoise enclosures with pesticides. Instruct owners to have their neighbors inform them when they apply pesticides so that their tortoises can be removed to a safer area.

Tortoises consume all the vegetation growing in their enclosure. Therefore, toxic plants should be removed. Plant toxicities are rare in tortoises. Most grasses, clover, perennial legumes, dandelions, and weeds are suitable for browsing. Tortoises also eat a variety of nonfood items in their cage. Enclosures should be regularly examined for scraps of metal, nails, wire, pieces of plastic, and other trash that blows in. Tortoises also consume small rocks and pebbles; generally these are no cause for concern unless present in large quantities. Large amounts of gravel or sand can cause intestinal impaction.

Indoor Housing

Indoor housing is usually mandatory for a good portion of the year, except in subtropical areas. Tortoises need more space than most reptiles. The New York Turtle and Tortoise Society recommends that the combined shell size of all tortoises present should not exceed a quarter of the floor surface area available to the tortoises.[31]

Aquariums, livestock troughs, concrete mixing containers, aquaculture containers, sweater boxes, or wading pools can be used for small tortoises. Cages can be constructed for larger tortoises with 1/2-inch to 3/4-inch plywood on the bottom and two 2 × 12–inch planks stacked on one another or plywood along the sides. The inner cage surfaces should be caulked and sealed with an undercoat of water sealant and two to three coats of polyurethane. Sealing exposed wood surfaces facilitates cleaning and disinfecting. Allow the cage to air out thoroughly (usually about a week) before placing any tortoises in it. Melamine tends to warp when wet and is no longer recommended. To prevent chilling, the cage bottom should not be in direct contact with cold concrete; a gap of 4 to 6 inches is advisable. An alternative to building a cage is to convert a garage or unfinished room into a tortoise pen.

Ambient indoor temperature should be 24°C to 32°C (75°F to 90°F) depending on the species. Rooms can be heated with thermostatically controlled space heaters. A thermogradiant should be provided with basking lights or heating pads (see temperature section in general considerations).

Substrates

Juveniles are often maintained on alfalfa pellets, crushed oyster shell, or newspaper and as they graduate to larger cages, a mixture of medium-to-large conifer bark nuggets and peat moss, cypress mulch, or top soil. Acceptable alternative substrates include indoor-outdoor carpeting (be sure to avoid

Table 7-4	Tortoise Diet[20,27,28]

Adults should be fed three times per week minimum, and hatchlings fed daily. For every feeding, dust food with calcium lactate, carbonate, citrate, or gluconate. Every 2 to 4 weeks, dust food with multivitamins (if vitamin-fortified foods are not available). To make salad, rinse, chop, and mix two or three types of dark leafy greens, some thawed frozen mixed vegetables, sprouts, and whatever other vegetables are available. This mixture can be fed directly or stored in a large sealable container and refrigerated for up to 6 days. Before feeding, add freshly chopped fruits and occasionally (not more than twice a month) some high-protein foods. Put the salad on a flat board, piece of newspaper, paper or metal plates, or trays. Disposable feeding trays cut down on cleaning. Salad mixture that has been refrigerated should be allowed to come to room temperature for 30 to 60 minutes before feeding. **Feed as much variety as possible!**

95% Vegetables. Most vegetables should be dark leafy greens (mustard, collard, radish and turnip greens or tops, kale, cabbage), dandelions (leaves, stems, and flowers), bok-choy, pak-choi, broccoli rape or rapina, backyard grasses (especially Bermuda and timothy grass), clovers, legumes, and weeds (freshly cut or as browse). Feed less of spinach, Swiss chard, beet greens, red leaf or romaine lettuce. Mulberry, hibiscus and grape leaves, roses, nasturtiums, hibiscus, carnation and squash flowers, cured moistened alfalfa or timothy hay, soaked alfalfa pellets, thawed frozen mixed vegetables (peas, corn, carrots, green and lima beans), peas in the pod, cauliflower, green beans are good; as are alfalfa, clover, radish, or soy bean sprouts, jicama, green peppers, radishes, summer and winter squashes, and prickly pear cactus (*Opuntia* spp.) pads (shave off spines).

<5% Fruits. Grapes, apples, oranges, pears, prickly pear fruit, peaches, plums, nectarines, dates, all types of melons, strawberries, raspberries, bananas, mangos, and tomatoes. Increase to 20% for Red-Footed and Yellow-Footed tortoises.

0 to 5% High-protein foods. Some genera (*Kinixys, Chersina,* and *Manouria*) are more omnivorous and may benefit from small amounts of high-protein foods. "High-protein foods" is a descriptive term that should not be taken literally. Many fruits and vegetables also have substantial protein content. Generally these foods are limited to once every 2 weeks in small amounts. These tortoises eat dry, maintenance low-fat dog food, commercial tortoise chows, whole mice, baby mice, and large carnivore diets. Dry chows should be soaked in lukewarm water until slightly soft. High-protein foods are widely assumed to promote rapid growth in young tortoises, which may result in pyramidal shell growth. These assumptions are controversial. The high-protein, fat, and multivitamin content of these foods can be dangerous in excess and may promote hepatic lipidosis, particularly in strict herbivores. In moderation, as a very small portion of the diet, they are not likely to be harmful. Others believe tortoises should not get any of these foods, thus the listing as 0 to 5%.

---

frayed edges) or corrugated cardboard. Remove fecal material from the enclosure several times per week, and replace the substrate several times per year. For very large enclosures and large species, smooth cement, top soil, or fine hay can be used, provided the room stays warm. Avoid sand, gravel, clay cat litter, and crushed corn cob or walnut shells. Many tortoises are reclusive animals. As with outdoor enclosures, a shelter or hide box should be provided.

Water

Water should constantly be available for indoor and outdoor tortoises. Shallow plastic plant saucers work well for small tortoises. Make sure the water is no deeper than chin deep or the tortoise may accidentally overturn and drown. Larger plastic containers, such as plant saucers or Pyrex cooking pans, work well for medium-sized tortoises. For large tortoises, one can notch the side of a plastic shoebox, or sink pan, and tortoises will use them. Tortoises often defecate in their water; thus, water bowls should be changed daily or every other day, or whenever dirty. Tortoises outdoors also drink from standing water, especially Desert Tortoises.

An alternative to water bowls is to soak the tortoises in chin-deep water three times per week. This option is less desirable in that invariably one occasionally forgets to soak tortoises. The resulting intermittent dehydration may contribute to formation of uroliths and gout (see Chapters 49 and 54).

Feeding

Diets for captive tortoises are an area of considerable uncertainty and variability. Wild tortoises often use forage of a relatively low nutritional value. In captivity, diets tend to have a much higher nutritional value that may not be beneficial in the long run. Empirically, the authors have had success with diets (see Tables 7-2, 7-3, and 7-4) that include 95% vegetables (mainly dark leafy greens, grasses, and weeds), less than 5% fruits, and 0 to 5% foods with a high protein content (except in herbivorous species).

Reproduction

Female tortoises must be in prime condition before egg production. This includes a well-balanced diet with adequate calcium. Additional calcium should be provided for females that produce large or multiple clutches. Chunks of cuttlebone can be placed in the enclosure or on food, or the food can be dusted with calcium. Small tortoises can be palpated in the inguinal fossa for eggs; this is much more difficult in larger tortoises. A large Leopard Tortoise can cause excruciating pain to the forefinger foolhardy enough to be caught between the shell and rear leg. Eggs show up well on radiographs. See Table 7-5 for clutch sizes, frequency, and length of incubation for common species of tortoises.

Gravid females feel heavier than normal and tend to be more active, often pacing in the cage. Nest areas are often selected in areas that get the most sun or late afternoon sun. If the keeper is not present during egg laying, the nest can be easily missed. A definite sign that a female has been digging is dirt packed onto her hind feet and rear margins of shell. Some females may excavate several nests before actually laying eggs. Indoors, one must provide a nesting substrate at least as deep as the female's carapace length. Oxytocin, at 2 to 10 IU/kg subcutaneously or intramuscularly in the rear legs, is effective in inducing oviposition within several hours in females reluctant to lay. The nest should be carefully excavated and the eggs removed for incubation.

Table 7-5	Captive Reproductive Data on Common Species of Captive Tortoises			
Species	Clutches Per Season	Clutch Size	Incubation Temperature (°C)	Length of Incubation (d)
Gopherus agassizii[2]	2-3	2-14	32-35	90-120
G. berlandieri[2]	NA	1-4	NA	90
G. polyphemus	1	1-9	NA	NA
Geochelone carbonaria	1-3	1-5, 2-15	26-27.5	105-202
G. denticulata	1+	1-8, 1-12	27-28	125-150
G. elegans	1-9	2-10	30	111-147, 120-150
G. nigra	1-3	1-24, 8-17	25-31	97-200
G. gigantea	1-2	18-20, 4-5, 12-14	29-40	97-113, 98-200
G. pardalis	3-5, 5-7	14-21, 5-30	27-28	120-140
G. sulcata	2	17-33	28	118-170, 212
G. radiata	1-6	3-12	28	121-271
Kinixys homeana	1-2	4-7	27-28	110-140, 150
K. belliana	1+	2-7	NA	90-110
Malacochersus tornieri	1-6, 1-3	1-2, 1-2	25-30, 26-31, 28	113-221, 122-190, 117-188
Manouria emys	2, 1	23-51, 39-42	26-28.9, 28	63-84, 66-71
Testudo graeca	1-3	1-24, 2-7	25-31	97-200
T. hermanni	2	3-12, 2-12	30.5-31	56-72, 90
T. horsfieldi	2-3, 4	3-5	30.5	60-75
T. graeca ibera	2+	4-12	31	60-80
T. marginata	2+	8-10, 3-11	31	60-70

Reference 2 lists data from wild populations. Considerable variation may exist between captive and wild populations.
NA, Data not available.

Neonatal Care

Once the neonate has pipped the eggshell with its caruncle, or eggtooth, it emerges from the shell within 1 to 4 days. During this time, the neonate's shell begins to unfold, facilitating yolk absorption. As the neonate's shell straightens and the tortoise begins to move, the eggshell breaks further.

Once out of the egg, the neonate may still have considerable yolk sac. The hatchling should be transferred to a container, such as a plastic shoe or sweater box, with clean, moist paper towels. The yolk sac slowly absorbs over the next few days.

Once the yolk sac is fully absorbed and the umbilicus sealed, the neonate can be transferred to a cage with previously mentioned substrates. Hatchlings usually begin feeding within 1 to 14 days of leaving the egg. Hatchlings are prone to dehydration; therefore, shallow water bowls should constantly be available. Make sure the water bowl is shallow or the hatchling may overturn and drown. Plastic plant saucers work admirably for water bowls. An alternative is to soak neonates in shallow water three times a week. This option is less desirable in that invariably one occasionally forgets to soak tortoises.

Ultraviolet lights should be provided for 12 hours per day. A thermal gradient should be provided. Ambient temperature should not get colder than 24°C (75°F) at night and gradually warm to 30°C (85°F) during the day. Temperatures cooler than this are devastating to hatchling tortoises and can quickly lead to respiratory problems, anorexia, and death. Temperate young tortoises should be given a carefully controlled, shorter brumation (hibernation) period or not hibernated at all for several years (see Brumation [Hibernation] section).

Hatchlings can be fed the previously described ration daily, finely chopped in a food processor. Hatchlings should develop a firm shell in the first year. A clutch of siblings commonly has different growth rates. Smaller timid individuals may eventually need to be separated to ensure adequate nutrition.

Aquatic Turtles

Aquatic turtles[27,28,32] are popular pets, but this does not mean they are easy to care for. In fact, they can be among the most labor intensive of all reptiles to maintain. Inadequate care often results in problems for turtles. To effectively treat these problems, the veterinarian must be able to evaluate and correct captive care. Keep in mind that exceptions are seen to most rules and no substitute exists for good information on the natural history.

Taxonomy

The most common genera seen in the pet trade in the United States include *Trachemys* spp. *(Sliders), Chrysemys* spp. (Painted Turtles), *Kinosternon* spp. and *Sternotherus* spp. (Mud and Musk Turtles), *Graptemys* spp. (Map Turtles), *Clemmys* spp. (Wood and Pond Turtles), *Apalone* spp. (formerly *Trionyx*, Softshell Turtles), *Pseudemys* spp. (River Cooters), *Chelydra* spp. (Snapping Turtles), *Malaclemys* spp. (Diamond-back Terrapins), *Macrochelys* spp. (Alligator Snapping Turtles), *Chelus* spp. (Matamatas), *Cuora* spp. (Asiatic Box Turtles), *Chinemys* spp. (Reeve's Turtle), *Geoemyda* spp. (Leaf Turtles), and *Platysternon* spp. (Big-headed Turtles) (Figures 7-27, 7-28, and 7-29).

Housing

Housing requirements vary according to the size of the turtle and the number being kept. A variety of enclosures can be used from glass aquaria, plastic cement mixing containers, stock watering tanks, and pond liners to elaborate outdoor ponds. Outdoor enclosures should have some shade available. Never place a plastic or glass aquarium in full sun

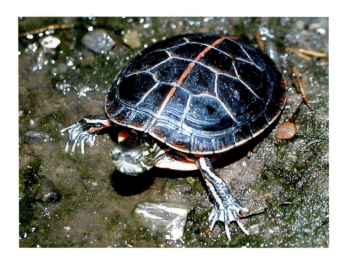

FIGURE 7-27 The Southern Painted Turtle (*Chrysemys picta dorsalis*), a colorful, hardy animal, is common in the pet trade. *(Photograph courtesy D. Mader.)*

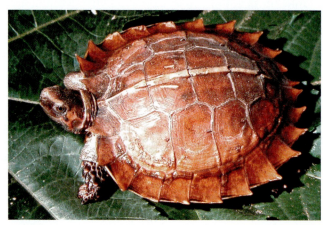

FIGURE 7-29 The Spiny Turtle from Southeast Asia (*Hosemys spinosa*) has been imported in large numbers during the past several years. *(Photograph courtesy R. Funk.)*

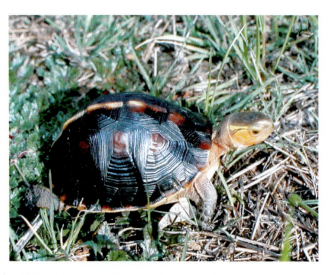

FIGURE 7-28 Asian Box Turtles (*Cuora flavomarginata*) are fast becoming a popular replacement for North American Box Turtles. *(Photograph courtesy D. Mader.)*

because it could easily overheat. A rule of thumb for minimum cage size is that the combined carapace size of all residents should not exceed 25% of the cage's floor surface area.[31] Floor surface area does not include any inaccessible areas that the turtle cannot rest on.

Water Quality

Water laden with bacteria and nitrogenous wastes smells and can quickly infect turtle shell or kill turtles. Aquatic turtles should have little odor (unless associated with feeding or musk glands). Turtle odor suggests a major water quality problem. Clean water is crucial to good health; several means are available to assure this.

Frequent full water changes are one method of keeping water clean. One can keep the water cleaner by feeding in a separate container because most foods foul the water quickly. If the turtles are fed in their regular enclosure, the water should be changed within 12 hours of feeding messy foods. Initially, some turtles may be reluctant to feed in the separate container, but they can be acclimated to this over time. Using the same water from the home container helps as does letting new water sit for 24 hours before feeding.

The frequency of water changes depends on the stocking density. For instance, for 3-inch or less than 4-inch turtles, a 10-gallon aquarium should be changed two to three times per week and a 50-gallon aquarium once a week. Full water changes are easier if no substrates are in the cage. Sand or gravel makes cleaning much more difficult. For smaller setups (10-gallon aquariums or less), one can carry the whole setup to a sink or bathtub for rinsing. Keep in mind that cleaning areas are a potential source of infectious bacteria, such as *Salmonella* (see *Salmonella* section). The 10-gallon storage container from Rubbermaid is easier to clean and more durable than a 10-gallon aquarium and is excellent for hatchlings.

For larger setups, one must drain the water. Portable electric submersible pumps can drain large volumes of water quickly and make cleaning much less labor intensive. These pumps are designed to drain swimming pools or flooded basements and are found in hardware departments of major department stores or pool supply stores. The Little Giant Pump Company (www.littlegiant.com) makes an excellent pump called the "Water Wizard," model 5-MSP, for about $65.00. Alternatively, one can use a siphon to drain the water, but this requires much more time. If one has the luxury of floor drains, one can install drains in the bottom of the cage, attach a hose, and drain the cage by gravity. Refill larger setups through a hose (with a nozzle) attached to a faucet. Separate drainage and refill hoses make cleaning much more convenient. When using a hose to drain or refill a cage, be sure to carefully secure the end of the hose or inadvertent flooding will occur.

Periodic scrubbing and rinsing of the cage well is important to remove residual bacterial growth on all sides. Abrupt changes in water temperature can kill turtles, so make sure the water temperature after cleaning is similar to what it was before cleaning. Thermometers facilitate this; with experience, one can gauge this with one's hand. Dechlorination of the water is generally not necessary; chlorinated water may help keep bacterial levels down. Obviously, with biologic filtration systems, water must be dechlorinated. Young turtles and those not accustomed to chlorinated water initially squint their eyes and have difficulty eating but quickly acclimate.

A partial alternative to the laborious task of full water changes is biological or chemical filtration. Filtration can decrease the time interval necessary for partial to full water changes but should not completely eliminate them. The authors' early impressions of fish filtration systems, used with turtles, was that filtration simply did not work. However, our knowledge and design of filtration systems for aquatic turtles have improved dramatically in the last few years (see Highfield[23] for a good review). Filtration is now feasible, especially for larger setups. Keep in mind that turtles produce considerably more solid fecal and urinary waste than fish. Most retail aquarium supply stores sell filters designed for biological breakdown of fish waste, not turtle waste. Even if the water looks clean, it can still have a lot of nitrogenous and bacterial waste in it. In general, select filters for turtles that are designed for large fish or high stocking densities.

As with all filtration systems, good aeration of water (through airstones or water agitated from falling into the surface, such as with a waterfall) is important to support aerobic bacterial growth in biological filters. For small setups, internal submersible filters are gaining in popularity. The best filters for turtles are large combination biological and mechanical filters, such as those designed for Koi fish, rapid sand filters, propeller driven fluidized bead filters, and external canister filters. In addition, ozone filtration and UV sterilization can be used. These types of filters tend to be expensive.

If the water level can be maintained within 8 inches of the top of the tank, powerlifting hanging filters are less expensive and simpler to maintain than canister filters but are also much less effective because of lower flow rates and filtration surface area. Under-gravel filters need a deep gravel bed (7.5 cm or more) or the turtle may dig and expose the filter plate.[23] Once exposed, water bypasses most of the gravel as it follows the path of least resistance, and the benefits of biological filtration are decreased. Foam rubber filters are essentially worthless. Disasters, such as die-offs, can result from poor water quality, particularly with low levels of oxygen saturation. Shell infections are the most common consequence of unclean water.

For the most part, turtles can be maintained in water with neutral pH. With exceptions for some species, knowledge of natural history becomes useful. For instance, some South American blackwater species, such as Red-headed River Turtles, *Podocnemis erythrocephala*; Snake-necked Turtle, *Hydromedusa tectifera*; Red Side-neck Turtle, *Phyrnops rufipes*; and other *Phyrnops* spp. need more acidic conditions.[23]

Water should be at least as deep as the width of the widest turtle's shell so that if overturned the turtle is able to right itself and avoid drowning. Diamond-back Terrapins live in brackish water and need addition of 2 tablespoons of aquarium salt and mineral mix per gallon of water (5 g per L).

Temperature
Water and air must be warm; 24°C to 28°C (75°F to 82°F) is recommended for most species. An incandescent 50-watt to 150-watt light bulb, with reflector, directed toward the basking area creates a hot spot for basking. Alternatively, one can keep the room temperature within this range. Submersible aquarium heaters are ideal for warming water.

Haul Out Area
A dry haul out area should be present so that turtles can crawl out of the water, dry off, and bask. Basking is a means of behavioral thermoregulation whereby turtles can achieve their preferred optimum body temperature. Basking areas can be as simple as a flat rock resting on submerged bricks or a cinder block. More elaborate platforms can be built into the cage above water level with access via a plastic ramp or piece of wood. One also can use floating pieces of cork, hardwood driftwood, or plastic floating platforms. Snapping Turtles and Mata Matas do not need basking areas.

Nesting Areas
Nesting areas should be provided for adult females, even if males are not present. If a sufficient nest area is provided, dystocia may be avoided and oviposition stimulated. The Columbus Zoo has a prodigious aquatic turtle breeding program and believes that temporarily rigging a nesting area, or shifting a gravid female to a cage with a nesting area, is far less successful than keeping a nesting area present year round.[34]

The nesting area should be approximately four to five times larger than the carapace of the female. Nest medium should be slightly moist sand or potting soil and two times deeper than the length of the carapace. Nest area containers can be made from a large plastic trash can cut in half or a variety of smaller plastic containers. The nesting area can double as a basking area.

Feeding
A balanced diet with adequate calcium is crucial to good health. A wide variety of foods should be provided (Table 7-6). Whole fish are better than gutted fish and can be fed chopped or whole. Most suppliers of feeder fish minimize their feeding to ensure good water quality in overcrowded setups. Ideally, fish should be well fed before being fed to turtles.

Freezing fish at −10°C (14°F) for more than 3 days may eliminate transfer of some, but not all, parasites.[35] Goldfish are not recommended because of the high incidence rate of mycobacteriosis. Wild-caught sticklebacks and mosquito fish

Table 7-6 Aquatic Turtle Diet[27,28,30,36]

Feed adults one to three times per week; hatchlings daily. Feed as much variety as possible.

Majority of the diet. Whole animals such as mice, earthworms, *Tubifex* worms, slugs, snails, shrimp (with shells) and thawed frozen guppies, trout, bait fish, shiners, and freshwater smelt.

Minority of the diet. Turtle brittle (Nasco, Fort Atkinson, Wis), trout or catfish chow (Ralston Purina), insects such as crickets, waxworms, mealworms, flies, moths, grasshoppers, small amounts of lean raw beef, liver, gizzards, or chicken.

In older omnivorous species, gradually increase dark leafy greens (kale, spinach, dandelion greens, romaine lettuce, cabbage, watercress, endive, bok choy, escarole), yams, carrots, duckweed, and fruits (apples, grapes, melons, bananas).

should not be fed because they are natural vectors for several serious parasites.[35,36]

Avoid large quantities of oil-laden species such as mackerel, and to a lesser extent smelt, that are known to induce steatitis. Saltwater smelt can have high levels of thiaminase (especially after freezing) that can induce thiamin or vitamin B1 deficiency if fed exclusively. If fed in moderation, as part of a balanced diet, frozen fish should not cause any problems.

Most aquatic turtles readily consume chopped, skinned mice and pinkies. GI impactions have been seen in turtles from fur, so skinned and chopped mice are recommended. Mata Matas refuse mice that are not skinned but can be trained to eat skinned mice. Older mice have more mineralized bone and are an outstanding source of calcium and phosphorus for shell growth. Mouse liver is also a good source of vitamin A.

A variety of insects in moderation also are good (see Table 7-6). Be aware that insects are calcium deficient. Earthworms are widely available and nutritious; small turtles often need them chopped. Some hatchlings do well with *Tubifex* worms. Snails and slugs can be fed but are a potential vector for trematodes. Desiccated invertebrates are nutritionally inadequate and should not be fed.

Small amounts of lean raw beef, liver, gizzards, or chicken occasionally can be fed but are severely calcium deficient unless bone is present. Hamburger is not recommended because it is calcium deficient and the high fat content leaves a greasy film on the surface of the water.

Many sliders and pond turtles become more herbivorous as they reach mature size and grow less rapidly. One can gradually increase greens and fruits (see Tables 7-2 and 7-3) for these species.

For larger collections, a prepared ration can be made by mixing several ingredients together and binding them with unflavored gelatin (see Table 7-3). Cut set gelatin into bite-sized pieces or strips. The strips can be tightly wrapped in plastic wrap, placed in self-sealing polyethylene plastic bags, and frozen. Remove as much air as possible before freezing to minimize freezer burn.[33] Do not refreeze the ration once thawed.

As much variety as is possible is needed to ensure a healthy diet. If a balanced diet with whole mice is provided, multivitamin and mineral supplementation is not necessary. Mineral blocks in the water do not help nutritionally. Encourage owners to experiment with turtles but be aware that it may take weeks to accustom turtles to new diets. Novel items may initially be tasted and spit out and accepted later. Persistence is important.

Neonatal Care

Hatchling aquatic turtles can be a challenge to raise. Avoid crowding neonate turtles. The Rubbermaid 10-gallon storage container works well for young turtles because it is easily cleaned and the nontransparent sides may offer additional security. Hatchlings may be shy and scramble for cover at your approach and can be reluctant to feed. Provide hatchlings with cover to retreat under such as floating pieces of cork, clay flower-pot pieces, plastic leaves (large enough that they cannot be ingested), or a small board or flat rock over bricks. Be certain that cage props are stable so that they do not shift and trap young turtles underwater and drown them.

To coerce young turtles to feed, try small live insects such as 2-week-old crickets, mealworms, waxworms, chopped pink mice, small chopped earthworms, or *Tubifex* worms. As the hatchlings begin to feed with more vigor, try a wider variety of foods. As soon as possible, try to get them eating finely chopped adult mice, pinkies, and guppies, which are all good sources of bone. UV lights, proper temperature, and a wide variety of foods are important to prevent metabolic bone disease and ensure proper growth.

As much variety as is possible is recommended to ensure a healthy diet for aquatic turtles. If a balanced diet with whole mice is provided, multivitamin and mineral supplementation is not necessary and could be detrimental in the long run. Encourage owners to experiment with their turtles. Reassure them that dietary changes are important, but acceptance on the part of the turtle can take weeks. The owner should not be discouraged if novel items are tasted and spit out initially; it can take weeks for turtles to accept new foods.

SPECIES INTERACTIONS

Some turtle species, such as Snapping Turtles, large Softshell Turtles, Mud and Musk Turtles, and Big-headed Turtles are aggressive toward other turtles. These species can cause severe lacerations, or kill other species, and should only be kept with others of the same species and size. Cannibalism is known to occur in the Chelydridae, Emydidae, Kinosternidae, and Trionychidae. In addition, many turtles can be carriers of *Entamoeba invadens*, which can cause serious GI disease in turtles and other reptiles.[37]

ACKNOWLEDGMENTS

Portions of this chapter have been previously published. We thank Stephen Barten, DVM, Jeffrey Jenkins, DVM, DABVP, Douglas Mader, MS, DVM, DABVP, Roger Klingenburg, DVM, Chuck Smith, Scott Stahl, DVM, and Brett Stearns for critical review of those portions. We thank John Tashjian and Stephen Barten for their pictures. Most of all, we thank our wives, Lilia and Sally, for help above and beyond the call of duty.

REFERENCES

1. Gibbon JW: Why do turtles live so long? *BioScience* 37-262, 1987.
2. Ernst CH, Barbour RW: *Turtles of the world*, Washington, DC, 1989, Smithsonian Institution Press.
3. Cogger HG, Zweifel RG, editors: *Encyclopedia of reptiles and amphibians*, ed 2, San Francisco, Fog City Press.
4. Boycott RC, Bourquin O: *The South African tortoise book*, Johannesburg, South Africa, 1988, Southern Book Publishers.
5. Iverson J: Checklist of turtles of the world with English common names, *SSAR Herp Circular* 14:1-4, 1985.
6. Zug GR: Age determination in turtles, *SSAR Herp Circular* 20:1-28, 1991.
7. Pritchard P: *Encyclopedia of turtles*, Neptune City, NJ, 1979, TFH Publications.
8. Highfield AC: *Keeping and breeding tortoises in captivity*, Portihead, England, 1990, R and A Publishing.
9. Jackson OF, Lawrence K: Chelonians. In Cooper JE, Hutchinson MF, Jackson OF, Maurice RJ, editors: *Manual of*

exotic pets, revised edition, Cheltenham, England, 1985, British Small Animal Veterinary Association.
10. Frye FL: *Biomedical and surgical aspects of captive reptile husbandry,* ed 2, vol II, Melbourne, Fla, 1991, Krieger Publishing.
11. Wood SC, Lenfant CJM: Respiration. mechanics, control, and gas exchange. In Gans C, editor: *Biology of the Reptilia,* vol 5, San Diego, 1976, Academic Press.
12. Fowler ME: Comparison of respiratory infection and hypovitaminosis A in desert tortoises. In Montali RJ, Migaki G, editors: *Comparative pathology of zoo animals,* Washington, DC, 1980, Smithsonian Institution Press.
13. Davies PMC: Anatomy and physiology. In Cooper JE, Jackson OF, editors: *Diseases of the Reptilia,* vol I, San Diego, 1981, Academic Press.
14. Girgis S: Aquatic respiration in the common Nile turtle, *Trionyx triunguis, Comp Biochem Physiol* 3:206, 1961.
15. Cann J: *Australian freshwater turtles,* Singapore, 1998, Beaumont Publishing.
16. Edwards MS: Dietary husbandry of large herbivorous reptiles the giant tortoises of Aldabra atoll *(Geochelone gigantea)* and Galapagos islands *(G. elephantopus), Proc Am Assoc Zoo Vets* 139, 1991.
17. Lawrence K, Jackson OF: Passage of ingesta in tortoises, *Vet Rec* 111:492, 1982.
18. Tothill A, Johnson J, Branvold H, Paul C, Wimsatt J: Effect of cisapride, erythromycin, and metoclopramide on gastrointestinal transit time in the desert tortoise, *Gopherus agassizii, J Herp Med Surg* 10(1):16-20, 2000.
19. Fitch H: *Sexual size differences in reptiles,* Lawrence, Kan, 1981, University of Kansas Museum of Natural History, Pub No 70.
20. Boyer DM, Boyer TH: Tortoise care, *Bull Assoc Reptil Amphib Vet* 4(1):16, 1994.
21. Jackson OF: Weight and measurement data on tortoises (*Testudo graeca* and *Testudo hermanni*) and their relationship to health, *J Small Anim Pract* 21:409, 1980.
22. Mader DR, Stoutenberg G: Assessing the body condition of the California desert tortoise, *Gopherus agassizii,* using morphometric analysis, *Proc Assoc Rept Amphib Vet* 103, 1998.
23. Highfield AC: *Practical encyclopedia of keeping and breeding tortoises and freshwater turtles,* London, England, 1996, Carapace Press.
24. Jarchow JL: Hibernating your turtle safely, *N Ohio Assoc Herp* XX(11):8, 1993.
25. Jacobson ER, Behler JL, Jarchow JL: Health assessment of chelonians and release into the wild. In Fowler ME, Miller RE, editors: *Zoo & wild animal medicine: current therapy 4,* Philadelphia, 1999, WB Saunders.
26. Boyer TH: Box turtle care, *Bull Assoc Reptil Amphib Vet* 2(1):14, 1992.
27. Boyer Th, Boyer DM: Biology: turtles, tortoises and terrapins. In Mader DR, editor: *Reptile medicine and surgery,* Philadelphia, 1996, WB Saunders.
28. Boyer TH: *Essentials of reptiles: a guide for practitioners,* Lakewood, Colo, 1998, AAHA Press.
29. de Vosjoli P: *The general care and maintenance of box turtles,* Lakeside, Calif, 1991, Advanced Vivarium Systems.
30. Swingland IR, Klemens MW, editors: *The conservation and biology of tortoises,* Gland, Switzerland, 1989, International Union for the Conservation of Nature and Natural Resources.
31. *Guidelines for the housing of turtles and tortoises: minimum standard housing guidelines for pet shops, wholesale animal dealers, and other commercial establishments,* vol XIX, no. 5, New York, 1990, New York Turtle and Tortoise Society.
32. Boyer TH, Boyer DM: Aquatic turtle care, *Bull Assoc Reptil Amphib Vet* 2(2):13, 1992.
33. Frye FL: *A practical guide for feeding captive reptiles,* Melbourne, Fla, 1991, Krieger Publishing.
34. Goode M: Breeding semi-aquatic and aquatic turtles at the Columbus Zoo. In Beaman KR, Caporaso F, McKeown S, Graff MD, editors: *Proceedings 1st international symposium on turtles and tortoises' conservation and captive husbandry,* Orange, CA, 1990, Chapman University.
35. Boyce W, Cardeilhac P, Lane T, Buergelt C, King M: Sebekiosis in captive alligator hatchlings, *JAVMA* 185(11): 1419-1420, 1984.
36. Boyer DM: *An overview of captive reptile diets,* Fort Collins, Colo, 1987, Student American Veterinary Medicine Association Symposium.
37. Bonner B, Denver M, Garner M, Innis C, Nathan R, moderator: *Entamoeba invadens* roundtable, *J Herpetol Med Surg* 11(3):17-22, 2001.
38. Barten SL: Clinical problems of iguanas and box turtles, *Proc Eastern States Vet Conf* 4:269, 1990.
39. Barten SL: *Reptile nutrition: herbivorous species,* Chicago, Ill, 1984, Chicago Herpetological Society Members Handbook.

8
CROCODILIANS
THOMAS LANE

EVOLUTION AND CLASSIFICATION

All living crocodilians belong to the clade called the "archosaurs," which, interestingly, also includes the birds. The remaining two clades are the "chelonians," the turtles and tortoises, and the "lepidosaurs," which includes the lizard, the snakes, and the Tuatara. The 28 species and subspecies of the crocodilians are divided into four subfamilies: the Alligatorinae, the Crocodylinae, the Gavialinae, and the Tomistominae (Table 8-1).

Many crocodilian species are considered to be either endangered or threatened, and as such, the status of any species can change over time. The Convention of International Trade in Endangered Species (CITES) has established the parameters for the inclusion of many species as being classified CITES–Appendix I or CITES–Appendix II. Appendix I includes all species that are threatened by extinction, whereas Appendix II includes: a, those that may become threatened by extinction unless regulated; and b, other species similar to those in Appendix IIa. (See Chapter 80 for more details regarding CITES.)

The hides of most species of crocodilians are in demand for the production of leather products. This worldwide demand is the primary reason many crocodilian species have been considered endangered in recent decades.

Crocodiles, alligators, caimans, and gharials are natural resources that are undergoing worldwide management efforts for the prevention of their extinction. Such successful management programs include crocodilian farming, captive breeding and rearing, artificial incubation of eggs, and the stocking of habitats. In recent years, limited hunting seasons with size and number limits has been successfully introduced under the control and regulation of federal and state wildlife management programs.

Members of the order Crocodylia are found in most tropical areas throughout the world.[1] They are the last survivors of the archosaurs or "ruling reptiles" and are descendants of the thecodonts of the early Triassic period of 200 million years ago. Fossil records indicate very little change between those that first appeared 160 million years ago and the modern crocodilians. Modern-day alligators, caimans, and crocodiles appear much as they did more than 65 million years ago. Although the dinosaurs of the world have come and gone, their crocodilian relatives are still with us and are likely the longest living reptile on earth. They are also the largest living reptiles in the world today.

The scientific names of members of the order Crocodylia are based on rules and guidelines of the International Commission of Zoological Nomenclature. Some taxonomists consider some animals to be subspecies, and as such, they are usually listed with a third name that is also lower case (Table 8-2).

Extinct species of crocodilians were of the marine type, probably reaching the size of 10 to 12 m. A crocodile of the species *Phobosuchus* has been reported from the Cretaceous straits of Texas and also Europe.[2]

Crocodilians are well adapted to an amphibious environment, with a streamlined body and a vertically compressed tail (Figure 8-1). The dorsal placement of the eyes and nostrils combined with long powerful jaws serve well the aquatic and predatory lifestyle of the crocodilian species of the world. Other adaptions that are unique to the order Crocodilia are the internal valvular mechanism of the nostrils that separates the respiratory system from the oral cavity, the ability to conserve metabolic energy when necessary, and the osteodermal armor, which has only minor differences among the species (Figure 8-2). The skin consists of an outer epidermis and scales.

Table 8-1 Crocodilians: Classification

Clade: Archosauria
Order: Crocodylia
Family: Crocodylidae

Subfamily	Genus (No. of Species)	Species
Alligatorinae	Alligator (2)	*Alligator sinensis*
		Alligator mississippiensis
	Caiman (5)	*Caiman crocodilus apaporiensis*
		Caiman crocodilus crocodilus
		Caiman crocodilus fuscus
		Caiman crocodilus yacare
		Caiman latirostris
	Melanosuchus (1)	*Melanosuchus niger*
	Paleosuchus (2)	*Paleosuchus palpebrosus*
		Paleosuchus trigonatus
Crocodylinae	Crocodylus (14)	*Crocodylus acutus*
		Crocodylus cataphractus
		Crocodylus intermedius
		Crocodylus johnstoni
		Crocodylus moreleti
		Crocodylus mindorensis
		Crocodylus niloticus
		Crocodylus novaeguineae
		Crocodylus palustris
		Crocodylus palustris kimbula
		Crocodylus porosus
		Crocodylus porosus porosus
		Crocodylus rhombifer
		Crocodylus siamensis
	Osteolaemus (2)	*Osteolaemus osborni*
		Osteolaemus tetraspis
Gavialinae	Gavialis (1)	*Gavialis gangeticus*
Tomistominae	Tomistoma (1)	*Tomistoma schlegelii*

Table 8-2   Twenty-Eight Species and Subspecies of Living Crocodilians

Species	Common Name	Location	Adult Length
Alligator sinensis	Chinese Alligator	East China	2 m
Alligator mississippiensis	American Alligator	Southeast United States	4.5 m
Caiman crocodilus	Speckled Caiman	South America	2 m
Caiman crocodilus apaporiensis-ss	Rio Apaporis Caiman	Colombia, South America	1.8 m
Caiman crocodilus fuscus-ss	Brown Caiman	Colombia to Mexico	1.8 m
Caiman crocodilus yacare-ss	Jacare	Paraguay, South America	2 m
Caiman latirostris	Broad-nosed Caiman	Brazil and Paraguay	3.5 m
Melanosuchus niger	Black Caiman	Amazon drainage, South America	6 m
Paleosuchus palpebrosus	Dwarf Caiman	Amazon and the Guinea	1.5 m
Paleosuchus trigonatus	Smooth-fronted Caiman	Amazon drainage	2 m
Crocodylus acutus	American Crocodile	Florida, South America, West Indies	4.5 m
Crocodylus cataphractus	Slender-nose Crocodile	West and Central Africa	2.3 m
Crocodylus intermedius	Orinoco Crocodile	Orinoco River, South America	5.5 m
Crocodylus johnstoni	Johnstone's Crocodile	North Australia	2.3 m
Crocodylus moreleti	Morelet's Crocodile	Yucatan to Guatemala	2.3 m
Crocodylus mindorensis	Mindoro Crocodile	Philippine Islands	2.3 m
Crocodylus niloticus	Nile Crocodile	Africa and Israel	5 m
Crocodylus novaeguineae	New Guinea Crocodile	New Guinea	2.5 m
Crocodylus palustris	Mugger Crocodile	India and Pakistan	3.5 m
Crocodylus palustris kimbula-ss	Ceylonese MCugger	Ceylon	3.5 m
Crocodylus porosus	Indopacific Saltwater Crocodile	Minikana, Ceylon	3.5 m
Crocodylus porosus porosus-ss	Saltwater Crocodile	Asia, Australia	6 m
Crocodylus rhombifer	Cuban Crocodile	Cuba and Isle of Pines	3 m
Crocodylus siamensis	Siamese Crocodile	Borneo, Siam, Java	3.5 m
Osteolaemus tetraspis	West African Dwarf Crocodile	West Africa	1.8 m
Osteolaemus tetraspis osborni-ss	Congo Dwarf Crocodile	Africa	1.2 m
Gavialis gangeticus	Gharial	India	6 m
Tomistoma schlegelii	False Gharial	Malay Penisula, Sumatra, Borneo	4.5 m

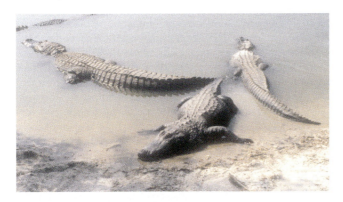

FIGURE 8-1 Crocodilians have long, sleek bodies covered with hard, bony scales that keep them well protected. The tail is powerful for propelling through water. When floating, the eyes, ears, and nostrils are all that is exposed above water.

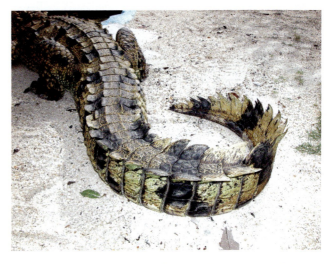

FIGURE 8-2 Crocodilians all share similar osteodermal armor. Scales, which are not shed as in other reptiles, consist of thickened keratin. *(Photograph courtesy D. Mader.)*

The scales are made up of thickened keratin of the epidermis. Crocodilian scales are not shed periodically as in some other reptilian species. The skin of the head is fused to the cranial and facial bones. These scales grow as the animal grows. The feet of the forelimbs have five digits, are not webbed, and are smaller than the hind feet. The hind feet have only four digits, are webbed, and have claws on the inner three toes. The medial three toes of the front feet are also clawed. All crocodilians have sharp conical teeth that do not have a root system and are shed periodically throughout life (Figure 8-3).

Crocodilians had existed in vast numbers throughout the tropical areas of the world until the last 80 years. The two factors that led to the reduction in crocodilian numbers are the worldwide demand for hides and meat and the widespread destruction of habitat.

Only in recent years, as the modern world recognized its obligation to endangered species, has crocodilian conservation received the necessary recognition and effort. Crocodilian conservation is now accomplished through the management of certain wild populations and farm production enterprises (Figure 8-4). A number of farms for a variety of crocodilian species exist throughout the world for the economic benefit of the owners and for conservation. The amazing fact is that crocodilians as unspecialized animals still

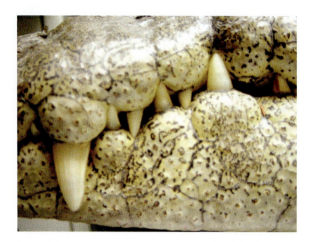

FIGURE 8-3 All crocodilians have conical teeth without a root system. These teeth are shed periodically throughout life. *(Photograph courtesy D. Mader.)*

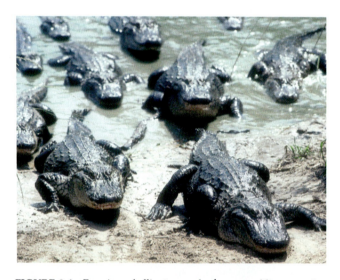

FIGURE 8-4 Farming of alligators and other crocodilians requires sufficient land and water areas and can enhance the value of wetlands habitat.

survive as an active group while more specialized groups have ceased to exist.

CROCODILIAN LIFE SPAN

Misconceptions abound about the size and age of crocodilians both in written accounts and rumors among the general populace. The wild tales of animals that are 1000 years of age or more are just that—tales! A well-recognized fact is that many reptiles have a more extensive life span than many common domestic animals. However, a great many factors can affect the longevity of any biologic species, and this is true also for crocodilians.

The life span of crocodilians is subject to such factors as the wild environment versus a captive situation. In the wild environment, the mortality rate is variable depending on

Table 8-3	Life Span and Longevity of Crocodilians	
Genus	No. of Species	Life Span (y)
Alligator	2	30-50
Caiman	5	12-20
Melanosuchus	1	5-10
Paleosuchus	2	15-30
Crocodylus	14	18-45
Osteolaemus	2	12-20
Gavialis	1	20+
Tomistoma	1	20+

available food, the numbers of animals in the location, and the amount of predation that occurs from year to year. In years when food is plentiful, population numbers and growth rates may be optimum. In those years when habitat or food sources become scarce, cannibalism may occur. Some researchers claim that cannibalism among crocodilians is rare, and others infer it is common. A third opinion on predation of wild populations is that it does not occur among adult crocodilians and among siblings or family members. Parents do not cannibalize offspring or members of the opposite sex in the same size category. However, reports show that under certain circumstances subadults do consume hatchlings and juveniles and, in adults, predation occurs on subadults. Such information concerning wild species is difficult to obtain. Natural predation of crocodilians larger than 1.5 m by other crocodilians is relatively rare. Reports do exist of predation by lions, elephants, and hippopotamuses on Nile Crocodiles *(Crocodilus niloticus)*, and in South America, anacondas have been known to kill small-size and medium-size caimans.

In captive populations, the life span and mortality rates are dependent to a great extent on the animals' environment and diet over a period of time. Severe changes in air and water temperature, water quality, noise influences, and diet can exert an effect that serves to shorten the life span of these animals. Shows that depict "alligator wrestling" have been stated, but not documented, to serve to shorten the animal's natural life. The frequent placing of the animal on its back has been theorized to deprive the brain of an adequate oxygen and blood supply. To the author's knowledge, this hypothesis has not been subjected to adequate study or documentation.

Current knowledge concerning the life span of crocodilians is limited and is related to known ages of animals that have been maintained in captive environments. Table 8-3 lists the ranges of life span of some species of crocodilians on the basis of available information.

Subfamily Alligatorinae

The 10 species of the subfamily Alligatorinae include two species of true alligators and five species of the genus *Caiman*, two species in the genus *Paleosuchus*, and one species in the genus *Melanosuchus*. The two species of alligators include the American Alligator *(Alligator mississippiensis)* and the Chinese Alligator *(Alligator sinensis)*.

The American Alligator is likely the most studied crocodilian of the entire family of Crocodylidae, probably because of its ready accessibility combined with the interest in commercial farming production that has occurred in the past 25 years.

The American Alligator is found in swamps, marshes, and lakes of the southeastern United States from the low areas of both North and South Carolina, Georgia, Florida, and westward to Texas. The range also includes the delta areas of Alabama and Arkansas and most of the Louisiana delta. Alligators have a broad, flat snout, and when the mouth is closed, only the teeth of the upper jaw are visible. They also have a nasal septum of bone that is not present in caimans. In adults, the nuchal scales are relatively large and number four to six.

The Chinese alligator is a severely endangered species and is found only in the valley of the lower Yangtze River in the Anhwei and Kiangsi provinces of the People's Republic of China.[3] This species is highly protected by both Chinese and United States law that prohibits importation. The endangered state has occurred as a result of illegal hunting and loss of habitat over time. The reproductive cycle is similar to that of the American Alligator. A number of captive breeding programs at zoos and wildlife refuges have been quite successful.

Caimans are closely related to alligators and include the following three genera: *Caiman* (five species), *Melanosuchus* (one species), and *Paleosuchus* (two species). They are located primarily in the northern area of South America and in Central America north to Mexico (Brown Caiman, *Caiman crocodilus fuscus*). Their habitat includes swamps, marshes, lakes, and freshwater streams. The Speckled Caiman (*Caiman crocodilus*) species were imported at one time into the southern United States for the pet trade. Caimans differ from alligators in that the snout is not as wide but is still flat (Figure 8-5). The skin of the caiman is not as useful for the hide trade because of the osteoderm or bony plate in the belly scales. At one time, juvenile caimans were stuffed and sold as curios to the tourist trade. The largest caiman species is the Black Caiman (*Melanosuchus niger*) at approximately 6 m, and the smallest species is the Dwarf Caiman (*Paleosuchus palpebrosus*) at 1.5 to 2 m. The genus *Paleosuchus* consists of two species: *P. palpebrosus* and *P. trigonatus*, which are frequently referred to as Smooth-Fronted Caiman. The *P. palpebrosus* is commonly noted as the Dwarf Caiman or Cuvier's Smooth-fronted Caiman as opposed to Schneider's Smooth-fronted Caiman (*P. trigonatus*). Cuvier's Smooth-fronted Caiman has a short broad snout; the snout of the Schneider's Smooth-fronted Caiman is comparatively longer and narrower. They are termed smooth fronted because they lack the bony ridge between the orbits that is common to all other caimans[4] (see Figure 8-5).

Subfamily Crocodylinae

Crocodilians are moderate to large in size and occur worldwide in tropical areas. Most species exist in fresh water, but some exist in marine and saltwater habitats in estuarine environments. The shape of the snout varies from short and blunt to long and narrow. Crocodiles can be differentiated from alligators and caimans by the visibility of the fourth mandibular tooth on each side of the mouth (Figure 8-6). These teeth fit into depressions or grooves between the teeth of the maxilla. (Members of the subfamily Alligatorinae have depressions on the upper jaw for the fourth mandibular tooth, but the teeth are not visible when the mouth is closed.) All members of the *Crocodylus* spp. have lingual salt glands that are absent in alligators and caimans. These lingual salt glands permit ionic water balance maintenance in a saltwater environment. The two Crocodylinae genera are *Crocodylus* and *Osteolaemus*.

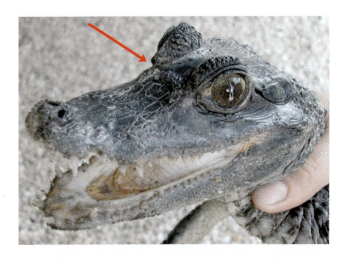

FIGURE 8-5 Caiman snouts are narrower than those of alligators but wider than those of crocodile species. Tapering of the snout gives some species a crocodile look. Caimans are readily differentiated from alligators by the bony ridge between eyes *(arrow)*. *(Photograph courtesy D. Mader.)*

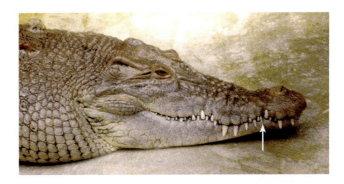

FIGURE 8-6 Alligators and crocodiles look very much alike. Crocodiles can be distinguished because the head is longer and more triangular. Also, the crocodile has a visible fourth mandibular tooth *(arrow)* on each side of the mouth.

Crocodylus acutus and *Crocodylus porosus* are the saltwater species. The remainder are freshwater species in both the Asian and North American continents. *Osteolaemus* spp. are the Dwarf Crocodiles from Africa.

The Orenoco Crocodile (*Crocodylus intermedius*) has a limited distribution in the Orinoco river basin of Venezuela and Colombia, South America. This animal is easily confused with the American Crocodile (*Crocodylus acutus*) because of its slender snout and size, which can exceed 5 m. The Nile Crocodile has a distribution in Central and South Africa.

The Indopacific Crocodile (*Crocodylus porosus*) is probably the largest member of the order Crocodylia. It has been reported to reach a length of 7 m and is widely distributed throughout the Pacific and Asian region. Although it is termed a Saltwater Crocodile, the animal is frequently found in freshwater environments. It is one of the most feared crocodilians because of its aggressive nature and reported attacks on humans.

Osteoaemus tetraspis and the subspecies, the Dwarf Crocodiles, are heavily armored small animals and are found

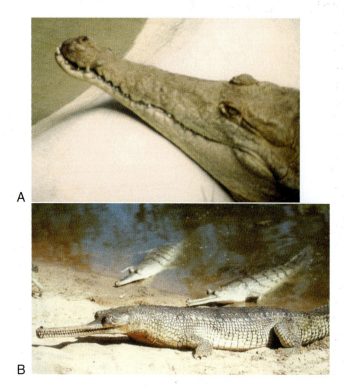

FIGURE 8-7 **A,** The Indian, or True, Gharial *(Gavialis gangeticus)* has a long slender snout and a bulb-like nose. All of the teeth are the same size, which differs from other crocodilians. Its diet is primarily fish. **B,** The False Gharial *(Tomistoma schlegelii)* is similar to the True Gharial in having a long slender snout but it is in a subfamily of its own. (*A, Photograph courtesy R. Funk.*)

in the tropical forest areas of central and west Africa. It has been reported to be primarily nocturnal, and only limited information is found on its biology and habits.

The Siamese Crocodile (*C. siamensis*) is a medium-size animal with a very limited distribution in Southeast Asia. Some reports indicate that this species is very close to extinction in the wild.

Subfamily Gavialinae

The one surviving species of this family, *Gavialis gangeticus*, also known as the Gharial, is considered the only true gavial and occurs only in the upper reaches of the Indus, Ganges, and Brahmaputra rivers of India and the Rapti-Narayani River of Nepal (Figure 8-7, *A*). This species is considered endangered. Most of the common day literature refers to this species as "the Gharial," although the scientific subfamily and genus remain Gavialinae and *Gavialis*, respectively. A distinctive long and slender snout identifies this Gharial from other members of the crocodilian family except for the False Gharial. When the mouth is closed, the fourth mandibular tooth and all the anterior teeth are visible on the outside of the jaw. In the True Gharial and the False Gharial (Tomistominae), the mandibular symphysis is extremely long and extends back to the level of the 14th or 15th mandibular tooth. This is not so in the other species of crocodilians.

The major diet of this crocodilian is fish, which the Gharial catches with rapid sideward swings of the jaw. The long jaws contain 100 interlocking teeth that are the same size and extremely sharp, which is efficient for catching fish and frogs.[5]

However, the long jaws are not well adapted for larger prey specimens. The Gharial is not well adapted to land but is adapted to a watery environment. The legs are weak, and on land, the animal uses a "belly slide" rather than a high walk like most other crocodilians. This belly slide movement on land is accomplished by propulsion of the body with the hind limbs.

Adult male Gharials have a conspicuous knob at the top of their snouts termed the narial excrescence. The function of this bulbous structure has not been determined. It is unlikely to be connected with the sense of smell or with breathing. It contains no apparent specialized cells and cannot be closed against water. One theory is that the male uses this bulb as a resonator during the breeding season. This nasal excrescence or bulb develops in the male at about 10 years of age. It is primarily cartilaginous, and the flaps on it allow the animal to make a hissing sound on exhalation. This hissing sound appears to be an important function during the breeding season. Reproduction occurs in this species when the male reaches approximately 4 m and the female reaches 2.5 m. Reproduction usually occurs with courtship maneuvers in December and breeding in January and February. Nesting occurs from late March through April. The Gharial is a hole nester and deposits between 35 and 50 eggs in a nest. Hatching of eggs occurs after incubation of 60 to 90 days depending on locale and environment. Normally the females are not aggressive except during this period when they guard the nest.

Subfamily Tomistominae

The subfamily Tomistominae includes a single species, the False Gharials (*Tomistominae schlegelii*), that exists in the swamps and rivers of the Malay Peninsula and the islands of Java, Borneo, and Sumatra (see Figure 8-7, *B*). The False Gharial is very similar to the True Gharial as it also has a long slender snout and also is considered an endangered species. Some confusion is seen in the phylogenetic relationship of the subfamilies Tomistominae and Gavialinae. The confusion arises because of the unresolved issue of whether Tomistominae is a member of the Crocodylinae or the Gavialinae. Both classifications have been proposed at one time or another. Therefore, we have for simplicity kept Tomistominae as a separate subfamily until a clear morphologic relationship is presented.

This False Gharial is considered a freshwater crocodilian and is found in fresh lakes, rivers, and swamps throughout its limited habitat range. The long slender snout contains from 80 to 100 sharp pointed teeth that interlock similar to those of the True Gharial.

The primary differences between the True Gharial and the False Gharial are in the body shape, nesting method, and world location. The False Gharial has a heavier and stouter body conformation, whereas the True Gharial is much slimmer in body conformation. The narial excrescence of the mature male Gharial does not occur in the False Gharial male. The sizes of mature males and females of both species are similar, with males reaching approximately 4 m in length (13 feet) and females attaining a length between 2 and 2.5 m (8 feet).

The coloration of the False Gharial is also much darker, with broad black bands, than the more northern counterpart. The False Gharial is a mound nester (rather than a hole nester like the True Gharial) and after laying eggs leaves the nest completely unguarded. This species shows no aggression and does not appear harmful to humans.

SKELETAL SYSTEM

The crocodilian skull is elongated and composed of 30 fused bones. All species of crocodilians have long, flattened, tooth-lined skulls of various sizes and shapes. Both upper and lower jaws have open-rooted teeth that are set in sockets via connective tissue. The upper and lower jaws articulate at the posterior aspect of the skull, which allows the wide opening of the jaws. The muscles that open the jaw, the depressor mandibular and the sternomandibularies, are quite weak, and therefore, the jaws can be held closed with a medium amount of effort (Figure 8-8). The muscles that close the jaws, the temporalis and the pterygoideus internus and externus, are very strong and close the jaws with extreme pressure. In adult animals, attempting to open the mouth can be dangerous because of this strength.[6] If one opens the mouth of an adult that has recently died, a point comes where the temporalis and the internus and the externus pterygoideus muscles are stimulated to close with tremendous force. The stimulatory effect may occur up to 24 hours after death.

The approximately 60 to 70 vertebrae consist of eight to nine cervical, 10 to 11 thoracic, four to five lumbar, 32 to 42 caudal, and two to three sacral. The distinction between the cervical, thoracic, and lumbar vertebrae is not clear, and disagreement is found among authorities about the exact points of change. Eight sets of true ribs and an additional eight pairs of gastralia or floating ribs are found. These are not true ribs but rather dermal bones in the ventral body wall superficial to the rectus abdominis muscles. The so-called sacral ribs are heavy bones that articulate with the transverse processes of the sacral vertebrae. A difference of opinion exists among authorities as to whether these are true ribs or merely thickened transverse processes. They are not fused to the vertebrae and so are frequently referred to as ribs. The pelvic girdle has a short ilium, a narrow pubis, and a short wide ischium. The front and hind limbs are anatomically similar to those of mammals and attach in an analogous fashion. The femur is longer than the humerus and holds the posterior portion of the body higher than the anterior. The front limbs have five digits with claws on the medial three digits, and the webbed hind limbs have four digits that are longer than the front limbs and also have claws on the medial three digits.

RESPIRATORY SYSTEM

The nostrils of all crocodilians are on a raised area at the end of their snouts and can be closed with muscular flaps when the animal submerges. The full development of a bony secondary palate is seen only in the crocodilians where the internal nostrils open at the back of the mouth in close proximity to the glottis. The glottis is the opening into the larynx from the pharynx. Valve-like flaps of tissue on the roof and floor of the mouth just in front of the internal nostrils and glottis enable the throat region to be sealed off from the oral cavity during submergence (Figure 8-9, *A, B*). This permits the animal to grab and hold prey underwater without drowning. The long nasal passage above the elongated palate allows air to pass through two openings in the pharynx, the posterior nasal choanae, and enter the trachea and lungs. The animal is also able to breathe via its nostrils even when the mouth is open and full of water. Water that is taken into the mouth can be swallowed but not inhaled.

The respiratory system is typical of most reptiles. Crocodilians have well-developed lungs located in the thoracic cavity. Air can be held in the lungs for an extended period by closure of the glottic valve, allowing submersion for extended periods. The lungs are nonlobulated and

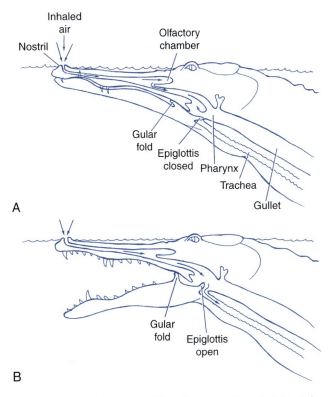

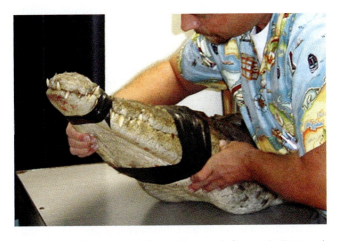

FIGURE 8-8 The jaws can be easily taped shut to facilitate safe handling. *(Photograph courtesy D. Mader.)*

FIGURE 8-9 A and **B,** Crocodilians have an anatomic fold at the back of the mouth, the gular fold, that allows the animal to breathe even when its mouth is open under water. The throat flap keeps water out of the lungs, enabling swallowing of food under water.

highly vascularized. Crocodilians are dependent on their lungs for respiration and gas exchange. Each lung is enclosed in the thoracic cavity and has a large surface area for oxygen and carbon dioxide exchange. Respiration is accomplished with the intercostal muscles and the diaphragm. Some disagreement exists about how long crocodilians can stay submerged. Factors such as animal size, the water and air temperature, amount of food in the stomach, and metabolic rate all have a bearing on the time any one individual animal can stay submerged.[7]

Crocodilians are well suited for their aquatic lifestyle. They have the ability to float in the water with just their nostrils and eyes above the surface. The elevated nostrils allow them to stay just below the surface of the water for great periods of time. The rate and depth of respiration increase with activity and metabolism. The American Alligator is reported to have a respiratory rate of 2.5 to 3 breaths per minute at rest at 28°C.

CIRCULATORY SYSTEM

Crocodilians are the only reptiles with a four-chamber heart (see Figure 10-5). Complete separation is seen of both the left and right atria and the left and right ventricles. The ventricular septum contains a small foramen (foramen of Panizza). This foramen is a high septal opening that connects the right and left aortic trunks and permits the mixture of oxygenated and deoxygenated blood. Crocodilians can make an adjustment in peripheral blood flow in response to being submerged for extended periods of time.

The foramen of Panizza permits the mixture of the right ventricular and left ventricular blood on the basis of the pressure in the left ventricle. When the animal is breathing, the left ventricle pressure is greater than the right ventricle pressure. A small amount of blood may go from the left side to the right side, but this is likely of no consequence. When the animal is submerged, the pressure in the lungs produces pulmonary hypertension and decreases the flow of blood to the lungs. This produces an increase in right ventricular pressure. This increase in right ventricular pressure causes the "opening" of the foramen and allows ventricular blood to enter the abdominal aorta. When the animal returns to the surface, the return of normal ventilation causes the reduction in the pressure in the lungs and in the right ventricle. This reduction allows the foramen to close so that only blood from the left ventricle enters both branches of the aorta. This mechanism apparently allows crocodilians to remain submerged for extended periods. By remaining inactive and using anaerobic metabolism, the lack of oxygen can be tolerated for as much as 5 or 6 hours.[8]

Crocodilian circulation and hemodynamics are difficult to determine in vivo. Therefore, much of the information regarding circulation is a result of physiologic models, dissections, and theory. Determination of borderline chemistries is also difficult on restrained animals and impossible on submerged animals under natural conditions. The theory is that the foramen of Panizza allows blood from the right ventricle to enter the left ventricle and be diverted to the abdominal aorta and this supposedly diverts deoxygenated blood from the lungs to non-oxygen-sensitive areas such as the stomach and liver. The oxygenated blood returning from the lungs to the left side of the heart is directed to the brain and heart, which are more oxygen sensitive. To date, no one has quantified the amount of blood that is shunted or the physiologic mechanism that regulates the foramen.

Crocodilian heart rates are slow and are temperature dependent. The rate at 10°C is 1 to 8 times per minute; at 18°C, 15 to 20 times per minute; and at 28°C, 24 to 40 times per minute. At 34°C, a wide variation in heart rate occurs. Irreversible cardiac damage occurs above 40°C.

NERVOUS SYSTEM

Crocodilians have small brains that account for less than 0.5% of their total body weight. The dorsal roots of the first two spinal nerves are absent but do occur on the remaining spinal nerves. The spinal cord of crocodilians extends almost to the tip of the tail. The dorsal and ventral caudal nerves leave the spinal cord in the same way as the body trunk nerves because of no cauda equina.[6]

Eye

Crocodilians are visually oriented and have eyes that are well suited for both day and night vision. Because the eyes are located high and lateral on the head, the eyes, like the nostrils, remain above the surface of the water when the animal is submerged. The eyes of caimans and alligators are more prominent than those of crocodiles. The bony orbits of the skull surround the eyes, and if the eyes are pressed, they sink into the orbit. Frequently, when handling large crocodilians, tape over the eyes and around the mouth is prudent. This lack of vision causes disorientation in the animal and stops movement and fighting.

The lateral placement of the eyes of crocodilians means that the anterior binocular vision is not well developed. In the American Alligator, the eyes are oriented to permit 25 degrees of binocular vision.[7] However, when working with large crocodilians in a capture environment, approach directly from the front is advisable and somewhat safer whenever feasible. The lack of binocular vision means that the defensive mechanism for the animal is better adapted to lateral approaches. In an approach on any crocodilian from the side, the rapid defensive movement of the head and tail is directed in the same direction, with an attempt to strike the individual with the head, tail, or both.

Crocodilians have a vertical slit-like pupil. This pupil dilates in a medial-lateral direction, and this pupil position remains vertical with the horizon even when the head is raised or lowered. It is postulated that when the animal is turned over on its back, it becomes disoriented because of this particular eye configuration. The muscles of the eye, the superior rectus, interior rectus, the internal rectus, and the inferior oblique serve to allow retraction of the eye into the orbit when the animal is threatened. Almost all crocodilians use vision to capture prey that is out of the water, but such vision under the water is limited and other sensations are used.

Crocodilian eyes, with more rods than cones, are well adapted for night vision. The tapetum lucidum is well developed; thus, one is able to locate the animals at night when a spotlight is used. The eyelids and nictitating membrane are well developed. The nictitating membrane is clear and covers the eye when the animal is under water. The degree of vision under water for crocodilians is unknown.

Apparently, crocodilians are able to recognize prey on land and in the water, their hatchlings, their environment, specific nests, and people. In alligator breeding houses, the daily caretaker is recognized as one individual. When two people enter the premises or when a strong vocalization occurs, such as people talking, the animals then become nervous and dive into the water or crowd into corners.

Crocodiles also possess a highly developed sense of smell. The raised nostrils at the end of the snout suggest an evolutionary dependence on the olfactory sense. Odor sensing likely has a role in food location. Olfactory nerve endings are located in the anterior end of the nasal cavity. The role of food odor in the raising and farming of crocodilians is unknown. Likewise, the effect of glandular secretions on animals in captivity or in the wild has not been thoroughly investigated.

Ear

The external auditory meatus are slit-like openings that are closed by a fibrous flap and are protected by a dorsal shelf of bone (Figure 8-10, A, B). The fibrous flap serves to close the external opening when the animal submerges. The middle ear is separated from the external ear by a tympanic membrane. Crocodilians have a well-developed hearing mechanism. They have only one bone in the middle ear, the stapes, that conducts sound to the inner ear.[6] How well crocodilians hear underwater is unknown and difficult to determine, but some of their behavior patterns suggest that they do hear when submerged. The possibility also exists that sounds and vibrations are detected underwater by the integumentary sense organs (ISO) located in the scales. The ability of crocodilians to detect sounds above water is well developed. A variety of sounds are used by crocodilians, such as grunts by hatchlings and hissing or snarling sounds when threatened. A characteristic bellowing sound is used during the mating season. Evidence of this is found in their behavior when strange sounds occur and in their ability to respond to vocalizations at specific times, such as the breeding season or when hatchlings are in the nest. It is not unusual for females to become disturbed when hatchlings are stimulated to make grunting sounds.

Homing Instinct

Crocodilians possess the homing ability or orientation to return home, but some limitation exists to the distance interval. This type of behavior is important in farm situations when animals raised in an area escape from the ponds. Frequently, when animals have been raised in captivity and then escape, they return to the area. Animals that have been brought into captivity from the wild, especially young adults, attempt to leave and return to their previous habitat. Homing has been studied in the American Alligator, the Saltwater Crocodile, the Spectacled Caiman, and the Freshwater Crocodile. Webb and associates[9] documented that the *C. johnstoni* was capable of returning to its habitat after being moved upstream a distance of 19 miles. After 15 months, from a group of 17 translocated animals, seven were located at the original capture site and one was midway between the capture site and the release site. None were at the release site.[9]

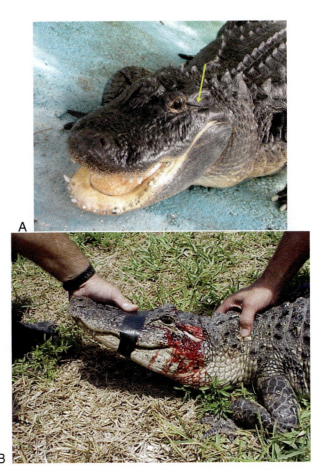

FIGURE 8-10 A, Crocodilians have a fibrous flap that covers the external ear opening when the animal submerges. **B,** The ear flap on this alligator was avulsed after an encounter with an automobile. *(Photographs courtesy D. Mader.)*

DIGESTIVE SYSTEM

Crocodilians are carnivorous predators, and their diet is variable depending on the species and the habitat. In the natural setting, crocodilians cease feeding at temperatures below 25°C or above 35°C. In farming operations, the temperatures are maintained in grow-out houses to encourage feeding and an active metabolic rate. The digestive system of crocodilians consists of the oral cavity, oropharynx, esophagus, stomach, small intestine, large intestine, colon, and cloaca.

The teeth of crocodilians are of a conical shape and are similar in their shape and size. Each tooth resides in a socket in the jawbone and is attached by connective tissue. Radiologic studies have indicated that each tooth has a life span of about 2 years and is lost as replacement teeth emerge. The replacement tooth develops from the germinal tissue in the tooth socket and migrates through the cylinder space of the mature tooth that is eventually dislodged. In aged animals, a permanent loss of some teeth may occur. The teeth and jaws of crocodilians are strong and are designed for grasping and tearing of prey. No provision is made for chewing or grinding of food. Tooth replacement decreases with the increasing age of the animal.

The tongue is attached to the floor of the mouth along the entire ventral surface, thereby preventing any protrusion of the organ. The posterior margin of the tongue is elevated into a large transverse fold that serves to partially shut off the oral cavity from the pharynx. Two large transverse folds (velum palatinum) from the bony palate between the oral cavity and the pharynx meet the transverse fold from the base of the tongue and serve to completely separate the oral cavity from the pharynx. Swallowing is accomplished by raising the snout after food is in the mouth. The tongue, because it is firmly attached to the mouth floor, has no part in moving food into the esophagus. The esophagus is a distensible organ with longitudinal folds of mucous epithelium and terminates at the cardiac sphincter of the stomach.

The crocodilian stomach is divided into two distinct regions, the corpus and the pars phylorica. The distinction is clear as the corpus forms the area that is comparable with an avian gizzard. This corpus or cardiac region also contains numerous glands that secrete mucus into the stomach. A thick collar of muscle and spongy tissue appears to serve as the gizzard and together with gastroliths is responsible for grinding the food into small particles in preparation for passage into the pyloris region.[10] The gastroliths or gizzard stones are a universal finding in large crocodilians in the wild. In farm-raised animals, foreign objects are seldom found in the highly muscular portion that serves to grind food. The stomach has a high acidic secretion and is capable of digesting the wide variety of dietetic materials consumed by the animal. Crocodilians swallow their food without chewing; therefore, the gizzard portion of the stomach serves a vital need in digestion. The stomach is separated from the small intestine by the thick pyloric sphincter.

The stomach has the most acidic environment of any vertebrate, which allows for the efficient digestion of the unchewed food. According to Coulson and Hernandez,[11] crocodilians have shifts in plasma pH levels on a frequent basis. They state that because of the high production of concentrated hydrochloric acid in the stomach, a shift of chloride ion from the plasma leaves a large amount of sodium to react with plasma carbonic acid. This results in large amounts of sodium bicarbonate, and they refer to this as the alkaline tide. Thus, a profound plasma alkalemia in crocodilians is associated with food ingestion. Digestion in the high-acid environment of the stomach must be highly efficient because mastication is minimal and whole segments or pieces of food are ingested. Appetite in crocodilians depends to a great extent on the environmental temperature. The most efficient temperatures for ingestion and digestion are between 25°C and 35°C. American Alligators in farm-raised conditions have been observed to not eat when the temperature is lower than 22°C. Temperatures above 35°C cause an undue amount of stress in crocodilians and cause inappetence as well.

The small intestine is supported by a dorsal mesentery, which also contains the spleen and ends at the ileocolic sphincter. The large intestine, although short, has a diameter at least two times the diameter of the small intestine. It is separated from the small intestine by the ileocolic sphincter and from the cloaca by a thick anal sphincter. The liver is divided into two lobes, and the gallbladder is contiguous with the liver. Three hepatic ducts join to form the common bile duct. The anus is the opening of the large intestine to the cloaca. The cloaca is the termination of the digestive, urinary, and genital system. The cloaca is divided into three chambers: the coprodeum, or anterior portion, is where the large intestine empties and feces are collected; the urodeum, the middle area, is the area of duct openings and the attachment of the penis; and the proctodeum, the posterior area, serves as the collection area for digestive and excretory waste before discharge. The cloaca opens externally through the longitudinal vent.

INTEGUMENTARY SYSTEM

The skin of all species of crocodilians is composed of separate, rough, leather-like scales. The separate scales are joined by elastic connective tissue. The skin on the head is fused tightly to the underlying bony skull. The dorsal hide is cornified and lies above bony plates (see Figure 8-2). Some crocodilian scales may appear to overlap, but they are distinct structures that form a continual epidermis. The skin of the back on the dorsal side of crocodilians is heavily cornified and has bony plates or osteoderms underneath. This part of the skin is not desirable in the leather trade. The lateral and ventral body covering are the areas of the skin that are used for manufacturing leather.

Each species has characteristic scales. The scales just posterior to the occipital area and the scales over the nuchal area are different to a greater or lesser degree for each species. The arrangement and number of scales or scutes is important in species identification. The tail has a double row of triangular scales that merge into a single row midway of the length. Two species of caimans and four species of crocodiles have bony plates in the ventral abdominal scales, which makes these skins of low economic value; therefore, they are not farmed or raised commercially to any extent.

Crocodilians possess two glands on the underside of the jaw for which the purpose is unclear. Also, two glands in the cloaca emit a musk-type odor. The excretion of these cloaca musk glands is likely used for mating and possibly defense.[12]

The crocodilian skin contains chromatophores or pigment cells. Skin color varies from black to gray to light brown or off green depending on the species. The abdominal and lateral sides tend to be lighter than the back and head. Hatchlings and young juveniles may have bands of light coloration, but this tends to disappear in adults. The ISO occur in the scales of all members of the Crocodylinae and Gavialinae families but are absent in the Alligatorinae. The purpose of the ISO is not definitely known, but it is theorized that they serve a sensory purpose related to underwater vibrations.

REPRODUCTIVE SYSTEM

Female

The ovaries of female crocodilians are located internally at the anteromedial border of each kidney. Each ovary is suspended by the mesovarium and is a solid, flat, convoluted gland with an inner medullary area composed of connective tissue, blood and lymphatic vessels, smooth muscle, and nerve fibers. The oviduct consists of the ostium, a muscular portion, an isthmus, and a uterine segment. The ostium is the funnel-like opening to the oviduct and is located anterior to the ovary. The muscular position is slightly convoluted with alveolar glands and ciliated columnar epithelium. The isthmus is much less glandular and muscular. The uterine segment consists of columnar epithelium with both muscular and glandular tissue. The oviducts in crocodilians are generally long to accommodate the large number of eggs. The oviducts open close together through the ventral wall of the posterior cloaca just anterior to the clitoris. The clitoris is similar in appearance to the penis but smaller.

Male

In the male crocodilian, the testes are elongated thin glands covered by a thick tunic and are suspended at the medial border of each kidney by the mesorchium. They lie on each side of the postcaval vein. The ductus vas deferens extend from the posterior end of the testes to the ventral surface of the cloaca where they open at the base of the penis. The penis is located on the ventroposterior surface of the cloaca near the vent. The dorsal surface of the penis has a single open groove that serves for conduction of spermatozoa. The penis is not elongated significantly during copulation. Two thick fibrous plates, the crus penis, are located at the base of the penis. The penile groove is the result of the fusion of the crus penis. The penis is primarily cartilaginous and has little erectile tissue (Figure 8-11). The penile groove is lined with cavernous tissue and the engorgement of this tissue may serve to move semen along the penile groove during copulation. Two accessory ducts are located bilaterally just distal to the fusion of the crus penis. The emission of accessory duct fluid during engorgement of the erectile tissue suggests a contribution to semen volume and sperm transport. The structure of the penis provides for sealing the cloaca when spermatozoa and accessory duct fluid are released at the openings of the oviducts.

REPRODUCTIVE ACTIVITY

Female

The reproductive cycle of most crocodilians is similar. The time of year and length of various stages of the reproductive cycle are somewhat variable depending on the species, habitat, and hemisphere of location. The reproductive cycle of the American Alligator has received considerable investigation in Florida and Louisiana and is used here to illustrate cyclic activity. Captive female alligators are capable of reproduction at 7 years of age. Females in the wild are reported to begin laying eggs at approximately 10 years of age. The development of the ovarian cycle in adult female alligators occurs once each year between March and May in the Northern Hemisphere. The introduction of reproductive activity is mediated via the pituitary hormones: follicle-stimulating hormone (FSH) and luteinizing hormone (LH). Stimulation of the pituitary gland results in an increase in gonadotropin hormone, which acts on the ovary. The increase in ovarian activity consists of follicular growth and an increase in estradiol and testosterone production. Vitellogenin, the yolk precursor protein, is produced as a result of the secretion of pituitary gonadotropin. Blood plasma collected from female alligators at this time of year has a characteristic white appearance as a result of the circulating vitellogenin.[13,14]

After activation of the ovary by FSH, the ovary produces estrogen, which is necessary for vitellogenesis. Vitellogenin travels via the vascular system to the developing follicles and is converted into yolk. The process of vitellogenesis results in the accumulation of yolk in preovulatory follicles. Yolk is a complex of protein, phospholipid, and fat within the ovum, which sustains the embryo during development. After ovulation, the plasma loses the white appearance and is similar to the plasma of males and nonreproductive females.

In the alligator, a hierarchy of follicle groups develops, with each group representing a clutch. The clutch to be fertilized may contain as few as 20 follicles or as many as 80 follicles. Approximately 40 eggs per clutch is considered an average and is most frequently reported. The stimulus for pituitary activity has been the subject of much study and speculation. The environmental conditions considered to be the stimulating factors that cause the initiation of pituitary activity are an increase in day length and an increase in water temperature in the Northern Hemisphere.

Observations support the concept that extraretinal photoreceptors may constitute part of an integrated photoendocrine system. Increasing day length in synergy with increasing water temperature is believed necessary for reproductive synchronization.

Another important factor in the reproductive capability of the female is diet. Dietary inadequacies or vitamin and mineral deficiencies adversely affect the ability of the female crocodilian to respond to pituitary stimulation and ovarian activity. Alligators and most of the crocodilian species go through a refractory period after ovulation. (An exception to this is the Indian Mugger [*Crocodylus palustris*], which produces two clutches per year under natural conditions.)

Evidence of the postovulatory refractory period exists because attempts to induce follicle development and ovulation with gonadotropin hormones have been unsuccessful. Likely both a reduced photoperiod and a decrease in water temperature are necessary for a variable period of time to enable the system to be responsive.

Male

Spermatogenesis occurs within the seminiferous tubules of the testes. Before the breeding season, the testes increase in vascularity. In the Northern Hemisphere, the production of spermatozoa begins in March, reaches a peak in mid-April to

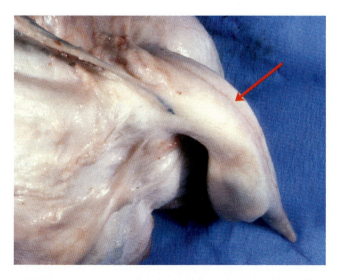

FIGURE 8-11 The ventral groove of the copulatory organ of the American Alligator (*Alligator mississippiensis*). Cartilaginous crura converge to form the groove.

mid-May, and ends in July. During the latter part of June, spermatogenesis is declining and connective tissue forms between the seminiferous tubules. By July, the seminiferous tubules are inactive and the testes are decreased in size. The testes remain in this regressed state until the following year. No evidence exists of prolonged sperm storage in crocodilians. The same factors that stimulate the female also affect the male. The increase in ambient temperatures and photoperiods is considered necessary for the initiation of the spermatogenic cycle on an annual basis.

Behavior During Reproduction

Crocodilians display advanced behavior patterns during the mating season. For most species, courtship behavior is extremely strong and dramatic over an extended period of time. The increased behavioral activity of the American Alligator has been described by Vliet.[15]

The two activities that are most observable in crocodilians are roaring or bellowing and head slapping (Figure 8-12). These displays are considered to be an important method of communication among members of a group. Such activities are increased dramatically during the breeding season; for both animals in the wild and those in farm ponds. Animals in zoos or close confinement pens only occasionally demonstrate such activity.

In breeding ponds or the wild habitat, the bellowing of one individual serves to stimulate the bellowing of others. This is most noticeable during the courting and breeding season. Both males and females engage in the bellowing and head-slapping performance. This behavior has been postulated as serving to synchronize some group activity and as indicating size and sex of members within the group. During a bellowing sequence, the animal holds its head above water and the tail is arched out of the water.

Mating

The female crocodilian must mate during the breeding season each year for fertilization to occur. The storage of spermatozoa does not occur. The greatest activity involving courtship and copulation occurs in the early morning hours. This is in contrast to the act of nest building and egg deposition that most often occurs during the nighttime.

Copulation follows the intense physical contacts displayed during the courtship period. The male approaches the female from behind and moves up over her body. Once mounted, the male must roll to one side to bring the base of his tail in juxtaposition with that of the female. When in the cloaca, the shaft of the penis is arched with the glans projecting posterior with the penile groove situated along the convex side of the arch. In the Northern Hemisphere, mating occurs during the latter part of May and early June. Multiple copulatory acts within a short period of time may occur.

Nesting and Egg Laying

Some species of crocodilians deposit their egg clutch in excavated holes, and others build mounds of surrounding vegetation. Crocodilian eggs contain the embryo, yolk, and albumen and are enclosed in shells that are incubated outside of the body. Females in the process of laying eggs become relatively docile. On completion of the egg-laying process, the female may become extremely broody and guard the nest (Figure 8-13, A, B).[16] The aggressiveness displayed by females at the nest site is extremely variable among individuals and among species. Egg collection from nests on farming and ranching operations is a common procedure.

After laying, the embryo orients toward the top of the egg. If a crocodilian egg is rotated after the embryo has attached to the yolk, a high propensity exists for early embryonic death. The critical period for egg handling is between day 1 and 15 after laying. For this reason, egg collectors always mark eggs on the top as they remove them from the nest. The period necessary for incubation of eggs is related to the temperature. In areas where temperatures are lower, the hatching of eggs requires a longer period of time. Average incubation time ranges from 40 to 100 days depending on the species and hemisphere.

Gender Determination

Crocodilian gender determination is not dependent on sex chromosomes. Temperature-dependent sex determination (TDSD) is now a well-established phenomenon in crocodilians. By the alteration of the temperature of eggs during incubation, the gender can be determined. TDSD has been shown in six species of crocodilians, and likely the same principle will be proven in the other species because they all lack sex chromosomes.

Temperature-dependent sex determination was first reported in the American Alligator in 1982.[17] The incubation temperature range is 28°C to 34°C. Temperatures greatly above 34°C result in a high proportion of embryonic deaths. In all species, when the incubation temperature is low (28°C to 30°C), the results are all females of the species. In the Common Caimans (*Caiman crocodilus*) and the American Alligator, males result from incubation temperatures of 32°C to 34°C. In crocodiles, the production of females predominates at temperatures of 33°C to 34°C. Male crocodiles predominate between 31°C and 33°C (Figure 8-14). The period of temperature sensitivity begins early in the embryonic development and continues throughout the first half of the incubation period. The small differences of 0.5°C to 1°C have a direct bearing on gender

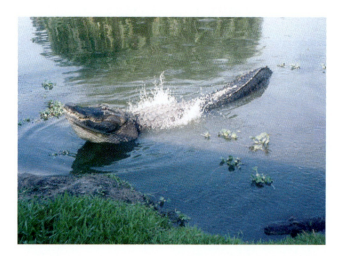

FIGURE 8-12 Bellowing and head slapping is a common activity at the beginning of the mating season and is shown by raising of the head and tail in this characteristic fashion.

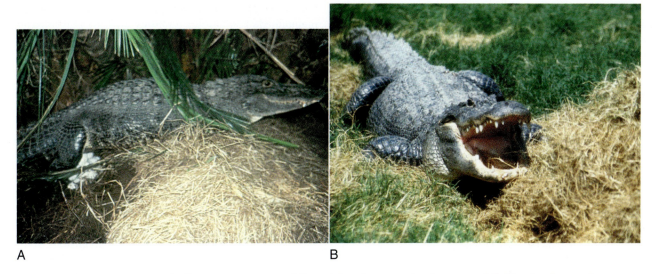

FIGURE 8-13 A, Female alligators prepare nests of dirt and decaying vegetation above ground. **B,** Most females guard their nests and stay in the vicinity until hatching occurs. Each nest may contain between 20 and 70 eggs, 50 to 90 mm in length. They hatch in approximately 65 days aided by heat generated by decaying vegetation making up the nest.

determination. In the wild populations, the climatic conditions in any given year combined with the next selection site have a great bearing on the sex of hatchlings that emerge from the nest (Figure 8-15). Specific temperature regulation is not yet a common practice on crocodile and alligator farms where eggs are collected for artificial incubation.

Birth Defects

Although birth defects do occur in any species, less available information is found regarding crocodilian birth defects, likely because of the almost certain mortality in most instances. The American Alligator, because of the large commercial production farms, has supplied the most information regarding birth defects. Serious birth defects include spina bifida, scoliosis, hydrocephalus, microphthalmia, and limb abnormalities.

A number of contributing factors can cause these defects and developmental malformations. Also, a higher percentage of birth defects is documented in the eggs from very young and older females. This is not unusual as this occurs in many species.

The factors that likely contribute to these defects include environmental conditions during egg incubation and maternal diet during the egg development stage. Female alligators fed a primarily fish diet have been reported to have more birth defects than those females that are fed a red meat diet. This is the result of the fish diet being deficient in vitamin E, a fat-soluble vitamin, and also a deficiency of trace minerals.

Nesting or incubation temperatures that are at the extreme ranges can also contribute to malformations. The result may be early embryonic death in the egg, hatchlings that hatch and are unable to survive, or a hatchling that survives but lacks the ability to grow and is stunted.

Mark W.J. Ferguson[17] has reported that incubation temperature does affect pigmentation patterns in American Alligators. Those incubated at 33°C have one extra stripe when compared with those incubated at 30°C. Ferguson has done

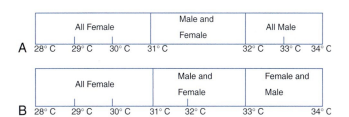

FIGURE 8-14 Temperature-dependent sex determination. **A,** Caiman and alligator eggs incubated at low temperatures produce females, and the upper extreme of incubation temperature results in males. A gradient of 31°C to 32°C results in production of both genders. **B,** Crocodiles follow the same pattern in the lower incubation range with females. At a high temperature range, some male production occurs, but predominance is with females. The opposite is true for the midrange, where males predominate over females.

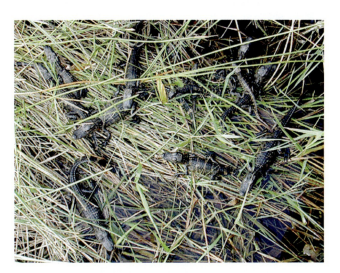

FIGURE 8-15 In wild populations, climatic conditions in any given year combined with nest selection site have great bearing on the gender of hatchlings that emerge from the nest.

extensive work with alligator embryos and reports that the alligator embryo is much more easily manipulated than mammalian embryos. Thus, they make good models for biomedical research in areas of sex determination, embryonic development, and certain birth defects.

LOCOMOTION

All crocodilians are well adapted for both an aquatic environment and a land environment. In the water, the limbs are carried against the body for efficiency but may be used to change direction. The tail, with its large muscle mass, is flattened laterally and is the main organ of propulsion in the water through lateral movement.

The limbs of most crocodilians are relatively small in relation to the size of their body. However, with the exception of the Gharial, these limbs are very effective for movement, which means that these animals can travel effectively on land and in the water. On land, as quadrupeds, crocodilians are capable of walking upright on all four legs. Three modes of land travel have been described: the high walk, the gallop, and the belly run.

In the high walk, the animal straightens the legs with its body completely off the ground and then strides in a leisurely fashion. Usually in this position, the posterior portion of the tail remains in contact with the ground as the animal moves. The hind legs appear to carry most of the weight. This mode of movement is usually used when the animal is exiting from water onto land or when moving on land. The animal does not move rapidly in this position but can traverse considerable distances.

The gallop is used for bursts of speed over short distances. In this movement, the reptile uses its front limbs to push forward and brings the hind limbs forward under the body. Most crocodilians are capable of great bursts of speed but only for a short distance. The exception to this is the Gharial, which has weak legs and can only move on land by crawling on its abdomen.

The belly run is commonly seen when the animal desires to move rapidly in an escape mode. The animal moves from side to side on its abdomen while making rapid rowing movements with its limbs. This type of movement is most commonly seen when crocodilians are entering water or going down steep banks. This movement is also used when the animal slips quietly into the water.

Juvenile and young adult crocodilians of many species are also capable of climbing. Instances of animals climbing as much as a 1-m fence have been recorded. This is especially so when young adults are captured in the wild, brought into captivity, and placed in a confined area.

The front feet have five toes, the inner three of which are clawed. The front limbs are smaller than the hind limbs. The hind feet have four webbed toes; the inner three toes are clawed. Although the hind feet are webbed, they are not used for swimming. When the crocodilian is startled, it can move the hind feet in a forward and upward pattern that causes the animal to go silently backward in a dive beneath the surface. Crocodilians are able to dive and stay underwater for long periods. They are also capable of moving underwater without causing surface disturbances. Therefore, the number of animals should be accounted for if people are going to be in the water of ranch and farm ponds where adult animals are maintained.

IDENTIFICATION

Identification of individual animals in a group of captive crocodilians is frequently advantageous. The use of collars, bands, or tattoos is considered unsatisfactory in most instances because collars and bands are frequently lost from the activity of the animals. The use of tattoos and banding is painful to the animal and produces enormous stress. Also, these marks tend to be of short duration even while disfiguring the animal.

Many farms and ranches use digit clipping or tags, tail notching, head tags, and microchips to identify individual animals (Figure 8-16, *A-D*). In present circumstances, digit clipping and tail notching are usually considered unsatisfactory. These procedures are painful and have the potential to cause infections. Also, the disfigurement of the animal is not desirable for animals on public display. These procedures can be accomplished correctly in young animals but are not always readily observable in adults.

Tags

Tags are commonly used for identification. Toe tags are used for hatchling alligators and crocodiles and are placed on the web of a hind foot. These are good only for a limited time, up to 1 year, and are frequently lost. The use of swine ear tags has been accomplished in the dorsal area of the mid-tail of larger animals. Although animals can be identified, they must be out of water to do so. The tags can also be lost or bitten off by other animals.

Another method that has been successfully used on some farms is the placement of a tag on the head. This method was devised and originated by the author for easy identification of animals in attractions and farm situations. The numbered half of the common swine tag can be attached to the head by passing a stainless steel surgical wire around the jugal bone midway between the eye and the auditory meatus. The jugal bones are elongated bones that form the lateral borders of the orbits. Each forms a part of the postorbital bar that separates the orbit from the lateral temporal fossa. The advantage of this method is that the tags are inexpensive, easily attached, and visible from a distance of 10 to 20 ft. The variety of tag colors allows the left or right side of the head to be used, depending on parameters of gender, clutch group, or age. The disadvantage of the head-tagging method is that the wire must be securely fastened or the tags come off. Also, if the wire is too tight, the jugal bone is weakened and scarred.

Transponders

The use of implanted microchip transponders offers a more expensive but satisfactory method of identification. The author has used microchips successfully in a group of alligators, which were still effective more than 1 year later. The main disadvantage of the transponder is that the scanner must be within a few centimeters of the microchip. The transponder is implanted with a needle in the 12-gauge range. The most satisfactory area for implantation is just

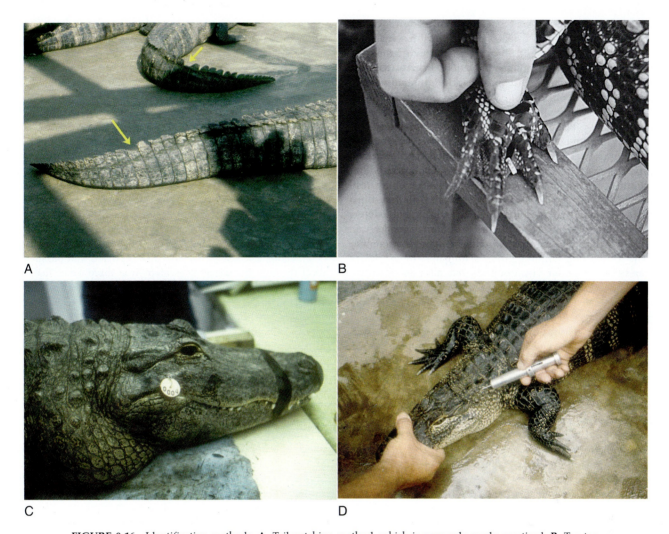

FIGURE 8-16 Identification methods. **A,** Tail-notching method, which is now only rarely practiced. **B,** Toe tag, which is satisfactory for hatchlings and young reptiles. **C,** Head tag, which can be used in young adults and larger crocodilians. Head tags allow identification even when the animals are in water. **D,** Microchips (transponders) are implanted with a 12-gauge needle. The most satisfactory area for implantation is just posterior to the dorsal plate of the head.

posterior to the dorsal plate of the head. These transponders have not been approved by the United States Food and Drug Administration for use in food animals, and some crocodilians are raised specifically for meat and hides. The application of hot branding or freeze branding on the jaw or the head has not proved to be satisfactory in crocodilians.

BEHAVIORS

Crocodilian behavior has fascinated man for several centuries. This can be attested to by the great variety of legends and myths about alligators and crocodiles that persist even today. Many of these myths are a result of partial fact and assumptive observation over a period of time. Much of this information, though incorrect, has affected the way the general public has feared and, therefore, treated crocodilians in the past.[2,18]

Animals in the wild are shy and elusive and difficult to study. Much of what is currently known about crocodilian behavior is based on the studies and observations of captive animals in artificial or seminatural environments. These animals seem to have a great array of behaviors even though they also exhibit extensive periods of inactivity.

Most of this information has been generated within the last 25 years and is a result of the widespread effort in population management and species conservation. Although all adult crocodilians are considered solitary predators, a complex set of behaviors is inherent to ectotherms. Factors that affect the type and degree of behavior are age, size, habitat, food source, season of year, and population density. Behaviors such as vocalization, aggressiveness, movement, dominance or submissiveness, and thermoregulation are all shown, depending on the previous factors.

Movements in and out of water are primarily for heat seeking or heat avoidance. This thermal regulatory mechanism is well developed in hatchlings and young crocodilians. These animals tend to form social groups, and no evidence is found of social dominance such as occurs in older animals.

Young crocodilians prefer to hide under any available cover, and in captivity, this causes them to pile together in groups in corners of the pens. In certain instances, this may result in suffocation or drowning of young hatchlings.

For this reason, special consideration is given to construction of pens and enclosures on crocodilian farms and public displays. An increased interest has been seen in the construction of round pens for the production of farm-raised crocodilians, and this has in many instances lessened the mortality of the young animals.

Alligators and caimans are much more vocal than most of the crocodile species. Hatchlings in all species are noted for their characteristic grunting, which appears to be a contact call. This grunting activity is a response to any stimulus and may also occur spontaneously.

Communication has been reported to begin in the egg. Eggs of both *A. mississippiensis* and *C. acutus* responded to sounds coming from nearby eggs during the last 2 weeks of incubation. Such communication has been theorized to help to synchronize the hatching of the entire clutch.

The social order within a group of alligators or crocodiles depends not only on vocal sounds but also on postures, odors, and physical contact. Some behaviors such as territorial dominance and courtship displays are somewhat species specific. Parental care at hatching and posthatching are universal traits in the wild. In captivity, however, some species such as *A. mississippiensis* become accustomed to repeated approaches to the nest and do not display a protective behavior. *C. porosus* is reported to aggressively defend the nest at all times.

THERMOREGULATION IN CROCODILES

The thermoregulatory mechanism is fairly well developed in crocodilians. This is true even for very young hatchlings. Crocodilians are considered ectotherms or poikilotherms, which refers to the fact that external sources of heat regulate their body temperature.

Behavior is the primary method that they use to control body temperatures. Studies indicate that heat exchange is influenced by heat conduction in the water and solar radiation in the air. Water is important because it serves as a heat reservoir and as a cooling medium. Methods of body temperature regulation are accomplished both in water and on land through heat-seeking or heat-avoidance behavior.

Significant differences are seen in the body temperatures of different species, and this accounts for changes in some behavior. As an example, alligators in temperate climates have a different thermal selection method than those species of crocodilians that are native to more tropical areas of the world. In captivity, the animals select the temperature best suited to their needs at any particular time.[19]

Thermophile or heat seeking occurs in all crocodilians after feeding. This increase in body temperature apparently benefits the animal by increasing the rate of digestion and absorption. The thermoregulatory mechanism is influenced by both internal and external factors. Internal factors include age, size, nutritional status, and infection. External factors include climatic conditions, circadian rhythms, social interactions, and reproductive status. Even though environmental temperature has an influence on their body temperature, crocodilians select behavior that enhances their activity in relation to the environment.

Evidence also shows that the particular temperature of incubation of an embryo may have an effect on selected body temperature later in life. The temperature range between 25°C and 35°C appears to be the most suitable for crocodilians in captivity. In these situations, captive facilities must have a variety of thermal environments that allow the animal to regulate body temperature. Sufficient water, dry area, shade, and access to heat should be available to allow the animals to acclimate easily. Maintaining crocodilians at constant temperatures and not providing an environment for thermal selection can be hazardous to the health of the animals. Temperatures below 25°C cause a low metabolic rate, resulting in limited food intake and reduced growth. Temperatures that are constantly high can result in stress and fighting within the group.

Lang[20] has reported that when *A. mississippiensis* are fed, they select the warmer area to increase mean body temperature. When not fed, the same animals move to a cooler area of the environment for lower body temperature.

Coulson and Hernandez[11] reported that digestion and absorption took twice as long at 20°C as they did at 28°C in *A. mississippiensis*. Diefenbach[21] also reported that passage of food through the digestive system was three times faster at 30°C than at 15°C in *Caiman crocodilus*. This selection in body temperature differential appears to occur in captive *A. mississippiensis* hatchlings and juveniles when given the opportunity. Adults living in the wild or in outside captive facilities also display this selection process. They come out of the water to bask in the sun. At this time, they may lie with their jaws open in an effort to obtain evaporative cooling of the head (Figure 8-17). Heating and cooling are accomplished by entering and leaving the water. Temperature compensation is also accomplished by adjustment of the metabolic rate.

Thermal selection also appears important in the maintenance of immune status and disease control. New hatchlings and youngsters with infections seek higher temperatures. Exposure to constant high temperatures of 33°C and above causes weight loss unless the animal is able to feed readily. Cooler temperatures cause a decrease in immune status and inhibit the desire for food. The requirement for heat is greater in hatchlings and juveniles than in adults. An experimental infection reported by Lang[20] caused an increase in selected body temperature within a short time and returned to normal by day 4. Increases in body temperature ranged from +1.6°C to +7.8°C. None of the animals showed ill effects in growth or behavior as a result.

In another study, Glassman and Bennett[22] reported that *A. mississippiensis* subjected to an induced infection and held at constant temperatures responded to the infection with increased white blood cells. The animals were maintained at 25°C, 30°C, and 35°C. The animals held at 30°C displayed the greatest hematologic response and recovered. Infected animals held at 35°C succumbed within 3 weeks, which was attributed to the stress of high temperature and an ineffective immune response.

Behavioral fever, which has been reported in other reptile species, appears to be an important factor in survival. However, an adequate thermal gradient must be available for the optimum immune response, which is temperature dependent. When temperatures are maintained at a constant, the stress combined with a reduced antibody response can lead to stunted growth or a high mortality in the group.

OSMOREGULATION

All members of the crocodilian species possess salt-excretory lingual glands, even those that are freshwater inhabitants.

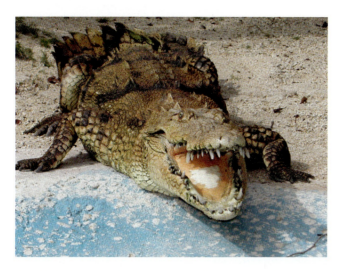

FIGURE 8-17 Crocodilians come out of the water to bask in the sun. They may lie with their jaws open in an effort to obtain evaporative cooling of the head. *(Photograph courtesy D. Mader.)*

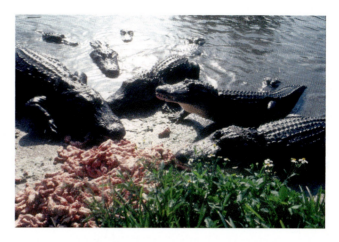

FIGURE 8-18 The diet of captive animals is highly variable, depending on the facility and the available food supply. Horse meat, beef, poultry, and nutria are potential food sources.

No totally marine species exist, but two species, the Saltwater Crocodile and the American Crocodile, are capable of spending a good deal of time in saltwater estuaries and are reported to travel great distances in the ocean. The lingual glands of members of Alligatorinae are much simpler in structure and have little ability to concentrate or secrete salt as compared with the other subfamilies.[23,24]

Periodic submergence in water is necessary for all crocodilians to counteract water loss. Water intake consists of incidental drinking and drinking when feeding. Water is also absorbed through the skin. Small crocodilians such as hatchlings and juveniles may lose up to 20% of body weight per day through dehydration. Daily movement between land and water is necessary to maintain the correct osmoregulation. Loss of sodium in fresh water is fairly low, and the main route of sodium loss is through the skin. Evaporative water loss occurs from the respiratory tract, the mouth, and the skin. The kidney and cloaca are the primary route for the excretion of nitrogenous waste but not for salt excretion. Some salt and water absorption is reported to occur in the cloaca. In dehydrated crocodilians, the nitrogen excretion occurs via uric acid. The kidneys are not able to regulate water and salt reabsorption.

The ability of crocodilians to tolerate saltwater is the result of their ability to retain water, the low rate of sodium absorption, and the sodium excretion ability. Alligators and caiman with their less-developed lingual glands are less tolerant of saltwater but can survive for a considerable time in a saltwater environment. This is probably because of their efficiency in regulation of water loss and sodium absorption.

Hatchling crocodilians of all species, because of their increased body surface in relation to body weight, are more susceptible to exposure to saltwater. Young crocodiles have a greater rate of water loss than larger crocodiles, and osmoregulation via behavior and movement between a dry and wet environment is especially important.

C. johnstoni and *C. niloticus* are noted for their ability to occupy esturine environments and spend time in saltwater. Apparently the salt-excreting lingual glands of these species are quite efficient. None of these estuarine species produce young in saltwater.

FEEDING AND NUTRITION

All crocodilians are indiscriminate carnivores that can consume live animals and carrion (Figure 8-18). In the wild environment, crocodiles and alligators are opportunistic hunters and efficient predators. Biochemical studies indicate that plant protein is not assimilated or digested. Most crocodilians are nocturnal in their native habitat.

Environmental temperature is also important in feeding behavior and the digestive process. Most crocodilians cease feeding when the temperature is below 25°C. The optimal feeding temperature is considered to be between 25°C and 35°C. When environmental temperature conditions become greater than 35°C, a stress is placed on the system and feeding is decreased. Prey size increases with age, and body size in relation to habitat.

Hatchling crocodilians' diet is primarily insects and a variety of small fishes. As the animals grow and become larger, the prey size increases and can include birds, larger fish, other reptiles, and even mammals for the larger adults. The American Alligator is reported to readily eat red meat, white meat, and fish. Switching from fish to red meat occurs quickly, but the reverse switch requires a period of fasting before the fish is accepted.[25]

Evolution has been generalized to have allowed the development of a narrow versus a broad snout based on the food availability in a particular natural environment. An example of this is the Gharial and the False Gharial with their narrow jaws designed for fish eating. However, studies of False Gharials feeding on primates suggest this generalization may not be valid.[26]

Digestion is temperature dependent to an extent and is compatible with the low metabolic rate. As the temperature increases, so does the metabolic rate. When food is plentiful and the animal can gorge itself, the digestive process may require 4 or 5 days. Many facilities with captive animals use a feeding regime of once or twice per week. In some alligator farming operations, this practice is used for breeding animals during the nonbreeding season. In farming operations where growth and production are of a primary concern, daily or every other day feeding schedules are more common.

Cannibalism has been reported both in wild animals and in captive situations. In the wild, such cannibalism is relatively rare as the number of captured animals with missing toes, legs, or tails is not great in comparison with the total number of animals. In captive situations, aggressive behavior and fighting are not uncommon if the animals are overcrowded. The ideal density, animals per square foot, has not been determined. Frequently, on farming operations, the densities are so great as to prevent adequate movement into and out of the water. In these situations, the fighting results in wounds and scars that decrease the value of the animal. In captive situations where animals are on public display, attention must be given to the total area and the number of animals that can be aesthetically contained.

Crocodilians are extremely efficient in the food conversion ratio. The highly acidic secretion of the stomach enables the digestion of a wide variety of protein materials. Most of the energy derived from digestion is stored as fat throughout the body. Fat stores include the tail, along the back, in the jowl area, and in the abdominal cavity. This fat storage capability allows the animal to survive, when necessary, for long periods without food.

In captive situations where animals are in a growth phase, the rate of growth can approach 0.3 m or more under the ideal environmental conditions. In the wild, this does not occur. Animals with good nutrition in grow-out facilities attain a length of 1.5 to 2 m between the second and third year of age. As animals attain a length of more than 2 m, the rate of growth decreases and the food conversion ratio increases.

The diet of captive animals is highly variable, depending on the facility and available food supply. In certain farming areas, nutria is used when available.[27,28] In other areas, horse meat, beef, and poultry are food sources. The crocodilian can use this material when it is not acceptable for human consumption. Other sources of food include fish offal and a commercially prepared pellet. The nutritional requirement of crocodilians in select environments or different stages of growth has not been well studied. Most feeding regimens and supplements are based on theoretic assumptions of the crocodilians' relationship to birds or to carnivorous animals. More work is necessary to determine the exact nutritional requirements of crocodilians.

RESTRAINT OF CROCODILIANS

The methods and requirements for the handling and restraint of crocodilians vary, depending on the size and the procedure to be accomplished. Animals from the hatchling stage up to 0.8 m can be physically restrained with one hand to hold the mouth closed and the other hand to control the lower body and tail. The muscles used to open the mouth are relatively weak, so the mouth is easily held closed (Figure 8-19). Gloves should be worn especially when handling crocodiles because the teeth that are exposed even when the jaws are closed can cause wounds to the handler. The tail must be controlled at all times to prevent vigorous lashing that is dangerous and can cause injury to the animal and to humans. In small animals, control can be maintained by grasping the head and cervical area if

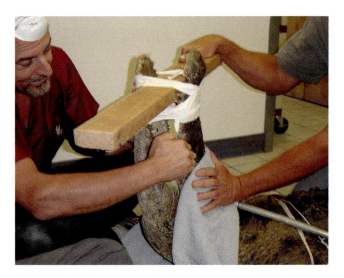

FIGURE 8-19 Proper restraint of the head of a crocodile. The snare restrains the head and neck while a strong, experienced handler sits on the animal's back. A bite block is placed in the mouth. The block and the jaws are taped securely. Finally, the eyes are covered to help calm the animal. *(Photograph courtesy G. Diethelm.)*

one wishes to examine the oral cavity. Animals between 1 and 3 m can be caught and handled with a catch pole and snare. The nature of the animal is to roll or twirl once the snare is around the neck. One must be prepared to rotate the snare to prevent injury or strangulation of the animal. The tail should be grasped as soon as possible because this serves to immobilize the animal to some extent until the mouth can be securely closed. The head can be swiftly moved from side to side even with a snare around the neck. One can then pin the head manually and secure the mouth with tape. Placing tape or a towel over the eyes tends to disorient and quiet the animal if the intended procedure is quite involved.

Caimans and alligators more than 3 m in length can be quite dangerous, and handling such animals requires the coordinated effort of two or three experienced individuals. These animals can be manually restrained by having one person control the head and the others control the tail and the hind legs. If the animal must be transported or restrained for a period of time, both the front and hind feet may be secured to the body by tying over the back.

Large crocodiles of any species are extremely dangerous to handle (more so than alligators). These animals are fast and more aggressive than alligators or caimans. Special nets and ropes should be used to secure these animals before any attempt is made to tape the mouth. In large crocodiles, tying the jaws shut with rope and then taping the jaws together may be prudent. The tail must be controlled because the flailing of the tail can cause severe injury. Crocodiles have exposed teeth on each side of the head. The swinging of the head from side to side can also cause severe injury. A pole snare around the neck and another around the jaw plus control of the tail and feet are necessary before tape can be applied to the jaws.

Transportation of these animals can be accomplished in crates or cages, depending on the size and circumstances. One must use caution because overheating is possible, especially if the animals continue to thrash about with the mouth closed. Removal of the tape from the eyes or mouth can also be dangerous. The usual procedure is to place a tie or rope around the tape on the ventral side of the jaws between the mandibles. A quick pull from a distance, after the other restraints have been removed, allows the animal to move off. Occasionally an animal escapes after all the restraints except the mouth tape are removed. In these instances, the animal must be recaptured to remove the tape to prevent starvation. Recapture is usually much more difficult.

The handling of large crocodilians in captivity is best accomplished by chemical injection whenever possible. Gallamine triethiodide is a muscle relaxant that is frequently used. Succinylcholine chloride has also been used in *A. mississippiensis*,[29] *C. crocodilus, C. acutus, C. palustris, C. porosus*, and *C. johnstoni*. Ketamine hydrochloride is an anesthetic and has also been used as an immobilization agent. Loveridge and Blake[30] reported that ketamine was unsatisfactory and unsuitable for *C. niloticus*.

One must remember that drug suitability and dosage differ for different species. Also, the environmental temperature has an effect on drug absorption, metabolism, and excretion in each individual animal. The following dosage chart is a guideline only, and the clinician is advised to consider the above factors in relation to the particular species of crocodilian:

Gallamine triethiodide: 0.5 to 2 mg/kg
  intramuscularly (IM)
Succinylchlorine chloride: 0.25 to 1.2 mg/kg IM
Ketamine hydrochloride: 50 mg/kg IM

Neostigmine methylsulfate at a dose of 0.03 to 0.06 mg/kg is used as an antidote to gallamine; however, some undesirable side effects have been reported with its use. The preferred method is to allow the animals to recover on their own. The animals must be kept warm, but do not allow the body temperature to go above 32°C. Care should be given at all times to maintain the airway and not block the nostrils.

A syringe should be used to administer drugs to crocodilians in captivity.[31] Dart guns can be used, but a pole syringe is much more satisfactory in most instances because penetration of the skin in a muscular area is not a problem. Once the drug has taken effect, the animal should have the mouth taped shut and be blindfolded.

REFERENCES

1. Darlington PJ: *Zoogeography: the geographical distribution of animals, reptiles*, New York, 1963, John Wiley & Sons.
2. Neill WT: *The last of the ruling reptiles: alligators, crocodiles, and their kin; two hundred million years of crocodilian history*, New York, 1971, Columbia University Press.
3. Chen B: The past and present situation of the Chinese alligator, *Asiat Herpetol Rec* 3:129, 1990.
4. Braziatis P: The identification of living crocodilians, *Zoologica* 58:59, 1973.
5. Levy C: *Crocodiles and alligators; hunting and feeding*, Secaucus, NJ, 1991, Chartwell Books.
6. Chiasson RB: *Laboratory anatomy of the alligator*, Dubuque, Iowa, 1962, Wm. C. Brown.
7. Mazzotte FJ: Evolution and biology: structure and function. In Ross CA, Garnett S, editors: *Crocodiles and alligators*, New York, 1989, Facts on File.
8. Lang JW: Crocodilian behavior: implications for management. In Webb GJW, Manolis SC, Whitehead PJ, editors: *Wildlife management: crocodiles and alligators*, Chipping Norton, Australia, 1987, Surrey Beaty and Sons Printing in Association with the Conservation Commission of the Northern Territory.
9. Webb GJW, Manolis SC, Whitehead PJ, editors: *Wildlife management: crocodiles and alligators*, Chipping Norton, Australia, 1987, Surrey Beaty and Sons Printing in Association with the Conservation Commission of the Northern Territory.
10. Brazaites P: The occurrence and ingestion of gastroliths in two captive crocodilians, *Herpetologica* 25:63, 1969.
11. Coulson RA, Hernandez T: *Alligator metabolism: studies on chemical reactions in vivo*, London, 1983, Pergamon Press.
12. Johnsen PB, Wellinton JL: Detection of glandular secretions by yearling alligators, *Copeia* 705-708, 1982.
13. Lang JW, Garrick LD: Alligator courtship, *Am Zoo* 15:813, 1975.
14. Lang JW, Garrick LD: The American Alligator revealed, *Nat Hist* 86:54, 1977.
15. Vliet KA: Social displays of the American Alligator, *Am Zoo* 29:1019, 1989.
16. Dietz DC, Hines TC: Alligator nesting in North Central Florida, *Copeia* 2:219, 1980.
17. Ferguson MWJ, Joanen T: Temperature dependent sex determination in *Alligator mississippiensis, J Zoo* 200:143, 1982.
18. Pooley AC, Gans C: The Nile crocodile, Sci Am 234:114, 1976.
19. Coulson RA, et al: Biochemistry and physiology of alligator metabolism in vivo, *Am Zoo* 29:921, 1989.
20. Lang JW: Crocodilian thermal selection. In Webb GJW, Manolis SC, Whitehead PJ, editors: *Wildlife management: crocodiles and alligators*, Chipping Norton, Australia, 1987, Surrey Beatty and Sons Printing in Association with the Conservation Commission of the Northern Territory.
21. Diefenbach CO: Thermal preferences and thermoregulation in *Caiman crocodilus, Copeia* 530-540, 1975.
22. Glassman AB, Bennett CE: Response of the alligator to infection and thermal stress. In Thorp JH, Gibbons JW, editors: *Energy and environmental stress in aquatic systems*, Washington, DC, 1978, Technical Information Center, U.S. Department of Energy.
23. Taplin L, Grigg GC: Salt glands in the tongue of the estuarine crocodile *Crocodylus porosus, Science* 212:1045, 1981.
24. Mazzote FJ, Dunson WA: Adaptations of *Crocodylus acutus* and alligator for life in saline water, *Comp Biochem Physiol* 79A:641, 1984.
25. Delaney FM, Abercombie CLP: American Alligator food habits, *J Wild Manage* 50:348, 1986.
26. Goldekas BMF, Yeager CP: Crocodile predation on a crab-eating macaque in Borneo, *Am J Prematol* 6:49, 1984.
27. Staton MA, McNease L, Joanen T, et al: Supplemented nutria (*Myocastor coypu*) meat as a practical feed for American alligators (*Alligator mississippiensis*), *Proceedings of 9th Working Meeting of the Crocodile Specialist Group of the Species Survival Commission of IUCN—The World Conservation Union* 2:199, 1988.
28. Joanen T, McNease L: Alligator farming programs in Louisiana, *Proceedings of 9th Working Meeting of the Crocodile Specialist Group of the Species Survival Commission of IUCN—The World Conservation Union* 2:6, 1988.
29. Spiegel RA, Lane TJ, Larsen RE, et al: Diazepam and succinylcholine chloride for restraint of the American Alligator, *JAVMA* 185(11):1335, 1985.
30. Loveridge JP, Blake DD: Crocodile immobilization and anesthesia. In Webb GJW, Manolis SC, Whitehead PJ, editors: *Wildlife management: crocodiles and alligators*, Chipping Norton, Australia, 1987, Surrey Beatty and Sons Printing in Association with the Conservation Commission of the Northern Territory.
31. Fowler, ME: *Restraint and handling of wild and domestic animals*, Ames, 1991, Iowa State University Press.

Section III
ANATOMY, PHYSIOLOGY, AND BEHAVIOR

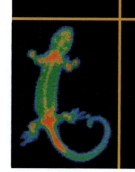

9
STRESS IN CAPTIVE REPTILES
DALE DENARDO

Stress and its detrimental effects on animal health are well known to the herpetocultural community. The phrase "died of stress" is frequently spoken by both owners and veterinarians and is often used for deaths in which no clear cause can be identified (Figure 9-1). Death from stress is particularly common for animals that were only recently acquired, especially from the wild (directly or through a commercial importer). Although stress may well play a vital role in many of these deaths, one should not blindly attribute death to stress. Such an action oftentimes fails to reveal the true cause of the problem and therefore can increase the chance of recurrence in the future.

WHAT IS STRESS?

Stress is usually used in broad terms and therefore often lacks a clear definition. Although most people can identify a stressful situation, few have a clear concept of the physiologic basis of the body's stress response. Of utmost importance is the realization that stress is not simply a tangible thing or condition but rather the perception or physiologic response to such a stimulus.[1] Thus, whether a stimulus induces a stressful response or not can vary among individuals and over time. What may be deemed a stressful situation by one individual may not be stressful to another individual or to that same individual at another time. For example, a rattlesnake (or merely its picture) invokes an intense stress response from a person who fears snakes,[2] but an experienced herpetophile might react with indifference or even euphoria. Furthermore, with increased exposure to rattlesnakes, an ophidophobic person likely adapts and eventually does not respond stressfully to the same situation in the future.

A stimulus that evokes a stress response is called a stressor. Broadly, stressors can be divided into two categories.[3] Physiologic stressors are those stimuli that induce hardship on the animal's ability to maintain homeostasis and include, but are not limited to, temperature extremes, food or water limitations, and oxygen deprivation. Clearly, any of these conditions can compromise normal body function and jeopardize survival. Physiologic changes are necessary to cope with such conditions.

Contrarily, psychologic stressors are those stimuli that do not pose a direct challenge to body physiology but rather may be indicative of imminent physiologic challenge. Social dominance, novel environments, confinement, and unmanageable situations can all induce a stress response without actual physiologic insult. For example, a child at school might initiate a stress response on the approach of the school bully. Although the bully's approach induces no harm and the interaction may pass without confrontation, the stress response prepares the individual for the possibility of physical insult (such as would occur should a fight ensue). Unfortunately, because psychologic stressors are perceptions of potential physiologic insult, misperception of danger from inoffensive stimuli can lead to an unnecessary initiation of the stress response. Phobias are simply misperceptions of innocuous stimuli that, as a result, stimulate the stress response.

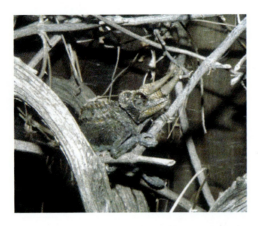

FIGURE 9-1 Stress of captivity, or "maladaptation syndrome," is often blamed for inexplicable death in captive reptiles. This originally wild-caught chameleon never adapted to caged life, refusing to eat and eventually succumbing to starvation. (*Photograph courtesy D. Mader.*)

WHY HAVE A STRESS RESPONSE?

One common misconception is that the stress response is detrimental to the individual. In actuality, the stress response is adaptive in that it physiologically prepares the individual for what has been perceived as a difficult situation. Both physical and psychologic stressors can indicate physiologic challenge. By making physiologic adjustments, the individual maximizes its chances of survival through a bad situation. Physiologic challenges, no doubt, vary among stressors, and therefore, the body's responses vary. However, common basic physiologic adjustments are made regardless of the specifics of the stressor. These common changes are induced by the stress response. A stressful situation typically requires the body to expend energy to cope with the physiologic challenge. Thus, the stress response is oftentimes referred to as a "fight-or-flight response." An organism must prepare itself to either cope with the challenge (i.e., fight) or distance itself from the challenge (i.e., flight). Either way, the individual likely needs to spend energy, and so one common need during all stressful situations is mobilization of energy reserves and reduction of energy utilization. The stress response diverts mobilized energy to those physiologic systems that are essential for life and reduces energy access to those systems that can be temporarily shut down.

HOW IS THE STRESS RESPONSE REGULATED?

The stress response is governed by a myriad of neural and hormonal inputs.[4,5] Once a stimulus is perceived as stressful, the brain triggers a neuroendocrine response that is composed of both an acute and a more chronic phase. The acute phase is regulated by the sympathetic nervous system and has direct action on most body tissues. Its signal throughout the body is enhanced by the stimulation of the adrenal medulla to rapidly release epinephrine. This combination of central nervous system activation and rapid hormonal release leads to a rapid and intense response.

In addition to the activation of the sympathetic nervous system, a perceived stress induces a slower onset but longer acting endocrine pathway: the hypothalamic-pituitary-adrenal (HPA) axis. Briefly, the HPA axis begins with the release of corticotropin-releasing factor (CRF) from the hypothalamus. CRF travels via the hypothalamic-pituitary portal system directly to the anterior pituitary where it stimulates the release of adrenocorticotropic hormone (ACTH). ACTH travels through the systemic blood circulation with its primary action the stimulation of the adrenal cortex to produce and release glucocorticoids. The predominant glucocorticoid in reptiles is corticosterone,[6] and an elevated serum corticosterone level is often used as an indicator that an animal has experienced stress. Stress or artificially increased corticosterone levels influence whole-body physiology and behavior by acting on numerous target organs. Glucocorticoids potentiate their effect by altering the circulating levels of sex steroid[7-10] and other hormones.[11] Combined, the direct and indirect effect of the sympathetic nervous system, epinephrine, and corticosterone rapidly induces substantial changes in physiologic condition that can be long lasting.

EFFECTS OF STRESS ON THE VARIOUS BODY SYSTEMS

As stated earlier, the role of the stress response is to maximize energy availability to vital body systems. Therefore, the stress response stimulates the mobilization of body reserves (e.g., lypolysis, gluconeogenesis)[12] and alters cardiovascular function.[13] In addition, the stress response is a potent inhibitor of systems that are nonessential. Specifically, growth[14] and reproduction[15] are oftentimes dramatically inhibited during times of stress. Although these processes are critical to long-term survival and fitness, they are nonessential for day-to-day survival.

The effect of the stress response on the immune system is complex; however, typically the inflammatory response and antibody production are inhibited.[12] Such changes minimize energy utilization and enhance immediate performance (e.g., reduced inflammation increases locomotor ability). Immune suppression also increases the incidence of disease, though.

The stress response also has a substantial effect on behavior. Behaviors that are energy demanding such as aggression are usually drastically inhibited. However, behavioral changes can be complex. Corticosterone inhibits reproductive behaviors that consume substantial amounts of energy, such as aggression[9,10] and territory maintenance,[16] yet copulation itself is unaffected.[10] For males, copulation is a relatively low-energy behavior with high fitness value, so with copulatory behavior maintained, stressed males remain able to produce offspring during challenging times. However, without the supportive behaviors associated with male-male competition, such opportunities for reproduction are likely to be rare.

The role of corticosterone in female reproduction appears complicated. Captivity-induced stress inhibits estrogen and therefore inhibits the production of vitellogenin.[17] This effect is likely the reason for the oftentimes inability to breed recently collected or purchased reptiles. However, corticosterone levels are frequently elevated during at least some stages of reproduction in wild female reptiles,[18-20] and this elevation is positively correlated with reproductive output.[20]

In fact, treatment with exogenous corticosterone implants increases reproductive output.[21] Therefore, corticosterone likely plays a constructive role in female reproduction rather than simply reflecting the stressful nature of reproduction. Corticosterone may simply increase the mobilization of energy reserves so that stored energy can be transferred into reproductive effort,[19,20] or corticosterone may have a more specific role in the regulation of the reproductive cycle. For example, in rats, corticosterone increases the secretion of follicle-stimulating hormone.[22]

WHEN DOES THE STRESS RESPONSE BECOME NONADAPTIVE?

Although the stress response is clearly an adaptive process, it also can lead to the death of an individual. Exposure to stressors is a common occurrence, and the stress response has evolved to help manage such situations. The stress response adjusts an individual's physiology to cope with a given situation, but this adjustment is designed to be relatively short term. The dramatic physiologic effects of the stress response provide a state in which the individual can overcome the stimuli or distance itself from it in a relatively short time frame. However, the extreme mobilization of energy and inhibition of other body systems cannot be supported for a lengthy period without detrimental effects. Repeated exposure to a stimulus leads to long-term adjustments in body physiology and or perception, and thus tolerance evolves of a stimulus previously recognized as a stressor. This process of acclimation applies to both physical and psychological stressors. For example, exposure to a temperature 10°C warmer than normal might induce a stress response in an animal, but a slow increase of the ambient temperature over a period of time allows for physiologic adjustments that lead to tolerance of this once stressful condition. Similarly, sudden changes in the social structure of a group of animals can lead to stress, but over time the animals within that group may adjust to the new structure. The concept of dominance and subordination reflects this adjustment.

THE STRESS OF CAPTIVITY

Reptiles live in a vast array of habitats throughout the world. Although environmental conditions vary greatly, each species has evolved behavioral and physiologic mechanisms that enable individuals to use the environment to meet both short-term and long-term needs. We may view many habitats as harsh or uninhabitable, but reptiles have evolved to a point where such conditions are not only bearable but perhaps optimal for physiologic performance. Captivity alters the balance between the environment and physiology. Inappropriate captive conditions may prohibit an animal from meeting its physiologic needs. Temperatures may be too hot or too cold, humidity too high or too low, or caloric intake insufficient. Each of these conditions, and others, can lead to physical stresses to a captive reptile. If unaltered, these conditions can lead to chronic stress and eventual decline of the individual.

Even when captivity provides proper physical conditions, no assurance exists that an animal may thrive in captivity. Not only should physical conditions be proper, but also they

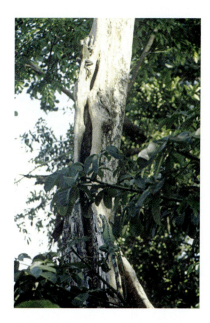

FIGURE 9-2 Although these two wild iguanas are seen near each other in a tree, it is likely a quest for prime basking space, NOT companionship, that brings them together. *(Photograph courtesy D. Mader.)*

should be provided in a means that is functional for the animal. An incandescent light as the sole heat source to a nocturnal animal, water in a bowl to a species that naturally only gets water from lapping morning dew, or inappropriate food items are all examples of providing for the animal's physiologic needs in an inappropriate manner that can lead to physical stress.

Even when reptiles are held in conditions that properly provide for physiologic needs, captivity can be quite stressful. Complex and generously sized enclosures rarely duplicate the complexity and size of the animal's natural home range. Thus, captivity clearly limits an animal's normal activity. Escape behaviors, foraging activity, and mate searching activity are all altered by captivity. Therefore, confinement in itself is usually a stressful situation.[23,24] However, this effect can be eliminated as the animal acclimates to the confinement.[25]

Another potential stressor that is unavoidable in captivity is handling. Handling leads to increases in both corticosterone[26,27] and adrenal catechloamines (epinephrine and norepinephrine).[28] In nature, direct restraint is usually closely tied to consumption by a predator, so handling as a stressor of reptiles is not surprising. As with confinement, reptiles likely can acclimate to handling as many long-term captive reptiles do not show a stress response to handling.[29]

Psychologic stress can also be induced by inappropriate social housing. Many reptile species are solitary, yet they are often group housed in captivity (Figure 9-2). A common mistake of novice herpetoculturists is to wrongly anthropomorphize the need to prevent loneliness in reptiles by cohousing them with another animal. Even species labeled as social normally are separated by territorial boundaries, and such a social arrangement can rarely be established in a captive setting. The importance of social interactions, whether the result be positive or negative, is unknown but clearly the complexity of social interaction seen in nature can rarely be duplicated in captivity.

Considering the dramatic changes between the natural and artificial environments, that so many animals survive the transition from the wild to captivity is somewhat surprising. Acclimation allows animals to adapt to novel environments provided the changes are reasonable and not too abrupt. Unfortunately, this situation is not always the case with commercially imported animals. Captive-born animals have much less dramatic environmental changes when they are transferred to a new owner, but change does occur and should be acknowledged.

HOW IS STRESS IMPORTANT TO REPTILE MEDICINE?

Because the stress response leads to a wide range of dramatic physiologic changes, veterinarians must understand and consider the role of stress relative to the patient's condition. A thorough understanding of stress and the physiologic changes associated with stress is vital for client education and patient treatment. In assessment of a case, stress should not be broadly blamed for an animal's decline, but also the contribution that stress may have made cannot be overlooked. A careful assessment must consider the animal's history, the current husbandry, physiologic changes associated with stress, and physiologic changes associated with any disease state that is present (e.g., bacterial infection, parasite infection, trauma). Treatment regimes must incorporate both the immediate treatment of the disease and the reduction or elimination of any stressors in the animal's home environment. Without consideration of both, long-term improvement in the animal's condition is unlikely.

In addition to recognizing the role of stress in the etiology of a patient's condition, veterinarians must recognize the potential for stress associated with medical care. Medical treatment can provide great benefits to an ill reptile, but it also unavoidably includes many potentially stressful stimuli. Minimally, animals need to be transported to the veterinary practice and handled for examination and treatment. Diagnostic procedures are also potential stressors. As discussed previously, stress is not the actual condition or event but rather the animal's perception of that experience. Therefore, the extent to which an animal is stressed during veterinary care depends on the state of the animal and how well it has acclimated to the captive environment. Historical information can aid in predicting the degree to which stimuli may induce the stress response in a patient. Recent acquisitions are more likely to perceive manipulations as stressors than are animals that are well established. Regardless, all manipulations associated with both diagnosis and treatment must be evaluated in terms of their potential for inducing stress versus their potential medical benefit.

Physiologic changes induced by the stress response (i.e., energy mobilization, alteration of the immune response) can be catastrophic to an already compromised animal. Therefore, minimization of stress associated with the trip to the veterinarian is critical. Animals should be transported to and from the veterinarian by a means that minimizes stress. Usually, a reptile travels best in a tightly confined dark enclosure rather than in an open cage where the animal can see the world whizzing by and be consistently jarred from its position. A dark confined enclosure (e.g., a small opaque box with a towel haphazardly folded in it) mimics a refuge where most reptiles escape to during threatening times. Thus, an animal more likely accepts an altered environment when it feels safely hidden from danger.

In addition, stress must also be minimized during examination and treatment. Most veterinarians have had experiences where patients are presented with chronic problems only to die acutely after the initiation of treatment, be it therapeutic or surgical. Proper preparation minimizes the duration of stress associated with handling. All instruments and equipment necessary for physical examination and possible treatments should be ready before an animal is removed from its transport enclosure.

One must also remember that other veterinary patients (e.g., dogs, cats) represent potential predators to most reptiles and that their presence can be detected with a keen sense of smell. Snake odor induces behavioral changes in rodents,[30] so one should reasonably expect that predator odors have an effect on snakes. Therefore, examination of reptile patients in a dedicated room or in a room that been properly sanitized since the last patient is optimal.

SUMMARY

Although the stress response is an adaptive response that maximizes immediate survival, it jeopardizes long-term survival, especially of compromised individuals. Critical to optimal veterinary care to reptiles is an understanding of the physiology of stress and the potential of seemingly innocuous stimuli to induce a stress response.

REFERENCES

1. Selye H: *The physiology and pathology of exposure to stress,* Montreal, 1950, Acta Inc Medical Publishers.
2. Fredrikson M, Sundin O, Frankenhaeuser M: Cortisol excretion during the defense reaction in humans, *Psychosomatic Med* 47(4):313-319, 1985.
3. Asterita MF: *The physiology of stress,* New York, 1985, Human Sciences Press Inc.
4. Axelrod J, Reisine TD: Stress hormones: their interaction and regulation, *Science* 224:452-459, 1984.
5. Rivier C, Rivest S: Effect of stress on the activity of the hypothalamic-pituitary-gonadal axis: peripheral and central mechanisms, *Bio Reprod* 45:523-532, 1991.
6. Sandor T, Mehdi AZ: Steroids and evolution. In Barrington EJW, editor: *Hormones and behavior,* vol 1, New York, 1979, Academic Press.
7. Licht P, Breitenbach GL, Congdon JD: Seasonal cycles in testicular activity, gonadotropin and thyroxine in the painted turtle *(Chrysemys picta)* under natural conditions, *Gen Comp Endocr* 59:130-139, 1985.
8. Lance VA, Elsey R: Stress induced suppression of testosterone secretion in male alligators, *J Exp Zool* 239:241-264, 1986.
9. Tokarz R: Effects of corticosterone treatment on male aggressive behavior in a lizard *(Anolis sagrei), Horm Behav* 21: 358-370, 1987.
10. DeNardo DF, Licht P: Effects of corticosterone on social behavior of male lizards, *Horm Behav* 27:184-199, 1993.
11. Lenihan DJ, Greenberg N, Lee TC: Involvement of platelet activating factor in physiological stress in the lizard *Anolis carolinensis, Comp Biochem Phys C* 81(1):81-86, 1985.

12. Norris DO: *Vertebrate endocrinology*, San Diego, 1997, Academic Press Inc.
13. Hailey A, Theophilidis G: Cardiac response to stress and activity in the armored legless lizard, *Ophisaurus apodus*; comparison with a snake and tortoise, *Comp Biochem Phys A* 88(2):201-206, 1987.
14. Hemsworth PH, Barnett JL, Hansen C: The influence of handling by humans on the behavior, growth, and corticosteroids in the juvenile female pig, *Horm Behav* 15:396-403, 1981.
15. Cunningham DL, van Tienhoven A, Gvaryahu G: Population size, cage and area, and dominance rank effects on productivity and well being of laying hens, *Poultry Sci* 67:399-406, 1988.
16. DeNardo DF, Sinervo B: Effects of corticosterone on activity and home-range size of free-ranging male lizards, *Horm Behav* 28:53-65, 1994.
17. Morales MH, Sanchez EJ: Changes in vitellogenin expression during captivity-induced stress in a tropical anole, *Gen Comp Endocr* 103:209-219, 1996.
18. Dauphin-Villemant C, Leboulenger F, Xavier F, Vaudry H: Adrenal activity in the female lizard *Lacerta vivipara* Jacquin associated with breeding activities, *Gen Comp Endocr* 8:399-413, 1990.
19. Grassman M, Crews D: Ovarian and adrenal function in the parthenogenic whiptail lizard *Cnemidophorus uniparens* in the field and laboratory, *Gen Comp Endocr* 76:444-450, 1990.
20. Wilson B, Wingfield JC: Correlation between female reproductive condition and plasma corticosterone in the lizard *Uta stansburiana*, *Copeia* 92:691-697, 1992.
21. Sinervo B, DeNardo DF: Cost of reproduction in the wild: path analysis of natural selection and experimental tests of causation, *Evolution* 50(3):1299-1313, 1996.
22. Baldwin DM, Srivastava PS, Krummen LA: Differential actions of corticosterone on luteinizing hormone and follicle-stimulating hormone biosynthesis and release in cultured rat anterior pituitary cells: interaction with estradiol, *Bio Reprod* 44:1040-1050, 1991.
23. Dauphin-Villemant, Xavier F: Nychthemeral variations of plasma corticosteroids in captive female *Lacerta vivipara* Jacquin: influence of stress and reproductive state, *Gen Comp Endocr* 67:292-302, 1987.
24. Moore MC, Thompson CW, Marler CA: Reciprocal changes in corticosterone and testosterone levels following acute and chronic handling stress in the tree lizard, *Urosaurus ornatus*, *Gen Comp Endocr* 81:217-226, 1991.
25. Manzo C, Zerani M, Gobbetti A, Di Fiori MM, Angelini F: Is corticosterone involved in the reproductive process of the male lizard, *Podarcis sicula sicula*? *Horm Behav* 28(2):117-129, 1994.
26. Lance VA, Lauren D: Circadian variation in plasma corticosterone in the American alligator, *Alligator mississippiensis*, and the effects of ACTH injection, *Gen Comp Endocr* 54:1-7, 1984.
27. Grassman M, Hess DL: Sex differences in adrenal function in the lizard *Cnemidophorus sexlineatus*: II. responses to acute stress in the laboratory, *J Exp Zool* 264:183-188, 1992.
28. Matt KS, Moore MC, Knapp R, Moore IT: Sympathetic mediation of stress and aggressive competition: plasma catecholamines in free-living male tree lizards, *Physiol Behav* 61(5):639-647, 1997.
29. Kreger MD, Mench JA: Physiological and behavioral effects of handling and restraint in the ball python *(Python regius)* and the blue-tongued skink *(Tiliqua scincoides)*, *Appl Anim Behav Sci* 38(3-4):323-336, 1993.
30. Dell'omo G, Alleva E: Snake odor alters behavior, but not pain sensitivity in mice, *Physiol Behav* 55(1):125-128, 1994.

10
CARDIOPULMONARY ANATOMY AND PHYSIOLOGY

MICHAEL J. MURRAY

A working knowledge of the anatomy and physiology of the reptilian cardiovascular and pulmonary systems is vitally important to the clinician. The reptile heart, although often described as "primitive" in comparison with the avian or mammalian organ, is actually quite complex in its structure and function. The physiologic changes that occur during various respiratory and environmental events are quite profound and appear to be ideally suited to the normal environment of the species of concern. An understanding of these changes during normal activity facilitates interpretation of a variety of clinical signs associated with cardiovascular disease. In addition, this understanding helps in the avoidance of serious consequences should important vital parameters, such as ventilation, be overlooked during anesthetic interventions or disease states.

CARDIOVASCULAR ANATOMY

The cardiovascular anatomy of reptiles varies with taxon. Each major structural pattern is discussed within taxonomic context. No single model exists for a generalized reptilian heart or ciruclation. However, two basic patterns of reptilian heart structure are seen. The first is found in squamates and chelonians, and the second is found in crocodilians.

NONCROCODILIAN REPTILES

The heart of the snake, lizard, and chelonian is essentially a three-chambered structure with two atria and one ventricle (Figures 10-1 to 10-3). Although this tends to suggest the potential for the mixing of well-oxygenated and poorly oxygenated blood from the lungs and systemic circulation, respectively, a series of muscular ridges and the timing of ventricular contractions tend to functionally separate the ventricle.

The right atrium receives deoxygenated blood returning from the systemic circulation via the sinus venosus, a large chamber located on the dorsal surface of the atrium. The wall of the sinus venosus is muscular but not as thick as the atrium. The sinus venosus receives blood directly from the

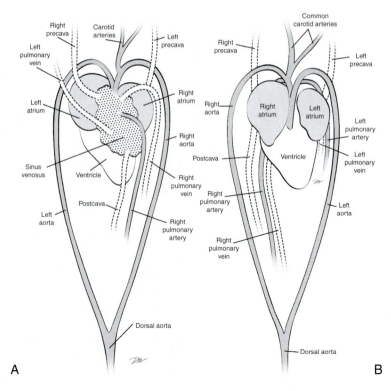

FIGURE 10-1 Snake heart. **A,** Dorsal view; **B,** ventral view. *(Diagrams courtesy J. Wyneken.)*

following four veins: (1) right precaval vein; (2) left precaval vein; (3) postcaval vein; and (4) left hepatic vein.[1] The left atrium receives oxygenated blood from the lungs via the left and right pulmonary veins.

The solitary ventricle is divided into three subchambers: the cavum pulmonale, the cavum venosum, and the cavum arteriosum. The cavum pulmonale is the most ventral chamber and extends cranially to the ostium of the pulmonary artery. The cavum arteriosum and cavum venosum are situated dorsal to the cavum pulmonale and receive blood from the left and right atria, respectively. The cavum venosum gives rise at its most cranial and ventral aspect to the left and right aortic arches (Figure 10-4).

A muscular ridge separates the cavum pulmonale from the cava arteriosum and venosum to some extent. The cava arteriosum and cava venosum are a continuous chamber connected by an interventricular canal.

The single-cusped atrioventricular valves arise from the cranial aspect of the interventricular canal. They are anatomically aligned in such a fashion that they partially occlude the interventricular canal during atrial systole. Their function during ventricular systole is the prevention of regurgitation of blood from the ventricle into the atria.

The series of muscular contractions and subsequent pressure variations within the noncrocodilian heart is timed in such a fashion as to create a functionally dual circulatory system.

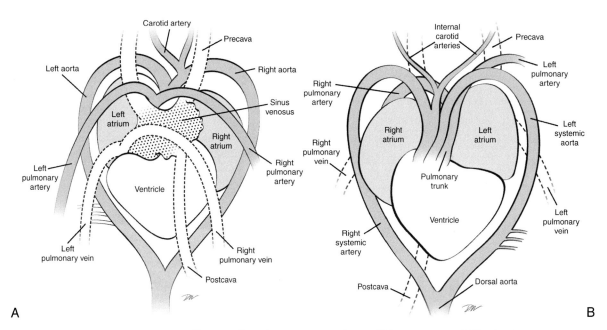

FIGURE 10-2 Lizard heart. **A,** Dorsal view; **B,** ventral view. *(Diagrams courtesy J. Wyneken.)*

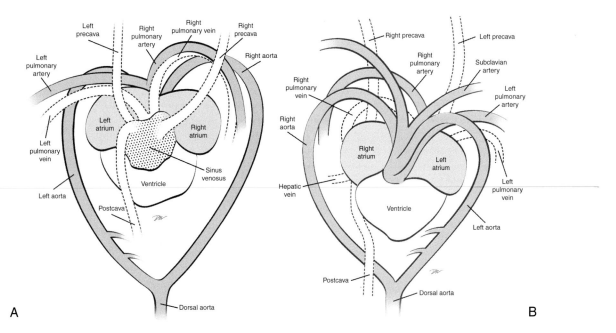

FIGURE 10-3 Turtle heart. **A,** Dorsal view; **B,** ventral view. *(Diagrams courtesy J. Wyneken.)*

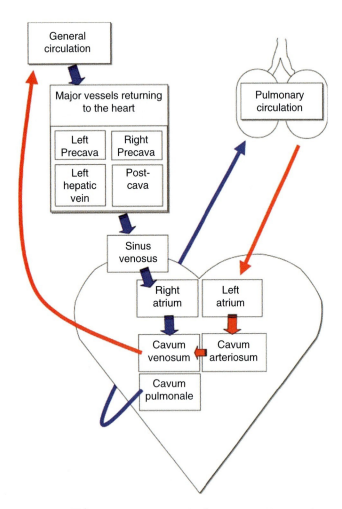

FIGURE 10-4 General circulation in the noncrocodilian reptile.

Atrial systole causes blood to flow into the solitary ventricle. The position of the atrioventricular valves across the interventricular canal results in systemic blood from the right atrium filling both the cavum venosum and the cavum pulmonale. Concurrently, pulmonary blood courses from the left atrium into the cavum arteriosum. The ventricular systole is initiated by the contraction of the cavum venosum. Sequential contraction of the cavum venosum and cavum pulmonale results in the propulsion of blood from these two areas of the ventricle into the low-pressure pulmonary circuit.

As systole proceeds, the cavum arteriosum initiates its contraction. This forces blood through the partially contracted cavum venosum and into systemic circulation via the left and right aortic arches. Ventricular contraction tends to bring a muscular ridge into close apposition with the ventral ventricular wall, thereby creating a barrier against the flow of blood from the cavum arteriosum into the cavum pulmonale.[2] Left and right atrioventricular valves prevent the regurgitation of ventricular blood into the atria.

The preceding series of events is applicable only during normal respiration. Such a blood flow system tends to create a left-to-right shunt on the basis of pressure differentials. During diving or other instances in which the pulmonary resistance and pressure are elevated, a right to left shunt occurs. Normal respiration in the Red-eared Slider (*Trachemys scripta elegans*) results in the blood flow favoring the pulmonary circulation, which receives 60% of the cardiac output; the remaining 40% enters the systemic circulation. During diving, the pulmonary circulation tends to be bypassed with most of the blood entering the systemic network.[3] Under such circumstances, the pressure of the pulmonary bed exceeds that in the periphery; therefore, blood enters the lowest pressure circuit available, the aortic arches. In lizards, this is primarily distributed through the left aortic arch.[2]

CROCODILIANS

The crocodilians have a cardiac structure quite similar to that of birds and mammals, except for the presence of the foramen of Panizza, a small aperture in the interventricular septum that separates the left and right ventricles, and a left aortic arch, which originates from the right ventricle (Figure 10-5).

The cardiac structure is essentially dual in nature. A small amount of mixing of oxygenated and deoxygenated blood may occur through the foramen of Panizza or in the dorsal aorta at the confluence of the left and right aortic arches. In normal breathing circumstances, such mixing does not occur because the pressures in the systemic side of the circulatory system exceed those in the pulmonary circuit. A left to right shunt does occur through the foramen of Panizza, and a small amount of oxygenated blood enters the right ventricle.

During diving or under other conditions that elevate pulmonary vascular resistance, the pressures within the pulmonary artery are significantly elevated. As a result, blood is diverted from its normal course through the pulmonary bed into the systemic circulation. Blood then enters the left aortic arch rather than the pulmonary artery. Speculation exists that the source of the high pulmonary resistance during diving that causes the right-to-left shunt resides in the outflow tract of the right ventricle itself.[2] The right ventricle has a separate "chamber," the subpulmonary conus, which as a result of its delayed depolarization and cog-like tooth-bearing valves, controls the flow of blood into the pulmonary vascular bed.[4]

The presence of right-to-left shunts during periods of apnea and elevated pulmonary vascular bed resistance may have significant clinical importance. Anesthetized or apneic reptiles without ventilatory support may not follow expected inhalant anesthetic protocols. The pulmonary bypass may result in inadequate transfer of anesthetic gases, such as isoflurane, to the systemic circulation for proper anesthetic management. The importance of prolonged right-to-left shunts, as may occur during chronic inflammatory disease of the lungs, has yet to be investigated. Significant changes within the cardiovascular system would not be surprising.

Renal Portal System

The renal portal system is a component of the venous system of reptiles that has raised numerous questions with potential clinical significance. The function of the renal portal system is to ensure adequate perfusion of the renal tubules when blood flow through the glomerulus is decreased as a water-conservation mechanism.

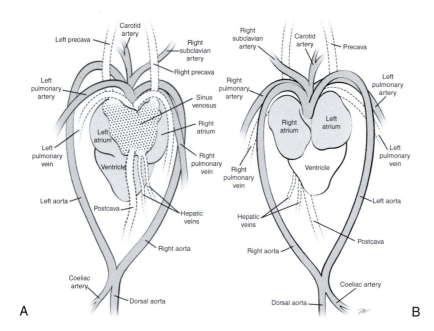

FIGURE 10-5 Crocodilian heart. **A,** Dorsal view; **B,** ventral view. *(Diagrams courtesy J. Wyneken.)*

The afferent renal portal veins do not perfuse the glomeruli; instead, they supply the proximal and distal convoluted tubules with blood. Like their mammalian counterparts, the reptilian tubular cells are also perfused by afferent arterioles leaving the glomeruli. Unlike the mammal, however, the reptile does not have a loop of Henle and therefore cannot concentrate urine. As a result, with the influence or arginine vasotocin, water is conserved by decreasing the afferent blood flow to the glomerulus. When this glomerular blood supply is decreased, the renal portal system is vitally important in supplying blood to the tubules to prevent ischemic necrosis.

Studies have shown that a great deal of variation exists in the anatomy of the renal portal system between reptilian orders and even within suborders.[5] For a thorough discussion of the renal portal system, see Chapter 11.

CARDIOVASCULAR PHYSIOLOGY

The heart rate of the reptile is dependent, often in a very complex fashion, on a number of variables, including body temperature, body size, metabolic rate, respiratory rate, and sensory stimulation.[6] The cardiac muscle has an inherent maximal efficiency, as measured by maximal twitch tension, within the species's preferred optimal temperature zone (POTZ).[2] In general, increased activity causes an increased heart rate. Such increases may actually exceed three times the animal's resting heart rate. In general, an inverse relationship exists between body size and heart rate at any given temperature.

Interesting variations in heart rate at a given environmental temperature are dependent on the temperature status of the reptile. Typically, animals that are warming up have higher heart rates than animals that are cooling down. Elevation of the heart rate during warm basking periods tends to maximize the rate of heat gain. Depression of the heart rate as environmental temperature decreases tends to slow the rate of heat loss from the reptile.

At lower temperatures, the cardiac output appears to be maintained by an increase in stroke volume.[2] The elevated heart rate associated with higher temperatures appears to have a complex relationship with metabolic rate. Theoretically, the increased heart rate should permit an increased oxygen transport. Studies of the oxygen pulses (mL O_2 consumed/heartbeat/g body weight) of various species suggest that no consistent pattern is found in the relationship between stroke volume, oxygen extraction, and heart rate as the need for increased oxygen in the face of an elevated metabolic rate.[2] Multiple mechanisms for increased oxygen delivery during periods of increased metabolism are suspected to be identified for a variety of reptilian species. Of particular significance is the fact that heart rates tend to elevate during active respiration and decrease during periods of apnea. This elevated heart rate coincides with the decreased pulmonary resistance and subsequent increased pulmonary blood flow. Increased pulmonary blood flow during the period of increased respiratory activity tends to maximize the efficiency of the gas exchange system.

The cardiovascular system is critically important in the thermoregulation of the reptile. As previously stated, heart rates tend to elevate as the animal warms and decrease as the animal cools. Although the exact control mechanism is not definitively known, cardiovascular changes are known to occur before alterations in the body core temperature are realized, suggesting a role for cutaneous thermal receptors or baroreceptors.

As the skin is heated, a cutaneous vasodilatation is noted. The pooling of peripheral blood tends to drop the central blood pressure. The declining peripheral vascular resistance supports the development of a right-to-left cardiac shunting of blood. Blood pressure is thereby maintained at a level adequate to supply blood to the brain and major sense organs via the right aortic arch. Meanwhile, pooled cutaneous blood is returning to central circulation, thereby elevating the body core temperature.

The decreased heart rate that accompanies cooling of the skin facilitates the conservation of body heat. Skin cooling causes cutaneous vasoconstriction and a relative vasodilatation of the vascular network within the muscle. Pooling of blood in this way tends to slow the loss of heat.

As seen in birds and mammals, cardiovascular changes are important in reptiles during diving. Reptiles have a distinct advantage over their warm-blooded diving counterparts: the ability to use an alternative metabolic pathway during periods of decreased oxygen, anaerobic glycolysis. Definite species differences are seen in the ability to tolerate anaerobiosis. Some lizards may only survive for 25 minutes without oxygen, whereas certain tortoises may exceed 33 hours.[2] The primary difference lies in the varying tolerance of the myocardium to hypoxia.

Typically, a bradycardia occurs during most instances of diving or submergence. In crocodilians, the bradycardia is induced by vagal inhibition of the heart with some influence by thoracic or intrapulmonary pressure.[6] During the dive, a sympathetically mediated vasoconstriction of the vascular bed of the skeletal muscle occurs, often to the point of ischemia. This elevation of peripheral resistance tends to support blood pressure for vital organ function.

Right-to-left cardiac shunting of blood occurs as the oxygen supply within the pulmonary parenchyma is exhausted. As the dive progresses, the right to left shunt predominates with almost complete bypass of the pulmonary circuit. Total cardiac output may fall to a level approaching only 5% of the predive level. It is this ability to minimize the work load on the heart by only supplying a limited portion of the systemic vasculature that provides the reptile with a distinct advantage over diving birds and mammals. The bradycardia associated with the dive is rapidly reversed with the first postdive breath; certain species even demonstrate an "anticipatory" elevation of the heart rate before surfacing.

The characteristics of the circulatory system as applied to gas exchange at the cellular level are applicable to any discussion of reptilian cardiology. Although the topic may appear rather esoteric, alterations in cardiac or pulmonary function as presented clinically may have profound effects on the circulatory system's ability to deliver oxygen and collect carbon dioxide.

Consistent with other more commonly encountered clinical species, the hemoglobin molecule is the compound responsible for the respiratory properties of the blood. Although the specific structure of reptilian hemoglobin has not been completely described, it is most likely very similar to that of other vertebrates. However, a number of significant differences do exist in the tendencies for hemoglobin to hold onto or unload oxygen. These variations have not shown any consistent pattern in relationship to environmental requirements or within the reptilian class.

In general, the affinity of the blood for oxygen is dependent on the reptile's species, age, body size, and temperature. In the whole animal, the total oxygen store is a function of the hematocrit, and the volume of blood. The oxygen-carrying capacity of the blood, a measure of the blood's ability to carry oxygen, is dependent on the number of red blood cells per unit volume (hematocrit). Published oxygen capacities in reptiles typically range from 5% to 11% in turtles, from 6% to 15% in crocodilians, from 8% to 12% in snakes, and from 7% to 8% in lizards.

Oxygen dissociation curves reveal the pressures (a measure of concentration) of oxygen that produce saturation or partial saturation of the hemoglobin. The hemoglobin molecules are responsible for the respiratory properties and color of the blood. These curves indicate how much oxygen is retained by the hemoglobin under specified conditions. Their shapes reflect how blood oxygen affinities are affected by temperature, pH, carbon dioxide, metabolites of glycolysis (DPG), and erythrocyte organic phosphates and by ions such as Na^+, K^+, Mg_2^+, Cl^- and SO_4^-.

Ontogenetic stage can impact oxygen saturation if hemoglobins change from those of neonates to those of adults. Oxygen dissociation curves are to be shifted right (meaning that the blood has a lower oxygen affinity, making delivery of oxygen easier) when metabolic rates are high. In reptiles, the oxygen dissociation curves are highly variable. Generalities about reptile O_2 dissociation curves are difficult to make because of the influences of variable temperature (and metabolic rate) and the other factors list previously.

Different reptiles have different forms of hemoglobins, and for some species, embryonic hemoglobins may have different oxygen affinity properties compared with adults. Hemoglobins differ in how they load and unload oxygen. These differences are often not detected at the clinical level within a species but are important to keep in mind to avoid "overextrapolating" from one species to another.

Oxygen affinity is a measure of how easily the hemoglobin gives up oxygen to tissues. Hemoglobins with higher affinities give up oxygen less readily. Low affinity means that the blood gives up oxygen readily. Reptiles generally have lower oxygen affinities than mammals. This adaptation allows reptiles to deliver oxygen to tissues even at very low blood oxygen levels.

During exercise or stress, reptiles can experience a metabolic acidosis that results from lactic acid production. This change in blood pH reduces blood oxygen affinity through the Bohr effect, which makes the blood hold less oxygen and makes oxygen release to tissues more readily.

Oxygen dissociation curves have been studied for a number of species. They have not shown any consistent pattern; however, several general concepts for individual groups of reptiles may be postulated.

In the lizards, as expected, the more active species (e.g., teids, anguids) have lower oxygen affinities. Higher oxygen affinities are seen in the slower or "sit-and-wait" predator species (e.g., chameleontids, gekkonids). Iguanid lizards (including *Iguana iguana*, *Anolis*, *Ctenosaura*) served as the baseline for comparison. A reported positive relationship exists between body size and oxygen affinity in iguanid lizards, measured at their preferred body temperatures. However, this measure is confounded by behavioral differences in the species and may not be clinically relevant.

In the chelonian, a significant difference appears to exist between aquatic and terrestrial species. In general, aquatic species have a lower oxygen affinity (i.e., they tend to unload oxygen more easily). Some turtles that live under typically hypoxic conditions have blood-buffering mechanisms that delay the Bohr effect. This may be an adaptation to the need for maximum unloading during the periods of submergence of these species. An unexpected exception to this rule is the Mud Turtle (*Kinosternum subrubrum*), whose O_2 dissociation curve is similar to that of a terrestrial turtle.

Snakes have a dissimilar pattern from turtles. When the aquatic Elephant Trunk Snake (*Acrochordus javanicus*) and the arboreal and terrestrial Boa Constrictors (*Constrictor constrictor*) were compared, the oxygen affinity was the opposite. The aquatic snake had a higher oxygen affinity than its terrestrial counterpart.

This difference may be in part the result of a greater Bohr effect seen in the aquatic snake. The role of this increased Bohr effect appears to facilitate increased oxygen availability during the apneic period of submergence when blood CO_2 levels increase. A dual system of blood respiration as seen in this species permits it to unload oxygen during the appropriate time, submergence, and load oxygen when it is most readily available, during ventilation.[6]

In snakes, the oxygen affinity tends to decrease with age, yet the oxygen capacity (the volume percentage of oxygen bound by fully saturated blood) increases as the snake matures. The effect of size on oxygen affinity is variable; whereas it decreases with body size in snakes (as they age), it increases with body size in lizards.

As one might expect, the oxygen-carrying capacity is at its maximum when reptiles are within their POTZ, the time of highest demand.[6] In snakes, which are episodic feeders, oxygen affinity goes down and oxygen consumption increases dramatically during postprandial digestion (a process that can be metabolically demanding).[7]

Not only does the oxygen consumption increase in carnivores after a large meal, so does heart size. Anderson et al[7] report that in Burmese Pythons (*Python molurus bivitattus*), metabolic rates increase up to 40% after eating. This increase in metabolism has been shown to last for up to 14 days.

To support this increase in metabolism, the python heart experiences a normal hypertrophy over the 48 hours immediately after ingestion of a meal. The reported 40% increase in cardiac mass is in response to an increased gene expression of muscle-contractile proteins. Heart size returns to normal once digestion of the current meal is complete.[7]

RESPIRATORY ANATOMY AND PHYSIOLOGY

A basic understanding of the normal anatomy and physiology of the reptilian respiratory tract is vitally important to the clinician. Although the basic structure and function of the lung has been relatively conserved between orders, important differences with clinical implications are found among the various groups of reptiles. Failure to completely understand reptilian pulmonary anatomy and physiology is likely to interfere with successful medical management of disease, such as pneumonia, and also impact management and monitoring of the anesthetized reptile.

Anatomy of the Respiratory Tract

The reptilian respiratory tract is anatomically and physiologically radically different from that of the mammal. Significant differences exist also among the various reptile orders and among species within an order. This is especially apparent in comparison of terrestrial and aquatic species. An attempt is made here to familiarize the clinician with the clinically important features of reptilian respiratory anatomy and physiology of the chelonians, lizards, snakes, and crocodilians. When appropriate, comments concerning intraorder differences are made.

Chelonians

The chelonian glottis is located at the base of the muscular fleshy tongue in a relatively caudal portion of the oropharynx (Figure 10-6, *A*). This location poses significant clinical problems in attempts to access the lower respiratory tract through the oral cavity in the awake individual. The trachea with its complete cartilaginous rings bifurcates after coursing a relatively short distance down the neck (Figure 10-7). The paired bronchi then enter the lung from a dorsal position within the rigid shell.

Chelonians have paired sac-like lungs (Figure 10-8). The air exchange structures, called falveoli (as opposed to alveoli in mammals) open into an open air space within the lung into which the bronchi terminate.[8] The gross anatomy of the lung reveals a structure with internal ridging and septae similar to the cross section of a sponge (see Figure 65-13).[9] The gross anatomy of the turtle's lower respiratory tract is clinically significant. Inflammatory exudates, particularly those associated with infectious disease, tend to accumulate in the dependent portion of the lung. This location precludes timely elimination through the bronchi and trachea as one expects in the mammalian patients.

Turtles accomplish the movement of respiratory gases across the gas exchange surface through a variety of methods. These differences vary depending on species and also on whether the animal is aquatic or terrestrial. In general, both inspiration and expiration are active processes. One must note, however, that the aquatic environment tends to make expiration a more passive process, and in some species, the terrestrial environment makes inspiration more passive. Although chelonians have no true diaphragm, most possess a membranous diaphragm-like structure that partially separates the thoracic and abdominal cavities called the *septum horizontale*.[10] This separation is not seen in the marine seaturtles (see Figure 65-14).

In the "classic aquatic turtle," four groups of muscles are involved in the respiratory cycle. Contraction of the diaphragmaticus and transversus abdominis muscles tends to compress the coelomic cavity, thus causing expiration. The testocoracoideus and obliquus abdominis muscles expand the cavity and cause inspiration.[11]

Interestingly, the repeated gular movements often interpreted by owners as respiratory in nature have no correlation with the respiratory cycle and are actually olfactory in function.[11] Significant differences have been noted in studies of the Greek Tortoise (*Testudo graeca*), a terrestrial chelonian. In this species, movements of the pectoral girdle are the primary muscles of respiration. Inspiration occurs with contraction of the serratus and obliquus abdominis muscles; expiration occurs with contraction of the transversus abdominis and pectoralis muscles.[11]

Lizards

The glottis of the lizard is variable in its location within the oral cavity. In many species, particularly carnivorous species, the glottis is found in the rostral aspect of the mouth (see Figure 10-6, *B*). In others, it is located ventrally, at the base of the fleshy tongue. The tracheal rings of the lizard, like those in the snake, are incomplete. Unlike in the turtle, the trachea

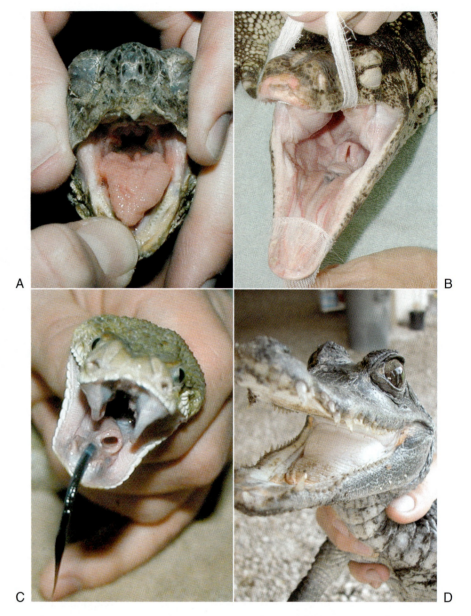

FIGURE 10-6 A, The turtle and tortoise glottis is situated behind the fleshy tongue. **B,** The position of the lizard glottis varies depending on species and can range from a rostral position that is readily visualized, as seen in this monitor, to a more caudal location behind the fleshy tongue, as is seen in the turtles. **C,** The snake glottis is located cranially on the floor of the oral cavity just caudal to the tongue. **D,** The crocodilian glottis is covered by a fleshy epiglottal flap, the *velum palati*, that allows the animal to remain partially submerged with the mouth open but still keep the nostrils above water to permit breathing. (*A, C, D, Photographs courtesy D. Mader; B, Photograph courtesy S. Barten.*)

does not bifurcate in the cervical region but remains a single structure until it enters the thoracic cavity near the base of the heart.

An exception to this is seen in some Old World Chameleons. Some chameleons have an accessory lung that is located in the ventral cervical region, cranial to the pectoral girdle (Figure 10-9). The function of this structure is not known, but it can be a site where pathology develops. Inflammatory exudates, parasites, and fluids can collect in this region, resulting in consolidation of the airspace (see Figure 65-17).

Here the trachea divides into the left and right bronchi.

The lungs of the lizard are approximately equal in size and volume and have an architectural structure similar to that seen in other reptiles (Figures 10-10 and 10-11). In many lizards, gas exchange occurs in the cranial portion of the lung. The caudal extension of the lung is analogous to the avian air sac. This is clinically important because inflammatory debris may accumulate within this nonrespiratory portion of the lung. Because this region is poorly vascularized, infectious material may persist and be relatively unaffected by parenteral antimicrobials.

As described in turtles, both inspiration and expiration are active processes in the lizard. In most species, both are facilitated by the intercostal muscles. Some species use smooth muscle within the lung to aid in the inspiratory process.[11] Most species complete the expiratory-inspiratory cycle with a nonventilatory period of varying length.

Some lizards, such as the monitors, possess a membranous separation between the heart and lungs and the rest of the coelomic viscera, which provides a separation similar to that seen by the diaphragm between the thorax and abdomen in mammals (Figure 10-12). This membrane has no respiratory function.

Snakes

The glottis of the snake is situated rostrally in the oral cavity, thereby permitting active respiration during food consumption. This also permits direct visualization and intubation of the

Cardiopulmonary Anatomy and Physiology

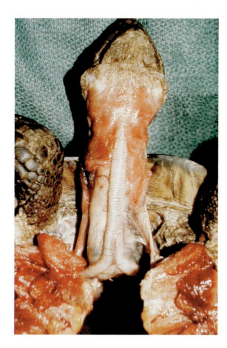

FIGURE 10-7 The turtle has a trachea that bifurcates into a left and right lung at the thoracic inlet, much the same as in a mammal. The chelonian trachea has complete cartilaginous rings. *(Photograph courtesy D. Mader.)*

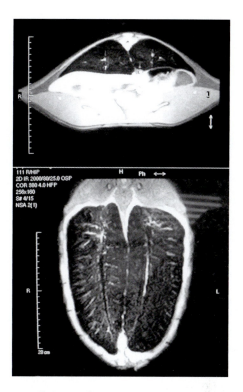

FIGURE 10-8 Chelonians have paired lungs similar to those seen in mammals. Magnetic resonance imaging of a turtle shows the lateral symmetry and shows the complete separation between the two lobes. *(Photograph courtesy D. Mader.)*

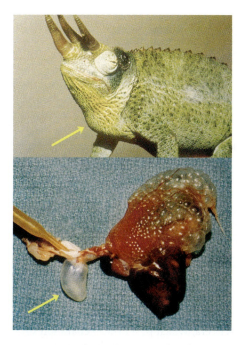

FIGURE 10-9 Most lizards have paired lungs similar to mammals. Some Old World Chameleons, such as this Jackson's Chameleon *(Chamaeleo jacksoni)*, also have an accessory lung lobe in the ventral cervical region, just cranial to the pectoral girdle *(yellow arrows)*. *(Photograph courtesy D. Mader.)*

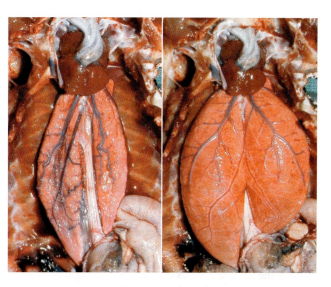

FIGURE 10-10 Lizards have paired, generally symmetrical lungs. The lungs are more like hollow sacs than like the typical mammalian alveolar lung. The image on the *left* shows the lung deflated, and the image on the *right* shows the lung during maximum inflation. No diaphragm exists in reptiles, so the view on the *right* is what is seen during a coeliotomy. Extreme care must be taken to ensure that the lungs are not overinflated during anesthetic ventilatory efforts; overinflation results in rupture of the delicate tissue. *(Photograph courtesy D. Mader.)*

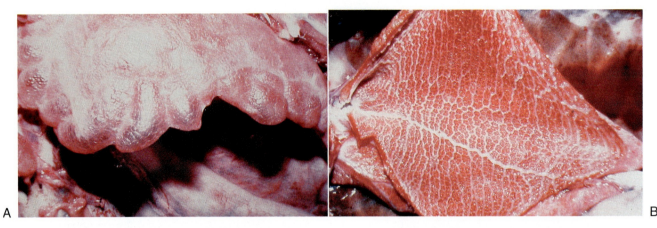

FIGURE 10-11 **A,** The normal lizard lung is a hollow, sac-like, diaphanous structure with most of the respiratory surfaces (falveoli) located toward the center of the structure. **B,** The peripheral margins function more like an air sac. *(Photographs courtesy D. Mader.)*

trachea in most snakes, even when awake (see Figure 10-6, C). The trachea, with its C-shaped incomplete tracheal rings, enters the lung at a level near the base of the heart (Figure 10-13). Some species have a "tracheal lung" that is located on the dorsal aspect of the trachea (see Figure 32-19). This structure is suggested to permit gas exchange when the lung has been compressed by ingested prey.[8]

Most snakes have only one functional lung, with the left side being vestigial or absent. In the more primitive species, such as the boids, both lungs are present, but the left is smaller. The lungs of most snakes are divided into two portions. The first one third to one half is a typical functioning reptile lung. The caudal portion is a relatively avascular sac-like structure similar to the avian air sac. The cranial, or alveolar lung, is typically located starting at 20% and ending at approximately 40% of the snout to cloaca length (Figure 10-14).[12] The caudal, or membranous, lung extends posteriorly for a variable length, potentially to the level of the cloaca, depending on the species.

The respiratory cycle of the snake involves both active and passive components. The expiration is controlled by dorsolateral (muscularis transversus dorsalis and muscularis costalis internus superior) and ventrolateral (muscularis transversus abdominis and muscularis obliquus abdominis internus) muscle sheets. Relaxation of the expiratory muscles results in the first component of inspiration, a passive process. Elevation of the ribs caused by contraction of muscularis levator costarum and retractor costarum decreases intrapulmonary pressure, resulting in the active component of inspiration. The final portion of the respiratory cycle, passive expiration, occurs as a result of the relaxation of the inspiratory muscles and the recoil of the lung.[11]

Crocodilians

The glottis of the crocodilians is located caudal to the prominent epiglottal flap (velum palati; see Figure 10-6, D; see also Figure 8-9). This membrane at the back of the mouth in conjunction with the basihyal valve permits respiration while the animal is partially submerged, despite an open mouth, by sealing off the oral cavity. These species have a coelomic

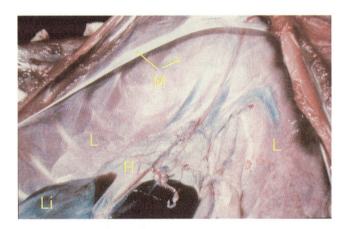

FIGURE 10-12 Although reptiles lack a functional diaphragm, the crocodilians have a membranous separation between the heart and lungs and the coelomic viscera. This image from a monitor lizard (*Varanus* sp.) shows a similar structure. The lung *(L)* and heart *(H)* can be seen through the membrane *(M)*. The liver *(Li)* is on top of the membrane on the *lower left side* of the image. *(Photograph courtesy D. Mader.)*

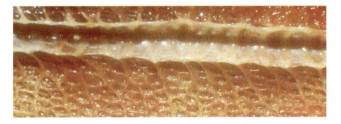

FIGURE 10-13 Snakes have a C-shaped trachea that courses through the entrance to the lung. *(Photograph courtesy D. Mader.)*

cavity that is bisected by a muscular septum analogous to the diaphragm. The cranial aspect of the liver is attached to this structure. Caudally, the liver is connected to the pelvic girdle by a pair of muscles, the diaphragmaticus. Contraction of these muscles, combined with the action of the intercostal

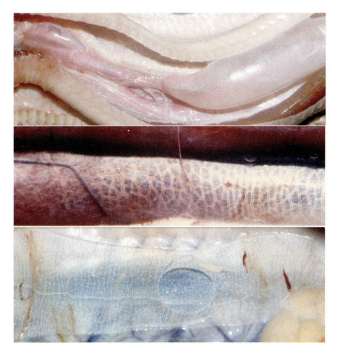

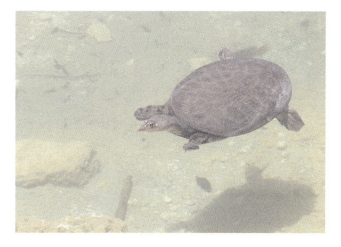

FIGURE 10-15 Several species of amphibians and reptiles are capable of nonrespiratory gas exchange. The aquatic Softshell Turtle (*Apalone* spp.) has both integumentary (through the shell) and buccopharyngeal gas exchange. These adaptations allow the animal to remain submerged for prolonged periods. *(Photograph courtesy D. Mader.)*

FIGURE 10-14 Most snakes have a single, long, tube-like lung, usually with the right side being the functional side. The cranial one third to one half of the lung *(top image)* serves as a functional respiratory exchange organ (the nonhyperinflated portion on the *left side* of the frame). Then, the lung tissue transitions into a membranous, nonrespiratory air sac *(middle image)*. The air sac is diaphanous and balloon-like. The purpose for this transition is not known, but one theory suggests that it serves as a mechanism for internally warming an animal during thermoregulation by inhaling large quantities of warm air. *(Photographs courtesy D. Mader.)*

muscles, supports active inspiration, often referred to as the "hepatic piston."[13] Active expiration occurs as a result of constriction of the body cavity by transverse muscles.[11] The lung of the crocodilian is more complex than that of the other reptiles. Parabronchi further divide the lungs into a series of chambers.[10]

Despite the tremendous variation in the gross anatomy of the reptilian respiratory tract, the microscopic anatomy is quite consistent. The trachea is lined with a pseudostratified, ciliated, columnar epithelium with varying numbers of goblet cells. The ciliated epithelium disappears on leaving the largest airways and is transformed into a more squamous profile.[14] The reticular falveolar lung is composed of thin-walled capillaries sandwiched between the epithelial cells of the falveolus. The caudal avascular lung of the snake is lined with a simple squamous epithelium.

Respiratory Physiology

In discussion of respiratory physiology, one must consider the three components of the respiratory mechanism: first, the movement of respiratory gases from the environment across the gas exchange surface; second, the movement of oxygen (O_2) and carbon dioxide (CO_2) across the respiratory epithelium; and third, the circulation of the O_2-bearing and CO_2-bearing blood from the lungs to the tissues and the subsequent diffusion of the gases to the cellular level.

Reptiles, as previously shown, have unique systems for the assimilation and elimination of respiratory gases. Although the techniques for these processes are quite varied within the reptile class, the remainder of the respiratory process is rather consistent.

Of particular clinical significance is the reptile's ability to function with anaerobic metabolism. The unique buffering systems present within the reptile circulatory system are able to handle the accumulation of lactic acid and hydrogen ions, which accumulate during these periods of anaerobiosis. This ability tends to facilitate the concealment of severe respiratory disease until it has advanced to a level beyond the compensatory abilities of the patient.

Reptiles are not limited to gas exchange through the pulmonary falveoli. Many aquatic species have shown an ability to exchange respiratory gases through the integument. Turtles, such as the Softshelled Turtle (*Apalone* spp.), may obtain up to 70% of their oxygen uptake during submergence through the leathery shell (Figure 10-15).[10]

The buccopharyngeal membranes also serve as a respiratory exchange surface in a variety of reptiles. The highly vascularized pharyngeal papillae are able to extract dissolved oxygen from the aquatic environment. The softshells are able extract sufficient oxygen by buccopharyngeal and cutaneous exchange during long-term submergences, such as during hibernation.

Numerous species of lizards are also capable of use of some degree of pharyngeal or cutaneous respiration.

As mentioned, certain snake species have a unique saccular diverticulum of open tracheal rings that acts as a "tracheal lung" for gas exchange when gastric contents preclude normal pulmonary function (see Figure 32-19).

Respiration in the poikilothermic reptile tends to be controlled by oxygen partial pressure (PO_2), CO_2, and temperature. As temperature increases, so does the body's demand for oxygen. This demand is generally not met by an increased respiratory rate but by an increased

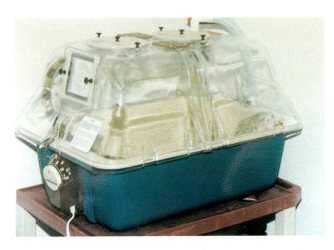

FIGURE 10-16 Placement of a reptile with severe pulmonary disease in an oxygen chamber may be detrimental because increased oxygen concentrations may actually depress respiratory efforts. *(Photograph courtesy D. Mader.)*

tidal volume.[11] Likewise, hypercapnia (an increase in CO_2) also causes an increase in tidal volume, whereas hypoxia causes an increase in respiratory rate. In reptiles, the stimulus to breath comes from low blood oxygen concentration.

This mechanism has limits, however, and in the face of significant pulmonary pathology, the ability of the patient to increase its functional tidal volume is compromised by inflammatory debris, cellular infiltrates, and loss of normal tissue elasticity.

Clinically significant is the fact that high oxygen–tension environments tend to suppress the reptile's spontaneous respiratory rate. Although the absence of a diaphragm and poor bronchociliary transport mechanism tend to inhibit the movement of inflammatory exudates from the lung, prolonged exposure to an environment of enriched oxygen tension may further inhibit this limited capacity by suppressing ventilation. Therefore, the use of hospital oxygen cages should be reserved for those cases in which hypoxemia is present or strongly suspected (Figure 10-16). The relative inefficiency of the lungs combined with the reptile's tendency to shift to anaerobic metabolism is clinically important in cases of pulmonary pathology.

Significant respiratory disease may result in an increase in pulmonary vascular resistance. Because this change tends to mimic the resistance changes that occur during apnea or diving, changes in cardiac output occur. During normal respiration, the noncrocodilian reptile heart directs most deoxygenated blood into the pulmonary artery. The increased pulmonary vascular resistance, which accompanies diving, and apnea cause blood to be preferentially shunted away from the lungs into the systemic circulation. The shunting that may occur from pulmonary pathology could decrease the oxygen delivery to peripheral tissues. Serious, life-threatening acidosis may result from overwhelming the blood's buffering systems as anaerobiosis becomes prolonged.

REFERENCES

1. Jackson CG Jr: Cardiovascular system. In Harless M, Morlock H, editors: *Turtles: perspectives and research*, Melbourne, Fla, 1979, Krieger Publishing.
2. White FN: Circulation. In Gans C, editor: *Biology of the reptilia*, vol 5, New York, 1976, Academic Press.
3. Williams DL: Cardiovascular system. In Beynon PH, Lawton MPC, Cooper JE, editors: *Manual of reptiles*, Cheltenham, United Kingdom, 1992, British Small Animal Veterinary Association.
4. Smith JA, McGuire NC, Mitchell MA: Cardiopulmonary physiology and anesthesia in crocodilians, *Proc Assoc Reptil Amphib Vet* 17-21, 1998.
5. Holz PH: The reptilian renal portal system—a review, *Bull Assn Reptil Amphib Vet* 9(1):4-9, 1999.
6. Davies PMC: Anatomy and physiology. In Cooper JE, Jackson OF, editors: *Diseases of the Reptilia*, vol 1, New York, 1981, Academic Press.
7. Anderson JB, Rourke BC, Caiozzo VJ, Bennett AF, Hicks JW: Postprandial cardiac hypertrophy in pythons, *Nature* (434): 37-38, 2005.
8. Stoakes LC: Respiratory system. In Benyon PH, Lawton MP, Cooper JE, editors: *Manual of reptiles*, Gloucestershire, England, 1992, British Small Animal Veterinary Association.
9. Junge RE, Miller RE: Reptile respiratory diseases. In Kirk RW, Bonagura JD, editors: *Current veterinary therapy XI*, Philadelphia, 1992, WB Saunders.
10. Marcus LC: *Veterinary biology and medicine of captive amphibians and reptiles*, Philadelphia, 1981, Lea & Febiger.
11. Wood SC, Lenfant CJ: Respiration: mechanics, control and gas exchange. In Gans C, editor: *Biology of the reptilia*, vol 5, San Diego, 1976, Academic Press.
12. McCracken HE: The topographical anatomy of snakes and its clinical applications, a preliminary report, *Proc Am Assoc Zoo Vet* 112-119, 1991.
13. Smith JA, McGuire NC, Mitchell MA: Cardiopulmonary physiology and anesthesia in crocodilians, *Proc Assoc Reptil Amphib Vet* 17-21, 1998.
14. Frye FL: *Biomedical and surgical aspects of captive reptile husbandry*, ed 2, vol II, Melbourne, Fla, 1992, Krieger Publishing.

11
RENAL ANATOMY AND PHYSIOLOGY

PETER HOLZ

GROSS ANATOMY

The reptilian urinary tract consists of paired kidneys, each connected to the urinary bladder or cloaca by a ureter. Depending on the species, a urinary bladder may be present and also enters (via the urethra) into the cloaca (Table 11-1). Although technically not part of the urinary system, the reproductive system (ovaries and testes) is also connected to the urinary tract via the cloaca and is discussed here in its relationship to the urinary tract.

Unlike mammals, reptiles do not have separate external orifices for the discharge of urinary and digestive waste products. The end products of the digestive and urinary tract and reproductive system all enter a single chamber, the cloaca, and are discharged through a single opening, the vent (Figure 11-1). The term "cloaca" is derived from Latin origins and means "sewer."

The cloaca is divided into three regions. The coprodeum is the most anterior section and receives the waste products of digestion from the rectum. The middle section, or urodeum, receives the ureters, urinary bladder, and genital ducts. In some species, the genital ducts and ureters penetrate the urodeum separately, but in others, they fuse before entering the urodeum (Figure 11-2). Posterior to the urodeum is the last section, or proctodeum, which is the final stop before waste and reproductive products are discharged to the exterior through the vent.

Order Squamata: Suborder Sauria

In most lizards, the kidneys are located deep in the pelvic canal (Figure 11-3). Monitors are the exception, and their kidneys rest in the caudal coelom (Figure 11-4).[1] The kidneys are paired, symmetrical, elongated, slightly lobulated, and flattened dorsoventrally. In many species, the caudal aspect of the kidneys is fused (Figure 11-5). The kidneys are fully separate in the Water Monitor (*Varanus salvator*) and some Chameleons (Figure 11-6).[2]

A fully developed bladder, connected to the urodeum by a urethra, is present in the Slow Worms, iguanas, geckos, chameleons,[2] and the Blue-tongued Skink (*Tiliqua scincoides*; Figure 11-7).[3] A rudimentary bladder exists in the Teiidae, which include the ameivas, tegus, and whiptails. The bladder does not connect to the ureters. Some monitors, such as the Water Monitor, do not have a bladder.[2,4] However, a bladder is present in the Savannah Monitor (*Varanus exanthematicus*; D. Mader, personal communication).

The vent appears as a fold of skin on the ventral side of the tail, just caudal to the attachment of the tail base to the pelvic girdle. Depending on the species, it may be slit-like, with the opening running transversely across the tail base, or round, placed centrally just caudal to the pelvis. The vent is covered by multiple single scales in iguanas, a single large scale on the anterior and posterior margin in skinks, or fleshy soft skin in geckos. In males, two copulatory structures, the hemipenes, open on either side of the vent. They are tucked caudally into the tail and evert when engorged during mating (see Figure 11-6).

Arterial blood is supplied by a variable number of renal arteries that branch off the aorta. Lizards, like all reptiles, have a renal portal system (Figure 11-8).[5] Blood flows from the tail via the caudal vein and the hind legs via the iliac veins and then enters two afferent renal portal veins that convey the blood to the kidneys. In the kidneys, the blood enters a series of capillaries that perfuse the renal tubule cells. From there, the blood leaves the kidneys via the efferent renal portal veins. These fuse to form the postcaval vein, which conveys the blood back to the heart. Pelvic veins connect to the iliac veins before their attachment with the afferent renal portal veins and can divert blood around the kidneys into the single ventral abdominal vein. From here, the blood flows to the liver (Figure 11-9).

Suborder Serpentes

Snake kidneys are paired, flattened, and elongated organs that contain 25 to 30 lobules,[6] except for the Dwarf Boas (*Trophidophis* spp.) and the Rough Boas (*Trachyboas* spp.) whose kidneys are not lobulated.[2] The right kidney lies cranial to the left (Figure 11-10).[1] Studies have calculated the position of snake kidneys as a proportion of the distance between the snout and the cloaca. For boids, this is 0.76 to 0.84; for colubrids, 0.84 to 0.96; for elapids, 0.80 to 0.92; and for crotalids, 0.84 to 0.96.[6,7] The kidneys occupy approximately 10% to 15% of the snake's body length.

Table 11-1	Reptile Species with Urinary Bladders[27]	
With Bladders	**Rudimentary Bladders**	**No Bladders**
Chelonians		Snakes
Rhynchocephalia		Crocodilians
Lizards		
Iguanidae	Agamidae	Anguidea
Lacertidae	Teeidae	
Some Varanidae		Some Varanidae
Chamaeleonidae		
Gekkonidae		
Scincidae		

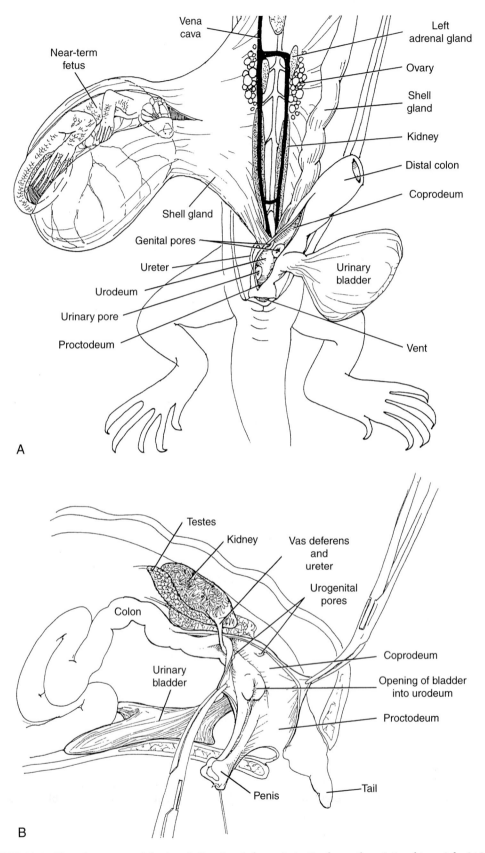

FIGURE 11-1 Cloacal anatomy of the female lizard and the male turtle shows the relationships of the kidneys, ureters, bladder, and reproductive sytems.

Renal Anatomy and Physiology

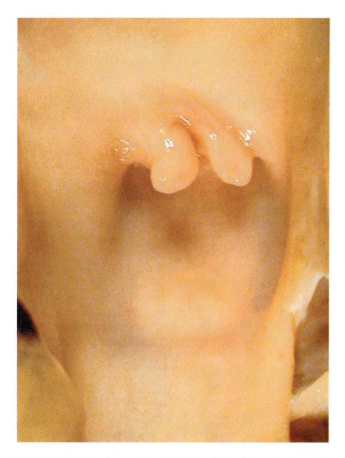

FIGURE 11-2 Urodeum of a male snake shows the ureteral papilla. *(Photograph courtesy D. Mader.)*

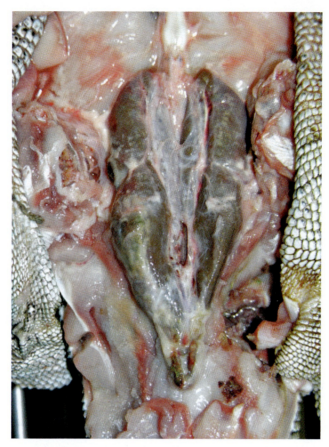

FIGURE 11-3 Normal kidneys in a Green Iguana *(Iguana iguana)*. Note how the kidneys are completely within the bony pelvis. In a healthy animal, the normal kidney is not visible on either a ventral or a lateral radiograph. *(Photograph courtesy D. Mader.)*

A ureter connects each kidney to the urodeum. No urinary bladder exists.[1] Urine is stored either in the distal colon or in flared ends in the distal end of each ureter, just before they enter the urodeum.

The vent is linear, with the slit-like opening running transversely across the tail base. Because no outwardly discernible pelvic girdle is found, except in boids, the vent is considered the beginning of the tail. A single scale covers the vent in boas, with paired scales in pythons. A pair of hemipenes, similar to that in lizards, is present (Figure 11-11).

Arterial blood supply is the same as for the Sauria. The venous blood flow is also similar except for the absence of iliac veins (Figure 11-12). Blood is able to bypass the kidneys through the mesenteric vein, which receives connections directly from the afferent renal portal veins (note: this vein is not pictured in Figure 11-12). The mesenteric venous blood is carried to the liver. The abdominal vein is present but is only connected to the afferent renal portal veins in the African Rock Python *(Python sebae)*. In other species, it has its origin in the fat bodies.[5]

Order Rhynchocephalia

The kidneys of the Tuatara *(Sphenodon punctatus)* are similar to those of lizards. They are paired, single-lobed, and crescentic in outline, tucked high up in the dorsal wall of the pelvic canal (R. Jakob-Hoff, personal communication). The two kidneys meet posteriorly, but they do not fuse.[2] The blood supply is also similar to lizards. However, no direct connection exists between the iliac veins and the abdominal vein. A connection to the abdominal vein has been postulated to exist within the body of the kidneys.[8] A bladder is present. The male does not have a copulatory organ.

Order Testudines

Chelonian kidneys are paired and lie in the caudal coelom just ventral to the carapace (Figure 11-13). In marine turtles, the kidneys are cranial to the pelvic girdle. The kidneys are flattened, lobulated, and symmetrical.[1]

Ureters leave the kidneys and enter the neck of the urinary bladder, similar to mammals. The bladder is connected to the cloaca via the urethra (Figure 11-14).[1] The bladder either is a single large structure or has a larger central structure with bilateral accessory bladders on either side (Figure 11-15).

The vent is circular and lies on the ventral aspect of the tail caudal to its attachment to the plastron. The skin is usually scaleless. The male chelonian has a single phallus situated cranial to the vent and ventral to the base of the tail (Figure 11-16, *A*). As a result, the vent in males is positioned

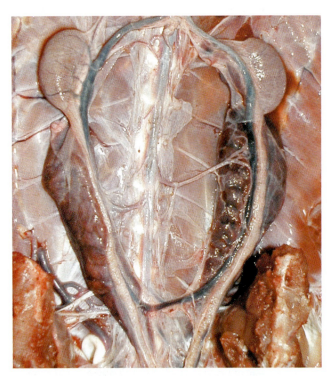

FIGURE 11-4 Normal kidneys in a Water Monitor *(Varanus salvator)*. Note that they are intraabdominal and not fused at the caudal pole. *(Photograph courtesy D. Mader.)*

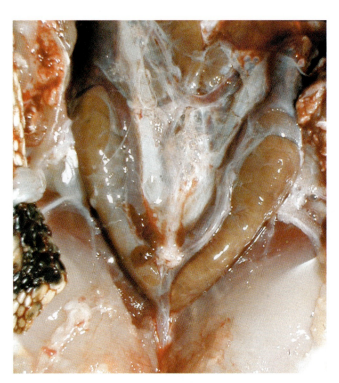

FIGURE 11-5 Fused kidneys at the caudal pole are common in many monitor species. *(Photograph courtesy D. Mader.)*

more caudally than in females. The female chelonian has a variably sized clitoris tucked into the cranioventral base of the tail (Figure 11-16, *B*).

In the female, the vent lies within the margins of the carapace. The vent in males is placed more distally on the tail such that it is beyond the outer margin of the carapace. This finding is consistent across chelonians and is a reliable method for sex determination.

Arterial and venous blood supply is similar to that of the lizards. However, two abdominal veins are found. These are linked by a transverse anastomosis (Figure 11-17).[5]

Order Crocodilia

Crocodilians have paired lobulated kidneys that lie against the dorsal body wall adjacent to the spinal column (Figure 11-18). The left kidney may be larger than the right kidney. Ureters enter the cloaca at the urodeum. No urinary bladder exists.[1] Crocodilians have a single phallus, similar to that described for chelonians.

Arterial and venous supply is similar to the lizards. However, two abdominal veins each connect to an iliac vein,[9] and as for snakes, a mesenteric vein originates from the afferent renal portal veins (Figure 11-19, in which this vein is not pictured).

MICROSCOPIC ANATOMY

Reptilian kidneys have no pelvis or pyramids and are not divided into a medulla and cortex. They contain a few thousand nephrons, compared with human kidneys that have about one million nephrons.[2] Where measured, reptilian

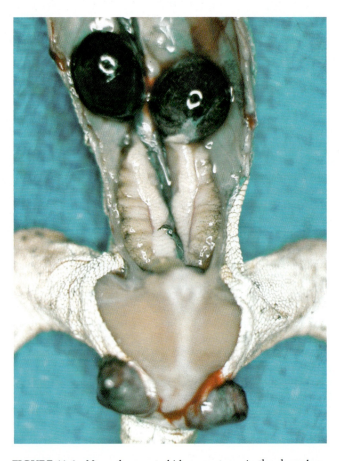

FIGURE 11-6 Normal separate kidney anatomy in the chameleon. Note the black round testes cranial to each kidney. In addition, in this male, the hemipenes can be seen extended bilaterally from the caudolateral margins of the vent (proctodeum). The head is toward the top. *(Photograph courtesy D. Mader.)*

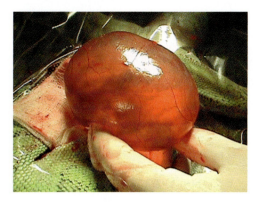

FIGURE 11-7 Fully distended bladder in the Green Iguana (*Iguana iguana*). The normal bladder is thin-walled and minimally vascular as in mammals. *(Photograph courtesy D. Mader.)*

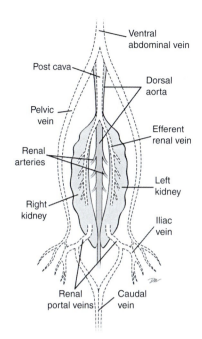

FIGURE 11-8 Renal and vascular anatomy of the generic lizard. *(Illustration courtesy J. Wyneken.)*

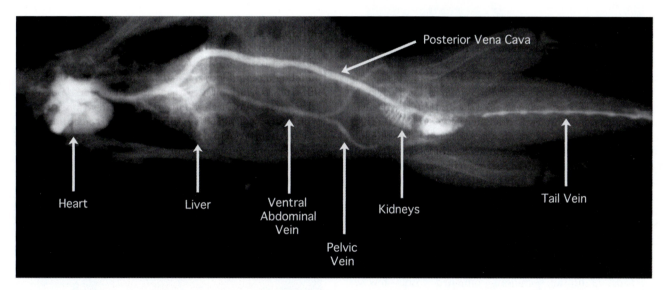

FIGURE 11-9 Contrast angiography showing the major vascular anatomy of the Green Iguana (*Iguana iguana*). Renografin-60 (Diatrizoate Megulime and Sodium, Squibb, New York), a high osmolar contrast medium (292 mgI/mL), was injected at a dose of 2 mL/kg body weight into the caudal tail vein. The radiograph was exposed immediately after the injection was administered (DV view). *(Photograph courtesy L. Pace.)*

nephrons are 2 to 8 mm long, compared with bird nephrons that are approximately 18 mm and human nephrons that are 30 to 38 mm.[10] Each nephron is oriented at right angles to the long axis of the kidney and enters the collecting duct at right angles. The renal corpuscles lie in a circular pattern near the midportion of each lobule.[11]

Structurally, reptilian glomeruli are poorly developed with a lower number of capillaries per gram body weight compared with birds.[10] The glomerulus is followed by the neck segment, proximal tubule, intermediate segment, and distal tubule (Figure 11-20). No loop of Henle is found. All of the segments, except the distal tubule, consist of ciliated cuboidal cells. The cells of the distal tubule lack cilia.

The distal tubule is followed by the sex segment. In all female reptiles, and male chelonians, this consists of columnar mucus-secreting cells. In male snakes and lizards, the cells are flat and filled with mucus during the nonbreeding season. During the breeding season, these cells increase in height two to four times and are filled with large refractile granules that stain brightly eosinophilic with hematoxylin and eosin (Figure 11-21).[12] They contain acid phosphatase, phospholipids, glycoprotein, mucoprotein, and amino acids.

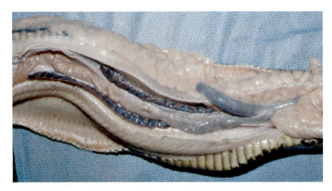

FIGURE 11-10 Normal kidney anatomy of the snake. Most all snakes have brown multilobulated kidneys, with the right cranial to the left. The dark structure to the immediate right of the left (upper) kidney is the cecum. *(Photograph courtesy D. Mader.)*

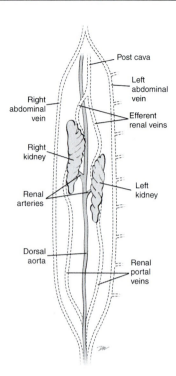

FIGURE 11-12 Renal and vascular anatomy of the generic snake. *(Illustration courtesy J. Wyneken.)*

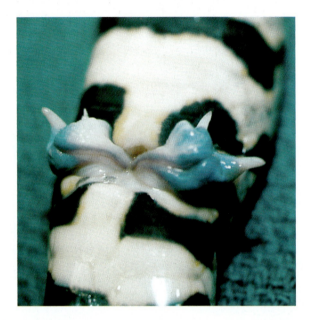

FIGURE 11-11 As seen in lizards, snakes have paired hemipenes that are normally inverted into the caudal wall of the proctodeum. In this case, the hemipenes have been manually everted for examination purposes. *(Photograph courtesy D. Mader.)*

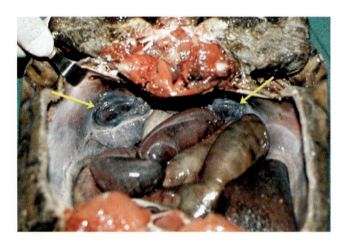

FIGURE 11-13 In the turtle, the kidneys are located immediately ventral to the carapace, just cranial to the rear legs *(yellow arrows)*. The plastron has been removed. The animal's head is toward the bottom of the photograph. *(Photograph courtesy D. Mader.)*

The function of the secretions contained within the sex segment is not known. A number of theories have been proposed. They may act to produce a copulatory plug to prevent rivals from mating successfully. Alternatively, they may block the tubules during copulation to keep the semen and the urine separate, or they may be a source of energy for the sperm.[10]

After the sex segment, the nephron finishes with the collecting duct. These cells are similar to those contained within the sex segment except mucus is only present at the tip of the cell. The collecting ducts are oriented at right angles to the long axis of the kidney. They originate on the dorsolateral surface of each lobule, wrap around the lateral margin of the lobule, and pass ventrally into the ureter, which lies on the ventromedial surface of the kidney.

Blood supply to the nephron consists of an afferent arteriole that forms the glomerular capillary tuft, which is surrounded by Bowman's capsule. Blood exits in the efferent arteriole, which supplies blood to the tubule cells. Venous blood, via the renal portal system, mixes with the arteriolar blood at the start of the proximal tubule.

RENAL PHYSIOLOGY

The metabolism of protein and amino acids results in the production of nitrogen, which must be excreted. The production

Renal Anatomy and Physiology

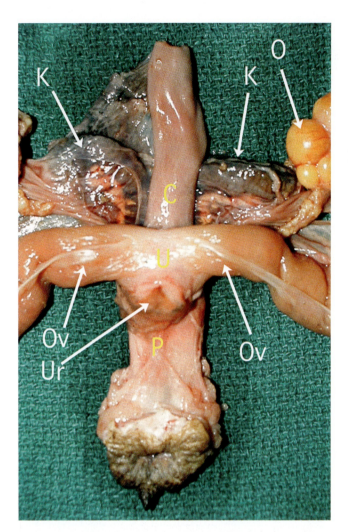

FIGURE 11-14 Normal relationship of the kidneys (K), ovaries (O), oviducts (Ov), and urethra (Ur) (note: the bladder has been removed) to the urodeum (U), corprodeum (C), and proctodeum (P). This photograph is a ventral view of the entire structure. (Photograph courtesy D. Mader.)

and excretion of ammonia is the simplest method for this task. However, ammonia is toxic to the central nervous system and requires large amounts of water for its excretion. Hence, its production in reptiles is limited to aquatic species such as marine turtles, alligators, and crocodiles.[13]

For mammals, the end product of protein metabolism is urea. This substance is less soluble than ammonia but 40,000 times more soluble than uric acid. Because it is dissolved in solution, it must also be excreted with water, which limits its production to species such as freshwater turtles. They produce 45% to 95% of their waste nitrogen as urea.[14] Because reptile kidneys lack a loop of Henle, they cannot produce a hypertonic urine. Consequently, other means of water conservation must be used. To facilitate this, terrestrial reptiles excrete predominantly uric acid.

Instead of dissolving in solution, like urea, uric acid complexes with protein and either sodium or potassium to form a suspension. A herbivorous diet leads to a greater amount of potassium complexing with urate, and a carnivorous diet favors sodium complexing with urate.[10] This suspension contains spheres that are composed of about 65%

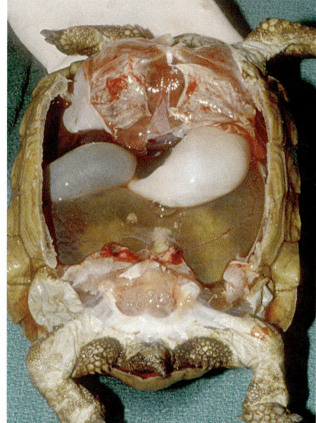

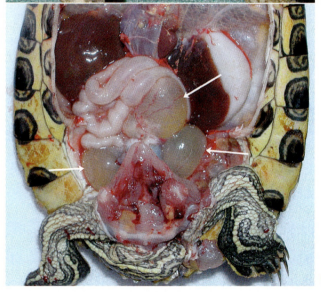

FIGURE 11-15 A, Tortoise bladder. B, Slider bladder. Note the two smaller accessory bladders off to either side of the main bladder in the center of the coelom. (Photograph courtesy D. Mader.)

uric acid and range in diameter from 0.5 to 15 µm. The kidney secretes mucoid substances that contain glycoprotein or mucopolysaccharides that aid in sphere formation and prevent clogging of collecting ducts with urates.[10] Consequently, ureteral urine in reptiles contains large amounts of protein, compared with that in mammals, which contains almost none. This is not lost to the animal because the ureteral urine,

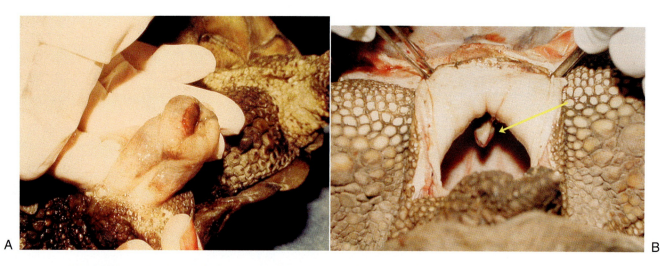

FIGURE 11-16 **A,** Normal phallus (penis) of the adult sexually active male tortoise. **B,** Normal phallus (clitoris) of the sexually active female tortoise. This latter structure is often misidentified as a penis. *(Photograph courtesy D. Mader.)*

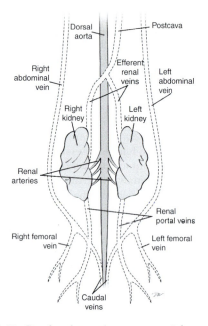

FIGURE 11-17 Renal and vascular anatomy of the generic turtle. *(Illustration courtesy J. Wyneken.)*

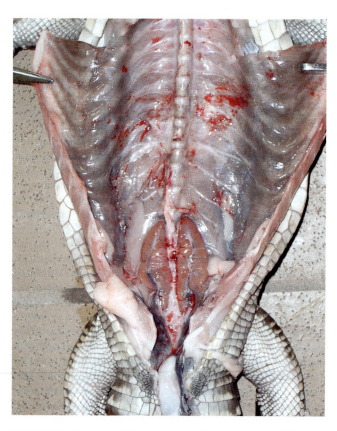

FIGURE 11-18 Normal kidney position in the alligator. *(Photograph courtesy J. Nevarez.)*

once it enters the urodeum, is moved via reverse peristalsis into the rectum. Here the protein is reabsorbed and recycled and the uric acid precipitates out, forms a semisolid white paste, and is excreted (Figure 11-22).[11]

Uric acid is actively secreted into the proximal tubule. This process requires potassium but is unaffected by a lack of sodium.[15] Urate secretion increases if blood pH increases but does not decrease if pH drops.[10]

Only 30% to 50% of the filtered water is absorbed in the proximal tubules, compared with 60% to 80% in mammals. The rest is absorbed in the distal tubules, colon, cloaca, and where present, bladder. Hydrogen ions are secreted into the bladder, which acidifies the urine and results in the precipitation of uric acid. Sodium, water, and bicarbonate can then be absorbed from the bladder.[10,16]

Water is conserved with the production of uric acid and with the decrease of glomerular filtration rate. Reptiles normally have a reduced glomerular filtration rate compared

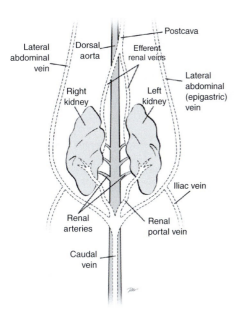

FIGURE 11-19 Renal and vascular anatomy of the alligator. *(Illustration courtesy J. Wyneken.)*

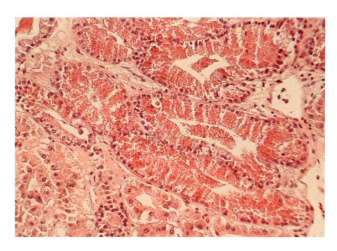

FIGURE 11-21 Histologic appearance of the sexual segment in a snake. During the breeding season, these cells increase in height two to four times and are filled with large refractile granules that stain brightly eosinophilic with hematoxylin and eosin. *(Photograph courtesy F.L. Frye.)*

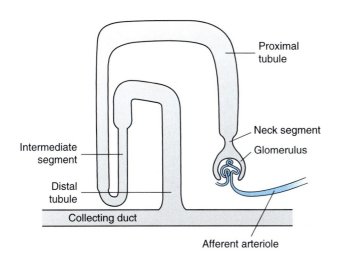

FIGURE 11-20 The reptilian glomeruli is poorly developed. The glomerulus is followed by the neck segment, the proximal tubule, the intermediate segment, and the distal tubule.

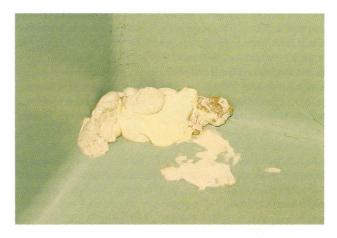

FIGURE 11-22 The end product of protein metabolism in the reptile is uric acid. To conserve body water, uric acid precipitates out and forms a semisolid whitish paste in the excrement. *(Photograph courtesy D. Mader.)*

with birds,[15] partly because of their lower blood pressure, 20 mm Hg diastolic as opposed to 120 mm Hg diastolic in birds.[17] The glomerular filtration rate is further decreased in times of dehydration through the action of arginine vasotocin, which is released by the posterior pituitary gland and causes constriction of the afferent arteriole. As a result, the glomerulus closes, the tubule collapses, and transport across the epithelium ceases.[18] Glomerular filtration rate decreases with dehydration or a salt load and increases with a water load.[16] In the freshwater turtle *(Pseudomys scripta)*, total anuria occurs if plasma osmolality exceeds 20 mOsm. For the Desert Tortoise *(Gopherus agassizii)*, this does not occur until osmolality exceeds 100 mOsm.[16] Prolactin increases glomerular filtration rate.[19]

The cessation of blood flow through the glomerulus means that no blood reaches the renal tubule cells, which places them at risk from ischemic necrosis. To prevent this from happening, renal portal blood continues to perfuse the tubules and keep the cells alive. As discussed previously, blood from the caudal regions of the body can be diverted through the kidneys or bypass the kidneys. Presumably more blood is shunted through the kidneys during times of water deprivation. A valve responsible for regulating the direction of blood flow has been identified in poultry[20] and tentatively described in Red-eared Sliders *(Trachemys scripta elegans)*.[21] What controls the valve in reptiles is unknown, but in poultry, adrenaline causes the valve to open, diverting blood around the kidneys, and acetylcholine causes it to close, shunting blood through the kidneys.[22]

The long-standing belief that drugs should not be injected in the caudal region of reptiles because the renal portal system conveys them to the kidney, leading to nephrotoxicity and subtherapeutic drug levels, has not been supported by experimental work in Red-eared Sliders and Carpet Pythons (*Morelia spilota*).[23,24] Injection site appears to be irrelevant to drug kinetics, and treatments may be administered anywhere in the body.

As well as functioning as an excretory organ, the reptilian kidney is also responsible for vitamin C synthesis[25] and the conversion of 25-hydroxycholecalciferol to the active forms, 1,25-dihydroxycholecalciferol or 24,25-dihydroxycholecalciferol.[26]

In conclusion, because reptiles represent the first group of animals to adapt to a wholly terrestrial lifestyle, their kidneys have evolved to maximize water conservation. This is accomplished with comparatively few nephrons, a low glomerular filtration rate, the production of uric acid as the end product of nitrogen metabolism, and the ability to cease glomerular filtration altogether in times of water stress.

REFERENCES

1. Canny C: Gross anatomy and imaging of the avian and reptilian urinary system, *Sem Avian Exotic Pet Med* 7:72-80, 1998.
2. Fox H: The urogenital system of reptiles. In Gans C, editor: *Biology of the Reptilia*, vol 6, New York, 1977, Academic Press.
3. Beddard FE: Contributions to the anatomy of the Lacertilia: (1) on the venous system in certain lizards, *Proc Zoo Soc* 436-450, 1904.
4. King D, Green B: *Goanna*, Kensington, NSW, Australia, 1993, New South Wales University Press.
5. Holz PH: The reptilian renal portal system: a review, *Bull Assoc Rept Amphib Vet* 9:4-9, 1999.
6. Kell R, Wissdorf H: Beiträge zur Organtopographie bei ungiftigen Schlangen der Familien Boidae (Boas und Pythons) und Colubridae (Nattern), *Tierärztl Prax* 20:647-656, 1992.
7. McCracken H: Organ location in snakes for diagnostic and surgical evaluation. In Fowler ME, Miller RE, editors: *Zoo and wild animal medicine, current therapy 4*, Philadelphia, 1999, WB Saunders.
8. Beddard FE: Some additions to the knowledge of the anatomy, principally of the vascular system, of Hatteria, Crocodilus, and certain Lacertilia, *Proc Zoo Soc* 461-489, 1905.
9. Rathke H: Von dem Herzen und den Blutgefassen. In: *Untersuchungen über die Entwickelung und den Körperbau der Krokodile*, Braunschweig, Germany, 1866, Vieweg.
10. Dantzler WH: Renal function (with special emphasis on nitrogen excretion). In Gans C, editor: *Biology of the Reptilia*, vol 5, New York, 1976, Academic Press.
11. Braun EJ: Comparative renal function in reptiles, birds, and mammals, *Sem Avian Exotic Pet Med* 7:62-71, 1998.
12. Zwart P: Anatomy, histology and physiology of the normal reptilian kidney. In: *Studies on renal pathology in reptiles*, Utrecht, Netherlands, 1963, Stichting Pressa Trajectina Lepelenburg 1.
13. Coulson RA, Hernandez T: Alligator metabolism, kidney, *Comp Biochem Physiol* 74(1):143-175, 1983.
14. Schmidt-Nielsen B, Skadhauge E: Function of the excretory system of the crocodile (*Crocodylus acutus*), *Am J Phys* 212:973-980, 1967.
15. Dantzler WH: Comparative aspects of renal function. In Seldin DW, Giebisch G, editors: *The kidney: physiology and pathophysiology*, New York, 1985, Raven Press.
16. Dantzler WH, Schmidt-Nielsen B: Excretion in fresh-water turtle (*Pseudemys scripta*) and desert tortoise (*Gopherus agassizii*), *Am J Phys* 210:198-210, 1966.
17. Rodbard S, Feldman D: Relationship between body temperature and arterial pressure, *Proc Soc Exp Biol Med* 63:43-44, 1946.
18. Schmidt-Nielsen B, Davis LE: Fluid transport and tubular intercellular spaces in reptilian kidneys, *Science* 159:1105-1108, 1968.
19. Brewer KJ, Ensor DM: Hormonal control of osmoregulation in the chelonia. I. The effects of prolactin and interrenal steroids in freshwater chelonians, *Gen Comp Endocrinol* 42:304-309, 1980.
20. Akester AR: Radiographic studies of the renal portal system in the domestic fowl (*Gallus domesticus*), *J Anat* 98:365-376, 1964.
21. Holz P, Barker IK, Crawshaw GJ, Dobson H: The anatomy and perfusion of the renal portal system in the red-eared slider (*Trachemys scripta elegans*), *J Zoo Wildl Med* 28:378-385, 1997.
22. Rennick BR, Gandia H: Pharmacology of smooth muscle valve in renal portal circulation of birds, *Proc Soc Exp Biol Med* 85:234-236, 1954.
23. Holz P, Barker IK, Burger JP, Crawshaw GJ, Conlon PD: The effect of the renal portal system on pharmacokinetic parameters in the red-eared slider (*Trachemys scripta elegans*), *J Zoo Wildl Med* 28:386-393, 1997.
24. Holz PH, Burger JP, Pasloske K, Baker R, Young S: Effect of injection site on carbenicillin pharmacokinetics in the carpet python, *Morelia spilota*, *J Herpetol Med Surg* 12(4):12-16, 2002.
25. Gillespie DS: Overview of species needing dietary vitamin C, *J Zoo Anim Med* 11:88-91, 1980.
26. Ilrey DE, Bernard JB: Vitamin D: metabolism, sources, unique problems in zoo animals, meeting needs. In Fowler ME, Miller RE, editors: *Zoo and wild animal medicine, current therapy 4*, Philadelphia, 1999, WB Saunders.
27. Fox H: The urogenital system of reptiles. In Gans C, Parsons T, editors: *Biology of the Reptilia*, vol 6, morphology E, New York, 1977, Academic Press.

12
GASTROINTESTINAL ANATOMY AND PHYSIOLOGY

ORLANDO DIAZ-FIGUEROA and
MARK A. MITCHELL

MORPHOLOGY AND PHYSIOLOGY

With more than 7500 different species of reptiles in the world, that the reptilian gastrointestinal tract is not only highly variable between orders but can also be highly variable between genera should not be unexpected. For this reason, reptiles that share similar ecologic niches can have completely different feeding strategies (e.g., insectivores and herbivores). Veterinarians who work with reptilian patients should become familiar with the anatomic and physiologic differences of the reptilian gastrointestinal tract to improve the management of diseases associated with this system. Gastrointestinal diseases are a common finding in captive reptiles and are commonly associated with infectious diseases, parasites, toxins, foreign bodies, and neoplasia.

The reptilian alimentary tract is anatomically simple in comparison with that of higher vertebrates.[1] The digestive system of reptiles is comprised of a mouth, buccal cavity, oropharynx, esophagus, stomach, small intestine, large intestine, colon, and cloaca. In some herbivorous species, a significant sacculated cecum is attached to the large intestine, and herbivores usually have a longer intestinal tract than do carnivores. Reptiles do not have a rectum-anus, as is found in mammals. Instead, reptiles have a cloaca, which is a combined excretory-reproductive organ. Other important organs associated with the digestive system of the reptile are the liver, gallbladder, and pancreas, the exocrine secretions of which empty into the duodenum. The gallbladder may be located at some distance from the liver in some reptiles.

Oral Cavity

The oral cavity of the reptile is lined by ciliated mucous epithelium with goblet cells.[2] The mucous membranes should be moist and can vary in color from grey to pale pink. A thick ropey discharge may indicate dehydration, and a pale coloration to the mucous membranes may be indicative of anemia and should be pursued. The oral cavity of squamates has skin folds, or lips, that seal the oral cavity. These structures are absent in crocodilians and chelonians.

Teeth are present in the squamates and crocodilians but absent in chelonians. Instead, chelonians use their tomia or keratinized beaks to acquire and tear their food. In the squamates, teeth may be located on the mandible, or specifically the dentary bones of the lower jaw, or the premaxillae, maxillae, palatine, or pterygoid bones of the upper jaw.

In crocodilians, the teeth are only located on the jaws. Reptilian teeth are generally cone-shaped, although variations to this scheme do occur. Marine Iguanas (*Amblyrhynchus cristatus*) have serrated teeth that enable them to scrape marine algae (Figure 12-1). Snake teeth are posteriorly curved and are invaluable for anchoring and holding prey. If a snake bites and attaches to a human, one must not pull the snake free because the bite victim's skin will tear. Instead, the snake should be gently extracted by pushing the head forward to "unlock" the teeth.

Crocodilian teeth are located in sockets within the jaws (thecodonts). Lizards are generally classified as acrodonts or pleurodonts; however, exceptions, like the *Uromastyx* spp., do occur. *Uromastyx* spp. have biting plates that are used to crush and tear plant material. The teeth of the acrodonts, such as the Bearded Dragon (*Pogona vitticeps*), are located on the biting edge of the jaw and are attached directly to the bone. The teeth of acrodonts are not necessarily replaced in mature lizards. For this reason, veterinarians must use caution when opening the oral cavity of these lizards to avoid damaging the teeth. The teeth of pleurodonts, such as the Green Iguana (*Iguana iguana*), are located in a groove in the jaw and are replaced throughout their life. Most reptiles use their teeth to acquire and hold their food, with little mastication.

Venomous snakes and helodermatid lizards have modifications to their teeth (fangs) to facilitate the delivery of venom. The fangs of venomous snakes may have an open or closed venom canal, and the fangs of the helodermatid lizards have an open groove to deliver the venom. Snakes may be either front or rear fanged, and their fangs may be fixed or retractable. In general, most rear-fanged snakes do not deliver potent venoms; however, several rear-fanged species do (Figure 12-2).

Snakes and lizards have well-developed oral multicellular mucous glands, and chelonians and crocodilians have poorly developed glands.[3] Reptiles, especially carnivores, rely on the mucous glands to lubricate prey items and facilitate swallowing. In addition to the mucous glands, reptiles also have labial, lingual, sublingual, palatine, and dental salivary glands. Reptiles can produce significant saliva that functions to lubricate the food and facilitate swallowing. The saliva of most reptiles appears to produce minimal proteolytic activity.[4] However, the helodermatid lizards, including *Heloderma suspectum* and *H. horriblum*, and snakes from the families Elapidae and Viperidae have modified labial salivary glands that produce venom. In addition to these

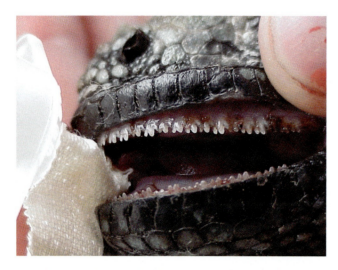

FIGURE 12-1 The serrated teeth of a Marine Iguana (*Amblyrhynchus cristatus*) enable the iguana to scrape marine algae.

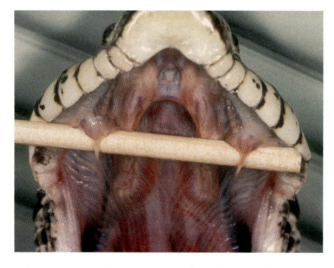

FIGURE 12-2 Rear-fanged Hog-nosed Snake (*Heterodon nasicus*). (Photograph courtesy S. Barten.)

families, some colubrid snakes produce venom too. Venoms may be comprised of various enzymes, polypeptides, inorganic ions, glycoproteins, or biologic amines.

A high degree of variation is found in the shape, size, and function of different reptile tongues. Most snakes have a thin, highly mobile protrusible tongue that has lost most of its mechanical capabilities in the interests of chemosensory specialization. Snake tongues are generally heavily keratinized and have few taste buds.[5] When a snake is introduced to a new environment, or hunts for prey, it "flicks" its tongue. The snake collects various chemical scents on the tongue, retrieves the tongue into the oral cavity, and inserts the tongue into the Jacobson's organ. The Jacobson's organ or vomeronasal organ is found in squamates and chelonians but is absent in crocodilians.[6] This olfactory structure is located in the nasal chamber in chelonians, and in squamates it is connected to the oral cavity via a duct. Lizard tongues are generally mobile and protrusible and are important mechanical aids in feeding and drinking. Lizards with large fleshy tongues generally have numerous taste buds,[7] and lacertids with heavily keratinized tongues may have relatively few taste buds.[5] The tongue of the chameleon is one of the most highly modified tongues in the animal kingdom. Chelonians generally have immobile fleshy tongues that have numerous taste buds and aid in swallowing food and water.

The glottis is located on the floor of the oral cavity of snakes. In lizards and chelonians, the glottis is located at the base of the tongue. The glottis is surrounded by two arytenoid cartilage and one cricoid cartilage. Unlike mammals, reptiles have conscious control over their glottis. The glottis is highly moveable in snakes, which enables these reptiles to breath while ingesting large meals that fill the oral cavity.

The openings to the eustachian tubes are located in the dorsal/dorsolateral pharynx. The eustachian tubes connect the oral cavity to the middle ear and regulate pressure within the ear. Aural abscesses are a common problem encountered in captive and wild chelonians and may be associated with ascending infections from the oral cavity. Snakes do not have eustachian tubes or a middle ear. Instead, snakes have a quadrate bone that connects from the mandible to the stapes and can receive low-frequency vibrations.

Crocodilians have evolved unique anatomic features associated with the oral and nasal cavities and pharynx that enable them to hunt and eat underwater and breathe at the water's surface with the mouth open. The cavum proprium nasi is a cavernous tissue that is located in the nasal sinuses and, when engorged, prevents water flow through the external nares and into the pharynx. When crocodilians hunt and feed underwater, the cavum proprium nasi engorges and the crocodilians consciously close the glottis to prevent aspiration of water. Crocodilians routinely float at the water's surface when they are thermoregulating, hunting, or avoiding predators. Because crocodilians cannot seal the oral cavity from the water, they have evolved unique structures to seal the pharynx from water. The basihyal valve and velum palati are muscular extensions from the base of the tongue and soft palate, respectively. When these two structures close together, they form a tight seal and prevent water from entering the pharynx (Figure 12-3).

The shape of a reptile's skull and the flexibility of the mandibular symphysis can affect the type and size of food that can be ingested by a reptile. In chelonians, the mandibular symphysis is fused and therefore has a limited range of movements. However, in some snakes and lizards, depending on the species, considerable modification exists of the bones and joints of the skull. These anatomic features allow for the movement of both the upper and lower jaws in relation to the cranium (called cranial kinesis). These changes in the kinetics of the jaws and skull increase the overall gape of a reptile and enable it to ingest prey that is larger than would be possible with a fused symphysis.[4]

Esophagus

The primary function of the reptile esophagus is to transport ingesta to the stomach. The esophagus may also serve as a temporary storage for food, as may be observed in species that ingest multiple meals (e.g., invertebrates or eggs). Both mechanical and enzymatic digestion may occur in the esophagus. Seaturtles and some species of tortoise use the strong

Gastrointestinal Anatomy and Physiology 147

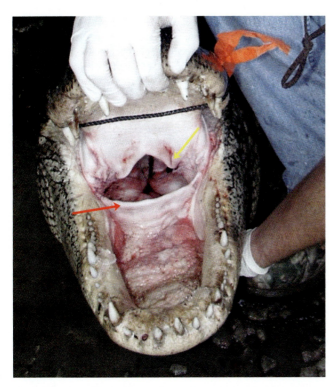

FIGURE 12-3 Oral cavity of a wild alligator. Note the velum palati (soft palate) fold on the top *(yellow arrow)* and the basihyal valve (basihyoid plate) on the bottom *(red arrow)*. Together the valves can close off the back of the oral cavity, thus preventing water from entering the pharynx. *(Photograph courtesy J. Nevarez).*

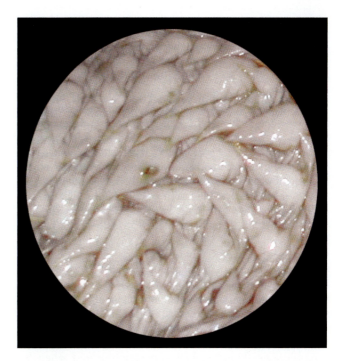

FIGURE 12-4 Endoscopic view of the conical papilla in the esophagus of a seaturtle. *(Photograph courtesy D. Mader.)*

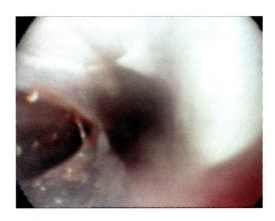

FIGURE 12-5 Endoscopic view of an esophageal tear (left side) in a snake from aggressive assist-feeding. *(Photograph courtesy D. Mader.)*

muscles of the esophagus to crush food and initiate mechanical digestion.[8] Enzymatic digestion may occur in the distal esophagus from gastric reflux or the production of pepsin.[8]

The anatomic and physiologic features of the reptile esophagus are fairly consistent between orders, with few exceptions. However, the length and proportion of the gastrointestinal tract represented by the esophagus can vary significantly. This is especially evident in snakes, which have a longer esophagus compared with chelonians, crocodilians, and lizards. The lining of the proximal esophagus is generally characterized by longitudinal folds, and the distal esophagus has broad and flat folds.[9] The width of these folds can be highly variable between species. Seaturtles have unique conical and cornified papillae that line the esophagus (Figure 12-4). The number and size of these papillae vary between species of seaturtles. The esophagus is lined with ciliated cells and goblet cells. The distribution of these cells can vary within different regions of the esophagus. The muscularis mucosae is generally located in the caudal esophagus but may be absent in chelonians. The tunica muscularis is comprised of both circular and longitudinal smooth muscle. The reptile esophagus is thin and fragile in comparison with the mammalian esophagus. It is not uncommon for the esophagus to tear when an animal is assist-fed by inexperienced handlers (Figure 12-5).

Stomach

All reptile stomachs are comprised of a fundic (corpus) and pars pylorica region, which may be grossly distinct or subtle in appearance. In addition, some chelonians, crocodilians, and lizards have a prominent cardiac region. Snake stomachs are generally the least prominent of all the reptiles and may appear as a benign extension of the esophagus and small intestine. The stomach of squamates is highly distensible, a trait that is important to accommodate the digestion of large prey. In crocodilians, the corpus is comprised of thick muscle and is gizzard-like, a trait that is developed further in avian species. The presence of rugae in the reptile stomach is variable between species, with prominent folds in some species and a complete absence of folds in other species. The stomach is similar to mammals and produces a variety of enzymes, hydrochloric acid and pepsin, by the gastric mucosa.[4]

The primary functions of the reptile stomach are the storage and digestion of ingesta. The highly distensible nature of the reptilian stomach enables these animals to store large meals.

Digestion of food occurs both via enzymatic and mechanical processes. The rate of digestion for reptiles may depend on a number of factors, including body temperature, hydration status, food type and meal size, and the general health of the reptile. Several studies have been published in reptiles and suggest that the rate of digestion can be highly variable.

The digestion of a rodent skeleton was found to require approximately 120 hours for a Boa Constrictor (*Constrictor constrictor*).[10] Unfortunately, the temperature at which the snake was maintained was not reported. When temperature is optimized, the digestive rate is approximately one third the time required at an inappropriate environmental temperature.[8]

Venom can also increase the rate of digestion significantly. *Bothrops jararacussu* can digest a rodent prey in approximately 4 to 5 days if the prey is injected with venom, and the same size and type of prey may take 12 to 14 days if not injected with venom.[11] The digestion of food occurs as a result of both enzymatic processes and the production of hydrochloric acid. Pepsinogen is important to the digestion of proteins, and its production is based on both temperature and gastric pH. The activity of pepsinogen is maximized when the pH is strongly acidic and the reptile is maintained at an optimal environmental temperature. In characterization of the gastric pH of a reptile, one should consider temperature and when the animal was last fed. Anorectic reptiles can have gastric pH levels of more than 3. Optimal gastric pH ranges for reptiles are likely between 2 and 2.5.[12,13] Because the secretion of acid, enzymes, and pepsinogen are temperature related, veterinarians should stress the importance of maintaining these animals at an optimal temperature. Failure to provide an appropriate environmental temperature could lead to decreased gastrointestinal motility and digestion and the putrefaction of digesta.

Intestine

The intestine continues the process of digesting food products started in the stomach but is also the primary site for absorption. The length of the reptilian intestine is highly variable. In general, the herbivore intestine is longer than the omnivore intestine, and the omnivore intestine is longer than the carnivore intestine. Herbivorous lizards also tend to be larger in size than their carnivorous counterparts. This physical difference has been attributed to several potential theories, including that large quantities of plant material are more readily accessible than small packets of energy (insects), that large carnivores that compete with mammals are unsuccessful, and that the large size of the herbivore coupled with a greater thermal inertia reduces the amount of energy necessary to expend to thermoregulation.[8]

Extensive longitudinal folds are often found in the reptilian alimentary tract, especially in snakes; this increases surface area for absorption and allows distention to accommodate large quantities of digesta. A range of enzymes and bile salts, similar to mammals, is produced by the pancreas and liver.[4,14] The pH (6.5 to 8) of the reptile intestine is generally slightly acidic to neutral to slightly alkaline. A gross distinction is usually found between the small intestine and colon in reptiles. The cecum is generally rudimentary in carnivorous reptiles, such as snakes, crocodilians, and monitors; however, it is present in herbivorous chelonians and lizards and serves as a site for postgastric fermentation. Diet is not the only predictor of the presence and size of a cecum, as a *Calotes jubatus*, an insectivore, and *Tupinambus teguixinm*, an omnivore, both have proportionally larger ceca than some herbivorous lizards.[15]

Gastrointestinal motility can be affected by a number of different extrinsic and intrinsic factors.[8] In fasted reptiles, gastric motility is characterized by two phases, single short duration contractions and a longer contraction dispersed over a greater duration. Gastric tone is generally unchanged during the fast. These effects can be diminished in hypothermic reptiles. Once the reptile has ingested a meal, contractions increase. The rate that food passes through the gastrointestinal tract can vary with the volume, type, and composition of the food; environmental and core body temperature; type and length of the gastrointestinal tract; and health of the reptile.[8] In small carnivorous squamates, food passage may occur within 2 to 4 days, and in large snakes, herbivorous chelonians, and lizards, it may require 3 to 5 weeks.

Cloaca

The cloaca and vent represent the terminus of the gastrointestinal tract. Although the cloaca is routinely considered nothing more than the terminus of the gastrointestinal, reproductive, and excretory systems, it also plays an important role in the active absorption of electrolytes and the passive absorption of fluids. The cloaca is comprised of the urodeum, coprodeum, and proctodeum. The excretory and reproductive systems empty directly into the urodeum. In lizards and chelonians, the urinary bladder also connects to the urodeum. Crocodilians and snakes do not have a urinary bladder and store urine in their ureters or colon. Even in chelonians and lizards, the potential exists for urine to become contaminated with feces. This is an important consideration in interpretation of the results of a urinalysis (see Chapter 66).

Gallbladder

In chelonians, crocodilians, and most lizards, the gallbladder is contiguous with the liver. In some lizards and most snakes, the gallbladder is located at some distance from the liver and conveys bile from the liver to the duodenum via a thin-walled cystic duct. The length of this cystic duct varies with the individual reptile and is longest in some snakes. Also, in chelonians, the pancreatic and bile ducts enter the pylorus instead of the duodenum.

Bile is stored in the gallbladder. Bile serves two primary roles in the reptile: as a method for excretion of fats and as an aid in the digestion and absorption of fat.[16] Triglycerides are digested with a mixture of lipases and bile into a solution of bile salts, monoglycerides, and fatty acids. The small molecular size of these products enables them to be absorbed via the enterocytes. Bile may also contain small concentrations of enzymes, such as amylase.

Pancreas

The reptilian pancreas functions in a similar manner to the mammalian pancreas. The pancreas is usually closely associated with the stomach and duodenum in chelonians and lizards. However, the snake pancreas is generally located caudal to the pylorus in the area of the gallbladder and spleen, and the three organs are generally referred to as the triad. In some snakes, pancreatic and splenic tissue are intermixed and form a splenopancreas. The reptilian pancreas is comprised of both exocrine and endocrine tissues (see Chapter 58).

The exocrine tissues secrete digestive enzymes, including amylolytic, proteolytic, and lipolytic enzymes. Chitinase is also produced in the pancreas in those species that feed on prey that use chitin in their exoskeleton. In addition to the enzymes, the pancreas secretes alkaline fluid to counter the low pH of the gastric juices. The functions of the enzymes produced by the pancreas are highly dependent on temperature and pH (>6). Amylolytic enzymes, such as amylase, are believed to be excreted in higher concentration in herbivores compared with carnivores. Chymotrypsin, trypsin, carboxypeptidase, and elastase are proteolytic enzymes that have been identified in reptiles.[8] The production of enzymes by the pancreas is tied to the feeding strategy of the reptile. Certain enzymes, such as chitinase and amylase, are produced in much higher concentrations in one reptile compared with another depending on the reptile's feeding strategy.

FEEDING ECOLOGY

The feeding ecology of reptiles varies from species to species. In general, reptiles can be classified into one of three primary feeding ecologies: herbivore, omnivore, and carnivore. Both anatomic and physiologic differences exist between reptiles that use different feeding ecologies. For example, the alimentary tract of herbivores is generally longer than that of an omnivore or carnivore. Because of the relatively short length of the carnivore alimentary tract, feeding these species high-quality foods is important to maximize nutrient uptake. Commercial diets for these animals generally use low-quality protein sources and may not be appropriate. A high degree of variation is found among carnivores, with some species exclusively insectivorous and others primarily ophiophagous (snake-eaters). In addition to the anatomic differences between feeding ecologies, physiologic differences exist as well.

Herbivorous reptiles are dependent on a functional intestinal microflora to facilitate the conversion of nondigestible cellulose to usable volatile fatty acids. The loss of this microflora could be detrimental to the health of an herbivorous reptile.

A basic understanding of the foraging strategy of a reptile is important in appropriate recommendations regarding feeding. For omnivores and carnivores that hunt prey, the two basic feeding strategies are ambush foragers and active foragers. Ambush foragers expend limited energy to hunt, whereas active hunters can use significant energies. Therefore, the caloric demands for these two different strategies can vary significantly. This is an important consideration for captive reptiles. Active forging reptiles should be provided ample area for hunting to ensure exercise and provide basic enrichment. Active foraging reptiles that are not provided exercise tend to have obesity and the health-related issues associated with obesity. In the wild, most varanids (monitors) are active foraging species and maintain body condition because of the high activity level. In captivity, these animals are frequently offered regular meals with minimal exercise, and they tend to have negative health affects as a result.

Reptiles may use different sensory methods to detect food, including visual detection, chemosensory detection, tactile detection, auditory detection, and thermal detection. The visual, chemosensory, and thermal sensory inputs are used most frequently in reptiles when foraging for food, and auditory and tactile sensory structures are not used heavily for foraging in reptiles.

Visual detection is the primary method for acquiring food used by crocodilians, chelonians, and lizards. Chameleons are unique in that they are the only group of reptiles that has two independently functioning eyes. This enables these lizards to scan a larger horizon for prey and potential predators than other species. When a chameleon identifies a potential prey, it generally focuses both eyes on the prey. Although chameleons have been suggested to do this because they require binocular vision to focus in on the prey, these lizards can catch prey with only uniocular vision.

Chemosensory detection of food is commonly used by squamates and chelonians. Although crocodilians are not considered to rely heavily on olfaction, they have been found to find food items that could not be visualized and also use olfaction for pheromone detection, suggesting that the system necessary for detection of various chemical cues is present. Chemosensory methods of food detection include olfactory, vomerolfaction, and gustation.[17] Olfaction is generally used for the detection of chemical cues that originate some distance from the reptile, and vomerolfaction occurs with those cues within close proximity to the animal. Vomerolfaction uses the Jacobson's organ to interpret chemical cues. Gustation is dependent on the presence of functional taste buds and is generally used to separate food items that are acceptable or unacceptable after ingestion.

Infrared-sensitive sensory structures are found on many species of snakes from the Families Boidae, Pythonidae, and Viperidae. These structures are located around the labial, loreal, and rostral scales on the head. Snakes with these pits can use them to characterize temperature changes associated with the environment. Because these pits are bilaterally symmetric, they enable the snake to characterize direction or location of prey.

GASTROINTESTINAL MICROFLORA

The gastrointestinal microflora of reptiles is generally composed of aerobic and anaerobic gram-positive and gram-negative bacteria, yeast, and protozoa. Several attempts have been made to characterize the aerobic and anaerobic bacterial flora of the alimentary tract in different species of reptiles. However, these studies are primarily based on oral or cloacal swabs and only represent the population of bacteria being shed. Johnson and Benson[18] isolated nine different species of aerobic bacteria from oropharyngeal swabs collected from Ball Bythons (*Python regius*). Five of the bacteria were gram-negative, including *Alcaligenes* spp., *Actinobacter* spp., *Flavobacterium* spp., *Pseudomonas* spp., and *Bordetella* spp., and four were gram-positive, including *Micrococcus* spp., *Corynebacterium* spp., *Staphylococcus* spp., and *Bacillus* spp.[18] Another study that attempted to characterize both aerobic and anaerobic microbes from the oral cavity of Ball Pythons cultured 14 different bacteria, 11 aerobes, and three anaerobes.[19] *Alcaligenes* spp., *Pseudomonas* spp., *Micrococcus* spp.,

Corynebacterium spp., and *Staphylococcus* spp. were again isolated from the Ball Python. In addition, six other aerobes, including *Brevundimonas* spp., *E. coli*, *Klebsiella* spp., *Kocuria* spp., *Shewanella* spp., and *Stenotrophomas* spp., and three anaerobes, *Anaerobiospirillum* spp., *Clostridium* spp., and *Eubacterium* spp., were also isolated. The findings of these two studies reinforce the importance of the environment on the colonization of microbes in animals. Many of these isolates are ubiquitous, and others were likely a specific product of the python's environment.

Because of the limited number of isolates retrieved from cultures of the oral cavity or cloaca, Salb et al[20] collected microbiologic samples directly from the intestinal tract of the Green Iguana to determine whether the flora within the intestine differed from that in the oral cavity and cloaca. Interestingly, 47 isolates were recovered from the intestine (39 aerobes and eight anaerobes). However, only 20 could be characterized, including *Alcaligenes* spp., *Bacillus* spp., *Bacteroides* spp., *Campylobacter* spp., *Candida* spp., *Clostridium* spp., *Citrobacter* spp., *Enterobacter* spp., *E. coli*, *Klebsiella* spp., *Pasteurella* spp., *Peptostreptococcus* spp., *Salmonella* spp., and *Staphylococcus* spp.. This result was not unexpected because other studies in both mammals and birds have also reported difficulty in characterizing isolates because of a limited number of biochemical test methods. Although a large number of isolates was identified in this study, it likely represents a small proportion of the actual number of bacteria that colonize the intestine of the iguana. The specific function or value that microbes provide to the host reptile is unknown in most cases, with the exception of the herbivores.

Green Iguanas are one of the few lizards that remain herbivorous throughout their life.[21] The diet of these arboreal lizards includes a variety of leaves, blossoms, and fruits.[22] The gastrointestinal tract of the Green Iguana is comprised of an esophagus, monogastric stomach, short small intestine, large partitioned colon, rectum, and cloaca. The partitioned colon is the location of hindgut fermentation. The functional significance of the partitioned colon is not well understood; however, it has been suggested to slow digest passage time and increase the absorptive surface area of the colon.[23] Mammalian herbivores feed constantly to satisfy caloric requirements. In contrast, the Green Iguana spends less than 10% of its active day feeding because it requires a short time to fill the gastrointestinal tract.[24]

Herbivorous mammals derive a portion of their caloric requirements from the fermentative activity of protozoa and bacteria that colonize the gastrointestinal tract. These microbes are responsible for the degradation of cellulose and components of vegetation into usable volatile fatty acids that can be incorporated into the Kreb's cycle. The domestic rabbit (*Oryctolagus cuniculus*) derives 4% to 12% of its caloric needs from the microbial processes in the hindgut,[25] whereas the beaver (*Castor canadensis*) derives approximately 19% of its maintenance energy from the hindgut.[26] The Green Iguana obtains a greater proportion of its daily caloric requirements, approximately 30%, from the activity of the microbial flora of the hindgut.[27]

Unlike mammals, reptiles must bask in radiant heat to maintain a core temperature to maximize fermentation in the hindgut. The primary volatile fatty acids produced in the colon of the Green Iguana include acetic, propionic, and butyric acids.[27] The production of acetic acid in the hindgut of the Green Iguana is consistent with mammalian endotherms. The reason for the high production of butyric acid, however, is not apparent.[27]

The gastrointestinal microflora responsible for hindgut fermentation in the Green Iguana is not well defined, although an unidentified complex of bacteria with *Lampropedia merismopedioides* as the principal species has been isolated from the colon of wild-caught individuals.[28] This organism has also been isolated from the rumen of cattle and sheep. Another microbe, an undescribed large ciliated protozoan that resembles the holotrichs of the rumen, has also been routinely identified in wild Green Iguana hatchlings.[28] *Clostridium* and *Leuconostoc* have also been predominant species identified in Green Iguanas,[27] and these microbes, and those yet undescribed, are considered important commensals in the digestion of plant products.

The transfer of the hindgut microbial flora in neonatal mammals occurs through close contact with the mother or fecal contents of other older conspecifics. The passage of the hindgut microbial flora in Green Iguanas does not occur through close contact because the female Green Iguana leaves the nesting grounds once the eggs are deposited.[29] When the hatchlings emerge during the spring (April to June), they inhabit different niches than adults. In areas where the adults and hatchlings do share a similar range, the adults are often located in the high canopy (15 to 30 m) and the hatchlings in the low vegetation (1 to 5 m).[28]

Hatchling Green Iguanas can consume a significant amount of soil within their nest and also lick eggshells, or each other.[28] Although this might be a potential source of microbial passage, a study that evaluated the colonic contents of hatchling Green Iguanas for *L. merismopedioides* and the ciliated holotrich protozoan found that animals exposed to the nest soil and eggshells were no more likely to be transfaunated with those microbes than captive hatched animals.[28] In the same study, no detectable fecal material was found in the nests. A comparison of the nest soil and surface soil for total microbe content was also unremarkable and suggested that maternal contamination of the nest was not a likely source of the organisms, although study results were limited by the total number of animals sampled.[28] The only technique found to consistently reproduce the microbial flora in hatchlings was reported when hatchlings were offered fresh adult fecal material or when the animals were housed with an older hatchling with a complete microflora.[28]

GASTROINTESTINAL TRACT DISEASE: DIAGNOSTICS

History and Physical Examination

A thorough history is essential in identification of a potential etiology or etiologies responsible for gastrointestinal disease in reptiles. Many of the disease processes associated with the gastrointestinal tract are related to a deficiency in the reptile's husbandry. For example, chronic hypothermia can lead to decreased gastrointestinal motility, which might be responsible for anorexia in a reptile. Historical questions should be directed at an understanding of the reptile's environment and nutrition and the owner's experience with reptiles and pet ownership in general. Specific questions may include, but are not limited to, the environmental temperature range and humidity, enclosure size, substrate, lighting and photoperiod, cage furniture, sanitation protocol, animal density, exposure to commercial products (toxins), diet, and water source.

The physical examination should be thorough and complete. The nares and eyes should be clear and free of discharge. The oral cavity should be examined closely (Figure 12-6). Depending on the species, mucous membranes should be moist (indicating proper hydration) and colored light grey (most snakes) to pale pink (most other reptiles). The tongue should be moist and evaluated for normal function. The openings to the Jacobson's organ, internal nares, and choanae should be free of discharge. The glottis should be moist and free of discharge. The dental arcade should be examined for fractured teeth. The jaws should be palpated for fractures or abnormal swellings.

The integument should be evaluated for the presence of ectoparasites, thermal injuries, trauma, or dermatitis. The cervical region and organ systems within the coelomic cavity should be palpated for abnormalities. Although the palpation of the chelonian coelomic cavity is limited by the shell, abnormal findings may be identified via palpation through the axillary or inguinal fossae. Palpation of the coelomic cavity in some species of lizards may be limited in those species that can inflate their lungs and air sacs.

Snakes provide the best opportunity for palpation of abnormalities in the coelomic cavity. Because snake anatomy is fairly consistent across genera, a basic knowledge of the location of different organs can be used to characterize normal and abnormal findings in snakes. Although auscultion of reptiles is difficult with a standard stethoscope, and some clinicians do not advocate auscultion of reptiles, the authors strongly recommend auscultion of all reptile patients. A moist paper towel should be placed on the animal in the general vicinity of the lungs to reduce the friction associated with the bell housing of the stethoscope on the scales or scutes of a reptile. A crystal ultrasonic Doppler scan can also be used to evaluate the heart (see Chapter 14).

DIAGNOSTIC TESTING

Diagnostic tests are an important consideration in evaluation of gastrointestinal disease in reptiles. In some cases, these diagnostic tests may assist in the confirmation of a specific etiology, such as an infectious agent, and in others, they may only provide a general direction to the diagnosis of a disease process. When evaluating gastrointestinal disease in a reptile, the authors generally pursue diagnostic tests in series. The initial series of tests includes complete blood counts (CBCs), plasma biochemistries, microbiologic testing, fecal examination, and survey radiographs. A second series of diagnostics may include a contrast radiographic examination, ultrasound, toxicologic/infectious disease testing, or endoscopy. The third series of diagnostics may include magnetic resonance imaging (MRI) or computed tomographic (CT) scans.

The first tier of diagnostic tests can provide important information regarding the physiologic status of the patient. These tests are also relatively inexpensive and noninvasive. Inflammatory leukograms are a frequent finding in reptiles with gastrointestinal disease and are generally characterized by a heterophilia and monocytosis. Anemia is also a frequent finding in chronic cases of gastrointestinal disease. Alterations in the enzymes, electrolytes, and proteins may be observed in reptiles with gastrointestinal disease. Reptiles that are regurgitating or have diarrhea may have alterations develop in the sodium, potassium, and chloride levels. Elevated aspartate aminotransferase (AST) and creatine kinase (CK) levels are a common finding in reptiles with gastrointestinal disease.

Microbiologic culture can be used to characterize primary bacterial disease. Veterinarians should use caution when interpreting these results because many of the indigenous microbes that colonize the gastrointestinal tract of reptiles are opportunistic pathogens. Feces should be collected from patients and screened for parasites with a direct saline smear and fecal flotation. Survey radiographs can be used to assess the gastrointestinal tract for foreign material, abnormal masses, or other disease processes.

The second tier of diagnostics provides the opportunity to characterize a specific disease process or etiology. These assays are generally more expensive and invasive. Contrast radiography and ultrasound allow the veterinarian to evaluate certain organs more closely. With a contrast series in a reptile, consideration of the gastrointestinal motility is important. **Reptiles that are not maintained at an optimal body temperature may have delayed emptying. In herbivores, such as iguanid lizards and tortoises, contrast can persist within the gastrointestinal tract for more than 25 days.** Endoscopic examination of the gastrointestinal tract provides the veterinarian with direct visualization of specific organs and the opportunity to collect samples for histopathologic evaluation.

Historically, very few reptilian diagnostic assays are available to the veterinarian. Fortunately, with the advent of new serologic and molecular assays, veterinarians can evaluate a reptile patient for a specific infectious disease.

The third tier of diagnostic assays is generally performed last because the tests are expensive and of limited availability to most practitioners. Advanced diagnostic imaging, such as CT and MRI, can provide valuable information regarding the

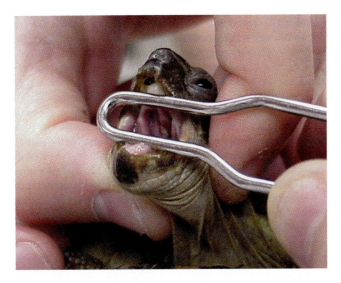

FIGURE 12-6 Oral examination in a Russian Tortoise (*Agrionemys horsfieldii*). Note the abscess that obstructs the right nasal cavity.

specific lesions within an organ. As these diagnostics become more available, and the expense associated with them decreases, their value to veterinarians who work with reptiles will increase.

COMMON GASTROINTESTINAL DISEASES

Infectious Diseases

Bacteria, viruses, fungi, and parasites are frequently associated with gastrointestinal disease in reptiles. Some of these infectious agents may be considered a component of the indigenous microflora of reptiles, and others are obligate pathogens. Whether these infectious agents can incite an inflammatory response and infect the reptile host is dependent on a number of host-specific and environmental factors.

Bacterial Diseases

Bacterial pathogens historically were blamed for the vast majority of all diseases reported in reptiles. Limited diagnostic assays, coupled with the fact that bacteria are an important component to the reptile microflora, frequently resulted in the diagnosis of bacterial diseases. Veterinarians should use multiple diagnostic results in combination in determination of a specific diagnosis. For example, the combination of culture and histopathology can be used to confirm the presence and isolation of a suspected pathogen. In cases where diagnostics are limited, the veterinarian must understand that isolation is possible of pure cultures of bacteria, especially Gram-negative bacteria, in both clinically normal and abnormal reptiles. These results should be combined with all the historical and physical examination findings and other diagnostic tests to determine the true value.

Infectious stomatitis, often referred to by lay individuals as "mouth rot," is a common finding in captive reptiles (see Chapter 72). Stomatitis is nothing more than a clinical finding and may be characterized by the presence of petechial or ecchymotic hemorrhages, damage to the mucous membranes, or abscesses (Figure 12-7). Many reptiles with stomatitis are maintained under inappropriate conditions and have hypothermia, crowding, poor sanitation, and inadequate nutrition.

A number of different bacteria may be isolated from the oral cavity of affected reptiles, including *Salmonella* spp., *E. coli*, *Pseudomonas* spp., *Aeromonas* spp., *Citrobacter* spp., *Pasteurella* spp., *Alcaligenes* spp., and *Klebsiella* spp. Infectious stomatitis associated with *Mycobacteria* spp. has been reported in Boa Constrictors.[30,31] Cases presented to the veterinarian should be pursued with tier 1 and tier 2 diagnostic testing. A CBC can be done to determine whether a systemic inflammatory response is occurring. Microbiologic culture and antibiotic sensitivity testing may be used to guide treatment. Survey radiographs are important for characterization of the extent of the disease and determination of whether surrounding soft tissue and bone are involved. Treatment for stomatitis should be based on the confirmation of an etiology.

Gastritis is defined as an inflammatory response to the lining of the stomach and may be classified into two forms: acute or chronic. Acute gastritis in reptiles has been associated with severe thermal burns, major surgery, antiinflammatory

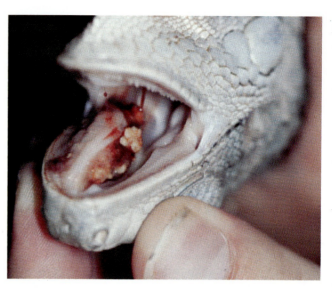

FIGURE 12-7 Severe infectious stomatitis in a Green Iguana (*Iguana iguana*).

agents, corticosteroid administration, toxins, and infectious diseases. Affected reptiles may be seen for anorexia, regurgitation, and melena. The symptoms usually abate after the causative agent has been removed. In contrast, chronic gastritis is more difficult to manage because of the pathologic changes that have occurred in the reptile, such as severe ulceration and granuloma formation. Chronic gastritis has been associated with chronic poor husbandry, neoplasia, and bacterial infections. Cases of diphtheritic necrotizing gastritis have been reported in a Rosy Boa (*Lichanura trivirgata*) associated with *Salmonella arizonae*.[32,33] In addition, atrophic gastritis has been reported in Red-eared Sliders (*Chrysemys scripta elegans*) and Hermann's Tortoises (*Testudo hermanni*). The disease is characterized by atrophy and inflammation of the glandular component of the gastric mucosa and loss of the oxynticopeptic cells with their subsequent replacement by mucus cells.[34]

Enteritis is one of the primary problems for which reptiles are presented to the authors' practice. Gram-negative bacteria are the most common agents associated with enteritis. Again, this may be because of the availability of microbiologic culture in combination with the ease of isolating these bacteria from reptiles. Common isolates from reptiles with enteritis include *E. coli*, *Klebsiella* spp., *Salmonella* spp., *Enterococcus* spp., *Pseudomonas* spp., *Serratia* spp., *Proteus* spp., *Citrobacter* spp., *Alcaligines* spp., and *Pasteurella* spp.[35] Gram-positive bacteria are also routinely isolated from reptiles with enteritis, including *Clostridium* spp., *Corynebacterium* spp., and *Staphylococcus* spp. Acid-fast bacteria, such as *Mycobacteria* spp., should also be considered when a reptile is seen for bacterial enteritis that is nonresponsive to antibiotics.[36] Veterinarians should not assume that enteritis is always associated with a bacterial pathogen because inappropriate diet, misuse of antimicrobials, stress, parasites, and foreign bodies can lead to the development of enteritis. The treatment for bacterial enteritis should include supportive care, with specific attention to the hydration status of the animal, an antibiotic based on sensitivity testing, and the optimization of the diet. Provision of adequate dietary fiber is important to encourage the growth of normal gastrointestinal flora when dealing with herbivorous reptiles. Transfaunating the intestine with indigenous microflora from a clinically normal reptile may be considered, but the true value of this procedure is unknown.

Viral Diseases

Viral pathogens associated with the reptilian gastrointestinal tract are diagnosed with increased frequency. Historically, few disease processes were associated with viral infection in reptiles. However, this was not because viruses are a recent finding but because our diagnostic abilities were limited. Acknowledgement that viruses are frequently identified in the microflora of vertebrates is important. Therefore, the presence of viruses, like the presence of bacteria, in the absence of concurrent pathology should be interpreted with caution. A number of viral diseases have been associated with gastrointestinal disease in different species of reptiles. However, these cases are all represented as case reports. For confirmation that a virus is responsible for a specific disease process, an experimental infection to fulfill Koch's postulate must be performed.

One suspected viral disease that has been associated with gastrointestinal disease in snakes is the retrovirus responsible for inclusion body disease (IBD; see Chapter 60). This disease primarily affects snakes in the families Pythonidae and Boidae (e.g., pythons and boas). The method of transmission of this virus is unknown, but snake mites (*Ophionyssus natricis*) may play a role in the dissemination of the disease. Affected snakes often are seen with chronic regurgitation but may have neurologic signs develop, including loss of righting reflex, tremors, and disorientation, as the disease progresses. Affected pythons have severe neurologic signs develop, similar to those described for the boas, and progressively worsen.

Many of the IBD snakes also have severe stomatitis develop, characterized by ulceration of the oral mucosa and the accumulation of caseous material in the oral cavity.[37] Animals typically die of this disease as a result of secondary infections and starvation. Diagnosis can be made antemortem from surgical biopsies of the pancreas, esophageal tonsils, or kidney and postmortem from histopathologic examination. Eosinophilic intracytoplasmic inclusions in visceral organs and the central nervous system are characteristic of this disease. No effective treatment exists for this virus. Affected animals should be euthanized to prevent the spread of the virus to other snakes.

Adenoviruses have been associated with high morbidity and mortality rates in reptile collections. The author has observed several devastating adenoviral outbreaks in Bearded Dragon collections. Although this virus was first reported in Australia in the early 1980s, the virus did not become problematic in the United States until the mid-1990s. Since that time, this virus has spread through numerous Bearded Dragon populations in the United States and should be considered endemic in the US population of Bearded Dragons. Transmission of the virus is presumed to be via the direct route (fecal-oral). Affected animals may have anorexia, weight loss, limb paresis, diarrhea, and opisthotonous. Concurrent dependovirus and coccidial infections have also been observed in neonatal Bearded Dragons.

Biopsies of the liver, stomach, esophagus, and kidney may be taken to confirm diagnosis (antemortem). Basophilic intranuclear inclusion bodies on histopathology are diagnostic. No effective treatment exists for adenoviral infections in these lizards, although supportive care (e.g., fluids, enterals, antibiotics) may be useful in stemming the secondary effects of the disease. Again, little is known regarding the epidemiology of this virus; therefore, special precautions should be taken when working with affected animals. Because no effective treatment exists, affected Bearded Dragons should be culled.

An adeno-like virus has been associated with esophagitis in a Veiled Chameleon (*Chamaeleo calyptratus*) and a Jackson's Chameleon (*C. jacksonii*). Electron microscopy revealed the presence of eosinophilic intranuclear inclusion bodies in the ciliated epithelial cells containing numerous viral-like particles in the mucosa of the esophagus.[38,39] Viral enteritis in crocodilians and a Rosy Boa has also been associated with adenovirus.[39] Diagnosis was made with description of adenoviral-like lesions and viral particles in the liver and intestine.[40]

Treatment for viral-related gastrointestinal disease is generally limited to supportive care, treatment of secondary pathogens, good husbandry, and most importantly, quarantine of the infected specimens to prevent further losses. Currently, no effective antiviral treatments exist.

The incidence rate of herpesvirus infections in chelonians has been on the rise since the virus was first isolated from Seaturtles in 1975. Herpesvirus infections have been identified in freshwater, marine, and terrestrial species of chelonians. Transmission of the herpesvirus is believed to be via the horizontal route, although a vertical route of transmission has also been suggested. Affected animals may have rhinitis, conjunctivitis, necrotizing stomatitis, enteritis, pneumonia, and neurologic disease. Molecular diagnostics (serum neutralization, enzyme-linked immunosorbent assay [ELISA], polymerase chain reaction [PCR], and reverse transcriptase [RT]–PCR), electron microscopy, and viral isolation have been used to diagnose herpes infections in chelonians. Affected animals should be provided appropriate supportive care (e.g., fluids, enterals, and antibiotics) to control clinical signs. Acyclovir has been used with some success by reducing viral replication. However, no effective treatment exists for this virus. Affected animals should not be released into the wild to prevent translocation of the virus to naïve chelonians.

Fungal Disease

A variety of mycotic diseases have been reported in captive chelonians, crocodilians, and squamates. Relatively few mycotic diseases have involved the gastrointestinal system in free-ranging reptiles. Mycoses are typically categorized as cutaneous or systemic mycosis. However, in reptiles, reports of cutaneous mycosis outnumbered cases of systemic mycosis.[41]

That most, if not all, of the reptile cases with systemic mycosis are diagnosed at necropsy is important to mention. Many factors can act as stressors to the reptile's immune system, including concurrent infectious disease, trauma, and toxicosis. Other factors that can increase the likelihood of infection with mycotic organism include high humidity or dampness, excessive dryness, and poor husbandry and sanitation.

Hyalohyphomycosis is used to describe any mycotic infection in the tissues associated with a fungal agent with septate hyphae and nonpigmented (hyaline) walls.[42] This description encompasses a large number of fungi, and several reports are found of these types of presentations in reptiles. *Paecilomyces lilacinus* has been isolated from the oral cavity, gastric mucosa, and liver of an Aldabra Tortoise (*Geochelone gigantean*),[43] a *Geotrichum* spp. was isolated from a cloacal lavage of a Honduran Milksnake (*Lampropeltis triangulum hondurensis*) with mucous colitis,[44] and *Chrysosporium keratinophilum* has been involved with necrotic stomach lesions of two Green Iguanas.[45]

Aspergillus spp. is a ubiquitous saprophytic fungus capable of causing severe and life-threatening illness in birds, mammals, and humans. In reptiles, *Aspergillus* spp. has been described in a Panther Chameleon (*Furcifer pardalis*) with periodontal osteomyelitis.[46] In a review of chameleons at the Oklahoma City Zoo, abscesses were noted to be common along the dental arcade, within the rostrum, and in the skin of the lips.[47]

Mucormycosis is caused most frequently by members of the family Mucoraceae. In snakes, mucormycosis has been isolated in a Diamond Python (*Morelia spilota spilota*) with clinical signs of hematochezia. *Rhizopus* spp. was isolated with cloacal lavage.[44]

Trichosporon beigeleii, the causative agent of trichosporonosis, has been isolated from a cloacal lavage of a Honduran Milksnake with mucous colitis. *Candida rugosa* was another isolate from the same snake.[44] In addition, *Candida albicans* has been isolated from necrotic esophageal lesions in a Crocodile Tegu (*Crocodilurus lacertinus*).[45]

Fungal etiologic agents are often opportunistic but are occasionally primary pathogens. Cutaneous, respiratory, or visceral granulomatous lesions must be differentiated from mycobacteriosis. Diagnosis is made on the basis of a complete physical examination, blood work, imaging techniques, fungal culture, and histopathology. Histopathologic examination of impression smears, biopsies, or necropsy specimens is required to identify and characterize the morphologic characteristics of the fungal elements. Characteristics such as the width of hyphae, presence or absence of septae, type and size of reproductive structures, colony morphology, and optimum incubation temperature are used to identify and classify fungi. Culture may require some specialization, and laboratories should be contacted to obtain instructions for specific sampling techniques to minimize bacterial overgrowth of cultures.

Because many fungal infections become encapsulated as a result of the reptile's immune response, excision of the entire lesion is necessary to increase treatment efficacy. The prognosis is poor to guarded with major organ involvement or disseminated disease.

Systemic antifungal chemotherapeutics are recommended along with surgical intervention to minimize reoccurrence. Amphotericin, fluorocytosin, nystatin, itraconazole, ketoconazole, fluconazole, and terbinafine are the primary antifungal drugs used by veterinarians to eliminate fungal infections in reptiles.[41] Few pharmacokinetic studies have been done to determine the pharmacokinetics of antifungals in reptiles (see Chapter 36).

The azole and the polyene macrolide derivatives are the most common antifungal drugs used in reptile medicine. The azole group has a broad spectrum of activity and is effective against many different classes of fungi. Itraconazole has been shown to have increased efficacy against *Aspergillus* spp. A preliminary report of itraconazole in Spiny Lizards (*Scleroporus* spp.) showed that the drug was absorbed from the gastrointestinal tract and achieved therapeutic levels in the blood at an oral dose of 23.5 mg/kg every 6 days.[48] Ketoconazole, another broad-spectrum antifungal agent, inhibits microsomal enzymes. A study that evaluated the kinetics of ketoconazole in Gopher Tortoises (*Gopherus polyphemus*) found that a 15 mg/kg dose every 24 hours for 2 to 4 weeks was appropriate.[49]

The group of polyene macrolide antibiotics commonly used to treat fungi includes amphotericin B and nystatin. Amphotericin B can be used for most systemic fungal diseases because of its wide range of fungicidal activity. In mammals, this drug can cause nephrotoxicity. No pharmacokinetic data are for amphotericin B in reptiles. Anecdotally, nystatin has been used to treat oral and gastrointestinal candidiasis infection at a dosage of 100,000 IU/kg daily for 10 days.[48] Nystatin must have direct contact with the yeast or fungus to be effective. Fluconazole has shown better activity against yeast. The use of terbinafine for cutaneous mycosis has also been considered; however, further studies need to be pursued for its use against deep mycosis.[41] Topical drugs are best used as an adjunct therapy against systemic mycosis. Treatment for a fungus should continue until complete resolution.

Parasitic Disease

Gastrointestinal parasitism is one of the most common reasons a reptile is seen at a veterinary hospital (see Chapter 21) and is especially common with imported reptiles. Affected reptiles may be seen for a variety of reasons, including anorexia, pica, prolapse, regurgitation, diarrhea, constipation, lethargy, and weight loss.

Reptiles serve as both definitive and intermediate hosts for a number of different parasites. Most clinicians are concerned with those parasites that the reptile serves as a definitive host because these are the parasites that are shed through the gastrointestinal tract. Reptiles can serve as the definitive host for nematodes, trematodes, cestodes, and protozoans.

Nematodes are frequently encountered during routine fecal examinations for snakes, chelonians, and lizards. One of the most common endoparasites in reptiles is the pinworm (e.g., oxyurids). The oxyurids are generally considered to be nonpathogenic in reptiles, although heavy burdens can lead to clinical disease. These parasites are found primarily in the lower gastrointestinal tract and show high host specificity. Oxyurids have a direct life cycle and can achieve significant population numbers within the colon, especially in herbivorous iguanids and chelonians, which puts them at risk for impaction (Figure 12-8).

Two families of ascarids commonly parasitize reptiles: Anisakidae and Ascarididae.[50] Larval nematodes from the family Anisakidae (*Anisakis* spp.) have been reported to cause gastric ulceration in Green Seaturtles (*Chelonia mydas*). The larvae were found coiled beneath the serosal surface of the stomach and duodenum. In this case, raw sardines fed to the turtles were considered the source of infection.[51]

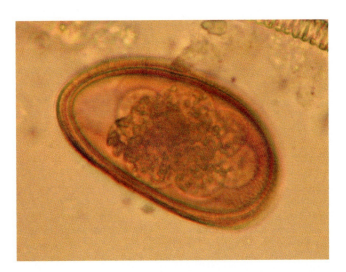

FIGURE 12-8 *Oxyurid* spp. ova from a Bearded Dragon (*Pogona vitticeps*).

From the family Ascarididae, three species has been shown to parasitize snakes. *Ophidascaris labiatopapillosa* has been reported in North American snakes after ingestion of frogs and rodents, which serve as intermediate hosts.[50] *Ophidascaris moreliae* and *Polydelphis anoura* have been found to infect pythons, especially if the larva are released into the water.[52] Two genera have also been found to affect crocodilians: *Dujardinascaris* and *Paratrichosoma*. High densities of these ascarids can cause gastrointestinal perforation and ulceration.[50]

Strongyloid nematodes can be found throughout the alimentary tract. Three genera of strongyles, including *Diaphanocephaloidea* spp., *Oswaldocruzia* spp., and *Kalicephalus* spp., have been found to infest lizards and snakes. These parasites can cause severe hemorrhagic ulceration, perforation, and gastrointestinal obstruction.[50,53] *Capillaria* spp. is the only known trichurid to infest squamates and crocodilians. These nematodes primarily infest the intestine but have been found in other organs such as the liver and gonads. This parasite also has a direct life cycle.

Treatment of nematodes in reptiles is readily accomplished with standard veterinary parasiticides. The authors generally use fenbendazole at 25 to 50 mg/kg by mouth once a day for 4 days and repeat in 10 days, ivermectin at 0.2 mg/kg intramuscularly (IM) every 2 weeks for a minimum of two treatments, or albendazole at 50 mg/kg once. Ivermectin should not be used to treat chelonians because it has been found to cause neurotoxicity and nephrotoxicity.

The three trematode orders are Monogenea, Aspidogastrea, and Digenea. Although these flukes are commonly reported in reptile medicine, limited data exist regarding the clinical course of disease in reptiles. One study has suggested a correlation of fluke infestation in a Green Seaturtle with gallbladder papilloma.[54] *Ochetosoma* spp., *Stomatotrema* spp., and *Pneumatophilus* spp. are flukes that are routinely found in the oral cavity of ophidians, and *Odhneriotrema* spp. is the most common fluke in alligators.[55] Trematodes of aquatic turtles are frequently found in the alimentary tract, liver, gallbladder, urinary bladder, and circulatory system; however, clinical disease associated with these infestations is rare.[55]

Anecdotally, praziquantel at 8 mg/kg orally or subcutaneous at 2-week intervals for two to three treatments has been shown to be effective against digenetic trematodes.

Three cestode orders are also important to reptiles: Proteocephalidae, Pseudophyllidae, and Mesocestoididea. The adult stages of these parasites are found within the lumen of small intestine. The life cycle of these cestodes is indirect and requires one or two intermediate hosts. Clinically, cestodes rarely cause significant disease; it all depends on the number of mature worms present. Proteocephalid cestodes are most commonly encountered in snakes and lizards. Three genera, *Ophiotaenia* spp. (snakes), *Proteocephalus* spp. (lizards), and *Crepidoboyhrium* spp. (boids), have been found to induce intestinal necrosis, epithelial loss, and round cell infiltrate within the tunica muscularis.[56,57] Members of the order Pseudophyllidae have also been isolated from snakes and lizards. Pathologic findings from these cestodes are frequently associated with ulceration of the intestinal mucosa, hemorrhage, and edema. Specific lesions associated with pseudophyllids have been documented in three genera, *Duthiersia* spp., *Scyphocephalus* spp. (both seen in monitors), and *Bothridium* spp. (boids).[56,57] Praziquantel has also been used to treat cestodes with the same regimen described for trematodes.

A variety of protozoa infests reptiles, and the infections are likely influenced by individual animal differences and the microecology of the intestine. Differences in pH and the passage of digesta can have major effects on the makeup of a protozoal community. Other factors that can affect protozoal density include antagonism between different species and predation. Protozoa can also affect the bacterial flora from substrate competition and predation. Most of the protozoal species recorded in reptiles are nonpathogenic. This must be taken into consideration in review of a fecal sample. Treatment for protozoal disease should only be done with clinical disease and an overgrowth of a species of protozoa.

Coccidia are an obligate pathogen in reptiles. These parasites are generally considered to be host specific. *Caryospora chelonian* is the common coccidial parasite found in Green Seaturtles, and *Eimeria carettae* is the coccidian parasite of Loggerhead Seaturtles (*Caretta caretta*).[58,59] Eight species of *Eimeria* and two species of *Isospora* have been reported in crocodilians.[60] Lizards have the most distinct coccidian species, followed by snakes.[61] Pathologic changes from many of these species are associated with sloughing of the intestinal lining, hyperplasia of the epithelium and enterocytes, and inflammatory cells in the mucosa.[61,62]

Isospora amphiboluri is a coccidian parasite of special interest because of its relatively recent introduction into the United States. This coccidian parasite appears to be host specific to the Bearded Dragon. These lizards have become very popular in the United States during the past decade, with some investigators suggesting that they are the most commonly bred lizards in captivity. The epidemiology of this parasite appears to mimic the spread of these lizards across the country, and they can be found in most breeding populations. This parasite can cause significant morbidity and mortality in juvenile dragons. Affected dragons may have anorexia, weight loss, and diarrhea. *Isospora amphiboluri* appears to retard the growth of infected dragons. This parasite has also been isolated concurrently in dragons infected with dependovirus and adenovirus (Figure 12-9). This parasite is

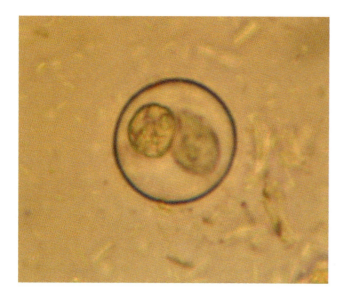

FIGURE 12-9 *Isospora amphiboluri* oocyst in the stool of a Bearded Dragon *(Pogona vitticeps)*.

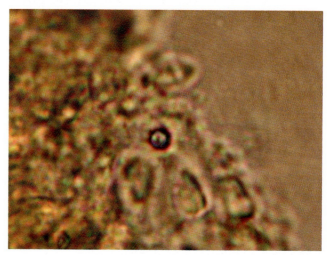

FIGURE 12-10 *Cryptosporidium saurophilus* in a direct wet smear prepared from fecal specimens of a clinically infected Leopard Gecko *(Eublepharis macularius)*.

difficult to eradicate in dragons. Sulfa-dimethoxine (50 mg/kg orally, once a day for 21 to 28 days) and trimethroprim sulfadiazine (30 mg/kg orally, once, followed by 15 mg/kg orally, once a day for 21 to 28 days) have been found to reduce shedding in infected dragons.

Cryptosporidium spp. has become a major concern in reptilian medicine because the infection usually results in a high mortality rate (see Chapter 48). Currently, two species of *Cryptospordium* spp. are known to parasitize reptiles: *Cryptosporidium serpentis* and *Cryptosporidium saurophilus*. Although no species has been speciated from chelonians, one report does exist of cryptosporidiosis in a Green Seaturtle.[63]

Anorexia, weight loss, and opportunistic bacterial infections are frequently reported in affected reptiles. Chronic regurgitation and hypertrophic gastritis are common findings in snakes. In snakes, the parasites infect mucin-secreting cells and their life cycle is hastened by the ingestion of food.[50] In contrast, *Cryptosporidium saurophilum* in Leopard Geckos *(Eublepharis macularius)* has been reported to be pathogenic and infect the intestines, rather than the stomach.[61,64] Patent infections are characterized by the shedding of large numbers of oocysts (Figure 12-10).

Currently, a number of different techniques are used to diagnose cryptosporidiosis. In humans, the modified acid-fast stain is the gold standard.[65] However, this does not always reflect the best sensitivity and specificity. The tests used in reptile medicine include acid-fast, immunofluorescence antibody (IFA), and PCR assay. Samples to be tested may be collected via cloacal/intestinal lavage or gastric lavage or from fresh feces or a regurgitated meal. Currently, *Cryptosporidium* spp. is resistant to many disinfectants, and no effective treatment exists for all species. However, one study published has found that bovine hyperimmune colostrum could be used to eliminate *Cryptosporidium saurophilum* from Savannah Monitors *(Varanus exanthematicus)*.[66] In the same study, the colostrum had no effect on *Cryptosporidium saurophilum* in Leopard Geckos.

Other case reports have evaluated the value of paromomycin, halifuginone, and spiromycin, but none of these compounds appear to be consistently effective. Prevention of cryptosporidiosis from entering a collection should be considered a priority for zoologic institutions and private collectors. Reptiles should be quarantined for a minimum of 90 days, and fecal samples collected at least monthly. Infected animals should be culled from a collection.

Noninfectious Diseases

Toxins

Few reports exist of toxicosis affecting the gastrointestinal tract of reptiles. A common Snapping Turtle *(Chelydra serpentina)* seen for anorexia was found to have fishing gear and lead weights in the gastrointestinal tract.[67] Blood lead levels confirmed a lead toxicosis. More recently, a Greek Tortoise *(Testudo graeca)* was reported to have neurologic signs after the ingestion of a lead shot.[68] The tortoise responded to chelation therapy with sodium calcium edetate at 35 mg/kg IM every 24 hours.

Reptiles may also have toxic episodes develop from diets that are offered in captivity. A group of captive alligators raised for leather was found to be neurologic and anorectic after being offered nutria. A thorough diagnostic work-up revealed that the alligators had had lead toxicosis develop as a result of ingesting lead shot used to kill the nutria.[69]

Feeding insectivorous reptiles wild-caught invertebrates can also lead to potential disaster. The common firefly, *Photinus* spp., produces steroidal pyrones (lucibufagans) that are highly toxic to Bearded Dragons and other species of lizards.[70] Ingestion of a single firefly is often fatal. Important to note, however, is that not all fireflies are fatal to all reptile species (see Chapter 83).

Animals exposed to environmental toxicants often have health effects similar to humans. Currently, in chelonians, researchers have not detected a measurable response to the exposure to toxic metals, although they still believe that elevated concentrations of toxic metals have contributed to chelonian morbidity and mortality.[71] With the anthropogenic influences, such as widespread pesticide and insecticide usage, placed on wild reptiles, and the large number of wild reptiles imported into the United States and Europe, the influence of toxins should be considered in management of cases with clinical disease.

Gastrointestinal Foreign Bodies

Pica or geophagy is a common practice in terrestrial reptiles. Some species are believed to ingest substrate to create gastroliths to assist with the mechanical digestion of foods, although this has not been proven. Substrate can also be found in wild reptiles not generally considered to be geophagic. In these cases, the substrate was suggested to be ingested because it was closely associated with the reptile's meal or because it was consumed nonselectively as the reptile ingested its meal.[8]

Foreign bodies of the gastrointestinal tract are not uncommon in captive reptiles. Inappropriate substrates are generally blamed for the development of gastrointestinal foreign bodies in captive reptiles. The most common signalment includes the smaller insectivorous lizards housed on sand or gravel substrate (Figure 12-11). Chelonians, especially omnivores and herbivores, are also prone to ingest woody materials and rocks (Figure 12-12). Snakes are not prone to ingest inanimate objects; however, the authors have seen ingestion of a cage item (coconut bark) during swallowing of prey (Figure 12-13). A less common presentation can be that of crocodilians with ingestion of fishing hooks during the wild harvest season (Figure 12-14).

Reptiles with gastrointestinal foreign bodies may have acute lethargy and anorexia. Regurgitation may be reported in the clinical history, especially in snakes. Snakes possess a poorly developed cardiac sphincter, thus permitting what can appear to be almost effortless regurgitation. Regurgitation is associated with pathology of the upper gastrointestinal tract, which includes the oral cavity, pharynx, esophagus, stomach, and small intestines. Consideration of regurgitation as only a symptom of the underlying disease is important. Episodes of vomiting as expected in a dog or a cat are very rare in reptiles. The history can also be much more chronic in nature, being characterized by gradual weight loss, lethargy, anorexia over several months, and constipation. Melena, hematochezia, reduced fecal production, and pain associated with eating may also be reported (see Chapter 74).

With an acute onset of clinical signs, reptiles are usually lethargic, dehydrated, and depressed on physical examination. Reptiles with a chronic history often are cachectic and dehydrated. Results of a CBC may reveal a decreased hematocrit (anemia), suggesting hemorrhage from the upper gastrointestinal tract; and a leukocytosis. Elevated hepatic and muscle enzymes, and electrolyte disturbances, may also occur with gastrointestinal foreign bodies.

Although not common, intestinal intussusception has been reported in a Green Iguana, a chameleon (*Chamaeleo* spp.), and a juvenile Blue Tongue Skink *(Tiliqua scincoides)* with a foreign body.[39] Lead poisoning and intestinal perforation from ingestion of fishing gear has also been documented in a Snapping Turtle.[67] In addition, volvulus of the proximal

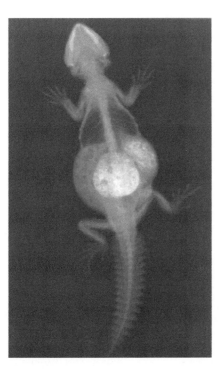

FIGURE 12-11 Radiopacity in the stomach and intestinal region of a *Uromastyx* spp. after ingestion of calcium carbonate from sand substrate.

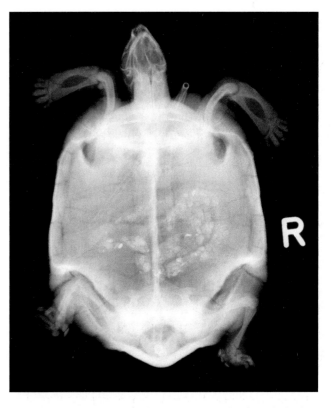

FIGURE 12-12 Radiograph of a Texas Tortoise *(Gopherus berlandieri)* depicts incidental ingestion of rocks.

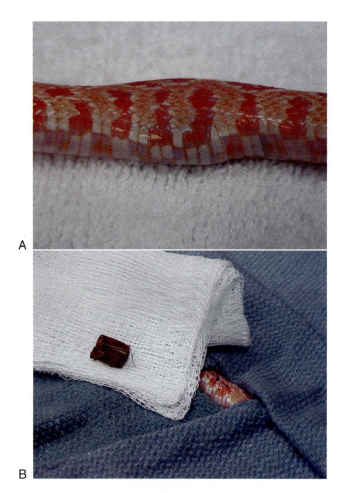

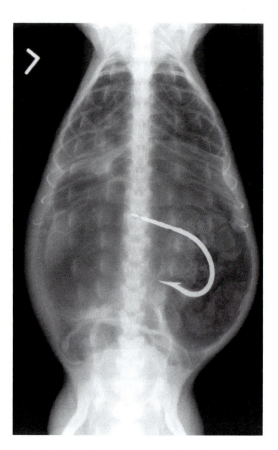

FIGURE 12-14 This alligator was seen with a history of anorexia. With radiography, the alligator was found to have a fishing hook in the gastrointestinal tract.

FIGURE 12-13 A, Large midbody swelling in a yearling Cornsnake *(Elaphe guttata guttata)*. **B,** Exploration reveals ingestion of a cage item (coconut bark), most likely during swallowing of prey.

colon has been reported in a Hawksbill Seaturtle *(Eretmochelys imbricata)* associated with foreign material.[72]

Diagnostic images are an important diagnostic tool to pursue in evaluation of a patient for a gastrointestinal foreign body. Metal and mineral foreign bodies can be detected with survey radiographs. Rubber and plastic materials may be more difficult to detect with survey radiographs. In these cases, a contrast series should be performed. Because the gastrointestinal motility of reptiles is longer than in mammals and birds, the contrast series may need to be extended over several days or weeks. Ultrasonography, CT, and MRI may be of significant value in the diagnosis of the reptile in which evidence of a foreign body is questionable.[73-78] Treatment generally requires surgical or endoscopic removal of the foreign body and recommendations to change the substrate to prevent reoccurrence.

Gastrointestinal Neoplasia

Although infectious diseases remain the major concern in treatment of reptile patients, gastrointestinal neoplasia is also becoming an important consideration in reptiles.[79-92]

Neoplasia is defined as any abnormal development of cells that can be either benign or malignant. Neoplastic disorders must always be considered with an unresolving or multifactorial symptom, no matter the age of the patient. Neoplastic diseases of the gastrointestinal system in reptiles may be a challenge to diagnose, even when a detailed diagnostic evaluation is performed.

Neoplasms of the gastrointestinal system have been reported in all of the major reptilian orders (see Chapter 19). Although our understanding behind the pathophysiology of reptile neoplasia is limited, we are beginning to unlock the mystery behind these aberrations. For example, some evidence now exists that a C-type oncorna virus may have an etiologic function in poikilotherm oncogenesis.[85,93] Although the virus was not associated with neoplasms of the gastrointestinal system, future attempts should be pursued to determine its role. Several malignant hepatic tumors have been reported in reptiles with no record of an underlying etiology of the tumors; however, a recent case report of a hepatoma in a Green Iguana was found to be associated with viral-like inclusions in the neoplastic hepatocytes.[94] Herpesvirus has recently been associated with the development of fibropapillomas in Green Seaturtles.[79]

Man-made and natural environmental toxins should also be evaluated as potentially carcinogenic. As yet, no reports link pollutants with gastrointestinal neoplasia. Currently, no reports exist of a genetic basis for neoplasm in reptiles because the role of specific genes in the neoplastic disease process has yet to be defined.[85] Also, no documented reports are found of parasite-induced neoplasm in reptiles; however,

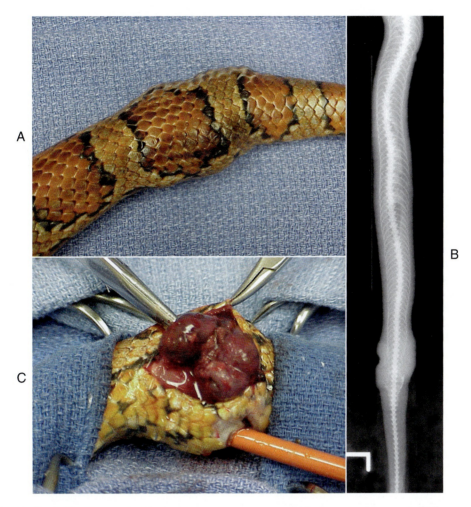

FIGURE 12-15 **A,** This Cornsnake *(Elaphe guttata guttata)* was seen with a firm cloacal mass. **B,** With radiography, a solid tissue mass was found associated with the ribs. Note the productive osteolysis along the segment. **C,** Note the infiltrative nature of the mass around the cloaca. With histology this was found to be a carcinoma.

some association may exist between a trematodes species and a papillomatous change observed in the gallbladder of a Green Seaturtle.[54]

Various physical agents including inanimate objects, trauma, and radiation are all suspected as possible causes of oncogenesis in man and laboratory animals; however, the role of these agents in the development of neoplasia in reptiles has yet to be documented.[85]

Clinical signs associated with gastrointestinal neoplasia are variable depending on the type and location of the tumor but may include emesis, hematoemesis, poor growth, anorexia, caudal coelomic distention, melena, minimal axial flexion of the posterior trunk, asymmetric cloacal enlargement, and constipation.[39,89] Physical findings have also included dysphagia, ptyalism, hemoptyalism, facial deformities, and palpable masses in the caudal coelom associated with distal intestine or cloaca (Figure 12-15, *A, C*). Survey radiographs, contrast radiographs, and ultrasonography can be useful in a diagnosis of gastrointestinal neoplasia (Figure 12-15, *B*).[89] Final diagnosis and confirmation of a neoplastic process must be done via fine-needle aspirate or biopsy and histopathology. Use of veterinary pathologists who are familiar with the unique histology of the reptile is important.

Treatment of gastrointestinal neoplasia is dependent on the size, location, and type of neoplasm (see Chapter 19 for more details regarding treatment). Surgical correction is the preferred treatment. Adjunctive therapy has been investigated but is limited. Radiation therapy is commonly used as an adjunctive therapy to manage soft tissue neoplasia in companion animals and humans. Reports suggest that lower vertebrates have a variable response to radiation and may be relatively resistant.[95] Cosgrove[96] found the lethal dose (LD_{50}) in the snake to be 300 to 400 roentgens, which is comparable with that in humans. With this taken into account, different methods of radiation therapy must be implemented to treat neoplasia in snakes.[95-100] In contrast, the LD_{50} dose for frogs and tortoises ranges from 700 to 3000 roentgens.[97] Further studies to evaluate the radiosensitivity of poikilothermic cells should be pursued.

Although chemotherapy is commonly used to treat a variety of neoplasms in companion animal medicine, it has inherent limitations in reptiles. Limited reports on the use of chemotherapy in reptiles are available. Cisplatin has been used in the treatment of fibrosarcomas.[79] Cytosine arabinoside was used to treat a subcutaneous lymphosarcoma in a Rhinoceros Viper *(Bitis nasicornia)*; however, the snake died within 24 hours of the first treatment.[98] Intravenous doxorubicin has been used to treat a Cornsnake *(Elaphe guttata guttata)* with a locally invasive sarcoma[101] and a Boa Constrictor with a renal fibrosarcoma.[102] In addition, carboplatin was injected into the body wall and subcutaneous space of a Boa Constrictor to treat a fibrosarcoma.[98] Further study is needed to determine the pharmacokinetics of chemotherapeutics for reptiles to ensure the most appropriate treatment regimens are designed.

REFERENCES

1. Guibé J: In Grasse PP, editor: *Traité de zoologie*, vol 14(2), Paris, 1970, Masson.
2. Frye FL: Euthanasia and necropsy: necropsy. In Frye FL, editor: *Reptile care: an atlas of diseases and treatments*, vol 2, Neptune City, NJ, 1991, TFH Publishing.
3. Kochva E: Phylogeny of oral glands in reptiles as related to the origin and evolution of snakes. In Rosenberg P, editor: *Toxins: animal, plant and microbial*, Oxford, 1978, Pergamon Press.
4. Skoczylas R: Salivary and gastric juice secretion in the grass snake, *Comp Biochem Physiol* 35:885-903, 1970.
5. Young BA: On the absence of taste buds in monitor lizards (*Varanus*) and snakes, *J Herpetol* 31:130-137, 1997.
6. Parsons TS: The nose and Jacobson's organ. In Gans C, Parsons TS, editors: *Biology of the Reptilia, vol. 2: morphology B*, London, 1970, Academic Press.
7. Schwenk K: Occurrence, distribution and functional significance of taste buds in lizards, *Copeia* 91-101, 1985.
8. Skoczylas R: Physiology of the digestive tract. In Gans C, Gans KA, editors: *Biology of the Reptilia, vol 1: physiology*, London, 1978, Academic Press.
9. Parsons TS, Cameron JE: Internal relief of the digestive tract. In Gans C, Parsons TS, editors: *Biology of the Reptilia, vol 7: morphology B*, London, 1977, Academic Press.
10. Blain AW, Campbell KN: A study of the digestive phenomena in snakes with the aid of a Roentgen ray, *Am J Roentgenol* 48:229-239, 1942.
11. Reichert E: *Bothrops jararacussu*, Bl Aquar Kunde 47:228-231, 1936.
12. Vonk HJ: Die biologische bedeutung des pH-optimums der verdauungsenzyme bei den vertebraten, *Ergebn Enzymol* 8:55-88, 1939.
13. Diefenbach CO: Gastric function in Caiman crocodiles (Crocodilia: Reptilia) I. Rate of gastric digestion and gastric motility as a function of temperature, *Comp Biochem Physiolo* 51A:259-265, 1975.
14. Davies PMC: Anatomy and physiology. In Cooper JE, Jackson OF, editors: *Diseases of Reptilia*, vol I, San Diego, 1981, Academic Press.
15. Lönnenberg E: On some points of relation between the morphological structure of the intestine and the diets of reptiles, *Bih Svensk Vet Ak Handl* 28:1-51, 1902.
16. Haslewood GAD: Bile salts evolution, *J Lipid Res* 8:535-550, 1967.
17. Zug GR, Vitt LJ, Caldwell JP: Foraging ecology and diets. In Zug GR, Vitt LJ, Caldwell JP, editors: *Herpetology: an introductory biology of amphibians and reptiles*, San Diego, 2001, Academic Press.
18. Johnson JH, Benson PA: Laboratory reference values for a group of captive ball pythons *(Python regius)*, *AJVR* 57(9):1304-1397, 1996.
19. Klarsfeld J, Mitchell MA, Futch R: *Characterization of the oral aerobic and anaerobic bacterial flora of royal pythons (Python regius)*, Reno, Nev, 2002, Proc ARAV.
20. Salb A, Mitchell MA, Riggs S, Diaz-Figueroa O: *Characterization of the aerobic and anaerobic intestinal flora of the green iguana (Iguana iguana)*, Reno, Nev, 2002, Proc ARAV.
21. Rand AS: Reptilian arboreal folivores. In Montgomery GG, editor: *Ecology of arboreal folivores*, Washington, DC, 1978, Smithsonian Institute.
22. Rand AS, Dugan BA, Monteza H, Vianda D: The diet of a generalized folivore, *Iguana iguana*, in Panama, *J Herpetol* 24:211-214, 1990.
23. Iverson JB: Adaptions to herbivory in iguanine lizards. In: Burghardt GM, Rand AS, editors: *Iguanas of the world: their behavior, ecology, and conservation*, Park Ridge, NJ, 1982, Noyes Publications.
24. Moberly WR: The metabolic responses of the common iguana, *Iguana iguana*, to activity under restraint, *Comp Biochem Physiol* 27:1-20, 1968.
25. Bailey J, McBee RR: The magnitude of the rabbit cecal fermentation, *Proc Montana Acad Sci* 24:35-38, 1964.
26. Hoover WH, Clarke SD: Fiber digestion in the beaver, *J Nutr* 102:4-16, 1972.
27. McBee RH, McBee VN: The hindgut fermentation in the Green Iguana, *Iguana iguana*. In: Burghardt GM, Rand AS, editors: *Iguanas of the world: their behavior, ecology, and conservation*, Park Ridge, NJ, 1982, Noyes Publication.
28. Troyer K: Transfer of fermentative microbes between generations in a herbivorous lizard, *Science* 216:540-542, 1982.
29. Rand AS: A nesting aggregation of iguanas, *Copeia* 552-561, 1968.
30. Olson GH, Hodgin C, Peckman R: Infectious stomatitis associated with *Mycobacterium* sp. in a boa constrictor, *Comp Anim Pract* 8:47-49, 1987.
31. Quesenberry KE, Jacobson ER, Allen JL, et al: Ulcerative stomatitis and subcutaneous granuloma caused by *Mycobacterium chelonei* in a boa constrictor, *J Am Vet Med Assoc* 189:1131, 1986.
32. Oros J, Rodriguez L, Herraez P, Santana P, Fernandez A: Respiratory and digestive lesions caused by *Salmonella arizonae* in two snakes, *J Comp Pathol* 115:185-189, 1996.
33. Garner MM, Raymond JT: *A retrospective study of gastritis in snakes*, Proceedings of the Association of Reptilian and Amphibian Veterinarians Annual Conferece 61-63, 2003.
34. Zwart P, van der Gaag I: Atrophic gastritis in a Hermann's tortoise *(Testudo hermanni)* and two red-eared sliders *(Chrysemys scripta elegans)*, *Am J Vet Res* 42:2191-2195, 1981.
35. Johnson JD: Enteritis in a pair of juvenile Aldabra tortoises (Geochelone gigantean), Proceedings of the American Association of Reptilian and Amphibian Veterinarians Annual Conference, 147-151, 2001.
36. Anderson NL: Diseases of *Iguana iguana*, *Comp Cont Educ/Small Anim Med* 14:1335-1343, 1992.
37. Schumacher J, Jacobson ER, Homer HL, et al: Inclusion body disease in boid snakes, *J Zoo Wildl Med* 25:511-524, 1994.
38. Jacobson ER, Gardiner CH: Adeno-like virus in esophageal and tracheal mucosa of a jacksons chameleon *(Chamaeleo jacksonii)*, *Vet Pathol* 27:210, 1990.
39. Benson KB: Reptilian gastrointestinal diseases, *Semin Avian Exotic Pet Med* 8:90-97, 1999.
40. Jacobson ER, Gardiner CH, Foggin CM: Adenovirus-like infection in two Nile crocodiles, *J Am Vet Med Assoc* 181:1325, 1984.
41. Paré JA: *Fungi and fungal diseases of reptiles*, Proceedings of the American Association of Reptilian and Amphibian Veterinarians Annual Conference, 128-131, 2003.
42. Jacobson ER, Cheatwood JL, Maxwell LK: Mycotic diseases of reptiles, *Semin Avian Exotic Pet Med* 9:94-101, 2000.

43. Heard DJ, Cantor GH, Jacobson ER, et al: Hyalohyphomycosis caused by *Paecilomyces lilacinus* in an Aldabra tortoise, *J Am Vet Med Assoc* 189:1143-1145, 1986.
44. Raiti P: *Mycotic gastroenteritis in a diamond python* (Morelia spilota spilota) *and two Honduran milk snakes* (Lampropeltis triangulum hondurensis), Proceedings of the American Association of Reptilian and Amphibian Veterinarians Annual Conference, 97, 1996.
45. Zwart P, Poelma FG, Strik WJ, et al: Report on births and deaths occurring in gardens of the Royal Rotterdam Zoo "Blijdorp" during the years 1961 and 1962, *Tijdschr Diergeneskd* 93:348, 1968.
46. Heatley JJ, Mitchell MA, Williams J, et al: Fungal periodontal osteomyelitis in a chameleon *(Furcifer pardalis)*, *J Herp Med Surg* 11:7-12, 2001.
47. Barrie MT, Castle E, Crow D: Diseases of chameleons at the Oklahoma City zoological park, *Proc AAZV* 1-6, 1993.
48. Gamble KC, Alvarado TP, Bennett CL: Itraconazole plasma and tissue concentration in the spiny lizard (*Sceloporus* spp.) following once-daily dosing, *J Zoo Wildl Med* 28:89-93, 1997.
49. Page CD, Mautino M, Derendorf H, et al: Multiple-dose pharmacokinetics of ketoconazole administered orally to gopher tortoise *(Gopherus polyphemus)*, *J Zoo Wildl Med* 22:191-198, 1991.
50. Lane TJ, Mader DR: Parasitology. In Mader DR, editor: *Reptile medicine and surgery*, Philadelphia, 1996, WB Saunders.
51. Burke JB, Rodgers LJ: Gastric ulceration associated with larval nematodes (*Anisakis* spp. type I) in pen reared green turtles *(Chelonia mydas)*, *J Wildl Dis* 18:41-46, 1982.
52. Marcus LC: *Veterinary biology and medicine of captive amphibians and reptiles*, Philadelphia, 1981, Lea & Febiger.
53. Bodri MS: *Common parasitic diseases of reptiles and amphibians*, Proceedings of the American Association of Reptilian and Exotic Veterinarian Annual Conference 11-17, 1994.
54. Smith GM, Coates C, Nigrelli R: A papillomatosis disease of the gallbladder associated with infection by flukes, occurring in the marine turtle *(Chelonia mydas)*, *Zoologica* 26:13, 1941.
55. Schell SC: *Trematodes of North America north of Mexico*, Moscow, 1985, University of Idaho Press.
56. Schmidt GD: *CRC handbook of tapeworm identification*, Boca Raton, Fla, 1984, CRC Press.
57. Khalil LF, Jones A: *Keys to the cestode parasites of vertebrates*, Wallingford, England, 1994, CAB International.
58. Leibovits L, Rebell G, Boucher GC: *Caryospora cheloniae sp.n.: a coccidial pathogen of mariculture-reared green sea turtle (Chelonia mydas)*, *J Wildl Dis* 14:269-275, 1978.
59. Upton SJ, Odell DK, Walsh MT: *Eimeria carettae sp.nov.* (Apicomplexa: Eimeriidae) from the loggerhead sea turtle, *Caretta caretta* (Testudines), *Can J Zool* 68:1268-1269, 1990.
60. McAllister CT, Upton ST: The coccidia (Apicomplexa: Eimeriidae) of Cocrodylia, with the description of two new species from *Alligator mississippiensis* (Reptilia: Alligatoridae) from Texas, *J Parasitol* 76:332-336, 1990.
61. Greiner EC: Coccidiosis in reptiles, *Semin Avian Exotic Pet Med* 12:49-56, 2003.
62. Ladds PW, Mangunwirjo H, Sebayand D: Diseases of young farmed crocodiles in Irian Jaya, *Vet Rec* 136:121-124, 1995.
63. Graczyk TK, Blazs GH, Work T, et al. *Cryptosporidium* sp. infection in green turtles, *Chelonia mydas*, as a potential source of marine waterborne cysts in the Hawaiian Islands, *Appl Envron Microbiol* 63:2925-2927.
64. Taylor MA, Geach MR, Cooley WA: Clinical and pathological observations on natural infections of cryptosporidiosis and flagellate protozoa in leopard geckos (*Eublepharis macularius*), *Vet Rec* 145:695-699, 1999.
65. Leav BA, Mackey M, Ward HD: *Cryptosporidium* species: new insights and old challenges, *Clin Infect Dis* 36:903-908, 2003.
66. Cranfield MR, Graczyk TK, Bostwick EF: *A comparative assessment of therapeutic efficacy of hyperimmune bovine colostrums treatment against* Cryptosporidium *infection in leopard geckos*, Eublepharis macularius, *and savannah monitors*, Varanus exanthematicus, Proceedings of the American Association of Reptilian and Amphibian Veterinarians Annual Conference, 119-121, 1999.
67. Borkowski R: Lead poisoning and intestinal perforation in a snapping turtle *(Chelydra serpentina)* due to fishing gear ingestion, *J Zoo Wildl Med* 28:109-114, 1997.
68. Chitty JR: *Lead toxicosis in a Greek tortoise* (Testudo graeca), Proceedings of the American Association of Reptilian and Exotic Veterinarian Annual Conference, 101, 2003.
69. Camus AC, Mitchell MA, Williams JF, Jowet PL: Elevated lead levels in farmed alligators consuming nutria meat contaminated by lead bullets, *J World Aquaculture Soc* 29(3):370-376, 1998.
70. Knight M, Glor R, Smedley SR, Gonzales A, et al: Firefly toxicosis in lizards, *J Chem Ecol* 25:1981-1986, 1999.
71. Homer BL, Domico LM, Williams JE, et al: *Desert tortoises as sentinels of environmental toxicants*, 26th Annual Meeting and Symposium of the Desert Tortoise Council, 2000.
72. Schumacher J, Papendick R, Herbst L, et al: Volvulus of the proximal colon in a Hawksbill turtle *(Eretmochelys imbricata)*, *J Zoo Wildl Med* 27:386-391, 1996.
73. Pennick DG, Stewart JS, Paul-Murphy J, et al: Ultrasonography of the California desert tortoise *(Xerobates agassizi)*: anatomy and application, *Vet Radiol* 23:112-116, 1991.
74. Raiti P, Haramiti N: *MR of bowel using mineral oil as a contrast agent: a viable option in reptiles with long transit times*, Proceedings of the Association of Reptilian and Amphibian Veterinarians, 59, 1994.
75. Rosenthal K, Kapatkin A: *Use of computed tomography as a diagnostic aid in the diagnosis of an abdominal mass in a box turtle*, Proceedings of the Association of Reptilian and Amphibian Veterinarians Annual, 45, 1994.
76. Sainsbury AW, Gili C: Ultrasonographic anatomy and scanning technique of the coelomic organs of the bosc monitor *(Varanus exanthematicus)*, *J Zoo Wildl Med* 22:421-433, 1991.
77. Isaza R, Ackerman N, Jacobson ER: Ultrasound of the coelomic structures in the boa constrictor *(Boa constrictor)*, *Vet Radiol Ultrasound* 34:445-450, 1993.
78. Holt PE: Radiological studies of the alimentary tract in two Greek tortoises *(Testudo graeca)*, *Vet Rec* 103:198-200, 1978.
79. Done LB: Neoplasia. In Mader DR, editor: *Reptile medicine and surgery*, Philadelphia, 1996, WB Saunders.
80. Harshbarger JC: *Activities report registry of tumors in lower animals, 1975 supplement*, Washington DC, 1976, Smithsonian Institute Press.
81. Harshbarger JC: *Activities report registry of tumors in lower animals, 1976 supplement*, Washington, DC, 1977, Smithsonian Institute Press.
82. Frye FL: Common pathologic lesions and disease processes: neoplasia. In Frye FL, editor: *Reptile care: an atlas of diseases and treatments*, vol 2, Neptune City, NJ, 1991, TFH Publishing.
83. Machotka SV: Neoplasia in reptiles. In Hoff GL, Frye FL, Jacobson ER, editors: *Diseases of amphibians and reptiles*, New York, 1984, Plenum Press.
84. Ramsay EC, Munson L, Lownestein L, et al: A retrospective study of neoplasia in a collection of captive snakes, *J Zoo Wildl Med* 27:28-34, 1996.
85. Jacobson ER: Neoplastic diseases. In Cooper JE, Jackson OF, editors: *Diseases of Reptilia*, vol 2, San Diego, 1981, Academic Press.
86. Elkan E, Cooper JE: Tumors and pseudotumors in some reptiles, *J Comp Pathol* 86:337-348, 1976.
87. Frye FL, Dutra F: Fibrosarcoma in a boa constrictor, *Vet Med/Sm Animal Clinician* 245-255, 1973.

88. Martin JC, Schelling SH, Pokras MA: Gastric adenocarcinoma in a Florida indigo snake *(Drymarchon corais couperi)*, *J Zoo Wildl Med* 25:133-137, 1994.
89. Latimer K, Rich GA: Colonic adenocarcinoma in a corn snake *(Elaphe guttata guttata)*, *J Zoo Wildl Med* 29:344-346, 1998.
90. Leonardi L, Grazioli O, Mechelli L, Frye FL: *Gastric mucinous adenocarcinoma in a diamond python* (Morelia spilotes spilotes), Proceedings of the Association of Reptilian and Amphibian Veterinarians Annual Conference 63, 2002.
91. Funk RS: *Cloacal adenocarcinoma in three juvenile diamond pythons* (Morelia spilotes spilotes), Proceedings of the Association of the Reptilian and Amphibian Veterinarians Annual Conference, 101-103, 2000.
92. Fickbohm BL, Kennedy GA: Gastric adenocarcinoma in a carpet python *(Morelia spilotes variegata)*, *J Herp Med Surg* 9:28-29, 1999.
93. Hardy WD, McClelland AJ: Oncogenic RNA viral infections. In Steele JH, editor: *CRC handbook series in zoonoses*, vol II, Cleveland, 1981, CRC Press.
94. Schillinger L, Selleri P, Frye FL: *Hepatoma in a Green Iguana* (Iguana iguana), *accompanied by viral-like inclusions*, Proceedings of the American Association of Reptilian and Amphibian Veterinarians Annual Conference, 75, 2002.
95. Leach MW, Nichols DK, Hartsell W, Torgerson RW: Radiation therapy of a malignant chromatophroma in a yellow rat snake *(Elaphe obsoleta quadrivettata)*, *J Zoo Wildl Med* 22(2):241-244, 1991.
96. Cosgrove GE: Reptilian radiobiology, *JAVMA* 159(11):1678-1684, 1971.
97. Robinson PT, von Essen CF, Benirschke K, Meier JE, Bacon JP: Radiation therapy for the treatment of an intraoral malignant lymphoma in an Indian rock python, *J Am Vet Radiol Soc* 19:92-95, 1978.
98. Langan JN, Adams WH, Patton S, et al: Radiation and intralesional chemotherapy for a fibrosarcoma in a boa constrictor *(Boa constrictor ortoni)*, *J Herp Med* 11:4-8, 2001.
99. Bryant BR, Vogelnest L, Hulst F: The use of cryosurgery in a Diamond python *(Morelia spilota spilota)*, with fibrosarcoma and radiotherapy in a common death adder *(Acanthophis antarcticus)* with melanoma, *Bull ARAV* 7(3):9-12, 1997.
100. Schumacher KL, Bennett RA, Fox LE, et al: Mast cell tumor in an eastern kingsnake *(Lampropeltis getulus getulus)*, *J Vet Diagn Invest* 10:101-104, 1998.
101. Rosenthal K: *Chemotherapeutic treatment of a sarcoma in a corn snake*, Proceeding of the Association of Reptilian and Amphibian Veterinarians Annual Conference, 46, 1994.
102. Orcutt C: Use of vascular access ports in exotic animals, *Proc ICE* 2(3):34-38, 2000.

13
BEHAVIORAL AND MORPHOLOGIC ADAPTATIONS

BRAD A. LOCK

The more than 11,000 species of extant reptiles and amphibians have a wide variety of behaviors and structural morphologies (Tables 13-1, 13-2, and 13-3) designed to allow them to escape notice or fight off enemies, reproduce, obtain food, and adapt to their environment. This chapter is meant to serve as an introduction and describes some commonly seen and some less commonly seen behaviors and morphologic adaptations in reptiles and amphibians. These behaviors and adaptations are normal for the particular species or group discussed but to the unfamiliar hobbyist or clinician may appear to be a sign of disease or trauma. Many more examples exist than can be presented in a single chapter, and research of some of the biology and natural history of unfamiliar species is important.

REPTILES

Defensive Behaviors

Catalepsy, Death Feigning, Tonic Immobility
This category describes a condition or state of external unresponsiveness to stimulation that can be seen as maintenance of a rigid posture or of a flaccid condition. This behavior occurs commonly in some groups of snakes (e.g., Hog-nosed Snakes, False Spitting Cobras) and has been described in lizards and crocodilians.

Hog-nosed Snakes (*Heterodon* spp.) are well known for their complex death-feigning behavior.[1] When first disturbed, the Hog-nosed Snake exhibits an elaborate bluff display that

Table 13-1	Behaviors in Reptiles	
Behavior	**Species**	**Comments**
Catalepsy, death feigning, tonic immobility	Many: Hog-nosed Snakes, False Spitting Cobras, Chameleons, Leaf-tailed Geckos, Caiman	Behavior reduced or absent with time in captivity
Squirting blood	Horned Lizards, *Tropidophis* sp. (Dwarf Boas), Long-nosed Snakes	Accurate up to 6 ft (2 m)
Tail display	Many: *Anilliidae* (Pipe Snakes), *Uropeltidae* (Shield-tailed Snakes), Ringnecked Snakes, Sand Boas, Rubber Boas, Coralsnakes	Often waves or strikes with tail; mimics head
Tail vibrating	Many: Kingsnakes, Pine Snakes, Ratsnakes, Racers, Coachwhip Snakes	Can be mistaken for Rattlesnake
Tail loss/autonomy	Some species in most families	Costly in terms of energy; may not reproduce first breeding season after tail loss
Caudal luring	Viperids (Vipers/Pit Vipers)	Can be mistaken for neurologic disease
Hemipenial eversion	Many: Blood Pythons, Coralsnakes, Monitors	Must differentiate from prolapse
Bluffs/threats	Many: *Uromastyx* (Spiny-tailed Agama), Bearded Dragons, Chameleons, Monitors, Asian Ratsnakes	Can resemble respiratory disease
Fragile skin	Various Gecko species	Usually no treatment necessary for skin defect
Balling behavior	Ball Python, African Burrowing Python, Rosy Boas, Rubber Boas	
Thermoregulation	Most species	
Reproductive behavior		Most common behaviors seen: head bobbing in lizards and chelonia, neck biting in snakes and lizards
Squamates	Most common species	
Chelonia	Tortoises, Box Turtles	
Incubation behavior	Pythons	Can resemble neurologic disease
Spectacle cleansing	Geckos	
Stargazing	Boas, Pythons, Rattlesnakes	Able to assume normal posture
Circumduction	Bearded Dragons, Asian Water Dragons	

Table 13-2	Morphologic Adaptations in Reptiles and Amphibians	
Adaptation	**Species**	**Comments**
Chelonians		
Plastral hinges	Mud, Musk, and Box Turtles, Spider Tortoises	Can be mistaken for fracture
Carapacial hinges	Hinge-backed Tortoises	Kinetic connection can feel like a fracture or one of the MBDs
Ligamentous connections	Asian Leaf, neotropical Wood Turtles, Big-headed, Mexican Musk Turtles	Can be mistaken for one of the MBDs
Open fontanels	Pancake Tortoise, Asian River Turtles	Can be mistaken for one of the MBDs
Bifurcate/Wormlike tongue	Alligator Snapping Turtle	Not a parasite or mass
Plastral fluid	Side-necked Turtles	Can resemble septicemia
Squamates/Crocodilians		
Tongue color	Iguanas, Blue-tongued Skink	Not tongue necrosis or disease
Breeding season color change	Many: Broad-headed Skink, Iguanas	Can resemble septicemia
Femoral pores	Many: Males of Iguanas, Bearded Dragons	Can be mistaken for abscess or mass
Ligamentous connection of mandible	Most snake species	Not fracture of mandible
Rostral growth	Male Gharial	Not tumor or granuloma
Amphibians		
Soak patch	Most toad species	Not defect in skin
Nutrient foramen/tibiotarsal bone	Many anurans	Not fracture
Transparent skin	Glass Frogs	Not defect in skin
Fourth segment in hind limb	All anurans	Not fracture
Hair-like modification of skin	Hairy Frog	Not fungal or parasitic disease
Tail	Tailed Frog	Modified cloaca

MBD, Metabolic bone disease.

Table 13-3	Behavior in Amphibians	
Behavior	**Species**	**Comments**
Defensive Behaviors		
Death feigning, tonic immobility	Anurans, salamanders	Not a nutritional or neurological disease
Lung inflation, puffing up	Anurans	Not respiratory disease
Unken reflex	Salamanders (many); Red-Belly Newt, Fire-Bellied Toad	Not neurological disease or pain
Head/neck posturing	Mole, Spotted, Spiny Salamanders, Casque-headed Frogs	Not musculoskeletal or neurological disease
Body posturing	False-eyed Frog	
Tail autonomy	Many salamander and newt species	
Predation		
Pedal luring	Horned Frogs	Not hypocalcemic tremors
Cocoon formation	Horned Frogs, African Bull Frogs	Appear dead or ill
Reproductive Behaviors		
Amplexus	Most anuran species	Not aggression
Brood pouches	Pouched Frog, Marsupial Tree Frog, Surinam Toad	Not injury or tumor/granuloma
Mouth brooding	Darwin's Frog	Not predation

consists of an exaggerated S-coil, loud hissing, and false strikes (Figure 13-1). The tail is often tightly coiled and can be elevated. If grasped or further harassed, the snake begins to writhe violently, with the mouth hung limply open, and defecate. Violent writhing continues for a short time, and then the snake assumes an inverted limp posture, usually with the mouth open and the tongue hanging out (Figure 13-2). If the snake is turned over onto its ventrum, it immediately turns back onto its dorsum. When the threat is removed, the Hog-nosed Snake slowly rights itself and crawls away (Figure 13-3). During the writhing display, Hog-nosed Snakes may regurgitate and defecate, which apparently serves to smear gastrointestinal and cloacal contents over the snake's body, making it distasteful to predators.

Pseudoxenodontines, closely related to the Hog-nosed Snakes and False Spitting Cobras (*Hemachatus* sp.) are also well known for their elaborate death feigning behavior that closely resembles that of the Hog-nosed Snakes. Assumption of a rigid posture that could be misinterpreted as an injury has been described in *Trachyboa* sp. and the Bandy Bandy (*Vermicllia anulata*).[2] Lizards and crocodilians, chameleons in the genus *Brookesia*, and Leaf-tailed Geckos (*Uroplatus* sp.) exhibit tonic immobility when threatened,[1] as does the microteiid, *Echinosaura horrida*.[3] Death feigning occurs in at least one teiid (*Callopistis flavipunctatus*),[1] one Cordylid (*Gerrhosaurus major*),[4] and three monitor species. Hatchling Spectacled Caimans (*Caiman crocodylus*) vocalize, bite, and struggle on land but feign death if grasped under water.[5,6]

Behavioral and Morphologic Adaptations 165

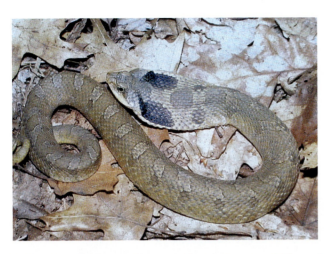

FIGURE 13-1 This Eastern Hog-nosed Snake, *Heterodon platirhinos*, is bluffing in response to the threat of the photographer before feigning death. Note that the cervical ribs are spread laterally, giving the appearance of a cobra-like hood. Many individuals of this species have dark cervical blotches that emphasize and draw attention to the hood. Bluffing Hog-nosed Snakes typically hiss and strike repeatedly, with either an open or closed mouth, but they almost never bite. People living within range of this species sometimes call it a "spreading adder" and incorrectly believe it to be deadly. *(Photograph courtesy S. Barten.)*

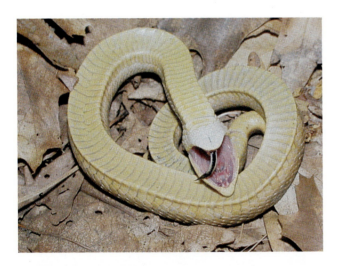

FIGURE 13-2 This Eastern Hog-nosed Snake, *Heterodon platirhinos*, is death feigning. Note the characteristic position of dorsal recumbency, with gaping mouth, protruding tongue, and gaped cloaca. If placed upright, the snake immediately rolls onto its back, as if to prove it is still dead. *(Photograph courtesy S. Barten.)*

The evolution of death feigning and tonic immobility may be related to removal of movement; a widespread class of stimuli among vertebrates that elicits killing behavior by a predator.[7,8] Reduction or elimination of the cues for killing might provide the potential prey animal with later opportunities for escape, especially from predators that transport whole immobile prey to their young (e.g., raptors, canids).[1]

Hemorrhage from Eyes, Nostrils, and Cloaca

A number of species of Horned Lizards (*Phrynosoma* sp.) and some snakes, Dwarf Boids (*Tropidophis* spp.),[9] Long-nosed Snakes (*Rhinocheilus* spp.), and some Kingsnakes (*Lampropeltis* spp.),

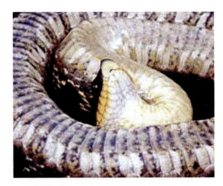

FIGURE 13-3 When the threat is removed, the Hog-nosed Snake slowly rights itself and crawls away. *(Photograph courtesy R.D. Bartlett.)*

squirt or exude blood from the eyes, nostrils, or cloaca as a defensive mechanism. Bags containing recently captured Long-nosed Snakes have been soaked with blood although the snake inside appeared to be fine. In Horned Lizards the ability to squirt blood is derived from modifications to the cephalic circulation. Restriction of blood flow from the head results in increased vascular pressure; subsequent contraction of the protrusure oculi muscles ruptures capillaries in and around the eyes and causes a thin stream of blood to be ejected up to 2 m.[10,11] This defensive mechanism seems to be an especially effective deterrent to some mammalian predators (e.g., Canids).[12]

Tail Displays

Tail displays as a defense mechanism are fairly common and are seen in Pipe Snakes (*Anilliidae* spp.), Shield-tailed Snakes (*Uropeltidae* spp.), Ring-necked Snakes (*Diadophis* spp.), Burrowing Pythons (*Calabaria* spp.), Sand Boas (*Eryx* spp.) and Rubber Boas (*Charina* spp.), Coralsnakes (*Micruroides* sp. and *Micrurus* spp.) and Shield-nosed Snakes (*Elapidae* spp.), and a few lizard species.[1,13,14] This behavior probably developed to divert a predator's attack away from the vulnerable head to the more disposable, less physiologically sensitive tail.

The display varies among the different species and families but usually involves hiding the head beneath the body (Coralsnakes, Shield-tailed Snakes) or within a coiled-up body (Sand Boas, Burrowing Python, Rubber Boas [Figures 13-4 and 13-5]). The tail is then waved around in the air, coiled tightly, or moved in a manner that mimics a striking head (Rubber Boas) (Figure 13-6). Many species (Pipe Snakes, Coralsnakes, Ring-necked Snakes) have a brightly colored contrasting ventrum that is exposed when the tail is displayed (Figure 13-7). This ventrum can startle the predator and give the snake a chance to escape; the tails of many of these individuals display scars from previous attacks that attest to the effectiveness of this behavior.[15,16] In many species, especially the Coralsnakes, the tail display is accompanied by writhing and cloacal discharge. These displays can be misinterpreted as an animal in pain or with possible neurologic disease.

Another defensive tail display often seen is tail vibrating. This is an almost universally known defensive behavior in a disturbed rattlesnake. Many other venomous and nonvenomous snakes also use tail vibrating as part of a defensive repertoire. Tail vibration as a behavior is usually seen as part of an overall defensive strategy that involves striking, writhing,

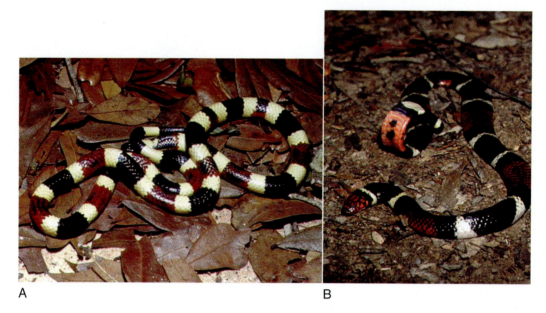

FIGURE 13-4 Coralsnake (*Micruroides* sp. and *Micrurus* spp.) defensive behaviors. **A,** Head hiding behavior. **B,** Tail display revealing the brightly colored ventrum. *(Photograph courtesy R.D. Bartlett.)*

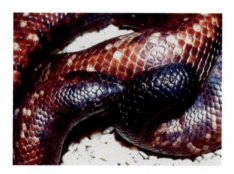

FIGURE 13-5 Head, *left*, and tail, *right*, of a Burrowing Python, *Calabaria reinhardtii*. Note the similar size and shape of the two, which allows the tail to serve as a decoy for the head when the snake rolls into a defensive ball. A small eye is visible on the head. *(Photograph courtesy S. Barten.)*

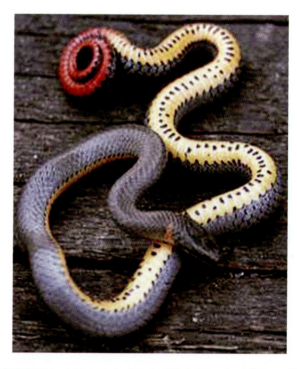

FIGURE 13-7 A Ring-necked Snake (*Diadophis* sp.) exhibits a coiled tail display and shows sharply contrasting coloration between the ventral and dorsal body scales. *(Photograph courtesy R.D. Bartlett.)*

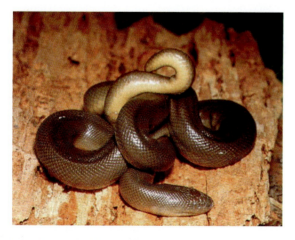

FIGURE 13-6 A Rubber Boa (*Charina bottae*) shows tail behavior. The tail is moved in a manner that mimics a striking head. *(Photograph courtesy R.D. Bartlett.)*

and emptying of the cloacal contents. A rapid tail movement or vibration characterizes this behavior. If performed in dry leaves, the vibration can produce a buzz that is audible to the human ear. This behavior is restricted to but widespread among snakes and is exhibited by many commonly kept colubrids such as Kingsnakes (*Lampropeltis* spp.), Bullsnakes and Pinesnakes (*Pituophis* spp.), Ratsnakes (*Elaphe* spp.),

Racers (*Coluber* spp.), and Whipsnakes (*Masticophis* spp.).[17,18] It is also a common behavior of many species of vipers. In the Bushmaster (*Lachesis* sp.), a large Central and South American viper, sound production is enhanced by the peculiar shape and arrangement of the terminal scales of the tail.[1] Although the behavior is most likely not to be misinterpreted as disease, a veterinarian may get a call because a person believes these various species of snakes to be rattlesnakes.

Tail loss or autotomy is a part of the broad category of defensive behaviors designed to divert an attack away from a vulnerable part of the body, such as the head, and allow escape. Although autotomy is common in invertebrates, it occurs in vertebrates only in some salamanders,[19] several rodents,[20] and most lizards. At least some species in all families except the *Agamidae, Chamaeleontidae, Helodermatidae, Lanthonodidae, Xenosauridae,* and *Varanidae* exhibit total or partial tail autotomy when grasped by a predator. After the tail is shed, it continues to wiggle, often vigorously, distracting the attacker and allowing the lizard an opportunity to escape.

In most species that exhibit this behavior, anatomic modifications are present in the tail that serve to direct where fractures occur (see Chapter 70). The ruptures occur at so-called fracture planes that are located within a single vertebral body and not between vertebral bodies.[21] This division in the vertebrae corresponds to a similar division between two muscle segments, and this zone of weakness is maintained even to the level of the skin.[21] Blood loss is minimal in autotomy, and for those lizards that escape an attack, the tail regrows over a period of months. A cartilaginous rod replaces the lost vertebrae, and the muscles and scales that regrow are irregular in shape and may differ somewhat in color (Figure 13-8).[22]

Tail loss, although not a sign of disease, has costs associated with it. The tail is often a common site for fat deposition, and some lizards use the tail in grasping or social interactions.[23-25] An owner should be informed that males may not breed without tails and that females may not have sufficient energy stores to produce viable young during the period between tail loss and regrowth.

Caudal luring, a term used to describe a behavior that is used to attract and capture food with the tail as a lure, is most common among vipers but has been suggested in boids (Madagascan Ground Boa [*Acrantophis madagascariensis*], Boa Constrictor [*Boa c. constrictor*] sp.) and elapids.[1] In most cases, the tip of the tail is a bright color (Figure 13-9) that contrasts with the rest of body. In *Bothriopsis bilineata,* the tip is swollen and pink.[26] In some instances, the tail tip is modified into the shape of an insect. The tail is waved in a rhythmic fashion and often imitates the movement of an invertebrate. Lizards, mice, frogs, and toads are attracted to within striking distance and captured and eaten. This behavior occurs in both juvenile and adult animals of various species.

Eversion of the Hemipenes

Another defense mechanism that is used by many reptiles and is especially well developed in some boids such as the Blood Python *(Python curtus),* elapids such as Coralsnakes (*Micurus* spp.), and monitors (*Varanus* spp.) is eversion of one or both hemipenes, or the phallus in chelonians. When harassed, these animals often writhe violently, empty the cloacal contents, and evert one or both hemipenes. Because this behavior is often associated with manipulation of the reptile, the novice owner may misinterpret this as an injury; the

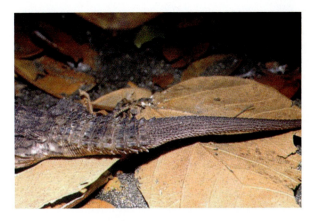

FIGURE 13-8 Regrown tail in a lizard. Note the difference in scalation and markings between the original and regrown portions. *(Photograph courtesy R.D. Bartlett.)*

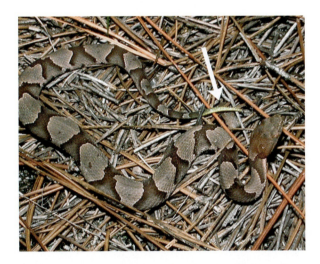

FIGURE 13-9 Many neonate snakes, like this Southern Copperhead, *Agkistrodon c. contortrix,* have brightly colored tails used in caudal luring. This snake's tail is fluorescent yellow. When it is waved rhythmically, small frogs and insects are attracted to within striking distance. The bright color fades with maturity and growth. *(Photograph courtesy S. Barten.)*

owner has caused the abdominal organs to prolapse. In the case of chelonians, owners often mistake the prolapsed organ for a parasite (leech) or tumor, and cage mates often bite at and cause trauma to the organ. In the vast majority of cases, the hemipenis or hemipenes reduces back into the cloaca on cessation of the stimuli. In those cases in which the prolapsed organ does not reduce back into the cloaca or in which obvious trauma to the organ has occurred, the animal should be seen by a veterinarian as soon as possible (see Chapter 64).

Bluff and Threat Displays

A portion of many defensive displays in reptiles involves bluffs and threats. One of the more common of these behaviors is increasing the body size by inflating the lungs and puffing up the body. Subsequently, the air is rapidly expelled from the lungs in a long loud hiss. This display behavior is common in many families of snakes and lizards. Pinesnakes have developed a septum at the glottal opening (glottal keel) that serves to amplify the sound produced during hissing. This category of behavior can deter attack by a predator by being extremely vigorous, as in many snakes and lizards, or by being passive, serving to increase the body size beyond the gape of many predators, as in the Spiny-tailed Agamas (*Uromastyx* sp.) and the Bearded Dragon (*Pogona vitticeps*) (Figure 13-10). For the herpetoculturist, this rapid influx and efflux of air may resemble an animal with respiratory disease. Inflation of the throat region in Bearded Dragons, chameleons, monitors, and snakes can look like excess fluid build up (Figure 13-11).

Another common threat display is gaping of the jaws. In many species of reptile, the oral mucosa may be a bright color that serves to distract the predator. Bearded Dragons have a bright-yellow oral mucosa that should not be interpreted as jaundice or other abnormality (Figure 13-12).

As an adjunct to the previous behavior, many reptiles, especially monitors and Asian Ratsnakes, flatten the caudal area of the head and the cranial area of the neck to increase size in a threat display. This display also has the effect of uncovering bright colors of the skin that are normally concealed by the scales.[1] These bright colors can startle an attacker and give the animal time to escape. Many of the Asian Ratsnakes and monitors also hold the head in a bent position and move the tongue slowly and stiffly during the display. This can be misinterpreted as respiratory disease or injury to the muscles or nerves of the head and neck.

Color Change

Many reptile species exhibit a circadian color change. Old World or True Chameleons are for the most part strictly diurnal animals that cease all movement as soon as the sun goes down or the cage lights are extinguished. Most species sleep at the ends of thin branches, and their color becomes blanched almost to a white. If they are disturbed in the wild or captivity at night, they drop as if dead from the branch. This is an effective escape behavior that allows the chameleon to avoid predation, but the uninformed owner may think the color change is abnormal or that the fall from the branch indicates a sick animal. Several snake species also exhibit a color change between day and night, including *Candoia carinata*, *Casarea dussumieri*, *Crotalus cerastes*, *Crotalus viridis*, several *Tropidophis* spp., and one crocodilian (*Crocodilus porosus*).[27]

Chameleons are also noted for and are especially adept at color change because of an elaborate system of chromatophores in the dermis. If two unfamiliar chameleons, two male chameleons, or a nonreceptive female are placed with a courting male, a violent color change can occur. Bearded Dragons rapidly darken their beard when threatened (see Figure 13-12), and a number of lizard species take on an overall dark coloration to the body after losing a fight with a conspecific. These color changes may be interpreted as illness. These changes are behaviorally and hormonally induced, and illness from stress can ensue if husbandry changes are not instituted.

Fragile Skin in Geckos

Most gecko species are nocturnal, have special scansorial foot pads for adhesion to walls and ceilings, and rely on crypsis (coloration and or body shape adaptations used to blend into the environment) or rapid locomotion for escape from predators such as snakes, owls, and bats. A number of species like the House Gecko (*Aristelliger hechti*), *Gehyra mutilata*, *Puchydactylus manquensis*, *Phelsuma* spp., *Teratoscincus scincus*, and *Ctenotus lenista* have evolved fragile skin.[28] These species lose large portions of epidermis even when handled gently. In species that have been studied, such as the Bronze Gecko (*Ailuronyx seychellensis*) of the Seychelles and the Madagascan

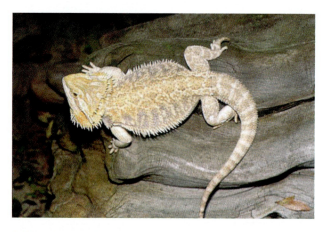

FIGURE 13-10 A Bearded Dragon (*Pogona* sp.) exhibits threat display. Puffing up the body serves to deter attack by increasing the body size beyond the gape of the predator. (*Photograph courtesy R.D. Bartlett.*)

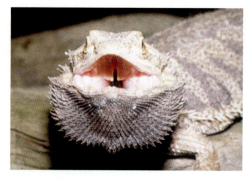

FIGURE 13-11 The inflated throat region in this Bearded Dragon (*Pogona* sp.) is part of threat display behavior and does not represent excess fluid buildup as might be seen with respiratory infection. (*Photograph courtesy R.D. Bartlett.*)

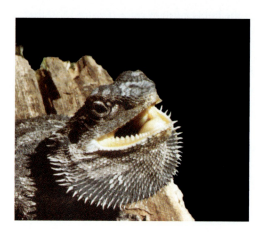

FIGURE 13-12 Bearded Dragons (*Pogona* sp.) are known for flashing their bright-yellow oral cavity as part of a defense mechanism. In addition, when threatened, their beards darken to near black. (*Photograph courtesy D. Mader.*)

genus *Geckolepis*, the skin on the animal's back is weakened by gaps in its fibrous structure. When predators grasp the lizard, most of the skin, except for a thin layer that remains to protect underlying tissues, tears away.[1] This is probably an escape mechanism similar in function to tail loss and does not indicate a nutritional, endocrine, or other similar disease.

Balling (Coiling Up) Behavior

Another defense mechanism similar to hiding the head under a loop of coils is hiding the head in the center of a ball of coils. A number of boids use this method of defense with the most well known of these being the Ball Python (*Python regius*) of West Africa. A number of other species including the African Burrowing Python (*Calabaria rehinhardii*), Rosy Boas (*Charina [Lichanura] trivirgatta*), and Rubber Boas (*Charina bottae*) exhibit this behavior (Figure 13-13).

When harassed, these boids roll into a tight ball with the vulnerable head in the middle of the coils. Protection from trauma is the obvious reason for this behavior. Field observations of *Charina (Lichanura) trivirgatta* support a less obvious reason for the behavior. On two separate occasions when these small boas were encountered under rocks, the animals balled up and rolled out of reach of the observer into nearby crevices.[1] This locomotor use of the balling behavior may be used to escape predators like ringtails (*Bassaricus astutus*), small raccoon-like mammals that live in the area and eat snakes.[29]

A similar behavior is exhibited by the Armadillo Girdled-tailed Lizard (*Cordylus cataphractus*) of Africa. When threatened in the open, this lizard grasps the heavily armored tail in its mouth and forms a circle to shield its more vulnerable underparts from attack.

Physiologic Behavior

Salt Glands

Accessory salt glands are present in all orders of reptiles including many commonly kept as pets such as Green Iguanas (*Iguana iguana*) and *Uromastix* sp. These glands function to rid the animals of excess salts accumulated, during feeding in the Marine Iguanas (*Amblyrhynchus* sp.), as a result of the environment (seaturtles), or as a way of conserving water (iguanas, desert species). Clinically, the excess salts are sneezed out of the nares, often in a fine spray, and white deposits are seen around the nares or on the glass of the caging. The owner may report this as respiratory or fungal disease to the practitioner. The Saltwater Crocodile (*Crocodylus porosus*) also has fairly extensive salt glands located in the tongue. These glands serve the same function as those glands located in the nares and can be seen as a discoloration of the tongue that may be misinterpreted as pathology.

The reptilian kidney cannot cope with excess salts absorbed from sea water. Sea Snakes and File Snakes possess a modified salivary gland located beneath the tongue. Excess salt is excreted into the tongue sheath, and when the snake protrudes the tongue, the salt is extruded into the sea. The homolopsines (South American Watersnakes) possess a similar gland located in the front of the roof of the mouth. The seaturtle's salt glands are modified tear glands, and excess salts are excreted from the corners of the eyes.

Thermoregulation

Reptiles do not have the ability to internally regulate their body temperature. Normally, the body temperature of an exposed reptile quickly approaches that of the environment. Because of this, a number of strategies are used to maintain the body temperature at a desired level. When too cool, reptiles bask in the sun and then shuttle between a cool shaded area and an open sunny one. Many nocturnal species expose portions of their body to the sunlight or hide under bark or rocks and absorb heat by transfer from these objects to themselves (thigmothermy). Some reptiles may also limit activity to certain times (morning and evening), thus avoiding extremes of temperature. Length of basking is controlled hormonally via the pineal gland, also known as the third, or parietal, eye.

A few of the behaviors associated with thermoregulation could be misinterpreted as disease, trauma, or pathology. Many reptiles begin morning basking by exposing only the head from a crevice or burrow (Figure 13-14). Heat uptake in

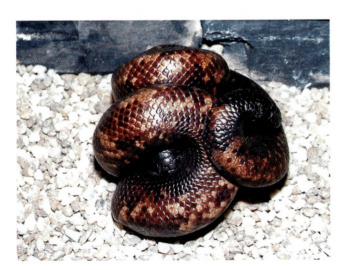

FIGURE 13-13 This Burrowing Python, *Calabaria reinhardtii*, has assumed a defensive balled position. The head is protected at the center of the ball, and the blunt tail, serving as a decoy of the head, is waved conspicuously on the outside of the ball. (*Photograph courtesy S. Barten.*)

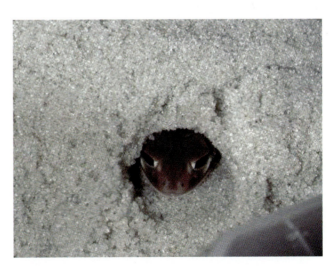

FIGURE 13-14 Thermoregulation in a gecko. The head is dark from hormonally controlled dispersal of melanin. Dark coloration allows the lizard to increase its whole body temperature by heating blood flowing to the head and only exposing a small portion of body.

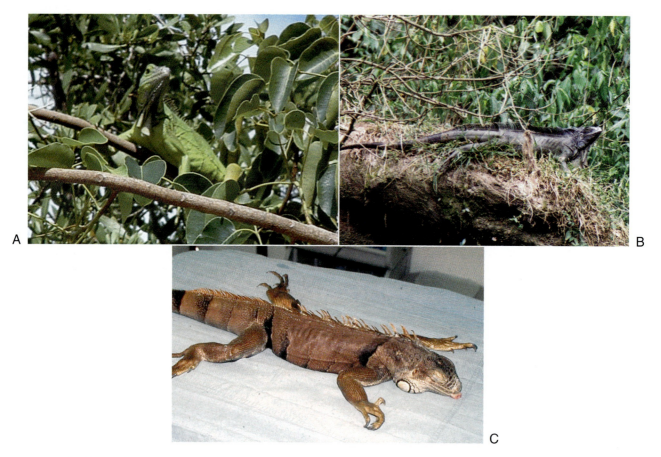

FIGURE 13-15 **A**, The Green Iguana (*Iguana iguana*) is generally bright green in early morning hours, before it thermoregulates and warms the core body temperature. **B**, Within minutes of positioning the body to incident rays of the sun, the skin darkens to help absorb radiant energy. **C**, Iguanas that are ill often exhibit this rust coloration; this is not normal and does not change with temperature or emotional status. (*A, Photograph courtesy C. Givens; B and C, Photographs courtesy D. Mader.*)

this situation is enhanced by hormonally controlled darkening of the skin through the dispersal of melanin.

The Green Iguana undergoes a dramatic color change during times of thermoregulation. Early morning colors are generally light bright green. When the animal ventures into the sun and starts to absorb the radiant energy its color darkens, almost to a black, within minutes. As the internal temperatures rise, the colors return back to their normal lighter color. These color changes are dramatic and rapid and should not be confused with the color change noted in sick iguanas that Mader refers to as "rust" (Figure 13-15).

Other strategies used are to move all or part of the body off the ground to avoid picking up heat radiated from the surface. As an example, a lacertid lizard (*Meroles anchietae*) that lives in the Namib Desert of Africa raises a foreleg and the opposite hind leg simultaneously, balancing on the other two legs. This allows the skin of the elevated feet to cool. The lizard then alternates the lifting and lowering of the diagonal pairs of legs as long as it is exposed to the hot sand.[30] This behavior could be interpreted as pain or neurologic disease. The pineal or third eye itself may be mistaken for a defective scale or an injury to the head. Lastly, many tortoises and some monitor species sun themselves with the head and neck fully extended and the forelimbs arranged limply. They can and do look as if they are dead.

Although not strictly associated with thermoregulation, Asian Water Dragons (*Physignathus concincinus*) commonly rest or sleep underwater (Figure 13-16). Although this behavior is normal, owners may believe their pet has drowned or is drowning.

Spectacle Cleaning in Geckos

Most gecko species lack eyelids and instead have evolved a spectacle analogous to that of snakes. A common behavior exhibited by most species is to clean the spectacle by licking it with their tongue (Figure 13-17). This behavior is normal, but one should rule out ulcers, retained spectacle, or any kind of irritation. However, those gecko species kept most commonly as pets, the Eublepharines (Leopard Geckos, Fat-tailed Geckos) do possess eyelids. Note the lack of spectacles in the skin being shed from the head (Figure 13-18).

Stargazing in Boids

An interesting behavior that has been noted in captive boids is the adoption of a posture where the neck is bent in such a manner as to cause the head to be tilted upwards (stargazing). A similar posture is seen in snakes with parasitic, viral, bacterial, or fungal central nervous system (CNS) disease. The difference between the two postures is that the animals without disease revert to a normal posture when disturbed or

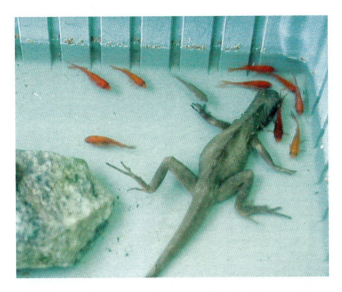

FIGURE 13-16 Asian Water Dragons (*Physignathus concincinus*) sometimes rest or sleep underwater. An owner may misinterpret this behavior as an ill or drowning animal. *(Photograph courtesy D. Mader.)*

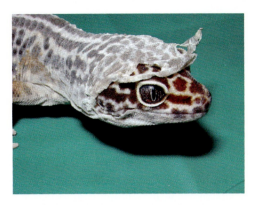

FIGURE 13-18 Most geckos have clear scales called spectacles protecting their eyes, as do snakes. They occasionally lick those spectacles to clean them. Eublepharine geckos, like this Leopard Gecko, *Eublepharis macularius*, are so named because they possess true eyelids and lack spectacles. Note that the shedding skin has eyeholes without spectacles. *(Photograph courtesy S. Barten.)*

Reproductive Behavior

Squamate (Lizards and Snakes) Reproduction and Courtship

Part of the behavioral repertoire in many iguanids includes social displays such as head bobbing, push-ups, dewlap extension, and aggression (biting, tail lashing). Head bobbing is used by both male and female iguanas, with males generally displaying this behavior more frequently and with greater variety. Females bob in a jerky erratic motion. They most commonly bob when irritated by a male iguana or when warning another iguana or owner away from food or a basking area.

Male iguanas have several different types of head bobs. All the different head bobs are executed in fluid smooth motions. The bobs are generally up and down in motion, can be fast or slow, and may include some side-to-side movement. The shudder bob is a warning and is characterized by a rapid vibration of the head in an up-down-sideways motion. At the completion of the movement, the head is held up for a few seconds and then a deliberate up-and-down bob is performed. Subordinate males tend to bob more like females.

Head bobbing in an aggressive territorial male is accompanied by a full rigid extension of the dewlap and extended legs that lift the body high off the ground. The body is presented laterally to the object in question, and the lungs are inflated. A characteristic stilted stiff gait is used by the animal. This behavior and posture serves to increase the size of the silhouette presented by the iguana to the offending object.

Another behavior associated with aggression is the open-mouth threat display (gaping). The mouth is opened wide, exposing the bright-pink oral mucosa. The tongue often is visible and in an extended arched configuration, and a low guttural hiss may accompany the display. These are strong warning and threat signs that may lead to full bites and tail lashing if not heeded. A modification of the gaping threat is used by some iguanas when involved in aggressive or dominance encounters. These animals sit with the body tensed and the mouth slightly opened. An iguana in this posture may bite at the slightest provocation.

Aggressive behavior in iguanas can be conveniently split into two categories: defensive and offensive aggression. **Defensive aggression** is most often associated with a threat

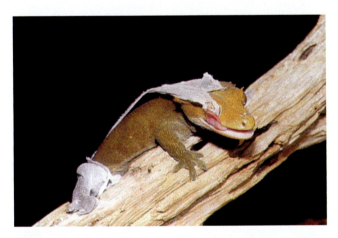

FIGURE 13-17 Many gecko species clean the spectacle with the tongue. This is normal behavior and does not indicate irritation of the eye or spectacle. *(Photograph courtesy R.D. Bartlett.)*

manipulated and the ones with disease do not. This behavior may be a feeding posture modified for captivity. Many animals are fed from top-opening cages. Even with those cages that are front opening, the prey items are often introduced from above. The snakes may have adapted to looking up for food in their search for prey.

Circumduction (Arm Waving)

Arm waving is seen in very young Bearded Dragons and Water Dragons and can be present within a few days of hatching. It seems to serve both as an intraspecies signal, for identification as a Bearded or Water Dragon, and as a submissive behavior. This behavior persists commonly in adult females and in subordinate males during aggressive encounters. This behavior could be misinterpreted as a painful or injured limb.

such as another iguana or human attempting to displace the animal from a basking site, perch, or food; grabbing the iguana; or invading its perceived territory. The behaviors most commonly associated with defensive aggression include the puffed-up sideways stance, extended dewlap, open mouth threat, and tail lashing; if provoked further, they may bite.

Offensive aggression is associated with the breeding season or in the establishment of dominance hierarchies and usually involves sexually mature males. These iguanas often stalk the human females in the household, biting them in an attempt to breed. Many of these attacks are directed at the neck and face because male iguanas bite and hold onto the neck of the female to achieve intromission. These male iguanas often view the human male in the household as competition and perform head bobs and tail lashing at an increased rate toward that person. Because the person does not leave the iguana's territory these displays often escalate into biting attacks. Although not the whole story, increases in aggression are generally associated with increases in testosterone. This breeding season aggression usually lasts for 3 to 4 months and can occur anytime of the year but generally is from November to April.

Suggested ways to deal with breeding season aggression are many and varied. Certain colors of clothing and (for female owners) the time of month (menses/ovulation) are suggested to trigger attacks. Owners should be aware of what they wear and do during attacks so they can become aware of a pattern if one exists. Adopting an aggressive stance or attitude can sometimes help to deter attacks. Reducing the photoperiod to 10 hours of light per day sometimes reduces the frequency and vigorousness of attacks. Changing the room or the cage the iguana lives in sometimes helps to reduce aggression, and providing a surrogate iguana, such as a towel, a stuffed toy, or a sock, to mate with has worked well for some iguana owners.

Castration can also be a helpful adjunct to one or more of the previously mentioned suggestions for reducing aggression in mature male Green Iguanas. In one recent study, 16 mature male Green Iguanas were randomly placed into one of three experimental groups. One group of five animals was castrated before the onset of breeding season aggression, a second group of five animals was castrated during the breeding season when exhibiting aggressive behavior, and a third group of six animals served as the control group; these animals were sham operated but were not castrated. **A statistically significant reduction was seen in aggressive behavior for the group castrated before breeding season. However, no significant reduction in aggression was found between the group castrated during breeding season and the control noncastrated group.** Subsequently, the author has castrated more than 60 male Green Iguanas. Follow-up information up to 3 years later has shown that castration has reduced or eliminated aggression in about 70% of the animals.[31]

Levels of conspecific aggression escalate between males during the breeding season. Ritualized combat is not uncommon in snakes, lizards, and turtles. In general, these combat displays end with the subordinate male fleeing the territory. However, the battles occasionally progress to actual physical injury. Attentive owners should be aware of the added stress of housing reproductive males in small captive enclosures during the breeding season and the necessity to keep them separate (Figures 13-19, 13-20, and 13-21).

The courtship behavior of many squamates involves the male grasping and biting the female in the neck and upper back region. This behavior can range from mild, causing the female no harm, to vigorous, with the creation of open bleeding wounds. In snakes, the males often grasp the female by the neck with an open mouth. This behavior can look like fighting or in the case of some snake species can appear as if one animal is trying to eat the other.

Boid Gestation and Incubation Behavior. During gestation, some female gravid boids exhibit an unusual behavior of lying on their backs or on their sides. The females appear

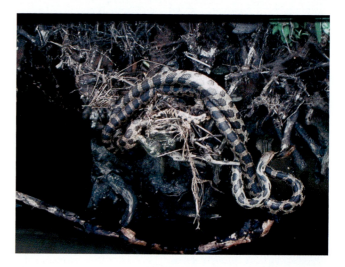

FIGURE 13-19 Two male Western Foxsnakes, *Elaphe vulpina*, engage in ritualized male combat. Combating snakes repeatedly intertwine and attempt to throw or topple their adversary to the ground until one individual withdraws. This pair was observed among the roots of a fallen tree adjacent to a river. Combat was well underway when they were discovered, and it continued for more than 30 minutes. *(Photograph courtesy S. Barten.)*

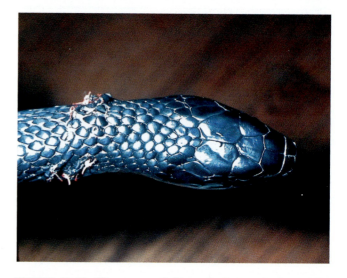

FIGURE 13-20 The owner of this male Eastern Indigo Snake, *Drymarchon couperi*, placed it with another male in hopes of stimulating combat and subsequent breeding behavior. Indigo Snakes are somewhat more violent than many colubrids, and the other male bit this one on the neck during a fight, inflicting bilateral wounds that needed sutures to close. *(Photograph courtesy S. Barten.)*

to be sleeping on their backs toward the end of the gestation period. If stimulated, they right themselves and appear completely normal. One explanation for this behavior is that these unusual positions may help with breathing during the time that the female's body is stretched to its maximum with eggs. To the untrained herpetologist, this bizarre behavior could easily be interpreted as evidence of neurologic disease.

Egg brooding or shivering thermogenesis is a phenomenon well known to herpetologists and herpetoculturists. This behavior is characterized by a female python coiled tightly around a clutch of eggs and exhibiting rhythmic muscular contractions (shivering) of the body that produce sufficient heat to maintain a relatively constant temperature in the egg mass over a fairly wide ambient temperature range (see Figure 23-3). This behavior has been reported for many different species and may be universal in pythons.[32]

In studies with captive pythons, rhythmic contractions begin when the temperature of the egg mass falls below the desired temperature (approximately 30°C).[33] At 30°C, no contractions occur and the female simply remains coiled around the egg mass. As the ambient temperature falls, the female python begins to shiver and the number of contractions increases as the temperature drops up to a maximum of approximately 30 contractions per minute.[33] Monitoring of the temperature of the egg mass revealed a constant differential of 5°C to 7°C (9°F to 15°F) between the egg mass and the surrounding environment and maintenance of the egg mass at 30°C.[33] The advantages to the species are that the eggs develop rapidly and the species that demonstrate egg brooding can reproduce successfully in cooler climates.[33]

This shivering behavior can resemble a parasitic infection (mites) or a nutritional (hypocalcemia) or neuromuscular disease especially as the female python often continues to shiver even if the egg mass is removed. This behavior is energetically expensive to the females who may lose up to half of their body weight during incubation and may need up to 3 years to regain enough body condition to breed again. To stop the shivering behavior, the animal should be moved to a clean cage and the old cage thoroughly cleaned and the substrate changed to remove all scent of the egg mass.

Chelonian Reproduction and Courtship

The social interactions of turtles and tortoises associated with reproduction and courtship usually involve head bobbing, males butting and biting the female's to immobilize them, and then mounting the female's shell from the rear. These behaviors are often accompanied by bellowing or whistling vocalizations.

To achieve intromission, the male must incline his body toward the vertical, to varying degrees in different species. The extreme is seen in the Box Turtles, which may incline beyond the vertical (Figure 13-22).

The reproductive and courtship behaviors described may be seen as fighting and the vocalizations as pain, respiratory disease, or injury by the owners. A Box Turtle inclined backwards may look as if he is stuck in the female's shell. The animals should NOT be separated during their mating encounter.

Morphologic Adaptations

Chelonia

A number of normal structures that are morphologic adaptations have evolved in reptiles that could be seen by an owner or practitioner as a disease process or traumatic injury.

Mud (*Kinosternon* spp.) and Musk Turtles (*Sternothernus* spp.), Box Turtles (*Terrepene* spp.), and Hinge-backed Tortoises (*Kinixys* spp.) have evolved a hinge or hinges in the plastron or carapace so that the animal can close itself in for protection from predators and, equally important, from loss of moisture (Figure 13-23). The hinges vary in number and location. In most species of Mud Turtles two hinges are present, one cranial and one caudal, that allow the turtles to completely close itself within the shell.

Musk Turtles have one cranially located hinge that serves to protect the front limbs and the head. Box Turtles also have one hinge in the plastron, but it is located further back than in Musk Turtles. This location allows the front and back halves of the plastron to close, completely sealing the animal within the

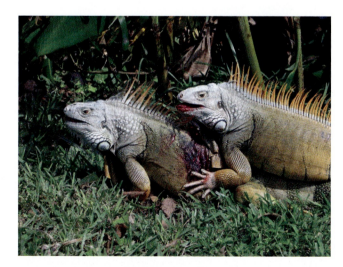

FIGURE 13-21 Two large male Green Iguanas (*Iguana iguana*) engage in combat. These encounters rarely escalate to actual injury. Rather the submissive animal usually retreats before participants suffer any damage. (*Photograph courtesy J. Wyneken.*)

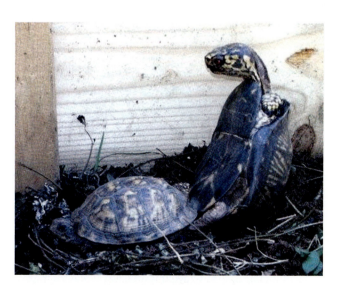

FIGURE 13-22 Male Box Turtles (*Terrepene* sp.) often incline the body beyond the vertical to achieve intromission during breeding.

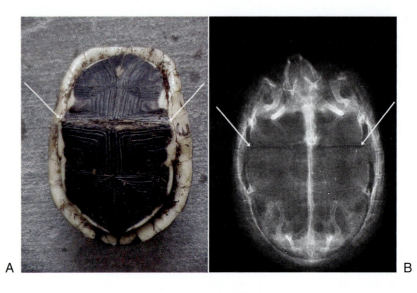

FIGURE 13-23 Asian Box Turtle (*Cuora flavomarginata*). **A,** Enclosed within its shell. **B,** Radiograph of same turtle as in **A**. Hinged plastron is a normal anatomic structure that allows for a tight seal between the plastron and carapace. This hinge does not represent a fracture of the plastron. *White arrows* point to the hinge.

shell. Spider Tortoises (*Pixys* spp.) have a hinge present in the gular area of the plastron, and Hinge-backed Tortoises have a hinge located on either side of the carapace that affords protection of the hindquarters (Figure 13-24). Other species that have had one or more hinges develop include African Mud Turtles, Asian Box Turtles, and Madagascan and Egyptian Tortoises.

A lesser degree of movement is found among certain species of pond and river turtles. Asian Leaf Turtles and neotropical Wood Turtles have a partial hinging of the plastron with ligamentous rather than bony connections between the plastron and the carapace. This gives flexibility to the plastron, but the shell cannot be closed. This adaptation appears to have evolved to allow these species to lay their exceptionally large eggs that could not otherwise fit through the shell opening. In a number of these species (Cane Turtle, Spiny Turtle) only mature females have the kinetic plastron.

Certain large-headed aggressive species such as Snapping Turtles (*Chelydra* spp.), Big-Headed Turtles (*Platysternon* spp.), and Mexican Musk Turtles (*Sternotherus* spp.) also have movable plastrons from ligamentous rather than bony connections between the plastron and the carapace. In these species, the flexibility of the plastron allows the large head to be retracted within the shell. With the jaws open and the head protected by the shell, a formidable and nearly impregnable defensive is provided.

Similarly, the Pancake Tortoise of East Africa (*Malachochersus tornieri*) has a flat, soft shell as an adult (Figure 13-25). This condition is the result of permanent open spaces, or fontanels, between the bony plates of the carapace and the plastron. These fontanels increase in size as the tortoises grow. These species live in rock outcroppings and are good climbers. When threatened, they wedge themselves in rock crevices and are difficult to extract. These are all normal structural modifications and should not be interpreted as traumatic injury or as a result of nutritional or other metabolic disease.

A morphologic adaptation for attracting and capturing prey is possessed by the Alligator Snapping Turtle (*Macrochelys temminckii*). This bifurcate modification of the tongue is worm-like in appearance and can be made to wiggle by contractions of the muscular base to which it is attached while the animal rests, mouth agape, under water. This appendage can look like an oral parasite to the layman.

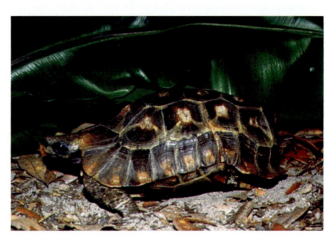

FIGURE 13-24 Hinge-backed Tortoises (*Kinixys* spp.) have bilateral hinges on the caudal carapace that serve to close the carapace against the plastron and protect from predators and loss of humidity.

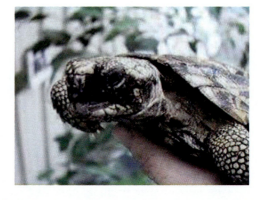

FIGURE 13-25 The Pancake Tortoise (*Malochochersus tornieri*) has open fontanels present in the carapace and plastron. This results in a soft, flat shell as an adult and is not indicative of metabolic bone disease.

Many species of Side-necked Turtles (*Phrynops* spp.) can exude fluid from the plastron, generally in the area of the bridge. Whether this fluid is for defense or a pheromone for courtship and reproduction is unknown. This process should not be mistaken for fluid loss from septicemia or trauma.

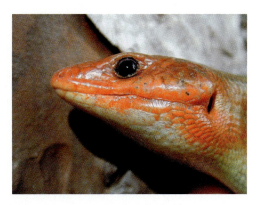

FIGURE 13-26 Male Broad-headed Skinks, *Eumeces laticeps*, develop broad jowls and bright-red head coloration during the breeding season. *(Photograph courtesy S. Barten.)*

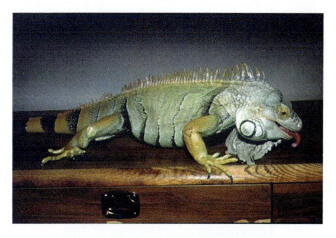

FIGURE 13-27 Male Green Iguanas *(Iguana iguana)* develop broad jowls and bright-red head coloration during the breeding season. Body color may change, depending on diet and country of origin, from bright green-blue to orange. *(Photograph courtesy R.D. Bartlett.)*

In juvenile Mata Mata *(Chelys fimbriata)* and some Side-necked Turtles the skin and plastron is bright red. This coloration in young animals is normal and does not represent dermatitis.

Squamates and Crocodilians

The tongues of many lizards are brightly colored or bicolored. Blue-tongued Skinks *(Tiliqua scincoides)* have a bright-blue tongue that they expose when harassed. Green Iguanas have a two-toned tongue, with the tip darker than the body. These colors do not represent cyanosis in the skink or an infection and necrosis in the iguana.

During the breeding season, many reptiles undergo a color or body shape change. Broad-headed Skinks develop an orange head (Figure 13-26) and Green Iguanas can have an overall orange or reddish appearance to the body, especially the head, dewlap, and forelimbs (Figure 13-27). These changes are associated with reproductive hormones and do not represent the reddening of the skin seen in septicemia. Many male lizards also have a hormonally induced increase in the size and activity of their femoral pore glands during the breeding season (see Figures 6-12 and 6-13). The femoral pores of male Green Iguanas increase greatly in size and exude a waxy material that contains pheromones. These waxy excretions, when applied to solid surfaces, reflect ultraviolet (UV) light. This is theorized to be another means of communication that serves to attract female iguanas. These pores can look like abscesses to the owner.

In snakes, the lower jaw is loosely connected by a ligament instead of a solid bony connection as is seen in most vertebrates (Figure 13-28). During feeding, the two halves of the mandible can move independently and stretch out of shape to aid in prehension and swallowing of food. After feeding, the snake manipulates the jaws by yawning to reposition the mandible back into normal position; this can take few minutes to accomplish. This should not be mistaken for a fracture of the mandibular symphysis.

Adult male Gharials *(Gavialis gangeticus)*, a slender-snouted crocodilian from India, develop a large bulbous growth on the tip of snout during the breeding season (Figure 13-29). This growth resembles a "ghara," the Hindi word for pot. Several functions attributed to it are: a resonator that produces a loud buzzing noise during vocalization; a visual stimulus to females; and production of bubbles associated with sexual

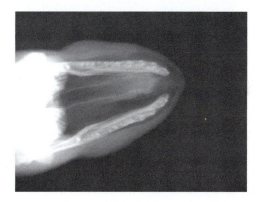

FIGURE 13-28 Open mouth radiograph of the mandibles of a Burmese Python *(Python molurus bivittatus)* shows that the two mandibles are not connected at the symphysis in snakes, as is the case in most other vertebrates. *(Photograph courtesy S. Barten.)*

behavior.[34] The growth is a normal structure and does not represent a granuloma or tumor.

AMPHIBIANS

Defensive Behaviors

Defensive Postures (Catalepsy, Death Feigning, Tonic Immobility, Unken Reflex)

Salamanders, newts, and anurans (frogs and toads) are attacked and eaten by many different types of predators including birds, reptiles, mammals, and other amphibians. This predatory pressure has led to the evolutionary development of antipredator mechanisms that often combine toxic secretions with unusual defensive postures and warning coloration. Death feigning and tonic immobility are widespread among frogs: some fold the limbs tightly against the body and lie motionless on their backs, and others assume a rigid posture with their limbs outstretched.[35,36]

Toads commonly inflate their lungs, puffing up the body and presenting a larger image to the predator, and at the same

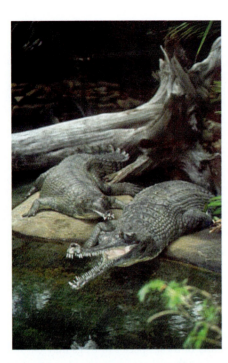

FIGURE 13-29 Adult male Gharials *(Gavialis gangeticus)* normally develop a bulbous growth on the tip of the snout during breeding season. *(Photograph courtesy R.D. Bartlett.)*

time often lift the body from the ground, tilting toward the predator.[35,36] Salamanders commonly practice tail autonomy as a defensive behavior (see tail displays in reptiles).[19]

The distribution on the body of the toxin-secreting glands and warning coloration correlates well with the defensive posture adopted by the species in question. Those species with well-developed parotid glands at the back of the head, such as the Mole, Spotted, and Spiny Salamanders *(Ambystoma* spp.), often adopt a posture where the head is bent down, thus presenting the attacker with a distasteful portion of the body.[35,36]

Some species (Mole and Spiny Salamanders) take this behavior a bit further. They hold the body high off the ground with the head bent down, and the back of the head is swung or butted into the attacker.[35,36] Other species that have skin glands concentrated on the upper surfaces of the tail tend to undulate the tail in defense, many in a vertical position. This presents a distasteful, nonvulnerable part of the body to a predator, and most of these species are capable of tail autonomy when harassed.[35,36]

Some species that tail undulate (Red-belly Newt, *Taricha vivularis*) when under intense attack adopt a rigidly immobile posture known as the **unken reflex**. This posture is characterized by having the tail and chin elevated, exposing the often brightly colored underside.[35,37] The attack reflex of predators may be inhibited by salamanders or anurans that exhibit the unken reflex. The Fire-bellied Toad *(Bombina* sp.) also exhibits this behavior for the same reason.[35,37] Most of the species that exhibit this behavior are well supplied with poison glands, and the ventrum usually exhibits warning coloration of bright reds or yellows. Imitators in many genera also mimic the unken posture and warning coloration of the abdomen *(Gyrinophilus, Pseudotriton, Desmognathus, Eurycea).* Similar to death feigning, the unken reflex serves to reduce the likelihood of receiving a mortal attack.[35,37]

The Sharp-ribbed Newt *(Pleurodeles waltl)* of eastern Asia adds an unusual component to this defense. The newt's ribs are long and sharp, and if the newt is grabbed, the tips of the ribs penetrate through the skin and its associated poison glands and, in effect, inject their toxin into the soft tissues inside the mouth of the predator.

Other species like the Casqued-headed Tree Frogs *(Hemiphractus* sp.) of the American tropics have the skin coossified to the underlying bones of the skull and have a greatly reduced blood supply to this area of skin.[35,38] During the dry season or if the humidity in the cage is not high enough, these frogs back into holes in trees or bromeliad plants containing small amounts of water to reduce water loss; they flex their heads at right angles to the body and block the holes with their heads (phragmosis), helping to conserve moisture and prevent dehydration.[35,38]

Another defensive posture is used by the False-eyed Frog *(Physalaemus bilogonigerus)* of South America, which has two large eye-like spots on its rump. When threatened, it aims its rump towards the predator.[35,38] These postures resemble an injured or sick animal, especially a musculoskeletal injury or CNS disease. Owners may think the animal is paralyzed or is distorted from pain.

Moisture Conservation

Two commonly kept genera of anurans, Horned Frogs *(Cerotophrys* sp.) and African Bullfrogs *(Pyxicephalus* sp.), along with the less commonly kept Water Holding Frog *(Cyclorana platycephala)*, form cocoons from layers of shed skin to conserve moisture in response to a dry environment. If the captive environment is too dry, these species can exhibit a similar behavior and form a cocoon. With encasement in a cocoon, movement is reduced and the frogs look and appear dead. In the wild, these frogs emerge from the cocoons when the environment becomes wet, as during the rainy season; similarly, a captive frog can often be stimulated to emerge from the cocoon by increasing the humidity in the cage and by soaking the frog in shallow water. The cocoon is usually peeled off the body of the frog with the front limbs and then eaten. When the frogs are encased in a cocoon, the client may think the animal has died or is sick.

Pedal Luring

Horned Frogs exhibit a behavior similar to caudal luring in viperids, termed **pedal luring**. The frog lifts the toes of one hind foot off the ground and curls them forwards and down in a rhythmic repeating wave. This species often eats smaller frogs, including siblings, and this behavior serves to attract these frogs close enough to be captured and eaten. This behavior can be exhibited with no prey species present in the enclosure and can be mistaken for hypocalcemic tremors.

Reproductive Behavior

With few exceptions, anurans (frogs and toads) fertilize eggs externally. The most common practice is to deposit sperm as the eggs are laid, with the male clasping the female from dorsally with his forelegs (amplexus). A number of Arrow Poison Frogs (Dart Frogs) do not use amplexus, but instead the male fertilizes the eggs after the female deposits them. In some

Behavioral and Morphologic Adaptations

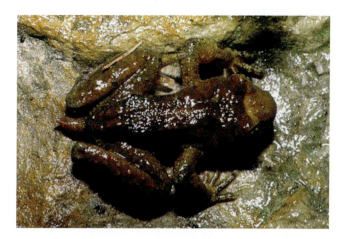

FIGURE 13-30 North American Tailed Frog *(Ascaphis truei)*. The tail is actually a modification of the cloaca used for sperm transfer during breeding. *(Photograph courtesy R.D. Bartlett.)*

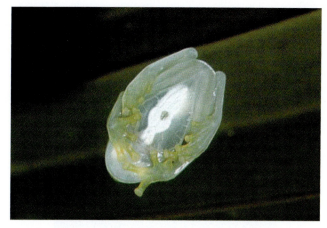

FIGURE 13-31 In Glass Frogs *(Centrolenidae)*, a normally transparent ventrum allows visualization of the abdominal organs. *(Photograph courtesy R.D. Bartlett.)*

species of Narrow Mouthed Frogs, the bodies of the male and female are glued together for a short period of time, and in other anurans, the male's cloaca is held next to the female's while sperm is transferred, resulting in internal fertilization, but no intromittent organ is present.[35,38] In the North American Tailed Frog *(Ascaphus truei)*, the tail is actually a modification or extension of the cloaca and is inserted into the female's cloaca to transfer sperm (Figure 13-30).[35,38] These behaviors and anatomic modifications could be interpreted as fighting (amplexus) in anurans in general or injury (prolapsed cloaca) in the Tailed Frog in particular.

Most herpetologists and herpetoculturists know that males (sometimes females) of many species of dendrobatids (Arrow Poison Frogs) carry their recently hatched tadpoles on their backs to water where they are released to complete their development.[35,38] However, a number of frog species carry eggs or newly hatched larvae in brood pouches, located on their sides or back, where the tadpoles develop into froglets, and others hold their tadpoles in sacks in their mouths or in the stomach to complete development.[35,38]

Several genera (subfamily *Hemiphractinae*) brood their eggs on the female's back (*Hemiphractus* sp.) or completely enclosed within a brood pouch (*Gastrotheca* sp.). The Pouched Frog *(Assa darlintoni)* of Queensland has a brood pouch located on each side of the body.[35,38] In the Marsupial Tree Frogs (*Gastrotheca* sp.), the male uses his feet to guide the eggs into the pouch as they are laid by the female. In the pouched frog, the male straddles the egg mass and the tadpoles wriggle into the pouches with the male assisting by swiping movements of the forelimbs.[35,38] The tadpoles undergo development in the pouches. As the tadpoles increase in size, the lumps they create resemble masses that could be interpreted as neoplasia or abscesses. As the froglets emerge, the pouch mucosa becomes visible and can look like a traumatic wound.

In the mouth-brooding frogs such as Darwin's Frog (*Rhinoderma darwin* and *Rhinoderma rufus*), the eggs are laid on land. When the tadpoles hatch, the males engulf them and then they go into the vocal sacs either to be brought to water or to undergo development to froglets in the sacs. Similarly, in two species of gastric-brooding frogs (which may now be extinct), the eggs are swallowed by the female and undergo development to froglets in the stomach; during development, the gastric digestive juices are suppressed. When development is complete, the froglets emerge from the mouth of the female. Keepers of any of these species of frogs may assume that the adults are eating the young.

The Surinam Toad (*Pipa pipa*) of South America has a peculiar method of carrying its eggs during development. The eggs become embedded in pockets in the skin of the female's back. The skin then hypertrophies, covering the eggs; the froglets emerge by burrowing out from under the skin to the outside.

Morphologic Adaptations

Many anurans such as the true toads and Spade Foot Toads (*Sped* spp.) possess a soak patch, which is an area of skin on the animal's ventrum that is thinner than the surrounding skin and is rich in blood vessels. These frogs place the patch in a shallow pool of water or damp ground and are able to absorb water through this structure. The soak patch can be mistaken for a defect in the skin or an area of infection or septicemia.

Healthy amphibians readily consume their shed skin. The amphibian often looks as if it gagging or is ill during the consumption period. This behavior is normal, and failure to consume the skin may be a sign of illness.

Another group of frogs, the Glass Frogs (*Centrolenidae*) of Central and South America, have a transparent ventrum that allows visualization of the internal organs (Figure 13-31). This is a normal condition for these species and does not represent a disease or injury state.

All anurans possess a fourth segment in the hind leg (all other limbed amphibians and reptiles have three segments). This fourth segment is created from the elongation of two of the ankle bones. This condition provides greater leverage for leaping and serves to distinguish the order Anura in which frogs and toads are placed.

Many species of frogs possess a prominent nutrient foramen in the tibiofibula bone of the hind limb. This foramen is often clearly visible on radiographs. This normal anatomic structure is often misinterpreted as a fracture (Figure 13-32).

Finally, males of the Hairy Frog (*Trichobatrachus robustus*) of Cameroon develop vascularized hair-like structures on the flanks and thighs during the breeding season. The males of

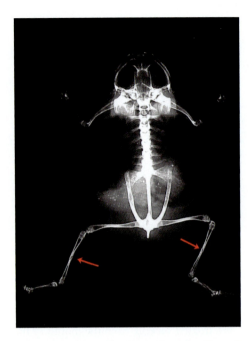

FIGURE 13-32 Dorsoventral radiograph of the Green Toad (*Bufo viridis*) shows a prominent nutrient foramen in the tibiotarsal bone of the hindlimb *(red arrows)*. This normal anatomic structure can be mistaken for a fracture especially in the lateral view where only one foramen may be visible. *(Photograph courtesy M. Stetter.)*

this species remain submerged and sit on and protect the egg masses during development. The hairs are actually extensions of the skin and serve to increase the surface area to allow greater respiration through the skin, increasing the time the frog can remain submerged[35,38]; these hairs can be mistaken for parasites or fungal infection.

ACKNOWLEDGMENTS

I thank Steve Barten, DVM, R.D. Bartlett, Eric Holt, and Mark Stetter for providing the photographs that greatly enhanced the usefulness of this chapter.

REFERENCES

1. Greene HW: Antipredator mechanisms in reptiles. In Gans C, Huey RB, editors: *Biology of the Reptilia, defense and life history, ecology B,* New York, 1988, Alan R. Liss.
2. Shine R: "Costs" of reproduction in reptiles, *Oecologia* 46: 92-100, 1980.
3. Leviton AE, Anderson SC: Further comments on the behavior of the Panamanian microteiid *Echinosaura horrida*, *Herpetologica* 22:160, 1966.
4. Schmidt KP: Contributions to the herpetology of the Belgian Congo based on the collection of the American Museum Congo Expedition, 1909-1915, Part I, turtles, crocodiles, lizards, and chameleons, *Bull Am Mus Nat Hist* 39:385-612, 1923.
5. Gorzula SJ: An ecological study of *Caiman crocodilus crocodilus* inhabiting savanna lagoons in the Venezuelan Guayana, *Oecologia* 35:21-34, 1978.
6. Gorzula SJ: Are caimans always in distress? *Biotropica* 17: 343-344, 1985.
7. Alcock J: *Animal behavior: an evolutionary approach,* ed 3, Sunderland, Mass, 1984, Sinauer Assoc.
8. Curio E: *The ethology of predation,* New York, 1976, Springer-Verlag.
9. Hecht MK, Walters V, Ramm G: Observations on the natural history of the Bahaman pigmy boa, *Tropidophis pardalis*, with notes on autohemorrage, *Copeia* 249-251, 1955.
10. Burelson GL: The source of blood ejected from the eye of horned toads, *Copeia* 246-248, 1942.
11. Heath JE: Venous shunts in the cephalic sinuses of horned lizards, *Physiol Zool* 39:30-35, 1966.
12. Cowles RB: *Desert journal,* Berkeley, 1977, University of California Press.
13. Obst FJ: Kroetenkoepfe, *Aquar Terrar Zoo* 12:187-188, 1959.
14. Dial BE: Tail display in two species of iguanid lizards: a test of the "predator signal" hypothesis, *Am Nat* 127:103-111, 1986.
15. Minton SA: A contribution to the herpetology of West Pakistan, *Bull Am Mus Nat Hist* 134:27-184, 1966.
16. Greene HW: Defensive tail display by snakes and amphisbaenians, *J Herpetol* 7:143-161, 1973.
17. Parker HW: *Natural history of snakes,* London, 1965, British Museum Natural History.
18. Radcliffe CW, Chiszar D, Smith HM: Prey-induced caudal movements in *Boa constrictor* with comments on the evolution of caudal luring, *Bull Maryland Herpetol Soc* 16:9-22, 1980.
19. Wake DB, Dresner IG: Functional morphology and evolution of tail autotomy in salamanders, *J Morphol* 122:265-306, 1967.
20. Mathews LH: *The life of mammals,* vol 2, London, 1969-1971, Weidenfeld & Nicolson.
21. Quattrini D: Piano di autotomia e rigenerazione della coda nei Sauri, *Arch Ital Anat Embriol* 59:225-282, 1954.
22. Arnold EN: Caudal autonomy as a defense. In Gans C, Huey RB, editors: *Biology of the Reptilia, vol 16, defense and life history, ecology B,* New York, 1988, Alan R. Liss.
23. Vitt LJ, Lacher TE: Behavior, habitat, diet, and reproduction of the iguanid lizard *Polychrus acutirostris* in the caatinga of northeastern Brazil, *Herpetologica* 37:53-63, 1981.
24. Carpenter CC, Ferguson GW: Variation and evolution of sterotyped behavior in reptiles. In Gans C, Tinkle DW, editors: *Biology of the Reptilia, vol 7, ecology and behavior A,* New York, 1977, Academic Press.
25. Vitt LJ, Cooper WE: Tail loss, tail color and predator escape in Eumeces (Lacertelia: Scincidae): age-specific differences in costs and benefits, *Can J Zool* 64:583-592.
26. Greene HW, Campbell JA: Notes on the use of caudal lures by arboreal green pit vipers, *Herpetologica* 28:32-34, 1972.
27. Cooper WE, Greenberg N: Reptilian coloration and behavior: In Gans C, Crews D, editors: *Biology of the Reptilia, vol 18, physiology,* Chicago, 1992, University of Chicago Press.
28. LaBarbera M: Why the wheels won't go, *Am Nat* 121:395-408, 1983.
29. Taylor WP: Food habits and notes on the life history of the ring-tailed cat in Texas, *J Mammal* 35:55-63, 1954.
30. Bauer AM: Lizards. In Cogger HG, Zweifel RG, editors: *Reptiles and amphibians,* New York, 1992, Smithmark Publishers.
31. Lock B, Bennett RA, Gross TS: *Changes in plasma testosterone and aggressive behavior in male green iguanas (Iguana iguana) following orchidectomy,* New Orleans, La, 2000, Proceedings Joint Conference, Am Assoc Zoo Vet, IAAAM.
32. Shine R: Parental care in reptiles. In Gans C, Huey RB, editors: *Biology of the Reptilia, vol 16, defense and life history, ecology B,* New York, 1988, Alan R. Liss.
33. Harlow P, Grigg C: Shivering thermogenesis in a brooding diamond python, *Python spilotes spilotes, Copeia* 959-965, 1984.
34. Maskey BGH, Bellairs ADA: The narial excresence and ptergoid bulla of the gharial, *Gavialis gangeticus,* (Crocodila), *J Zoo London* 82:541-558, 1977.

35. Halliday T, Adler K: *The encylcopedia of reptiles and amphibians*, New York, 1987, Facts on File.
36. Duellman WE, Carpenter CC: Reptile and amphibian behavior. In Cogger HG, Zweifel RG, editors: *Reptiles and amphibians*, New York, 1992, Smithmark Publishers.
37. Lanza B, Vanni S, Nistra A: Salamanders and newts. In Cogger HG, Zweifel RG, editors: *Reptiles and amphibians*, New York, 1992, Smithmark Publishers.
38. Zweifel RG: Frogs and toads. In Cogger HG, Zweifel RG, editors: *Reptiles and amphibians*, New York, 1992, Smithmark Publishers.

Section IV
MEDICINE

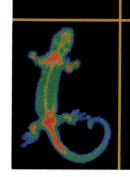

14
CARDIOLOGY

MICHAEL J. MURRAY

Reptilian clinical cardiology is a subject that has been poorly documented in the veterinary literature. Although the scientific data regarding cardiac anatomy and physiology in various reptilian species are relatively voluminous, the accessibility and applicability of the data to the veterinary clinician is questionable. Despite this deficit, the ability to diagnose and treat various forms of cardiac disease in the reptile remains critically important for the practitioner.

Clinical cardiac disease may be primary (e.g., idiopathic cardiomyopathy, congenital defects, and degenerative disease) or caused by metabolic or nutritional diseases. In addition, many systemic, infectious, and parasitic diseases may affect the cardiovascular system and thus manifest clinical signs referable to this system. Patients with peripheral edema, ascites, ecchymotic hemorrhages, weakness, or dyspnea undergo complete physical and laboratory evaluations, with an emphasis on the cardiovascular system. Ancillary diagnostic techniques, such as radiography, ultrasonography, and electrocardiography (ECG), may be used to detect cardiac disease.

Of particular clinical interest is the use of cardiac monitoring during anesthetic periods (see also Chapter 27). The advent of the use of isoflurane and sevoflurane anesthesia with their inherent increased margin of safety in clinical reptile medicine has increased the frequency of reptile anesthetic interventions. ECG, Doppler technology, and pulse oximetry are all ideally suited for managing the anesthetic period because respiratory rate, cardiac rhythm and rate, and anesthetic depth tend to be variable in reptiles undergoing anesthesia.

CLINICAL CARDIAC DISEASE

Cardiac disease may manifest itself in a variety of forms, dependent on its etiopathogenesis. The clinical signs of cardiovascular disease are typically quite nonspecific and rarely, if ever, pathognomonic. Swelling in the area of the heart, pleural or peripheral edema, ascites, cyanosis, and ecchymoses are all clinical signs that should stimulate investigation of the cardiovascular system (Figure 14-1). A variety of nonspecific clinical signs, such as generalized weakness, apparent exercise or activity intolerance, anorexia, weight loss, change in skin color, and sudden death, can also be seen.

Regardless of the inherent limitations in examining these challenging patients, a complete cardiovascular examination should be performed on all reptiles seen for veterinary care. Experience with as many different species as possible has more value than the most expensive piece of diagnostic equipment. **The more reptiles examined, the easier for the practitioner to recognize the abnormal when it presents.**

In snakes, the heart is typically located at a point one third to one fourth the length of the patient caudal to the head.[1] Placing the patient in dorsal recumbency in a quiet well-lit room and observing for movement of the ventral scutes is usually an effective way to locate the heart. A crude estimation of the cardiac size may be obtained through observation

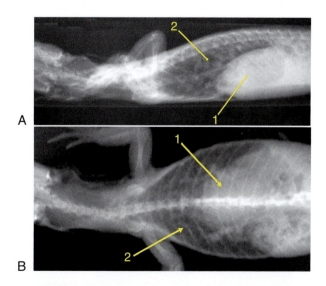

FIGURE 14-1 Swelling in the area of the heart, pleural and peripheral edema, ascites, cyanosis, and ecchymoses are all clinical signs that suggest cardiovascular disease. This monitor presented with weakness, obvious cardiomegaly, and ascites. Marked cardiomegaly was noted radiographically (1), as well as pulmonary edema (2). (Photographs courtesy B. Okimoto.)

of the movements of the ventral scutes under the heart associated with the cardiac cycle (Figure 14-2).

The peripheral pulse may be difficult to palpate; however, digital examination of the artery at the base of the glottis may be useful. Use of a Doppler flow detector may enhance the clinician's ability to realize an arterial pulse. Auscultation of the heart is best accomplished in a quiet area because heart sounds are typically of low amplitude. Use of a moistened towel or gauze sponge aids in the elimination of extraneous sounds that occur when the stethoscope diaphragm rubs against the scales.

In other reptile species, such as lizards, crocodilians, and turtles, the heart is located on the ventral midline either within or just caudal to the pectoral girdle. Its location tends to preclude observation of the cardiac movements; however, cardiac movements may be palpable in certain lizard species. Auscultation is again enhanced with the damp towel or gauze sponge placed against the scales (Figure 14-3). Peripheral pulses are frequently difficult to identify, and the use of the Doppler flow detector is recommended (Figure 14-4).

The heart rate should be determined and noted in the record for all species examined. One must remember that the heart rate is dependent on a number of noncardiac factors, especially temperature. Therefore, an accurate assessment of the animal's core body temperature is always warranted as part of any reptilian physical examination. Likewise, the patient's core body temperature should also be recorded in the record. This helps when comparing findings at future dates. Many inexpensive electronic digital thermometers are available that produce reliable immediate core readings that are effective in all reptile species (see Figure 31-2).

The entire length of the patient should be palpated for evidence of edema or swelling, which may accompany cardiac disease. Examination of the oral mucous membrane and the lining of the vent may reveal pallor or cyanosis in cardiovascular disease. The cloacal vent is oftentimes the only reliable mucous membrane that can be evaluated in reptiles. A simple Capillary refill time (CRT) test can be performed by blanching the mucous membrane with a gentle pinch or digital pressure. The time needed for the tissue to return from pale to pink should be less than 2 seconds. A CRT longer than 2 seconds suggests cardiovascular or some other disease process affecting circulation (patient temperature is critical in this evaluation).

NUTRITIONAL DISEASES

Several nutritional diseases may have direct and substantial effects on the cardiovascular system. Muscle tremors with hypocalcemia are often encountered in a variety of reptilian species. Hypocalcemia affects not only the peripheral nerves and skeletal muscle but also the striated cardiac muscle. Delayed cardiac muscular repolarization, as shown by increased S-T and Q-T intervals in mammals,[2] probably occurs in reptiles as well. For this reason, chemical or protracted physical restraint should be avoided or used with extreme caution until the hypocalcemia can be resolved.

Dietary deficiency of vitamin E may result in cardiac muscle abnormalities. The classic "white muscle disease," as described in ruminants, has been diagnosed in a variety of reptilian species.[3] In addition to skeletal muscle disease, cardiac muscle shows changes commensurate with cardiomyopathy. Typically, affected animals have received inappropriate diets

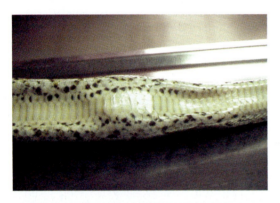

FIGURE 14-2 A crude estimation of cardiac size may be obtained through observation of movements of the ventral scutes under the heart associated with the cardiac cycle. Emaciated patients may give a false impression of cardiomegaly because the cardiac shape is so readily identified. (*Photograph courtesy D. Mader.*)

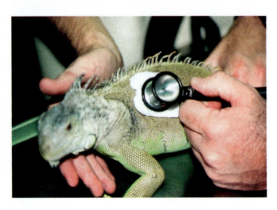

FIGURE 14-3 Auscultation is enhanced with a dampened gauze sponge between the scales and stethoscope head, which helps eliminate the typical scratching sounds associated with hard scales. (*Photograph courtesy D. Mader.*)

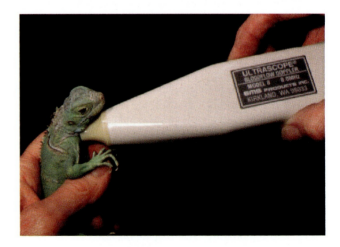

FIGURE 14-4 Peripheral pulses are frequently difficult to identify, and the use of a Doppler flow detector is recommended. This handheld unit can be used to identify both vascular flow and abnormalities in cardiac hemodynamics. (*Photograph courtesy F. Frye.*)

of excessively oily fish or obese laboratory rodents. Clinical signs of affected reptiles are nonspecific and may mimic hypocalcemia or be associated with steatitis. Diagnosis is difficult, with a reliance primarily on history and physical examination. Biopsy of skeletal muscle may support the diagnosis.

Unless disease is too advanced, treatment with the commercially available vitamin E (12.5 mg/kg) and selenium products (0.05 mg/kg) is generally curative.

A common vascular condition seen in reptiles is calcification of the tunica media of the large vessels (Figure 14-5).[4] Although the exact etiopathogenesis is unclear, a distinct association appears to exist between this condition and diets containing excessive levels of vitamin D_3 and calcium, such as primate chows. The mineralization is often an incidental finding during radiographic examination.

Sudden death may occur should the myocardium be affected or an aneurysm develop in a major vessel with subsequent rupture (Figure 14-6). Onset of clinical signs is usually peracute with death as the endpoint. Treatment is rarely successful because the progression to death is usually immediate.

INFECTIOUS DISEASE

A number of infectious agents have been associated with cardiac pathology. Most do not affect the cardiovascular system as a primary target organ but tend to cause systemic illnesses; thus, their affects on the cardiovascular system are secondary. A variety of bacterial pathogens have been associated with and recovered from the cardiovascular system of several reptile species. Many of the aerobic gram-negative bacteria have the potential for producing a septicemia.

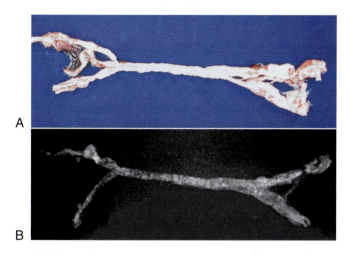

FIGURE 14-5 **A,** Resected aorta and large vessels from a Green Iguana *(Iguana iguana).* **B,** Radiograph of the same vessel in **A**. Note the calcified wall structure. *(Photographs courtesy K. Rosenthal.)*

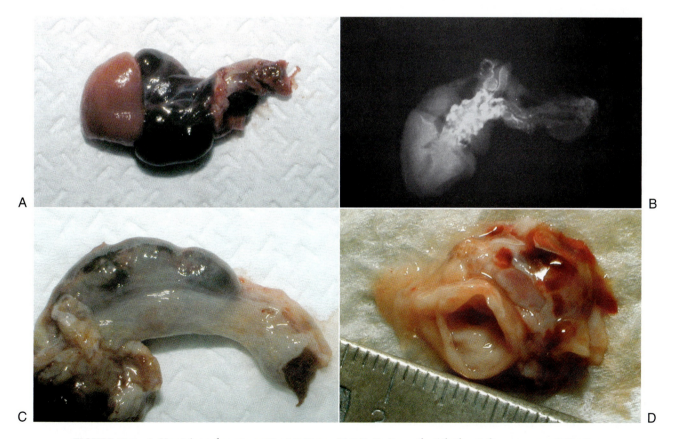

FIGURE 14-6 **A,** Heart from the same patient in Figure 14-5. **B,** Radiograph of the heart shows severe calcification of the aortic trunk. **C,** A large aneurysm in the aortic arch from a different Green Iguana *(Iguana iguana).* **D,** Aneurysm removed shows a large defect in the curvature of the arch. This patient died peracutely when the aneurysm ruptured, with no premonitory signs. *(A and B, Photographs courtesy K. Rosenthal; C and D, Photographs courtesy D. Mader.)*

The potential for a secondary endocarditis exists with any of the commonly seen gram-negative bacterial pathogens. As a result, routine blood cultures should be performed on all cases of bacterial sepsis. Blood sample collection for culture via cardiocentesis (with aseptic technique) is the preferred method. *Vibrio damsela* was recovered from an endocardial thrombus in a stranded Leatherback Seaturtle (*Dermochelys coriacea*).[5] Because the diagnosis was made postmortem, the exact circumstances surrounding the etiopathogenesis are unclear.

Septic endocarditis was diagnosed in a Burmese Python (*Python molurus bivittatus*) with a combination of angiography and ultrasonography. Both *Salmonella arizona* and *Corynebacterium* sp. were recovered from the affected snake.[6] A pure culture of *Escherichia coli* was recovered postmortem from a myocardial abscess in a Green Iguana (*Iguana iguana*), likely another example of a secondary cardiac manifestation of systemic illness.[7]

A chlamydial infection in Puff Adders (*Bitis arietans*) resulting in a granulomatous pericarditis and myocarditis, pneumonia, and hepatitis has been reported.[8] Although a specific *Chlamydia* sp. was not recovered, the light and electron microscopy results found changes consistent with the life-cycle stages of Chlamydia. Because the diagnosis was made at postmortem examination, the possibilities of control, treatment, and zoonosis remain speculative. An outbreak of mycoplasmosis in captive American Alligators (*Alligator mississippiensis*) caused pneumonia, pericarditis, and arthritis.[9] Granulomatous myocarditis associated with a systemic *Mycobacterium* sp. infection has been identified in a Frilled Lizard (*Chlamydosaurus kingi*).

PARASITIC DISEASE

Several parasitic diseases have been identified in association with the cardiovascular system. Postmortem examination of a number of reptile species has shown focal pathology of the aortic arch and pulmonary trunk. These lesions were primarily scar tissue accumulations associated with presumed parasitic infections.[4] The pathology was clinically insignificant without any antemortem signs of affliction.

Several species of filarid nematodes have been identified in almost all major groups of reptiles. Little host specificity appears to exist for the most important filarid genera, *Oswaldofilaria*, *Foleyella*, and *Macdonaldius*.[10] The adult worms are capable of living in the vascular system where they release microfilaria into the circulation. Transmission occurs via blood sucking arthropods, primarily mosquitoes and the ticks (*Ornithodoros talaje* and *Amblyomma dissimile*).[11] Most infections are asymptomatic and are diagnosed at autopsy; however, ischemic necrosis may occur should microfilaria obstruct peripheral capillaries. Such cases may be seen with a vesicular or necrotizing dermatitis. Diagnosis is based on the microfilaria in the peripheral blood of the adults at autopsy. Chemotherapeutic therapy has not been well described. Reports have been made that maintaining infected individuals at an environmental temperature of 35°C to 37°C for 24 to 48 hours has been adulticidal.[10] Reptiles maintained at these elevated temperatures should be monitored closely for evidence of thermal stress.

Digenetic spirorchid flukes may be encountered in the cardiovascular system of reptiles. Although a variety of reptiles is susceptible, the turtle is most commonly infested. In such cases, trematodes of the genera *Spirorchis*, *Henotosoma*, *Unicaecum*, *Vasotrema*, and *Hapalorhynchus* are most often encountered.[9] The small, 1-mm to 3-mm, adults are typically found in the heart or the great vessels exiting the heart. Minimal clinical disease is associated with the adult stage of the life cycle; however, some focal endothelial hyperplasia may occur in response to their presence.

In chelonians, the primary clinical concern associated with the presence of the spirorchid flukes is attributable to the release of the fluke eggs within the vascular compartment. Accumulation of eggs may occlude terminal vessels in a variety of locations, including the gastrointestinal tract, spleen, liver, heart, kidneys, and lungs.[10] A severe granulomatous inflammatory response typically ensues in these locations. Affected turtles are often listless and anorectic. Vascular occlusion of vessels to the carapace and plastron may result in focal and coalescing ulcerative lesions of the shell.

Diagnosis of fluke infestation is difficult. Adult spirorchids are infrequently identified at necropsy, but identification of the eggs in tissue specimens is diagnostic. Eggs may be identified in a "squash" preparation of pulmonary tissue. Antemortem detection of eggs may be accomplished with direct or sedimentation examination of stool specimens or occasionally on direct saline solution mounts of lung washes.[9]

Treatment of spirorchid infections is difficult and has limited success. Use of praziquantel orally or intramuscularly (8 mg/kg) may prove effective.[9] Other authors suggest that no chemotherapeutic measures are effective but suggest use of drugs used for treatment of human schistosomiasis.[10] In a study performed in the Green Seaturtle (*Chelonia mydas*), praziquantel was safe and effective in eliminating cardiovascular trematodes. In contrast to earlier published reports, the dosage administered was 50 mg/kg orally for a single day at hours 0, 7, and 9.[12] No observable effect was noted on trematode egg-induced granulomata, the primary pathology-causing component of spirorchid trematode infestation. In most instances, control of the parasite is relatively simple. This digenetic trematode requires a small snail to act as an intermediate host. Elimination of the snail breaks the life

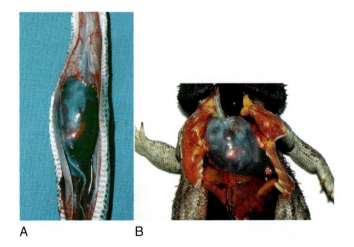

FIGURE 14-7 Many cases of cardiomyopathy are diagnosed at necropsy. This python **(A)** and Bearded Dragon (*Pogona vitticeps*) **(B)** each had hemopericardium. This is not an uncommon finding. The cause is not known but may be related to dietary imbalances, neoplasia, trauma, clotting disorders, and as-yet-undetermined causes. (*Photographs courtesy D. Mader.*)

cycle. Therefore, most infections occur in wild-caught specimens or those maintained in outside habitats with significant invertebrate populations.

OTHER CARDIAC DISEASES

A number of congenital cardiovascular anomalies have been reported in a variety of reptile species. In most cases, abnormalities of the myocardium or great vessel were detected postmortem.

As the husbandry, nutrition, and medical management of reptiles continues to improve, the reported incidence rate of geriatric cardiovascular disease is certain to increase. At this time, most cases of myocardial degeneration are diagnosed at necropsy (Figure 14-7). Congestive heart failure has been diagnosed in association with infectious disease and with cardiomyopathy.[6,13] With the aid of color Doppler echocardiography, ECG, and radiography, right atrioventricular (A-V) valve insufficiency and subsequent bilateral congestive heart failure was diagnosed in a Carpet Python (Morelia spilota variegata).[14] As such advanced technologies continue to be applied to reptile patients, the rate of diagnosis of cardiac insufficiency and failure is likely to increase (Figure 14-8). Hopefully, an increased diagnostic rate will result in development of therapeutic regimen.

Exceptional care should be exercised in the use of cardiac glycosides, sympatholytics, vasodilators, and diuretics in reptiles. The pharmacokinetics and pharmacodynamics of these agents have not been well researched in reptiles. Direct extrapolation of data from mammals is probably inappropriate, partly owing to the unique anatomy and physiology of the cardiorespiratory systems of the reptile. For example, the effects of atropine and glycopyrrolate, blocking the negative chronotropic effects of vagal stimulation of the heart, as is seen in mammals, have been shown to be ineffective in the Green Iguana.[15] Despite these differences, many similarities do exist, such as the presence of beta-adrenergic receptors that mediate the positive ionotropic and chronotropic effects of the catecholamines.

Because specific dosage calculations have yet to be determined for most drugs and species, the use of allometric scaling is recommended (see Chapter 25). For obvious physiologic reasons, no indication is seen for the use of loop diuretic therapy, as reptiles do not possess a loop of Henle within their kidney.

RENAL PORTAL SYSTEM

The renal portal system is a component of the venous system of reptiles that has raised numerous questions with potential

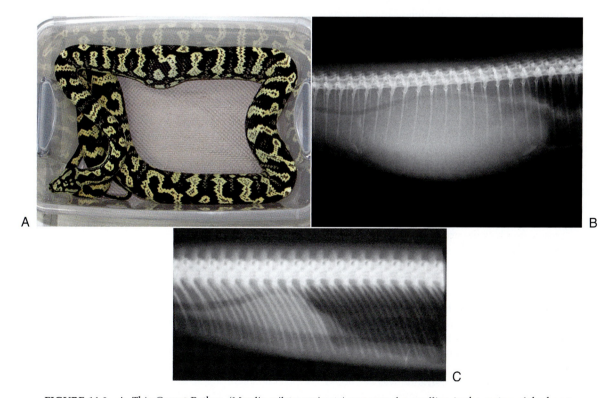

FIGURE 14-8 **A,** This Carpet Python (Morelia spilotes variegata) was seen for swelling in the region of the heart. **B,** Radiograph of the patient shows an enlarged heart. **C,** Radiograph from a normal python for comparison. As diagnostics and therapeutics become more sophisticated, these cases will no longer carry a grave prognosis. (*A and B, Photographs courtesy S. Barten; C, Photograph courtesy D. Mader.*)

clinical significance (see Chapter 11). The function of the renal portal system is to ensure adequate perfusion of the renal tubules when blood flow through the glomerulus is decreased as a water conservation mechanism. The afferent renal portal veins do not perfuse the glomeruli and instead supply the proximal and distal convoluted tubules with blood. Like their mammalian counterparts, the reptilian tubular cells are also perfused by afferent arterioles leaving the glomeruli. Unlike the mammal, however, the reptile does not have a loop of Henle and so cannot concentrate urine. As a result, under the influence of arginine vasotocin, water is conserved by decreasing the afferent blood flow to the glomerulus. When this glomerular blood supply is decreased, the renal portal system is vitally important in supplying blood to the tubules to prevent ischemic necrosis.

Studies have shown a great deal of variation in the anatomy of the renal portal system between reptilian orders and even within suborders.[16] Typically, however, blood flows from the tail via the caudal vein and from the pelvic limbs via the femoral or iliac veins. Blood may then enter the kidney via the afferent renal portal vein, through the kidneys into efferent renal portal veins, and back into general circulation via the post cava. Blood from the caudal portion of the body may, however, bypass the kidneys through alternative routes via the abdominal vein or the mesenteric vein. Blood flow through the renal portal system is controlled by a valve located within the external iliac vein in the bird. The presence of such a valve was shown in Red-eared Sliders (*Trachemys scripta elegans*)[17] but was not recognized in the Green Iguana.[18]

Several studies have evaluated the effect that the renal portal system may have on the pharmacokinetics of drugs administered into the caudal portion of the reptile's body. In the Green Iguana avoidance of the use of the hind limb musculature and vasculature for drug administration was unnecessary.[18] However, the caudal tail vein was shown to be a direct route to the renal portal system. This is obviously of little consequence for chemotherapeutics cleared by glomerular filtration. A slight effect appears to be seen on those compounds with a high first pass tubular excretory rate (e.g., penicillins). The exact significance of this potential impact is unknown at this time but is likely to be inconsequential in most cases.

Similarly, site of administration was shown to have no significant effect on the pharmacokinetics of gentamicin in the Eastern Box Turtle (*Terrapene carolina*).[19] A study in the Red-eared Slider with carbenicillin and gentamicin supported the findings published earlier in the Eastern Box Turtle.[17] A significant difference in the serum concentration of the carbenicillin administered was seen when the administration was in the front legs versus the rear legs, with the caudal administration serum concentrations lower than the value obtained from the front legs. However, the serum concentration that remained after the rear administration was still above therapeutic levels. Therefore, the authors of the study concluded that no evidence exists to support avoidance of the caudal aspect of the body for the administration of chemotherapeutic agents.

Mader (personal communication) points out that a significant difference in serum levels was, in fact, noted in this study. Even though the ultimate serum concentration was still above therapeutic levels, the difference should not be overlooked. This single study should remind the clinician that a massive amount of information is still lacking regarding pharmacokinetics, pharmacodynamics, and the renal portal system.

Mader recommends that cranial administration is still warranted with use of a novel drug and no knowledge of how it is eliminated or metabolized.

DIAGNOSTIC TECHNIQUES

Electrocardiography

Despite several significant limitations, the reptilian ECG does have some clinical applications for the practitioner. Its use may enhance other diagnostic methods in cases of clinical cardiac disease (Figures 14-9 and 14-10). In addition, the ECG may play an adjunctive roll in the monitoring of the reptile patient during anesthetic episodes. Keep in mind, however, that a reptile's heart continues to beat after it is dead. So, the mere presence of an apparent sinus rhythm should not be relied on as the sole means of monitoring vitality during anesthesia.

One of the most important limitations in the use of the ECG is the paucity of clinically relevant published material on the subject available to the practitioner. A few values have been published, but the data are few and the values vary from species to species and within individual species.

Consistent with its use in small animal practice, the ECG is described as a recording of the heart's electrical activity as detected at the skin level. An important clinical assumption is made when the ECG is used—that the recorded electrical activity is truly an accurate reflection of the muscular action of the organ.

The components of the reptilian ECG are quite similar to those described for the mammal with three primary wave complexes, the P, QRS, and T, comprising most of the recording. Both the terminal posterior vena cava at its termination at the sinus venosus and the sinus venosus itself have been observed participating in the systolic action of the atria. Such activity may be detected with the ECG and be observed as a wave preceding the P wave, the SV wave.[20]

The P wave is associated with the depolarization of the atria; the QRS complex is associated with the depolarization of the ventricle; and the T wave is associated with the repolarization of the ventricle. The SV wave, if present, represents the depolarization of the posterior vena cava and the sinus venosus. The heart contraction appears to initiate in the right atrium in the region of the sinus venosus and then proceed to the left and caudally. The ventricle is depolarized starting at the base and then proceeding to the left. Repolarization tends to progress from the base to the apex, equally deviating to the left and the right.[21]

The placement of the surface electrodes is critically important in the recording of the reptilian ECG. The electrical amplitude of many reptilian waveforms is frequently quite small, often less than 1 mV; therefore, equipment with good sensitivity or preamplification is required. In addition, the background interference associated with skeletal muscle activity may obscure the cardiac waveforms.

Leads are generally applied to the body surface in one of several techniques. Subcutaneous leads may be created by placing a stainless steel hypodermic needle through the skin and then attaching the lead to the metallic portion of the needle (Figure 14-11). Loops of stainless steel suture material passed through the skin in the appropriate locations provide a more durable location for lead attachment.

Cardiology

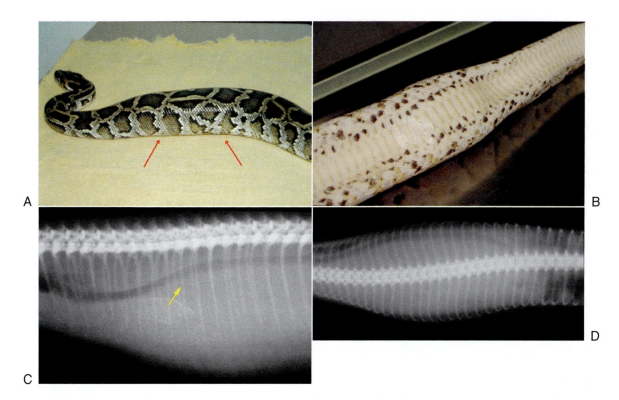

FIGURE 14-9 **A** and **B,** Burmese Python *(Python molurus bivittatus)* with cardiomegaly (between arrows). **C** and **D,** Radiographs of the patient show calcification at the base of the aorta *(arrow)*. Aortic stenosis resulted in ventricular hypertrophy. *(Photographs courtesy D. Mader.)*

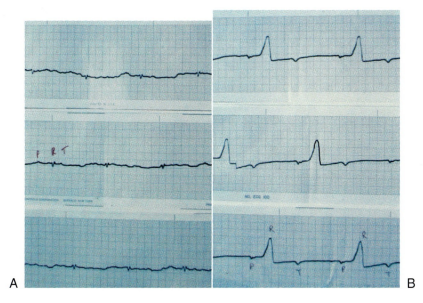

FIGURE 14-10 Electrocardiographic tracing from the patient in Figure 14-9. **A,** Normal ECG from age, size, and temperature matched conspecific. **B,** Tracing from the patient. Note the enlarged and widened QRS, typical of ventricular enlargement seen in mammal patients. *(Photographs courtesy D. Mader.)*

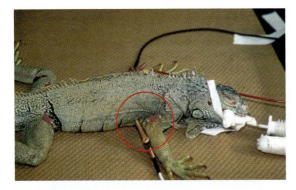

FIGURE 14-11 Electrocardiographic lead placement in a Green Iguana (*Iguana iguana*). Recording of potentials can be enhanced with fine hypodermic needles through the skin and attachment of the ECG clips to the bare metal portion of the needle. (*Photograph courtesy K. Rosenthal.*)

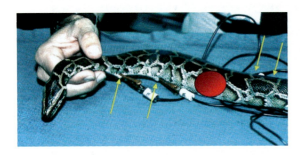

FIGURE 14-12 Lead placement in a snake can be a challenge because of the lack of limbs. Placing the two forelimb leads cranial to the heart (shown as a *red circle*) and the rear limb leads caudal to the heart yields a tracing similar to a standard lead II in dogs and cats. (*Photograph courtesy D. Mader.*)

Table 14-1	Electrocardiographic Results of American Alligator (*Alligator mississippiensis*)
Temperatue = 25°C	Heart rate = 37.6 ± 4.79 bpm
R-R interval	1.71 s
QRS duration	0.10 s
Q-T interval	1.18 s
T duration	0.33 s
Q amplitude	0.09 mV
R amplitude	0.25 mV
S amplitude	0.16 mV
T amplitude	0.13 mV
Mean electrical axis	82.95 ± 13.85

Note: P-R interval and P-wave duration/amplitude were inconsistently recorded and not evaluated.
From Heaton-Jones TG, King RR: Characterization of the electrocardiogram of the American alligator (*Alligator mississippiensis*), J Zoo Wildl Med 25(1):40, 1994.

Table 14-2	Evaluation of Reptile Electrocardiographic Results
Heart rate	Use standard techniques (at 50 mm/s, 1 mm = 0.02 s)
Identify components	P-wave, QRS-complex, T-wave, SV-wave (if present)
Rhythm	P-wave for each QRS?/QRS for each P-wave?
Evaluate components	Intervals uniform in length?
Normal for species?	Consider temperature and heart rate differences
	Compare with "normal" control patient
Integrate into clinical setting	Is it consistent with patient findings and ancillary examinations?

In snakes, the use of the self-adhering cutaneous skin electrodes designed for human use provide excellent electrical contact; however, the use of the traditional limb leads is obviously impossible (Figure 14-12). In chelonians it has been suggested that better electrical contact may be made by drilling holes in the carapace and attaching the leads to the dermal bone. Such a technique is probably excessively invasive and not indicated in the clinical setting. In most species, the tendency is to attach electrodes in the traditional four limb positions. Such positioning may not provide adequate wave deflections in many species with low signal voltages.

In lizards with hearts located caudal to the pectoral girdle (e.g., monitors and Tegus) and in crocodilians, use of either limb electrodes or torso electrodes appears appropriate. In those lizards with a heart located at the level of the pectoral girdle (e.g., skinks, iguanas, chameleons, and Water Dragons), he use of electrodes placed in the cervical region, rather than on the forelimbs, is preferable. Snakes should have electrodes placed approximately two heart lengths cranial and caudal to the heart. Placement of the electrodes in the turtle is often problematic. Although the traditional four-limb placement is often adequate, surface voltages are frequently so small that ECG interpretation is not possible. Placement of the cranial leads on the skin lateral to the neck and medial to the forelimbs is frequently more rewarding.

Electrocardiograms are traditionally interpreted in a systematic fashion: calculating heart rate and rhythm; determining interval and segment values; and determining the mean electrical axis. Such an evaluation is based on the ability to recognize not only the various components of the ECG but also the presence of normal values for the species under question. Currently such a technique is not practical, nor possible, for most reptiles.

Clinically relevant parameters for the ECG of the American Alligator collected at 25°C and 38 bpm have been published (Table 14-1).[22] **Not only is the size of the recorded electrical potentials dependent on electrode placement, but the various ECG parameters are also dependent on several environmental factors, such as temperature, body size, age, and state of excitement.**

The heart rate is dependent on the body temperature, and the intervals, such as the P-R segment and Q-T segment, are dependent on the heart rate.[21] If at all possible, the clinician is advised to use an ECG from a "normal" similarly sized individual of the same species at the same temperature for comparison with the reptile in question. All reptilian ECGs should be evaluated in a consistent organized fashion to maximize their clinical value (Table 14-2).

The mean electrical axis is difficult, if not impossible, to determine. With the low surface electrical potentials of many reptiles, identification of the isoelectric lead may not be feasible. Lead placement is frequently inconsistent from individual to individual, thereby altering the surface voltages recorded. Normal parameters are not well established for most species. Therefore, the cardiac vector is not of significant clinical importance.

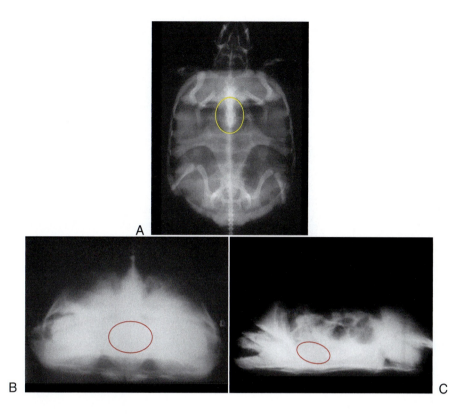

FIGURE 14-13 In chelonians, standard radiographic survey films include **A**, VERTICAL beam dorsoventral *(DV)* view, **B**, HORIZONTAL beam anterior-posterior *(AP)* view, and **C**, HORIZONTAL beam lateral *(L)* view. Because the heart is soft tissue and is generally surrounded by bony shell *(DV* and *L)* or heavy tissue *(AP)*, visualization of the heart on any of the views is limited. *(Photographs courtesy D. Mader.)*

In mammals, the ECG can be used to diagnose a variety of cardiac lesions, including arrhythmias, congenital heart disease, chamber enlargements, pacemaker dysfunction, and the effects of cardiac drugs used for cardiac monitoring during and after anesthesia.[23] Although some of these maladies may be identified in the reptilian patient with the aid of ECG, they have been poorly described in the veterinary literature. In the published literature, the ECG has proven beneficial as an adjunct in the diagnosis of chronic aortic valvular stenosis and ventricular hypertrophy in a Children's Python (*Liasis childreni*),[4] congestive heart failure from a dilated cardiomyopathy in a Black Kingsnake (*Lampropeltis niger*),[13] and aortic stenosis and atrioventricular dilatation in a Green Iguana.[24] In all three cases, the ECG changes were dramatic and supported by clinical, radiographic, and other diagnostic means.

The reptilian ECG has a great deal of potential as an aid in the diagnosis of cardiac disease in the reptile. Unfortunately, significant limitations do exist and must be addressed by the clinician before the diagnosis of any condition. Of particular importance is the collection of a variety of "normal" ECGs for use as reference in the interpretation of the clinical ECG. Despite these limitations, the clinician is advised to use this ancillary technique as an aid in the management of disease with signs that may be attributed to the cardiovascular system.

Radiography

Radiography is a valuable tool for diagnosis of cardiac disease. Some limitations to the standard techniques do exist, but once understood, the benefits gained are paramount.

In chelonians the standard radiographic survey films include a VERTICAL beam dorsoventral (DV) view, a HORIZONTAL beam anterior-posterior (AP) view, and a HORIZONTAL beam lateral (L) view (Figure 14-13). Because the heart is soft tissue and is generally surrounded by boney shell (DV and L) or heavy tissue (AP), visualization of the heart on any of the views is limited to none. Generally, the terminal trachea and bronchi can be visualized on the DV, which gives an approximation of the location of the heart, but the cardiac silhouette is not visible. If pathology is present (Figure 14-14), the heart may be more readily observed.

Clear visualization of the heart is possible with nonselective angiography (Figure 14-15). This technique is easy and readily performed with injection of 1 to 2 mL of either a high-osmolar (ionic) contrast medium (e.g., Diatrizoate Meg & Na, 292 mg I/mL) or a low-osmolar (nonionic or ionic) contrast medium (e.g., Iohexol 240/300 mg I/mL) via a large-bore jugular catheter.

Survey (plain) films must be taken to establish technique. Radiographs should be taken with a vertical beam DV view. The kVp should be increased by 5 to 10 over the survey film setting. The first film should be exposed when 50% to 80% of the calculated contrast has been injected. Ideally, additional exposures should be made every second for 5 seconds. The normal transit time for contrast in small mammals is approximately 6 to 8 minutes. This has not been established for reptiles, but in general one can usually take several images before the contrast is no longer effective.

The best imaging for chelonian hearts is via magnetic resonance imaging (MRI) or computed tomography (CT) scans (Figure 14-16). The three-dimensional technology allows for multiview images of the heart without the imposition of the

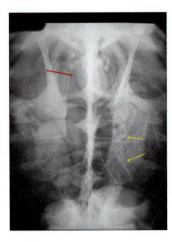

FIGURE 14-14 Generally a normal chelonian heart cannot be seen on a DV view. However, when certain pathologies are present, as is the case in this seaturtle with dystrophic mineralization, both the heart *(red arrow)* and intestinal walls *(yellow arrows)* are readily visualized. *(Photograph courtesy D. Mader.)*

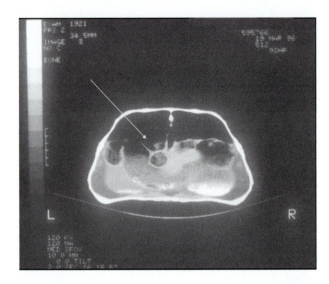

FIGURE 14-16 The best imaging for chelonian hearts is via an MRI or, as pictured here, a CT scan. Three-dimensional technology allows for multiview images of the heart *(arrow)* without imposition of the carapace, bony pelvic and pectoral girdles, soft tissue, and ingesta. *(Photograph courtesy K. Rosenthal.)*

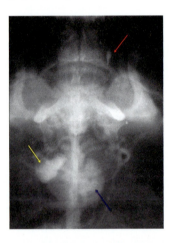

FIGURE 14-15 Clear visualization of the heart with nonselective angiography is possible. Contrast media, 1 to 2 mL, are injected through a large-bore catheter *(red arrow)*. Note the clear image of the heart and great vessels *(yellow arrow, right atrium)* *(Photograph courtesy D. Mader.)*

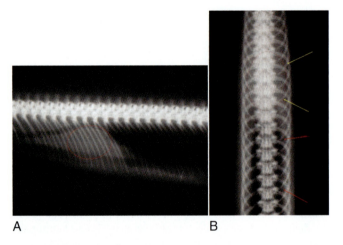

FIGURE 14-17 A and B, In snakes, standard survey radiographic views include the vertical beam L and the vertical beam DV. Heart position is noted with *dashed red line*. *Yellow arrows* define the cranial and caudal borders of the heart on the DV. *Red arrows* point to the lungs. The L view gives the best image of the cardiac silhouette without superimposition of the spinal vertebrae. *(Photograph courtesy D. Mader.)*

carapace, bony pelvic and pectoral girdles, soft tissue, and ingesta.

In snakes, the standard survey radiographic views include the vertical beam L and the vertical beam DV. The L view gives the best view of the cardiac silhouette without superimposition of the spinal vertebrae (Figure 14-17). This also allows the best visualization of the lung fields (although these are superimposed in species with two separate lungs) without interference of the underlying liver and viscera. The heart is generally obscured by the vertebrae on the DV view.

Lizards have the widest range of body forms and ultimate placement of the heart. As a result, no one best view is used for cardiac evaluation. Lizards that have their heart located within the pectoral girdle (such as the iguanids and chameleodontids) are difficult to image. The heart silhouette is lost in the surrounding bone on the lateral and the DV views (Figure 14-18). Visualization of the great vessels is possible, however, and every attempt should be made to evaluate position and radiodensity (see Figure 14-5, A, B).

In lizards with a more caudally placed heart, both the L and DV views are useful, with the former giving the best image (Figure 14-19). **Although a vertical beam lateral works for lizards, a HORIZONTAL beam lateral affords a better anatomic assessment of cardiac size, shape, and location** and anatomic position.

Crocodilian hearts image similar to lizards. In larger specimens, the osteoderms in the skin may make visualization of the heart difficult.

Additional cardiac imaging is possible in all species with the aforementioned CT and MRI scans. Radioisotope scans are possible and have a place in evaluating blood flow and renal perfusion (Figure 14-20).

Cardiology

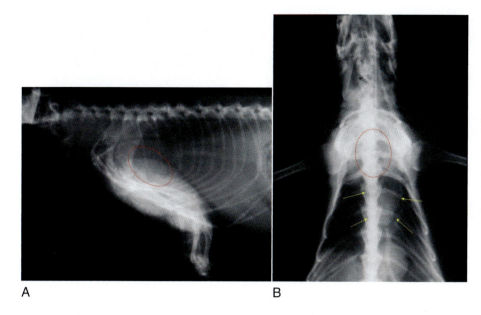

FIGURE 14-18 A and B, Lizards that have their heart located within the pectoral girdle (e.g., iguanas and chameleons) are difficult to image. The heart silhouette *(dashed red circle)* is lost in the surrounding bone on the L and DV views. The bony sternum *(yellow arrows)* on the DV view is often confused with the cardiac silhouette. Visualization of the great vessels is possible, however, and every attempt should be made to evaluate position and radiodensity. *(Photograph courtesy D. Mader.)*

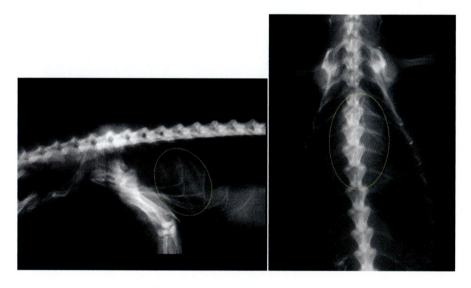

FIGURE 14-19 In lizards with a more caudally placed heart (e.g., varanids, monitors), both the L and DV views are useful, with the former giving the best cardiac image *(dashed yellow circle)*. *(Photograph courtesy D. Mader.)*

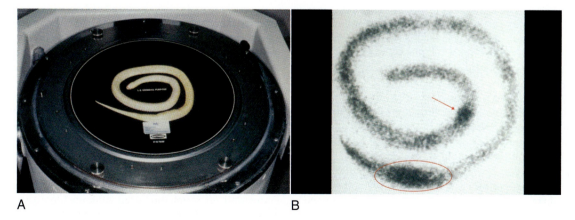

FIGURE 14-20 A, Radioisotope scans are possible and have use in evaluating blood flow and renal perfusion. B, The vascular phase of the scan readily shows the heart *(red arrow)* and kidneys *(red oval)*. *(Photograph courtesy R. Funk.)*

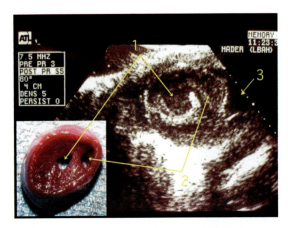

FIGURE 14-21 Transverse (short axis) echocardiographic view of a typical snake heart. Note the apparent thickened ventricle, which is a normal finding in snakes. Both *1* and *2* show chambers in the ventricle separated by a large muscular ridge; *3* points to a small amount of pericardial fluid, which is a normal finding. *(Photograph courtesy D. Mader.)*

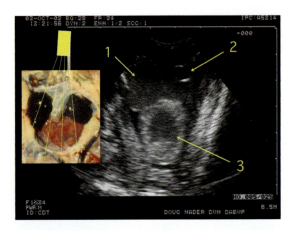

FIGURE 14-22 Cranial transverse view of a tortoise heart. The window is between the neck and forelimb. *1, 2,* Right and left atria; *3,* ventricle. *(Photograph courtesy D. Mader.)*

Echocardiography

Echocardiography (cardiac ultrasound) is frequently used in the diagnosis of mammalian cardiac disease because it is noninvasive, identifies specific cardiac anatomy, and estimates and quantifies cardiac function.[23] Its use in the reptile provides similar advantages, with the distinct disadvantage being the lack of well-described normal values for most species. Echocardiography may be most useful in the evaluation of heart valve motion and in the identification of mural thrombi; pericardial effusion; structural defects, such as outflow stenosis; and valvular disease.[25]

In most reptiles, a water bath is preferable to a traditional coupling gel to minimize the artifactual effects of air trapped between scales. Minimization of movement is critically important, particularly in smaller specimens, as the footprint size (surface area) of the transducer and depth of field is often quite small in reptilian patients.

In the Burmese Python, sagittal plane scanning was most effective in identifying major vessels, cardiac chambers, septae, and valves.[26] The entry point of the caudal vena cava into the right atrium via the sinus venosus valve may serve as a good landmark for sagittal plane scanning. The transverse plane is less effective in identification of important cardiovascular structures; however, it does provide imaging of the ventricular trabeculae and the horizontal septum (Figure 14-21). Important landmarks in this plane are the position of the pulmonary artery and aortic arches. In this species, the cranial vena cava, left atrium, vertical septum, and smaller pulmonary veins were inconsistently visualized.[26]

Much work has been done on the use of ultrasonography in chelonia. In most species, visualization of the heart and major vessels is obtained via one of two windows. The best access to image the heart is from a cranial perspective, between the base of the neck and the humerus (from either side). Alternately, you can image the heart through a small window behind the axilla (Figure 14-22).[27] In the Soft-shelled Turtles (*Apalone* sp.), good cardiac visualization is obtained between the plastral callosities through the median vacuity.

In lizards, because of the variable anatomic location of the heart, the windows for ultrasonography also vary. Lizards with

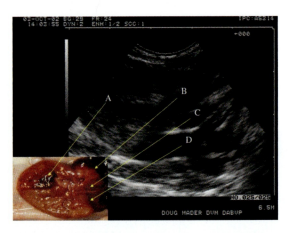

FIGURE 14-23 Long axis view of a Green Iguana (*Iguana iguana*) heart. The window is through the axilla behind the right forelimb. *A,* Ventricle; *B,* right atrium; *C,* aortic trunk; *D,* left atrium. *(Photograph courtesy D. Mader.)*

hearts located within the pectoral girdle are best visualized through a window in the axillary region on either the right or left side (Figure 14-23). Animals with a more centrally located heart can be scanned with a window just caudal to the xiphoid.

Without species and temperature specific normal values, the measurement of chamber wall thickness and changes in cardiac contractility is questionable. In addition, the highly trabeculated ventricular muscle of the reptile makes such measurements difficult.

The changes detected in a reported case of cardiac disease in a Green Iguana were advanced enough to support the diagnosis.[24] A Burmese Python with clinical and radiographic evidence of cardiac disease and cardiomegaly was diagnosed with endocarditis and congestive heart failure with the aid of echocardiography. The technique revealed a mass within the right atrium that was later identified as a septic thrombus.[6] Pericardial effusion and atrial dilation were detected in a posthibernation Spur-thighed Tortoise (*Testudo graeca*).[28] These cases suggest the circumstances in which echocardiography may be most useful—intracardiac masses, cardiomegaly, and cardiac function visualization. As in ECG, the availability of a clinical "normal" may be critical in the evaluation of the echocardiogram.

Cardiac Monitoring During Anesthesia

One of the most important aspects of reptilian cardiology is its application in the monitoring of anesthesia. The tendency of many reptiles to exhibit prolonged apnea and the ability to use prolonged anaerobic respiration complicates the maintenance of adequate cardiopulmonary function during anesthetic episodes. Traditional techniques for the monitoring of cardiac function during anesthesia are generally ineffective in reptiles.

Heart rate may be determined in snakes with observing the movement of the ventral scutes adjacent to the heart. Such a determination may not be possible in other species. The anatomy of the heart does not lend itself to auscultation; therefore, the stethoscope is of limited use. Placement of an esophageal stethoscope may enhance physical monitoring of heart sounds.[29] Regardless of the type of cardiac monitoring used, establishment of baseline norms is important for every patient before the induction of anesthesia. Allometric scaling has been used to predict a variety of physiologic parameters based on body weight (kg) and a series of mathematical formulas. The formula for the prediction of heartbeat frequency (hbf) per minute is[30]:

$$hbf = 33.4 \, (Wt_{kg}^{-0.25})$$

with Wt_{kg} = weight in kilograms; 33.4 is a constant called the k factor.

This formula assumes that the reptile under consideration is within its preferred optimal temperature zone (POTZ).

The purpose of this portion on reptilian cardiology is to discuss the applications of cardiology in the monitoring of anesthesia. The basic concepts of anesthetic selection, induction, and support are assumed to be already understood (see Chapter 27).

Electrocardiographic Monitoring

Although the ECG is being rapidly replaced by more technologically advanced monitoring equipment, it remains a valuable and useful method for monitoring circulation during an anesthetic event (Figure 14-24). As previously described, specific changes in the ECG are not well described, especially during anesthetic procedures. The ECG can, however, facilitate management of the anesthetic period by providing a record of the heart rate of the patient. Unfortunately, no direct, predictable relationship is found between anesthetic depth and ECG appearance.[31] In addition, the ECG shows electrical activity but does not ensure normal myocardial function and hence, circulation.

Electrocardiographic leads are attached in the normal fashion with alligator clips, hypodermic needles, or stainless steel sutures. Leads placed cranial and caudal to the heart in the snake are typically adequate (previously discussed, see Figures 14-11 and 14-12). **Because lead II is the most commonly used lead for anesthetic monitoring, one may use a simple modification of the base-apex lead.** In this case, the left leg lead is caudal to the heart apex, the right arm lead cranial to the heart base, and the left arm lead on the head or

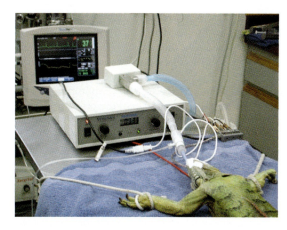

FIGURE 14-24 Although few normals are available for reptile patients, ECG still has value in monitoring anesthetized patients. This Green Iguana (*Iguana iguana*) is being monitored with a sophisticated multimodal monitor that includes ECG, SPO$_2$, end tidal CO$_2$, and core body temperature (Vet Advisor, Surgivet, Waukesha, Wis). (*Photograph courtesy D. Mader.*)

neck. The appearance of the ECG tracing is similar to that of a traditional lead II when the controls are set to lead II.[31] In smaller patients, one may merely construct an esophageal base-apex lead with a red-rubber feeding tube. In this case, a positive lead is caudal to the heart and a negative lead cranial to the heart.

Particularly important is the establishment of "norms" before and immediately after the induction of anesthesia. Variations from the anticipated cardiac values during the anesthetic period suggest increasing depth of anesthesia, excessive loss of body temperature, or hypoxemia.

In mammals, the ECG is used to monitor not only heart rate but also arrhythmias and conduction abnormalities. In addition, myocardial hypoxia may be implied with the ECG by the presence of changes in the S-T segment, reversal of the T-wave polarity, and increase in T-wave amplitude.[32] Because reptilian ECG is not so well described, such inferences are nebulous at best. The clinician should, however, be cognizant of changes from the initial "normal" as the anesthetic period progresses. Changes in the ECG suggest the need to evaluate depth of anesthesia, anesthetic concentrations, increase oxygenation, or start chemotherapeutic manipulation of cardiac function.

Doppler Ultrasonic Flow Detector Monitoring

The Doppler ultrasonic flow detector has tremendous potential for the monitoring of anesthesia in reptiles. Its primary advantage over the ECG is the ability to use the technology in very small patients. The extremely low surface electrical potential generated by small reptiles may render the ECG essentially useless in anesthesia. The ultrasonic flow detector uses two piezoelectric crystals, one of which is stimulated by an electric voltage. When stimulated, the crystal emits a wave of ultrasonic energy at a constant rate and frequency. On transfer through the skin, the wave is either reflected by stationary tissue or by moving red blood cells. In the first instance, the reflected signal is identical to the transmitted one.

When the signal strikes moving cells, a different frequency, which varies according to the velocity of the blood, is reflected. The differences between the two, the Doppler shift frequency, are then measured electronically and amplified.[33] The Doppler flow detector provides an audible representation of the arterial pulse. The character and amplitude of this signal vary with changes in the character of the pulse and, indirectly, the heartbeat.

The Doppler probe may be placed over any artery located near the surface of the skin. In snakes, the probe is typically situated just cranial to the heart at the base of the glottis or under the ventral tail vein. In lizards, an arterial pulse may be monitored with the Doppler flow detector in the lateral cervical region, over the carotid artery, on the medial aspect of the thigh, over the femoral artery, or at the thoracic inlet. In chelonians, the Doppler probe appears to be most practical when placed over the carotid artery.

Use of the Doppler flow detector allows the anesthetist and surgeon to monitor heart rate through an audible signal. In addition, an indirect subjective measure of the arterial pulse pressure may be made. This last parameter should not be overinterpreted because motion or decreased contact between the probe and skin may alter the intensity of the signal.

Pulse Oximetry

Pulse oximetry was originally designed for use in human medicine to detect hypoxemia in anesthesia and critical care settings. This noninvasive and user-friendly technology has great potential as an adjunct in the anesthetic management of reptiles (Figure 14-25). The pulse oximeter uses a two-wavelength spectrophotometer to determine the color of pulsating blood, which is then equated to an oxygen saturation estimate.[34] The primary limitations to its use in veterinary medicine, and reptiles in particular, relates to the inability to adapt the sensor to the veterinary patient. The vascular bed being measured needs to be positioned between the red and infrared light-emitting diodes and the photodetector. The placement should ensure absence of air gaps that interfere with accurate interpretation of the light signals.

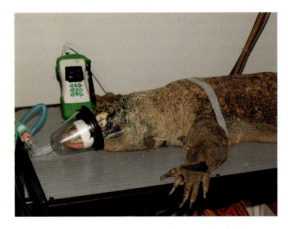

FIGURE 14-25 The pulse oximeter has been validated in the Green Iguana (*Iguana iguana*). Even for those species that have not been tested, such as this Komodo Dragon (*Varanus komodoensis*), the pulse oximeter provides excellent trend monitoring during anesthesia. The instruments work well as long as the patient is properly warmed during the anesthetic episode, and the probe is applied across a mucous membrane. (*Photograph courtesy D. Mader.*)

In the Green Iguana, no significant difference has been shown between SaO_2 (as measured with arterial blood gas analysis) and SpO_2 (as measured with a properly positioned pulse oximeter).[35,36] Pulse oximetry does not, however, ensure adequate blood flow or oxygen delivery, as only 4% to 8.6% of normal blood flow is necessary for pulse oximeter function.[31]

As the technology is refined, the probes may be modified to permit their application in reptilian medicine. In most species, the most practical probe used is a pencil-shaped reflectance probe for insertion into either the esophagus or the cloaca. The ability to manage not only anesthetic depth but also oxygen saturation of the blood has distinct advantages.

CARDIOCENTESIS

Cardiocentesis, as a tool for blood collection, is frequently used in snakes, and less so in other species of reptiles. Controversy has surrounded this technique, suggesting that it could be damaging to the heart muscle, and ultimately, the patient.

Cardiocentesis has historically been the method of choice in snakes since blood collection via the ventral coccygeal tail vein, dorsal buccal veins, and jugular veins can be challenging and often unrewarding. With proper technique cardiocentesis, even repeated cardiocentesis, has proven safe.

Isaza et al collected 39 blood samples via cardiocentesis from Ball Pythons (*Python regius*) over a 120-day period. No clinically apparent complications were noted in any of the snakes after the cardiocentesis procedures. Minimal gross lesions were noted at necropsy. Microscopic findings were limited to moderate and regularly arranged collagen fibrosis and focal thickening of the epicardium. The pericardial sac in all the snakes had a mild infiltrate of hemosiderin-laden macrophages and small numbers of heterophils. The results suggest that serial cardiocentesis is well tolerated in Ball Pythons.[37]

Similar studies have not been performed in other reptilian species. Although cardiocentesis has been reported in other reptiles, the ease of blood collection from various non–cardiac sites in most non–snake species precludes cardiocentesis as the first method of choice for blood collection.

SUMMARY

Reptilian cardiology is yet in its infancy. As the interest in the clinical medicine and surgery of this interesting and diverse class of animals progresses, the clinician's need to understand the ramifications of cardiac disease will increase. A side effect of improved clinical capabilities is the increased longevity of the reptile. As life spans in captivity become longer, the incidence of geriatric disease will increase. One of the challenging aspects of reptile geriatric medicine is certain to be cardiovascular disease.

REFERENCES

1. McCracken HE: The topographical anatomy of snakes and its clinical applications: a preliminary report, *Proc Am Assoc Zoo Vet* 112-119, 1991.

2. Ettinger SJ: Weakness and syncope. In Ettinger SJ, editor: *Textbook of veterinary internal medicine,* ed 4, Philadelphia, 1995, WB Saunders.
3. Frye FL: *Biomedical and surgical aspects of captive reptile husbandry,* ed 2, Melbourne, Fla, 1991, Krieger Publishing.
4. Williams DL: Cardiovascular system. In Beynon PH, Lawton MPC, Cooper JE, editors: *Manual of reptiles,* Cheltenham, UK, 1992, British Small Animal Veterinary Association.
5. Obendorf DL, Carson J, McManus TJ: Vibrio damsela infection in a stranded leatherback turtle *(Dermochelys coriacea), J Wild Dis* 23(4):666, 1987.
6. Jacobson ER, Homer B, Adams W: Endocarditis and congestive heart failure in a Burmese python *(Python molurus bivittatus), J Zoo Wildl Med* 22(2):245, 1991.
7. Innis CJ: Myocardial abscess and hemopericardium in a green iguana, Iguana iguana. In *Proceedings of the Association of Reptilian and Amphibian Veterinarians,* 2000.
8. Jacobson ER, Gaskin JM, Mansell J: Chlamydial infection in puff adders *(Bitis arietans), J Zoo Wildl Med* 20(3):364, 1989.
9. Conboy GA, Laursen JR, Averbeck GA et al: Diagnostic guide to some of the helminth parasites of aquatic turtles, *Compend Cont Ed Pract Vet* 15(10):1217, 1993.
10. Jacobson ER: Parasitic diseases of reptiles. In Fowler ME, editor: *Zoo and wild animal medicine,* ed 2, Philadelphia, 1986, WB Saunders.
11. Wallach JD, Boever WJ: *Diseases of exotic animals,* Philadelphia, 1983, WB Saunders.
12. Adnyana w, Ladds PW, Blair D: Efficacy of praziquantel in the treatment of green sea turtles with spontaneous infection of cardiovascular flukes, *Aust Vet J* 75(6):405-407, 1997.
13. Wagner RA: Clinical challenge case 1, *J Zoo Wildl Med* 20(2):238, 1989.
14. Rishniw M, Carmel BP: Atrioventricular valvular insufficiency and congestive heart failure in a carpet python, *Aust Vet J* 77(9):580-583, 1999.
15. Pace L, Mader DR: Atropine and glycopyrrolate, route of administration and response in the Green iguana *(Iguana iguana),* Reno, Nev, 2002, Proc ARAV.
16. Holz PH: The reptilian renal portal system—a review, *Bull Assoc Reptl Amphib Vet* 9(1):4-9, 1999.
17. Holz PH et al: The effect of the renal portal system on pharmacokinetic parameters in the red-eared slider *(Trachemys scripta elegans), J Zoo Wildl Med* 28(4):386-393, 1997.
18. Benson KG, Forrest L: Characterization of the renal portal system of the common green iguana *(Iguana iguana)* by digital subtraction imaging, *J Zoo Wildl Med* 30(2):235-241, 1999.
19. Beck K et al: Preliminary comparison of plasma concentrations of gentamicin injected into the cranial and caudal limb musculature of the eastern box turtle *(Terrapene carolina carolina), J Zoo Wildl Med* 26(2):265-268, 1995.
20. McDonald HS: Methods for the physiological study of reptiles. In Gans C, editor: *Biology of the reptilia,* New York, 1976, Academic Press.
21. White FN: Circulation. In Gans C, editor: *Biology of the reptilia,* vol 5, New York, 1976, Academic Press.
22. Heaton-Jones TG, King RR: Characterization of the electrocardiogram of the American alligator *(Alligator mississippiensis), J Zoo Wildl Med* 25(1):40, 1994.
23. Tilley LP, Smith FWK Jr, Miller MS: *Cardiology pocket reference,* Denver, 1990, American Animal Hospital Association.
24. Clippinger TL: Aortic stenosis and atrioventricular dilatation in a green iguana *(Iguana iguana), Proc Am Assoc Zoo Vet* 390-393, 1993.
25. Stoskopf MK: Clinical imaging in zoological medicine: a review, *J Zoo Wildl Med* 20(4):396, 1989.
26. Snyder PS, Shaw NG, Heard DJ: Two-dimensional echocardiographic anatomy of the snake heart *(Python molurus bivittatus), Vet Radiol Ultrasound* 40(1):66-72, 1999.
27. Schildger BJ et al: Technique of ultrasonography in lizards, snakes, and chelonians, *Semin Av Exotic Pet Med* 3(3):147-155, 1994.
28. Redrobe SP, Scudamore CL: Ultrasonographic diagnosis of pericardial effusion and atrial dilation in a spur-thighed tortoise *(Testudo graeca), Vet Rec* 146(7):183-185, 2000.
29. Bennett RA: A review of anesthesia and chemical restraint in reptiles, *J Zoo Wildl Med* 22(3):282, 1991.
30. Sedgwick CJ: Allometrically scaling the data base for vital sign assessment used in general anesthesia of zoological species, *Proc Am Assoc Zoo Vet* 360-369, 1991.
31. Bailey JE, Pablo LS: Anesthetic monitoring and monitoring equipment: application in small exotic pet practice, *Semin Av Exotic Pet Med* 7(1):53-60, 1998.
32. Sawyer DC: *The practice of small animal anesthesia,* Philadelphia, 1982, WB Saunders.
33. Hagood CO, Mozersky DJ, Tumblin RN: Practical office techniques for physiologic vascular testing, *So Med J* 68(1):17, 1975.
34. Saint John BE: Pulse oximetry: theory, technology, and clinical considerations, *Proc Assoc Wild Vet* 223-229, 1992.
35. Diethelm G, Mader DR, Grosenbaugh DA, Muir WW: Evaluating pulse oximetry in the green iguana *(Iguana iguana), Proc Assoc Reptl Amphib Vet* 11-12, 1998.
36. Diethelm G. The effect of oxygen content of inspiratory air (FiO_2) on recovery times in the green iguana *(Iguana iguana),* Zurich, 2001, Inaugural-Dissertation, University of Zurich.
37. Isaza R, Andrews G, Coke R, Hunter R: Assessment of multiple cardiocentesis in Ball Pythons *(Python regius), Contemp Top Lab Anim Sci* 43(6):35-38, 2004.

15
DERMATOLOGY

JOHN E. COOPER

"Skin for skin, yea, all that a man hath will he give for his life"
Job 2:4

The skin has played a key part in the evolutionary success of reptiles, especially in their assumption of a terrestrial (as opposed to an aquatic) lifestyle.[1-3] The skin is the largest and most accessible organ of the body, and this, coupled with the fact that changes in the integument often reflect more systemic ill health, makes an understanding of its biology vital to veterinarians and herpetologists. Reptile skin has also attracted the interest of research workers, especially in the fields of comparative neurology, oncology, and repair.[4,5]

Pathology of the skin (integument) is common in reptiles, especially but not exclusively when they are kept in captivity.[3,6-12] Such diseases can be broadly divided into two groups: *infectious*, the result of viruses, bacteria, fungi, metazoan, and protozoan parasites; and *noninfectious*, the result of trauma, hyperthermia, hypothermia, and other physical factors.

Overlap is often seen between the two categories; for example, a skin wound may permit the entry of bacteria, which can initiate dermatitis. Environmental factors frequently predispose to, or exacerbate, other dermatologic conditions. Investigation of management is, therefore, always necessary. The veterinarian must be familiar with the requirements of the species in captivity, especially temperature, relative humidity (RH), and substrate, and should be prepared to visit the premises where the reptiles are kept to investigate these. The role of the environment is discussed in more detail later.

NORMAL REPTILE SKIN

Keratinized skin is a characteristic feature of the Class Reptilia (Figure 15-1). It fulfills the usual functions of a vertebrate animal's integument but in reptiles plays a particularly important role in protecting the animal from desiccation, from abrasion, and from ultraviolet radiation and in providing an impermeable barrier to exogenous organisms, including potential pathogens (Figure 15-2). The skin is protected by scales that, in contrast to those of fish, are of ectodermal origin with scale pockets between them. They can vary greatly in shape and size as shown in Figure 15-3. The epidermis is usually thin over joints, but elsewhere on the body it is modified to form such structures as horns, crests, spines, rattles, and dewlaps, most of which have a behavioral (defense, warning, or communication) role. The dermis is composed of mesenchymal (mainly connective) tissue that encompasses blood and lymphatic vessels, nerves, and chromatophores. The amount of elastin present varies considerably. The mechanical behavior of snake skin has attracted the interest of researchers[13,14] and is relevant not only to locomotion but also to dermal disease (see later).

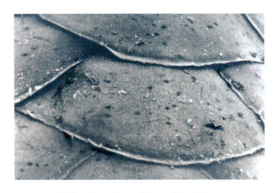

FIGURE 15-1 Low-power scanning electron microscopy (SEM) of the skin of a skink, *Leiolopisma telfairii*, shows overlapping scales. *(Courtesy J.E. Cooper.)*

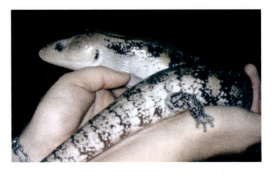

FIGURE 15-2 Live skink, *Tiliqua* sp., shows external barrier provided by keratinized epithelium. *(Photograph courtesy M.E. Cooper.)*

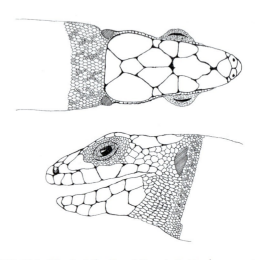

FIGURE 15-3 Head of the lizard *Lacerta lepida* shows variation in size and appearance of scales. *(Courtesy Edward Elkan Collection.)*

Chelonians have a well-defined shell, which comprises a plastron and carapace that consist of both osseous (dermal bone) and epithelial elements.[15]

Osteoderms are bony structures in the dermis. They are well developed in some species (e.g., crocodilians and certain lizards) and vary considerably in shape and size. They are seen on radiography and can hamper surgery (Figure 15-4).

The skin of crocodilians is thick and often bears osteoderms but is more permeable to water than that of other species of reptiles.[16]

Many interspecific differences are seen in skin structure. Some species, mainly squamates, were studied in detail a century ago.[17] The histologic features of the skin and other organs of the Tuatara, *Sphenodon punctata*, were described by Gabe and St. Girons.[18] The Edward Elkan Reference Collection of Lower Vertebrate Pathology[19] contains an extensive series of fine drawings of the histology of many reptiles, most of which have never been published (Figure 15-3).

Skin glands are generally rare in reptiles. Small cloacal glands and nuchal glands are found in a few species, and the males of some lizards (e.g., members of the Iguanidae) have femoral pores (see Figure 6-12). The structure of the latter and some of the medical problems that may involve them have been discussed.[20] Secretory sacs (scent glands) are found in the base of the tail of all known species of snake (see Figure 5-21). They produce malodorous secretions that are probably defensive.[21] Two pairs of glands are found in crocodiles, one nuchal and the other cloacal, and both produce musk.

Lipid production by the skin is important, primarily to maintain the permeability barrier and secondarily, in a few desert saurian species, so that water can be collected as droplets for drinking.

Chromatophores are often abundant, and they make color changes possible. Color changes are visually mediated and neuroendocrinologically controlled and are primarily a feature of four families of lizards.[2] Some dermatologic disorders of reptiles cause changes in coloration and either hypopigmentation or hyperpigmentation (Figure 15-5). These are features of wound repair and sometimes are induced by ketamine or other caustic injectable medication.

The skin of reptiles serves also as a sense organ as it is well innervated and often associated with bristles, tubercles, and depressions, including heat-sensitive pits that differ considerably, histologically and embryologically, in some snakes (e.g., Pit Vipers [*Crotalus* spp.]) and boids. The skin sense organs of iguanian lizards have been studied with histology and scanning electron microscopy (SEM),[22] and they were postulated to serve various functions: mechanoreception and thermoreception and, possibly, sensitivity to humidity.

Some species of lizard have "mite pockets," or invaginations of the skin in the neck, axillary, or crural regions (Figure 15-6) that appear to have evolved to contain ectoparasites and thus to limit the amount of damage they cause.[23] This interesting aspect of host–parasite relations is discussed again subsequently.

Remarkably little is known of the normal flora and fauna of the skin of most reptiles, with a few exceptions.[24] Studies on the bacterial flora of other organs, such as the cloaca[25] and gular and paracloacal glands,[26] have thrown some light on species' differences, but clearly far more work is needed. Changes in bacterial flora occur in some reptiles when they come into captivity,[27] which may be relevant to the health of these animals and to others with which they come into contact.

Host–parasite relations are the key to most infectious diseases of reptiles, and this balance can be upset by a variety of factors, especially environmental changes that reduce host resistance. Most environmental bacteria, for example, probably can be associated with skin disease; whether they are so,

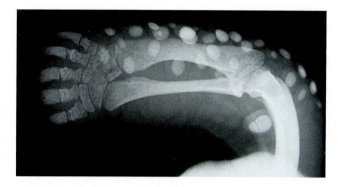

FIGURE 15-4 Radiograph shows osteoderms in the forelimb of a tortoise. (*Courtesy S. Barten.*)

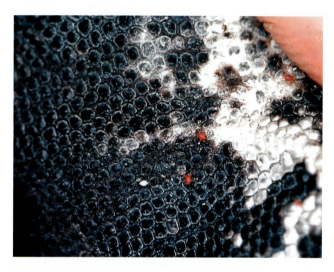

FIGURE 15-5 Chronic dermatitis from mite infestation (red spots on skin) has resulted in depigmentation of the skin of this Chuckwalla, *Sauromalus obesus*. (*Photograph courtesy D. Mader.*)

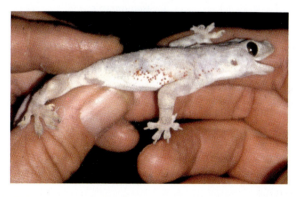

FIGURE 15-6 Tropical gecko, *Hemidactylus* sp., with a cluster of mites behind the forelimb. (*Photograph courtesy M.E. Cooper.*)

however, depends on the size of the challenge, the integrity of the integument, and the ability of the host to mount a humoral or cellular response.

All reptiles are ectothermic, and thus metabolic processes, including the immune responses and those that more specifically involve the skin, such as wound healing,[28] are temperature-dependent. The ambient temperature (and RH) can also have a profound effect on the microclimate and biology of the skin surface.

ECDYSIS AND OTHER FORMS OF REGENERATION AND HEALING

Regeneration and healing are well-recognized features of the Reptilia, and awareness of this has given rise to many traditions and myths relating to these animals, especially snakes and lizards.

Skin shedding (sloughing or ecdysis) is a normal characteristic of most reptiles. It is usually periodic and complete in snakes and some lizards but often only partial in other species (Figure 15-7). For example, in most chelonians, the epidermis covering the dermal shell is not shed; layers of keratin-containing cells, each layer broader than the previous one, are continually added to the lower surface of the epidermis to build up the characteristic protruding scales that cover the dermis and form tortoiseshell. Some aquatic turtles, however, shed pieces of scute from their carapace and plastron. The sloughing pattern is a useful guide to health in snakes and lizards (see subsequent, Dysecdysis).

Normal sloughing is part of a cycle and has been described and summarized by various authors.[29,30] The process is depicted in Figure 15-8. The resting phase follows a slough and is essentially the norm. The renewal phase is characterized by mitotic divisions of the stratum germinativum, resulting in a new generation of epidermis that ultimately replaces the outer generation. Separation of the two epidermal generations occurs by enzyme-induced lysis of the inner layer of the outer

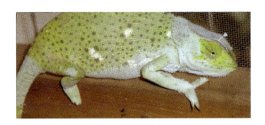

FIGURE 15-7 Partial sloughing in a Flap-necked Chameleon, *Chamaeleo dilepis*. (Photograph courtesy M.E. Cooper.)

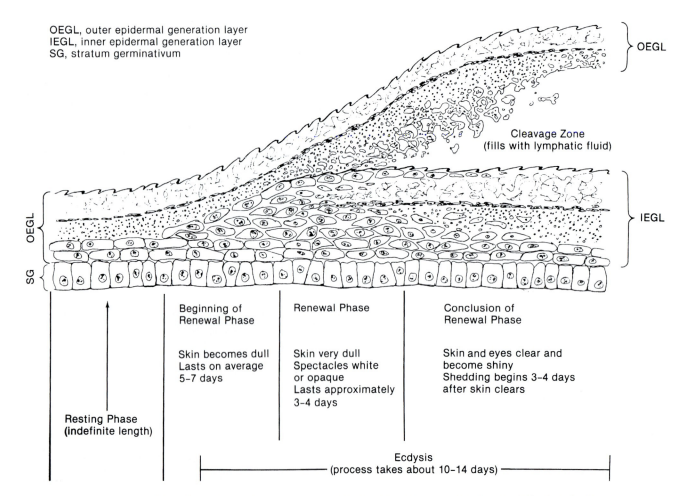

FIGURE 15-8 Normal shedding cycle of reptilian skin. (Modified from Landman L: In Bereiter-Hahn J, et al, editors: *Biology of the integument*, vol 2. New York, 1986, Springer-Verlag.)

generation, together with diffusion into the space of lymph. Cardiovascular changes facilitate the separation, which occurs along a cleavage plane, and the external layers are then shed, including the spectacles of snakes that initially become opaque and sometimes distended (Figure 15-9).

During sloughing, the skin is particularly vulnerable to traumatic injury (Figure 15-10) and to infection.[31] An increased sensitivity to toxicity occurs during this time (for example, the absorption of parasiticidal agents).[32] Other features of sloughing may include changes in protein, carbohydrate, lipid, and enzyme histochemistry,[33] which might in turn affect skin defense mechanisms. A need exists for more work on this.

Loss and regeneration of the tail (autotomy) occurs readily in certain lizards and was studied and described in some detail more than 200 years ago by John Hunter. His specimens survive in the Hunterian Museum in London. Autotomy is a remarkably complex process that has attracted much research in recent years (see Chapter 70).[34] The severed tails or limbs of other reptiles usually heal but do not regenerate, in contrast to the situation in some amphibians.

THE ROLE OF THE ENVIRONMENT

The famous bacteriologist Louis Pasteur is alleged to have stated on his deathbed, "The germ is nothing, the terrain is everything." This comment is true *par excellence* of reptiles where the ingress of infective agents and the development of infectious diseases are closely linked with the animal's environment. The skin plays a key role in protecting the reptile from insults, but its ability to do so can be hampered by such factors as a suboptimal temperature/RH or an unsuitable (too wet, too dry, too abrasive) substrate. The design of the

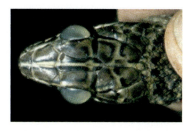

FIGURE 15-9 Sand Snake, *Psammophis* sp., about to slough. The spectacles are opaque and distended. *(Photograph courtesy M.E. Cooper.)*

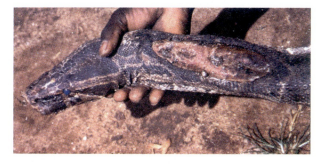

FIGURE 15-10 Damage to the skin of a recently captured Rock Python, *Python sebae*. *(Photograph courtesy M.E. Cooper.)*

vivarium is also most important. Arboreal species need to be able to climb and fossorial species to burrow. Appropriate temperature and RH ranges are important, but how these are attained is also critical (see Chapter 4).

Monitoring of the environment is part of maintaining the health of captive reptiles and is crucial in the prevention and control of skin diseases. Hygiene (sanitation) is a key component, but creation of a sterile vivarium is impossible (and probably undesirable). In any case, as emphasized already, pathogenic organisms are only one part of the mosaic that influences the health and well-being of the reptile.

Environmental monitoring includes appraisal of cage design; positioning of "furniture"; type of substrate; presence of shelter and hiding places; measuring of temperature and RH in various areas of the cage, including such microenvironments as burrows; evaluation of food including, where appropriate, microbiological and toxicological analysis; assessment of hygiene (sanitation), including culturing of surfaces, air, and water; examination and laboratory investigation of shed skin; water-testing chemicals; and other investigations, in addition to culture.

The investigation and assessment of water can be important, especially when aquatic or semiaquatic species are kept, and yet is often overlooked by herpetologists. Basic aquarium kits can be used, as can more sophisticated equipment that analyzes both chemical and biological parameters.[35]

CLINICAL TECHNIQUES: OBSERVATION AND EXAMINATION

Evaluation of skin diseases necessitates thorough investigation, with attention paid to the whole animal and its environment and not just the presenting signs or lesions. Assessment of management is vital. Before the reptile is handled, it should be observed, preferably from a distance, because subtle clinical signs such as muscle fasciculations, pruritus, or eye closure, which are sometimes hidden by the reptile, may provide valuable diagnostic information.

Figure 15-11 illustrates the approach recommended by the author.

The clinical examination of a reptile is covered elsewhere in this book and is not repeated here. Standard systematic techniques are essential. The fingers (and sometimes the nose) and the eyes are important in the investigation of skin diseases. A useful adjunct to clinical work that is often overlooked by veterinarians is examination of the skin with a hand lens or magnifying loupe. Also helpful is the inclusion on the patient's clinical record sheet of an outline drawing on which the distribution and size of lesions are recorded (see subsequent). Digital images can be used in a similar way and can also be sent to colleagues for a second opinion on the lesions.

SAMPLE COLLECTION

The collection of skin samples from live reptiles for laboratory investigation plays an important part in diagnosis.[36] Some methods are listed in Table 15-1.

Occasionally, especially when working with large, active, free-living reptiles, such as crocodiles, a minimally invasive

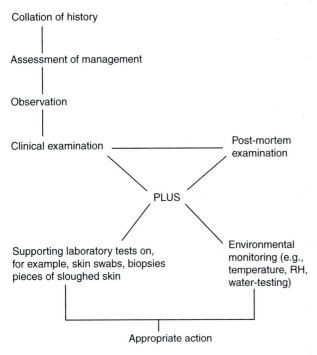

FIGURE 15-11 Algorithm.

method of sampling is helpful. The remote method of taking skin biopsy specimens from wild mammals with a darting system as described by Karesh and colleagues[37] might be applicable here.

Laboratory investigations are of great importance in dermatologic diagnosis and prognosis because few clinical signs are pathognomonic.[38,39] One should assume from the outset that samples are likely to be necessary for microbiological and histopathologic examination and that other tests (e.g., hematology) may be necessary.

Interpretation of laboratory findings is not always easy. The culture of bacteria or fungi from skin lesions, for example, need not indicate that they are the etiologic agents; contamination from the environment, together with secondary infection, can complicate the picture. Whether a pure or mixed growth was obtained may be relevant, as is the species isolated and any correlation with the results of other tests (e.g., hematology). These and other questions that form a part of clinical interpretation were discussed in an earlier publication.[40] As was mentioned previously, virtually all species of microorganism possibly can, if the conditions are correct, prove pathogenic in reptiles. Whether they do so or not is probably a measure of host resistance and the size of the challenge.

Table 15-1 Sample-Taking from Skin of Reptiles and Amphibians

Species	Sample	Technique and Comments
Reptiles (all species)	Skin biopsy (soft tissue)	Surgical excision of representative portion of skin with scalpel, skin biopsy instrument, or even sterilized paper punch.[9] Remove biopsy with general anesthesia or local analgesia. Clean skin beforehand with methanol or (if microbiological samples to be taken, see subsequent) sterile saline solution. Insert sutures or seal with glue, if necessary.
Crocodiles and lizards with osteoderms	Skin biopsy (soft tissues)	Can prove difficult because of osteoderms. If necessary, use similar technique to that for chelonians (see subsequent).
Chelonians	Shell biopsy	Excision of wedge with saw (hand or rotary power) or bone trephine. Fill defect temporarily with dental paste, more permanently with epoxyresin (as in shell repair). Grind biopsy before culture.
Reptiles (all species)	Fine needle aspirate	Use for proliferative lesions (masses). Insert 22-gauge needle attached to 5-mL or 10-mL syringe.
	Touch preparations (impression smears)	Apply microscope slides to exposed lesion. If necessary, remove excess exudate or blood from lesion first or take series of preparations.
	Swabs (for microbiology)	Use moistened swabs, preferably alginate-coated, for small lesions. If necessary, roll swab in or across lesion.
	Washings	Irrigate ulcerative/erosive lesions with sterile saline solution. Centrifuge saline solution and examine pellet cytologically.
	Brushings/scrapings	Brush (with endoscopy brush or soft toothbrush) or scrape (with scalpel blade) appropriate lesions, especially those that readily exfoliate.
Amphibians (all species)	Skin biopsy	As for reptiles but minimize size of incision/punch hole. Never use alcoholic preparations on (sensitive, mucous) amphibian skin.
	Fine needle aspirate Touch preparations (impression smears) Swabs Washings Brushings/scrapings	As for reptiles.
All species but especially aquatic amphibians (particularly gill-breathing larval forms) and some aquatic reptiles	Water samples	Water in vivarium or enclosure may provide information that is relevant to skin disease. Remove samples, at different depths, with sterile syringe and subject to full water-quality testing, including pH, hardness, nitrates/nitrites, and microbiological examination. Water samples may also yield sloughed skin and other specimens.

CLINICAL SIGNS

In human and conventional (domestic animal) dermatology, the use of well-defined descriptions of skin disease is standard and does much to promote consistency in terminology and thus improve efficiency in diagnosis. As Rossi[41] wisely pointed out, in reptile work, "Proper identification and description of skin lesions are necessary for assessment of treatment..." And yet herpetologic medicine abounds with terms that are often descriptive and sometimes colorful but that may or may not relate to the etiology/pathogenesis of the condition and that only rarely are in line with standard dermatologic nomenclature.

In this chapter, such popular terms are perpetuated because the clinician must be aware of what is heard in herpetologic circles; however, whenever possible, a more precise description of the lesion is appended. The need is urgent for an internationally approved glossary of terms for reptile dermatology, and until that is available, more precise descriptions are vital. In particular, lesions should be characterized as to whether they are degenerative (e.g., an ulcer) or proliferative (e.g., papillomatosis) and their color and texture.

Changes in the integument also must be quantified. For example, measurement of skin wounds should be taken each time the patient is seen and scoring systems should be used to evaluate and subsequently reassess the severity of lesions.

The recognition of clinical signs of skin disease in reptiles requires sound knowledge of what is normal. The integument of different species can differ in gross appearance, in color, and in texture, and changes may be associated with behavior, with breeding, and with stages of the sloughing cycle. Some conditions produce generalized skin changes (for instance, a loss of sheen, malformed carapace, or dysecdysis), and many others result in localized lesions that can include discoloration, petechiation, erosion/ulceration, inflammation, proliferation, scute/scale loss, and developmental abnormalities.

Ecto (macro) parasites may be visible as can fungi such as *Saprolegnia* and algae.

SPECIFIC DISEASES

Although this book is primarily concerned with captive reptiles, brief mention is often made of free-living animals, not only because the author is involved in projects concerning the latter but because diagnosis and control of skin disease in captive reptiles can benefit from an understanding of the situation in the wild. Behavioral changes may be present but are often only subtle, requiring careful observation, preferably without the patient's awareness of the presence of an observer. The skin of most reptiles is richly innervated, and therefore, pain or pruritus are assumed to occur; they are associated with clinical signs such as writhing, skin rubbing, and scratching. Rossi[41] reported pruritus and self trauma in iguanas recovering from spinal cord trauma or nerve damage and postulated that nerve regeneration might be the cause.

Abrasions

Captive and free-living reptiles are liable to abrasions (defined by Rossi[41] as "the traumatic removal of the superficial epidermis") as a result of damage by substrate. In captivity, rostral abrasions are commonly caused by rubbing on a glass or wire surface (Figure 15-12); social competition and sexual activity may be exacerbating factors or even the cause of such damage (Figure 15-13).

Attention to management is necessary to prevent such injuries. Topical therapy reduces the risk of a deeper wound or entry of pathogenic organisms, which in turn may result in the development of dermatitis, cellulitis, or abscesses.

Persistent trauma can lead to hyperkeratosis, callus formation, and localized dysecdysis.

Abscesses

The lesions in reptiles that are usually termed abscesses generally appear as raised, hard, and well-circumscribed subcutaneous swellings[42,43] (Figures 15-14 and 15-15). Histologic examination of such lesions usually reveals a central core containing bacteria surrounded by fibrosis and inflammatory cells. Huchzermeyer and Cooper[44] suggested that such lesions might be better termed "fibriscesses" and postulated that the fibrinous core might entrap bacteria and thus discourage systemic spread. Other swellings are more cellular and essentially granulomas. Elkan and Cooper[43] coined the term "pseudotumours" for some such lesions on the grounds that they superficially resemble neoplasms.

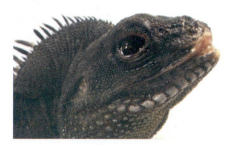

FIGURE 15-12 Rostral damage in a Water Dragon, *Physignathus* sp., caused by rubbing on glass. *(Photograph courtesy M.E. Cooper.)*

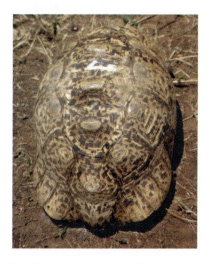

FIGURE 15-13 Bilateral abrasions on the carapace of a female Leopard Tortoise, *Geochelone pardalis*, caused during copulation. *(Photograph courtesy M.E. Cooper.)*

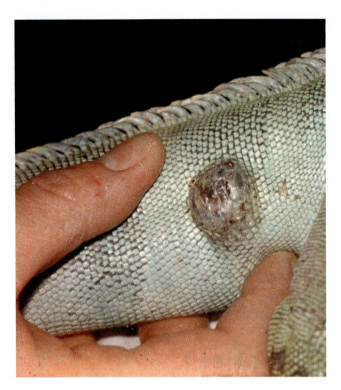

FIGURE 15-14 Abscess on the base of the tail of a Green Iguana, *Iguana iguana*. (*Photograph courtesy M. Cooper.*)

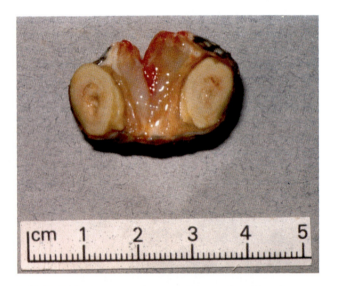

FIGURE 15-15 Lesion in Figure 15-14 bisected to show the central core of laminated caseous material. (*Photograph courtesy J. Cooper.*)

The cause of abscesses is usually a bacterial infection, often after trauma such as a bite wound or an injection. A mixed infection may occur, particularly by two or more gram-negative bacteria. *Aeromonas* and *Pseudomonas* are commonly involved, but other organisms may be isolated, amongst them *Actinobacillus*,[10] *Arizona*,[10,45] *Corynebacterium*,[41] *Edwardsiella*, *Escherichia (coli)*, *Klebsiella*, *Neisseria*, *Pasteurella*, *Proteus*, and *Providencia* spp. *Serratia* was first reported as a cause of abscesses in reptiles more than 60 years ago[46] and is one of the most common organisms isolated and an initiating factor in septicemic cutaneous ulcerative disease (SCUD; see subsequent). Anaerobes are sometimes isolated and may be significant. Mycobacteria and salmonellae are discussed subsequently.

Definitive diagnosis of an abscess usually requires aspiration and culture and either cytologic or histopathologic examination. Differentiation from fungal, parasitic, and neoplastic lesions is vital.

Abscesses are best excised *in toto* (see Figures 15-14 and 15-15), and this procedure must include removal of the fibrous capsule. Recurrence may be discouraged by the use of an appropriate antibacterial agent (systemic) and local antiseptics, coupled with high standards of hygiene.

Cellulitis (referred to by Rossi[41] as "carbuncles") is an underrunning of the skin by an infective process and can result in a whole network of infected sinuses and tracts within the dermis. Various organisms may be involved, among them some of those listed previously. Such lesions are often difficult to treat, and repeated surgery with antibiotics may be necessary.

Mycobacterium spp. can on occasion cause localized abscess-like lesions but are more often associated with deep infections, including those of bone and digits.[12,47-49] *Salmonella* spp. are sometimes isolated from abscesses or other skin lesions of reptiles.[10,50] Appropriate precautions may need to be instigated in view of the zoonotic potential of some of these organisms. Nevertheless, the risk must be seen in the context of other dangers, including the fact that other apparently less pathogenic bacteria may cause disease in immunocompromised humans.

For a thorough discussion of reptilian abscess, see Chapter 42.

Beak and Claw Deformities

Deformities and overgrowth of the beak are common in chelonians and are usually the result of overgrowth/damage or a developmental abnormality. Nutritional and genetic factors are possibly also involved. Clipping and shaping are necessary, together with appropriate management changes (Figure 15-16; see also Figure 72-5).

Claw overgrowth and distortion occur in lizards and chelonians and often necessitate regular clipping and manicuring.

Blister Disease

Diseases of reptiles that produce blisters, properly termed vesicles and bullae, are well recognized by herpetologists.

The condition most frequently seen in captive snakes, and occasionally lizards, is characterized by raised subcutaneous fluid-filled lesions (Figure 15-17). Histologic studies[38] confirm the presence of intraepidermal bullae. Predisposing factors appear to be poor ventilation or wet substrate, both of which can produce too high an RH.

The initial lesions are usually apparently sterile. As secondary infection occurs, the fluid becomes cloudy and a subsequent bacteremia may result.[38]

Treatment necessitates changes to the environment and prompt attention to infected lesions. The application of an adhesive drape (to cleaned lesions) can help prevent secondary infection.[51]

Other causes of vesicular/bullous disease of reptiles are recognized, including thermal and chemical burns and

Dermatology

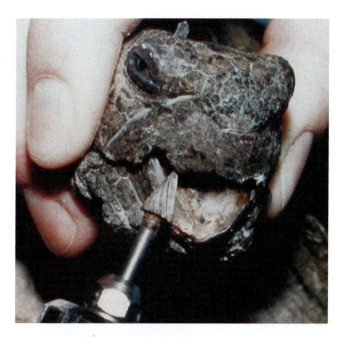

FIGURE 15-16 Beak lesions are common in turtles and tortoises. When left untreated, the animals often lose the ability to prehend food. A high-speed motor tool is used here to grind the beak back to its normal appearance. This is the same animal as in Figure 72-5. *(Photograph courtesy D. Mader.)*

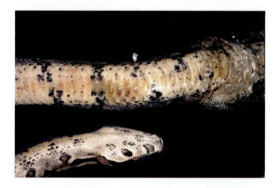

FIGURE 15-17 Boa Constrictor, *Constrictor constrictor*, with blister disease and retained slough. *(Photograph courtesy R. Norman.)*

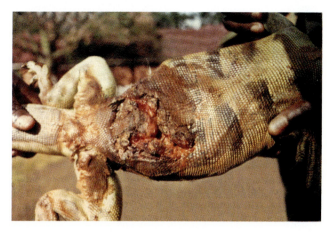

FIGURE 15-18 Green Iguana, *Iguana iguana*, with severe ventral burns. *(Photograph courtesy M.E. Cooper.)*

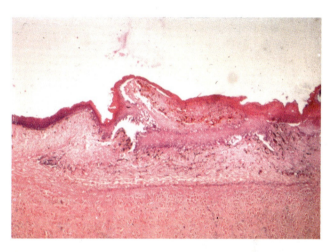

FIGURE 15-19 Histologic appearance of a minor burn in an Indian Python, *Python molurus*, shows raised damaged epidermis, edema, and granulocytic infiltration. *(Photograph courtesy J.E. Cooper.)*

epidermal damage by migrating nematodes (e.g., *Kalicephalus* spp.; see subsequent).

Cysts are sometimes seen in the skin of reptiles and differ from vesicles and bullae in that they have a lining—often of epithelial, sometimes of fibrous—tissue. These are usually parasitic or developmental in origin.

Burns

Thermal burns usually occur in captivity because of contact with a poorly protected heat source, either within the vivarium or when an iguana or other species is at liberty in the home and gains access to lights or electric heaters (see Chapter 71).

In the wild, burns may be caused by grass or forest fires. Surprisingly deep lesions sometimes occur, and the abdominal (coelomic) cavity may be perforated as a result of tissue necrosis (Figure 15-18). Even minor burns cause substantial cellular damage, as illustrated by histologic examination (Figure 15-19). Initially a burn wound is sterile, but infections rapidly supervene and, as in endothermic animals, the ubiquitous *Pseudomonas* is one of the most frequent isolates. Healed burns can be a cause of dysecdysis (see subsequent) on account of fibrosis (Figure 15-20) and disruption of normal scalation (Figure 15-21). See Chapter 71 for greater detail.

Chemical burns are less commonly seen but may occur. Disinfectants that have not been diluted correctly are often a cause (Figure 15-22). Accidentally spilled irritant chemicals can produce lesions in both captive and free-living reptiles, and occasionally a case in a zoo is attributable to malicious behavior by an aggrieved person.

Immediate treatment of any burn, thermal or chemical, should involve repeated irrigation of the lesion with normal saline solution. Subsequent management may include debridement, reconstructive surgery, and appropriate supportive therapy. Transparent adhesive drapes[51] applied to clean wounds protect and discourage reinfection. They also permit regular inspection of the lesions without any need to remove the dressing (Figure 15-23).

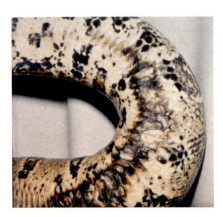

FIGURE 15-20 Healed burn in a *Boa Constrictor* 2 months after incident. Fibrosis and scarring are apparent. *(Photograph courtesy J.E. Cooper.)*

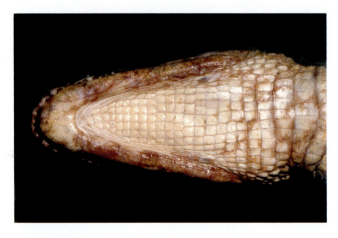

FIGURE 15-22 Chemical burns in a Caiman, *Caiman* sp. *(Photograph courtesy M.E. Cooper.)*

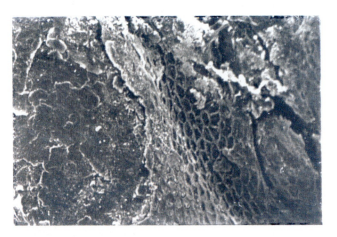

FIGURE 15-21 Low power scanning electron microscopy (SEM) of the previous case. Disruption of normal scalation is found. *(Courtesy J.E. Cooper.)*

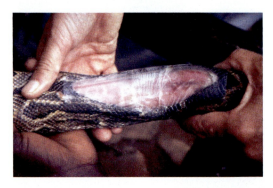

FIGURE 15-23 Extensive wound in a Rock Python, *P. sebae*, has been cleaned and dressed with a transparent adhesive drape. *(Photograph courtesy M.E. Cooper.)*

In all cases of burn, preventive measures must be instigated to prevent repetition.

Scute Loss in Chelonians

Abnormal sloughing of scutes of chelonians is most commonly a result of poor husbandry, especially in environments that are too humid or wet. In East Africa, tortoises (*Geochelone* and *Kinixys* spp.) that are kept out of doors with inadequate cover may show such signs, usually after the rainy season. Infection can supervene. Correction of the environment, coupled with appropriate local and systemic treatment, is usually successful. Scute loss can also be a sequel to renal disease and is considered to carry a poor prognosis.[41]

Shell Damage

The shell (carapace and plastron) of chelonians may be damaged by trauma, burning,[52] adverse environment, nutritional/metabolic/genetic factors, and infection (see subsequent). Such lesions need careful examination and evaluation before treatment commences. Radiography is necessary if bone damage is suspected, and laboratory tests, especially bacteriology and histopathology, are advisable.

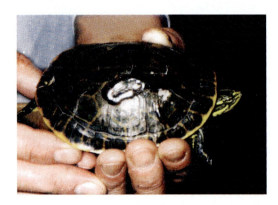

FIGURE 15-24 Epoxy resin repair of a shell injury in a freshwater turtle. *(Photograph courtesy M.E. Cooper.)*

Lesions can be repaired by cleaning, disinfection, and application of plastic skin dressings (mild lesions) or epoxy resin (severe lesions; Figure 15-24). Where the latter is not available (in poorer countries, for example) local car repair material may be used (Figure 15-25). Healing can be prolonged, and temperate species may need to be stopped from hibernating during this period.[53,54] Untreated injuries often resolve leaving marked damage (Figure 15-26).

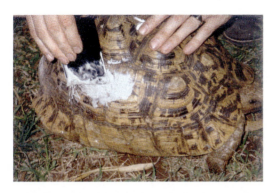

FIGURE 15-25 Field repair. Use of local East African materials to fill a defect in the shell of a Leopard Tortoise, *G. pardalis*. *(Photograph courtesy M.E. Cooper.)*

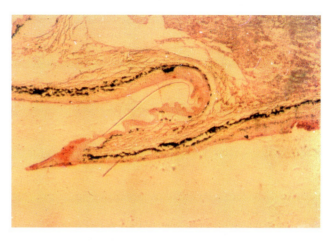

FIGURE 15-27 Early scale lesion in a snake. Pitting and hyperchromia of areas of keratin are seen. *(Photograph courtesy J.E. Cooper.)*

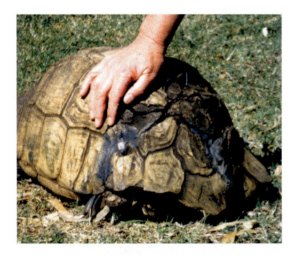

FIGURE 15-26 Severe untreated carapacial damage in a Leopard Tortoise, *G. pardalis*. *(Photograph courtesy M.E. Cooper.)*

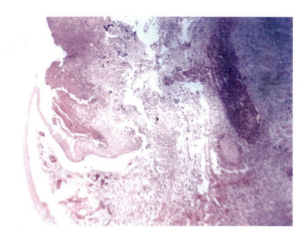

FIGURE 15-28 More severe lesion shows tissue destruction, hyperemia, and infection. *(Photograph courtesy J.E. Cooper.)*

Before embarking on the treatment of shell damage, the practitioner should be familiar with the normal anatomy, particularly the relationship between the keratinized nonviable outer layers and the underlying live bone (see Chapter 67).

Dermatitis

Dermatitis is an inflammation of the skin and can be infectious or noninfectious in origin, or sometimes a mixture of the two. Specific dermatitides are discussed here, but inflammatory changes can be a feature of many other conditions that are covered in this chapter. The cells involved in inflammation in reptiles include granulocytes (especially heterophils) and agranulocytes (especially lymphocytes and macrophages).[55]

Foreign-body dermatitis (FBD) is mentioned later.

Skin lesions variously described as necrotic dermatitis, ulcerative dermatitis, or ventral dermal necrosis are commonly referred to by lay herpetologists as "scale rot."

Infectious dermatitis can take several forms, especially when it is caused by trauma or environmental factors. Many genera and species of bacteria may be involved. *Aeromonas* and *Pseudomonas* are particularly common isolates, but others that have been isolated include *Flavobacterium*,[56] *Staphylococcus*,[41] and *Morganella*,[10] and sometimes anaerobes such as *Bacteroides*, *Fusobacterium*, and *Clostridium* spp.[57] Some overlap is found with abscesses (see previous discussion); many of the same organisms can be involved in both types of infection.

The early clinical signs of dermatitis in snakes and lizards include discoloration of the skin (see previous). Care must be taken to distinguish this from the normal coloration of some species (e.g., the [North American] Redbelly Watersnake [*Nerodia erythrogaster*]). In chelonians, patches may be seen.[41,58] Histologic study results on early cases reveal minor changes that affect the superficial keratin (Figure 15-27), but these can rapidly deteriorate. Erosive changes follow, and severe cases become ulcerated. Inflammation and necrosis may extend deep into underlying musculature (Figure 15-28). Septicemia can be a sequel. Conversely, some cases of dermatitis appear to follow a blood-borne infection. Gram-negative bacteremia and septicemia cause petechiation, possibly thrombosis, of small vessels, and degenerative changes in the skin follow.

Affected reptiles should be placed in a clean, dry vivarium and investigated fully. Treatment is usually with topical disinfectants, topical or systemic antibiotics (after sensitivity tests), and application of adhesive drapes.[51] Scarification and debridement are important when necrosis is present.

Foreign-Body Dermatitis

Foreign-body dermatitis (FBD) can occur as a result of exposure to fiberglass from the cage[59] and to talc from gloves and other sources.[60] FBD usually manifests itself as one or more areas of chronic inflammation, but early cases may be characterized by behavioral changes suggestive of localized pain or pruritus. Treatment is with excision of the lesions or, in superficial cases, with repeated soaking or bathing of the affected reptile.

Contact Dermatitis

Contact dermatitis occurs when reptiles are exposed to certain chemicals in the environment. The lesions seen are erythema and sometimes vesicle formation. Treatment is as for chemical burns (see previous), coupled with removal of the source of the irritation.

Dermatophilosis

This condition is caused by infection with the actinomycete *Dermatophilus congolensis*,[48,61,62] and although generally considered to be a disease of lizards, it can also affect other species, including chelonians.[63] It is also a potential zoonosis. Dermatophilosis is characterized by raised skin lesions or subcutaneous abscesses over the skin of the body and limbs.

Diagnosis is by culture or histopathologic examination of a biopsy. Characteristic gram-positive filaments and coccoid bodies are seen. The application of a povidone iodine, coupled with keeping the animals in a drier environment, often proves successful in treatment.

Developmental/Genetic Abnormalities

Various conditions have been described, including scale agenesis, scale irregularities, cleft scutes, and various abnormal color patterns.[41,64,65] Captive breeding, especially if there is a high inbreeding coefficient, may result in a higher prevalence.

Discoloration

The chromatophores of reptiles are remarkably sensitive to metabolic disturbances, and as a result, changes in color of skin can follow local insults or systemic disease. Brown coloration to scales is often an early sign of dermatitis; other colors (depending on the species) may indicate bruising, inflammation, vasodilatation, jaundice, or bile-staining. Hyperpigmentation of the skin is a feature of some reptiles (e.g., melanistic individuals) but may also follow wounds. Burns can result in either hyperpigmentation or hypopigmentation (see Chapter 71). The latter, leukoderma, may also be a normal feature.

Dysecdysis

Dysecdysis (difficulty in sloughing or an abnormal sloughing process) is primarily a condition of captive reptiles but is occasionally seen in free-living snakes and lizards. It can be caused by a number of factors, both in isolation and in combination. The usual cause in captivity is a suboptimum environment (e.g., low relative humidity [RH] or no bathing facilities). Other predisposing factors include malnutrition (protein deficiency), systemic disease, old scars, and possibly endocrinologic disorders. Viral infections have been postulated to be associated with the syndrome.[66]

Dysecdysis may be followed by retention of slough, either generally or in certain areas (e.g., digits, head eyecaps [spectacles]). Histologic examination may reveal several layers of keratinized epidermis (Figure 15-29), and pockets of such material may provide a focus for infection (Figure 15-30).

Diagnosis of sloughing disorders demands systematic and detailed evaluation of the reptile and its environment. The owner's records relating to feeding, temperature, and previous skin shedding can prove useful.

Treatment of dysecdysis is attempted initially by increasing the RH or by soaking the reptile in tepid water. Retained spectacles should be treated with great care; repeated irrigation with saline solution for 24 hours usually permits removal with a cotton-tipped swab.

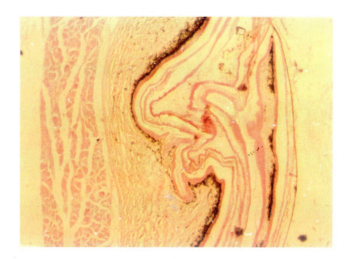

FIGURE 15-29 Case of dysecdysis. Histologic examination reveals layers of unsloughed material. *(Photograph courtesy J.E. Cooper.)*

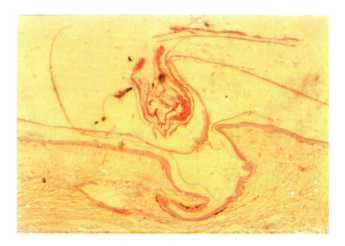

FIGURE 15-30 Same case as in previous figure. Pocket of keratin is the focus of infection. *(Photograph courtesy J.E. Cooper.)*

If dysecdysis persists or recurs despite treatment, full clinical investigation of the reptile is indicated.

In aquatic chelonians, failure to shed scutes may be the result of poor basking facilities or osteodystrophy. Inadequate lighting may also contribute. Abnormal (excessive) sloughing of scutes is discussed subsequently.

Excessive sloughing may be the result of endocrine disorders or hypervitaminosis A (see subsequent). See Chapters 52 and 59 for more detailed discussion.

Edema

Subcutaneous edema is a feature of many disorders, ranging from hypovitaminosis A that mainly affects the eyelids to cardiovascular or renal disease that causes generalized fluid accumulation (Figure 15-31). Edema warrants full diagnostic investigation.

Fibrosis or Cicatrization

This condition follows burns or other deep healed wounds (see previous) and is important because it is unsightly and can impair ecdysis. Differentiation from fibrosarcoma and other neoplastic lesions is important; if necessary, biopsies should be taken.

Macroparasites

Using modern ecologic terminology, macroparasites are metazoan organisms that survive on or within another animal. Those that affect the skin are primarily ectoparasites, as mentioned previously, but some endoparasites can also cause skin lesions (Figure 15-32), including the nematodes *Kalicephalus*[67] and *Paratrichosoma*,[10] cestodes,[41] and trematodes.[68] Filaroid worms that inhabit the vascular system may cause a sloughing dermatitis.[41]

Mites and ticks (Acarina) of various species are prevalent on free-living terrestrial reptiles and may be brought with them into captivity (Figure 15-33). Concern has been expressed over the introduction of exotic ticks with imported reptiles and the pathogens (microparasites) that they might transport with them.[69] *Amblyomma* and *Aponomma* ticks are perhaps of particular concern and may transmit *Cowdria ruminantium*, the cause of heartwater of ruminants (Figure 15-34).

Although ticks are usually readily visible on reptiles, mites can be difficult to locate, especially when present in small numbers. Careful searching may be necessary, particularly under the scales, with a hand lens. Mites can be picked up with a moistened cotton-tipped swab, with methanol if the mites are to be killed and with saline solution if they are to be kept alive. Manual removal of ticks should be carried out with care; if mouthparts remain in the skin, inflammation and infection may occur. Rossi advocated applying ivermectin to ticks in sensitive or inaccessible sites, such as the eyelid, but not in chelonians where this product can be dangerous.[41]

Dichlorvos can be used for treatment of ticks and mites but with care. Alternatively, reptiles can be sprayed with a dilute solution of trichlorphon or pyrethrum-based products may be applied. Ivermectin is effective via injection or as a spray[70] but, as mentioned previously, should not be used on chelonians.

Treatment of ectoparasites must be coupled with cleaning and disinfection of the vivarium or, in some cases such as zoological collections, the whole reptile house.

The mite *Ophionyssus natricis* is probably the most significant ectoparasite of reptiles (Figure 15-35) and has been reported in captive reptiles in most continents. The mite can

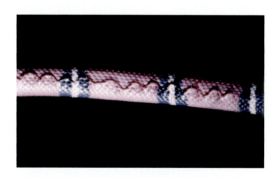

FIGURE 15-32 Subcutaneous nematode in a Kingsnake, *Lampropeltis* sp. (*Photograph courtesy M.E. Cooper.*)

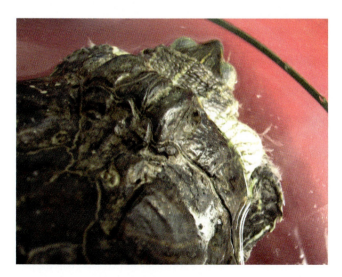

FIGURE 15-31 Generalized edema and skin sloughing in a freshwater terrapin. Also seen are ulcerated lesions of the shell. (*Photograph courtesy D. Mader.*)

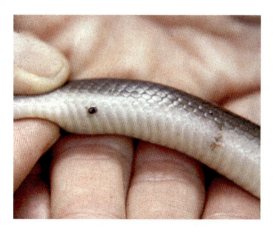

FIGURE 15-33 A tick on a newly captured Brown House Snake, *Boaedon fuliginosus*. (*Photograph courtesy M.E. Cooper.*)

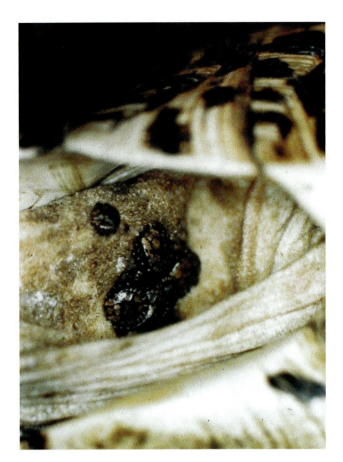

FIGURE 15-34 The African ticks, *Ambylomma* spp., are commonly found on recent imports such as this Leopard Tortoise, *G. pardalis*. These ticks can act as vectors for mammalian diseases such as heartwater. *(Photograph courtesy D. Mader.)*

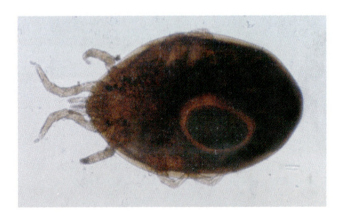

FIGURE 15-35 Snake mite, *Ophionyssus natricis*. *(Photograph courtesy J.E. Cooper.)*

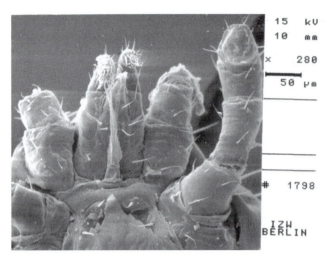

FIGURE 15-36 Low-power scanning electron microscopy (SEM) of the mite in the previous figure shows its sucking mouthparts. *(Photograph courtesy J.E. Cooper.)*

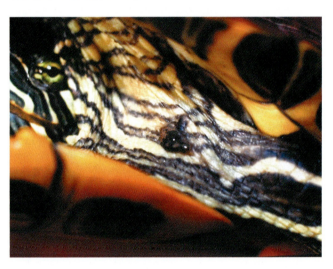

FIGURE 15-37 Leeches are commonly found on wild-caught fresh and marine turtles. These have been shown to transmit organisms, such as blood parasites and *Aeromonas* spp., between animals. *(Photograph courtesy D. Mader.)*

be readily spread when reptiles are moved, especially if health monitoring and hygiene are poor. *O. natricis* is found mainly on snakes where it uses its sharp mouth parts (Figure 15-36) to pierce the skin between scales and as a result can cause poor shedding, anemia, and death. More than 50 years ago, mechanical transmission by the mite of *Aeromonas hydrophila* was reported.[71] *O. natricis* may, on occasion, be transmitted to humans where it has been reported to cause skin hypersensitivity.[72]

Other mites are also found on reptiles. Within the Cheyletoidea, two families are found, one living under the scales of snakes (Ophioptidae) and the other in the cloaca of turtles (Cloacaridae). Trombiculid mites are found on reptiles but are not species-specific. See Chapter 43 for more details.

Leeches (Hirudinea) are found on free-living, sometimes captive, aquatic chelonians and crocodilians and are occasionally seen (usually in the nasal and buccal cavity or attached to the cloaca) on snakes and lizards (Figure 15-37). They have been reported to cause ulcers in aquatic turtles.[41] Leeches may also transmit blood parasites[73] and in theory can introduce *Aeromonas* as this organism is part of the normal bacterial flora of some leeches.[74] Leeches drop off the host once they have engorged with blood. Removal can be effected by touching the leech with a cotton-tipped swab that has been dipped in ivermectin or in (chelonians) saturated salt solution.

Myiasis, the infection of live tissues by maggots (dipterous larvae), is sometimes seen in reptiles (Figure 15-38).

Dermatology

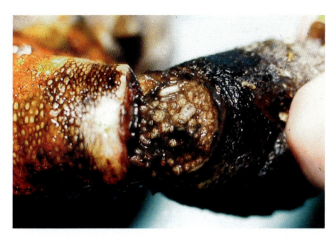

FIGURE 15-38 Myiasis, or Fly Strike, is common around wounds in outdoor or wild chelonians or cloaca in animals with chronic diarrhea. *(Photograph courtesy D. Mader.)*

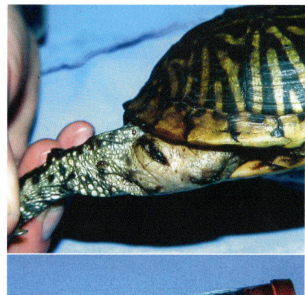

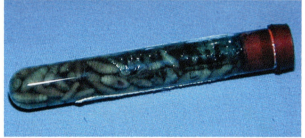

FIGURE 15-39 **A**, This Box Turtle, *Terrapene* sp., has fly larva infestation in a wound on the rear leg. Usually, all that is seen is a small breathing hole surrounded by black, oily discharge. **B**, All of these fly larvae were removed from the thigh of the turtle in **A**. *(Photographs courtesy D. Mader.)*

Flies of certain species may lay their eggs on skin lesions, especially around the cloaca, if the patient has diarrhea or cloacitis, or following an attack by rodents. A crusty black discharge from the skin/shell is often a feature in chelonians (Figure 15-39).[75]

Diagnosis of myiasis is by detection of the larvae. Treatment is attempted by cleaning (flushing); warm soapy water sprayed with a syringe appears to be efficacious and inexpensive and is regularly used in Africa by the author, followed by disinfection and cautious application of insecticidal agents. Supportive therapy may be necessary, and further attacks must be prevented with vigilance and regular inspection.

Much remains to be learned about host-parasite relations in reptiles. Therefore, every effort should be made to (1) quantify parasite burdens (by counting them), (2) attempt to relate parasite numbers to such parameters as body condition, blood counts, etc., and (3) save specimens of parasites for identification and future reference. In some cases, mites and ticks may need to be kept alive so that they can metamorphose or lay eggs.

Macroparasites are a normal feature of many reptiles in the wild, and a mistake may be for the veterinarian to assume that they are a primary cause of ill health and to attempt to eliminate them. Reptiles can probably develop resistance to certain parasites, as has been shown in studies on *Amblyomma* on tortoises.[76]

Mycotic Fungal Diseases

Fungal lesions of the skin have been described in many reptiles, especially aquatic species (see Chapter 16).[9] The fungi involved are often not isolated or accurately identified, but various species have been reported, including *Aspergillus*, *Basidobolus*, *Geotrichum*, *Mucor*, *Saprolegnia*, and *Candida*. An outbreak of fungal dermatitis in Watersnakes, *Nerodia harteri harteri*, was associated with various species of fungi, including *Phialophera*, *Alternaria*, and *Fusarium* spp. and *Trichophyton mentagrophytes*; a link with slugs was postulated.[77] Another dermatophyte, *T. terrestre*, was implicated in skin disease of Madagascar Day Geckos, *Phelsuma* spp.[78]

The relationship of fungal lesions to scale rot (see Dermatitis) is often unclear because the clinical signs are

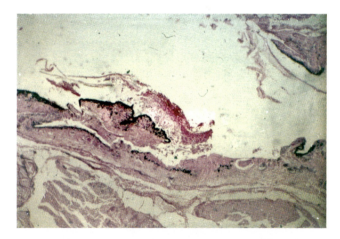

FIGURE 15-40 Histologic section of early mycotic infection in a Grass Snake, *Natrix natrix*. The epidermis has been infiltrated by fungal hyphae. *(Photograph courtesy J.E. Cooper.)*

often similar. The fungi initially attack superficial areas of skin (Figure 15-40) and can quickly develop into a subcutaneous mycelial growth. Fungi can also cause mycotic granulomas, which need careful differentiation from bacterial abscesses.[79]

Diagnosis is usually based on the detection of fungi in scale samples, touch preparations, squash preparations (following treatment with potassium hydroxide [KOH] to dissolve keratin), or biopsies.

Treatment can be attempted with topical agents or oral agents, such as nystatin[80] or ketoconazole,[81] coupled with excision of badly affected tissues but often proves unsuccessful. Attention to management is always important because fungal infections frequently follow trauma and poor hygiene.

A useful review of fungal infections of reptiles, which among other things stressed the importance of distinguishing pathogens from environmental contaminants, was by Austwick and Keymer.[82] Jacobson[9] subsequently expressed the belief that many mycoses in reptiles are the result of secondary invasion, especially if the reptile's immunity is reduced (e.g., by low temperatures).

Algae are sometimes present on the skin of aquatic chelonians and crocodilians and are occasionally suspected of causing erosions and ulceration.[83] Removal of algae with a toothbrush was recommended by Rossi.[41]

Necrosis

Necrosis is not a disease *per se* but can be a feature of dermatitis, of thermal and chemical burns, and of skin neoplasia. In addition, a vascular necrosis may occur after constriction of digits or tail by bands of retained slough or cage substrate. Exposure to extreme cold can also be a cause.

Necrotic lesions provide a focus for bacterial multiplication, including anaerobes, that may cause local or systemic infection. They should be debrided, if necessary with incision, and the resultant wound protected from infection until healing has taken place by first intention or by granulation.

Neoplasms

Neoplastic lesions involving the skin are not uncommon in reptiles (see Chapter 19)[38,84] and include fibrosarcomas (Figures 15-41 and 15-42), melanomas, and squamous cell carcinomas. In chelonians, the shell may be directly or indirectly involved[85] (Figures 15-43 and 15-44).

Papillomatosis, characterised by the presence of raised proliferative lesions, is particularly prevalent in European Green Lizards (*Lacerta viridis*; Figure 15-45, *A, B*) and is probably caused by a virus.[86,87] The lesions vary in distribution. In female lizards, they predominate around the tail, and in

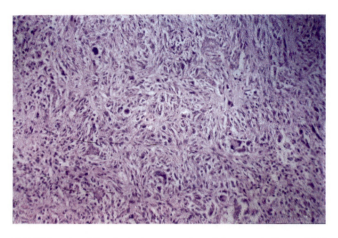

FIGURE 15-42 Histological presentation of the mass in Figure 15-41 before treatment. Poorly differentiated fibrosarcoma. *(Photograph courtesy J.E. Cooper.)*

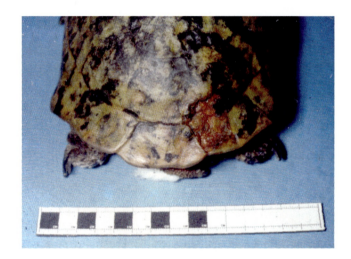

FIGURE 15-43 Shell lesion in a tortoise, *Testudo hermanni*, associated with neoplasm. *(Photograph courtesy J.E. Cooper.)*

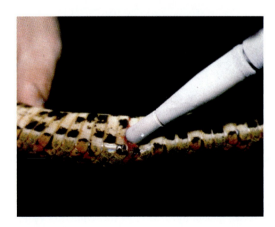

FIGURE 15-41 Fibrosarcoma of the skin of a Cornsnake, *Elaphe guttata*, that is being treated with a cryoprobe. *(Photograph courtesy J.E. Cooper.)*

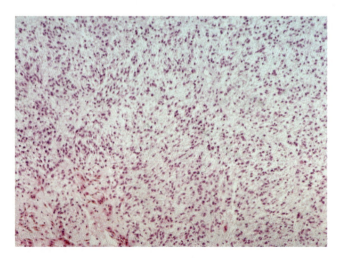

FIGURE 15-44 Histologic section of the lesion in Figure 15-43; this was considered to be neurilemmal sarcoma. *(Photograph courtesy J. Harshbarger.)*

Dermatology

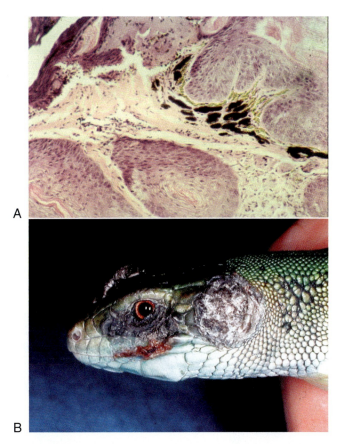

FIGURE 15-45 **A**, Histologic appearance of a papilloma in a Green Lizard, *Lacerta viridis*. Marked epithelial proliferation is found. **B**, Gross papilloma lesions on the head of a Green Lizard. (*A, Photograph courtesy J.E. Cooper; B, Photograph courtesy S. Barten.*)

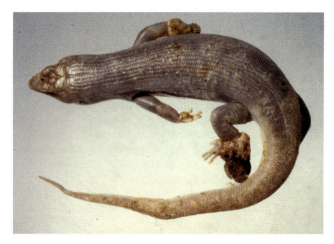

FIGURE 15-46 Round Island Skink, *Leiolopisma telfairi*, with squamous cell carcinomas on both right fore and left hind feet. (*Photograph courtesy J.E. Cooper.*)

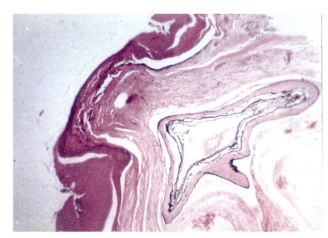

FIGURE 15-47 Hypovitaminosis A in a Common Lizard, *Lacerta vivipara*. The eye has been occluded by proliferation of hyperkeratotic and parakeratotic epidermis. (*Photograph courtesy J.E. Cooper.*)

males, the base of the head appears to be the predilection site. Papillomata should be removed by excision, cryotherapy, or laser.

Fibropapillomatosis was first reported in Green Seaturtles (*Chelonia mydas*) more than 60 years ago, and currently is known to affect all species of marine turtles. It is characterized by external and internal tumors of epithelial and fibrous origin. A herpesvirus is suspected to be the cause, and the animal's immune status may play a part in the development and severity of fibropapillomatosis.[88]

A papillomatosis of Bolivian Side-neck Turtles (*Platemys platycephala*) has also been reported.[89] Other species of reptiles may be affected.

Prompt and thorough investigation of skin lesions is essential if a neoplasm is to be diagnosed at an early stage. A biopsy is usually necessary to distinguish a neoplasm from other lesions such as abscesses and granulomas (see previous), but cytologic examination (impression smears/touch preparations) can sometimes provide a rapid and less expensive method of diagnosis.

Treatment of tumors is usually by surgical excision, but cryotherapy or laser ablation may be of value.[90]

Neoplasia may be a particular problem in small (inbred) populations of threatened reptiles, as was postulated when squamous cell carcinomas were diagnosed in a captive group of the rare Round Island Skink, *Leiolopisma telfairii*[91] (Figure 15-46).

Nutritional Disorders

Lesions associated with nutritional secondary hyperparathyroidism (NSHP) are discussed in Chapters 18 and 61.

The skin is an important indicator of health. A reptile that is in poor condition because of inadequate nutrition may show color changes, abrasions, and secondary infection.

Hypovitaminosis A has been recognized in reptiles for at least four decades and is primarily a disease of chelonians. The upper alimentary and respiratory tract are particularly affected, but the eyelids may become swollen and sometimes abraded. Abnormal keratin is a feature. Both hyperkeratosis and parakeratosis may be seen (Figure 15-47). Other areas of skin can show lesions, including dermatitis, but these lesions may be secondary rather than a direct effect of the deficiency. The role of hypovitaminosis A in other dermatologic conditions of reptiles is generally unclear, but many clinicians include vitamin A supplement in nonspecific therapy.

Other vitamin deficiencies may play a part in skin disease (see subsequent, Skin Wounds), but the administration of fat-soluble vitamins without careful evaluation of their need is potentially dangerous.[92]

Hypervitaminosis A in terrestrial chelonians, after the administration of the vitamin via injection, was excellently described by Frye.[92] The clinical signs are those of a subacute xeroderma followed by necrotizing dermatitis, especially (but not exclusively) on the neck and limbs. The histologic features of early cases are a flattening of the epithelium leading to exposure of dermis and muscle. More severe cases have severe skin destruction and may die.

Patches

Rossi[41] defined a patch as "a flat, circumscribed change in color and texture of the skin" and pointed out that such lesions are relatively common in reptiles (e.g., in grey-patch disease of seaturtles and other dermatitides). Patches of uncertain cause are commonly seen in farmed crocodiles (*Crocodylus niloticus*) in East Africa.[93] Cytology and biopsy may be necessary to diagnose the etiology of the patches.

Skin Wounds

A wound is any breach of the integrity of the skin. Examples have been discussed elsewhere in this chapter. Wounds may be inflicted by physical damage during handling or from the substrate.[94] Another important cause is bites from other reptiles and predators (Figure 15-48), including bites by live food such as rodents.[95] As a general rule, the use of live food should be discouraged and when this is deemed necessary, strict protocols should be enforced in the interests of both reptile and its prey. In reptiles, any skin wound is a significant breach in the integument and serves as a portal of entry for bacteria.

Wounds should be treated as in other species. Immediate attention to hygiene is important. Povidone iodine disinfection helps to reduce the risk of secondary infection and also serves to mark the lesions, facilitating subsequent inspection (Figure 15-49). The application of an adhesive drape assists.[51] Skin wounds may take several weeks to heal. The process is temperature-dependent, repair being more rapid at higher temperatures.[28] Nutritional status, especially protein but also probably vitamin intake, is also likely to influence wound repair.

Abnormal fragility of the skin of snakes has been reported by Jacobson[9] and seen by others.[96,97] The syndrome is sometimes associated with poorly organized collagen, and a vitamin C deficiency has been postulated as the possible cause. Care must, however, be taken in diagnosing such a condition. Variations exist in skin elasticity in different regions of the body, certainly in some snakes,[33] and this must be borne in mind when assessing dermal integrity. It must be distinguished from skin-tearing from malnutrition or rough handling with "snakesticks" during sloughing.[31] Separation and tearing of the skin in boas have been attributed to hypovitaminosis C,[12] but little scientific evidence is found for such deficiencies. Such wounds need careful management. Suturing may be helpful if healing by first intention is feasible. Hygiene is vital to minimize the risk of infection. See Chapter 18 for more information on vitamin C deficiency.

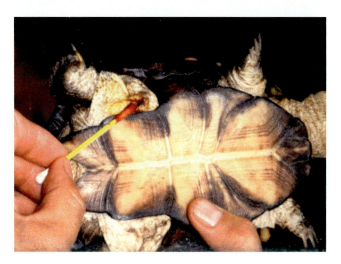

FIGURE 15-49 Skin wounds on a terrapin are treated topically with a povidone iodine preparation. (*Photograph courtesy M.E. Cooper.*)

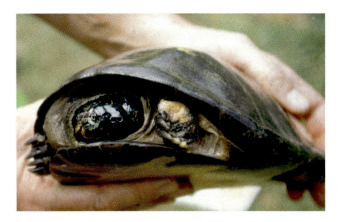

FIGURE 15-48 Injury to the skin of the foot of a freshwater terrapin caused by the bite of a Nile Crocodile, *Crocodylus niloticus*. (*Photograph courtesy M.E. Cooper.*)

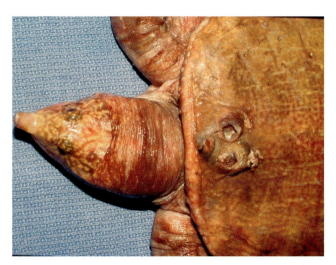

FIGURE 15-50 Carapacial lesions are common in freshwater turtles. These ulcers can be confined to the shell or may become septicemic. A number of different organisms may be involved. (*Photograph courtesy D. Mader.*)

Ulcerative Lesions

Ulceration (defined by Rossi[41] as "a break in the continuity of the epidermis with loss of substance and exposure of underlying dermis or deep tissue") is a common sequel to infectious dermatitis and burns. Ulcers can also be caused by the gnawing of invertebrates (e.g., if cockroaches provided as food remain too long in the cage or if hibernating chelonians are attacked by soil-dwelling species).

Ulcerative shell disease of chelonians, mainly aquatic species,[98,99] is associated with poor hygiene, intraspecies aggression, low temperature, or dysecdysis (Figure 15-50). It can be confined to the shell or become septicemic. A number of different organisms may be involved; culture and sensitivity should be performed.

Topical treatment of all ulcers consists of cleaning, debridement, and application of antimicrobial agents (ranging from iodine preparations to antibiotics) as necessary. Prevention of further infection is vital. Ulcers that fail to heal may contain foreign material, such as talc (see previous), or be chronically infected. Scarification and irrigation with 1% saline solution encourages granulation.

A specific condition termed septicemic cutaneous ulcerative disease (SCUD) has been reported in terrapins (freshwater turtles, *Pseudemys,* and *Trachemys* spp.) in North America and Europe. It probably occurs elsewhere; an apparently identical condition has been seen in terrapins in East Africa.[93] The lesions, which usually follow trauma or other insults, consist of necrotic ulcerations of the shell and skin. A number of different bacteria are possibly involved, including *Citrobacter, Serratia,* and *Beneckea* spp., and synergism may occur. Improvement of water quality and topical attention to the lesions are the recommended treatment.

Viral Diseases

A number of viral diseases may affect the skin of reptiles.[9] Papillomatosis was discussed previously. Other dermal conditions of viral etiology include grey-patch disease of Green Seaturtles and poxvirus skin disease of crocodilians[100-102] and certain other reptiles.[103]

Diagnosis of viral infections usually requires the examination of biopsies, with light and electron microscopy, and attempted virus isolation.

Other diseases of reptiles caused by viruses are likely to be described in due course. The clinician should be aware of the possibility of viral involvement and, especially in cases where conventional therapy proves ineffective, consider submitting material for laboratory investigation.

TREATMENT

As will be apparent from the foregoing text, treatment of dermatologic disorders can be medical, surgical, managemental, environmental, or a combination of these.

Both medical and surgical treatment of dermatologic disorders are facilitated by the accessibility and visibility of the skin, which also makes it relatively easy to assess progress and to initiate changes in therapy or management. Sloughing often contributes to healing as it results in a reduction of bacteria and fungi, coupled with regeneration of underlying epithelium. Shed skins should therefore always be saved, stored, and inspected as part of health monitoring (Figure 15-51). The clinician should ask the client to save and to bring in any recent sloughed skins as part of the patient examination; these sloughs should be sealed in plastic bags to retain any parasites (e.g., mites) that may be present and to enhance the value of bacteriologic or mycologic culture.

A range of medicinal agents can be used for skin diseases, including antibiotics, antimycotics, and parasiticides. Because dermatologic disorders often reflect other (systemic) conditions, diverse treatments have a part to play. For the same reason, a careful decision has to be made as to whether to treat a reptile with skin disease topically, systemically, or both. Each case has to be assessed individually; much depends on evidence (as a result of, for example, hematologic findings) of involvement of internal organs and the integument. In the author's experience, both topical and systemic therapy are often wise. The clinician who is managing a reptile with a skin disease must be prepared to be involved in internal medicine and dermatology.

Immunotherapy is, in theory at any rate, an important part of treating skin diseases, but little scientific information is available. Immunostimulants, such as levamisole, have been tried but usually with equivocal results. Thermotherapy (warming the patient to the top of its preferred optimal temperature zone [POTZ]) is often of more value. Immunoglobulin production and the mobilization of lymphocytes and macrophages, cell-mediated responses, are likely to be optimal at such temperatures.

Immunization may have potential, as in some skin diseases of fish. Bacterins have been used in an attempt to protect

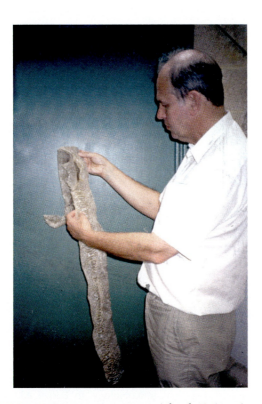

FIGURE 15-51 Routine examination of the shed skin of a captive snake. *(Photograph courtesy M.E. Cooper.)*

reptiles against certain organisms.[31,104] Vaccines against *Aeromonas* and other organisms have been used successfully in fish, and some of the technology might be usefully applied to reptiles.

Surgical treatment includes excision, cryotherapy, and other standard techniques. Wound closure in some species, such as crocodilians, may require special materials. Shell repair in chelonians is covered elsewhere in this book (see Chapter 67).

Managemental therapy relates to such matters as nutrition, access to ultraviolet light, and reduction of stressors. There is overlap with attention to environmental factors, which also includes reduction of pathogen challenge by such measures as cleaning and disinfection. Hygiene, coupled with the correct use of disinfectants, plays an important part in the prevention of skin diseases and is an area where the veterinarian and herpetologist must work closely together.

ACKNOWLEDGMENTS

I am grateful to Dr Douglas Mader for inviting me to write this chapter, to my wife Margaret Cooper for taking most of the photographs, and to veterinary and herpetological friends and colleagues, in many countries, with whom I have collaborated over the years.

REFERENCES

1. Cloudsley-Thompson JL: *Predation and defence amongst reptiles*, Bristol, 1994, RSA Publishing.
2. Davies PMC: Anatomy and physiology. In Cooper JE, Jackson OF, editors: *Diseases of the Reptilia*, London, 1981, Academic Press.
3. Elkan E, Cooper JE: Skin biology of reptiles and amphibians, *Proc Royal Soc Edinb* 29B:115-125, 1980.
4. Whimster IW: The natural history of endogenous skin malignancy as a basis for experimental research, *Trans St John's Hosp Dermatol Soc* (59):195-224, 1973.
5. Whimster IW: Nerve supply as a stimulator of the growth of tissues including skin: II animal evidence, *Clin Exp Dermat* (3):389-410, 1978.
6. Brogard J: *Les maladie bactériennes et virales des reptiles étude bibliographique*, Thesis, 1980, L'Ecole Nationale Vétérinaire de Toulouse, France.
7. Cooper JE, Jackson OF, editors: *Diseases of the Reptilia*, London, 1981, Academic Press.
8. Marcus LC: *Veterinary biology and medicine of captive amphibians and reptiles*, Philadelphia, 1981, Lea & Febiger.
9. Jacobson ER: Diseases of the integumentary system of reptiles. In Ackerman L, Nesbitt G, editors: *Dermatology for the small animal practitioner*, Trenton, NJ, 1991, Veterinary Learning Systems Company.
10. Jacobson ER: Reptile dermatology. In Kirk RW, Bonagura JD, editors: *Kirk's current veterinary therapy XI, small animal practice*, Philadelphia, 1992, WB Saunders.
11. Ippen R, Schröder H-D, Elze K, editors: *Handbuch der Zootierkrankheiten, Band 1, Reptilien*, Berlin, 1985, Akademie-Verlag.
12. Frye FL: *Biomedical and surgical aspects of captive reptile husbandry*, ed 2, Malabar, Fla, 1991, Krieger.
13. Brown CH: *Structural materials in animals*, New York, 1975, John Wiley & Sons.
14. Jayne BC: Mechanical behaviour of snake skin, *J Zool London* 214:125-140, 1988.
15. Zangerl, R: The turtle shell. In Gans C, Bellairs A d'A, Parsons TS, editors: *Biology of the Reptilia, vol 1, morphology: A*, London, 1969, Academic Press.
16. Bentley PJ, Schmidt-Nielsen K: Cutaneous water loss in reptiles, *Science* 151:1547-1549, 1966.
17. Schmidt WJ: *Studien am Integument der Reptilien*, Leipzig, 1912, Wilhelm Engelmann.
18. Girons G, Saint H: *Contribution à L'Histologie de Sphenondon punctatus*, Paris, 1964, Gray Editions du Centre National de la Recherche Scientifique.
19. Cooper JE: The guiding hand ... foundations of lower vertebrate pathology, the first Edward Elkan memorial lecture, *Herpetopathologia* 11:1-4,1989.
20. Klaphake E: Femoral gland biology and possible medical concerns in the green iguana, *Iguana iguana*, *Proc ARAV*, 31: 2000.
21. Weldon PJ, Sampson HW, Wong L, et al: Histology and biochemistry of the scent glands of the yellow-bellied sea snake (*Pelamis olaturus*): Hydrophiidae, *J Herpetol* 25:367-374, 1991.
22. Ananjeva NBD, Imuchanedov ME, Matveyeva TN: The skin sense organs of some iguanian lizards, *J Herpetol* 25:186-199, 1991.
23. Benton MJ: The mite pockets of lizards, *Nature* 325:391-392, 1987.
24. Hulse AC: Carapacial and plastral flora and fauna of the Sonoran mud turtle *Kinosternon sonoriense*, *J Herpetol* 10:45, 1975.
25. Cooper JE, Needham JR, Lawrence K: Studies on the cloacal flora of three species of free-living British reptiles, *J Zool London* 207:521-526, 1985.
26. Williams PA, Mitchell W, Wilson GR, et al: Bacteria in the gular and paracloacal glands of American alligator *Alligator mississippiensis*; Reptilia, crocodilia, *Lett Appl Microbiol* 10: 73-76, 1990.
27. Cooper JE, Needham JR: Isolation of bacteria from healthy mambas (*Dendroaspis* species), *Vet Rec* 113:135-136, 1983.
28. Smith DA, Barker IK, Allen OB: The effect of ambient temperature and type of wound on healing of cutaneous wounds in the common garter snake (*Thamnophis sirtalis*), *Can J Vet Res* 52:120, 1988.
29. Maderson PFA: The skin of lizards and snakes, *Br J Herpetol* 3:151-154, 1964.
30. Maderson PFA: Histological changes in the epidermis of snakes during the sloughing cycle, *J Zoo London* 146:98-113, 1965.
31. Cooper JE, Leakey JHE: A septicaemic disease of East African snakes associated with Enterobacteriaceae, *Trans Royal Soc Trop Med Hyg* 70:80-84, 1976.
32. Boyer DT, Boyer TH: Trichlorfon spray for snake mites (*Ophionyssus matrices*), *Bull Assoc Reptl Amphib Vet* 11:2, 1991.
33. Singh JPN, Mittal AK: Structure and histochemistry of the dermis of a chequered water snake, *Natrix piscator*, *J Zool London* 219:21-28, 1989.
34. Arnold N: The throwaway tail, *N Scientist* 42-45, 1990.
35. Stirling HP: *Chemical and biological methods of water analysis for aquaculturalists*, United Kingdom, 1985, Institute of Aquaculture.
36. Cooper JE: Biopsy techniques, *Semin Avian Exotic Pet Med* 33:161-165, 1994.
37. Karesh WB, Smith F, Frazier-Taylor H: A remote method for obtaining skin biopsy samples, *Conservation Biol* 13:261-262, 1987.
38. Cooper JE, Lawrence L: Pathological studies on skin lesions in reptiles. In Vago C, Matz G, editors: *Proceedings of the 1st International Colloquium on Pathology of Reptiles and Amphibians*, Angers, France, 1982.
39. Cooper JE: The role of pathology in investigation of diseases of reptiles, *Acta Zoologica at Pathologica Antiverpiensia* 2:15, 1986.
40. Cooper JE: Reptilian microbiology. In Fudge AM, editor: *Laboratory medicine: avian and exotic pets*, Philadelphia, 2000, WB Saunders.

41. Rossi JV: Dermatology. In Mader DR, editor: *Reptile medicine and surgery,* Philadelphia, 1996, WB Saunders.
42. Boam GW, Sanger VL, Cowan DF, et al: Subcutaneous abscesses in iguanid lizards, *J Am Vet Med Assoc* 157:617, 1970.
43. Elkan E, Cooper JE: Tumours and pseudotumours in some reptiles, *J Comp Path* 86:337-348, 1976.
44. Huchzermeyer FW, Cooper JE: Fibriscess, not abscess, resulting from a localised inflammatory response to infection in reptiles and birds, *Vet Rec* 147:515-517, 2000.
45. Hoff GL, Hoff DM: *Salmonella* and *Arizona*. In Hoff GL, Frye FL, Jacobson ER, editors: *Diseases of amphibians and reptiles,* New York, 1984, Plenum Book Co.
46. Duran-Reynals F, Clausen HJ: A contagious tumor-like condition in the lizard *(Anolis equestris)* as induced by a new bacterial species *Serratia anolium, J Bacteriol* 33:369, 1937.
47. Frye FL: *Biomedical and surgical aspects of captive reptile husbandry,* Edwardsville, Kan, 1981, Veterinary Medicine Publishing Co.
48. Ryan TP: Dermatophilosis in a Savannah monitor *Varanus exanthematicus,* Bull Assoc Reptl Amphib Vet 22:7, 1992.
49. Rossi J, Frye FL, Dutra FR: Two cases of turtle leprosy, *Annual Proc Am Assoc Zoo Vet* 102, 1976.
50. Mader DR, DeRemer K: Salmonellosis in reptiles, *Vivarium* 4:12, 1993.
51. Cooper JE: Use of a surgical adhesive drape in reptiles, *Vet Rec* 108:56, 1981.
52. Bourdeau P: Pathologie des tortues. 2e partie: affections cutanées et digestives, *Le Point Veterinaire* 20:871, 1989.
53. Jackson OF: Tortoise shell repair over two years, *Vet Rec* 102:104, 1978.
54. Holt PE: Healing of a surgically induced shell wound in a tortoise, *Vet Rec* 108:102, 1981.
55. Montali RJ: Comparative pathology of inflammation in the higher vertebrates (reptiles, birds and mammals), *J Comp Path* 99:1-26, 1988.
56. Barten SI, Jacobson ER, Gardiner CH: Infection of aquatic turtles with *Flavobacterium meningosepticum, Proc Third Int Colloquium Pathol Reptl Amphib* 33, 1989.
57. Stewart JS: Anaerobic bacterial infections in reptiles, *J Zoo Wildlife Med* 212:180, 1990.
58. Witham R: Focal necrosis of the skin in tank-reared sea turtles, *J Am Vet Assoc* 163:656, 1973.
59. Frye FL, Myers MW: Foreign-body dermatitis in a snake, *Mod Vet Pract* 63(3):102, 1985.
60. Cooper JE: Ulcerative skin lesions of snakes: a diagnostic challenge, *UK Vet* 43:54-56, 1999.
61. Anver MR, Park JS, Rush HG: Dermatophilosis in the marble lizard *(Calotes mystaceus), Lab Anim Sci* 26:817, 1976.
62. Montali RJ, Smith EE, Davenport M, et al: Dermatophilosis in Australian beaded lizards, *J Am Vet Med Assoc* 167:553, 1975.
63. Ramsay EC, Bernis DA, Patton CS: Dermatophilus infections in a tortoise collection, *Proc AAZV/AAWV Joint Conf* 279, 1998.
64. Millichamp NJ: Congenital defects in captive bred Indian pythons *(Python molurus molurus), Proc Third Int Colloquium Pathol Reptl Amphib* 103, 1989.
65. Hammack SH: New concepts in colubrid egg incubation: preliminary report, *Proc 15th Int Symp Captive Propagation Husbandry* 103-108, 1991.
66. Wright K: Dysecdysis in boid snakes with neurologic diseases, *Bull Assoc Rept Amphib Vet* 22:7, 1992.
67. Cooper JE: Disease in East African snakes associated with *Kalicephalus* worms (Nematoda: Diaphanocephalidae), *Vet Rec* 89:385-388, 1971.
68. Wright K, Tousignant A, Overstreet R, et al: Mesocercariae infections in a Texas indigo snake and red-sided garter snakes, *Proc Third Int Colloquium Pathol Reptl Amphib* 54, 1989.
69. Burridge MJ: Significance and control of exotic ticks on imported reptiles, *Proc ARAV* 121-122, 2000.
70. Abrahams R: Ivermectin as a spray for treatment of snake mites, *Bull Assoc Reptl Amphib Vet* 21:8, 1992.
71. Camin JH: Mite transmission in snakes, *J Parasitol* XXXIV: 345-354, 1948.
72. Schultz H: Human infestation by *Ophionyssus natricis* snake mite, *Br J Dermatol* 93:365, 1975.
73. Sawyer RT: *Leech biology and behaviour,* New York, 1986, Oxford Science Publications.
74. Cooper JE: A veterinary approach to leeches, *Vet Rec* 127: 226-228, 1990.
75. Boyer TH: Common problems of box turtles *(Terrapene* spp) in captivity, *Bull Assoc Reptl Amphib Vet* 21:9, 1992.
76. Fielden LJ, Rechau Y, Bryson NR: Acquired immunity to larvae of *Amblyomma marmoreum* and *A. hebraeum* by tortoises, guinea-pigs and guinea-fowl, *Med Vet Entomol* 6:251-254, 1992.
77. Rossi J, Rossi R: Fungal dermatitis in a large collection of Brazas water snakes, *Nerodia harteri harteri,* housed in an outdoor enclosure, and a possible association with slugs, *Proc ARAV* 81: 2000.
78. Schilcher F, Kübber-Heiss A, Breuer-Strosberg, et al: Dermatomy kose durch Trichophyton terrestre bei madegassischen Taggeckos *(Phelsuma m madagascariesis), Wien Tierärtzliche Mschr* 85:131-135, 1998.
79. Schildger BJ, Frank H, Gobel T, et al: Mycotic infections of the integument and inner organs in reptiles, *Proc Third Int Colloquium Pathol Reptl Amphib* 4, 1989.
80. Jacobson ER: Necrotizing mycotic dermatitis in snakes: clinical and pathologic features, *J Am Vet Med Assoc* 1779:838, 1980.
81. Page CD, Mantion M, Derendorf H, et al: Multiple dose pharmacokinetics of ketoconazole administered to gopher tortoises *(Gopherus polyphemus), J Zoo Wildl Med* 22:191, 1991.
82. Austwick PCK, Keymer IF: Fungi. In Cooper JE, Jackson OF, editors: *Diseases of the Reptilia,* London, 1981, Academic Press.
83. Hunt TJ: Notes on disease and mortality in Testudines, *Herpetologica* 14:45, 1958.
84. Elkan E: Malignant melanoma in a snake, *J Comp Pathol Ther* 84:51, 1974.
85. Cooper JE, Jackson OF, Harshbarger, JC: A neurilemmal sarcoma in a tortoise *(Testudo hermanni), J Comp Pathol* 93: 541, 1983.
86. Raynaud A, Adrian M: Lesions cutanées a structure pilomateuse associees à des virus chez lezard vert *(Lacerta viridis* Laur), *CR Acad Sci Paris,* 283 Series D: 845, 1976.
87. Cooper JE, Gschmeissner S, Holt PE: Viral particles in a papilloma from a green lizard *(Lacerta viridis), Lab Anim* 16:12-13, 1982.
88. Work TM, Rameyer RA, Balazs GH, et al: Immune status of free-living green turtles with fibropapillomatosis from Hawaii, *J Wildlife Dis* 37:574-581, 2001.
89. Jacobson ER, Gaskin JM, Clubb S, et al: Papilloma-like virus infection in Bolivian side-neck turtles, *J Am Vet Med Assoc* 181(11):1325, 1982.
90. Baxter JS, Meek R: Cryosurgery in the treatment of skin disorders in reptiles, *Br Herpetol J* 1:227, 1988.
91. Cooper JE: Tumours (neoplasms) of reptiles: some significant cases from Jersey Zoo, *Dodo* 36:82-86, 2000.
92. Frye FL: Vitamin A sources, hypovitaminosis A, and iatrogenic hypervitaminosis B in captive chelonians. In Kirk RW, editor: *Current veterinary therapy,* vol X, Philadelphia, 1989, WB Saunders.
93. Cooper, JE: Personal observation.
94. Cooper JE: Physical injury. In Fairbrother A, Locke LN, Hoff GL, editors: *Non-infectious diseases of wildlife,* ed 2, Ames, 1996, Iowa State University Press.

95. Rosskopf WJ, Woerpel RW: Rat bite injury in a pet snake, *Mod Vet Pract* 62:871, 1981.
96. Cooper JE, Dutton CJ: A skin disorder in captive snakes at the Jersey Zoo, British Channel Isles. In preparation.
97. Frye FL, personal communication, 1998.
98. Wallach JD: The pathogenesis and etiology of ulcerative shell disease in turtles, *J Zoo Anim Med* 6:11, 1975.
99. Wallach JD: Ulcerative shell disease in turtles: identification, prophylaxis and treatment, *Int Zoo Yearbook* 17:170, 1977.
100. Buoro IBJ: Pox-like virus particles in skin lesions of five Nile crocodiles in Kenya, *Discovery and Innovation* 41:117-118, 1992.
101. Horner RF: Poxvirus in farmed Nile crocodiles, *Vet Rec* 122:459, 1988.
102. Huchzermeyer FW, Huchzermeyer KDA, Putterill JF: Observations on a field outbreak of pox virus infection in young Nile crocodiles *(Crocodylus niloticus)*, *J South Afr Vet Assoc* 621:27-29, 1991.
103. Stauber E, Gogolewski R: Poxvirus dermatitis in a tegu lizard *(Tupinambis teguixin)*, *J Zoo Wildl Med* 21:2,228, 1990.
104. Jacobson ER: Chemotherapeutics in reptile medicine. In Jacobson ER, Kollias G, editors: *Exotic animals*, New York, 1988, Churchill Livingstone.

16

MICROBIOLOGY: FUNGAL AND BACTERIAL DISEASES OF REPTILES

JEAN A. PARÉ, LYNNE SIGLER, KAREN L. ROSENTHAL, and DOUGLAS R. MADER

FUNGAL DISEASES

Jean A. Paré and Lynne Sigler

Fungal disease has been documented worldwide and in all orders and suborders of the Reptilia, with the exception of the Rhynchocephala (Tuataras). Both yeasts and filamentous fungi have been incriminated in cutaneous and systemic mycosis in reptiles. A number of fungi are true pathogens of mammals but, until recently, none had yet been clearly identified as a true pathogen of reptiles.[1-4] Infection of reptiles by fungi has been regarded as opportunistic, caused by normally saprophytic organisms that invade living tissue strictly under favorable circumstances.[2,5] Although such opportunistic infection is the rule, the recent evidence that two fungi consistently and reproducibly initiate disease in a given reptile species under seemingly normal environmental conditions casts a novel perspective in mycopathology of reptiles. *Fusarium semitectum* has been implicated as the agent of necrotizing scute disease in both captive and wild Texas Tortoises (*Gopherus berlandieri*)[6] and the *Chrysosporium* anamorph of *Nannizziopsis vriesii* (CANV) induces dermatomycosis in Veiled Chameleons (*Chamaeleo calyptratus*) under experimental conditions,[7] fulfilling all of Koch's postulates and further supporting the role of some fungi as primary pathogens.

The CANV is consistently isolated from pet inland Bearded Dragons (*Pogona vitticeps*) affected with a newly described contagious dermatomycosis called yellow fungus disease.[8,9] In contrast to ubiquitous omnipresent saprophytic fungi such as *Aspergillus* or *Paecilomyces* species, the CANV is rarely found on normal reptile integument[10] and yet has been firmly incriminated in a disproportionately high number of reptilian mycoses in lizards, snakes, and crocodiles,[9,11-14] suggesting it carries a substantial pathogenic potential for reptiles. As our knowledge of the interactions between fungi and reptiles expands through better understanding of the fungal species involved, further evidence to support the concept of other fungi being unusually pathogenic for reptiles may be disclosed.

Although mycosis in captive reptiles is less commonly encountered than bacterial disease, it does occur with regularity and is likely both underestimated and underdiagnosed because fungal lesions and clinical signs of fungal disease often are indistinguishable from those of bacterial disease. Isolation of bacteria from a lesion or from diseased tissue may further mislead the clinician because it does not rule out primary or secondary fungal involvement. As a result, fungal infections in reptiles are too often diagnosed at necropsy, usually on observation of fungal elements on histologic sections.[2] The literature is replete with case reports of mycoses in reptiles in which the agent was never identified because fungal disease was not suspected by either the clinician or the prosector and therefore specimens were not available for culture.[2] In practically all documented cases of systemic mycoses in reptiles, the chronicity of lesions, as determined histopathologically, attested to the insidious nature of fungal disease. Reptiles with signs of systemic illness or with cutaneous lesions need to be investigated aggressively if a timely diagnosis of mycosis is to be established and the chances of therapeutic success are to be optimized.

Fungal disease may present as dermatomycosis (cutaneous infection) or as disseminated (systemic) mycosis. Several review articles that focus on mycotic diseases in reptiles have been published.[1-4] Austwick and Keymer[2] compiled a particularly exhaustive list of documented case reports and observed that a fungus was isolated or identified in less than 50% of these documented cases and that histopathologic examination was not performed in more than 50% of cases. Often, when the fungal agent was not cultured, a tentative identification was risked based solely on histologic features of the fungal elements in tissues.[2] Case reports that establish a causal relationship between the fungal isolate and lesions observed in the reptile are the exception rather than the rule, and therefore, the extant literature should be interpreted with caution.[2] In addition, many case reports that describe mycoses in reptiles are dated, with fungal nomenclature that is obsolete. *Cephalosporium*, for example, incriminated in pulmonary and disseminated mycosis in spectacled caimans,[15] is the older name for fungi now accommodated within the genus *Acremonium*.[16,17] Reexamination of the yeast-like fungus *Trichosporon beigelii*, often implicated in cutaneous and systemic mycoses in reptiles,[2,18-21] showed that it encompassed several *Trichosporon* species, and the name *T. beigelii* is no longer in use.[16] Some reports fail to mention the species of reptile affected,[2] and the reptile nomenclature used by earlier authors who are cited in review articles[1,2] is often outdated.[22] The disease terminology for mycoses also has undergone revision according to current classification so that, for example, the term *phycomycosis* has now been replaced by the more descriptive zygomycosis.[16] All the previous reasons make definitive conclusions difficult to draw from the literature about the role of specific fungi in reptile infections. In this chapter, we aim to review the basics of fungal-reptile interactions and the clinical presentation of dermatomycoses and systemic mycoses, identify clinical entities, assess the pathogenic potential of fungi reported in earlier case reports through a critical review of the literature, and describe diagnostic procedures and modalities, as well as therapeutic options.

THE FUNGUS-REPTILE INTERACTION

Fungi are ubiquitous eukaryotic organisms that exist in an anamorph (asexual, mitotic, imperfect) or a teleomorph (sexual, meiotic, perfect) stage and reproduce by means of asexual (e.g., conidia, budding cells) or sexual (e.g., ascospores, zygospores) spores.[23] Dissemination of spores, whether airborne, water-borne, via fomites or other, is governed by environmental factors. On an appropriate substrate and under the right environmental conditions, spores germinate to produce a hyphal filament that grows in an apical fashion and rapidly branches to form a submerged mycelium. The mycelium produces aerial structures that bear the reproductive spores.[23] Most of the organisms associated with documented reptile mycoses are heavily sporulating fungi, and if conditions are favorable (i.e., large amounts of organic debris, high humidity), spore contamination in a closed environment may quickly reach sufficient levels to challenge the reptiles housed within it. Although little is known about the relationship between environmental exposure to spores and reptile disease, the magnitude of exposure to fungal spores in a captive environment remains largely a function of husbandry (temperature, humidity, ventilation, hygiene).

Saprophytic molds and yeasts are commonly isolated from reptile material. Surveys of skin and intestinal and oropharyngeal tracts have yielded different populations of organisms depending on the focus of the investigation. Freshly shed skins of captive reptiles examined for the presence of the *Chrysosporium* anamorph of *Nannizziopsis vriesii* have been shown to harbor a varied and complex fungal biota[10] (Figure 16-1). Fungi belonging to 50 different genera were cultured from skin samples obtained from 127 apparently healthy squamate reptiles. Species belonging to the ubiquitous genera *Aspergillus* and *Penicillium* were grown from almost 70% of the samples.[10] *Paecilomyces lilacinus*, an occasional pathogen of reptiles,[2,9,24-27] was recovered at high frequency (24% of sampled animals).[10] The gastrointestinal mycobiota of reptiles is as varied and complex as the cutaneous flora. Species of *Aspergillus*, *Penicillium*, *Basidiobolus*, *Fusarium*, *Mucor*, and numerous other fungi were isolated from the intestines and feces of healthy reptiles.[28-30] The intestinal contents of 29 wild-caught African Dwarf Crocodiles (*Osteolaemus tetraspis*) slaughtered for market yielded 20 different species of fungi and up to five fungi per individual crocodile.[31] Yeasts belonging to the genera *Candida*, *Torulopsis*, *Trichosporon*, *Rhodotorula*, and *Geotrichum* were recovered from the pharynx and feces of healthy tortoises (*Testudo hermanni*, *T. horsfieldi*, and *T. graeca*).[32] From these 23 tortoises, 23 *Candida* isolates were isolated and speciated as *C. tropicalis* (n = 13), *C. albicans* (n = 9), and *C. parapsilosis* (n = 1). In a different study, yeasts were isolated from swabs of the oral cavity and cloaca in 40.2% of reptile patients that were cultured.[33] *Candida* species and *Trichosporon* species were most frequently isolated, but *Torulopsis* and *Rhodotorula* species were also present. In that study, yeasts were isolated significantly more frequently from the guts of herbivorous than carnivorous reptiles.[33] Interestingly, *Basidiobolus*, a chitinophilic fungus, is commonly isolated from the guts of insectivorous reptile species,[28-30] further illustrating that the gut mycobiota may vary according to the feeding strategy. The pulmonary mycobiota of reptiles has not received as much attention but, in one study, *Aspergillus niger* and *A. fumigatus*, *Pseudallescheria boydii*, and members of the genera *Penicillium*, *Paecilomyces*, *Cladosporium*, and others were isolated with regularity from the lungs, and rarely but surprisingly from the spleen, of healthy free-ranging Agama Lizards (*Agama agama*), and Wall Geckos (*Hemidactylus* sp.).[29] A study of human lungs, cultured at necropsy from patients who died of extrapulmonary causes, also yielded fungal isolates in 81% of the samples, predominantly *Aspergillus* and *Penicillium* species.[34]

Because the previous evidence supports the concept that spores are omnipresent and unavoidable both on and within healthy reptiles, to infer that host response to fungal invasion is the key to the outcome of fungal spore–reptile interaction appears logical. Because they are ectotherms, the core body temperature of reptiles is more prone to fluctuate than that of mammals or birds. This range in body temperatures is more likely to allow mesophilic fungi, unable to grow at 37°C, to infect reptiles, especially if the animal is kept at suboptimal temperatures.[2] The immune system, coupled with mechanical barriers such as the integument, protects the reptile from fungal invasion. In mammals, the first line of defense to invasive fungi typically includes activation of the alternate pathway of the complement system, with attraction of neutrophils, followed by the recruitment of macrophages, natural killer (NK) cells, T cells, and other mononuclear cells.[35] Reptiles have a functional and complex immune system that is comparable with that of other vertebrates.[35-38] The efficiency of the reptilian immune system is influenced by a combination of factors that include health and nutritional

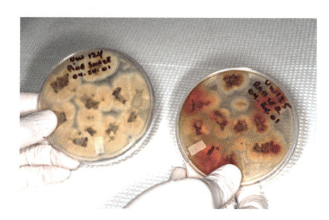

FIGURE 16-1 Profuse fungal growth around specimens of shed skin from a healthy Pinesnake (*Pituophis melanoleucus mugitus*) and a Mojave Rattlesnake (*Crotalus s. scutulatus*) plated onto Mycosel agars. (*Photograph courtesy J. Paré.*)

status, environmental temperature, brumation (hibernation) or estivation, seasonal changes, age, and stress. In virtually all outbreaks or individual cases of reptile mycosis, inadequacies in husbandry, poor sanitation, overcrowding, stressful procedures, or heating system mechanical failures were identified as potential predisposing factors.[2,4,12-14] When a reptile is diagnosed with mycosis, each of the previously mentioned immune-modulating factors needs to be thoroughly assessed. If deficiencies are identified, appropriate corrections need be made so that the patient may mount an adequate immune response, with fully functional healing mechanisms.

In reptiles, the whole skin is periodically shed, which helps in the control of early fungal invasion of the cornified epithelial layer. The epithelia of reptiles are comparable with those of other vertebrates, but the epidermal keratins are similar to those of mammals and birds and are substantially different from those of amphibians.[39] This similarity in keratins suggests that agents of dermatomycoses are likely to be similar in mammals, birds, and reptiles and may explain why recognized amphibian pathogens such as *Basidiobolus ranarum*, *Mucor amphibiorum*, and *Batrachochytridium dendrobatidis* rarely, if ever, infect reptilian integument.[2,4] Although a breach in the integrity of epidermal or epithelial barriers undoubtedly facilitates opportunistic infections, fungi that elaborate enzymes such as collagenases, elastases, and keratin-degrading proteases have the potential to invade intact nonkeratinized and keratinized epithelial surfaces. Reptiles may ward off fungal tissue invasion partially or completely depending on the timeliness and vigor of the immune response and the virulence of the invading fungus. Once established, infection may later resolve or may progress to a deeper-seated mucosal or dermal infection and eventually to disseminated disease. Histologically, a substantial inflammatory response to fungal elements can typically be shown.[36] Heterophils usually dominate in the acute phase of inflammation, followed by a gradual recruitment of mononuclear cells. Within a week, macrophages and multinucleated giant cells may wall off fungal elements within granulomata. Mature granulomata, with a thick connective tissue capsule, develop within a month. Systemically administered antifungal drugs cannot access the core of mature granulomata, where live fungal elements may persist. Such lesions require surgical exeresis. On the basis of published reports, the skin and the respiratory tract, and to a lesser extent the gastrointestinal tract, are the usual fungal portals of entry in reptile mycoses.[2]

CUTANEOUS AND SUBCUTANEOUS MYCOSES

Dermatophytes are the agents of dermatophytosis in mammals but are extremely rare in reptiles. The term *dermatophytosis* is restricted to infections caused by fungi belonging to the genera *Trichophyton* and *Microsporum*, both of which include anthropophilic, zoophilic, and geophilic species, and the strictly anthropophilic *Epidermophyton*.[16,17] Of the known mammalian pathogens, only *Trichophyton mentagrophytes* has been implicated as the cause of dermal lesions in a Ball Python (*Python regius*),[40] but the fungus has not been reexamined to confirm its identification. All other reports involve geophilic keratinophilic fungi[17] that may be isolated as contaminants and for which demonstration of a pathogenic role was not well established. *Trichophyton terrestre*, a geophilic fungus usually considered nonpathogenic,[17] was isolated from the scales of an apparently healthy Boa Constrictor (*Boa constrictor*)[2] and was associated with progressive digital necrosis in Eastern Blue-tongued Skinks (*Tiliqua scincoides*).[41] Although numerous hyphae were seen histologically in the necrotic toes of these skinks, a causal relationship could not be ascertained. Unspeciated *Trichophyton* isolates were recovered from granulomatous lesions on the feet of an American Alligator (*Alligator mississipiensis*) with pododermatitis[3] and from the cutis and muscles of one of several Day Geckoes (*Phelsuma* sp.) with multiple nodular skin lesions.[18] The latter was likely a misidentified isolate of the *Chrysosporium* anamorph of *Nannizziopsis vriesii*,[9] a fungus that has microscopic features similar to *Trichophyton* species, raising the possibility that the previous reports may also be based on misidentified isolates. Some evidence exists to suggest that zoophilic dermatophytes are rarely found on the skin of reptiles. A survey of keratinophilic fungi from Australia only showed the presence of *Microsporum cookei*, a geophilic species, and a *Chrysosporium* species from epidermal scales of clinically normal monitor lizard (*Varanus* sp.) and from a skink, *Egernia bungana*.[42] Two geophilic species of *Microsporum*, *M. boullardii* and *M. gypseum*, were recovered at a frequency of less than 3% in shed skin from 127 captive squamate reptiles.[10] The survey failed to recover any *Trichophyton* dermatophyte from these reptiles. Reptiles therefore do not appear to pose a significant zoonotic threat for dermatophytosis.

Although the evidence concerning true dermatophytosis is questionable, dermatomycoses occur commonly. In squamate reptiles, blisters may be the first manifestation of fungal skin infection.[11] Such lesions are easily misinterpreted as bacterial and relegated as "blister disease," a syndrome for which etiology is believed to be multifactorial. However, the presence of blisters should always evoke the possibility of fungal involvement.[1,11,12,43-46] In lizards, blisters may occur anywhere on the body, but in snakes, lesions tend to occur more often on the ventral scutes (Figure 16-2). Blisters may be filled with serous colorless or brownish blood-tinged fluid. Fluid should be cultured for bacteria and for fungi and examined microscopically for the presence of microorganisms. Gram-stained smears can be examined for the presence of fungal elements, or specific fungal stains may be used. Blisters may be subtle and overlooked. They also are short-lived and soon rupture to form a yellowish or brown crust over the exposed dermis. Dermatomycosis may also manifest as focal skin discoloration, proliferative growths, hyperpigmentation, or hyperkeratosis, papules or pustules, ulcers, granulomata, or nodules (Figures 16-3 and 16-4). Lesions of dermatomycosis are often described as "necrotic." In snakes, thickened yellow to orange-brown discolored scales are rather suggestive of fungal epidermal disease,[41] and lesions may be quite extensive along the ventrum.[1,12,45,46] Sometimes, a rather suggestive white or pigmented cottony growth covers or surrounds the lesion. Various species of fungi have been isolated from cutaneous lesions in snakes and lizards.[1-3,9,18,27,46-49] Of these fungi, species belonging to the genera *Aspergillus*, *Trichosporon*,[2,18] *Geotrichum*, and the CANV have been repeatedly and reliably incriminated. If misdiagnosed or left untreated, dermatomycosis may lead to death from extensive disruption of the integument or from dissemination to internal viscera.[8-14,27,46,47]

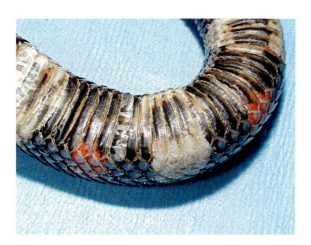

FIGURE 16-2 Fungal dermatitis in a Pueblan Milksnake (*Lampropeltis triangulum campbelli*). The ventral scutes are turgid with fluid. *Chaetomium* sp., *Penicillium* sp., *Mucor* sp., and *Alternaria* sp. were isolated from biopsy samples. Hyaline fungal hyphae were shown histologically and were morphologically incompatible with *Mucor* or *Alternaria* species. *Chaetomium*, growing circumferentially around three separate biopsy pieces, was the most likely suspect. (*Photograph courtesy S. Barten.*)

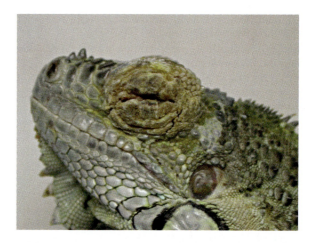

FIGURE 16-4 Severe histologically confirmed fungal blepharitis and periocular dermatomycosis in a Green Iguana (*Iguana iguana*). Samples collected after initiation of itraconazole failed to grow the causative agent. (*Photograph courtesy G. Rich.*)

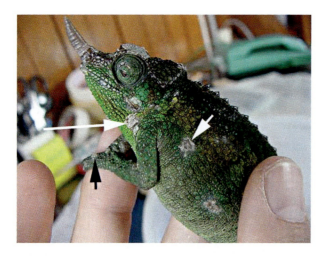

FIGURE 16-3 Exfoliative *(long arrow)*, ulcerative *(short arrow)*, and bullous *(black arrow)* dermatomycotic lesions in a Jackson's Chameleon (*Chamaeleo jacksonii*). (*Photograph courtesy B. Strand.*)

Single or multifocal, fluctuant to firm, caseous to granulomatous subcutaneous nodules, or "mycetomas," occur in snakes[2,9,24,49,50] and less often in lizards,[3,50,51] with or without concomitant epidermal or systemic fungal disease. The etiopathogenesis is unknown, but fungi may gain entrance through punctiform (or other) skin wounds. Of the published reports of subcutaneous mycetomas, most have involved colubrids, and especially Cornsnakes (*Elaphe guttata*) from which *Geotrichum* sp., an unknown *Chrysosporium* species, and the CANV were isolated.[2,9,50] Nuchal hematomas in Green Anoles (*Anolis carolinensis*) are often infected with fungi (e.g., *Trichosporon cutaneum*).[3,50] Such hematomas are believed to be the result of bites inflicted during fights among lizards. Subcutaneous mycetomas in reptiles may grossly be indistinguishable from chronic bacterial abscesses or from mesenchymatous tumors and should be included in the list of differential diagnoses for subcutaneous swellings in squamates, particularly ophidians. They often remain quiescent but may eventually lead to disseminated disease.

Very few fungal clinical syndromes have been recognized in squamates. *Cladosporium*, a dematiaceous (darkly pigmented) fungus, has been linked to a condition dubbed "black spot disease" in captive and wild geckoes (*Hoplodactylus* sp.) in New Zealand.[52] Initial epidermal infection progresses to dermal invasion, causing multifocal dark lesions. Without information from culture, evaluation of the fungus involved is difficult. *Cladosporium* species are among the most ubiquitous environmental fungi and occur commonly on plant litter. Human infections formerly attributed to *Cladosporium* species are now considered to have been caused by members of the genus *Cladophialophora*.[16] In Spain, a *Penicillium* species has been persistently isolated from cutaneous lesions in a wild population of the Wall Lizard, *Podarcis bocagei*.[48] These lizards have dermatomycotic lesions in winter that regress and disappear in summer. In the last few years, a progressive, contagious, deep granulomatous dermatomycosis dubbed "yellow fungus disease" by herpetoculturists has been documented in inland Bearded Dragons (*Pogona vitticeps*).[8,9] The CANV has been isolated from all cases of yellow fungus disease investigated to date. The disease may be precipitated by the use of antibiotics. Lesions consist of single or multiple areas of coalescing necrotic hyperkeratotic epidermis over the head, limbs, or body and may become disfiguring. The necrotic tissue may slough, exposing an ulcerated dermis. Yellow fungus disease typically undergoes a protracted course, and infection often progresses to involve underlying muscles and bones.

In crocodilians, documented cases of systemic mycosis outnumber the rare documented cases of dermatomycoses.[2] Fungal skin lesions in crocodilians have been described in various terms: skin discoloration, necrotic, creamy or caseous to leathery thickenings or plaques[13,53] locally or over the whole body. Various fungi have been isolated from these skin lesions[2,53] with little evidence of a causative role, except for the CANV.[13] This fungus caused outbreaks of highly fatal dermatomycosis in farmed Saltwater Crocodiles (*Crocodylus porosus*) housed in a laboratory setting.[13] Animals that were spared from the disease were housed in different pens, and the CANV was absent from these crocodiles on the basis of culture results.

The CANV merits further attention because it is emerging as the cause of many individual cases and outbreaks of severe dermatomycosis both in squamates and crocodilians worldwide.[7-14] *Nannizziopsis vriesii* is an ascomycetous fungus that belongs to the order Onygenales, family Onygenaceae.[11] Before isolation from sick reptiles, *N. vriesii* was known only from one original lizard (*Ameiva* sp.) isolate and one other isolate from soil in California.[11] In culture, *N. vriesii* produces an anamorph, described in the genus *Chrysosporium*, that is morphologically indistinguishable from the isolates recovered from various reptiles with fungal infection. Therefore, the name for the anamorph is currently used for these isolates. The taxonomic relationship between the teleomorphic *N. vriesii* and the reptile isolates is still under investigation, but preliminary molecular genetic evidence suggests that the CANV represents a species complex and that its members may be allied to specific hosts. Infection with this fungus begins as a cutaneous disease often characterized by vesicular lesions and bullae but can and often does disseminate, with a fatal outcome. Reported or known infections of reptiles with the CANV include three species of chameleons (*Chamaeleo jacksonii*, *C.* [*Furcifer*] *lateralis*, and *C.* [*Calumna*] *parsoni*)[11] and Tentacled Snakes (*Erpeton tentaculatum*)[14] in Canada; Saltwater Crocodiles[10] and a File Snake (*Acrochordus* sp.)[9] in Australia; a Ball Python in the United Kingdom[9]; Day Geckoes in the Netherlands[9]; and inland Bearded Dragons,[8,9] Brown Tree Snakes (*Boiga irregularis*),[12] cornsnakes,[9] a milksnake (*Lampropeltis* sp.),[9] and a gartersnake (*Thamnophis* sp.)[9] in the United States. The CANV forms solitary single-celled conidia similar to the microconidia of dermatophytes, and arthroconidia formed by fragmentation of the hyphae, and thus may easily be confused with other species of *Chrysosporium* or even with *Geotrichum* when the arthroconidia are predominant. For example, in the first documented mycosis, the fungus isolated from lesions in chameleons was first identified as an atypical strain of *Trichophyton verrucosum* by a veterinary laboratory and then as an atypical *T. terrestre* by a human reference laboratory before its final determination as the CANV.[11] Similarly, the fungi isolated from a gartersnake[54] and from sick Saltwater Crocodiles[13] were first identified as a *Geotrichum* species, a *Chrysosporium* species, or a *Trichophyton mentagrophytes*–like fungus, before being recognized as the CANV. The morphologic features and the growth characteristics of the CANV have only been recently described[11,12] and are not in current mycology identification manuals. Because lack of knowledge of this fungus has led to its misidentification, previously reported cases of reptile fungal disease attributed to unspeciated *Trichophyton*, *Chrysosporium*, or *Geotrichum* should be interpreted with caution.

In chelonians, dermatomycosis affects mostly the shell, and less often the feet and skin. Marine, and freshwater turtles and tortoises are all susceptible.[2,6,18,55] Outbreaks of fatal dermatomycosis in chelonians have only been seen in hatchlings or very young captive Florida Softshell Turtles (*Apalone ferox*)[55] and Wood Turtles (*Clemmys insculpta*).[56] Multiple, sometimes coalescing, raised, grayish or yellowish to tan papules and plaques were present on the carapace and plastron[55,56] and on the head and limbs.[56] In both instances, *Mucor* sp. was isolated, and wide aseptate hyphae consistent with those of zygomycetous fungi were observed histologically. Overcrowding and other captivity-related stressors were believed to be contributory. Fungal shell disease in adult tortoises and turtles is somewhat insidious, and initial lesions may be subtle.[6,18] Focal to extensive discoloration of the shell, dyskeratosis, scute necrosis, ulceration, and pitting may be present, alone or as a continuum of lesions. *Trichosporon* sp. has been repeatedly incriminated in various chelonians in Europe,[18] and *Fusarium semitectum* has been convincingly implicated as the cause of necrotizing scute disease in Texas Tortoises (Figure 16-5).[6] This condition is encountered in both wild and captive tortoises, and although shell lesions may be extensive, dissemination to the viscera does not occur.[6] The condition is reproducible experimentally, fulfilling Koch's postulates. Experimentally challenged Western Box Turtles (*Terrapene ornata*) failed to develop lesions, suggesting some degree of host specificity. Diagnosis of skin or shell fungal disease is ideally based on histopathologic examination of biopsies, although shell biopsies may be challenging (Figure 16-6). Hypovitaminosis A was suspected as an underlying factor in several cases of chelonian dermatomycoses, on the basis of apparent clinical response to vitamin A supplementation.[18]

Dermatomycosis has rarely been documented in wild reptiles, but this may be more a reflection of the lack of data pertaining to diseases of free-ranging reptiles. Cold and humid winter months coincided with the annual cyclical onset of fungal dermatitis in the previously mentioned population of wild Wall Lizards in Spain,[48] and unusually inclement climactic conditions were linked with an outbreak of dermatomycosis in a population of Dusky Pigmy Rattlesnakes (*Sistrurus miliarius barbouri*) in Florida.[57] Several individual accounts of fungal disease in a Pigmy Rattlesnake (*S. miliarius*),[49] a Timber Rattlesnake (*Crotalus horridus*),[58] a Green Seaturtle (*Chelonia mydas*),[59] and a Loggerhead Seaturtle (*Caretta caretta*)[60] were similarly attributed to adverse environmental conditions, or to primary debilitating injuries (Figure 16-7). In contrast, the prevalence of carapacial fungal infection with *Fusarium semitectum* in wild Texas Tortoises appears linked to the distribution of the fungus within this tortoise's range, and predisposing stressful environmental factors have not yet been identified.[6] As herpetologic studies of wild populations intensify, fungi may well be increasingly identified as a cause of disease in wild reptiles.

SYSTEMIC MYCOSES

Fungal disease also presents as focal or disseminated systemic mycoses, which carry a graver prognosis than dermatomycoses. Clinical signs are nonspecific and range from subclinical infections to animals that are simply found dead. More often, however, a chronic course of intermittent anorexia with progressive weight loss, lethargy, and weakness precedes death. When present, other clinical signs reflect the affected organ system. Pneumonia and disseminated granulomatous disease are the most common manifestations of systemic mycosis in reptiles. The literature suggests that mycotic pneumonia is particularly prevalent in chelonians[2,25,59,61] and in crocodilians.[2,62] Giant Tortoises (*Geochelone* [*Megalochelys*] *gigantea* and *G. elephantopus*) account for a substantial

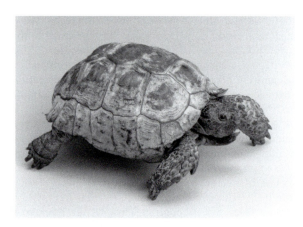

FIGURE 16-5 A Texas Tortoise *(Gopherus berlianderi)* with necrotizing scute disease, a slow and progressive infection of the carapacial scutes caused by *Fusarium semitectum*. (Photograph courtesy F. Rose.)

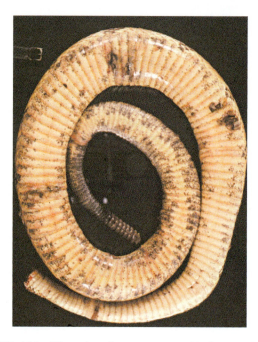

FIGURE 16-7 Ulcerative dermatitis in a Timber Rattlesnake *(Crotalus horridus)*. The lesions developed after the snake came out of its hibernaculum early and faced inclement weather. *Paecilomyces lilacinus* was isolated from skin and liver lesions. (Photograph courtesy K. Coyle.)

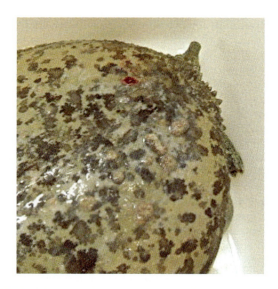

FIGURE 16-6 Brown to tan, granular, raised cutaneous lesions on the shell of an Eastern Spiny Softshell Turtle *(Apalone (Trionyx) s. spiniferus)*. Histology showed a multifocal hyperkeratotic fungal dermatitis, with marked keratolysis and intralesional fungal elements. Culture attempts were unsuccessful. Note the freshly biopsied site. (Photograph courtesy R. Boily.)

number of documented chelonian pulmonary mycoses.[2,25,61] Wheezing, tachypnea, or dyspnea may or may not occur with fungal pneumonia or tracheitis. Lesions in chelonians practically always consist of nodular caseous to firm masses within the pulmonary parenchyma or over the mucosa or serosa. Sometimes, pale plaques or fungal mats are present over tracheal and bronchial mucosae, but rarely is there caseous exudate within air passages unless secondary bacterial pneumonia is present. In severe cases, a whole lung or part of the lung may be consolidated and emphysematous bullae may be observed. In several published cases of chelonian pulmonary mycoses, lesions were also found in the myocardium. *Aspergillus*, *Penicillium*, *Beauveria*, and *Paecilomyces* have been isolated from tortoises. These fungi are extremely prevalent environmental saprobes that probably gain entrance to the lung on a regular basis, and mycosis likely develops exclusively under unfavorable conditions or in immunosuppressed individuals. In seaturtles, hypothermia (cold stunning) leading to immune compromise appears to be a common predisposing factor to systemic mycosis. *Colletotrichum acutatum*, a phytopathogenic fungus, was isolated from the lungs and kidneys of a Kemp's Ridley Seaturtle *(Lepidochelys kempi)*,[63] further illustrating the susceptibility of debilitated seaturtles to severe mycotic disease from opportunistic molds. *Penicillium griseofulvum* caused a systemic mycosis in an Aldabra Tortoise.[64] In crocodilians, pneumonia also presents as multifocal necrotic to granulomatous foci in the substance of the lung. Often, fungal mats cover the surface of air sacs. The same genera as listed for tortoises are associated with pneumonia in crocodilians, along with fungi belonging to *Metarhizium*, *Fusarium*, *Mucor*, and *Acremonium* (formerly *Cephalosporium*).[2,62] *Metarhizium*, *Beauveria*, and *Acremonium* are known insect pathogens with an affinity for chitinous exoskeletons. A repeat offender in crocodilians is *Paecilomyces*, chiefly *P. lilacinus*, isolated in several cases of pneumonia affecting alligators, caimans, and crocodiles.[2,26] *Paecilomyces lilacinus* thrives in the aquatic environment, particularly when water is contaminated or soiled with meat and fat.[13] Regular cleaning of the water and feeding of crocodilians out of the water onto haul-out surfaces may help to reduce its growth in the water and possibly minimize the risk of *Paecilomyces* pneumonia. Although pneumonia has regularly been reported in squamate reptiles, lesions are seldom restricted to the lungs and disseminated fungal infection is more common.[2] Nodules are scattered across viscera and coelomic surfaces (Figure 16-8). Dissemination often represents a late manifestation of untreated dermatomycosis or pulmonary mycosis. Diarrhea, slimy feces, and hematochezia have been associated with rare cases of candidiasis or other

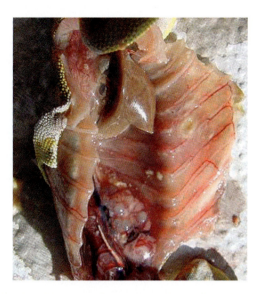

FIGURE 16-8 Disseminated mycosis in a Lesser Chameleon *(Furcifer minor)*. Caseous, tan to yellow plaques are visible in the lung and over the coelomic wall. *(Photograph courtesy B. Strand.)*

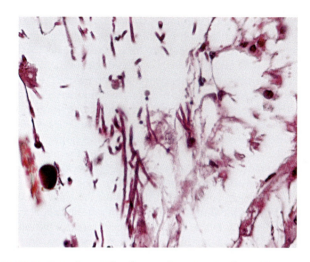

FIGURE 16-9 Fungal hyphae proliferating in the yolk sac of a dead-in-the-egg Mexican Beaded Lizard *(Heloderma horridum)* embryo. A *Fusarium* was isolated from the egg. Periodic acid-Schiff stain, 400×. *(Photograph courtesy H. Simmons.)*

fungal gastrointestinal disease, mostly in squamates.[2,21] In one Green Iguana *(Iguana iguana),* a cystic urolith was associated with fungal cystitis.[20] *Fusarium solani* and *F. oxysporum* were implicated in two cases of ischemic necrosis of the tail in snakes.[65] In reptiles, histologic examination sometimes reveals the presence of hyphae in association with neoplastic lesions,[2,66] but the relationship is unclear.

The dimorphic fungi *Blastomyces dermatitidis, Histoplasma capsulatum, Paracoccidioides brasiliensis,* and *Coccidioides immitis* are primary pathogens of humans and other mammals and are restricted to specific endemic areas. Of these, only *C. immitis* has been documented as causing naturally occurring systemic mycosis in a reptile.[67] Raised, white, 3-mm to 4-mm lesions were present in the lung of a captive Sonoran Gophersnake *(Pituophis catenifer [melanoleucus] affinis)* that died with no premonitory clinical signs. Isolation of *C. immitis* from the lungs and observation of typical thick-walled spherules in histologic sections of the pulmonary lesions left no doubt as to causality.[67] This captive snake was believed to be originally wild caught in the Sonoran desert, an area where *C. immitis* is endemic.[67] Otherwise, experimental infection trials with *C. immitis* in various lizards[68,69] and in rattlesnakes[69] have been inconsistent. The pathogenic yeast *Cryptococcus neoformans,* a cause of pneumonia and meningitis in mammals, has the potential to cause disease in reptiles. A captive Green Anaconda *(Eunectes murinus)* died of granulomatous pneumonia and meningoencephalitis, and budding cells morphologically consistent with *Cryptococcus* were observed histologically within granulomata.[70] Specific fluorescent antibodies were used to confirm that they were *Cryptococcus neoformans.* In the only other documented case of reptilian cryptococcosis, an Eastern Water Skink *(Eulamprus quoyii)* had a discrete subcutaneous swelling develop over the caudal dorsum.[51] Biopsy results disclosed the presence of budding yeasts consistent in morphology with *Cryptococcus.* The subcutaneous mycetoma in this lizard constituted an unusual presentation for cryptococcosis. At necropsy, no other lesions were seen.[51]

The impact of fungi as pathogens of reptilian eggs has received only minimal attention.[2] Causes of embryonic death or poor hatchability in reptiles have not been investigated systematically, but decreased gas exchange from fungal growth over the egg shell has been hypothesized as a cause of embryonic mortality in seaturtles.[71] In ovo embryos may succumb to mycosis, but reptile eggs are often buried or laid among rotting vegetation and therefore appear innately resistant to fungal invasion.[2] Fungi isolated from dead embryos, or from the yolk sacs of egg membranes in rotting eggs, may be secondary invaders. Only when inflammation around fungal elements can be shown histologically in embryo tissue sections can a diagnosis of mycosis be made (Figure 16-9).

DIAGNOSIS

Lesions of dermatomycosis are typically obvious but are nonspecific, and a diagnosis can only be made on the basis of histopathologic examination of a biopsy from a representative, preferably early, lesion. The presence of inflammatory cells around fungal elements attests to the fungus invading living tissue, supporting a primary pathogenic role and ruling out secondary or postmortem invasion of necrotic or dead tissues.[71] Culture of scrapings from cutaneous lesions or, preferably, culture of a biopsy usually grows the causative fungus. The microscopic features of the isolated fungus need to be consistent with the microscopic features of fungal elements identified histologically if it is to be incriminated.[72] This is especially important when culture yields more than one fungal species. Culture of a fungus in the absence of diagnostic elements in scrapings or tissue should be interpreted with caution, and a repeat specimen obtained if a mycosis is strongly suspected. Ideally, reptiles with dermatomycotic lesions should be investigated for the presence of concurrent disseminated fungal disease.

Reptiles with deep or disseminated mycotic disease often present with nonspecific signs such as prolonged or progressive lethargy, poor appetite, and weight loss. A thorough physical examination, a complete blood count, and biochemistry panel, combined with radiographs, echography, and other imaging modalities help detect and locate lesions, which should then be biopsied and cultured. Visceral lesions may be accessed via coeliotomy, laparascopy, or ultrasound-guided fine-needle aspiration. If pulmonary disease is suspected, a transtracheal lung wash with saline solution can easily be performed in most species and the collected fluid submitted for cytology and culture. In the larger reptiles, a small bronchoscope may allow access to the pulmonary lumen and to biopsy lesions. A transcarapacial technique may be used to perform a lung lavage in chelonians and collect cytologic specimens.[73] The most affected lung is selected radiographically, on the basis of a craniocaudal view with a horizontal beam. The same transcarapacial technique may later be used for intrapulmonary instillation of antifungal medication.[73] In ophidians, a technique for pulmonary intraluminal endoscopy through the air sac via a caudal flank approach has been used to visualize lesions and collect biopsies.[74] Stomatitis, or mouth rot, is commonly encountered in reptiles. Culture and cytology of scrapings from oral lesions are always indicated to rule in or dismiss fungal involvement. Culture of a cloacal or rectal swab is also indicated in reptiles with suspected gastrointestinal mycoses, but because reptiles harbor fungi in the digestive tract, results need be interpreted with caution. Cytology of a cloacal or rectal swab is suggestive of intestinal mycosis when fungal hyphal filaments or budding yeasts and, ideally, heterophils and other inflammatory cells are present. Guidelines and instructions as to submission of samples should be obtained from the laboratory before actual collection of specimens to optimize preservation of the samples during shipping.

Cutaneous or systemic lesions should be biopsied with general or local anesthesia. Care is taken to collect the biopsy at the edge of the lesion so that the interface of normal and diseased tissue can be examined histologically. Hematoxylin and eosin (H&E) stain best allows for the demonstration of tissue response to fungal elements, and special stains (e.g., periodic acid-Schiff, Gomori) may be necessary to disclose the presence of hyaline fungi on histopathological examination.[72,75,76] Structures in tissues will vary according to the fungal taxa involved.[72,75,76] Spherical or ovoid budding cells with or without pseudohyphae or capsules are characteristic of yeasts. Although speciation of yeasts is generally not possible on the basis of microscopic morphology in tissue, the presence of oval single budding yeast cells surrounded by a capsule is diagnostic for a *Cryptococcus* species. The hyphae of zygomycetous fungi (e.g., *Absidia*, *Mucor*, *Rhizopus*, or *Syncephalastrum* species) are often found in short segments and within lumina or walls of blood vessels. The hyphae are wide (up to 10 to 12 µm) with uneven walls because of their propensity to collapse, and they often take up the stain rather poorly. The hyphae of other molds are septate and narrow (commonly 2 to 4 µm wide), typically nonpigmented, usually with parallel walls but sometimes showing irregular swellings, and are dichotomously (*Aspergillus* sp.) or randomly branched. Dematiaceous fungi (*Cladosporium*, *Alternaria*, and *Curvularia* sp.) are characterized by brown pigmented hyphae. However, some fungi that are darkly pigmented in culture may show hyaline hyphae in tissue (e.g., *Scedosporium* or *Pseudallescheria*) and then be suggestive of *Aspergillus*. Identifiable spore forms may occasionally be seen. *Fusarium*, *Aspergillus*, *Acremonium*, and other fungi may sporulate in

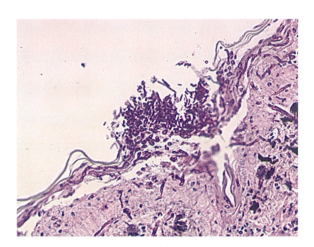

FIGURE 16-10 CANV infection. Fungal proliferation in the epidermis and superficial dermis of a Veiled Chameleon (*Chamaeleo calyptratus*). Note the dense arthroconidial tuft at the epidermal surface. Periodic acid-Schiff stain, 400×.

tissue, usually but not always at the air-tissue interface, allowing for recognition of the etiologic agent at least to the genus. The presence of arthroconidia can be consistent with geotrichosis, but in reptiles, arthroconidia have been repeatedly observed in lesions caused by the CANV (Figure 16-10).[8,10-14]

At necropsy, lesions suggestive of a granulomatous or abscedative process should be submitted for culture. Stained impression smears of the cut surface of lesions may disclose fungal elements. Freezing a portion of representative lesions or select tissues is useful to allow later fungal culture of specimens if clinically unsuspected mycosis is diagnosed histologically. Pathologists may resort to immunohistochemistry or fluorescent antibody techniques to identify fungi in histologic sections, but only if suitable reagents are available.[76] Molecular probes have been developed for the diagnosis of some fungal infections, with use of DNA extraction from clinical specimens followed by polymerase chain reaction (PCR) amplification,[77] but are not commercially available.

The isolation of a fungus from submitted material is sometimes difficult. Treatment of the animal with antifungal drugs, inadequate processing of submitted material, or bacterial contamination may all result in negative culture results, even if the fungal nature of the lesion is clearly shown on histology. Biopsies should therefore be collected before onset of antifungal therapy and be submitted fresh for culture. Alternatively, freezing the sample until shipment is acceptable and does not typically affect the viability of the fungus. Bacterial contamination can be minimized with treatment of the submitted material in an acidified broth or dipping it in a wide spectrum antibiotic suspension before inoculation. Antibiotics are also present in some commercially available selective fungal culture media but are not always sufficient to prevent bacterial growth. Recovery of a fungus may also be hampered by the presence of fast-growing contaminants, such as aspergilla and zygomycetes, that quickly overrun slower growing fungi. This can be avoided by including a medium containing cycloheximide, a compound that completely inhibits or severely restricts the growth of these contaminants.

Identification of fungal isolates from specimens should ideally always be carried out to the species. This is especially important in gaining a better understanding of the fungi involved in reptile disease. Isolation of the same fungal species from multiple animals with fungal disease carries a different meaning than isolation of fungi belonging to the same genus or order. A number of factors make identification to species difficult. As with bacterial classification, many recent changes have occurred in fungal classification. Genera and species are being reexamined with molecular and other approaches, sometimes resulting in taxonomic changes or discovery of new species not yet described in standard texts. In culture, many fungi adopt remarkably distinct morphologies under different growth conditions. Sometimes challenging is determination of whether these morphologies represent the same or different species. Mesophilic saprophytic fungi that would be ruled out as agents of mammalian mycoses are not uncommonly isolated from reptile material. These factors result in medical laboratories sometimes being unable to identify or speciate a fungal isolate, or worse, misidentifying it. One is prudent to forward unspeciated and unknown isolates to mycologists so that progress in understanding reptile mycoses may be achieved. Ideally, all reptile fungal isolates reasonably incriminated in reptile mycosis should be deposited in a publicly available culture collection to ensure that they remain available for later studies.

THERAPY

Because fungal disease in reptiles is almost always secondary to some form of immune suppression, investigation of reptiles diagnosed with mycosis for underlying disease and critical assessment of captive conditions for any perceived inadequacy are crucial. Nonspecific supportive measures such as fluid therapy and thermal and nutritional support are practically always indicated. Antibiotics are given if an underlying or concurrent bacterial disease is suspected. Concurrent vitamin A supplementation has been advocated, chiefly in chelonians.[18] Treatment of mycosis in a reptile may be prolonged because of the chronicity of the disease and the state of debilitation of the animal by the time of diagnosis. Patients should be monitored for possible adverse reactions to antifungal drugs by means of close observation for new clinical signs and serial blood sampling for complete blood counts and serum biochemistry. Maintaining reptiles within and preferably toward the higher spectrum of the species' optimal (preferred) temperature range is likely to hasten recovery and may impede the growth of fungal species that exhibit limited thermotolerance such as the CANV, most isolates of which do not grow at 35°C. Ideally, patients should be examined thoroughly before medications are discontinued. Currently no guidelines exist as to how long antifungal therapy should be administered, in the absence of adverse effects. Lesions may take weeks or months to regress.[11,18] The decision to stop is left to the clinician and is made on the basis of complete regression of lesions. Treatment for an additional 2 weeks to cover for persistent but clinically undetectable lesions or disease may be advisable.

Treatment of dermatomycoses depends somewhat on the presentation. Contrary to dermatophytosis in mammals, reptile fungal skin infection is rarely restricted to the epidermis. Lesions of dermatomycosis may be solitary but are

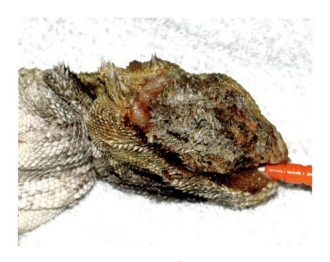

FIGURE 16-11 Hyperkeratosis, with epidermal necrosis covering the right aspect of the face of an inland Bearded Dragon (*Pogona vitticeps*). The CANV was isolated in pure culture from biopsy material. *(Photograph courtesy J. Paré.)*

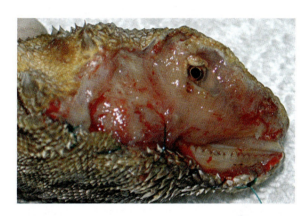

FIGURE 16-12 Same lizard as in Figure 16-11, after surgical debridement and cleansing of the lesion. *(Photograph courtesy J. Paré.)*

more often multiple. If solitary, cutaneous lesions are best addressed surgically. A wide-margined excision is preferred, and systemic antifungals are administered. Lesions may be too numerous or extensive to be amenable to excision, so that medical treatment with topical and systemic antifungal therapy is the only option. In such cases, and because epidermal lesions are often necrotic or hyperkeratotic, with fungal elements extending to the subjacent dermis and musculature, topical treatment alone is bound to fail. Removal of epidermal debris and adherent sloughed or necrotic skin, debridement, and cleansing of the resulting wound are essential before institution of topical therapy (Figures 16-11, 16-12, and 16-13). Even then, however, topically administered compounds may not penetrate deeply enough to reach affected muscles or bones, and therefore, combined topical and systemic antifungal therapy is advocated. In farming or captive rearing situations where animals are too numerous to be treated individually, overcrowding and other stressors should first be eliminated. Medicated food may be used as long as palatability is not altered, or in the case of aquatic chelonians, medication may be mixed with the tub water. Dry-docking

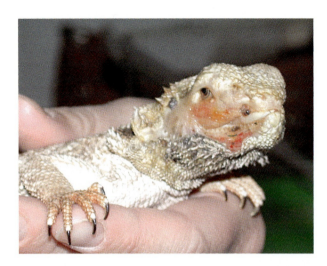

FIGURE 16-13 Same lizard as in Figure 16-11, after 5 weeks of systemic itraconazole and topical silver sulphadiazine. *(Photograph courtesy J. Paré.)*

of pond turtles for a few hours daily may discourage the growth of aquatic molds and allow wound cleansing and more effective topical treatment of fungal skin lesions.

Pulmonary and deep mycoses are rarely amenable to exeresis and are best addressed through aggressive systemic antifungal therapy, ideally on the basis of in vitro sensitivity testing. Transcarapacial intraluminal instillation of antifungal medication has been described in chelonians, and nebulization with amphothericin or other antifungal drugs may be useful. Lesions are usually too numerous or the animal too weak to contemplate surgery. Prolonged systemic antifungal therapy may be the only practical option and may allow for stabilization of the patient for eventual surgical excision or debulking of visceral lesions, should it be considered. Ophthalmic mycoses, typically reported in snakes, have responded to little else but enucleation.[78,79] Mycotic disease that affects the oropharyngeal mucosa or the gastrointestinal tract can be treated with orally administered antifungal agents. Because it is not absorbed systemically, nystatin is the drug of choice in such cases. Chlorhexidine-based solutions may also be used for oral candidiasis.

A number of antifungal drugs are available to the clinician,[80] but very few have been evaluated in even fewer reptile species. Fungi are eukaryotic organisms, with cellular structure and physiology more similar to those of vertebrates than the prokaryotic bacteria. Antifungal drugs therefore generally carry a lower therapeutic index than most antibacterial drugs. Because mycoses are seldom diagnosed ante mortem, treatment with antifungals has rarely been reported in the literature. For dermatomycoses, soaks in dilute organic iodine solution, alone or in combination with topical nystatin, enilconazole, miconazole, or tolnaftate, have yielded varying results. Malachite green in the water has been used to treat aquatic turtles with dermatomycosis. Griseofulvin failed to bring any improvement in two snakes with dermatomycosis, possibly because lesions in these snakes were not confined to the epidermal stratum corneum.

The systemic drugs of choice for use in reptiles include ketoconazole, itraconazole, and fluconazole. Oral administration of ketoconazole to Gopher Tortoises (*Gopherus polyphemus*),[81] of itraconazole to Spiny Lizards (*Sceloporus* sp.)[82] and Kemp's Ridley Seaturtles,[83] and fluconazole to Loggerhead Seaturtles[84] yielded therapeutic serum levels or adequate tissue concentrations, suggesting the same can be achieved in other reptile species. Given the broad spectrum of the triazoles, and low toxicity when compared with other antifungals, their use appears justified. Of the three, ketoconazole is associated with more side effects in mammals, and its spectrum of activity offers no advantage over itraconazole. Fluconazole remains an excellent choice against yeasts but has virtually no activity against filamentous fungi and as such should not be used when infections with *Aspergillus*, *Paecilomyces*, the CANV, or any mold are suspected. Itraconazole is currently the drug of choice in reptiles diagnosed with infection caused by a filamentous fungus. Ideally, in vitro susceptibility testing dictates the use of one over the other. This has long been the standard of practice for yeast infections in human medicine. For example, *Candida krusei*, increasingly involved in cases of candidiasis in immunocompromised humans, is inherently resistant to fluconazole and warrants the use of other antifungal drugs. Testing of filamentous fungi isolates for in vitro susceptibility has become available and may prove extremely useful in selection of the right antifungal treatment. All molds are not alike in their susceptibility pattern. Most *Fusarium* species, for example, and zygomycetous fungi (e.g., *Mucor*) are resistant to available azoles. *Paecilomyces* isolates may also be resistant. A newer azole, voriconazole, is now available and has extended activity against various molds, including fusaria, but has not been used yet in reptiles. Terbinafine is an allyamine compound with a wide spectrum of activity that is safely and successfully used in the treatment of onychomycoses and dematophytoses in children, and its use in reptiles is worthy of investigation. Other novel antifungals such as ravuconazole, posaconazole, echinocandins, and chitin synthase inhibitors may in the future prove to be useful but are as of yet unproven, and the development of newer formulations of current antifungal drugs, such as liposomal amphotericin and intravenous itraconazole, opens unexplored avenues for treatment of mycoses in reptiles.

CONCLUSION

Clinicians need to maintain a higher index of suspicion for mycosis when confronted with a patient with cutaneous lesions or clinical signs of nonspecific systemic illness. Only through fungal cultures and histopathologic examination of biopsies can a diagnosis of fungal disease be truly established or dismissed. The epidemiology of fungal infection in reptiles is still poorly understood, and more work is needed to determine both the factors and the conditions that lead to onset of disease and the scope of fungi that are potential etiologic agents. The deposit of case isolates from published reports into public culture collections allows for reexamination of unspeciated isolates, for strain typing of common isolates, or for reevaluation of the taxonomy.

BACTERIAL DISEASES

Karen L. Rosenthal and Douglas R. Mader

Infectious diseases, as a group, are one of the largest causes of morbidity and mortality in reptiles. Many of these diseases can be treated successfully if recognized in time. Infectious disease is almost always the result of immunosuppression in reptiles,[85] and this is often associated with the stress of captivity. Gram-negative bacterial infections from parasitism are known to occur.[86] Management and husbandry problems are often at the root of the problem, but knowledge of microbiology is an essential aid to the husbandry of captive reptiles.[87]

Gram-negative bacteria are the most common bacterial pathogens.[88-91] This fact is not surprising because gram-negative bacteria are common isolates in healthy reptiles.[92] Gram-positive bacteria are infrequently associated with disease.[93] *Salmonella* spp., ubiquitous reptilian bacteria, have been cultured from more than 90% of selected reptile colonies.[94] In addition, anaerobic bacteria and pathogenic fungi may be important components of reptilian disease.

DIAGNOSTIC TECHNIQUES

Gram Stain

The Gram stain is an underutilized, convenient, and inexpensive procedure. While one is waiting for the results of bacterial culture and sensitivity testing, a Gram stain is used to identify and quantitate the presence of gram-positive and gram-negative bacteria collected from the site of infection. In addition, fungal and yeast elements can be identified. This information allows the clinician to formulate a presumptive diagnosis to initiate therapy. For example, if gram-negative bacteria predominate, antibiotics effective against negatives should be chosen.

In the event that the culture is lost or the results indicate no growth, the Gram stain provides a record of the type of microbes that were present at the culture site before treatment. The results also provide the microbiologist with information crucial to identifying pathogens and selecting appropriate culture media. Finally, if clients cannot afford microbiologic culture and sensitivity testing, Gram stain results assist the clinician toward empirical antimicrobial selection.

Miscellaneous Staining

In addition to the Gram stain, two other techniques could prove helpful to the clinician. Acid-fast and periodic acid-Schiff staining for the detection of mycobacteria and fungi, respectively, should be submitted at the same time that a specimen is submitted for microbiologic culture and sensitivity testing. Both of these organisms grow slowly in their respective media, and positive staining results allow the clinician to recommend appropriate treatment long before culture results are available.

Sampling Techniques

Proper specimen collection is the key to identification of the pathogen and, therefore, diagnosis of an infectious disease. Improperly collected samples may lead to erroneous results and the wrong choice of an antimicrobial. Although swabs are the most convenient commonly used device for specimen collection, they provide the poorest conditions for survival and transport of microbes. A swab should not be submitted if fluid, purulent discharge, or infected tissue is otherwise available. Swabs are most effective when premoistened with sterile nonbacteriostatic saline solution before sampling. After thorough swabbing of infected areas, the inoculated swab should be protected in a suitable transport medium.

A minimum of 5 to 10 mL of infected fluid or tissue is an optimum volume for proper testing. Tissue is transported in sterile saline solution. In collection of limited amounts of fluid or purulent exudate, the site is irrigated with a small amount of sterile nonbactericidal saline or lactated Ringer's solution.

Blood

Blood cultures are warranted if septicemia is suspected. The skin should be disinfected with alcohol and air dried for 30 seconds (Figure 16-14). Both aerobic and anaerobic cultures can be obtained from a minimum sample size of 0.5 to 1 mL of blood with a pediatric lysis-centrifugation tube.[95]

Skin and Body Surfaces

Sampling discharges from the nasal or oral cavities is not recommended. These specimens contain inflammatory exudates that have passed through anatomic locations known to be colonized with normal flora. As a result, cultures often reveal a mixed growth of bacteria, which leads to misinterpretation of the true pathogen.

For dermatophytes, the skin should be precleansed with alcohol to decrease the likelihood of bacterial contamination

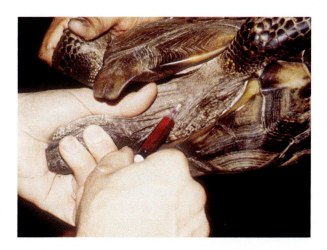

FIGURE 16-14 Blood cultures are underutilized in reptilian medicine. The skin should be disinfected with alcohol and air dried for 30 seconds. Both aerobic and anaerobic cultures can be done from a minimum sample size of 0.5 to 1 mL of blood with a pediatric lysis-centrifugation tube. (*Photograph courtesy D. Mader.*)

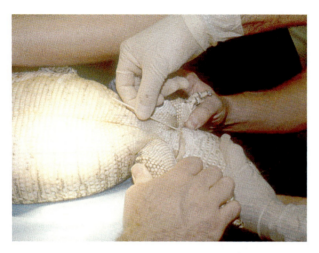

FIGURE 16-15 Placement of a sterile swab into the cloaca or rectum of a patient is sure to produce a plethora of bacterial growth. Distinguishing the normal from the pathogenic flora can be hard because of overlap in normal flora and opportunists. *(Photograph courtesy D. Mader.)*

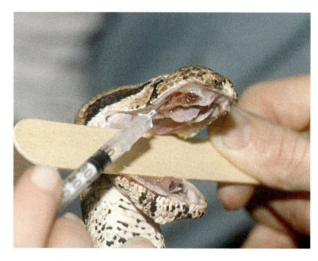

FIGURE 16-16 Culturing from deep within the affected site, as opposed to sampling from superficial tissues, results in a more accurate assessment of the bacteria involved in the abscess. Here a small amount of sterile saline solution is injected and massaged into the lesion; then the aspirate is used for bacterial culture and sensitivity testing. *(Photograph courtesy D. Mader.)*

of the fungal culture medium. This is essential if ointments or creams have been used. A better chance of successful fungal culture exists if the site is scraped rather than swabbed.

Open abscesses are debrided and specimens taken from deep within the lesion, preferably from the lining or capsule of the lesion (see Chapter 42). Closed abscesses are sampled with aspiration of material with sterile technique. Cystic and vesicular fluid is cultured in a similar manner.

Gastrointestinal Tract

A common practice is to culture both the oral cavity and the cloaca. This is often called a "combo culture" and is used as a screening tool. Although this method may be easy, it does not always give specific information regarding bacterial pathogens. Oral cavity flora is a reflection of environmental bacteria. Although the actual pathogen might be included in the culture sample, it may be obscured by a myriad of other incidental microorganisms. A similar problem is encountered in random culture of the cloacal region.

Placement of a sterile swab into the cloaca or rectum of a patient is sure to produce a plethora of bacterial growth (Figure 16-15). Distinguishing the normal from the pathogenic flora can be difficult because of overlap in normal flora and opportunists (see subsequent). In addition, practitioners may commonly get a "no growth" result when these samples have been submitted. This is a sign of obvious sample mishandling or laboratory error because a sterile cloaca is impossible.

Site-specific bacterial sampling is preferable to random sampling. Snakes with infectious stomatitis benefit from appropriate antimicrobial therapy on the basis of proper bacterial isolation. However, a specimen collected with swabbing a culturette over the affected gingiva yields a mixed bag of oral cavity and environmental flora. A gram-negative isolate is almost always found, but its significance is nebulous at best. A better technique is to prepare the area with alcohol or similar antiseptic, make a small stab incision through the infected area with a no. 11 scalpel blade, and then, with either a syringe or a premoistened microculturette swab, sample the affected tissue from within the incision (Figure 16-16). A pathogen isolated in this manner has far greater clinical significance.

Cloacal cultures may be warranted and are occasionally performed in patients with diarrhea or other gastrointestinal signs. Proper diagnostics, such as fecal examinations for ova and parasites including protozoal pathogens, should always be done before bacterial cultures. Interpretation of the culture results can be confusing because many different bacteria are normally present. However, certain isolates in large numbers should be cause for immediate concern (discussed subsequently).

Respiratory Tract

Proper sampling is imperative in patients that display respiratory signs. Again, random culturing of the saliva or tracheal exudate within the oral cavity is nondiagnostic. If time and cost restraints are imposed, the preferable sampling site is high within the choanal slit. Because this is juxtaposed to the opening of the glottis, a true pathogen is more likely to be found (Figure 16-17).

A preferred technique is to perform a tracheal wash. An appropriately sized, sterile, red-rubber catheter is inserted transglottally and directed into the lung (Figure 16-18; also see Figure 65-11, *A-F*). Sterile saline solution (approximately 1% of the patient's body weight) is infused through the catheter. The patient is then gently inverted, rolled side to side, or in some way rocked to allow mixing and washing of the saline solution within the lung, then as much fluid as possible is withdrawn. Not uncommon is a return of only a small portion of the infused saline solution. One should not be alarmed if all the fluid is not retrieved. Any remaining fluid is readily absorbed through the lungs. Occasionally, in cases of severe pneumonia, quantities greater than the amount infused are retrieved. The fluid collected is used for both cytologic examination and bacterial culture and sensitivity testing.

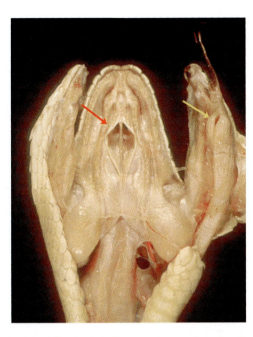

FIGURE 16-17 The glottis *(yellow arrow)* opens from the floor of the oral cavity into the choana *(red arrow)* on the dorsal surface of the mouth. This prosected snake head shows the relationship between these two important anatomic locations. If culture of the lungs or the trachea is not possible, high within the choanal slit is the next best alternative. *(Photograph courtesy D. Mader.)*

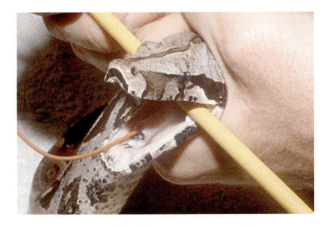

FIGURE 16-18 Retrieval of only a small amount of the fluid infused during the lung wash is not uncommon. This fluid can now be used for cytologic examination and microbial culture and sensitivity testing. *(Photograph courtesy D. Mader.)*

Sample Handling

Proper handling after a specimen has been collected is most important so that the laboratory is given the best opportunity to culture pathogenic microorganisms. The following are general rules and guidelines for the handling and transportation of microbiologic specimens. Each laboratory has its own requirements, and one should be familiar with these before specimens are collected.

Laboratory samples are routinely submitted in one of three ways—in the container in which it was collected

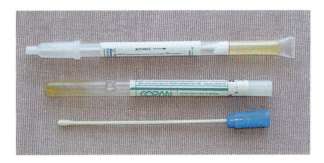

FIGURE 16-19 Appropriate transport media should be used when shipping to a diagnostic laboratory. Most transport media are buffered fluid or semisolid media with addition of minimally required nutrients. Once the transport medium has been inoculated, it must be allowed to remain at room temperature for approximately one half hour to establish growth or provide nutrients to the bacteria before it is refrigerated. *(Photograph courtesy D. Mader.)*

(e.g., syringe), in transport media, or directly inoculated onto a plate. Specimens collected in a sterile syringe and needle can be sent directly to the laboratory in the same syringe. Handling of the specimen is kept to a minimum, which decreases the chances of sample contamination. Transit time to the laboratory is critical because no support medium is in the syringe. The specimen may desiccate, killing the collected microbes.

Appropriate transport media should be used in shipping to a diagnostic laboratory (Figure 16-19). Most transport media are buffered fluid or semisolid media with addition of minimally required nutrients. Their function is to sustain the microbes in the sample until it is plated, and thus, they are designed to prevent drying, maintain a neutral pH, and support minimal growth or prevent death. Most transport media allow anaerobes to survive in the depths of the liquid or semisolid media. The best transport media for anaerobes include a reducing agent such as thioglycolate. Once the transport medium has been inoculated, it must be allowed to remain at room temperature for approximately one half hour to establish growth or provide nutrients to the bacteria before it is refrigerated. Refrigeration helps decrease growth so that bacterial colonies do not outgrow the transport medium.

Specimens can be inoculated onto a media plate immediately after they are taken from the patient. This bypasses the transport media step and is the most efficient process for rapid identification of bacterial pathogens. A disadvantage to this method is that if the plate does not reach the laboratory within a short period of time, the plate may be overgrown with bacterial colonies and identification of a pathogen may not be possible. This method may also be cost prohibitive for many clinicians because it requires that different types of media be available in the clinic. If an anaerobe is suspected, an anaerobic environment (e.g., a candle jar) must be provided. Also, plastic petri dishes are not suitable for mailing.

Certain organisms require specialized transport media. *Salmonella* spp. are best sent to the laboratory in an enrichment medium such as selenite broth or tetrathionate.[96] *Mycobacterium* spp. can be cultured from normal transport media, but the clinician should check with the laboratory before submitting specimens. *Mycoplasma* spp. and

Ureaplasma spp. can be cultured from bacterial transport media, but use of specialized enrichment broth is best for transport if these bacteria are suspected.

Contact the clinical laboratory for proper instructions. Most laboratories provide these specialized collection media if requested.

Selection of Culture Media

The clinician must anticipate the type of pathogen that might be isolated from the cultured area. You do not find what you do not culture for. Meaning, if one does not ask for a salmonella or anaerobic culture, one will not find these organisms. FOR ALL REPTILE PATIENTS, ALWAYS ASK FOR SALMONELLA! Studies have shown that in some reptilian collections more than 93% of the animals may harbor *Salmonella* spp.[10]

In the clinical laboratory, a common practice is placement of a sample in a nutrient broth. Broth selects for and detects small numbers of bacteria and allows nonselective growth of both aerobes and anaerobes.

Laboratory samples may also be inoculated onto media plates. Unlike broth, media plates facilitate rapid isolation of pure colonies. Good communication between the veterinarian and the laboratory is essential at this point. A history and a list of suspected pathogens aid the laboratory in selection of the appropriate plate media to inoculate. Hundreds of media are used by laboratories, but only a few are used on a routine basis. Blood agar plates are useful for growing most microorganisms and are also used to identify pathogenic *Streptococcus* spp. (Figure 16-20). Chocolate agar plates are used for growth of fastidious bacteria. MacConkey agar plates inhibit the growth of gram-positive organisms while simultaneously selecting for the gram-negative bacteria. Brilliant green MacConkey agar has been suggested as the best selective medium for *Salmonella* spp. growth.[96] Anaerobic media are partially composed of reducing agents and are kept in a low oxygen environment. Typically, aminoglycosides are also added to inhibit the growth of aerobic bacteria.

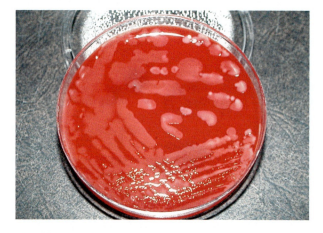

FIGURE 16-20 Blood agar plates are useful for growing most microorganisms, including gram-negative bacteria, and are also used to identify pathogenic *Streptococcus* spp. *(Photograph courtesy K. Rosenthal.)*

INITIAL THERAPEUTICS: WHAT TO DO WHILE CULTURE AND SENSITIVITY DATA ARE PENDING

That most bacterial pathogens of reptiles are gram-negative bacteria has been well established. Proper bacterial isolation and subsequent evaluation of the resulting laboratory data can be somewhat confusing. The practice of treatment of all patients from which gram-negative bacteria has been isolated is no longer acceptable because many reptiles harbor gram-negative bacteria as part of the normal flora. These microbes are either commensal or opportunistic. The decision to treat or not to treat depends on many factors, including the source of the isolate, the type of patient, the patient's physical and clinical condition, the pharmaceuticals available, owner compliance, experience of the clinician, and, of course, the isolate itself.[97]

Common practice is the collection of a specimen for bacterial culture, and then while one awaits the results, the patient is started on an empirically selected antibiotic. This practice is prudent because it gives the clinician a head start in treatment. See Chapter 36 for guidelines.

Interpretation of Culture Results

When the culture results are available, correlation of the culture results with the response to treatment is important. If the patient is not responding favorably, the laboratory data can be used to help modify the therapeutics. The two areas of the culture results that must be evaluated are the quantitative results and the antibiotic sensitivity patterns.

Reporting of the laboratory culture results in quantitative terms is useful. Quantitation is used to differentiate between the normal flora and the pathogens. This is especially true in reptilian clinical microbiology because gram-negative bacteria are normally part of that indigenous flora. Isolation of organisms from the normal flora in a disease outbreak is most difficult to interpret because determination of whether the organism is causing clinical disease or is only a secondary invader is not always possible.[87] Sometimes the only indication that a bacterial infection is the cause of disease is heavy growth of bacteria that are normally present in smaller numbers. In reptiles, gram-negative bacteria are part of the resident flora, but during times of illness (e.g., pneumonia), the numbers of these bacteria rise significantly. This may be reported by the laboratory as moderate to heavy growth. This is useful in determining whether an organism should be considered a pathogen. A common organism found in low numbers may not be the cause of an infection. A common organism found in large numbers in a sick reptile may be important.

The clinician should request that bacterial sensitivity results be reported as mean inhibitory concentrations (MIC) in addition to the traditional information on sensitivity and resistance to antibiotics. An MIC is a quantitative measurement of the concentration of antibiotic in the patient's serum necessary to inhibit the growth of the bacteria.

The antibiotic disc diffusion method is the older method of determination of antibiotic sensitivity and is based on human clinical data. This does not indicate the degree of susceptibility that the cultured bacteria has to different antibiotics.

If the clinician knows the range of serum concentrations for an antibiotic that corresponds to the dosage used, then MIC data can be better used and the drug dosed more rationally. Thus, MIC data allow the clinician to select not only a sensitive antibiotic but, specifically, the most sensitive.

The MIC results are reported as an actual number. If the number is low for a certain antibiotic, a comparatively low concentration of that antibiotic is needed to inhibit bacterial growth, and the antibiotic may be a good choice for treatment. If the number is high for a certain antibiotic, achievement of the necessary serum concentration of that antibiotic necessary to inhibit growth of the bacteria may be impossible. The highest achievable concentration of an antibiotic in a patient is independent of culture results and depends on the volume of distribution and clearance time of the antibiotic in the patient.

The value of use of MIC results is that the clinician can tailor the dosage of the antibiotic to the sensitivity of the specific pathogen and not have to generalize treatment rationale to a type of bacteria. If the MIC number is relatively low in the sensitivity range for that antibiotic, then the antibiotic may be effective at a lower dosage than if the MIC number were higher. A result that just says "sensitive" does not tell the clinician how sensitive. Thus, use of MIC data allows a clinician to avoid prescribing an antibiotic in the high end of the dosage range when a smaller dosage might be as effective. This is important with potentially toxic drugs such as the aminoglycosides. For example, *Proteus penneri* is cultured from an abscess in a box turtle. The MIC for amikacin is less than 0.5 µg/mL, and the MIC for gentamicin is 8 µg/mL. Both would be reported as sensitive according to the older system, but amikacin is shown to be the better choice on the basis of MIC values. *Pseudomonas aeruginosa* is cultured from a bite wound in a snake and a bite wound in an iguana. Piperacillin is reported as sensitive in both cases, but the MIC for piperacillin for the *Pseudomonas* infection in the snake are less than 8 µg/mL and in the Iguana is 16 µg/mL. From these MIC data, clearly the bacteria cultured from the snake is more sensitive to the effects of piperacillin, and a lower dosage can be used. Within an expected MIC range of an antibiotic, a smaller number is more desirable than a larger number. In a situation in which MIC data for two drugs are the same, the antibiotic choice should be for the drug that is less expensive, easier to administer, and less toxic.

Interpretation of "No Growth" Sample Results

A number of factors explain why a "no growth" occurs out of a sample collected from an obviously infected site. A study of the bacterial flora of ill reptiles revealed that approximately 50% of cultured specimens yielded anaerobic bacteria.[98] This could account for laboratory results of "no growth" if anaerobic culture is not requested.

"No growth" reports also occur as a result of submission of an inoculated swab on which the bacteria die before it arrives at the laboratory for plating. If a sample is taken from an aggressive infection, collection of too much bacteria is actually possible. When this happens, the bacteria grow so fast in the transport tube that they actually outgrow the food supply and die. Another problem with sampling large abscesses is that the center of the abscess may be necrotic, and essentially sterile (Figure 16-21). Sampling from the center of a large abscess or fluid pocket may not be of any diagnostic value. Other possibilities include prolonged storage, overheating of the specimen, inappropriate or outdated culture media, and laboratory error.

MICROORGANISMS

The following section refers to Table 16-1.

Gram-Positive Isolates

Most gram-positive bacteria are not considered pathogenic in reptiles. They are common inhabitants, especially of the skin. However, some gram-positive bacteria can cause disease. A report identified *Corynebacterium* sp. as a cause of a liver abscess in a Desert Tortoise (*Gopherus agassizii*).[99]

Coagulase-positive staphylococci are usually pathogenic (Figure 16-22). The production of coagulase and pathogenicity has a 95% correlation. Treatment should be considered in any reptile that has clinical signs and has had coagulase-positive staphylococci cultured from its lesion.

Streptococci are grouped by the ability to hemolyze blood agar. The two main types of hemolysis are alpha and beta. More than 90% of beta-hemolytic streptococci are pathogenic; thus, treatment should be considered whenever this type is present. *Streptococcus* sp. has been implicated as one cause of osteoarthritis of the spine in snakes.[100]

All gram-positive bacteria have the potential to be pathogenic, especially in an immune-compromised animal. Treatment should be considered when the patient does not respond to therapy for gram-negative bacteria or when an infection is present but no gram-negative bacteria are cultured. For example, a report exists of three Emerald Monitors (*Varanus prasinus*) with fatal septicemia caused by *Streptococcus agalactiae*.[101] This organism may have come from the feeder mice. Anytime a coagulase-positive staphylococcus or a beta-hemolytic streptococcus is cultured, treatment, as directed by MIC results, should be considered.

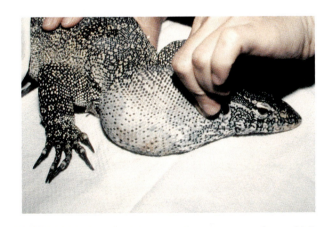

FIGURE 16-21 Samples taken from large abscesses often yield "no growth." The large abscesses can have necrotic, sterile centers. Alternately, if too many bacteria are added to the transport media, they may overgrow the nutrients available and kill the sample before it gets to the laboratory to be plated. (*Photograph courtesy K. Rosenthal.*)

Table 16-1	Common Bacterial Isolates, Pathogenicity, and Antimicrobials Recommended for Treatment	
Organism	Pathogenic	Antibiotic of Choice
Acinetobacter spp.	+++	F
Actinobacillus spp.	+++	A,F
Aeromonas spp.	++++	A
Bacteroides spp.	+++	P,C,M,Az
Chlamydophila spp.	+++	D,Az
Citrobacter freundii	++++	A,F
Clostridium spp.	+++	P,C,M
Corynebacterium spp.	++++	P,C
Edwardsiella spp.	+++	A,F
Enterobacter spp.	+++	A,F
Escherichia coli	++	A
Klebsiella spp.	++++	A,C
Micrococcus spp.	No	Nn
Morganella spp.	++++	A,F
Mycobacterium	++++	Tx NOT recommended
Mycoplasma spp.	+++	F,D,Az
Pasteurella spp.	+++	F
Proteus spp.	++++	F
Providencia spp.	+++	A
Pseudomonas spp.	++++	A,C
Salmonella spp.	? to ++++	Treatment questionable
Serratia spp.	++++	A
Staphylococcus spp. (coagulase positive)	+++	F,C,Az
Staphylococcus spp. (coagulase negative)	No	Nn
Streptococcus spp. (alpha-hemolytic)	No	Nn
Streptococcus spp. (beta-hemolytic)	+++	F,C,Az

+++, Pathogenic; *No*, not pathogenic; *+ to +++*, opportunistic to varying degrees of pathogenicity; *F*, fluoroquinolone; *A*, aminoglycoside; *P*, penicillin; *C*, cephalosporin; *M*, metronidazole; *Az*, azithromycin; *D*, doxycycline or tetracycline; *Nn*, none needed; *Tx*, treatment.

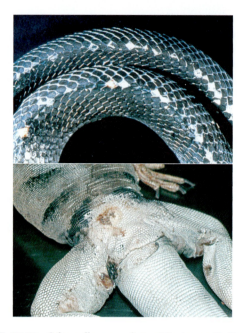

FIGURE 16-23 *Salmonella* spp. dermatitis in an Indigo Snake (*Drymarchon couperi*; top) and Green Iguana (*Iguana iguana*; bottom). (Photograph courtesy D. Mader.)

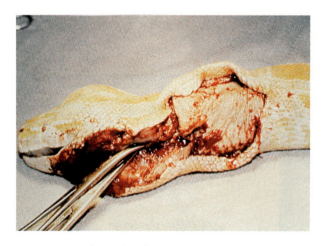

FIGURE 16-22 This python had a severe coagulase-positive infection develop after a traumatic wound was sutured with nonsterile technique. *(Photograph courtesy D. Mader.)*

Gram-Negative Isolates

Salmonella

Most serotypes of *Salmonella* spp. and the *Salmonella arizonae* group (formerly *Arizona arizonae*) are considered pathogenic (see Chapter 68).[102] Variations in the lipopolysaccharide structure confer different degrees of virulence to each serotype and also help define each serotype.[103] Many reptiles harbor these organisms as part of their normal flora, and interpretation of their presence can be difficult.[104,105] Animals affected (as opposed to merely carrying the organism) with salmonella bacteria usually do not show clinical signs. Rather, they may present as poor doers or die acutely. Recently, a report showed that salmonella was cultured from bone and blood from six of 15 snakes with bacterial vertebral disease.[100] One overt clinical sign that the authors have noticed is a weeping, crusting, vesicular dermatitis in both lizards and snakes (Figure 16-23). This group of bacteria has public health importance because of the zoonotic potential (see Chapter 79).[106]

Pseudomonas

Pseudomonas spp., especially *P. aeruginosa*, are commonly found as part of the normal flora in the oral cavity and intestinal tracts of reptiles.[87,104,107,108] As such, they are often considered opportunistic pathogens. Poor husbandry, including suboptimal environmental temperature and malnutrition, can predispose reptiles to *Pseudomonas* infections. *Pseudomonas* spp. are frequently isolated from lesions associated with ulcerative stomatitis (see Figure 72-10), pneumonia, dermatitis, and septicemia (Figure 16-24).[109] Healthy reptiles from which *Pseudomonas* spp. are cultured in light numbers from the oral cavity or gastrointestinal tract probably need not be treated. However, a pure culture of *Pseudomonas* spp. from a lung wash is considered significant, and treatment is warranted.

Aeromonas

Aeromonas spp. are associated with pneumonia, lesions of the oral cavity, cutaneous lesions, and septicemia (Figures 16-25

Microbiology: Fungal and Bacterial Diseases of Reptiles 233

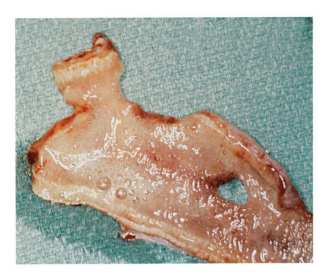

FIGURE 16-24 Chronic *Pseudomonas aeruginosa* pneumonia in a prosected lung. Note the heavy, thick, edematous appearance of the lung tissue (compare with Figures 10-13 and 10-14). *(Photograph courtesy D. Mader.)*

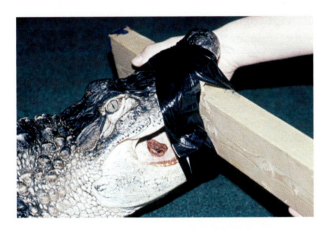

FIGURE 16-25 *Aeromonas hydrophila* was cultured from this lingual lesion. Treatment failed in spite of sensitivity data that supported the choice of antibiotics. After sedation and thorough examination, a small wooden foreign body was found imbedded in the tissue. Once removed, recovery was uneventful. *(Photograph courtesy S. Barten.)*

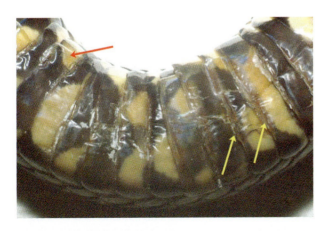

FIGURE 16-26 "Blister disease," or vesicular dermatitis, in a Florida Kingsnake (*Lampropeltis getulus floridana*) caused by *Aeromonas* sp. These bacteria may be carried from snake to snake by the mite *Ophionyssus natricis*. *(Photograph courtesy D. Mader.)*

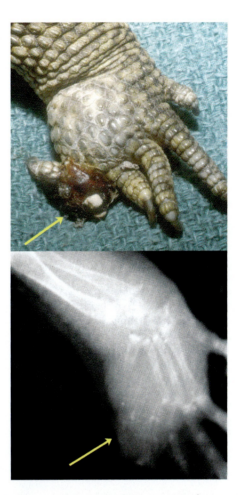

FIGURE 16-27 Caseated abscess *(yellow arrow)* in the foot of a lizard *(top)*. This was induced from bite trauma. Radiograph shows severe lysis of the affected digits *(yellow arrow; bottom)*. The culture revealed a pure growth of *Serratia marcescens*. *(Photograph courtesy D. Mader.)*

and 16-26).[110] *Aeromonas* spp. have been found in the oral cavity of snakes.[111] The snake mite, *Ophionyssus natricis*, is a vector of these bacteria. *Aeromonas* spp. isolated from healthy animals in light numbers may be part of the normal flora.[87,107,112] However, if growth is significant or in patients with clinical signs, treatment should be considered.

Serratia

Serratia spp. are part of the normal flora of the oral cavity in reptiles.[113] They are commonly isolated from cutaneous lesions and appear to be introduced by traumatic events, such as bite wounds. Cutaneous infection with *Serratia* spp. typically causes caseated abscesses that require surgical curettage and antibiotic therapy for resolution (Figure 16-27).

Providencia

Providencia spp. are commonly isolated from the oral cavity of healthy snakes. These are believed to be opportunistic pathogens. In a group of thermally stressed American Alligators (*Alligator mississippiensis*), *Providencia rettgeri* caused septicemia and meningoencephalitis.[114] In this outbreak, approximately 30% of the more than 1000 animals died before treatment was instituted. Treatment is considered if the patient has a poor clinical status.

Escherichia coli

Culture of *Escherichia coli* from the feces of reptiles is not unusual. These organisms are a normal component of the bacterial flora of the reptilian intestinal tract.[115] The challenge to the clinician is determining whether the cultured *E. coli* is an incidental finding or whether this isolate is involved in a disease process. The clinician is further challenged by deciding whether this is a primary or secondary infection.

Klebsiella

Klebsiella spp., especially *K. pneumoniae*, are commonly associated with pneumonia and hypopyon (Figures 16-28 and 16-29). These organisms are considered normal flora by some clinicians. When they are isolated in pure culture, or from clinically ill reptiles, the patient should be treated.

Chlamydia

This class of organisms is becoming more recognized as an infectious agent of reptiles.[116] The order Chlamydiales consists of four families, and the family Chlamydiacea is known to infect reptiles. *Chlamydia* infections have been reported in various reptiles including Emerald Tree Boas (*Corralus caninus*), Puff Adders (*Bitis* spp.), Green Seaturtles, and Nile Crocodiles (*Crocodylus niloticus*).[116]

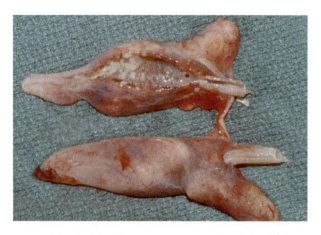

FIGURE 16-28 *Klebsiella pneumoniae* pneumonia in a chameleon. Note the thick gelatinous exudate. (*Photograph courtesy D. Mader.*)

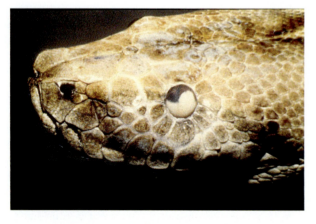

FIGURE 16-29 *Klebsiella* sp. hypopyon in a snake.

In a retrospective study of 90 tissue samples from various reptile species, 5.6% tested positive with immunohistochemistry with monoclonal antibodies for chlamydial LPS antigens, but 64.4% of the tissues were positive with Chlamydiales order-specific PCR testing. Ten percent of the *Chlamydia*-positive cases showed similarity to *Chlamydophila* (Cp.) *pneumoniae*, and 54.4% showed similarity to newly described "*Chlamydia*-like" microorganisms *Parachlamydia acanthamoebae* and *Simkania negevensis*.[117]

Chlamydia, specifically, *Chlamydophila* (Cp.) *pneumoniae*, should be considered in the differential for any granulomatous lesions in reptiles.[117,118] *Chlamydophila* (Cp.) *pneumoniae* was once considered solely a human pathogen. Because it has been identified in reptiles, specifically snakes, chameleons, and iguanas,[119] it obviously has the potential for zoonotic transmission from reptiles to humans.[117,119]

Mycoplasma

Within the last 10 years, a number of species of mycoplasma have been identified as pathogens in reptiles. Some of the first reports concerned *Mycoplasma agassizii* infection in the Gopher Tortoise (*Gopherus polyphemus*) and the Desert Tortoise (*G. agassizii*; see Chapter 73).[120,121] A mycoplasma species that caused respiratory disease was identified in a Burmese Python.[122] *Mycoplasma* spp. have been identified in crocodilians.[123,124] In all reports, mycoplasma is reported as a cause of pneumonia and tracheitis. It is also a cause of polyarthritis. It can be cultured from areas of the respiratory tract or synovial fluid.[124]

Mycobacterium

Mycobacterium spp. are ubiquitous in the environment. Potentially pathogenic species in reptile patients include *M. marinum*, *M. chelonae*, and *M. thamnopheos*.[125] Although commonly isolated from cutaneous lesions, mycobacteria can also cause systemic illness accompanied by nonspecific signs such as anorexia, lethargy, and wasting. *Mycobacterium chelonae* has been shown to cause osteoarthritis and systemic disease in Seaturtles.[126]

Acid-fast organisms are readily identified in skin scrapings or tissue biopsy (Figure 16-30). A Ziehl-Neelsen (ZN) stain is used on the tissue samples for identification of acid-fast bacilli. A broad-range PCR has also been used to identify mycobacteria in reptilian tissue samples.[117]

In a retrospective study that involved tissue sample from 90 reptiles, mycobacteria were detected in 15.6% of the cases with ZN staining, and 25.6% with PCR. Sequencing of these isolates revealed that the mycobacteria were other than *Mycobacterium tuberculosis* complex (MOTT). The authors concluded, on the basis of their results, that MOTT is an important consideration for any granulomatous inflammation in diseased reptiles.[117]

No successful treatment of infection with *Mycobacterium* spp. has been reported in reptiles. In a recent case involving a Kemp's Ridley Seaturtle, *M. chelonae* was isolated from an osteoarthritic joint. Even in this endangered species, because of apparent systemic involvement, euthanasia was elected.[126] In addition to the inherent difficulty in treatment, indication exists that the mycobacteria may have zoonotic potential.[127] Euthanasia of clinically affected animals is an option that should be discussed with the client.

Anaerobic Bacteria

A study of the bacterial flora of infirmed reptiles revealed that approximately 50% of all cultured specimens yielded anaerobic bacteria.[98] *Bacteroides* spp. are the most common obligate anaerobes isolated from reptiles.[128] A survey of the oral flora of Royal (Ball) Pythons *(Python regius)* revealed three genera of anaerobic bacteria, including *Clostridium* sp.[129] *Clostridium perfringens* has been associated with diarrhea in a Red-footed Tortoise *(Geochelone carbonaria).*[130] These facts should play a part in empirical selection of antibiotics (Figure 16-31).

These findings explain why some patients fail to respond to properly selected antibiotics. For instance, microbiologic culture and sensitivity data indicate that an aminoglycoside is the best antibiotic for a *Pseudomonas* spp. infection in the lungs. The drug is administered with standard protocols, but the patient fails to recover. That a secondary anaerobic infection is also present is possible. Aminoglycosides are not effective against anaerobes and are not expected to be effective. For proper therapy, an antimicrobial with action against anaerobes is needed. Combination therapy is necessary in many situations.

SUMMARY

Bacteria are the most common cause of disease in reptiles. As with most health problems in herpetology, this is generally the result of underlying husbandry and nutritional issues that lead to an immunocompromised patient. An understanding of the normal bacterial flora of reptiles helps the clinician decide what does and what does not need treatment.

Clinicians are encouraged to perform bacterial cultures and sensitivities whenever evaluating ill reptile patients, and especially before initiating antimicrobial therapy.

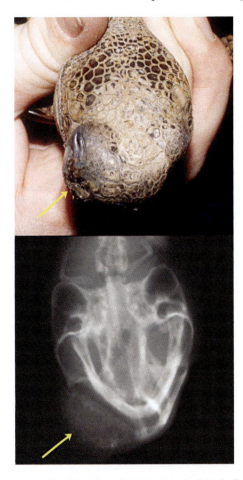

FIGURE 16-30 *Mycobacterium chelonei* osteomyelitis *(yellow arrow)* in a Desert Tortoise *(Gopherus agassizii; top)*. Radiograph shows lysis of the maxilla *(yellow arrow; bottom)*. *(Photograph courtesy D. Mader.)*

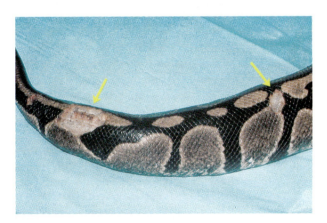

FIGURE 16-31 This Ball Python *(Python regius)* was bitten by its prey. Findings of anaerobes such as *Bacteroides* spp., *Peptostreptococcus* spp., and *Fusobacterium* spp. are common in these wounds. Antibiotic selection should consider the need to treat anaerobes. *(Photograph courtesy D. Mader.)*

REFERENCES

1. Frank W: Mycotic infections in amphibians and reptiles. In Page LA, editor: *Wildlife diseases,* New York, 1976, Plenum Press.
2. Austwick PKC, Keymer IF: Fungi and actinomycetes. In Cooper JE, Jackson OF, editors: *Diseases of the Reptilia,* vol 1, New York, 1981, Academic Press.
3. Migaki G, Jacobson ER, Casey HW: Fungal diseases in reptiles. In Hoff GL, Frye FL, Jacobson ER, editors: *Diseases of amphibians and reptiles,* New York, 1984, Plenum Press.
4. Jacobson ER, Cheatwood JL, Maxwell LK: Mycotic diseases of reptiles, *Semin Avian Exotic Pet Med* 9:94-101, 2000.
5. Rossi JV: Dermatology. In Mader DR, editor: *Reptile medicine and surgery,* Philadelphia, 1996, WB Saunders.
6. Rose FL, Koke J, Koehn R, Smith D: Identification of the etiological agent for necrotizing scute disease in the Texas tortoise, *J Wildl Dis* 37:223-228, 2001.
7. Paré JA, Coyle KA, Sigler L, Maas AK III, Mitchell RL: Pathogenicity of the *Chrysosporium* anamorph of *Nannizziopsis vriesii* for veiled chameleons *(Chamaeleo calyptratus), Med Mycol,* In press, July 2005.
8. Bowman MR, Naeser JP, Paré JA, Sigler L, Phillips LA, Sladky KK, et al: Mycotic dermatitis and stomatitis in bearded dragons *(Pogona vitticeps)* caused by the *Chrysosporium* anamorph of *Nannizziopsis vriesii,* In preparation.
9. Sigler L, Paré JA: Unpublished data.
10. Paré JA, Sigler L, Rypien K, Gibas CF: Cutaneous mycobiota of captive reptiles with notes on the scarcity of the *Chrysosporium* anamorph of *Nannizziopsis vriesii, J Herpetol Med Surg* 13(4): 10-15, 2003.
11. Paré JA, Sigler L, Hunter DB, Summerbell RC, Smith DA, Machin KL: Cutaneous mycoses in chameleons caused

by the *Chrysosporium* anamorph of *Nannizziopsis vriesii* (Apinis), [Currah] *J Zoo Wildl Med* 28:443-453, 1997.
12. Nichols DK, Weyant RS, Lamirande EW, Sigler L, Mason RT: Fatal mycotic dermatitis in captive brown tree snakes *(Boiga irregularis)*, *J Zoo Wildl Med* 30:111-118, 1999.
13. Thomas AD, Sigler L, Peucker S, Norton JH, Nielan A: *Chrysosporium* anamorph of *Nannizziopsis vriesii* associated with fatal cutaneous mycoses in the salt-water crocodile *(Crocodylus porosus)*, *Med Mycol* 40:143-151, 2002.
14. Bertelsen MF, Crawshaw GJ, Sigler L, Smith DA: Fatal cutaneous mycosis in tentacled snakes *(Erpeton tentaculatum)* caused by the *Chrysosporium* anamorph of *Nannizziopsis vriesii*, *J Zoo Wildl Med* 36:82-87, 2005.
15. Trevino GS: Cephalosporiosis in three caimans, *J Wildl Dis* 8:384-388, 1972.
16. de Hoog GS, Guarro J, Genè J, Figueras MJP: Atlas of clinical fungi, ed 2, 2000, Centraalbureau voor Schimmelcultures, Utrecht, The Netherlands, and Universitat Rovira I Virgili, Reus, Spain. Universitat Rovira I Virgili.
17. Kane J, Summerbell RC, Sigler L, Krajden S, Land G: *Laboratory handbook of dermatophytes. A clinical guide and laboratory manual of dermatophytes and other filamentous fungi from skin, hair and nails*, Belmont, Calif, 1997, Star Publishing.
18. Schildger BJ, Frank H, Göbel Th, Weiss R: Mycotic infections of the integument and inner organs in reptiles, *Herpetopathol* 2:81-97, 1991.
19. Reddacliff GL, Cunningham M, Hartley WJ: Systemic infection with a yeast-like organism in captive banded rock rattlesnakes *(Crotalus lepidus klauberi)*, *J Wildl Dis* 29:145-149, 1993.
20. Anderson NL: Successful treatment of a urolith associated with a fungal cystitis in *Iguana iguana*, *Proc Assoc Rept Amphib Vet* 52-56, 1994.
21. Raiti P: Use of nystatin to reduce suspected overgrowth of enteric fungal organisms in a diamond python *(Morelia spilota spilota)* and two Honduran milksnakes *(Lampropeltis triangulum hondurensis)*, *Bull Assoc Rept Amphib Vet* 8: 4-8, 1998.
22. Obst FJ, Richter K, Jacob U: *The completely illustrated atlas of reptiles and amphibians for the terrarium*, Neptune City, NJ, 1998, TFH Publications.
23. Deacon JW: *Introduction to modern mycology*, ed 3, Malden, Mass, 1997, Blackwell Science.
24. Austwick PKC: Some mycoses of reptiles, *Proc VII Congress Int Soc Human Anim Mycol* 383-384, 1982.
25. Heard DJ, Cantor GH, Jacobson ER, Purich B, Ajello L, Padhye AA: Hyalohyphomycosis caused by *Paecilomyces lilacinus* in an Aldabra tortoise, *J Am Vet Med Assoc* 189: 1143-1145, 1986.
26. Maslen M, Whitehead J, Forsyth WM, McCracken H, Hocking AD: Systemic mycotic disease of captive crocodile hatchling *(Crocodylus porosus)* caused by *Paecilomyces lilacinus*, *J Med Vet Mycol* 26:219-225, 1988.
27. Cork SC, Stockdale PHG: Mycotic disease in the common New Zealand gecko *(Hoplodactylus maculatus)*, *N Z Vet J* 42:144-147, 1994.
28. Gugagni HC, Okafor JI: Mycotic flora of the intestine and other internal organs of certain reptiles and amphibians with special reference to characterization of *Basidiobolus* isolates, *Mykosen* 23:260-268, 1980.
29. Enweani IB, Uwajeh JC, Bello CSS, Ndip RN: Fungal carriage in lizards, *Mycoses* 40:115-117, 1997.
30. Feio CL, Bauwens L, Swinne D, DeMeurichy W: Isolation of *Basidiobolus ranarum* from ectotherms in Antwerp zoo with special reference to characterization of the isolated strains, *Mycoses* 42:291-296, 1999.
31. Huchzermeyer FW, Henton MM, Riley J, Agnagna M: Aerobic intestinal flora of wild-caught African dwarf crocodiles, *Osteolaemus tetraspis*, *Onderstepoort J Vet Res* 67: 201-204, 2000.
32. Milde K, Kostka V, Kaleta EF, Willems H, Jäger C: Multiplex-PCR-based differentiation and characterization of *Candida*-isolates derived from tortoises (Testudinidae), *Vet Microbiol* 76:395-402, 2000.
33. Kostka VM, Hoffmann L, Balks E, Eskens U, Wimmershof N: Review of the literature and investigations on the prevalence and consequences of yeasts in reptiles, *Vet Rec* 140: 282-287, 1997.
34. Okudaira M, Kurata H, Sakabe F: Studies on the fungal flora in the lung of human necropsy cases: a critical survey in connection with the pathogenesis of opportunistic fungus infections, *Mycopathologia* 61:3-18, 1977.
35. Tizard IR: *Veterinary immunology, an introduction*, ed 5, Philadelphia, 1996, WB Saunders.
36. Montali RJ: Comparative pathology of inflammation in the higher vertebrates (reptiles, birds and mammals), *J Comp Path* 99:1-26, 1988.
37. Klingenberg RJ: Therapeutics. In Mader DS, editor: *Reptile medicine and surgery*, Philadelphia, 1996, WB Saunders.
38. Gliÿski Z, Buczek J: Aspects of reptile immunity, *Medycyna Wet* 55:574-578, 1999.
39. Wyld JA, Brush AH. The molecular heterogeneity and diversity of reptilian keratins, *J Mol Evol* 12:331-347, 1979.
40. Frye FL: *Biomedical and surgical aspects of captive reptile husbandry*, Edwardsville, Kan, 1981, Veterinary Medicine Publishing.
41. Hazell SL, Eamens GJ, Perry RA: Progressive digital necrosis in the eastern blue-tongued skink, *Tiliqua scincoides* (Shaw), *J Wildl Dis* 21:186-188, 1985.
42. Rees RG: Keratinophilic fungi from Queensland: I: isolations from animal hair and scales, *Sabouraudia* 5:165-172, 1967.
43. Branch S, Hall L, Blackshear P, Chernoff N: Infectious dermatitis in a ball python *(Python regius)* colony, *J Zoo Wildl Med* 29:461-464, 1998.
44. Jacobson ER: Diseases of the integumentary system of reptiles. In Rosenthal KL, editor: *Practical exotic animal medicine, the compendium collection*, Trenton, NJ, 1997, Veterinary Learning Systems.
45. McKenzie RA, Green PE: Mycotic dermatitis in captive carpet snakes, *J Wildl Dis* 12:405-408, 1976.
46. Jacobson ER: Necrotizing mycotic dermatitis in snakes: clinical and pathologic features, *J Am Vet Med Assoc* 177: 838-841, 1980.
47. Tappe JP, Chandler FW, Liu SK, Dolensek EP: Aspergillosis in two San Esteban chuckwallas, *J Am Vet Med Assoc* 185:1425-1428, 1984.
48. Martinez-Silvestre A, Galán P. Dermatitis fúngica en una población salvaje de *Podarcis bocagei*, *Bol Assoc Herpetol Esp* 10:39-43, 1999.
49. Crispens CG Jr, Marion KR: Granulomas in reptiles: a report of four cases, *J Alabama Acad Sci* 52:48-52, 1981.
50. Frye FI, Williams DL: *Self-assessment color review of reptiles and amphibians*, Ames, 1995, Iowa State University Press.
51. Hough I. Cryptococcosis in an eastern water skink, *Aust Vet J* 76:471-472, 1998.
52. McGall PG: *Studies on "black spot," a disease of New Zealand geckoes*, unpublished BSc Honours thesis, Palmerston, North, NZ, 1981, Massey University.
53. Jasmin AM, Baucom J: *Erysipelothrix insidiosa* infections in the caiman *(Caiman crocodilus)* and the American crocodile *(Crocodilus acutus)*, *Am J Vet Clin Pathol* 1:173-177, 1967.
54. Vissienon Th, Schüppel K-F, Ullrich E, Kuijpers AFA: Case report: a disseminated infection due to *Chrysosporium queenslandicum* in a garter snake *(Thamnophis)*, *Mycoses* 42:107-110, 1999.

55. Jacobson ER, Calderwood MB, Clubb SL: Mucormycosis in hatchling Florida softshell turtles, *J Am Vet Med Assoc* 177:835-837, 1980.
56. Lappin PB, Dunstan RW: Difficult dermatologic diagnosis, *J Am Vet Med Assoc* 200:785-786, 1992.
57. Cheatwood JL, Jacobson ER, May PG, Farrell TM: An outbreak of fungal dermatitis and stomatitis in a wild population of pigmy rattlesnakes, *Sistrurus miliarius barbouri*, in Volusia County, Florida, *Proc Assoc Reptil Amphib Vet* 19-20, 1999.
58. McAllister CT, Goldberg SR, Holshuh HJ, Trauth SE: Disseminated mycotic dermatitis in a wild-caught timber rattlesnake, *Crotalus horridus* (Serpentes: Viperidae), from Arkansas, *Texas J Sci* 45:279-281, 1993.
59. Lewbart GA, Medway W: A case of mycotic lung disease in a wild caught juvenile sea turtle, *J Small Exotic Anim Med* 2:58-59, 1993.
60. Cabanes FJ, Alonso JM, Castellá G, Alegre F, Domingo M, Pont S: Cutaneous hyalohyphomycosis caused by *Fusarium solani* in a loggerhead sea turtle (*Caretta caretta* L.), *J Clin Microbiol* 35:3343-3345, 1997.
61. González Cabo JF, Espejo Serrano J, Bárcena Asensio MC: Mycotic pulmonary disease by *Beauveria bassiana* in a captive tortoise, *Mycoses* 38:167-169, 1995.
62. Frelier PF, Sigler L, Nelson PE: Mycotic pneumonia caused by *Fusarium moniliforme* in an alligator, *J Med Vet Mycol* 23:399-402, 1985.
63. Manire CA, Rhinehart HL, Sutton DA, Thompson EH, Rinaldi MG, Buck JD, et al: Disseminated mycotic infection caused by *Colletotrichum acutatum* in a Kemp's Ridley turtle (*Lepidochelys kempi*), *J Clin Microbiol* 40:4273-4280, 2002.
64. Oros J, Ramirez AS, Poveda JB, Rodriguez JL, Fernandez A: Systemic mycosis caused by *Penicillium griseofulvum* in a Seychelles giant tortoise (*Megalochelys gigantea*), *Vet Rec* 139:295-296, 1996.
65. Holz PH, Slocombe R: Systemic *Fusarium* infection in two snakes, carpet python, *Morelia spilota variegata*, and a red-bellied black snake, *Pseudechis porphyriacus*, *J Herpetol Med Surg* 10:18-20, 2000.
66. Jacobson ER: Chromomycosis and fibrosarcoma in a mangrove snake, *J Am Vet Med Assoc* 185:1428-1430, 1984.
67. Timm KI, Sonn RJ, Hultgren BD: Coccidioidomycosis in a Sonoran gopher snake, *Pituophis melanoleucus affinis*, *J Med Vet Mycol* 26:101-104, 1988.
68. Swatek FE, Plunkett OA: Ecological studies on *Coccidioides immitis*. In Ferguson MS, editor: *Proc symp coccidioidomycosis*, Atlanta, Ga, 1957, Department of Health, Education, and Welfare.
69. Egeberg RO: Socioeconomic impact of coccidioidomycosis. In Einstein HE, Catanzaro A, editors: *Coccidiomycosis: proc 4th int conf coccidioidomycosis*, Washington, DC, 1985, National Foundation for Infectious Diseases.
70. McNamara TS, Cook RA, Behler JL, Ajello L, Padhye AA: Cryptococcosis in a common anaconda (*Eunectes murinus*), *J Zoo Wildl Med* 25:128-132, 1994.
71. Philott AD, Parmenter CJ: Influence of diminished respiratory surface area on survival of sea turtle embryos, *J Exp Zool* 289:317-321, 2001.
72. Migaki G: Mycotic diseases in captive animals: a mycopathologic overview. In Montali RJ, Migaki G, editors: *The comparative pathology of zoo animals*, Washington, DC, 1980, Smithsonian Institution Press.
73. Hernandez-Divers SJ, Hernandez-Divers SM: Pulmonary candidiasis caused by *Candida albicans* in a Greek tortoise (*Testudo graeca*) and treatment using intrapulmonary amphotericin B, *J Zoo Wildl Med* 32, 2001.
74. Paul-Murphy J: Unpublished data, 2002.
75. Chandler FW, Watts JC: *Pathologic diagnosis of fungal infections*, Chicago, 1987, ASCP Press.
76. Kwong-Chung KJ, Bennett JE: Histopathologic diagnosis of mycoses. In *Medical mycology*, Philadelphia, 1992, Lea & Febiger.
77. Sandhu GS, Kline BC, Stockman L, Roberts GD: Molecular probes for the diagnosis of fungal infections, *J Clin Microbiol* 33:2913-2919, 1995.
78. Zwart P, Verwer MAJ, De Vries GA, Hermanides-Nijhof EJ, De Vries HW: Fungal infection of the eyes of the snake *Epicrates cenchria maurus*: enucleation under halothane narcosis, *J Small Anim Pract* 14:773-779, 1973.
79. Collette BE, Curry OH: Mycotic keratitis in a reticulated python, *J Am Vet Med Assoc* 173:1117-1118, 1978.
80. Andriole VT: Current and future antifungal therapy: new targets for antifungal therapy, *Int J Antimicrob Agents* 16:317-321, 2000.
81. Page CD, Mautino M, Derendorf H, Mechlinski W: Multiple-dose pharmacokinetics of ketoconazole administered orally to gopher tortoises (*Gopherus polyphemus*), *J Zoo Wildl Med* 22:191-198, 1991.
82. Gamble KC, Alvarado TP, Bennett CL: Itraconazole plasma and tissue concentrations in the spiny lizard (*Sceloporus* sp.) following once-daily dosing, *J Zoo Wildl Med* 28:89-93, 1997.
83. Manire CA, Rhinehart HL, Pennick GJ, Rinaldi MG: Plasma and tissue concentrations of itraconazole in the Kemp's Ridley sea turtle, *Lepidochelys kempi*, *Proc Int Assoc Aquatic Anim Med* 167, 2001.
84. Bartlett KM, Harms CA, Lewbart GA, Papich MG: Single- and multiple-dose pharmacokinetics of fluconazole in loggerhead sea turtles (*Caretta caretta*), *Proc Int Assoc Aquatic Anim Med* 80, 2001.
85. Tangredi B, Evans R: Organochlorine pesticides associated with ocular, nasal, or otic infection in the eastern box turtle (*Terrapene carolina carolina*), *J Zoo Wildl Med* 28:97-100, 1997.
86. Raidal S, Ohara M, Hobbs R, et al: Gram-negative bacterial infections and cardiovascular parasitism in green sea turtles (*Chelonia mydas*), *Aust Vet J* 76:415-417, 1988.
87. Needham J: Microbiology and captive reptiles, *Acta Zoo Pathol Antverpiensia* 79:33-38, 1986.
88. Cooper J: Bacteria. In Cooper JE, Jackson OF, editors: *Diseases of Reptilia*, San Diego, 1981, Academic Press.
89. Draper C, Walker R, Lawler H: Patterns of oral bacterial infection in captive snakes, *J Am Vet Med Assoc* 179:1223, 1981.
90. Jacobson E: *Biology and diseases of reptiles: laboratory animal medicine*, San Diego, 1984, Academic Press.
91. Ross R: *The bacterial disease of reptiles*, Palo Alto, 1984, The Institute for Herpetological Research.
92. Johnson J, Benson P: Laboratory reference values for a group of captive ball pythons (*Python regius*), *Am J Vet Res* 57:1304-1307, 1996.
93. Plowman C, Montali R, Phillips L, et al: Septicemia and chronic abscesses in iguanas (*Cyclura cornuta* and *Iguana iguana*) associated with a *Neisseria* species, *J Zoo Anim Med* 18:86-93, 1987.
94. Chiodini R, Sundberg J: Salmonellosis in reptiles: a review, *Am J Epidemiol* 113:494-499, 1981.
95. Paisley J, Lauer B: Pediatric blood cultures, *Clin Lab Med* 14:17, 1994.
96. Harvey R, Price T: Salmonella isolation from reptilian faeces: a discussion of appropriate cultural techniques, *J Hygiene* 91:25-32, 1983.
97. Mader D: Antibiotic therapy in reptile medicine. In Frye F, editor: *Biomedical and surgical aspects of captive reptile husbandry*, ed 2, Melbourne, Fla, 1990, Krieger Publishing.
98. Stewart J: Anaerobic bacterial infections in reptiles, *J Zoo Wildl Med* 21:180, 1990.
99. Berschauer R, Mader D: Hepatic abscess due to *Corynebacterium* sp. in desert tortoise, *Gopherus agassizii*, *Bull Assoc Reptil Amphib Vet* 8:13-15, 1998.

100. Isaza R, Garner M, Jacobson E: Proliferative osteoarthritis and osteoarthrosis in 15 snakes, *J Zoo Wildl Med* 31:20-27, 2000.
101. Hetzel U, Konig A, Yildririm A, et al: Septicaemia in emerald monitors (*Varanus prasinus* Schlegel 1839) caused by *Streptococcus agalactiae* acquired from mice, *Vet Microbiol* 95:283-293, 2003.
102. Olsen S, Bishop R, Brenner F, et al: The changing epidemiology of salmonella: trends in serotypes isolated from humans in the United States, 1987-1997, *J Infect Dis* 183:753-761, 2001.
103. Fierer J, Guiney DG: Diverse virulence traits underlying different clinical outcomes of *Salmonella* infection, *J Clin Invest* 107:775-780, 2001.
104. Dickinson V, Duck T, Schwalbe C, et al: Nasal and cloacal bacteria in free ranging desert tortoises from the western United States, *J Wildl Dis* 37:252-257, 2001.
105. Mitchell M, Shane S: Preliminary findings of *Salmonella* spp. in captive green iguanas *(Iguana iguana)* and their environment, *Prevent Vet Med* 45:297-304, 2000.
106. Woodward D, Khakhria R, Johnson W: Human salmonellosis associated with exotic pets, *J Clin Microbiol* 35:2786-2790, 1997.
107. Hilf M, Wagner R, Yu V: A prospective study of upper airway flora in healthy boid snakes and snakes with pneumonia, *JZWM* 21:318-325, 1990.
108. Blaylock R: Normal oral bacteria l flora from some southern African snakes, *Onderstepoort J Vet Res* 68:175-182, 2001.
109. Branch S, Hall L, Blackshear P, et al: Infectious dermatitis in a ball python *(Python regius)* colony, *J Zoo Wildl Med* 29:461-464, 1998.
110. Keymer I: Diseases of the chelonians: (2) necropsy survey of terrapins and turtles, *Vet Rec* 103:577-582, 1978.
111. Jorge M, Nishioka S, De Oliveira R, et al: *Aeromonas hydrophila* soft tissue infection as a complication of snake bite, *Ann Trop Med Parasitol* 92:213-217, 1998.
112. Flandry F, Lisecki E, Domingue G, et al: Initial antibiotic therapy for alligator bites: characterization of the oral flora of *Alligator mississippiensis*, *S Med J* 82:262-266, 1989.
113. Hsieh S, Babl F: *Serratia marcescens* cellulitis following an iguana bite, *Clin Infect Dis* 28:1181-1182, 1999.
114. Camus A, Hawke J: *Providencia rettgeri*-associated septicemia and meningoencephalitis in juvenile farmed American alligators *(Alligator mississippiensis)*, *J Aquatic Anim Health* 14:149-153, 2002.
115. Gopee N, Adegiyum A, Caesar K: A longitudinal study of *E. coli* strains isolated from captive mammals, birds and reptiles in Trinidad, *J Zoo Wildl Med* 31:353-360, 2000.
116. Jacobson E, Origgi F, Heard D, et al: An outbreak of chlamydiosis in emerald tree boas, *Corallus caninus*, Association of Reptilian and Amphibian Veterinarians 47-48, 2002.
117. Soldati G, Lu ZH, Vaughan L, Polkinghorne A, Zimmermann DR, Huder JB, et al: Detection of mycobacteria and chlamydiae in granulomatous inflammation of reptiles: a retrospective study, *Vet Pathol* 41(4):388-397, 2004.
118. Pospischil A: *Novel chlamydiae in cats and reptiles,* General Meeting of the American Society for Microbiology 2003.
119. Bodetti T, Jacobson E, Wan C, et al: Molecular evidence to support the expansion of the hostrange of *Chlamydophila pneumoniae* to include reptiles as well as humans, horses, koalas and amphibians, *Systematic Applied Microbiol* 25: 146-152, 2002.
120. Brown M, McLaughlin G, Klein P, et al: Upper respiratory tract disease in the gopher tortoise is caused by *Mycoplasma agassizii*, *J Clin Microbiol* 37:2262-2269, 1999.
121. Brown M, Schumacher I, Klein P, et al: *Mycoplasma agassizii* causes upper respiratory tract disease in the desert tortoise, *Infect Immun* 62:4580-4586, 1994.
122. Penner J, Jacobson E, Brown D, et al: A novel *Mycoplasma* sp. associated with proliferative tracheitis and pneumonia in a Burmese python *(Python molurus bivittatus)*, *J Comp Pathol* 117:283-288, 1997.
123. Kirchhoff H, Mohan K, Schmidt R, et al: *Mycoplasma crocodyli* sp. nov., a new species from crocodiles, *Int J Syst Bacteriol* 47:742-746, 1997.
124. Helmick K, Brown D, Jacobson E, et al: In vitro drug susceptibility pattern of *Mycoplasma alligatoris* isolated from symptomatic American alligators *(Alligator mississippiensis)*, *J Zoo Wildl Med* 33:108-111, 2002.
125. Matlova L, Fischer B, Kazda J, et al: The occurrence of mycobacteria in invertebrates and poikilothermic animals and their role in the infection of other animals and man, *Veterinarni Medicina* 43:115-132, 1998.
126. Greer L, Strandberg J, Whitaker B: *Mycobacterium chelonae* osteoarthritis in a Kemp's Ridley sea turtle *(Lepidochelys kempii)*, *J Wildl Dis* 39:736-741, 2003.
127. Hernandez-Divers SJ, Shearer D: Pulmonary mycobacteriosis caused by *Mycobacterium haemophilum* and *M. marinum* in a royal python, *J Am Vet Med Assoc* 220(11):1661-3, 2002.
128. Jang S, Hirsh D: Identity of *Bacteroides* isolates and previously named *Bacteroides* spp in clinical specimens of animal origin, *AJVR* 52:738-741, 1991.
129. Klarsfeld J, Mitchell M, Futch R: *Characterization of the oral aerobic and anaerobic bacterial flora of royal pythons* (Python regius), ARAV Ninth Annual Conference 53-54, 2002.
130. Weese J, Staempfli H: Diarrhea associated with enterotoxigenic *Clostridium perfringens* in a red-footed tortoise *(Geochelone carbonaria)*, *J Zoo Wildl Med* 2000:265-266, 2000.

17
NEUROLOGY
R. AVERY BENNETT and STEPHEN J. MEHLER

A variety of clinical syndromes in reptiles have neurologic manifestations. Trauma, nutritional deficiencies, neoplastic conditions, and degenerative diseases are examples of conditions that affect the nervous system of reptiles. In addition, infectious diseases (bacterial, parasitic, and viral) may cause neurologic abnormalities. A paucity of information is available on clinical neurology in reptiles. Information is primarily extrapolated from that of the more familiar mammalian species. Reptiles have been said to function more from spinal segmental reflexes than cerebral stimulation, which implies that body movements are more autonomous from the brain in reptiles than in higher vertebrates.[1] Reflexes useful in a neurologic examination on a reptile patient have not been established. Reptile reflexes may differ from mammalian reflexes, although anatomically, segmental reflex arcs are known to exist in all amniote vertebrates. For example, in mammalian neurology, the anal sphincter reflex is a segmental reflex that does not require an intact spinal cord for proper function. In reptiles, a loss of tone to the vent has been reported with spinal cord injury[1,2]; however, spinal cord injury in mammals causes hyperreflexia of the anal sphincter.

Diagnostic aids used in mammalian neurology, such as cerebrospinal fluid (CSF) analysis, myelography, and electrodiagnostic evaluations, may be of limited value in reptile neurology on the basis of patient size and anatomic and physiologic differences. Clinical signs associated with neurologic disease are often nonspecific, which makes localization of the source or the cause of the disease difficult. A basic knowledge of the reptile nervous system and syndromes commonly encountered helps the clinician develop a diagnostic and therapeutic plan. Unfortunately, many diagnoses are still made at necropsy with the aid of microbiology and histopathology.

NEUROANATOMY

A basic understanding of reptile neuroanatomy helps the clinician understand the clinical manifestations of neurologic diseases and provides an opportunity for the clinician to determine the location of a focal lesion.[3-5] Ascending the phylogenetic scale, reptiles are the first vertebrates to have enlargement of the cerebral hemispheres, optic lobes, and a cerebellum. They are lissencephalic (having no cerebral gyri and sulci) but are the first group to have a developed cerebral cortex with two hemispheres that are separated by a deep median fissure. Reptiles are also the first group of animals with a cephalic flexure such that the brain lies off-line with the spinal cord and grows back to partially cover the diencephalon. With this development of the brain, an increase is seen in the brain-to-body weight ratio. The midbrain continues to be the center for nervous integration; however, the corpus striatum begins to take over this function in reptiles.

Two meninges are found in reptiles. The pia-arachnoid layer is vascular and lies in close contact with the surface of the brain and spinal cord. The dura mater is quite thick and relatively nonvascular. The space between the pia-arachnoid layer and the dura mater is the subdural space. Reptiles do not have a true subarachnoid space, an important fact in attempts to collect CSF because in mammals fluid is collected from the subarachnoid space.

The spinal cord of reptiles extends to the limit of the osseous spine (the tip of the tail), and no cauda equina exists. Locomotor centers are found within the spinal cord, giving it a degree of functional autonomy from the brain. Because of this, reptiles with spinal cord injury have been said to have a better prognosis for recovery than higher vertebrates.[1]

Peripheral nerves are composed of dorsal nerve roots that are primarily sensory and ventral roots that contain visceral motor and somatic motor roots, comprising the reflex arc that is normal amniote neuroanatomy. Nerve endings in the skin of reptiles are similar to those identified in mammals and serve the same function. They are acutely tuned for cutaneous sensation. Some lizards have hair-like structures in the skin with sensory function as well.[3] Reptiles are the first group phylogenetically to have 12 cranial nerves (CNs).

NEUROLOGIC EXAMINATION

Before the reptile patient is restrained, the clinician should observe the patient in its environment and evaluate its mental status, degree of alertness, and the presence of any abnormal postures. Stimulating the patient to move is helpful so it can be evaluated for postural or ambulatory abnormalities, such as paresis or hemiparesis, that could indicate the presence of a neurologic condition.

Head tilt, opisthotonos, dysequilibrium, circling, and seizure activity are indications of central nervous system disorders. Dysecdysis is commonly observed in reptiles with central nervous system disease. Because of the loss of motor control, they are unable to complete ecdysis by rubbing off the old skin. Snakes with central nervous system disease often have fine motor tremors and are unable to strike at prey with accuracy. Some snakes are unable to constrict prey because of the loss of muscle tone or may be unable to move the prey accurately toward their mouth after a kill. As a snake ambulates across the hand and arm, the gastropedges gripping the skin provide an indication of muscle tone. Palpation is also useful for evaluation of general body muscle tone. When a healthy snake is suspended by its midbody, it should be able to lift its head straight and steady to search for a substrate. With neurologic disease, jerky irregular movements as the snake seeks a substrate may be observed.[1]

In most cases, tortoises are able to walk with their plastron suspended off the ground. With loss of muscle tone or paresis, they may no longer be able to do so. Chelonians with neurologic disease frequently circle and are unable to hold up their head or hold their head with cervical hyperextension. They may be unable to prehend food properly and may show dysphagia. With chelonians, the head and legs should be pulled from within the shell to evaluate the muscle tone of the extremities. In evaluation of seaturtles or other aquatic species that are swimming in circles in one direction, one must remember that the most common cause of asymmetric buoyancy in the water is a mass or uneven gas distribution in the lungs or coelomic cavity and not vestibular disease.[6]

Phylogenetically, reptiles are the first vertebrates with 12 CNs; lower vertebrates have only 10.[5] Olfaction (CN I) is a chemosensory system in reptiles mediated by sensory cells in the nasal cavity and by the Jacobson's organs, which have ducts that open into the mouth. The tongue brings odoriferous particles to the Jacobson's organ where the vomeronasal branch of the olfactory nerve is stimulated providing input to the brain. The Jacobson's organ is absent in crocodilians and modified or absent in chelonians. Testing the patient's response to noxious odors such as alcohol may assess the functional status of the olfactory nerve. A healthy patient recoils or moves away from an alcohol-soaked pledget or cotton-tipped applicator. A history of a normal ability to locate food may also indicate a functional CN I, although other sensory functions may also play a role in food recognition.

The optic nerve (CN II) is sensory and responsible for vision. Most reptiles have eyelids and nictitating membranes; however, in snakes and some lizards (especially geckos and skinks), the eyelids are fused and transparent, forming the spectacle, and the nictitans is absent. Movement of the upper eyelid closes the eyes of crocodilians, and the eyes are closed by movement of the lower lid in other reptiles. Reptiles with eyelids show a menace reflex confirming optic nerve (CN II) and facial nerve (CN VII) function (Figure 17-1). The functional status of this nerve may also be assessed by observing the patient's ability to react to movement within the environment. One must not create air movement or vibrations in the substrate or enclosure because many reptiles are able to sense vibrations that are imperceptible to humans. Some reptiles use vibrations or thermal sensors to locate prey and may not rely on their visual senses.

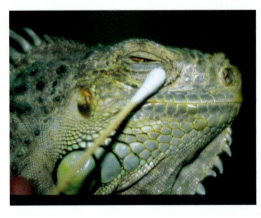

FIGURE 17-1 This Green Iguana (*Iguana iguana*) shows a normal menace reflex by closing its eyelids. (*Photograph courtesy D. Mader.*)

Some reptiles (chameleons) are capable of moving their eyes independently, which makes assessment for the presence of strabismus difficult. CNs III, IV, and VI are involved in coordination of ocular movements. Normal and coordinated eye movements indicate healthy function of these nerves. Strabismus may indicate dysfunction. A branch of the abducens (CN IV) supplies the nictitans.

The iris is composed entirely of skeletal muscle, which provides voluntary control of pupil size. Pupillary light response, which evaluates CNs II and III in mammals, is not reliable in reptiles. They are not responsive to traditional mydriatics; however, topical neuromuscular blocking agents produce mydriasis. Intracameral injection of neuromuscular blocking agents, such as d-tubo curare, produces mydriasis but is somewhat invasive (see Figure 20-3). Topical application of nondepolarizing neuromuscular blocking agents, such as vercuronium, on the cornea of species without a spectacle may produce good mydriasis.[7]

The trigeminal nerve (CN V) is composed of both sensory and motor fibers with mandibular, maxillary, and ophthalmic branches. The mandibular branch supplies motor fibers to the muscles responsible for mouth function. The presence of normal jaw function indicates healthy nerve function. The ophthalmic branch provides sensory innervation to the skin surrounding the eye and the mucosa of portions of the nasal and oral cavities. The maxillary branch is sensory to the upper jaw, nose, and lower eyelid. Its function may be tested by determining the patient's ability to feel a cotton-tipped applicator around the face. If necessary, a painful stimulus such as a 27-gauge needle may be used.

Sensory pits that act as thermoreceptors are present in some reptiles (especially snakes). The pit membrane of pit vipers is innervated by the ophthalmic and maxillary branches of the trigeminal nerve. In these snakes, the sensory fields overlap creating three-dimensional heat perception used to locate prey. In boas and pythons, smaller simpler pits are present along the upper and lower labial scales and are innervated by the ophthalmic, maxillary, and mandibular branches of the trigeminal nerve (CN V).

The facial nerve (CN VII) is motor to the structures of the face. In reptiles, the only moveable portions of the face are the eyelids. In patients with eyelids, the functional status of the facial nerve may be assessed (see Figure 17-1). The facial nerve also supplies sensory fibers to the taste buds of the cranial two thirds of the tongue. These fibers form part of the chorda tympani, which is a branch of the facial nerve that passes through the middle ear.

Hearing is well developed in most reptiles, especially those with an externally visible tympanum. Snakes were once thought to be deaf and only able to sense vibrations in the substrate; however, they have been shown to perceive low-frequency airborne sound. Many reptiles may not have a pronounced response to auditory stimuli. This, coupled with their ability to sense vibration, makes assessment of the cochlear portion of the acoustic nerve (CN VIII) difficult. A defect in the vestibular system may manifest itself as nystagmus, head tilt, rolling, and an abnormal righting reflex.

Reptiles also have a chemosensory system analogous to taste with taste buds and sensory papillae throughout the oral mucosa. This system is innervated primarily by the glossopharyngeal nerve (CN IX). Assessment of the ability of reptiles to taste is difficult. Many patients have a negative reaction to bitter substances placed into their mouth by holding their mouth open, writhing, and pawing at their mouth.

Cranial nerves IX, XI, and XII are involved in normal tongue movement, swallowing, and jaw strength. Dysfunction is manifested as dysphagia. Deviation of the tongue may indicate damage to the hypoglossal nerve (CN XII). The spinal accessory nerve (CN XI) supplies motor fibers to the larynx, pharynx, and the superficial cervical musculature. The vagus nerve (CN X) is primarily composed of preganglionic visceral motor fibers of the parasympathetic nervous system.

The righting reflex is frequently used to evaluate the neurologic status of reptile patients. Squamate reptiles and crocodilians placed on their back should turn their head over first and then roll the body over to the normal position (Figure 17-2). Chelonians placed on their back generally try to right themselves by pushing their head against the substrate and attempting to get their legs onto the surface. This provides a good opportunity to evaluate movements of the head, neck, and limbs as the patient attempts to right itself. In snakes, the righting reflex is useful in identifying the location of a spinal cord injury. The snake rights itself to the level of the injury and is unable to right caudal to the lesion. Some animals, especially crocodilians and lizards, when placed on their back with their abdomen gently stroked become sedate or flaccid, inhibiting the righting reflex.[4,8]

Foot withdrawal and response to tail or vent stimulation are also used to evaluate the neurologic status of reptile patients. A healthy animal has a brisk withdrawal reflex and a quick righting reflex.[4] However, these reflexes are known to be temperature dependent.[1] With a decrease in environmental temperature, a corresponding decrease is seen in conduction velocity within the peripheral nerves. During brumation (hibernation), conduction along peripheral nerves almost ceases.[9] Assessment of the patient's body or environmental temperature in conjunction with an evaluation of reflexes is therefore important. Reflexes are best evaluated with the animal in its optimum temperature range.

The panniculus reflex is present in reptiles and is particularly useful in snakes. A hypodermic needle may be used to stimulate the patient's skin along the lateral margins of the body. A healthy patient responds with a twitch of the skin. With spinal cord injury, the panniculus response is present cranial to the lesion and absent caudal to the lesion.

A vagal-vagal response is present in most lizards and crocodilians.[2] When digital pressure is applied to both eyes for several minutes, the patient responds with a decrease in heart rate and blood pressure. They also become inactive, and in this state, minor procedures such as radiography can be accomplished. They may be aroused from this condition by either a loud noise or physical stimulation.

ELECTRODIAGNOSTIC AND IMAGING TECHNIQUES

Because of their relative unavailability, these methods have not been used extensively in clinical reptile neurology. Reptiles are poikilothermic, and their nerve conduction velocity varies with the ambient temperature. Information regarding normal velocity for a given temperature and reptile species is lacking. If a conspecific control is available for comparison, a difference might support a tentative diagnosis of a conduction disturbance. Still, the size of many patients and difficulty finding a nerve to evaluate make this diagnostic tool of limited value.

Spinal cord evoked potentials (SCEPs) may be useful in assessment of the severity of spinal cord injury (Figure 17-3, A, B). SCEPs are evaluated with electrical stimulation of peripheral nerves and recording of the activity in various regions of the spinal cord.[10] Conduction time and conduction velocity can be calculated for the spinal cord and peripheral nerves from the tracings produced. SCEPs have shown promise in evaluation of chelonians with dorsal carapace injury and hindlimb paresis. A stimulating electrode is placed in a hindlimb and evoked potentials are measured at the base of the skull. The presence of potentials indicates an intact spinal cord and may indicate a better prognosis for return of neurologic function.

Electromyography is used to determine whether muscle dysfunction is the result of nerve injury or a primary myopathy. If the dysfunction is from a neuropathy, fibrillation potentials and positive sharp waves are generated.

Plain radiographs are useful for locating a spinal or cranial fracture that may cause neurologic dysfunction. Currently, a lack of scientific evidence exists to the presence of a subarachnoid space in reptiles. With no subarachnoid space, myelography should not be possible. However, clinical reports indicate that CSF collection and myelography are useful in examining the central nervous system of reptiles.[11,12] Scientific investigation into the existence of a subarachnoid space and the ability to collect CSF and perform myelography is warranted to determine the value and efficacy of these diagnostic techniques.

Computed tomography (CT) is useful for locating anatomic abnormalities such as masses and fractures. CT scan uses radiographs and computer technology to create cross-sectional images of the patient.[13,14] CT scan provides superior soft tissue imaging with no superimposition of structures when compared with conventional radiography and provides good contrast images of calcified structures.[15] Contrast enhancement allows for better visualization of soft tissue structures with increased blood flow. This is especially

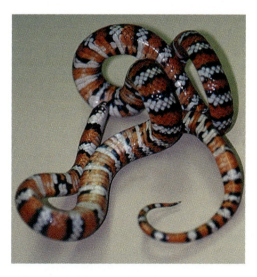

FIGURE 17-2 A snake placed in dorsal recumbency shows a normal righting reflex by turning its head over first.

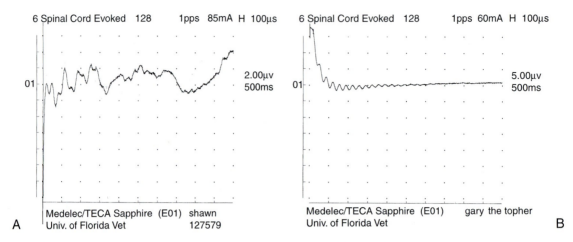

FIGURE 17-3 A, Spinal cord evoked potential (SCEP) in a healthy Gopher Tortoise *(Gopherus polyphemus).* Electrical activity is recorded with an electrode placed at the base of the skull indicating that electrical impulses are conducted along the spinal cord. **B,** SCEP in a Gopher Tortoise with a transected spinal cord. The initial spike is seen but no electrical activity is noted after electrode stimulation.

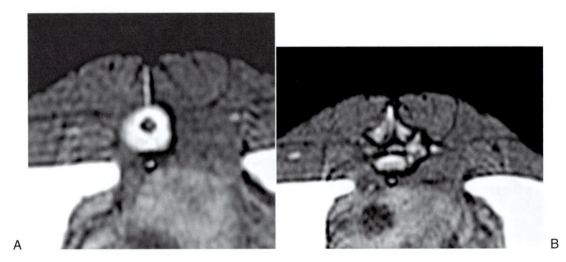

FIGURE 17-4 A, Magnetic resonance imaging (MRI) of a Savannah Monitor Lizard *(Varanus exanthematicus)* with spinal cord trauma. This image is in a normal section of the spine. The white surrounding the spinal cord represents fat or fluid (cerebrospinal fluid [CSF]), which is normal. **B,** This image shows a loss of the white perimeter of fluid and fat and attenuation of the canal with no visible spinal cord present. Neurologic function was not improving after several weeks, and the lizard underwent euthanasia after this study.

helpful and superior to magnetic resonance imaging (MRI) in imaging acute intracranial hematomas within 2 days of the trauma.[16] CT scan also helps to reveal changes in bony tissues and provides greater detail of imaged structures than conventional radiography.[17]

Magnetic resonance imaging not only identifies anatomic abnormalities but also identifies changes in the microscopic structure such as occurs with inflammation or vascular injury (Figure 17-4, *A, B*). MRI uses a pulsating external magnetic field that produces radiofrequency signals used to generate images.[14,15] The natural frequency of the hydrogen ion is used as the frequency for the magnetic pulse because of the high content of hydrogen ions in biological tissues.[18] Tissues with high hydrogen ion content are imaged, and regions of bone and air appear void. Contrast may also be used with this imaging method. The main advantages of MRI over CT include the ability to image the entire brain, an increase in soft tissue detail, and the creation of true images in various planes (Figure 17-5).[17]

Nuclear scans help identify active bone lesions and are safe and relatively inexpensive (Figure 17-6). Newer imaging methods have become increasingly more available to veterinarians and are useful neurodiagnostic tools.

Cerebral Spinal Fluid

Analysis of CSF is an important diagnostic tool in the evaluation of patients with neurologic disorders. Currently, no normal values are reported for reptilian CSF. In a study with American Alligators *(Alligator mississippiensis),* CSF was collected percutaneously from the dorsal midline near the base of the skull with a spinal needle (Bennett RA, unpublished data).

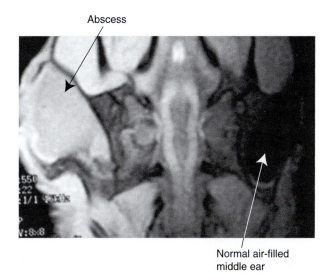

FIGURE 17-5 Magnetic resonance imaging of the head of an aquatic turtle with a middle ear abscess.

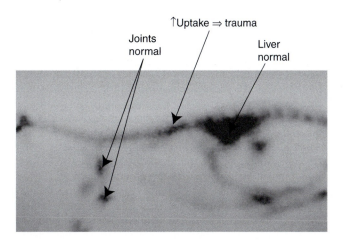

FIGURE 17-6 A nuclear scan of a Savannah Monitor Lizard (*Varanus exanthematicus*) shows a "hot spot" in the thoracic spine indicative of inflammation in the bone in this location.

The animals consistently showed gross body movement or a muscle twitch when the tip of the needle was in the proper position for fluid collection. The fluid was confirmed to be CSF on the basis of its constitution. Healthy alligator CSF was found to have a higher protein content compared with mammalian CSF.

CSF was reportedly collected from the lumbar region of a Green Iguana (*Iguana iguana*) with a spinal osteopathy. Only a few drops were collected, but cytology was consistent with an inflammatory response.[12] Further research is needed to identify the meningeal layers of the nervous system of various reptiles to determine the best way to consistently collect CSF.

NUTRITIONAL NEUROPATHIES

When dealing with a patient with neurologic disease, evaluation of the patient's nutritional status is important. Animals being fed intact whole prey diets rarely have nutritional deficiencies.

Hypothiaminosis (Leukoencephalopathy)

Thiamine deficiency may be observed in animals fed thawed frozen fish, clams, and some types of vegetation.[1,2,19] Freezing fish decreases the amount of available thiamine and increases the activity of thiaminases. Snakes of the genus *Thamnophis* and *Natrix* are piscivorous as are some crocodilians and chelonians, which makes them more prone to leukoencephalopathy if fed thawed frozen fish. Some houseplants contain phytothiaminase.[2] Herbivorous reptiles fed a diet high in vegetation containing phytothiaminases could have thiamine deficiency develop.

Clinical signs are generally nonspecific and include muscle twitching, incoordination, blindness, seizure activity, torticollis, abnormal posture, spiral locomotion, jaw gaping, dysphagia, and potentially death.[1,2,19] Snakes frequently are unable to accurately strike prey. In chelonians, the most striking clinical sign is a sinking of the eye within the bony orbit (enophthalmos).[2] At necropsy, usually no gross lesions are seen. Histologically, cerebral cortical necrosis with peripheral neuritis and cardiomyopathy is frequently encountered.[1,2,19] Histologic lesions also include a diffuse eosinophilia with severe demyelination and axon sheath fragmentation. Generally inflammatory cells are absent.

Treatment involves oral or subcutaneous supplementation of vitamin B_1 (thiamine) at 25 mg/kg/d.[1,2] A dramatic response to therapy is usually seen. The longer the duration of clinical signs, the more severe the neurologic compromise and the less likely it is to completely resolve.[2] In addition to supplementation, the diet should be evaluated and, if possible, the patient should be placed on a fresh fish diet. If frozen fish must be used, they should be supplemented with thiamine. Fish may also be boiled to denature the thiaminase.

Herbivores fed plant material containing phytothiaminase should be placed on an appropriate diet containing alternative plant sources. From a theoretical standpoint, long-term antibiotic therapy has been suggested to induce clinical signs of thiamine deficiency by decreasing the intestinal microflora responsible for producing vitamin B_1.[2,19] Although this theory has not been confirmed scientifically, some believe placing patients receiving long-term antibiotic therapy on a thiamine supplement may be prudent.

Biotin Deficiency

Biotin is a B vitamin readily supplied in most food sources. Raw egg whites contain avidin, which has antibiotin activity.[2] Deficiency may be induced in reptiles (usually in egg-eating snakes and lizards; for example, varanids) by feeding a diet of whole raw eggs.[1,2,19] Because of the ubiquitous nature of biotin, the entire diet must consist of raw eggs to induce deficiency. Free-ranging egg-eating reptiles do not generally have biotin deficiency because they eat fertile eggs, often with some degree of embryonic development. Embryonic tissue contains biotin, and the avidin in the egg is used up during embryonic development.[2,19] In addition, most egg-eating reptiles also consume small animals that contain biotin.

Clinical signs of biotin deficiency consist of muscle tremors and generalized muscle weakness. Treatment involves supplementing vitamin B complex orally or via injection and correcting the dietary deficiency with supplementing with biotin or diversifying the diet to include other items that contain adequate biotin.

Hypocalcemia

Hypocalcemia is generally observed as the result of nutritional secondary hyperparathyroidism. The reader is referred to Chapter 61 on nutritional secondary hyperparathyroidism for a detailed discussion of calcium metabolism in reptiles.

The neurologic manifestation of hypocalcemia is muscle twitching or tetany, which may be seen in any class of reptiles. Lizards frequently have a deficiency of vitamin D_3 and an improper calcium-to-phosphorus ratio in the diet. In chelonians and crocodilians, the deficiency is usually from a diet of exclusively red meat, which is deficient in calcium. Early in the course of the disease, fine twitching of the digits may be observed either unilaterally or bilaterally. This may progress to generalized tetany. In some cases, heart failure from hypocalcemia results in the patient's death. Treatment of hypocalcemic tetany entails the parenteral administration of a calcium solution (see Chapter 61).

TRAUMA-INDUCED NEUROPATHIES

Reptiles are susceptible to traumatic neuropathies from a variety of causes including direct trauma (e.g., head trauma that can cause seizures and opisthotonos) or indirect trauma (e.g., chelonians with egg binding that can cause paraparesis).[1] A chelonian dropped on its back may show signs of paraparesis as a result of spinal cord injury because it is contained within the carapace.[1] Pathologic spinal fractures can occur as the result of metabolic bone disease.[1,20-23] Reptiles with spinal cord injury generally have a loss of panniculus response caudal to the site of injury and a loss of tail or vent stimulation reflex.[1,2] In some cases, they have hypertonia cranial to the site of the injury.[2]

Fractures of the extremities can injure peripheral nerves, causing peripheral neuropathy. Paraparesis occurs in reptiles, especially chelonians, with egg binding presumably as a result of nerve compression. Such patients may have excessive wear on the hind limb claws and the plastron because of their digging behavior.[1]

Treatment of acute central or peripheral nerve trauma is primarily supportive.[10] External support of spinal fractures should be implemented.[21,23] The use of steroids in head or spinal cord trauma is controversial. The original rationale for use of glucocorticoids in central nervous system trauma came from the thought that they would reduce edema and intracranial pressure and counteract oxidative damage.[24,25] Methylprednisone sodium succinate may exert further actions such as preventing progressive ischemia and reversing intracellular calcium accumulation.[26] Current human and veterinary literature indicates that the use of steroids in central nervous system and spinal cord trauma shows no specific benefit and their use may actually increase morbidity.[27,28] Some of the side effects observed in patients with head trauma or spinal cord trauma treated with steroids include increased blood pressure, lowered seizure threshold, decrease in platelet aggregation, muscle weakness, and gastric ulceration. Glucocorticoids stimulate gluconeogenesis, and hyperglycemia has been associated with increased mortality rates in humans with severe head injury.[27] A recent report of 109 dogs with intervertebral disc disease indicates that the use of methylprednisolone sodium succinate concurrently with surgical intervention is associated with an increased postoperative complication rate and, consequently, an increased cost to the client.[28]

Spinal Osteopathy

Lytic proliferative spinal osteopathy has been reported in boids, *Crotalus,* and Southern Copperhead Snakes (*Agkistrodon contortrix*)[2,15,29,30]; however, clinically it appears to be more widespread among species of snakes. The exact cause of this condition is unknown. Because it occurs in snakes fed mice, speculation is that a virus of mouse origin may induce this disease in the snakes.[2] Some believe it may be caused by a virus of snakes that is transmitted by mice.[2] Another theory is that this is the manifestation of a slow neoplasm.[2] Hypovitaminosis D and prolonged inactivity from cage confinement have also been suggested as the cause.[30] Septicemia has also been implicated as a cause because often these lesions culture positive for bacterial organisms.[22,30] The blood flow in the area of the intervertebral discs may favor seeding of infection in this location during episodes of septicemia. Another theory is that it is an immune-mediated disease caused by a septicemia that stimulates a polyclonal B cell proliferation.[29] *Pseudomonas fluorescens, Salmonella arizonae,* and *Staphylococcus* sp. have been implicated in inducing this type of gammopathy.

The potential role of bacteria in proliferative osteoarthritis and osteoarthropathy of the spine has been reported.[30] Ten of the 15 snakes with histologic evidence of bacterial osteoarthritis had positive bone cultures, and eight of 10 snakes with positive bone cultures had corresponding positive blood cultures. *Salmonella* sp. and *Streptococcus* sp. were cultured from these patients. Three distinct groups were identified. Group 1 had strong evidence of active bacterial osteoarthritis, both histologically and on bone cultures. Group 2 was identified as having a noninflammatory osteoarthrosis without histologic evidence of bacteria but with positive culture results of the bone. Group 3 had degenerative osteoarthrosis and ankylosis with minimal to no inflammation and lack of positive bone or blood culture results.

Early in the course of the disease, focal or multifocal swellings may be identified along the dorsum associated with the spine. Palpation of the spine may reveal segmental areas of ankylosis and kyphosis.[30] Digital pressure usually induces a pain response. The patient may be hyperreflexic cranial to the lesion.[2] Motor deficits, trembling, torticollis, and spinal deformity may be manifested.[22,30] Radiographically, in the early stages of the disease, sclerosis of the vertebral endplates is seen with evidence of bone proliferation that does not involve the adjacent ribs.[2] The condition progresses with remodeling of vertebrae. The bony proliferation is usually periarticular at the costovertebral joints and the dorsolateral articular facets.[12] As the disease progresses, the ribs may become affected and the costovertebral articulations often show evidence of ankylosis, making this condition different from spondylosis deformans or ankylosing spondylosis.[30]

With time, ankylosis of the spine occurs, often affecting large segments of the spinal column (Figure 17-7). Eventually,

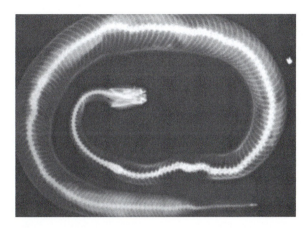

FIGURE 17-7 Spinal ankylosis in a Boa Constrictor *(Boa constrictor)* with spinal osteopathy.

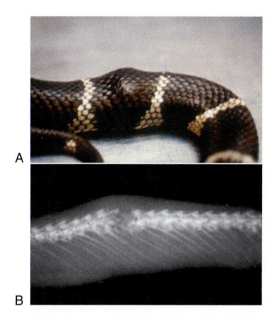

FIGURE 17-8 A, Obvious swelling is present in this California Kingsnake *(Lampropeltis getula)* with vertebral osteomyelitis. **B,** Radiographically, bone lysis is pronounced. This snake was neurologically healthy.

the animal becomes unable to move, constrict, or swallow prey. Histologically, the bone trabeculae in the vertebrae are thickened with irregular cement lines and the intertrabecular spaces are usually filled with blood vessels and fibrous connective tissue.

Blood cultures are recommended for evaluation for septicemia; however, evidence shows that the lesions develop 22 to 36 months after an episode of septicemia.[22] Local cultures may be obtained with fine needle aspirate or surgical exploration for debridement and sample collection. Cultures should be submitted for aerobic and anaerobic evaluation and acid-fast staining. One case was reported with *Mycobacterium* sp. isolated from an osseous spinal lesion causing paralysis.[2]

In a California Kingsnake *(Lampropeltis getula)* with vertebral osteopathy at the San Francisco Zoo, *Salmonella* sp., *Proteus mirabilis,* and *Bacteroides* sp. were isolated from samples collected during surgical debridement of the lesion (Figure 17-8, *A, B*). A section of the spinal column was removed, and the snake remained neurologically healthy after surgery. This snake was followed radiographically for 6 months, during which time no evidence of reossification was found in the area where the vertebrae were removed.

A condition characterized by progressive proprioceptive deficits of all four limbs leading to a state of immobility has been described in a Green Iguana.[12] No evidence of pain was seen on palpation, and the iguana continued to eat, defecate, and urinate. Survey radiographs indicated a lesion at the fourth cervical vertebra (C_4). CSF was collected and suggestive of an inflammatory response. Bacterial culture results of CSF and blood were negative. A myelogram confirmed a lesion at C_4. The iguana did not respond to supportive care and underwent euthanasia. Alhough bacterial culture results were negative, this condition was suspected to be similar to that reported in snakes.

Where spinal cord injury has occurred, the cord is repaired by ingrowth of connective tissue and nerve fibers do not regenerate.[23] Any loss of motor or sensory function is permanent. Because of the high degree of suspicion that this disease is related to septicemia, any patient having undergone an episode of sepsis should be monitored closely for evidence of spinal osteopathy. In addition, snakes with radiographic evidence of spinal osteopathy should be evaluated with blood cultures and local aspirates to identify bacteria present within the lesion or systemically. Treatment involves appropriate long-term antibiotic therapy and surgical debridement if lysis predominates.

Chapter 69 discusses spinal osteopathy in detail.

METABOLIC NEUROPATHIES

Circulatory Disturbances

Gout may cause neurologic dysfunction caused by circulatory abnormalities and directly by the formation of tophi within nervous tissue. A decrease in blood flow to the central nervous system as a result of gout may result in neurologic signs (see Chapter 54).

Granulocytic leukemia in a Gophersnake *(Pituophis melanoleucus)* at the San Francisco Zoo caused thrombus formation and infarction of the spinal cord. The patient showed paralysis caudal to the site of the infarction, which was identified histologically.

Hypoglycemia

A syndrome caused by hypoglycemia that appears to be stress induced has been reported in crocodilians.[1,19] Clinical signs include muscle tremors, loss of righting reflex, and mydriasis. The pathophysiology of this syndrome is unknown. Animals respond to oral glucose administered at 3 g/kg and elimination of the inducing stress factor.

Xanthomatosis

Xanthomatosis has been reported in captive female Leaf-tailed Geckos *(Uroplatus henkeli)* with hydrocephalus and encephalopathy. Clinical signs are stargazing, torticollis, dorsal recumbency, and seizures.[31,32] Xanthomas are cholesterol-laden granules that develop in various organs and are thought to be caused by hypercholesterolemia and hyperlipidemia. Xanthomatosis is suspected to be frequently accompanied and exacerbated by renal disease. Metabolic derangements associated with hyperuricemia, hypercholesterolemia, and hyperlipidemia are suspected in cases of xanthomatosis. A dietary correlation is suspected but currently unable to be identified. Most cases occur in females, and the condition is thought to be exacerbated by folliculogenesis, follicular degeneration, and yolk coelomitis. By the time animals are seen with neurologic signs, they appear to be unresponsive to supportive care.

Freeze Damage

This condition is most commonly observed in tortoises coming out of brumation (hibernation).[1] The cause is unknown but may be related to fatty liver syndrome or to a bacterial infection causing microabscessation within the brain. Clinical signs include circling, head tilt, and blindness with hyphema. Ocular lesions include lenticular change and retinal damage. These lesions may improve with vitamin A supplementation.[1] Many cases improve clinically with time; however, a head tilt usually does not resolve.

CONGENITAL NEUROPATHIES

Congenital neuropathies in reptiles are frequently associated with poor maternal and sometimes paternal husbandry or improper gestational incubation conditions. Most embryonic neuropathies lead to an early fetal or neonatal death.

Coiling Syndrome

Congenital neuropathic anomalies reported in snakes include axial bifurcation, kyphosis, and fusion of adjacent coils.[33] A congenital neurologic conditon exists in newborn Boa Constrictors (*Constrictor constrictor*) that grossly appears like a vertebral malformation. Though the vertebrae are normal, these snakes appear to have kyphosis, scoliosis, or lordosis. Affected snakes are seen with single to multiple coils of their spine, compromised locomotion, abnormal posturing, and anorexia. The conditon frequently affects only the caudal half of the snake and has been termed caudal coiling syndrome. Radiographically, the vertebral bodies themselves appear to be normal and not the cause of the condition. When anesthetized, the snake's body is able to be manually stretched and uncoiled. The condition can be a cause of acute mortality in neonates or a chronic debilitating syndrome in juveniles. Affected animals have shown no response to assist-feeding and supportive care, ultimately progressing and succumbing to the disease. The unaffected portions of the snake's body appear to function normally, and normal voluntary muscle contractions are observed as the snake attempts to drag its disfigured body. The disorder does not appear to involve the brain or CNs and structures caudal to the lesion maintain sensory and motor function.

Necropsy examination confirms the radiographic findings; no gross abnormalities of the vertebrae are identified. Histologically, the dorsal epaxial musculature contains multiple leukocytic infiltrates surrounding the nerves and vessels within the perimysium.[33] Potential causes of this condition include infectious agents, an inflammatory process, neoplasia, and improper incubation conditions. All attempts to culture or isolate an infectious organism have been unsuccessful, and the husbandry associated with the gestation of the neonates is reportedly appropriate.[33] Further investigations into the cause of this condition are indicated.

TOXIC NEUROPATHIES

Chlorhexidine

Reports are seen of a 0.024% chlorhexidine solution as a topical medication or soaking solution in reptiles with cutaneous disease.[34] At this concentration, the agent appears to be safe. However, the use of the 2% stock solution as a therapeutic bath has caused acute neurologic disease and death in reptiles. Chelonians appear to be extremely sensitive to the toxic affects of the solution.

Clinical signs include acute flaccid paralysis and improve to loss of the righting reflexes and diminished withdrawal reflexes. Signs do not resolve, and death from neurologic and respiratory collapse readily ensues.

Insecticides

Reptiles appear to be especially sensitive to insecticide toxicosis. Birds are reportedly 10 to 20 times more sensitive to insecticides than mammals, and reptiles appear to be more sensitive than birds. Many forms of insecticides, including sprays, powders, and pesticide strips, have been used to control external parasite problems in reptiles. Their use may result in neurologic signs from pesticide toxicity.[1]

Clinical signs are generally nonspecific and include head tilt, circling, opisthotonos, and seizure activity. Treatment is generally supportive and includes fluid therapy for hydration and renal support. Respiratory support may be necessary in some patients. Atropine is beneficial in treatment of organophosphate or carbamate intoxication.[1] Diazepam or other benzodiazepines may help control seizures. Mild cooling of the patient has been recommended to decrease nerve conduction velocity and lessen the severity of seizure activity[1]; however, this also slows the patient's ability to metabolize the drug and eliminate the toxin.

Ivermectin

Ivermectin is a macrocyclic lactone derived from *Streptomyces avermitilis*, which acts at gamma-aminobutyric acid (GABA) synapses to stimulate excess release of GABA.[35] In nematodes, GABA is an inhibitory neurotransmitter. It binds irreversibly to the receptors, thus requiring that it be metabolized before its effects diminish. In mammals, ivermectin is not able to cross the blood-brain barrier and therefore shows no effect in the patient animal. Ivermectin has been used successfully in a variety of reptilian species; however, it appears to be toxic primarily in chelonians. Ivermectin has been postulated as able to cross the blood-brain barrier in chelonians or GABA may be a more important peripheral neurotransmitter in chelonians.[35]

Clinical signs associated with ivermectin intoxication are primarily related to general neuromuscular weakness. Death is a function of paralysis of the respiratory muscles. Some variation appears in species susceptibility, and Leopard Tortoises (Geochelone pardalis) are especially sensitive with paresis occurring at a dose as low as 0.025 mg/kg.[35] Because ivermectin binds irreversibly, it takes at least 7 days for reversal of clinical signs. Further, a cumulative effect may be observed if the drug is administered at frequent intervals. Treatment is primarily supportive, with particular attention paid to the respiratory, hydration, and nutritional status. Most animals need ventilatory support for several days. In general, the use of ivermectin in chelonians is best to avoid.

Milbemycin (Interceptor; Ciba-Geigy Corp, Greensboro, NC) is safe and effective for use in some chelonians.[36] This agent acts similar to ivermectin on the GABA receptors and was effective in Red-eared Sliders (Trachemys scripta elegans), Gulf Coast Box Turtles (Terrepene carolina major), and Ornate Box Turtles (Terrepene ornata). No toxic side effects have been observed, but the drug has not been evaluated in chelonians, which appear to be more sensitive to ivermectin. Milbemycin was effective at 0.5 to 1 mg/kg subcutaneously.

Metronidazole

Metronidazole is an antibiotic and antiprotozoal agent commonly used in reptile medicine. The half life of metronidazole in iguanas is longer (12.7 ± 3.7 hours) than that reported for mammalian species (dogs, 4 to 5 hours; humans, 6 to 10 hours).[37] At high doses, metronidazole may induce clinical signs of vestibular disease with head tilt, circling, and dysequilibrium.[1] In snakes, severe neurologic signs and death have been associated with administration of metronidazole above 100 mg/kg. Treatment is supportive and clinical signs are reversible.

Other Antibiotics

Polymyxin and the aminoglycocides (streptomycin, kanamycin, gentamicin, and neomycin) at high doses cause neuromuscular blockade and may induce neurologic signs such as paralysis.

Heavy Metal Intoxication

Plumbism was diagnosed in a tortoise after ingestion of lead-based paint chips.[1] Diagnosis was made on the basis of clinical signs of generalized central nervous system disease and supported by high blood lead levels. Blood samples from a control animal must be submitted for comparison purposes. Treatment should involve eliminating the lead from the gastrointestinal system with gastric lavage and catharsis in conjunction with calcium ethylenediamine tetraacetic acid therapy at 10 to 40 mg/kg intramuscularly twice a day.

Apparent zinc toxicity was observed in a Green Iguana that had ingested pennies. The patient was seen with anorexia, weakness, and anemia. Blood zinc levels were elevated compared with normal ranges published for other species. The iguana recovered uneventfully after chelation therapy and surgical removal of the pennies from the cecum (Figure 17-9, A, B).

Other Toxins

A variety of other environmental agents are potentially toxic to reptiles including iodoforms, nicotine, naphthalene, paraffin, and paint solvents.[1] Wood shavings with high resin content such as cedar shavings may cause a reversible ataxia.

Ingestion of fireflies of the genus Photinus is lethal to inland Bearded Dragons (Pogona vitticeps).[38] These fireflies contain lucibufagins, a steroidal pyrone, and ingestion of one insect is enough to be fatal to an adult Bearded Dragon. The toxin is actually thought to be cardiotoxic, but affected animals show signs of focal facial seizures, violent head shaking, mouth gaping, and protrusion and biting of the tongue.

Although fireflies have been shown to be nontoxic in certain lizards (see Chapter 83), it is recommended *not* to use fireflies as food items.

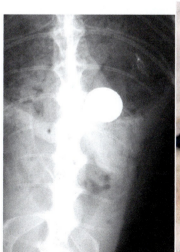
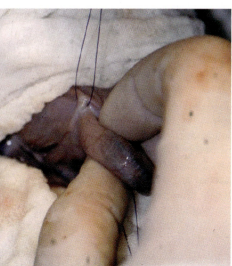

FIGURE 17-9 A, Radiograph of a Green Iguana (*Iguana iguana*) with coins in the cecum believed to be causing zinc intoxication. **B,** Intraoperative view of the coins found at surgery. The iguana recovered after removal of the coins.

INFECTIOUS NEUROPATHIES

Bacterial, viral, fungal, and protozoan infections are known to cause neurologic signs in reptiles. In some cases, although an infectious agent is suspected, definitive determination may not be possible. For example, in a Burmese Python (*Python molurus bivittatus*) with opisthotonos the meninges were infiltrated by small lymphocytes at necropsy. Perivascular cuffing was evident, indicating a possible viral cause; however, no definitive diagnosis for this lymphocytic meningitis was determined.[2]

Parasitic

Acanthamebic Meningoencephalitis

Species of *Acanthamoeba* are generally pathogenic to humans but can infect any soft tissue of reptiles.[2,39] Human infections are most commonly the result of contamination of recreational water sources. Organisms enter via the nasal mucosa and migrate through the cribriform plate or are transported to tissues by the vascular system.[1,2] Frank[40] reported a free-living *Acanthameba* encountered during necropsies of amphibians and reptiles. In his studies, he was able to induce infection both in the central nervous system and in other organs. In a Boa Constrictor and a Pacific Coast Rattlesnake (*Crotalus viridis oreganus*) with spasmodic opisthotonos, acanthamebic encephalitis was diagnosed.[2] Organisms were contained within the CSF in both snakes. Environmental stimulus exacerbated the clinical sign of opisthotonos. The drinking water was proposed as the source of contamination. A diagnosis of acanthamebic meningoencephalitis is difficult antemortem, and no successful treatment has been reported.

Toxoplasmosis

Nosema sp. and *Toxoplasma gondii* have been reported to be associated with meningoencephalitis in reptiles. *Toxoplasma* is generally a parasite of homeotherms that can develop in reptiles when their body temperature is maintained near 37°C (99°F). Insects may serve as vectors or fomites for the transmission of toxoplasmosis, emphasizing the need for pest control. Diagnosis is based on histopathology, and no predictably successful treatment has been identified. Clindamycin has appeared to be beneficial in treating mammals with toxoplasmosis.[41] The recommended dose in reptiles is 5 mg/kg by mouth daily[42]; however, no studies are found regarding its efficacy in reptiles with toxoplasmosis.

Bacterial

Bacterial infections may be a primary cause of nervous system disorder or may secondarily affect the nervous system as exemplified by spinal osteopathy causing paresis in snakes.[1,2] After septicemia, especially from respiratory infections, microabscesses or macroabscesses can develop within the brain. Histologically, these abscesses consist of areas of necrosis usually associated with a large numbers of mononuclear leukocytes. Granulocytic leukocytes are usually not found in brain and spinal cord inflammation in reptiles.[2] Clinical signs of bacterial encephalitis are generally nonspecific. Treatment consists of systemic antibiotic therapy with an agent with the potential to cross the blood-brain barrier.

Mycobacterium generally produces a multisystemic disease that can involve the nervous system. It induces a granulomatous inflammation with granulomas containing caseous cellular debris and acid-fast organisms. Cytologic preparations of granulomatous debris may be acid fast stained to determine the presence of the organisms. Treatment of mycobacteriosis in reptiles is controversial because of the zoonotic potential of the infection.

Viral

Paramyxo-like Virus

A progressive central nervous system disorder manifesting clinically as head tremors and loss of equilibrium with opisthotonos has been described in Rock Rattlesnakes (*Crotalus lepidus*).[21] These snakes also lost the righting reflex and had irregular and slow tongue flick responses. The disease was linked to a paramyxo-like virus that was identified with electron microscopy. The disease was believed to have been introduced to the private collection with the addition of two wild-caught snakes that had signs develop within 14 days of their capture. Because colubrid snakes maintained within the same collection were unaffected, not all genera of snakes are believed to be susceptible to this virus.

Histologically, gliosis and perivascular cuffing were identified in a variety of locations within the hind brain. Demyelination, axon degeneration, and ballooning of axon sheaths were seen in the brain stem and spinal cord. In addition to the central nervous system lesions, the lungs also showed pathology consisting of cellular debris and exudate filling the primary bronchi and air spaces. This proliferative interstitial pneumonia was characteristic of squamous metaplasia of the lining of the air spaces with interstitial thickening.

See Chapter 63 for more information on paramyxovirus.

Inclusion Body Disease of Boids

This condition is believed to be caused by a retrovirus and affects boas and pythons; however, the clinical syndrome is distinct between these two groups.[1,2,43-45] The severity is significantly worse in pythons than in boas, underscoring the recommendation to not mix boas and pythons in the same collection. Boas may be inapparent carriers. The snake mite, *Ophionyssus natricis*, is suspected as one of the vectors incriminated in the spread of the disease. Other modes of transmission include direct contact and venereal spread.[45-46]

Clinical signs are generally multisystemic, including gastrointestinal, respiratory, and neurologic signs. In juvenile boas, the condition is often quickly fatal with an acute onset of flaccid paralysis. Adult boas have a different, more chronic manifestation of the disease develop, with central nervous system signs occurring only in the terminal stages. Early in the course of the disease, chronic regurgitation, profound cachexia, and chronic pneumonia are common. Neurologic signs are generally manifest as an inability to strike, constrict, and prehend food items. Dysecdysis may occur as a result of an inability to control body movements to rub off the shed skin.[43]

In pythons, the clinical course is much more rapid, progressing to a fatal CNS disturbance. Pythons also have multisystemic disease, with pneumonia and infectious stomatitis common. Neurologically, they have a loss of righting reflex, hyperreflexia, disorientation, and loss of motor coordination. Some animals have central blindness develop.[2,45]

Currently, no serologic test is available to diagnose inclusion body disease. Biopsy results of the liver, kidney, esophageal lymphoid tissue, and skin may show the typical eosinophilic intracytoplasmic inclusions. Histologically, eosinophilic intracytoplasmic inclusion bodies have been identified within epithelial cells of the pancreas, kidney, esophagus, stomach, and liver. A nonsuppurative encephalitis with neuron degeneration and mononuclear cell infiltrates characterizes the lesions within the brain and spinal cord. In the white tracts of the spinal cord, areas of gliosis with extensive myelin degeneration and axon loss are seen. Intracytoplasmic eosinophilic inclusion bodies have been found within the neurons of the brain and the gray tracts of the spinal cord. The degree of inflammation is much greater in pythons compared with that found in boas. Perivascular cuffing with degenerative myelopathy is evidence of a viral etiology; however, some bacterial infections also stimulate perivascular cuffing.[1,2] Electron microscopy has shown viral particles suspected of being in the retrovirus family.[1,2,43,45]

No treatment has been shown to be successful for this viral disease. It may be mild in boas and may go undiagnosed. Therefore, prevention of exposure of pythons to boas is best as they may be inapparent carriers. Identification and elimination of animals with known positive disease are recommended.

See Chapter 60 for more information on inclusion body disease.

Other Viral Infections

Reptiles may serve as reservoir hosts for western equine encephalitis and Venezuelan equine encephalitis; however, the clinical significance is unknown.[2] West Nile virus has been reported in reptiles as early as the 1960s in Israel.[47] More recently, West Nile virus has been found to occur in crocodilians in the United States.[48,49] The mode of transmission to reptiles is thought to be from the ingestion of or a bite from the insect carrier or from ingestion of infected horse meat.[49] Affected animals have an acute onset of loss of leg control, neck spasms, and a star gazing appearance before death. In reptiles with neurologic disease, the presence of perivascular cuffing within the brain and spinal cord is indicative of viral infection, yet in many instances no agent has been identified.

SUMMARY

Much remains to be learned about neurologic diseases of captive reptiles. In many instances, neurologic manifestations are caused by improper husbandry, trauma, or infectious disease. Clinical signs associated with neurologic disease in reptiles are often nonspecific, and localization of the site of the lesion and the etiology may be difficult. Evaluating the patient for known causes of neuropathies in reptiles helps the clinician develop a diagnostic and therapeutic plan appropriate for the patient. A complete diagnostic evaluation both antemortem and postmortem is vital especially in treatment of animals within a collection.

REFERENCES

1. Lawton MPC: Neurological disease. In Benyon PH, editor: *Manual of reptiles,* Kingsley House, Gloucestershire, England, 1992, British Small Animal Veterinary Association.
2. Frye FL: Viral diseases. In *Biomedical & surgical aspects of captive reptile husbandry,* ed 2, Malabar, Fla, 1991, Krieger Publishing.
3. Davies PMC: Anatomy and physiology. In Cooper JE, Jackson OF, editors: *Diseases of the Reptilia,* New York, 1981, Academic Press.
4. Marcus LC: *Veterinary biology and medicine of captive amphibians and reptiles,* Philadelphia, 1981, Lea & Febiger.
5. Weichert LK, Presh WW: Integrating system: nervous system. In *Elements of cordate anatomy,* New York, 1975, McGraw Hill.
6. Chrisman CL, Walsh M, Meeks JC, Zurawka H, LaRock R, Herbst L, et al: Neurologic examination of sea turtles, *J Am Vet Med Assoc* 211(8):1043-1047, 1997.
7. Williams DL: Ophthalmology. In Mader DR: *Reptile medicine and surgery,* Philadelphia, 1996, WB Saunders.
8. Jacobson ER: The evaluation of the reptile patient. In Jacobson ER, Kollias GV, editors: *Exotic animals,* New York, 1988, Churchill Livingstone.
9. Rosenberg ME: Temperature and nervous conduction in the tortoise, *J Physiol (Lond)* 270(1):50, 1977.
10. Sims MH: Electrodiagnostic evaluation. In Braund KG, editor: *Clinical syndromes in veterinary neurology,* ed 2, St Louis, 1994, Mosby.
11. Schumacher J, Toal RL: Advanced radiography and ultrasonography in reptiles, *Semin Avian Exotic Pet Med* (10)4: 162-168, 2001.
12. Divers SJ, Lawton MPC: Spinal osteomyelitis in a green iguana, *Iguana iguana*: cerebospinal fluid and myelogram diagnosis, *Proc ARAV* 77: 2000.
13. Hathcock JT, Stickle RL: Principles and concepts of computed tomography, *Vet Clin North Am Small Anim Pract* 23(2):400-415, 1993.
14. Rubel A, Kuoni W, Augustiny N: Emerging techniques: CT scan and MRI in reptile medicine, *Semin Avian Exotic Pet Med* 3(3):156-160, 1994.
15. Stoskopf MK: Clinical imaging in zoological medicine: a review, *J Zoo Wildl Med* 20(4):396-412, 1989.
16. Rosenthal K, Stefanacci J, Quesenberry K, Hoefer H: Computerized tomography in 10 cases of avian intracranial disease, *Proc Annu Conf Assoc Avian Vet* 305, 1995.
17. Clippinger TL, Bennett RA, Platt SR: The avian neurologic examination and ancillary neurodiagnostic techniques, *J Avian Med Surg* 10(4):221-247, 1996.
18. Shores A: New and future advanced imaging techniques, *Vet Clin North Am Small Anim Pract* 21(3):461-469, 1993.
19. Frye FL: Feeding and nutritional diseases. In Fowler ME, editor: *Zoo and wild animal medicine,* ed 2, Philadelphia, 1986, WB Saunders.
20. Russo EA: Anorexia and spinal fracture in a boa constrictor, *Avian Exotic Pract* 2(3):7, 1985.
21. Jacobson ER, et al: Paramyxo-like virus infection in a rock rattlesnake, *J Am Vet Med Assoc* 177(9):795-799, 1980.
22. Kiel JL: Spinal osteoarthropathy in two southern copperheads, *J Zoo Am Med* 8(2):21-24, 1977.
23. Peary GM: A non-surgical technique for stabilizing multiple spinal fractures in a gopher snake, *VM/SAC* 72:1055, 1977.
24. Braughler JM, Hall ED: Current application of "high dose" steroid therapy for CNS injury, *J Neurosurg* 62:806-810, 1985.
25. Alderson P: Corticosteroids in acute traumatic brain injury: systematic review of randomised controlled trials, *Br Med J* 314:1855, 1997.
26. Hall E: The neuroprotective pharmacology of methylprednisone, *J Neurosurg* 76:13-22, 1992.
27. Dewey CW: Emergency management of the head trauma patient, *Vet Clin North Am Small Anim Pract* 30(1):207-225, 2000.
28. Boag AK, Otto CM, Drobatz KJ: Complications of methylprednisolone sodium succinate in dachshunds with

surgically treated invertebral disc disease, *J Vet Emerg Crit Care* 11(2):105-110, 2001.
29. Kiel JL: Paget's disease in snakes, *Proc Am Zoo Vet* 201-207, 1983.
30. Isaza R, Garner M, Jacobson E: Proliferative osteoarthritis and osteoarthrosis in 15 snakes, *J Zoo Wildl Med* 31(1): 20-27, 2000.
31. Raiti P, Garner M: Uremic encephalopathy in a leaf-tailed gecko, *Uroplatus henkeli*, *Proc ARAV* 29:30, 2000.
32. Garner M, Lung NP: Xanthomatosis in geckos: five cases, *Proc ARAV* 61: 1997.
33. Fitzgerald SD, Janovitz EB, Burnstein T, Axthelm MK: A caudal coiling syndrome associated with lymphocytic epaxial perineuritis in newborn boa constrictors, *J Zoo Wildl Med* 21(4):485-489, 1990.
34. Lloyd M: Chlorhexidine toxicosis from soaking in red-bellied short necked turtles, *Emydura subglobosa*, *Bull Assoc Reptl Amphib Vet* (6)4:6,7, 2000.
35. Teare JA, Bush M: Toxicity and efficacy of ivermectin in chelonians, *J Am Vet Med Assoc* 183(11):1195-1197, 1983.
36. Bodri MS, Nolan TJ, Skeeba SJ: Safety of milbemycin (A_3-A_4 oxime) in chelonians, *J Zoo Wildl Med* 24(2):171-174, 1993.
37. Kolmstetter CM, Frazier D, Cox S, Ramsay EC: Pharmacokinetics of metronidazole in the green iguana, *Iguana iguana*, *Bull Assoc Reptl Amph Vet* (8)3:4-7, 1998.
38. Glor R, Means C, Weintraub MJH, Knight M, Adler K, Eisner T: Two cases of firefly toxicosis in bearded dragons, *Pogona vitticeps*, *Proc ARAV* 27-29, 1999.
39. Frank W: Non-hemoparasitic protozoans. In Hoff GL, Frye FL, Jacobson ER, editors: *Diseases of amphibians and reptiles*, New York, 1984, Plenum Press.
40. Frank W: *Limax* - amoebae from cold-blooded vertebrates, *Ann Soc Belg Med Trop* 54(4,5):343-349, 1974.
41. Plumb DC: *Veterinary drug handbook*, ed 4, Ames, 2002, Iowa State University Press.
42. Carpenter JW, Mashima TY, Rupiper DJ: Antimicrobial agents used in reptiles. In *Exotic animal formulary*, ed 2, Philadelphia, 2001, WB Saunders.
43. Wright K: Dysecdysis in boid snakes with neurologic diseases, *ARAV* 2(2):7, 1992.
44. Schumacher J, Jacobson ER, Gaskin JM: Inclusion-body disease in boid snakes: a retrospective and prospective study, *Proc Am Assoc Zoo Vet* 289: 1990.
45. Schumacher J, Jacobson ER, Homer BL, Gaskin JM: Inclusion body disease in boid snakes, *J Zoo Wildl Med* 25(4):511-524, 1994.
46. Jacobson ER: An update on inclusion body disease of boid snakes, *Proc ARAV* 165, 1997.
47. Nir Y, Lasowski Y, Avivi A, Goldwasser R: Survey for antibodies to arboviruses in the serum of various animals in Israel during 1965-1966, *Am J Trop Med Hyg* 18(3):416-422, 1969.
48. Miller DL, Mauel MJ, Baldwin C, Burtle G, Ingram D, Hines ME, et al: West Nile Virus in farmed alligators, *Emerging Infect Dis* 9(7):794-799, 2003.
49. Steinman A, Banet-Noach C, Tal S, Levi O, Simanov L, Perk S, et al: West Nile Virus infection in crocodiles, *Emerging Infect Dis* 9(7):887-888, 2003.

18
NUTRITION

SUSAN DONOGHUE

Diet and feeding management play key roles in reptile medicine and surgery, at times causing disease and at others aiding recovery. Diet attracts more attention, but inappropriate feeding management, regardless of diet quality, has killed many reptiles. In the case of venomous reptiles and giant snakes, it has even killed their keepers.

Nutritional disorders arise from imbalanced or unsuitable diets and from poor husbandry. Each species has an ideal habitat, optimal ranges of temperature and humidity, specific preferences for food, and a nutritional heritage manifested as digestive and metabolic adaptations that influence its requirements for water, calories, and nutrients. Captive management strives for but rarely achieves conditions identical to the animal's natural habitat. Stress from captivity may negatively impact food intake and nutrient utilization, and in turn, diet and feeding management can be used effectively to minimize untoward effects of stress from captivity, illness, and surgery.

Common nutritional problems in captive reptiles include starvation and malnutrition; dietary deficiencies of calcium, cholecalciferol (vitamin D_3), and vitamin A in certain lizards and chelonians; obesity in large sedentary snakes and lizards; and nutrient toxicities from oversupplementation. In addition, complex and challenging nutritional problems can be found in collections managed by experienced and knowledgeable keepers. Extensive questioning about diet, feeding management, and overall husbandry is a critical part of history taking for every reptile patient.

NUTRITION AND METABOLISM

For reptiles, as for all species, metabolism significantly impacts nutritional needs and vice versa. Metabolic rates and food preferences dictate food intakes, fuel (energy) sources, metabolic responses to disease, and diets for nutrition support. Energy requirements or metabolic rates for captive reptiles are usually expressed as calories (kcal) of estimated metabolizable energy (ME) for specified conditions.

Energy

Reptiles are *ectothermic* (older terms are *poikilothermic* and *cold-blooded*). Their body temperature depends on the environment (and their behavior within the environment) rather than on internal metabolism. Also, reptiles are *heterothermic*, exhibiting a wide range of body temperatures in line with environmental conditions. Ambient environmental temperature affects core body temperature; activity such as food procurement, digestion, and absorption of nutrients; and metabolic rate.

Wild reptiles maintain body temperature within an optimal range through behavioral choices such as basking on a rock, digging into forest floor litter, entering or exiting water, and changing their color and body shape to facilitate heat uptake. Heart rates increase during heating and decrease during cooling, serving to heat reptiles quickly and cool them slowly.[1] Many have evolved body shapes that improve surface-to-volume ratios to improve heat uptake (Figures 18-1 and 18-2). Some change colors to achieve faster heating and slower cooling (Figure 18-3). Temperature gradients and appropriate habitat furnishings allow captive reptiles to effectively regulate body temperature.

Failure to provide appropriate temperature gradients and sufficient basking spots is a common problem with inexperienced keepers. Reptiles housed in pairs or groups are especially vulnerable to cold conditions. For example, research with Green Iguanas (*Iguana iguana*) has shown that social hierarchies develop in group-housed iguanas; the dominant males gained twice as much exposure to heat sources and as a result showed greater digestive efficiency.[2] A cold reptile cannot maintain an active metabolism, which leads to low intakes of food and water and poor utilization of what is taken in (Figure 18-4). Immune suppression and dehydration often follow and lead to life-threatening infections or renal failure.

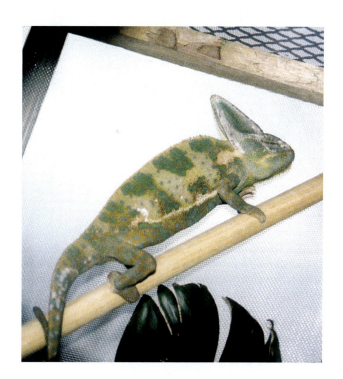

FIGURE 18-1 Reptiles use morphology and behavior to warm their body temperature. This young male Veiled Chameleon, *Chamaeleo calyptratus*, has a high casque on his head that increases the surface area-to-volume ratio, facilitating warm-up. In addition, he has moved to the top of a 6-ft-high enclosure to be close to the basking light.

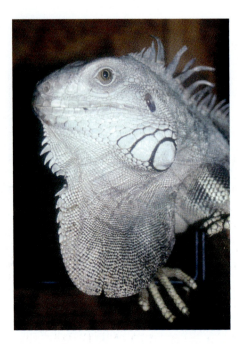

FIGURE 18-2 This Green Iguana's *(Iguana iguana)* dewlap not only serves as a mode of communication but also increases the surface area-to-volume ratio, hastening warm-up.

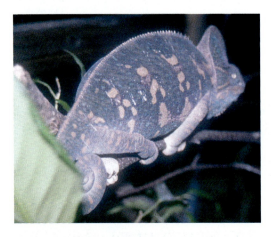

FIGURE 18-3 Some reptiles turn dark colors to warm more quickly. These dark warming colors may be confused with stress coloration in chameleons such as this female Veiled Chameleon *(Chamaeleo calyptratus)*. She is reacting to a male that has entered her habitat.

Reptiles underfed in warm environments lose weight rapidly because of relatively high metabolic rates. By the time of presentation, however, prolonged underfeeding may have led to starvation evidenced by cachexia and *decreased* metabolic rate (despite warm temperatures).

Calorie intakes often must be estimated in reptile patients as part of the medical examination, with suggesting appropriate food intakes and with providing nutrition support. Metabolic rate in reptiles relates to metabolic body size—the smaller the animal, the greater its metabolic rate per unit body weight (BW). However, metabolic rates in reptiles average only 25% to 35% those for mammals (Table 18-1).[3-5]

Daily energy needs are estimated from research data and clinical experience. Calorie intakes are often based on

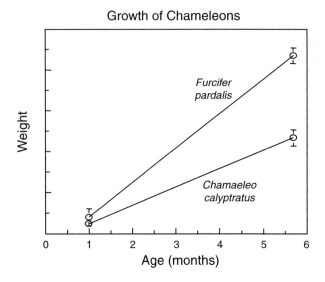

FIGURE 18-4 Panther *(Furcifer pardalis)* and Veiled Chameleons *(Chamaeleo calyptratus)* are lowland species that grow quickly under optimal conditions. These data from the author's feeding trials show slow growth in Veiled Chameleons kept at cool temperatures. Low temperatures decrease metabolic rate, slowing growth.

calculations of average standard metabolic rate (SMR), usually measured on fasting animals at rest in a dark temperature-controlled environment (see Table 18-1). These equations are starting points only because as more data are published, differences between species and groups become known. For example, Australian Pythons have been shown to maintain lower preferred body temperature and lower SMR than other boids, which are already lower than most other snakes.[6] The slower metabolism is thought to better conserve energy for pythons' "sit and wait" predatory behavior. Variations in energy have been measured in Green Iguanas *(Iguana iguana)*, monitors, Rock Iguanas *(Cyclura* spp.), Komodo Dragons *(Varanus komodoensis)*, seaturtles, and Tuatara *(Sphenodon punctatus)*.[7-10] Variations between seasons, gender, age, diet, and habitat have also been noted in a variety of species.[11-16] Lower metabolic rates are found in montane species, relative to lowland species (Figure 18-5).

Equations for turtles are similar to other reptiles, even though the shell comprises 15% to 30% of BW. Calorie utilization rates specifically for turtle shell are unknown, but the carapace and plastron are undoubtedly metabolically active tissue.[17] Shells (carapace and plastron) of turtles (aquatic and semiaquatic) and tortoises (terrestrial) are vascularized, growing, and serve as buffering organs in hypoxic and acidotic specimens. The total weight of turtles and tortoises should be used for calorie calculations, and shell trauma may be expected to raise their calorie needs.

Energy requirements likely increase with eating, activity, reproduction, growth, protein synthesis (as in wound healing), and certain disorders. Crocodiles that consumed a meal equivalent to 7.5% of their BW increased their metabolic rate four-fold.[18] Blood lactate rose slightly, indicative of aerobic metabolism contributing to the large increases in metabolic rate. Daily energy intakes should be calculated with multiplying the SMR by a factor that ranges from 1.1 to about 3 or 4,

Table 18-1	Estimates of Standard Metabolic Rate and Fractional Decreases and Increases for Feeding and Activity[3-5]					
Body Weight (g)	0.5 SMR (kcal/d)	0.75 SMR (kcal/d)	1.0 SMR (kcal/d)	1.5 SMR (kcal/d)	2.0 SMR (kcal/d)	3.0 SMR (kcal/d)
1	0.09	0.14	0.18	0.28	0.38	0.57
5	0.30	0.45	0.60	0.90	1.2	1.8
10	0.50	0.75	1.0	1.5	2.0	3.0
15	0.68	1.0	1.4	2.1	2.8	4.2
20	0.85	1.3	1.7	2.6	3.4	5.1
25	1.0	1.5	2.0	3.0	4.0	6.0
30	1.2	1.7	2.3	3.4	4.6	6.9
40	1.4	2.2	2.9	4.4	5.8	8.7
50	1.7	2.6	3.4	5.1	6.8	10
75	2.3	3.4	4.6	6.9	5.2	14
100	2.8	4.3	5.7	8.6	11	17
150	3.8	5.8	7.7	12	15	23
200	4.8	7.2	9.6	14	19	29
300	6.5	9.8	13	20	26	39
400	8.0	12	16	24	32	48
500	9.5	14	19	28	38	57
1000	16	24	32	48	64	96
1500	22	32	43	64	86	129
2000	27	40	54	81	108	162
3000	36	54	73	110	146	219
4000	46	69	91	136	182	273
5000	54	81	107	161	214	321
10,000	90	135	180	270	360	540
20,000	152	228	303	454	606	909
40,000	254	382	509	764	1018	1527
60,000	345	518	690	1035	1380	2070
80,000	428	642	856	1284	1712	2568

Values at 86°F (30°C).
SMR = 32 (BW$^{0.75}$), where *SMR* is standard metabolic rate in kcal/d and *BW* is body weight in kg.

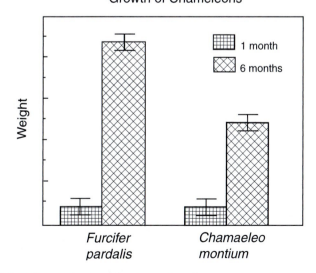

FIGURE 18-5 Lowland species of chameleon grow faster than montane species because they inhabit warmer climes, thus maintaining faster metabolic rates and consuming more food. Genetics may also contribute to differences in growth rates. These data from the author's feeding trials show slower growth in montane *Chamaeleo montium* compared with the lowland *Furcifer pardalis*.

according to activity and other conditions that increase metabolic rate (Figure 18-6; see Table 18-1). Energy needs decrease in cold temperatures, unlike in endotherms.

Some reptiles change their behavior when ill, selecting temperatures at the upper end of their preferred temperature range. These *behavioral fevers* are thought to aid the patient's response to the disease and may be replicated for sick reptiles in captivity.

With so much emphasis on heat, clients need to know that reptiles can heat up much faster than they can cool down and that overheating is a frequent cause of death. Reptiles placed in sun (behind glass especially, but also in wire habitats) without shade, tortoises that have become upended in the sun, and montane species maintained in temperatures greater than about 85°F (29°C) can die quickly.

Calorie Sources

Reptilian digestive tracts range from relatively short and simple for hydrolysis in small intestines (carnivores) to relatively large for fermentation in the lower bowel (herbivores). In practice, optimal proportions of fuel sources (dietary protein, fat, and carbohydrate [starch and fiber]) are estimated from information on natural history, including feeding habits, habitat, and digestive morphology. Carnivores (including

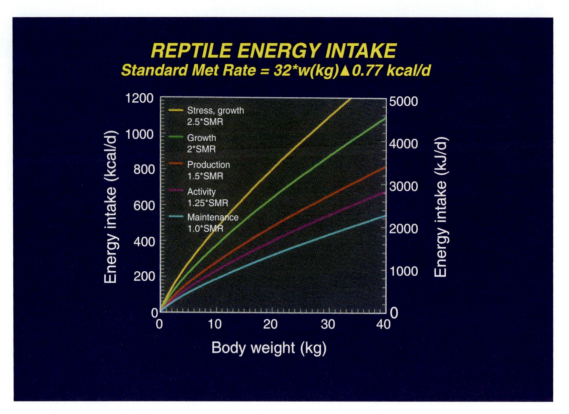

FIGURE 18-6 Energy intakes (kcal/d) increase above standard metabolic rate (SMR) for activity and production (new tissue, eggs).

insectivores) use primarily fat and protein as fuel sources; herbivores use relatively more soluble carbohydrate and fermented fiber (Figure 18-7). Omnivores use all three fuel sources (Figure 18-8).

Carnivores

Snakes, alligators, caimans, crocodiles, many species of monitors, many juvenile aquatic turtles, and many lizards are carnivores. Healthy carnivorous reptiles consume high intakes of protein and fat, about 25% to 60% of ME as protein and 30% to 60% of ME as fat. Juvenile American Alligators (*Alligator mississippiensis*) were found to grow best when fed diets containing 42% of ME from protein.[19] Optimal levels are likely to be similar for other carnivorous reptiles.

Carbohydrate intake for carnivorous reptiles is often limited to that found in digesta from herbivorous prey, but a few exceptions exist. The popular Veiled Chameleon, *Chamaeleo calyptratus*, is an insectivore that consumes small amounts of leaves, greens, or fruit in captivity. The behavior is thought to ensure adequate water intake during times of scarcity in its native Yemen.

Carnivores require protein of high quality. This issue is usually irrelevant when whole prey are fed but critical when assist-feeding patients. Data are limited, but research in alligators suggests that proteins from nonmeat sources, including corn gluten, soy, casein, and gliadin, are inadequate.[20] Genuinely "all-meat" pet foods are rare; most canned meat dinner pet foods contain corn gluten and soy flour, which lowers protein quality and decreases the appropriateness of these products for carnivorous reptiles. In studies of nutrition support of carnivorous reptiles in the author's laboratory, protein sources of egg and isolated soy protein have maintained BW.

Omnivores

Many aquatic turtles, wood turtles, forest tortoises, and lizards consume both animal and plant matter. Energy sources for omnivores such as Box Turtles (*Terrapene* spp.) and Bearded Dragons (*Pogona vitticeps*) are a mix of protein, fat, and carbohydrates (see Figure 18-8). Wild omnivorous reptiles tend to eat more protein and fat during juvenile growth than during adulthood (slow growth). For example, omnivorous aquatic turtles consume more fish (high in protein and fat) than vegetation (high in carbohydrate) when young. Also, aquatic turtles grow faster when fed diets containing 25% and 40% rather than 10% crude protein.[21,22] Similarly, wild Bearded Dragons eat prey when young and plants when older and in captivity thrive when fed prey as juveniles, a mix of prey and salads during years of reproductive activity, then salads in old age, their "salad years."[23]

The shift from carnivorous as juveniles to omnivorous as adults is observed in many aquatic turtles, Bearded Dragons, and other reptiles. The evolutionary and functional significance of the shift is unclear. Conventional thought is that the higher caloric density from a meat-based diet is the only way to meet energy needs for growth when gut capacity is limited. However, recent studies with Red-eared Sliders (*Trachemys scripta elegans*) show that juveniles (28 g BW) can meet their energy and nitrogen needs with a plant diet.[24]

In contrast, other omnivorous species appear to retain a meat-based dietary component to meet energy needs.

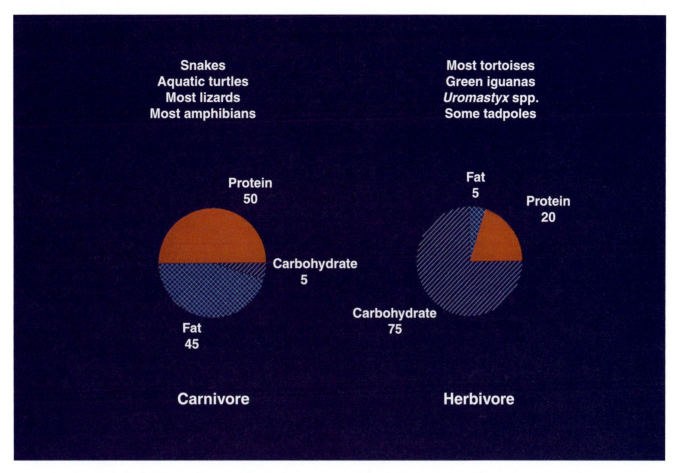

FIGURE 18-7 Fuel sources are mainly fat and protein for carnivores, and mainly carbohydrate and protein for herbivores.

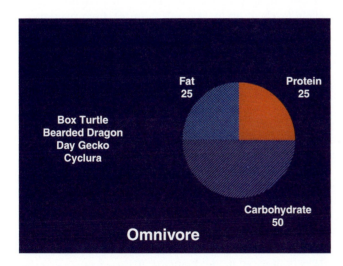

FIGURE 18-8 Omnivores use substantial quantities of fat, protein, and carbohydrate as energy sources.

For example, studies with the Australian aquatic turtle *Emydura macquarii* showed significant differences in rates of food consumption and digesta passage with body temperature.[25] As a result, digestive efficiency of a plant-based diet was only 49% at 85°F (30°C), yet of a meat-based diet was 91%. The data suggest that this omnivorous species cannot meet its calorie needs with a plant-only diet.

Until further data are available, current recommendations maintain meat-based diets for juveniles and gradual introductions of increasing amounts of plant-based diet as growth begins to slow. A small component of meat-based foods can remain in diets of omnivores throughout their lives.

Herbivores

Tortoises, Green Iguanas, *Uromastyx* lizards, Chuckwallas (*Sauromalus* spp.), and Prehensile-tail Skinks (*Corucia zebrata*) are among the herbivorous reptiles kept as pets and in large collections. In the author's experience, healthy herbivorous reptiles consume about 15% to 35% of ME from protein, less than 10% from fat, and more than 50% from carbohydrate (see Figure 18-7). Crude fiber intakes range from about 15% to 40% of dry matter (DM).

Herbivores use hydrolytic digestion in the small intestine for protein (about 3.5 kcal ME/g DM) and fat (about 8.5 kcal/g) absorption. Fibers are fermented in the lower bowel, yielding short-chain fatty acids such as acetate, proprionate, and butyrate. These acids nourish enterocytes in the lower bowel and provide energy. Fibers average about 2 kcal/g.

Fibers in the lower bowel hold water. Estimates in mammalian hindgut fermenters suggest 5 to 10 g water held for every gram of fiber. Partial availability of this water for absorption and prevention of dehydration is usually assumed.

Herbivores generally have digestive upset when dietary fat is greater than about 12%, regardless of the source. Herbivorous reptiles are unlikely to thrive on diets containing more than 12% fat, which limits the role of commercial pet foods for these species. Thus, commercial pet foods may occasionally suffice for some carnivorous reptiles, but they contain too much fat to be the sole diet for herbivorous and many omnivorous species.

Factors Affecting Calorie Sources

Genetics. Studies show that food preferences are heritable in some reptiles. The Common Gartersnake (*Thamnophis sirtalis*) is a generalist carnivore, consuming fish, worms, and other prey. Preferences for fish (but not earthworms) and changes in dietary preferences from worms to fish, and subsequent growth rates, were found to be heritable.[26] Herpetoculturists refer to certain food preferences and feeding behaviors as "hard wired." Genetics may place immovable limits on types of diets and feeding practices that succeed with captive reptiles (Figure 18-9).[27]

Ontogenic Shifts. In addition to the classic ontogenic shifts observed in omnivorous reptiles, smaller shifts may occur with carnivores and herbivores. Crocodiles, for example, shift prey selection as they grow larger, from spiders, insects, and frogs to fish, turtles, and snakes.[28] Juvenile herbivores may select tender shoots and new leaves rather than the fibrous browse consumed. The greatest ontogenic shift, however, is seen with hatchling herbivores (Figure 18-10).

Species Variations. These categorizations (carnivorous, herbivorous, and omnivorous) serve as guides, but many species fall into gray areas between categories. Day Geckos (*Phelsuma* spp.), for example, are enthusiastic insectivores but also consume nectar and, in captivity, infant foods made from fruit. Moreover, although all reptiles can be assigned to one of the three general categories, many are such specialized feeders that only a few foods may be recognized as such and consumed. For example, with few exceptions, Eastern Hog-nosed Snakes (*Heterodon platirhinos*) eat only toads, the lizard *Eumeces okadae* discriminates between queen ants (palatable) and worker ants (unpalatable), and the Impressed Tortoise (*Manouria impressa*) eats mostly forest mushrooms (see Figure 18-9).[27,29]

Seasonal Variations. Fuel utilization also varies within species according to season (e.g., temperature, day:night cycles, and perhaps food supplies). Aquatic turtles, for example, use anaerobic glycolysis for energy during active periods in cold temperatures (spring) but use oxidation in the citric acid cycle and beta-oxidation of fatty acids in warmer (autumn) temperatures.[30,31] Wild snakes are known to alter their diets seasonally, shifting, for example, from spring diets of mostly birds to summer diets of mostly rodents.[32] The changes are thought to reflect prey availability. Current recommendations call for diet changes by season when shifts in the wild reflect metabolic changes for species undergoing winter cool-down or summer estivation. For some species, diet shifts in the wild may need replication in captivity.

Nitrogen

Sources of nitrogen are amino acids from proteins in plants and animals, and a nonprotein source in chitin from exoskeletons of invertebrates. Protein quality is a measure of efficiency. As protein quality improves, less nitrogen has to be excreted by the kidney and bowel.

The chemical form in which excess nitrogen is excreted varies, depending in part on the reptile's habitat, aquatic or terrestrial. Aquatic and semiaquatic turtles excrete more ammonia and urea than uric acid. Terrestrial tortoises, snakes, and lizards excrete more uric acid (Figure 18-11). Crocodiles excrete ammonia. The systems for nitrogen excretion are designed to conserve water in terrestrial species. Thus, nitrogen balance affects water balance, and vice versa.

Herbivores and Protein

Domestic herbivores such as horses and rabbits tolerate protein levels of up to 20% to 25% of ME from plant-based

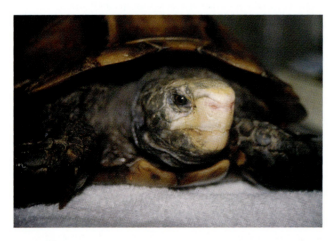

FIGURE 18-9 Many reptiles are specialized feeders, complicating their care in captivity. The Impressed Tortoise, *Manouria impressa*, is a montane species from southeast Asia that feeds on forest mushrooms. Its long-term refusal of food in captivity, except for oyster mushrooms, contributes to nearly 100% mortality rate observed in new imports.

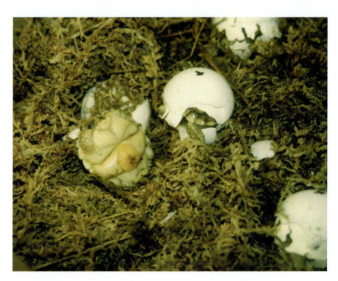

FIGURE 18-10 The Sulcata Tortoise (*Geochelone sulcata*) is a grassland herbivore and hindgut fermenter. Remnants of resorbed yolk sac can be seen on plastron of this Sulcata hatchling. The hatchling was nourished throughout incubation with yolk sac contents, a mix of fats and protein. Absorbed yolk sustains the tortoise for another 4 weeks, while it transitions from prehatching carnivory to posthatching herbivory. The phenomenon is not unlike that of weaning in a mammalian herbivore.

sources. Generalizations about protein limits for reptiles are less well documented. Protein requirements relate to quantity and quality. Studies in the author's laboratory show that iguanas grow poorly when fed diets of less than 25% protein (DM basis; Figure 18-12).[33,34]

Concerns about nitrogen excretion and its effect on renal function have led to conservative estimates of dietary protein requirements for terrestrial herbivorous and omnivorous reptiles. Such recommendations may be inadequate to support growth, reproduction, immune function, and tissue regeneration. Because of the system-wide untoward effects of low protein intakes, a more effective strategy for maintaining water balance and preventing uricemia may hinge on sustaining adequate water balance, which is helped by the use of higher quality protein.

Plant proteins often lack sufficient essential amino acids (lysine, methionine, cystine, tryptophan, and threonine). Plant species vary in amino acid content; for example, cereals often lack lysine, whereas legumes (such as beans and alfalfa) often lack methionine. Animal proteins often contain more optimal proportions of amino acids and so are considered higher quality than many plant proteins. However, meats contain other substances, such as fat, phosphorus, and purines, which may cause problems and in effect negate advantages of higher quality protein. Many plants also contain high levels of purines (50 to 150 mg/100 g), such as asparagus, whole grain cereals, cauliflower, beans and peas, spinach, mushrooms, and wheat germ.

Chitin

The exoskeleton of invertebrates contains chitin, a nitrogen-containing polysaccharide. Enzymes that digest chitin, termed *chitinases* and *chitobiases,* have been quantified in the stomach, intestine, pancreas, and liver of insectivorous and omnivorous reptiles, including lacertid, limbless, and *Uromastyx* lizards; anoles; chameleons; and chelonians (Table 18-2).[35]

Nitrogen released during the metabolism of chitin represents nonprotein nitrogen (NPN). It must be excreted via kidneys yet fails to provide the benefits typical of protein-associated nitrogen. Because of the risks of NPN to water balance and renal function, invertebrates are not recommended for assist-feeding diets.

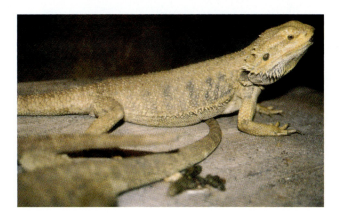

FIGURE 18-11 Normal feces for many reptiles contain a formed brown fecal fraction and a hard white urate fraction, as seen for these omnivorous Bearded Dragons (*Pogona vitticeps*). Herbivorous lizards and tortoises produce relatively more fecal matter because they consume diets of higher fiber and lower digestibility.

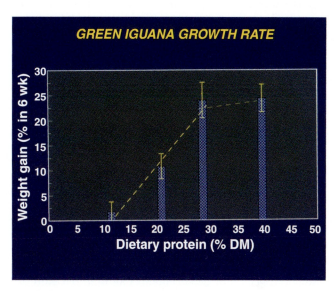

FIGURE 18-12 Juvenile Green Iguanas (*Iguana iguana*) grow optimally when fed diets containing more than 25% protein, dry matter basis.[34] For an iguana eating chopped fresh salads, this corresponds to about 5% to 8% protein, as-fed basis.

Table 18-2	Activities of Chitinases and Chitobiases in Reptiles[35]							
	Chitinases				Chitobiases			
Species	Stomach	Intestine	Pancreas	Liver	Stomach	Intestine	Pancreas	Liver
Emerald Lizard (*Lacerta viridis*)	7400	0-3	12,000	0	0	45	0-160	80
Slow Worm (*Anguis fragilis*)	2440	NA	NA	NA	0	NA	0	0
Uromastyx acanthinurus	1840	0	NA	NA	50	0	NA	NA
Green Anole (*Anolis carolinensis*)	9400	NA	5320	NA	0	NA	0	0
Chamaeleo vulgaris (*C. chamaeleo*)	1470	0	4280	0	96	10	0	10
Pond Turtle (*Clemmys capsica rivulata*)	5800	NA	7700	0	0	NA	0	NA
Pond Turtle (*Emys orbicularis*)	3470	60	4150	0	60	44	0	82
Hermann's Tortoise (*Testudo hermanni*)	0	0	0	0	45	57	NA	35

Chitinases, µg chitin hydrolyzed/h/g tissue; and chitobiases, µg acetylglucosamine produced/h/g tissue.
NA, Not available.

Water

All captive reptiles should have access to wholesome water. Acceptance of water, however, depends on several factors. Certain lizards may need to see light reflectance from dripping water to begin drinking (Figure 18-13). Turtles, snakes, and many lizards willingly drink from bowls, but turtles and snakes sip and lizards lap.[36] Anoles, chameleons, and Day Geckos lap from droplets sprayed or dripped onto foliage. Other lizards, such as iguanids, learn to drink from bowls; smaller reptiles drink from lids (such as the plastic caps for pet food cans). Plastic containers for holding water should be approved for food use. Some reptiles reject water held in plastic, presumably because of off-odors or taste. A switch to glass, ceramic, or stainless steel usually corrects the situation.

Most tortoises, snakes, and many lizards soak in large shallow bowls (Figure 18-14). Soaking enhances water uptake, stimulates excretion, and aids shedding of skin. Tortoises use their bladders as sinks for electrolytes (especially K^+) and nitrogen during times of drought. Typically, tortoises in the wild drink water, void their urine, then refill their bladders with dilute urine.[37] Thus, soaking of terrestrial tortoises in captivity is usually necessary for many species to maintain water balance.

Soaking can be voluntary, in deep-set soaking trays within habitats, or performed every 5 to 10 days (daily for hatchlings) in soaking chambers. While soaking, turtles and tortoises may take up water into their cloacas, termed *cloacal drinking*. Recent studies with the aquatic Slider *(Trachemys scripta)* showed that turtles dehydrated by 10% to 12% of maximum body mass exhibited increased hematocrit and extracellular fluid (ECF) osmolality but still osmoregulated by reabsorbing water from their bladders. The turtles drank readily via the oral route and were able to lower ECF osmolality. In contrast, turtles with cloacas submerged were unable to correct their ECF osmolality.[38] Therefore, cloacal drinking should not replace opportunities for oral drinking in captive chelonians.

Dehydration is common, especially in sick reptiles. It may result from water provided in improper form or from anorexia, or occur secondary to the pathologic process of a disease.

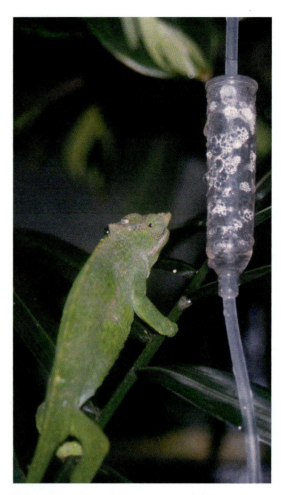

FIGURE 18-13 All reptiles depend on maintenance of positive water balance to maintain health. Certain species need exacting techniques for delivery of water. Chameleons, for example, need slow consistent delivery of water dripping onto foliage. Drippers can be simple (such as a pinhole in the bottom of a plastic container of water set on top of the cage) or complex (commercial dripper systems). In this set-up, intravenous tubing is used to deliver water droplets.

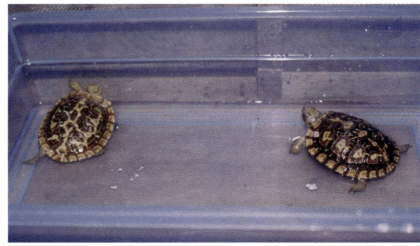

FIGURE 18-14 Hatchling tortoises should be soaked daily in tepid water to a depth that approximates one third the height of the shell. Most juveniles urinate and defecate at this time.

Uricotelic species need large amounts of water to sustain normal excretion, and dehydration in these species may result in urinary stasis, uricemia, and gout (see Chapter 54).[39]

Clinical impressions suggest that inadequate humidity may contribute to dehydration, stress, and dysecdysis. Likewise, excessive humidity may contribute to skin infections and hyperkeratinization.

Desert animals need less water than temperate and tropical species. Some species receive enough water from food to meet requirements. For example, a 27-g mouse contains 17 g water, a 200-mg cricket contains about 140 mg water, and a cupful (about 35 g) of chopped romaine contains 33 g water.

Empirically, daily parenteral doses of water for rehydration are 10 to 30 mL/kg BW. Saline solution and replacement fluids work well. When providing nutrition support, a useful approximation is that 1 mL should be given for each kcal provided.

Water quality comes into question for collections of water-inhabiting or water-loving reptiles, such as aquatic turtles, alligators, and water snakes. It should probably be a concern for all reptiles, especially juvenile tortoises that soak frequently.

Hard water contains the bicarbonate and sulfate salts of calcium and magnesium. It is safe for reptiles. Softened water has calcium and magnesium replaced by sodium; it is a danger to patients on sodium-restricted diets. **Demineralized and distilled waters have minerals removed; these types of water are not necessarily beneficial to reptiles.**

Fluoridated water contains 0.5 to 1 ppm fluoride, usually as the sodium salt.[40] Fluoride has a narrow safety range. In mammals, deficiency is associated with dental caries and with osteoporosis in the aged. Fluoride toxicity (fluorosis), as a result of accumulation from long-term consumption of high levels, is associated with deformed bones and soft, mottled, and irregularly worn teeth. Animals fed diets deficient in protein, calcium, and vitamin C are more susceptible to fluorosis. Water sources that contain high levels of fluoride are found in parts of Arkansas, California, South Carolina, and Texas and may be a risk for fluorosis.

Water should be free of coliform bacteria. Until specific data for reptiles are available, data from the World Health Organization may be used as a guideline for water quality (Table 18-3). Water may be chlorinated (to destroy bacteria) at home by adding 8 to 16 drops of bleach to 1 gallon (2 to 4 drops/L) of water.[40]

Table 18-3	Upper Limits for Metals and Contaminants in Water[40]

Metal or Contaminant	Concentration (mg/L)	
	WHO	USPHS
Arsenic	0.05	0.05
Cadmium	0.01	0.01
Cyanide	0.20	0.05
Lead	0.05	0.05
Mercury	0.001	NA
Selenium	0.01	0.01
Nitrates	NA	10.0
Polycyclic hydrocarbons	0.0002	NA

WHO, World Health Organization; *USPHS*, United States Public Health Service; *NA*, not available.

Salt Glands

A number of species have nasal salt glands for excretion of sodium and chloride in response to an osmotic load. White crusty deposits may be seen around the nares of Green Iguanas, chameleons, and other lizards and are normal findings. Certain species, such as the Desert Iguana (*Dipsosaurus dorsalis*), also secrete potassium and sodium, and chloride or bicarbonate.[41]

Metabolic States

Published research suggests that reptiles partition energy similarly to endotherms. For example, insectivorous lizards (*Anolis limifrons*) assimilated about 88% of calories consumed.[42] Of that absorbed, adults allocated 68% to respiration, 23% to production, and 9% to urinary waste. Juveniles allocated relatively more calories to production (growth) compared with adults. The Racerunner (*Cnemidophorus sexlineatus*) fed crickets absorbed 88% lipids, 84% soluble carbohydrates, and 83% protein. Calories per cricket averaged 0.30 for protein, 0.21 for fat, and 0.01 for carbohydrate.[43]

Growth

The author's 10 years of feeding trials show typical sigmoid growth responses for reptiles, with relatively flat curves immediately after hatching and when adult size is neared and rapid linear growth between the two plateaus (Figures 18-15 through 18-17).

Both food and water affect the growth of juveniles. Lack of calories or protein, poor-quality protein, and deficiencies of vitamins or minerals may retard growth. Red-eared Sliders grew poorly on high-calcium diets, for example, whereas vitamin C had no effect on growth.[44,45] Snapping Turtles (*Chelydra serpentina*) hatched in a dry substrate were smaller than those hatched in a wet substrate or those that entered a wet environment immediately after hatching.[46]

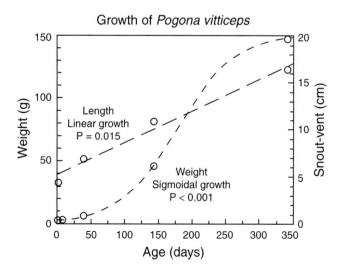

FIGURE 18-15 In the author's feeding trial with Bearded Dragons (*Pogona vitticeps*) from hatchling to 1 year of age, increases in body weight showed sigmoidal growth curves and increases in body length, termed *snout-vent length*, were linear.

Juveniles pushed for rapid growth are also vulnerable. The author has observed nutrition-related metabolic bone diseases (NMBDs), shell deformities, obesity, and high mortality rates in lizards and chelonians overfed as juveniles.

Vitellogenesis and Embryo Nutrition

Hepatic synthesis of egg yolk protein requires calories, nitrogen, and micronutrients. Failure to provide adequate nutrition reduces egg yolk synthesis, compromising reproduction.[47,48] Use of energy and nutrients by reptile embryos has been quantified. Few differences are found between oviparous species and those species that are viviparous with simply structured placentas. However, those species that are viviparous with complex placentas showed a significant increase in dry mass and nutrients in the neonates (Figure 18-18). In oviparous species, nutrients from eggshell (calcium) and yolk (lipids, calcium, magnesium) are transferred to the embryo.[49]

In the Australian Lizard, *Eulamprus tympanum*, maternal metabolic rates during pregnancy increased 29% over nongravid rates. Embryos from these viviparous simple-placenta lizards consumed 20 kJ (5 kcal) per g compared with 16 kJ (4 kcal) per g for oviparous embryos.[50] The SMRs of gravid Mountain Spiny Lizards (*Sceloporus jarrovii*), a viviparous species, increased in early, mid, and late gestation 80%, 98%, and 140%, respectively, compared with nongravid controls.[51]

Some snakes and lizards eat less when gravid, but conclusions and supporting data about the nutritional significance are varied. For example, gravid Gartersnakes (*Thamnophis elegans*) eat less than controls when presented with ample food, whereas gravid pythons eat readily when food is presented.[52] Other species, such as chameleons, appear to lower food intake because of coelomic fill from a large number of eggs. Anecdotal observations suggest that heavy feeding during vitellogenesis results in excess numbers of eggs that stress coelomic capacity. Veiled Chameleons, for example, typically produce about 25 eggs in the wild, yet may produce more than 60 eggs in captivity. Research has shown that skinks decreased food intake when carrying large numbers of eggs or embryos; the phenomenon is termed a fecundity-dependent cost of reproduction.[53]

Fasting and Torpor

Several species fast for weeks or months in the wild as an adaptation to excess heat or cold, drought, or lack of food. Fasting may persist in captive specimens (American Box Turtles, Bearded Dragons) even if kept in warm temperatures with adequate food and water. The Ball Python (*Python regius*) may fast for prolonged periods, perhaps because of stress from handling and captivity and not because of inborn behaviors.

Normal periods of fasting are accompanied by metabolic slow down that results in little weight loss. However, prolonged fasts or multiple fasts in less than ideal conditions (too warm, for example) can debilitate captive specimens. Acceptance of anorexia accompanied by weight loss, or fasting in a species not known to brumate (hibernate) in the wild, as a "normal fast" is rarely advisable.

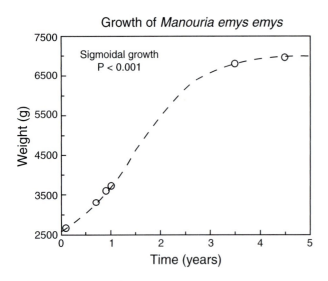

FIGURE 18-16 This 5-year feeding trial of young Burmese Mountain Tortoises, *Manouria emys emys*, shows sigmoidal growth curves. This popular tortoise is a herbivorous forest species, thriving on high-fiber, high-fruit diets that often require careful formulation to ensure good growth and bowel health.

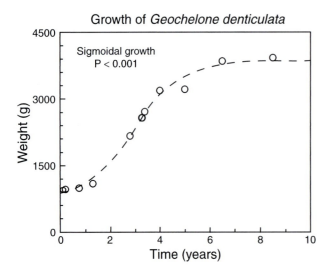

FIGURE 18-17 The author's 10-year feeding trials with the Yellow-foot Tortoise, *Geochelone denticulata*, show sigmoidal growth curves. This South American forest tortoise thrives on standard tortoise diets of high-fiber salads and tropical fruits, with occasional (twice monthly) meals of meat-based foods.

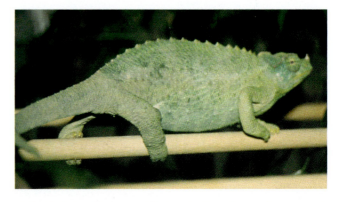

FIGURE 18-18 This gravid Jackson's Chameleon (*Chamaeleo jacksonii*) is a live-bearer, with embryos receiving nutrition from yolk sacs. Proteins for egg yolk formation are synthesized in the liver, in a process termed *vitellogenesis*. The entire process is nutritionally demanding, and studies show that gravid chameleons in poor condition have high mortality rates.[137]

Very little energy is consumed in reptiles that undergo true brumation (hibernation). Gartersnakes *(Thamnophis sirtalis)* that weigh about 53 g and brumate (hibernate) for 165 days used only 3 kcal when submerged in water and about 7 kcal when in air.[54] Box turtles that weigh about 400 g may lose less than 5% of their BW during brumation (hibernation). Reptiles that truly brumate (hibernate) (such as Box Turtles) or have normal winter cool-down periods (such as Bearded Dragons) should not be expected to lose much weight. Unfortunately, Box Turtles and tortoises of the *Testudo* genus that are kept by inexperienced owners can be brumated (hibernated) improperly, only to emerge from winter half awake and starved. These chelonians are susceptible to pneumonia, anorexia, and high mortality rates.

Routine weighing is recommended for animals that are fasting. Box Turtles are accessible if brumated (hibernated) in cold rooms or refrigerators. Bearded Dragons often go through winter cool-down in their usual habitats. Veterinarians have provided brumation (hibernation) and cool-down services, maintaining clients' reptiles in a cold room until spring, with frequent checks on weight.

Aquatic turtles in temperate climates brumate (hibernate) underwater by means of two extraordinary physiologic changes: metabolic rate reduction and enormous buffering capabilities. Painted Turtles, *Chrysemys picta*, can survive submerged in an anoxic state for up to 5 months at 37°F (3°C). Their metabolic rate lowers to 10% of what it is at the same temperature in a normoxic state. Moreover, carbonates (sodium, calcium, and magnesium) are released from bone and shell and lactic acid moves into shell and bone for buffering and storage.[55,56] Turtle species with less shell mineralization, such as the Softshell *Apalone spinifera*, are less able to compensate for high lactate levels and thus are less tolerant of anoxia.[57] The role of nutrition and dietary calcium has yet to be explored with regard to buffering capacity and health in chelonians.

Senescence

Reptiles show three types of aging: rapid senescence (seen in the Skink *Mabuya buettneri*), gradual senescence (most lizards, such as the Agama *Calotes versicolor*, and snakes, such as the Grass Snake *Natrix natrix*), and slow or negligible senescence (turtles, tortoises, and crocodiles).[58] Gradual senescence is associated with increased stability of collagen, accumulation of altered enzyme molecules, and decreased metabolic rate, but unlike data for mammals, lipofuscin accumulation and reproductive senility are not yet clearly documented for aging lizards and snakes.[59,60] Clinical experience suggests reproductive senescence occurs in some lizards, such as Bearded Dragons. Metabolic changes for middle-aged and geriatric lizards include reduced hepatic glucose uptake, slowed responses in glucose uptake after starvation and cold stress, and low levels of vitamin C and renal succinic dehydrogenase.[61,62]

In contrast, chelonians and crocodiles show few signs of aging. Long-term studies with the Three-toed Box Turtle *(Terrapene carolina triunguis)* documented similar reproductive rates and clutch sizes in females 66 to 74 years old as in females less than 60 years.[63]

On the basis of these findings, diets for older turtles, tortoises, and crocodiles are recommended to remain identical to diets for younger specimens. Diets for lizards and snakes can be adjusted for old age. In feeding trials in the author's laboratory, diets with lower calorie concentration but unchanged nutrient concentrations, and higher fiber contents, have performed well for aged Bearded Dragons and Green Iguanas. For old snakes, one may try feeding lean well-fed prey, to minimize calories from fat while maintaining nutrient intakes.

Sarcopenia is the loss of muscle mass and strength observed in senescent animals. Of particular concern are high mortality rates in older individuals termed "the fat frail" who are obese but sarcopenic.[64] Care should be taken in examination of older reptiles prone to obesity (such as confined monitors and sedentary snakes) to detect sarcopenia. Although cytokines and decreased anabolic hormones play roles in the development of sarcopenia, nutritional intervention to reduce the degree of obesity may help to avoid functional impairments.

FOODS

Because of the diversity of species in herpetoculture, a variety of foods must be considered. Most foods are available commercially (Table 18-4).

Table 18-4 Commercial Suppliers of Foods, Supplies, and Services

Company	Contact	Goods
Beneficial Insectary	www.insectary.com	Green lacewings, housefly pupae
Big Apple Herpetological Supply	www.bigappleherp.com	Commercial diets, dry goods and supplies
Connecticut Valley Worm Farm	www.ctvalley.com	European earthworms, red wrigglers
Grubco	www.grubco.com	Crickets, mealworms, superworms, waxworms
HerpNutrition at Walkabout Farm*	www.HerpNutrition.com	Enterals, dusts, complete diets, invertebrate foods, salad mixes
Mulberry Farms	www.mulberryfarms.com; 760-731-6088	Silkworms
Oxbow Hay	www.oxbowhay.com	Grass and legume hays, enterals
Southern Cricket	www.southerncricket.com	Crickets, mealworms, superworms, waxworms, earthworms, red wrigglers
That Pet Place	www.thatpetplace.com	Commercial diets, dry goods and supplies
The Bean Farm	www.beanfarm.com	Specialized reptile supplies, feeding tongs
The Gourmet Rodent	www.gourmetrodent.com; 352-495-9024	Live and frozen mice, rats, rabbits, chicks
Woodson-Tenent Laboratories	www.wtlabs.com; 901-521-4500	Feed analyses

*Owned by author.
This list provides information on vendors that have provided good service to the author and is not meant to be all-inclusive. Additional companies can be located with Internet searches and perusal of reptile-related magazines.

Vertebrate Prey

The most common feeder vertebrates are mice and rats of various ages and sizes (Figure 18-19; Table 18-5).[65] Fed less frequently, but often important to the overall health and well being of the predator, are fish, frogs, toads, lizards, snakes, chicks, finches, gerbils, rabbits, and other mammals. Whole vertebrate prey, whether mammalian, avian, reptilian, amphibian, or piscine, provides essential amino acids and high-quality protein from muscle and organs, lipids from adipose, vitamins and trace minerals from liver, macrominerals from bone, iodine from thyroid, and vitamins K and B_{12} from ingesta. Well-nourished, healthy vertebrate prey may be considered complete and balanced (Table 18-6).

General recommendations call for small prey to be fed to small predators and larger prey to larger predators. However, ratios of prey mass to predator mass vary between types of predators, with certain species preferring remarkably smaller prey. For example, ratios (prey mass:predator mass) for colubrid snakes (such as Cornsnakes [*Elaphe* spp.]) average 0.18 and for vipers, 0.36.[32] Analysis of stomach contents in the wild report prey mass equivalent to about 10% to 30% of the snake's BW.[32,66]

A few snakes are known to eat carrion in the wild. These include the Brown Treesnake (*Boiga irregularis*) and a Mediterranean island-dwelling colubrid *Coluber hippocrepis nigrescens*.[66,67]

Factors That Affect Nutritional Composition

The age and health of prey animals and their diet and environment can affect nutritional composition. Older spent laboratory rodents may be obese or underweight. Obese prey usually contain over 50% fat. In fat prey, nutrient content relative to calories is decreased, placing the predator at risk for development of multiple insidious secondary nutrient deficiencies. Conversely, underfed prey lack fat and protein relative to ash. These prey provide excess minerals relative to calorie intake and reduce energy intake for the predator.

Mineral and fat-soluble vitamin contents of neonatal prey (termed *pinkies*) have been in question. Generally, suckled newborn mice and rats are likely to contain enough calcium and vitamin A for reptiles, but more data are needed. Reptiles fed pinkies are often fed additional prey such as dusted invertebrates, older vertebrates, or meat-based pet foods to ensure dietary completeness.

Risks

Wild and commercial prey may transmit parasites and pathogenic organisms to reptiles.[68] As an aid to controlling foodborne illness, freezing and subsequent thawing of prey is recommended before feeding out. Live prey, especially rodents, may seriously injure reptiles from bites and scratches, so feeding dead prey is preferred. Rodents that are older than about 2.5 weeks (furred and eyes open) should be killed before feeding out. The only exception is the rare snake that does not take dead prey when healthy and properly

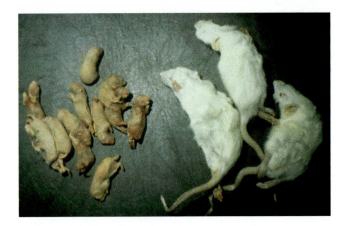

FIGURE 18-19 Prekilled pinkie (*left*) and adult mice may be purchased and thawed before feeding out. Dead rodents are safer for snakes than live mice and rats.

Table 18-5 Average Weight and Length of Rodent Prey Fed to Reptiles[65]

Food	Weight (g)	Length (cm)
Mouse (*Mus musculus*)		
Pinkie	1.7	3.0
Fuzzy	3.8	3.7
Crawler	6.5	4.7
Small	7.4	5.2
Medium	15	7.0
Large	36	8.2
Rat (*Rattus norvegicus*)		
Pinkie	10	5.2
Small	54	13
Medium	117	14
Large	257	20

Table 18-6 Proximate Nutrient Composition of Vertebrate Prey

Species (g)	Water (%)	Energy (kcal/g) AF	Energy (kcal/g) DM	Protein (% kcal)	Fat (% kcal)	Carbohydrate (% kcal)
Meadow vole (32)	64	1.3	3.6	63	15	22
Mouse, adult (27)	65	1.7	4.8	48	47	5
Mouse, pup (1.5)	81	0.8	4.2	57	40	3
Mouse, pup (4)	71	1.7	5.9	29	69	2
Rat, adult (330)	66	1.6	4.7	55	43	2
Chicken (380)	66	1.6	4.7	47	49	4
Chick, day old (40)	73	1.3	4.8	52	44	4
Atlantic herring (100)	69	1.8	5.7	39	58	3
Atlantic smelt (100)	77	1.0	4.3	63	31	6

Energy is presented as calories (kcal) of metabolizable energy per gram, on as-fed (*AF*) and dry matter (*DM*) bases.

managed. In these rare cases, the rodent can be stunned, then offered head first in feeding tongs.

Fresh-killed prey are equal nutritionally to live prey, and freezing for short periods does not destroy nutrients. Freezing for more than 6 months results in deterioration of odor, taste (presumably), and texture. Moreover, labile nutrients may be lost as well. Fresh-killed prey that are not yet stiff from rigor mortis (and frozen prey that have been thawed) cannot attack snakes and lizards (see Chapter 46) and pose less danger of scratches to the feeding reptile's esophagus from toenails and incisors. Owners may need information regarding optimal care for live prey and humane methods for killing.[69]

Offering Food to Reptiles

Some carnivores take prey from tongs; for others, prey are left in the habitat. For large carnivorous snakes and lizards, dead prey is always presented on tongs (head first for hand feeding) and never presented from the human hand. A mistake by inexperienced keepers is to place prey into a snake's habitat by hand when the snake is small. The snake becomes habituated to the hand, associating it with food. As the snake grows, it then strikes when hungry at any hand entering the habitat. If a large species, the snake then becomes a threat to human safety and the learned behavior prevents safe snake handling and habitat maintenance. Some keepers remove snakes into separate cages for feeding, to reduce the association of food and hands in the home habitat. **For giant snakes, the keeper must be free of all prey odors and always have a second person in attendance.**

Newborn and juveniles rodents can be offered to smaller predators from tongs or left in habitats. For nocturnal carnivores, prey are fed out late in the day.

Scenting

Few differences in nutrient contents appear to exist between the vertebrate species for which nutrient values are known. Thus, disguising one vertebrate prey species to smell as another, such as smearing frog or lizard scent onto mice, is acceptable nutritionally. Scenting is essential for neonatal snakes of some species offered pinkie mice; certain kingsnakes, for example, begin life as lizard feeders.[70] **Nutritional problems from long-term feeding of scented prey have not been reported. However, the practice may risk deficiencies of essential nutrients, fatty acids for example, that could be prevalent in amphibians but not rodents.**[71-73]

Invertebrate Prey

Commercially available invertebrate prey include crickets, mealworms, superworms, waxworms and wax moths, silkworms and silk moths, hornworms, cockroaches, houseflies, fruit flies, springtails, earthworms (Canadian and European), and red wriggler worms (Figure 18-20).[74] Others wild-caught and fed to reptiles include stick insects and mantids, lacewings, May beetles and June bugs, grasshoppers, locusts, katydids, sow bugs, and snails. Knowledge in the biology and captive care of invertebrates is essential for successful management of these prey.[74]

Calorie and Nutrient Contents

Proximate analyses for common prey species allow comparisons on energy bases. Many species provide ME of at least 30% from protein, 40% from fat, less than 15% from carbohydrate, and more than 3 kcal/g DM (Table 18-7).[75-85] Invertebrates that are starved (such as those for sale in some pet shops) are likely to contain less than optimal levels of fat, protein, and other nutrients.

Invertebrates lack an endoskeleton and thus most contain little calcium. Reptiles that consume land snails take in calcium carbonate from the shells. Calcium is inadequate in most other invertebrate species, less than 0.5 mg/kcal or 0.2% DM (Table 18-8).[75-78] The few insect species that contain more calcium have calcified exoskeletons that may limit their acceptance and consumption. Although variation is found within species and among geographic areas in the United States, generally invertebrates, whether commercial or wild-caught, require supplementation with calcium. Phosphorus contents are usually adequate, and the mineral appears to have high biologic availability.

Protein Quality

Protein quality of many invertebrates is good, equal to or better than soy protein, although lower than the quality of the milk protein lactalbumin, which is the gold standard.[80,81] In comparative studies with rats and chickens, house cricket protein was higher quality than Mormon cricket and soy, which in turn were of higher quality than tent caterpillar protein.

Data on protein quality are unavailable for reptiles; however, estimates from chickens may pertain to reptiles because both consume insects naturally and both have altered uric acid metabolism. In chickens fed insect-based diets, arginine and methionine were colimiting amino acids.[80] Arginine may assume similar importance in reptiles because slow synthesis in the uric acid cycle may limit endogenous supply (M. Finke, personal communication). Arginine content is about 45 and 62 mg/g protein for crickets and mealworms, respectively. This level is slightly above minimal levels for strict carnivores and for growing poultry, but data are needed for reptiles before recommendations can be made.

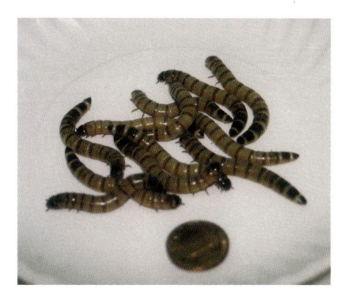

FIGURE 18-20 Superworms (*Zophobas mori*) are a superior invertebrate for species large enough to eat them. Adult Bearded Dragons (*Pogona vitticeps*), Water Dragons (*Physignathus cocincinus*), Cyclura iguanids, small monitors, and Tegus (*Tupinambus* spp.) thrive on these invertebrates.

Table 18-7	Proximate Nutrient Composition of Commercial Invertebrate Prey							
Species	Water (%)	Crude Fat (% DM)	Total Nitrogen (% DM)	Crude Protein (% DM)	ADF-N (% DM)	NDF (% DM)	Ash (% DM)
Commercial cricket (Acheta domestica)							
Adults	62-73	19-44	10	40-68	0.7	19	2.7-5.1
Juvenile	67	10	9	40-50	0.6	16	9.1
Mealworm (Tenebrio molitor)	56-66	31-60	8-9	35-55	14	4	3-7
Superworm (Zophobas morio)	57-59	41-44	6.9	40-50	0.4	13	2.9-3.5
Waxworm (Galleria mellonella)	62-63	51-73	5.5	27-41	0.4	12	2.7-3.3
Silkworm (Bombyx mori)	61-80	4-21	8.7-10	65	NA	NA	5.2
Fruit fly (Drosophila melanogaster)	67	18	9.0	NA	1.0	16	5.2
May beetle (Lachnosterna sp.)	69	16	11	NA	NA	NA	5.2
Grasshopper (Melanophus spp.)	NA	7.2	12	NA	NA	NA	5.6
Housefly pupae (Musca domestica)	68	9-24	10	49	NA	NA	4-12
Brazilian termite (Velocitermes paucipilis)							
Worker	70	NA	7.3	NA	NA	NA	13
Soldier	70	NA	9.3	NA	NA	NA	11
Brazilian ant (Carebara sp.)	60	8-60	1-10	NA	NA	NA	NA
Earthworm (Lumbricus terrestris)							
Wild-caught	74-85	6-13	5-11	NA	0.2	51.2	9-46
Commercial	76-84	11-13	8-13	73	0.3	20.9	25

Acid-detergent fiber-nitrogen (ADF-N) was used as measure of nitrogen in chitin (nonprotein nitrogen), and neutral detergent fiber (NDF) was used as measure of complex carbohydrates.[81]
NA, Not available.

Table 18-8	Mineral Concentrations (Dry Matter Basis) of Commercial Invertebrate Prey						
Species	Ca (%)	Mg (%)	P (%)	Cu (mg/kg)	Fe (mg/kg)	Mn (mg/kg)	Zn (mg/kg)
Cricket (Acheta domesticus)							
Adults	0.1-0.2	0.08	0.8-1.4	8.5	112	30	186
Juvenile	0.1-1.3	0.16	0.8	9.6	197	53	159
Mealworm (Tenebrio molitor)	0.04-0.12	0.28	0.9-1.4	18	40	6.8	131
Superworm (Zophobas morio)	0.03-0.12	0.18	0.6-0.8	14	50	1.5	88
Waxworm (Galleria mellonella)	0.06-0.07	0.09	0.6-1.2	3.1	77	3.3	79
Silkworm (Bombyx mori)	0.21	0.24	0.54	NA	NA	NA	NA
Fruit fly (Drosophila melanogaster)	0.14	0.13	1.1	8.7	454	16	147
Earthworm (Lumbricus terrestris)							
Wild-caught	0.97	0.31	0.79	33	11,087	199	271
Commercial	1.2	0.19	0.86	8.1	5802	113	231

High iron (Fe) concentrations in earthworms reflect soil intake.

The relatively high but variable protein quality of insect species suggests that protein quality is an important consideration when feeding insectivorous reptiles. For example, when feeding a postoperative patient, a diet for assist-feeding should contain very high-quality protein. Diets of low-quality protein result in higher nitrogen excretion because of inefficient use of amino acids. Thus, feeding high-quality proteins to insectivores with questionable hydration status or renal function is prudent.

Factors That Affect Nutritional Composition

Diets that contain 8% calcium have been fed to crickets to increase calcium content of the insects from 0.2% to 1.3% DM.[86] When fed these supplemented crickets, Fox Geckos (Hemidactylus garnoti) increased total body calcium 17%, but Cuban Treefrogs (Osteopilus septentrionalis) showed no calcium increase. High-calcium diets are unpalatable and imbalanced for crickets. Studies on the nutrient requirements of crickets suggest that dietary calcium levels above 1366 ppm (0.14%) had deleterious effects on growth and reproduction.[87] If used, high-calcium diets should be fed to crickets for about 48 hours but not longer before feeding out.

Gut-Loading

In the early studies and subsequent research that showed increased calcium content in invertebrates fed high-calcium diets, the term *gut-loading* was used.[86,88,89] It referred to invertebrate diets containing about 8% calcium. The extra calcium was not absorbed into the cricket but instead remained within its intestines.

The term gut-loading is now used to mean the feeding of any nutritious diet to any invertebrate. The term is currently misleading because it implies nutrients remain within the intestinal tract when they are instead absorbed. For example, protein found in a cricket's intestines is not dietary but part of shed cells, secreted enzymes and mucus, microbes, and

Table 18-9	Nutrient and Energy Composition of Mulberry *(Morus nigra)* and Silkworm *(Bombyx mori)* Larvae[79]		
Component	Mulberry Leaves	Silkworm Ingesta intact	Silkworm Ingesta removed
Moisture (%)	63	76	70
Nitrogen (%)	2.7	10.4	10.0
Protein (%)	17	65	63
Fat (%)	3.5	21	14
Calcium (%)	0.69	0.21	0.24
Phosphorus (%)	0.17	0.54	0.57
Magnesium (%)	0.70	0.24	0.26
Energy (kcal/g)	NA	5.74	5.69

NA, Not available.

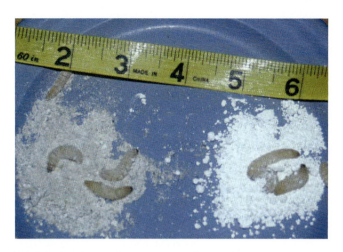

FIGURE 18-21 Supplements may fail to stick to certain invertebrates, risking nutritional deficiencies in the predator. In these instances, prey can be offered in dishes or bowls containing a shallow level of supplement. These waxworms are in a vitamin-mineral supplement *(left)* and in calcium carbonate *(right)*.

the like. Sound diets improve the nutritional content of prey, compared with diets that are incomplete, imbalanced, or in short supply, but effects are from changes within the prey, such as increased muscle and adipose, and changes, if any, in gut contents.

Proposed effects of gut-loading on nutritional contents of prey need confirmation. In a study of silkworm *(Bombyx mori)* larvae, no differences in composition were found with intestinal contents intact or removed (Table 18-9).[83] Moreover, nutrient composition of the silkworms had no discernible similarity to the nutrient composition of their diet of mulberry leaves (see Table 18-9).

Nutritious diets for invertebrates should contain fuel sources in amounts appropriate for the species (see Table 9). Most need a water source. Because many invertebrates drown in pooled water, moisture is provided by fresh produce or from a diet with high moisture content, such as mulberry leaves for silkworms.

Supplementation of Invertebrates

Applying nutritional supplements to the external surface of invertebrates is recommended before feeding out. This process, often termed *dusting*, is intended to supply the nutrients missing from invertebrates that may be needed by the reptilian predator. Dusting may be accomplished by placing prey in a container with the powdery supplements and shaking gently (termed a "shake-and-bake" technique). Supplements may fail to stick to certain invertebrates, risking nutritional deficiencies in the predator. In these instances, prey can be offered in dishes or bowls containing a shallow level of supplement (Figure 18-21).

Although calcium is often included in commercial vitamin-mineral supplements, it may not be present in quantities sufficient to meet requirements. Moreover, many supplements fail to provide essential nutrients other than vitamins and trace minerals.

Invertebrates contain little calcium, except for snails with shells and earthworms that ingest calcium-rich soil. Dusting of prey with calcium and vitamin supplements is commonly recommended, but it is a risky venture nutritionally. Too little calcium risks deficiency. Much of the supplement may be dislodged by movement and grooming if prey are not eaten readily. Too much calcium risks conditioned deficiencies of trace minerals. In one study, crickets were dusted with an unnamed product containing 11% calcium and 3.2% phosphorus, with $1/8$ tsp/100 crickets.[88] Immediately after dusting and 3 hours later, the dusted crickets contained only 0.12% calcium. By 22 hours after dusting, calcium levels were only 0.08%. In other circumstances, however, calcium levels of dusted crickets may be higher.

Studies in the author's laboratory show that the amount of dust sticking to invertebrate prey varies with products, as does the rate at which dust is dislodged from prey. Moreover, significantly more dust (all products) sticks to fruit flies, gram per gram, than to crickets. Absolute values differ with products used, but generally twice as much dust sticks to fruit flies. This is likely because of differences in surface structures and in surface area:volume ratios. Values for pinhead crickets ($<1/8$ inch long) are between those for fruit flies and older ($1/2$ inch) crickets. Thus, a dust that delivers appropriate levels of nutrition when applied to older crickets may deliver toxic levels of nutrients when applied to fruit flies. In our feeding trials, Poison Dart Frogs *(Dendrobates bicolor)* that consumed dusted fruit flies had a high mortality rate compared with Treefrogs *(Pelodryas caerulea)* that consumed the same dust applied to $1/4$-inch crickets (unpublished data). Mortalities disappeared when the dust for dart frogs was changed to one formulated to account for the greater amounts of dust ingested.

Dusting is recommended because it helps prevent nutrient deficiency in insectivorous reptiles, but it should be applied with care and its limitations appreciated. Generally, invertebrate prey are dusted once or twice weekly, if the reptile is fed daily. Rates of supplementation decrease as the animal matures. A history of dusted food items should not rule out nutritional deficiencies or toxicities.

Risks

Chitinous exoskeletons found in crustaceans, spiders, and insects reduce digestibility. Chitin is a water-soluble polymer of acetylglucosamine, with a structure similar to cellulose but containing nitrogen as well. Digestion of chitin occurs by intestinal symbionts and in some species by chitinolytic enzymes (see Table 18-2).[35,90]

Firefly toxicity has been reported in Bearded Dragons (*Pogona vitticeps*).[91] The poisonous principle is thought to be lucibufagins (steroidal pyrines). Enough toxin is found in one firefly to kill a Bearded Dragon within moments of ingestion. A study suggests fireflies may not be toxic to Fence Lizards (*Sceloporus undulatus*) and Broadhead Skinks (*Eumeces laticeps*).[92] Venomous spiders and stinging bees should probably be avoided.

Safety of the Eastern tent caterpillar (*Mallacosoma americanus*) is in question because rats fed this invertebrate as a protein source have had diarrhea develop and several have died. At necropsy, the rats were noted to have distended stomachs and colons.[80,81] Humans handling the dried tent caterpillar meal had allergic reactions. Because tent caterpillars frequently feed on cherry leaves, the caterpillar meal was tested for cyanide but none was detected (M. Finke, personal communication). Until the safety of tent caterpillars is better established, these invertebrates cannot be recommended as food for reptiles.

One should avoid invertebrates in contact with pesticides or herbicides. Diets fed to invertebrate prey should be balanced energetically and nutritionally. Finely ground commercial dry pet foods sustain growth and reproduction of most invertebrates (Table 18-10). Water is provided with moist slices of fruits and vegetables. Some invertebrates (such as crickets) thrive in warm temperatures, whereas others (such as mealworms) do better in cool temperatures.

Feeding to Reptiles

Invertebrate prey typically are fed alive because insectivorous reptiles key on prey movement to stimulate feeding behavior. Many captive invertebrate-eating reptiles appear to do well when fed only commercial prey, such as crickets and mealworms. Captive lizards and small snakes are sometimes fed only one or two species of prey throughout their life in captivity. Snails are especially relished by omnivorous and carnivorous turtles and many species of mid-sized ground-dwelling lizards. Earthworms and garden worms are taken by many forest-dwelling species, especially Box and Wood Turtles, and many aquatic turtles.

Although reptiles such as the Leopard Gecko (*Eublepharis macularius*) and Tokay Gecko (*Gekko gecko*) grow and reproduce on diets of supplemented well-fed crickets and mealworms, other species may not thrive. For example, studies suggest that wild lizards selected prey on the basis of the species of prey, not size of prey.[93] These data suggest that in addition to feeding the appropriate size of prey for insectivorous reptiles, the species of prey should be considered as well. For collections of less-common lizards, old world chameleons, and small snakes, and especially for individuals that are eating poorly, a variety of appropriately sized invertebrates should be offered, including snails, slugs, moths, flies, beetles, and mantids.

A general guideline for invertebrate size is to offer prey no longer than the width of the predator's head. Many lizards are more comfortable with slightly smaller prey, about 75% of the predator's head width. Other species, in contrast, show preferences for very large invertebrates. One such species is the Helmeted Iguana, *Corytophanes cristatus*, often available in petshops and notoriously difficult to feed long term. This Central American lizard in the wild consumes prey as long as one half the body length of the predator, although it does take smaller prey in captivity.[94] Generally, however, inexperienced keepers err by offering prey that are too large for their lizard.

Anecdotal evidence suggests that young dragons can develop fatal paralysis when large prey is ingested; pathogenesis is unclear. Feeding smaller prey reduces the surface area-to-volume ratio, thus reducing the percentage of chitin and nonprotein nitrogen relative to calories and amino acids in meals.

Invertebrates may be offered as free-roaming prey or confined to a bowl or cup within the habitat. The author prefers the former technique because hunting provides behavioral enrichment and stimulates cognitive function. However, food intake is more difficult to quantify when prey are free roaming, and prey may escape the habitat. Reptiles have to be taught to bowl feed, and some never feed from containers. Underfeeding can be the result of owners bowl feeding to prevent escaped prey.

Plants

Free-ranging herbivorous reptiles are quite specialized and selective in food choices.[95] In practice, the tendency is to lump all of these species as generalized herbivores. For better results, recognition is necessary of specialized types of herbivores, such as folivores, frugivores, and the like.

Proportions of greens, fruits, and vegetables to feed vary by species. For example, reptiles from desert and arid environments tend to accept and better metabolize hays, cacti, and drier foods. Any fruit offered to these reptiles must be countered with adequate chopped dried forages to maintain crude fiber intakes greater than 15% (DM). Fruits are fermented rapidly and to do otherwise risks lactic acidosis and diarrhea. In contrast, reptiles from tropical habitats prefer moist sweet foods and tolerate greater levels of fruits and lower fiber intakes; some accept occasional intakes of carrion or other meat-based foods.

Many herbivorous reptiles are color oriented toward food. They enjoy diets containing bits of red, yellow, and orange and seem to relish strawberry, apple, squash, banana, sweet potato, and mango.

Greens

Readily available salad greens include endive, escarole, and romaine lettuces, amaranth, collards, dandelion, kale, mustard, and spinach. Packages of chopped mixed greens are sold in groceries; one of the tastiest for reptiles is spring mix.

According to human taste buds, lettuces, spinach, and beet greens provide subtle flavors, and others may be classified as bitter, spicy, or peppery. For example, kale is bitter to our taste buds, and collards are slightly sweeter. Palatable greens

Table 18-10 Diet Characteristics of Commercial Invertebrate Prey

Prey	Diet
Cricket	Omnivore
Mealworm	Herbivore (granivore)
Superworm	Omnivore
Waxworm	Specialized feeder
Fruit fly	Herbivore (frugivore)
Silkworm	Herbivore (mulberry leaves)
Housefly	Omnivore
Mantid	Carnivore (insectivore)
Stick insect	Herbivore (foliavore)

include romaine and other leaf lettuces. These often serve as the main ingredient of salads, but other greens and high-fiber items, such as hay, should be fed as well. To these staples are added sources of vitamins and minerals, and sometimes protein, with an adequate level of fiber maintained. Commercial premixes are available.

Lettuce is commonly referred to as unsuitable for tortoises and iguanids because of nutritional inadequacies. Nutritionally, lettuce is no worse or better that most greens and is better nutritionally than most fruits (Table 18-11).[96] Romaine, for example, contains 35% protein and 0.7% calcium (DM basis). It is palatable and readily available throughout the United States. All produce, including romaine, needs supplementation to provide a complete diet.

Other Vegetables

Zucchini, shredded carrot, mild peppers, pumpkin, and shredded sweet potato are colorful tasty additions to greens. Legumes are good sources of calcium and plant protein. Legumes include beans (butter, green, lima, snap, and soy) and peas (green, snow, and sugar).

Sprouts may be added to salads. Commercially grown sprouts include legumes (alfalfa, mung bean) and grasses (barley, oats, radish). The *Salmonella* bacterium has been found in commercially grown sprouts, so homegrown sprouts may be safer and fresher.

Fruit

Most herbivorous reptiles from the tropics eat fruits (Figure 18-22). Favorites are banana, mango, and papaya. Others include apple, fig, guava, kiwifruit, melon, peach, pear, pineapple, plantain, and watermelon. Many enjoy a variety of berries: blackberries, blueberries, boysenberries, mulberries, raspberries, and strawberries.

Leaves and Blossoms

Homegrown plants that are well washed and free of herbicides and pesticides may be fed. Clover, dandelion, grape leaves (and fruit), hibiscus, kudzu, nasturtium, pothos, and rose are just a few readily consumed by Green Iguanas, *Uromastyx*, and tortoises.

Hay

Hays generally provide about 25% to 40% (DM) crude fiber, whereas supermarket produce generally provides less than half that amount. Commercial hays are available in pet shops and on the Internet (see Tables 18-4 and 18-11). Fiber-containing products may be purchased from supermarkets and pharmacies; most contain cellulose, bran (which can irritate bowels), or psyllium. Enterocytes use volatile fatty acids that arise from fermentation of fiber in the lower bowel as energy sources. Fiber is therefore useful when promoting wound healing in the intestine and recovery from enteritis.

Graze and Browse

Tortoises thrive on appropriate pastures of mixed swards. In the author's experience, most are generalist grazers with minor selectivity. Tortoises readily consume legumes (alfalfa, clover, kudzu, lespedeza, vetch) and grasses (johnsongrass, bluegrass, orchardgrass, timothy, crabgrass; see Table 18-11). Daily manure removal and periodic mowing maintain tortoise pastures in optimal condition (Figure 18-23).

The larger tortoise species (*Geochelone sulcata* and *Manouria emys*, for example) also browse cactus, bushes, shrubs, and vines such as rose, grapevine, and kudzu.

Nutritional Contents

Protein requirements of herbivorous reptiles are likely to range from about 14% to 35% DM, with the higher end of the range suited for growth and stress (see Figure 18-7). Protein contents of plants selected by free-ranging iguanas tend to have higher protein contents (13% to 33%) than those rejected (7% to 17%).[97] In a study of juvenile Green Iguanas (*Iguana iguana*) in Costa Rica, BW of those fed diets containing 28% crude protein (DM basis) were 30% and 300% greater than BW for iguanas fed 20% and 15% protein, respectively. In our studies that compared growth in juvenile Green Iguanas fed diets ranging from 13% to 31% protein (DM basis), growth rates were greatest for the 31% protein diet (Figure 18-24).[33] Further research showed that iguanas grow best when fed diets containing more than 25% DM (see Figure 18-12).[34] This level corresponds to about 5% to 8% protein on an as-fed (wet) basis for fresh salads. Protein requirements are likely to decrease as growth slows, perhaps by 24 months of age.

Plants with protein contents likely to be adequate for juvenile herbivores include romaine; spinach; legumes such as alfalfa sprouts, clover, and bean sprouts; dandelion; bamboo shoots; and mushrooms (see Table 18-11).[96] The foods listed vary in acceptance by different species; not all of these foods are accepted equally by all herbivores.

Fiber provides calories through hindgut fermentation and aids gut motility. Excessive fiber, however, limits calorie intake and inhibits trace mineral absorption. Relatively wide ranges of fiber intakes, perhaps from 4% to 40% DM, are found in diets for reptile collections. Both extremes may cause medical problems.

Risks

Oxalates occur in spinach, rhubarb, cabbage, peas, potatoes, and beet greens. Oxalates bind calcium and trace minerals, inhibiting their absorption. Conditioned trace mineral deficiencies may occur if diets contain mostly these foods and mineral intakes are marginal. Goitrogens occur in cabbage, kale, mustard, and other cruciferous plants. Large intakes of these foods with marginal iodine intake may lead to hypothyroidism.

Although green plants provide needed essential nutrients and fuels, herbage contains nonnutritive substances too. Secondary plant compounds are stored by most plants and used as deterrents to bacteria, fungi, and herbivores. Many are toxic, such as saponins, phenols, and alkaloids. Most herbivores are selective feeders in the wild, but plants with potentially toxic substances are consumed in variable quantities. Little work has been done on identifying secondary plant compounds in diets for reptiles, and the roles of these substances in clinical nutrition are unknown.

Goitrogens bind the trace mineral iodine, with risk of goiter or hypothyroidism. Goitrogens are found in highest quantities in cabbage, kale, mustard, turnip, rutabaga, and other cruciferous plants. These foods can be fed as part of a varied diet along with provision of a supplement that contains iodine such as iodized table salt; iodized "lite" salt containing iodine, sodium, potassium, and chloride; and kelp. Many commercial supplements contain adequate levels of iodine.

Table 18-11 Calorie and Nutrient Contents of Foods for Herbivorous Reptiles[91,95]

Food	Weight (g)	Water (%)	Energy (kcal/g) AF	Energy (kcal/g) DM	Protein (% DM)	Fat (% DM)	Carbohydrate (% DM)	Fiber (% DM)	Ca (% DM)	P (% DM)
Greens										
Lettuce										
Romaine	100	94	0.18	3.0	36	7	50	11	1.1	0.4
Iceberg	100	63	0.13	3.2	25	0	59	11	0.4	0.5
Spinach	100	91	0.26	2.9	36	3	48	7	1.0	0.6
Dandelion	100	86	0.44	3.1	18	5	61	11	1.3	0.4
Beet	100	91	0.24	2.7	24	3	51	14	1.3	0.4
Sprouts										
Alfalfa	100	88	0.39	3.2	37	4	39	12	0.3	0.8
Mung bean	100	89	0.35	3.2	31	2	54	6	0.1	0.5
Other vegetables										
Frozen mixed	100	83	0.47	2.8	28	1	51	13	0.2	0.2
Lima beans	95	62	1.0	2.6	19	1	67	6	0.1	0.3
Mushrooms	100	90	0.27	2.7	30	6	49	9	0.1	1.3
Sweet potato	180	64	0.82	2.8	5	1	84	2	0.1	0.2
Squash	100	94	0.18	3.0	17	2	65	9	0.4	0.4
Fruits										
Apple	128	84	0.51	3.2	1	2	86	4	Trace	Trace
Blueberries	145	85	0.51	3.4	4	2	80	12	0.1	0.1
Banana	114	74	0.82	3.2	4	2	86	2	Trace	Trace
Cantaloupe	160	90	0.32	3.2	8	2	79	4	0.1	0.2
Strawberries	149	92	0.28	3.5	6	4	77	6	0.2	0.2
Forages										
Alfalfa hay	100	10	2.2	2.5	17	2	45	27	1.2	0.2
Timothy hay	100	11	2.2	2.5	15	3	45	28	0.5	0.2
Orchardgrass hay	100	11	2.2	2.5	15	3	41	31	0.4	0.4
Graze and browse										
Kentucky Bluegrass	100	65	0.9	2.5	5.2	2	75	8.1	0.1	0.1
Prickly pear	100	83	0.4	2.0	4.8	2	69	14	9.6	0.1
Clover	100	80	0.5	3.0	19	1	47	23	1.7	0.4

DM, Dry matter; *AF*, as-fed.

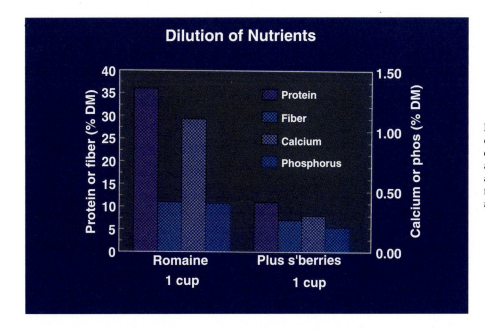

FIGURE 18-22 Additions of fruit to chopped salads significantly reduce nutrient concentrations. Fruit should be added at about 5% of diets for grassland tortoises and up to 20% of diets for certain tropical forest tortoises and Green Iguanas (*Iguana iguana*).

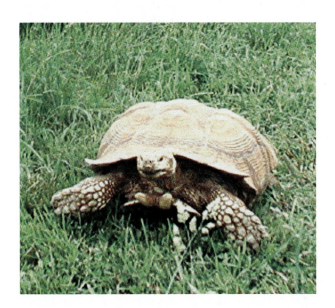

FIGURE 18-23 This pasture for Sulcata Tortoises (*Geochelone sulcata*) is mowed at least monthly to maintain the sward at a relatively short length suited for tortoise grazing. Manure is removed daily. Patches of sward are allowed to grow tall to provide visual barriers. Sturdy fencing prevents escapes.

The mineral iodine is itself toxic in large quantities (also acting as a goitrogen), so care should be taken not to overdose.

Many other secondary plant compounds exist, and that oxalates and goitrogens receive more attention than needed, and other substances are ignored, is unfortunate. For example, many plants contain substances with hormone-like activity (such as phytoestrogens in soybeans) that may affect reproduction and health. A large number of different plant fibers may affect digestion and intestinal health. Other compounds in plants influence cognitive function, acting as stimulants or sedatives. Other potentially harmful secondary plant compounds include alkaloids, phenolics, tannins, and terpenoids. Potentially beneficial secondary plant compounds include bioflavonoids, glucosinolates, and alliins (alk[en]yl cysteine sulphoxides).[98]

Care must be taken to restrict access of herbivorous reptiles to poisonous plants, yet limited data on dose responses in reptiles preclude the presentation of lists of known plant offenders. Presumably safe plants include clover, dandelion, and alfalfa for reptiles grazing outdoors. Outdoor plants that have caused illness in mammals or birds include cherry, rhododendron, oleander, lupine, foxglove, yew, privet, and lantana. Presumably safe houseplants for use in natural vivaria include pothos (*Scindapsus* spp.), snakeskin plant (*Sansevieria* spp.), and umbrella tree (*Schefflera* spp.). Pothos is especially tolerant of heat and wet and dry conditions. Houseplants that have caused illness in mammals or birds include dumbcane (*Diffenbachia* spp.), Easter lily, and *Euphorbia* spp.) All plants in contact with reptiles should be free of pesticides and herbicides.

Tolerances for poisonous plants are mostly unknown for reptiles. Studies with the Whiptail Lizard (*Cnemidophorus arubensis*) showed that plants were not eaten in proportion to their prevalence in the environment, but rather certain rare plants were selected and other common plants were ignored. Moreover, plants with relatively large quantities of phenolics, saponins, and alkaloids were avoided, but a plant with a cyanogenic compound was eaten.[99] Large quantities of oral cyanide doses had no effect on the lizards. Nevertheless, avoidance of plants with cyanogenic substances (such as wilted wild cherry leaves) and invertebrates that eat cyanogenic plants (such as Eastern tent caterpillars that consume fresh wild cherry leaves) is recommended.

Feeding to Reptiles

Clients should be counseled to wash greens and remove wilted leaves before feeding out. Greens can be washed in cold water,

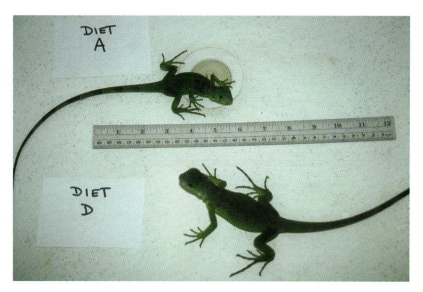

FIGURE 18-24 Growth in juvenile Green Iguanas (*Iguana iguana*) is affected by dietary protein. Diet A provided only 13% protein (dry matter basis), and Diet D provided 35% protein.[33]

and commercial products designed for washing salad greens destined for human consumption may be used. Soaking leaves in cold water revitalizes limp leaves. After soaking, leaves may be patted dry with paper towels or a salad spinner can be used to remove excess water. Greens and mixed salads should be stored at cool temperatures until feeding out.

Salads should be comprised of bite-sized portions. Flat plates are preferred to bowls for many species. Many herbivores soil their food, so care should be taken to minimize fecal contamination of salads.

Commercial Diets

Commercial diets offer an efficient and usually safe means of providing calories and essential nutrients if formulated and produced properly, if fed appropriately, and if the calorie and nutrient contents are within the animal's range of nutritional needs.

Pellets for Carnivores

Many carnivores need vertebrate prey, but some aquatic and Box Turtles may be fed pelleted diets. Formulations are based on pellets for fish and may be very high in protein and fat (diets for trout) or moderately high in protein and fat (diets for catfish and koi). Fish meal is a major ingredient of both pellet types. A few products fail to add essential vitamins and minerals. Processes used in extrusion and pelleting involve high temperatures that partially destroy labile vitamins. Mineral and vitamin contents of fish meals vary with species, season of harvest, and processing.

Pellets for Omnivores and Herbivores

These products are typically comprised of plant-based and animal-based ingredients usually in the form of extruded (and occasionally compressed) pellets. Most contain dyes to enhance colors, and many have sprayed-on odors (marketed erroneously as flavors) to enhance acceptance (by owners as much as reptiles). Many of these products are relatively new, and information about testing in feeding trials is limited or lacking.

Several characteristics, however, are common to all plant-based pellets, regardless of the formulation or quality control in manufacture (Figure 18-25). Pellets contain minimal water, about 10% to 12%. In contrast, the water content of fresh salads is about 85% to 92% and the water content of invertebrates is about 60% to 70%. A reptile fed only pellets receives much less water from its food than what it is used to and evolved on.

Plant-based pellets use the ingredients and production techniques of the commercial livestock and pet food industries. Although these features are not inherently bad for reptiles, they limit the scope and breadth of formulations. The ingredients in pellets include corn, soy, poultry meal, tallow, alfalfa, and wheat, for example. The deficiencies in ingredient variety in pellets is compensated for by differing shapes and dyes, which may please the eye of the owner more than the palate of a reptile.

Plant-based pellets contain relatively low fat; about 10% or 12% is the limit for commercial pellets sold in paper and cardboard containers. Salads contain even less fat. In contrast, invertebrates contain 30% to 60% fat. This fat is essential for omnivores, providing needed calories for growth, reproduction, and good health and essential fatty acids for development of vital tissues, especially brain. The author has worked with Bearded Dragon breeders who observed poor growth in juvenile dragons fed pellets of low fat and relatively low protein; growth improved markedly once the pellet was changed to a product with more fat.

Other products are marketed as treats, such as dried flies, sometimes dusted with a few vitamins. Potencies of the vitamins are likely to be limited to no more than a few months from date of production. These diets are rarely complete or balanced.

Pet Foods for Reptiles

Diets produced for domestic species have been fed to reptiles. Most are wholesome; some are cost-effective for large collections. Some diets, such as most pet foods for dogs and cats, are formulated to be complete and balanced for the intended species. Others, such as many hay-based pellets, are intended

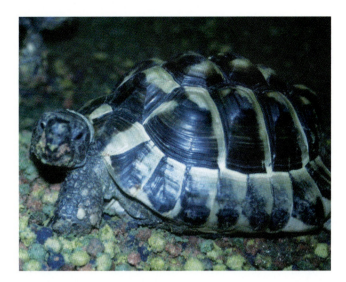

FIGURE 18-25 Soaking pellets before feeding out improves water intake and food acceptance. This juvenile Hermann's Tortoise (*Testudo hermanni*) significantly increased its water intake when fed pellets (even when soaked), raising concerns about maintenance of water balance in reptiles fed pellet-based diets.

to serve as only one part of a diet for the intended species. Although variation in nutritional requirements between species is not huge, differences between reptiles and mammals in food preferences, metabolism, stress from captivity, and nutrient requirements suggest that commercial diets for mammals in most instances should not be used as the sole source of nutrients for reptiles.

Carnivores
Commercial pet foods are marketed in canned, dry, frozen, and semimoist forms, with animal-based and plant-based ingredients. Wide ranges of protein, fat, and carbohydrate are available. A statement of nutritional adequacy on labels of dog and cat foods refers to standards of the Association of American Feed Control Officials (AAFCO) for maintenance, growth, reproduction, or all stages of the life cycle. These claims may be established by nutrient profile (laboratory analysis) or by trials according to AAFCO protocols. Protein in pet foods ranges from 16% to 40% of ME; many pet foods provide more than 22% of ME from protein and more than 25% of ME from fat. These protein levels per se are unlikely to harm most reptiles. Most cat foods are formulated to produce acid urine (for urinary health) in cats. Acidic urine increases the excretion of calcium in urine. Thus, juvenile reptiles fed cat foods risk calcium deficiency. Controlled data for reptiles are scarce and anecdotal reports are rarely documented, but long-term feeding of commercial pet foods has appeared to be associated with problems, such as shell deformities in growing tortoises. Anecdotal reports also suggest that Box Turtles (*Terrepene carolinensis*) fed commercial pet foods for long periods (years) suffer shell deformities and soft tissue calcification.

Forages
Commercial forages include legumes, primarily alfalfa, marketed as a meal, pelleted, cubed, and chopped. Grinding and pelleting of forage fed to ruminants increases both food intake and utilization of digestible energy. Most tortoises and herbivorous lizards, however, show limited interest in processed forages, eating these items only when disguised with fresh produce or when no other foods are available. Exceptions include some of tortoises from arid lands that enjoy hay, such as African Sulcata Tortoises, *Geochelone sulcata*.

Hay can be purchased from feed stores, farms, pet shops, and the Internet (see Table 18-4). Alfalfa cubes sold in pet shops are readily available and consistent but expensive. The same cubes can be purchased from feed stores in 50-lb bags and stored in metal trash cans in a cool dry room. About half the vitamin A activity from beta-carotene is lost within a year.

Hay-based pellets are marketed for a variety of species and may be supplemented to be complete feeds. Most range from 12% to 28% crude protein and 14% to 19% crude fiber.[100] Occasionally, nutritional problems are reported in mammalian species fed pellets, such as vitamin A deficiency or intoxication. Problems arise from use of old hay or errors in mixing. Some success has been noted in the use of hay-based pellets as **bedding** for juvenile herbivorous reptiles. Although these products are safe if wholesome, in the authors' experience, most pellets are quick to mold. Risks of mold-related respiratory disease and digestive upset may be a high price to pay for the convenience of bedding with pellets.

When purchasing or recommending commercial herbivore diets, read labels with extreme care. Some may contain low-level antibiotics and other growth promotants that have unpredictable and potentially deleterious effects on reptiles.

Supplements
Vitamins and minerals are added to diets made up of invertebrates, mixed salads, and boned or eviscerated vertebrates. Preparations should contain the fat-soluble and water-soluble vitamins and trace minerals known to be essential for other species. Vitamin D_3 should be included unless the reptile is outdoors most of the time with exposure to unfiltered sunlight or has adequate access to appropriate commercial bulbs (Table 18-12; also see Chapter 84).

Thought should be given to how the supplement is provided. Addition of a supplement to the animal's water may speed the decomposition of vitamins and also deter water consumption. Additions to salads may decrease palatability. Certain vitamins decompose in light or moisture, and the shelf life of most preparations is restricted to a few months after manufacture. Most commercial preparations have traveled from point of manufacture to a distributor, then to a retail outlet, before purchase. For this reason, use of products without expiration dates on labels is discouraged. Commercial supplements should be stored in a cool dark place. Invertebrates, muscle meat, and salads require supplementation with calcium. Additional calcium may be provided as limestone (38% calcium) or as calcium salts: carbonate (40% calcium), lactate (18% calcium), and gluconate (9% calcium). Calcium and phosphorus are supplied in bone meal (24% calcium, 12% phosphorus) and dicalcium phosphate (18% to 24% calcium, 18% phosphorus). Bone meal tablets vary in size. A small (aspirin-size) tablet weighs 0.75 g and provides about 180 mg calcium and 90 mg phosphorus. Products vary, so labels should be read carefully. Supplemental calcium, phosphorus, and vitamin D_3 are available for humans, livestock, companion animals, and reptiles and amphibians (Table 18-13). Calcium salts are available in tablet form from groceries and pharmacies. These can be placed into thoracic and abdominal cavities of vertebrate prey or ground and dusted onto prey and plants.

Recent interest has focused on eggshell powder (ESP) and its safety. Analyses of chicken ESP for minerals, amino acids, and hormones determined that it contained high levels of calcium (401 mg/g) and strontium (372 µg/g).[101] Low levels were found for lead, aluminum, cadmium, mercury, vanadium, boron, iron, zinc, phosphorus, nickel, fluorine, selenium, copper and chromium. Large differences between products were found for fluorine, selenium, copper, chromium, and strontium. These differences were thought to be the result of differences in chicken diets and environments. Protein was low; high levels of glycine and arginine were found. Detected hormones included transforming growth factor–beta 1 (up to 7.28 ng/g ESP), calcitonin (up to 25 ng/g ESP), and progesterone (up to 0.33 ng/g ESP). Below detection limits were estradiol-17 beta and calcitriol.[101] The authors concluded that chicken ESP is safe and effective as a calcium supplement for humans, but it has not undergone controlled trials in reptiles. Clients often ask about the value of hard (high-calcium) drinking water for their reptiles. Comparative trials in reptiles are lacking. Investigators used metaanalysis to examine a body of data from multiple papers published from 1966 to 1998 on calcium bioavailability of calcium-rich mineral water. The authors found that absorption of calcium from mineral water was significantly greater ($p = .03$) than calcium absorption from dairy products. In light of new recommendations for humans (up to 1500 mg calcium/d), the authors suggest that mineral waters that are calcium rich are a useful addition to diets of humans trying to achieve intakes of 1500 mg calcium/d.[102] Concerns about lead levels in calcium supplements are justified because analyses for lead can often be erroneously low, by up to 50%, or erroneously below detection limits.[103] In one study, 136 brands of calcium supplements were analyzed,

Table 18-12 Examples of Ultraviolet A and Ultraviolet B Emission from Commercial Bulbs

Light Source	UVA (µW/cm²)			UVB (µW/cm²)		
	Surface	1 ft	3 ft	Surface	1 ft	3 ft
Sunlight 9/27/00 3 pm at Bronx, NY	132			51		
Verilux 40W	23	2	0	10	1.6	0
Verilux 30W (4 mo old)	43	7		14.2	1.7	
New Industrial True Lite	12	1	0	7	0	0
Metal Halide 400W (~2 y old)	1800+	230	113	360	35	18
Sylvania BL 350 20W	1023	135	60	658	78.5	36
Sylvania BL 350 30W	594	25	5	222	11	2
Sylvania BL 350 40W (4 mo old)	1800+	298	70	1212	123	35.1
Zoo Med Iguana Light 5.0 40W	65	5	1	84	6	1
Zoo Med Reptisun Desert 40W	70	4	1	22	1	0
GE infrared spot 250W	120	2	2	11	0	0
Phillips spot 150W	6	2	0	5	0	0
ESU Super UV Daylight 3% UVA/7% UVB	8	1	0	12	1	0
Westron 100W spot		1800+	660		308	97
Westron 100W flood	1207	223	160	134	21.5	4.4
Westron 160W spot		1800+	1080		400	269
Westron 160W spot (1.5 y old)		370			57	
Westron 160W flood		221	89		91.5	61
Westron 300W spot			1800+	1800+	1033	190
Westron 300W flood	1800+	600	180	205	39	15
Lumichrome F40WIxx 6500 K	143	15	14	50	3.3	0.4
Aquasun VHO 60" (140W)	6	3	1.3	3.4	1.4	0
Ottlite 40W (new)	11	1.4		4.7	0.9	
Ottlite 40W (3 mo old)	24	14	6.4	10.4	6.4	4.4

Note: Ultraviolet-B (*UVB*) sensor calibrated at 310 nm; range, 260 to 310 nm; ultraviolet-A (*UVA*) sensor calibrated at 370 nm; range, 310 to 400 nm.
Data were collected and summarized by Sam Lee and Bill Holmstrom from Wildlife Conservation Society, New York. Data are reproduced here with their permission. Measurements were made with UVX Radiometer (UVP, Inc., 2066 W 11th Street, Upland, Calif 91786; (800) 452-6788; fax (909) 946-3597; uvp@uvp.com). Although effectiveness of equipment to measure absolute values for UV-A and UV-B is questionable, these data are useful for comparing relative emissions between bulbs.

Table 18-13 Commonly Available Calcium Supplements

	Calcium (%)	Phosphorus (%)	Calcium in 1 tsp (5 g)	Phosphorus in 1 tsp (5 g)
Calcium carbonate	40	0	2000 mg	0 mg
Limestone	38	0	1900 mg	0 mg
Calcium lactate	18	0	900 mg	0 mg
Calcium gluconate	9	0	450 mg	0 mg
Bone meal	24	12	1200 mg	600 mg
Dicalcium phosphate ("Dical")	24	18	1200 mg	900 mg

with calcium originating from bonemeal, dolomite, and oyster shell, and calcium that was synthesized, refined, chelated, or nonchelated.[103] Two thirds of the calcium supplements failed to meet 1999 California criteria for acceptable lead levels (1.5 μg/daily dose of calcium). The pharmaceutical, synthesized, and refined products had lowest lead levels (from nondetectable to 2.9 μg Pb/g calcium) and had the largest proportion of brands that met criteria for acceptable levels (85% of antacids and 100% infant formulas). Calcium supplements sometimes include vitamin D. Cholecalciferol (vitamin D_3) may be listed on food labels as cholecalciferol, animal sterol, D-activated animal sterol, irradiated animal sterol, or vitamin D_3. Do not assume that the term vitamin D in the label ingredient list is actually D_3 because it may be D_2 and unusable by reptiles.

Nutritional Support

Diet selection for nutritional support is determined by fuel source and nutrient contents, digestibility, form, and degree of sterility. Fuel source proportions should match patient needs: high protein and fat for carnivores, more complex carbohydrate for herbivores.

Enterals are appropriate for reptiles in need of nutritional support and are offered commercially (see Table 18-4). Because of their formulations and ingredients, enterals are superior nutritionally and make better sense medically than baby foods, commercial fat-containing nutritional boosters, homemade diets, and sports drinks that have historically been tube-fed to sick reptiles. Food boluses for carnivores may be balls of canned pet food or oiled prey. Reports of a sausage diet and a paste diet for snakes deserve further attention because the products could facilitate nutrient manipulations, such as low purine or low fat, for snakes and monitors.[104,105] For tube-feeding, carnivores may receive diets of blended whole prey or enterals containing high protein and fat, each more than 25% of ME calories. Diets made with enterals can be manipulated, so that animals with gout may be fed low-purine diets and those with hepatoencephalopathy or renal disease, for example, may be fed lower-protein or lower-phosphorus diets, respectively. Juvenile omnivores are fed as carnivores. Older omnivores and all herbivores should receive diets lower in protein and fat. Tolerance of herbivores to the higher fat contents found in many enterals is encouraging because it enables meeting calorie needs without volume overload.

All foods should be gently warmed before administration. Foods warmed in a microwave should sit for a few minutes and be stirred to avoid thermal burns from hot spots.

FEEDING MANAGEMENT

In practice, most nutritional problems arise from imbalanced diets, unpalatable food items, malnourished prey, and poor feeding management. Specific nutrient requirements for each reptile species are for the most part unknown, but some generalities may be addressed. As for other species, an optimal range of intake likely exists for each essential nutrient below which deficiency occurs and above which intoxication occurs (Figure 18-26).

Signs of deficiency or intoxication depend in part on the specific intake, the patient's vulnerability, and the nature of the nutrient in question. Vitamin A, selenium, and fluoride, for example, kill animals when fed in high enough quantities. Thiamin and vitamin E, in contrast, may cause little duress when fed in large quantities. The benign characteristics of some nutrients, B vitamins for example, are often lost when the nutrients are administered intravenously. Although little controlled research has been done on specific nutrient requirements of reptiles, anecdotes abound. For example, reptiles do need vitamin D_3 and apparently make inadequate use of vitamin D_2, but little consensus and fewer data exist on optimal methods for ensuring vitamin D status in captive reptiles. Some anecdotal legends are disproved once research is accomplished. One example is the suggestion that snakes with ulcerative stomatitis have vitamin C deficiency; research has shown that snakes synthesize adequate amounts of ascorbate in the kidneys.[106] Similarly, snakes synthesize adequate niacin, and this vitamin likely has no influence on necrotic enterohepatitis.[107] Also, lipid metabolism and fatty acid absorption were thought to differ between fresh-water and

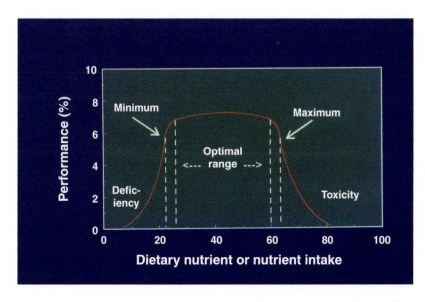

FIGURE 18-26 Each reptile has a dietary intake of each essential nutrient that may vary from deficient to toxic. Our goal is to have each nutrient within the optimal range. Determining optimal ranges for essential nutrients is currently based on clinical experiences, feeding trials, and extrapolation from other species, pending controlled laboratory research.

marine alligators, but recent research suggests otherwise.[108] As more work is done, recommendations for feeding healthy reptiles, preventing and treating nutritional diseases, and providing nutrition support are likely to advance. With time and effort, many (but not all) captive specimens become accustomed to unnatural food items. Many snakes, for example, learn easily to accept fresh-killed domestic mice, although newly captured specimens may still need movement, either from live prey or through simulation. Certain species, however, recognize few items as food, which makes adaptation to a captive diet difficult. Examples are small lizards that accept only flies or ants and hognose snakes that eat only toads. Timing and frequency of feeding are important. Certain species eat at any time, others eat only in daylight, and still others eat only in darkness. Small reptiles usually eat often, daily or every second day. Juveniles with rapid growth rates, such as very young chameleons (*Chamaeleo* spp.) and Bearded Dragons, may be fed two or three times daily. Older larger animals eat less frequently. Large boids and pythons, for example, may eat once every few weeks. Chronic starvation occurs in reptiles fed in less than optimal intervals or in the wrong part of the light-dark cycle.

Snakes

All snakes are carnivores, with the smallest eating invertebrates and the largest consuming adult rabbits and other large prey. Feeding of venomous and constrictor snakes can be dangerous to keepers, and precautions must be taken to avoid bites or entrapment. Large snakes can be moved to feeding habitats; others are usually fed in their usual cage. Many snakes are nocturnal or crepuscular (active at dusk and dawn), and for these species prey should be offered in late afternoon or evening. Snakes are adapted to eating relatively large meals infrequently.

Snakes that feed on rodents and chicks include pythons, boas, ratsnakes, cornsnakes, gophersnakes, bullsnakes, and pinesnakes.[109] Although these generalizations are helpful, subtle differences may exist between species. For example, Rubber Boas (*Charina bottae*) in the wild take 66% mammals, 17% lizards, 7% birds, and 5% lizard eggs. In contrast, Sand Boas (*Eryx* spp.) feed mainly on mammals.[110] One may wish to make appropriate adjustments to diets in captivity.

Snakes that feed on amphibians, crayfish, fish, and small lizards or snakes include kingsnakes, indigo snakes, watersnakes, gartersnakes, and hog-nosed snakes.[109] Those that take insects and other small invertebrates include wormsnakes and ring-necked and other fossorial snakes.

Lizards

Most lizards are insectivorous, including anoles, chameleons, geckos, Water Dragons, most skinks, swifts, ameivas, lacertas, and smaller monitors and tegus.[109] Day Geckos (*Phelsuma* spp.) take invertebrates and nectar or, in captivity, fruit baby food. Large monitors, tegus, Gila Monsters (*Heloderma suspectum*), and Beaded Lizards (*Heloderma horridum*) take vertebrate prey. Some tegus also eat fruit in addition to prey.

Omnivores include Bearded Dragons, Blue-tongue and Pink-tongue Skinks and *Cyclura* iguanids. *Uromastyx* spp. eat greens and seeds (peas, lentils, bird seed) and the occasional invertebrate.

Herbivorous lizards include Green Iguanas, Chuckwallas, and Prehensile-tail Skinks. Determination of appropriate diets can be a difficult task when faced with a petshop lizard known only by its common name.

Chelonians

Aquatic turtles begin life as carnivores, and most spend adult lives as omnivores. True carnivores include Snapping Turtles (*Chelydra* spp.) and Softshell Turtles (*Apalone* spp.), yet studies of stomach contents reveal plant matter (acorns, persimmon, wild grape) and foreign bodies (rock, fish hook).[111] Other species are characterized as generalist omnivores, yet their stomach contents can contain all animal matter.[112] Many species thrive on pelleted foods formulated for fish (such as various brands of trout, catfish, and koi pellets). Box Turtles, Wood Turtles and Marsh Turtles are mostly omnivorous and consume earthworms, mushrooms, fruits, and small invertebrates such as sow bugs and slugs. Aquatic and Box Turtles may be fed in separate feeding tanks to avoid fouling their home habitat with uneaten food.

Tortoises (terrestrial turtles) are primarily herbivorous. Grassland varieties (Sulcata, Leopard, and Star Tortoises as well as *Testudo* spp.) thrive on mixtures of grasses and forages that are grazed in warm weather and mixed into salads when housed indoors. Forest varieties (Redfoot, Yellowfoot, Elongate) may consume more fruit and occasionally (about once monthly) animal-based foods.

Nutrition Support

For nutrition support to succeed in reptiles, attention must be given to provision of the patient's optimal environmental conditions and to energy and nutrients (Figure 18-27). Gradients of temperature and humidity, delivery of water, and provision of substrates, hiding places, and cage furniture should be considered; all impact a patient's attitude and recovery.

Endotherms with severe infection or trauma or certain malignant diseases are hypermetabolic, with increased use of fat and protein for energy and hormonal changes, including peripheral insulin resistance. The role of hypermetabolism in sick reptiles deserves more attention. For example, the degree of a fever response (if any) to infection is questionable, perhaps present in some lizards but not in others and perhaps absent in tortoises.[113-115] However, data from geckos that regenerate tails suggested hypermetabolism. These reptiles exhibit elevated blood glucose, T_4, and T_3 concentrations during periods of wound healing and tissue regeneration (Figure 18-28).[116,117]

Nutritional Assessment

With mammalian guidelines, nutrition support is started when the patient loses 10% BW acutely or 20% chronically or when anorexia or injury precludes the consumption of sufficient calories to meet about 85% of nutrition goals. Ideal weights are not published for reptile species, so in addition to weighing, nutritional status is assessed by means of diet history, body condition assessment, and laboratory analyses. Of these methods, body condition evaluation is likely to be most convenient and effective.

Reptiles in optimal body condition have muscle and fat over bony protuberances (Figures 18-29 and 18-30). Vertebral

Nutrition

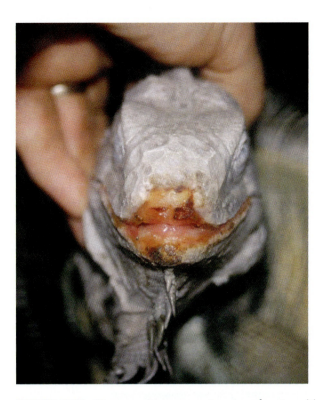

FIGURE 18-27 Disease and trauma can impair prehension of food and decrease the appetite because of pain. This Green Iguana *(Iguana iguana)* traumatized his rostrum from rubbing on the screened sides of his habitat. He responded well to nutritional support with liquid enterals (with antibiotics and a move to another habitat).

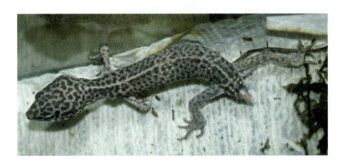

FIGURE 18-28 Lizards can drop their tails (autotomy) when fearing capture, so care must be taken when examining patients. For species that regenerate tails, requirements for calories and nutrients increase during tissue growth. This emaciated Leopard Gecko *(Eublepharis Macularis)* was provided too few calories to sustain body weight and tissue repair. Note the loss of muscling on the limbs.

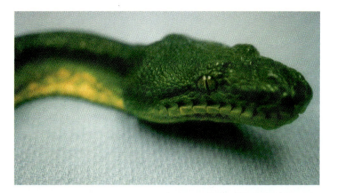

FIGURE 18-29 This emaciated Emerald Tree Boa *(Corallus caninus)* shows loss of muscling that occurs with low calorie intake and disease. The muscle has been mobilized, with amino acids transported to the liver to produce glucose via gluconeogenesis. Glucose is the fuel of choice for the brain, red blood cells, and renal medullary cells. *(Photograph courtesy S. Stahl.)*

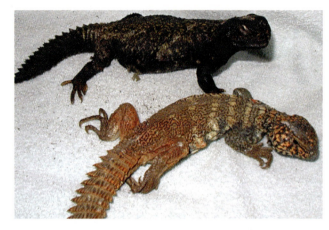

FIGURE 18-30 This thin juvenile Rainbow Uromastyx *(Uromastyx benti; bottom)* exhibits muscle loss in its limbs, fat loss from the tail, and loose folds of skin. Mali Uromastyx *(U. malienensis; top)* is of similar age and in good condition. Originating from the deserts of northern Africa, *Uromastyx* spp. in captivity consume supplemented salads, dried legumes (lentils, peas), and small seeds. In the healthy Mali, note the coelomic paunch (from hindgut fermentation) and fat tail (a store of fat and water developed for arid habitats).

processes, ribs, and pelvic girdles may be palpated but not readily seen in snakes and lizards. Folds of skin running vertically along the trunk should be minimal, perhaps one or rarely two, in well-fleshed lizards. Turtles and tortoises should have heft when lifted.

Studies with free-ranging tortoises report allometric relationships between BW and shape or size, often carapace length (Figure 18-31).[118-122] Because dimensional analysis (assuming similar shapes and weight proportional to volume) indicates that weight is a function of the cube of length, we looked for a correlation between BW and cube of carapace length (L):

$$\text{Predicted BW (g)} = 0.15(L^3_{cm}) r^2 - 0.99$$

Our data were obtained on 42 tortoises from nine species, ranging from 214 to 21,338 g BW and 9.4 to 51.4 cm length (Figure 18-32, *A*).[123] In another study, BW of 220 healthy California Desert Tortoises *(Gopherus agassizii)* were compared with volume measurements:[124]

$$\text{Predicted BW (g)} = 0.588(L \times W \times H) + 388 r^2 = 0.89, \\ p < .001$$

This formula, validated against water displacement measurements, allows prediction of optimal BW for Desert

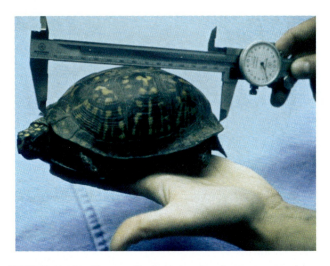

FIGURE 18-31 Allometry in chelonians involves measures of carapace length and sometimes carapace width, plastron length, and scute size. *(Photograph courtesy S. Stahl.)*

Tortoise patients and aids in determining body condition of ill, postsurgical, or prebrumation (prehibernation) animals (Figure 18-32, *B*). Additional studies to assess body condition have used allometry, body condition scoring, and bioelectrical impedance in snakes, lizards, and chelonians.[125-131]

Laboratory testing holds promise for assessment of body condition. For example, plasma triglycerides correlated positively with body condition in female Gartersnakes (*Thamnophis sirtalis parietalis*) emerging from brumation (hibernation).[132]

Laboratory data, such as low concentration of serum albumin, may suggest malnutrition, but generally the markers of poor nutritional status that are measured in other species, such as transthyretin and retinol-binding protein, are not measured in reptiles.

Techniques

Nutrition support is provided by voluntary and involuntary means. When additions of just a few nutrients are indicated and appetite is good, supplements are added to the usual diet. Liquids can be injected into vertebrate prey. Large prey, such as whole fish, rabbits, and chickens, can be supplemented by placing tablets into the abdominal cavity, esophagus, or

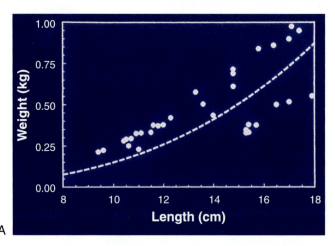
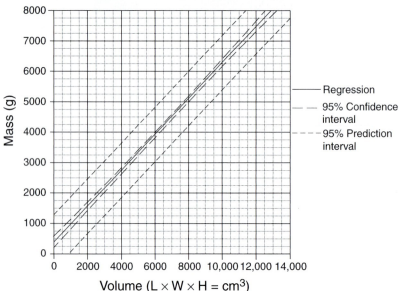

FIGURE 18-32 A, Data from the author's laboratory showed a relationship between body weight and the cube of carapace length. **B,** In another study, a prediction of mass from volume was evaluated in 220 healthy Desert Tortoises (*Gopherus agassizii*). (Predicted BW (g) = 0.588 (L × W × H) + 388r^2 = 0.89, $p < .001$, with *BW*, body weight; *L*, length; *W*, width; *H*, height.)

gill slits before feeding out. These methods suffice for administration of supplemental calcium, thiamin, and vitamin E. Invertebrate prey can be dusted or soaked in nutrient preparations, but odor and taste may affect intake. Some reports have success injecting invertebrates with supplements, but the author has observed limited effectiveness with this technique. (Note: Many of the injectable vitamin formulations are not intended for enteral administration, and no evidence exists that they are even absorbed when given via that route.)

Sluggish carnivores may respond to a process where prey are gently tapped or slapped alongside the mouth of the reptile. The goal is for the patient to strike at the prey then grasp and swallow it. Handlers should use tongs with this technique.

Involuntary feeding is managed by assist-feeding or with indwelling feeding tubes. It should be attempted only after dehydration and electrolyte imbalances have been corrected.

Assist-feeding is accomplished by gently opening the patient's mouth with a speculum (laboratory spatula, credit card, radiographic film) or by gently applying downward pressure on dewlap (iguanas, chameleons, anoles). A speculum may be used to hold the mouth open, and care is taken to avoid injuring teeth or keratin surfaces in (toothless) chelonians. Food is passed as boluses, or more commonly as slurries administered via syringe, metal feeding tube, or catheter of plastic or red rubber. Some patients may be lightly sedated for this procedure. Prey should have incisors and claws trimmed to avoid lacerations of the patient's esophagus. For snakes and lizards, the bolus may be "milked" down the esophagus to the stomach. For tortoises and turtles, the bolus may be gently pushed down the tract with a blunt instrument. The author prefers less-traumatic slurries to bolus feeding.

Care should be taken when working with small reptiles to avoid causing harm to the patient. Care should be taken when working with large reptiles to avoid causing harm to personnel. Reptiles are strong, and their bites, even unintentional ones from tortoises, are frequently painful and occasionally damaging.

Tubes may be passed into the distal esophagus or stomach at each feeding or may be indwelling (Figure 18-33). With passing of tubes, a mouth speculum may be needed, especially for tortoises who can bite through tubes. Stainless steel feeding needles of appropriate diameter are recommended for many species (Figure 18-34).

Feeding tubes placed in the distal esophagus and stomach can be relatively wide bore. Feeding tubes can be adapted from intravenous or urinary catheters or made specifically for gavage feeding. The latter may be especially useful in larger reptiles because of their length (often about 36 in), weighted tips (to avoid migration), and radiopaque marks (to ascertain correct location). Tubes may double back on themselves so placement should be checked with small doses of water or radiography before feeding.

Indwelling pharyngostomy and gastrostomy tubes are indicated when the patient's mouth is difficult to open, restraint is causing untoward levels of stress, and the patient is aggressive (Figure 18-35). Tubes are relatively wide bore, and diets can be slurries or enterals. Jejunostomy tubes are indicated for patients with loss of function or disease in the upper gastrointestinal tract and should work well in reptiles (although no reports have been published). Jejunostomy tubes are small bore, and only enterals should be fed.

Hypermetabolic patients are fed frequent small meals of a diet that uses highly digestible ingredients and emphasizes protein and fat. Provision of adequate calories and protein minimizes the use of endogenous protein for calories. However, until hypermetabolic responses are better understood in reptiles, care should be taken not to overfeed patients because they may be susceptible to refeeding syndrome.

Feeding Schedules

Meal size varies with the patient's disease, the method of feeding, and the chosen diet. Feeding schedules and routes of diet administration depend on the patient's metabolic state and the availability of materials, nursing care, and special diets. Patients in good condition receive 75% to 100% of their daily energy need over the first 24 to 48 hours; debilitated

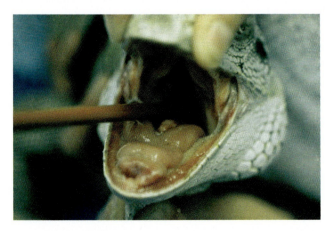

FIGURE 18-33 Soft feeding tubes are passed relatively easily in most reptiles. Relatively rostral placement of the glottis lowers the risk of accidental tracheal intubation. Care must be taken to not harm teeth, nor be bitten. *(Photograph courtesy S. Stahl.)*

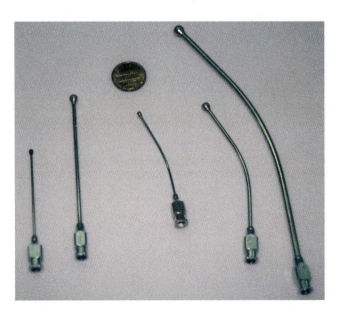

FIGURE 18-34 Ball-tipped stainless steel feeding needles facilitate assist-feeding. The author uses a variety of straight and curved needles of varying lengths in feeding trials and in clinical care of herps ranging from hatchling lizards and dart frogs weighing less than a gram to adult tortoises weighing more than 50 kg.

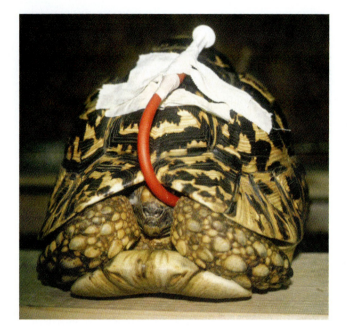

FIGURE 18-35 Indwelling pharyngostomy tubes are especially useful when access to the head is limited in strong tortoises. This Leopard Tortoise's *(Geochelone pardalis)* red rubber feeding tube is plugged with a small syringe and secured with tape to the carapace. Feeding tubes allow multiple small daily meals of an enteral, facilitating nutritional support and recovery.

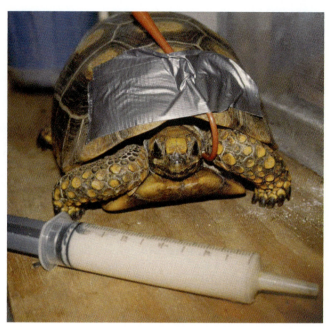

FIGURE 18-37 This Yellow-foot Tortoise *(Geochelone denticulata)* refused to eat because of stomatitis. Placement of a pharyngostomy tube permitted daily feeding with enterals and treatment with antibiotics.

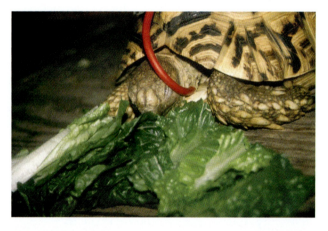

FIGURE 18-36 Tortoises are able and willing to eat voluntarily even while a pharyngostomy tube is in place. This allows a gradual transition from assist-feeding to voluntary intake of natural foods.

patients should receive only 40% to 75% of their daily energy requirement to avoid digestive and metabolic upsets.

In providing nutrition support, all changes should be gradual. A patient is brought gradually (over 2 to 5 days, usually) up to full nutritional goals and then is gradually tapered off nutrition support as voluntary food intake commences (Figures 18-36 through 18-38). Times may be found when support is stopped abruptly. Fractious patients, for example, may resist handling once recovery has begun. Also, patients that eat infrequently when healthy, such as large boids, never achieve the feeding rates of, say, a young iguana that normally eats several times daily.

As data collection proceeds and reports are published, we will gain better understanding of appropriate schedules for feeding various species. For example, regurgitation can be a problem in snakes. Perhaps multiple small meals of a high-protein/low-fat diet would aid gastric emptying in snakes, as in carnivorous mammals, and improve patient responses to nutrition support. Whereas mammals that receive nutrition support often receive meals four times daily, perhaps only once or twice daily will suffice for some reptiles, and once weekly for others.

Continuous feeding of liquid diets, administered via pump, is not recommended. Continuous feeding has been shown in mammals to disrupt the natural hormonal rhythms of the feeding cycle. Such disruptions delay the metabolic recovery of sick patients.

To date, nutritional support has had positive results in reptiles.

Snakes

Questions about meal sizes and feeding schedules remain unanswered for snakes that need assist-feeding. Snakes eat relatively large meals infrequently, whereas one of the primary tenets of nutritional support is to feed relatively small meals frequently. Studies of Burmese Python *(Python molurus bivittatus)* small intestines show that the enormous changes in size (up to three times fasting values by 2 days after feeding) were completely reversible and repeatable because of transitional epithelium, which allows size changes without cell proliferation.[133] Intestinal villi are inflated with a fluid pressure-pump system that uses blood and lymph. The system requires little metabolic investment and functions even when a snake is starved and without calorie reserves. These data suggest that snakes may be assist-fed, even when

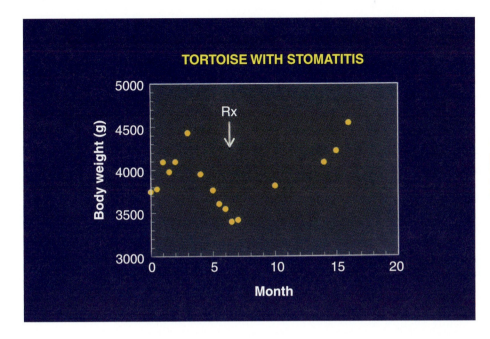

FIGURE 18-38 This is a body weight graph of the patient in Figure 18-37. Recovery graph shows timing of placement of pharyngostomy tube and rapid weight gain immediately thereafter.

Commercial Liquid Products for Nutritional Support

Product Name	Manufacturer	Target Species	Use in Reptiles
Enteral Carnivore	Nutrition Support Services (author's business), Pembroke, Va	Carnivorous reptiles and amphibians	Carnivores, including snakes, large monitors, Snapping and Softshell Turtles
Clinical Care Feline	Pet-Ag, Elgin, Ill	Domestic cats	Carnivores
Enteral Insectivore	Nutrition Support Services	Insectivorous reptiles and amphibians	Insectivores, including many lizards, small snakes
Enteral Omnivore	Nutrition Support Services	Omnivorous reptiles and amphibians	Omnivores, including Bearded Dragons, Box Turtles
Clinical Care Canine	Pet-Ag	Domestic dogs	Omnivores
Ensure	Ross Laboratories, Columbus, Ohio	Humans	Omnivores
Ensure Plus	Ross Laboratories	Humans	Omnivores, herbviores
Enteral Herbivore	Nutrition Support Services	Herbivorous reptiles	Herbivores, including tortoises, Green Iguanas, *Uromastyx*
Critical Care	Oxbow Hay Co, Murdock, Neb	Herbivorous small mammals and reptiles	Herbivorous reptiles

severely debilitated, with minimal gastrointestinal upset and reasonable tolerance of relatively large infrequent meals.

Ongoing research in the author's laboratory is looking at effects of frequent assist-feeding (daily small meals) in Ball Pythons (*Python regius*) and Cornsnakes (*Elaphe* spp.). Healthy snakes tolerate daily tube feeding with maintenance of BW and few side effects. Further work is ongoing. Healthy feeding snakes (Sidewinder Rattlesnakes [*Crotalus cerastes*]) show remarkable metabolic changes, including peak metabolic rates of 8 times fasting levels by 2 days after feeding, peak concentrations of amino acid transporters up to 22 times fasting levels 1 to 3 days after feeding, and a two-fold increase in intestinal mass within 1 day of feeding.[134] Daily feeding of smaller meals is likely to blunt these responses, but to date no untoward effects have been seen with a variety of schedules (tested on healthy snakes).

Comparisons between smaller snakes that eat relatively frequently and large snakes that eat less often show that the larger snakes have lower metabolic rates and organ masses when fasting, followed by higher metabolic rates and organ masses after consuming a large meal.[135] A downward adjustment in calories fed to sick large snakes may facilitate the initiation of nutrition support.

Snakes are true carnivores, and feeding trials show ratios of intestinal uptake of amino acids to glucose of 104 mg/dL.[134] Thus, snakes should be assist-fed diets of high protein with protein sources of high biologic value, with minimal carbohydrate. In the author's studies, protein sources for snakes that need assist-feeding are egg, isolated soy protein, and amino acids. Snakes fed a paste diet for 19 weeks maintained weight and shed cycles; protein sources were high quality: beef, liver, and eggs.[105]

More than 85% of snake species have a hinged jaw that increases gape size.[110] The hinged jaw is thought to be an evolutionary advance that allowed primitive snakes to add bulkier prey (mammals and birds) to their typical elongated prey.

Risks

Aspiration during assist-feeding is rare in conscious patients. Regurgitation may result from administration of large or hyperosmolar meals. Generally, feeding is continued if a patient regurgitates, with smaller more dilute meals offered. Elevation of the patient's front end helps reduce regurgitation. Prokinetic agents (cisapride, erythromycin, metoclopramide) may aid gastric emptying in reptiles. Metoclopramide was given by the author to one tortoise with recurrent regurgitation during feeding via a pharyngostomy tube, with no untoward effects. One study showed no effect of prokinetic agents on gastrointestinal transit times in the Desert Tortoise.[136]

Parenteral Nutritional Support

For domestic mammals, less than 2% of patients in need of nutrition support need parenteral administration of calories and nutrients. The development of enterals has diminished the need for parenteral support of reptiles, but the parenteral route is still preferred in patients with gut failure or when anesthesia (for tube placement) causes serious risk to a patient with uncontrolled vomiting.

Calories are delivered as amino acids (solutions of 2% to 10%), dextrose (solutions of 25% or 50%), and fatty acids (emulsions of 10% or 20%) into large central veins. Water volume is about 1 mL/kcal. Generally, total calorie delivery does not exceed maintenance. Solutions of vitamins and trace minerals may be added.

Intravenous amino acids are used with low efficiency in omnivorous mammals; nitrogen losses may be as bad in reptiles and perhaps worse for carnivorous species. Dextrose should be administered cautiously because peripheral insulin resistance may occur in critical patients, especially those with hypermetabolism from sepsis, burns, or severe trauma. Lipid emulsions are well tolerated by mammals. Lipids may be administered into a peripheral vein; a schedule of alternating replacement fluids (18 hour) with lipid emulsions (6 hour) has been successful in nonreptilian species.

Proportions of fuel sources vary, depending in part on the species (more protein and fat for carnivores), disease (more protein and fat for hypermetabolism), and venous access (central veins for amino acids and dextrose). Generally, for omnivores and carnivores, protein comprises about 20% to 30% of ME, lipids about 25% to 45%, and carbohydrate makes up the difference.

Complications of intravenous nutrition include sepsis, phlebitis and thrombosis, fatty liver, hyperglycemia, and hypokalemia. Intravenous nutrition is expensive, starves enterocytes, and requires intensive nursing care and attention to detail, coupled with thorough patient evaluation and monitoring.

Care must be taken to assess patient responses to nutrition support and to plan transitions back to the patient's usual feeding management. Overall, however, nutrition support provides a successful adjunct to medical and surgical care that improves recovery and reduces mortality.

NUTRITIONAL DISEASES

The prevalence of nutritional disorders varies with species and feeding management. For example, large snakes that consume whole prey are more likely to have generalized starvation than a deficiency of only one nutrient. In contrast, iguanas and other herbivorous reptiles are more likely to have calcium deficiency from imbalanced homemade diets. Large lizards and snakes may be obese from overfeeding and inactivity. Small aquatic turtles fed lettuce and meat are seen with calcium and vitamin A deficiencies.

Water Disorders

Hypohydration

Cases of hypohydration in reptiles are seen in clinics, pet shops, reptile shows, recent imports, and long-standing collections. The condition should be considered whenever water balance has been threatened. Signs are subtle if present; however, any information in the history suggestive of impaired water balance should be treated with aggressive rehydration.

Because reptiles lack a loop of Henle, urine cannot be concentrated when water intake is low or water loss high. Instead, complete nephrons shut down in succession until water balance is restored.[137] Urine is resorbed from the distal tubules (under control of vasotocin), cloaca, and bladder when present. The dynamics relate to many factors, including status of potassium and sodium, acid-base balance, metabolic rate, and corticosteroid levels.

Water intake is markedly lowered in reptiles switched from salads to pelleted diets and when humidity fails to be maintained, water bowls are allowed to dry, and reptiles are kept too cold. For example, large adult iguanas kept at room temperature with one basking light often fail to reach optimal temperature and as a result drink little, lower food (and hence food water) intake, and suffer chronic stress, adrenal exhaustion, and lowered circulating corticosteroid. Hypohydration is often unobserved until clinical signs of dehydration occur.

Dehydration

Reptiles may become dehydrated for the same reasons as they become hypohydrated; the difference is one of degrees, clinical signs, and prognosis. Reestablishment of individual glomerular function depends on circulating corticosteroids (and other factors) and may fail in reptiles with chronic stress. Less than optimal body temperature lowers metabolic rate, which in turn lowers glomerular filtration rate and inhibits reestablishment of functional glomeruli. Treatment of dehydration is thus critical in reptiles. If oral fluids fail to correct the problem, intravenour, intracoelomic, or intraosseous fluids should be considered.

Dehydrated reptiles have sunken eyes, dry loose skinfolds, depression, and anorexia (Figure 18-39).

Renal Failure

Although cause and effect have yet to be determined in controlled trials, the association between water balance and kidney disease is strong in reptiles. Other factors may play a role, too, such as acidogenic diets, which increase precipitation of urate crystals and cause renal failure in other animals. Low-quality protein leads to excessive nitrogen excretion, and excretion of absorbed NPN from chitin (invertebrate exoskeletons) is via the kidneys, too. Excessive potassium excretion can also cause precipitation of urates. These factors coupled with limited water intake and secondary components such as cold temperatures and chronic stress may cause kidneys to fail.

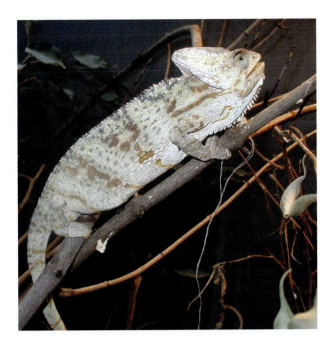

FIGURE 18-39 A dehydrated Veiled Chameleon (*Chamaeleo capyptratus*) showing sunken eyes. This degree of dehydration is best treated with parenteral replacement fluids.

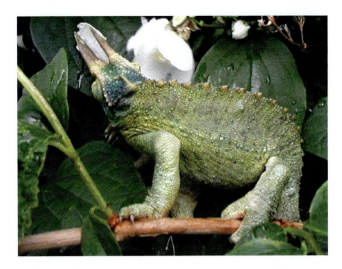

FIGURE 18-40 This male Jackson's Chameleon (*Chamaeleo jacksonii*) had dehydration in a pet store and subsequently developed articular gout, immune suppression, cellulitis, and sepsis. In the author's opinion, most chameleons fail to survive long term, even with aggressive treatment, if they have a bout of severe dehydration.

In the author's opinion, the key to limiting renal failure is through diet (high water content; high-quality protein; carefully formulated intakes of sodium, potassium, and fiber; control of acidogenic ingredients), water (adequate intakes), feeding management and scheduling (to regulate urine pH), and husbandry (temperature, humidity, and controlling stress).

Until data from controlled trials are available, dietary management of reptiles with renal disease should follow mammalian guidelines: moderate protein of high quality, restricted phosphorus, appropriate levels of insoluble fibers, and altered ratios of omega-6:omega-3 fatty acids (from 6:1 to approximately 3:1).

Specific dietary changes for reptile patients with renal disease depend on the animal's feeding management. Herbivores and omnivores may be supplemented with additions of soy protein isolate, calcium carbonate, flax seed (whole or oil), and psyllium to salads. Insectivores and vertebrate-eating carnivores can be assist-fed appropriate enterals.

Gout

Deposition of urates (termed *tophi*) on visceral and articular surfaces, termed *gout*, is found in reptiles (see Chapter 54). Gout has been reported in tortoises, snakes, lizards, and alligators. Etiopathologic theories include inappropriate dietary protein levels and dehydration. Gout is associated clinically with many other disorders, especially those that affect water balance (Figure 18-40). Recent case reports link gout with renal disease and, in one iguana, the subsequent development of hypertrophic osteopathy.[138,139] Most likely, any disturbance in renal excretion of uric acid in uricotelic species predisposes an individual to precipitation of urate crystals.

Treatment of gout includes supportive therapy and diuresis. Uric acid inhibitors, such as allopurinol, may be helpful. Diet management may be tried, but in other species with disordered purine metabolism, support and drugs are considered to be more effective than changes in diet. For dietary management, use foods that are low in purine and promote acidification.

Cystic Calculi (see Chapter 49)

Nutritionally related calcium-containing bladder stones may be related to: (1), dietary excesses of vitamin D, vitamin C, calcium, sodium, phosphorus, or magnesium; (2), low moisture content of food, such as pellets; (3), urine retention; (4), abnormalities in the excretion of calcium, sodium, or phosphorous; and (5), altered pH (acidic for calcium oxalate, alkaline for calcium phosphate). Dietary management may include sodium restriction to less than 0.4% DM, phosphorus restriction to less than 1% DM, and carefully metered levels of dietary calcium (1% to 1.4% DM), magnesium (0.2% DM), vitamins C (1 mg/kcal ME), and vitamin D_3 (1000 to 3000 IU/kg DM). Efforts to avoid bladder stones should include frequent soaking and full-time access to water (see Chapter 49).

Energy Disorders

Cachexia

Starvation may arise from stress-induced failure to eat, provision of too little food, inappropriate foods or feeding management, and diseases that affect appetite and metabolism. Like starved mammals, starved reptiles lose lean tissue (protein) and adipose (Figure 18-41). Loss of protein from skeletal muscle is readily evident as atrophied musculature. Loss of protein from heart, liver, intestines, and other organs is less evident but impairs function and threatens life.

Ectotherms have remarkable abilities to withstand fasts but are debilitated by long-term starvation. Metabolic rates may decrease by 50%. Degree of weight lost with fasting is variable. Snakes starved for up to 100 days at 82°F (28°C) lost up to 37% of their BW and catabolized their fat bodies.[140] Juvenile aquatic turtles fasted for 19 days lost from 1% to 16% of BW and oxygen consumption (VO2) decreased to about one third prefast levels.[141] Underfed female chameleons allocate their energy reserves to egg production, resulting in increased mortality at egg deposition, higher incidence of

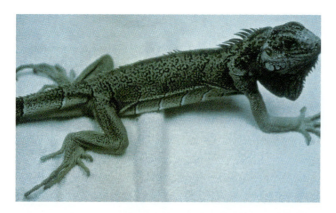

FIGURE 18-41 This thin Green Iguana (*Iguana iguana*) has lost all visible body fat and muscling from the limbs and tail. Its body condition may be from poor husbandry or feeding management, dietary imbalance, or illness resulting in anorexia. (*Photograph courtesy S. Stahl.*)

retained eggs, and poorer physical condition after nesting, compared with fed chameleons.[142] Laboratory diagnosis of starvation may be difficult, for in at least one species, the Green Lizard (*Ameiva ameiva*), ketone bodies were unaltered (acetoacetate) or decreased (3-hydroxybutyrate) with starvation.[143]

To treat starvation, first restore fluids and electrolytes. Then, provide judicious amounts of calories and nutrients, with assist-feeding if necessary, until appetite returns. Deficiencies in management must be identified and corrected. Common husbandry errors include low temperatures, inappropriate food items, and stress from excessive crowding, noise, and light.

To initiate voluntary feeding in starved reptiles, place the patient in a warm environment, over 85°F (30°C) for most reptiles but cooler for montane species, especially *Chamaeleo* spp. Include a basking light and a gradient toward cooler temperatures. Many patients respond to warm (80°F [26°C]) water soaks.

Offer small amounts of food frequently. Foods should be fresh, and dead vertebrate prey should be warmed. If possible, natural food items should be offered. A low dose of metronidazole (12.5 to 25 mg/kg PO) may initiate feeding, although the likely mechanism is unknown and the drug's efficacy has not been established in controlled trials.

Some products sold for nutritional rehabilitation of veterinary patients contain too much fat and almost no protein. These products, usually in gel or paste forms, fail to meet the immediate nutritional needs of starved or hypermetabolic animals.

Refeeding Syndrome

For starved patients that are critically ill, overfeeding may lead to life-threatening hypokalemia and hypophosphatemia. Starved patients contain low total body contents of nutrients such as phosphorus and potassium. Blood concentrations are maintained within normal ranges at the expense of cellular levels. With refeeding, these electrolytes move with glucose from blood into cells. Too rapid administration of calorie sources, especially carbohydrate, predisposes to hypophosphatemia and hypokalemia.

Data in turtles (*Phrynops* sp.) suggest a similar response in starved reptiles. With refeeding, after a 30-day fast, insulin levels increased five fold for 72 hours. With radiolabeled glucose, researchers found several-fold increases in the rates of incorporation of substrates into cells.[144] These data suggest that reptiles may be susceptible to refeeding syndrome.

For patients at risk for refeeding syndrome, initially feed about 50% of calculated energy needs for the patient's real (not optimal) BW over a 24-hour period. This energy level may be repeated for several days until clinical improvement is noted. Serum levels of phosphorus, potassium, and glucose should be monitored. Calories are increased in increments of 10% to 50% only when patients show improvements, such as stabilized electrolytes, improved hydration, decreased depression and immobility, and increased alertness. Increases in BW at this time are likely to be the result of increased body water and adipose, not lean tissue.

Obesity

Excess calorie intake may lead to rapid growth in juveniles and obesity in adults. In juvenile mammals, overfeeding refers usually to excess intakes of calories, protein, calcium, and phosphorus, but few dietary associations have been shown to be causative for growth-associated problems. Information for reptiles is for the most part anecdotal. For example, shell deformities have been noted in hatchling tortoises fed diets deficient in calcium or diets of pet foods containing relatively high protein and fat of animal origin. Excess calories, and fermented ingredients, may play a role, along with deficiencies of calcium or vitamin D_3. However, calorie-restricted diets for juveniles, fed at levels that severely restrict growth, are inhumane and often lead to deficiencies of protein and micronutrients. Rather, diets of natural food items are fed in measured amounts for moderate growth, and time outdoors with exercise is encouraged.

Some reptiles, such as the Gecko (*Gekko japonicus*) and the Brown Watersnake (*Nerodia taxispilota*), store fat for subsequent use during brumation (hibernation) and reproduction.[145] Maintenance of such reptiles without brumation (hibernation) or reproduction, when warm ambient temperatures and appetites are sustained and without the opportunity to mobilize the fat stores, may lead to obesity.

Obese reptiles store fat in deposits located in coelomic, subcutaneous, and parenchymatous sites. Fatty infiltration of organs may occur. Lack of exercise, especially that necessary for food procurement, is a likely factor in obese patients. Some species are more sedentary than others. Pythons, boas, vipers, Tegu lizards, monitors, and other heavy-bodied lizards, crocodiles, Snapping Turtles, and Alligator Snappers tend to be sedentary (Figure 18-42). Food intake should be monitored in these species. Obesity is less likely in active reptiles, such as gartersnakes, racers, many cobras, anoles, and many aquatic turtles.

Weight-reduction programs for vertebrate-eating reptiles consist of feeding very lean prey in restricted amounts. Calorie restriction is achieved for invertebrate-eating animals with limiting the number of prey offered. For both, habitat enlargement, cage enrichment, and improved feeding strategies are used to increase activity.

Weight-reduction diets for obese herbivorous reptiles are formulated to reduce fat or increase fiber or both. Foods to be

Case Report: Weight Loss and Low Activity

Signalment: Wild-caught (Hawaiian) young adult male Jackson's Chameleon (*Chamaeleo jacksonii*).

Presenting Symptom: The chameleon had exhibited weight loss and a decrease in activity over the past 4 weeks. Onset appeared to be gradual.

History: The chameleon had been purchased from a pet shop 8 months earlier. At that time, the chameleon had been examined and dewormed by a veterinarian and found to be in good health. The chameleon was housed in a birdcage that measured 18 × 18 × 24 in (length × width × height). The cage was furnished with horizontal wood dowel perches and one pothos plant. Water was provided from a commercial dripper jar, and the chameleon was misted once daily. Crickets were offered daily, free-choice, in a glass bowl placed at the bottom of the cage. A commercial vitamin-mineral dust was added once weekly.

Clinical Examination: The chameleon showed signs of mild muscle wasting in his tail and limbs. His eyes were slightly sunken, and remains of shed skin were seen on his feet and tail. No signs of respiratory disease were found. Feces appeared normal, and subsequent fecal examination results were unremarkable. The chameleon showed strong grip with his feet and tail, and mobility appeared normal. His weight was 37 g.

Diagnosis: Because the chameleon was not critically ill and because several husbandry errors were identified that could have caused or contributed to this chameleon's problem, it was decided to address the husbandry first before attempting further testing. The chameleon was hypothesized to be bored and stressed from the absence of behavioral enrichment and monotony of prey.

Treatment Plan: The chameleon was adminstered an over-the-counter oral rehydration solution by mouth (15 mL Pedialyte [Ross Laboratories]/kg body weight [BW]). The following husbandry issues were reviewed with the owner.

Housing: The use of a bird cage as chameleon habitat was believed to be the source of several problems. The small cage size limited this patient's opportunities to select from a gradient of temperature and humidity. Because prey could escape between the cage bars and the owner did not want prey loose in the house, the chameleon was fed only crickets in a bowl. The bird cage was replaced with a screened habitat measuring 24 × 24 × 48 in. This type of habitat allowed for vertical climbing, tall leafy plants with woody stems, and gradients of temperature and humidity.

Furnishings: Commercial bird perches of smooth wood doweling and uniform diameter provided no variation in foot-holds, rough bark for aid in shedding, and few opportunities for behavioral enrichment. The dowels were replaced with natural wood branches and grape vine. The pothos was replaced with several upright plants with woody or strong stems, such as schefflera, ficus, and small palms. These provided shelter and visual barriers and leaf surfaces for drinking and helped create gradients of light, temperature, and humidity.

Prey presentation: Although some chameleons seem to tolerate the monotony of eating just one prey species, most benefit from the opportunity to consume a variety of invertebrates (and for some of the large species, small vertebrates). Jackson's chameleons particularly enjoy houseflies and other flying insects. All chameleons benefit from the natural activity of hunting food, rather than feeding from a bowl. The owner purchased fly larvae for pupating into flies and used a bug-trap to gather moths and other flying insects at night. Crickets were offered twice weekly, free-ranging in the cage. Other invertebrates were offered on the remaining days. The crickets were dusted with a commercial supplement once every 7 to 10 days.

Water: Misting once daily was inadequate for this chameleon, as evidenced by his mild dehydration and retained shed. The owner was instructed to mist two to three times daily. The drip jar was used at least once daily, usually twice daily. The owner was shown how to give water by mouth with a small syringe. She was shown the characteristic signs of dehydration (sunken eyes, dry skin, mucus strands in mouth) and instructed to administer water by mouth (up to 15 mL/kg BW) when needed.

Outcome: This chameleon responded well to the changes in habitat. The owner reported increased interest in food, especially flies, and the chameleon's weight increased by 10% (up to 41 g). No recurrence was seen of retained shed skin.

---

avoided, which are rich in fat, include all pet foods; commercial diets for fish, aquatic turtles, and other carnivorous animals; vertebrates; and many invertebrates. Low-fat high-fiber foods include grasses and hays, berries, fruits, and vegetables. To these ingredients are added sources of plant protein, calcium, vitamins, and trace minerals to balance the diets.

For all obese reptiles, complete physical examination is needed first to rule out signs of diseases or conditions that mimic obesity, such as ascites, pregnancy, and large tumors. After examination, calories are restricted progressively to no less than 60% of usual intake. Increased activities, especially food foraging, should accompany calorie restriction. Weight loss should not exceed 1% BW weekly, and because of low metabolic rates, perhaps less than 0.5% BW weekly is preferable.

Weight reduction results in loss of lean tissue as well as fat, so for each patient the risk of protein loss should be weighed against the risks of obesity. In species that do not have atherosclerosis and mature-onset diabetes mellitus, a medical risk may be difficult to assign to patients that are only moderately overweight (Figure 18-43). This is especially true for pets that are not part of breeding programs. Decisions on weight loss should be in the best interest of the patient.

Leptin

Interest in human obesity has focused recently on the hormone leptin, which regulates energy expenditure, thermoregulation, BW, and onset of puberty. Leptin has been identified with immunoassay in the Fence Lizard, *Sceloporus undulatus*.[146] Moreover, Fence Lizards given recombinant murine leptin exhibited temperatures 0.6°C higher than controls, ate 30% less food, were 14% less active, and maintained a 250% increase in resting metabolic rate.[146]

Hepatic Lipidosis

Fatty livers are caused by excessive accumulation of triacylglycerides in hepatocytes. In mammals, the problem is

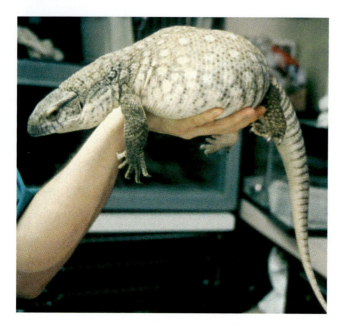

FIGURE 18-42 Obesity is more prevalent in species that are relatively sedentary, such as this Savannah Monitor (*Varanus exanthematicus*). (Photograph courtesy S. Stahl.)

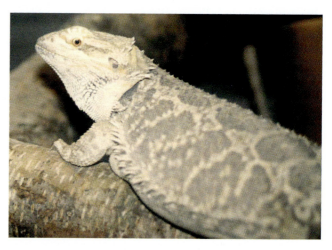

FIGURE 18-43 Obesity also is seen in overfed pet Bearded Dragons (*Pogona vitticeps*). Decisions about weight loss include considerations of health risks and goals for the animal. Risks from obesity tend to be low in dragons kept as pets.

associated with alterations in mitochondrial oxidation.[147] Starvation exacerbates mitochondrial oxidative injury, with decreased hepatic ATP synthesis. Hence, the problem is seen most often in patients that have been starved, especially if obese. Species prone to stress-induced anorexia seem to be especially vulnerable to hepatic lipidosis (see Chapter 56).

Patients with hepatic lipidosis should be checked for a history of recent anorexia or neglect and examined for obesity. Best responses in mammals are found with assist-feeding of diets containing typical levels of fat, protein, and carbohydrate for long periods (1 to 2 months). A key to successful treatment is provision of sufficient but not excessive calories each day. If calorie intakes meet energy needs, peripheral fat lipolysis and amino acid mobilization for gluconeogenesis are minimized. If calorie intakes are not excessive, further hepatic triacylglyceride accumulation is avoided.

Pyramiding

Tortoises and occasionally turtles are afflicted by a growth disorder termed pyramiding. It is characterized by excess growth of scutes on the carapace, with a resultant pyramid shape on each scute (Figures 18-44 and 18-45). Much speculation, but few facts, is found concerning the role of nutrition in pyramiding. For now, the author considers the disorder to be multifactorial in origin, with humidity and energy intake/output playing key roles.

Concerns center on overfeeding, which is defined for most species as excessive intakes of protein, fat, calcium, and phosphorus. Such overfeeding per se rarely causes growth disorders. Rather, specific nutrient imbalances, such as copper, vitamin A, zinc, and so on, have caused growth disorders in many species of mammals and birds.

A study with Red-eared Sliders (*Trachemys scripta elegans*) showed no effects of excess dietary calcium or phosphorus on pyramiding.[44] Anecdotes abound, but only one controlled trial has been published that shows a specific cause and effect between nutrient(s), humidity, and pyramiding (Figure 18-44).

This author's opinion is that the cause of pyramiding is multifactorial and that a number of factors are both necessary and sufficient to cause the disorder. These factors are calorie intake, calorie output, body temperature, acid-base balance, hydration, and environment. In general, a young tortoise provided a high-fiber (hence, low-calorie) diet, all-day access to food (instead of meal feeding), much opportunity to exercise through behavioral enrichment, exposure to unfiltered sunlight, a temperature gradient that includes highest preferred temperatures for that species with proper humidity, and continual access to water with weekly soaking has a low risk for pyramiding. The diet and feeding schedule may be critical to lowering risk through regulation of blood and urine pH and thus control of shell buffering capacity.

Nutrient Disorders

Protein Deficiency

The prevalence of protein deficiency in reptiles is unknown, but it may be a likely component of many cases of malnutrition (Figure 18-46). The patient may have had poor food intake or consumption of low-protein foods (such as fruits and many vegetables) or fatty foods (such as goldfish or obese mice). Laboratory analyses may aid diagnosis but not always.

Signs of protein deficiency tend to be generalized and nonspecific for most species. Often the patient is seen with a history of "poor doing," exhibiting poor growth if a juvenile and perhaps failed reproduction if an adult. Anorexia, listlessness, mild bouts of diarrhea, and recurrent infections may be seen. Protein deficiency should be considered in animals with histories of poor diets. Likewise, other diseases should be ruled out before a diagnosis of protein deficiency.

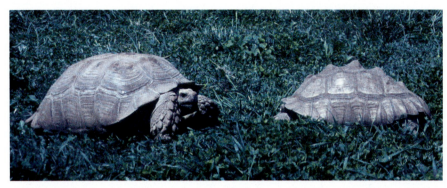

FIGURE 18-44 Pyramiding is notable in the captive-reared Sulcata Tortoise (*Geochelone sulcata*) on the right. The animal on the left is a wild-caught, mature adult. Hatchling grassland Sulcatas, raised for five months in environments of low or high humidities and fed diets of low, medium, or high protein developed significant pyramidal carapacial growth in the low-humidity environment. Dietary protein (14%, 19%, or 30% crude protein, dry matter basis) had little effect on carapacial growth. It is theorized that wild hatchling tortoises consume little food during dry periods with resultant slow growth. During rainy periods, in contrast, the tortoises consume much food and grow rapidly. Only in captivity are young tortoises raised with excess food in an environment of low humidity. This scenario is thought to predispose to pyramidal growth. Future studies should replicate and then clarify the effects of environmental humidity on carapacial growth. Until then, hatchling tortoises, even those from arid environments, should be raised with hide-boxes containing moist substrate and relative humidities of at least 50%. (Wiesner CS, Iben C: Influence of environmental humidity and dietary protein on pyramidal growth of carapaces in African spurred tortoises [*Geochelone sulcata*]), *J Anim Physiol Anim Nutr* 87:66-74, 2003.)

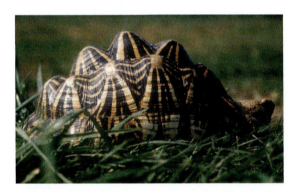

FIGURE 18-45 A few tortoise species grow naturally conical scutes, mimicking pyramiding. The appearance of the carapace in this adult Star Tortoise (*Geochelone elegans*) is normal.

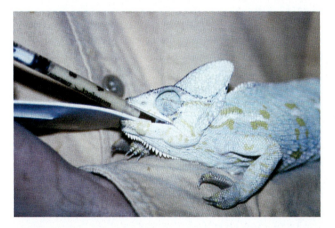

FIGURE 18-46 In insectivores such as this young Veiled Chameleon (*Chamaeleo calyptratus*), protein deficiency results from low food intake compounded by diet of only waxworms. Although waxworms are excellent food for reptilian carnivores, insectivores, and omnivores, their high fat (and thus relatively lower protein content on an energy basis) precludes their use as the sole source of calories (see Table 18-7). This chameleon also had parasites and responded well to worming, rehydration, and an assist-feeding of a diet containing more than 25% of calories from protein.

Treatment includes supportive therapy and change to a diet with appropriate protein content in the authors' experience: greater than 25% of calories (ME) for carnivores, about 15% to 25% of calories for omnivores, 25% to 30% for juvenile herbivores, and 15% to 20% for adult herbivores.

Protein quality should be addressed. Amino acid contents of vertebrate and invertebrate prey are usually adequate for species that are by nature carnivorous and insectivorous. The amino acid content of plant-source ingredients, such as soybean and gluten meals, is not adequate for carnivores and insectivores but should suffice for herbivores. Ingredients that provide animal-source protein, however, may contain high levels of other substances such as fat and purine that may be excessive for herbivorous reptiles.

Protein supplements used successfully in reptile nutrition include dried whole egg and soy protein isolate and ingredients for herbivores such as legumes, wheat germ, and debittered brewer's yeast.

Calcium and Vitamin D_3 Deficiencies

Deficiencies of calcium or vitamin D_3 lead to one form of MBD, termed *nutritional secondary hyperparathyroidism* (NSHP; see Chapter 61). Typically associated clinically with juveniles, NSHP can be seen also in adults and newly acquired or long-term specimens and with a variety of diets. Patient histories are varied, but results of diet evaluations are consistent. The condition arises from consumption of diets low in calcium and sometimes vitamin D_3, occasionally diets high in phosphorus (with a reversed Ca:P ratio), and lack of exposure to ultraviolet-B (UV-B) wavelengths from unfiltered sunlight or UV-B–generating bulbs. NSHP may be the most common problem in reptiles seen at veterinary clinics.

In carnivores, calcium deficiency is usually associated with diets of skeletal muscle and viscera but not bone; diets of neonatal prey, such as pinkie mice and day-old chicks; or diets of unsupplemented insects. In herbivores, deficiency arises from diets devoid of legumes and calcium supplements. Calcium absorption is impaired in diets containing phytates (especially soy ingredients), oxalates (spinach), high fat (certain "performance" pet foods), or acid (certain commercial cat foods), and in diets deficient in vitamin D.

Signs

Low intakes of calcium (directly or from vitamin D_3 deficiency) stimulate parathyroid hormone (PTH) secretion and calcium is mobilized from bone to maintain normal blood calcium levels. Signs are related to demineralized bone (fractures, deformities), demineralized eggs (incomplete calcification, weak eggshells), and eventually hypocalcemia (muscle tremors, seizures). Bone lesions are common in the long bones, mandible, skull, and vertebrae (Figures 18-47 through 18-49). Chelonians often exhibit shell deformities (Figures 18-49 and 18-50). Radiographs show loss of mineralized bone and usually multiple old and new fractures.

In some reptiles, the earliest signs of NSHP involve subtle nerve and muscle dysfunction. Baby Bearded Dragons show tremors and twitches before bone changes. Chameleons show tongue dysfunction when catching prey and a crouching stance (belly hugging) on perches (Figures 18-51 and 18-52). Veiled chameleons have a wrinkled and crooked casque develop. Intestinal (or cloacal) prolapses are a frequent sign of developing hypocalcemia in the young Green Iguana.

Treatment

The owner must correct any underlying husbandry and management problems if the overall treatment plan is to be successful (Figure 18-53). In particular, therapy consists of attending to the patient's medical needs, rehydration, and specific calcium supplementation. Intravenous calcium is given if the patient is hypocalcemic or showing muscle tremors or paresis. Subcutaneous or intramuscular calcium gluconate is effective in less critical patients. Oral calcium may also be given if vitamin D status is adequate.

Specific calcium and vitamin D_3 requirements are poorly determined for most reptiles. General recommendations are

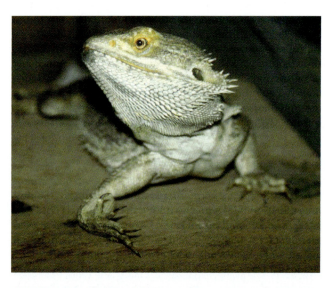

FIGURE 18-47 This Bearded Dragon (*Pogona vitticeps*) has a permanently deformed right carpus as a sequela to nutritional secondary hyperparathyroidism.

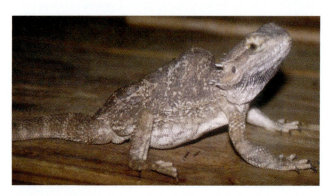

FIGURE 18-48 This female Bearded Dragon (*Pogona vitticeps*) has permanent scoliosis as a sequela to nutritional secondary hyperparathyroidism. She lived many years and successfully produced several clutches each year.

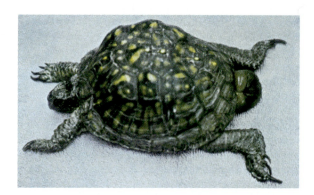

FIGURE 18-49 Nutritional secondary hyperparathyroidism in chelonians can result in shell deformities and dystocia. Nutritional secondary hyperparathyroidism in Box Turtles often results from long-term feeding of unsupplemented lettuce and ground meat. (*Photograph courtesy S. Stahl.*)

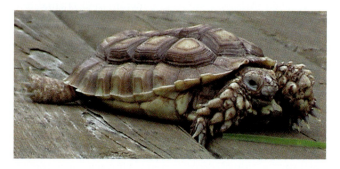

FIGURE 18-50 This 16-month-old *Geochelone sulcata* was fed a diet of unsupplemented fruits and lettuce and housed in a tank without access to sunlight or ultraviolet-B–generating bulbs. His severely deformed carapace is a result of multiple nutrient deficiencies, most notable calcium and vitamin D_3. See Figure 18-44 for appearance of normal carapacial structure in Sulcata Tortoises. (*Photograph courtesy D. Senneke.*)

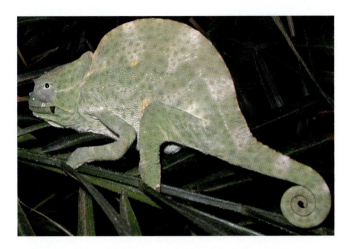

FIGURE 18-51 This young *Chamaeleo deremensis* suffered a fracture of the left radius and ulna because of nutritional secondary hyperparathyroidism. His invertebrates had been coated with dust containing low levels of calcium and vitamin D_3, and the chameleon had limited access to ultraviolet-B during a period of several months of rapid growth.

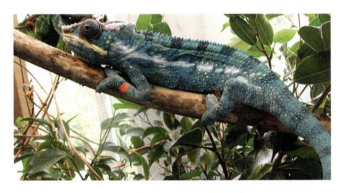

FIGURE 18-52 This Panther Chameleon *(Furcifer pardalis)* exhibits the belly-hugging, crouching stance characteristic of early nutritional secondary hyperparathyroidism in chameleons. Another early sign of calcium deficiency in chameleons is tongue dysfunction during prehension of prey.

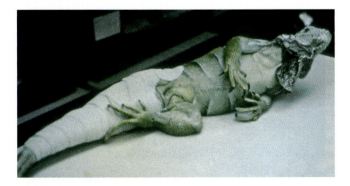

FIGURE 18-53 This Green Iguana *(Iguana iguana)* with nutritional secondary hyperparathyroidism has its fractured limb splinted to its tail for stability. Changes in husbandry and diet are also essential parts of treatment. *(Photograph courtesy S. Stahl.)*

calcium, 1.8 to 3 mg/kcal or 0.6% to 1.5% DM (perhaps higher for breeding tortoises); phosphorus, 0.5% to 0.8%; and vitamin D_3, 200 to 2000 IU/kg DM. Specific recommendations for the Crag Lizard *(Pseudocordylus melanotus melanotus)* suggest 1.4% of DM, with no added benefit from greater amounts.[148] A calcium:phosphorus ratio of 1:1 to 2:1 minimizes the vitamin D requirement. For many species, maximum tolerances are about 2.5% for calcium, 1.6% for phosphorus, and 5000 IU/kg for vitamin D_3.[149,150]

Calcium requirements for turtles may be higher because of shell tissue, but care must be taken to avoid excessive dietary phosphorus through additions of bone meal or dicalcium phosphate. Excess phosphorus may cause secondary hyperparathyroidism, bone resorption, and calcification of kidney and heart. In ongoing long-term feeding trials conducted by the author, juvenile tortoises *(Geochelone* spp.) have done well for 10 years on diets containing 1.4% calcium and 0.7% phosphorus.

Extraosseous calcium storage exists in some reptiles. Female Day Geckos *(Phelsuma* spp.) store calcium in endolymphatic sacs, visible as whitish swellings on the neck. This calcium is mobilized for deposition in eggshells. Calcium requirements for female Day Geckos are likely to be higher than for males. Studies with wild-caught Day Geckos suggest that calcium sources include coral sand and shells from land snails, marine molluscs, and gecko eggs.[151] For *Phelsuma* spp., calcium, and other nutrients, may be provided with the addition of supplements to peach infant food.

As for many nutrients, vitamin D is toxic when fed in excess. Toxicity most commonly occurs from overly zealous supplementation with vitamin-mineral products. Toxicity also occurs from the ingestion of certain types of rat and mouse poisons. Signs of toxicity often involve multiple organ systems because of widespread soft tissue calcification. The active form of vitamin D (1,25-$[OH]_2$-cholecalciferol) is made with a series of chemical transformations in liver and then kidney. Thus, diseases of the liver or kidney affect vitamin D metabolism and can lead to signs of deficiency or, occasionally, toxicity.

Blood values were compared in wild and captive Komodo Dragons *(Varanus komodoensis)*. Blood was sampled from 33 lizards from five localities at Komodo National Park, Indonesia, and from 44 captive Komodos from zoos in the United States and Indonesia. Analyses included complete blood counts and blood chemistries, selected minerals, and fat-soluble vitamins (A, D_3, E). Blood was screened for chlorinated pesticides and several toxins. Komodo Dragons housed indoors had significantly lower levels of circulating vitamin D_3 compared with Komodos exposed to sunlight, whether captive or wild. Circulating vitamin D_3 increased to levels found for wild Komodos for four dragons exposed to UV-permeable skylights, direct sunlight, or self-ballasted mercury vapor UV lamps.[152]

Husbandry should include exposure to unfiltered sunlight or to appropriate artificial UV sources. While basking lizards relish direct sunlight, other species, such as woodland turtles and many snakes, need shelter from strong sunlight but still need exposure to UV light. Species housed indoors should be able to choose to spend time under full-spectrum lamps.[153] The UV-B output varies between bulbs (see Table 18-12). Unfiltered sunlight is always preferred. Reptiles should not be exposed to sunlight while in glass housing because of blocked beneficial UV radiation and life-threatening high temperatures. Humans with Crohn's disease were able to synthesize vitamin D and increase blood levels 400% to normal range with use of tanning bed UV-B radiation for 10 minutes three times weekly.[154] The technique may show promise in reptiles.

Much of the clinical nutritional work with dietary calcium is straightforward. Dietary calcium deficiencies are obvious from histories, as are husbandry errors that reduce vitamin D_3 synthesis. However, calcium-related disorders are complex in other species, and the future may hold surprises as we aim for positive calcium balance in our patients. In the past 2 years, negative calcium balance or nutritional MBD has been precipitated in mammals by dietary phytates (found in soy), small intestinal bacterial overgrowth, and magnesium deficiency.[155-157] Genetics also plays a role in bone health. Foods

Case Report: Crouching and Belly-Hugging

Signalment: Eight-month-old captive-bred Veiled Chameleon clutch-mates, one male and one female.

Presenting Symptom: The chameleons had begun crouching on their branches, seemed reluctant to walk, and kept their ventral body wall in contact with branches (belly-hugging). Onset appeared to be sudden.

History: The chameleons had been purchased from a breeder when 8 weeks old. They were housed separately in large screened cages. Furnishings included many large plants and natural wood branches. They were misted daily and watered with drip systems (enteral bags with tubing) once daily. Meals consisted of crickets, waxworms, zophobas superworms, flies, and fresh greens. A commercial vitamin-mineral dust was dusted onto the prey once weekly.

Clinical Examination: The chameleons appeared to be well fleshed, perhaps slightly overweight, and well hydrated. They were reluctant to walk, but once moving, they appeared tentative in their movements but otherwise normal. When at rest on branches, both chameleons crouched on the branches and exhibited signs of belly-hugging. The chameleons showed weaker than typical grip with their feet and tails. Occasional twitching of large muscle groups was noted in both chameleons. The owner declined the opportunity to radiograph the chameleons.

Differential Diagnoses: The chameleons' problems appeared to be centered in their neuromusculoskeletal systems. Toxic reactions from spider bites and trauma from falls could not be ruled out. Without radiographs, metabolic bone disease of nutritional origin could not definitively be ruled in or out. However, the signs were consistent with early nutritional secondary hyperparathyroidism, and the feeding program was examined more closely.

Diet Evaluation: The chameleons were fed daily, and a commercial vitamin-mineral dust was applied to prey once weekly. The product's label guaranteed analysis showed calcium level to be 4.8% and vitamin D_3 to be 52,000 IU per pound. If the dust stuck to prey in amounts that increased weight by 25% (a generous but unlikely amount), intakes of both calcium and vitamin D_3 would be inadequate. At usual rates that dusts stick to prey, the levels of calcium and vitamin D_3 would have been deficient. Although the crickets were fed a commercial cricket food, the value of this gut-load product was limited by the capacity of the crickets' gastrointestinal tract. The product was unable to make up the deficits provided with infrequent use of a poorly formulated dust. The gut-load likely prevented an earlier onset of advanced metabolic bone disease but could not meet the needs of rapidly growing heavily fed young Veiled Chameleons. Further questioning of the owner revealed that the chameleons were kept inside, with no exposure to natural unfiltered sunlight. Each had access to reputable full-spectrum fluorescent bulbs, with no further lighting. Each cage was placed in a window, so much natural lighting in daytime was filtered through glass.

Diagnosis: Intakes of calcium and vitamin D_3 were hypothesized to be deficient. Other nutritional components to this problem were possible and could not be ruled out without further testing, which the owner declined. Deficiencies of vitamin E, choline, many of the B-complex vitamins, magnesium, selenium, manganese, sulfur, and copper may have contributed to the signs observed.

Pathogenesis: Metabolic bone disease of nutritional origin is multifactorial in origin. Dietary intakes of calcium, phosphorus, and vitamin D_3 need to be adequate but not excessive. Many other nutrients are involved with normal bone growth, and acid-base balance likely plays a role. Ambient temperatures affect activity and food acquisition, food intake, digestion and absorption, and rate of growth. Species differences and degrees of inbreeding influence growth rates and subsequently utilization of calories and nutrients. Importance of the contributions of yolk sac nutrients is unknown for chameleons, as are the relative contributions of ultraviolet-B and diet for supply of vitamin D_3. Observations and experience suggest that yolk sac contents help to maintain adequate vitamin D_3 levels in hatchlings and that ultraviolet-B may be essential for adequate vitamin D_3 in juveniles during phases of rapid growth. Marginal intakes of calcium and vitamin D_3 may sustain an animal until it reaches a life stage of increased need. Rapidly growing 4-month-old to 8-month-old juveniles and heavily producing females are especially vulnerable. Not only are the quality of dusts and prey diets critical, but management factors such as lighting and temperature are also important parameters. In this case, an inappropriate dust combined with cool temperatures because of the absence of basking lights interacted with rapid growth rates from heavy feeding to produce the early stages of metabolic bone disease.

Treatment Plan: The owner was counseled to use true full-spectrum (ultraviolet B–providing) fluorescent bulbs and to allow the chameleons time outside in partial shade but with opportunities to bask in unfiltered sun. The dust was switched to an interim product with a full complement of vitamins and minerals and high-optimal levels of calcium and vitamin D_3.

The goals were to provide a calcium (Ca) intake of 1.4% to 2.0% of diet dry matter (DM), limit phosphorus (P) to less than 1.2% DM, and provide a vitamin D_3 intake of 2 to 5.5 IU/g DM. This was accomplished with an interim dust containing about 11% Ca, 0.59% P, and 32 IU D_3/g with approximately 7% dust sticking to half-inch crickets.

Outcome: After several months, all signs had resolved and the chameleons were switched to a maintenance dust that provided a balanced intake of vitamins and minerals. The maintenance dust provided a dietary Ca intake of 1.2% to 1.8% DM, P of 0.9% DM, and vitamin D_3 2 to 3 IU/g DM. The interim dust contained 9% Ca, 0.59% P, and 19 IU D_3/g with approximately 7% dust sticking to half-inch crickets.

can affect bone health by provision of nutrients such as amino acids, zinc, copper, iron, fluoride, and vitamins A, C, and K and by provision of nonnutrients such as phytoestrogens.[158]

Research in the turtle *Trachemys scripta* has detected a novel dual-binding protein for both vitamin D and thyroxin.[159] Injections of thyroxine into hatchlings increased the circulation of the protein and subsequently vitamin D. Increases in the circulating protein are associated with increased thyroidal activity. Interactions with vitamin D metabolism remain to be determined. Research in humans has identified and cloned the gene responsible for 1-alpha-hydroxylase, which controls vitamin D activation and impacts vitamin D–dependent rickets.[160] The link between genetics and NSHP has not yet been examined in reptiles.

Vitamin A Deficiency

Hypovitaminosis A has been historically most prevalent in young aquatic turtles fed diets of unsupplemented greens (lettuce), meat, and poorly formulated commercial diets (see Chapter 59). Affected turtles are seen with a history of anorexia and poor growth; examination often reveals edema and inflammation and infection of the eyes, resulting from squamous metaplasia of Harderian glands (see Figure 59-1).

Vitamin A deficiency has been linked to aural abscesses in American Box Turtles, although supporting data are scarce. Clinical observations suggest that *Terrapene* spp. inefficiently convert beta-carotene to retinol and likely need a dietary source of retinyl esters.

More recently, clinical cases of vitamin A deficiency have been diagnosed in chameleons, especially the Veiled Chameleon.[161] Dietary histories reveal minimal or no supplementation with vitamin A. Instead, feeder crickets have been dusted with products that contain calcium and vitamin D_3 only or beta-carotene (vitamin A precursor found in plants).

In the early 1990s, a magazine article suggested that chameleons are susceptible to vitamin A intoxication. After this unsubstantiated claim, commercial dusts were marketed with only carotene as a vitamin A source. Cases of vitamin A deficiency in chameleons then began to appear. Affected Veiled and Panther Chameleons show ocular lesions, respiratory dysfunction, spinal kinking, dysecdysis, and increased formation of hemipenal plugs.[161,162]

Green Anoles (*Anolis carolinensis*) have also had hypovitaminosis A develop in captivity.[163] Three of 18 in a colony had focally thickened lips, ulcerative cheilitis, lethargy, depression, and weight loss develop. The diet was crickets fed fruits and leafy vegetables and mealworms coated with a liquid vitamin supplement. Histopathologic results showed squamous metaplasia of mucus-secreting glands and epithelial surfaces.

A dietary source of vitamin A is needed by all vertebrates. It can be in the form of animal-based retinyl esters (preformed dietary vitamin A), such as retinyl acetate and retinyl palmitate. Also, it can be in the form of its plant-based precursor, beta-carotene. Species differ in their ability to convert carotene to vitamin A. Herbivores are efficient converters, and carnivores tend to be poor converters, needing retinyl ester in their diets to meet their needs for vitamin A.

Chameleons appear to need dietary vitamin A, as do all vertebrates. Recommendations include 37.5 IU orally for panther chameleons.[162] Because they eat diets of living prey, they likely respond as do other carnivores, with less than optimal abilities to convert enzymatically carotene to retinol. The cases of vitamin A deficiency seen in chameleons fed dusts containing no preformed vitamin A support this hypothesis. Vitamin A is stored primarily in liver, and crickets lack livers. Moreover, assays of vitamin A content in crickets suggest markedly low levels, less than 1 IU/g as fed.[165] Thus, chameleons fed diets of crickets and other invertebrates appear to need a dietary source of retinyl ester, which is provided most easily through dusts containing vitamin A, not beta-carotene.

Treatment of reptiles includes injectable and oral preparations of vitamin A.[164] Concentrations are higher in water-miscible products, but hepatic storage may be lower than with use of emulsified or oil-based products.

With treatment of vitamin A deficiency, care must be taken to avoid inducing vitamin A intoxication. It occurs after dosages about 100 times recommended intake and is characterized by anorexia; in turtles, erythematous and sloughing skin also occurs (Figure 18-54). Chameleons overdosed with vitamin A may have a type of nutritional MBD from interference with vitamin D and disorders of liver and kidney with resultant anorexia and edema.[161]

Reptiles with vitamin A deficiency are likely to be deficient in other nutrients as well. In particular, adequate intakes of vitamin E, zinc, and protein are essential for metabolism of retinol. Patients should be placed immediately on a balanced diet. Aquatic turtles are fed commercial diets formulated for trout and other farmed fish; for pet aquatic turtles, the diet is supplemented, preferably, with fresh prey (small fish, earthworms).

Thiamin and Vitamin E Deficiencies

Aquatic carnivorous reptiles are susceptible to deficiencies of thiamin because of thiaminases and of vitamin E because of high levels of polyunsaturated fatty acids in fish.[166] Care should be taken to ensure that fish are fresh (or fresh-frozen and thawed in cool temperatures) and wholesome, with no evidence of rancidity. Varieties of fish species should be

Injectable and Oral Vitamin A Dosages for Reptiles

Species	Recommended Treatment Dose	Recommended Dietary Levels
Aquatic turtles	50-50,000 IU/turtle; start with 200-300 IU/kg BW	2-8 IU/g diet DM
Box turtles	Parenterally 1000-2000 IU/kg every 1 wk × 2-6 doses[164]	3-6 IU/g diet DM
Chameleons	2000 IU/30 g BW by mouth every 7 d × 2 doses[161] Dusts containing 86 IU retinyl ester/g DM, followed by 60 IU/g DM	Dusts providing up to 60 IU/g DM or 5-9 IU/g cricket DM

BW, Body weight; *DM,* dry matter.

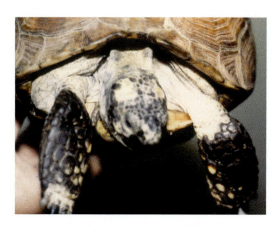

FIGURE 18-54 High doses of parenteral vitamin A in tortoises cause erythema and eventual sloughing of skin on the forelimbs and neck. Light areas of skin in this tortoise represent healed areas of sloughing from parenteral vitamin A. *(Photograph courtesy D. Mader.)*

offered, and fatty fish, such as goldfish, should not comprise the entire diet.

Signs of thiamin deficiency are similar to those in mammals. They include ataxia, muscle tremors, blindness, and bradycardia. Signs of vitamin E deficiency include anorexia and painful swollen nodules under the skin. Steatitis occurs in crocodiles and other aquatic species.[167] The role of selenium in these cases is unknown.

For treatment, thiamin is given parenterally and orally. Dosages are not determined rigorously; 25 mg/kg BW may suffice. Dosages for vitamin E are even less specific. Mammalian dosages may be appropriate, about 1 IU/kg BW suffices in the absence of conditioning factors (such as high fat or low selenium) that affect the vitamin. Diets should be balanced and patients fed involuntarily if anorexia persists. **Selenium** is mentioned rarely in reptile nutrition, yet it is critical in all domestic species and likely affects captive reptiles. Signs of selenium deficiency vary with species but are usually similar to those for vitamin E deficiency. Depending on the species, muscles, immune function, vision, or nervous system may be affected. Selenium requirements may be reported as 0.1 ppm (mg/kg) because this was a limit set by the government, which was eased a bit and then reimposed in 1993. Most animals do best when diets contain about 0.3 ppm selenium, but the optimal range is narrow and should never exceed 0.5 ppm.

Iodine Deficiency

The first nutrient to be recognized as essential for animals and humans, iodine plays a critical role in metabolism as a component of thyroxine (T_4) and triiodothyronine (T_3). Iodine joins with the amino acid thyronine (monoiodothyronine [MIT] and diiodithyronine [DIT]), and is part of triiodothyronine (T_3), thyroxine (T_4), and thyroglobulin (the storage form of thyroid hormones). These hormones (T_3 and T_4) are under control of thyroid, pituitary, brain, and feedback messages from peripheral tissues. The hormones influence rates of oxidation in cells, thus affecting physical and mental functions including growth, brain and nerve tissue, muscles, and so on. Iodine influences the metabolism of every other nutrient. Deficiency of iodine (goiter—enlarged thyroid gland as it tries to compensate for low iodine levels) leads to stillbirths and abortions in mammals and prolonged gestation, congenital malformations, mental retardation, dwarfism, stunted growth, skin problems, reduced metabolic rates, and increased mortality. Iodine is an essential (necessary in diet) trace mineral. Dietary iodine is absorbed in the small intestine. In the species studied (mammals), about 30% of absorbed iodine is taken up by the thyroid gland. The remaining iodine is mostly excreted in urine, with a small amount excreted in feces and, in mammals, sweat.

Anything that affects the availability of iodine may induce goiter. Iodine-deficient soils occur worldwide, but other causes of goiter include the presence of dietary goitrogens. Goitrogens are found in bok choy, broccoli, cabbage, cauliflower, kale, mustard seed, rapeseed, and turnips. These plants do not have to be avoided entirely but should be fed only intermittently. The specific amounts of these foods that can be tolerated safely in diets for reptiles require further study.

Iodine intoxication presents as goiter, identical in appearance to iodine deficiency, because of impaired utilization of iodine. In domestic mammals, clinical cases of goiter are seen in offspring after overdosage of the dam. Goiter occurs in tortoises and reportedly is more prevalent in the giant species from Galapagos and Aldabra Islands. This has led to anecdotal reports that the giant tortoises need more than usual amounts of dietary iodine or sea salt. Few data exist to support or refute these claims. This is especially unfortunate because iodine is toxic in large doses, and iodine intoxication has been reported for human populations treated for goiter with dietary modification. Veterinarians should be aware of the potential liability incurred from recommending iodine supplementation (or any other nutrient) that may lead to illness or death of animals.[168] A daily intake of iodine is recommended; hence, the development of iodized salt for iodine-deficient areas. Humans need to "trap" 60 µg of iodine daily to meet their needs; recommendations for growth are 50 to 150 µg, depending on age, and for reproduction 175 to 200 µg daily for humans. Safe levels of iodine intake in reptiles are unknown. Given the markedly lower metabolic rate of reptiles, an adequate daily level of dietary iodine might approximate one quarter to one third of levels for humans, or about 0.3 g/kg BW. Iodine-deficient soils in the United States were associated with goiter before the development of iodized salt and when only local foods were consumed. These areas include the Appalachian Mountain chain from New York to West Virginia, the Great Lakes area, and the Pacific Northwest and Rocky Mountain states.

A feature of sick animals sometimes includes low thyroid activity. These animals are not truly hypothyroid but are responding to their disease and to lack of adequate food intake. Serum concentrations of thyroid hormones thus can reflect levels of metabolism and serum concentrations of thyroid hormones influencing levels of metabolism.

Circulating thyroid hormones in the Desert Tortoise (*Gopherus agassizii*) were measured over 2 years. Levels of T_4 cycled with the seasons and was lowest during brumation (hibernation), increasing as emergence drew near. Females exhibited one peak of circulating T_4 in early spring. Adult males exhibited two peaks, in early spring and late summer. These periods corresponded to high activity levels from feeding, mating, locomotion, and fighting. When food was withheld for 2 weeks, T_4 levels decreased, then increased within 36 hours of feeding.[169]

Iodine may be supplemented as iodized salt and as kelp in powder or tablet form. Iodized salt contains 0.01% potassium iodide or 76 µg iodine/g; 1 tsp of salt weighs about 4 g. About 13% of the salt sold in the United States derives from the sea; other sources are mines and brine wells. Sea water that has been evaporated by the sun is often marketed as solar salt. Salt from the sea has minerals removed to be sold as table salt; these minerals are then reinserted to market the product as sea salt, which increases product cost. Low-sodium salts contain potassium chloride mixed with sodium chloride.

Kelp is one of a confusing list of names applied to seaweed. Used for centuries as a food item, kelp contains a wide variety of trace minerals, including iodine. Dried kelp for human or livestock consumption contains about 5% protein (low biologic value), 7% fiber, 1.9% calcium, and 0.2% phosphorus. Average iodine content is 0.062% or 620 µg/g, about eight times the iodine content of iodized salt.

In Norway and Japan, the kelp industry is well organized, with product regulation. However, products sold in the United States, in health food stores for example, may have escaped such regulation and one cannot assume that quality control has been achieved. Product contamination may have occurred, as could have errors in labeling. Kelp products should be used with care, with specific intakes calculated, to avoid risk of toxicity.

A form of hypothyroidism has been associated with selenium deficiency. The deiodinase that converts T_4 to T_3 contains selenium. This condition is characterized by changes in plasma concentrations such as increased T_4 and decreased T_3. It has been described only in mammals but needs to be kept in mind for reptiles raised on foods from selenium-deficient regions.

Deficiencies of Additional Vitamins and Minerals

Reptiles likely need the same vitamins and minerals as mammals and birds. Carnivorous reptiles may need additional nutrients, such as the amino acid taurine and fatty acid arachidonate. Herbivorous reptiles may be at greater risk for deficiencies, however, because of difficulties owners encounter in providing balanced salads.

Few vitamin-mineral supplements contain all essential vitamins (about 14, depending on species) and trace minerals (about 11, with an additional eight necessary at ultratrace levels). Compensation for product inadequacies is achieved with a mixture of supplements and ingredients; indeed, variety is the basis of balance in most human diets. If nutritional completeness is a goal, however, provision of micronutrients is best not left to chance.

In veterinary clinical nutrition, deficiencies of micronutrients are seen secondary to diet imbalance. Common problems are deficiencies of zinc, copper, or iodine from excessive calcium supplementation and conditional vitamin E deficiencies from excess polyunsaturated fatty acids. Other deficiencies are from drug interactions, such as vitamin K deficiency with long-term use of oral antibiotics or consumption of poisoned rodents.

In practice, most deficiencies are diagnosed with history, clinical signs, and responses to appropriate therapy. Few clinical laboratories assay for vitamins and most trace minerals. In addition, with many nutrients, blood levels remain within normal limits even after deficiency signs occur.

For immediate treatment of sick patients, administration of one or two vitamins or minerals is not recommended. Most of the micronutrients function best when in balance with other nutrients, and many, working as coenzymes, require fuels to work effectively. Dosing with one or two vitamins, without administration of a complete diet, risks intoxication of those nutrients, secondary and acute deficiencies of other nutrients, and poor patient responses. That said, instances do occur when only a few nutrients are likely to be given to reptiles seen in practice, for example, vitamins A and D_3 to aquatic turtles or vitamin K to species on long-term oral antibiotics. Because of marked differences from product to product in concentrations, forms, and vehicles, specific doses are not provided here. Rather, labels and package inserts should be consulted, and generally, doses are scaled downward because of lowered metabolic rates.

Case Report: Goiter in a Giant Tortoise Housed in the Great Lakes Area

Presentation: A Galapagos Tortoise was seen with a swelling in its neck typical of goiter.

History: The tortoise was one of three Galapagos fed a salad supplemented with iodine along with locally grown hay. The goiter appeared after the feeding of salad was reduced from 3 days weekly to 2 days weekly and hay feeding was increased. Two other tortoises fed identically showed no symptoms.

Laboratory Tests: Blood levels were 0.4 for T_4 and less than 7 for T_3 in the affected tortoise, versus 0.8 and 0.9 (T_4) and 13 and less than 7 (T_3) for the unaffected tortoises.

Diet Evaluation: Iodine concentration of the supplemented salad averaged 1.2 mg/kg DM. Iodine in hays, according to published analyses, would average less than 0.1 mg/kg.

Diagnosis and Treatment: A diagnosis of iodine deficiency was made, and the tortoises were returned to their original feeding program of supplemented salads three times weekly. In this instance, that only one of the three tortoises was clinically ill was not a surprise, for rarely a nutritional disorder affects 100% of a population. For example, in iodine-deficient areas, only 10% of untreated humans exhibit clinical goiter.

Intoxication with Additional Vitamins and Minerals

Cases of intoxications are documented only rarely for reptiles, but the potential exists for overdosage. Generally, vitamin and mineral intoxications from natural food items are rare. Selenium-accumulating plants such as *Astragalus* and *Stanleya* grow in western states and have poisoned grazing mammals. No such poisonings have been published for reptiles, but plants in areas maintaining tortoises should be identified, especially in areas with native mineral accumulators.

Intoxications from oversupplementation are likely to be more common. Nutrients with the most narrow ranges of safe intakes (established in other species) include calcium, selenium, vitamin A, and vitamin D_3.

Maximal calcium tolerances depend on many variables and, in practice, are presumed to be only three to five times corresponding minimums (e.g., three to five times 0.6% DM). Higher intakes of calcium may lead to conditioned deficiencies of trace minerals and, if combined with a high-fat diet, formation of calcium soaps in the digestive tract.

Selenium intoxication in mammals leads to abnormalities in hair, nails, hooves, and skin, and in humans, a garlic odor to the breath from dimethyl selenide. Fluorosis results in soft bones and mottled teeth.

Hypervitaminosis A leads to depression, anorexia, headache and vomiting, sloughing skin, and bone lesions. The condition is treated symptomatically; glucocorticoids prolong the elevated levels of circulating retinol and retinyl esters and so are contraindicated.

Hypervitaminosis D produces soft tissue calcification. Vitamin D intoxication has followed ingestion of rodenticides that contain cholecalciferol. Clinical signs in mammals are depression, anorexia, polyuria/polydipsia, and weight loss. Treatment regimens for reptiles have not been tested with controlled clinical trials; currently, treatment should follow guidelines for other species, which often include glucocorticoids and calcitonin and, most recently, pamidronate.[170]

Vitamin K intoxication has followed overzealous treatment of dogs that have ingested rodenticides that contain warfarin. Hemorrhage and hemolysis are associated with hypoprothrombinemia. Reptiles should be protected from poisonings by rodenticides.

Fiber Disorders

Dietary fiber is a concern when feeding herbivorous reptiles because its role is critical for maintenance of gut motility and production of volatile fatty acids. Tortoises on low-fiber diets (less than about 12% DM) have loose feces (Figure 18-55). Although not well-documented, low-fiber diets may also predispose herbivores to bloat or lactate-induced diarrhea from too-rapid fermentation of carbohydrate.

Fiber relates to diet digestibility and transit times. In tortoises, research on digestibility and transit times produced varying results. Most seem to be in agreement, however, that transit times are slow relative to those of other species. In Galapagos (*Geochelone elephantopus*) and Aldabran (*G. gigantea*) Tortoises, transit times ranged from 3 to 45 days, and for the Greek Tortoise, 55 days.[171,172] This compares with about 1 day for rats, 2 for dogs, and 5 for ruminants.

For Galapagos tortoises free-ranging on Santa Cruz island, diet digestibility averaged 52% for DM, 70% for protein, 41% for cellulose, 28% for acid-detergent fiber, and 22% for neutral-detergent fiber.[171] These values suggest that tortoises are less efficient at digesting food than horses or sheep and are similar to swine.[171] Observations of scat on the island verified the laboratory data.

In our feeding trials, long-stem fiber sources, such as hay or grass, are readily apparent in feces (Figure 18-56). This should not be considered an abnormality, especially in larger species such as Galapagos, African Spur (*G. sulcata*), or other grassland tortoises.

Diet affects digestibility in tortoises. Trials with Aldabran tortoises grazing Aldabra atoll showed cellulose digestibility of 24% to 45%.[172] Transit times averaged 10 days when tortoises grazed turf and 14 days when they grazed coastal grass. Transit times varied with age, size, and diet but not gender or season.

Smaller species of tortoise show differences because of diet. Digestibility trials on two species of forest-dwelling tropical tortoises (Red-footed and Yellow-footed) fed diets of all guava, all mango, or all lantana foliage found transit times of 4 to 7 days and digestibility ranging from negative 14% (for protein on an all fruit diet) to 71% (for organic matter on an all fruit diet). Digestibility of cell walls ranged from 7% for guava to about 40% for mango and lantana. The authors suggest that these data indicate digestive flexibility in these two common pet species.[173] The negative apparent digestibility of protein suggests negligible digestion of exogenous nitrogen and substantial entry of endogenous nitrogen into the digestive tract, an extreme associative effect or an abnormal condition.

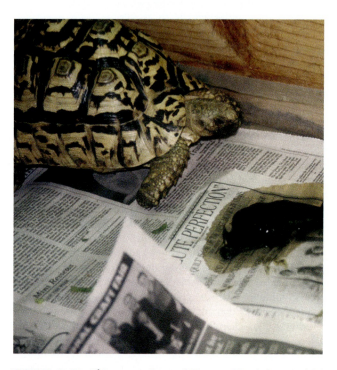

FIGURE 18-55 This young Leopard Tortoise (*Geochelone pardalis*) was fed salad without fiber supplementation. Note the unformed watery stools.

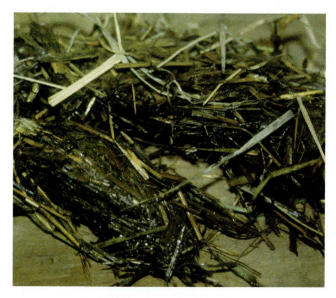

FIGURE 18-56 Typical feces from grassland tortoises (Leopard, Sulcata, Star, most *Testudo* species) are formed, with visible strands of fibrous foods such as hay and grasses. Hay strands shown here on the surface of feces are from bedding.

In studies of the Gopher Tortoise (*Gopherus polyphemus*) fed either a succulent (*Erodium cicutarium*) or dry forage (*Schismus barbatus*), transit times ranged from 13 to 33 days. As food intake increased, transit times and digestibility decreased. DM digestibility ranged from about 40% to 60% and was higher for the succulent diet.[174]

The data concerning diet digestibility and transit times are belabored here because fiber most likely plays a critical role in the nutritional health of herbivorous reptiles, yet we know little about it in these species. The data collected to date and notations on anatomic differences among species suggest that tortoises show species differences in fiber digestion and that diets, age, and size affect fiber nutrition.

The data from iguanas are even more limited. Free-ranging Green Iguanas tend to select plants that contain not only high protein but also relatively high fiber, yet very high-fiber diets suppress growth of juvenile Green Iguanas.[33] In a study of iguana growth and commercial diets, the best growth was observed from the diet containing not only the highest protein (31%) but also the highest fiber (13%).[34] Digestibility in Green Iguanas decreased with increasing dietary lignin and cutin, and transit times ranged from 4 to 9 days. With increasing environmental temperature (from 30°C to 36°C), transit time decreased from 10 to 3 days, with no change in digestibility.[175] These data add further evidence that iguanas do best when maintained at warm temperatures on relatively high-fiber diets.

Fiber should be considered when making nutritional recommendations concerning tortoises and iguanas and when providing nutrition support. Fibers include cellulose, hemicellulose, gums, mucilages, pectins, lignins, and a variety of polysaccharides such as galactan. Cell-wall fibers include lignin, cellulose, and some hemicelluloses. These are measured by Dairy Herd Improvement Association (DHIA) laboratories servicing the dairy industry. Less commonly quantitated are soluble fibers from the cell interior, hemicelluloses, gums, mucilages, and pectins.

Each type of fiber varies in its action and beneficial properties. Because food ingredients contain different fibers in varying proportions, comparisons between studies are difficult. Generally, until more data are available for reptiles, fiber sources that are standard for mammalian herbivores are recommended.

Hays may be fed to large herbivorous reptiles. Many tortoises and iguanas prefer clover, timothy, and mixed hays to alfalfa. Hays may be chopped and added to diets of produce. Hays have been used as bedding and consumed along with a produce diet, but care must be taken to keep the hay clean and wholesome. Pellets and meals contain short-stem fibers, which may be less effective in regulating gut motility.

Stress Disorders

Stress in reptiles is associated with elevated plasma catecholamines and corticosterone, elevated platelet-activating factor, lowered testosterone, decreased hepatic protein synthesis, decreased hepatic vitellogenin synthesis, hyperthermia, tachycardia, lowered food intake, fewer breeding displays, and other suppressed or detrimental behavioral changes. Studies have documented that these markers of stress are elevated in reptiles after capture, restraint, handling, excessive heat or cold, chemical or visual exposure to a dominant male, and deprivation of water or food. The previous changes have been studied in lizards, snakes, turtles, sea turtles, and Tuatara.[176-192]

The Bearded Dragon has been one of the success stories for herpetoculture, with multiple successive generations bred in captivity. Remarkably, wild Bearded Dragons in Australia show minimal increases in corticosterone after capture.[193] Researchers suggest that low adrenocortical responses to capture may be an excellent predictor of adjustment to captivity. Plasma corticosterone was used as a predictor of survival in Galapagos marine iguanas facing starvation.[181]

Nutritional management of stress centers on provision of diets that are nutritionally balanced, readily digestible, and highly palatable. For stress-induced anorexia, a first step is to sustain the patient with assist-feeding. This may necessitate placement of a pharyngostomy tube to minimize handling. A next step is to encourage the patient to eat *anything* that is edible. Then, a diet is built around this food item, slowly and gradually, with monitoring of food intake and BW.

In mammals, several nutrients are depleted during stress. To date, vitamin C has been tested in reptiles and found to decrease in stressed lizards (*Calotes versicolor*).[62] Current trials with reptiles by the author (unpublished data) have focused on providing these nutrients—vitamin E and selenium, vitamin C and bioflavonoids, zinc, potassium, and magnesium—and medium chain triglycerides as an alternative energy source. To date, the dietary changes are well tolerated by carnivores, omnivores, and herbivores.

Neurotransmitters

Studies with lizards and turtles suggest that neurotransmitters in reptiles respond to stress similarly to mammals.[192-197] Thus, use of diet to alter levels of serotonin, dopamine, and endogenous opiates may be possible.

Feeding trials in the author's laboratory have included dosing reptiles and their prey with several herbs known to impact specific areas of metabolism affected negatively by stress. Trials are investigating chamomile (*Matricaria recutita*), echinacea (*Echinacea spp.*), ginkgo (*Ginkgo biloba*), ginseng (*Panax ginseng*), kava kava (*Piper methysticum*), and valerian (*Valerian officinalis*). Each herb has been shown in mammals to affect neurotransmitters, thus improving cognition and reducing anxiety, depression, and insomnia in controlled clinical trials.[198,199]

In the author's work with valerian, for example, daily intakes for invertebrates are 0.12% DM for crickets and house flies, 0.10% for superworms, and 0.08% for mealworms. Dosages are lowest for mealworms because they appear to be most affected by the tranquilizing effect of the herbs. Concentrations of valerian in invertebrate dusts are adjusted to provide intakes for a chameleon, for example, of 0.018% on an as-fed basis. No untoward effects from the herbs have been noted in the reptiles (20+ species), but feeding for no more than 3 weeks at a time is recommended.

Although kava kava shows no impact on the opioid pathways, habituation and hepatic disorders are found in humans taking large doses for extended periods. For humans, suggestion is that kava kava can be used 3 months without a physician, but patients need physician counsel if using kava kava more than 3 months.[199] The author has tested the herb for 3-week periods only, with no untoward effects, although liver function tests were not performed.

The goal of this work is to lessen stress from captivity, handling, and interaction with conspecifics or humans by improving cognition and reducing anxiety and depression, thereby improving somatic health.[198,199] To date, the work is promising, with no ill effects noted from judicious use of selected herbs. Future investigations by others will hopefully include study of pharmacologic agents such as selective serotonin reuptake inhibitors (SSRIs).

Foreign Bodies, Lithophagy, Geophagy, Dermatophagy, and Cannibalism

Gastrointestinal blockage may occur after ingestion of foreign objects. Grazing tortoises readily consume plastic objects, especially those that are white or red. Reptiles fed produce discarded from supermarkets may consume twist ties, plastic bags, and rubber bands.

Tortoises, iguanas, and crocodiles have been reported to consume stones (lithophagy) and sand (geophagy).[200,201] Although attempts have been made to attach physiologic and nutritional significance to stone consumption, the risk from intestinal blockage is of greater importance to veterinarians. Because significant amounts of time may pass before the intestinal blockages are diagnosed and corrected, patients are frequently debilitated. For these reptiles, nutritional support is recommended.

Consumption of the shed epidermis (dermatophagy) from oneself or a conspecific is common in lizards, especially geckos, and has also been reported in aquatic turtles, tortoises, and snakes.[202] The value of dermatophagy in reptiles remains unknown, but theories concerning nutrition, grooming, and behavior have been put forth. Dermatophagy is considered normal and not indicative of nutritional deficiencies or aberrant behavior (Figure 18-57).

Cannibalism has been reported for some reptiles, such as juvenile Bearded Dragons. It may be considered a sign of hunger or stress, and efforts should be made to provide more food and a more hospitable environment. Some species grow very rapidly and need feeding two or three times daily when young. In one of our feeding trials, for example, Bearded Dragons from a few days to 14 days of age increased their BW by 63%. This rate of growth is much higher than rates observed in most animals; it is perhaps 10 times greater than that seen for neonatal puppies. Rapid growth creates an extraordinary demand for calories and nutrients, and calories fed must be sufficient in quantity to prevent cannibalism.

REFERENCES

1. Seebacher F: Heat transfer in a microvascular network: the effect of heart rate on heating and cooling in reptiles (*Pogona barbata* and *Varanus varius*), *J Theor Biol* 203:97, 2000.
2. Phillips JA, Alberts AC, Pratt NC: Differential resource use, growth, and the ontogeny of social relationships in the green iguana, *Physiol Behav* 53:81, 1993.
3. Kleiber M: *The fire of life*, ed 2, Melbourne, Fla, 1975, Kreiger Publishing.
4. Bennett AF, Dawson WR: Metabolism. In Gans C, editor: *Biology of the reptilia*, vol 5, San Diego, 1976, Academic Press.
5. Schmidt-Nielsen K: *Animal physiology: adaptation and environment*, ed 5, New York, 1997, Cambridge University Press.
6. Bedford GS, Christian KA: Standard metabolic rate and preferred body temperatures in some Australian pythons, *Austral J Zool* 46:317, 1998.
7. Green B, King D, Bratsher M, et al: Thermoregulation, water turnover and energetics of free-living Komodo dragons, *Varanus komodoensis*, *Comp Biochem Physiol* 99A:97, 1991.
8. Maxwell LK, Jacobson ER: Intraspecific allometry of standard metabolic rate in the green iguana, *Iguana iguana*, *Proc Assoc Rept Amphib Vet* 1999:113.
9. Davenport J, Scott CR: Individuality of growth, appetite, metabolic rate and assimilation of nutrients in young green turtles (*Chelonia mydas* L), *Herp J* 3:26, 1993.
10. Thompson GG, Deboer M, Pianka ER: Activity areas and daily movements of an arboreal monitor lizard, *Varanus tristis* (Squamata : Varanidae) during the breeding season, *Austral J Ecol* 24:117, 1999.
11. Nagy KA, Girard IA, Brown TK: Energetics of free-ranging mammals, reptiles, and birds, *Annu Rev Nutr* 19:247, 1999.
12. Thompson MB, Daugherty CH: Metabolism of tuatara, *Sphenodon punctatus*, *Comp Biochem Physiol A* 119:519, 1998.
13. Kohel KA, MacKenzie DS, Rostal DC, et al: Seasonality in plasma thyroxine in the desert tortoise, *Gopherus agassizii*, *Gen Comp Endocrinol* 121:214, 2001.
14. Christian KA, Conley KE: Activity and resting metabolism of varanid lizards compared with 'typical' lizards, *Austral J Zool* 42:185, 1994.
15. Christian K, Green B: Seasonal energetics and water turnover of the frillneck lizard, *Chlamydosaurus kingii*, in the wet-dry tropics of Australia, *Herpetologica* 50:274, 1994.
16. Nagy KA, Morafka DJ, Yates RA: Young desert tortoise survival: energy, water, and food requirements in the field, *Chelonian Conserv Biol* 2:396, 1997.
17. Kuchling G: Restoration of epidermal scute patterns during regeneration of the chelonian carapace, *Chelonian Conserv Biol* 2:500, 1997.
18. Busk M, Overgaard J, Hicks JW, et al: Effects of feeding on arterial blood gases in the American alligator *Alligator mississippiensis*, *J Exp Biol* 203:3117, 2000.
19. Staton MA, Edwards HM, Brisbin IL, et al: Protein and energy relationships in the diet of the American alligator (*Alligator mississippiensis*), *J Nutr* 120:775, 1990.

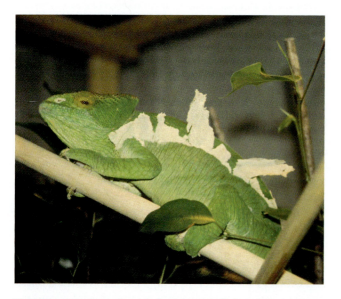

FIGURE 18-57 Lizards and chelonians shed their skin in pieces. Consumption of their own shed skin or that of a conspecific has been noted for more than 100 species, including the Parson's Chameleon (*Chamaeleo parsonii*) shown here.

20. Coulson RA, Coulson TD, Herbert JD, et al: Protein nutrition in the alligator, *Comp Biochem Physiol* 87A:449, 1987.
21. Davenport J, Wong TM, East J: Feeding and digestion in the omnivorous estuarine turtle *Batagur baska* (Gray), *Herpetol J* 2:133, 1992.
22. Avery HW, Spotila JR, Congdon JD, et al: Roles of diet protein and temperature in the growth and nutritional energetics of juvenile slider turtles, *Trachemys scripta*, *Physiol Zoo* 66:902, 1993.
23. MacMillen RE, Augee ML, Ellis BA: Thermal ecology and diet of some xerophilous lizards from western New South Wales, *J Arid Environ* 16:193, 1989.
24. McCauley SJ, Bjorndal KA: Response to dietary dilution in an omnivorous freshwater turtle: implications for ontogenetic dietary shifts, *Physiol Biochem Zool* 72:101, 1999.
25. Spencer RJ, Thompson MB, Hume ID: The diet and digestive energetics of an Australian short-necked turtle, *Emydura macquarii*, *Comp Biochem Physiol A* 121:341, 1998.
26. Burghardt GM, Layne DG, Konigsberg L: The genetics of dietary experience in a restricted natural population, *Psychol Sci* 11:69, 2000.
27. Chanard T, Thirakhupt K, van Dijk PP: Observations on *Manouria impressa* at Phu Luang Wildlife Sanctuary, northeastern Thailand, *Chelonian Conserv Biol* 2:109, 1996.
28. Tucker AD, Limpus CJ, McCallum HI, et al: Ontogenetic dietary partitioning by *Crocodylus johnstoni* during the dry season, *Copeia* 1996:978, 1996.
29. Hasegawa M, Taniguchi Y: Visual prey discrimination of queen and worker ants by a generalist lizard, *J Ethol* 11:55, 1993.
30. Costanzo JP, Litzgus JD, Iverson JB, et al: Seasonal changes in physiology and development of cold hardiness in the hatchling painted turtle *Chrysemys picta*, *J Exp Biol* 203:3459, 2000.
31. Olson JM: The effect of seasonal acclimatization on metabolic-enzyme activities in the heart and pectoral muscle of painted turtles *Chrysemys picta marginata*, *Physiol Zoo* 60:149, 1987.
32. Capizzi D, Luiselli L: The diet of the four-lined snake *(Elaphe quatuorlineata)* in Mediterranean central Italy, *Herp J* 7:1, 1997.
33. Donoghue S: Growth of juvenile green iguanas *(Iguana iguana)* fed four diets, *J Nutr* 124:2626S, 1994.
34. Donoghue S, Vidal J, Kronfeld D: Growth and morphometrics of green iguanas *(Iguana iguana)* fed four levels of dietary protein, *J Nutr* 128:2587S, 1998.
35. Jeuniaux C: *Chitine et Chitinolyse*, Paris, 1963, Masson et C Editeurs.
36. Cundall D: Drinking in snakes: kinematic cycling and water transport, *J Exp Biol* 203:2171, 2000.
37. Jorgensen CB: Role of urinary and cloacal bladders in chelonian water economy: historical and comparative perspectives, *Biol Rev Cambr Philosph Soc* 73:347, 1998.
38. Peterson CC, Greenshields D: Negative test for cloacal drinking in a semi-aquatic turtle *(Trachemys scripta)*, with comments on the functions of cloacal bursae, *J Exp Zool* 290:247, 2001.
39. Dantzler WH: *Comparative physiology of the vertebrate kidney*, New York, 1989, Springer-Verlag.
40. Ensminger AH, Ensminger ME, Konlande JF, et al: Foods and nutrition encyclopedia, ed 2, Boca Raton, Fla, 1994, CRC Press.
41. Hazard LC: Ion secretion by salt glands of desert iguanas *(Dipsosaurus dorsalis)*, *Physiol Biochem Zool* 74:22, 2001.
42. Andrews RM, Asato T: Energy utilization of a tropical lizard, *Comp Biochem Physiol* 58A:57, 1977.
43. Witz BW, Lawrence JM: Nutrient absorption efficiencies of the lizard, *Cnemidophorus sexlineatus* (Sauria, Teiidae), *Comp Biochem Physiol A* 105:151, 1993.
44. Stancel CF, Dierenfeld ES, Schoknecht PA: Calcium and phosphorus supplementation decreases growth, but does not induce pyramiding, in young red-eared sliders, *Trachemys scripta elegans*, *Zoo Biol* 17:17, 1998.
45. McRobert SP, Hopkins DT: The effects of dietary vitamin C on growth rates of juvenile slider turtles *(Trachemys scripta elegans)*, *J Zoo Wildl Med* 29:419, 1998.
46. Packard GC, Packard MJ, Birchard GF: Availability of water affects organ growth in prenatal and neonatal snapping turtles *(Chelydra serpentina)*, *J Comp Physiol B* 170:69, 2000.
47. Bonnet X, Naulleau G, Mauget R: The influence of body condition on 17-beta estradiol levels in relation to vitellogenesis in female *Vipera aspis* (Reptilia, Viperidae), *Gen Comp Endocrinol* 93:424, 1994.
48. Deeming DC, Ferguson MWJ, editors: *Egg incubation: its effects of embryonic development in birds and reptiles*, New York, 1991, Cambridge University Press.
49. Ji X, Sun P, Fu S, et al: Utilization of energy and nutrients in incubating eggs and post-hatching yolk in a colubrid snake, *Elaphe carinata*, *Herp J* 7:7, 1997.
50. Roberts KA, Thompson MB: Energy consumption by embryos of a viviparous lizard, *Eulamprus tympanum*, during development, *Comp Biochem Physiol A Mol Intregr Physiol* 127:481, 2000.
51. Demarco V: Metabolic rates of female viviparous lizards *(Sceloporus jarrovi)* throughout the reproductive cycle: do pregnant lizards adhere to standard allometry? *Physiol Zool* 66:166, 1993.
52. Gregory PT, Crampton LH, Skebo KM: Conflicts and interactions among reproduction, thermoregulation and feeding in viviparous reptiles: are gravid snakes anorexic? *J Zool* 248:231, 1999.
53. Schwarzkopf L: Decreased food intake in reproducing lizards: a fecundity-dependent cost of reproduction? *Austral J Ecol* 21:355, 1996.
54. Costanzo JP: A physiological basis for prolonged submergence in hibernating garter snakes *Thamnophis sirtalis*: evidence for an energy-sparing adaptation, *Physiol Zoo* 62:580, 1989.
55. Jackson DC: Living without oxygen: lessons from the freshwater turtle, *Comp Biochem Physiol A* 125:299, 2000.
56. Jackson DC, Crocker CE, Ultsch GR: Bone and shell contribution to lactic acid buffering of submerged turtles *Chrysemys picta bellii* at 3 degrees C, *Am J Physiol Regul Integr Comp Physiol* 278:R1564, 2000.
57. Jackson DC, Ramsey AL, Paulson JM, et al: Lactic acid buffering by bone and shell in anoxic softshell and painted turtles, *Physiol Biochem Zool* 73:290, 2000.
58. Patnaik BK: Ageing in reptiles, *Gerontology* 40:200, 1994.
59. Das K, Patnaik BK: Effect of age and short-term cold stress on SDH activity and oxygen consumption of lizard brain, *Gerontology* 26:68, 1980.
60. Manibabu PV, Patnaik BK: Lipofuscin concentration of the brain shows a reduction with age in male garden lizard, *Comp Biochem Physiol C* 117:229, 1997.
61. Jena BS, Patnaik BK: Age-related responses of hepatic glucose uptake to starvation and cold stress in male garden lizards, *Gerontology* 36:262, 1990.
62. Padhi SN: Effect of age, starvation and circadian rhythm on the ascorbic acid content and succinic dehydrogenase activity of the kidney of male garden lizard, *Calotes versicolor*, *Exp Gerontol* 19:101, 1984.
63. Miller JK: Escaping senescence: demographic data from the three-toed box turtle *(Terrapene carolina triunguis)*, *Exp Gerontol* 36:829, 2001.
64. Morley JE, Baumgartner RN, Roubenoff R, et al: Sarcopenia, *J Lab Clin Med* 137:231, 2001.
65. Douglas TC, Pennino M, Dierenfeld ES: Vitamins E and A, and proximate composition of whole mice and rats used as feed, *Comp Biochem Physiol* 107A:419, 1994.

66. Capula M, Luiselli L, Rugiero L, et al: Notes on the food habits of *Coluber hippocrepis nigrescens* from Pantelleria Island: a snake that feeds on both carrion and prey, *Herp J* 7:67, 1997.
67. Jojola-Elverum SM, Shivik JA, Clark L: Importance of bacterial decomposition and carrion substrate to foraging brown treesnakes, *J Chem Ecol* 27:1315, 2001.
68. Stoskopf MK, Hudson R: Commercial feed frogs as a source of trematode infection in reptile collections, *Herp Rev* 13:125, 1982.
69. Mader DR: Rodents and rabbits as food animals, *Proc Assoc Rept Amphib Vet* 2000:89.
70. Mills T: To scent or not to scent: techniques for feeding baby snakes, *The Vivarium* 2:8, 1990.
71. Martin RE, Hopkins SA, Steven Brush R, et al: Docosahexaenoic, arachidonic, palmitic, and oleic acids are differentially esterified into phospholipids of frog retina, *Prostaglandins Leukot Essent Fatty Acids* 67:105-111, 2002.
72. Herman CA, Hamberg M, Granstrom E: Quantitative determination of prostaglandins E1, E2 and E3 in frog tissue, *J Chromatogr* 394:353, 1987.
73. L'vova AP: [Characteristics of energy metabolism in tissues of edible frog in different seasons], *Ukr Biokhim Zh* 50:744, 1978.
74. Abate A, editors: *Thoughts for food*, 2000, Chameleon Information Network.
75. Finke MD: Complete nutrient composition of commercially raised invertebrates used as food for insectivores, *Zoo Biol* 21:269, 2002.
76. Studier EH, Sevick SH: Live mass, water content, nitrogen, and mineral levels in some insects from south-central lower Michigan, *Comp Biochem Physiol* 103A:579, 1992.
77. Reichle DE, Shanks MH, Crossley DA Jr: Calcium, potassium, and sodium content of forest floor arthropods, *Ann Entomol Soc Am* 62:57, 1969.
78. Carter A, Cragg JB: Concentrations and standing crops of calcium, magnesium, potassium, and sodium in soil and litter arthropods and their food in an Aspen woodland ecosystem in the Rocky Mountains (Canada), *Pedobiologia* 16:379, 1976.
79. Dashefsky HS, Anderson DL, Tobin EN, et al: Face fly pupae: a potential feed supplement for poultry, *Environ Entomol* 5:680, 1976.
80. Finke MD: *The use of nonlinear models to evaluate the nutritional quality of insect protein*, Madison, 1984, PhD Thesis, University of Wisconsin.
81. Finke MD, DeFoliart GR, Benevenga NJ: Use of a four-parameter logistic model to evaluate the quality of protein from three insect species when fed to rats, *J Nutr* 119:864, 1989.
82. Barker D, Fitzpatrick MP, Dierenfeld ES: Nutrient composition of selected whole invertebrates, *Zoo Biol* 17: 123, 1998.
83. Frye FL, Calvert CC: Preliminary information on the nutritional content of mulberry silk moth *(Bombyx mori)* larvae, *J Zoo Wildl Med* 20:73, 1989.
84. Redford KH, Dorea JG: The nutritional value of invertebrates with emphasis on ants and termites as food for mammals, *J Zool Lond* 203:385, 1984.
85. Pennino M, Dierenfeld ES, Behler JL: Retinol, alpha-tocopherol and proximate nutrient composition of invertebrates used as feed, *Int Zoo Yearbook* 30:143, 1991.
86. Allen ME, Oftedal OT, Ullrey ED: Effect of dietary calcium concentration on mineral composition of fox geckos *(Hemidactylus garnoti)* and Cuban tree frogs *(Osteopilus septentrionalis)*, *J Zoo Wildl Med* 24:118, 1993.
87. McFarlane JE: Dietary sodium, potassium and calcium requirements of the house cricket, *Acheta domesticus* (L.), *Comp Biochem Physiol* 100A:217, 1991.
88. Trusk AM, Crissey S: Comparison of calcium and phosphorus levels in crickets fed a high-calcium diet versus those dusted with supplement, *Proc 7th Dr Scholl Conf Nutr Capt Wild Animals*, 93, 1987.
89. Anderson SJ: Increasing calcium levels in cultured insects, *Zoo Biol* 19:1, 2000.
90. Skoczylas R: Physiology of the digestive tract. In Gans C, editor: *Biology of the reptilia*, vol 8, San Diego, 1978, Academic Press.
91. Glor R, Means C, Weintraub MJH, et al: Two cases of firefly toxicosis in bearded dragons, *Pogona vitticeps, Proc Assoc Rept Amphib Vet* 27, 1999.
92. Sydow SL, Lloyd JE: Distasteful fireflies sometimes emetic, but not lethal, *Florida Entomol* 58(4), 1975.
93. Magnussen WE, Da Silva EV: Relative effects of size, season and species on the diets of some Amazonian savannah lizards, *J Herpetol* 27:380, 1993.
94. Andrews RM: The lizard *Corytophanes cristatus*: an extreme "sit-and-wait" predator, *Biotropica* 11:136, 1979.
95. Iverson JB: Adaptations to herbivory in Iguanine lizards. In Burghardt GM, Rand AS, editors: *Iguanas of the world: their behavior, ecology, and conservation*, Park Ridge, NJ, 1982, Moyes Publishing.
96. Souci SW, Fachman W, Kraut H: *Food composition and nutrition tables*, ed 6, Boca Raton Fla, 2000, CRC Press.
97. Allen ME, Oftedal OT, Baer DJ, et al: Nutritional studies with the green iguana, *Proc 8th Dr Scholl Conf Nutr Capt Wild Animals*, 73, 1989.
98. Rhodes MJC: Physiologically-active compounds in plant foods: an overview, *Proc Nutr Soc* 55:371, 1996.
99. Schall JJ, Ressel S: Toxic plant compounds and the diet of the predominantly herbivorous whiptail lizard, *Cnemidophorus arubensis, Copeia* 111, 1991.
100. National Research Council: United States: Canadian tables of feed composition, revision 3, Washington, DC, 1982, National Academy Press.
101. Schaafsma A, Pakan I, Hofstede GJ, et al: Mineral, amino acid, and hormonal composition of chicken eggshell powder and the evaluation of its use in human nutrition, *Poult Sci* 79:1833, 2000.
102. Bohmer H, Muller H, Resch KL: Calcium supplementation with calcium-rich mineral waters: a systematic review and meta-analysis of its bioavailability, *Osteoporos Int* 11:938, 2000.
103. Scelfo GM, Flegal AR: Lead in calcium supplements, *Environ Health Perspect* 108:309, 2000.
104. Burchfield PM: An experimental artificial diet for captive snakes, *Int Zoo Yearbook* 17:172, 1977.
105. Panizzutti MHM, de Oliveira MM, Barbosa JL, et al: Evaluation of a balanced fresh paste diet for maintenance of captive neoptropical rattlesnakes used for venom production, *JAVMA* 218:912, 2001.
106. Vosburgh KM, Brady PS, Ullrey DE: Ascorbic acid requirements of garter snakes: plains *(Thamnophis radix)* and eastern *(T. sirtalis sirtalis)*, *J Zoo Anim Med* 13:38, 1982.
107. Bartkiewicz SE, Ullrey DE, Trapp AL, et al: A preliminary study of niacin needs of the bull snake *(Pituophis melanoleucus sayi)*, *J Zoo Anim Med* 13:55, 1982.
108. Davenport J, Andrews TJ, Hudson R: Assimilation of energy, protein and fatty acids by the spectacled caiman *Caiman crocodilus crocodilus* L, *Herpetol J* 2:72, 1992.
109. Stahl S: Feeding carnivorous and omnivorous reptiles, *Proc Assoc Rept Amphib Vet* 2000:177.
110. Rodriguez-Robles JA, Bell CJ, Greene HW: Gape size and evolution of diet in snakes: feeding ecology of erycine boas, *J Zool* 248:49, 1999.
111. Sloan KN, Buhlmann KA, Lovich JE: Stomach contents of commercially harvested adult alligator snapping turtles, *Macroclemys temminckii, Chelonian Conserv Biol* 2:95, 1996.

112. Jackson DR: Meat on the move: diet of a predatory turtle, *Deirochelys reticularia* (Testudines: Emydidae), *Chelonian Conserv Biol* 2:105, 1996.
113. Zurovsky Y, Mitchell D, Laburn H: Pyrogens fail to produce fever in the leopard tortoise *Geochelone pardalis*, *Comp Biochem Physiol* 87A:467, 1987.
114. Hallman GM, Ortega CE, Towner MC, et al: Effect of bacterial pyrogen on three lizard species, *Comp Biochem Physiol* 96A:383, 1990.
115. Ortega CE, Strane DS, Casal MP, et al: A positive fever response in *Agama agama* and *Sceloporus orcutti* (Reptilia: Agamidae and Iguanidae), *J Comp Physiol* 161B:377, 1991.
116. Menon J, Shah RV, Hiradhar PK: Effect of thyroidectomy on carbohydrate metabolism during tail regeneration in the gekkonid lizard *Hemidactylus flaviviridis*, *Indian J Exp Biol* 19:1018, 1981.
117. Ramachandran AV, Swamy MS, Abraham S: Serum T3 and T4 levels during tail regeneration in the gekkonid lizard *Hemidactylus flaviviridis*, *Amphibia-Reptilia* 14:149, 1993.
118. Mahmoud ZN, El Naiem DA, Hamad DM: Weight and measurement data on the grooved tortoise *Testudo sulcata* (Miller) in captivity, *Herpetol J* 1:107, 1986.
119. Meek R, Avery RA: Allometry in *Testudo sulcata*: a reappraisal, *Herpetol J* 1:246, 1988.
120. Lambert MRK: On growth, sexual dimorphism, and the general ecology of the African spurred tortoise, *Geochelone sulcata*, in Mali, *Chelonian Conserv Biol* 1:37, 1993.
121. Lambert MRK, Campbell KLI, Kabigumila JD: On growth and morphometrics of leopard tortoises, *Geochelone pardalis*, in Serengeti National Park, Tanzania, with observations on effects of bushfires and latitudinal variation in populations of eastern Africa, *Chelonian Conserv Biol* 3:46, 1998.
122. Seidel ME: Morphometric analysis and taxonomy of cooter and red-bellied turtles in the North American genus *Pseudemys* (Emydidae), *Chelonian Conserv Biol* 1:117, 1994.
123. Donoghue S: Nutritional status of tortoises, *Vivarium* 8:46, 1996.
124. Mader DR, Stoutenberg G: Assessing the body condition of the California desert tortoise, *Gopherus agassizii*, using morphometric analysis, *Proc Assoc Rept Amphib Vet* 1998:103.
125. Davenport J, Scott CR: Individual growth and allometry of young green turtles (*Chelonia mydas* L), *Herpetol J* 3:19, 1993.
126. Helminski G, DeNardo D: Bioelectrical impedance analysis as a non-destructive measure of energy stores in the leopard gecko (*Eublepharus macularius*), *UBEP 7th Ann Undergrad Res Symp*, Abstr 19, 2000.
127. Bonnet X, Naulleau G: Utilisation d'un indice de condition corporelle (BCI) pour l'etude de la reproduction chez les serpents, *C R Acad Sci III* 317:34, 1994.
128. Hailey A: Assessing body mass condition in the tortoise *Testudo hermanni*, *Herp J* 10:57, 2000.
129. Lestrel PE, Sarnat BG, McNabb EG: Carapace growth of the turtle *Chrysemys scripta*: a longitudinal study of shape using Fourier analysis, *Anat Anz Jena* 168:135, 1989.
130. Ernst CH, Wilgenbusch JC, Boucher TP, et al: Growth, allometry and sexual dimorphism in the Florida box turtle, *Terrapene carolina bauri*, *Herp J* 8:72, 1998.
131. Smallridge CJ, Bull CM: Prevalence and intensity of the blood parasite *Hemolivia mariae* in a field population of the skink *Tiliqua rugosa*, *Parasitol Res* 86:655, 2000.
132. Whittier JM, Mason RT: Plasma triglyceride and beta-hydroxybutyric acid levels in red-sided garter snakes (*Thamnophis sirtalis parietalis*) at emergence from hibernation, *Experientia* 52:145, 1996.
133. Starck JM, Beese K: Structural flexibility of the intestine of Burmese python in response to feeding, *J Exp Biol* 204:325, 2001.
134. Secor SM, Stein ED, Diamond J: Rapid upregulation of snake intestine in response to feeding: a new model of intestinal adaptation, *Am J Physiol* 266:G695, 1994.
135. Secor RM, Diamond JM: Evolution of regulatory responses to feeding in snakes, *Physiol Biochem Zool* 73:123, 2000.
136. Tothill A, Johnson J, Branvold H, et al: Effect of cisapride, erythromycin, and metoclopramide on gastrointestinal transit time in the desert tortoise, *Gopherus agassizii*, *J Herp Med Surg* 10:16, 2000.
137. Dantzler WH: *Comparative physiology of the vertebrate kidney*, New York, 1989, Springer-Verlag.
138. Antinoff N: Renal disease in the green iguana, *Iguana iguana*, *Proc Assoc Rept Amphib Vet* 2000:61.
139. Ball RL, Dumonceaux G, MacDonald C: Hypertrophic osteopathy associated with renal gout in a green iguana, *Iguana iguana*, *Proc Assoc Rept Amphib Vet* 1999:49.
140. Blem CR, Blem LB: Lipid reserves of the brown water snake *Nerodia taxispilota*, *Comp Biochem Physiol* 97A:367, 1990.
141. Sievert LM, Sievert GA, Cupp PV Jr: Metabolic rate of feeding and fasting juvenile midland painted turtles, *Chrysemys picta marginata*, *Comp Biochem Physiol* 90A:157, 1988.
142. Blazquez MC, Diaz-Paniagua C, Mateo JA: Egg retention and mortality of gravid and nesting female chameleons (*Chamaeleo chamaeleon*) in southern Spain, *Herp J* 10:91, 2000.
143. Pontes RCQ, Cartaxo ACL, Jonas R: Concentrations of ketone bodies in the blood of the green lizard *Ameiva ameiva* (Teiidae) in different physiological situations, *Comp Biochem Physiol* 89A:309, 1988.
144. Da Silva RS, Migliorini RH: Effects of starvation and refeeding on energy-linked metabolic processes in the turtle (*Phrynops hilarii*), *Comp Biochem Physiol* 96A:415, 1990.
145. Ji X, Peichao W: Annual cycles of lipid contents and caloric values of carcass and some organs of the gecko, *Gekko japonicus*, *Comp Biochem Physiol* 96A:267, 1990.
146. Niewiarowski PH, Balk ML, Londraville RL: Phenotypic effects of leptin in an ectotherm: a new tool to study the evolution of life histories and endothermy? *J Exp Biol* 203:295, 2000.
147. Vendemiale G, Grattagliano I, Caraceni P, et al: Mitochondrial oxidative injury and energy metabolism alteration in rat fatty liver: effect of the nutritional status, *Hepatology* 33:808, 2001.
148. Van der Wardt ST, Kik MJ, Klaver PS, et al: Calcium balance in Drakensburg crag lizards (*Pseudocordylus melanotus melanotus*; Cordylidae), *J Zoo Wildl Med* 30:541, 1999.
149. National Research Council: *Vitamin tolerance of animals*, Washington, DC, 1987, National Academy Press.
150. Arnaud CD, Sanchez SD: Calcium and phosphorus. In Brown ML, editor: *Present knowledge in nutrition*, ed 6, Washington, DC, 1990, Nutrition Foundation.
151. Gardner AS: The calcium cycle of female day geckos (*Phelsuma*), *Herpetol J* 1:37, 1985.
152. Gillespie D, Frye FL, Stockham SL, et al: Blood values in wild and captive Komodo dragons (*Varanus komodoensis*), *Zoo Biol* 19:495, 2000.
153. Gehrmann WH: Ultraviolet irradiances of various lamps used in animal husbandry, *Zoo Biol* 6:117, 1987.
154. Koutkia P, Lu Z, Chen TC, et al: Treatment of vitamin D deficiency due to Crohn's disease with tanning bed ultraviolet B radiation, *Gastroenterology* 121:1485, 2001.
155. Grases F, Prieto RM, Simonet MB, et al: Phytate prevents tissue calcification in female rats, *Biofactors* 11:171, 2000.
156. Di Stefano M, Veneto G, Malservisi S, et al: Small intestine bacterial overgrowth and metabolic bone disease, *Dig Dis Sci* 46:1077, 2001.
157. Saris NE, Mervaala E, Karppanen H, et al: Magnesium: an update on physiological, clinical and analytical aspects, *Clin Chim Acta* 294:1, 2000.

158. Ilich JZ, Kerstetter JE: Nutrition and bone health revisited: a story beyond calcium, *J Am Coll Nutr* 19:715, 2000.
159. Whitworth DJ, Hunt L, Licht P: Widespread expression of the mRNA encoding a novel vitamin D/thyroxine dual binding protein in the turtle *Trachemys scripta*, *Gen Comp Endocrinol* 118:354, 2000.
160. Miller WL, Portale AA: Genetics of vitamin D biosynthesis and its disorders, *Baillieres Best Pract Res Clin Endocrinol Metab* 15:95, 2001.
161. Stahl SJ: Captive management, breeding, and common medical problems of the veiled chameleon (*Chamaeleo calyptratus*), *Proc Assoc Rept Amphib Vet* 1997:29.
162. Ferguson GW, Jones JR, Gehrmann WH, et al: Indoor husbandry of the panther chameleon *Chamaeleo (Furcifer) pardalis*: effects of dietary vitamins A and D and ultraviolet irradiation on pathology and life history traits, *Zoo Biol* 15:279, 1996.
163. Miller EA, Green SL, Otto GM, et al: Suspected hypovitaminosis A in a colony of captive green anoles (*Anolis carolinensis*), *Contemp Top Lab Anim Sci* 40:18, 2001.
164. de la Navarre BJS: Diagnosis and treatment of aural abscesses in turtles, *Proc Assoc Rept Amphib Vet* 2000:9.
165. Finke MD: Complete nutrient composition of commercially raised invertebrates used as food for insectivores, *Zoo Biol* 21:269, 2002.
166. National Research Council: *Nutrient requirements of warmwater fishes and shellfishes*, Washington, DC, 1983, National Academy Press.
167. Larsen RE, Buergelt C, Cardeilhac PT, et al: Steatitis and fat necrosis in captive alligators, *JAVMA* 183:1201, 1983.
168. Hannah HW: Grounds for recovery and defenses in feed liability cases, *JAVMA* 210:1604, 1997.
169. Kohel KA, MacKenzie DS, Rostal DC, et al: Seasonality in plasma thyroxine in the desert tortoise, *Gopherus agassizii*, *Gen Comp Endocrinol* 121:214, 2001.
170. Rumbeiha WK, Kruger JM, Fitzgerald SF, et al: Use of pamidronate to reverse vitamin D3-induced toxicosis in dogs, *AJVR* 60:1092, 1999.
171. Hintz HF: Observations on the nutrition of Galapagos tortoises, personal communication.
172. Hamilton J, Coe M: Feeding, digestion and assimilation of a population of giant tortoises (*Geochelone gigantea* (Schweigger)) on Aldabra atoll, *J Arid Environ* 5:127, 1982.
173. Bjorndal KA: Flexibility of digestive responses in two generalist herbivores, the tortoises *Geochelone carbonaria* and *Geochelone denticulata*, *Oecologia* 78:317, 1989.
174. Meienberger C, Wallis IR, Nagy KA: Food intake rate and body mass influence transit time and digestibility in the desert tortoise (*Xerobates agassizii*), *Physiol Zoo* 66:847, 1993.
175. Lichtenbelt WDV: Digestion in an ectothermic herbivore, the green iguana (*Iguana iguana*): effect of food composition and body temperature, *Physiol Zoo* 65:649, 1992.
176. Mohamed MI, Rahman TA: Effect of heat stress on brain 5-hydroxytryptamine and 5-hydroxyindoleacetic acid in some vertebrate species, *Comp Biochem Physiol C* 73:313, 1982.
177. Tyrrell CL, Cree A: Relationships between corticosterone concentration and season, time of day and confinement in a wild reptile (tuatara, *Sphenodon punctatus*), *Gen Comp Endocrinol* 110:97, 1998.
178. Tyrell C, Cree A: Plasma corticosterone concentrations in wild and captive juvenile tuatara (*Sphenodon punctatus*), *N Z J Zool* 21:407, 1994.
179. Kothari RM, Patil SF: Protein metabolism in *Calotes versicolor* (Daud) exposed to various stresses, *Radiat Environ Biophys* 13:267, 1976.
180. Morales MH, Sanchez EJ: Changes in vitellogenin expression during captivity-induced stress in a tropical anole, *Gen Comp Endocrinol* 103:209, 1996.
181. Romero LM, Wikelski M: Corticosterone levels predict survival probabilities of Galapagos marine iguanas during El Nino events, *Proc Natl Acad Sci U S A* 98:7366, 2001.
182. Moore MC, Thompson CW, Marler CA: Reciprocal changes in corticosterone and testosterone levels following acute and chronic handling stress in the tree lizard, *Urosaurus ornatus*, *Gen Comp Endocrinol* 81:217, 1991.
183. Mahmoud IY, Licht P: Seasonal changes in gonadal activity and the effects of stress on reproductive hormones in the common snapping turtle, *Chelydra serpentina*, *Gen Comp Endocrinol* 107:359, 1997.
184. Cabanac M, Bernieri C: Behavioral rise in body temperature and tachycardia by handling of a turtle (*Clemmys insculpta*), *Behav Processes* 49:61, 2000.
185. Moore IT, Greene MJ, Mason RT: Environmental and seasonal adaptations of the adrenocortical and gonadal responses to capture stress in two populations of the male garter snake, *Thamnophis sirtalis*, *J Exp Zool* 289:99, 2001.
186. Lance VA, Morici LA, Elsey RM, et al: Hyperlipidemia and reproductive failure in captive-reared alligators: vitamin E, vitamin A, plasma lipids, fatty acids, and steroid hormones, *Comp Biochem Physiol B* 128:285, 2001.
187. Gregory LF, Gross YS, Bolten AB, et al: Plasma corticosterone concentrations associated with acute captivity stress in wild loggerhead sea turtles (*Caretta caretta*), *Gen Comp Endocrinol* 104:312, 1996.
188. Lance VA, Elsey RM: Plasma catecholamines and plasma corticosterone following restraint stress in juvenile alligators, *J Exp Zool* 283:559, 1999.
189. Ray PP, Maiti BR: Adrenomedullary hormonal and glycemic responses to high ambient temperature in the soft-shelled turtle, *Lissemys punctata punctata*, *Gen Comp Endocrinol* 122:17, 2001.
190. Alberts AC, Jackintell LA, Phillips JA: Effects of chemical and visual exposure to adults on growth, hormones, and behavior of juvenile green iguanas, *Physiol Behav* 55:987, 1994.
191. Lenihan DJ, Greenberg N, Lee TC: Involvement of platelet activating factor in physiological stress in the lizard, *Anolis carolinensis*, *Comp Biochem Physiol C* 81:81, 1985.
192. Summers CH, Larson ET, Ronan PJ, et al: Serotonergic responses to corticosterone and testosterone in the limbic system, *Gen Comp Endocrinol* 117:151, 2000.
193. Cree A, Amey AP, Whittier JM: Lack of consistent hormonal responses to capture during the breeding season of the bearded dragon, *Pogona barbata*, *Comp Biochem Physiol A* 126:275, 2000.
194. Bennis M, Ba m'hamed S, Rio JP, et al: The distribution of NPY-like immunoreactivity in the chameleon brain, *Anat Embryol* 203:121, 2001.
195. Bennis M, Gamrani H, Geffard M, et al: The distribution of 5-HT immunoreactive systems in the brain of a saurian, the chameleon, *J Hirnforsch* 31:563, 1990.
196. Bennis M, Versaux-Botteri C: Catecholamine-, indoleamine-, and GABA-containing cells in the chameleon retina, *Vis Neurosci* 12:785, 1995.
197. Mahaptra MS, Mahata SK, Maiti B: Effect of stress on serotonin, norepinephrine, epinephrine and corticosterone contents in the soft-shelled turtle, *Clin Exp Pharmacol Physiol* 18:719, 1991.
198. McMillan FD: Influence of mental states on somatic health in animals, *JAVMA* 214:1221, 1999.
199. *PDR for herbal medicines*, ed 2, Montvale, NJ, 2000, Medical Economics Co.
200. Sokol OM: Lithophagy and geophagy in reptiles, *J Herpetol* 5:69, 1971.
201. Fitch-Snyder H, Lance VA: Behavioral observations of lithophagy in captive juvenile alligators, *J Herpetol* 27:335, 1993.
202. Weldon PJ, Demeter BJ, Rosscoe R: A survey of shed skin-eating (dermatophagy) in amphibians and reptiles, *J Herpetol* 27:219, 1993.

19
ONCOLOGY

G. NEAL MAULDIN and LISA B. DONE

The clinical practice of oncology is the same for reptilian species as it is for mammals:

- Establish an accurate diagnosis.
- Perform complete staging.
- Choose an appropriate therapy (local versus systemic).
- Identify and deal with any toxicities or complications caused by the treatment.

Many case reports of reptiles with cancer can be found in the literature (Tables 19-1 to 19-4).[1-25] Punitive causative agents have been identified for a few species, such as a herpesvirus as a cause of fibropapillomas in Green Seaturtles (*Chelonia mydas*) (see Figure 24-1) and a C-type oncornavirus related to the Rous sarcoma virus of chickens identified in the tumors of some snakes.[2,26-28] However, no known causal agent has been found for most spontaneous tumors diagnosed in reptiles.

Most of the reported cases of reptiles with malignant tumors have had minimal therapy, and symptomatic care followed by euthanasia is a typical course of action. The only way to significantly impact the survival of reptiles with cancer is an early diagnosis and intervention with aggressive treatment when possible. As our experience with treatment of cancer in these species grows, safe administration of several different chemotherapy agents without unacceptable toxicity appears possible. The challenge now lies in the proof that our treatments are not only safe but effective for the treatment of cancer in reptiles.

PRINCIPLES, DIAGNOSTICS, AND STAGING

Important to remember is that not all abnormal growths are neoplastic. This is especially true in reptiles, where chronic granulomatous or caseous inflammation may mimic a tumor by causing growths or swellings with secondary deformity and tissue destruction (Figure 19-1). Some parasites of reptiles, such as plerocercoids, larval dracunculids, acanthocephalans, and spiruroids, can mimic tumors but rarely cause clinical disease.[29] Other conditions associated with poor husbandry, such as gastric hypertrophy from cryptosporidium, steatitis, or infectious stomatitis, may also mimic neoplastic diseases (Figure 19-2). Fine needle aspiration of these masses is often difficult to interpret and is frequently unrewarding. Therefore, any suspected neoplasm must be biopsied and definitively diagnosed before the initiation of anticancer therapy. A good rule to remember is that **if a growth is worth removing, it is worth sending in for histopathology.**

Once a definitive diagnosis has been obtained, a treatment option must be chosen that has the best chance of inducing a response in the tumor while minimizing the risk of unacceptable toxicity in the patient. For example, one would not choose aggressive chemotherapy (a systemic treatment) to treat a solitary low-grade sarcoma (a localized disease). **The oncologic adage to remember is that systemic therapy is used for systemic disease and local therapy for local disease.** Practically speaking, we use chemotherapy for the treatment of lymphomas, leukemias, myeloproliferative diseases, and epithelial tumors with a high metastatic potential, such as renal carcinoma (Figure 19-3). For most other tumors, especially sarcomas and low-grade carcinomas, we choose some form of local therapy (Figure 19-4).

The process of staging refers to the performance of tests to assess the tumor burden present in a cancer patient. Common staging tests include radiographs, ultrasound, bone marrow evaluation, and routine hematologic and biochemistry tests (Figure 19-5). Vascular access may pose a problem for routine testing, but catheter placement may facilitate both blood acquisition and chemotherapy administration. Bone marrow evaluation can be performed when warranted.

Advanced imaging, such as computed tomographic (CT) scans, magnetic resonance imaging (MRI), and nuclear scintigraphy, may also be of benefit in these patients, with a noninvasive evaluation of coelomic structures before surgery is attempted. Unfortunately, little is known about the significance of tumor stage and prognosis in reptilian cancer patients. Practically speaking, one can assume that a patient with a more advanced stage of disease warrants a worse prognosis and needs a more aggressive course of therapy. For example, a boa constrictor with renal carcinoma that has metastasized to the liver should be treated with a combination of surgical resection of the mass and chemotherapy, which warrants a grave prognosis. This same snake without metastasis may benefit from surgical resection of the primary, without adjuvant chemotherapy. Unfortunately, many reptile patients are not presented for evaluation until they have an advanced stage of tumor that causes clinical illness, which may severely limit the treatment options available.

TREATMENT OPTIONS

Local Therapy

Many different options are available for the treatment of reptiles diagnosed with malignant tumors. The clinical challenge is to choose an appropriate treatment option for the histologic type and stage of tumor in a particular patient. Local treatment options include surgery, radiation therapy, intralesional chemotherapy, photodynamic therapy (PDT), laser surgery, and cryosurgery. Each of these methods may prove useful for the treatment of an individual tumor. One should realize the limitations of each and be familiar with the potential complications associated with their use. For most locally aggressive nonmetastatic tumors, surgery is the preferred method of treatment. However, incomplete surgical

(Text cont'd. on p. 315)

Table 19-1 Tumors by Body Systems in Chelonians

Organ	Tumor Type	Metastasis	Treatment	Species	Comments	References
Integumentary System						
Skin on flippers, neck, head, tail	Papillomas; fibromas; fibropapillomas	NR	Surgical	*Chelonia mydas* (Green Seaturtle)	Viral etiology suspected; tiny warts to cauliflower-like masses; multiple cases	1-5
Skin, foot	Squamous cell carcinoma	NR	NR	*Geomyda trituga* (Ceylon Terrapin)		6
Intermandibular space	Squamous cell carcinoma	Liver	NR	*Emys orbicularis* (European Pond Turtle)		1
Hematopoietic System						
Multiple organs	Lymphosarcoma	Disseminated	NR	*Testudo hermanni* (Greek Land Tortoise)	Lymphoblastic	2
Multiple	Lymphoreticular neoplasia	NR	NR	*Apalone ferox* (Florida Soft-shelled Turtle)		7
Multiple	Leukemia	Disseminated	NR	*Pelomedusa subrufa* (Helmeted Turtle)	Myelogenous	8
Multiple	Leukemia	Disseminated	NR	*Pseudemys elegans* (Mobile Terrapin)	Moribund after 12-h to 14-h episode of epistaxis; large myeloblasts on blood smears	9
Multiple	Multicentric, lymphoblastic, lymphoma	Thymus, plastron, thyroid, heart, aorta, left lung, spleen, liver, kidneys, stomach, small intestine	NR	*Caretta caretta* (Loggerhead Seaturtle)	Anorexia and lethargy for 2 wk before death	10
Endocrine System						
Thyroid	Adenoma	NR	NR	*Pseudemys geoffronamus* (Freshwater Turtle)		2
Parathyroid	Adenoma	NR	NR	*Geochelone carbonaria* (South African Red-footed Tortoise)	Lethargy, anorexia, carapace soft, demineralized skeleton, decreased blood Ca, increased phosphorus	11
Parathyroid	Adenoma	NR	NR	*Testudo graeca* (Greek Tortoise)		12
Parathyroid	Adenoma	NR	NR	*Gopherus (Xerobates) agassizii* (Desert Tortoise)		12
Thyroid	Carcinoma	NR	NR	*G. trijuga* (Ceylon Terrapin)		6
Respiratory System						
Lungs	Fibroma	NR	NR	*C. mydas* (Green Seaturtle)	Multiple cases	13
Lungs	Fibroadenoma	NR	NR	*Testudo horsfieldi* (Horsefield's Tortoise)		2

Lungs	Fibroadenoma	NR		*E. orbicularis* (European Pond Turtle)	2
Gastrointestinal System					
Stomach	Carcinoma	NR		*Pelusios subniger* (Black Side-necked Turtle)	6
Stomach	Carcinoma	Widespread, especially intestinal		*Trachemys scripta elegans* (Red-eared Slider Turtle)	12
				30 y old	
Gallbladder	Papilloma	NR		*C. mydas* (Green Seaturtle)	13
				Associated with presence of trematodes	
Digestive tract mucosa	Lymphosarcoma	Disseminated	Supportive	*Geochelone sulcata* (African Spurred Tortoise)	14
				Five adult males, with depression, lethargy, anorexia; terminally septicemic; herpesvirus suspected	
Intestine	Leiomyoma	No	Surgical, exploratory, excision	*C. mydas* (Green Seaturtle)	15
				Clinical signs of gastrointestinal obstruction; 540-degree intestinal volvulus with stricture (leiomyoma); successful outcome	
Reproductive System					
Testes	Interstitial tumor	NR		*G. (Xerbates) agassiz* (Desert Tortoise)	16
				Incidental finding: testes normal on gross; presented with chronic respiratory distress, anorexia	
Urinary System					
Kidney	Adenocarcinoma	Liver		*Terrapene carolina* (Box Turtle)	2
Kidney	Myxofibroma	Possibly		*C. mydas* (Green Seaturtle)	4
				Multiple fibropapillomas; was thought to be renal myxofibroma primary lesion	
Musculoskeletal System					
Under plastron	Neurilemmal sarcoma	NR	Surgical, excision, cryosurgery	*T. hermanni* (Hermann's Tortoise)	17
				Found after surgery on infected plastron; subsequent mass hindered leg	

Incidence rate is one individual unless mentioned otherwise under Comments.
NR, Not reported.

Table 19-2 Tumors by Body Systems in Crocodilians

Organ	Tumor Type	Metastasis	Treatment	Species	Comments	References
Hematopoietic System						
Liver	Lymphosarcoma	Heart, cerebellum	NR	*Crocodylus porosus* (Porose Crocodile)	Ataxic, recumbent	2
Integumentary System						
Skin	Papilloma	NR	NR	*Crocodylus sp.*		18
Nasal area	Papilloma	NR	NR	*Alligator mississippiensis* (American Alligator)		18
Reproductive System						
Testes	Seminoma	NR	NR	*A. mississippiensis* (American Alligator)	Found in same alligator with papilloma; football-sized mass obscured adrenal gland	18
Gastrointestinal System						
Liver	Lipoma	NR	NR	*Crocodylus acutus* (American Crocodile)	Thought was that it could have been fat-storage disease	8
Musculoskeletal System						
Periosteum, oral cavity	Fibrosarcoma	NR	NR	*Crocodylus Siamensis* (Siamese Crocodile)	22-yr-old male captive	19

Note: Few reports of neoplasia have been made in this group, which is interesting considering the longevity of these animals.
NR, Not reported.

Table 19-3 Tumors by Body Systems in Lizards

Organ	Tumor Type	Metastasis	Treatment	Species	Comments	References
Hematopoietic System						
Multiple	Lymphoma	Diffuse	NR	*Uromastix acanthinus* (Egyptian Spiny-tailed Lizard)	Eight lizards of group of 15; concurrent leukemic blood profile; infectious disease etiology suspected	20
Multiple	Lymphoma	Disseminated	NR	*Iguana iguana* (Green Iguana)		21
Multiple	Lymphoma	Neck, tail	NR	*Lacerata sicula* (Ruin Lizard)	Presented with large neck bulge, growth in tail followed	22
Multiple	Lymphoma	Diffuse	NR	*Hydrasaurus amboinensis* (East Indian Water Lizard)	Present in heart, spleen, kidneys, lungs, liver	23
Multiple	Lymphosarcoma	Disseminated	NR	*Varanus salvator* (Malaysian Monitor)	No signs of illness before death; present in liver, spleen, kidneys, heart, testes	23
Lower neck, jaw	Lymphosarcoma	NR	NR	*Varanus salvator* (Water Monitor)		2
NR	Lymphosarcoma	NR	NR	*Uromastix acanthinuis* (Spiny-tailed Agamid)		24
NR	Leukemia	NR	NR	*Varanus bengensis* (Indian Water Monitor)		21
NR	Acute lymphoblastic leukemia	NR	Prednisone radiation	*Cordylus giganteus* (Sungazer Lizard)	Diagnosis: anemia, elevated WBC (80,000) with 87% lymphoblasts; 11 mo after radiation treatment: normal Hct, WBC; died; necropsy: no evidence of leukemia	25
Multiple	Myelogenous leukemia	Disseminated multiple, including bone	NR	*Pogona vitticeps* (Bearded Dragon)	Presented with lethargy, swollen right elbow joint, inability to move rear limbs normally, marked leukocytosis	26
NR	Plasma cell tumor	NR	NR	*Varanus niloticus* (Nile Monitor)		7
Multiple	Plasma cell tumor	Disseminated	NR	*H. amboinensis* (East Indian Water Lizard)	Present in lung, liver, stomach	27
Left mandibular labial fold	Reticulum cell sarcoma	NR	NR	*Anolis carolinensis* (American Anole)		28
Gastrointestinal System						
Liver	Adenocarcinoma	NR	NR	*P. vitticeps* (Bearded Dragon)	Biochemical values indicated liver disease	29
Liver	Hepatoma	NR	NR	*I. iguana* (Iguana)	Two reports	2
Liver	Hepatoma	NR	NR	*Tupinambis rufescens* (Golden Tegu)		2
Liver	Hepatoma	NR	NR	*Chamaeleo dilepis* (Two Flapped Chameleon)		7
Liver	Hepatoma	NR	NR	*C. dilepsis* (Chameleon)		30
Colon	Carcinoma	NR	NR	*Varanus komodoensis* (Komodo Dragon)	Had multiple other tumors	8

Continued

Table 19-3 Tumors by Body Systems in Lizards—cont'd

Organ	Tumor Type	Metastasis	Treatment	Species	Comments	References
Liver	Hepatocarcinoma	Serous membrane of body cavity	NR	*Eumeces fasciatus* (Five-lined Skink)		2
Gallbladder	Biliary adenoma	NR	NR	*Cyclura ricordii* (Ricard's Iguana)		23
Gallbladder	Cholangioma	NR	NR	*I. iguana* (Green Iguana)		31
Gallbladder	Cholangiocarcinoma	NR	NR	*Varanus* sp. (Monitor Lizard)		12
Gallbladder	Cholangiocarcinoma	Widespread dissemination	NR	*Eublepharis macularius* (Leopard Gecko)	Very aggressive tumor	12
Gallbladder	Cholangiosarcoma	NR	NR	*Phrynosoma* sp. (Horned Lizard)		12
Bile duct	Adenoma	NR	NR	*Basiliscus plumifrons* (Plumed Basilisk)		32

Integumentary System

Organ	Tumor Type	Metastasis	Treatment	Species	Comments	References
Skin	Papilloma	NR	NR	*Lacerta viridis* (Emerald Lizard)	Three cases reported	7,21
Skin	Papilloma	NR	NR	*Lacerta muralis* (Wall Lizard)	Multiple cases	2
Skin	Papilloma	NR	NR	*Lacerta agilis* (Sand Lizard)		2
Skin	Squamous cell carcinoma	NR	NR	*L. agilis* (Sand Lizard)	Seven cases reported	2
Skin, right forefoot	Squamous cell carcinoma	NR	NR	*Tupinambis teguixin* (Common Tegu)		2
Feet	Squamous cell carcinoma	NR	Antibiotics	*Leiolopisma telfairi* (Round Island Skink)	Swollen inflamed feet that bled readily, missing digits; two separate individuals	32
Skin	Squamous cell carcinoma	NR	NR	*Heloderma suspectum* (Gila Monster)		2,33
Oral	Squamous cell carcinoma	NR	NR	*Tupinambis nigropunctatus* (Black Spotted Tegu)		2
Tail	Melanoma	NR	NR	*H. suspectum* (Gila Monster)	For more than 5 yr, this tail mass slowly enlarged	2,33
Palpebra	Melanoma	NR	Antibiotics, CO_2 surgical laser	*I. iguana* (Green Iguana)	Clear for 6 mo after surgery	34
Skin, subcutaneous, left scapula	Lymphosarcoma	Multiple in all parenchymal organs	Euthanized	*Varanus exanthematicus* (Savannah Monitor Lizard)	FNA: lymphosarcoma; blood: marked lymphocytosis with lymphoid blast cells	35
Subcutaneous tissue, base of tail	Liposarcoma	NR	NR	*Trachydosaurus rugosus* (Shingleback Skink)	Three sequential biopsies done: 1st: fat cell tumor 2nd: granuloma 3rd: liposarcoma	36
Subcutaneous tissue right shoulder to right hemithorax	Lymphosarcoma	Muscle, spleen, liver, ovaries, kidneys		*I. iguana* (Green Iguana)	FNA: diagnostic necropsy confirmed	37

Location	Tumor type	Metastasis	Species	Notes	Ref
Soft tissue	Fibrosarcoma	NR	*Basiliscus plumifrons* (Basilisk Lizard)		38
Left foreleg	Fibrosarcoma	NR	*L. sicula* (Ruin Lizard)		39
Left foreleg	Mesenchymosarcoma	Thoracic cavity	*L. sicula* (Ruin Lizard)	Surrounded humerus, radius, ulna, and spread into thoracic cavity	40
Endocrine System					
Thyroid gland	Adenoma	NR	*V. komodoensis* (Komodo Dragon)	Also had colon carcinoma	8
Thyroid gland	Adenoma	NR	*Cordylus polyzonus* (African Sungazer Lizard)		7
Pancreas	Islet cell tumor	NR	*V. komodoensis* (Komodo Dragon)	Also had colon carcinoma, thyroid gland adenoma	8
Adrenal gland	Pheochromocytoma	NR	*V. komodoensis* (Komodo Dragon)	Also had colon carcinoma, thyroid gland adenoma, pancreatic islet cell tumor	8
Musculoskeletal System					
Multiple bones	Enchondroma	Yes	*Varanus dracoena* (Indian Monitor)	In distal metaphysis right humerus, left humerus, metacarpal bones, hyoid; two cervical vertebrae described as having rickets; tumor thought to be nutritionally related	2,33
Neck	Osteochondroma	NR	*Varanus bengalensis* (Bengal Monitor)		12
Multiple	Osteosarcoma	Yes	*Lacerta viridis* (Emerald Lizard)	Numerous small tumors	2
NR	Chondroosteofibroma	NR	*Cyclura cornuta* (Rhinoceros Iguana)		2,33
Reproductive System					
Ovary	Adenocarcinoma and ovarian teratoma	NR	*I. iguana* (Green Iguana)	Adenocarcinoma was huge polycystic structure with ovarian teratoma inside	7
Ovary	Teratoma	NR	*Aspidoscelis [Cnemidophorus] uniparens* (Desert Grassland Whiptail Lizard)	Two separate lizards; coelomic distention	41
Testes	Interstitial cell tumor (cystic)	NR	*V. komodoensis* (Komodo Dragon)	Same individual with multiple other tumors	8
Urinary System					
Kidney	Adenocarcinoma	NR	*Dipsosaurus dorsalis* (Desert Iguana)	Presented with firm ventral swelling at base of tail, dorsal to cloaca; cloaca was stretched	42
Kidney	Adenoma	NR	*I. iguana* (Green Iguana)	Slight swelling at base of tail	42
Kidney	Adenoma	NR	*D. dorsalis* (Desert Iguana)	Slight swelling at base of tail	42
Nervous System					
Peripheral nerve	Malignant peripheral nerve sheath	?	*Pogona vitticeps* (Bearded Dragon)	?	43

NR, Not reported; *WBC*, white blood cell; *Hct*, hematocrit; *FNA*, fine-needle aspiration.

Table 19-4 Tumors by Body Systems in Snakes

Organ	Tumor Type	Metastasis	Treatment	Species	Comments	References
Gastrointestinal System						
Oral cavity	Transitional cell carcinoma	NR	NR	*Elaphe obsoleta quadrivittata* (Yellow Ratsnake)		44
Oral cavity	Transitional cell carcinoma	NR	NR	*Bittis gabonica* (Gaboon Viper)	Presented with bloody exudate from glottis swelling on left ramus, size of pigeon egg	18
Oral cavity	Squamous cell carcinoma	NR	NR	*E. inornatus* (Puerto Rican Boa)	In lingual sheath	45
Oral cavity	Squamous cell carcinoma	NR	NR	*Agkistrodon piscivorus* (Water Moccasin)	In lower mandible	2
Oral cavity	Squamous cell carcinoma	NR	NR	*Lampropeltis getulus californiae* (California Kingsnake)	Presented as firm ulcerated mass with enlargement of right maxilla	46
Oral cavity	Squamous cell carcinoma	NR	Photodynamic therapy (two treatments)	*B. constrictor* (Boa Constrictor)	Two tumors on lip margins; no reoccurrence after second treatment	47
Oral cavity	Rhabdomyosarcoma	NR	NR	*Pituophis melanoleurus musitus* (Pinesnake)	On left anterior portion of palate	48
Oral cavity	Adenoameloblastoma	NR	NR	*Python molurus* (Indian Python)	On buccal mucous membranes	48
Oral cavity	Carcinoma	NR	NR	*P. m. bivittatus* (Burmese Python)	Erosion of dorsal palate, maxilla, nasal, and suborbital tissue occurred	49
Oral cavity	Lymphoma	NR	NR	*P. m. bivittatus* (Burmese Python)	Presented with ulcerative stomatitis	29
Oral cavity	Fibroma	NR	Successful surgical excision	*P. molurus* (Indian Python)	Very large mass that occluded pharynx	50
Oral cavity	Fibrosarcoma, ossifying	NR	Surgical excision	*Morelia [Chondropython] viridis* (Green Tree Python)	Affected rostral portion of mandible, surrounding teeth; died several months later; necropsy unable to be done	Unpublished data (personal experience)
Oral cavity	Fibrosarcoma, ossifying	NR	Surgical excision	*Python regius* (Ball Python)	Rostral mandible and teeth; lost to follow-up	Unpublished data (personal experience)
Oral cavity	Fibrosarcoma	NR	NR	*Morelia spilotus* (Carpet Python)		29
Oral cavity	Fibrosarcoma	NR	NR	*Crotalus viridis viridis* (Prairie Rattlesnake)	Retropharyngeal area	51
Oral cavity, palatine gland	Adenocarcinoma	NR	Photodynamic therapy, surgical resection	*P. m. bivittatus* (Burmese Python)	4 mo after first, palatine bone resected, PDT repeated; snake died of bacterial pneumonia unrelated to PDT; necropsy: no signs of tumor	47
Oral cavity	Lymphosarcoma	Uterus, ovary, spleen		*P. m. bivittatus* (Burmese Python)	Type C-like retroviral particles in tumors	52

Oncology

Site	Tumor	Metastasis	Treatment	Species	Comments	Ref
Esophagus	Lymphosarcoma	Stomach	NR	*Elaphe guttata guttata* (Red-tailed Ratsnake)		53
Stomach	Adenoma	NR	NR	*Python sebae* (African Rock Python)	Presented with midbody swelling	2
Stomach	Sarcoma	NR	NR	*A. piscivorus* (Water Moccasin)		6
Stomach wall, intestine	Adenocarcinoma	NR	Surgically excised	*Drymarchon corais couperi* (Florida Indigo Snake)	Presented with large swelling in cranial third of body; died 8 wk after surgery; no necropsy done	54
Pylorus	Leiomyoma	NR	NR	*Elaphe guttata* (Cornsnake)		29
Intestine	Papilloma	NR	NR	*Pituophis melanoleucus sayi* (Bullsnake)		8
Intestine	Adenoma	NR	NR	*Crotalus horridus* (Rattlesnake)		18
Intestine	Adenocarcinoma	Also in colon	NR	*Crotalus horridus atricaudatus* (Canebrake Rattlesnake)		18
Intestines	Adenocarcinoma	NR	NR	*Elaphe obsoleta* (Black Rat Snake)		2
Colon	Adenocarcinoma	Possibly	NR	*E. obsoleta* (Ratsnake)	Adenocarcinoma also found in liver	45
Colon	Adenocarcinoma	NR	NR	*P. sayi* (Bullsnake)		6
Intestine	Leiomyosarcoma	NR	Surgically resected (successfully)	*Drymarchon corais erebennus* (Texas Indigo Snake)	Presented with large coelomic mass; also had subcutaneous myxoma; died after future resection of this mass	54
Colon	Carcinoma	NR	NR	*Python reticulatus* (Reticulated Python)		33
Colon	Adenocarcinoma	NR	Surgical resection	*E. guttata guttata* (Cornsnake)	History of constipation; snake lost to follow-up 4 mo after surgery	55
Colon	Adenocarcinoma	NR	Surgical resection	*P. m. bivittatus* (Burmese Python)	Euthanized after complications; type C-like retroviral particles in tumor	52
Cloaca	Leiomyosarcoma	Liver	NR	*Naja naja* (Egyptian Cobra)		7
Cloaca	Squamous cell carcinoma	NR	NR	*Thamnophis sirtalis* (Eastern Gartersnake)		2
Cloaca	Carcinoma	NR	NR	*E. g. guttata* (Cornsnake)		2
Cloaca	Sarcoma	NR	NR	*Heterodon nasicus* (Hog-nosed Snake)		2
Cloaca	Hemangioma	NR	NR	*Crotalus viridis helleri* (Southern Pacific Rattlesnake)	Tumor was cystic, enlargement on one side of cloaca	33
Cloaca	Melanophroma	NR	NR	*Drymarchon cornis* (Indigo Snake)		45
Cloaca	Adenocarcinoma	NR	NR	*Pituophis melanoleucus* (Gopher Snake)	Had been passing bloody, mucus-covered stools	12

Continued

Table 19-4 Tumors by Body Systems in Snakes—cont'd

Organ	Tumor Type	Metastasis	Treatment	Species	Comments	References
Cloaca, external	Adenocarcinoma	Adrenal gland	Surgically debulked, photodynamic therapy	*Viper ammodytes* (European Viper)	Also had adenocarcinoma of oviduct; died 4 days after PDT	47
Liver	Adenoma	NR	NR	*Lampropeltis getulus holbrooki* (Speckled Kingsnake)		56
Liver	Adenoma	NR	NR	*L. g. californiae* (California Kingsnake)		56
Liver	Adenoma	NR	NR	*Sistrurus catenatus* (Massasauga Rattlesnake)		56
Liver	Adenoma	NR	NR	*E. obsoleta obsoleta* (Pilot Black Snake)		56
Liver	Hepatoma	NR	NR	*Pseudoboa cloelia* (Massurana)		6
Liver	Hepatoma	NR	NR	*Epicrates inornatus* (Puerto Rican Boa)		45
Liver	Hemangioendothelioma	NR	NR	*B. cookii* (Cook's Tree Boa)	Euthanized for whole body paralysis and found to have this tumor in liver	56
Liver	Carcinoma	NR	NR	*L. g. californiae* (California Kingsnake)		56
Liver	Carcinoma	NR	NR	*Sitrurus catenatus* (Pygmy Rattlesnake)		12
Liver	Carcinoma	Kidneys, lungs	NR	*B. gabonica* (Gaboon Viper)		45
Liver	Adenocarcinoma	Yes, multiple	NR	*Naja sp.* (Black Cobra)		45
Liver	Adenocarcinoma	Possibly	NR	*E. obsoleta* (Ratsnake)		45
Bile duct	Adenoma	NR	NR	*Naja naja* (Asian Cobra)		45
Bile duct	Adenoma	NR	NR	*P. melanoleucus musitus* (Pinesnake)		45
Bile duct	Adenoma	NR	NR	*Naja nigricollis* (Black-necked Cobra)		6
Bile duct	Adenoma	NR	NR	*Pseudechis porphyriacus* (Red-bellied Black Snake)		2
Bile duct	Adenoma	NR	NR	*Dispholidus typhus* (Boomslang)		2
Gallbladder	Cholangioma	NR	NR	*T. sirtalis* (Gartersnake)		7
Bile duct/gallbladder	Adenocarcinoma	NR	NR	*Bothrops atrox* (Fer-de-lance)		30
Bile duct/gallbladder	Adenocarcinoma	NR	NR	*Agkistrodon halys brevicaudus* (Korean Viper)		24
Bile duct/gallbladder	Adenocarcinoma	NR	NR	*B. gabonica* (Gaboon Viper)	Adenocarcinoma also found in colon	23

Location	Tumor Type	Metastasis	Species	Notes	Ref
Bile duct/gallbladder	Adenocarcinoma	NR	*Vipera palenstine* (Palestine Viper)		1
Gallbladder	Cholangiocarcinoma	Aggressively to multiple organs	*L. g. californiae* (California Kingsnake)		12
Gallbladder	Cholangiocarcinoma	NR	*Morelia spilotes variegata* (Carpet Python)	Lobulated mass attached to pylorus	12
Pancreas	Adenocarcinoma	NR	*Elaphe vulpina* (Ratsnake)	Presented with signs of indigestion, foul-smelling stools	12
Pancreas	Adenocarcinoma	NR	*P. melanoleurus musitus* (Pinesnake)	Pancreas was greatly enlarged	57
Pancreas	Adenocarcinoma	NR	*Crotalus horridus* (Timber Rattlesnake)		1
Pancreas	Adenocarcinoma	NR	*Spilotes pullatus* (Tiger Ratsnake)		24
Pancreas	Adenocarcinoma	NR	*B. atrox* (Fer-de-lance)		24
Pancreas	Adenocarcinoma	NR	*Crotalus mitchelli pyrrhus* (Southwestern Speckled Rattlesnake)		2
Pancreas	Adenocarcinoma	NR	*S. pullatus* (Tiger Ratsnake)		12
Integumentary System/Subcutaneous Tissue					
Back skin/subcutaneous	Fibrosarcoma	NR	*C. horridus* (Timber Rattlesnake)		7,51
Side skin/subcutaneous	Fibrosarcoma	Skeletal muscle	*B. constrictor* (Boa Constrictor)		12
Skin/subcutaneous	Fibrosarcoma	NR	*Viper russelli* (Russell's Viper)		24
Skin/subcutaneous	Fibrosarcoma	NR	*Crotalus atrox* (Western Diamondback Rattlesnake)		18
Skin/subcutaneous	Fibrosarcoma	NR	*C. v. viridis* (Prairie Rattlesnake)		18
Skin/subcutaneous	Fibrosarcoma	NR	*B. gabonica* (Gaboon Viper)		12
Intermandibular subcutaneous mass	Fibrosarcoma	Liver, heart, spleen, kidney	*Boiga dendrophila* (Mangrove Snake)	Died after biopsy done; concurrent chromomycosis in mass	58
Right side upper jaw	Melanoma	NR	*Python reticulatus* (Reticulated Python)	Also two other small black masses close to head, tip of tail melanoma	59
Skin	Melanoma	NR	*L. g. californiae* (California Kingsnake)	Malignant	45
Skin	Melanoma	NR	*B. constrictor* (Boa Constrictor)	Malignant	38
Skin	Melanoma	Kidney	*Elaphe obsolete rossalleni* (Florida Ratsnake)	2 mo after first tumor excised, multiple small black tumors arose from various parts of skin, hemipenes, fat bodies	60
Upper labial fold	Melanoma	NR	*P. melanoleucus musitus* (Pinesnake)		48
Tail skin/subcutaneous	Melanoma	Liver	*P. m. musitus* (Pinesnake)	Surgically excised; 2 yr after excision, swelling occurred anterior to cloaca;	48

Continued

Table 19-4 Tumors by Body Systems in Snakes—cont'd

Organ	Tumor Type	Metastasis	Treatment	Species	Comments	References
Skin/subcutaneous	Squamous cell carcinoma	NR	NR	*Boa constrictor occidentalis* (Argentine Boa)	this snake was paired with previous one	45
Skin/subcutaneous	Squamous cell carcinoma	NR	NR	*Eryx conicus* (Sand Boa)		45
Skin	Sarcoma	NR	NR	*Crotalus ruber* (Red Diamond Rattlesnake)	Undifferentiated sarcoma found dorsal and lateral to spinal column	39
Skin	Sarcoma	Lung, kidneys, stomach, colon, spleen, esophagus, pharynx	Euthanized	*P. m. molurus* (Indian Rock Python)	Multiple nodules, undifferentiated sarcoma	61
Deep dermis	Malignant chromatophoroma	NR	Resected	*Pituophis catenifer* (Gophersnake)	Integument ulcerated, tumor reoccurred	12
Skin/subcutaneous	Malignant chromatophoroma	NR	NR	*Thamnophis elegans terrestris* (Western Terrestrial Gartersnake)	Presented as blisters but were firmly attached subcutaneous nodules	62
Skin	Histiocytoma	Muscle	NR	*Epicrates cenchri* (Rainbow Boa)	Ulcerated mass covering dorsal spine	12
Skin/subcutaneous	Myxosarcoma	NR	NR	*Lampropeltis triangulum sinaloae* (Sinaloan Milksnake)	Oval mass on lateral/cranial portion of coelomic wall, external to coelom with skin attached, inclusion bodies in neoplastic cells	64
Skin/subcutaneous	Hemangioendothelioma	NR	Surgically excised	*B. constrictor* (Boa Constrictor)	Raised red ulcerated lesion, successfully excised	65
Skin/subcutaneous	Lipoma	NR	NR	*B. constrictor* (Boa Constrictor)		2
Skin/subcutaneous	Lipoma	NR	NR	*E. guttata* (Corn Snake)	Four cases, three infiltrative (can invade muscle, common clinical signs, obstipation)	66
Subcutaneous left lateral abdomen	Chromatophoroma			*Crotalus horridus* (Rattlesnake)	Malignant	67
Hematopoietic System						
Multiple	Lymphosarcoma	Disseminated	NR	*Heterodon platyrhinos* (Hognose Snake)		6
Multiple	Lymphosarcoma	Disseminated	NR	*N. naja* (Egyptian Cobra)		6
Multiple	Lymphosarcoma	Disseminated	NR	*Naja nigricollis* (Spitting Cobra)		24
Multiple	Lymphosarcoma	Disseminated	NR	*Eunectes murinus* (Anaconda)		2
Multiple	Lymphosarcoma	Disseminated	NR	*L. g. califorriiae* (California Kingsnake)		2
Multiple	Lymphosarcoma	Disseminated intestines, kidney, liver	NR	*P. reticulatus* (Reticulated Python)		44
Multiple	Lymphosarcoma	Intestines	NR	*E. g. guttata* (Red Rat Snake)		53

Multiple	Lymphosarcoma	Spleen, kidney, mesentery	NR	*Corallus enydris* (Cook's Tree Boa)	45
Intermandibular	Lymphosarcoma	NR	NR	*P. molurus* (Indian Python)	68
Multiple	Lymphosarcoma	Coelomic mass	Surgical excision, chemotherapy, cytosine arabinoside	*Bitis nasicornis* (Rhinoceros Viper)	69
Multiple	Lymphosarcoma	Disseminated	NR	*Lampropeltis mexicana greeri* (Grey-banded Kingsnake)	12
Air sacs, liver	Lymphosarcoma	Disseminated	NR	*L. getulus* (Eastern Kingsnake)	69
Multiple	Malignant lymphoma	Disseminated (liver, spleen, kidney)		*Epicrates subflavus* (Jamaica Boa)	32
NR	Leukemic lymphosarcoma	NR	NR	*Acanthophis antarcticus* (Death Adder)	24
NR	Leukemic lymphosarcoma	NR	NR	*Bitis arietans* (African Puff Adder)	24
NR	Leukemic lymphosarcoma	NR	NR	*B. nasicornis* (Rhinoceros Viper)	24
Multiple	Leukemia	Disseminated (liver, spleen, kidney)	NR	*E. subflavus* (Jamaican Boa)	32
Blood	Leukemia	Disseminated	NR	*B. nasicornis* (Rhinoceros Viper)	24
Blood	Leukemia	Disseminated	NR	*Lampropeltis triangulum hondurensis* (Honduran Milksnake)	70
Blood	Leukemia	Disseminated	NR	*C. horridus* (Timber Rattlesnake)	40
Blood	Leukemia	Disseminated	NR	*Vipera russelli* (Russell's Viper)	56,70
Blood	Leukemia	Disseminated	NR	*B. constrictor* (Boa Constrictor)	12
Blood	Leukemia	All major organs	NR	*P. molurus* (Indian Python)	71
Body Cavity: Mesentery					
Mesentery and/or body wall	Fibrosarcoma	NR	NR	*Boiga dendrophilis* (Mangrove Snake)	45
Mesentery and/or body wall	Fibrosarcoma	NR	NR	*V. russelli* (Russell's Viper)	45

Comments (by row):
- Row 3 (Lymphosarcoma, *Bitis nasicornis*): Two separate cases: one case presented with subcutaneous mass; later coelomic mass appeared after surgery, chemotherapy
- Row 5 (Lymphosarcoma, *L. getulus*): Bloody discharge from glottis; lung washings showed lymphocytic cells; radiographs showed soft tissue densities in air sacs, liver
- Row 14 (Leukemia, *Vipera russelli*): Poorly differentiated myelogenous leukemia
- Row 15 (Leukemia, *B. constrictor*): Presented with weakness, postural abnormalities, unilateral blindness, anemia; blood smears showed all stages of mitosis in lymphocytes
- Row 16 (Leukemia, *P. molurus*): Blood smears: numerous lymphoblastic infiltrates, lymphocytic-type cells

Continued

Table 19-4 Tumors by Body Systems in Snakes—cont'd

Organ	Tumor Type	Metastasis	Treatment	Species	Comments	References
Mesentery and/or body wall	Fibrosarcoma	NR	NR	*E. murinus* (Green Anaconda)		45
Body wall	Fibrosarcoma	NR	NR	Unknown		45
Body wall	Fibrosarcoma	NR	NR	Unknown		45
Abdomen	Adenocarcinoma	NR	NR	*Coluber flagellum testaceus* (Coach Whip Snake)		2
Mesentery	Adenocarcinoma	NR	NR	*B. constrictor* (Boa Constrictor)	Also had cardiac rhabdomyosarcoma	40
Abdomen	Mesothelioma	NR	NR	*C. horridus* (Timber Rattlesnake)	15-y-old snake	2
Abdomen	Mesothelioma	NR	NR	*P. melanoleurus musitus* (Pine Snake)	Possible diagnosis, not definitive	2
Intracoelomic	Spindle cell tumor	NR	NR	*Echis carinatus* (Saw-scaled Viper)		45
Reproductive System						
Ovary	Hemangioma	NR	NR	*S. catenatus catenatus* (Massasauga Rattlesnake)		24
Ovary	Hemangioma	NR	NR	*C. horridus* (Timber Rattlesnake)		24
Ovary	Granulosa cell tumor	NR	NR	*Trimeresurus albolabri* (Green Tree Viper)		24
Ovary	Granulosa cell tumor	NR	NR	*E. murinus* (Anaconda)		24
Ovary	Granulosa cell tumor	NR	NR	*T. sirtalis* (Gartersnake)	2 y previous to death, passed large quantities of yellow sticky mucus; 1 wk later, passed large amount of blood from cloaca; lost muscle tone just before death	72
Ovary	Fibroma	NR	NR	*A. piscivorus* (Water Moccasin)		7
Ovary	Fibroma	NR	NR	*Aerochordus javanicus* (Elephant Trunk Snake)		7
Oviduct	Leiomyosarcoma	NR	NR	*E. inornatus* (Puerto Rican Boa)		45
Ovary	Carcinoma	NR	NR	*Naja naja oxiana* (Oxus Cobra)		45
Ovary	Carcinoma	NR	NR	*B. c. constrictor* (Red Tailed Boa Constrictor)	Presented with midbody enlargement and mild weight loss; died 1 d later of exsanguination of hemorrhagic follicular cyst caused by palpation, handling of snake	73
Reproductive tract	Carcinoma	NR	NR	*P. m. catenifer* (Gophersnake)		45
Reproductive tract	Adenocarcinoma	NR	NR	*N. naja* (Asian Cobra)		44
Testes	Sertoli cell tumor	NR	NR	*T. sirtalis* (Gartersnake)		7

Location	Tumor type	Metastases	Species	Notes	Ref
Testes	Interstitial cell tumor	?	*P. m. bivittatus* (Burmese Python)		45
Musculoskeletal System					
Mandible	Lymphoma	NR	*P. m. bivittatus* (Burmese Python)	Partial mandibulectomy done	29
Mandible	Osteosarcoma	NR	*P. m. bivittatus* (Burmese Python)		12
Intermandibular	Fibrosarcoma	NR	*P. m. bivittatus* (Burmese Python)	Recurred; Type C-like retroviral in tumor	52
Spinal area	Osteosarcoma	NR	*R. rostralus* (Rufous-beaded Snake)		2
Spinal column, dorsal aspect	Osteochondrosarcoma	NR	*Naja melanoleuca* (Black Cobra)		51
Skeletal	Chondrosarcoma	NR	*E. guttata* (Cornsnake)		7
Musculoskeletal	Adenocarcinoma	Multiple organs	*Naja sp.* (Black Cobra)		45
Striated muscle	Sarcoma	NR	*Lampropeltis sp.* (Kingsnake)		45
Dorsal musculature	Fibrosarcoma	NR	*E. obsoleta* (Pilot Black Snake)		56
Urinary System					
Kidney	Adenoma	NR	*P. m. catenifer* (Gophersnake)		45
Kidney	Adenoma	NR	*Naja naja* (Asian Cobra)		45
Kidney	Adenoma	NR	*P. m. annectens* (San Diego Gophersnake)		24
Kidney	Adenoma	NR	*Bitis arietans* (African Puff Adder)		24
Kidney	Adenocarcinoma	NR	*P. m. annectens* (San Diego Gophersnake)	Same snake with adenoma	45
Kidney	Adenocarcinoma	NR	*B. constrictor* (Boa Constrictor)		8
Kidney	Adenocarcinoma	NR	*N. natrix* (Ring Snake)		51
Kidney	Adenocarcinoma	NR	*P. reticulatus* (Reticulated Python)		74
Kidney	Carcinoma	Liver, lungs	*B. gabonica* (Gaboon Viper)		44
Kidney	Renal cell carcinoma	Liver, lung	*E. guttata* (Cornsnake)	Kidney removed. Presented with intracoelomic mass 8 cm cranial to cloaca; euthanized when second mass appeared after kidney removal	75
Kidney	Sarcoma	Eye, mesentery, liver	*L. triagulum annulata* (Mexican Milksnake)		45
Kidney	Mixed cell tumor	Widespread	*E. coricus* (Sand Boa)		45
Kidney, right	Transitional cell carcinoma	NR	*P. m. bivittatus* (Burmese Python)	Type C-like retroviral particles in tumor	52

Continued

Table 19-4 Tumors by Body Systems in Snakes—cont'd

Organ	Tumor Type	Metastasis	Treatment	Species	Comments	References
Cardiovascular System						
Heart	Rhabdomyosarcoma	NR	NR	*B. constrictor* (Boa Constrictor)	Also had mesenteric adenocarcinoma	40
Heart	Fibrosarcoma	Lung	NR	*B. gabonica* (Gaboon Viper)		56
Precardiac region	Myofibroma	NR	NR	*V. russelli* (Russell's Viper)		2
Endocrine System						
Adrenal gland	Pheochromocytoma	NR	NR	*Arizona elegans occidentalis* (California Glossy Snake)		1
Adrenal gland	Pheochromocytoma	NR	NR	*Walterinnesia aegyptia* (Sinai Desert Cobra)		53
Parathyroid or thyroid gland	Carcinoma	Reproductive tract	NR	*P. m. catenifer* (Gophersnake)	Also had renal adenoma and renal adenocarcinoma	45
Respiratory System						
Lung	Adenocarcinoma	NR	NR	*Naja nivea* (Cape Cobra)	Considered bronchogenic	24
Lung	Adenocarcinoma	NR	NR	*L. g. California* (California Kingsnake)	Considered to be of tracheal origin	2
Trachea	Chondroma	No	Two snakes; removal of mass via rigid laparoscopy; systemic antibiotics, nebulization	*P. regius* (Ball Python)	Severe dyspnea due to partial tracheal obstruction occurred in three snakes; one died; histologic confirmation	76
Nervous System						
Spinal cord	Neurofibrosarcoma	NR	NR	*Agkistrodon halys brevicaudus* (Korean Viper)		24
?	Peripheral nerve sheath tumor	NR	NR	*Agkistrodon piscivorus*	Malignant	77
Ocular						
Eye	Sarcoma	NR	NR	*L. triangulum annulata* (Mexican Milksnake)		44

Note: Most cases of neoplasia have been reported in snakes. Often, collections have a prevalence of snakes compared with chelonians and lizards; this should be taken into consideration when looking at the incidence rate of neoplasia in this group.
NR, Not reported; *PDT*, photodynamic therapy.

resection results in local tumor recurrence and may allow time for a tumor to become metastatic. Therefore, if complete surgical resection is not possible, then some adjuvant form of therapy, such as radiation therapy, intralesional chemotherapy, or other treatment designed to enhance local tumor control, should be considered as part of the treatment protocol.

Radiation therapy is an appropriate choice for the treatment of residual tumor after surgery. Reptiles tolerate radiation therapy with minimal effects, but very few reports of the use of this treatment in the species exist.[30]

Intralesional chemotherapy, typically involving the use of a platinum-based chemotherapy agent such as cis-Platin suspended in oil, may also serve to improve the local control of an incompletely resected tumor. Because the platinum compound is dissolved in oil, little systemic absorption or toxicity is associated with this treatment. These oil-based compounds have a limited diffusion distance through tissue, typically only 3 to 5 millimeters, and are not appropriate for the treatment of large bulky tumors. The use of intralesional cis-Plat has been reported in reptilian species without apparent adverse effect.[31] Minimal efficacy data are currently available for this treatment method.

Photodynamic therapy involves the systemic administration of a photoactive compound, followed by application of a controlled wavelength of coherent (laser) light to the area of interest, which results in the formation of oxygen radical species locally. As with intralesional chemotherapy, PDT is primarily indicated for the treatment of superficial tumors. Because the photoactive compounds are potent photosensitizers, care must be taken to keep the patient out of direct sunlight, sometimes for several weeks after the systemic administration of these compounds.[32-34] Newer topical photosensitizers may help decrease the chance of significant patient morbidity during PDT therapy.[35] PDT has been used to treat several different reptiles with cancer, with variable results.[36]

Other surgical techniques, such as electrocautery, cryosurgery, and laser surgery may be appropriate for individual patients. Specialized equipment and training are necessary with each of these techniques, and a definitive diagnosis with surgical biopsy before their use is important because they cause severe disruption in tissue architecture and may not allow for an accurate histologic diagnosis.[37]

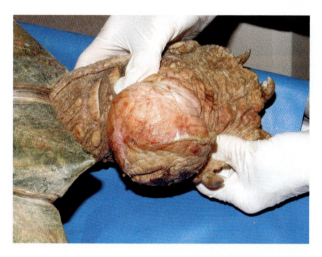

FIGURE 19-1 An Alligator Snapping Turtle (*Macrochelys temminckii*), 56.8 kg (125 lb), with a fibroid mass on the plantar surface of the hind foot caused by a rough concrete surface and an enclosure too small for the size of the turtle. Reptiles commonly have large tissue reactions that mimic neoplasia development. (*Photograph courtesy S. Barten.*)

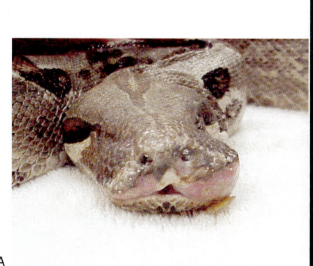 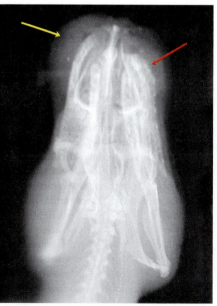

FIGURE 19-2 **A,** A Red Tailed Boa (*Boa constrictor*) with chronic infectious stomatitis. **B,** The granulomatous tissue, which is secondary to tissue infection and inflammation, has grossly disfigured the maxillary region (*yellow arrow*). The inflamed tissue on the lower jaw has displaced the mandible medially. Diagnosis in presentations like these can be difficult but ultimately depends on biopsy with microbiologic testing. (*Photograph courtesy L. Pace.*)

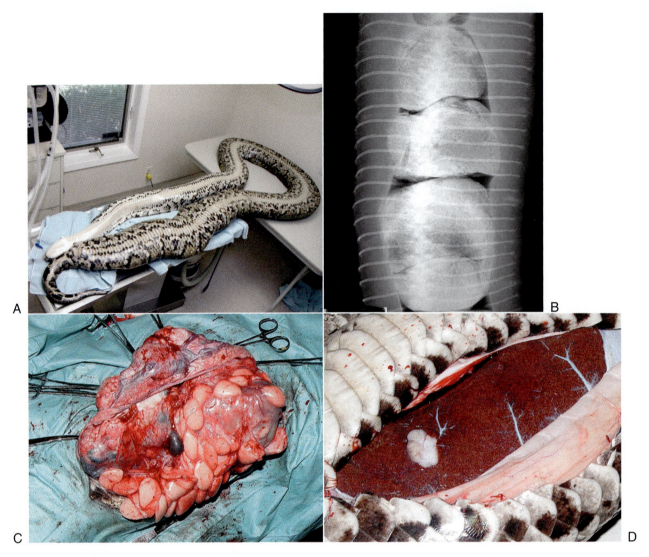

FIGURE 19-3 **A,** A Burmese Python *(Python molurus bivittatus)* with renal adenocarcinoma. The snake was 26 years old, 5.56 m (18 ft, 3 inches), and 90 kg (198 lb). It presented for anorexia, weight loss, and a visible coelomic mass. **B,** Lateral radiograph of massive chronic constipation caused by gastrointestinal obstruction by a metastatic lesion in the cloaca. **C,** This is the primary tumor seen during celiotomy. It obliterates the left kidney and measures 28 × 20 × 20 cm (11 × 8 × 8 inches). Coelomic fat bodies are adhered to the ventral half of the tumor in this view, and the oviduct is adhered as it crosses the middle of the tumor. Virtually no normal kidney tissue remains. **D,** A large, pale metastatic lesion is seen in the liver at necropsy. *(Photographs courtesy S. Barten.)*

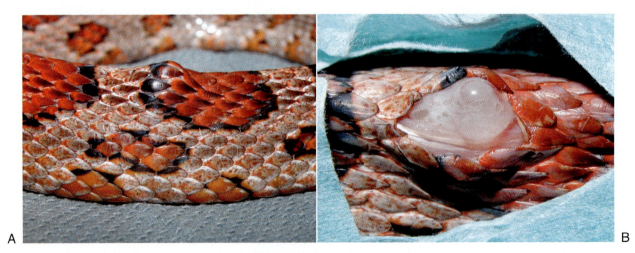

FIGURE 19-4 **A,** A Cornsnake, *Elaphe guttata*, 12 years old, with a subcutaneous mass. **B,** The mass consisted of multilobular cysts filled with clear gelatinous fluid that were nestled between, but not attached to, bands of muscle. Simple surgical excision was used to remove the mass, which was diagnosed as a myxosarcoma. *(Photographs courtesy S. Barten.)*

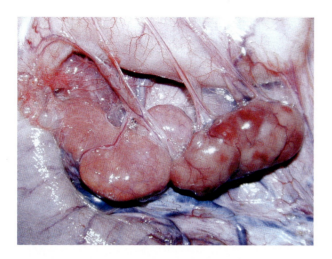

FIGURE 19-5 A Savannah Monitor, *Varanus exanthematicus*, 5 years old, with lymphoma. The lizard presented for anorexia and lethargy. It had a white blood cell count (WBC) of 100,000/mm^3 with 97% lymphocytes including young and blast forms. Massive hepatomegaly was visible on dorsoventral radiographs and was also confirmed at necropsy (see Figure 39-15, *A, B*). All the parenchymatous organs, such as the pancreas *(left)* and spleen *(right)*, were grossly enlarged and heavily infiltrated with neoplastic lymphocytes. *(Photograph courtesy S. Barten.)*

Chemotherapy

As mentioned, chemotherapy should be reserved for those patients with metastatic disease at the time of presentation or patients with tumors that are known to have a high metastatic rate. Little is known about most chemotherapeutic agents in reptilian species. However, several different classes of antineoplastic agents do appear to be safely used in reptiles. Efficacy data are not currently available for most tumor types and can only be accrued over time with the clinical use of these drugs.

The systemic administration of antineoplastic drugs is associated with some significant risks, many of which have been poorly defined in reptilian species. Most chemotherapy agents are immunosuppressive and myelosuppressive, which can result in opportunistic infections and clinical disease. In mammalian species, most of the chemotherapy agents have well-defined nadirs of leucopenia, which coincide with an increased susceptibility to normal gastrointestinal or genitourinary, respiratory, and skin bacterial flora. The effects of chemotherapy on heterophil, lymphocyte, and monocyte counts, with concomitant changes in immunity, have not been documented in reptiles. Bacterial species such as *Salmonella* may pose a risk of opportunistic infection to the reptilian patient and a zoonotic risk to its owner. The patient's hemogram should be followed during any chemotherapy events.

Other gastrointestinal inhabitants, such as *Cryptosporidium*, may also cause disease in a previously asymptomatic reptile patient undergoing chemotherapy. The zoonotic potential of reptilian *Cryptosporidium* for mammals has not been established. However, a reptile shedding *Cryptosporidium* during chemotherapy is a risk to other captive reptiles.[38]

Finally, one must remember that many chemotherapy drugs require either activation or elimination by the liver. Therefore, a general recommendation, until more research has been done, is to administer all parenteral solutions in the cranial portion of the body, to avoid any possible complications with the hepatic-portal or renal-portal circulation system. One should also remember that many chemotherapy agents are excreted as active metabolites in the urine and feces and may pose an exposure risk to the owners. Appropriate care and hygiene are essential to minimize client exposure to chemotherapeutic agents with treatment of reptile cancer patients.

Table 19-5 Partial List of Chemotherapy Drugs, Dosages, and Routes of Administration

Chemotherapy Agent	Dose	Routes of Administration	Tumors
Prednisone or equivalent corticosteroid	0.5-1 mg/kg	PO, SQ, IM, IV	Lymphoma, leukemia, myeloproliferative
Cyclophosphamide (Cytoxan)	10 mg/kg	IV, SQ, IM, IC	Lymphoma, leukemia, myeloproliferative
Chlorambucil (Leukeran)	0.1-0.2 mg/kg	PO	Lymphoma, leukemia, myeloproliferative
Melphalan (Alkeran)	0.05-0.1 mg/kg	PO	Lymphoma, leukemia, myeloproliferative
Doxorubicin (Adriamycin)	1 mg/kg	IV	Lymphoma, carcinomas, high grade sarcomas
Cisplatin	0.5-1 mg/kg	Intralesional (in oil), IV (requires prehydration), IC	Carcinomas, osteosarcoma, infiltrative sarcomas (intralesional), mesothelioma, carcinomatosis
Carboplatin (Paraplatin)	2.5-5 mg/kg	IV, IC	Carcinomas, osteosarcoma, mesothelioma, carcinomatosis
L-Asparaginase (Elspar)	400 U/kg	SQ, IM, IC	Lymphoma, leukemia, myeloproliferative
Vincristine (Oncovin)	0.025 mg/kg	IV	Lymphoma, leukemia, myeloproliferative
Methotrexate (Methotrexate)	0.25 mg/kg	IV, SQ, PO	Lymphoma, leukemia, myeloproliferative

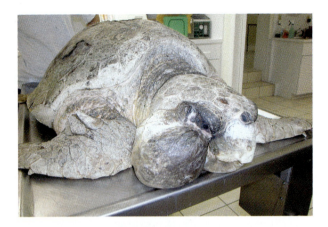

FIGURE 19-6 An Adult Loggerhead Seaturtle (*Caretta caretta*) with a histiosarcoma effacing the maxillary region below the eye. Similar lesions were noted in the heart, liver, and kidneys on necropsy. (*Photograph courtesy D. Mader.*)

One of the most commonly used antineoplastic agents in veterinary oncology is prednisone. This and other glucocorticoids have significant lympholytic activity and may be used as powerful induction agents for the treatment of lymphoid tumors. However, the remissions achieved with single agent prednisone are usually short lived in duration. With treatment of lymphoid tumors, such as lymphoma or multiple myeloma, a combination chemotherapy approach is preferable. Other drugs that could be considered for the treatment of lymphoid tumors include alkylating agents, such as Cytoxan or Leukeran, and the anthracycline antibiotics, such as adriamycin. Cytosine arabinoside has been used to treat a Rhinoceros Viper diagnosed with lymphoma, but the snake died acutely after the administration of this purine antimetabolite.[15] The cause of death was thought to be severe renal tubular necrosis and may have been coincidental to the administration of cytosine arabinoside.

However, antimetabolites are designed to take advantage of specific biochemical pathways, which may differ from species to species. For example, 5-fluorouracil is an antimetabolite that is well tolerated in man and dogs but causes a fatal neurotoxicity in cats. **Owners should always be warned about the possibility of an idiosyncratic, potentially fatal, toxicity with an untested chemotherapy agent in a new species.**

Route of administration can be a significant complicating factor for many of the chemotherapy agents in reptiles. Several of the alkylating agents are available as oral formulations. Unfortunately, many of the other classes of antineoplastic agents are only available as parenteral solutions. Some of these injectable solutions may be administered subcutaneously, intramuscularly, or intracoelomically. However, other injectable agents such as Adriamycin or vincristine cause significant tissue necrosis if administered extravascularly and may require euthanasia if the extravasation is severe. Table 19-5 is a partial list of chemotherapy drugs, dosages, and possible administration routes for use in reptiles.

Recently, the use of subcutaneously implanted vascular access ports has been described for repeated blood sampling and drug administration.[39] The use of these surgically implanted ports may make antineoplastic chemotherapy

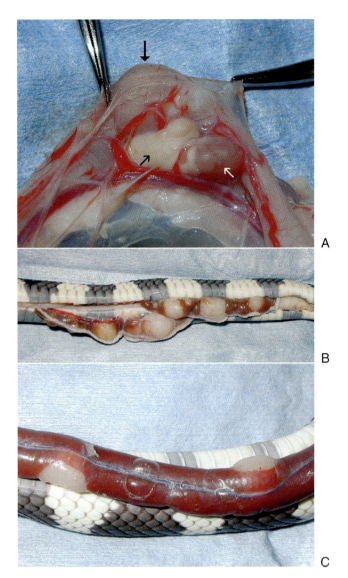

FIGURE 19-7 **A,** The primary neoplastic lesion in this California Kingsnake (*Lampropeltis getula californiae*) was an intestinal adenocarcinoma (*large black arrow*). The light-colored pancreas (*small dark arrow*) is just ventral to the tumor, and the spleen (*white arrow*) is to the right. **B,** Metastatic lesions are visible throughout both kidneys. **C,** Two metastatic lesions are visible in the liver. (*Photographs courtesy S. Barten.*)

administration and hematologic monitoring much more practical in reptilian species. The author has administered adriamycin to a cornsnake (*Elaphe* spp.) with a vertebral body osteosarcoma via a surgically placed vascular access port with no significant toxicities noted from either the port or the chemotherapy (Mauldin GN, et al: unpublished data).

In summary, cancer affects reptiles in much the same manner as it does mammalian species. A survey of reptilian neoplasms is presented in Tables 19-1 to 19-4. Reptiles are affected, as is readily apparent, by many of the same neoplastic processes that are seen in mammals (Figures 19-6 to 19-12).

Little is known about the prognostic factors and treatment options available for the different tumors, especially with regards to intraspecies variation. However, if we practice good oncologic technique, choose appropriate therapies on

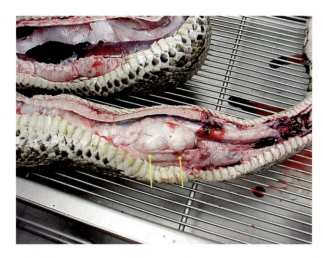

FIGURE 19-8 This Red Tailed Boa *(Boa constrictor)* presented with a large firm mass firmly attached to the ribs. Necropsy and tissue analysis revealed a chondrosarcoma *(between yellow arrows)*. *(Photograph courtesy D. Mader.)*

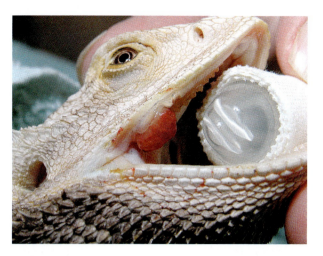

FIGURE 19-9 Bearded Dragon, *Pogona vitticeps*, with a mass arising from the mucocutaneous junction of the right upper lip. Biopsy of the lesion confirmed a nerve-sheath tumor. *(Photograph courtesy S. Barten.)*

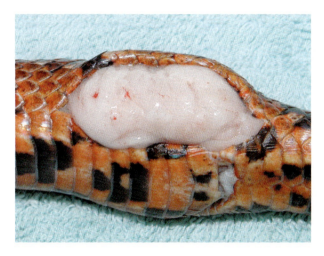

FIGURE 19-10 Older captive Cornsnakes *(Elaphe guttata)* sometimes have lipomas and liposarcomas develop. These tumors are usually located subcutaneously on the lateral aspect of the trunk adjacent to and anterior to the cloaca. They may be locally invasive but rarely metastasize. *(Photograph courtesy S. Barten.)*

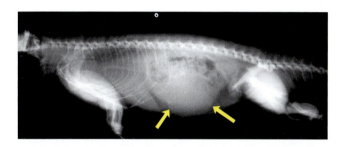

FIGURE 19-11 This Green Iguana *(Iguana iguana)* presented with a swollen abdomen. The lateral radiograph shows a large circular mass in the caudal coelom. A 7-cm-diameter *(yellow arrows)* mass was removed. The diagnosis was ovarian carcinoma. The contralateral ovary was not removed, and the patient had a complete recovery. *(Photograph courtesy D. Mader.)*

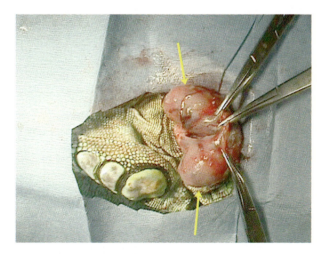

FIGURE 19-12 Bilateral thyroid adenomas *(yellow arrows)* in a Green Iguana *(Iguana iguana)*. *(Photograph courtesy D. Mader.)*

the basis of the stage and biologic behavior of the tumor in question, and document our results, we should be able to add rapidly to our knowledge of reptile oncology.

TEXT REFERENCES

1. Helmick KE, et al: Intestinal volvulus and stricture associated with a leiomyoma in a green turtle (*Chelonia mydas*), *J Zoo Wildl Med* 31(2):221, 2000.
2. Schultze AE, Mason GL, Clyde VL: Lymphosarcoma with leukemic blood profile in a Savannah monitor lizard (*Varanus exanthematicus*), *J Zoo Wildl Med* 30(1):158, 1999.
3. Lackovich JK, et al: Association of herpesvirus with fibropapillomatosis of the green turtle *Chelonia mydas* and the loggerhead turtle *Caretta caretta* in Florida, *Dis Aquat Organ* 37(2):89, 1999.
4. Drew ML, et al: Partial tracheal obstruction due to chondromas in ball pythons (*Python regius*), *J Zoo Wildl Med* 30(1):151, 1999.
5. Schumacher J, et al: Mast cell tumor in an eastern kingsnake (*Lampropeltis getulus getulus*), *J Vet Diagn Invest* 10(1):101, 1998.
6. Ramis A, et al: Malignant peripheral nerve sheath tumor in a water moccasin (*Agkistrodon piscivorus*), *J Vet Diagn Invest* 10(2):205, 1998.
7. Latimer KS, Rich GA: Colonic adenocarcinoma in a corn snake (*Elaphe guttata guttata*), *J Zoo Wildl Med* 29(3):344, 1998.
8. Janert B: A fibrosarcoma in a Siamese crocodile (*Crocodylus siamensis*), *J Zoo Wildl Med* 29(1):72, 1998.
9. Gregory CR, et al: Malignant chromatophoroma in a canebrake rattlesnake (*Crotalus horridus atricaudatus*), *J Zoo Wildl Med* 28(2):198, 1997.
10. Gravendyck M, et al: Renal adenocarcinoma in a reticulated python (*Python reticulatus*), *Vet Rec* 140(14):374, 1997.
11. Machotka SV, et al: Report of dysgerminoma in the ovaries of a snapping turtle (*Chelydra serpentina*) with discussion of ovarian neoplasms reported in reptilians and women, *In Vivo* 6(4):349, 1992.
12. Goldberg SR, Holshuh HJ: A case of leukemia in the desert spiny lizard (*Sceloporus magister*), *J Wildl Dis* 27(3):521-5, 1991.
13. Jacobson ER, et al: Renal neoplasia of snakes, *J Am Vet Med Assoc* 189(9):1134, 1986.
14. Hruban Z, Maschgan ER: A hepatocellular adenoma in a rattlesnake, *J Comp Pathol* 92(3):429, 1982.
15. Jacobson E, et al: Lymphosarcoma in an Eastern king snake and a rhinoceros viper, *J Am Vet Med Assoc* 179(11):1231, 1981.
16. Barten SD, Frye FL: Leiomyosarcoma and myxoma in a Texas indigo snake, *J Am Vet Med Assoc* 179(11):1292, 1981.
17. Onderka DK, Zwart P: Granulosa cell tumor in a garter snake (*Thamnophis sirtalis*), *J Wildl Dis* 14(2):218, 1978.
18. Wilhelm RS, Emswiller BB: Intraoral carcinoma in a Burmese python, *Vet Med Small Anim Clin* 72(2):272, 1977.
19. Schmidt RE: Plasma cell tumor in an East Indian water lizard (*Hydrosaurus amboinensis*), *J Wildl Dis* 13(1):47, 1977.
20. Hill JR: Oral squamous cell carcinoma in a California king snake, *J Am Vet Med Assoc* 171(9):981, 1977.
21. Frye FL, Dutra FR: Reticulum cell sarcoma in an American anole, *Vet Med Small Anim Clin* 69(7):897, 1974.
22. Elkan E: Malignant melanoma in a snake, *J Comp Pathol* 84(1):51, 1974.
23. Frye FL, Dutra F: Fibrosarcoma in a boa constrictor, *Vet Med Small Anim Clin* 68(3):245, 1973.
24. Frye FL, Carney J: Myeloproliferative disease in a turtle, *J Am Vet Med Assoc* 161(6):595, 1972.
25. Dawe CJ: Neoplasms of blood cell origin in poikilothermic animals: a status summary, *Bibl Haematol* (36):634, 1970.
26. Lunger PD, Hardy WD Jr, Clark HF: C-type virus particles in a reptilian tumor, *J Natl Cancer Inst* 52(4):1231, 1974.
27. Svet-Moldavsky GJ, Trubcheninova L, Ravkina LI: Sarcomas in reptiles induced with Rous virus, *Folia Biol (Praha)* 13(1):84, 1967.
28. Drury SE, et al: Detection of herpesvirus-like and papillomavirus-like particles associated with diseases of tortoises, *Vet Rec* 143(23):639, 1998.
29. Russo E: Diagnosis and treatment of lumps and bumps in snakes, *Compend Cont Ed Pract Vet* 9(8):797, 1987.
30. Leach MW, et al: Radiation therapy of a malignant chromatophoroma in a yellow rat snake (*Elaphe obsoleta quadrivittata*), *J Zoo Wildl Med* 22(2):241, 1991.
31. Ramsay EC, Fowler M: *Reptile neoplasms in the Sacramento zoo, 1981-1991*, Oakland, Calif, 1992, Joint Conference of the American Association of Zoo Veterinarians and American Association of Wildlife Veterinarians.
32. De Rosa FS, Bentley MV: Photodynamic therapy of skin cancers: sensitizers, clinical studies and future directives, *Pharm Res* 17(12):1447, 2000.
33. Fritsch C, et al: Photodynamic diagnosis and therapy in dermatology, *Skin Pharmacol Appl Skin Physiol* 11(6):358, 1998.
34. Roberts DJ, Cairnduff F: Photodynamic therapy of primary skin cancer: a review, *Br J Plast Surg* 48(6):360, 1995.
35. Szeimies RM, et al: Topical photodynamic therapy in dermatology, *J Photochem Photobiol B* 36(2):213, 1996.
36. Roberts WG, et al: Photodynamic therapy of spontaneous cancers in felines, canines, and snakes with chloro-aluminum sulfonated phthalocyanine, *J Natl Cancer Inst* 83(1):18, 1991.
37. Landthaler M, Szeimies RM, Hohenleutner U: Laser therapy of skin tumors, *Recent Results Cancer Res* 139:417, 1995.
38. Graczyk TK, Cranfield MR: Experimental transmission of *Cryptosporidium* oocyst isolates from mammals, birds, and reptiles to captive snakes, *Vet Res* 29(2):187, 1998.
39. Orcutt C: Use of vascular access ports in exotic animals, *Exotic DVM* 2(3):34, 2000.

TABLE REFERENCES

1. Billips LH, Harshbarger JC: Neoplasia: reptiles. In Melby EC, Altman NH, editors: *Handbook of laboratory science*, vol III, Cleveland, 1976, CRC Press.
2. Machotka SV: Neoplasia in reptiles. In Hoff CL, Frye FL, Jacobson ER, editors: *Diseases of amphibians and reptiles*, New York, 1984, Plenum Press.
3. Jackson ER, Mansell JL, Sundgerg JP, et al: Cutaneous fibropapillomas of green turtles (*Chelonia mydas*), *J Comp Pathol* 101:39, 1989.
4. Norton TM, Jacobson ER, Sundberg JR: Cutaneous fibropapillomas and renal myxofibroma in a green turtle, *Cheloriia mydas*, *J Wildl Dis* 26(2):265, 1990.
5. Aguirre AA: Green turtle fibropapillomatosis: in search of an etiology. *Proc Joint Conf Am Assoc Zoo Vet Am Assoc Wildlife Vet* 167, 1992.
6. Cowan DF: Diseases of captive reptiles, *J Am Vet Med Assoc* 153:848, 1968.
7. Harshbarger JC: *Activities report registry of tumors in lower animals: 1965-1973*, Washington, DC, 1974, Smithsonian Institute Press.
8. Harshbarger JC: *Activities registry of tumors in lower animals*, 1975 supplement, Washington, DC, 1976, Smithsonian Institute Press.
9. Frye FL, Carney J: Myeloproliferative disease in a turtle, *J Am Vet Med Assoc* 161:595, 1972.

10. Oros J, Torrent A, Espinosa de los Monteros A, Calabuig P, Deniz S, Tucker S, et al: Multicentric lymphoblastic lymphoma in a Loggerhead Sea Turtle (Caretta caretta), Vet Pathol 38(4):464, 2001.
11. Frye I, Carney J: Parathyroid adenoma in a tortoise, Vet Med Sm Anim Clin 70:582, 1975.
12. Frye FL: Common pathological lesions and disease processes: neoplasia. In Frye EL, editor: Reptile care: an atlas of diseases and treatments, vol 2, Neptune City, NJ, 1991, TFH Publishing.
13. Smith GM, Coates C, Nigrelli R: A papillomatous disease of the gallbladder associated with infection by flukes, occurring in the marine turtle, Chelonia mydas, Zoologica 26:13, 1941.
14. Duncan M, Dutton CJ, Junge RE: Lymphosarcoma in African Spurred tortoise (Geochelone sulcata), Proc Conf Am Assoc Zoo Vet 71, 2002.
15. Helmick KE, Bennett RA, Ginn P, DiMarco N, Beaver DP, Dennis PM: Intestinal volvulus and stricture associated with a leiomyoma in a green turtle (Chelonia mydras), J Zoo Wildl Med 31(2):221, 2000.
16. Frye FL, Dybal NO, Harshbarger JC: Testicular interstitial tumor in a desert tortoise (Gopherus agassizii), J Zoo Anim Med 19(1-2):55, 1988.
17. Cooper JE, Jackson OF, Harshbarger JC: A neurilemmal sarcoma in a tortoise (Testudo hermanrii), J Comp Pathol 93:541, 1983.
18. Wadsworth JR, Hill WCO: Selected tumors from the London zoo menagerie, Univ Pa Vet Ext Quart 141:70, 1956.
19. Janert B: A fibrosarcoma in a Siamese crocodile (Crocodylus siamensis), Zoo Wildl Med 29(1):72, 1998.
20. Gyimesi ZS: High incidence of lymphoid neoplasia in a colony of Egyptian spiny tailed lizards (Uromastyx aegyptus), Proc Assoc Reptil Amphib Vet 7, 2003.
21. Harshbarger JC: Activities report registry of tumors in lower animals, 1976 supplement, Washington, DC, 1977, Smithsonian Institute Press.
22. Lawson R: A malignant neoplasia with metastasis in the lizard, Lacerta siculai cetti, Br J Herpetol 322, 1962.
23. Zwart P, Harshbarger JC: Hematopoietic neoplasms in lizards: report of a typical case in Hydrosaurus ambinensis and of a probable case in Varanus salvator, Int J Cancer 9:548, 1972.
24. Effron M, Griner L, Berirschke K: Nature and rate of neoplasia in captive wild mammals, birds, and reptiles at necropsy, J Nat Cancer Inst 591, 1977.
25. Martin J: Successful radiation treatment of leukemia in a sungazer lizard (Cordylus giganteus), Proc Assoc Reptil Amphib Vet 8, 2003.
26. Tocidiowski ME, McNamara PL, Wojcieszyn JW: Myelogenous leukemia in a bearded dragon (Acanthodraco vitticeps), J Zoo Wildl Med 32(01):90, 2001.
27. Schmidt RE: Plasma cell tumor in an East Indian water lizard Hydrosaurus amboinensis, J Wildl Dis 13:47, 1977.
28. Frye FL, Dutra F: Reticulum cell sarcoma in an American anole, Vet Med Sm Anim Clin 69:897, 1974.
29. Hernandez-Divers SM, Garner MM: Reptile neoplasia, Exotic DVM 43:91, 2002.
30. Marcus LC: Specific diseases of herpetofauna: neoplastic diseases. In Marcus LC, editor: Veterinary biology and medicine of captive amphibians and reptiles, Philadelphia, 1981, Lea & Febiger.
31. Well M, Rodiger KS: Cholangioma in a green iguana, Kleintierpraxis 93:415 1992.
32. Cooper JE: Tumors (neoplasms) of reptiles: some significant cases from Jersey Zoo, Dodo 36:82, 2000.
33. Jacobson ER: Neoplastic diseases. In Cooper JE, Jackson OF, editors: Diseases of the Reptilia, vol 2, San Diego, 1981, Academic Press.
34. Johnson JD: Laser removal of a palpebral melanoma in a green iguana, Proc Assoc Reptil Amphib Vet 41, 2003.
35. Schutze AE, Mason, GL, Clyde VL: Lymphosarcoma with leukemic blood profile in a Savannah monitor lizard (Varanus exanthematicus), J Zoo Wildl Med 30(1):158, 1999.
36. Garner MG, Johnson C, Funk R: Liposarcoma in a shingleback skink (Trachydosaurus rugosus), J Zoo Wildl Med 25(1):150, 1994.
37. Romagnano A, Jacobson ER, Boon GD, Broeder A, Ivan A, Homer BL: Lymphosarcoma in a green iguana (Iguana iguana), J Zoo Wildl Med 27:83, 1996.
38. Harshbarger JC: Activities report registry of tumors in lower animals, 1974 supplement, Washington, DC, 1980, Smithsonian Institute Press.
39. Harshbarger JC: Activities report registry of tumors in lower animals, 1974 supplement, Washington, DC, 1975, Smithsonian Institute Press.
40. Elkan E, Cooper JE: Tumors and pseudotumors in some reptiles, J Comp Pathol 86:337, 1976.
41. Tocidiowski ME, Merrill CL, Loomis MR, Wright JF: Teratoma in Desert Grassland whiptail lizards (Cnemidophorus uniparens), J Zoo Anim Med 32(2):257, 2001.
42. Burt DG, Chrisp CE, Giller CS, et al: Two cases of renal neoplasia in a colony of desert iguanas, J Am Vet Med Assoc 185(11):1423, 1984.
43. Mikaelian I, Levine BS, Smith JC, et al: Malignant peripheral nerve sheath tumor in a bearded dragon (Pogona vitticeps), J Herpetol Med Surg 11(1):9, 2001.
44. Harshbarger JC: Activities report registry of tumors in lower animals, 1978 supplement, Washington, DC, 1979, Smithsonian Institute Press.
45. Ramsay EC, Fowler M: Reptile neoplasms at the Sacramento zoo, 1981-1991, Oakland, Calif, 1992, Proceedings Joint Conference of American Association of Zoo Veterinarians and American Association of Wildlife Veterinarians.
46. Hill JR: Oral squamous cell carcinoma in a California king snake, J Am Vet Med Assoc 171:81, 1977.
47. Roberts WG, Klein MK, Loomis M, et al: Photodynamic therapy of spontaneous cancers in felines, canines, and snakes with chloroaluminum sulfonated phthlocyanine, Natl Cancer Inst 83(1):18, 1991.
48. Ball HA: Melanosarcoma and rhabdomyoma in two pine snakes (Pituophis melanoleucus), Cancer Res 6:134, 1946.
49. Wilhelm RS, Emswiller BB: Intraoral carcinoma in a Burmese python, Vet Med Sm Anim Clin 72:272, 1977.
50. Idowu AL, Golding KR, Ikede BO, et al: Oral fibroma in a captive Indian python (Python molurus), J Wildl Dis 11:210, 1975.
51. Machotka SV, Whitney GD: Neoplasms in snakes: report of a probable mesothelioma in a rattlesnake and a thorough tabulation of earlier cases. In Montali RJ, Migaki G, editors: Pathology of zoo animals, Washington, DC, 1980, Smithsonian Institute Press.
52. Chandra AM, Jacobson ER, Munn RJ: Retroviral particles in neoplasms of Burmese pythons (Python molurus bivittatus), Vet Pathol 38(5):561, 2001.
53. Kollias GV, Jacobson ER, Norton TM, et al: Unusual cases of neoplasia in snakes from the Central Florida zoological park collection, Orlando, Fla, 1989, Proceedings Third International Colloquium Pathology of Reptiles and Amphibians.
54. Martin JC, Schelling SH, Pokras MA: Gastric adenocarcinoma in a Florida indigo snake (Drvmarchon corais couperi), J Zoo Wildl Med 25W:133, 1994.
55. Latimer KS, Rich GA: Colonic adenocarcinoma in a corn snake (Elaphe guttata guttata), J Zoo Wildl Med 29(3):344, 1998.
56. Hruban Z, Carter WE, Meehan T, et al: Neoplasia in reptiles and amphibians in the Lincoln Park zoological garden, Orlando, Fla, 1989, Proceedings Third International Colloquium Pathology of Reptiles and Amphibians.
57. Ratcliffe HL: Carcinoma of the pancreas in Say's pine snake (Pituophis sayi), Am J Cancer 24:78, 1935.

58. Jacobson ER: Chromomycosis and fibrosarcoma in a mangrove snake, *J Am Vet Med Assoc* 185(11):1428, 1984.
59. Schlumberger HG, Lucke B: Tumors of fishes, amphibians and reptiles, *Cancer Res* 8:657, 1948.
60. Elkan E: Malignant melanoma in a snake, *J Comp Path* 84:51, 1974.
61. Abou-Madi N, Jacobson ER, Buergelt CD, et al: Disseminated undifferentiated sarcoma in an Indian rock python *(Python molurus molurus)*, *J Zoo Wildl Med* 25(1):143, 1994.
62. Frye F, Larney J, Harshbarger J, et al: Malignant chromatophoroma in a Western terrestrial garter snake, *J Am Vet Med Assoc* 167(7):557, 1975.
63. Ewing PJ, Setser MD, Stair EL, et al: Myosarcoma in a Sinaloan milk snake, *J Am Vet Med Assoc* 199(12):1775, 1991.
64. Frye F, Lane IR: Hemangioendothelioma in a boa constrictor, *J Zoo Anim Med* 15:78, 1984.
65. Reavill DR, Schmidt RE: *Lipomas in corn snakes (Elaphe guttata guttata): a series of four cases*, Minneapolis, 2003, Proceedings Association of Reptilian and Amphibian Veterinarians.
66. Gregory CR, Harmon BG, Latimer KS, Hafner S, Campagnoli RP, McManamon RM: Malignant chromatophoroma in a canebrake rattlesnake *(Crotalus horridus atricaudatus)*, *J Zoo Wildl Med* 28(2):198, 1997.
67. Harshbarger JC: *Activities report registry of tumors in lower animals*, 1977 supplement, Washington, DC, 1978, Smithsonian Institute Press.
68. Jacobson E. Calderwood MB, French TW, et al: Lymphosarcoma in an Eastern kingsnake and a rhinoceros viper, *J Am Vet Med Assoc* 179:1231, 1981.
69. Hruban Z, Vardimani. Meehan T, et al: Haematopoietic malignancies in zoo animals, *J Comp Pathol* 106:15, 1992.
70. Finnie EP: Lymphoid leukosis in an Indian python *(Python molurus)*, *J Pathol* 107:295, 1972.
71. Onderka DK, Zart P: Granulosa cell tumor in a garter snake *(Thamnophis sirtalis)*, *J Wildl Dis* 14:218, 1978.
72. Michaels SJ, Sanecki R: Undifferentiated carcinoma in the ovary of a boa constrictor *(Boa constrictor ortoni)*, *J Zoo Anim Med* 19(4):237, 1988.
73. Gravendyck M, Marschang RE, Schroder-Gravendyck AS, Kaleta EF: Renal adenocarcinoma in a reticulated python *(Python reticulatus)*, *Vet Rec* 140(14):375, 1997.
74. Barten SL, Davis K, Harris RK, et al: Renal cell carcinoma with metastases in a corn snake *(Elaphe guttata)*, *J Zoo Wildl Med* 25(1):123, 1994.
75. Drew ML, Phalen DN, Berridge BR, Johnson TL, Bouley D, Weeks BR, et al: Partial tracheal obstruction due to chondromas in ball pythons *(Python regius)*, *J Zoo Wildl Med* 30(1):151, 1999.
76. Ramis A, Pumarola M, Fernanadez-Moran J, Anor S, Majo N, Zidan A: A malignant peripheral nerve sheath tumor in a water moccasin *(Agkistrodon piscivorus)*, *J Vet Diagn Invest* 10(2):205, 1998.

20
REPTILIAN OPHTHALMOLOGY

MARTIN P.C. LAWTON

Reptilian ophthalmology (indeed, like much of reptilian medicine) is still very much in its infancy but is slowly becoming more of an established and appreciated discipline. In 1978, a paper stated that "The veterinary clinician does not routinely find himself examining the eyes of snakes"[1]; a mere 5 years later, disease of the eye and the adnexal structures was considered commonly encountered in reptiles.[2] The difference in these statements probably has more to do with the lack of a full and thorough ophthalmic examination as part of the standard clinical examination of all reptile cases than with a sudden advance in knowledge within such a short period of time.

The eye is a barometer that reflects the health of the animal, and therefore, that many diseases produce ocular symptoms even though they are not primary ocular diseases is not surprising. On occasion, the reptilian eye can also be an environmental barometer because toxicity can affect many aspects of the eye. Organochlorine pesticides have been associated with ocular discharge, conjunctivitis, and blepharitis in Eastern Box Turtles (*Terrapene carolina carolina*).[3] Always to remember that the ocular responses to injury vary between different species and have a profound influence on the type of inflammatory responses and healing powers that may be expected.[4]

The eye is considered[5] to clearly show how various species have modified their basic structures to current conditions and evolutionary opportunities. The anatomy of the reptilian eye (with the exception of snakes) has many general anatomic similarities with only minor variations between the groups.[2,6] In snakes, many structural differences are seen in comparison with the rest of the reptiles and are covered separately.

EXAMINATION

The examination of any body system requires knowledge of the normal before the abnormal can be appreciated. Reptilian ophthalmology is no exception. The veterinarian who wants to be proficient in reptilian medicine should perform a full ophthalmic examination of all cases, not only to gain the experience of the normal but also because systemic disease often can be seen or suspected from lesions noted in the eyes and related structures (Figure 20-1).

The ophthalmic examination of reptiles should be systematic in much the same way as for any other animal. The examination should start with an assessment of the eyelids (fused or mobile), the tear film, and then the globe as a whole and then with a more detailed examination of the cornea, anterior chamber, iris, lens, and finally fundus. Both eyes should always be examined so that they can be compared and contrasted. If an obvious or suspected problem is seen with one eye, a good policy is to examine the other eye first because many subtle changes or early lesions associated with disease processes may be more noticeable in the apparently normal eye than in an eye with well-established disease.

A brief examination with some form of focal illumination should be used (pen light, auroscope, etc.). This allows a simple assessment of the clarity of the cornea and anterior chamber and highlights any adnexa abnormalities. Any pupillary light response should be noted. Although the presence of striated muscles within the reptilian iris could prevent a pupillary light reflex, it is seldom absent unless substantial ocular disease exists[7]; indeed, a rapid direct light response is noted. Reptiles do not have a consensual light response, although they show a normal direct pupillary light response.[8]

A more detailed examination of the eye is not possible without some form of magnification (magnifying loupe, slit-lamp biomicroscope, or +10 to +15 diopter lens of the direct ophthalmoscope). The small size of the reptile eye leads to a high likelihood of subtle changes being missed if magnification is not used. Magnification is essential to also aid the clinician, in examination of snakes and lizards with spectacles, to distinguish between the anterior chamber and the subspectacular space, which is essential in reaching an accurate diagnosis of the site of any pathology.[9,10]

Fundoscopy is often best achieved with indirect ophthalmoscopy with a 90 diopter lens (Figure 20-2) or a panophthalmoscope (Welch Allen) that allows vision even through a small, often undilated pupil as found in reptiles. The striated muscle in the iris allows voluntary control of the pupil size,

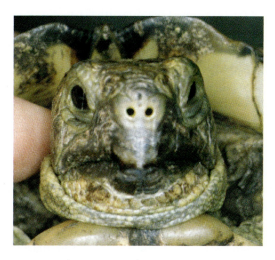

FIGURE 20-1 The left eye shows Horner's syndrome in a Mediterranean Tortoise (*Testudo graeca*).

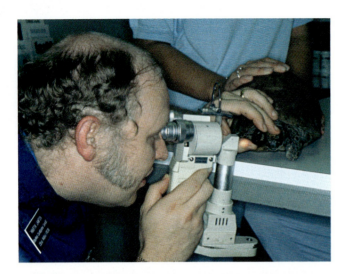

FIGURE 20-2 Indirect ophthalmoscopy with 90 diopter lens in a Mediterranean Tortoise *(Testudo graeca)*.

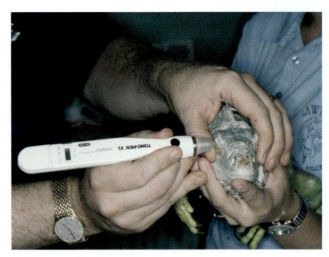

FIGURE 20-4 Tonometry in a Green Iguana *(Iguana iguana)*.

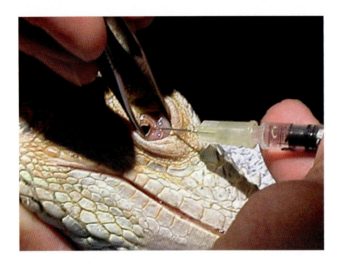

FIGURE 20-3 Intracameral injection of atracurium to dilate the iris of a Green Iguana *(Iguana iguana)*. This patient is anesthetized. *(Photograph courtesy of D. Mader.)*

which is unaffected by topical mydriatics routinely used in mammals.[2] Two ways of inducing mydriasis are with general anesthesia or with intracameral injection of neuromuscular blocking agents. Mitchell and others[11] have shown that topical application of neuromuscular blocking agents is not effective in achieving mydriasis and concluded that this may be related to a lack of corneal penetration of the drugs. The intracameral injection is performed with local anesthesia (proxymetacaine, applied topically to species without a spectacle) or with sedation (for those with spectacles). The technique requires a 27-gauge to 30-gauge needle to be advanced through the limbal conjunctiva and the cornea, into the anterior chamber where the neuromuscular blocking agent is administered, but in small volumes (Figure 20-3). Reports of 0.05 to 0.1 mL of d-tubocurarine[12] or 0.1 mL of 20 mg/mL curare have been found.[2] The resulting mydriasis may last from 30 minutes to several hours for d-tubocurarine[12] to even days for curare.[2] In snakes and lizards that have a spectacle (see subsequent), an injection into the subspectacular space should not be confused with an intracameral injection, and such an injection has been found not to cause mydriasis.[2]

Ancillary ophthalmic aids, such as tonometry (Figure 20-4), stains, bacteriology, cytology, histopathology, or electronmicroscopy, should not be overlooked nor should routine investigatory tools such as hematology, biochemistry, and radiography. Special mention should be made of the usefulness of ultrasound (a 10-mHz probe is necessary) for the assessment of the globe or retroorbital evaluation,[7,13] which is easily performed, in most species, with manual restraint alone.

PARIETAL EYE

Anatomy

The parietal eye is also known as the third eye, median eye, or pineal accessory apparatus. It is found in two distinct groups of reptiles (order Squamata, suborder Sauria [Lacertillia], and order Rhynchocephalia). This is the remnant of the median eye of provertebrates, which was originally a paired visual organ on the roof of the head.[6] In reptiles, it still appears as an eye-like structure, on the top of the head, situated in a hole beneath the parietal bone.[14] Supporting evidence has shown that dinosaurs had a pineal foramen that was thought to have contained a parietal eye.[15] The overlying scales show varying degrees of transparency (almost clear in *Sphenodon punctatus*) and are described as a cornea-like apparatus.[15] Lactertilla, which have a prominent parietal eye, include Slow Worms, monitors, lacertids, some iguanids, and skinks.[16]

Histologically, the parietal eye is variable in complexity and design but has been shown to always have a neurologic input and to contain a primitive retina. In the Tuatara (*Sphenodon punctatus*), *Anguis* spp., *Varanus* spp., and *Sceloporus* spp. the retina is cup shaped and surrounded by a fibrous capsule with a lens-like structure above and attached to the retina on both sides.[6,16] The posterior space between the lens and the retina is filled with a material that resembles the vitreous of the lateral eyes. No irises, lids, or muscles are found.[16] The retina of the parietal eye, unlike that of the lateral eye, has few but larger ganglion cells, and the photoreceptoral processes protrude forward into the lumen.[15] The retinal innervation leads to the parietal nerve, which is a small nonmyelinated structure that may have two branches and a not entirely known distribution of the fibers.[15]

Physiology

Although the true function of this organ remains a mystery,[17] a relationship and connection exists between the parietal eye, the pineal body,[15] the diencephalons of the forebrain, and especially the Habenular nucleus.[6,16] With no parietal eye (Gekkonids), the pineal body has been noted to be reduced in size.[15] The parietal eye is thought to play a role in both hormone production and thermoregulation[6] by acting as a dosimeter[14,16] to the presence and intensity of solar irradiation and allowing optimal timing for reproduction and other activities.[15] Electroretinographic (ERG) studies suggest that the parietal eye has a slower response to light than do lateral eyes and that this is irrespective of the light wavelength.[15] The experimental effects of removal of the parietal eye in various lizards have shown changes in basking behavior and activity cycles[16] and a lower thermal tolerance.[15] This is probably because of the close physiologic relationship between the parietal eye and the pineal body. The pineal body is responsible for producing melatonin and serotonin, both of which have marked effects on the sleep and awake cycles, and the parietal eye has been reported as having high levels of melatonin-forming enzymes (hydroxyindole O-methyltransferase).[15] This connection between the parietal eye acting as a dosimeter is further supported by the natural absence of the parietal eye in nocturnal lizards,[15] although exceptions exist, such as in Teiids and some geckos.

EYELIDS

Anatomy

Eyelids within the class Reptilia could well fill a chapter in itself. Reptiles are divided into those with functional eyelids with a normal palpebral fissure, to those with immobile and fused eyelids (spectacle) with no palpebral fissure, and all the possible variations in between.[18] The variation, however, does not just stop there because even that group of reptiles with functional eyelids and normal palpebral fissures can be further divided on the basis of the various adaptations and changes that occur within the lower eyelid. Chelonia and Crocodilia all have functional eyelids with normal palpebral fissures, and the main variation to functionality of the eyelids and size of the palpebral fissure is mainly found in the squamates. Reptiles with spectacles are not dealt with in this section but have a separate heading of their own (Spectacles).

In most reptiles, the upper eyelid is the smaller and less mobile of the two,[14] which is the reverse of the mammalian situation. The lizards are no exception, with the lower eyelid being the more moveable.[2] Most species have a third eyelid. In Lacertidae, Teiidae, Scincidae, Cordylosaurus, Lanthanotus, and Anolis, some of the lower eyelid has become transparent,[2,19] with reduced or absent scales.[19] Some iguanids just have a few scales that are semitransparent when the eyelid is closed but are hidden within folds when the eyelid is open.[19]

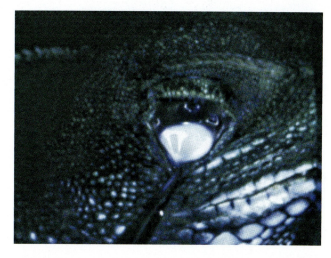

FIGURE 20-5 Tarsal plate of a Water Dragon (*Physignathus* sp.).

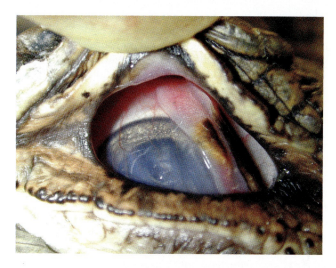

FIGURE 20-6 Transparent third eyelid in a Caiman (*Dracaena* sp.).

These are a protective mechanism to allow varying degrees of vision when the eyelids are closed, providing protection from sand or grit.[2,19] Some lizards have a tarsal plate in the lower eyelid that offers support and is made of fibrous tissue[19] (Figure 20-5). Ablepharus and ground geckos often have fused eyelids that form a spectacle, which is dealt with under the heading Spectacle. If any doubt exists as to the presence of true mobile eyelids or not, one should look for a nictitating membrane because whenever the eyelids are mobile, it is present.[19]

Similar to most lizards, the lower eyelid of Chelonia is larger and more mobile than the upper eyelid.[19] The presence of a transparent window in the eyelid is rare in Chelonia and is only found in Chelodina or Emyda.

In crocodilians, the upper eyelid is more mobile and, like humans, has a well-developed tarsal plate (tarsus),[12,19] although this may often become ossified with age.[20] The nictitating membrane (third eyelid) of crocodilians is well developed but semitransparent (Figure 20-6) with a cartilaginous plate.[19] The presence of this third eyelid and the ability to close it across the eye even when the eyelids are open can make examination difficult[2] but is a highly desirable protective feature. In aged alligators, calcium or other salt deposits can lead to an opacification of the normally clear third eyelid.[2]

Trauma

Trauma frequently affects the eyelids and may occur in all species. Trauma is particularly noted in Red-eared Sliders (*Trachemys scripta elegans*) as a result of fighting frenzy at the time of feeding.[21]

In most cases, traumatized lids need only topical antiseptic treatment (povidone-iodine) and cleaning to allow healing. More substantial lesions need surgical intervention, as was the case in which substantial damage to the eyelids as a result of heatlamp burns resulted in loss of function, requiring a blepharoplasty to return some normal function.[22] Often simple repair to return normal anatomic apposition is all that is necessary.

Blepharedema and Blepharitis

Swollen eyelids can be the result of a fluid edema (blepharedema) or more solid swelling (blepharitis). Often one can lead to the other. A blepharospasm is often the presenting clinical sign. Blepharospasm may be present in association with other ocular pathology or disease (see subsequent). Only primary blepharedema and blepharitis are dealt with here. As always, samples should be taken for further investigation and to allow a definitive diagnosis for the correct treatment.

Blepharedema is a common finding in reptiles, especially aquatic Chelonia,[23] and is often associated with hypovitaminosis A (also see Lacrimal System, subsequently, and Chapter 59). Hypovitaminosis A is the most common problem that affects the ocular adnexa.[2,23] The lack of vitamin A leads to changes that result in squamous metaplasia of the orbital glands and their ducts. This leads to a replacement of the mucus-secreting cells by flattened keratinized squamous epithelium and the gland lamina become dilated and filled with keratinaceous and cellular debris.[24] Once the cells have undergone squamous metaplasia, they no longer perform their protective functions and opportunistic bacterial infection is easier. As a direct effect of the lack of tears and formation of these metaplastic cells, blepharedema, and a secondary blepharitis and conjunctivitis, occurs.[2,23] A good clinical history often allows the diagnosis to be suspected and response to treatment used to confirm a diagnosis. Where treatment does not improve the condition, biopsies for histopathology prove useful. Treatment with vitamin A is dose related, and care must always be taken to prevent iatrogenic hypervitaminosis A. Daily injections of 10,000 IU vitamin A for 20 days have failed to cause a response, but 100,000 IU vitamin A/kg in food each third day brought about an improvement.[23] Swollen eyelids are not just seen in Chelonia with hypovitaminosis A but also in a colony of Green Anoles (*Anolis carolinensis*).[24] Blepharitis (closure of the eyelids) associated with hypovitaminosis A is partly the result of the increase in bulk of the eyelids caused by enlargement of the ophthalmic glands.[23] Blepharitis can also be associated with a wide range of bacteria and can result in granulomata or abscess formation. Blepharitis can also be associated with parasitic infestations, and five parasites (genus *Foleyella*) removed surgically from a newly imported Oustalet's Chameleon (*Chamaeleo oustaleti*) have been described with such a cause.[25] Eyelid scrapes for cytology should always be the first approach. Where bacteria are shown, samples for culture and sensitivity are advised. Where granuloma or abscess formation has occurred, surgical removal is necessary but with care to preserve the anatomic position of the eyelids. Sliding graft for eyelid surgery in reptiles is possible but is more involved than in mammals and is a reason for referral.

Neoplasia

Viral neoplasia of the eyelids has frequently been reported in a number of species of reptiles. No reports are found of non-viral-related neoplasia of the eyelids; however, these can occur (Figure 20-7). Viral neoplasia reported includes fibropapilloma in Green Seaturtles (*Chelonia mydas*) (see Figure 76-34, C), papillomata in Green Lizards (*Lacertillia* spp.) (Figure 20-8), and papillomata associated with poxvirus in the Speckled Caiman (*Caiman crocodilus*).[2,12] Poxvirus in the caiman can be seen as lesions anywhere on the skin, including the eyelids, as focal raised papules.[2]

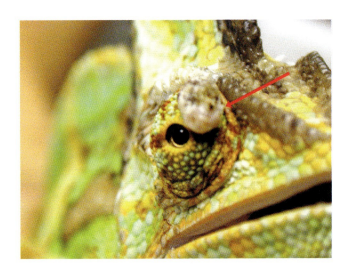

FIGURE 20-7 Papilloma on a chameleon eyelid.

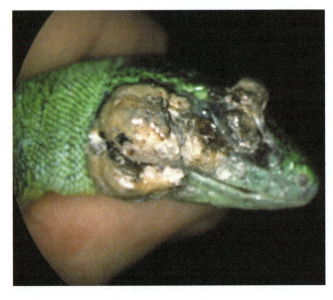

FIGURE 20-8 Papillomata (viral related) around the face in a European Lizard (*Lacerta* sp.).

The herpesvirus infection of Green Seaturtles may cause severe cutaneous and multisystemic visceral involvement other than the eyes.[26] The lesions have been reported as affecting the cornea, eyelids, periocular skin, and conjunctiva[2,26] and are seen as proliferative ulcerative lesions[2] that are typically pedunculated or polypoid with verrucous surface composed of hyperplastic epithelium overlying a collagenous stroma containing reactive fibroblasts[26] (see Chapter 76). This condition is often made worse by secondary bacterial infections, usually gram negative. In all these cases, surgery may be attempted, although because the tumors are associated with viruses, recurrence is common and any infected individuals are a potential source of infection for others in a colony.

Diagnosis can often be made on the basis of gross appearance, but histopathologic examination is definitive for the typical lesions.

SPECTACLES

Anatomy

When the eyelids are fused, they form a transparent membrane over the globe, which is known by many terms, including *spectacle, brille, eyecap, eye scale, watchglass,* and *goggle.*[6,14,27] The *spectacle* is the term that is used here. Three types of spectacles have been described[6]; the type found in squamates are the tertiary spectacle. Embryologically, a circular lid fold forms for all vertebrates, but in squamates (that have spectacles) this gradually closes over the globe, with the aperture moving dorsally and shrinking until it vanishes.[6,19] This dorsal movement of the aperture means that most of the squamate spectacle is composed of the lower eyelid. In the uropeltid snake *(Rhinophis* spp.) a small horizontal slit-like palpebral fissure is present in the newborn.[6,19]

All snakes, Amphisbaenidae, some geckos, some Lacertilia (*Ablepharus* sp., *Ophisops* sp., *Aniella* sp., Dibamidae, Anelytropidae, Euchirotidae), some Teiidae, Uroplatus, Pygopodidae, and Xantusiidae have fused eyelids with no palpebral fissure.[6] Although sometimes incorrectly reported as having spectacles, *Eublepharis* spp. and *Coleonyx* spp. have normal eyelids, confirmed by the existence of the nictitating membranes.

The spectacle is composed of skin and therefore is a dry horny scale that is transparent. The spectacle has been referred to as a fixed window covered by the *stratum corneum* of the epidermis.[5] The surface of the spectacle is insensitive. Lizards with spectacles often are seen cleaning this surface with their tongues.[14] Microsilicone injection of the spectacle has shown it to be highly vascular,[2] and although in normal circumstances these vessels are not readily seen, they become apparent with underlying inflammation (Figure 20-9).[18,27] The vascularity increases during ecdysis, when a change in color of the spectacle is brought about by the separation of the new and old layers of the epidermis by a fluid layer between. The spectacle becomes transparent again just before molting.[2]

The most important point to remember is that the spectacle is not part of, nor is it attached to, the cornea.[18] A space separates the spectacle and the cornea—the subspectacular space. This space has also been referred to as the intraconjuctival space.[6] The spectacle functions like a contact lens[19] under which the eye is fully mobile and independent. The subspectacular space is the equivalent of the conjunctival sac or space in mammals, except it is enclosed by the spectacle (Figure 20-10).[18] The space is filled with the secretions of the Harderian gland (see Lacrimal System), which provides lubrication and easy movement of the globe (although this is limited) beneath the spectacle. Despite this anatomic arrangement to allow movement, spontaneous movements of the globe are not frequently noted because the bursalis and retractor bulbi muscles are absent.[19] The thick, oily Harderian secretions do have a high reflective index and are thought to have some optical importance.[6]

Abrasions and Ulcers

The spectacle is an important evolutionary development that protects the delicate cornea in animals that live in an environment or have a lifestyle that would otherwise risk substantial trauma to this sensitive structure with risk of sight damage or blindness.[18] The spectacle is a physical barrier, and as such it is also impervious to most topical medicaments,[2] making treatment of the underlying cornea or globe difficult if not impossible without a subspectacle injection or application (Figure 20-11).

Spectacles are protective in function, therefore some trauma naturally occurs and is noted on routine examination. Damage to the spectacles of snakes may occur from a variety of causes. Factors that can lead to damage include the hazards of feeding live prey, especially to captive breed species,

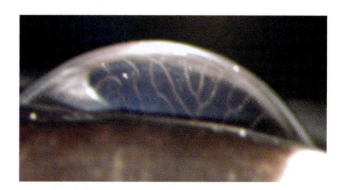

FIGURE 20-9 Normal spectacle vascularization.

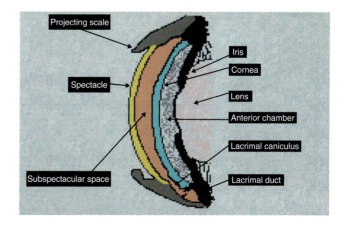

FIGURE 20-10 Diagram of the tertiary spectacle of reptiles.

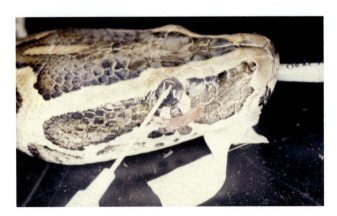

FIGURE 20-11 Flushing the subspectacular space as part of the treatment of an abscess of the space.

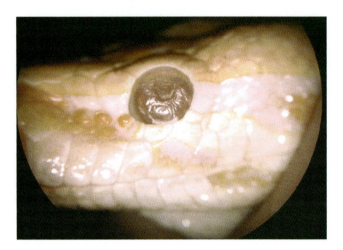

FIGURE 20-13 Ulcerated spectacle.

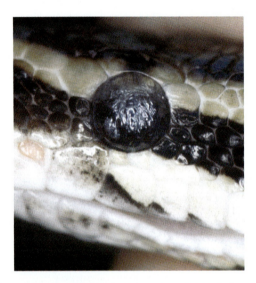

FIGURE 20-12 Abraded spectacle in a Royal (Ball) Python *(Python regius).*

inappropriate environment, dysecdysis, and incorrect treatment of retained spectacles.[18] The spectacle is also subject to infectious or parasitic conditions. Only after a full ophthalmic examination can the degree of damage be assessed. Further investigations may also be necessary, including the use of scrapings for cytology or bacterial culture and sensitivity. In severe or chronic conditions, biopsy may be necessary for histopathologic examination.

In most circumstances, damage to the spectacle is normal and is of no adverse consequence, especially as on shedding, any damage to the surface is rectified by the loss of that old surface. Excessive rubbing can be seen on the surface of the spectacle. Scratches and minor abrasions regularly occur without any discomfort (Figure 20-12). If loss of transparency of the spectacle occurs, then the underlying cause should be assessed; causes include ecdysis, inflammatory deposits on the inner surface,[28] exposure to chemicals, or retention of spectacles and any bacterial or fungal infection. The use of organophosphate insecticide or volatile polyurethane organic solvents for chemical fogging of the vivaria has been implicated in a thickening of the deeper cellular layers of the spectacle and a resulting loss of transparency in *Lampropeltis* sp.[29]

Deeper abrasions can, in some circumstances, be more correctly referred to as ulcers once the epidermis has been breached (Figure 20-13).[18] These more noticeable abrasions are always secondary to an underlying problem with husbandry or disease, such as low humidity, parasites, or dysecdysis. The increased and often constant rubbing of the face against rocks, trees, or other objects in the vivaria results in abrasions to the spectacle. This appears as loss of clarity of the spectacle, with abrasions varying from superficial scratches to deep ulcers. The accumulation of substrate (particularly sawdust) also may be forced under the superficial layers of the spectacle. Once the spectacle is damaged, associated neovascularization or secondary infection may also be seen.

Providing the abrasions are not full thickness (see Loss of Spectacle), treatment is with topical antibiotics (ophthalmic or dermal) and correction of the underlying problem usually leads to no permanent damage. Steroidal combinations should be avoided because these could lead to delayed healing or predisposition to secondary infection, particularly fungal. Surgical debridment may be necessary with excessive roughness or pocketing or looseness of the edges of the skin or with accumulation of substrate under the surface layer of the spectacle. Any debridement is best performed with the aid of an operating microscope to allow reliable removal of all the foreign material, especially when organic, to prevent the possibility of foreign body reaction or granuloma formation. If the development of scarring should occur during the healing stage, this usually disappears after the next or subsequent slough. Very rarely does damage or treatment of abrasions result in permanent opacity to the spectacle.

Loss of Spectacle

More substantial trauma to the spectacle usually involves avulsion, which is serious because it may result in corneal desiccation from a lack of continuity of the tear film and may ultimately result in loss of the eye, despite topical antibiotic therapy.[1,18] The spectacle is important for maintaining the tear film within the subspectacular space. The loss of a small part of the spectacle may have only minimal effects by increasing overflow (through the deficit) or evaporation of tears. If total loss of the spectacle occurs, this leads to the loss of the tear film and eventual desiccation of the cornea (Figure 20-14) or a panophthalmitis. The loss of the protective spectacle and

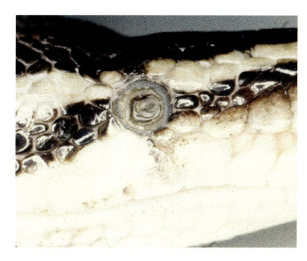

FIGURE 20-14 Desiccated eye through loss of the right spectacle.

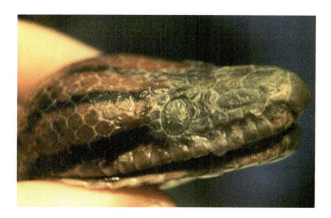

FIGURE 20-15 Dermal fungal infection that affects the spectacle.

the underlying fluid leads to damage of this single delicate layer of corneal epithelium (see Cornea). The resulting damage to the cornea by drying probably leads to infection, ulceration, scarring, and permanent opacity with loss of vision. In severe cases, shrinking of the globe (phthisis bulbi) occurs.

Loss of the spectacle can occur from a number of causes. The most common cause of the loss of the whole spectacle is associated with an inexperienced herpetologist (or veterinarian) attempting to remove a normal spectacle (wrongly diagnosed as a retained spectacle) with cellophane tape or forceps.[18] Other causes of loss include trauma (particularly as a sequel to long-term abrasion of the spectacle) or infection (see subsequent). Feeding of live prey (rodents) could also result in injury or penetration of the spectacle and should be avoided.

Treatment may be attempted with topical antibiotics and artificial tears, a cut-down soft contact lens, or transposition of an oral mucosa flap over the eye.[30] The use of a mucosal flap may save the eye but seldom allows normal vision, even though (like conjunctival grafts to the cornea in mammals) some long-term clearing may be seen. Some success has recently been achieved with a collagen graft material.[31]

Infection: Bacterial and Fungal

Although it is transparent, the spectacle is dermal and this fact should not be forgotten at any stage of the assessment. Swabs, scrapes, and even biopsies can be performed to allow assessment with cytologic, histopathologic, bacterial, or fungal examinations, as they would for any other dermal abnormality on the body.[18] Topical dyes routinely used for the examination of the cornea (such as Rose Bengal or fluorescein) have little advantage for assessment of the spectacle. For infection beneath the spectacle, see Subspectacular Abscess.

Infections of the external surface of the skin are a common problem. Bacterial infections usually involve opportunistic gram-negative bacteria. In some cases, the epidermal layer may become infected with bacteria and result in an intraspectacular dermatitis.[32] In severe cases, such an infection may be noted to spread beyond the margins of the spectacle.[18] This is often caused by retained spectacles or poor hygiene. Such an infection, in itself, could lead to retained spectacles or even the loss of a spectacle or the eye. Treatment may require surgical incision to allow debridement and application of a suitable antibiotic agent. Where systemic spread is suspected, parenteral antibiotics may also be necessary.

Fungal infections are often encountered and are considered to be a reflection of poor management.[2] They are usually slower to develop, with the resulting infection causing more deformity of the spectacle, particularly thickening and pigmentary changes.[18] The changes are seldom restricted to just the spectacle and often involve surrounding scales or even the whole head (Figure 20-15). Fungal infections need to be identified and treated at an early stage or they spread further. Diagnosis is based on cytology, culture, and sensitivity. These infections, if diagnosed early enough, can be treated with topical dermal antifungal creams, lotions, or ointments. A fungal infection from *Fusarium oxysporum* was reported[33] as penetrating the spectacle, and treatment required enucleation of the eye.

Subspectacular Abscess

Infection under the spectacle, involving the subspectacular space, is a common problem.[2] Infection is thought to occur either from a penetration wound, from the mouth via the nasolacrimal ducts, or from systemic infection and hematogenous spread.[2,12,28,34] It can also be associated with conjunctivitis.[35] Although with a primary infection only one eye is affected, with septicemic spread the infection could be unilateral or bilateral.

The spectacle appears cloudy or white (leukoria) and may sometimes, but not always, be distorted.[18] In cases of unilateral involvement, whether the infection is local or secondary to septicemia is important. White blood cell counts and sometimes blood cultures are necessary for differentiation. If the infection is secondary to septicemia, then locating the site of origin of the primary infection and undertaking treatment of this at the same time as dealing with the subspectacular abscess is important.

Treatment and obtaining material for cytology or culture requires a small wedge resection of the spectacle (spectaculotomy) and removal of the material. This should be performed with anesthesia for greatest control and comfort to the reptile. On opening the subspectacular space, a swab should be taken of any material (Figure 20-16) and submitted for culture and sensitivity; a stained smear may be useful in confirming a bacterial infection. The subspectacular space should then be flushed out with balanced salt solution or another suitable

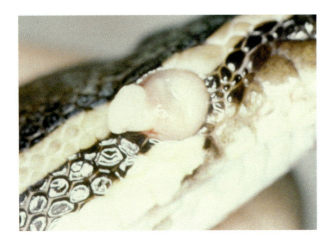

FIGURE 20-16 Subspectacular abscess after lancing.

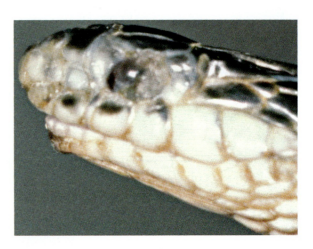

FIGURE 20-17 Retained spectacle in a Gartersnake (*Thamnophis sirtalis*).

solution and an ophthalmic antibiotic solution such as ciprofloxacin or gentamicin (see Figure 20-11). Depending on the culture and sensitivity results, systemic antibiotic treatment may also be necessary.

Parasites

Parasites, especially mites or ticks, are not uncommonly found around the adnexa.[36] Mites (*Ophionyssus* spp.) are commonly found between the thin skin in the area of the sulcus formed by the periorbital scales and the spectacle. Ticks (*Ixodidae*) are only found on newly imported species. Although ticks may be found anywhere on the body, they are more usually found around the cloaca or head of snakes. They usually attach to the softer skin between scales or at the junction where the spectacle meets the scales of the head.

Parasitic infestation can lead to retained spectacles and the possibility of spread of bacterial or viral disease. Slit-lamp biomicroscopy is often necessary for detection of the presence of the mites, but even then detection may prove difficult as they are deep within the sulcus. Parasites may be physically removed (to thus confirm the diagnosis) by flushing with a suitable solution (such as balanced salt solution) via a fine 24-gauge cannula.[18] They may also be noted after the removal of a retained spectacle.

One must remember that parasites are always an environmental problem and removal is not sufficient to eliminate the problem and prevent recurrence. Flushing with ivermectin (Ivomec; MSD Agvet) is a good method of physical removal of mites from the sulcus of the spectacle.[18] This technique requires the instillation of a small amount (0.2 mL) of undiluted ivermectin flushed around the sulcus, which is then 2 minutes later followed by a thorough flushing with saline solution to remove the parasites. Although a possibility of transdermal absorption exists, the small volume of ivermectin and the thorough flushing seem to remove any potential toxic effects.

Retained Spectacle

Retained spectacle is the most common ocular problem of snakes.[18,37,38] Geckos may also, less commonly, develop problems with retained spectacles, but this is almost entirely associated with bacterial infection and is considered secondary to this. The rest of this section concentrates only on the condition in snakes. Although the etiology is multiple, usually environmental conditions are contributory if not the cause.[21] The condition arises because of a failure of the old spectacle to be shed during ecdysis.[18,21,39] The most common cause is a dry environment or dehydration (such as associated with systemic illness).[2] Other factors, such as inadequate nutrition or systemic disease, may also be contributory.[12] Scarring and the presence of mites may also lead to dysecdysis and retained spectacles. Not unusual on the removal of a retained spectacle is finding the mite (*Ophionyssus natricis*) still clinging to the spectacle or within the sulcus formed from the spectacle and the protruding scales of the orbit ridge. Any cause of skin disease could also lead to the retention of spectacles,[18] including a suggestion of thyroid dysfunction.[10]

Temporary visual impairment may result from the retention of several spectacles (Figure 20-17). The retained spectacles may become secondarily infected, resulting in permanent blindness. If not removed, subsequent shedding is also inhibited and the spectacles build up to form a thickened mass of dead skin that affects the snake's vision and may affect its willingness or ability to feed.[18] The more retained layers, the easier is diagnosis of the retained spectacle. A single retained spectacle may have only limited effects on the vision of the snake and is often missed by the owner, being picked up only during routine clinical examination at the time of presentation for other reasons. Often an associated creasing of the spectacle is seen as a dent in the surface when a spectacle has been retained but subsequently was shed. Royal (Ball) Pythons seem to be particularly prone to this phenomenon (Figure 20-18). Even a single retained spectacle has this effect after a while. Although the absence of denting cannot be used to eliminate the possibility of a retained spectacle, the denting of a healthy spectacle (without a retained spectacle) is in itself pathognomonic of a previously retained spectacle. The denting decreases with time and usually disappears after the next slough, providing the spectacle is shed easily at that stage. This creasing or indenting of the new spectacle appears to have no effect on vision.

Diagnosis of a retained spectacle requires more than examining a slough and failing to find spectacles. Where dysecdysis is seen with retained skin still on the head and around, or

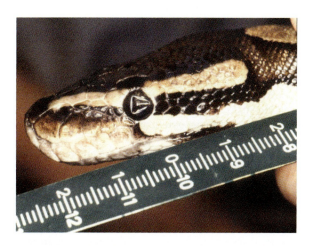

FIGURE 20-18 Indented spectacle in a Royal (Ball) Python (*Python regius*).

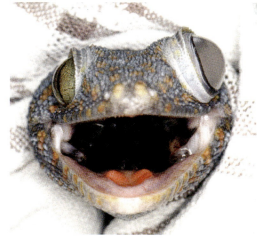

FIGURE 20-19 Left increased subspectacular space from failure of tear drainage in a Tokay Gecko (*Gekko gecko*).

leading to, the spectacle, the diagnosis is easy. Diagnosis is also easily made when multiple retained layers are found. The difficulty arises with the possibility of only one retained layer, when no indentation or opacification is seen. Examination with magnification, ideally with a slit lamp, allows visualization of the increased thickness of the spectacle associated with the extra layers.[18] A look at the edges of the spectacle is useful because often tags of skin may be in this area, especially if the head skin has been sloughed but only the spectacle is retained. Failure to confirm a spectacle is indeed retained before attempting treatment may lead to iatrogenic damage to the spectacle (see subsequent). If any doubt exists as to whether or not a spectacle is retained, no treatment should be attempted but to wait until after the next slough and reexamine at that time.

Treatment involves soaking the retained spectacle to aid its removal. This is best done with a wet cotton swab and rubbing from the medial and lateral canthi toward the center of the spectacle. If the spectacle does not detach after gentle manipulation with a cotton swab, then artificial tears (hydromellose, Tears Naturale; Alcon) are applied several times daily for a few days to soften the spectacle and the technique is repeated. Although Frye[40] advises the use of forceps or other instruments to remove a retained spectacle, this author considers that this technique should not be the first course of treatment and should only be used by an experienced veterinarian and with magnification because of a great risk of damage to, or even avulsion of, the underlying spectacle. The inadvertent removal of a new spectacle, as opposed to a retained spectacle, leads to exposure keratitis[1,2] and eventual loss of the eye. If the retained spectacle cannot be removed easily, then waiting until the next slough to try again is best.

Pseudobuphthalmos

Blockage of the nasolacrimal system is more commonly encountered as a clinical problem in snakes and geckos (Figure 20-19) than in any other reptile.[2,8] Any fluid not draining down the nasolacrimal ducts is incapable of overflowing the eyelid margin and accumulates in the subspectacular space. If an accumulation of fluid is in the subspectacular space because of a failure to drain through the nasolacrimal duct, then the spectacle is seen to bulge. This is correctly referred to as *pseudobuphthalmos*.[41] The resultant stretching of the spectacle has also been referred to in the literature as a *bullous spectaculopathy*.[32,42] This term was used because of the considered similarity to bullous keratopathy seen in mammals, where bullae or vesicles form within the epithelial cells of the cornea and can become large and even pendulous with the possibility of rupture.[43,44] The definition of a bulla is a cavitation, larger than a vesicle, within the epidermis.[45] The buildup of fluid within the subspectacular spaces cannot, therefore, be referred to as bullous, nor indeed does it involve the spectacle per se. It should not, therefore, be referred to as bullous spectaculopathy but pseudobuphthalmos.

This condition was first described[1] in an Indigo Snake (*Drycmarchon corais*) as an "acute proptosis," but examination confirmed the accumulation of a clear, colorless fluid between the spectacle and the cornea causing the spectacle to protrude with a noticeable enlargement in the subspectacular space that was evident on slit-lamp biomicroscopy.[21] Pseudobuphthalmos is differentiated from subspectacular abscesses in that the fluid is clear.

Investigation of the patency of the nasolacrimal duct is possible with injection of a small amount of fluorescein dye through the lateral canthus of the spectacle into the subspectacular space, as mentioned previously. However, when blockage is present, the increased pressure is likely to push fluid out through even the smallest hole in the spectacle. Chronic increase in pressure can eventually lead to damage of the cornea or even the globe itself.[18]

This condition may be only a temporary problem, and in one case, the eye returned to normal within 3 days without any therapy.[1] However, if it persists, then it is an abnormality that needs treatment. The distension has been suggested to be treated with a small wedge-shaped area in the ventral spectacle,[10] but recurrence with this technique has been reported when the wedge is too small.[8] Even with a 30-degree wedge section removed from the inferior quadrant, recurrence was noted and eventually led to the rupture of the lacrimal duct and fluid forming within the face.[28] This author considers that irrespective of the size of the wedge removed, a high risk of recurrence always exists and if too big a wedge is removed, problems can develop from exposure keratitis or secondary infection. The critical and essential part of the treatment is to either treat the blocked nasolacrimal duct or create a new drainage canal.[18] A new drainage canal (conjunctivoralostomy) should be formed between the medial aspect of the inferior fornix of the subspectacular space and the mouth, emerging between the palatine and maxillary teeth. This is performed with an 18-gauge needle; the conjunctivoralostomy should be prevented from closing too quickly with a 0.635-mm Silastic/silicon tube,[27,28] which should be sutured in place on the periorbital scales and left in situ for a suitable period of time, such as up to 6 weeks.[18] Any fluid removed from the subspectacular space should always be examined with the microscope (fresh and stained) as it has been reported that numerous flagellates have been found in subspectacular exudates.[28]

LACRIMAL SYSTEM

Anatomy

The lacrimal (also cited as lachrymal or ophthalmic) glands are variable within the class Reptilia.[23] Most Sauria and Chelonia have a Harderian (Harder's) gland in the orbitonasal (medial) region[23,46] and a lacrimal gland in the orbitotemporal (lateral) region.[23] Conjunctival glands are also found and are mainly associated with the upper lid.[19]

The Harderian gland is firmly fixed in the medial part of the orbit, with the duct normally opening on the surface of the nictitating membrane (where present).[46] This is common to all groups of terrestrial vertebrates and was first described by Johan Harder in 1694, after whom the gland was named. Histologically, an enormous similarity is seen in reptiles between the lacrimal and Harderian glands that prevents them from being identified on sections only.[23] In Chelonia, confusion exists over which is the Harderian gland and which is the posterior lacrimal gland; the literature names both.[46] This has caused much doubt on claims such that the Harderian gland is absent in many geckos and chameleons.[2,19] In various Chelonia (*Testudo graeca*, *Trachemys scripta*, and *Chelonia mydas*), salt-secreting cells have been shown within the Harderian glands; these play a part in osmoregulation.[2] A large number of immunocompetent cells are also in the Harderian gland.[46]

Snakes are generally accepted as having no lacrimal gland,[5,6,12,14] and Williams[32] appears to be alone in considering that snakes have both lacrimal and Harderian glands. This lack of a lacrimal gland in snakes is an odd arrangement because the lacrimal glands are usually associated with the upper and lower lids and the Harderian gland is usually associated with the nictitating membrane,[46] which is absent in snakes. The Harderian gland is mainly posterior to the orbit and is large except in sea snakes, where it is reduced but still present.[2] The Harderian gland produces an oily secretion, and the lacrimal gland produces a watery secretion. The tear production in snakes is from the Harderian gland, which enters and fills the subspectacular space. The oily Harderian secretion is superior in lubrication properties to the watery lacrimal tears, and thus, the retention of the Harderian gland and loss of the lacrimal gland is of advantage to the squamates with spectacles, where the globe may otherwise run on the dorsal aspect of the spectacle. The duct of the Harderian gland opens directly into the lacrimal duct in *Natrix natrix*, but in more primitive snakes, it opens into the subspectacular space by several small ducts with a main duct opening into the lacrimal duct direct.[2] This oily secretion flows from the subspectacular space through the nasolacrimal duct first to the nose and then to the mouth.[6] In the family Dasypeltis (egg-eating snakes), the large Harderian gland contributes to the lubrication that is essential in swallowing the eggs whole.[46]

The nasolacrimal duct is absent in all Chelonia.[14] In crocodilians, the lacrimal ducts open in the front section of the nose, similar to mammals.[14]

Testing Patency

The lacrimal system can be tested with fluorescein. In reptiles with a palpebral fissure, the stain is placed into the eyes and where it drains into the mouth is noted. In squamates with a spectacle, the patency of the lacrimal ducts can still be shown with injection of 0.05 mL of fluorescein through a 30-gauge needle into the subspectacular space.[28] The technique requires the needle to pass through the spectacle near the lateral canthus with visualization of the eye with some form of magnification to prevent damage to the underlying (and very thin) cornea and examination of the mouth near Jacobson's organ for evidence of patency.[18] One must remember that tear staining syndrome seen in some species of tortoises (*Testudo* spp.) is the result of the lack of a functional nasolacrimal system and is not indicative of an abnormality.[35] The tears of Chelonia naturally spill over the eyelids and down the side of the face to eventually evaporate away, and any fluorescein placed into the eye does the same.

Keratoconjunctivitis Sicca (Dry Eye)

Keratoconjunctivitis sicca (dry eye) is seen in reptiles (Figure 20-20). It is related to a reduction or failure of production of the aqueous phase of the tear film and is usually associated with changes in the lacrimal and Harderian glands associated with vitamin A deficiency.[23] The deficiency also causes conjunctival and corneal epithelial metaplasia and

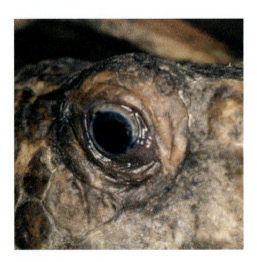

FIGURE 20-20 Kerratoconjunctivitis sicca (dry eye) in a Mediterranean Tortoise (*Testudo graeca*).

hyperkeratosis. Changes are reversible, but this is dependent on the length of time that the deficiency has existed. Often by the time the condition is presented to the veterinarian, permanent changes may have developed. Definitive diagnosis of the dry eye is made with cut down Schirmer tear test strips or phenol red thread placed into the conjunctival fossa to measure the aqueous phase of the tear film. Treatment of keratoconjunctivitis is similar to that used in mammals, with artificial tear preparations, and when xerothalmia (no tear production) is from vitamin A deficiency, administration of vitamin A on a weekly basis is advised.[35]

GLOBE

Anatomy

The globe of most reptiles, unlike that of birds, is almost spherical. The scleral bones (scleral ossicles), when present, number between 6 to 17, with *Testudo* spp. having 6 to 9, chameleons 11, and Spenodon 16 or 17.[6] The bones are compactly placed and overlap their neighbors such that they form an almost immobile cup. In Chelonia, in addition to the scleral ossicles that may extend to the corneal rim,[6] a scleral cartilage is seen, up to 1 cm thick. In chameleons, the scleral cartilage is reduced to the foveal region, but in most other lizards it extends from the posterior pole of the globe to beyond the equator.[19] The scleral ossicles serve to maintain the convexity of the globe, allowing the ciliary body to be close to the lens and play an important part in accommodation by changing the shape of the eye, therefore altering the distance between the cornea and fundus.

Scleral ossicles are absent in crocodilians, but scleral cartilage extensions are found well into the ora serrata,[2,19] forming a cartilaginous cup.[6]

The snake eye is totally different from all other reptiles in that it is slightly elongated along the visual axis.[19] The eye also has no scleral ossicles or cartilage but retains the spherical shape with the presence of tendinous connective tissue.[6] Pigmentary cells are found throughout the sclera.

Movement of the eye (except in chameleons) is limited because of the poor development of the rectus muscles, although, unlike birds, the retractor bulbi muscle is well developed. Chameleons have well-developed ocular muscles that allow a wide range of vision both monocular and binocular with 180 degrees in the horizontal plane and 90 degrees in the vertical plane.[14] Crocodilia have eyes situated dorsally so that even when they are in the water they can see as if they were placed above water level.[19] Land tortoises, crocodiles, and many diurnal lizards have narrow binocular vision of 25 degrees or less and thus rely on monocular vision.[14] Binocular vision is better in freshwater Chelonia (up to 30 degrees) and is most marked in the snapping turtle.[14]

The position of the eye in relation to the body has been shown[47] to affect the intraocular pressure in juvenile Loggerhead Seaturtles (*Caretta caretta*). In dorsoventral and ventrodorsal positions the turtle has lower intraocular pressures than when the head is in down position; this is a response that is also seen in humans and is the result of venous pressure gradients within the eyes and the head. The normal intraocular pressure of reptiles is far lower than in mammals, with an average of about 6 mm Hg.[47] A nonlinear negative relationship between body length and intraocular pressure was found in American Alligators (*Alligator mississippiensis*).[48] The intraocular pressure was found to decrease as the body length increased, with a relationship to length and age; therefore, a direct correlation may exist between the age and the intraocular pressure as has been found in some mammals.

The snake eye does not follow the normal reptilian format. Paleontologists and researchers generally agree that the snake evolved from the Varanidae.[18] Because of evolutionary changing lifestyles to involve a nocturnal, burrowing, or subterrestrial existence, modification to the serpentine eye occurred. The changes involved were many, but of particular importance were the formation of the spectacle and development of a yellow lens and loss of the scleral ossicles. These changes in the eye occurred at the same time as the loss of limbs, parietal eye, and ears. The eye is considered to have degenerated to a vestigial organ, and later the vertebrate eye was reinvented all over again to form its present structure, as the snakes came back to the surface.[6] This certainly explains the major differences (not just the spectacle) of the snake eye when compared with other reptilian species.

Congenital Abnormalities

Of the congenital abnormalities described for the reptilian globe, microphthalmia is the most common disorder and seems most common in snakes,[2,20] although cyclopia and anophthalmia have been noted.[2] Five cases of bilateral and two of unilateral microphthalmia in a clutch of 16 eggs from two Red-headed Ratsnakes (*Elaphe moellendorfii*) have been reported.[1] On histopathologic examination, normal structures were found within the small globes with the only abnormalities noted being the absence of lenses.[1] Factors that can cause microphthalmia include genetic factors, nutrition or incubation temperatures, and oxygen concentrations. Anophthalmia is rare but has been reported in several Northern Pinesnakes (*Pituophis melanoleucus melanoleucus*).[2] The occurrence of true anophthalmia is rare, and a reptile that appears not to have eyes should always be considered as a case of microphthalmia unless histopathology confirms the absence of an eye[27] (Figure 20-21).

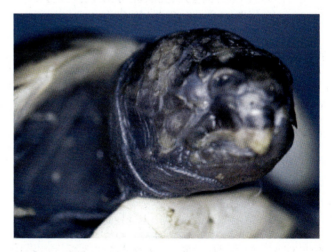

FIGURE 20-21 Microphthalmos in a hatchling Mediterranean Tortoise (*Testudo graeca*).

Exophthalmos

Any retro-orbital mass or swelling can result in exophthalmia. Ultrasonographic examination with a 10-mHz probe is a useful tool to investigate and allow a diagnosis of the cause of exophthalmos and even allows guided biopsy for the collection of samples for cytology, histopathology, and culture. Abscessation is the most common cause of exophthalmos or periorbital swelling, and surgery is always indicated.[13] An orbital varix (pathologic enlargement of one or more venous channels) has been described as a cause of an acute progressive swelling of one eye associated with an aneurysm of the retrobulbar vein, probably as a result of trauma.[7] Exophthalmia is often misdiagnosed in snakes and is really pseudobuphthalmos,[1] with the subspectacular space being enlarged and causing a magnification of the globe. A true unilateral congenital exophthalmia has been described,[37] with histopathologic results showing it to be a cyst-like structure with abundant eosinophils.

Infection: Bacterial and Fungal

Bacterial infection can lead to a widespread degeneration within the globe that can lead to granulomatous responses, often with the infection spreading beyond the globe itself.[49] Orbital infections can occur from hematogenous infection, penetrating injury, or foreign body.[50] The granulomatous response usually causes an enlargement of the globe, but as in other animals, severe trauma, inflammation, or infection can also lead to a shrinking of the eye (phthisis bulbi). A fungal infection in a Rainbow Boa (*Epicrates chenchria maurus*) has been reported as a cause of phthisis bulbi.[33]

Enucleation

With severe infection, inflammation, or trauma of the globe with little chance of a successful outcome (Figure 20-22), enucleation can be performed. In species with nonfused eyelids, the approach is the same as that described for mammals, where after removal of the globe, the eyelid margins are removed and then sutured together to form a permanent tarsorrhaphy over the empty orbit. In snakes, suggested treatment is that the whole of the spectacle and the globe be removed, the optic blood vessels sealed with hemostatic pressure, and the wound allowed to granulate over a period of 4 weeks.[33]

CONJUNCTIVA

Foreign Bodies

The examination of the conjunctivia should be routine in all reptiles with nonfused eyelids. Visual examination can still be performed (especially with magnification) in reptiles with a spectacle, but this is often limited because most of the conjunctiva is hidden from view. The frequent occurrence of foreign bodies within the conjunctival fornix is often linked to environmental conditions. In tortoises (*Testudo* spp.), ocular foreign bodies are a common finding in those that hibernate in hay[35] (Figure 20-23) or sand (Figure 20-24). Lizards kept on peat or sand may occasionally get these materials into their eyes, resulting in blepharospasm.[35] Treatment is the removal of the foreign body by grasping it, with the aid of magnification,

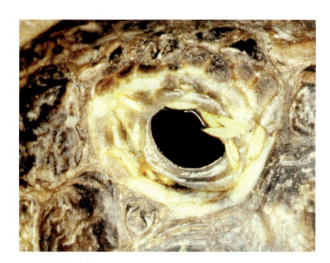

FIGURE 20-23 Grass seed foreign body after brumation (hibernation) in the eye of a Mediterranean Tortoise (*Testudo graeca*).

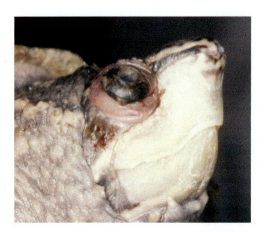

FIGURE 20-22 Prolapsed and ruptured globe in a Musk Turtle (*Sternotherus* sp.).

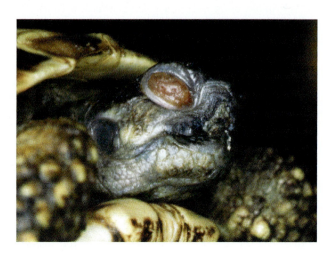

FIGURE 20-24 Conjunctival hyperplasia associated with foreign body (sand substrate) in a juvenile Mediterranean Tortoise (*Testudo graeca*).

with fine forceps or by physically flushing it out with a suitable solution (such as balanced salt or Hartmann's [lactated Ringer's] solution) via a soft fine gauge intravenous cannula. Any ulceration or abrasion of the cornea should be treated with topical antibiotic.

Conjunctivitis

Conjunctivitis is a common problem, although primary bacterial conjunctival infections are considered to be rarely reported[2] and secondary opportunistic bacteria are frequently encountered. In a survey of bacteria isolated from nondomesticated species with eye infections at a zoological collection,[51] five of the 19 reported cases involved reptiles and included infections associated with *Aeromonas* spp., *Pasteurella* spp., and *Pseudomonas* spp. In a laboratory colony of mixed lizards, an outbreak of conjunctivitis (with some developing respiratory disease) was associated with *Aeromona liquefaciens*.[52] A catarrhal conjunctivitis in a large group of Horsfield Tortoises (*Testudo horsfieldi* [*Agrionemys horsfieldi*]) was associated with *Proteus vulgaris* and *Citrobacter intermedium* but also had a heavy infestation with oxyurids and so thought was that the general debilitation of the tortoise resulted in an opportunistic bacterial infection.[53]

Bacterial conjunctivitis in mammals is frequently suggested by a mucopurulent discharge, but reptiles, as in birds, have a lack of lysosomes in the heterophils and therefore a mucopurulent discharge is not usually seen. Infectious conjunctivitis usually results in caseous plaques that are often retained within the conjunctival fornix but more commonly are involved with the corneal surface (see subsequent).[21,35] Cases of keratoconjunctivitis (where both the cornea and conjunctiva are involved) are more likely to be associated with poor hygiene.[10] Ocular discharge has been noted with bacterial infections of the conjunctiva in lizards and is associated with closure of the eyelids (blepharospasm) and accumulation of the discharge under the eyelids causing a bulging of the eyelids and a clear or opaque exude noted when the eyelids are stretched open.[52] Local extension of any infection could result in panophthalmitis and loss of the eye or even eventual septicemia and death (Figure 20-25).

The presence of plaques within the conjunctival fornix can cause a foreign body reaction. Any caseous material within the conjunctival fornix should be examined carefully with a microscope and, where indicated, for culture and sensitivity (Figure 20-26). Occasions also exist where conjunctival biopsies should be taken for histopathologic or electron microscopic examination to see whether it is of an infectious cause or the more common reaction associated with vitamin A deficiency. In hypovitaminosis A, the conjunctiva is displaced by desquamated cells that lead to the production of an amorphous mass forming a pseudoabscess and multiple retention cysts.[23] The material that accumulates in the conjunctival sac is a mixture of keratinous lamellae and eosinophil granulocytes.[23] One should always remember that the ocular changes are not all that occur and that this condition is a systemic disease (the kidneys and pancreas are also affected).

Caseous conjunctivitis is part of the herpesvirus-related lung, eye, and trachea disease (LETD) reported in Green Seaturtles.[54] An underlying secondary infection often involves gram-negative bacteria and a resultant keratoconjunctivitis. All turtles that are affected also have respiratory signs and are noted to have gasping sounds when they are surfaced and may often be unable to dive.[54]

Where conjunctivitis was noted in a survey of reptiles in a zoological collection,[51] it was found to be associated with blepharitis (blepharoconjunctivitis), corneal disease, or other problems. Any reptile (except those with spectacles) found with closed eyelids (blepharospasm) warrants a careful examination of the conjunctival fornix with magnification and wetted endodontic paper points to remove any caseous plaques and routine flushing with an appropriate solution via a fine soft cannula (24-gauge). Antibiotics, such as ciprofloxacin (Cilloxin, Alcon), usually control bacterial infections.[35] Conjunctivitis in snakes presents as a subspectacular abscess[35] and has been covered previously.

Infections: Viral

Fibropapilloma, the herpesvirus infection of Green Seaturtles, may cause proliferative or ulcerative lesions of the conjunctiva.[2,26]

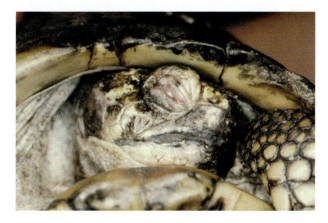

FIGURE 20-25 Orbital cellulitis and an ear abscess in a Mediterranean Tortoise (*Testudo graeca*).

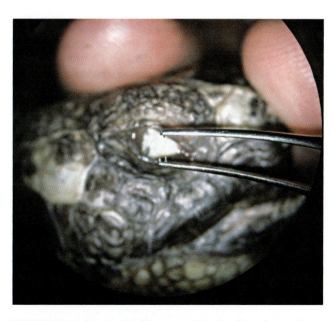

FIGURE 20-26 Pus in a Mediterranean Tortoise (*Testudo graeca*) eye.

Parasites

Parasitic conjunctivitis is well reported. Leeches *(Ozobrancus* sp.) have been found to parasite the conjunctiva of Green Seaturtles.[2] Six species of *Neopolystoma* spp. were isolated from the conjunctival sac of freshwater Chelonia, with a prevalence rate of 80% in one study,[55] although the intensity was low (one to three worms per animal).

CORNEA

Anatomy

The reptilian cornea is usually thin with no Bowman's membrane (layer). The crocodilian cornea is typically reptilian and thin.[19] In squamates with spectacles, only a single layer of corneal epithelium is found,[6,19] which is all that is necessary with the protection provided by the presence of the spectacle. In lizards, the Descemet's membrane is present in all but a few geckos.[19] In land Chelonia, the cornea is thick with a prominent Descemet's membrane.[6]

The corneas of Chelonia have small radii of curvature and are therefore optically powerful in air, contributing dioptric power to the eye. In aquatic species, the cornea is optically ineffective when in water, but they are able to overcome this loss and still focus properly.[56] Freshwater turtles have exceptionally well-developed ciliary and iris musculature and a highly flexible lens that provides a wide dioptric range, giving high visual acuity in both air and water despite the loss of the corneal refraction.[57] They are able to squeeze the lens (which is soft) through the pupil aperture,[6,19,56] which is similar to the accommodative changes seen in some diving birds. Two investigations have been undertaken of the visual acuity of the various Chelonia. The first was a retinoscope assessment of Green Seaturtles, which were compared with a Freshwater Turtle *(Clemmys insulpta)* and a Gopher Tortoise *(Gopherus polyphemus)*[57]; the second study involved anatomic dissection, the use of a streak retinoscope, and schematic eye calculations in a Red-eared Slider *(Trachemys scripta elegans)* and marine turtles *(Chlonia mydas, Dermochelys cariacea,* and *Eretmochelys imbricata)*.[56] Both studies came to the conclusion that the eyes of the marine turtles varied significantly compared with those of the freshwater turtles and land tortoises. The severe hyperopia of underwater is compensated by the accommodative changes of the lens.[56] The Green turtle was found to be emmetropic in water but extremely myopic when out of the water by Ehrenfeld and Kock.[57] It was still considered emmetropic by Northmore and Granda[56] such that marine turtles are able to see coastlines and out of water well, which they could not if they were myopic out of water. The difference in opinion was considered by Northmore and Granda[56] to be made on observations made from the actively accommodating eye. The land tortoises were found to be similar to humans in that they are not able to overcome the loss of the corneal refraction when they are in water.

As part of the normal aging process of *Testudo* spp., arcus lipoides cornea, seen as a white infiltration of cholesterol crystals into the peripheral cornea,[35] is not unusual (Figure 20-27). Corneal cholesterol dystrophy can also occur in reptiles (such as terrapins) on a high polysaturated fat diet and is usually noted in the center of the cornea (Figure 20-28).

Ulceration

Ulceration of the cornea may be associated with foreign bodies, prolonged infection, and trauma, as encountered in other taxa (Figure 20-29). Corneal ulceration in snakes is very rare because of the protection afforded by the spectacle; only infection may cause this problem. Diagnosis of a corneal ulceration is made with the uptake of fluorescein dye (Figure 20-30). In reptiles with spectacles, topical fluorescein is pointless and meaningless to apply unless it is injected into the subspectacular space. Corneal lacerations are usually traumatic[58] and can be repaired with a fine suture material (8/0 or 10/0 Mersilene, Ethicon) with the aid of magnification and prophylactic topical antibiotic provided. Severe ulcerations in Chelonia and lizards may be treated with performing a third eyelid flap (Figure 20-31).

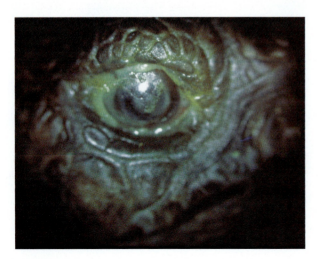

FIGURE 20-27 *Acrus lipoideus corneae* in an aged Mediterranean Tortoise *(Testudo graeca)*.

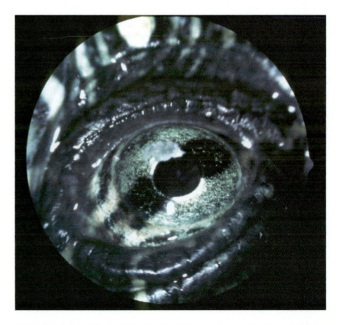

FIGURE 20-28 Corneal cholesterol dystrophy in a Red-eared Slider *(Trachemys scripta elegans)*.

Keratitis

Corneal infection (keratitis) in tortoises (*Testudo* spp.) is diagnosed with the presence of a white corneal mass and may be the result of infection with *Moraxella* spp., *Pseudomonas* spp., or *Aeromonas* spp. (Figures 20-32 and 20-33).[35] Such keratitis is infectious and contagious and should be considered a herd problem. Treatment consists of removal of the plaque from the cornea with general anesthesia. This requires magnification and the use of a 27-gauge needle to lift the mass off; sometimes a superficial keratectomy needs to be performed. Samples should be routinely sent for culture and sensitivity. Topical treatment with a suitable antibiotic such as ciprofloxacin (Ciloxan, Alcon) usually successfully treats the infection but may need to be continued for several months. Severe keratitis can lead to scarring and pigmentation of the cornea, similar to that seen in mammals (Figure 20-34).

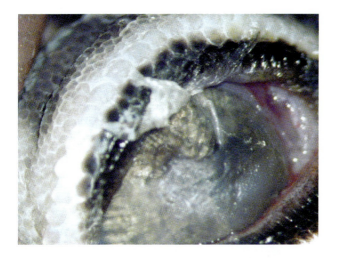

FIGURE 20-29 *Pseudomonas* infection in a Leopard Gecko (*Eublepharis macularius*) that causes sloughing of the cornea.

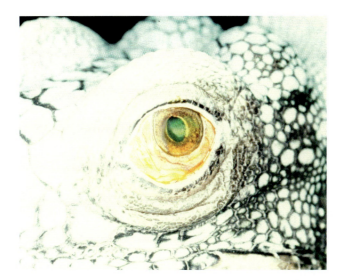

FIGURE 20-30 Corneal ulceration shown with flourescein dye in a Green Iguana (*Iguana iguana*).

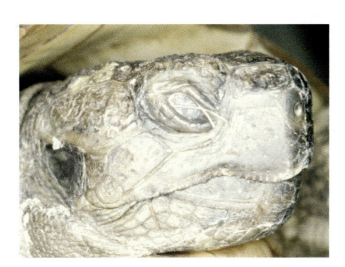

FIGURE 20-31 Third eyelid flap for treatment of corneal ulceration in a Mediterranean Tortoise (*Testudo graeca*).

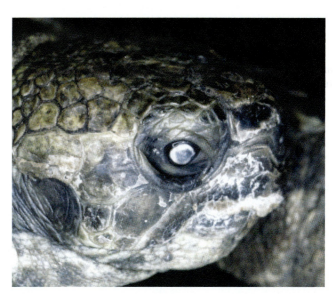

FIGURE 20-32 Bacterial keratitis in a Mediterranean Tortoise (*Testudo graeca*).

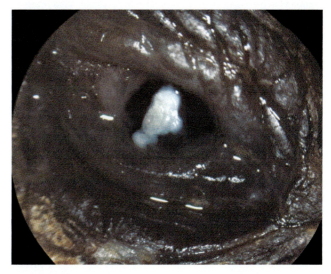

FIGURE 20-33 Bacterial keratitis in a Mediterranean Tortoise (*Testudo graeca*).

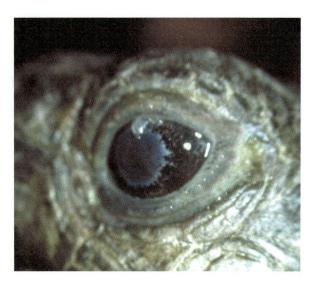

FIGURE 20-34 Postinflammatory pigmentation of the cornea in a Mediterranean Tortoise *(Testudo graeca)*.

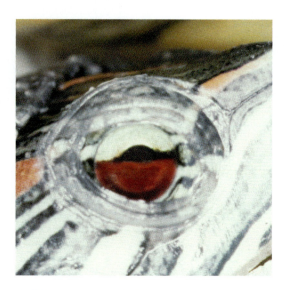

FIGURE 20-35 Hyphema after hibernation in an outside brumated (hibernated) Red-eared Slider *(Trachemys scripta elegans)*.

The presence of the spectacle in snakes does not preclude the development of corneal disease. A mycotic keratitis in a Reticulated Python has been described[59] where a firm mass was palpated under the spectacle and required enucleation together with the removal of some surrounding tissue. Histopathologic examination showed the corneal stroma to be infiltrated with spores and mycelia with branching filaments and septation. If a diagnosis is made with the find of fungal hyphae on corneal scrapings, then treatment with topical miconazole is a possibility. Fungal keratitis, however, can cause a panophthalmitis,[8,33] which is only treatable with enucleation.[33] Topical corticosteroid therapy[8,33] and trauma[8] are considered as possible underlying causes of fungal keratitis.

Infection: Viral

Fibropapilloma, a herpesvirus infection of Green Seaturtles, may cause proliferative or ulcerative lesions of the cornea[2,26,60] that can be so extensive as to involve the entire cornea.[26] The lung-eye-trachea (LET) disease also causes changes to the cornea, usually involving a white plaque or opacification.[61]

ANTERIOR CHAMBER AND UVEAL TRACT

Anatomy

The reptilian iris has a well-developed sphincter of striated muscles that allows rapid control over papillary movement[2] and is resilient to the effects of mydriatics. Voluntary control of the iris is important where the sphincter iris is responsible for accommodation by deforming the lens, such as in Chelonia.[6] A peculiar sexual dimorphism is shown in the color of the iris of most (but not all) *Terepene carolina*, where the male has a red iris and the female a brown iris.[19]

In lizards, often a difference is seen in the shape of the pupils, depending on whether a reptile is nocturnal (slit pupil) or diurnal (round pupils). In lizards, Heloderma are the exception as they have a round pupil.[19] In the Gekkonidae, often several tiny notches are paired off along the opposite margin of the iris.[6] In bright light, the pupil (normally a single slit) closes completely, leaving a series of pin holes (stenopeic openings)[19] that are very small oval pupils formed by these apposed notches. These stenopeic openings form a sharp image irrespective of distance and a far sharper image than that of a single aperture.[6] Stenopeic openings are most obvious in the Tokay Gecko *(Gekko gecko)*, in which its presence is considered to allow the formation of a clear image without any other accommodative adjustments.[19] The crocodilian iris, although more mobile and responsive than in lizards or Chelonia, is also able to form a stenopeic slit in bright sunlight.[19]

The snake iris is generally a thick, heavily pigmented structure. It is highly mobile as, with the absence of eyelids, it plays a more important role in light protective function.[19] The East Indian Long-nosed Treesnake *(Dryophis mycterizans)* and the African Bird Snake *(Thelotornis kirtlandi)* have a horizontal keyhole-shaped pupil with the slot of the keyhole pointing forward beyond the rim of the lens. This is to position the slot of the keyhole (nasally) in line with the fovea (two of only three genera that have a fovea).[6] These two snakes are thought to have the sharpest sight and most accurate judgment of distance of any snakes.[6]

Uveitis

Uveitis may result from trauma or infection (bacteria, fungi, or virus) or be associated with neoplasia. The clinical signs and treatment are similar to those noted in mammals. Hyphema (Figure 20-35) and hypopyon are often present after exposure to freezing temperatures in Chelonia.[62] Hypopyon is considered to be a secondary feature of reptiles with an underlying systemic infection[2] such as a bacterial septicemia; *Klebsiella pneumoniae* has been associated as one possible cause.[9] All reptiles with hypopyon should have a thorough investigation to rule out or diagnose a potential

Reptilian Ophthalmology

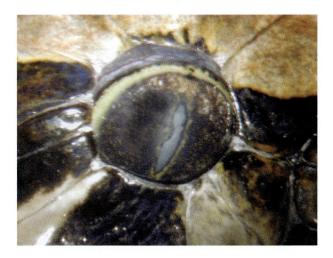

FIGURE 20-36   Dense cataract.

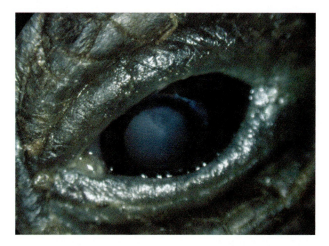

FIGURE 20-38   A dense cortical cataract in a Mediterranean Tortoise *(Testudo graeca)*.

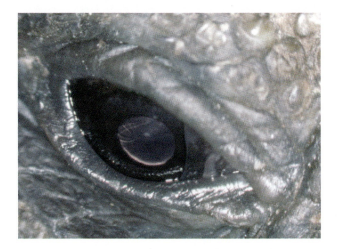

FIGURE 20-37   The early start of a cataract in a Mediterranean Tortoise *(Testudo graeca).*

infectious cause. Where septicemia is found, a guarded prognosis should always be given.

LENS

Anatomy

Most reptiles have some sort of annular pad (ringwulst or annular ring), which is a thickened area of epithelial cells, usually at or near the equator, that allows the lens to connect directly to the ciliary body, usually by zonular fibers. The lizards have a thick equatorial annular pad formed by radial growth of the subcapsular epithelium that is largest in chameleons.[19] The ciliary body has a broad zone of firm contact with the lens in lizards.[6] Unlike lizards, Chelonia have well-formed ciliary processes that attach to the lens,[19] although a small but weakly developed annular pad is found.[6,19] The Crocodilia have ciliary processes that connect with the equator of the lens, where a small annular pad is found.[19] The snake has no equatorial annular pad,[6,19] but an anterior pad is formed from the subcapsular epithelial cells on the anterior surface.[19]

The lenses of lizards are soft.[2] A larger lens is seen in nocturnal species.[19] In lizards, accommodation depends on the deformation of the lens.[19] Nocturnal and diurnal gekkonids differ in the biochemical composition of their lenses.[63] Nocturnal animals have colorless lenses, and yellow crystalline (water soluble protein) is found exclusively in lenses of diurnal geckos and gives their lenses a yellow coloration.[63]

The lens capsule is thin in Chelonia, and the lenses are extremely soft and almost fluid-like in consistency.[6,19] The land tortoise has a flat lens that is less flat in the terrapins and more spherical in seaturtles.[6] Turtles are able to accommodate when submerged by squeezing the soft lens through the pupil aperture.[6,19,56]

The snake lens is pigmented yellow, is spherical, and is firmer than that of other reptilian lenses.[19] In snakes, the oil droplets in the rod cells of the retina do not have any color, so the yellow lenses take over this function of ultraviolet protection.[6] Accommodation in the snake is unique compared with other reptiles[19] because it relies on the lens moving backward and forward in response to pressure changes within the vitreous and aqueous.[17] This is aided by the ciliary muscles having migrated into the root of the iris where they can apply pressure onto the lens, helping it to move forward or backward within the eye but not able to alter the shape of the lens.[14]

Cataracts

As in all taxa, cataracts may occur for a variety of reasons (Figure 20-36). Cataracts in tortoises *(Testudo* spp.) have been associated with freezing episodes[62,64] (Figures 20-37 and 20-38). They are hypothesized to be particularly prone to damage from low temperatures because of the soft and fluid-like nature of the lenses.[19] In some cases, these changes are reversible, although up to 18 months may be necessary for the lens to clear.[62]

Cataract surgery in reptiles can be performed in a similar manner to that described for birds. Cataract surgery in reptiles with spectacles is more difficult because of the necessity of cutting through the spectacle to expose the cornea before an incision is made into the anterior chamber.

RETINA

Anatomy and Visual Tracts

Reptiles, like birds, have an anangiotic (avascular) retina. Nutrients are supplied and metabolic wastes removed by choroidal blood vessels or modified vessels protruding into the vitreous. All reptiles have a choriocapillaris and, during development, had a hyaloid vascular system.[65] The major differences found in the various reptile orders occurred as the hyaloid system regressed.

Chelonia have had a total regression of both the hyaloid system and the choriocapillaris and rely solely on remaining choroidal blood vessels. An early avascular conus did develop above the optic disc in some turtles, but this regressed and is absent in all adults.[19]

The conus is absent in Amphisbaenidae.[19]

In lizards, a structure similar to the avian pecten develops but is known as the conus papillaris. The conus papillaris usually protrudes into the vitreous from the optic disc,[2] consists of a vascularized glial tissue,[65] and is ectodermal in origin.[6] As for the avian pecten, the inner limiting membrane (vitreoretinal border) covers the conus papillaris.[66] It consists mainly of tiny blood vessels that are heavily pigmented.[6] The conus papillaris entirely obscures the fundoscopic view of the optic disc.[19]

In snakes, the conus has regressed in all but a few species and is replaced by a preretinal vascular meshwork derived from the hyaloid vessels known as the membrana vasculosa retinae,[65] which is mesodermal in origin.[6] This is a branching array of vessels derived from the choroid running into the posterior vitreous near and originating from the optic disc but just above the retina. In colubrids, the capillaries of the membrana vasculosa retinae penetrate the retina and become an intraretinal vessel.[19,65]

In adult crocodilians, the conus papillaris is functionless and is reduced to a glial pad consisting of one or two capillary loops that scarcely protrude into the vitreous and are on the optic nerve head.[2,6,19] In alligators, the conus has regressed even more into a layer of melanocytes found on the optic nerve head.[65]

The reptile retina has rods and cones.[2,14] The New World Chameleon (*Chamaeleo* sp.) also has a cone-rich retina.[67] In Chelonia, cones predominate the retina.[19] In diurnal reptiles, yellow oil droplets are associated with the rod or certain cone cells (except for snakes), which act as ocular filters and are able to absorb ultraviolet and shortwave blue radiation with a protective effect on the underlying cells[68] and reduction of glare.[14] Where colored oil droplets are not found in the rod cells of the retina (such as in snakes) this function can be undertaken by yellow lenses.[6] Extraretinal photoreceptors allow circadian rhythms to be initiated and controlled and the eyes have an inhibitory role.[69]

An area centralis is found in most species where the cones are smaller and more densely packed. Vision in all animals is improved by the presence of areae centrales or foveae. The area centralis, despite its name, is not always in the center of the fundus other than in man (macula lutea). The area centralis is an area that has a marked increase in resolving power compared with the rest of the retina. A foveal depression in the retina is associated with a thinning of the retina and allows for a magnifying action and thus increased visual acuity; however, it is only present in a small number of reptiles.[6]

Fovea are present in *Amyda* spp. (the only turtles to have a fovea), the *Sphenodon punctatus* (a medium, pure rod fovea), some diurnal skinks and *Varanus,* and three genera of snakes (*Dryophis, Dryophiops,* and *Thelotornis*). The fovea is absent in all crocodilians.[6] In nocturnal species of lizard, the fovea is absent (Heloderms and most geckos) or reduced to the remnant of a foveal pit *(Xantusia)*.[19] In diurnal species of lizards with a fovea, it has elongated cones that are closely packed, and some species (mainly arboreally diurnal) may have a second fovea temporally as is also seen in some bifoveate birds.[19]

The crocodilian retinal epithelium has a tapetum formed by guanine crystals[6,19] that is hyperreflective at night when lights are shone into their eyes and is often used while hunting them. Rods greatly outnumber the cones in the periphery, with the cones resuming in the tapetal area. Near the ventral border of the tapetum a horizontal oval area centralis, mainly of rods, exists.[19]

The optics and ocular physiology of the *Trachemys scripta elegans* have been extensively studied.[56,70,71] They were found to have good fine vision; with the photoreceptors being 90% cones, they are able to see colors[71,72] and are particularly sensitive in the red region of the spectrum.[71] Although they have a high number of cones, they are thought to have a similar optic range to the duplex system of man.[56]

Nearly complete crossover occurs of the optic nerves at the optic chiasm in the *Trachemys scripta*.[70] This allows an accurate panoramic vision and the ability to have a high detection of movement, although only limited binocular vision is present, restricted to directly in the front (25 to 30 degrees). The more lateral the eye, the more independence for each eye and provision of the panoramic field of vision. Optokinetic studies in the *Trachemys scripta*[70] showed that transection of the tectal commissure caused no significant change in vision, suggesting that visual movement detection is a relatively independent function of the two eyes.

Many differences are seen in the neural pathways of reptiles. Blind snakes (which despite their names are sensitive to light and therefore not blind) of the families Typhlopidae and Leptotyphlopidae have been shown to have a different retinal efferent system from that of the higher snakes.[73] The blind snakes were found to lack the retinotectal connections, and the nucleus rotundus (the major thalamic nucleus receiving tectal efferens in reptiles and birds) is barely distinguishable.[73]

Boidae and Crotalinae have two electromagnetic radiation imaging systems, which are very similar although they evolved independently.[74] The first is the lateral eyes, responsible for visible light, and the second is the pit organ, responsible for seeing infrared radiation. These are the only animals known to image two distinct parts of the electromagnetic spectrum at the same time. Both the visual and infrared information obtained are probably involved in prey targeting. Experiments have shown that although vision is not necessary for accurate targeting (shown in experimentally blinded snakes), it is necessary for precise targeting in association with the infrared perception.[74] The infrared and visual information merge in the optic tectum where the individual neurons are found to be sensitive to both stimulation of the eyes (by visible light) and stimulation of the pit organs (by infrared radiation) from the same points in space.[74] A lateral descending nucleus of the medulla oblongata also is unique to infrared-imaging snakes.

Retinal Disease

Our knowledge of retinal disease in reptiles is still very much in its infancy and is sadly lacking when compared with that of mammalian and avian species. Retinal damage associated with vitamin A deficiency, and after freezing episodes, has been reported in tortoises (*Testudo* spp.).[64] In certain circumstances, treatment with vitamin A may result in a clinical improvement. Retinal degeneration has been reported in Tokay Geckos (*Gekko gecko*),[9,75] although it is also thought to be a sporadic finding in most reptile families.[28]

REFERENCES

1. Ensley PK, Anderson MP, Bacon JP: Ophthalmic disorders in three snakes, *J Zoo Anim Med* 9:57-59, 1978.
2. Millichamp NJ, Jacobson ER, Wolf ED: Disease of the eye and ocular adnexae in reptiles, *J Am Vet Med Assoc* 183(11):1205-1212, 1983.
3. Tangredi BP, Evans RH: Organochlorine pesticides associated with ocular, nasal or otic infection in the Eastern Box turtle (*Terrapene carolina carolina*), *J Zoo Wildl Med* 28(1): 97-100, 1997.
4. Millichamp NJ: Management of ocular disease in exotic species, *Semin Avian Exotic Pet Med* 6(3):152-159, 1997.
5. Underwood G: The eye. In Gans C, Parsons TS, editors: *Biology of the Reptilia*, vol 2, morphology B, London, 1970, Academic Press.
6. Walls GL: *The vertebrate eye and its adaptive radiation*, Bloomfield Hills, Mich, 1942, Cranbrook Institute of Science, Bulletin No. 19.
7. Whittaker CJG, Schumacher J, Bennett RA, Neuwirth L, Gelatt KN: Orbital varix in a Green iguana (*Iguana iguana*), *Vet Comp Ophthalmol* 7(2):101-104, 1997.
8. Cullen CL, Wheler C, Grahn BH: Diagnostic ophthalmology, *Can Vet J* 41:327-328, 2000.
9. Bonney CH, Hartfiel DA, Schmit RE: *Klebsiella pneumoniae* infection with secondary hypopyon in Tokay Gecko lizards, *J Vet Med Assoc* 173(9):1115-1116, 1978.
10. Davidson MG: Ophthalmology of exotic pets, *Compendium Continuing Educ Pract Vet* 9:724-736, 1985.
11. Mitchell MA, Hamilton H, Smith JA, Tucci TR: Evaluation of the effects of three neuromuscular blocking agents on pupil size in the red-ear slider (*Trachemys scripta elegans*). In Willette MM, editor: Columbus, Ohio, 1999, Proceedings of the 1999 annual conference of the Association of Reptilian and Amphibian Veterinarians.
12. Millchamp NJ, Jacobson ER: Ophthalmic diseases of reptiles. In Kirk RW, editor: *Current veterinary therapy IX*, Philadelphia, 1986, WB Saunders.
13. Schumacher J, Pellicane CP, Heard DJ, Voges A: Periorbital abscess in a three-horned chameleon (*Chamaeleo jacksonii*), *Vet Comp Ophthalmol* 6(1):30-33, 1996.
14. Bellairs A: Nervous system, psychology and sense organs. In *The life of reptiles*, vol II, London, 1969, Weidenfeld & Nicholson.
15. Quay WB: The parietal eye-pineal complex. In Gans C, Northcutt RG, Ulinski P, editors: *Biology of the Reptilia*, vol 9, *neurology A*, London, 1979, Academic Press.
16. Stebbins RC, Eakin RM: The role of the "third eye" in reptilian behavior, *Am Museum Novitates* 1870:1-40, 1958.
17. Davies MPC: Anatomy and physiology. In Cooper JE, Jackson OF, editors: *Diseases of the Reptilia*, vol 1, London, 1981, Academic Press.
18. Lawton MPC: *The spectacle in health and disease*, London, 1999, Diploma of Zoological Medicine Thesis, RCVS Wellcome Library.
19. Duke-Elder S: The eyes of reptiles. In *Systems of ophthalmology*, vol 1, London, 1958, Kimpton.
20. Dupont C, Murphy CJ: Ocular disorders in reptiles. In Ackerman L, editor: *The biology, husbandry and health care of reptiles*, vol III, *health care of reptiles*, Neptune City, 1998, TFH Inc.
21. Lawton MPC: Ophthalmology. In Beynon PH, Lawton MPC, Cooper JE, editors: *Manual of reptiles*, Cheltenham, 1992, BSAVA.
22. Frye FL: Blepharoplasty in an iguana (a case report), *Vet Med Small Anim Clin* 67:1110-1111, 1972.
23. Elkan E, Zwart P: The ocular disease of young terrapins caused by vitamin A deficiency, *Vet Pathol* 4(3):201-222, 1967.
24. Miller EA, Green SL, Otto GM, Bouley DM: Suspected hypovitaminosis A in a colony of captive green anoles (*Anolis carolinensis*), *Contemp Top Am Assoc Lab Anim Sci* 40(2):18-20, 2001.
25. Thomas CL, Artwohl JE, Pearl RK, Gardiner CH: Swollen eyelid associated with *Foleyella* sp infection in a Chameleon., *J Am Vet Med Assoc* 209(5):972-973, 1996.
26. Brooks DE, Ginn PE, Miller TR, Bramson L, Jacobson ER: Ocular fibropapillomas of green turtles (*Chelonia mydas*), *Vet Pathol* 31:335-339, 1994.
27. Lawton MPC: *Introduction to reptilian ophthalmology*. In Frahm MW, editor: Kansas City, Mo, 1998, Proceedings of the Association of Reptilian and Amphibian Veterinarians Annual Conference.
28. Millichamp NJ, Jacobson ER, Dziezyc J: Conjunctivoralostomy for treatment of an occluded lacrimal duct in a blood python, *J Am Vet Med Assoc* 189(9):1136-1138, 1986.
29. Frye FL, Gillespie DS: Tracing the etiology of ocular opacities, *Vet Med* 79:1385-1387, 1984.
30. Lawton MPC: Ophthalmology of exotic species. In Petersen-Jones SM, Crispin SM, editors: *Manual of small animal ophthalmology*, Cheltenham, 1993, BSAVA.
31. Divers SJ, Lawton MPC: The use of lyophilised skin grafts for the treatment of integumental disease in birds and reptiles, *Proc BSAVA Congress* 48:279, 2000.
32. Williams DL: Ophthalmology. In Mader DR: *Reptile medicine and surgery*, Philadelphia, 1996, WB Saunders.
33. Zwart P, Verwer MAJ, de Vries GA, Hermanides-Nijhof EJ, de Vries HW: Fungal infection of the eyes of the snake *Epicrates chenchria maurus*: enucleation under halothane narcosis, *J Small Anim Pract* 14:773-779, 1973.
34. Cooper JE: Bacteria. In Cooper JE, Jackson OF, editors: *Diseases of the Reptilia*, vol 1, London, 1981, Academic Press.
35. Lawton MPC: Common ophthalmic problems seen in chelonia. In Frahm MW, editor: *ARAV*, Texas, 1997, Proceedings of the 4th Annual Conference of the Association of Reptilian and Amphibian Veterinarians.
36. Jacobson ER: The evaluation of the reptile patient. In Jacobson ER, Kollias GV, editors: *Exotic animals*, New York, 1988, Churchill Livingstone.
37. Cooper JE: Exophthalmia in a rhinoceros viper (*Bitus nasicornis*), *Vet Rec* 97:130-131, 1975.
38. Cooper JE, Jackson OF: Miscellaneous diseases. In Cooper JE, Jackson OF, editors: *Diseases of the Reptilia*, vol 2, London, 1981, Academic Press.
39. Lawton MPC: *Disease of the spectacle*, Kansas City, Mo, 1998, Proceedings of the Association of Reptilian and Amphibian Veterinarians 1998 Annual Conference.
40. Frye FL: Traumatic and physical diseases. In Cooper JE, Jackson OF, editors: *Diseases of the Reptilia*, vol 2, London, 1981, Academic Press.
41. Boniuk M, Luquette GF: Luekokoria and pseudobuphthalmos in snakes, *Invest Ophthalmol* 2:283, 1963.

42. Frye FL: *Biomedical and surgical aspects of captive reptile husbandry*, ed 2, Melbourne, 1991, Kreiger.
43. Blogg JR: *The eye in veterinary practice, extraocular disease*, vol I, Philadelphia, 1980, WB Saunders.
44. Dice PF: The canine cornea. In Gelatt KN, editor: *Textbook of veterinary ophthalmology*, Philadelphia, 1981, Lea & Febiger.
45. Smith HA, Jones TC, Hunt RD: *Pathology*, ed 4, Philadelphia, 1972, Lea & Febiger.
46. Payne AP: The Harderian gland: a tercentennial review, *J Anat* 185:1-49, 1994.
47. Chittick B, Harms C: Intraocular pressure of juvenile Loggerhead Sea turtles (*Caretta caretta*) held in different positions, *Vet Rec* 149:587-589, 2001.
48. Whittaker CJG, Heaton-Jones TG, Kubilis PS, Smith PJ, Brooks DE, Kosarek C, et al: Intraocular pressure variation associated with body length in young American alligators (*Alligator mississippiensis*), *Am J Vet Res* 56(10):1380-1383, 1995.
49. Leonard JL, Shields RP: Acid-fast granuloma in a turtle's eye, *J Am Vet Med Assoc* 157(5):612-613, 1970.
50. Hamilton HL, Mitchell MA, Williams J, Tully TN, Glaze MB: Orbital abscess in a Green iguana, *Iguana iguana*, *Bull Assoc Reptl Amphib Vet* 9(3):27-31, 1999.
51. Williams DL, MacGregor S, Sainsbury AW: Evaluation of bacteria isolated from infected eyes of captive, non-domestic animals, *Vet Rec* 146:515-518, 2000.
52. Cooper JE, McClelland MH, Needham JR: An eye infection in laboratory lizards associated with an *Aeromonas* sp, *Lab Anim* 14:149-151, 1980.
53. Hanuskova Z, Tilc K: Problems of veterinary significance concerning imported tortoises after unsuitable wintering with regard to the incidence of ophthalmic affects and oxyuridosis, *Acta Vet BRNO* 44:407-412, 1975.
54. Jacobson ER, Gaskin JM, Roelke M, Greiner EC, Allen J: Conjunctivitis, tracheitis and pneumonia associated with herpesvirus infection in Green Sea turtles, *J Am Vet Med Assoc* 189(9):1020-1023, 1986.
55. Platt TR: Helminth parasites of the Western Painted turtle, *Chrusemys picta belli* (Gray), including *Neopolystoma elizabethae* N. Sp. (Monogenea: Polystomatidae), a parasite of the conjunctival sac, *J Parasitol* 86(4):815-818, 2000.
56. Northmore DPM, Granda AM: Ocular dimensions and schematic eyes of freshwater and sea turtles. *Vis Neurosci* 7:627-635, 1991.
57. Ehrenfeld DW, Kock AL: Visual accommodation in the Green turtle, *Science* 155:827-828, 1967.
58. Northway RB: Repair of a fractured shell and lacerated cornea in a tortoise, *Vet Med Small Anim Clin* 65:944, 1970.
59. Collette BE, Curry OH: Mycotic keratitis in a reticulated python, *J Am Vet Med Assoc* 173(9):1117-1118, 1978.
60. Norton TM, Jacobson ER, Sundberg JP: Cutaneous fibropapillomas and renal myxofibroma in a Green Turtle, *Chelonia mydas*, *J Wildl Dis* 26(2):265-270, 1990.
61. Jacobson ER, Gaskin JM, Roelke M: Conjunctivitis, tracheitis, and pneumonia associated with herpes-virus infection in green sea turtles, *J Am Vet Med Assoc* 189:1020-1023, 1985.
62. Lawton MPC, Stoakes LC: Post hibernation blindness in tortoises (*Testudo* spp.). In Jacobson ER, editor: *Third International Colloquium on Pathology of Reptiles and Amphibians*, Orlando, Fla, 1989.
63. Roll B: Evidence for diurnality from an eye lens crystalline in *Cnemaspis* (Reptilia, Gekkonidae), *Herpetol J* 11:75-77, 2001.
64. Lawton MPC: Neurological problems of exotic species. In Wheeler SJ: *Manual of small animal neurology*, Cheltenham, 1989, BSAVA.
65. Bellhorn RW: Retinal nutritive systems in vertebrates, *Semin Avian Exotic Pet Med* 6(3):108-118, 1997.
66. Heegaard S: Structure of the animal vitreoretinal border region: a comparative study, *Vet Comp Ophthalmol* 4:1:13-22, 1994.
67. McGinnis JF, Stepanik PL, Jariangprasert S, Lerious V: Functional significance of recoverin localization in multiple retina cell types, *J Neurosci Res* 50:487-495, 1997.
68. Lythgoe JN: *The ecology of vision*, Oxford, 1979, Clarendon Press.
69. Underwood H: Extraretinal photoreception in the lizard *Sceloporus occidentalis*: phase response curve, *Am J Physiol* 248:R407-414, 1985.
70. Hertzler DR, Hayes WN: Effects of monocular vision and midbrain transection on movement detection in the turtle, *J Comp Physiol Psychol* 67:4:473-478, 1969.
71. Zwick H, Holst GC: Experimental alteration of the red cone photoreceptor process. Colour vision deficiencies III, international symposium, Amsterdam 1975, *Mod Prob Ophthalmol* 17:257-263, 1976.
72. Granda AM, Dvorak CA: Vision in turtles. In Crescitelli F, editor: *The visual system in vertebrates: handbook of sensory physiology*, New York, 1977, Springer-Verlag.
73. Halpern M: Retinal projections in blind snakes, *Science* 182:390-391, 1973.
74. Grace MS, Woodward OM, Church DR, Calisch G: Prey targeting by the infrared-imaging snake python: effects of experimental and congenital visual deprivation, *Behav Brain Res* 119:23-31, 2001.
75. Schmidt RE, Toft JD: Ophthalmic lesions in animals from a zoological collection, *J Wildl Dis* 17:267-275, 1981.

21
PARASITOLOGY
ELLIS C. GREINER and DOUGLAS R. MADER

Parasites are animals that live in or on other species of animals (**hosts**), gain their nourishment from the host, and use the host as the environment in which they spend most, if not all, of their life. All vertebrates including reptiles have parasites, and usually multiple species of parasites infect each species of host. Some parasites cause outright disease, and others peacefully coexist with their hosts. The balance between the host and the parasite sometimes is tipped in favor of the parasite and sometimes in favor of the host and other times is neutral. Thus, a continuum exists ranging from the relationship in which the host is totally in charge and eliminates the parasite to the one in which the parasite is in charge and causes illness or even death of the host. We know little about most parasites of reptiles, and for many, we have no idea whether the parasite is normally a pathogen (causes disease) or a benign symbiont that does nothing obvious to the host. Host-parasite relationships that are long standing usually have evolved to a point where little or no damage is done to the host; usually when disease is caused by the parasite, the host and parasite have not been in a long evolutionary relationship.

Different types of hosts have developed through time. A **definitive host** (DH) is one in which the sexually mature form of the parasite develops. An **intermediate host** (IH) harbors immature parasites that might undergo morphologic changes or increase in number through an asexual means or both. **Vectors** are usually IHs that have direction and force as they take the parasite to the next host rather than passively wait to shed their infective parasite stages into the environment or be eaten by the DH. **Paratenic** or **transport hosts** are those in which the parasite lives and is a source of infection to the DH but in which limited or no development takes place. This could be considered an extra, but nonessential, route of access to the DH. A final grouping is **aberrant hosts** in which the host may be a **dead end** for the parasites as little or no hope exists that the parasite will be passed along to another host. The parasite may develop normally in the aberrant host or may develop to a certain point and stop, before it is infective to the next host.

The host might be viewed as a series of niches and habitats rather than a single individual in the community in which it lives. If one is to view the host in this light, the potential for a community (multiple species) living in the host can best be visualized. Some parasites live inside the host and are **endoparasites**, and some live on the surface of the host and are considered **ectoparasites**. With the gastrointestinal tract as an example, different parasites live in the oral cavity, esophagus, stomach, small intestine, cecum (if present), and large intestine. Furthermore, considering the small intestine, some parasites live unattached in the lumen, some attach to the mucosa but are still lumen dwellers, some penetrate into the mucosa as extracellular parasites, and yet others live as intracellular parasites in various cells of the gut wall. Usually the parasite is restricted to a single region of the gut. To take this to another step, the distribution in the gut may be influenced further by the presence of other parasites that share the tubular habitat. Most organ systems in the host may have their own parasites or specific stages of parasites. This is important to understand to find the parasites that occur in the host.

Life cycles are important to determine because this is the means in which the parasite perpetuates its gene pool. The simplest of these is the **direct life cycle** in which only one host is needed to complete the cycle. Some coccidians use this model; the intracellular parasite develops in the cells that line the host gut and then produces the stage to be passed out of the host, which is infective to the next host, called the oocyst. These parasites may need to develop in the **abiotic** (outside of the host) environment before becoming infective. So, part of the parasite's development is in a free-living nonparasitic phase of the life cycle. Some of the roundworms (nematodes) do this as well.

Indirect life cycles require at least two different species of host to complete the life cycle (Figure 21-1). These cycles use both DHs and IHs. The parasite has adapted to move between the necessary hosts for completion of the life cycles. The DH usually passes stages that become the infective stage to the next host (eggs or first-stage larvae for worms and cysts or oocysts for gut-inhabiting protozoans). The IH then ingests the stage infective to it, and the parasite changes its morphology or reproduces asexually. Once the stage infective to the DH is developed, the IH is eaten by the DH or, in the case of vector-borne parasites, the vector takes a blood meal from the vertebrate host and the infective stage is either deposited on the skin or injected by the feeding vector. In captivity, some reptile parasites do not have the opportunity to develop because the correct IHs are not available in the facility housing the reptiles.

Through these different life cycles, it becomes apparent that parasites gain access to their reptilian hosts in different manners. Most parasites are obtained with ingestion of the infective stage of the parasite. This can be through ingestion of eggs, oocysts, or larvae in the environment (fecal-oral contamination), or by eating IHs that contain infective stages. Other means include penetration of intact skin by infective larvae, deposition on the skin of infective stages by the vector, or direct inoculation by the vector.

Understanding life cycles is important in trying to control the parasite. If the animal is continuously reinfected in its environs, then what appears to be drug failure is really the parasite outsmarting the veterinarian. If one is feeding naturally infected IHs to the DH, the problem can explode and result in deaths of reptiles in the collection.

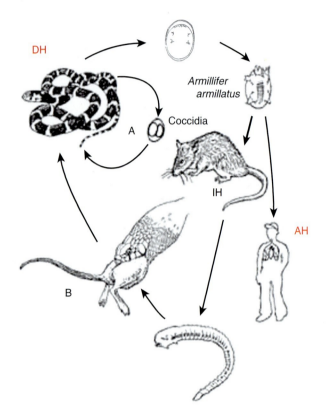

FIGURE 21-1 **A,** In a direct life cycle, such as with coccidia, parasites that are passed from definitive host (DH) are capable of directly reinfecting either the same host or a host animal of the same species. **B,** In an indirect life cycle, such as seen here with the parasite *Armillifer armillatus*, the parasite must pass through an intermediate host (IH) to develop its infective stage. If the parasite accidentally is ingested by an incorrect intermediate host, such as a human, the parasite cannot reproduce. In this case, man is considered an aberrant host (AH).

DIAGNOSIS OF PARASITES

This diagnosis is most often performed on the living reptile. Parasites are at times diagnosed with necropsy, usually when a major mortality occurs and the collection loses multiple individuals. Parasite recovery must be built into necropsy procedures. A problem that is becoming more apparent is untrained people performing diagnostic tests for parasites and then guessing what parasite is represented with the findings. We have very few documented cases with reptile parasitology in which the worm eggs have been matched to their adults. Need for cooperation between reptile collection management, reptile veterinarians, and parasitologists is essential for progress in diagnostic capabilities.

Many parasites may be detected with fecal examinations in living reptiles. **Reptilian feces are normally brown to black and should not be confused with the whitish urates. The parasitic stages are mainly in the feces.** A variety of examinations are done, and some of these for detection of specific parasites.

The most common procedure is the fecal flotation. This is used to detect nematode eggs, cestode eggs (if they have been released from the proglottids), nematode larvae, many acanthocephalan eggs, pentastome eggs, mites and their eggs, coccidian oocysts, and enteric protozoan cysts. Different flotation media are used; some are concentrated salts and others are sugars. The senior author primarily uses sodium nitrate (Fecasol, Evsco Pharmaceuticals, Buena, NJ) because it has as broad a spectrum of activity as any flotation media he has used. With coccidian oocysts in which measurements are made, sugar flotation is used because it allows the use of oil immersion due to its viscosity and does not dry out nearly as rapidly as do salt solutions.

Flotations need to stand for at least 10 minutes before they are read. They should be read systematically so the entire cover slip is examined under the 10× objective. If questionable items are found, then the high dry lens should be used to enhance characterization and to make measurements. Some parasitologists prefer to use a double centrifugation because this cleans up the eggs and concentrates them better than a standing flotation. However, if few eggs or cysts are found and the technician is well trained, hundreds of eggs are not necessary for a diagnosis.

Too often too much is made of the number of diagnostic stages present, usually with helminth eggs. Too many factors come into play that influence the number of eggs in the feces to make it meaningful in estimating worm populations. In the opinion of the senior author, the only time that counts are warranted is when an individual animal is examined before and after treatment to see whether a significant difference in egg counts has occurred. Although some eggs do not change with time after collection, some do, and therefore, collection of the feces and examination within a few hours of collection is best unless the search is for motile protozoan trophozoites.

The best way to detect motile protozoa that live in the gut is with the direct smear. This is performed with the simple addition of a small amount of feces to a drop of normal saline solution on a microscope slide. The feces is mixed with an applicator stick, and then a coverslip is added. One should scan the slide with the 10× objective lens and be sure to have a good amount of contrast or the smaller motile forms will be missed. If anything is found, then higher magnification should be used for a better look that may allow a proper diagnosis. The slide should not have so much feces on it that the technician cannot read newsprint through it. Remember, this is not a cleaning or a concentration method but is intended to allow detection of moving ciliates, flagellates, or amoebae.

If the collection occurs in another city from the laboratory, one may try fixing the feces in polyvinyl alcohol (PVA). Feces fixed in this way can be stained with a trichrome stain or iron hematoxylin stain to show the characteristics of the protozoa present. Not all flagellates tolerate this method of fixation.

Another fecal examination technique is sedimentation. This system is usually used to detect trematode eggs. Other eggs and cysts are cleaned and concentrated with this procedure, but if the stage can be floated, more success should be found in detection of those stages in the flotation than in the sediment. Fluke eggs normally do not float. Although a formalin ethyl acetate centrifugation procedure could be used, one can also use a soapy water solution to clean the eggs. In the latter case, the feces is mixed in a specimen cup with less than 50 mL of soapy water (<0.5%) and mixed thoroughly. The solution is passed through two layers of gauze into a 50-mL centrifuge tube and then allowed to stand for 5 minutes. One should decant the fluid but not dispose of the sediment at the bottom of the tube. Refill the tube with soapy water, and resuspend the sediment and allow it to stand for 5 minutes, and then decant. Repeat this process until the

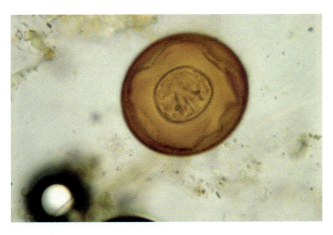

FIGURE 21-2 *Hymenolepis diminuta*, pseudoparasite. Photomicrograph magnification, 400×.

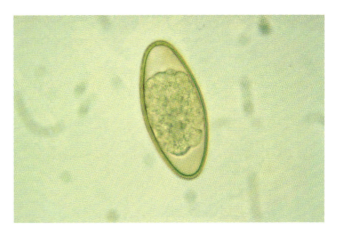

FIGURE 21-4 *Aspicularis tetraptera*, pseudoparasite. Photomicrograph magnification, 400×.

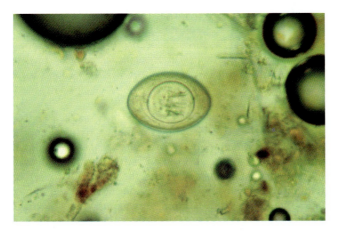

FIGURE 21-3 *Hymenolepis nana*, pseudoparasite. Photomicrograph magnification, 400×.

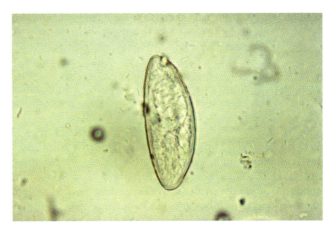

FIGURE 21-5 *Syphacia muris*, pseudoparasite. Photomicrograph magnification, 400×.

water remains clear. Decant the fluid and transfer the sediment onto a microscope slide, add a coverslip, and scan as a flotation slide would be scanned. This washes debris away from the fluke eggs and concentrates them.

Examples of helminth eggs (all photographed at 400×, unless stated otherwise) and protozoa are illustrated throughout the chapter. Individual figures are called out under specific sections.

Pseudoparasites are parasites found during patient or fecal examinations of a reptile, but the parasite is actually from another host. For example, if reptiles are fed mice, four helminth eggs might appear in fecal examinations that are parasites of the mice (prey) and not the reptile (Figures 21-2 to 21-5). Pseudoparasites are common and can be easily confused with true parasites, an important distinction because the former do not need treatment.

Blood parasites can be detected with blood smears stained with Wright's or Giemsa stain or a combination. Some blood parasites are intracellular, and some are extracellular. See Chapter 55 for photomicrographs and a complete discussion of the medical significance.

For the diagnosis of *Cryptosporidium* in snakes, gastric biopsies are the gold standard. In lizards, the biopsy should be from the intestines. If animals in a collection are dying, necropsy and histopathologic examination of gastric and intestinal tissue are helpful in determination of the cause.

Reptiles fed mice may have false-positive fecal examination results because mice harbor their own *Cryptosporidium* species and these cause problems for diagnosis based on the similarity in size to those that are parasites of the reptile (Figure 21-6). For more information on cryptosporidiosis, see Chapter 48.

Recovery of metazoan parasites at necropsy is done with sectioning the gut by organ and then slitting one section at a time to open the full length of that section. The opened gut should be stripped between gloved fingers into a catch vessel, and all contents and mucus should be washed into the container. Examine the stripped mucosa and remove any parasites still attached. The container contents then can be washed into a #50 standard sieve, or a #100 sieve if the search is for tiny nematodes, and washed with a steady stream of water. Once the water comes through clear, backflush the material into a flat Pyrex casserole dish and view for worms. These can be picked and placed into normal saline solution in Petri dishes that then can be prepared for fixation (Table 21-1).

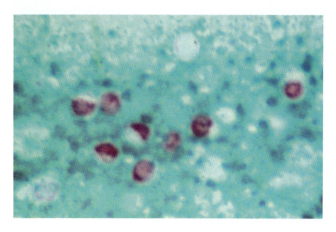

FIGURE 21-6 *Cryptosporidium muris* from a Cornsnake (*Elaphe* sp.), pseudoparasite. Photomicrograph magnification, 400×.

Table 21-1	Fixatives for Helminths Recovered from Reptiles

Nematodes. Glycerine alcohol: 90 parts 70% ethanol and 10 parts glycerine after straightening in stock glacial acetic acid
Trematodes and **Cestodes.** AFA: 85 parts 85% ethanol, 5 parts stock glacial acetic acid, and 10 parts stock formalin after they have been relaxed in tap water or slightly flattened.
Acanthocephala. AFA: after placing adults in tap water to allow proboscis to evert.

AFA, Acetic acid–formalin–alcohol.

Specimens are best kept from different parts of the host in separate vials labeled with the complete collection data (host species and common name, organ of origin, date, locality, and name of collector). Specimens should be sent to a parasitologist after contact with that person to ensure acceptance of the specimens.

ECTOPARASITES

Ectoparasites include a variety of arthropod parasites such as primarily ticks and mites, occasionally larval flies that live in tissue and result in myiasis, and, in aquatic circumstances, leeches. A complete listing of the arthropod ectoparasites of reptiles (excluding mites) is that of Barnard and Durden.[1]

Ticks

Ticks are hematophagous (feed on blood). As a result, they may induce blood loss, they may transmit etiologic agents, and they may open the skin for other agents to breach this primary defense mechanism. The two major groups of ticks are the hard ticks (Ixodidae) and the soft ticks (Argasidae).

Most ticks seen on reptiles are ixodids. Ixodid ticks typically remain on the host, and during each life cycle stage (larvae, nymphs, and female adults) they feed once to engorgement on their host's blood. The argasids feed and then leave the host. These ticks have five nymphal stages, unlike the single one in the ixodids. They spend more time off of the host in the abiotic environment than do the ixodids.

Some of the tick genera that feed on reptiles include *Amblyomma, Aponomma, Haemophysalis, Hyalomma,* and *Ixodes.* Some species feed on reptiles only as immature stages, rather than as adults. Argasids include species of *Ornithodoros* and *Argas.* They often feed more quickly than do the hard ticks. A good summary of the tick and dipteran parasites of reptiles is the book by Barnard and Durden.[1]

Recently, an exotic tick capable of feeding on ruminants and transmitting an exotic disease to the ruminants has been found on imported African tortoises in Florida.[2] Most biologists did not realize the potential significance of these reptilian ticks and thought that they were restricted to reptiles. When animals are imported into a country, they must undergo examination for external parasites such as ticks and all specimens must be removed and submitted for identification to experts who can take appropriate action to preclude establishment of new problems no country needs. A permethrin (Provent-a-Mite, Pro Products, Mahopac, NY) has been shown to be effective in eliminating ticks from reptiles and still not be toxic to the hosts.[2] See Chapter 43 for a thorough discussion of the clinical significance of ticks.

Mites

The most common mite on reptiles is *Ophionyssus natricis* (see Figure 43-4, *A, B*). It is a common pest of captive snakes and lizards. Infested hosts rub against items in their environment or remain in their water bowls. The benefit of this is that the mites release or die. Chiggers are the larvae of free-living mites and normally are found on outdoor reptiles (see Figure 43-6, *A, B*). Species of *Pterygosoma, Geckobiella,* and *Hirstiella* are found on lizards (see Figures 43-5, *A, B,* and 43-7, *A, B*). See also Chapter 43.

Myiasis

This condition is detected in captive tortoises kept outside or in free-ranging individuals. The female fly deposits larvae into an open wound (see Figure 15-37). The larvae begin to grow and molt two times before the mature larvae leave the host to pupate on the ground. Development time from the time larvae enter the wound until the mature larvae leave the wound to pupate was 43 to 52 days.

The area around this wound becomes swollen from the mass of maggots under the skin and possibly secondary invaders that cause a host response. The common species that causes this condition in terrestrial chelonians such as the Gopher Tortoise (*Gopherus polyphemus*) and Box Turtles (*Terepene* sp.) is *Cistudinomyia cistudinis*[3] (see Figure 15-38, *A, B*). Other species of dipteran larvae cause myiasis in reptiles as well.

Leeches

These hematophagous annelids are found on aquatic reptiles such as turtles and crocodilians (see Figure 15-36). The leeches on American Alligators (*Alligator mississippiensis*) are *Placobdella multilineata* and *P. papillifera*.[4,5] They are able to transmit nonpathogenic hemogregarines, such as *Haemogregarina crocodilinorum*.[6] Infestations of large numbers of leeches have been reported to cause anemia in young crocodilians.

When leeches feed on aquatic animals, the resultant lesion may allow secondary bacteria to invade and establish infections. Marine leeches *(Ozobranchus margoi)* are found in massive numbers on Green Seaturtles *(Chelonia mydas)*, Atlantic Hawksbill *(Eretomochelys imbricata)*, Loggerhead Seaturtles *(Caretta caretta)*, and Atlantic Ridleys *(Lepidochelys kempi)*. High populations of this leech usually are seen on severely emaciated turtles (see Chapter 76).

ENDOPARASITES

Endoparasites live throughout the bodies of most reptiles. Some are pathogens, and some are benign (commensals). These parasites range in size from unicellular intracellular parasites that measure a few microns to tapeworms that measure 15 to 20 centimeters in length. These are considered infections and not infestations. Each has its peculiar aspects of its life cycle, physiology, behavior, and anatomy to assist in its success as a parasite.

Because of some of the needs of many life cycles, the infections may be self-limiting, although some parasites appear to be long lived. In efforts to approach a natural-appearing setting, zoologic collections sometimes mix species, which might allow continuity of an indirect life cycle without knowledge. Some invertebrate hosts gain access to such natural settings with addition of plants in which the invertebrates are living. Thus, care must be taken to monitor the animals for parasitic infections as outlined earlier in this chapter.

Protozoa[7]

Amoebiasis, caused by *Entamoeba invadens,* in reptiles is an important disease in captive snakes, lizards, and chelonians (Figure 21-7). This is a protozoan that moves and feeds by forming pseudopodia, thus changing shape while in the **trophozoite** stage. The **cyst** is a resting stage in which a wall is produced by the trophozoite to encapsulate and protect the parasite while it is in the abiotic environment.

The cyst is the infective stage and enters the host via ingestion. It has a direct life cycle. Once in the host, it becomes a feeding motile trophozoite in the large intestine where it begins to reproduce (Figure 21-8). Some become cysts and leave the host in the feces. This parasite can move quickly through collections, resulting in large numbers of infected individuals. In one example of a major snake mortality, multiple deaths occurred within 10 weeks of the indicator case.[8] In another case involving Red-footed Tortoises *(Geochelone carbonaria)* imported into south Florida, 200 of 500 tortoises died over a 6-week period. The deaths began after a cold snap, and the tortoises became depressed, listless, and dehydrated and had watery diarrhea.[9] Histologic examination of the gut and the liver revealed *Entamoeba.*

Depending on the trophozoite's host immune status, this parasite may burrow into the mucosa and cause ulcerations. In immune-competent animals, the infection may stay in the lumen of the large intestine. Moving animals between reptile collections has been suggested to potentially result in outbreaks of amoebiasis as individuals are introduced to strains of *E. invadens* that they are not protected against.[10] Although this has not been proven, it is a logical explanation for acute outbreaks.

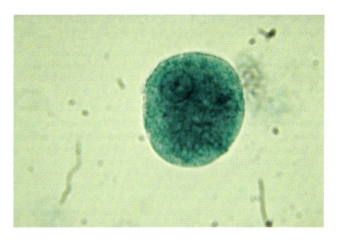

FIGURE 21-7 Ameba, *Entomoeba invadens* trophozoite. Photomicrograph magnification, 1000×.

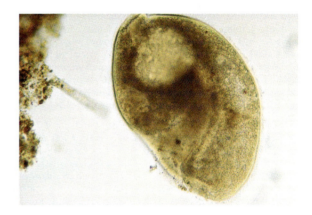

FIGURE 21-8 Ciliate trophozoite from a Star Tortoise *(Geochelone elegans)*. Photomicrograph magnification, 160×.

Signs of amoebiasis include anorexia, dehydration, and wasting. Ulcerative gastritis develops, as does colitis, inducing dysentery with mucus and blood. The liver and kidney may be reached via trophozoites in the blood. The parasite then colonizes these organs, and further damage is done, leading to necrosis and abscess formation. Diagnosis may be aided with direct smear of feces, but the best method is examination of histologic sections of the gut and liver at necropsy. The sections should be stained with trichrome or iron hematoxylin stain for better demonstration of the vesicular nucleus in the trophozoites than with the standard hematoxylin and eosin (H&E) stains.

Trophozoites are found in extracellular spaces near the ulcers or necrotic portions of the tissues. They also are found in other organs such as liver, kidney, and lung. During epizootics of amoebiasis, performance of necropsies on freshly dead or moribund animals is essential.

These parasites damage the host tissue and provide portals of entry for opportunistic bacteria and other pathogens. Therefore, one may have bacterial overgrowth along with amoebiasis simultaneously in a reptile collection.

Coccidiosis

The protozoans that may cause this disease produce an oocyst from development in the epithelial cells that line the

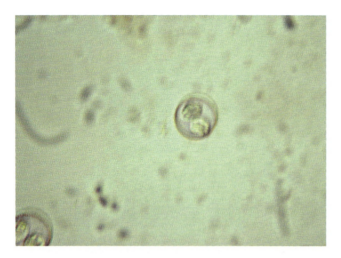

FIGURE 21-9 *Isospora amphiboluri* from a Bearded Dragon *(Pogona vitticeps)*. Photomicrograph magnification, 400×.

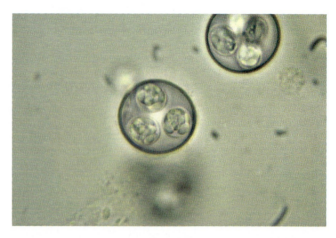

FIGURE 21-11 *Eimeria tokayae* from a Tokay Gecko *(Gekko gecko)*. Photomicrograph magnification, 1000×.

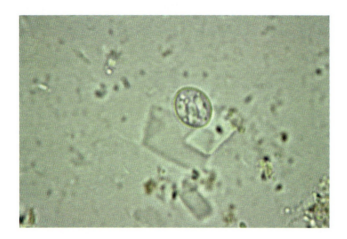

FIGURE 21-10 *Sarcocystis* sp. sporocyst from a viper. Photomicrograph magnification, 1000×.

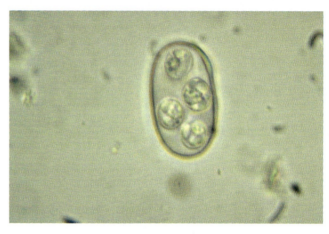

FIGURE 21-12 *Eimeria* sp. from a Bearded Dragon *(Pogona vitticeps)*. Photomicrograph magnification, 1000×.

gut. Not all infections with coccidians cause disease, and sometimes this condition is correctly called **coccidiasis** (infection with coccidians, but not disease). This is opposed to **coccidiosis,** in which the parasite causes disease.

An example of coccidiasis is seen in the Bearded Dragons. It is not uncommon to find coccidia in clinically healthy Bearded Dragons on routine fecal examinations. Many healthy individuals shed large numbers of *Isospora amphiboluri* oocysts. **These animals are infected, not diseased. There is no reason to treat these animals.**

In many cases in which coccidian oocysts are seen in the feces, whether disease or simply infection exists is unknown. Some coccidians (species of *Isospora, Eimeria,* and *Cryptosporidium*) have direct life cycles with a single host with the oocysts produced and passed in the feces (Figures 21-9 to 21-12). Others such as *Sarcocystis* spp. are obligate two host cycles normally with a predator-prey relationship and potentially with a reptile for either IH or DH. An exception to the norm was shown with a species of lizard that was able to function as both hosts.[11]

Oocysts are the infective stages to the next host. Most oocysts can be identified to genus by the number of **sporocysts** and **sporozoites** per sporocyst per **oocyst** (Table 21-2).

Table 21-2 Generic Oocyst Morphology

	Sporocyst No.	Sporozoites/Sporocyst No.
Cryptosporidium	0	4/oocyst
Caryospora	1	8
Isospora	2	4
Sarcocystis	2	4*
Eimeria	4	2

*Oocysts of *Sarcocystis* rupture while passing though the gut; thus, one typically sees sporulated sporocyst.

Only species of *Sarcocystis* and *Cryptosporidium* pass fully infective when they exit the host that produced them. Species of the other genera need to develop (sporulate) in the abiotic environment. In no instance has anyone proven that the coccidia that infect reptiles can go vertically through the egg into the progeny. In general, once the sporulated oocyst is ingested, the sporozoites leave the oocyst and penetrate into epithelial cells that line the mucosa. The development is intracellular, and with each phase of the cycle, more host cells are killed as the parasites exit the host cells in which they were produced and enter other cells.

Set numbers of asexual generations exist within one life cycle, and then the sexual phase ensues and produces gametes and zygotes. A wall is produced by the parasite around the zygote that is now an oocyst. It is expelled from the host cell and passes in the feces.

Whether disease is caused by the developing coccidian depends on the number of oocysts initially ingested, the ability of the host to replace the cells killed quickly enough to preclude clinical disease, the genetics of the parasite itself, and the host immune status. Coccidiosis is usually a disease of young animals.

Clinical signs are usually not detected, but a stunting or slowing of growth and maturation may be seen in lizard hosts. Coccidiosis apparently is important in rearing captive crocodilians in Zimbabwe. To compound this problem, oocysts are rarely found in the feces of these hosts, and diagnosis is with histopathologic examination of the gut tissues. This coccidian evidently develops in other organs than the gut as well. Signs in this case are hemorrhagic enteritis with swelling and congestion of the small intestine.

Cryptosporidiosis

Cryotosporidiosis is caused by species of *Cryptosporidium*. In reptiles this tiny coccidian (oocysts less than 8 microns in diameter) is caused by two species: *C. serpentis* in snakes and *C. saurophylum* in lizards.[12] The former develops on the gastric mucosa, and the latter develops on the mucosa of the small intestine.

This disease is usually fatal in snakes, but the diagnosis is confused by oocysts of rodents fed to the snakes as rodents have their own species of *Cryptosporidium*. These species are not infective to reptiles, but because they are so close in size, they cause serious confusion. **The gold standard for proving a snake is infected with *Cryptosporidium* is by gastric biopsy.**

If the stages are present in classic manner as little round bodies sitting on the surface of the mucosa, the snake is infected. Gastric lavages, direct or fecal flotation examinations, and enzyme-linked immunosorbent assays (ELISAs) to date are insufficient proof for euthanasia of a snake.

Clinical signs in snakes include a midbody swelling and regurgitation of food items 2 to 3 days after eating. Lizards are harmed by their form of cryptosporidiosis and become stunted and sometimes die. Reports of *Cryptosporidium* developing aural-pharyngeal polyps in the ear canal of Green Iguanas are bizarre but do represent an unusual site for development of this coccidian genus.[13] See Chapter 48 for a thorough discussion of reptilian cryptosporidiosis, diagnosis, and management.

HEMOPARASITES OF REPTILES

Species of blood parasites of lizards represent several genera. All of these reside in the blood, and some of these genera are common, with others rarely reported.

Hemoparasites have indirect life cycles. Most are arthropod transmitted, at least in the terrestrial reptiles. Some of the blood parasites of aquatic blood parasites are transmitted by leeches. Most hemoparasites are intracellular, but one genus remains extracellular and is found free in the plasma. Most of these are not considered to be pathogens even though they are killing cells in circulation.

The genera most commonly found are *Plasmodium, Haemoproteus, Haemogregarina, Hepatozoon,* and *Trypanosoma,* and the remainder are minor players that include *Schellackia, Lankesterella, Fallisia,* and *Saurocytozoon*. The most complete summary of these parasites is that of Telford,[14] and although this publication is somewhat dated, it is still the best starting place for these parasites. Telford[14] indicated that reptiles in some areas were commonly infected with these parasites, whereas in other places, either the prevalence was low or the parasites were not detected. For the most part, these infections are of little significance because most are considered nonpathogenic. Schall[15] has shown that some species of *Plasmodium* do have an impact on their lizard host reproductive capabilities as infected females have smaller clutch sizes and infected males may not be able to defend their territories as well as uninfected males.

The diagrammatic figures in *A Veterinary Guide to the Parasites of Reptiles: Protozoa* by Barnard and Upton[7] illustrate the basic morphology of these parasites. The clinical significance and the management of the hemoparasites are discussed in Chapter 55.

GUT-INHABITING FLAGELLATED PROTOZOA

All parasites in this group have direct life cycles and include species of *Hexamita, Monocercomonoides, Proteromonas, Monocercomonas,* and *Giardia*. The arrangement of the flagella on these motile forms is characteristic of the genera. Many of these have not been proven to be pathogens for their reptilian hosts (*Monocercomonoides* and *Proteromonas*). Some are pathogens at times but are apparently not under other circumstances.

Intestinal flagellates may be disconcerting because permanent slides for staining are nearly impossible. Most of these must be examined in the fresh condition. This is aided with examination of the slides after the flagellates begin to slow down. *Hexamita* is smaller than the rest, usually less than 8 microns in length, and quickly swims directly out of the field of view at high magnifications (Figure 21-13).

If one has the potential to process these for scanning electron microscopy, then the identification is more easily determined. Hexamitiasis in tortoises is caused by *Hexamita parva*, which normally resides in the lumen of the intestines but sometimes enters the biliary tract and the urinary tract in which changes are caused. Pale and enlarged kidneys were seen in some cases. Collecting tubules were dilated. In the liver, bile ducts were thickened and the lumen was dilated. Trophozoites were present in the lumen of tubules in both organs. No specific signs were recognized.[16]

Giardia is a graceful swimmer, and as it rolls over, one can see the concave sucking disc (Figure 21-14). No proof exists that species of this genus cause disease in reptiles.

Monocercomonas has a stiff axostyle running its length, three anterior flagella, and a single trailing flagellum. Monocercomoniosis has been reported in snakes and lizards. Clinical signs include anorexia, wasting, and behavioral changes; individuals may become aggressive. Occasionally, the

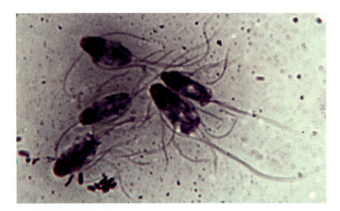

FIGURE 21-13 *Hexamita* from *Clemmys marmorata*. *(Photograph courtesy F.L. Frye.)*

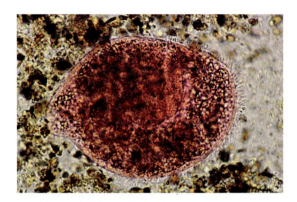

FIGURE 21-15 Nyctotherus (merthiolate stain). *(Photograph courtesy F.L. Frye.)*

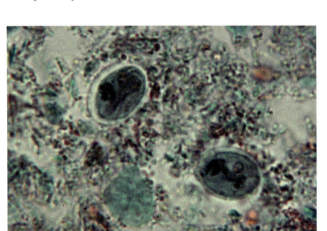

FIGURE 21-14 *Giardia lamblia*. *(Photograph courtesy F.L. Frye.)*

flagellates are found in the reproductive tract, liver, and lungs. The most common lesion is an undermining of the intestinal epithelium and a separation from the underlying propria. Ronidazole (Ridzol, Merck, Iselin, NJ) has been used orally at 10 mg active ingredient/kg 8 to 10 days or 150 mg/liter of drinking water. Supportive therapy may be needed.

CILIATED PROTOZOA

Ciliated protozoa are more commonly found in herbivorous reptiles such as tortoises and some species of lizards. The more common genera are *Balantidium* and *Nyctotherus* (Figures 21-15 and 21-16). These are large ciliates, usually more than 60 microns in length, uniformly covered with cilia. The trophozoites are hard to miss on a direct smear, and the cysts are the means of transmission to the next host via fecal-oral contamination. If stained, the large macronucleus is obvious, but the micronucleus is rarely seen. No indication is seen that these cause disease in reptiles.

MICROSPORIDIOSIS

Although this group of complex protozoans is rarely a problem in reptiles, now and then reptiles are infected and these

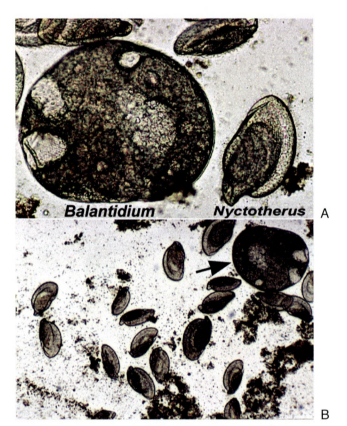

FIGURE 21-16 A, *Balantidium* (left), *Nyctotherus* (right). Note size difference. **B,** *Balantidium* (larger, *upper right, arrow*), *Nyctotherus* (numerous). *(Photographs courtesy F.L. Frye.)*

parasites may lead to the death of the infected host. Most of the infections in reptiles (snakes, turtles, and lizards) are caused by species of *Pleistophora*. These are usually represented by cyst-like masses of the spores in muscles but may occur in other tissues as well. Little is known about their biology in their reptilian hosts.

Bearded Dragons were recently found to be infected with microsporidians. The spores were found mainly in the livers of the dragons.[17] This group of parasites is becoming recognized more commonly in various classes of vertebrates, whereas most of them are parasites of invertebrates, predominantly arthropods.

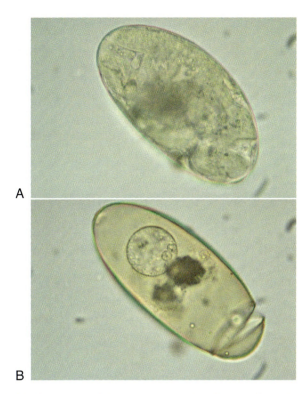

FIGURE 21-17 **A,** Fluke egg *(Lophotaspis vallei)* containing larva. **B,** *L. vallei* egg that has hatched from a Loggerhead Seaturtle *(Caretta caretta).* Photomicrograph magnification, 400×.

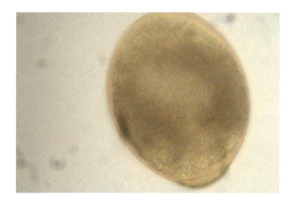

FIGURE 21-18 *Nematophila* sp. egg from a Yellow-footed Tortoise *(Geochelone denticulata).* Photomicrograph magnification, 400×.

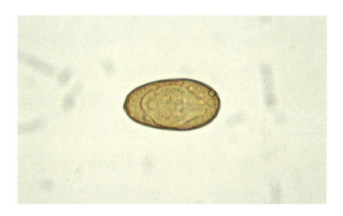

FIGURE 21-19 *Euparadistomum* sp. from a Green-eyed Gecko *(Gekko smithii).* Photomicrograph magnification, 400×.

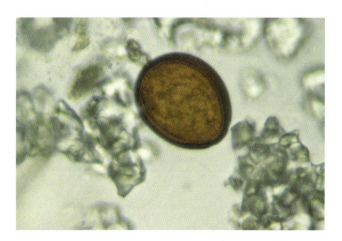

FIGURE 21-20 *Orchidasma amphiorchis* from a Loggerhead Seaturtle *(Caretta caretta).* Photomicrograph magnification, 400×.

TREMATODES

These metazoans are all parasitic flatworms. Some have direct life cycles (**monogenetic flukes** and aspidobothrid flukes), and the remainder have indirect life cycles (**digenetic flukes**). The latter is commonly found in all groups of reptiles, and some are extremely pathogenic.

Monogenetic trematodes are primarily found as ectoparasites of fish. A few species parasitize fresh water turtles. They reside in the urinary bladders, oral cavity, and associated spaces of their turtle hosts. They are not known to be pathogenic to their reptilian hosts and are included here for completeness.

Aspidobothrid trematodes have the ventral surface subdivided as a holdfast organ. These are considered intermediate between the monogenetic and digenetic flukes. Most of these are parasites of molluscs, but a few species are parasites of turtles. *Lophotaspis vallei* resides mainly in the stomach and upper small intestine of Loggerhead Seaturtles (Figure 21-17). They are not known to cause any damage to their hosts.

Digenetic trematodes are the most diverse group of trematodes (Figures 21-18 to 21-24). They all require at least one IH to complete their cycles, and some require two or more. These live in nearly every soft tissue organ in the body of their reptilian hosts, although most reside in the gastrointestinal tract. They all have the potential to alternate between generations of sexual reproduction and asexual reproduction. The former occurs in the DH, and the latter occurs in the first IH, which is normally a mollusc. Some use terrestrial gastropods for their IHs and are therefore not tied to an aquatic habitat.

Other digenetic trematodes need aquatic snails for their first IH, and thus, flukes have different potentials to be found in captive reptilian collections kept in natural settings.

Most digenetic trematodes have evolved to a level of mutual coexistence, and little or no pathology is inflicted. However, when a reptile keeper opens the mouth of a snake and sees worms attached to the oral mucosa and in the esophagus, they are a problem that needs to be eliminated for aesthetic reasons. These flukes include *Haplometroides, Ochetosoma, Pneumatophilus, Stomatrema,* and *Zeugorchis.* They are acquired with eating a vertebrate second IH that contains encysted metacercariae.

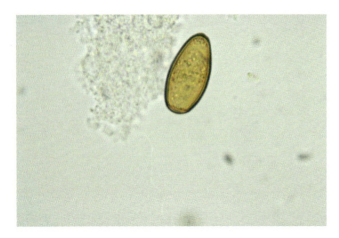

FIGURE 21-21 *Enodiotrema* sp. from a Loggerhead Seaturtle *(Caretta caretta)*. Photomicrograph magnification, 400×.

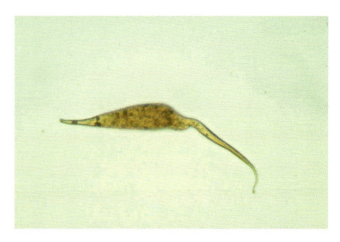

FIGURE 21-24 *Learedius learedi* from a Green Seaturtle *(Chelonia mydas)*. Photomicrograph magnification, 400×.

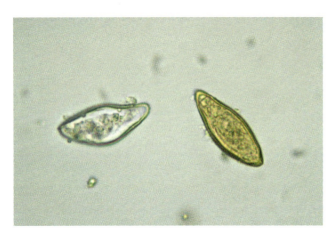

FIGURE 21-22 *Pachypsolus irroratus* from a Loggerhead Seaturtle *(Caretta caretta)*. Photomicrograph magnification, 400×.

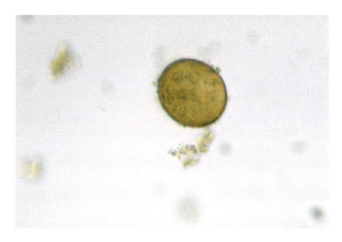

FIGURE 21-25 *Neospirorchis* sp. from a Loggerhead Seaturtle *(Caretta caretta)*. Photomicrograph magnification, 400×.

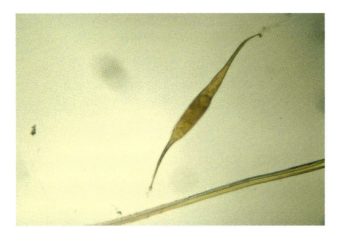

FIGURE 21-23 *Hapalotrema loossi* from a Loggerhead Seaturtle *(Caretta caretta)*. Photomicrograph magnification, 400×.

Spirorchiidae, a group of flukes whose adults live in blood vessels and the heart, are pathogenic. As for all parasites that are going to exist in nature, they have to get their offspring (eggs) out of the host as a source of infection to another host and perpetuation of the species. Because no direct means exists to eliminate eggs from the blood, the eggs are trapped in capillary beds and then essentially are worked passively through the host tissue into the gut where they may be shed in the feces. Sometimes the adults may be numerous enough to block smaller vessels (capillaries) and cause ischemia and damage to the tissue not being fed or oxygenated. Sometimes the eggs can pile up and cause the same problem, and some of those eggs that leave the gut are trapped by the host and form granulomas. These can be found in most soft tissues of the body, and the more of these that develop in an organ, the less functional that organ becomes.[18] Marine turtles may be seriously affected by these flukes (Figure 21-25; see Chapter 76).

Other flukes, such as *Styphlodora* spp., live in the excretory system. This is a common parasite in free-ranging snakes with up to 66% of some snakes infected. A captive boa died after about 6 months of anorexia, and the adults of *Styphlodora horrida* were recovered from the preserved kidneys.[19] The flukes were believed to be the cause of death.

TAPEWORMS

Tapeworms are flatworms comprising a scolex (holdfast organ) and a chain of repetitive sections (proglottids).

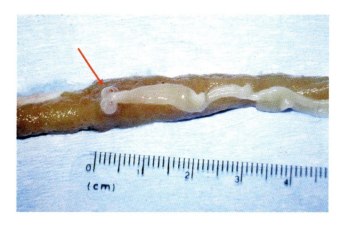

FIGURE 21-26 *Bothridium* sp. tapeworm in the intestine of a Ball Python (*Python regius*). Note the scolex on the left side of the photograph (*arrow*). (Photograph courtesy S. Barten.)

Each proglottid increases in maturity as they move farther from the scolex with budding of new sections. The adults reside in the small intestine of their DH, and they all have indirect life cycles (Figure 21-26). Tapeworms parasitize all groups of reptiles except crocodilians.

Tapeworms can outcompete the host for basic nutrients, but if the host is on a good plane of nutrition, tapeworms are not considered to be pathogens. Reptiles may serve as an IH as the larvae tapeworms, not the adult, are found in the reptiles. These larvae are often subcutaneous, causing bumps or ridges in the skin, and make a reptile less attractive for display purposes.

Many of the adult tapeworms of reptiles are in the families Anoplocephalidae, Diphyllobothriidae, and Proteocephalidae. Anoplocephalidae typically use a mite or an insect as the IH. Diphyllobothriidae life cycle uses two IHs, typically an aquatic crustacean as the first and a vertebrate as the second (Table 21-3).

Proteocephalidae cycles have the eggs eaten by copepods in which the procercoid larva develops, and these are infective to the DH. But they first develop into plerocercoids, and these develop in the solid organs, such as the liver. The parasite then wanders through the host, and if it reaches the lumen of the intestine, it attaches and matures. Adult tapeworms may be diagnosed with fecal flotation if the eggs are released from the proglottids or with visualization of free proglottids in the feces and then a search for eggs in normal saline solution. All of the tapeworm eggs (except species of the Diphyllobothriidae) from reptile feces should contain a fully formed oncosphere with six hooks (Figures 21-27 to 21-33).

Larval tapeworms of *Spirometra* (spargana) may be found in the viscera (see Figure 72-11) or subcutaneously in snakes and lizards, and the same is true for the tetrathyridia of *Mesocestoides*. The latter should contain an inverted scolex with four suckers, but this is not always obvious in the experience of the senior author.

ACANTHOCEPHALA

The spiny headed worms are the acanthocephala, and the adults all live within the small intestines. They have a

Table 21-3	Tapeworm Genera and Reptile Hosts	
Genus	**Reptiles Infected**	**Intermediate Hosts**
Anoplocephalidae		Mites and insects
Oorchistica	Snakes, lizards, turtles	
Panceriella	Varanids	
Diochetos	Lizards	
Semenoviella	Lizards	
Diphyllobothriidae		Freshwater crustaceans then vertebrates
Scyphocephalus	Varanids	
Bothridium	Varanids, boids	
Duthiersia	Varanids	
Proteocephalidae		Freshwater crustaceans
Ophiotaenia	Snakes, lizards	
Macrobothriotaenia	Snakes	
Kapsulotaenia	Varanids	
Acanthotaenia	Varanids	
Crepidobothrium	Snakes	
Deblocktaenia	Snakes	
Tejidotaenia	Lizards	

From Schmidt GD: *Handbook of tapeworm identification*, Boca Raton, Fla, 1984, CDC Press.

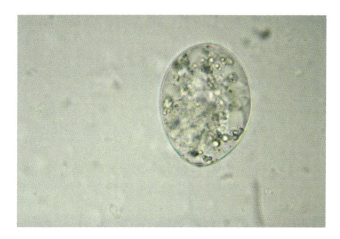

FIGURE 21-27 Cestode eggs as passed in feces from a python (*Python* sp.). Photomicrograph magnification, 400×.

retractable proboscis armed with spines that is inserted into the mucosa as a holdfast. They have separate sexes and lack a digestive system. These helminths have indirect life cycles, usually with an arthropod as the IH, but occasionally they use a terrestrial reptile (usually a lizard) as a paratenic host.

Cystacanth larvae are encysted usually in the abdominal cavity, and these are infective to the DH as the cystacanths in the normal arthropod IHs.

The eggs of acanthocephalans are usually complex with multiple layers enclosing the acanthor larva (Figure 21-34). Some of these rise on fecal flotation, and others must be detected with a sedimentation procedure. Perhaps the best examples of acanths in reptiles are the species of

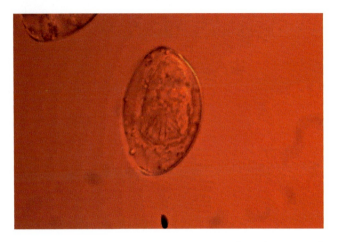

FIGURE 21-28 Cestode larva from a python (*Python* sp.). Photomicrograph magnification, 400×.

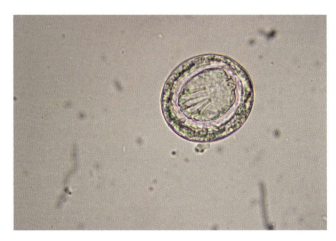

FIGURE 21-30 Unknown tapeworm egg from a Rhinocerous Iguana (*Cyclura cyclura*). Photomicrograph magnification, 400×.

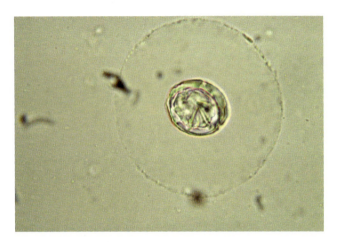

FIGURE 21-29 *Oochoristica* from a Tokay Gecko (*Gekko gecko*). Photomicrograph magnification, 400×.

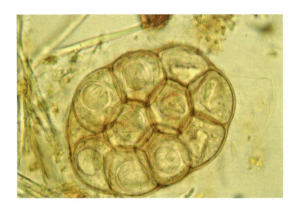

FIGURE 21-31 Unknown tapeworm egg from a boa. Photomicrograph magnification, 400×.

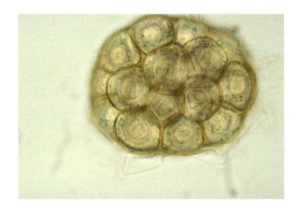

FIGURE 21-32 Unknown tapeworm egg from a Green Tree Python (*Morelia viridis*). Photomicrograph magnification, 400×.

Neoechinorhychus, which infect freshwater turtles. The proboscis spination of these is reduced, and they are unlikely to cause much damage.

NEMATODES

Nematodes are tubular worms and are round in cross section and thus called round worms. They are parasites of all groups of reptiles. Adults live in tubular organs such as the gut, free in the body cavity, in the lungs and nasal passages, and subcutaneously in their reptilian hosts (see Figure 15-31). They may have either direct or indirect life cycles. They have separate sexes and complete digestive systems.

Some are pathogenic, and some may be beneficial. The effects of most nematodes are unknown, and many could be neutral in their influence on their hosts. Nematodes are the most diverse group of helminths that infect reptiles. Some produce eggs, some release L_1 larvae, and some produce microfilariae that are actually motile embryos. Those that produce eggs are diagnosed with fecal flotation, and those that release larvae are easily diagnosed with a Baermann funnel. These larvae do float but are greatly distorted by the flotation medium. Those nematodes that produce microfilariae can be detected with a finding of microfilariae in the blood. Members of the Rhabditida, Strongylida, Spirurida, Ascarida, and Oxyurida, and superfamilies Trichuroidea and Filarioidea will be discussed.

The order **Rhabditoidea** includes *Strongyloides* and *Rhabdias* (Figures 21-35 and 21-36). These tiny nematodes are represented as parthenogenetic females in the homogonic cycle and also have a free-living phase called the heterogonic phase. Both have direct life cycles, and the infective stages

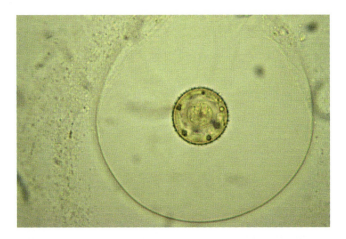

FIGURE 21-33 Unknown tapeworm egg from a python (*Python* sp.). Photomicrograph magnification, 400×.

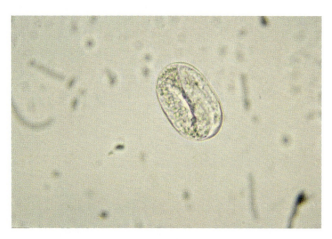

FIGURE 21-36 Nematode egg from a Blue-tailed Monitor (*Varanus doreanus*). Photomicrograph magnification, 400×.

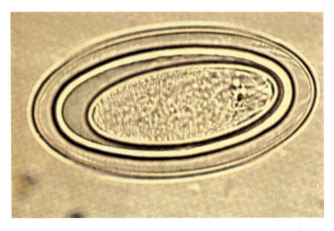

FIGURE 21-34 Acanthocephalan egg from a monitor lizard. Note the multiple layers enclosing the acanthor larva. (*Photograph courtesy F.L. Frye.*)

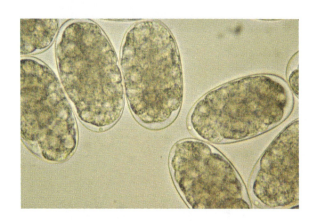

FIGURE 21-37 *Kalicephalus* sp. eggs from a Black Racer (*Coluber constrictor*). Photomicrograph magnification, 400×.

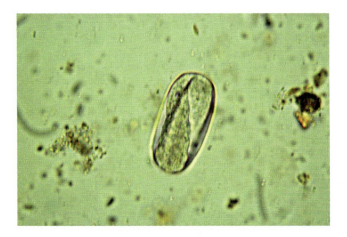

FIGURE 21-35 Nematode egg (*Rhabdias* sp.) from a Red Ratsnake (Cornsnake) (*Elaphe guttata*). Photomicrograph magnification, 400×.

can penetrate intact skin and move to the site of adult development. Adults of *Rhabdias* spp. reside in the lungs, and infections may be benign or they may induce great quantities of mucus production, pneumonia, and gasping for air. This may be fatal if the hygiene is poor and high temperature and humidity exist, which are ideal for the free-living heterogonic cycle to increase the populations of infective larvae.

The eggs are larvated when shed by the females, and these may hatch as they exit the host. Adults of *Strongyloides* reside in the small intestine and may become entwined in and out of the mucosa. In a case of a Burmese Python (*Python molurus bivitattus*) infected with *Strongyloides*, the python became anorexic and died. On necropsy, the ureters were obstructed and distended and ureteritis, nephritis, and gastroenteritis developed. Multiple sections of worms were found in these tissues. Whether the entire problem was caused by the nematode infection or merely associated with it is unresolved.[20]

The Strongylida has some important blood-sucking nematodes. These include *Kalicephalus* of snakes (Figure 21-37). They normally reside in the small intestine but have been presented to the senior author from the mouth and esophagus of snakes (Figure 21-38). The oral cavity is fairly distinctive (Figure 21-39), and the males have a prominent copulatory bursa (Figure 21-40).

Another genus found in stomachs of tortoises is *Chapiniella* (Figure 21-41). This species has a different oral appearance because of a large oral cavity that is preceded by two rows of sensory papillae that compose the leaf crowns.[21] They have direct life cycles, and the infective larvae are eaten and usually

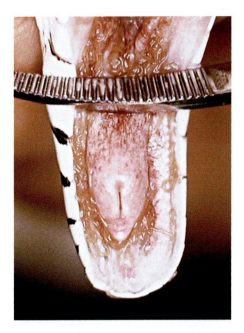

FIGURE 21-38 *Kalicephalus* sp. larva in the oral cavity of a snake. (*Photograph courtesy D. Mader.*)

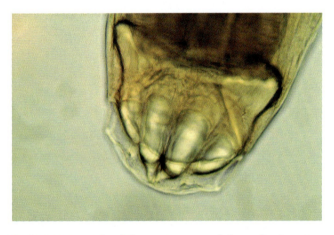

FIGURE 21-39 *Kalicephalus* sp. Anterior end shows the distinctive oral cavity (from *Bothrops* sp.). Photomicrograph magnification, 160×.

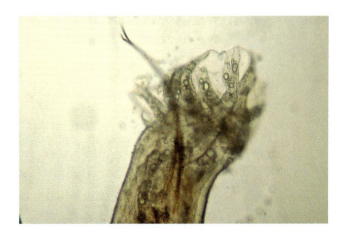

FIGURE 21-40 *Kalicephalus* sp. Prominent copulatory bursa (from a Black Racer). Photomicrograph magnification, 100×.

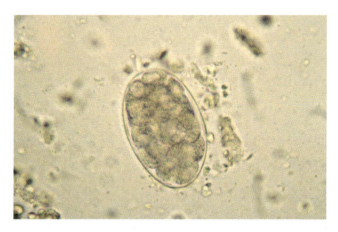

FIGURE 21-41 *Chapiniella* sp. egg from an Ornate Box Turtle (*Terrapene ornata*). Photomicrograph magnification, 400×.

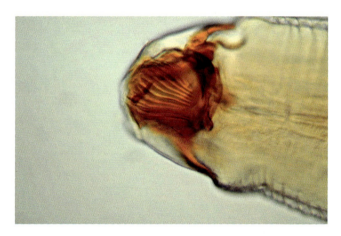

FIGURE 21-42 *Serpinema* sp. Common Spirurid from a freshwater turtle. Note the distinctive buccal capsule. Photomicrograph magnification, 160×.

enter the wall of the stomach or intestines, mature, and then return to the lumen and attach to the mucosa.

The Spirurida are a group of nematodes that use an IH (usually an arthropod) and live in the upper digestive system, primarily in the stomach. *Serpinema* is common in freshwater turtles. The distinctive buccal capsule helps identify species of this genus (Figure 21-42). *Spiroxys* lives in the stomachs of freshwater turtles, and their mouths are also distinctive (Figure 21-43). Species of this genus use microcrustaceans as IHs and then in *Spiroxys* are able to use a variety of aquatic organisms ranging from fish and amphibians to snails and dragonfly naiads as paratenic hosts.

Another important order is the Ascarida. These are large worms with three prominent lips (Figure 21-44). The species of *Hexametra, Amplicaecum, Ophidascaris,* and *Polydelphis* primarily infect the stomachs and intestines of snakes and have indirect life cycles (Figure 21-45). *Dujardinascaris* is a genus of stomach worm of crocodilians (Figure 21-46). They use amphibians, reptiles, and small mammals as IHs. Some of these induce deep pits where the worms attach, and sometimes many worms can be attached in a single crater-like lesion.

Sulcascaris sulcata is a parasite of the stomach of Loggerhead Seaturtles and uses oysters as its IH (Figures 21-47 and 21-48).

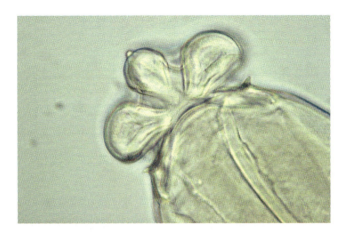

FIGURE 21-43 Distinctive mouth parts of *Spiroxis* sp. from a freshwater turtle. Photomicrograph magnification, 400×.

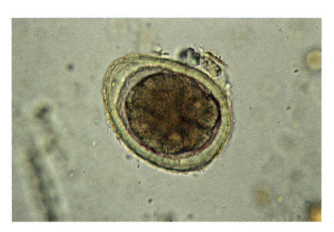

FIGURE 21-46 *Dujardinascaris* sp. from an American Alligator (*Alligator mississippiensis*). Photomicrograph magnification, 400×.

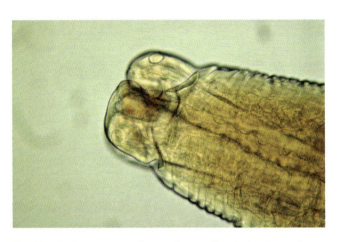

FIGURE 21-44 Prominent lips on the mouthpart of an Ascarid nematode. Photomicrograph magnification, 100×.

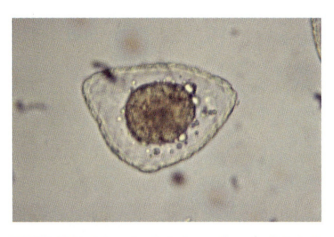

FIGURE 21-47 *Sulcascaris sulcata* from a Loggerhead Seaturtle (*Caretta caretta*). Photomicrograph magnification, 400×.

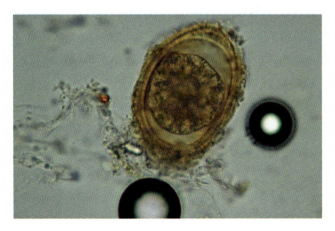

FIGURE 21-48 *Sulcascaris sulcata* from a Loggerhead Seaturtle (*Caretta caretta*). Photomicrograph magnification, 400×.

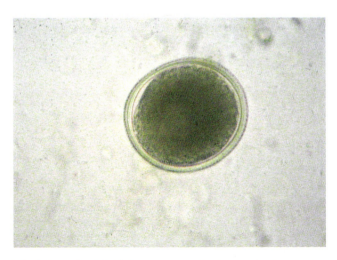

FIGURE 21-45 *Polydelphis* sp. from a Reticulated Python (*Python reticulatus*). Photomicrograph magnification, 400×.

The eggs of all of these are large and pitted or roughened on the shell.

The order Oxyurida has many genera (Table 21-4) that infect reptiles. The eggs are smooth and elongate, with a straight side and a lens-shaped plug at one end (Figures 21-49 to 21-51). Most lizards have at least one species, and some have

Table 21-4	Genera of Oxyurida (Pinworms) of Reptilian Hosts
Genus	**Definitive Hosts**
Ozolaimus	Iguanids
Paraleuris	Iguanids
Parapharyngodon	Lizards
Pharyngodon	Lizards
Skrjabinodon	Lizard
Spauligodon	Lizards and tortoises
Tachygonetria	Uromastix and tortoises
Aleuris	Lizards and tortoises
Thelandros	Lizards and tortoises
Mehdiella	Tortoises
Ortleppnema	Tortoises
Thaparia	Tortoises

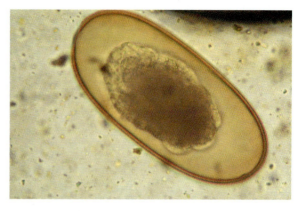

FIGURE 21-51 Unknown pinworm from a spur-thighed (Greek) Tortoise *(Testudo graeca)*. Photomicrograph magnification, 400×.

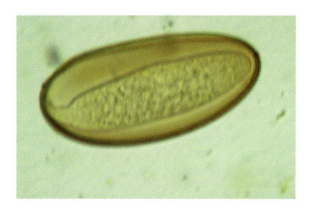

FIGURE 21-49 *Ozolaimus* sp. from a Green Iguana *(Iguana iguana)*. Photomicrograph magnification, 400×.

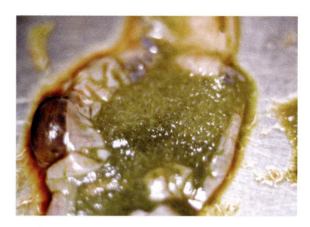

FIGURE 21-52 Large colon from a Desert Tortoise *(Gopherus agassizii)* impacted with Oxyurid larva. *(Photograph courtesy D. Mader.)*

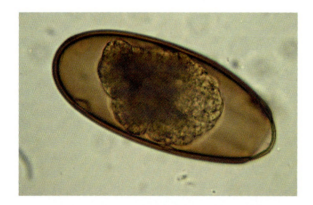

FIGURE 21-50 Unknown pinworm from a Spur-thighed (Greek) Tortoise *(Testudo graeca)*. Photomicrograph magnification, 400×.

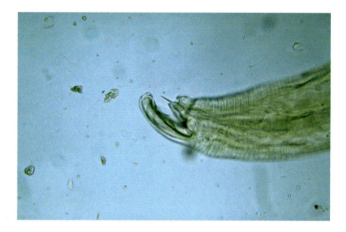

FIGURE 21-53 Posterior end of male *Ozolaimus* sp., lateral view. This is an important distinction for identification of different species of pinworms.

several. The tortoises often have a community of multiple species of these short worms (Figure 21-52). These worms all have an esophageal bulb that helps to distinguish them. They are short worms, and the females have a long tapering tail that gives them their name. The male posterior ends are all important in identification, and two such tails are illustrated: *Ozolaimus* lateral view (Figure 21-53) and *Aleuris* sp. ventral view (Figure 21-54). They live in the lumen of the large intestine (Figure 21-55). They all have direct life cycles, and for the main part, these should be left intact. Many people have tried to eliminate them and have not had great success. Sometimes harm is done to the host with the drugs whose application is unwarranted.

The Trichuroidea of reptiles are in two genera. *Capillaria* spp. are tiny worms that live mainly in the small intestine, and the

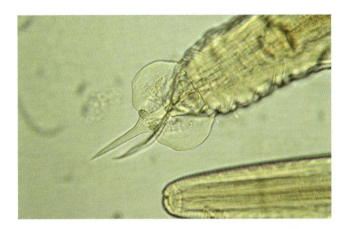

FIGURE 21-54 Posterior end of a male *Aleuris* sp., ventral view.

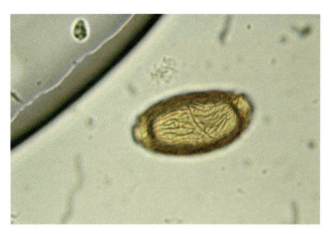

FIGURE 21-57 *Capillaria* sp. egg from a Green Tree Python *(Morelia viridis)* (same egg as in Figure 21-56—focus is on the shell surface). Photomicrograph magnification, 400×.

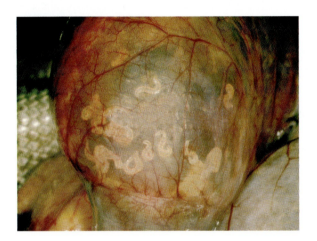

FIGURE 21-55 Oxyurids in the distended colon of a Green Iguana *(Iguana iguana)*. *(Photograph courtesy S. Barten.)*

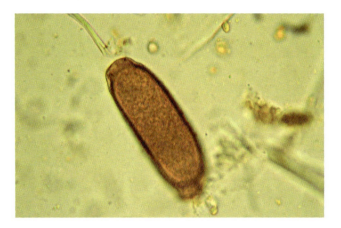

FIGURE 21-58 *Capillaria* sp. egg from a boa. Photomicrograph magnification, 400×.

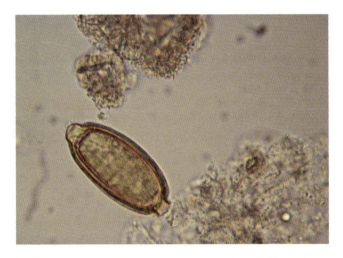

FIGURE 21-56 *Capillaria* sp. egg from a Green Tree Python *(Morelia viridis)*. Photomicrograph magnification, 400×.

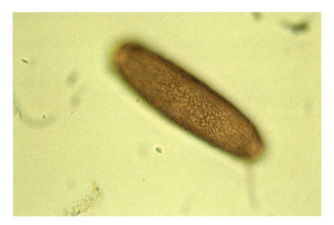

FIGURE 21-59 *Capillaria* sp. egg from a boa (same egg as in Figure 21-58—focus is on the shell surface). Photomicrograph magnification, 400×.

females contain the bipolar eggs as illustrated previously (Figures 21-56 to 21-59). The second genus is *Paratrichosoma*; these worms live under the abdominal skin of crocodilians in Asia and make black tracks in the skin as they migrate.[22]

Members of the final order, Filarioidea, all require some sort of vector to deliver the infective larvae to the DH. Adults live in blood vessels, in body cavities, subcutaneously, and in connective tissues. *Foleyella furcata* resides in the subcutaneous tissues and body cavity of chameleons (Figure 21-60). *Macdonaldius oschei* adults live in the major arteries of Pythons, and the microfilariae are in the blood. Frank[23] found necrotic lesion in the muscle that he attributed to being

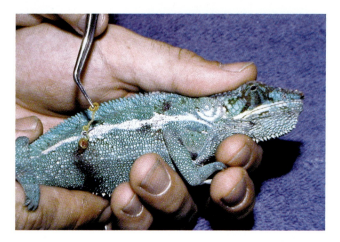

FIGURE 21-60 *Foleyella furcata* being removed from the subcutaneous tissue of a chameleon. *(Photograph courtesy D. Mader.)*

Table 21-5	Genera of Filarioidea in Reptilian Definitive Hosts
Hosts	**Genera**
Crocodilians	*Oswaldocruzia*
Crocodilians and lacertid lizards	*Befilaria*
	Conispiculum
	Gonofilaria
	Piratuba
	Piratuboides
	Solafilaria
Chameleons and lacertid lizards	*Foleyella*
Chelonians and lacertid lizards	*Cardianema*
	Pseudothamugadia
	Madathamugadia
	Thamugadia (gecko)
Lacertid lizards	*Saurocitus*
Snakes and lizards	*Macdonaldius*

Table 21-6	Pentasomids and Reptilian Hosts
Host	**Genera**
Crocodilians	*Sebakia* spp.
Monitor Lizards	*Elenia* spp. and *Sambonia* spp.
Lizards, snakes	*Raillietiella* spp.
Nonpoisonous snakes in the United States	*Kiricephalus* spp.
Rattlesnakes and Cottonmouth	*Porocephalus* spp.
African Python	*Armillifer* spp.

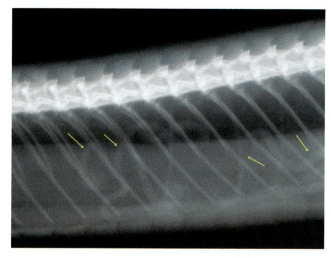

FIGURE 21-61 Radiograph of a wild Indigo Snake (*Drymarchon couperi*). Note the radiodense serpiginous pattern within the lungs *(yellow arrows)*. These are internal pentastomid parasites. *(Photograph courtesy D. Mader.)*

caused by occluded arteries. Five species of *Oswaldocruzia* reside in different locations in their DHs (Table 21-5).

PENTASTOMIDS

About 70 species of pentastomids are recognized worldwide. These primitive arthropods, which look like a cross between a helminth and an insect, belong to their own phylum. The majority of pentastomids are found as adult worms (as opposed to larval stages) in reptiles. The adult worms are segmented and worm-like, measuring from 0.5 to 20 cm in length, and are exclusively internal and usually occur in the lungs of snakes, lizards, and crocodilians (Table 21-6).[10] Evidence of the adult worms living in the lungs on survey radiographs is not uncommon (Figure 21-61).

Turtles may be occasionally infected. The most common genera of reptilian Pentastomes are *Raillietiella*, *Porocephalus*, *Kiricephalus*, *Armillifer*, and *Sebekia*.

Raillietiella spp. occur in lizards and snakes, and *Kiricephalus* spp. may be found in nonpoisonous snakes of the United States. The American Rattlesnake and the Cottonmouth Moccasin harbor the *Porocephalus crotali*. *Armillifer* spp. infect the vipers and African Python, and *Sebekia* spp. have the crocodilians as hosts.

Pentastomids have an ability to bore through tissue, and adult worms occasionally may pierce through the lung and body and protrude from the skin. Pentastome infections may be asymptomatic with little inflammatory response, but in other instances, significant damage and destruction of tissue of the host may be seen.

The life cycle consists of the adult parasites in the lung depositing eggs that contain larvae and have four leg-like appendages (see Figure 21-1). These eggs are coughed up, swallowed, and then passed in the fecal material. A fecal examination reveals characteristic pentastomid ova: a distended thin-walled capsule that measures up to 130 micrometers in diameter. Larvae, with four hooklets, are seen within the egg (Figures 21-62 to 21-65).

The eggs develop to an infective stage and are swallowed by an IH where larval development takes place. The larvae develop into infective nymphs in the IH and then into adults in the reptile host after ingestion of the IH. The infective larvae perforate the intestinal wall of the host and migrate through the body to enter the lungs. The major pathology in the host is the local tissue damage that results from attachment in the lung (Figure 21-66).

The severity and nature of the host's response are dependent on the immune status of the host, the number and stage of the invading parasite, and presence or absence of concurrent disease. Despite the migratory passages, most

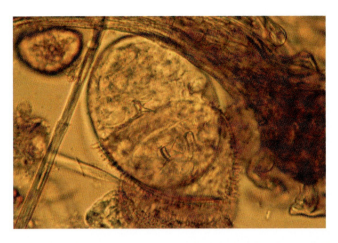

FIGURE 21-62 Pentastome eggs are characteristically thin walled and can measure up to 130 µm in diameter. Larvae with four hooklets are typically seen within eggs. This is an unidentified pentastome from a Water Monitor (*Varanus* sp.).

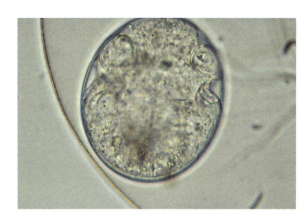

FIGURE 21-65 Unknown pentastome from a Narrowhead Softshell Turtle *(Chitra indica)*. Photomicrograph magnification, 400×.

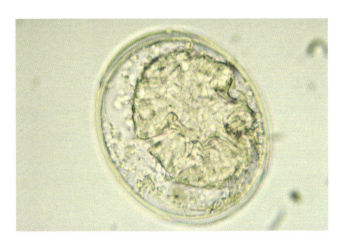

FIGURE 21-63 *Railietiella frenatus* from a Tokay Gecko *(Gekko gecko)*. Photomicrograph magnification, 400×.

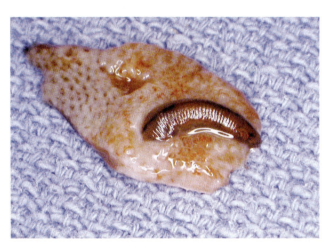

FIGURE 21-66 Close-up of a pentastomid parasite adhering to the inside of the lung tissue from a python (*Python* sp.). *(Photograph courtesy D. Mader.)*

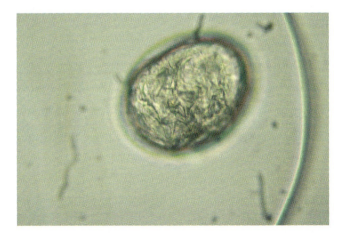

FIGURE 21-64 *Sebekia* sp. from a Softshell Turtle (*Apalone* sp.). Photomicrograph magnification, 400×.

infections with pentastomids, especially in wild reptiles, are asymptomatic.

Young hatchling crocodilians in captivity seem the most susceptible, and severe tissue and pulmonary damage may result from a *Sebekia* spp. infection. Usually, focal tissue damage in the lungs is seen at the site of attachment. Cherry and Ayer[5] report a prevalence of 93% *Sebekia oxycephala* in their survey of alligators. Diagnosis can be accomplished with the finding of eggs in feces. The eggs contain a larva form with hooks, which can be seen inside the egg.

Deakins[24] ascribed the death of American Alligators (*A. mississippiensis*) to an infection with *S. oxycephala*. Cause of death was pulmonary damage and intestinal hemorrhage. The pentastomid hooks, besides serving to hold the adult parasite to the lung tissue, may facilitate the entry of bacteria into the tissue and result in chronic pneumonia.

Boyce and coworkers[25] reported an infestation of *Sebekia* in captive hatchling alligators. The hatchlings were infected with *S. oxycephala* with ingestion of live mosquito fish

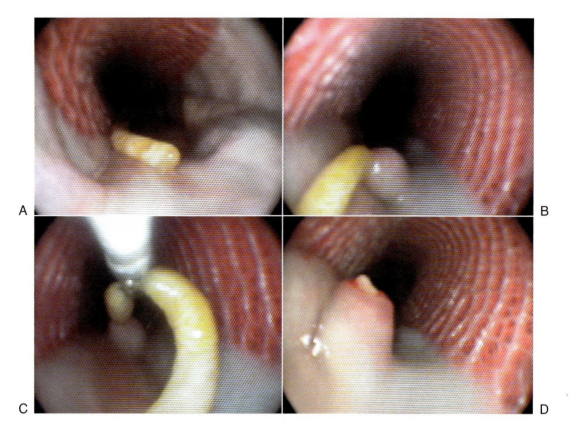

FIGURE 21-67 **A,** Adult pentastomid in the lung of an Indigo Snake *(Drymarchon couperi)*. **B,** Attachment of the mouth part to the lung tissue. Note the raised inflammatory response associated with attachment. **C,** Grasping the pentastomid near the attachment so as not to allow the parasite to break into pieces when traction is applied. **D,** Inflamed tissue left behind after the parasite has been removed. *(Photographs courtesy D. Mader.)*

(Gambusia affinis). Anorexia, weight loss, and respiratory distress were reported for the 4-week-old hatchlings. *S. oxycephala* larvae were recovered from lung tissue. Freezing the mosquito fish at 10°C for 72 hours was found to kill the *S. oxycephala* larvae in the fish. In most situations, control of *Sebekia* infections can be accomplished through hygiene and the control of dietary materials.

Treatment is controversial. Because an IH is necessary for completion of the life cycle, infections in animals in captivity should be self-limiting and treatment may not be needed.

Reports are found with use of levamisole and ivermectin, but because infections may be self-limiting, without controlled studies, conclusion that the chemotherapeutics were effective is difficult. Surgical or endoscopic retrieval of the adult parasites offers a viable option for removal of parasites from animals with high intensities (Figures 21-67 and 21-68).[26]

PARASITE TREATMENT

An important consideration in treatment of parasites is the nature of the parasite's life cycle. Remember that a parasite with a direct life cycle has the potential of reinfecting its host over and over again. A parasite with an indirect life cycle requires an IH, such as a mouse, before it can once again reinfect its original host or others in the same enclosure. Because of this, eradication of parasites with a direct life cycle is much more difficult.

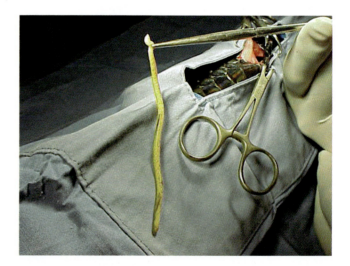

FIGURE 21-68 Extracted adult pentastomid from the lung of an Indigo Snake *(Drymarchon couperi)*. Endoscopy allows simple, safe extraction of the typically low worm burden. *(Photograph courtesy D. Mader.)*

An animal infected with a parasite that has an indirect life cycle can be rid of the parasite with treatment with the appropriate antiparasite drug and then ensuring that it does not have access to any IHs that are affected by the same parasite. For instance, if a snake is infected with roundworms, it should be dewormed (or "wormed" as it is called by herpetologists) and then fed only parasite-free mice.

A knowledge of a parasite's direct life cycle is helpful in eradication from a reptile's environment. For instance, the hookworm has a direct life cycle. It passes from one snake to the next, or back to itself, with either food, such as a plate of vegetables, contaminated with infected feces or with direct contamination and infection through the skin (as happens when a lizard steps in infected feces within its cage).

If these types of transmission can be stopped, then the parasite's life cycle can be broken. This process involves cleaning of the cage on a frequent basis. For instance, if a pet is dewormed and then any fresh feces from within the cage is immediately removed, the parasite cannot reinfect the host. After the appropriate treatment is finished, no parasites are left to reinfect or pass along to another host.

Medical treatments vary depending on the type of parasite present. Because of the anatomic location of some parasites, treatment may not be possible or may not be attempted. The spiny-headed worms are an example. They live in various locations throughout the abdominal cavity, but in general do no harm to the host. Because deworming drugs may not be effective at some of these locations and little risk of danger exists, these parasites are often left untreated.

Treatment times and amounts also vary depending on the type of parasite identified. Research in Ball Pythons suggests that reptiles parasitized with roundworms should be treated a minimum of three consecutive times, separated each time with a 2-week interval. Some protozoan, or one-celled parasites, can be effectively treated with a single dose. Certain protozoans (such as ciliates in tortoises or herbivorous lizards such as the Green Iguana [*Iguana iguana*]) need not be treated, and others may need to be treated daily for 3 weeks (coccidia).

Many different types of deworming medications are found. Most are in the form of a paste or pill given orally. Oral fenbendazole has been shown effective when given **per rectum** for difficult-to-eradicate parasites. Injectable dewormers have the advantage of ease of administration. For instance, opening the mouth of a large tortoise to pass a stomach tube full of deworming medicine is often impossible; however, administration of an injection under the skin is usually easy.

Prevention is always better than treatment. All deworming medications used in reptiles are drugs that have been developed and evaluated in other species. Little toxicity, safety, and pharmacokinetic research has been conducted in reptiles, and as a result, veterinarians are constantly learning more and more about the side effects of the drugs used to treat parasites.

For instance, ivermectin, a drug used extensively in cattle and other species, has proven to be effective in snakes and lizards for the treatment of various common parasites. However, **ivermectin has been proven lethal in chelonians and should never be used in any of these species.** Although this has been common knowledge for almost 20 years, improperly trained individuals still use this drug to treat parasites in turtles.

A simple technique frequently used to help decrease or eliminate parasites from prey items is to feed previously frozen dead meals or prey. Some research indicates that freezing a prey item for at least 30 days before thawing and feeding kills or destroys any parasites that it might be harboring.[25,27]

Some herpetologists recommend feeding alternate prey. For instance, if a snake normally eats lizards, the parasite life cycle can be broken by switching from lizard prey to mouse prey. Be careful with this technique because some reptiles may refuse alternate prey species. Also, the risk always exists for induction of subtle nutrient deficiencies with a nonnormal prey item.

A reptile's parasite burden can be decreased by feeding parasite-free prey only. If a need exists for large numbers of mice or rats, herpetologists might be wise to raise their own. Advise breeder clients to start out with a pair of parasite-free breeders, which should result in all of the offspring being free of parasites.

Chapter 89 lists the more common antiparasiticides used in reptile medicine.

CONCLUSION

All wild reptiles have a normal parasite burden. Some are truly parasitic; some are commensals. In the balance of nature, these organisms coexist. In captivity, however, when stress, poor nutrition, crowding, and more are added, even a "normal" parasite load can be a serious problem. Some apparent parasites (such as ciliates in tortoises) should not be treated because they are as much a part of the digestive process as the flora in a hind gut. However, others, because of complications of biologic concentration (in captivity) and stress, must be treated or death of the host might result.

As with most anything in captive reptile husbandry, the parasite load is almost always the result of husbandry and management imbalances. In addition to the medical intervention needed to treat the parasites, problems with husbandry must also be addressed.

Parasites are a real threat to captive reptiles. Whether the client's animals are pets or commercial breeders, an effective parasite treatment/prevention program is essential. Parasitized animals have poor growth rates, are unthrifty, have reproductive problems, and are generally more susceptible to disease than parasite-free animals. Because complete avoidance of parasites is almost impossible, especially for those reptiles that eat live food, evaluation of animals at least on a yearly basis is wise.

The most important control practice is quarantine of all new animals for at least 30 days. This allows diagnosis of most parasite infections and infestations and works to remove them before they become fully established. Precluding a parasite from entering a facility should be easier than eliminating it.

REFERENCES

1. Barnard SM, Durden LA: *A veterinary guide to the parasites of reptiles, vol 2, arthropods (excluding mites)*, Malabar, Fla, 2000, Krieger Publishing.
2. Burridge MJ, Simmons L-A: Control and eradication of exotic tick infestations of reptiles, *Proc Assoc Reptil Amphib* 21-23, 2001.
3. Knipling EF: The biology of *Sarcophaga cistodinis* Aldrich (Diptera), a species of Sarcophagidae parasitic on turtles and tortoises, *Proc Ent Soc Wash* 39:91-101, 1937.
4. Forrester DF, Sawyer RT: *Placobdella multilineata* from the American alligator in Florida, J Parasitol 60:673, 1974.

5. Cherry RH, Ayer AL: Parasites of American alligators, *A. mississippiensis*, in South Florida, *J Parasitol* 68:509, 1982.
6. Khan RA, Forrester DJ, Goodwin TM, Rose CA: A haemogreegarine from the American alligator (*Alligator mississippiensis*), *J Parasitol* 66:324-328, 1980.
7. Barnard SM, Upton AJ: *A veterinary guide to the parasites of reptiles, vol, protozoa*, Malabar, Fla, 1994, Krieger Publishing.
8. Donaldson M, Heyneman D, Dempster R, Garcia L: Epizootic of fatal amebiasis among exhibited snakes: epidemiologic, pathologic, and chemotherapeutic considerations, *Am J Vet Res* 36(6), 1975.
9. Jacobson E, Clubb S, Greiner E: Amebiasis in red-footed tortoises, *J Am Vet Med Assoc* 183:1192-1194, 1983.
10. Telford SR Jr, Campbell HW Jr: Parasites of the American alligator, their importance to husbandry and suggestions toward their prevention and control. Cardeilhac P, Lane T, Larsen R, editors: Proceeding First Annual Alligator Production Conference, Gainesville, Fla, 1981, College of Veterinary Medicine, University of Florida.
11. Matuschka FR: Reptiles as intermediate and/or final hosts of Sarcosporidia, *Parasitol Res* 73:22-332, 1987.
12. Koudela B, Modry D: New species of *Cryptosporidium* (Apicomplexa: Cryptosporidiidae) from lizards, *Folia Parasitol* 45:93-100, 1998.
13. Uhl EW, Jacobson E, Bartick TE, Micinilio J, Schmidt R: Aural-pharyngeal polyps associated with *Cryptosporidium* infection in three iguanas (*Iguana iguana*), *Vet Path* 38:239-242, 2001.
14. Telford SR Jr: Hemoparasites of reptiles. In Hoff GL, Frye FL, Jacobson ER, editors: *Diseases of amphibians and reptiles*, New York, 1984, Plenum Press.
15. Schall JJ: The ecology of lizard malaria, *Parasitol Today* 6:264-269, 1990.
16. Zwart P, Truyens EHA: Hexamitiasis in tortoises, *Vet Parasitol* 1:175-183, 1975.
17. Jacobson ER, Green DE, Undeen AH, Cranfield M, Vaughn KL: Systematic microsporidiosis in inland bearded dragons (*Pogona vitticeps*), *J Zoo Wildl Med* 29:315-323, 1998.
18. Gordon AN, Kelly WR, Cribb TH: Lesions caused by cardiovascular flukes (Digenea: Spirorchiidae) in stranded green turtles (*Chelonia mydas*), *Vet Pathol* 35:21, 1998.
19. Kazacos KR, Fisher LF: Renal styphlodoriasis in a boa constrictor, *JAVMA* 171:876-878, 1977.
20. Veasy RS, Stewart RB, Snider RC: Ureteritis and nephritis in a Burmese python (*Python mourus bititattus*) due to *Strongyloides* sp infection, *J Zoo Wildl Med* 25:119-122, 1994.
21. Lichtenfels JR, Stewrt TB: Three new species of *Chapiniella yamaguti*, 1961 (Nematoda: Strongyloidea) from tortoises, *Proc lm Soc Wash* 48:137-147, 1981.
22. Ashford RM, Muller R: *Paratrichosoma crocodilus* n.gen, n.sp. from the skin of the New Guinea crocodile, *J Helminth* 52:215-220, 1978.
23. Frank W: Die pathogenen Wirkungen von *Macdonaldius oschei* Chaubaud et Frank 1961 (Filarioidea. Onchocercidae) bei verschiedenen Arten von Schlangen (Reptilia, Ophidia), *Zeitschrift fur Parasitenkunde* 24:249-275, 1964.
24. Deakins DE: Pentastomes from Blackbeard Island, Georgia with notes on North American pentastomes, *J Parasitol* 57:1197, 1971.
25. Boyce WM, Cardeilhac P, Lane TJ, et al: Sebekiosis in captive alligator hatchlings, *J Am Vet Med Assoc* 185(11):1419, 1984.
26. Mader DR: Treating pentastomids in an Eastern Indigo Snake (*Drymarchon corais*), *Proc Assoc Rept Amphib Vet* 105-106, 2000.
27. Frye FL: *Reptile care: an atlas of diseases and treatments*, vol I, Neptune City, NJ, 1991, THF Publishing.

22
PERINATOLOGY

DOUGLAS R. MADER

In human medicine pediatrics refers to the treatment of children and their associated diseases. In avian medicine, this term is applied to the treatment of chicks and their associated diseases. The term pediatrics can only be loosely applied to reptilian medicine, however, because reptiles, unlike most other vertebrates, are born precocious. Neonates are essentially "little adults" and are fully capable of independence and survival from birth (Figure 22-1). Adult reptiles rarely provide any special provisions or care for their neonatal young.[1]

More and more is learned as captive breeding increases. As the availability of wild-caught animals diminishes and as herpetoculture moves away from the acquisition of animals from the wild, the importance of neonatal care takes on more significance.

Most therapeutics used in reptilian pediatric medicine are merely scaled-down versions of treatments used in adults of the same species. Because numerous sources are available for this information,[2] this discussion concentrates on the description of normal and frequently encountered abnormal findings.

EMBRYONIC/FETAL DEVELOPMENT

Development

Before a discussion on reptilian pediatrics is begun, some important differences need to be pointed out between reptilian and avian procreation. Whereas all avian species are oviparous (egg-laying), reptiles can be either oviparous, ovoviviparous, or viviparous (live-bearing; Figure 22-2).[1,3]

Viviparity implies some sort of exchange between the embryonic and maternal bloodstreams and is usually reserved for higher placental mammals. However, a correlation between viviparity and cool high altitude or latitude habitats has been pointed out in lizards and snakes.[3] Viviparity has been documented in 11 families of the order Squamata, of which nine show some sort of placentation.[4,5]

Ovoviviparity is probably a more appropriate term to use in reptiles.[1] Ovoviviparity refers to the condition in which the fertilized ova develops to varying degrees within the oviduct of the female and either "hatches" in the oviduct or shortly after delivery.[4] The embryo is surrounded by a thin membrane that tears off at birth, and the fully formed juvenile begins its independent life. Unlike true viviparity in placental mammals, this form of reproduction requires no special organs for supplying the embryo with food and thus resembles ordinary egg production.[1]

Although this is not a discussion on reproduction, one should point out that a number of factors determine the length of gestation. Season, ambient temperature, housing, and food supply are a few. The length of time between fertilization and oviposition, or egg-laying, occurs on a regular basis within a given species but can be affected by any of these factors.[2]

The point is made to distinguish the difference between the *time of fertilization* and oviposition and the *time of mating* and oviposition. *Amphigonia retardata*, or sperm storage, has been shown in turtles and snakes.[1-8] This is similar to, but more elaborate than, the sperm storage phenomena seen in birds.[6] This adaptation allows mating to occur in one season and reproduction in subsequent seasons. This also allows for a female to produce several clutches from a single mating in one season if the conditions are favorable. However, sperm viability is not indefinite and, depending on the species, can range from several months to up to 6 years.[3]

An alternate strategy to reproduction without mating in a given season (i.e., sperm storage) is parthenogenesis.[3] Parthenogenesis in reptiles occurs when females of the species become gravid and produce young in the absence of males. In reptiles, the females produce only female offspring, whereas in birds (turkeys), the females produce only male offspring.[2] Parthenogenesis has been documented in a number of reptile genera. Common examples include members of the genera *Aspidoscelis* (*Cnemidophorus*) (Whiptails) and *Hemidactylus* (Geckos).[2]

Ambient temperature plays an important role in reptilian reproduction.[2] In adult reptiles, seasonal changes in the ambient temperature stimulate gametogenesis. Ambient incubation temperature also has a direct effect on the length of incubation and, in some species, the gender of the developing embryo. When the incubation temperature is abnormal, either high or low, an effect can be seen on the health of the emerging hatchling.

Examples of this temperature effect on gender determination in reptiles are well-documented in Leopard Geckos (*Eublepharis macularius*) and numerous species of turtles.

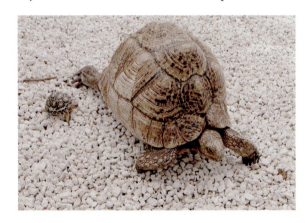

FIGURE 22-1 Most neonatal reptiles are born precocious, as is this Leopard Tortoise (*Geochelone pardalis*).

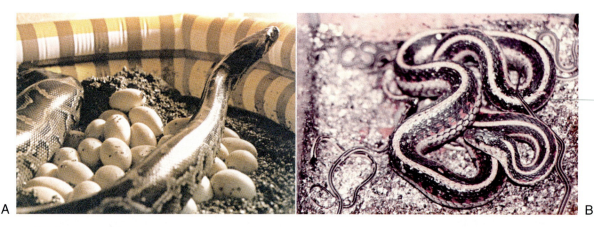

FIGURE 22-2 Whether hatched from an egg like the Burmese Python (*Python molurus bivitattus*), **A**, or live-born like the California Giant Red-sided Gartersnake (*Thamnophis sirtalis*), **B**, all reptiles are precocial and are capable of independent life without parental care.

In the gecko, incubation temperatures that ranged from 26.7°C to 29.4°C resulted in 99% female offspring. When the incubation temperature was greater than 32.2°C, 90% of the hatchlings were male.[2]

Temperature has the opposite effect on some of the water turtle species. A skewing of the sex ratios toward females was found when the incubation temperature was greater than 31°C, but a preponderance of males was seen when the temperatures were between 24°C and 27°C.[9]

Gender determination in snakes is based on genetics rather than incubation temperature. Sex chromosomes have been identified in many snake taxa.[10]

Reptilian ova are telolecithal, that is, they contain large amounts of yolk.[4] The embryonic developmental stages resemble those of birds. The eggs are deposited on land, usually in a warm but moist environment. The eggs have an outer protective leathery shell in snakes and most lizards and a calcareous shell in turtles. All have three internal membranes: the amnion, the chorion, and the allantois. These membranes retard outward diffusion of water but still allow embryonic respiration to occur.[3] The soft-shelled eggs of snakes and most lizards and, to some extent, the hard-shelled eggs of turtles, crocodilians, and geckos take up water from their environment and swell in size during development.[1]

The nutrition necessary for the entire development of the embryo is obtained from the yolk and the white.[1] Any remaining yolk in the egg is incorporated into the hatchling's coelomic cavity.[11] This provides enough energy to the animal until it takes its first meal.[3] At hatching, the umbilical attachment to this yolk sac spontaneously separates. Occasionally, the remnants of the yolk sac may remain attached to the umbilicus and subsequently tethered to the hatchling. These remnants can be removed with ligating the umbilicus near the animal's ventrum and severing the remaining tissue.[2] Sterile technique should be used. The umbilical scar closes spontaneously and heals rapidly.[2]

PARENTAL CARE

Most reptiles deposit their eggs at a given site and then leave. As previously mentioned, minimal parental care is seen among the reptile species. Some of the best known examples of prenatal care in reptiles are found in pythons (see Figure 23-3).[12]

Female pythons are known to brood their eggs during incubation.[12] The female has been reported to incubate her eggs for up to 65 days[13,14] and maintain a mean body temperature of 7.3°C over the mean ambient surface temperature the entire time.[4] This is accomplished by periodic rhythmic contractions of her abdominal musculature. In other examples of brooding, some snakes sun themselves and then return to their nests, thus taking the heat back to the eggs.[3] Once the eggs hatch, little, if any, parental care or protection of the young is seen. Likewise, in the ovoviviparous and viviparous snake species, no known examples of parental care are found.[3]

Parental care in the lizard seems to be more elaborate than in the snake. Female lizards deposit their eggs in various natural crevices or cracks, dig burrows, or build nests. Often these nests are covered and left. Most oviparous lizards show little or no maternal care. A remarkable exception to this is the female *Anolis*, which retrieves scattered eggs to the nest and then buries them in the substrate.[15] Some skinks incubate their eggs, and they have been known to protect their nests against predators.[3] In the Skink, *Eumeces obsoletus*, the female assists in the hatching of the young and then subsequently licks their cloacas. She also supplies them with food up until about the 10th day.[1,15]

The most extreme case of parental care reported is in *Xantusia vigilis*, the viviparous Yucca Night Lizard.[3,15] The attention displayed by the parent to the offspring has been likened to almost mammal-like maternal behavior.[3] When the fetus with its surrounding membranes first appears, the female grasps the fetal envelope with her teeth and rips it open. This tends to excite the newborn into activity. If the neonate does not show signs of life, the female then nips at its flank and legs, causing it to thrash violently and extricate itself from the parental cloaca. The female then collects and eats the placental membranes and carefully licks up any remaining fluid that spilled on the ground. This entire procedure lasts only a couple of minutes, and the actual expulsion of the fetus takes only about 1 minute.[3] In general, parental care is more the exception than the rule.[3,4,15]

EGG MANAGEMENT

A thorough discussion on egg management and care extends beyond the scope of this chapter. However, both artificial incubation and manual pipping merit a brief review.

Most incubators are relatively simple in design. Commercially available chick incubators work well with minor modifications. The three basic requirements for most reptile incubators are[10]: they should be well-insulated to prevent loss of heat and humidity; the heat should be evenly dispersed throughout the incubator with no hot spots; and the heat should be controlled with a reliable thermostat. Back-up thermostats are recommended.

Various substrates have been used in incubators (Figure 22-3; Table 22-1). Commonly used substrates include vermiculite, potting soil, sand, sphagnum moss, and shredded paper. Check with someone who has experience with your species for the best type to use.

Most incubators are designed with a double-chamber principle (Figure 22-4). The eggs are placed in the incubation substrate within a small inner container, which is then suspended within a larger container. This smaller inner chamber can be suspended in air or, in some cases, in water, as is done in a water bath. Elevation of the inner chamber above the heat source ensures an even distribution of heat to the eggs inside. When water is used, the evaporation of the water also helps maintain the necessary high humidity within the incubation chamber.

Plastic waterproof containers such as sweater or shoe storage boxes make an excellent inner chamber. This chamber can then be suspended within a larger plastic or styrofoam ice chest.

Numerous heat sources are available to maintain incubator temperature. Heating coils, strips, and pads work well, but each has its limitations. A submersible aquarium heater in the water bath is another excellent method for warming the incubator. These heaters can be adjusted to precisely maintain an accurate incubation temperature within the inner chamber. The incubator should have a reliable thermostat. Professional breeders often have "back-up" thermostats in case the primary regulator fails.

The incubator should be set up and operational several days before the expected arrival of the eggs to allow for equilibration of the temperature within the entire system. Once the ambient temperature within the incubator has been adjusted and established, frequent opening of the unit should be avoided. A window in the top of the incubator allows for monitoring the eggs and observation of the hatching process and, ultimately, the neonates (Figure 22-5).

The eggs are collected after oviposition. Although no scientific studies have recommended otherwise, care should be taken not to rotate or change the spatial orientation of the egg during transport or when placed in the incubator (Figure 22-6).[10] A small pencil mark on the top of the egg helps maintain orientation when the egg is moved. One should note that alteration of the position of the egg is a controversial issue and that not all herpetologists agree that it can cause damage.[2]

The egg is half-buried within the substrate. Water is added to the substrate to make it very moist but not liquid. The author prefers bottled spring water, but excellent results have been obtained with ordinary tap water.[10] If questions exist regarding the safety of the municipal water source, either have the water quality commercially tested or use bottled or filtered water.

After the eggs are placed into the moist substrate, a thin layer of dampened sphagnum moss can be used to cover the tops of the eggs to help prevent desiccation. Some herpetologists disagree with this step because visual checking of the viability of the eggs is made more difficult.

A thermometer should be placed into the substrate, level with the bottom of the eggs (see Figure 22-5). This should be clearly readable from the outside of the incubator. Inner chamber incubation temperature should be checked at least

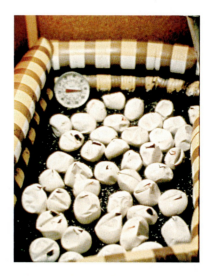

FIGURE 22-3 Various substrates have been used in artificial incubators. Here, the eggs are set into moistened vermiculite.

Table 22-1	Substrates for Incubation of Reptile Eggs

Vermiculite
Perlite
Sphagnum moss
Potting soil
Peat moss
Sand (chemical free)
Dirt (sanitized)*
Pea gravel
Paper towels

*Dirt can be baked in a conventional oven at 93°C (200°F) for 1 hour.

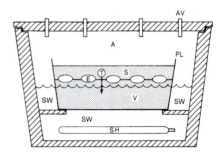

FIGURE 22-4 Design of the standard reptile incubator. *A,* Air; *AV,* air vent; *E,* egg; *PL,* plastic liner; *S,* sphagnum moss; *SH,* submersible heater; *SW,* spring water; *T,* thermometer; *V,* moist vermiculite.

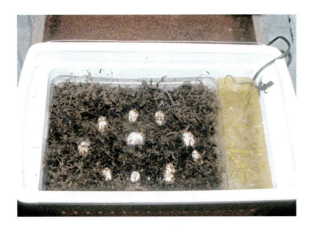

FIGURE 22-5 The eggs should be placed in a prewarmed incubator. A thermometer should be placed in the vermiculite at the level of the eggs, and the temperature checked daily. A clear top permits easy observations of egg or neonatal activity.

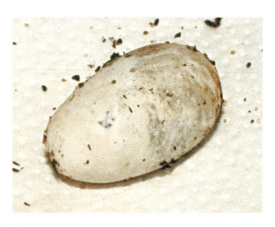

FIGURE 22-6 A small wax pencil mark on the top of the egg helps maintain orientation when the egg is moved. One should note that altering the position of the egg is a controversial issue and that not all herpetologists agree that it can cause damage. Avoid use of inks that may prove toxic to the developing embryo.

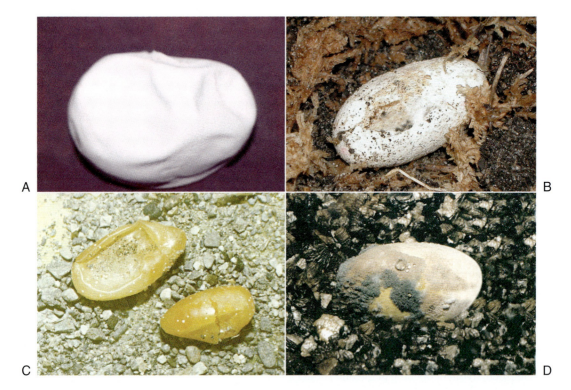

FIGURE 22-7 Egg viability should be checked on a daily basis. **A,** Collapsed eggs are a sign of dehydration and not necessarily egg death. These eggs can often be salvaged with rehydrating the substrate with warm spring water. **B,** Mottling or partial discoloration, although appearing lethal, can be normal in many cases. **C,** Waxy yellow "slugs" may be passed from either viviparous or oviparous animals. These are discarded unfertilized ova and usually signify some underlying disease problem with the female. **D,** Mold on the surface of the egg is a sign of egg death.

daily. Graphing of daily temperatures is wise because it helps to identify problems should any abnormalities be seen at hatching.

The inner chamber with the eggs and sphagnum moss should be misted daily to maintain a high humidity. Inexpensive thermometers/hygrometers are available from most garden stores and are worth the modest investment. The spray bottle should be kept within the incubator so that the temperature of the mist is the same as the incubator temperature.[10]

Many amateur herpetologists have had success in incubating eggs with placing the collected eggs in a chicken egg crate and leaving it in a dark closet for a few months. Different methods work for different people and different species. Investigation of the appropriate way to incubate the eggs from the specific species with which you are working is best.

Table 22-2	Potential Causes of Egg Death

Diapause*
Infertile eggs
Incorrect incubation temperatures (high or low)
Incorrect incubation humidity (high or low)
Insufficient ventilation†
Excessive handling or trauma

*Some eggs do not develop unless all the environmental conditions are correct (temperature, humidity, substrate). In some cases, a short developmental delay may exist, only with subsequent continued normal incubation.
†Incubators without air holes, eggs stuck on the bottom of an egg mass.

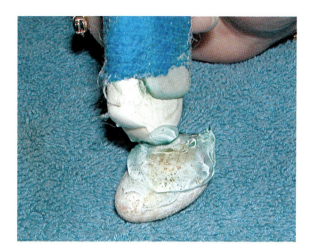

FIGURE 22-9 An 8-MHz ultrasound transducer is used to evaluate the viability of this snake egg.

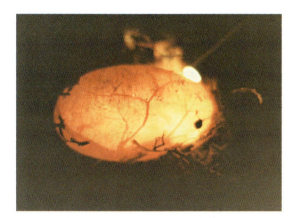

FIGURE 22-8 Egg viability can be easily checked with candling with a bright light, such as this ophthalmic transilluminator. Healthy eggs readily show developing vasculature. As the embryo develops in later stages, movement can be seen within the egg.

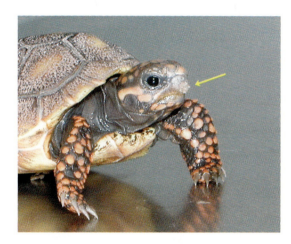

FIGURE 22-10 Most of the oviparous species have a caruncle, or egg tooth, that they use to pip through the egg. The egg tooth usually disappears after the first shed or within a couple of weeks.

The eggs should be monitored daily. A slight mottling to the surface of the egg may not be significant; however, marked changes in color or texture or growth of fuzzy mold usually indicate that the egg has either died or was nonfertile (Figure 22-7; Table 22-2). Egg viability can be easily checked with a high-intensity light source, such as an ophthalmic transilluminator, placed in direct contact with the side of the egg in a darkened room. Egg viability can be confirmed by the presence of a developing vascular pattern as the embryo grows (Figure 22-8). Nonviable eggs have a homogenous diffuse yellow-white luminescence. Alternately, for noncalcified eggs, a high-frequency (7.5 to 10 MHz) ultrasound transducer can be used to evaluate the developing embryo (Figure 22-9). A water-soluble gel should be used as an interface. Ultrasound gel has been reported to potentially damage the egg by clogging the pores, thus preventing oxygen exchange.

Egg incubation times vary with the species and the incubation temperature (see Appendix C).[2] In general, the warmer the incubation temperature, the shorter the gestation period. When working with breeders, one is wise to be familiar with the expected normals for the species they are cultivating. Species-specific indices can be found in the herpetologic literature.[2]

Most young of oviparous species possess a small caruncle or egg tooth, similar to that seen in birds, that is used for pipping the egg at term (Figure 22-10). The actual process of emergence takes from 24 to 48 hours.[13] Most eggs within a clutch hatch within a couple of days of each other.

The egg has only a limited life span. It cannot support the life of the embryo indefinitely. If hatching does not occur within the appropriate time period, the embryo dies. The herpetoculturist must monitor this time frame accurately to maximize the number of viable hatchings.

Hatchlings do not always pip on the top of the egg. Although it is the norm, many reports exist of hatchlings attempting to pip out the bottom or the side of the egg.[10] In species in which eggs are deposited in a mass, pipping on the sides can cause a problem if the snake pips into the inside of an adjacent egg. The hatchlings that pip in an inappropriate direction usually die of exhaustion if the herpetoculturist does not intervene and assist in removal (Figure 22-11).

Only the following few instances exist in which an egg should be manually pipped: when most eggs in a clutch have pipped and still some remaining eggs are unpipped; when no eggs have pipped by the estimated due date; or when no due date is known and pipping is necessary to determine viability or stage of gestation.[10]

A small slit is made in the top of the egg with either a sterile scalpel or sharp clean scissors (Figure 22-12, A). The tip of a delicate scissor is inserted into the slit, and the cut is extended. The cut should be made with a series of small snips, with the scissor point kept adjacent to the inside of the egg surface to avoid cutting any of the internal vessels (Figure 22-12, B). A second cut is made at approximately a 45-degree angle to the first to make a wedge incision. This incision is then gently retracted and cut off to expose the embryo inside. Extreme care is necessary to prevent damage to any of the egg vessels. If this procedure has been performed properly, the shell membranes should be intact. At this time, the embryo should be fully developed. If gently stimulated with a blunt probe, it should react with movement. The neonate should be allowed to remain in the egg and exit on its own. It is not uncommon even for natural hatchings that naturally pip to remain in their egg for 12 to 24 hours (Figure 22-13).[10]

If the hatchling requires manual removal from its egg, it must be stimulated to breathe on its own immediately. This can be accomplished with gentle tapping with a sharp instrument until the snake is breathing regularly.[10] The author has used 1 to 2 drops of 0.2% doxapram HCl, administered with an oral dropper, to assist with initiation of breathing in some fatigued hatchlings.

The yolk can be gently teased away with a saline solution–moistened cotton-tipped applicator and forceps. The umbilicus can be severed and ligated (Figure 22-14).

In most cases, the yolk sac has been absorbed into the coelomic cavity before hatching.[2,10] If this sac is still attached when the hatchling emerges, the animal should be maintained on a clean damp surface, such as a moistened paper towel, until the umbilicus breaks on its own. Alternately, the umbilicus can be ligated with heavy gauge suture and then severed. Light gauge suture may cut through the yolk stalk.[10] The umbilical stump can be coated with an iodinated or chlorhexidine solution.

Occasionally, this umbilicus and yolk sac become entangled around an emerging hatchling and strangulate the animal.[10] Careful monitoring of the hatching events can prevent this occurrence. Also, Frye[2] reported a retained umbilicus that adhered to the substrate, acting as a tether to the animal and accidentally eviscerating the hatchling when it tried to crawl away.

HOUSING THE NEONATE

Many different housing requirements are seen for the various species of reptiles. Species-specific literature should be investigated. In general, for the first few days after hatching, the neonate should be maintained at or near the incubation temperature. Many breeders leave the animals in the incubator for the first few days of life (Figure 22-15). Because hatchlings are prone to dehydration and desiccation at these higher temperatures, the relative humidity should be maintained near 100%. In snakes, the risk of dehydration lessens after the first ecdysis, or shed.[10]

Moistened paper towels are a good substrate to use for hatchlings. Paper towels are inexpensive, clean, and easily replaced. Regardless of the substrate chosen, it should be one that is easily cleaned to minimize the risk of infection to the hatchling, especially during the first few days of life before the yolk sac has fully absorbed into the coelomic cavity.

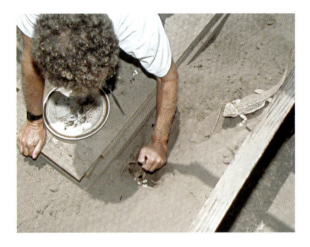

FIGURE 22-11 Harvesting eggs from a nest may be necessary when the anticipated hatch date has past, when only a portion of the nest has emerged, or when concern exists that the nesting conditions may not be ideal.

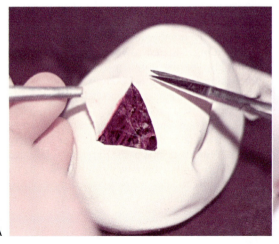
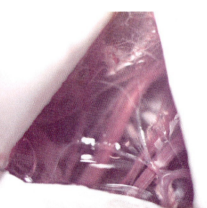

A   B

FIGURE 22-12 Occasionally, artificial pipping of the egg becomes necessary. **A,** A triangular wedge is cut into the egg. **B,** Extreme care is taken to avoid cutting or damaging the vessels of the underlying membrane.

Neonatal lizards and snakes can be aggressive immediately after hatching (Figure 22-16). This aggression is normal and may represent either an instinctive defense mechanism or a predator-prey behavior.[10,16] If the aggression is directed at conspecifics, the hatchlings should be separated.[10]

If a number of hatchlings are housed within an enclosure, separation may be necessary to ensure that each is feeding properly and has equal access to food. After feeding, the hatchlings can be returned to their groups.

FEEDING THE NEONATE

The yolk provides nutritional support for the neonate for the first few days of its life and, in some instances, enough to last through its first brumation (hibernation).[3] Most neonatal snakes do not eat until after their first shed, which occurs between 1 and 3 weeks after hatching.[10]

If many animals are in a clutch, one may be wise to separate the animals into smaller groups to monitor the health status and assess the appetite of each animal. Weekly weights are good indicators of each animal's progress. Most neonates eat spontaneously when offered appropriate foods (this includes appropriately sized food items) for the given species (Figure 22-17).

Insects, baby mice (pinkies), small lizards, chicks, small eggs, wingless fruit flies, termites, slugs, small fish, and grubs can be offered to carnivorous and insectivorous snakes and lizards (Table 22-3).[2,10,16] Dead baby mice with the cranium cut open, mouse parts such as limbs or tails, chick legs, and frogs can also be used to stimulate hatchlings that are slow to start eating.

Herbivorous reptiles do well on a proper mix of fresh vegetables grated to the appropriate size. Certain herbivorous species, such as the Green Iguana *(Iguana iguana)*, have shown that inoculation into the stomach of the neonate with microbes from the feces of adults from the same species helps in stimulating the appetite and increases the efficiency of digestion.[17]

The nutritive value of the offered food items can and should be enhanced for the rapidly growing hatchling. Vegetarian diets can be dusted with commercially available vitamin and mineral products. Mealworms, waxworms, crickets, and the like can also be dusted with these powders. An alternative to dusting is to allow these insects to feed off an enriched media for a few days before being fed to the reptiles. Frye[2] recommends a medium of wheat bran middlings supplemented with alfalfa flakes, high protein baby cereal, and a small amount of dry poultry mash. A powdered vitamin/mineral supplement can be added to this mash.

In some, but not all, species, the feeding habits of the young are different than the adults. A common misconception is that juvenile Green Iguanas shift their dietary preferences from carnivory to herbivory as they age. In fact, one should emphasize that the Green Iguana is born into herbivory and remains a herbivore throughout life.[18,19] Herpetoculturists must have a thorough understanding of the dietary requirements of the species they are raising.

In some instances, particular food preference items may not be readily available. For example, certain snakes have a preference for frogs, but because of geographic limitations, the appropriate prey items cannot be obtained. In these situations, one may possibly train the neonate to eat alternate food items by "scenting" the proffered food with the scent from the appropriate prey species.[2] Scenting can be accomplished with "sliming" a mouse pup with a fish or frog, or washing the outside of a dead pup and placing it in a sealed plastic bag with a dead chick.[2,10] Although this is often quite

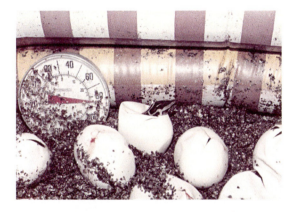

FIGURE 22-13 The neonate often remains inside the egg for 24 to 48 hours after pipping.

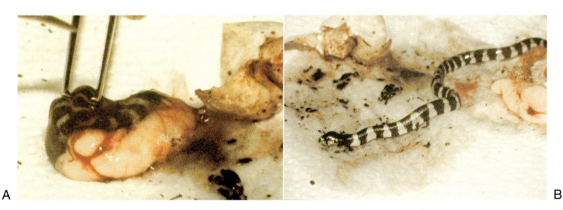

FIGURE 22-14 If the embryo has to be removed from the egg, separating the yolk is necessary. **A,** This can be done with forceps and a saline solution–moistened cotton swab. **B,** The umbilical stalk should be severed and ligated with aseptic technique. The neonate can be left on a clean moistened substrate such as paper towels.

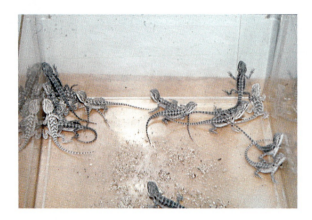

FIGURE 22-15 Neonates should be left in their incubators at their incubation temperature for a few days after hatching.

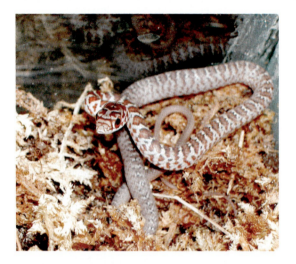

FIGURE 22-16 Hatchling reptiles are often aggressive immediately after emerging from the egg. Care must be taken when handling these animals. This aggression often abates within a few days.

effective, potential problems may occur with nutrient deficiencies if the hatchling is deprived of the proper diet for prolonged periods.

Regardless of the fitness of the hatchlings, some always refuse to eat voluntarily. A number of techniques can be used to help stimulate reluctant animals to eat. In snakes, getting them to eat is often possible with gentle tapping of the snake on the nose with a small prey item. This tends to initiate the snake's strike reflex with the intention that the snake will then grasp the prey item during the strike. This technique is often referred to as "slap feeding."[10] Placing the food item in the neonate's mouth and warming the food items are other techniques that can be used to stimulate poor appetites. In cases in which danger exists of losing an animal from anorexia, assist feeding and tube feeding may be necessary. In assist feeding an animal, extreme care should be taken to avoid damaging the delicate young tissues of the oropharynx and esophagus of the neonate. A puree of appropriate food items (mouse parts, eggs, vegetables, etc.) can be easily administered through an infant feeding tube and is often times less stressful than actual assist feeding of whole or partial prey items.

CONDITIONS THAT AFFECT THE NEONATE

Most of the medical conditions that affect the neonate are a result of a genetic mutation or a developmental aberration within the egg. Although both true genetic mutations and mutagenic agents that can induce developmental defects exist, most defects in hatchling reptiles are a direct result of abnormal incubation temperatures during embryonic development.[2] Developmental anomalies are frequently seen in snakes and turtles but only rarely in lizards, crocodilians, and the Tuatara.[2]

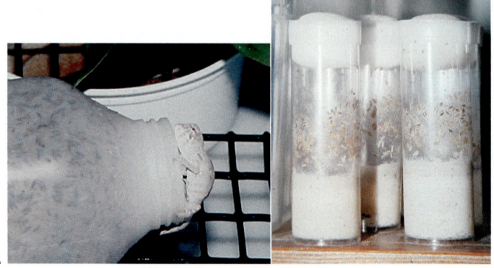

FIGURE 22-17 A, This chameleon is feeding off wingless fruit flies. The nutritive value of the fruit flies can be augmented with adding vitamin and mineral supplements to the nectar that the fruit flies consume. **B,** One is wise to plan ahead and either purchase or cultivate the proper food items needed before hatching.

Table 22-3	Foods for Carnivorous Neonatal Reptiles

Pinky mice (dead; preferably with milk in their stomachs)
Small (dead) lizards (anoles or geckos)
Small frogs (caution: do not use toads because they are potentially poisonous)
Small fish (guppies or comets)
Chick legs
Hatchling quail
Mouse (adult) parts
Various insects (crickets, meal worms, grubs, etc)
Canned cat food*
Meat baby (human) food*

*When assist or tube feeding is necessary.

Changes in the color, pigment, or pattern of animals are controlled by genetic influence. Variations from albinism to heavily pigmented (melanistic) animals can be seen in most reptiles.[2] In many cases, these defects or recessive traits are selected for in an attempt to create more attractive animals for the pet trade.

Abnormalities of scales, shells, and scutes and fetal monsters, animals with duplicate body parts and hatchlings with severe internal abnormalities, have all been well documented (Figure 22-18).[2] Although many of these animals may appear quite unusual or even grotesque, some, such as the double-headed snakes, can survive. Most of the fetal monsters either fail to hatch or die shortly thereafter.

MORBIDITY AND MORTALITY OF NEONATES

Neonatal reptiles are susceptible to numerous diseases and adversity, much as is seen in adults (Table 22-4). All of the pathogens also affect neonates, but because their immune systems are not yet developed, these can be rapidly lethal. Routine diagnostic techniques should be applied in investigation of diseases in newly hatched reptiles. Culture and sensitivity testing, fecal analysis, blood panels, and urinalysis can all be performed, depending on the needs of the practitioner and the size of the patient.

Treatments for neonates are similar to those used in larger adult reptiles. Reported adult drug dosages and therapeutic regimens can be scaled down for the neonate's small size, with principles of metabolic scaling.[20] Unfortunately, because most of the information in the literature on reptilian therapeutics is still empirical, the scaled dosages are nothing more than mathematic guesswork. Until further work is done specifically with neonatal reptiles, scaling and trial-and-error therapeutics have to suffice.

The obtaining of samples for hematology and clinical chemistry in neonatal reptiles can be a clinical challenge. Standard sampling techniques such as cardiocentesis and jugular, axillary, femoral, buccal, and tail vein venipuncture can be adapted to many of the smaller neonates. Cardiocentesis with a 27-gauge or 30-gauge needle can be attempted in animals that weigh just a few grams. However, even if a sample can be obtained, the sample size may be so prohibitively small that adequate diagnostics cannot be conducted.

The risk of injury to the patient during sampling must be considered when diagnostics are of limited value because of small sample size.

Blood volumes for reptiles vary from 5% to 8% of total body weight (TBW).[21] Of this amount, 10% can be collected for analysis without harm to the patient. For a rough approximation, consider that the sample size should not be larger than 1% of the animal's TBW.

The standard capillary tube holds 70 μL, which means that for any patient that weighs at least 7 g, one full capillary tube of blood can be safely taken. Although this is a small sample, enough exists to yield some valuable diagnostic information. The total protein, packed cell volume, and icterus index are easily measured from a single capillary tube. If a thin blood smear is made, an estimated white blood cell count with a differential can be performed and the red cells can be evaluated for abnormalities. After the cells have been spun down, the remaining serum can be used for a limited number of chemistries. In reality, with very small patients, a single drop of blood may be all that can be safely collected. A thin well-prepared blood smear can still be of value as a diagnostic aid.

The choana and the cloaca are routinely cultured for bacterial screening and disease investigation. Interpretation of the culture results, however, can often be difficult. The author has cultured *Pseudomonas* and *Salmonella* spp. from the cloacas of apparently healthy hatchling pythons immediately on emergence from the eggs. These animals had no exposure to other snakes at the time of the cultures, but they were born from infected females. Neither hatchling showed any signs of illness, and as a result, neither was treated. Both snakes remained clinically healthy when rechecked at 6 months of age. Obviously, bacterial culture and sensitivity data are important, but the data need to be interpreted in light of pertinent clinical symptoms and history.

Ectoparasites, such as mites, can be a serious problem to neonatal snakes, especially in large colonies. The snake mite, *Ophionyssus natricis*, is hematophagous, and aside from acting as a vector for diseases such as aeromoniasis, they can exsanguinate hatchlings in a short time.[2]

Treatment of acariasis in neonates can be difficult because of their small size. Desiccants used against the mites can result in dehydration of the patient if not used properly. Insecticides, such as pyrethrins, can be too potent for the small neonates and can cause toxicity problems. Herpetologists often use a dichlorvos strip or a small piece of impregnated flea collar placed inside or on top of the affected reptile's cage. This practice can often have lethal outcomes for the hatchling if it remains exposed to high concentrations of the toxins from the strips for too long. The author does NOT recommend any type of insecticidal or pest strip (or dog/cat flea collar) in or around any reptile cage.

The author has had mixed success in treatment of mites in snakes and lizards by a number of methods. Spraying the affected animal with a dilute synthetic pyrethrin spray (0.03%) followed by an *immediate and complete* rinsing has proven to be effective in removing the mites. Extreme care must be taken to avoid contact of the poison with the animal's oral cavity. Pyrethroids have a quick-kill property, which is why they are effective in removing the mites, but the spray must be washed off the host before the toxins have any deleterious effects.[21,22]

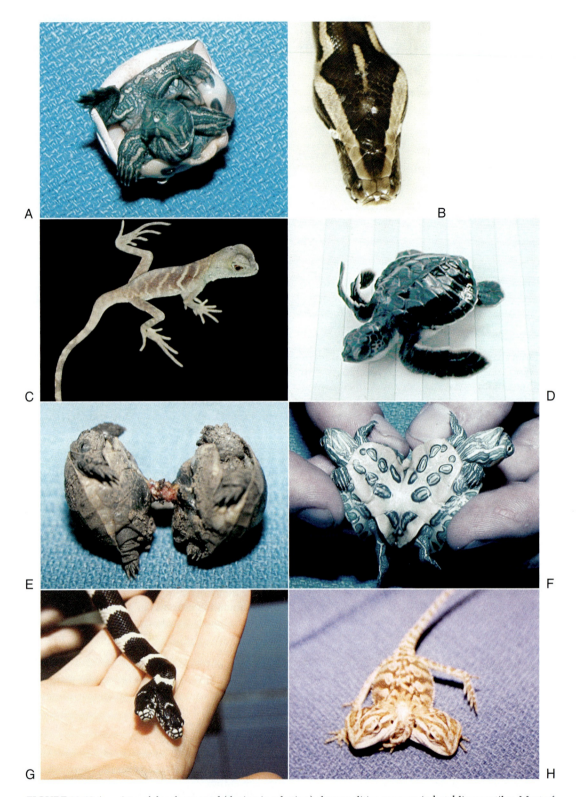

FIGURE 22-18 A variety of developmental (during incubation) abnormalities are seen in hatchling reptiles. Most of these are related to improper incubation temperatures or moisture levels. However, some are the result of severe inbreeding. In some cases, the abnormalities result in fetal death; in other cases, fetal monsters that die shortly after hatching; and in others, missing or duplication of body parts, scales, or pigmentation. **A,** Slider Turtle (*Trachemys* sp.), died in the egg. **B,** Bilateral anophthalmia (technically, microphthalmia, vestigial eyes located under the scales) in a Burmese Python (*Python molurus bivitattus*). **C,** Scoliosis and hydrocephalus in a Chinese Water Dragon (*Physignathus cocincinus*). **D,** Duplicate flipper in a Loggerhead Seaturtle (*Caretta caretta*). *(Photograph courtesy J. Wyneken.)* **E,** Twin California Desert Tortoises (*Gopherus agassizii*). **F,** Red-eared Slider (*Trachemys scripta elegans*) Siamese twin, conjoined at the pelvis. **G,** Bicephalic (two-headed) California Kingsnake (*Lampropeltis getulus getulus*). **H,** Two-headed Bearded Dragon (*Pogona vitticeps*).

Table 22-4 Causes for Neonatal Morbidity and Mortality

Genetic or congenital conditions
Environmental temperatures too high or too low
Environmental humidity too high or too low
Dehydration (lack of proper drinking water or delivery of water source)
Exteriorized yolk sac or infected yolk sac
Sepsis
Cannabilism
Mites
Miaisis (fly strike; especially hatching eggs)
Predation from prey species (crickets)

The author has also used ivermectin, 200 µg/kg subcutaneous, in both lizards and snakes as a treatment for mites in large collections.[23] The advantage is that the ivermectin has a residual effect in the host's body, thus protecting the animal against future attacks from the pesty mites. The ivermectin injection is repeated 2 to 3 weeks after the initial treatment.

Numerous reports exist of ivermectin causing paralysis and death in various turtle and tortoise species. Ivermectin can be *lethal* in chelonians and should *never* be used.[24]

QUARANTINE AND HYGIENE

As with any reptile husbandry, proper hygiene when working with eggs and neonates is critical. Good sanitary practices take on even more significance when dealing with neonates because their immune systems are not yet developed. Refer to Chapter 85 for more information regarding disinfectants and cleaning.

Many diseases that affect neonates have yet to be fully described. However, viral infections, such as adenovirus in Bearded Dragons (*Pogona vitticeps*) and inclusion body disease in the Boidae, may have horizontal transmission that could be significant in breeder situations. The reader is encouraged to review Chapter 78 for working with large collections and especially instituting quarantine procedures.

CONCLUSION

Reptilian pediatrics is a new concept in nondomestic medicine. Fortunately, because reptiles are born precocious, most of the medical problems encountered are similar to those seen in adults of the same species, just in a scaled-down fashion.

Proper management and husbandry remain the major obstacles to maintaining healthy reptilian collections. Learning what is the normal for a given species and then duplicating that in the captive environment are the keys to successful propagation and rearing of healthy specimens. Veterinary practitioners are encouraged to get involved with local herpetology clubs and organizations to familiarize themselves with the peculiarities of the more common reptile species and to gain a better understanding of the reptilian reproductive process in general.

REFERENCES

1. Grzimek HCB: *Animal life encyclopedia*, vol 6, reptiles, New York, 1968, Van Nostrand Reinhold.
2. Frye FL: *Biomedical and surgical aspects of captive reptile husbandry*, ed 2, Melbourne, Fla, 1991, Krieger Publishing.
3. Porter KR: *Herpetology*, Philadelphia, 1972, WB Saunders.
4. Goin CJ, Goin OB, Zug GR: *Introduction to herpetology*, San Francisco, 1978, WH Freeman.
5. Yaron Z: Endocrine aspects of gestation in viviparous reptiles, *Gen Comp Endocrinol Suppl* 3:663, 1972.
6. Gans SC: *Biology of the reptilia*, vol 6, San Diego, 1977, Academic Press.
7. Mertens R: *The world of amphibians and reptiles*, London, 1960, George C Harrap.
8. Trauth SE: Testicular cycle and timing of reproductive in the collard lizard (*Crotophytus collaris*) in Arizona, *Herpetologica* 35:184, 1978.
9. Bull JJ, Vogt RC: Temperature-dependent sex determination in turtles, *Science* 206:1186, 1979.
10. Ross RA, Marzec G: *The reproductive husbandry of pythons and boas*, Stanford, 1990, Institute for Herpetological Research.
11. Bellairs A: *The life of reptiles*, New York, 1970, Universe Books.
12. Boos HEA: Some breeding records of Australian pythons, *Intl Zoo Yb* 19:87, 1979.
13. Tryon BW: Reproduction in captive forest cobras, *Naja Melanoleuca* (Serpentes:Elapidae), *J Herp* 13:499, 1979.
14. Van Meirop LHS, Barnard SM: Observations on the reproduction of *Python molurus bivittatus* (Reptilia, Serpentes, Boidae), *J Herp* 10:333, 1976.
15. Tokarz RR, Jones RE: A study of egg-related maternal behavior in *Anolis carolinensis*, *J Herp* 13:282, 1979.
16. Mader DR: Captive propagation of the Chinese water dragon (*Physignathus cocincinus*), *Proc North Calif Herpetol Soc, Special Publication* #4:67, 1987.
17. Troyer K: Transfer of fermentive microbes between generations in a herbivorous lizard, *Science* 216:540, 1982.
18. Iverson JB: Adaptions to herbivory in iguanine lizards. In Burghardt GM, Rand AS, editors: *Iguanas of the world: their behavior, ecology and conservation*, Park Ridge, NJ, 1982, Noyes Publications.
19. McBee RH, McBee VH: The hindgut fermentation in the green iguana, *Iguana iguana*. In Burghardt GM, Rand AS, editors: *Iguanas of the world: their behavior, ecology and conservation*, Park Ridge, NJ, 1982, Noyes Publications.
20. Mader DR: Antibiotic therapy. In Frye FL, editor: *Biomedical and surgical aspects of captive reptile husbandry*, ed 2, Melbourne, Fla, 1991, Krieger Publishing.
21. Mader DR: Herpetological medicine: mites and the herpetologist, *The Vivarium* 1(4):27, 1988.
22. Mader DR, Houston RH, Frye FL: *Hirstiella trombidiiformis* infestion in a colony of chuckwallas, *J Am Vet Med Assoc* 189:1138, 1986.
23. Funk RS: Herp health hints and husbandry: parasiticide dosages for captive amphibians and reptiles, *Bull Chicago Herpetol Soc* 23(2):30, 1988.
24. Jacobson ER: Use of chemotherapeutics in reptile medicine. In Jacobson ER, Kollias GV, editors: *Exotic animals*, New York, 1988, Churchill Livingstone.

23
REPRODUCTIVE BIOLOGY
DALE DENARDO

Although an increasing interest has been seen in reptiles simply as personal pets, a significant interest remains in breeding them. Captive propagation of many reptile species has become common. However, for successful reproduction, one must understand the animal's general reproductive physiology and critical husbandry techniques. Many people turn to their veterinarian for such information. Therefore, a practitioner who sees reptile patients must know much of this information and provide services such as sex and pregnancy determination. This knowledge and these skills instill clients with confidence in their veterinarian's overall knowledge of this group of animals and in the veterinarian's ability to successfully treat them.

More directly, knowledge in the reproductive biology of reptiles is essential in accurate and effective diagnosis and treatment of many patients. Although reproduction is quite natural, clinical problems associated with reproducing captive reptiles are relatively common. This chapter is designed to provide a simple overview of reptile reproductive biology and to furnish information that is critical to understanding captive reptile reproduction and evaluating reptilian patients.

CLINICAL REPRODUCTIVE ANATOMY

Male Reproductive Anatomy

The reptile testis is an ovoid mass of seminiferous tubules, interstitial cells, and blood vessels encased in a connective tissue sheath. The testes are located dorsomedially within the coelomic cavity but may vary in location depending on species. The right testis is located cranial to the left, especially evident in snakes. The epididymis is absent in snakes.

The copulatory organ is either a single median penis originating from the cranioventral aspect of the cloaca (chelonians and crocodilians) or a pair of hemipenes located laterally in the cloaca and inverting into the base of the tail (lizards and snakes). The hemipenes are maintained in the tail base by a retractor muscle. In all instances, the ureters do not flow through the copulatory organ but instead empty directly into the cloaca.

Female Reproductive Anatomy

The ovaries are similarly located as the testes and consist of epithelial cells, connective tissue, nerves, blood vessels, and germinal cell beds encased in an elastic tunic. The variable gross appearance is dependent on the stage of oogenesis, ranging from small and granular in an inactive ovary to a large lobular sac filled with spherical vitellogenic follicles in an active ovary. The oviducts have both an albumin-secreting and shell-secreting function, and no true uterus exists. The oviducts empty directly into the cloaca through genital papillae.

REPRODUCTIVE CYCLES OF REPTILES

Onset of Sexual Maturity

Sexual maturity in reptiles is determined primarily by size, with age possibly playing a less significant role.[1] Although standard ages of sexual maturity can be found in the literature, these numbers are usually based on free-ranging animals where all individuals in a population have similar environmental influences. However, in captivity, care and, more importantly, diet can vary dramatically, and as a result, captive reptiles may sexually mature at dramatically different ages. For example, Boas (*Boa constrictor*) can be quickly "pushed" to almost 2 m, breeding at 18 months of age and producing young at 23 months.[2] In contrast, the author has seen healthy 10-year-old boas less than a meter in length and reproductively immature.

The interspecific variation in maturation size is greater than the intraspecific variation in growth rate. This makes any discussion on specific maturation sizes impossible in such a general text. **To provide the reader with some sort of reference, the following rough generality is probably warranted. Snakes raised in optimal conditions usually mature in 2 to 3 years, and small lizards take 1 to 2 years and large lizards 3 to 4 years. Chelonians take much longer to mature, usually needing 5 to 7 years.**

Follicle and Egg Development

A major step in the maturation of the reptilian follicle is the accumulation of yolk, or vitellogenesis. Estrogen stimulates the liver to convert lipid from the body's fat stores to vitellogenin. During this time, the liver enlarges dramatically and takes on a yellowish color. The vitellogenin is selectively absorbed from the bloodstream by the follicles. The mature ovum is 10-fold to 100-fold larger than its previtellogenic size.[3] In most reptiles, calcium is predominantly supplied to the offspring in the yolk. Therefore, plasma calcium levels are extremely high during vitellogenesis.

Once ovulation occurs, usually little transfer of nutrients occurs between the female and the ova (but see subsequent discussion under viviparity). The ovum becomes an egg when albumin and a shell are added in the oviduct. The degree of shell calcification varies between species, ranging from pliable (snakes, most lizards, and some turtles) (Figure 23-1) to rigid (crocodilians, tortoises, and many geckos) (Figure 23-2).

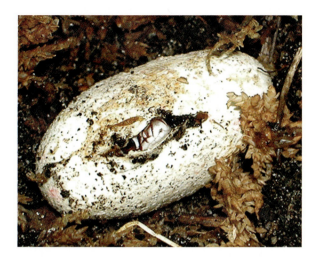

FIGURE 23-1 Snake hatchling shows a pliable egg typical of snakes, most lizards, and some turtles. Hatchlings often remain in the egg with only the head emerged for 24 hours or more while they absorb yolk. (*Photograph courtesy D. Mader.*)

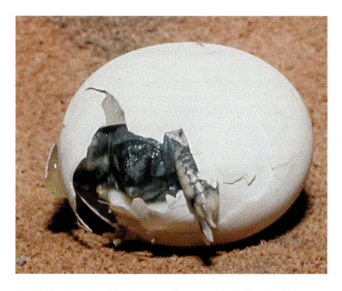

FIGURE 23-2 Hatching tortoise shows rigid shell typical of crocodilians, tortoises, and many geckos. (*Photograph courtesy D. Mader.*)

Clinically, ultrasonography can be used to distinguish the general stages of follicle development, including gonadal inactivity, early previtellogenic follicle growth, vitellogenesis, ovulation, and either shelling or fetal development (see Chapter 37). Birth can be reasonably predicted with ultrasonographic monitoring of the loss of yolk. Birth usually occurs about a week after yolk is no longer detectable.

Viviparity

Although most reptiles lay eggs (oviparous), some bear live young. Live-bearing reptiles are often subdivided into ovoviviparous and viviparous, depending on the degree to which the female contributes nutrients to the developing embryos. In this chapter, the author uses viviparous synonymously with live-bearing.[4,5] In addition, although the term pregnant is oftentimes reserved for viviparous species and gravid for oviparous species, in this chapter, for simplicity, the term pregnant encompasses females with either developing fetuses or oviductal eggs.

The means by which nutrients are provided to the developing embryos can be through lecithotrophy (i.e., yolk) or matrotrophy (i.e., postovulatory, such as across a placenta). The degree of matrotrophy can be variable, with the most extreme example being some skinks (*Mabuya* spp.) that contribute more than 99% of the neonatal mass through a chorioallantoic placenta.[6] Besides providing gas and possibly nutrient exchange to the developing offspring, viviparity provides some protection to the developing embryos and permits a female to easily adjust the developmental temperature.[4] By simply moving between warm and cold locations, optimal developmental temperatures can be consistently maintained.

Viviparity also has costs. By retaining the developing fetuses within the body for an extended period of time, the female is limited to, at most, a single clutch per year.[4] In addition, the space occupied by the fetuses limits the function of the gastrointestinal tract, and as a result, **reptiles usually limit or cease feeding during the latter stages of pregnancy**. Postpartum females are often in poor condition, having mobilized virtually all energy stores for production of their offspring. Because sufficient lipid stores are necessary for reproduction, reptiles that are unable to rapidly restore lipid stores often reproduce biannually.[7] In captivity, however, extensive postpartum feeding may allow for naturally biannual breeding species to produce annually. **Oviparous species may also suspend feeding during the latter stages of egg development; however, the length of time during which feeding is reduced is much shorter** (weeks versus months) and has a less significant effect.

Although all viviparous species cannot possibly be listed, Table 23-1 provides a list of common viviparous and oviparous species. Clearly, reproductive mode has a phylogenetic component (e.g., all pythons are oviparous, all rattlesnakes are viviparous). However, reproductive mode is a plastic trait that evolved independently 45 times in lizards alone,[6] and both viviparity and oviparity can be present within a genus (e.g., *Chamaeleo*, *Eryx*, *Charina*) and even a single species (e.g., *Sceloporous aeneus*).

Parthenogenesis

Although not widespread, parthenogenesis, or asexual reproduction, has been reported in about 30 species of lizards. It has been most widely studied in Whiptail Lizards (*Aspidoscelis* [*Cnemidophorus*] spp.) where parthenogenic species have evolved from the hybridization of two species. These animals reproduce asexually, but females still show courting and pseudocopulation, and these behaviors have a positive effect on reproductive output.[8]

Parthenogenesis has also been discovered in snakes. One known parthenogenic species, the Blind Snake (*Rhamphotyphlops braminus*), is triploid,[9] but recent work suggests that some sexually reproducing snakes can also reproduce asexually.[10]

Table 23-1	Reproductive Mode of Commonly Kept Reptiles

Oviparous
All crocodilians
All chelonians
Most lizards
    All monitors (*Varanus* spp.)
    Most iguanids
        Iguanas (*Iguana* spp.)
        Water Dragons (*Physignathus* spp.)
    All geckos
    Most chameleons
        Veiled Chameleon (*Chamaeleo calyptratus*)
        Panther Chameleon (*C. pardalis*)
Some snakes
    All pythons
    Most colubrids
        Kingsnakes and Milksnakes (*Lampropeltis* spp.)
        Ratsnakes and Cornsnakes (*Elaphe* spp.)

Viviparous
Some lizards
    Some skinks
        Blue-tongued Skinks (*Tiliqua* spp.)
        Shingle-backed Skink (*Trachysaurus rugosus*)
        Prehensile-tailed Skink (*Corucia zebrata*)
    Some chameleons
        Jackson's Chameleon (*C. jacksonii*)
Some snakes
    Most boas (NOT *Charina reinhardti, Eryx jayakari*)
    Most vipers
        All rattlesnakes (*Crotalus* spp.)
    Some colubrids
        Gartersnakes (*Thamnophis* spp.)

Clutch Dynamics

A limited amount of energy is available for reproduction, and consequently, a trade-off is seen between offspring size and clutch size. A small amount of energy can be allocated to each of many offspring, or large amounts of energy may be allocated to only a few offspring. The total amount of energy allocated to reproduction can be extraordinary in reptiles, especially in snakes where more than 40% of a female's body mass can be allocated to reproduction. Such a maternal investment would coincide with a woman producing a 40-pound to 60-pound baby.

Clutch size is extremely variable in reptiles ranging from one (Anoles [*Anolis* spp.], Pancake Tortoise [*Malocochersus tornieri*]) to 200 (Green Seaturtle [*Chelonia mydas*]) in oviparous species and one (Shingleback Skinks [*Trachysaurus rugosus*]) to 92 (Gartersnake [*Thamnophis radix*]) for viviparous species.[1] Experimental techniques have been developed to alter the clutch size of reptiles. Ablating some of the developing follicles during early vitellogenesis reduces clutch size and allows for a greater allocation of energy to the remaining ova.[11] Therefore, gigantized offspring are produced. Although this technique is not yet used clinically, the benefits of such a manipulation could be great in species where neonates are extremely small and difficult to maintain, as is the case for some boids (e.g., Solomon Island Ground Boa [*Candoia carinata*]) and many lizards.

Alternatively, treatment at the onset of the reproductive cycle with the gonadotropin follicle-stimulating hormone increases clutch size while decreasing offspring size.[11] Such treatment could be of value in cases where offspring are large but few in number. Such a manipulation must be used with caution, but it may prove worthy for endangered species or in head-start programs.

Timing of Reproduction

Although some reptiles reproduce throughout the year, most species have a distinct breeding season. The onset of the reproductive season is usually triggered by one or more environmental stimuli. **The most common stimulus of reproduction is a change in temperature.** For most reptiles (especially temperate species), reproductive behavior commences in spring after a period of seasonal cooling.[12] As with most generalities applied to a group as diverse as reptiles, exceptions do exist. One noteworthy exception is tropical boids (boas and pythons). Tropical boids, such as the Boa (*Boa constrictor*) and Burmese Python (*Python molurus*), tend to breed during the cooler period, which does not have as dramatic a temperature decrease as for temperate species (see section on Captive Breeding for further discussion on seasonal cooling). In addition, **in habitats where rainfall is seasonal, many species key their reproduction cycle to rainfall rather than temperature.**[13]

Even when environmental cues are appropriate, reproduction may still be inhibited because of other limiting factors. The role of the male in influencing the reproductive cycle of females is not well understood but seems to vary between species. In some species (*Iguana iguana*, parthenogenic species), females can proceed through the entire oogenic cycle in the absence of a male, but some female snakes require the male's presence, and possibly the act of copulation, to proceed beyond previtellogenic follicular growth.[14,15] Although the requirement for male presence before vitellogenesis is premature for fertilization, it assures the female of a mate before mobilizing substantial energy stores into reproduction.

In addition, reproduction may be inhibited by the lack of sufficient energy stores. Many reptiles, especially snakes, are capital breeders in that the energy necessary for reproduction is derived from fat stores rather than food intake. If females have insufficient energy stores, they forego reproduction that season. Such regulation assures that a female can complete a reproductive effort without consuming a meal,[16] which is critical when food availability is unpredictable.

Frequency of Reproduction

The frequency in which a reptile reproduces is dependent on the species in question, environmental conditions, and the nutritional status of the specific individual. The bottom line is that a female must be in good health with adequate energy stores to reproduce. Reproduction is costly and nonessential for individual survival, so it can be, and usually is, bypassed when body condition is poor.

Many oviparous species have the ability to produce more than one clutch per year. This is true for many turtles and lizards but is less common in snakes. Some tropical gecko species produce a clutch of two eggs once a month throughout the year. More commonly, however, only two to three clutches are laid during a more defined breeding season, lasting only a few months. Whether a second clutch is laid is

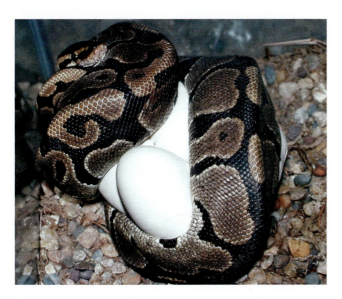

FIGURE 23-3 Many pythons coil around eggs until hatching, thus providing eggs with protection from predators and temperature and humidity regulation. *(Photograph courtesy R. Funk.)*

especially crocodilians (virtually all species). Crocodilians not only guard their nest but also assist the neonates in emerging from the nest and guard them for some time after hatching.

Some viviparous species also show some maternal care. Rattlesnakes remain with their offspring until the neonates first shed (approximately 1 week).[19] In addition, some females assist neonates in escaping from their amniotic sacs (skinks [*Mabuya* spp.] and Night Lizards [*Xantusia* spp.]) and consuming infertile yolk sacs (boas *[Boa constrictor]* and Sand Boas [*Eryx* spp.]). The latter behavior is questionable in terms of its value to the young. Consumption of infertile yolks may reduce the attraction of predators to a birthing site or may simply be performed for the energy value of the yolk.

SEX DETERMINATION IN REPTILES

Reptiles do not possess external genitalia, so sex determination is not always obvious. The proper method to determine the sex of a reptile varies among species and age classes. In some species, sex can be determined with various methods that differ in simplicity or accuracy. When choosing a method, one must realize the accuracy of that method. If the sex of an individual is merely a curiosity or the basis for naming a pet, simplicity may play an important role in choosing a method. However, when captive breeding is intended, one must choose a sex determination method that provides virtually 100% accuracy. Obviously, accuracy of a given procedure is dependent on the ability of the individual performing the procedure. Proper training and experience greatly enhance one's ability to determine the sex of reptiles.

The following material provides a description of the various methods used to determine sex in reptiles and points out when each method is applicable. Table 23-2 provides a quick reference to the preferred method of sex determination of common species.

dependent on the time of year and the condition of the female. Although females may not attain the weight they were before producing the first clutch, females must regain sufficient energy stores after oviposition to commit to another clutch. **Reinsemination is not necessary between clutches, but it can lead to increased fertility.**

As stated previously, species that are viviparous commit a greater amount of time to a single reproductive event. Gestation lasts from 1.5 to 6 months, and the female feeds sparingly or not at all during this time. As a result of this lengthy investment, viviparous reptiles are limited to the production of a single clutch per year.

Maternal Care

Most reptiles show no maternal care of their eggs or offspring beyond choosing an appropriate nesting site and concealing the eggs. However, some degree of parental care has been documented in at least 100 species of reptiles.[17] In the few cases of maternal care in reptiles, the investment is usually limited and nonessential for survival of the offspring.

Many pythons coil around their eggs until hatching, thus providing the eggs with protection from predators and with temperature and humidity regulation (Figure 23-3). During warmer parts of the day, the female python loosens her coils, allowing the eggs to gain heat. As night ensues and temperatures drop, the female python tightens her coil to provide an insulation barrier and reduce heat loss from the egg. Some python species, but not all, have the ability to twitch muscles to generate heat.[18] Although pythons have brooded eggs for thousands of years, python eggs can hatch equally successfully with artificial incubation methods similar to those used for other reptile eggs.

Nest guarding has been documented in several species of reptiles, including turtles (e.g., Burmese Mountain Tortoise [*Manouria emys*]), lizards (e.g., skinks [*Eumeces* spp., *Mabuya* spp.] and Glass Lizards [*Ophiosaurus* spp.]), snakes (e.g., King Cobra *[Ophiophagus hannah]* and cobras [*Naja* spp.]), and

Secondary Sexual Characteristics

In some species, sex determination can be made with a quick glance based on secondary sexual characteristics that anatomically distinguish males from females. This is most prevalent in lizard species and to a lesser extent in chelonians. Other than a possible difference in maximal body size, secondary sexual characteristics are rare in snakes and crocodilians. The accuracy of using secondary sexual characteristics for sex determination varies dramatically, depending on the species in question, the characteristic being examined, and the experience of the observer.

Some species have obvious coloration or ornamentation that distinguishes the sexes. This is best exemplified in chameleons, such as Jackson's Chameleons *(Chamaeleo jacksoni)* where the male possesses three large rostral horns. These horns are conspicuously absent in female *C. jacksoni*. Unfortunately, most secondary sexual characteristics, even when they do exist, are more subtle, involving either minor differences between the sexes or the observation of small inconspicuous features.

Male reptiles often have a larger more robust appearance, especially of the head. However, in most species, this difference is minor and large females can easily be confused with

Table 23-2	Preferred Technique for Sex Determination of Common Reptiles						
Taxonomic Group	**2° Sex**	**Pop**	**Probe**	**Hydro**	**Hyd+**	**Other**	**None**
Lizards							
Juveniles (most species)							X
Adults							
Most geckos	1						
Iguanas	2				X		
Large skinks					X		
Monitors			X		X	A	
Snakes							
Boas and Pythons							
Juveniles	3			X			
Adults	3		X		X		
Colubrids							
Juveniles (most species)		X					
Adults			X				
Turtles (most species)							
Juveniles							X
Adults	4						
Crocodilians (most species)							
Juveniles							X
Adults						B	

1, Hemipenal bulge in tail base.
2, Enlarged femoral pores, dorsal spines, and dewlap in males.
3, Larger cloacal spurs in males of most species.
4, Concaved plastron and larger tail in males of many species.
A, Radiographs of hemipenes in many species (see Table 18-3).
B, Digital palpation of cloaca for penis.
2° *Sex*, Secondary sexual characteristics; *pop,* manual eversion of hemipenes; *probe,* cloacal probing; *hydro,* hydrostatic eversion of hemipenes; *hyd+,* hydrostatic eversion with anesthesia; *none,* no reliable method available.

small males. Vast experience with a given species is essential for using size differences as a sex determinant. Common species in which general appearance and head size are frequently used, but not always with high accuracy, in sex determination include iguanas and Gila Monsters *(Heloderma suspectum)*.

In chelonians, the plastron of males is often concaved. This concavity, in part, allows the males to more closely appose its cloaca to the female's during mounting. Like most secondary sexual characteristics in reptiles, the degree of the concavity and the amount to which it varies from the female shows considerable amounts of both intraspecific and interspecific variation.

Many inconspicuous but notable secondary sexual characteristics are located near the cloaca. Many iguanid and gekkonid lizards possess either femoral or preanal pores that excrete a waxy substance used for marking territory. Although present in both sexes, these pores are more pronounced in males. In males, the size of the pores and the active excretion of wax are seasonally variable, being most pronounced during the breeding season and superficially similar to females during the remainder of the year.

Many boid snakes possess spurs located just lateral to the vent. The spurs are vestigial hind limbs, and in males, they are used for tactile stimulation of the female during courtship. Therefore, spurs are usually larger in males, but the difference in size is highly dependent on the species. In some species, such as the Rosy Boa *(Charina trivirgata)* and the Sand Boas *(Eryx* spp.), spur size is a highly reliable predictor of sex. However, in other boids, the reliability is not as good. All male Boas *(Boa constrictor)* have large spurs, but so does an occasional female. In the Ball Python *(Python regius)*, spur

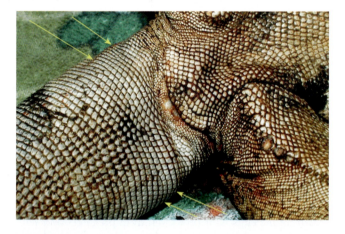

FIGURE 23-4 Ventral view of a male Green Iguana *(Iguana iguana)* shows the large femoral pores and enlarged tail base characteristic of many male lizards (between *yellow arrows*). (Photograph courtesy D. Mader.)

size is extremely variable in both sexes and therefore has little value as a sex determinant.

The tail is a critical reproductive organ for many male reptiles because it provides both a storage location for hemipenes (in snakes and lizards) and a muscular appendage to help position the male's cloaca adjacent to the female's (in most reptiles). Because of these traits, the size and shape of the tail is often sexually dimorphic. The presence of hemipenes within the base of the tail causes this area to be enlarged (Figure 23-4). The symmetrical bulging can often be quite dramatic, sometimes visible without picking up the individual in question. The extent of the dimorphism is usually greater in lizards than snakes, especially the smaller species (particularly geckos).

Chelonian tails, while not basally enlarged because of the presence of a phallus, are usually much larger and longer in males than in females. In addition, the vent is usually located more distally on the tail of males. The larger tail provides better access to the female's cloaca, which with the presence of the shell cannot be taken for granted. Some tortoises also use the tip of the tail for tactile stimulation of the female's cloacal region.

Other secondary sexual characteristics located near the tail but specific to individual species include enlarged postanal scales of many iguanid lizards (e.g., Spiny Lizards [*Sceloporus* spp.]) and the pelvic protruberances of the Banded Geckos (*Coleonyx* spp.).

In addition to the problems of species specificity and sometimes only minor differences between the sexes, secondary sexual characteristics are usually not developed in juvenile specimens. As a result, juveniles of many species that as adults may possess obvious sexual dimorphism must have their sex determined with other methods or, to the misfortune of many reptile breeders, sex frequently cannot be determined until later in life.

Manual Eversion of Hemipenes

The most common method used for determining the sex of neonatal colubrid snakes is to manually evert the hemipenes. This procedure, frequently referred to as popping, entails firmly rolling one's thumb proximally up the tail base toward the cloaca. The pressure forces the hemipenes, if present, to evert through the cloaca (Figure 23-5). To avoid injury to the hemipenes, care must be taken to roll the thumb rather than simply apply pressure.

The presence of everted hemipenes obviously identifies a male. In females, the oviductal papillae can sometimes be identified during popping as two small reddish openings located laterally in the cloaca. This is especially visible in the Kingsnakes (*Lampropeltis* spp.); however, females of most species are determined merely by the lack of hemipenes. The diagnosis of females simply from negative results can lead to the misdiagnosis of males as females, especially for people with limited experience in the procedure. In general, with experience, the sex of most neonatal colubrids can be determined with nearly 100% accuracy with this technique.

For heavy-bodied juvenile snakes, including most of the boids and some colubrids (e.g., the Hog-nosed Snakes [*Heterodon* spp.]), everting the hemipenes is not possible with manual pressure, and therefore, alternate sex determination techniques must be used.

Cloacal Probing

Probing the cloaca with a slender blunt instrument is the most common method of sex determination in adult snakes and many large lizards (e.g., Monitors [*Varanus* spp.]). This procedure, like manual eversion, uses the presence of the hemipenes in the base of the tail. The particular instrument used is not critical as long as it is long, smooth, and blunt on the probing end. Commercially manufactured probes are available in various sizes from several sources (Figure 23-6, *A*). In the author's opinion, plastic-tipped bobby pins that have been straightened and lubricated are the best probes because they are inexpensive and disposable after a single use. This eliminates the possibility of transferring microorganisms between individuals.

Cloacal probing is a simple technique that can be quickly mastered. With the animal properly restrained, the probe is inserted into the cloaca and directed caudally. With gentle maneuvering of the probe just lateral to midline, the probe enters the inverted hemipenis in a male and freely inserts into the tail base (Figure 23-6, *B*). The depth to which the probe enters the tail is dependent on the species in question. Probing females results in the total inability or a limited ability to insert the probe into the tail base.

The ability to insert the probe in the tail base of some females is the result of the presence of a pair of blind diverticula. These diverticula, when present, are shorter in depth and smaller in diameter than hemipenes. A properly sized probe (versus one that is too small) allows the probe to enter the inverted hemipenis but reduces its ability to enter the diverticula of females. Common species in which these diverticula are well-developed and misidentification of sex is therefore common include the Monitors (*Varanus* spp.) and the Blood Python *(Python curtus)*.

Hydrostatic Eversion of the Hemipenes

Hydrostatic eversion, commonly referred to as saline injection, involves more effort but is extremely accurate and sometimes the only way to accurately determine the gender of certain reptile species. The technique, like manual eversion, relies on the eversion of the hemipenes from the base of the tail to diagnose males, making it only applicable to lizards and snakes. However, unlike manual eversion, the technique provides a definitive anatomic indicator of females rather than the mere absence of the male sex character.

Procedurally, sterile fluid, preferably isotonic saline solution, is injected into the tail just distal to where the hemipenes is located if the individual is a male. The fluid, as much as 100 mL

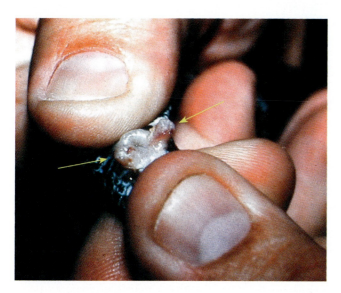

FIGURE 23-5 Popping technique to evert the hemipene in a hatchling snake. *(Photograph courtesy D. Mader.)*

in large specimens, is injected into the tail until either sufficient eversion has occurred or resistance can be felt at the plunger (Figure 23-7, A). Placement of the needle too proximally on the tail may direct the fluid into a hemipenis rather than behind it, therefore making the procedure not only ineffective but also potentially injurious (Figure 23-7, B).

The hydrostatic pressure created within the tail not only forces the hemipenes to evert but also causes swelling of the tissue surrounding the cloaca. This swelling partially everts the cloaca through the vent, allowing for easy visualization of the oviductal papillae in females. For large specimens, including boids, monitors, iguanas, and Gila Monsters, the strength of the retractor penis muscle can counteract the hydrostatic pressure, preventing eversion of the hemipenes. For this technique to be accurately performed, in these larger species, the muscle must be relaxed with a surgical level of anesthesia. Although anesthesia use complicates the procedure by requiring both the proper equipment and more time, it should be willingly used when necessary because it greatly increases the accuracy of the procedure and reptiles are excellent gas anesthetic patients.

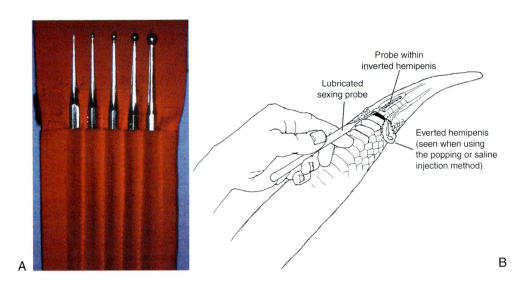

FIGURE 23-6 A, Sexing probes can be made or purchased commercially. B, Probing method for sex determination. (A, Photograph courtesy D. Mader.)

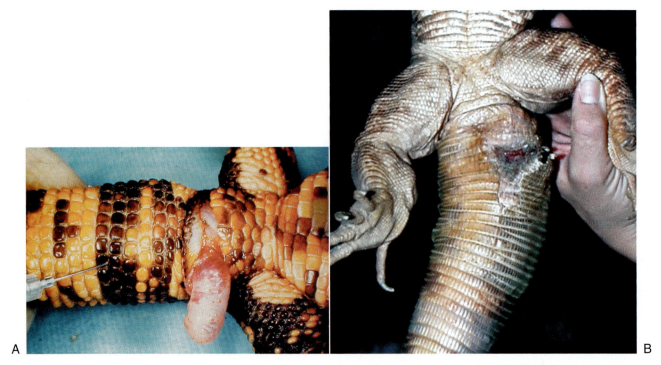

FIGURE 23-7 A, Saline solution injection technique to evert the hemipenes. The head is to the right. B, This Tegu (*Tupinambis* sp.) had a severe infection develop around and in the hemipenis after saline solution injection. The hemipenis was rendered useless for breeding even after the infection was treated. (A, Photograph courtesy C.J. Murphy; B, Photograph courtesy D. Mader.)

The use of hydrostatic pressure to determine sex is the procedure of choice for neonatal snakes in which manual eversion is ineffective and for many of the large lizard species.

Noteworthy, the blind diverticula may, on eversion, appear quite similar to hemipenes. Close examination may be necessary in some species to differentiate them from hemipenes, especially in neonatal specimens. Hemipenes are more ornate and larger in length and diameter compared with the diverticula of females.

Digital Palpation of Cloaca

The preferred method for sex determination of crocodilians involves digitally palpating the ventral aspect of the cloaca for the presence of a penis. With the animal thoroughly restrained in dorsal recumbency, the cloaca can be easily explored with a gloved finger. The presence of a penis is obvious because it is the only structure that can be felt in the otherwise smooth-walled cloaca. If desired, the penis can be everted through the vent for visualization (Figure 23-8).

Ultrasonography

Ultrasound can be used to monitor the reproductive condition of many female reptiles. For many breeding programs, such monitoring is invaluable not only to aid in pregnancy diagnosis and the prediction of parturition date but also to reveal early reproductive events to maximize breeding success. The value of ultrasound as an aid to sex determination is limited because ovarian follicles are the only easily recognized reproductive structures. Therefore, only reproductively active females can be diagnosed with confidence, leaving immature females, acyclic females, and all males oftentimes undistinguishable.

Radiography

Many but not all species of monitors (*Varanus* spp.) possess mineralized hemibacula within their hemipenes, which are easily recognizable on radiographs. Species in which these structures occur are listed in Table 23-3.[20] In addition, recent work has indicated that pelvic measurements from radiographs can be used to determine the sex of Gila Monsters.[21] The accuracy and universality of this technique is still unclear, but it warrants further investigation.

Surgical Sex Determination

Visualization of the gonads via surgery or endoscopy is a definitive method for determining the sex of reptiles. However, the procedure is complicated in terms of time and equipment requirements. In addition, difficulties can arise from the presence of large amounts of adipose tissue and regression of the gonads during the nonbreeding season. A flank approach usually provides the best access to the gonads, but it may leave an obvious scar.

Temperature-Dependent Sex Determination

Many reptile species have temperature-dependent sex determination, where the sex of the developing fetus is determined by the temperature at which the eggs are incubated. Temperature-dependent sex determination occurs in all crocodilians, many turtles, and a few species of lizards, most notably the Leopard Gecko (*Eublepharis macularius*).

The exact temperatures at which each sex is produced is dependent on the species. In some species, warmer temperatures produce males, and in others, warmer temperatures produce females. In still other species, a bimodal breakdown is seen, with one sex produced at moderate temperatures and the other sex produced at extreme temperatures. In all cases, the shift from one sex to the other is not absolute, but instead a range of temperatures exists at which both sexes are produced at varying proportions.

Because these intermediate temperature ranges exist and because most incubators, and even thermometers, used by reptile breeders are not accurate, one must be careful in predicting sex on the basis of incubation temperatures.

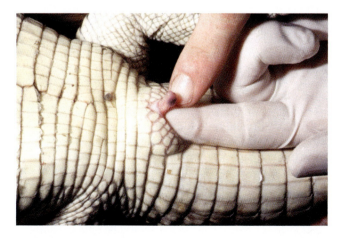

FIGURE 23-8 Penis of a male Caiman (*Caiman* sp.) everted with digital palpation. (*Photograph courtesy F.L. Frye.*)

Table 23-3	Species of Monitors (*Varanus* spp.) in Which Mineralized Hemibacula Are Present within Hemipenes
Mineralization Present	**Mineralization Absent**
V. acanthurus (Spiny-tailed)	*V. bengalensis* (Bengal)
V. beccarii (Black Tree)	*V. dumereli* (Dumeril's)
V. caudolineatus (Stripe-tailed)	*V. exanthematicus* (Savannah)
V. eremias (Desert Pygmy)	
V. giganteus (Perenty)	*V. griseus* (Desert)
V. gilleni (Gillen's Pygmy)	*V. mertensi* (Merten's water)
V. gouldii (Gould's)	*V. niloticus* (Nile)
V. indicus (Mangrove)	*V. rudicollis* (Roughneck)
V. karlschmidti (Peach-throat)	*V. salvator* (Water)
V. komodensis (Komodo)	*V. timorensis* (Timor)
V. olivaceus (Gray's)	
V. panoptes (Argus)	
V. prasinus (Green Tree)	
V. salvadori (Crocodile)	
V. storri (Storr's)	
V. tristis (Freckled)	
V. varius (Lace)	

Structures are easily visualized on radiographs and can be used for sex determination.

One should confirm the sex in these species using one of the previously mentioned techniques.

GENOTYPING

For species where sex is determined genetically, determination of the sex of an individual using a genetic code unique to the heterogametic chromosome is possible.[22] Unlike mammals where the male is the heterogametic sex in all species, the heterogametic sex varies among species of reptile. Although this technique is feasible, it has received little attention.

CAPTIVE BREEDING

An understanding of the reproductive physiology of reptiles and the ability to determine the sex of a reptile are important to the reptile practitioner. However, this information alone is not sufficient to understand these animals and be able to deal with the problems often associated with them. Although the anatomy and physiology of reptiles is a science, captive reproduction of these animals in many ways is an art. The ability to combine the science and the art is critical for properly educating clients and effectively treating their animals. References on captive breeding of reptiles are readily available, but an overview is warranted here.

The Breeding Stock

The three obvious, yet often overlooked, components of good breeding stock are: at least one individual of each sex is needed, the individuals in question must be adults, and they must be healthy. Although these points are obvious, finding breeding pairs consisting of individuals of the same sex or of emaciated individuals is not uncommon. These requirements are essential for captive breeding, but they are not sufficient to ensure positive results. Breeding reptiles involves a series of events that occur in succession, and failure at any one of these points leads to poor results.

Seasonal Cooling

As discussed previously, a period of cool temperature is necessary for most species to initiate reproductive behavior. This seasonal cooling is commonly referred to as hibernation, brumation, or even "being put down" (lay term). The latter term must not be confused with the mammalian equivalent that infers euthanasia. A few clinically important aspects exist regarding the seasonal cooling period of captive reptiles.

A reptile's physiology is greatly affected by the imposed cooler ambient temperature and, therefore, cooler body temperature. Most body systems, including the digestive and immune systems, operate best at a certain temperature referred to as the optimal temperature. When body temperature differs substantially from optimal temperature, such as during seasonal cooling, these systems are much less efficient. The greater the difference between optimal and body temperature, the more drastic the effect. To stimulate reproductive activity in the following spring, temperate species are usually subjected to a constant winter temperature of 10°C to 13°C (50°F to 55°F) for 8 to 12 weeks. High latitude and high elevation species may need lower temperatures. Subtropical and tropical species need less drastic temperature drops, usually 20°C to 24°C (68°F to 75°F), and these species are often offered limited periods (4 to 8 hours) each day when ambient temperature is warmer and a supplemental heat source is provided. The existence of a substantial nighttime cooling appears to be the critical component to stimulating reproduction in many subtropical and tropical species. A similar cool night and limited heat during the day approach to seasonal cooling can also be used for small temperate lizards, providing a reproductive stimulation that is equally effective yet safer than a constant cool environment.

Because of the physiologic effects of suboptimal body temperatures, care must be taken in preparing animals for extended periods of cool temperatures and in maintaining proper temperatures during this time. The immune system functions best at the optimal body temperatures, so unhealthy animals should not be cooled for significant lengths of time. All captive reptiles should undergo a careful physical examination before seasonal cooling.

The only unhealthy condition to which seasonal cooling may actually be beneficial is anorexia. Many reptiles, especially wild-caught individuals, have a circannual rhythm to their feeding, and even if kept warm during the naturally cooler months, they may cease feeding. Oftentimes, these animals respond to a short cooling period and emerge with a voracious appetite. A similar scenario is true for neonates that do not feed. A short cooling period often triggers finicky eaters to accept a more varied diet. Before cooling any nonfeeder, one must be certain that the anorexia is behaviorally motivated, rather than a complication of a more serious condition. Thorough examinations, including a fecal examination, are mandatory before cooling a nonfeeding reptile.

Like the immune system, the digestive system is dramatically affected by body temperature. For temperate reptile species experiencing a quite dramatic and constant temperature reduction, first ensuring that the digestive tract is empty is essential. Digesta left in the gut may cause serious and sometimes fatal results. The lower body temperature reduces the ability of the digestive tract to digest food; therefore, any material in the gut can lead to severe and sometimes fatal enteritis. Snakes should have food withheld for at least 2 weeks before extended constant cooling, and lizards and chelonians usually clear their gut within several days to a week.

Seasonal cooling is usually coordinated with the natural weather pattern, but animals can be phase-shifted to respond at other times. The required duration of the cooling period to assure reproductive conditioning is unknown. Common lengths range from 4 to 12 weeks. Novice breeders usually prefer shorter cooling periods, because, to them, this is a period of uncertainty. On the contrary, experienced herpetoculturists lean toward longer cooling periods, because, for them, this is a period of reduced colony maintenance. Energy demands of a cooled reptile are variable; however, losses in body weight during seasonal cooling are usually less than 10%.[7]

Within the herpetocultural community, disagreement exists as to how seasonal cooling should be initiated and terminated. Should the temperature be gradually lowered and raised over a period of time, or should the change be abrupt, immediately converting the animal from optimal body temperature to cooling temperature? One may assume that a gradual change in temperature is more natural because the change in ambient temperature from one season to another is gradual. However, one must examine the microhabitat and the behavior of the animal to properly define the natural condition. The onset of the winter climate involves a change in behavior, from one of actively foraging and thermoregulating to one of inactivity and seclusion. Although the ambient temperature may change only slightly or not at all, the change in body temperature in an animal that switches from active thermoregulation to inactivity in a deep burrow is dramatic.

Similar dramatic temperature change also occurs when a reptile emerges from its hibernaculum and recommences an active life. This is true for turtles surfacing from the mud at the bottom of a cold pond to bask on a rock at the pond's edge or a snake emerging from a deep crack in a rock outcrop to situate itself under a flat rock in the warm sun. Therefore, **based on the natural history of these animals, the dramatic temperature shift is more natural and probably more appropriate.**

This is not to deny the fact that many herpetoculturists successfully use gradual temperature changes, but caution must be taken during these transition times. Intermediate body temperatures, those between the optimal temperature and target cooling temperature, may be deleterious because such temperatures are nonconducive to feeding and reduce immunocompetence yet dictate still rather moderate metabolic rates and allow for relatively rapid bacterial growth. As a result, animals at intermediate body temperatures experience sufficient weight loss and are prone to opportunistic infections.

All reptiles seasonally cooled at a constant low temperature should be checked weekly or biweekly. Although the animals should be quite sluggish, they should not show any physical or behavioral signs of illness. In addition, water, if not offered ad libitum, should be offered during these checks. If water is to be offered continuously at this time, precautions must be taken to assure that it does not spill. High humidity during seasonal cooling is a frequent cause of respiratory infections in all groups of reptiles. Reptiles showing any signs of potential illness must be returned to an environment that is optimal for activity.

Similar to the precooling period, the postcooling period is a time of careful observation. Many problems that were developing during seasonal cooling fulminate on the return to active temperatures. Quick detection and correction of such problems are essential for maximizing the reproductive potential, and even survival, of the animal.

Other Stimuli of Reproduction

Because temperature change is the predominant stimuli of reproduction, seasonal cooling is the most commonly used method to induce reproduction in captive reptiles. However, other environmental parameters can also affect reproductive activity, so other techniques are sometimes used in conjunction with or as an alternative to seasonal cooling to stimulate captive breeding. Such stimuli include increased cage humidity, artificial raining, increased feeding, repeated introduction to multiple potential mates, and male-male combat. Although these methods seem to provide benefits in certain species, the details and the universality of their use are not well known.

Copulation

Fertilization in reptiles is internal with either the penis or a single hemipenis being inserted into the female's cloaca. Copulation may last from seconds to in excess of a day depending on the species. Before copulation, some form of courtship is usually seen. Male snakes use their bodies and especially their tail for tactile stimulation of the female, and male lizards more commonly use species-specific postures and movements to impress the female. Chelonians use both visual and tactile stimulation in the form of head bobs (tortoises), forepaw fluttering (turtles), and biting.

Injuries are relatively common during courtship and copulation, especially in lizards and chelonians. Chelonians often bite at the limbs and shell of females to discourage them from walking or swimming. These attacks can be quite intense, and if the female cannot escape from the male's assault, the resulting wounds can be severe and even fatal.

To secure a position on the back of the female, male lizards often bite and hold the nape of the female's neck while attempting copulation. In addition, like chelonians, lizards bite at a female's limbs and tails if she is avoiding his pursuit. These injuries, although often not as severe as those seen in chelonians, may need medical attention. This is especially true for Green Iguanas (*Iguana iguana*), whose courtship and copulation can be quite a physical battle.

The brunt of injury is levied on the female from the male, but males are not free of risk. Blue-tongued Skinks (*Tiliqua* spp.) are especially noted for the aggressiveness of females toward advancing males. Injury during courtship is not totally an artifact of captivity; however, the confinement of captive reptiles in a cage limits the ability of an individual to escape and therefore increases the risk of serious injury.

The timing of fertilization in terms of the female's reproductive cycle is not well understood. Copulation frequently occurs during mid vitellogenesis but also may be required before vitellogenesis in some species. Because many observers use copulation as the onset of gestation, estimated gestation times are often exaggerated.

To further complicate the issue of gestation time, multiple breedings are commonplace in reptiles. This is especially true for boid snakes, where a pair may repeatedly copulate over a period of 1 to 2 months. In these instances, copulation is obviously occurring at varied stages of the female's reproductive cycle. To accurately determine the gestation of a reptile, more advanced techniques such as ultrasonography must be used.

Because copulation occurs before ovulation, sperm must be stored by the female. **Some reptiles have the ability to store sperm for up to 6 years**[1]; however, fertility is highest when copulation occurs in concert with the female's reproductive cycle. Similarly, second clutches can be produced without second matings, but again, fertility is much greater if copulation occurs during the development of the second clutch. Artificial insemination has been used in reptiles with limited success.[23,24] To maximize success, artificial insemination should be coordinated with the female's follicular cycle, a point that is often overlooked.

Determination of Pregnancy

Pregnancy, which is used loosely to include both fetal development in viviparous species and postovulatory egg development in oviparous species, can usually be determined by observing the appearance and behavior of a female. Usually, a combination of indicators is used to assess an individual. Mid-body swelling is apparent in pregnant snakes and lizards; however, obese animals can cause both false-negative and false-positive pregnancy assessments. The change in appearance is more obvious in smaller and less robust species. In geckos, the eggs can usually be seen through the semitransparent skin of the abdomen. Realizing that the right ovary is located more cranial to the left aids in differentiating developing eggs from similarly colored but symmetrically located fat bodies.

Behavioral signs can be used in conjunction with appearance to aid in pregnancy determination. Classic behaviors of pregnant reptiles include an increase in basking time that correlates with an increase in selected body temperature, partial or complete anorexia, and a change in body positioning. In snakes, body positioning changes often include looser coiling and lying in semilateral or even dorsal recumbency. Later in pregnancy, restlessness and nesting behavior can be observed.

Although the above indicators of pregnancy are frequently used, they are not definitive. More conclusive evidence is usually warranted. Abdominal palpation can be used to provide such evidence in many cases. Palpation is easiest in snakes (exclusive of the boids), but with practice it can also be used with certainty in lizards. In chelonians, the shell makes palpation difficult but not impossible. Fingers directed craniomedially through the hind limb fossae can sometimes reveal eggs in a chelonian. Success can be increased using gravity to direct the eggs toward the fossae by holding the turtle vertically, with the head pointed upward.

In snakes, a firm but careful thumb run down the ventrum from approximately midbody to the cloaca reveals not only the presence but also the number of follicles, eggs, or fetuses. Follicles are firm and easily differentiated from the softer eggs or fetuses. Lizards are palpated with a thumb and forefinger placed ventrolaterally on the relaxed abdomen. As with snakes, follicles are differentiated from eggs by their firmness. As mentioned previously, lizards are more difficult to palpate than snakes, leading to an increase in both false-negative diagnoses and iatrogenic injury, most commonly follicle or egg rupture.

The most exact methods of pregnancy determination use radiography and ultrasonography. Radiology is useful in determining pregnancy of chelonians because the hard calcium-rich eggshells are clearly visible on radiographs and alternative methods are quite limited (Figure 23-9). **No evidence is found that limited radiographic exposure has any detrimental effects on the eggs.**

For lizards and snakes, the lack of calcium in the eggshell makes radiographic identification more difficult. Therefore, ultrasonography is preferred in these animals. Ultrasonography reveals all stages of ova development, including early previtellogenic follicular growth. In snakes, the gallbladder can be used as a marker because it is readily identified as a large echolucent sphere about three fifths down the body. The right ovary is located just distal to the gallbladder, and the left ovary just distal to the right. Early previtellogenic follicles are recognized as either a chain or grape-clustering of small echolucent spheres (6 to 20 mm) (Figure 23-10). Vitellogenesis is signified by the follicles becoming larger and progressively more echogenic but remaining clustered (Figure 23-11). Ovulated follicles and eggs are linearly arranged, occupying nearly the entire caudal half of the snake. With practice, egg shelling can also be detected (Figure 23-12).

The ultrasonographic appearance of viviparous species is similar in appearance to oviparous species until after ovulation. Immediately after ovulation, developing fetuses are dominated mostly by yolk and, therefore, appear similar to ovulated eggs. However, as the embryo grows, an amniotic sac can be seen as a small echolucent sphere on the periphery of the larger echogenic yolk mass (Figure 23-13). Eventually, in

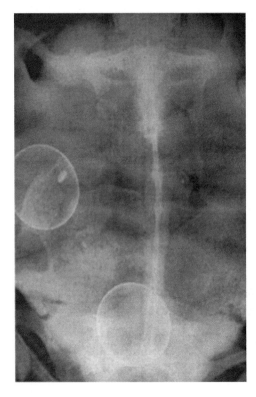

FIGURE 23-9 Radiograph of a Desert Tortoise *(Gopherus agassizii)* shows two eggs.

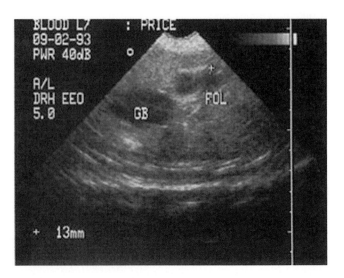

FIGURE 23-10 Echolucent previtellogenic follicles *(FOL)* of the right ovary in a Blood Python *(Python curtis)*. The easily visualized gallbladder *(GB)* can be used to locate the right ovary. The left ovary (not shown) lies slightly caudal to the right.

larger specimens, fetuses can be seen (Figure 23-14). The ultrasonic appearance of lizards is very similar to snakes except for the lack of the linear arrangement of the ovaries and ova.

Gestation and Oviposition

Gestation is a critical time for both the female and the developing offspring. A great demand is placed on a pregnant female because pregnancy requires energy output but oftentimes limits energy intake. The drastic imbalance between energy intake and energy demand is satisfied by energy reserves, including the breakdown of muscle mass.

In addition, pregnancy has an inhibitory effect on the immune system.[25] The combined effect of the energy deficit and impaired immune function often leads to clinical disease during pregnancy. Persistent, low-grade infections often fulminate during pregnancy, jeopardizing both the female and the offspring. **No reports have been found nor has the author observed any negative effects of antibiotics on pregnancy, neither as an abortifacient nor a teratogen.**

True gestation time can be difficult to determine in reptiles for a multitude of reasons. Among these are the separation in time between copulation and ovulation, the prevalence of multiple copulations, and the temperature-dependent effect in which warmer temperatures decrease gestation time. Reported gestation lengths for viviparous reptiles range from 1.5 to 6 months. Most snakes undergo ecdysis before oviposition. This "pre-lay shed," as it is commonly termed, provides a relatively reliable predictor of oviposition date. Colubrid snakes usually oviposit 8 to 14 days after this shed, and pythons tend to take 18 to 26 days. Although these ranges are not absolute and variation does occur, they are a useful guide. The pre-lay shed date is used by many herpetoculturists as the time to offer the female a nesting site.

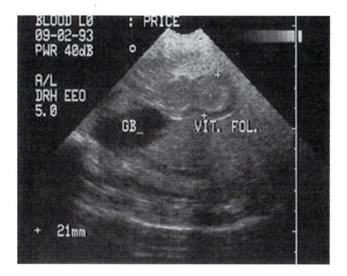

FIGURE 23-11 Echogenic vitellogenic follicles *(VIT. FOL.)* in a Blood Python *(Python curtis)*. Gallbladder *(GB)* is also identified.

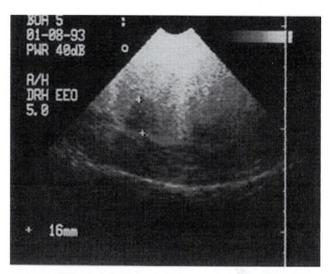

FIGURE 23-13 Echolucent germinal disc surrounded by echogenic yolk in a viviparous Boa *(Boa constrictor)*. Visualization of germinal discs confirms fertility in viviparous species.

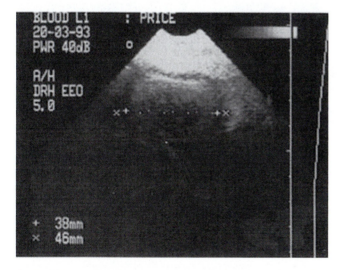

FIGURE 23-12 An echogenic egg in the oviduct of a Blood Python *(Python curtis)*. Note the oblong shape. Fertility of the egg cannot be assessed.

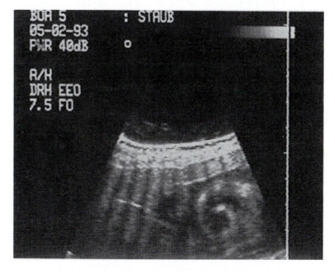

FIGURE 23-14 Ultrasound image of the caudal end of a well-developed fetus in a Boa *(Boa constrictor)*.

Provision of an appropriate oviposition site is critical in many species. Not providing a female with the proper laying conditions can lead to dystocia in an otherwise healthy animal. Many reptiles use an ovipositorium or "lay-box." Ovipositoria can simply consist of an opaque container with a small entrance hole in the side (for lizards) or top (for snakes; Figure 23-15). The container should be half filled with any of a number of lightly moistened substrates, the most commonly used are vermiculite and green moss. The ovipositorium should be situated so that the temperature inside is 28°C to 30°C (82°F to 86°F). Although snakes usually always use the provided ovipositorium, lizards oftentimes ignore it, laying their eggs in another area of the cage where they rapidly dessicate. To avoid this, gravid lizards can be moved to a separate cage that is set up entirely as an ovipositorium. In such set ups, the substrate, moistened vermiculite or peat, should be reasonably deep and a basking platform should be provided. The platform, a tray that covers approximately one quarter to one third of the substrate, allows the lizard to get off of the moist substrate and provides the lizards with an object under which to dig. A basking light is provided over the platform. Properly designed large-scale ovipositoria can house lizards for extended periods and greatly increase the success in obtaining viable eggs.

Oftentimes the nest site is more for the benefit of the herpetoculturist (to harvest viable eggs) rather than for the female (to prevent dystocia), but this is not always the case. Dystocias are common in Green Iguanas *(Iguana iguana)* and frequently are a result of an inadequate nesting site. In nature, gravid iguanas exhibit extensive nesting behavior, including migration to a suitable nest site and digging a relatively deep nest for the eggs. In captivity, homologous conditions to allow such behavior are difficult to provide. Minimally, gravid iguanas should be provided a large ovipositorium with substantial amounts, 30 to 60 cm (1 to 2 ft), of substrate.

Chelonians lay their eggs in excavated holes, which they then carefully cover. Unless nesting is observed, chelonian nest sites can be difficult to locate. A week or two before oviposition, chelonians usually show increased activity, commonly digging several incomplete nest holes before selecting the ultimate nest site. This preovipository behavior can be used to signify that a female is gravid.

To avoid the possibility that the nest site is not located, chelonians can be easily induced to oviposit by administering 10 IU/kg oxytocin intramuscularly (IM) or intracoelomically (ICe). Oxytocin is reliable and effective in initiating oviposition in chelonians, with oviposition of the first egg usually within 1 hour. Eggs may be laid continuously or at intervals of 15 minutes or more. Although usually not necessary, a radiograph can be taken to confirm that oviposition is complete. Females injected with oxytocin exhibit stereotypical digging motions with their hind legs, but a hole is not dug. Therefore, females should be closely monitored and eggs removed immediately on oviposition to prevent the eggs from being crushed. Aquatic chelonians, which usually take longer than terrestrial species to respond to oxytocin, may be placed in a shallow tub of water after injection to reduce the chance of crushing the eggs. Eggs should be removed from the water as soon as possible but can survive several hours of submersion.[26]

Egg Incubation

Viable eggs are usually firm, dry, and chalky white (Figure 23-16). The egg shells of all snakes, most lizards, and some turtles are pliable, and the shells of crocodilians, many chelonians, and some lizards (many geckos) are rigid. Incubation requirements for the eggs of most reptile species are similar, although some are more sensitive to perturbations. Incubation substrate is variable, with vermiculite and perlite, two generic materials commonly used for potting plants, being the most common substrates used. These products are

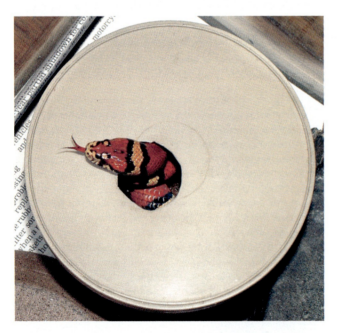

FIGURE 23-15 Red Milksnake *(Lampropeltis triangulum syspila)* in a simple ovipositoria made from a disposable plastic container and slightly dampened vermiculite. Opening can be either on the side or through the top, as in this case. *(Photograph courtesy S. Barten.)*

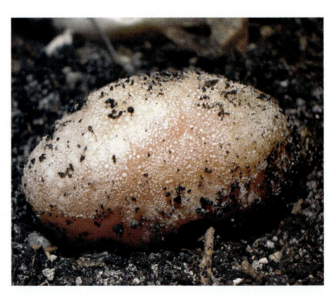

FIGURE 23-16 Viable eggs are usually firm, dry, and chalky white. When an egg changes color, develops a coating of fungus, or collapses prematurely, embryonic death is likely. *(Photograph courtesy D. Mader.)*

manufactured by numerous companies and are routinely available at nurseries and garden shops. The substrate should be slightly moistened with filtered water but not wet. Excessive moisture frequently leads to fungal growth, and low moisture can lead to water loss (and eventual embryonic death) in porous eggs. Proper incubation temperatures range from 26°C to 32°C (80°F to 90°F). Higher temperatures reduce incubation length but increase the risk of congenital defects, most commonly abnormal color or pattern.

The eggs of most snakes and small lizards hatch in 45 to 70 days, and eggs of larger lizards (e.g., iguanas and many monitors) usually need 90 to 130 days of incubation. Chameleon eggs can also take extended in periods of time to hatch (e.g., several months). Incubation times of chelonian eggs show great variation, both among species (ranging from 28 days for *Trionyx sinensis* to 540 days for *Geochelone pardalis*[27]), within species (240 to 540 days for *G. pardalis*[27]), and even within a clutch (30-day to 40-day variation for *G. pardalis*[28]).

At the time of hatching, the neonate uses its caruncle or egg tooth to incise the eggshell. The neonate usually remains in the egg with only its head protruding for 12 to 72 hours (see Figures 23-1 and 23-2). During this time, the remaining yolk is absorbed. Neonates need no assistance during hatching, and efforts to aid this process are usually detrimental.

COMMON REPRODUCTIVE DISORDERS

Dystocia

Dystocia, abnormal labor or retained eggs/fetuses, is the most common reproductive malady in reptiles and therefore is discussed separately in Chapter 53.

Calcium Deficiencies

Calcium deficiency is common in captive reptiles and has numerous causes (see Chapter 61). However, it is worth noting as a reproductive disorder because reproduction imposes high calcium demands on the body and females in a marginal calcium state oftentimes show clinical signs of calcium deficiency during reproduction, predominantly from the production of massive amounts of calcium-rich yolk. Plasma levels of calcium are extremely high during vitellogenesis because of the mobilization of calcium stores primarily from the bones. Rapid depletion of bone calcium can lead to lameness, abnormal locomotion, and deformation of the mandibles. Such conditions are most prevalent in herbivorous and insectivorous species and are best prevented by actively supplementing the diet with calcium. Treatment of calcium deficiency during reproduction should follow that which is standard for all calcium deficiencies, plus consideration should be given to terminating the reproductive event to reduce further calcium demand.

Oviductal and Cloacal Prolapse

Oviductal or cloacal prolapse can occur during normal oviposition or parturition. However, most cases are iatrogenic, resulting from owners attempting to manually correct dystocias. Externalized tissues should be kept moist and clean. Treatment depends on the severity of the prolapse and the tissue involved. Most cloacal prolapses and mild oviductal prolapses can be replaced through the cloaca. Care must be used to avoid traumatizing the tissue and to assure proper replacement. Externalized tissue must be inverted and not simply placed back through the cloaca. If the inversion is properly performed, a purse-string suture around the cloaca is unnecessary. In fact, a purse-string suture may be contraindicated because it prevents improperly replaced tissue from reverting through the cloaca and, therefore, going undetected. Inversion of tissue is best accomplished by placing a relatively large diameter blunt instrument through the exteriorized opening and carefully working the tissue back through the cloaca. This procedure should be repeated several times. Prolapse of larger lengths of oviduct are best treated with resection of the tissue after ligation of both ends.

Hemipenile and Penile Prolapse

Penile prolapse occurs as a result of trauma while the penis or hemipenis is everted for copulation (Figure 23-17; Chapter 64). Traumatized tissue quickly swells, making retraction back through the cloaca impossible. The exposed tissue is then subjected to further trauma with bleeding, sometimes substantial, resulting. Because of the extensive trauma, desiccation, and oftentimes necrosis, penile prolapses are best treated with amputation. Amputation of the penis does not affect excretion of urates because the ureters empty into the cloaca. In addition, the reproductive potential of squamates is unaffected because they possess a second hemipenis. Double ligation of the base of the hemipenis before amputation is essential because this tissue is highly vascularized. Fluid therapy (e.g., saline or Ringer's solution) may be warranted if excessive bleeding occurred.

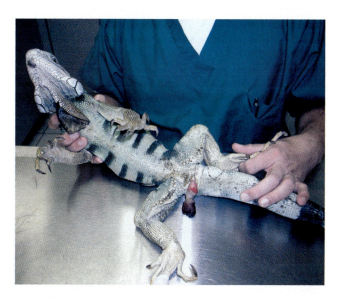

FIGURE 23-17 Green Iguana (*Iguana iguana*) with a chronic prolapsed hemipenis. (*Photograph courtesy D. Mader.*)

REFERENCES

1. Porter KR: *Herpetology*, Philadelphia, 1972, WB Saunders.
2. Staub R: Personal communication.
3. Zug GR: *Herpetology: an introductory biology of amphibians and reptiles*, San Diego, 1993, Academic Press.
4. Tinkle DW, Gibbons JW: The distribution and evolution of viviparity in reptiles, *Misc Pub Mus Zoo, Univ Mich* 154, 1977.
5. Blackburn DG: Convergent evolution of viviparity, matrotrophy, and specializations for fetal nutrition in reptiles and other vertebrates, *Am Zoo* 32:313, 1992.
6. Blackburn DG: Evolutionary origins of viviparity in the reptilia. I. Sauria, *Amphibia Reptilia* 3:185-205, 1982.
7. Derickson WK: Lipid storage and utilization in reptiles, *Am Zoo* 16:711, 1976.
8. Crews D, Moore MC: Psychobiology of reproduction of unisexual whiptail lizards. In Wright JW, Vitt LJ, editors: *Biology of whiptail lizards (genus Cnemidophorus)*, Norman, Okla, 1993, Okla Mus Nat His.
9. Wynn AH, Cole CJ, Gardner AL: Apparent triploidy in the unisexual Brahminy blind snake, *Rhamphotyphlops braminus*, *Am Mus Nov* 2868:1-7, 1987.
10. Schuett GW, Fernandez PJ, Gergits WF, Casna NJ, Chiszar D, Smith HM, et al: Production of offspring in the absence of males: evidence for facultative parthenogenesis in bisexual snakes, *Herp Nat His* 5:1-10, 1997.
11. Sinervo B, Licht P: Hormonal and physiological control of clutch size, egg size, and egg shape in side-blotched lizards (*Uta stansburiana*): constraints on the evolution of lizard life histories, *J Exp Zoo* 257:252, 1991.
12. Seigal RA, Ford NB: Reproductive ecology. In Seigal RA, Collins JT, Novak SS, editors: *Snakes: ecology and evolutionary biology*, New York, 1987, McGraw Hill.
13. Saint Girons H: Reproductive cycles of male snakes and their relationships with climate and female reproductive cycles, *Herpetologica* 38:5, 1982.
14. Garstka WR, Tokarz RR, Diamond M, et al: Behavioral and physiological control of yolk synthesis and deposition in the female red-sided garter snake (*Thamnophis sirtalis parietalis*), *Horm Behav* 19:137, 1985.
15. DeNardo DF, Autumn K: The effect of male presence on reproductive activity in captive female blood pythons, *Python curtus, Copeia* 2000(4):1138-1141, 2000.
16. Bonnet X, Naulleau G, Shine R, Lourdais O: Short-term versus long-term effects of food intake on reproductive output in a viviparous snake *Vipera aspis, Oikos* 92:297-308, 2001.
17. Shine R: Parental care in reptiles. In Gans C, Huey RB, editors: *Biology of the Reptilia, vol 16 (ecology B, defense and life history)*, New York, 1988, Alan R Liss Inc.
18. Ellis TM, Chappell MA: Metabolism, temprature relations: maternal behavior, and reproductive energetics in the ball python *(Python regius)*, *J Comp Physiol B* 157:392-402, 1987.
19. Price AH: Observations of maternal behavior and neonate aggregation in the western diamondback rattlesnake, *Crotalus atrox* (Crotalidae), *Southwest Nat* 33(3):370-373, 1988.
20. Card W, Kluge AG: Hemipeneal skeleton and varanid lizard systematics, *J Herp* 631, 1995.
21. Card W, Mehaffey D: A radiographic sexing technique for *Heloderma suspectum, Herp Rev* 25:47, 1994.
22. Halverson J, Mader DR: DNA testing for sex identification in the green iguana *(Iguana iguana). Proc Assoc Reptl Amphib Vet* 2:80, 1995.
23. Larsen RE, Cardeilhac PT: Artificial insemination, semen handling, and assessment of reproductive status in alligators. *Proc Am Assoc Zoo Vet* 159, 1984.
24. Quinn H, Blaseedel T, Platz CC Jr: Successful artificial insemination in the checkered garter snake, *Thamnophis marcianus, Int Zoo Yearbook* 28:177, 1989.
25. Saad AH, Deeb SE: Immunological changes during pregnancy in the viviparous lizard, *Chalcides ocellatus, Vet Immunol Immunopathol* 25:279, 1990.
26. Kennett R, Georges A, Palmer-Allen M: Early developmental arrest during immersion of eggs of a tropical freshwater turtle, *Chelodina rugosa*, from North America, *Aust J Zoo* 41:37, 1993.
27. Ewert MA: The embryo and its egg: development and natural history. In Harless M, Morlock H, editors: *Turtles: perspectives and research*, New York, 1979, Wiley Interscience.
28. Fife RJ: Observations on incubation, diet, and sex determination in hatchling tortoises, *Proc Int Herpetol Symp Captive Propagation Husbandry* 16: 1992.

24
VIROLOGY
BRAN RITCHIE

During the last century, viral infections have been associated with overt signs of disease in most species of living organisms, including some of the most severe and devastating of all diseases in humans and other animals. In addition to the readily detectable changes that have been associated with viral infections, improved techniques for detection of viral proteins or viral genetic material (DNA or RNA) implicate subclinical viral infection in debilitating diseases, neoplasms, and immune system damage and as a predisposing factor in recurring bacterial, fungal, and parasitic infections. In many cases, the damage to the infected host caused by concurrent infections with bacterial, parasitic, and fungal agents may disguise initial pathology induced by a primary viral pathogen.

Research data on viruses in reptiles are few. For entire families of viruses, little or no information exists about their ability to infect captive or free-ranging reptiles or about what types of disease they may cause in these species. Integral to viral outbreaks may be the mixing of reptile species from numerous sources, the shift in herpetoculture to high-density confined breeding operations, and the frequent relocation of reptiles into established collections with insufficient quarantine.

The global movement of numerous reptile species to meet the demands of the various commercial markets results in the exposure of immunologically naïve animals to widely varying endogenous microflora (viruses, bacteria, fungi, and parasites) that may be endemic to geographically isolated reptile populations. The ease of intercontinental mass transportation through airline travel continues to favor the dissemination of highly pathogenic viruses into naïve populations of all types of animals, including humans and reptiles. Mixing reptiles from various herpetariums can create a similar portal for widespread dissemination of infectious agents.

Twenty-four families of animal viruses have been described. Of these, 17 families have been documented in domestic fowl, 14 families in psittacine birds, 9 families in snakes, 6 families in chelonians, 6 families in lizards, and only 4 families in crocodilians (Table 24-1). Either commonly maintained species of reptiles are tremendously resistant to viral infections or the veterinary community has a limited understanding of the association between viruses and disease in reptiles. The latter is certainly more likely. As investigations into reptilian diseases of suspected viral etiology increase, many families of viruses that have not previously been documented will undoubtedly emerge.

In many reptiles, a virus may cause cellular damage that allows other pathogens (particularly bacteria and fungi) to colonize unhealthy tissues. The reptile may clear the viral infection that initiated the disease process, and bacteria or fungus is recovered from the clinically ill animal. The relative lack of experimental infection studies in reptiles makes determination of which pathogen causes which problem difficult. Detection of an abnormality in a reptile that is a member of a collection should alert the attendant to scrutinize each and every management technique that may predispose other reptiles to the same problem. Aggressive pursuit of the factors that have contributed to a viral-induced disease when the first affected reptile is identified can help prevent the virus from spreading to multiple animals within the herpetarium. Waiting to determine why a reptile is abnormal or has died until a second or third animal is also affected gives a virus time to infect multiple animals, which makes control of a virus-associated disease outbreak more difficult.

Some viruses are present in a reptile for only a brief period, and detection is easiest if diagnostic samples are collected early in the infectious process. If samples are not collected during the correct period, then direct demonstration (cell culture, microscopic evaluation, DNA probes, electron microscopy) that a virus is present may not be possible. In these cases, however, documentation that a viral infection has

Table 24-1 Comparison of Documented Virus Activity in Some Birds and Groups of Reptiles

Virus	Affected Groups					
	1	2	3	4	5	6
Adenoviridae	X	X	–	X	X	X
Arenoviridae	?	–	–	–	–	–
Astroviridae	–	–	–	–	–	X
Birnaviridae	–	–	–	–	–	X
Bunyaviridae	–	–	–	–	–	–
Caliciviridae	–	X	–	–	–	–
Circoviridae	X	–	–	–	–	X
Coronaviridae	X	–	–	–	–	X
Filoviridae	–	–	–	–	–	–
Flaviviridae	X	X	?	–	X	X
Hepadnaviridae	–	–	–	–	–	–
Herpesviridae	X	X	X	X	X	X
Iridoviridae	–	–	X	X	–	–
Ortheomyxoviridae	X	–	–	–	–	X
Papillomavirus	X	–	X	X	–	–
Papovaviridae	–	–	–	?	–	–
Paramyxoviridae	X	X	–	X	–	X
Parvoviridae	?	X	–	?	–	?
Picornaviridae	X	–	–	–	–	X
Pneumovirus	–	–	–	–	–	X
Polyomavirus	X	–	–	–	–	X
Poxviridae	X	–	–	X	X	X
Reoviridae	X	X	X	X	–	X
Retroviridae	X	X	X	X	–	X
Rhabdoviridae	–	–	–	?	–	X
Rotavirus	–	–	–	–	–	–
Togaviridae	X	X	X	X	–	X
Toroviridae	–	–	–	–	–	–

1, Psittaciformes; 2, snakes; 3, chelonids; 4, lizards; 5, crocodilians; 6, galliformes (chickens and turkeys); ?, indicates some data to suggest that infection could occur.

occurred still may be possible with indirect techniques (antibody detection methods).

Annual losses in a properly managed group of reptiles should be minimal. Any reptile that dies, whether a neonate or an adult, should be immediately refrigerated and necropsied as soon as possible. Reptiles should not be frozen before necropsy. Many of the microscopic changes that differentiate certain diseases are subtle. Freezing causes damage to tissues that may reduce a pathologist's ability to make a proper diagnosis.

A complete necropsy and histologic examination of tissues of any animal that dies are the most important tools for evaluation of problems and development of programs to prevent infectious diseases. A properly performed necropsy and histologic examination by an experienced pathologist serve as a repository of data concerning the general health of a group of reptiles and may facilitate detection of specific or recurring problems that can be resolved.

For diseases for which an etiologic agent has not been confirmed, the clinician is encouraged to collect, process, and store serum, whole blood, formalin-fixed tissues, and fresh-frozen tissues. These archival samples may prove valuable in determination of the etiologies of common syndromes as more advanced investigative techniques are applied to identification of viruses that may be associated with diseases in reptiles.

Catastrophic outbreaks with high levels of morbidity and mortality can occur if infectious viruses are introduced into young or highly susceptible animals. Until more effective vaccines are available, reptiles can be maintained in the best health with combining the principles of quarantine, avoiding direct or indirect contact with reptiles outside the established flock, providing animals with an excellent environment, paying close attention to sanitation methods, maintaining a high plane of nutrition, and maintaining reptiles in a low-stress environment.

Any reptile with signs of illness should be immediately isolated to prevent exposure of other reptiles to an infectious disease–causing organism. The common practice of placing a hospital or "sick" room in the same building or air space with other animals is contrary to sound preventative medical practices.

Reptiles maintained in less crowded areas with sufficient air circulation, reduced exposure to excrement, and frequent exposure to sunlight are less likely to be exposed to, or succumb to, viral infections than are reptiles maintained in crowded indoor areas with poor hygiene and poor ventilation. Mixing reptiles from different sources (multiple breeding facilities, multiple pet retailers, or multiple overseas sources) increases the risk of a virus-associated disease.

If a reptile must be added to an established collection or household, careful and critical scrutiny of the source of the new animal is extremely important. Care in choosing the source for a new reptile is just as important for the individual who has only one or two other reptiles as it is for the herpetoculturist with a large facility. The addition of only one reptile from a questionable source that is shedding an infectious agent can cause a severe disease outbreak in a naïve population of animals.

Reptile enthusiasts must design and implement a quarantine program for new arrivals (see Chapter 78). Although a quarantine program does not eliminate the possibility of introduction of an infectious agent to other reptiles, it does provide an evaluation period that may prevent some infected animals from being added to a group. Before placement in quarantine, new reptiles should be given thorough physical examinations by a knowledgeable veterinarian.

A newly obtained reptile that was raised in captivity should be quarantined for a minimum of 90 days. All other reptiles should be quarantined for a minimum of 180 days. Ideally, reptiles in quarantine should be maintained in an area that is completely separate from the established group. Reptiles in quarantine should be attended by a different individual than the person who provides care to the established group. If a separate facility is not available, then quarantined reptiles should be placed in an area where they are physically separated from the established group (different air, supplies, and feeding utensils) and the quarantined reptiles should not be fed and cleaned on the same day as the established group. Once daily contact with a quarantined reptile has occurred, the herpetoculturist must not approach the area where the established group is housed without a shower and a change of all garments, including shoes. Any reptile that has been removed from a group and exposed to any other reptiles that might be shedding a pathogen should be quarantined before reintroduction to the group.

Herpetoculturists and conservationists from every geographic area of the world should be concerned about the movement of reptiles between continents. Reptiles that are moved from remote regions of the earth can be subclinically infected with indigenous microbial flora to which reptilian species in the importing country may have no immunity. Currently, assurance that reptiles imported from other continents are free of potentially dangerous pathogens is not possible, nor is it likely to be possible.

The susceptibility of viruses to inactivation varies among families, and different virus particles of the same type can exhibit varying susceptibility to inactivation. Most (but not all) viruses that have a lipoprotein envelope are unstable and are inactivated by most disinfectants. Viruses that do not have a lipoprotein envelope generally are resistant to harsh environmental conditions and many disinfectants. The health hazards associated with frequent exposure of reptiles and hospital or herpetarium personnel to harsh disinfectants or their fumes are rarely considered in choice of disinfectant. Any disinfectant that inactivates viruses is toxic, and care should be used to prevent the unnecessary exposure of facility personnel or reptiles to the residues or fumes of these disinfectants. Perfumes and scents designed to hide the noxious odor of many disinfectants do not decrease the damage that these agents cause if the fumes are inhaled. When any disinfectant solution is used, treated surfaces must be thoroughly rinsed to prevent contact of potentially tissue-toxic solutions with the delicate tissues of reptiles (see Chapter 85).

HERPESVIRUS

Herpesvirus virions are enveloped and are pleomorphic. Their size ranges from 120 to 200 nm in diameter. Replication occurs in the nucleus, and the envelope is acquired when new virus particles are released from an infected cell by budding through the nuclear membrane. As a group, herpesviruses tend to be well adapted to a particular species and are ubiquitous in a population of these animals. Most herpesviruses are host specific, but some can infect many different species, either naturally or experimentally. Varying types of herpesviruses tend to cause lifelong latent infections that are characterized by the periodic recurrence of viral shedding with or without detectable clinical signs. Depending on the strain of virus and the species of infected animal, various herpesviruses have a propensity to infect lymphatic tissue, epithelial cells, or nervous tissue and may cause neoplastic, hemorrhagic, or necrotic lesions.

In general, host-adapted herpesviruses cause a mild, subclinical, latent infection in their natural host; however, severe, often life-threatening, disease can occur when a nonadapted herpesvirus enters a new host.[1,2] Herpesvirus infections are typically associated with the formation of intranuclear inclusion bodies. These inclusion bodies represent areas where damaged portions of the cell's nucleus accumulate.

Clinical Features

Herpesviruses have been recovered from reptiles with a variety of clinical or pathologic changes including hepatomegaly, hepatic necrosis, and pulmonary edema in aquatic turtles; necrotizing oral and pharyngeal lesions in tortoises; papillomatous skin lesions in seaturtles; liver necrosis in boas and lizards; gastrointestinal necrosis in snakes and lizards; and necrotizing venom gland infections in cobras, kraits, and rattlesnakes.[3-10]

Tortoises

A herpes-like virus was reported in association with upper respiratory disease in a Gopher Tortoise (*Gopherus polyphemus*) that had been in captivity since hatching.[11] Since this initial report, herpesviruses have been associated with hepatic, respiratory, and gastrointestinal disease in many species of tortoises (see Chapter 57). Disease may occur in young or mature tortoises, and herpesvirus-associated respiratory disease was described in a 60-year-old captive Desert Tortoise (*Gopherus agassizii*).[11-15]

The clinical lesions associated with herpesvirus infections in tortoises are generally necrotizing and involve ulceration of the mucosa in the upper respiratory or gastrointestinal tract.[13] Some authors consider herpesvirus stomatitis to be the most common cause of upper alimentary tract disease in tortoises (see Figure 57-1).[14] Affected tortoises often have anorexia, lethargy, regurgitation, serous to mucopurulent nasal and ocular discharge, and labored breathing from rhinitis, conjunctivitis, pharyngitis, glossitis, pneumonia, and pharyngeal abscesses.[9,11,14,15] Ataxia may be noted in tortoises with central nervous system (CNS) involvement.[15]

Coalescing lesions near the glottis can cause severe respiratory distress, particularly when secondarily infected with bacteria or fungi.[16,17] Untreated bacterial infections can progress to septicemia, osteomyelitis, and death.[14] Severe respiratory lesions are fatal. Mortality rates in outbreaks that involve naïve populations may approach 100% as has been reported in a colony of Hermann's (*Testudo hermanni*) and Leopard Tortoises (*Geochelone pardalis*).[18,19]

The most common lesions that are likely to occur vary by species. Changes in Hermann's Tortoises are typically associated with glossitis, stomatitis, enteritis, and meningoencephalitis. Affected Afghan Tortoises (*Testudo horsfieldi*) were seen with stomatitis and enteritis, and Desert Tortoises typically have stomatitis, tracheitis, and pneumonia develop. Stomatitis was the predominate lesion reported in affected Argentine Tortoises (*Geochelone chilensis*). Stomatitis and encephalitis occur in some Spur-thighed Tortoises (*Testudo graeca*), and epizootics of seromucoid rhinitis are common in large groups of this tortoise.[20,21]

Herpesvirus infections have also been documented in Yellow-footed Tortoises (*Geochelone denticulata*) and Leopard Tortoises.[19,21] An irido-like virus was shown in two Hermann's Tortoises with stomatitis lesions that appeared clinically similar to those associated with herpesvirus infection.[21] An unidentified agent that caused lysis of TH-1 cells was recovered from Leopard Tortoises, Hermann's Tortoises, and Spur-thighed Tortoises that had clinical lesions consistent with herpesvirus-associated stomatitis.[21]

Tortoises are also susceptible to *Mycoplasma* infections, which are characterized by conjunctivitis and rhinitis with only rare occurrence of stomatitis and glossitis (see Chapter 73). The similar symptoms can easily be confused. The two diseases can occur simultaneously.

Pond Turtles

On the basis of electron microscopic findings, herpesvirus-associated disease has been reported in Pacific Pond Turtles (*Clemmys marmorata*), Painted Turtles (*Chrysemys picta*), and Map Turtles (*Graptemys* spp.).[7,22] The initial report involved a wild-caught Pacific Pond Turtle that had been in captivity for 3 weeks when it had a sudden onset of lethargy, anorexia, and muscular weakness. The turtle died within a day of development of recognizable clinical changes. Numerous subcutaneous petechial to ecchymotic hemorrhages were noted on the limbs, neck, and plastron. A second Pacific Pond Turtle died 3 weeks after the index case.[22] In another outbreak, several Map Turtles that had been in captivity for more than 8 years died 5 months after the introduction of two Western Painted Turtles (*Chrysemys picta belli*).[7] Lethargy, anorexia, and subcutaneous edema were noted in these turtles for up to a week before death.[7]

Marine Turtles

Herpesviruses of undetermined relationship have been associated with three distinct syndromes in marine turtles: circular papular skin lesions (grey-patch disease); ulcerative lung, eye, and tracheal (LETD) lesions; and external and internal fibropapillomas.

Green Turtle fibropapilloma (GTFP) was first described by Lucke in 1938.[23] This disease is associated with proliferative or ulcerative skin lesions in seaturtles, particularly Green Seaturtles (*Chelonia mydas*).[24,25] These papillamotous growths vary in number and may be gray to black and range in size from 2 to 20 cm in diameter. Lesions may be focal or multifocal and involve the head, neck, limbs, tail, plastron, carapace, and cornea (Figure 24-1). Periocular or corneal lesions are particularly debilitating for free-ranging turtles because the mass may inhibit vision and prevent food acquisition. Flipper lesions may reduce swimming ability. Once ulcerated, these lesions are readily infected with secondary bacteria or fungi. Although skin lesions are most common, internal fibropapillomas also have been reported. Affected turtles are usually

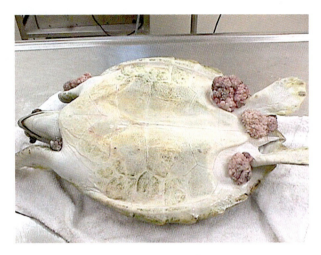

FIGURE 24-1 This Green Seaturtle *(Chelonia mydas)* is covered with cauliflower-like papillomas. A herpesvirus has been isolated from these lesions. *(Photograph courtesy D. Mader.)*

cachectic when removed from the wild.[6,25,26] See Chapter 76 for more details on GTFP.

Grey-patch disease primarily affects 56-day-old to 1-year-old captive-raised Green Seaturtles.[25] In the first reported outbreak, most affected turtles were 8 to 10 weeks old.[24] Skin lesions are characterized by small nonspreading papules or, more typically, raised coalescing areas of raised grey patches that frequently ulcerate.[24,27] In one study, 90% to 100% of at-risk turtles had lesions develop during a several month period. Lesions spontaneously resolved in mildly affected turtles, and the mortality rate in those with severe lesions ranged from 5% to 20%.[24] Overcrowding and high temperature are considered precipitating factors in the development and severity of lesions in captive turtles.[24]

A herpesvirus-associated disease characterized by ulceration and accumulation of caseous debris over the globe and in the oropharynx, lungs, and trachea has been described in marine turtles.[5] One of the first reported epizootics involved 1-year-old to 2-year-old Green Seaturtles maintained in a breeding facility in Grand Cayman, the British West Indies.[5] The clinical changes noted in these turtles included a 2-week to 3-week period of harsh respiratory signs, buoyancy abnormalities, caseated keratitis, conjunctivitis, tracheitis, and pneumonia. Affected turtles typically died from several weeks to several months after the onset of clinical signs. During a decade-long incidence study, most epizootics were found to occur between January and August. Most affected turtles had secondary gram-negative bacterial infections of the virus-damaged epithelial tissues.[5]

Other Species

A herpesvirus was detected in young Boas *(Boa constrictor)* that were born and raised in a European zoologic facility. The affected animals were from a female that had produced 16 young, nine that were stillborn and six that died within 1 year.[28] Subclinical herpesvirus infections have also been documented in Boa Constrictors with hepatic necrosis.[29]

Herpesviruses have been shown in association with venom gland infections in Indian Cobra *(Naja naja)*, Banded Krait *(Bungarus fasciatus)*, Siamese Cobras *(N. n. kaouthia)*, and Mojave Rattlesnakes *(Crotulus scutulatus)*.[8,30,31] Affected snakes produced poor-quality venom that contained inflammatory cells. Thick tenacious venom was reported in 80 of 400 Siamese Cobras imported from Thailand. Herpesvirus particles were described in the surgically excised venom glands of two of these cobras.[31]

A herpes-like virus was recovered in primary iguana cells inoculated with tissues from an adult Iguana that originated from a zoologic collection. Once isolated, the virus also replicated in primary cells collected from Box Turtles. The virus isolates were antigenically distinct from the avian and mammalian herpesviruses with which they were compared. Virus was recovered from the tissues of experimentally infected animals when they were necropsied 15 days after inoculation.[32] Although the initial isolates were made from subclinical iguanas, herpesvirus infections have been implicated, but poorly documented, as a cause of anorexia, lethargy, brilliant green coloration, and lymphocytosis in some iguanas. Spontaneous hemorrhage was reported in one affected iguana.

A herpesvirus is the suspected cause of renal adenocarcinomas (Lucke's renal tumor), renal failure, and ascites in Northern Leopard Frogs *(Rana pipiens)*. Tumor growth was most rapid during the spring and summer, and virus production was reported as highest in the fall when tumors reached their largest size. Viral shedding occurred during spawning the following spring, which continued the infectivity cycle. Affected frogs typically died within months of spawning in a severely cachectic state. Neoplastic cells may be noted in ascitic fluid. Eosinophilic intranuclear inclusions bodies can be found in the kidneys from affected frogs.[33]

Nine wild-caught Agamas *(Agama agama)* that were introduced to a zoologic collection died during a 6-month period. Eight of the lizards died within 38 days, and one died 6 months after arrival at the facility. Histologic examination of tissues indicated that one affected lizard had random foci of necrosis in the liver and spleen and another had mild exudative pneumonia. Intranuclear inclusion bodies were present in the liver or lung of the affected lizards, and these inclusions contained virus particles morphologically consistent with herpesvirus.[34]

A herpesvirus was shown in the papillomatous tissues of Lacerta lizards. The papillomas ranged in size from 2 to 20 mm and varied from two to 25 in number. Lesions were most common on the caudal lumbar area of females and the dorsocranial area around the base of the head in males. The lesion distribution was theorized to represent areas of trauma associated with mating behavior. In addition to herpesvirus, electron microscopy of the papillomas also revealed virus particles that resembled papovavirus and reovirus.[35]

Epizootiology

The global distribution of herpesviruses in respective populations of reptiles has been poorly documented. Herpesviruses have been isolated from tortoises in Europe,[14,18,21,36] the United States,[4,11,12] and Africa.[37] Herpesviruses have been documented in both wild-caught and long-term captive tortoises.[2,11]

Fibropapillomas were not reported in the Caribbean until the 1930s and in Hawaii until 1958.[38] Lesions have now been documented in Green Seaturtles in both the Atlantic and the

Pacific Oceans. In one study, 57% of the Green Seaturtles collected in the Indian River Lagoon System of east central Florida from 1985 to 1986 had suggestive lesions, and prior to 1982, none of the evaluated turtles in the same system had lesions.[26] In another study, up to 10% of female Green Seaturtles evaluated during nesting activities in Hawaii had fibropapillomas.[39] This disease is theorized to involve both infectious (possibly a herpesvirus and a retrovirus) and environmental factors.[40]

The relationship of the herpesviruses recovered from reptiles has been insufficiently studied. Typically, herpesviruses have a restricted host range. Numerous, serologically distinct, host-adapted herpesviruses likely occur in specific families or genera of reptiles. In birds and mammals, herpesviruses can infect any aged animal; however, susceptibility to disease has been shown to vary among genera and between individuals. By example, in a mixed shipment of tortoises, Argentine Tortoises died and Red-footed Tortoises remained unaffected.[4] Whether the Red-footed Tortoises were subclinically infected with a host-adapted herpesvirus that exhibited increased virulence for Argentine Tortoises or whether the Red-footed Tortoises were resistant to the strain of herpesvirus that caused severe disease in the Argentine Tortoises was undetermined.

In another mixed population of tortoises, Afghan Tortoises died acutely and Hermann's, Spur-thighed, and Red-footed Tortoises remained unaffected.[13] Two Side-neck Turtles inoculated with liver suspensions from affected Map Turtles remained clinically normal.[7]

On the basis of apparent host susceptibility, some of the isolates from chelonids have been designated as follows: grey-patch disease virus (ChHV-1), Pacific Pond Turtle virus (ChHV-2), Painted Turtle virus (ChHV-3), and Argentine Tortoise virus (ChHV-4).[20] On the basis of serologic testing and restriction endonuclease analysis, an isolate of herpesvirus from Afghan Tortoises was shown to be genetically and antigenically distinct from six other tortoise herpesviruses.[13,41,42] The nucleic acid sequence coding for the UL 5 protein is sufficiently conserved among tortoise herpesvirus isolates from the United States and Europe to allow for in situ hybridization detection of viral nucleic acid in affected tissues.[20]

Transmission

Most herpesviruses are transmitted from one susceptible individual to another through direct contact. Although poorly documented, reptiles with respiratory signs likely shed large quantities of virus in respiratory secretions, and those with gastrointestinal or liver disease shed large quantities of virus in their feces or saliva.[4,11,14] In one study, herpesvirus was isolated from pharyngeal swabs of affected Afghan Tortoises.[13] As is the case for most herpesviruses, horizontal transmission is probably most common in reptiles, although the finding of viral particles in testicular epithelium of tortoises supports the possibility of vertical transmission, at least in some species.[17,43]

Herpesviruses generally persist in a population of animals with induction of latent infections with periodic shedding of virus following stressful factors such as concomitant disease, malnutrition, temperature changes (high or low), movement of animals, introduction of new animals to an established group collection, or breeding activity. Virus shedding may or may not be associated with concurrent signs of disease. In infected tortoises, herpesvirus-associated lesions have been suggested to be most common in the spring as animals come out of brumation (hibernation).[2] Latently infected tortoises, possibly *T. graeca*, are also theorized to serve as a reservoir for at least some strains of herpesvirus.[19,20]

Hygiene in the herpetarium, the species of exposed reptile, the distance between enclosures, the strain of the virus, and the condition of the collection are all expected to influence the transmission of herpesvirus. Crowding, poor air or water quality, accumulation of excrement, and stacking of enclosures is expected to increase the likelihood of herpesvirus transmission from infected to susceptible reptiles.

Transmission studies with reptilian herpesviruses are limited. Grey-patch disease was experimentally reproduced in 6-week-old to 8-week-old Green Seaturtles through inoculation of a scratch in the skin. Characteristic lesions developed within 2 to 3 weeks.[24] Fibropapillomas have been experimentally reproduced in green turtles with cell-free extracts.[44]

Pathology

Chelonians

The pathologic changes in infected tortoises vary by species and among individuals but may include ulcerative lesions of the gastrointestinal and respiratory mucosa, diphtheritic plaques with necrotizing stomatitis and glossitis, necrotizing bronchitis, pneumonia with emphysema, enteritis, and hepatomegaly.[4,11,14,45] Other changes include hepatitis, fatty degeneration of the liver, and serous atrophy of fat. Histologically, diffuse areas of epithelial necrosis are frequently infiltrated with mixed inflammatory cells and bacteria, particularly gram-negative bacteria.[4,11,14,25] In one study that involved 142 affected tortoises, the most common lesion was ulcerative diphtheroid-necrotizing stomatitis and glossitis.[2]

Large eosinophilic intranuclear inclusion bodies are common in degenerating epithelial cells and have been documented in the tongue, palatine mucosa, esophagus, intestines, stomach, cloaca, liver, trachea, bronchi, alveoli, endothelial cells of capillaries, glomeruli, and spinal cord and within neurons and glial cells in the brain of affected tortoises.[2,4,11,14,15,17,18,21,25] Lymphoproliferative lesions that primarily involve the liver and spleen have been documented in some affected tortoises.[18,19,46]

In one European study, eosinophilic intranuclear inclusion bodies suggestive of a herpesvirus infection were documented in 142 of 914 postmortem samples (15.5%). Affected species included 99 Spur-tailed Tortoises, 29 Spur-thighed Tortoises, 8 Leopard Tortoises, 4 Marginated Tortoises (*Testudo marginata*), 1 Four-toed Tortoise, and 1 Yellow-footed Tortoise.[2]

Gross lesions in herpesvirus-positive Map Turtles (*Graptemys* sp.) included subcutaneous edema and swollen diffusely pale livers.[7] Pacific Pond Turtles were described with acute hepatic necrosis and moderate splenic hyperplasia.[22] Herpesvirus particles have been shown with electron microscopy in association with intranuclear inclusion bodies in the liver, spleen, lungs, kidneys, and pancreas of various pond turtles with hepatomegaly, hepatic necrosis, and pulmonary edema.[7,22,47]

In Green Seaturtles, grey-patch disease is characterized by papular skin lesions that coalesce to form ulcerated patches. Basophilic intranuclear inclusion bodies are common in affected cells.[24,27]

Lung, eye, and tracheal disease has been associated with periglottal necrosis, necrotizing tracheitis, and severe bronchopneumonia in marine turtles. Accumulation of caseous exudates and laminated necrotic debris with infiltrates of mixed inflammatory cells is common in the lumen of the trachea and lungs.[5] Granulomatous lesions have been described in the liver. Amphophilic intranuclear inclusions are common in cells of the trachea and lungs.[5]

Fibropapillomas may be noted on the skin and in the lung, liver, kidneys, and gastrointestinal tract of affected seaturtles. Microscopically, these lesions are characterized by hyperplasia of the epidermis, vacuolation of cytoplasm, ballooning degeneration of epidermal cells, and proliferation of fibroblasts in the dermis. Eosinophilic intranuclear inclusion bodies have been described in spongiotic epidermal cells of some affected turtles.[6]

Other Reptiles

Herpesvirus infections of the venom gland have been associated with multifocal necrosis of columnar glandular epithelium and infiltration of mixed inflammatory cells that can be detected in the venom. Both naked and enveloped herpesvirus-like particles were detected with electron microscopy among accumulations of desquamated and necrotic epithelial cells within the lumen of affected glands.[8,30,31]

Herpesvirus was shown in amphophilic intranuclear inclusion bodies in young boa constrictors with fatty degeneration and multifocal hepatic necrosis. One of the boas also had pancreatic necrosis, and the other had exudative glomerulonephritis.[28]

In iguanas, a herpes-like virus has been implicated as the cause of lymphocytosis, splenic hyperplasia, and histocytic lymphoid infiltrates of liver, spleen, myocardium, and bone marrow.[22,32]

Immunity and Diagnosis

As is the case with herpesvirus infections in mammals, the primary spread of virions inside an infected reptile's body is thought to occur with direct cell-to-cell contact. Thus, the spaces outside the cell are not exposed to the virus.[1] This mechanism protects the virus from circulating antibodies. Herpesviruses are able to use this mechanism to establish infections that persist in a host even after antibodies are developed to the virus.

Reptiles that survive a herpesvirus infection probably have latent infections develop and protective long-lasting immunity against the severe changes that can be induced by the same strain of virus. These reptiles are likely to have detectable levels of virus-neutralizing antibodies develop that probably persist for at least several months. Although undocumented in reptiles, in birds, an increase in antibodies may occur in some latently infected animals when they are actively shedding virus.[48,49] However, a decrease in the antibody level with no detectable increase in viral shedding has been shown to occur in other latently infected birds.[50]

In tortoises, a virus neutralizing antibody assay can be used to document a previous infection. However, virus neutralizing assays are typically epitope specific, and an animal tested may have been infected with a strain of virus that varies antigenically from the one used in the assay.[1,9,13,41,42,51]

Detection of an antibody titer in a single sample suggests a previous infection. The finding of a rising antibody titer in paired serum samples collected 8 to 12 weeks apart is necessary to confirm an active infection.[17,52] An enzyme-linked immunosorbent assay (ELISA) with a high sensitivity and specificity has been developed for tortoises.[52,53] In one study that involved 175 plasma samples from Mediterranean Tortoises kept in France, 35 tortoises had positive results with a serum neutralization assay and 38 had positive results with ELISA.[17] Finding of a repeatable antibody titer is an indication of prior infection, and assumption that a seropositive animal is latently infected is safest.

A herpesvirus infection should be suspected in any reptile with suggestive clinical signs. In any species, suspect lesions should be biopsied, and samples submitted for virus isolation, electron microscopic evaluation, and histologic examination.[25] Finding of intranuclear inclusion bodies in association with species-specific pathology should raise the index of suspicion.[16,29] Because the inclusion bodies associated with herpesviruses can appear similar to those caused by other viruses, confirmation of an infection requires the finding of virus particles with electron microscopy or the finding of viral antigen or nucleic acid with specific staining techniques. A rapid diagnosis may be possible with fresh fluids collected from vesicular lesions, washes of the epithelium of oral or tracheal lesions, intestinal contents, or fresh biopsy samples from acute lesions for electron microscopic evaluation.[4,11,14,16,25,29,45] Electron microscopy services are available through many state diagnostic laboratories, or samples can be sent to the Electron Microscopy Laboratory at the University of Georgia, College of Veterinary Medicine, Athens, GA 30602-7371.

Virus isolation in TH-1 cells has been used to confirm the presence of a herpesvirus in tortoises. Virus has been isolated from pharyngeal swabs, tongue, liver, spleen, esophagus, intestines, lung, brain, and trachea from affected animals.[13,19,21] In tortoises, polymerase chain reaction (PCR)–based testing may prove of benefit in screening for target segments of viral nucleic acid in secretions or excretions.[20] Nucleic acid probes for in situ hybridization have proven effective in detection of herpesvirus nucleic acid in the tissues of affected tortoises.[20] Restriction endonuclease analysis has been used to genetically characterize herpesvirus isolates from tortoises.[41,42]

In marine turtles with internal fibropapillomas, radiographs may be helpful in detection of internal masses.[6] A PCR-based assay has been developed for detection of target segments of nucleic acid from the herpesvirus associated with fibropapillomas in marine turtles.[8] Sequences used for primers appear to detect nucleic acid sequences from other chelonid herpesviruses as well.[17,54] At the time this assay was described in the literature, it had a sensitivity of 10,000 copies of plasmid DNA.[17]

Electron microscopy has been used to detect herpesvirus-like particles in the venom of infected Mojave Rattlesnakes, Indian Cobra, and Banded Krait.[8,30] The initial herpesvirus isolate from the venom gland of an infected cobra was recovered through coculture with a mouse oncornavirus.[55]

Control and Prevention

Most reptiles are probably infected with herpesvirus after they inhale or ingest contaminated secretions or excretions. Thus, hygiene is critical in prevention of herpesvirus outbreaks.

Herpesviruses are enveloped and are generally unstable when outside of a reptile's body and can be easily inactivated. Although insufficient studies are found with the reptilian herpesviruses, most herpesviruses are sensitive to common disinfectants, high heat (56°C for 5 to 10 minutes or 37°C for 22 hours), or acid conditions (pH less than 5).[1] Sodium hypochlorite (3%) was recommended for disinfection after an outbreak of herpesvirus in Pond Turtles.[7] Organic debris such as blood, soil, substrates, or feces is expected to protect herpesvirus from disinfectants that do not contain detergents.[1]

Because affected reptiles likely shed large quantities of virus in their respiratory secretions or feces, any reptile suspected of having a herpesvirus infection or that has been exposed to herpesvirus should be maintained in strict isolation.[1] The common practice of placing a hospital or "sick" room in the same building or air space with the main herpetarium area is contrary to good medical practices.

Herpesvirus outbreaks have been difficult to manage in herpetariums because of limited methods for identification of latently infected reptiles. One should attempt to prevent latently infected individuals from being introduced to a collection through a strict quarantine program of at least 6 months' duration with use of available serologic and nucleic acid detection assays at the beginning and end of the quarantine period.[17,52,53]

Use of a sentinel program is expected to be of limited value in detection of latently infected reptiles because of varied susceptibility among species, the intermittent nature of virus shedding, and the uncertainty that a sentinel reptile is sufficiently exposed to a latently infected animal when the latter is shedding infectious virus.

Treatment and Vaccination

Reptiles with suspected herpesvirus infections should be maintained in isolation while awaiting results of specific diagnostic testing. Supportive care should include fluid maintenance, supportive nutrition, increasing the ambient temperature, and use of topical or systemic antibiotics to treat or prevent secondary bacterial infections.[5,6] Animals with upper respiratory tract lesions may respond to removal of caseated debris, an increase in humidity, and nebulization of appropriate antimicrobials based initially on results of cytologic samples and confirmed with results of sensitivity testing.[16,29] Any reptile that survives a herpesvirus infection should be considered latently infected and should be restricted from direct or indirect exposure to susceptible individuals.

Some marine turtles with external fibropapillomas respond to supportive care and surgical removal of applicable lesions (see Chapter 76). Turtles with mild cutaneous disease may recover spontaneously. The prognosis for turtles with internal lesions is grave.[6] Affected individuals should be isolated during treatment. Supportive care should include decreasing stress and improving immune system function with providing a well-maintained pool with exceptional hygiene and proper water temperature for the affected species.[24,27]

In humans, treatment with acyclovir has been shown to shorten the duration of viral shedding, decrease the degree of morbidity, and reduce the redundancy of some herpesvirus infections. Acyclovir is widely distributed in most tissues, including the brain, and is excreted principally through the kidneys. Unfortunately, acyclovir has not been shown to eliminate latent infections in humans.[56]

Only a few reports describe the use of acyclovir in reptiles, but subjective data suggest that it is clinically useful. However, the role that acyclovir may play in producing or preventing the development of latent infections in reptiles has not been reported. Therapy is expected to be most effective when initiated before herpesvirus-infected reptiles have clinical signs of disease develop. Both acyclovir and gancyclovir have been shown to have in vitro activity against some strains of tortoise herpesvirus and should be considered in affected animals.[13] Acyclovir at a dose of 80 mg/kg orally every 72 hours has been suggested for treatment of herpesvirus-associated ulcerative stomatitis in California Desert Tortoises.[29] Systemic acyclovir has been recommended for marine turtles.[5] Five percent acyclovir ointment has been suggested for treatment of herpesvirus-associated dermal lesions.[22] Application of 5% acyclovir ointment appeared to improve oral lesions in Spur-thighed Tortoises.[29] Because acyclovir has been associated with kidney damage in some species, this drug should be used with caution and only when specifically indicated.

ADENOVIRUS

Adenoviruses are nonenveloped and 70 to 90 nm in diameter. Replication occurs in the cell nucleus, where viral particles accumulate and typically form intranuclear inclusion bodies (Figure 24-2). Various strains of adenovirus have been isolated from mammals and birds. The strains that infect mammals have been placed in the genus *Mastadenovirus*, and the strains that affect birds have been placed in the genus *Aviadenovirus*. This classification is based on unique group-specific characteristics.[1] The strains recovered from reptiles have been insufficiently studied, but they have been suggested to be placed in their own genus.[29,57]

As a family, adenoviruses are commonly recovered from persistently infected asymptomatic birds. Some strains of avian adenovirus are host-specific; others can infect various species of birds.[58] The host specificity of reptilian adenoviruses has not been determined. Although adenovirus infections have been associated with a number of syndromes in birds and mammals, experimental infections are usually asymptomatic or mild, which suggests that a diseased animal from which an adenovirus is isolated may have concomitant problems or immunosuppression.[1] Epizootiologic data suggest a similar scenario for reptiles.

Clinical Features

In birds and mammals, the morbidity and mortality rates associated with adenovirus infections appear to vary with the host and the strain of infecting virus. Asymptomatic infections that are not detected until an animal becomes immunocompromised are most common. Adenoviruses have been documented in 12 different species of reptiles, including crocodiles, snakes, and lizards.[59] Clinical and pathologic changes vary among species, and individuals but have included gastroenteritis, hepatitis, nephritis, pneumonia, and encephalitis.[59]

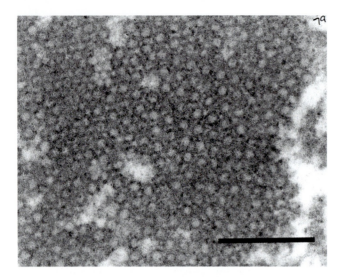

FIGURE 24-2 The liver of a Bearded Dragon *(Pogona vitticeps)*. Intranuclear paracrystalline array of hexagonal viral particles is typical of adenovirus. Uranyl acetate and lead citrate; bar = 640 nm. *(Photograph courtesy M.M. Garner, Northwest ZooPath.)*

Disease has been documented in reptiles with and without detectable concurrent diseases, but the role that immunosuppression plays in the pathogenesis of reptile adenovirus infections is poorly defined.

Snakes

Adenovirus infections have been implicated in fatal hepatitis or gastrointestinal disease in boids, colubrids, and viperidae and should be on the rule-out list for snakes with regurgitation, diarrhea, or CNS signs.[3,57,59-62] Adenoviral-associated gastrointestinal disease was reported in a Four-lined Rat Snake *(Elaphe quatuorlineater)*, Boa Constrictor, Aesculpian Snake *(E. longissima)*, and Gaboon Viper *(Bitis gabonica)*. All affected snakes had concomitant infections with viruses that morphologically resembled parvovirus, picornavirus, or herpesvirus.[3] Paramyxovirus has also been documented in snakes with concurrent adenovirus-associated enteritis.[60] An adenovirus was isolated from a Royal Python *(Python regius)*.[63]

Adenovirus-associated disease in an adult boa was characterized by an unreported period of antibiotic unresponsive lethargy, dehydration, anorexia, and dermatitis before death. The boa had concurrent enterohepatic amebiasis, bacterial-associated ulcerative enteritis, and a severe retroviral infection.[59] In other Boa Constrictors, adenovirus infections have been loosely associated with either death with no premonitory signs or death after a short period of neurologic signs. One affected boa began to regurgitate 2 weeks before development of a head tilt followed in 36 hours by death.[61] Another affected boa was anorectic for 2 months before dying 24 hours after regurgitating a force-fed meal.[64] Infection in Rosy Boas *(Lichanura trivirigata)* was associated with hepatic necrosis and enteritis or death with no premonitory signs.[57]

Adenovirus was recovered from a Mojave Rattlesnake that died the day after an abdominal mass was detected. This snake had concurrent intestinal amoebosis and a renal carcinoma.[59] Young Kingsnakes *(Lampropeltis zonata multicincta)* infected with an adenovirus and a suspected dependovirus (Parvoviridae) presented with acute gastroenteritis with emesis and dehydration before death.[65] Necrotic enteritis associated with gram-negative bacteria or *Clostridium* spp. has been implicated in the death of snakes with adenovirus-associated hepatitis.[64]

Lizards

Adenoviruses have been implicated in fatal hepatitis or gastrointestinal disease in monitors, Bearded Dragons, and Rankin's Dragon *(Pogona henrylawsoni)*.[60,66,67] A Rankin's Dragon died shortly after exhibiting signs of inappetence, lethargy, and limb paresis. Hepatitis was the dominant change in affected Water Dragons *(Physignathus cocincinus)*. A Savannah Monitor *(Varanus exanthematicus)* died without premonitory signs.[68]

Clinical changes are most common in young dragons and include an acute onset of depression and anorexia followed by death.[65,66] Others fail to thrive and may exhibit intermittent inappetence and limb paresis followed by death. Adenovirus infections have been documented in some young Bearded Dragons that died with no premonitory signs.[69] Many affected dragons have concomitant parasitic infections, particularly coccidia and microsporidia.[70] Although disease is most common in young Bearded Dragons, adenovirus was implicated in the death of several mature dragons with listlessness, anorexia, and coelomic distention.[70]

Some chameleons with adenovirus infections remain subclinical, and others have signs of disease that indicate pathology in the digestive tract, trachea, or CNS. Reported changes include anorexia, tracheitis, and opisthotonos followed by death, frequently within 3 days of the onset of clinical signs.[71-73] In one case, adenovirus was shown in enterocytes of a Mountain Chameleon *(Chamaeleo montium)* that died after 28 days of anorexia. However, the adenovirus infection was considered subclinical on the basis of the absence of pathologic changes.[73] Intranuclear inclusion bodies similar to those associated with adenovirus were found in the intestinal tract of American Anoles *(Anolis carolinensis)*.[68]

Crocodiles

A virus with morphologic characteristics suggestive of an adenovirus was detected in two 8-month-old Nile Crocodiles *(Crocodylus niloticus)* from a farm in Zimbabwe. Except for being underweight for their age and size, the animals died without clinical signs.[74]

Epizootiology

Any aged bird or mammal is considered susceptible to adenovovirus infection, but disease is most common in young animals or adults with concurrent infections or severe immunosuppression.[1] Age susceptibility of reptiles to adenovirus associated disease has been poorly documented. However, most reports of affected lizards and snakes document disease in immature animals.

Relationship of Virus Strains

In birds, adenoviruses are divided into serotypes on the basis of differences in virus neutralization.[1] Chickens, turkeys, geese, and ducks have been shown to be infected with species-specific adenoviruses; however, the adenovirus that infects chickens may also infect pigeons and quail. Some adenoviruses recovered from budgerigars, pigeons, and ducks were found to be serologically similar to those found in gallinaceous birds.[75,76] Nucleic acid analysis indicated that an adenovirus isolated from budgerigars was unique, even though this virus shared antigenic characteristics with strains recovered from chickens.[1] Although the serologic relationship of reptilian isolates has not been reported, a neonatal boa was susceptible to experimental infection with virus isolated from a Savannah Monitor.[68]

Incubation

In chickens, the incubation period after a naturally acquired adenovirus infection is considered to be 24 to 48 hours. Although avian adenovirus infections are associated with a relatively short incubation period, the rate of horizontal spread through a flock can be slow.[77] In the only reported transmission study in reptiles, a neonatal boa died from hepatic necrosis 14 days after intracoelomic injection with an adenovirus that contained suspension derived from a Savannah Monitor.[68]

Transmission

In birds, some adenoviruses can be transmitted via both horizontal and vertical routes, and others are transmitted only horizontally.[75,77] Viral particles are commonly identified in hepatocytes, pancreatic cells, and enterocytes of infected birds, and virus is shed principally in the feces.[1,75,77] Because adenoviruses are relatively durable outside the host, environmental persistence of the virus is common, and transmission can occur through indirect contact with objects contaminated with feces or respiratory secretions from infected birds.[1]

The routes of viral transmission in reptiles have not been determined, although the presence of lesions predominately in the liver and gastrointestinal tract suggests fecal-oral transmission.[66-69] Adults with persistent subclinical infections have been suggested to serve as reservoirs for virus transmission to highly susceptible young, particularly among Bearded Dragons. Vertical transmission is also suspected in some reptiles.[60,66-69] Because species susceptibility to reptilian adenoviruses is undefined, Bearded Dragons with chronic subclinical infections have been suggested as a potential risk to other reptiles. Diagnosis of adenovirus in a recently captured Mountain Chameleon maintained in strict quarantine suggests naturally acquired infections can occur.[73]

Pathogenesis

The pathogenesis of reptilian adenoviruses is poorly documented. In mammals, many adenoviruses cause asymptomatic infections that persist even though neutralizing antibodies develop to the virus. Disease is rare in individuals with a functional immune system; however, severe pathologic changes can occur if the host is immunocompromised.[1] Adenoviruses that infect birds appear to vary widely in their ability to cause morbidity or mortality. Some strains are mildly pathogenic and primarily cause persistent infections. Others are considered sufficiently virulent to induce disease in an otherwise healthy bird.

Generally, adenoviruses are considered to be opportunistic pathogens.[1] Affected birds often have concomitant chlamydial, fungal, bacterial, parasitic, or other viral infections, which suggests that immunosuppression is occurring in the affected bird.[78-80] Because adenoviruses are frequently recovered from birds that die of other causes, the role, if any, that adenoviruses may play in a disease process is difficult to define. Aviadenoviruses are thought to be more virulent in non-host-adapted species than they are in their typical host.[1]

Pathology

Lesions associated with adenovirus in snakes and lizards occur predominately in the liver and gastrointestinal tract and are characterized by nuclear swelling, ballooning degeneration, necrosis of affected tissues, and hemorrhage. Both eosinophilic and basophilic intranuclear inclusion bodies have been described in affected reptiles.[3,61,63,64,69]

In boas, adenovirus infections have been associated with edema of the small intestines with excessive mucus in the lumen, lung congestion, and mottling of an enlarged liver. Severe multifocal to coalescing hepatic necrosis with infiltration of mononuclear cells and heterophils is common, and basophilic intranuclear inclusion bodies were present in hepatocytes.[61,64] In another affected boa, basophilic intranuclear inclusion bodies were detected in hepatocytes, Kupffer cells, and endothelial cells, and eosinophilic inclusion bodies consistent with those described with retrovirus were detected in renal tubular cells, tracheal mucosa, lung, and gastric mucosa.[57]

An adenovirus-positive Mojave Rattlesnake had severe intestinal lesions including multifocal hemorrhage and ulceration with intralesional amoebae and renal carcinoma.[59]

Lesions in Rosy Boas included hepatitis and multifocal hemorrhage in the serosa of the gastrointestinal tract. Basophilic intranuclear inclusion bodies were detected in the liver and renal epithelial cells with occasional inclusions in the endothelium of the heart and epithelial cells lining the lungs.[57]

In Kingsnakes coinfected with adenovirus and parvovirus, pathologic changes occurred primarily in the intestines and included segmental mucosal necrosis and hyperplasia, villus blunting, and fusion. Basophilic Cowdry type A intranuclear inclusion bodies were noted in enterocytes peripheral to necrotic areas.[65]

With an aviadenoviral nucleic acid probe, adenoviral DNA was detected in hepatocytes, Kupffer cells, endothelial cells, and enterocytes of affected snakes.[59,64]

In Bearded Dragons, adenovirus infections have been characterized by petechial to ecchymotic subcutaneous, coelomic, intestinal, and perirenal hemorrhage. The liver is frequently enlarged and may be reddish or yellowish and mottled (Figure 24-3).[69] Hemorrhage is theorized to occur secondary to liver damage. Although severe hepatic necrosis is the most common lesion, pancreatitis, vacuolar hepatic lipidosis, interstitial and peritubular nephritis, and vacuolar renal tubular lipidosis have been described in some dragons.[60] Large basophilic intranuclear inclusion bodies have been found in hepatocytes, proximal convoluted tubules, enterocytes, pancreas (principally exocrine pancreas), and epithelium of intrahepatic bile ducts of some affected dragons (Figure 24-4).[66-69] In one report, intranuclear inclusion bodies

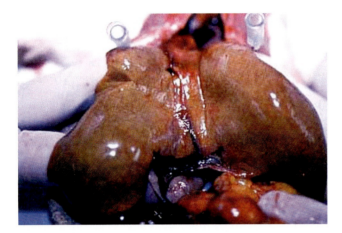

FIGURE 24-3 Liver of a Bearded Dragon *(Pogona vitticeps)*. Note the swelling of the hepatic lobes and the pale, mottled appearance of the parenchyma (necrosis). *(Photograph courtesy T. Boyer.)*

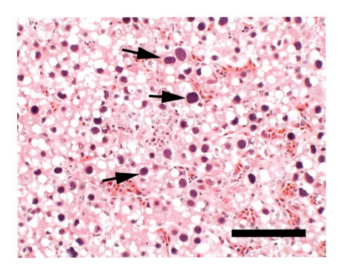

FIGURE 24-4 Liver of a Bearded Dragon *(Pogona vitticeps)*. Note the large numbers of hepatocytes with large intranuclear basophilic or amphophilic inclusions. The hepatocytes also have moderate lipidosis. Hematoxylin and eosin; bar = 250 μm. *(Photograph courtesy M.M. Garner, Northwest ZooPath.)*

were found in the liver of one dragon and in the mucosa of the small intestines of three others. These dragons were coinfected with a dependovirus.[69]

In affected Rankin's Dragons, the lungs were congested and the liver was diffusely swollen and pale. Multifocal hepatic necrosis was the most consistent histologic change in Rankin's Dragons and a Savannah Monitor.[67,69]

Basophilic intranuclear inclusion bodies with virus particles characteristic for adenovirus have been detected in enterocytes of chameleons with and without pathologic changes.[73] The absence of pathologic changes in some individuals suggests that adenovirus can cause subclinical nonpathogenic infections. Adenovirus was detected in eosinophilic intranuclear inclusion bodies of affected tissues of Jackson's Chameleons *(Chamaeleo jacksonii)* with esophagitis and tracheitis characterized by proliferation of mucosal epithelium.[71] Esophagitis was the predominate lesion in a Veiled Chameleon *(Chamaeleo calyptratus)* with adeno-like virus infections.

Affected Nile Crocodiles had enteritis and hepatitis with congestion of the intestines, lung, and kidneys. One of two affected crocodiles had scattered pale areas throughout the liver and fatty liver degeneration. Basophilic intranuclear inclusion bodies were present in the hepatocytes and crypt epithelial cells.[74]

Immunity

The immune response that occurs to an adenovirus infection in reptiles has been insufficiently studied. Adenovirus neutralizing antibodies can be detected within 1 to 2 weeks in experimentally infected chickens.[77] Adenoviruses are commonly recovered from young asymptomatic chickens, and surveys for antibodies suggest that most adult birds have been exposed to numerous strains of adenovirus.[75,77] The activation of latent adenovirus infections in birds and mammals appears to be cyclic. High concentrations of antibodies are associated with low levels of viral shedding, and as the antibody concentrations decrease, a subsequent increase is seen in the level of viral shedding.[75] Maternal antibodies may be passed to the developing embryo through the yolk. Chicks from hens with antibodies are refractory to severe disease for up to 3 weeks after hatching but become susceptible after 4 weeks, suggesting a decay in the protective maternally derived antibodies.[75,81] Chicks with maternally derived antibodies remain susceptible to infection; however, mortality rate in chicks with maternal antibodies is low compared with chicks without maternal antibodies.[81,82]

Diagnosis

Intranuclear inclusion bodies suggestive of an adenovirus infection are routinely seen in association with necrosis of cells in infected birds. One should note, however, that inclusion bodies are also found in asymptomatic birds.[75,79] During one survey of budgerigars, 170 of 293 birds (58%) examined were found to have suggestive inclusion bodies, but none of these birds showed any specific lesions or disease that could be associated with these inclusion bodies.

Adenovirus infections should be suspected in reptiles with large basophilic intranuclear inclusion bodies in the liver, biliary ductular epithelium, pancreatic acinar epithelium, renal tubular epithelium, gastrointestinal epithelium, Kupffer cells, splenic macrophages, and endothelium.[59] Infections can be confirmed with isolation of virus in cell culture, electron microscopic detection of 70-nm to 80-nm virus particles, or finding of viral nucleic acid with in situ hybridization.[59,64] In situ hybridization testing is available through the In Situ Hybridization Laboratory at the University of Georgia, College of Veterinary Medicine, Athens, GA 30602-7371. Biopsy samples of liver tissue may be used for antemortem diagnosis. Although a positive biopsy sample is confirmatory, a negative result does not indicate the absence of infection.[66,67]

Control

A 6-month quarantine period coupled with attempts to find virus shedding should be used to reduce the chances of introduction of a subclinically infected reptile to a group.[74] Characteristic virus particles may be detected in the feces of some animals with electron microscopy, and a PCR-based assay may prove of benefit in detection of animals shedding viral nucleic acid.

No studies have reported on the stability of adenoviruses recovered from reptiles. However, adenoviruses from birds and mammals are resistant to inactivation when outside a host and can remain infectious for long periods in litter, food, water, or contaminated feces. Adenoviruses are resistant to extremes of heat, organic solvents, and extremes in pH (pH3 and pH9). The precise heat susceptibility varies with the strain of virus. Some isolates are resistant to 56°C for 20 minutes, and others can withstand this temperature for 22 hours. Some strains are inactivated after 30 minutes of exposure to 60°C or 1 hour of exposure to 50°C. Many commonly used disinfectants are ineffective. The adenoviruses that have been studied can be inactivated with treatment for more than 1 hour with formalin, aldehydes, or iodophors.[1]

Treatment

No specific therapy exists for most adenovirus infections. Supportive care that includes reducing stress, providing a proper thermal gradient, maintaining adequate hydration, assisted feeding, and broad-spectrum antibiotics to prevent secondary infections may reduce the level of mortality.[70]

PARAMYXOVIRIDAE

Viruses in the family Paramyxoviridae are enveloped and can vary in shape and size from 150 to 300 nm. These viruses replicate in the cytoplasm of an infected cell, but virus-induced inclusion bodies can be found in the nucleus and cytoplasm of some hosts. The genera included within the Paramyxoviridae (*Paramyxovirus, Pneumovirus,* and *Morbillivirus*) are thought to be closely related to the rhabdoviruses and the orthomyxoviruses. Paramyxoviruses have been associated with influenza-like diseases in birds and mammals, including humans. Pneumoviruses have been associated with upper respiratory disease in turkeys and in mammals, including humans. Morbilliviruses have been described only in mammals; they cause measles in humans and canine distemper in dogs. Classification of the Paramyxoviridae isolates from reptiles has not been reported.[1]

Clinical Features in Snakes

In birds and mammals, multiple strains of paramyxovirus may infect closely related species with substantial variation in clinical signs, pathologic changes, and prognosis.[1] Multiple strains of paramyxovirus likely infect differing reptiles, resulting in similar variations in host response on the basis of the infected species and the individual response to infection.[83]

A paramyxovirus was documented as the cause of disease in a group of captive Fer-de-lance (*Bothrops lanceolatus*) in Switzerland in the mid 1970s.[84] Although poorly defined strains of paramyxovirus are considered important pathogens in viperids, clinical changes and death have also been documented in non-viperid snakes, including Elapidae, Colubridae, Boidae, and Pythonidae.[83,85-88]

Paramyxovirus infection should be considered in susceptible species with nasal discharge, open-mouth breathing, accumulation of caseous debris in the oral cavity, and harsh respiratory sounds.[29] In addition to respiratory signs, paramyxovirus infections should also be considered in snakes with emaciation, loss of muscle tone, unwillingness to move, head tremors, stargazing, heat-seeking behavior, recurring unresponsive bacterial or fungal pneumonia, mucoid diarrhea, malodorous stools, bowel distention, and severe protozoal infections.[16,83,89-91]

The clinical progression may be peracute, acute, or chronic.[92] Some snakes appear clinically normal in the evening and are dead the following morning.[85] More typically, affected snakes have an acute onset of severe respiratory disease characterized by open-mouth breathing and discharge of a blood-tinged or brownish mucus from the trachea, pharynx, or oral cavity. These snakes may exhibit opisthotonos, head tremors, terminal loss of righting reflex, and convulsions within 1 to 3 days of development of respiratory signs.[85,92] Others may die within several weeks of development of anorexia followed by an acute onset of head tremors and stargazing.[83,90] The chronic form of paramyxovirus is characterized by an onset of mild respiratory disease that progresses to severe respiratory disease and pneumonia (open-mouth breathing, nasal discharge, periglottal accumulation of caseated material, and harsh respiratory sounds) followed by progressive neurologic disease.[87,91] Other snakes may have anorexia, hypophagia, and regurgitation develop followed from weeks up to 7 months by a progressive onset of respiratory or neurologic signs.[91] Stargazing, paralysis, and convulsions have been noted in some snakes with advanced disease.[90] See Chapter 63 for a detailed clinical discussion.

In one outbreak, several affected vipers regurgitated mice or passed greenish mucoid feces for 1 to 3 weeks before the development of respiratory signs.[85] A Rock Rattlesnake had head tremors and loss of righting reflex develop 3 days after introduction to the collection followed by death 11 days later.[93] Six other exposed animals died with similar signs during the next 2 months. Only one at-risk rattlesnake survived.[93] Severe neurologic signs are particularly common in rattlesnakes and other viperids and may include writhing, head tremors, slowed tongue flicking, loss of righting reflex, and opisthotonos.[83,85,93]

The severity and duration of an outbreak can vary, but several outbreaks have continued from months to more than a year. Once clinical signs are noted, disease is usually progressive and the prognosis is guarded to poor, particularly when the CNS is affected. Mortality rates are highest in large collections of highly susceptible families of naïve snakes.[83] In the initial outbreak of paramyxovirus in captive Fer-de-lance, 25% of 431 at-risk snakes died.[84] In an outbreak that involved Viperidae in a zoologic collection, 35 of 438 at-risk snakes (8%) died during a 3-month period.[85]

As is true for most diseases in reptiles, improper husbandry, particularly suboptimal temperatures, is expected to weaken a snake's immune response and increase the severity of infection.[91] Geriatric snakes may be more susceptible to disease and death than younger conspecifics.[83] Secondary bacterial pneumonia is common in affected snakes, and concomitant adenovirus enteritis has been reported.[83,87]

Epizootiology

The global distribution of paramyxoviruses in captive and free-ranging reptiles has been insufficiently studied. However, various paramyxovirus isolates should be considered infectious for any aged captive or free-ranging representative of a homologous species of reptile. Infections are most common in viperid snakes but have been documented in *Crotalus, Vipera, Bothrops, Trimeresurus, Bitis, Ophiophagus, Agkistrodon, Cyclagras,* Elapidae, Colubridae, Boidae, and Pythonidae.[29,85,91] The finding of serologically positive free-ranging Copperheads (*Agkistrodon contortrix*) indicates virus activity in this species. The impact of paramyxoviruses on free-ranging individuals or representative populations is undefined.[87]

The paramyxoviruses that infect birds and mammals differ in host range. Some strains cause disease in only specific species, and others can infect a wide variety of avian and mammalian hosts with varying clinical diseases.[1] Similarly, epizootiologic evidence suggests that strain variation in reptilian paramyxoviruses may control host specificity or virulence, with most strains having a relatively restricted host range.[88] The most severe outbreaks may occur when a non–host-adapted strain of paramyxovirus is introduced to a naïve population of susceptible reptiles.[85] As an example, pit vipers are considered particularly susceptible to paramyxovirus-associated disease, but in one outbreak, exposed rattlesnakes died and adjacent Copperheads remained clinically normal.[89] In most outbreaks, only a few species considered at risk have been affected.

The serologic relationship and variation in virulence among paramyxoviruses recovered from differing species of reptiles has been insufficiently studied. When compared, isolates from a Puff Adder (*Bitis arietans*) and Rock Rattlesnake (*Crotalus lepidus*) were found to be antigenically similar but did exhibit varied cytopathic effects in cultured viper heart cells.[85] A paramyxovirus that indirect fluorescent antibody testing suggested was related to parainfluenza virus-2 was recovered from the lungs of two dead Ottoman Vipers (*Vipera xanthina xanthina*) maintained in a zoologic collection.[94]

Comparison of partial nucleic acid sequences from the hemagglutinin-neuraminidase and polymerase genes from 15 reptilian paramyxoviruses to that of the Fer-de-Lance paramyxovirus indicated a phylogenetic relationship with two distinct subgroups. The nucleotide divergence within a subgroup was less than 2.5%, and the divergence between the two subgroups was 20% to 22%. The phylogenetic groupings suggested some correlation with geographic distribution and showed that the viruses had a low level of host specificity.[95]

The incubation period for reptilian paramyxovirus isolates is poorly defined because of relatively few experimental transmission studies in only a few species.[96] Experimentally infected rattlesnakes died by 21 days after inoculation.[96] Field observations suggest that acute infections can result in death within 6 to 10 weeks after exposure.[91] In most cases, the incubation period is theorized to be greater than 90 days.[87]

Transmission

In birds, paramyxoviruses can be shed in all secretions (but primarily respiratory) and excretions (but primarily feces) for varying lengths of time. Ingestion of contaminated materials or inhalation of contaminated aerosols is the most common method by which birds are exposed to the virus. Aerosolized fecal dust and contaminated bedding are considered potential sources for indirect exposure to paramyxoviruses.[1]

Although insufficiently studied in reptiles, direct contact with contaminated respiratory secretions is considered the primary method of transmission.[85] Shedding probably starts with the earliest signs of disease and is expected to continue with chronic forms of infection, although the quantity of virus exiting the body at any particular time may vary.[91,92] Development of hemagglutination inhibiting (HI) antibodies does not correlate with cessation of virus shedding.[91] Shedding may be detected before seroconversion, which can take up to 8 weeks.[85] Transmission may vary among species. In one outbreak, a Northern Copperhead (*A. mokasen*) remained clinically normal and serologically negative after 6 weeks of being housed next to a seropositive Bushmaster (*Lachesis mutus*).[90]

In birds, Newcastle disease virus is stable outside the host and contaminated fomites, and insects, rodents, and humans are considered potential mechanical vectors for the dissemination of this virus between flocks. Chicken-to-chicken transmission by the feather mite has been reported.[1] Although unproven in reptiles, contaminated fomites or ectoparasites have been implicated in indirect spread of the virus.[83,97]

In birds, vertical transmission of some paramyxoviruses is possible but is considered unlikely because viremic hens generally stop laying eggs.[1] The effect of nonfatal infections on reproduction and whether vertical transmission can occur have been insufficiently studied in reptiles.

Persistently infected snakes have been suggested to remain subclinical and shed virus for at least 10 months.[90] Boas and pythons have been specifically mentioned as persistently infected hosts that may serve as a reservoir for a paramyxovirus, with increased virulence for vipers.[85] Stress, shipping, temperature fluctuation, and overcrowding may precipitate an otherwise subclinical infection.

Pathology

Caseous pneumonia with secondary bacterial infections is common, particularly in snakes with more chronic forms of disease. Many of the gross lesions associated with respiratory tract infections, including the accumulation of caseous debris in the trachea and nasal passages associated with secondary bacterial colonization of virus-affected mucosal tissues, may be confirmed endoscopically.[85] At necropsy, the lungs may be edematous and hemorrhagic frothy exudates, and caseous material may be noted in the lungs and air sacs.[29,97] Hemorrhagic pneumonia with bloody discharge from the trachea is considered a common lesion with acute phase infections.[83] Granulomas that contain bacteria were reported in the lungs of paramyxovirus-positive Rock Rattlesnakes, and gram-negative pneumonia is considered common in many affected animals.[16,29]

Histologically, paramyxovirus-associated lesions may be seen in the respiratory, intestinal, and nervous tissues of affected snakes (see Figure 63-3). Proliferation of alveolar type II cells in the lungs with infiltrates of heterophils and lymphocytes is suggestive.[87] Syncytial cells may be noted in some patients, and interstitial fibrosis has been described in some snakes with chronic infections.[87] Respiratory epithelial cells are frequently hypertrophied, and eosinophilic intracytoplasmic inclusions have been reported in some snakes.[85] Some snakes have an enlarged pancreas with ductal epithelial necrosis or hyperplasia of the pancreatic ducts and acinar cells with cystic dilation.[83,97] Hepatic necrosis, pyogranulomatous hepatitis, and necrosis of the bile ducts with interstitial fibrosis have been noted in some cases.[87] Neurologic lesions are characterized by multifocal gliosis and perivascular cuffing in the brain and ballooning degeneration of axonal fibers in the brain stem and proximal spinal cord.[88,93]

Diagnosis and Immunity

Diagnosis of an active paramyxovirus infection can be accomplished with paired plasma (preferable to serum) samples to find an increase in antibody titer, with the electron microscopic identification of paramyxovirus particles in respiratory secretions or feces, or with culturing the virus from diseased tissues, feces, or respiratory secretions. Although culture is the gold standard for diagnosis, multiple samples of respiratory secretions or feces may be necessary for successful virus isolation, and to date, virus has not been cultured from a live snake.[91] PCR-based testing of secretions, excretions, and tissues from suspect patients is being validated for accuracy and clinical value by the Emerging Diseases Research Group at the University of Georgia College of Veterinary Medicine, Athens, GA 30602-7371. This assay may also be of value for screening reptiles during quarantine.[98] In snakes that are regurgitating, vomitus should be submitted for electron microscopic evaluation and PCR-based testing for detection of viral nucleic acid.

Postmortem diagnosis requires isolation of the virus from infected tissues, use of transmission electron microscopy to detect virus in either fresh tissue homogenates or fixed tissues, fluorescent antibody staining to find viral proteins in affected tissues (particularly lung), or detection of viral nucleic acid in tissues with in situ hybridization.[96,98,99]

Samples of lung and pancreas should be submitted for histologic evaluation in suspect patients. Any tissue samples for immunohistochemistry should be fixed initially in 10% formalin and then either sectioned or transferred to 70% ethanol within 24 hours.[99] Finding of eosinophilic intracytoplasmic inclusion bodies is presumptive. Specific staining for antigen or nucleic acid, or electron microscopic finding of virus particles, is necessary for a confirmed diagnosis.

Ophidian paramyxovirus, hemagglutinated chicken erythrocytes, and an HI assay can be used to document seroconversion. Seroconversion confirms that a snake has been previously infected. Documentation of an active infection requires finding of a rising antibody titer in paired plasma samples collected 10 to 12 weeks apart.[83] Seroconversion requires a minimum of 8 weeks. Plasma (at least 0.5 mL) has been suggested for testing in place of serum because the latter has a tendency to clot. Survivors of paramyxovirus infection may have titers greater than 10,240.[100] Serologic testing is currently available through the University of Florida, University of Tennessee, and the Texas State Diagnostic Laboratory (see Chapter 91). The antigens used for testing vary with each laboratory, and titers are not comparable.

Some snakes have reportedly died before development of detectable antibodies to the virus.[91] Alternatively, these snakes could have been infected with a strain of paramyxovirus that is not detected with currently available serologic assays. Because the immune response in reptiles is temperature dependent, proper husbandry may play an important role in helping infected snakes respond appropriately.[83] Shedding has been documented to continue in affected snakes despite the development of HI antibodies.[91]

Some asymptomatic seropositive snakes are considered persistently infected shedders, and others appear to have an appropriate immune response develop and clear an infection.[90] In one fatal outbreak in viperids, antibody titers were detected in some surviving vipers and nonvipers that remained subclinical, including a Reticulated Python (*Python reticulatus*), Cornsnake (*Elaphe guttata guttata*), and Gulf Hammock Ratsnake (*E. obsoleta williamsi*).[85] In another outbreak, a Bushmaster remained seropositive, but clinically normal, for 9 months.[90]

A seropositive snake that is not shedding virus and remains clinically normal for more than a year has been considered prognostically encouraging.[91] Alternatively, detection of antibody titers in snakes that remain clinically normal could indicate a persistent low-grade infection that has not been documented.[83,90] In one study, 17 of 22 snakes maintained detectable levels of HI antibodies at 5 months after an outbreak.[85]

Treatment and Control

The prognosis in affected snakes is grave, and the treatments that have been recommended are limited to controlling clinical signs while confirmatory diagnostic testing is being completed.[91] Suspect patients should be maintained in strict isolation while awaiting the results of diagnostic tests. Seizures can be controlled with diazepam 0.5 mg/kg intramuscularly (IM) or general anesthesia. In patients with severe respiratory disease, the nasal passages and trachea can be cleared with a combination of flushing and suction. Atropine at 0.2 mg/kg subcutaneously may help reduce respiratory secretions.[101] Secondary bacterial of fungal infections should be treated appropriately.

Reptiles in direct or immediate indirect contact with a confirmed positive animal should be placed in isolation and serologically tested immediately and again 4 to 6 months later.[83,97] Reptiles that remain serologically negative are considered relatively safe. IM administration of 2 mL/kg of body weight of hyperimmune serum has been suggested to protect exposed birds if they are treated before the development of clinical signs.[102] Correlative data have not been reported for reptiles.

One should attempt to reduce the introduction of paramyxovirus to a group by serologically testing all snakes at the beginning and end of at least a 4-month quarantine period. Serial electron microscopic or PCR-based screening of tracheal washes or feces may prove useful for detection of subclinical shedders during quarantine.[98] Husbandry during isolation and quarantine should include maintenance of a proper thermal gradient, air quality, humidity, and reduction of physical and social stress. Mites should be eliminated from snakes early in the quarantine period.[83]

Although paramyxoviruses are enveloped, and are expected to be rapidly inactivated when outside of the host, the viruses that occur in birds and mammals are in fact relatively stable in the environment and are resistant to many commonly used disinfectants.[1] The stability of reptilian paramyxoviruses has been insufficiently evaluated, but consideration of them as at least as stable as the isolates recovered from birds seems clinically prudent. Newcastle disease virus is stable at 50°C for 134 days, 40°C for 30 days, and 27°C for 4 weeks.[1] The virus has been found to remain active in moist soil for 22 days, on feathers at 20°C for 123 days, and in lake water for 19 days.[103-105] The virus can be inactivated by extremes of pH (<2 and >11), high temperatures (56°C), sunlight, detergents, chloramine (1%), sodium hypochlorite (bleach), lysol, phenol, and 2% formalin.[1,103-105]

Jacobson et al[85] have shown that ophidian paramyxovirus that is not protected by organic debris is rapidly inactivated by 3% sodium hypochlorite or quaternary ammonium. When organic debris is present, a detergent should be used for cleaning, and thorough rinsing should occur before a snake is placed back in contact with disinfected items.[85]

Vaccination

Both modified-live and inactivated vaccines have been successfully used to reduce the impact of paramyxoviruses in birds and mammals.[1] Preliminary studies with an inactivated vaccine in Western Diamondback Rattlesnakes (*Crotalus viridis*) provided inconsistent results.[106]

OTHER PARAMYXOVIRUSES

Paramyxoviruses have been documented in various species of lizards. In some lizards, isolates have not been associated with any specific pathology, and lesions in others suggest that the demonstrated paramyxovirus was associated with disease.[83,107] A paramyxovirus with proteins that cross-reacted with antibodies directed against ophidian paramyxovirus was recovered from recently imported Caiman Lizards (*Dracaena guianensis*) with proliferative pneumonia. The virus was detected with electron microscopy in tissue homogenates. In addition, syncytial cell formation was noted in viper heart cells within 10 days of inoculation with lung, liver, and kidney homogenates from affected lizards.[107]

A virus with morphologic characteristics suggestive of paramyxovirus was detected with electron microscopy in ascitic fluid collected from a Bearded Dragon with hepatitis.

RETROVIRIDAE

No group of viruses is as diverse as the Retroviridae. This family contains viruses that exhibit markedly different behaviors that range from subclinical infections to rapid formation of tumors and death. Many of these viruses have the ability to integrate into the genome of host cells and cause tumors or otherwise permanently alter the function of infected cells.[1]

In birds and mammals, retroviruses have been associated with cancers, chronic weight-loss diseases, neurologic disease, damage to the immune system, and persistent infections. These viruses are frequently difficult to control because they change rapidly, thus avoiding the host defense systems, or specifically damage the immune system, allowing unrestricted replication. Host-specific retroviruses have been shown to cause neoplasms (leukemias, lymphomas, sarcomas, and carcinomas), immunodeficiencies, and autoimmune diseases in humans, livestock, companion animals, and poultry.[1]

Clinical Features

Retroviruses were first implicated as a cause of lymphoid tumors in the early 1900s, when the Rous-sarcoma virus was shown to cause neoplastic changes in the B-lymphocytes of young chickens. This virus induces tumors by inserting oncogenes into the nucleic acid of an infected cell. In chickens, the avian leukosis/sarcoma viruses (ALSV) have been associated with a range of tumors including lymphoid leukosis (most common), erythroid leukosis (erythroblastosis), myeloid leukosis (myeloblastosis), renal neoplasms, hemangiomas, and osteopetrosis.[108] The same retrovirus may cause widely varying neoplastic changes depending on the source of the virus, the route of exposure, and the age and strain of the chicken. Generally, a particular retrovirus causes one type of neoplasia in most cases and only occasionally causes a different neoplasia.[108]

Some ALSV are endogenous, which means they are spread from infected parent to offspring directly in the transferred genetic material. Others of this group are exogenous, being acquired after hatching through contact with an infected bird.[1]

Many retroviruses are recovered from subclinical hosts. Some groups of chickens have natural resistance to infection or to the development of tumors after infection, and these traits can be enhanced in a flock through selective breeding.[108]

Inclusion Body Disease

The retrovirus associated with inclusion body disease (IBD) was first associated with CNS signs including head tremors, opisthotonos, and loss of righting reflex in pythons, particularly Burmese Pythons (*Python molurus bivittatus*), in the late 1970s.[109,110] IBD remained common in captive pythons throughout the 1980s. Starting in the 1990s, the incidence rate of disease appeared to decrease in pythons and increase in Boa Constrictors.[109,110] See Chapter 60 for a clinical review of IBD.

The clinical changes associated with IBD vary with the species and individual. However, IBD should be considered in any snake, particularly boids, with chronic wasting, regurgitation, loose feces, stomatitis, dermatitis (ulcerative or necrotizing), pale mucous membranes, respiratory disease (particularly pneumonia), cutaneous neoplasias, and leukemias. These changes may be noted with or without concurrent CNS signs.[29,109,110] Secondary bacterial and protozoal infections are common.[29,110] Most young snakes have an acute infection develop, with a mortality rate that approaches 100%. Infections in adults tend to be more protracted and debilitating.[111]

Some clinicians consider recurring infections in chronic poor doers as the most common clinical change.[29,109,110] Other snakes may have slowly progressive CNS signs develop that start with an inability to strike and constrict prey followed by dysecdysis, presumably secondary to incoordination and an inability to initiate or control the refined body movements necessary for successful shedding.[110,112] Subtle head tremors, depressed tongue flicking, and dull mentation have been described as early signs, followed by anorexia, lethargy, weight loss, and dehydration as the disease progresses.[29,110] Early CNS signs progress to a slowed righting reflex, hyperreflexia, head tremors, head tilt, rolling, disorientation, blindness, and stargazing that, depending on species, may quickly lead to death or persist for 4 to 5 years.[110,112,113] Lymphoproliferative disorders and secondary bacterial stomatitis, pneumonia, and dermatitis may occur in chronically infected boas and pythons.[29,114]

Disease progression is typically more rapid and severe in pythons than boas.[29,110] Regurgitation is frequently the first sign in Boas, followed by slowly progressive CNS signs that worsen during 1 to 2 years.[114] Other affected boas may regurgitate partially digested food and then die within several weeks. Some clinicians report that young boas are most likely to have regurgitation develop, with an acute onset of flaccid paralysis, and mature boas are more likely to have recurring or chronic infections develop, particularly pneumonia.[109,114] Other authors consider CNS signs as a late change in boas, with chronic regurgitation, pneumonia, and cachexia occurring in early stages of the disease.[112]

Pythons frequently have an acute onset of severe CNS signs, and CNS signs appear to be more severe in pythons than boas. The typical disease in pythons has been described as stomatitis and pneumonia that progresses rapidly to fatal CNS signs.[113] IBD has been suggested to be on the rule-out list for chronic respiratory disease in mature pythons.[109,114]

An outbreak of IBD in a group of Diamond and Carpet Pythons (*Morelia* spp.) resulted in the death of six of 33 at-risk snakes.[115] The collection had a history of mite infestation. The clinical signs varied among affected individuals. One Diamond Python had a history of mid-body bloating, and an affected Carpet Python had a 4-month to 5-month history of anorexia, lethargy, head tilt, writhing, and bloating. No regurgitation or diarrhea was noted in these snakes despite the presence of bloating.[115] Another Carpet Python had a history of anorexia and restlessness, followed by respiratory signs that included mucus discharge from the trachea and gurgling sounds that recurred several times during a 4-month period. In this snake flaccid paralysis of the caudal third of the body developed a year after initial presentation, but whether this lesion was a result of viral damage or secondary to a thrombi in the caudal vena cava was undetermined.[115]

Although IBD has been most commonly reported in snakes in the family Boidae, infections have recently been described in other species as well. An outbreak of IBD occurred in a collection of Palm Vipers (*Bothriechis marchi*) and affected both captive raised and wild-caught individuals. Three of eight at-risk vipers died with no premonitory signs, and five died after development of signs that included anorexia, dehydration, regurgitation, and paresis. All affected snakes were adults at the time of death, with a mean age of 8.6 years.[116]

Inclusion body disease was diagnosed in two captive Pythons (*Morelia spilota variegata* and *M. s. spilota*) in Australia,[117] in a captive Boa Constrictor in the Canary Islands,[118] and in an Eastern Kingsnake (*Lampropeltis getulus*) that was housed with an infected boa.[114]

Other Clinical Presentations of Retroviruses

In addition to IBD, retroviruses have also been recovered from neoplasms from snakes and were found with electron microscopy in the venom of Jararacussu Vipers (*Bothrops jararacussu*).[119] A virus with characteristics typical for a type-C retrovirus was recovered from the spleen of a Russell's Viper (*Vipera russelli*) with a pericardial myxofibroma.[120] Similar virus particles were detected in an embryonal rhabdomyosarcoma from a Cornsnake. Retrovirus particles were found with electron microscopy within intranuclear inclusion bodies in a California Kingsnake with lymphosarcoma.[121,122] Similar viral particles were reported in the spleens of tumor-free Cornsnakes.[123] C-type oncogenic retroviruses have been associated with mesenchymal tumors in other snakes.[122] Retroviruses were also detected in a Boa Constrictor with erythroleukosis,[124] in a Brazilian Lancehead Viper (*Bothrops moojeni*) with renal tumors,[119] and in a Four-lined Chicken Snake (*E. obsoleta quadrivittata*) with lymphoid leukemia.[125]

A type-C retrovirus was detected in the neoplasms of four Burmese Pythons from the same collection. One affected snake was a 7-year-old with recurring tan nodular masses in the lower left distal mandible and soft palate. These masses were diagnosed as undifferentiated mesenchymal round cell tumor (lymphosarcoma), and similar neoplasms were detected in the uterus, ovary, and spleen. Retrovirus was also detected in a 4.5-year-old with segmental colonic adenocarcinoma and fulminant fibrinosuppurative coelomitis, in a 19-year-old with recurring intermandibular fibrosarcoma, and in a 5-year-old with transitional cell carcinoma originating from the pelvis of the right kidney.[126]

Neither in vivo transmission nor in vitro transforming capacity of retroviral particles has been reported, and the role that a retrovirus may have played in the formation of neoplasms in the affected snakes described previously has not been determined.[114,126]

Other Reptiles

Retrovirus nucleic acid sequence of undetermined clinical importance has been detected in Green Seaturtles from the Hawaiian Islands.[40] Viral nucleic acid was detected with amplification procedures in apparently healthy turtles and in those with fibropapillomas.[40] Reverse transcriptase activity was lower in clinically unaffected turtles that were hatched and raised in captivity compared with affected free-ranging turtles. Virus was also found in heart and lung tumors from affected turtles. Retroviruses have been suggested as a possible precipitating factor in Green Seaturtle fibropapillomatosis. These benign tumors could be experimentally reproduced through inoculation with cell-free tumor filtrate.[44] Nucleic acid studies suggest that retroviral activity is widespread in Hawaiian Green Turtles.[40]

An endogenous retrovirus has been identified in Tuatara (*Rhynchocephalia* sp).[127]

Epizootiology

Inclusion body disease has been diagnosed in snakes maintained in the United States, Africa, Australia, Europe, and the Canary Islands.[114] Although IBD is considered most common in boids, infections have also been diagnosed in vipers and a Kingsnake. Why an apparent increase was seen in the incidence rate of IBD in boas and a reduction was seen in the incidence rate of IBD in pythons during the 1990s has not been determined. Theory exists that many exposed pythons developed resistance to disease or alternatively the virulence of the virus changed for pythons.[29,110] On the basis of epizootiologic data collected during outbreaks in mixed species collection, Rosy Boas have been described as resistant to disease and Ball Pythons may be less susceptible than other pythons.[29,110]

In birds, avian leukosis viruses are divided into subgroups on the basis of differences in the proteins found in the virus envelope. These differences restrict the host range. With a few exceptions, neutralizing antibodies to each subgroup of viruses do not cross-react with those of other subgroups. One study showed that the retrovirus associated with IBD in two boids was antigenically similar.[114] A pedigree analysis in a group of affected Palm Vipers suggested a familial susceptibility.[116]

Transmission

In chickens, retroviruses may be transmitted vertically or horizontally, although horizontal transmission is probably more important.[108] These viruses are transmitted through direct contact with contaminated blood, saliva, respiratory secretions, semen, or feces or can be transmitted with indirect contact with contaminated insects. Virus is shed from the oviduct of an infected hen and can enter the albumen of the developing egg. Infected males can infect hens during copulation. The subgroup E viruses are endogenous and are transmitted from parent to offspring through the genome.[128]

In chickens, clinical signs of disease and increased shedding of virus are most common during periods of stress or after damage or suppression of the immune system.[108] Correlative data have not been reported for reptiles.

Although the routes of virus transmission in reptiles are poorly documented, contaminated aerosols or excrement have been implicated in the transmission of the IBD retrovirus in snakes. Infections spread rapidly when an infected snake is introduced to a susceptible group.[29,109] Pythons typically show signs within weeks, and *Boa* spp. may require months.[29] Epizootiologic data support that snake mites may be involved in virus transmission in large groups of infested snakes. Alternatively, retrovirus may be an opportunistic pathogen that takes advantage of a host that is weakened by mites.[29]

Vertical transmission is also suspected to occur but is unproven.[29,109] Pythons frequently have disease develop after exposure to clinically normal boas, suggesting the latter may serve as persistently infected reservoirs.[29] Naïve pythons may have signs develop within 2 weeks of infection.[29]

Inclusion body disease in boids is one of the few virus-associated diseases that has been experimentally reproduced in reptiles. Virus-containing suspensions have been used to reproduce characteristic lesions in snakes.[29,110,129]

Pathology

Snakes with IBD typically have eosinophilic intracytoplasmic inclusion bodies in epithelial cells of affected tissues. Although the number and location of inclusion bodies vary between species and among individuals, inclusions have been described in hepatocytes, pulmonary epithelial cells, glial cells, ependymal cells, neuronal cells, heart, spleen, kidney, stomach, and pancreas.[114] Inclusion bodies are particularly common in the pancreas, kidneys, brain, and spinal gray matter (Figure 24-5).[29]

In one study, inclusion bodies were found in the pancreas of all affected snakes, 70% of liver and kidney samples, and the gastrointestinal mucosa of only 30% of diseased animals.[29] Other reported lesions have included ulcerative dermatitis, hepatic lipidosis, subacute periportal hepatitis, interstitial pneumonia, subacute myocarditis, splenic fibrosis, depletion of splenic lymphocytes, diffuse spongiosis, and neuronal degeneration.[111,114] Splenic fibrosis, pancreatic fibrosis, pancreatic atrophy, loss of fat bodies, and loss of muscle mass are common with chronic forms of the disease.[29]

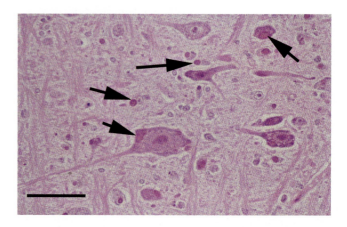

FIGURE 24-5 Inclusion body disease. Cerebrum of a Red Tailed Boa *(Boa constrictor)*. Note single variably sized inclusions in the cytoplasm of glial cells and neuron cell bodies. Hematoxylin and eosin; bar = 150 μm. *(Photograph courtesy M.M. Garner, Northwest ZooPath.)*

The most common lesions in boids with IBD-associated CNS signs are nonsupportive meningoencephalitis characterized by neuronal degeneration and mononuclear cell infiltrates in the brain and spinal cord. Gliosis, myelin degeneration, and perivascular cuffing are also common. In general, inflammatory lesions are more severe in pythons than in boas.[113]

Chronic proliferative pneumonia with massive alveolar cell proliferation, usually with the absence of inflammatory cells, was a common lesion described in affected Burmese Pythons with respiratory signs. Neuronal degeneration and spongiform changes in the absence of inflammatory cells were consistent in a group of snakes with CNS signs.[111]

In Palm Vipers with IBD, the most consistent pathologic changes were urate nephrosis, septic thrombi, and hepatocellular degeneration. Other lesions included biliary hyperplasia, granulomas, hepatitis, gastroenteritis, aortic mineralization, interstitial pneumonia, and hepatic melanosis. In addition, all eight affected vipers in the index outbreak had round to oval, intracytoplasmic eosinophilic inclusion bodies in hepatocytes and renal tubular epithelial cells. In some infected vipers, inclusion bodies were also noted in respiratory epithelium, bilary ductal epithelium, gastric mucosa, intestinal mucosa, striated myofibers, thyroid follicular cells, glomerular mesangial cells, myenteric ganglia, oviductal epithelial cells, pancreatic acinar cells, and esophageal mucosal cells.[116]

Pathogenesis, Immunity, and Diagnosis

In birds, retroviruses can be recovered from plasma, serum, feces, vaginal swabs, pharyngeal secretions, feather pulp, or albumen of freshly laid eggs. Because retrovirus infections are common in chickens, antibodies to the virus are frequently detected during seroprevalence studies. Chicks and adults infected through an exogenous route have neutralizing antibodies develop; however, the immunologic response that occurs may not prevent tumor formation.[1]

Inclusion body disease should be on the rule-out list in any susceptible snake with a white blood cell (WBC) count of more than 30,000 cells/dL, particularly with lymphocytosis.[109] However, leukocytosis may be phasic, and chronically infected or severely affected snakes may have a normal WBC count.[29,109] Some authors report the detection of sky blue inclusion bodies in circulating blood cells, particularly erythrocytes, but these inclusions may be found in only 1% of the cells.[109] These inclusions have not been found to contain virus, and their relationship to infections is undetermined.[29]

The index of suspicion of IBD is increased with the finding of characteristic intracytoplasmic inclusion bodies in biopsy samples collected from the liver, kidney, esophageal tonsils, and gastric mucosa.[109,110] In one study, the pancreas was the only tissue in which inclusion bodies were detected in 100% of affected snakes.[110] The liver and kidney were the next most commonly positive tissues.[109,110] One should note that a lack of detectable inclusion bodies does not rule out infection, and inclusion bodies may be detected in snakes that are clinically normal.[114] A confirmatory diagnosis of IBD requires finding of virus particles in affected tissues with electron microscopy or with culturing the virus in primary kidney or brain cells.[111] Serologic, immunohistochemical, and PCR-based assays are likely to prove of clinical value in the antemortem diagnosis of IBD.[98,99] A PCR-based assay is being validated by the Emerging Diseases Research Group at the University of Georgia for its accuracy in detection of viral nucleic acid in clinical samples collected from diseased animals and subclinical reptiles exposed to them.

Control and Vaccination

Control of retrovirus transmission in birds requires excellent hygiene and prevention of exposure to the virus with identification and removal of infected hens from the breeding flock. Selective breeding can be used to produce strains of chickens that are resistant to avian leukosis virus.[1]

Rapid identification and removal of affected snakes in combination with strict quarantine procedures, particularly with Boa Constrictors, are currently the most effective control measures available. Some authors have suggested that boas may be subclinically infected and serve to transmit the virus to more susceptible pythons.[29,109] Thus, restriction of exposure between boas and pythons may be prudent. Control of snake mites may help reduce the spread of retrovirus in large collections. Antibiotics, fluids, and increased temperatures may help stabilize snakes with septicemia and pneumonia; however, these snakes should be isolated pending histologic examination of biopsy samples. Diazepam may be useful in decreasing the frequency of seizures, but IBD should be considered fatal.

The use of Ball Pythons as sentinels to detect subclinically infected snakes during quarantine is considered unreliable.[29,109] Injection of susceptible pythons with the blood from test animals followed by a 6-month quarantine has been suggested to reduce the chances of introduction of the virus to valuable collections.

Avian and mammalian retroviruses are relatively unstable outside of a host. Infectivity is destroyed by most disinfectants and detergents and by temperatures of 37°C (4 hours) and 50°C (1 minute).[1] No correlative data are available for the retroviruses isolated from reptiles. However, the housing unit, furniture, and handling equipment used for an affected snake should be repeatedly cleaned, disinfected, rinsed, and sun dried or discarded.[29]

REOVIRIDAE

The respiratory, enteric, orphan (Reo) viruses were so-named because they were initially isolated from the respiratory or enteric systems in animals with no specific signs of disease. The Reoviridae family consists of three genera that have been shown to infect birds: orthoreoviruses, orbiviruses, and rotaviruses. Most viruses in the Reoviridae are considered nonpathogenic; however, a few strains have been associated with high levels of morbidity and mortality in specific populations of susceptible birds and mammals. In many cases, animals infected with these viruses have clinical changes develop attributable to secondary infectious agents that take advantage of the immunosuppressed host.[1]

Currently 11 serotypes of avian orthoreoviruses (heretofore called reoviruses) are antigenically distinct from each other and antigenically distinct from the strains that infect mammals.[1] Reoviruses are commonly recovered from subclinical birds. The type and degree of pathology that occurs appear to vary with the age of the host, virulence of the virus strain, and the route of exposure.[1] The morbidity and mortality rate associated with reovirus infections in birds is usually highest in those with concurrent bacterial or other viral infections.[1]

Clinical Features

A reovirus was found in two of four Chinese Vipers (*Azemiops feyi*) that died with no premonitory signs shortly after their arrival in the United States.[130] The primary pathologic changes were hepatic necrosis, vacuolar degeneration of hepatocytes, and enteritis. Leukocytes had infiltrated the intestines in response to nematodiasis. Virus particles with characteristics suggestive of reovirus were found with electron microscopy in the cytoplasm of affected intestinal cells and in viper heart cells inoculated with suspensions of liver and spleen.[130]

A reovirus was found in the brain of a rattlesnake that died after progressive neurologic changes that included incoordination, proprioceptive deficits, and convulsions. The affected snake had no gross or microscopic lesions in the brain or spinal cord.[131]

A reo-like virus was isolated from the tongue, esophagus, lung, liver, and kidney of a Spur-thighed Tortoise. The virus caused syncytium formation in chicken embryo fibroblasts but no cytopathic effect in TH-1 cells.[21]

A virus morphologically consistent with reovirus was found in papillomas from a European Green Lizard (*Lacerta viridis*).[35,87] A reovirus was isolated from *Python regius*.[132]

Transmission

The incubation period for reoviruses in reptiles has not been reported. In birds, the experimental incubation period is generally from 2 to 9 days.[1] Routes of reovirus transmission in reptiles have been insufficiently studied. In chickens, reoviruses are primarily transmitted via horizontal routes after direct or indirect contact with contaminated feces.[1]

Diagnosis

Confirmation of the presence of a reovirus requires its isolation from the feces or affected tissues of a reptile.

Electron microscopy may be helpful in finding virus particles in the feces of suspect patients. However, reovirus is commonly found in the feces of normal birds and mammals, and finding of the virus does not necessarily indicate that an animal will develop disease.

Control

Reoviruses, in general, are stable in the environment and are resistant to pH3, lipolytic agents (ether and chloroform), 2% lysol, 3% formalin, 3% formaldehyde, 1% hydrogen peroxide, 1% phenol, quaternary ammonium, and heating to 56°C for 120 minutes or 60°C for 8 to 10 hours.[1,102] These viruses are extremely stable in contaminated organic materials as long as they remain moist. Infectivity can be reduced by prolonged contact (up to 2 hours in some cases) with phenols, aldehydes, 70°C, halides, formalin, 70% ethanol, beta-propiolactone, and 0.5% iodine.[1,102]

Control of reovirus in chickens is difficult because it can be vertically transmitted, it is resistant to inactivation, and infected birds may intermittently shed the virus. Vaccination of breeding birds, which confers temporary protection to the chicks, is the best method to reduce reovirus infections in gallinaceous birds.[1]

POXVIRIDAE

Poxviruses are one of the largest and most complex of all animal viruses. With a brick-shaped virion that measures up to 400 nm in diameter, these viruses are only slightly smaller than many common bacteria. Unlike most DNA viruses that replicate in the nucleus, poxviruses replicate in the cytoplasm of infected cells. Currently seven genera of poxviruses infect vertebrates. In birds and mammals, some poxviruses are antigenically similar, and others have mutated to become immunologically distinct.[1,120] Some poxviruses have a limited host range, and others are capable of infecting a wide range of related animals. These viruses are generally placed into specific groups largely on the basis of the type of animal they infect.[1]

Clinical Features

A poxvirus was found with electron microscopy in proliferative epidermal lesions in young captive Spectacled Caiman (*Caiman sclerops*).[133] Focal 1-mm to 3-mm gray-white papular skin lesions were present over much of the skin (see Figure 41-3). In two of three caimans, the lesions resolved during a 1-month period. In the other caiman, lesions were particularly common on the palpebrae, phalanges, and skin over the mandibles and maxillae. These lesions coalesced to form gray-white patches, and the animal was ultimately euthanized.[133] Microscopic changes were characterized by edematous dermis with mononuclear cell infiltrates and large eosinophilic intracytoplasmic inclusion bodies within hypertrophied epithelial cells. Small inclusions resembled Borrel bodies, and larger ones resembled Bollinger's bodies. Electron microscopy confirmed virus particles morphologically consistent with poxvirus in affected epithelial cells.

An outbreak of poxvirus characterized by 2-mm to 6-mm yellowish to brownish proliferative skin lesions was reported in Nile Crocodiles from a farm in Zambia. Of 4000 animals of various ages that were at risk, only yearlings were affected. Eighty-two of 300 affected yearlings died. Skin lesions were diffuse but were particularly common around the eyes, nostrils, mouth, ventral neck, ventral belly, limbs, and base of the tail.[134]

In 9-month-old farm-raised Nile Crocodiles, poxvirus lesions were particularly common on the head and neck but were reported on all parts of the body, except the tail.[135] Lesions varied from 2-mm to 3-mm flat spots to 8 mm in diameter raised nodules. Periocular lesions were particularly large and caused blindness in severely affected animals. Two-mm to 5-mm, flat, irregular, brownish blotches were noted on the gums and tongue of some animals.[135] Approximately 400 of 1000 crocodiles had lesions develop within 21 days after the initial cases were identified. In most animals, the lesions regressed during a 3-week to 4-week period, leaving a gray translucent scar.[135] Histologic lesions were characterized by focal areas of hyperkeratosis and parakeratosis with large numbers of eosinophilic intracytoplasmic inclusion bodies. Virus particles were not documented in the oral lesions. Lesions were not reported in any animals in an adjacent pond or in the adult breeding population, and stress associated with poor water quality was considered a factor in the outbreak.[135]

Poxvirus was associated with brown papular dermatitis in a captive Tegu (*Tupinambis teguexin*). The lesions in this animal spontaneously resolved during a 3-month to 4-month period.[136]

Virus particles with morphologic characteristics consistent with a poxvirus were found in circulating monocytes of Flap-necked Chameleons (*Chamaeleo dilepis*) trapped in Tanzania (Figure 24-6). One lizard became ill 46 days after initial examination and was euthanized at day 56. In this animal, inclusion bodies that contained either poxvirus-like particles or chlamydia-like particles were found in the liver and spleen (Figure 24-7).[137]

Poxvirus has been mentioned as a cause of dermal changes in frogs.[138]

Transmission

As a group, poxviruses survive by being extremely durable outside of the host. This durability increases the likelihood that viable virus particles come in contact with a susceptible host. In other species, poxvirus transmission can occur through direct contact with an infected animal or through indirect contact with contaminated objects, water containers, or insects. However, in other species, poxviruses are not capable of penetrating intact epithelium and must enter the body through abraded skin or mucus membranes.[1]

In one outbreak that involved captive crocodiles, animals that originated from a farm with a previous history of similar problems were speculated to have been persistently infected and to have had lesions develop after environmental stressors.[135]

Diagnosis

The presence of poxvirus in suspect lesions can be confirmed with the finding of virus particles with electron microscopy or microscopic identification of intracytoplasmic inclusion bodies (Bollinger bodies) in a biopsy sample.[1]

Control and Treatment

Poxviruses are environmentally stable; can survive for years in dried organic debris such as feces, blood, soil or scabs; and are resistant to many commonly used disinfectants. Fowlpox virus remains infectious when placed in 1% phenol or a 1:1000 dilution of formalin for up to 9 days but can be inactivated with 1% potassium hydroxide, heating to 50°C for 30 minutes, or 60°C for 8 minutes, steam, 2% NaOH, and 5% phenol.[1,120] Correlative disinfection data have not been reported for reptilian poxviruses.

To prevent the spread of poxvirus through a group, animals with active lesions, and those exposed to them, should be housed separately from other reptiles. Provision of appropriate low-stress environments may prevent poxvirus outbreaks or minimize their impact.

Papules usually resolve without scarring if no secondary invaders are involved. However, once opened, poxvirus-associated vesicles are susceptible to secondary infections, and the severity and duration of lesions are determined by the presence or absence of bacterial or fungal agents. Severe scarring with loss of pigmentation may occur as infected erosions heal. Focal poxvirus-induced lesions can be treated with gentle removal of devitalized tissue, thorough cleansing of the wound, and application of topical antimicrobial agents to prevent secondary bacterial and fungal infections. Systemic antibiotics are indicated in reptiles that have signs of systemic infections.

In one study, crocodiles vaccinated with an autogenous vaccine healed at least 15 days earlier than unvaccinated controls; however, the vaccination procedure resulted in severe stress and anorexia.[135]

IRIDOVIRUS

A virus with morphologic characteristics consistent with an iridovirus was found with electron microscopy in tortoises with hepatitis and respiratory disease.[139] The virus was found in basophilic intracytoplasmic inclusion bodies of a Hermann's Tortoise with multifocal hepatic necrosis. The affected tortoise died with no premonitory signs. Gross lesions included multifocal gray spots throughout the liver and splenic congestion with small white foci on the cut surface. Virus-containing inclusion bodies were also found in intestinal epithelial cells.[140] An irido-like virus was recovered in TH-1 cells and chicken embryo fibroblasts from the tissues of several Hermann's

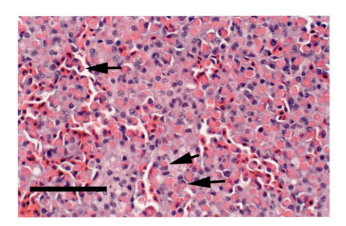

FIGURE 24-6 Spleen of Flap-necked Chameleon *(Chamaeleo dilepis)*. Note the multiple histiocytes and erythrocytes with intracytoplasmic eosinophilic inclusions. Hematoxylin and eosin; bar = 170 μm. *(Photograph courtesy M.M. Garner, Northwest ZooPath.)*

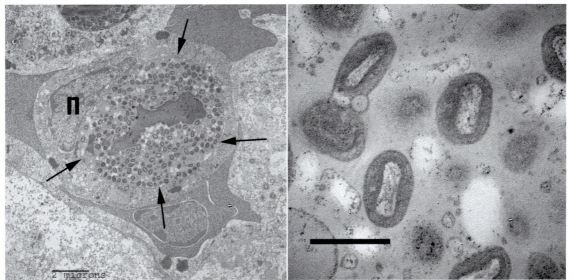

FIGURE 24-7 A, Spleen of a Flap-necked Chameleon *(Chamaeleo dilepis)*. Nucleus *(n)* of a macrophage in splenic sinusoid displaced by intranuclear inclusion *(arrows)* composed of numerous viral particles and some central electron-dense material. Uranyl acetate and lead citrate; bar = 2 μm. **B,** Higher magnification of viral particles from inclusion in **A,** showing elongated particles with a dumbbell-shaped core, typical of poxvirus. Uranyl acetate and lead citrate; bar = 300 nm. *(Photographs courtesy M.M. Garner, Northwest ZooPath.)*

Tortoises with stomatitis lesions similar to those associated with herpesvirus infection.[21] Iridovirus-like particles of undetermined clinical importance were detected with electron microscopy in a Spur-tailed Tortoise.[141] Iridovirus was implicated as the cause of upper respiratory disease in a free-ranging Gopher Tortoise from Florida.[142] Basophilia has been reported in some turtles with iridovirus infections.[143]

Iridovirus was recovered from a moribund Box Turtle (*Terapene carolina*). This isolate and one from a Hermann's Tortoise were antigenically related to frog virus 3, the type-specific genus of *Ranavirus*.[144] Some ranaviruses have been shown to infect both fishes and frogs, suggesting the possibility of cross transmission.[145] Virus particles morphologically consistent with iridovirus were found within intranuclear inclusion bodies of circulating red blood cells collected from Geckos (*Gehyra variegata*).[146] Similar intracytoplasmic inclusions were found in the erythrocytes of *Chamaeleo* spp. in Tanzania.[147] Infection was suggested to be associated with anemia, but inclusion bodies seem to be common in the circulating red blood cells of some clinically normal free-ranging reptiles.

An iridovirus has been implicated as the cause of edema and subcutaneous hemorrhage in tadpoles and metamorphosing froglets. Infections are subclinical in adult anurans but fatal in young. Intranuclear inclusion bodies can be detected within erythrocytes. Affected animals frequently have secondary bacterial infections.[148] This virus may be responsible for reducing populations of free-ranging frogs in Australia.[149]

A PCR-based assay has been developed that can be used to detect target segments of iridovirus nucleic acid in frogs and turtles.[144]

PARVOVIRIDAE

Parvoviruses are 18-nm to 26-nm nonenveloped virions that replicate in the nucleus of rapidly dividing cells and produce large intranuclear inclusion bodies. Depending on the genus of virus, replication may occur autonomously or a helper virus (usually an adenovirus or herpesvirus) may be required. The progression of disease is linked with its requirement for rapidly growing cells in which to replicate. The rapidly dividing cells that line the intestinal tract are the principal site of parvovirus replication and disease.[1]

Clinical Features

To date, all reptiles with parvoviruses have had concomitant infections with other viruses, particularly adenovirus and herpesvirus.[3,69,150] Virus particles with morphologic characteristics suggestive of parvovirus have been suggested as a cause of diarrhea in colubrids.[3]

In juvenile California Mountain Kingsnakes, coinfection with an adenovirus and dependovirus was associated with severe acute gastroenteritis.[151] Individually housed, 6-week-old captive-raised snakes began regurgitating, followed by dehydration and death within 48 to 72 hours. Seven of eight at-risk young died within 2 weeks of the index case, and other snakes, including the parents, that were housed in the same room remained unaffected. The affected snakes had been fed wild-caught Western Fence Lizards (*Sceloporus occidentalis*), which were considered a possible, but unproven, source of the viruses.[151]

The pyloric region and small intestines of affected snakes were dilated and partially filled with pasty yellow digesta. Multifocal petechial hemorrhages were evident on the serosa of the gastrointestinal tract. Microscopic changes included edema of the intestinal mucosa, segmental mucosal necrosis, crypt distention with sloughed enterocytes and degenerative heterophils, hyperplasia, and villus blunting. Basophilic Cowdry type A intranuclear inclusions were found in occasional enterocytes, peripheral to areas of mucosal necrosis. Viruses morphologically consistent with adenovirus (65 to 70 nanometers nonenveloped) and parvovirus (15 to 18 nanometers nonenveloped) were found with electron microscopy in affected cells.[151]

Adenovirus and dependovirus infections were documented in a group of four young Bearded Dragons that originated from two different locations. Intranuclear inclusion bodies were documented in the liver of one dragon and in the mucosa of the small intestines in the other.[69]

Parvoviruses are resistant to many common disinfectants and to a pH range of 3 to 9. They are heat stable at 37°C for 1 hour, 56°C for 30 minutes to 3 hours, and 60°C for 10 to 30 minutes.[1] Formalin and oxidizing agents (sodium hypochlorite and stabilized chlorine dioxide) inactivate the parvoviruses that have been studied. A solution of 0.5% formaldehyde destroys the virus in 15 minutes. In mammals, parvoviral-associated disease is best prevented through vaccination.[1]

TOGAVIRUSES AND FLAVIVIRUSES

Historically, the term *arbovirus* has been used (without regard for taxonomic classification) to describe any virus that is transmitted in nature by an arthropod vector. Hundreds of viruses, principally within the families Togaviridae, Flaviviridae, Reoviridae, Rhabdoviridae, and Bunyaviridae, can be transmitted from host to host by arthropods.[152] Many of the viruses within the Togaviridae and Flaviviridae families can cause encephalitis in humans and birds. Reptiles have been implicated in the maintenance and transmission of many of these viruses including Western equine encephalomyelitis (WEE), Eastern equine encephalomyelitis (EEE), Venezuelan equine encephalomyelitis (VEE), and West Nile viruses (WNV).[1,153]

Characteristically, animals involved in the transmission of arboviruses have a high level of viremia develop that provides an opportunity for insects that feed on blood to ingest the virus with a blood meal. The ingested virus then replicates inside the insect and is transmitted to a new host when the infected insect bites a susceptible host.

In birds, togaviruses and flaviviruses typically cause subclinical infections in species native to an area where the virus naturally occurs. The apparent resistance to disease exhibited by indigenous birds is thought to be the result of centuries of natural selection in which native birds have coevolved with these viruses and now function as reservoirs. In some non-native bird species, these viruses have been associated with encephalitis or enteritis.[1] A similar adaptation to infection probably occurs in reptiles. Reptiles have been shown to be naturally and experimentally susceptible to EEE, WEE, and Japanese encephalitis (JE) viruses.[32,154-156] One summary report suggested serologic evidence of togavirus infections in 25 species of snakes, 14 lizards, 12 turtles, and one crocodilian. Infected species originate from North and South America, Europe, Asia, and Australia.[32]

Togaviruses have been recovered from the blood of subclinical tortoises in Texas.[157] Ticks that transmit the flavivirus responsible for transmitting Russian spring-summer encephalitis have been recovered from reptiles in Europe and Asia. California black-legged ticks (Ixodes sp.) have been recovered from lizards and snakes from the Pacific regions of North America. This genus of ticks has been linked to transmission of European tick-borne encephalitis.[158] Western equine encephalitis virus was recovered from the blood of 34 of 84 snakes (44%) collected in Utah in May and July, before seasonal mosquito activity, which suggests the virus overwintered in the snakes. Virus was isolated from Gartersnakes (Thamnophis spp.), Gophersnakes (Pituophis catenifer), and Blue Racers (Coluber constrictor). Snakes born in captivity to wild-caught mothers had positive results, which suggests vertical transmission and maintenance of the virus.[159] Viremia in snakes appears to be cyclic with temperature changes. Culex tarsalis became infected when allowed to feed on naturally infected snakes.[154-157]

In experimental infections in multiple species of snakes and turtles, approximately 50% were susceptible to EEE virus infection, with gartersnakes particularly susceptible. One gartersnake and three Spotted Turtles (Clemmys guttata) inoculated and maintained in hibernation conditions maintained viremia for more than 6 months.[156] Gartersnakes naturally infected with WEE through mosquito exposure had viremia develop that lasted up to 36 days.[155]

Reptiles may serve as a reservoir for the overwintering of WEE, EEE, and VEE viruses.[153-156,159] In one study, posthibernation viremia was shown to persist up to 70 days.[155] The interval from inoculation to infection was found to be the most important factor in development of postbrumation viremia. Snakes that entered brumation (hibernation) 11 days after infection with WEE virus were viremic after brumation, and those that were brumated 19 days after infection were not viremic.[159] In a Canadian study, WEE virus was recovered from the blood of snakes (Thamnophis sp.) and frogs (Rana pipiens).[160] Reptiles housed outdoors and those exposed to vector mosquitos could be infected and potentially serve as a reservoir. One might consider moving reptiles indoors during seasonal increases in mosquito and virus activity.

The serologic response to EEE or WEE viruses in reptiles has been insufficiently studied. Birds that survive EEE and WEE virus infections become solidly immune and have HI, complement-fixation, and virus-neutralizing antibodies develop. The viremia that is associated with EEE virus infections ceases rapidly after the production of antibodies. Antibodies may be detected as soon as 5 days to 2 weeks after infection in gallinaceous and passerine birds.[161-162] Complement fixation and HI antibodies may persist for several weeks to months, and virus-neutralizing antibodies may persist for months to years after natural or experimental infections.[1] Serologic activity has been documented in free-ranging reptiles.[154-157,159]

Active or recent alphavirus infections can be diagnosed with finding of rising antibody levels in paired serum samples, complement fixation, HI, agar-gel immunodiffusion, or virus-neutralizing assays.

Alphaviruses are unstable outside of the host and are easiest to recover from fresh blood, liver, and spleen. Most disinfectants are expected to inactivate these viruses rapidly. Inactivated vaccines licensed for use in horses have been used successfully in birds, but no correlative studies in reptiles have been found.[1]

West Nile virus was linked to an outbreak of CNS disease in a group of farmed alligators (Alligator mississippiensis) in Florida.[163] The first cases were noted in October in 1-m-long yearlings. Approximately 300 of 9000 animals died during September and October of 2002. Clinical changes included depression, lethargy, and signs of neurologic disease. Three affected animals were necropsied, and gross changes included mild coelomic effusion, fibrinonecrotic oral mucosal exudate, and enlarged pale livers with red mottling. The most significant microscopic lesions were a moderate heterophilic to lymphoplasmacytic meningoencephalomyelitis, necrotizing hepatitis and splenitis, myocardial degeneration with necrosis, mild interstitial pneumonia, hepatic lipidosis, adrenalitis, heterophilic necrotizing stomatitis, and glossitis.[163] West Nile virus was recovered from neural tissues, and viral nucleic acid was found with a PCR-based assay. Immunoperoxidase staining with monoclonal antibodies confirmed the presence of West Nile virus proteins in diseased tissues. Viremia was documented in tested animals, and alligators were suggested to serve as an amplification host for the virus.[163]

CALICIVIRUS

Caliciviruses that were antigenically indistinguishable were recovered from both subclinical and clinically affected Aruba Island Rattlesnakes (Crotalus unicolor) and from clinically affected Bell's Horned Frogs (Ceratophrys ornata), a Rock Rattlesnake, and an Eyelash Viper maintained in a zoologic collection.[164] The viruses recovered from these animals were designated reptilian calicivirus Crotalus type 1. The calicivirus was recovered in Vero cells from animals with a high mortality rate associated with enteritis and hepatitis. However, the isolated virus was not definitively associated with any particular disease. Virus was recovered from cloacal swabs of clinically normal animals and from small intestines, liver, and kidney of animals seen for postmortem examination. One of two experimentally infected Rattlesnakes (C. viridis helleri) died 61 days after inoculation. Experimentally infected pigs remained clinically normal but seroconverted, as did contact controls. A chronically infected reptile suspected to be shedding virus in the feces was responsible for introducing the virus to the index collection. Keepers were implicated as mechanical vectors.[164]

PAPOVAVIRIDAE

The Papovaviridae family of viruses consists of two subfamilies, Papillomavirinae and Polyomavirinae, which vary in virion size and biologic features and in genome size and organization.[1] Viruses in the Papillomavirinae subfamily are generally associated with the formation of benign skin tumors commonly referred to as papillomas (warts). Papillomaviruses have been identified in a wide variety of animals, including reptiles, birds, and mammals. These viruses tend to be highly host-specific.

Only a few of the human papillomaviruses have been replicated in cell culture, but other advanced techniques have been used to study these viruses. The characteristics and pathobiology of papillomaviruses in mammals and birds have been determined principally with molecular biology evaluation techniques (sequencing, cloning, and hybridization) with viral nucleic acid derived from infected tissues.[1]

Clinical Features

Papillomavirus-associated skin lesions have been documented in Bolivian Side-neck Turtles (*Platemys platycephala*) and European Green Lizards.[35,72,165] Papillomas in European Green Lizards were characterized by firm, gray to black, 2-mm to 20-mm proliferative masses that were most common on the base of tail of females and neck of males (see Figure 15-45).[35] Severely affected lizards had lesions that involved most of the dorsum. Lizards with mild or early cases were generally subclinical, and anorexia, lethargy, and death occurred in lizards with more chronic changes. Interestingly, lesions were not reported on the ventral scales of any affected lizards. Viruses with characteristics consistent with herpesvirus and reovirus have also been detected in papillomatous lesions on European Green Lizards.[35]

In Bolivian Side-neck Turtles, papillomatous lesions are typified by flat, white, oval skin lesions that can be focal or coalesce into patches. Lesions were particularly common on the head of affected turtles. Early lesions on the plastron appeared similar to those on the head but were prone to ulceration and secondary infections.[165]

Papillomatous growths of undetermined cause have been reported around the eyes of iguanas.[72] Papillomavirus-like particles were detected with electron microscopy in a lung wash from a Horsfield's Tortoise (*Testudo horsfieldi*) with stomatitis.[19]

Transmission

In other species, papillomaviruses are transmitted with direct or indirect contact with epithelium. Although unconfirmed in lizards, biting activities focused on the tail base of females and neck of males are theorized to be involved in virus transmission.[35] Because the incubation period in reptiles is unknown, determination of when, where, and how an affected reptile was infected by a papillomavirus is usually difficult.

Pathology

The microscopic changes associated with papillomas in reptiles are similar to those in other species and include a thickened stratum corneum with hyperplastic, acanthotic epidermis (see Figure 15-45). Nuclei are typically vacuolated and enlarged with peripheral margination of chromatin. Intranuclear inclusion bodies were described in the hyperkeratotic, hyperplastic epidermal cells in tissues of European Green Lizards.[35]

Immunity and Diagnosis

Most papillomas are raised, but papillomavirus infections should be considered with flat, proliferative, discolored lesions that cannot be linked to bacterial or fungal causes and that do not respond to antimicrobials.[29] Confirmation that suspicious lesions are caused by a papillomavirus requires electron microscopic examination of affected tissues to find the 45-nm to 50-nm virus particles that are commonly contained in intranuclear inclusion bodies.[1]

Control and Treatment

Generally, papillomas on the skin of birds and mammals need no treatment unless they cause specific problems. Some lesions can be debilitating if they are damaged, allowing secondary infections to occur; if they inhibit an animal's ability to move; or if they interfere with grasping or chewing food. Mild lesions can be observed for changes that necessitate their removal. Severe lesions should be radiosurgically or laser removed to make the patient more comfortable and treated with appropriate antimicrobials to prevent secondary infections. However, lesions that are surgically removed usually recur.

In humans, isolated lesions usually respond to prolonged treatment with salicylic acid, and this therapy may prove helpful in reptiles. Affected animals should be isolated during treatment, and at least a 6-month quarantine period should be used to help prevent the introduction of an infected animal to a collection.

In some mammals, the use of autogenous vaccines has been shown to be effective in stimulating an immune response that results in cessation of clinical lesions. Whether an autogenous vaccine is effective in treatment of papillomavirus-induced skin lesions in reptiles has not been determined.

OTHER VIRUSES

Antigenically distinct viruses with morphologic characteristics consistent with rhabdovirus were isolated from *Ameiva ameiva* lizards. The potential pathogenicity of this virus has not been reported.[32]

DISEASE OF PROBABLY VIRAL ETIOLOGY

Gross lesions in a group of affected *Morelia* sp. included pale livers and gaseous distention of the proximal small intestines. Gliosis was the most consistent microscopic lesion, with intranuclear eosinophilic to amphophilic inclusions in glial cells. Multiple areas of coalescing vacuolar change in the brain were most severe between the white and gray matter (Figure 24-8).

One Carpet Python (*Morelia* sp.) had epicardial, mesenteric, and facial ganglioneuritis. Two pythons had mild lymphocytic myocarditis, and one had pulmonary lymphofollicular hyperplasia and nonsupportive interstitial pneumonia.[115]

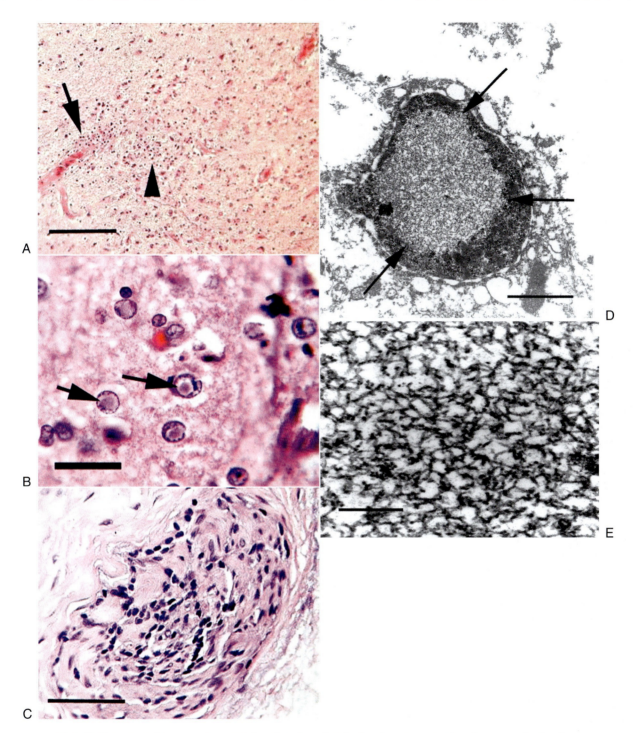

FIGURE 24-8 **A,** Midbrain of a Carpet Python (*Morelia* sp.). Note the gliosis *(arrowhead)* and perivascular lymphoid cuff *(arrow)*. Hematoxylin and eosin (H&E); bar = 380 μm. **B,** Midbrain of a Carpet Python. Note intranuclear inclusions *(arrows)* in glial cells. H&E; bar = 25 μm. **C,** Myenteric ganglion of a Carpet Python. Note the lymphocytic inflammation within the ganglion. H&E; bar = 225 μm. **D,** Glial cell from the midbrain region of a Carpet Python. Note the intranuclear inclusion *(arrows)* composed of filamentous material. Uranyl acetate and lead citrate; bar = 3.5 μm. **E,** Glial cell from the midbrain region of a Carpet Python. Note reticular pattern of filamentous material. Uranyl acetate and lead citrate; bar = 300 nm. *(Photographs courtesy M.M. Garner, Northwest ZooPath.)*

SUMMARY

Although thorough research data are lacking for many reptilian viruses, the reality is that these animals are highly susceptible to viral disease. Because of the omnipresent problems associated with hygiene and nutrition of captive reptiles and the resultant immunosuppression, viruses continue to be a threat.

Proper husbandry, appropriate nutrition, physical screening, and quarantine procedures are still the best ways to prevent viral disease. For a summary of reptilian viruses, see the Appendix A.

REFERENCES

1. Ritchie BW: *Avian viruses: function and control*, Lakeworth, Fla, 1995, Wingers Publishing.
2. Posthaus H, Marschang RE, Gravendyck M, et al: Study on herpesvirus infections in land tortoises in Switzerland, *Proc Am Assoc Zoo Vets* 17, 1997.
3. Heldstab A, Bestetti G: Virus-associated gastrointestinal disease in snakes, *J Zoo Anim Med* 15:118, 1984.
4. Jacobson ER, Clubb SL, Gaskin JM: Herpesvirus-like infection in Argentine tortoises, *J Am Vet Med Assoc* 187:1227, 1985.
5. Jacobson ER, Gaskin JM, Roelke M, et al: Conjunctivitis, tracheitis, and pneumonia associated with herpesvirus infection in green sea turtles, *J Am Vet Med Assoc* 189:1020, 1986.
6. Jacobson ER, Buergelt C, Williams B, et al: Herpesvirus in cutaneous fibropapillomas of the green sea turtle *Chelonia mydas*, *Dis Aquatic Organ* 12:1, 1991.
7. Jacobson ER, Gaskin JM, Wahlquist H: Herpesvirus-like infection in map turtles, *J Am Vet Med Assoc* 181:1322, 1982.
8. Jacobson ER: Venom gland herpesvirus infection of snakes, *Proc Assoc Rept Amphib Vet* 93, 2000.
9. Jacobson ER: Causes of mortality and diseases in tortoises: a review, *J Zoo Wildl Dis* 25:2, 1994.
10. Barten SL: Infectious diseases in reptile patients, *Proc North Am Vet Conf* 923, 2000.
11. Harper PAW, Hammond DC, Heuschele WP: A herpes-like agent associated with a pharyngeal abscess in a desert tortoise, *J Wildl Dis* 18:441, 1982.
12. Pettan-Brewer KC, Drew ML, Ramsay E, et al: Herpesvirus particles associated with oral and respiratory lesions in a California desert tortoise *(Gopherus agassizii)*, *J Wildl Dis* 32:521, 1996.
13. Marschang RE: Evidence for a new herpesvirus serotype associated with stomatitis in Afghan tortoises, *Testudo horsfieldi*, *Proc Assoc Rept Amphib Vet* 77, 1999.
14. Cooper JE, Gheschmeissner S, Bone RD: Herpes-like virus particles in necrotic stomatitis of tortoises, *Vet Rec* 123:554, 1988.
15. Heldstab A, Bestetti G: Herpesviridae causing glossitis and meningoencephalitis in land tortoises *(Testudo hermanni)*, *Herpetopathologia* 1:5, 1976.
16. Schumacher J: Respiratory diseases of reptiles, *Sem Avian Exotic Pet Med* 6(4):209, 1997.
17. Origgi F, Jacobson ER, Romero CH, et al: Diagnostic tools for herpesvirus detection in chelonians, *Proc Assoc Rept Amphib Vet* 127, 2000.
18. Drury SEN, Gough RE, McArthur S, et al: Detection of herpesvirus-like and papillomavirus associated disease of tortoises, *Vet Rec* 143:639, 1998.
19. Drury SE, Gough RE, McArthur SDJ: Isolation and identification of herpesvirus and papillomavirus from tortoises in Great Britain, *Proc Assoc Reptil Amphib Vets* 69, 1999.
20. Teifke JP, Lohr V, Marschang RE, et al: Detection of chelonid herpesvirus DNA by nonradioactive in situ hybridization in tissues from tortoises suffering from stomatitis-rhinitis complex in Europe and North America, *Vet Pathol* 37:377, 2000.
21. Marschang RE, Posthaus H, Gravendyck M, et al: Isolation of viruses from land tortoises in Switzerland, *Proc Am Assoc Zoo Vets* 281, 1998.
22. Frye FL, Oshiro LS, Dutra RF, et al: Herpesvirus-like infection in two Pacific pond turtles, *J Am Vet Med Assoc* 171:882, 1977.
23. Lucke B: *Studies on tumors in cold-blooded vertebrates*, Washington, DC, 1937-1938, Annu Rep Tortugas Laboratory Carnegie Institute.
24. Rebell H, Rywlin A, Haines H: A herpesvirus-type agent associated with skin lesions of green sea turtles in aquaculture, *Am J Vet Res* 36:1221, 1975.
25. Jacobson ER: Diseases of the integumentary system of reptiles. In Nesbitt GH, Ackerman LJ, editors: *Dermatology for the small animal practitioner*, Lawrenceville, NJ, 1991, Vet Learning Systems.
26. Jacobson ER, Mansell JL, Sundberg JP, et al: Cutaneous fibropapillomas of green turtles, *J Comp Path* 101:39, 1989.
27. Haines HG, Rywlin A, Rebell G: A herpesvirus disease of formed green sea turtles *(Chelonia mydas)*, *Proc World Mariculture* 5:183, 1974.
28. Hauser B, Mettler F, Rubel A: Herpesvirus-like infection in two young boas, *J Comp Pathol* 93:515, 1983.
29. Schumacher J: Viral diseases. In Mader DR, editor: *Reptile medicine and surgery*, Philadelphia, 1996, WB Saunders.
30. Monroe JH, Shibley GP, Schidlovsky T: Action of snake venom on Rauscher virus, *J Natl Cancer Inst* 40:135, 1968.
31. Simpson CF, Jacobson ER, Gaskin JM: Herpesvirus-like infection of the venom gland of Siamese cobras, *J Am Vet Med Assoc* 175:941, 1979.
32. Clark HF, Lunger PD: Viruses. In Cooper JE, Jackson OF, editors: *Diseases of the Reptilia*, New York, 1981, Academic Press.
33. Hoff GL, Frye FL, Jacobson ER, editors: *Diseases of amphibians and reptiles*, New York, 1984, Plenum Press.
34. Watson GL: Herpesvirus in red-headed (common) agamas *(Agama agama)*, *J Vet Diagn Invest* 5:444, 1993.
35. Raynaud A, Adrian M: Lesions cutanees a structure papillomateuse associees a des virus chez le lezard vert (Lacerta viridis Laur), *CR Acad Sci Paris* 283:845, 1976.
36. Heldstab A, Bestelli G: Spontaneous viral hepatitis in a spur-tailed Mediterranean land tortoise *(Testudo hermanni)*, *J Zoo Anim Med* 13:113, 1982.
37. Oettle EE, Steyfler YGM, Williams MC: High mortality in a tortoise colony, *S Afr J Wild Res* 20(1):21, 1990.
38. Herbst LH: Fibropapillomatosis of marine turtles, *Annu Rev Fish Dis* 4:389, 1994.
39. Balazs GH: Current status of fibropapillomas in the Hawaiian green turtle, *Chleonia mydas*. In Balazs GH, Pooley SG, editors: *Research plan for marine turtle fibropapilloma*, 1991, US Dept Commer, NOAA Tech Memo NMFS-SWFSC-156.
40. Casey RN, Quackenbush SL, Work TW, et al: Evidence for retrovirus infections in green turtles *Chelonia mydas* from the Hawaiian Islands, *Dis Aquatic Org* 31:1, 1997.
41. Marschang RE, Gravendyk M, Kaleta EF: New investigations on herpesviruses in tortoises, *Verh ber Erkrg Zootiere* 38:29, 1997.
42. Marschang RE, Gravendyck M, Kaleta EF: Investigation into virus isolation and the treatment of viral stomatitis in *T. hermanni* and *T. graeca*, *J Vet Med Series B* 44(7):385, 1997.

43. Muller M, Sachsse W, Zangger N: Herpesvirus-epidemic bei der Griechschen *(Testudo hermanni)* and der Maurischen Landschildkrote *(Testudo graeca)* inder Schneiz, *Schneiz Arch Tierheilk* 132:199, 1990.
44. Herbst LH, Jacobson ER, Moretti R, et al: Experimental transmission of green turtle fibropapillomatosis using cell-free tumor extracts, *Dis Aquat Org* 22:1, 1995.
45. Lange H, Herbest W, Wiechart JM, et al: Elektronen mikos kopischer nachweis von herpesviren bei einem mussessterben von griechischen landschildkroten *(Testudo hermanni)* and vierzehenschildkroten, *Tieraztl Prax* 17:319, 1989.
46. McArthur SDJ: Lymphoproliferative disease in *Testudo hermanni* and *Geochelone pardalis* tortoises associated with herpesvirus-like infection, *Br Chelonia Group Testudo* 4(5):1998.
47. Cox WR, Rapley WA, Barker IK: Herpesvirus infection in a painted turtle, *J Wildl Dis* 16:445, 1980.
48. Gaskin JM: Psittacine viral disease: a perspective, *J Zoo Wildl Med* 20:249, 1989.
49. Hitchner SB, Calnek BW: Inactivated vaccine for parrot herpesvirus infection (Pacheco's disease), *Am J Vet Res* 41:1280, 1980.
50. Gaskin JM: The serodiagnosis of psittacine viral infections, *Proc Assoc Avian Vet* 7, 1988.
51. Frost JW, Schmidt A: Serological evidence of susceptibility of various species of tortoises to infections by herpesviruses, *Verh ber Erkrg Zootiere* 38:29, 1997.
52. Jacobson ER: Diagnosis of reptilian viral disease, *Proc Assoc Reptil Amphib Vet* 189, 2000.
53. Origgi FC, Jacobson ER: Development of an ELISA and an immunoperoxidase based test for herpesvirus exposure detection in tortoises, *Proc Assoc Reptil Amphib Vet* 65, 1999.
54. Lackovich JK, Brown DR, Homer BL, et al: Association of herpesvirus with fibropapillomatosis of the green turtle, *Chelonia mydas*, and the loggerhead turtle, *Caretta caretta*, in Florida, *Dis Aq Org* 37:89, 1999.
55. Padgett F, Levine AS: Fine structure of the Rauscher leukemia virus as revealed by incubation in a snake venom, *Virol* 30:623, 1966.
56. O'brien JJ, Campolin-Richards DM: Acyclovir: an updated review of its antiviral activity, pharmacokinetic properties, and therapeutic efficacy, *Drugs* 37:233, 1989.
57. Schumacher J, Jacobson ER, Burns R, et al: Adenovirus infection in two rosy boas *(Lichanura trivirgata)*, *J Zoo Wildl Med* 25:461, 1994.
58. McFerran JB, Conner TJ, McCraken RM: Isolation of adenoviruses and reoviruses from avian species other than domestic fowl, *Avian Dis* 20:519, 1976.
59. Perkins LEL, Campagnoli RP, Harmon BG, et al: Detection and confirmation of reptilian adenovirus infection by in situ hybridization, *J Vet Diagn Invest* 13:365, 2001.
60. Boyer TH, Garner MM, Jacobson ER: Intranuclear inclusion disorder in *Morelia* spp, *Proc Assoc Reptil Amphib Vet* 85, 2000.
61. Jacobson ER, Gaskin JM: Adenovirus-like infection in a boa constrictor, *J Am Vet Med Assoc* 187:1226, 1985.
62. Juhasz A, Ahne W: Physicochemical properties and cytopathogenicity of an adenovirus-like agent isolated from a corn snake *(Elaphe guttata)*, *Arch Virol* 130:429, 1992.
63. Ogawa M, Ahne W, Essbauer S: Reptilian viruses: adenovirus-like agent isolated from royal python *(Python regius)*, *J Vet Med Ser B* 39:732-736, 1992.
64. Ramis A, Fernandez-Bellon H, Majo N, et al: Adenovirus hepatitis in a boa constrictor *(Boa constrictor)*, *J Vet Diagn Invest* 12:573, 2000.
65. Wozniak EJ, DeNardo DF, Brewer A, et al: Identification of adenovirus- and dependovirus-like agents in an outbreak of fatal gastroenteritis in captive born California Mountain kingsnakes, *Lampropeltis zonata multicincta*, *J Herp Med Surg* 10:4, 2000.
66. Julian AF, Durham JK: Adenoviral hepatitis in a bearded dragon *(Amphibolurus barbatus)*, *N Z Vet J* 30:59, 1985.
67. Frye FL, Munn RJ, Gardner M, et al: Adenovirus-like hepatitis in a group of related Rankin's dragon lizards *(Pogona henrylawsoni)*, *J Zoo Wildl Med* 25:167, 1994.
68. Jacobson ER, Kollias GV: Adenovirus-like infection in a savannah monitor, *J Zoo Anim Med* 17:149, 1986.
69. Jacobson ER, Kopit W, Kennedy FA, et al: Coinfection of a bearded dragon, *Pogona vitticeps*, with adenovirus- and dependovirus-like viruses, *Vet Pathol* 33:343, 1996.
70. Stahl SJ: Update on diseases of bearded dragons *(Pogona vitticeps)*, *Proc North Am Vet Conf* 822, 2001.
71. Jacobson ER, Gardiner CH: Adeno-like virus in esophageal and tracheal mucosa of a Jackson's Chameleon *(Chamaeleo jacksonii)*, *Vet Pathol* 27:210, 1990.
72. Benyon PH, Lawton MP, Cooper JE, editors: *Manual of reptiles*, Gloucestershire, England, 1992, British Small Animal Vet Assoc.
73. Kinsel MJ, Barbiers RB, Manharth A, et al: Small intestinal adeno-like virus in a mountain chameleon *(Chameleo montium)*, *J Zoo Wildl Med* 28:498, 1997.
74. Jacobson ER, Gardiner CH, Foggin CM: Adenovirus-like infection two Nile crocodiles, *J Am Vet Med Assoc* 185:1421, 1984.
75. McFerran JB, McNulty MS: *Virus infections of birds*, London, 1993, Elsevier Science Publishers.
76. Takase N, Yoshinaga N, Egashira T, et al: Avian adenovirus isolated from pigeons affected with inclusion body hepatitis, *Jpn J Vet Sci* 52:207, 1990.
77. McFerran JB: Adenovirus infections. In Calnek BW, et al, editors: *Diseases of poultry*, ed 9, Ames, 1991, Iowa State University Press.
78. Lowenstine LJ, Fry M: Adenovirus-like particles associated with intranuclear inclusion bodies in the kidney of a common mure *(Uria aalge)*, *Avian Dis* 29:208, 1985.
79. Mori F, Touchi A, Suwa T, et al: Inclusion bodies containing adenovirus-like particles in the kidneys of psittacine birds, *Avian Pathol* 18:197, 1989.
80. Ward JM, Young DM: Latent adenoviral infections of rats: intranuclear inclusions induced by treatment with a cancer chemotherapeutic agent, *J Am Vet Med Assoc* 169:952, 1976.
81. McFerran JB: Immunity to adenoviruses. In Rose ME, et al, editors: *Avian immunology*, Edinburgh, 1981, British Poultry Science.
82. Grimes TN, King PJ: Effect of maternal antibody on experimental infections of chickens with a type 8 avian adenovirus, *Avian Dis* 21:97, 1977.
83. Jacobson ER, Flanagan JP, Rideout B, et al: Ophidian paramyxovirus, *Bull Assoc Rept Amphib Vet* 9(1):15, 1999.
84. Foelsch DW, Heloup P: Fatale endemische infection in eineum serpentorium, *Tieraerzth* 4:527, 1976.
85. Jacobson ER, Gaskin JM, Page D, et al: Illness associated with paramyxo-like virus infection in zoologic collections of snakes, *J Am Vet Med Assoc* 179:1227, 1981.
86. Ahne W, Neubert WJ, Thomson I: Reptilian viruses: isolation of myxovirus-like particles from the snake *Elaphe oxycephala*, *J Vet Med* 34:607, 1987.
87. Jacobson ER: Viruses. In Fowler ME, editor: *Zoo and wild animal medicine*, Philadelphia, 1993, WB Saunders.
88. Clarke HF, Lief FS, Lunger PD, et al: Fer-de-Lance virus: a probable paramyxovirus isolated from a reptile, *J Gen Virol* 44:405, 1979.
89. Jacobson ER, Gaskin JM, Simpson CF, et al: Paramyxo-like virus infection in a rock rattlesnake, *J Am Vet Med Assoc* 177:796, 1980.
90. Cranfield MR, Ialeggio DM, O'Donnell D: Ophidian paramyxovirus, *Proc Avian Exotic Symp*, 1991, Davis, CA.

91. Cranfield MR, Graczyk TK: Ophidian paramyxovirus. In Mader DR, editor: *Reptile medicine and surgery*, Philadelphia, 1996, WB Saunders.
92. Lloyd ML, Flanagan J: Recent developments in ophidian paramyxovirus research and recommendations on control, *Proc Am Assoc Zoo Vet* 151, 1991.
93. Jacobson ER, Gaskin J: Paramyxo-like virus associated respiratory disease of viperid snakes, *Proc Assoc Zoo Vet* 17, 1981.
94. Potgieter LND, Sigler RE, Russell RG: Pneumonia in Ottoman vipers *(Vipera xanthena xanthena)* associated with a parainfluenza 2-like virus, *J Wildl Dis* 23:355, 1987.
95. Ahne W, Batts WN, Jurath G, et al: Comparative sequence analysis of sixteen reptilian paramyxoviruses, *Virus Res* 63:65, 1999.
96. Jacobson ER, Adams HP, Geisbert TW, et al: Pulmonary lesions in experimental ophidian paramyxovirus pneumonia of Aruba Island rattlesnakes, *Crotalus unicolor*, *Vet Pathol* 34:450, 1997.
97. Jacobson ER, Gaskin J, Wells S, et al: Epizootic of ophidian paramyxovirus in a zoological collection: pathological, microbiological and serological findings, *J Zoo Wildl Med* 23:318, 1992.
98. Sand MA, Smith KG, Gregory CR, et al: *Paramyxovirus infection in snakes*, at www.vet.uga.edu/vpp/Undergrad/Sand/.
99. Homer BL, Sandberg JP, Gaskin JM, et al: Immunoperoxidase detection of ophidian paramyxovirus in lungs using a polyclonal antibody, *J Vet Diag Invest* 7:72-77, 1995.
100. Gaskin JM, Haskell M, Keller N, et al: Serodiagnosis of ophidian paramyxovirus infections, *Proc Third Int Colloq Pathol Rept Amphib* 21, 1989.
101. Rossi JV: Emergency medicine of reptiles, *Proc North Am Vet Conf* 799, 1998.
102. Gerlach H: Viruses. In Ritchie BW, et al, editors: *Avian medicine: principles and application*, Lake Worth, 1996, Wingers Publishing.
103. Boyd RJ, Hanson RP: Survival of Newcastle disease virus in nature, *Avian Dis* 2:82, 1958.
104. Moses HE, Barndly CA, Jones EE: The pH stability of the viruses of Newcastle disease and fowl plague, *Science* 105:477, 1947.
105. Olesink OM: Influence of environmental factors on viability of Newcastle disease virus, *Am J Vet Res* 12:152, 1951.
106. Jacobson ER, Gaskin JM, Flanagan JP, et al: Antibody responses of western diamondback rattlesnakes *(Crotalus atrox)* to inactivated ophidian paramyxovirus vaccines, *J Zoo Wildl Med* 22:184, 1991.
107. Jacobson ER, Origgi F, Pessier AP, et al: Paramyxo-like virus infection in caiman lizards, *Draecena guianensis*, *Proc Assoc Reptil Amphib Vet* 59, 2000.
108. Payne LN, Purchase HG: Leukosis/aracoma group. In Calnek BW, et al, editors: *Diseases of poultry*, ed 9, Ames, 1991, Iowa State University Press.
109. Jacobson ER, Klingenberg RJ, Homer BL, et al: Inclusion body disease, *Bull Assoc Rept Amphib Vet* 9(2):18, 1999.
110. Schumacher J, Jacobson ER, Homer BL, et al: Inclusion body disease in boid snakes, *J Zoo Wildl Med* 25:511, 1994.
111. Axthelm MK: Clinicopathologic and virologic observations of a probable viral disease affecting boid snakes, *Proc Assoc Zoo Vet* 108, 1985.
112. Wright K: Dysecdysis in boid snakes with neurologic diseases, *Bull Assoc Reptil Amphib Vet* 2:7, 1992.
113. Frye FL: *Biomedical and surgical aspects of captive reptile husbandry*, ed 2, Melbourne, Fla, 1991, Krieger Publishing.
114. Jacobson ER, Oros J, Tucker SJ, et al: Partial characterization of retroviruses from boid snakes with inclusion body disease, *Am J Vet Res* 62:217, 2001.
115. Boyer TH, Garner MM, Jacobson ER: Intranuclear inclusion disorder in *Morelia* spp, *Proc Assoc Reptil Amphib Vet* 85, 2000.
116. Garner MM, Raymond JT, Nordhausen RW, et al: Inclusion body disease in captive palm vipers, *Bothriechis marchi*, *Proc Assoc Reptil Amphib Vet* 95, 2000.
117. Carlisle-Nowak MS, Sullivan N, Carrigan M, et al: Inclusion body disease in two captive Australian pythons *(Morelia spilota variegata* and *Morelia spilota spilota)*, *Aust Vet J* 76:98, 1998.
118. Oros J, Tucker S, Jacobson ER: Inclusion body disease in two captive boas in the Canary Islands, *Vet Rec* 143:283, 1998.
119. Carneiro SM, Tanaka H, Kisielius JJ, et al: Occurrence of retrovirus-like particles in various cellular and intracellular compartments of the venom glands from *Bothrops jararacussu*, *Res Vet Sci* 53:399, 1992.
120. Zeigel RF, Clark HF: Electron microscopic observations on a C-type virus in cell cultures derived from a tumor-bearing viper, *J Natl Cancer Inst* 43:1097, 1969.
121. Jacobson ER, Calderwood WB, French TW, et al: Lymphosarcoma in an Eastern kingsnake and a rhinoceros viper, *J Am Vet Med Assoc* 179:1231, 1981.
122. Lunger PD, Hardy WD, Clark HF: C-type particles in a reptilian tumor, *J Natl Cancer Institute* 52:1231, 1974.
123. Hardy WD, McClelland AJ: Oncogenic RNA viral infections. In Steele JH, editor: *CRC handbook series in zoonoses*, vol II, Cleveland, 1981, CRC Press.
124. Konstantinov A, Ippen R. Erythroleukosis with presence of virus particles in two boa constrictors, *Proc Int Colloquim Pathol Rept Amphib* 123, 1982.
125. Zshiesche W: Lymphoid leukemia with presence of C virus particles in a four-lined chicken snake: *Elaphe obsoleta quadrivittata*, *Verh Int Symp Erkrank Zoot* 30:275, 1988.
126. Chandra AMS, Jacobson ER, Munn RJ: Retroviral particles in neoplasms of Burmese pythons *(Python molurus bivittatus)*, *Vet Pathol* 38:561, 2001.
127. Tristem MT, Myles T, Hill F: A highly divergent retroviral sequence in a tuatara *(Sphenodon)*, *Virol* 210:206, 1995.
128. Crittenden LB, Astrin SM: Genes, viruses and avian leukosis, *Bioscience* 31:305, 1981.
129. Jacobson ER, Tucker S, Oros J, et al: Studies with retroviruses isolated from Boa constrictors *(Boa constrictor)* with inclusion body disease, *Proc Assoc Reptil Amphib Vet* 5, 1999.
130. Jacobson ER: Viral diseases of reptiles: a review, *Proc Assoc Zoo Vet* 107, 1985.
131. Vieler E, Baumgartner W, Herbst W, et al: Characterization of a reovirus isolated from a rattlesnake, *Crotalus viridis*, with neurological dysfunction, *Arch Virol* 138:341, 1994.
132. Ahne W, Thomsen I, Winton J: Isolation of a reovirus from the snake *Python regius*, *Arch Virol* 94:135, 1987.
133. Jacobson ER, Popp JA, Shields RR, et al: Pox-like skin lesions in captive caimans, *J Am Vet Med Assoc* 175:937,1979.
134. Pandey GS, Inoue N, Ohshima K, et al: Poxvirus infection in Nile crocodiles *(Crocodylus niloticus)*, *Res Vet Sci* 49:171, 1990.
135. Horner RF: Poxvirus in farmed Nile crocodiles, *Vet Rec* 122:459, 1988.
136. Stauber E, Gogolewski R: Poxvirus dermatitis in a tegu lizard *(Tupinambis teguizin)*, *J Zoo Wildl Med* 21:228, 1990.
137. Jacobson ER Telford SR: Chlamydial and poxvirus infections of circulating monocytes of a flap-necked chameleon, *J Wildl Dis* 26:572, 1990.
138. Cunningham AA, et al: Unusual mortality associated with poxvirus-like particles in frogs *(Rana temporaria)*, *Vet Rec* 133:141, 1993.

139. Mueller M, Sachsse W, Zangger N: Epidemic herpesvirus infection in spur-tailed *(Testudo hermanni)* and spur-thighed Mediterranean land tortoises *(Testudo graeca)* in Switzerland, *Schweiz Arch Tierheilk* 132:199, 1990.
140. Heldstab A, Bestetti G: Spontaneous viral hepatitis in a spur-tailed Mediterranean land tortoise *(Testudo hermanni)*, *J Zoo Anim Med* 13:113, 1982.
141. Ahne W: Viruses of chelonia, *J Vet Med* 40:35, 1993.
142. Westhouse RA, Jacobson Er, Harris RK, et al: Respiratory and pharyngo-esophageal iridovirus infection in a gopher tortoise *(Gopherus polyphemus)*, *J Wildl Dis* 32:682-686, 1996.
143. Sypek J, Borysenko M: Reptiles. In Rowley AF, Ratcliffe NA, editors: *Vertebrate blood cells*, Cambridge, 1988, Cambridge University Press.
144. Moa J, Hedrick RP, Chinchar VG: Molecular characterization, sequence analysis, and taxonomic position of newly isolated fish iridoviruses, *Virology* 229:212, 1997.
145. Moody NJG, Owens L: Experimental demonstration of the pathogenicity of a frog virus, Bohle iridovirus, for a fish species, barramundi, *Lates calcarifer*, *Dis Aquat Org* 18:95, 1994.
146. Stehbens WE, Johnson MRL: The viral nature of *Pirhemacyton tarentolae*, *J Ultrastruct Res* 15:543, 1966.
147. Telford SR, Jacobson ER: Lizard erythrocytic virus in east African chamaeleons, *J Wildl Dis* 1993.
148. Gruia-Gray J, Desser SS: Cytopathologic observations and epizootiology of frog erythrocytic virus in bullfrogs *(Rana catesbeiana)*, *J Wildl Dis* 28:34, 1992.
149. Green DE: Are virus infections contributing to amphibian declines? *Frog Log* 9:3, 1994.
150. Kim DY, Bauer RW, Poston R: Adenovirus-like virus and dependovirus infection in hatchling bearded dragons, *CL Davis Foundation Southcentral Division*, Galveston, Tex, 10, 1999.
151. Wozniak EJ, DeNardo DF, Brewer A, et al: Identification of adenovirus- and dependovirus-like agents in an outbreak of fatal gastroenteritis in captive born California mountain kingsnakes, *Lampropeltis zonata multicincta*, *J Herp Med Surg* 10:4-7, 2000.
152. Karabatsos N: International catalogue of arboviruses 1985 including certain other viruses of vertebrates, *Am Soc Trop Med Hyg* 1985.
153. Karstad L: Arboviruses. In Davis JW et al, editors: *Infectious and parasitic diseases of wild birds*, Ames, 1971, Iowa State University Press.
154. Gebhardt LP, Stanton JG, Hill WD, et al: Natural overwintering hosts of the virus of Western equine encephalitis, *N Engl J Med* 271: 172, 1964.
155. Thomas LA, Eklund CM: Overwintering of Western equine encephalomyelitis virus in garter snakes experimentally infected by *Culex tarsalis*, *Proc Soc Exp Biol Med* 109:421, 1962.
156. Hayes RO, Daniels JB, Maxfield HK, et al: Field and laboratory studies on eastern encephalitis in warm and cold-blooded vertebrates, *Trop Med Hyg* 13:595, 1964.
157. Bowen GS: Prolonged Western equine encephalitis viremia in the Texas tortoise *(Gopherus berlandieri)*, *J Trop Med Hyg* 26:171, 1977.
158. Flynn RJ: *Arthropods: in parasites of laboratory animals*, Ames, 1973, Iowa State University Press.
159. Gebhardt LP, St. Jear SC, Stanton GJ, et al: Ecology of Western equine encephalitis virus, *Proc Soc Exp Biol Med* 142:731, 1972.
160. Acha PN, Szyfres B: *Zoonoses and communicable diseases common to man and animals*, ed 2, Washington, DC, 1987, Pan American Health Organization, WHO.
161. Lamotte LC, Crane GT, Shriner RB, et al: Use of adult chickens as arbovirus sentinels: I: viremia and persistence of antibody in experimentally inoculated adult chickens, *Am J Trop Med Hyg* 16:348, 1967.
162. Stamm DD, Kissling RE: The influence of reciprocal immunity on eastern and western equine encephalomyelitis infection in horses and English sparrows, *J Immunol* 79:342, 1957.
163. Jacobson ER, Troutman JM, Ginn P, et al: *Outbreak of West Nile virus in farmed alligators in Florida*, West Nile Virus Wildlife Health Workshop, 2003, at www.serc.si.edu/migartorybirds/WNV_wkshop.
164. Smith AW, Anderson MP, Skilling DE, et al: First isolation of calicivirus from reptiles and amphibians, *Am J Vet Res* 47:1718, 1986.
165. Jacobson ER, Gaskin JM, Clubb S et al: Papilloma-like virus infection in Bolivian side-neck turtles, *J Am Vet Med Assoc* 181:1325, 1982.

Section V
CLINICAL TECHNIQUES/ PROCEDURES

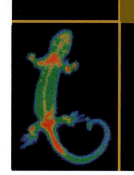

25
ALLOMETRIC SCALING

JOERG MAYER, GRETCHEN KAUFMAN, and MARK POKRAS

The principles of scaling have been known and used by physiologists for many decades.[1-3] Physiologic processes that vary with body size and mass are thought to be easily predicted with the help of simple mathematic expressions (e.g., surface area increases with length to the power of 2, volume increases with length by the power of 3). Numerous equations describing the rate and duration of various physiologic processes have been produced by observation and measurement of chemical and mechanical processes, both in individuals of varying body size and in individuals of different species.[3] The purpose of this chapter is not to provide an in-depth discussion of the fundamental theories of allometric scaling but to provide a critical review of applications from a physiologic and pharmacologic point of view to show the broad-ranging scientific uses of these principles. For a more detailed description of the fundamentals of veterinary applications of allometric scaling, the following publications can be recommended: Sedgwick et al, 1986, 1988, 1990, 1996; Gibbons et al, 1989; Pokras et al, 1993; and Jacobson, 1996.[4-10] Discussion of the origin and validity of the equations used in allometric scaling is active in veterinary medicine and in the human medical literature.[10-13] Kleiber[1] first introduced the general formula used in allometric scaling as aM^b, with **a** being a scaling constant, **M** the body mass, and **b** the scaling exponent. The scaling exponent **b** was considered to be 0.75 for physiologic rates (e.g., metabolic rate) and –0.25 for physiologic durations (e.g., gestation, elimination). This exponent has been accepted and used by many researchers; however, it has also been the focus of dispute over the validity of the unique equation. In a number of physiologic trials, the observed results produced an exponent that varied from the predicted value of 0.75. As discussed subsequently, many experimentally derived equations differ somewhat from Kleiber's original equation; however, the general principle that allometric relationships can be derived from this equation is valid. No doubt, much more research is needed to define the limitations of these "universal" equations. Some considerations might include:

The quality of the data: Measurement of metabolic rates is an extremely delicate procedure, and normal standard measurement techniques for reptilians might not be available. In addition, for ectotherms, environmental temperatures have a profound effect on metabolic rates and need to be careful documented.

Taxonomic uncertainty: Currently, certain species are considered for reclassification of family or even genus within the Class Reptilia. This might have a significant impact on the use of scaling because significant differences in allometric relationships have been observed between different families of reptiles.[14] In addition, calculations derived from only a few individuals may add bias the calculations. This bias may be further enhanced by lack of uniform representation of all taxonomic groups within the class.

Limitations of data range: Certain calculations might be based on a group of specimens that do not vary significantly in body weight because of their naturally narrow range in body mass. Alternatively, gender or age may not have been determined for experimental animals. Thus, small databases might lead to significant biases when conclusions are drawn and extrapolated to larger specimens, as with giant snakes.[15]

After all, a formula that applies to every physiologic aspect of every species of reptile is unlikely when dealing in the life sciences. Applying these equations to ectothermic animals also brings additional uncertainty with it in regard to providing a predictable outcome. Gillooly et al[16] showed that the metabolic rate (the transformation of energy and materials) is governed by two factors: the Boltzman factor (a factor used to describe the temperature dependence of biochemical processes) and the specific allometric relation used to describe the change of biologic processes with the change in body size. Because the body temperature in reptiles is environmentally dependent and therefore not constant, prediction of the metabolic rates have to be made with the specific temperature optimal for the species. Berner[17] was able to show the significance of this by measuring the oxygen consumption of mitochondria in reptiles at different temperatures. Mader and colleagues[18] were able to show the importance of temperature for pharmacokinetics in the Gophersnake (*Pituophis* sp.) dosed with amikacin. Caligiuri et al[19] also showed the same effect of temperature on pharmacokinetics in Gopher Tortoises (*Gopherus* sp.) given amikacin.

Another significant consideration in the use of scaling has to be differentiating between scalable and nonscalable variables. Schmidt-Nielson[2] points out that most chemical and physiologic constants belong to the latter category. Such factors as atomic weight and surface tension are not altered by changes in body size. To what effect these might influence physiology has yet to be determined. On the other hand, variables considered to be nonscalable functions might be significantly influenced by different physiologic factors. Oxygen diffusion, an example of a nonscalable factor, can be accelerated by the presence of hemoglobin.[2]

The advantages of familiarity with certain allometric equations is obvious when dealing with a complex situation such as drug clearance or pharmacokinetic studies. In spite of their limitations, these formulas help to summarize data and gain information about basic anatomic and physiologic facts.

CONTROVERSIES RELATING TO ALLOMETRY

A definition of scaling has been proposed by Schmidt-Nielson[20]: "Scaling deals with the structural and functional consequences of changes in size or scale among otherwise similar organisms." The words "deals" and "similar" in this definition clearly indicate both the aim and the limitation of this principle. Individual allometric equations should not be regarded as laws of nature, predicting exact results, but more like general predictions of approximate expected outcomes. Many opponents of allometric scaling use this uncertainty to argue against the use of it for drug dosage calculation.[11,12] Making the jump from descriptive physiologic formulas to pharmacologic data appears both logical and, at the same time, incredible. Having already seen the problems created when trying to express "normal" physiologic patterns in straightforward mathematical expressions, how could it be possible to create meaningful, user-friendly formulas involving pharmacokinetics?

Adding new variables such as variations in drug absorption, drug metabolism, drug binding, and drug excretion to the calculations must also be considered in pharmacokinetic predictions. The introduction of more variables may appear to make it impossible to accurately predict the dosage of a new drug in a new species. However, more and more publications examining physiologic phenomena suggest that allometric scaling does apply and they therefore support the idea of using allometrics for calculation of drug dosages.[21-23] In addition to the physiologic data, pharmacologic studies examining individual drug scaling or multiple drugs scaled between different species suggest that scaling can be a useful tool for the clinical application.[23-28]

In human medicine, the application of allometric scaling to calculate drug dosages is also much discussed. The issue of the "first-time-in-man" (FTIM) dose selection remains without a clear solution. Factors influencing this dose selection include: toxicology, toxicokinetics, allometric scaling, and the integration of preclinical pharmacology data. The guidelines of the Association of Food and Drug officials of the United States delineates the FTIM maximum dose as: $1/10$ of the largest, no observable effect dose of a chronic rodent toxicity study; $1/6$ of the largest, no observable effect dose of a chronic dog toxicity study; $1/3$ of the largest, no observable effect dose in monkeys.

This method appears to be rather random and has been criticized by scientists.[29] In contrast to this method, more and more scientific publications are showing that allometric scaling is a useful tool for retrospective pharmacologic studies.[30-33] One such retrospective study examined the clearance of 115 xenobiotics in at least three different species. In 91 cases (79%), clearance was successfully predicted via allometric scaling.[27] The study suggests that allometric scaling appears to be a useful tool for retrospective studies, but because of the lack of complete accuracy of prediction (and perhaps our lack of knowledge), caution should be used when applying it to prospective applications. In this same study, the authors noticed a significant difference in the allometric scaling exponent when applied to the drug clearance pathway. When drug clearance was achieved via metabolism alone, or via metabolism plus renal excretion, the scaling exponent value was 0.75. However, if the drug was excreted exclusively via the renal pathway, they found that this value needed to be adjusted to 0.67. Interesting to note is that Schmidt-Neilsen[2] equates the 0.67 exponent directly with surface area of organisms. In addition to this finding, pharmacokinetic publications show that in drugs excreted mainly via the bile, allometric dosage predictions are unsuccessful.[34,35]

Unfortunately, none of these pharmacologic studies include reptiles. The vast anatomic and physiologic differences seen within the Class Reptilia have to be a serious consideration regarding the use of allometric scaling for drug dosages. At the least, the different methods of nitrogen elimination in reptiles, which include the excretion of ammonia, urea, and uric acid in various combinations, probably significantly affect the elimination of some drugs.

Physiologic Application of Scaling

As mentioned previously, the principles of allometric scaling have been known to physiologists for many decades, and the methods are still used and applied to a wide range of biologic and physiologic functions, ranging from the growth of plants, to the allometry of the kidney in lizards, to diving behavior of Green Turtles, to the application of scaling in whole ecosystems.[36-39] The fundamental need to apply allometric scaling according to body size has been explicitly published by Kirkwood.[40] The author uses the example of a 1-g tissue sample from a shrew and a blue whale, pointing out that the tissue sample of the shrew has a 100 times higher metabolic rate than the tissue sample of the whale. Experimental application of this idea in reptiles has been published in the past.[41,42] The authors were able to show a significantly lower molecular activity of the sodium pumps (in ATP/min) of different tissues from ectotherms when compared with endotherms. The tissues of the ectotherm and endotherm specimens were found to have a similar sodium pump number expressed as the approximate density in pmol/g. In a different trial, the authors compared the oxygen consumption of different tissues from rats and Bearded Dragons (*Pogona vitticeps*). The authors were able to show the mammalian brain tissue used three to six times the energy for Na$^+$-K$^+$ transport than the reptilian tissue.[41]

The physiologic applications of allometric scaling play a much more significant role in the future for determining pharmacologic doses. The problems facing predictability in human pharmacology has led researchers to believe that the current methods of predicting a drug dose are not accurate enough and that using a combination of different methods might be more successful. An example includes using the combination of allometric scaling renal clearance and brain weight to successfully predict drug clearance of various drugs in humans.[43]

With allometric scaling, one has to keep in mind that all equations are merely descriptive in nature; they should NOT be considered biologic laws. Equations such as these are probably most useful when they are seen as tools to detect general patterns or used for estimations where data on physiologic normals or pharmacokinetics are not available.

In the following list, a few reptile-specific formulas are compiled that might be of use to the reptile-oriented practitioner. Knowing physiologic rules, such as maximum oxygen consumption (mL/min/kg) in reptiles with varying body temperature, can help to monitor anesthetic procedures in controlled (surgery suite) or uncontrolled (field) environments. Growth rate and home range predictions can also be useful in the clinical setting.

Examples, with W as bodyweight in kilograms and L as length in centimeters, include:

- $13W^{0.8}$ = minimum energy (ME in kcal/d) requirements for free-living existence in lizards[44]
- $6.5W^{0.75}$ = ME requirements for maintenance (kcal/d) in snakes[45]
- $6W^{0.75}$ = ME requirements for maintenance (kcal/d) in chelonia[46]
- $14.6W^{0.23}$ = life span in captivity (years) in reptiles[3]
- $W = 0.0003 L^{2.85}$ bodyweight in relation to carapace length in *Testudo greaca*[47]
- $0.0012W^{0.61}$ = growth rate (g) of reptiles[3]
- $4.8W^{0.95}$ = area (ha) home range of lizards[48]

Maximum oxygen consumption (mL/min/kg) in reptiles at varying body temperature[3]:

$3.1W^{0.81}$ Lizards at 20°C $\quad$ $3.3W^{0.83}$ Reptiles at 20°C
$6.2W^{0.76}$ Lizards at 30°C $\quad$ $6.1W^{0.77}$ Reptiles at 30°C
$9.5W^{0.76}$ Lizards at 35°C $\quad$ $8.1W^{0.71}$ Reptiles at 35°C
$8.1W^{0.64}$ Lizards at 40°C $\quad$ $8.1W^{0.64}$ Reptiles at 40°C

Pharmacologic Application of Scaling

Allometric scaling can be extremely useful with calculation of a dose for a drug that has not been used in a reptile species before. Allometric data can provide additional information that may help narrow down the guess work and bring a greater level of rationality to the process of determining a dose that might actually work, be effective, and not prove toxic. As mentioned previously, allometric scaling is a crude approximation even within its own scope. The formulas used may vary from species to species, between different aged animals of the same species, for individuals kept at different environmental temperatures, and between healthy and ill animals.[10] Use of formulas incorporating species-specific data, when available, may help to decrease error in prediction, but we are only at the earliest stages in the development of such models. The technique described for drug calculation depends on metabolic rate alone and does not take into account differences in metabolism that may affect the uptake, modification, distribution, elimination, and thus the activity of a drug in a particular individual. This level of uncertainty is very real and must be kept in perspective when proceeding with the technique. *However*, **as a tool, allometric scaling is still useful in derivation of a rational dose of a novel medication in the absence of specific pharmacokinetic information.**

Allometric scaling is also extremely useful, and appears to be reliable, when used to calculate a dose from a very small to a very large animal (and vice versa) within the same or closely related taxonomic group. If a pharmacokinetically derived dose is available for a small snake, this information might be used to extrapolate a more accurate dose for a very large snake, instead of merely using the mg/kg dose (Figure 25-1). This principle is illustrated subsequently with the use of ceftazidime in a large snake.

Review of Technique

Allometric scaling, as described by Sedgwick,[4-7] uses a simple ratio comparing established data from a well-known animal with the unknown patient to derive a logical dose. The energy formula is used as a point of comparison between two subjects to establish predictable data.

$$\text{Minimum energy cost} = K \times \text{bodyweight}_{kg}^{0.75}$$

K = 10	Reptiles
K = 49	Marsupial mammals
K = 70	Placental mammals
K = 78	Nonpasserine birds
K = 129	Passerine birds

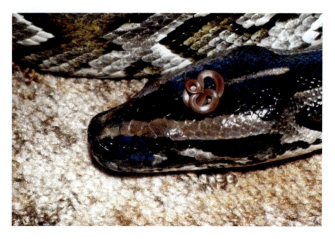

FIGURE 25-1 Allometric scaling allows extrapolation of dosages between animals of different sizes and between individuals of different species. Here, a full-grown Sharp-tailed Snake (*Contia tenuis*) has a body mass $1/1000$ of that of an adult Burmese Python (*Python molurus bivittatus*). (Photograph courtesy D. Mader.)

With this formula, the minimum energy cost (MEC) can be predicted for both the well-known animal and the patient. With the addition of the drug dose information for the well-known animal, the drug dose can be predicted for the patient with a ratio:

$$\frac{\text{Well-known animal dose}}{\text{Well-known animal MEC}} = \frac{\text{Patient dose}}{\text{Patient MEC}}$$

The dose derived through this formula gives a suggested one-time or therapeutic dose for a particular drug in a novel patient. Sedgwick suggests a similar manipulation to calculate the periodicity, or frequency of dose administration. This manipulation uses the mass specific minimum energy cost (SMEC).

$$\text{Specific minimum energy cost} = K \times \text{bodyweight}_{kg}^{-0.25}$$
$$= \text{MEC}/\text{bodyweight}_{kg}$$

Again, the ratio is used to develop the frequency of administration on the basis of a well-known animal.

$$\frac{\text{Well-known animal frequency (times per day)}}{\text{Well-known animal SMEC}}$$
$$= \frac{\text{Patient frequency (times per day)}}{\text{Patient SMEC}}$$

Following these two procedures results in a therapeutic dose and a frequency of administration. This dosage regimen may have to be adjusted for practical application. For example, a dose prediction of 4.2 mg to be given 0.4 times per day might be adjusted to 5 mg every 3 days. Adjustments must be made with safety and efficacy and practicality in mind and necessarily involve adequate knowledge of the drug in question. In addition, maintenance of careful and detailed records of the outcome after the use of allometrically scaled doses is always prudent. In this way, experience builds confidence in the safety and efficacy of the estimated dose for future reference.

As more and more pharmacokinetic studies are published and accurate information becomes known, certain drugs, such as enrofloxacin, are shown not to scale accurately. Replacement of estimated doses with more accurate information is important, as is comparison of this information when it becomes available, either as validation or invalidation of the technique for future use.

Choosing a Model

One can attempt to minimize metabolic and physiologic differences between the well-known animal and the patient by basing the comparison on a pharmacokinetically derived dose of a closely related species as a model. For example, to determine a dose of ceftazidime for a 30-kg snake, an allometrically scaled dose based on the pharmacokinetically derived dose in a 2-kg snake is more accurate than a direct dose from a human or a dog or even the mg/kg dose established in the small snake. The 2-kg snake dose is 40 mg (20 mg/kg) every 3 days.[49] The 30-kg snake dose, based on allometric scaling from the smaller snake, is 307 mg (10.4 mg/kg) every 5 days.

Unfortunately, pharmacokinetic data are often not available on a closely related species and calculations must be based on a disparate model. Some remarkable examples exist, however, where even a far distant species can still predict a reasonable dose.

Derivation of a Completely New Application

Considering the use of a new drug for the very first time in a species is a complicated process. Drug discovery is currently moving at a dramatic pace, and newer and better therapies are being released for humans and domestic animals all the time. Many of the antibiotics, antifungal agents, antiprotozoal drugs, and others are proving useful in reptile medicine. Investigation into the use of one of the newer neuromuscular blockers by the author provides an excellent example of how useful allometric scaling can be in starting to consider an appropriate dose.[28] Rocuronium was chosen for this study because in humans it was shown to be reversible, relatively short acting, and associated with minimal side effects. This was considered a great improvement over other neuromuscular blockers used in reptiles and also would have application in place of injectable general anesthetics and tranquilizers in instances where their full effects might not be necessary or may carry greater risk.

Rocuronium had been used in humans for several years and was widely available. The dose in humans was reported to be 0.6 to 1.2 mg/kg, given once. Setting up the ratio based on data for a 70-kg human, a range of doses was determined for a 450-g box turtle as follows:

70-kg human MEC = $70 \times 70^{0.75}$ = 1694 kcal/d
70-kg human low dose = 0.6×70 = 42 mg
70-kg human high dose = 1.2×70 = 84 mg
450-g Box Turtle MEC = $10 \times 0.45^{0.75}$ = 5.5 kcal/d

$$\frac{\text{Well-known animal dose}}{\text{Well-known animal MEC}} = \frac{\text{Patient dose}}{\text{Patient MEC}}$$

$$\frac{42 \text{ to } 84 \text{ mg}}{1694} = \frac{\text{Turtle dose}}{5.5}$$

This predicted dose was then used to establish a range of reasonable doses to evaluate for efficacy and safety. The final dose recommendations based on the experimental findings were 0.25 to 0.5 mg/kg. The experimentally derived dose is close to the predicted allometrically scaled dose and quite different from the human dose of 0.6 to 1.2 mg/kg.

The use of allometric scaling to derive drug doses in reptiles has been well described and shown.[7,50,51] It continues to be useful in situations where pharmacokinetic information and empirical or experiential data are not available. This occurs most often with the application of new therapies, established in mammals or humans but not yet tried in reptiles. In these situations, a clinician must synthesize knowledge of the particular species involved, the medical condition at hand, and the various options for therapy used in other species with similar conditions. At some point, a leap of faith is required to try a particular dosing regimen, hoping that safety is preserved and that efficacy is maintained.

CONCLUSION

Despite the controversies over the accuracy of allometric scaling in reptiles, the clinician dealing with reptiles finds that the methodology of scaling has distinct advantages, not the least of which is that it encourages us to think in detail about our patient's metabolism. We have tried to highlight limitations and applications of allometric scaling relevant to the clinician. Without a doubt, much more research on the physiology and pharmacokinetics in reptiles is needed. As is well documented in mammalian species, allometric scaling is a valuable tool when used in retrospective studies to predict drug doses for novel pharmaceuticals in different species. Once more pharmacologic studies in reptiles are published, a similar analysis of the use of allometric scaling as a retrospective tool in reptilians will be possible. As has been pointed out for humans and other mammals, some drugs appear to be scalable and others do not seem to be predicable with current methods. In mammals, the drug-kidney interaction appears to be a significant factor limiting the accuracy of allometric predictions. To what degree this is applicable to the wide variations of the reptile excretory system is unknown.

The need for more physiologic data even within the suborder Serpentes has been documented by Shine et al[15] in their discussion of giant snakes in comparison with smaller snakes and shows that we are just at the beginning of understanding the potential applications of allometric scaling in a wide variety of taxa.

We believe that we must restate that the method of allometric scaling should not be regarded as a substitute for pharmacology but more as an addition to the problem-solving tool kit that all clinicians must use when choosing the proper dosage for extra label pharmaceuticals. Even Boxenbaum,[29] a pioneer in the application of allometric scaling in human pharmacology, does not rely solely on allometric scaling when selecting a dose. In human and veterinary medicine, one of the most widely accepted uses of allometric scaling is in dosing chemotherapeutic drugs with a narrow margin of safety using the body surface area to derive dosages instead of the standard mg/kg rate. Oncologists have long used body surface area (a rough approximation of metabolism) to derive dosages instead of the standard mg/kg rate. Even in this instance of a widely accepted dose calculation method, the method is not 100% reliable and care must be exercised because of the toxicity seen in patients at the small end of the scale.[52]

Despite all the criticism, the need for allometric scaling is clear. Utmost importance when dosing a novel drug for a novel species is to be conservative for safety reasons and aggressive for efficacy reasons. The development of techniques for the use of the neuromuscular blocking agent in box turtles by Kaufman et al[28] is a prime example of deriving a reptile dose from the human pharmacologic data with allometric techniques.

The efficacy of antibiotic therapy will become more and more important as the number of resistant strains of bacteria continue to outstrip the introduction of novel antibiotics to the market. Which method would you use if you had to treat a 1-ton saltwater crocodile with a potentially nephrotoxic antibiotic?

Tables 25-1 through 25-3 list an MEC/SMEC–body weight conversion, an allometric scaling formulary, and an allometric scaling worksheet, respectively. Clinicians are encouraged to use these simple tools to help with formulating therapeutic plans for novel drugs in novel patients.

Table 25-1 Body Weight Conversion Table for Reptiles (K=10)

BW (kg)	MEC	SMEC	BW (kg)	MEC	SMEC
0.01	0.316	31.623	1.20	11.465	9.554
0.02	0.532	26.591	1.30	12.175	9.365
0.03	0.721	24.028	1.40	12.871	9.193
0.04	0.894	22.361	1.50	13.554	9.036
0.05	1.057	21.147	1.60	14.226	8.891
0.06	1.212	20.205	1.70	14.888	8.758
0.07	1.361	19.441	1.80	15.540	8.633
0.08	1.504	18.803	1.90	16.183	8.517
0.09	1.643	18.257	2.00	16.818	8.409
0.10	1.778	17.783	2.50	19.882	7.953
0.15	2.410	16.069	3.00	22.795	7.598
0.20	2.991	14.953	3.50	25.589	7.311
0.25	3.536	14.142	4.00	28.284	7.071
0.30	4.054	13.512	4.50	30.897	6.866
0.35	4.550	13.001	5.00	33.437	6.687
0.40	5.030	12.574	5.50	35.915	6.530
0.45	5.494	12.209	6.00	38.337	6.389
0.50	5.946	11.892	6.50	40.708	6.263
0.55	6.387	11.612	7.00	43.035	6.148
0.60	6.817	11.362	7.50	45.321	6.043
0.65	7.239	11.137	8.00	47.568	5.946
0.70	7.653	10.933	8.50	49.781	5.857
0.75	8.059	10.746	9.50	54.112	5.696
0.80	8.459	10.574	10.00	56.234	5.623
0.85	8.852	10.415	15.00	76.220	5.081
0.90	9.240	10.267	20.00	94.574	4.729
0.95	9.623	10.129	25.00	111.803	4.472
1.00	10.000	10.000	30.00	128.186	4.273

BW, Body weight; *MEC*, minimum energy cost; *SMEC*, specific minimum energy cost.
MEC = K × $BW_{kg}^{0.75}$ = kcal/d
SMEC = MEC/BW = K × $BW_{kg}^{-0.25}$
K = 10, Reptiles (37°C)
K = 49, Marsupial mammals
K = 70, Placental mammals
K = 78, Nonpasserine birds
K = 129, Passerine birds

Table 25-2 Allometric Scaling Formulary for Reptiles

Drug	Model	Model Dose	Universal MEC Dose (yields mg/dose)	Frequency Coefficient (yields times/day)	Comments
Allopurinol	Human	300 mg sid	0.18	0.04	
Amikacin	Gophersnake[1]	5 mg/kg IM, then 2.5 mg/kg q 72 h	0.4 (loading) 0.2	0.024	PK dose available for Gophersnake, Alligator, Water Turtle
Ampicillin	Dog	22 mg/kg tid	0.665	0.09	
Calcium edetate (CaEDTA)	Avian	35 mg/kg bid	0.333	0.019	Scaled dose used successfully for Snapping Turtle (Borkowski, personal communication)
Carbenicillin	Dog	15 mg/kg PO, IV tid	0.453	0.091	PK dose available for snake, tortoise
	Snake[2] (1 kg)	400 mg/kg IM q 24 h	40	0.1	
	Tortoise[3] (1 kg)	400 mg/kg q 48 h	40	0.05	
Carprofen	Dog	4 mg/kg IV once	0.12	One time only	
		2.2 mg/kg PO bid	0.07	0.06	
Ceftazadime	Small snake[4]	20 mg/kg q 72 h	2.4	0.04	PK dose available for small snake; scaled dose recommended for large snakes
Cephalexin (Keflex)	Dog	22 mg/kg PO tid	0.665	0.091	PK dose available for Gophersnake, Indigo Snake, Ratsnake, and Kingsnake, Boas, Rattlesnakes
Cephalothin (Keflin)	Dog	15-35 mg/kg IM, SQ, IV tid	0.453-1.0	0.091	
Chloramphenicol	Dog	25-50 mg/kg PO IM, IV tid	0.755-1.5	0.091	
	Snake[5] (1kg)	50 mg/kg SQ q 12-72 h	10.6	0.063-0.4	
Ciprofloxacin	Human	500 mg bid	0.3	0.08	PK dose available for chicken
Cisapride	Child	0.2 mg/kg qid-tid	0.006	0.1	Used successfully in tortoise (Kaufman, unpublished)
Clindamycin	Dog	10 mg/kg bid	0.271	0.054	Antiinflammatory for articular gout
Colchicine	Macaw	0.01 mg/kg bid	0.00013	0.025	Based on 3-kg dog; manufacturer's dose; successfully used in many herp species (Kaufman, unpublished)
Drontal PLUS Small (Praziquantel/pyrantel pamoate/febantel)	Dog	1 tab (22.7/22.7/113.4 mg)	0.0064 tab/kcal (0.14/0.14/0.73)	Single treatment	
Enrofloxacin	Does *not* scale well across species		Does *not* scale well across species		PK dose available for many reptile species
Fenbendazole	Dog	50 mg/kg sid × 3 d	1.5	0.03	Toxicities reported in birds and reptiles; use with CAUTION; many empirical doses available
Fluconazole	Human	200 mg sid	0.12	0.04	
Flunixin meglumine	Horse	1.1 mg/kg sid	0.074	0.068	Used with good effect in reptiles (Kaufman, unpublished)

Gentamicin	Gophersnake[6]	2.5 mg/kg q 72 h	0.03	MEC dose recommended for large snakes; PK dose available for Gophersnake, Red-eared Slider, Alligator, many bird species
Itraconazole	Dog	2.5 mg/kg bid	0.06	
Ketoprofen	Horse	2.2 mg/kg sid	0.066	Used IM or IV, follow-up with oral carprofen for long-term therapy; successfully used in many reptile species (Flo Tseng, unpublished)
Metronidazole	Dog	7.5 mg/kg tid	0.08	
	Iguana[7] (1.5 kg)	20 mg/kg PO q 24-48 h	0.055-0.1	Based on canine antibacterial dose; PK dose available for Iguana
Praziquantel	Dog	5-10 mg/kg	Single dose	
Probenicid	Human	250-500 mg bid	0.08	
Rocuronium	Box Turtle[8]	0.3-0.5 mg/kg IM	Single dose	For immobilization only, NOT ANALGESIC; reverse with glycopyrrolate/neostigmine (Kaufman, 2003)
Trimethoprim-Sulfa	Dog	15 mg/kg bid	0.06	

To calculate a patient's dose:
1. Multiply the universal MEC dose by patient's MEC = mg/treatment
2. Multiply frequency coefficient by patient's SMEC = number of times/day

[1]Mader DR, Conzelman GM, Baggot JD: Effects of ambient temperature on the half-life and dosage regimen of amikacin in the gopher snake, *JAVMA* 187(11):1134-1136, 1985.
[2]Lawrence K, et al: A preliminary study on the use of carbenicillin in snakes, *J Vet Pharmacol Ther* 7:119-124, 1984.
[3]Lawrence K: Use of carbenicillin in two species of tortoise, *Res Vet Sci* 40:413-415, 1986.
[4]Lawrence K, Muggleton PW, Needham JR: Preliminary study on the use of ceftazadime, a broad spectrum cephalosporin antibiotic, in snakes, *Res Vet Sci* 36:16-20, 1984.
[5]Clark CH, Rogers ED, Milton JL: Plamsa concentrations of chloramphenicol in snakes, *AJVR* 46(12):2654-2657, 1985.
[6]Bush M, et al: Biological half-life of gentamicin in gopher snakes, *AJVR* 39(1):171-173, 1978.
[7]Kolmstetter CM, et al: Pharmacokinetics of metronidazole in the green iguana, *ARAV* 8(3):4-7, 1998.
[8]Kaufman GE, et al: Use of rocuronium for endotracheal intubation of North American Gulf Coast box turtles, *JAVMA* 222(8):1111-1115, 2003.

MEC, Minimum energy cost; *sid*, once daily; *IM*, intramuscularly; *q*, every; *tid*, three times a day; *bid*, twice daily; *PO*, orally; *IV*, intravenously; *SQ*, subcutaneously; *qid*, four times daily.

Table 25-3 Allometric Scaling Worksheet to Calculate the Universal Minimum Energy (MEC) Cost Dose from Published Dosages in the Literature

Required Data

Drug: _____
Source: _____
Model Animal: _____
Body Weight (BW; kg): _____
Dose: _____
Model Animal MEC = $K \times BW_{kg}^{0.75}$ = _____
Single Dose: _____mg (mg/kg × kg)

Universal MEC Dose Calculation

Divide known single dose (mg) by Model Animal MEC
Universal MEC Dose = _____

Frequency Coefficient Calculation

Divide frequency (per 24 h) by (Model Animal MEC/BW [kg])
Frequency Coefficient = _____

REFERENCES

1. Kleiber M: Body size and metabolism, *Hilgardia* 6:3125-3153, 1932.
2. Schmidt-Nielsen K: *Scaling: why is animal size so important?* New York, 1984, Cambridge University Press.
3. Calder WA III: *Size, function and life history*, Cambridge, Mass, 1984, Harvard University Press.
4. Sedgwick CJ, Haskell A, Pokras MA: Scaling drug dosages for animals of diverse body sizes, *Proc Natl Wildlife Rehabil Assoc* 5:3-11, 1986.
5. Sedgwick CJ, Pokras MA: Extrapolating rational drug doses and treatment periods by allometric scaling, *Proc 55th Annu Meeting Am Anim Hosp Assoc* 156-157, 1988.
6. Sedgwick CJ, Pokras MA, Kaufman G: Allometric scaling: using estimated energy costs to extrapolate drug doses between different species and different individuals of diverse body sizes, *Proc Am Assoc Zoo Vet* 249-254, 1990.
7. Sedgwick CJ, Borkowski R: Allometric scaling: extrapolating treatment regimens for reptiles. In Mader DR, editor: *Reptile medicine and surgery*, Philadelphia, 1996, WB Saunders.
8. Gibbons G, Pokras MA, Sedgwick CJ: Allometric scaling and veterinary medicine, *Aust Vet Pract* 8:160-164, 1989.
9. Pokras MA, Karas A, Kirkwood J, Sedgwick CJ: An introduction to allometric scaling and its uses in raptor medicine. In Redig PT, Cooper JE, Remple D, editors: *Raptor biomedicine*, 1993, University of Minnesota Press.
10. Jacobson E: Metabolic scaling of antibiotics in reptiles: basis and limitations, *Zoo Biol* 15:329-339, 1996.
11. Bonate PL, Howard D: Prospective allometric scaling: does the emperor have clothes? *J Clin Pharmacol* 40:335-340, 2000.
12. Bonate PL, Howard D: Rebuttal to Mahmood, *J Clin Pharmacol* 40:345-346, 2000.
13. Mahmood I: Prospective allometric scaling: does the emperor have clothes? *J Clin Pharmacol* 40:341-344, 2000.
14. Galvano PE, Tarasantchi J, Guertzenstein P: Heat production of tropical snakes in relation to body weight and body surface, *Am J Physiol* 209:501-506, 1965.
15. Shine R, Harlow PS, Keogh JS, Boeadi: The allometry of life-history traits: insights from a study of giant snakes, *J Zoo* 244:405-414, 1998.
16. Gillooly JF, Brown JH, West GB, Savage VM, Charnov EL: Effects of size and temperature on metabolic rate, *Science* 293:2248-2251, 2001.
17. Berner NJ: Oxygen consumption by mitochondria from an endotherm and an ectotherm, *Comp Biochem Physiol B Biochem Mol Biol* 124:25-31, 1999.
18. Mader DR, Conzelman GM Jr, Baggot JD: Effects of ambient temperature on the half-life and dosage regimen of amikacin in the gopher snake, *J Am Vet Med Assoc* 187:1134-1136, 1985.
19. Caligiuri R, Kollias GV, Jacobson E, McNab B, Clark CH, Wilson RC: The effects of ambient temperature on amikacin pharmacokinetics in gopher tortoises, *J Vet Pharmacol Ther* 13:287-291, 1990.
20. Schmidt-Nelson K: *Animal Physiology*, Cambridge, UK, 1997, Cambridge University Press.
21. Else PL, Hubert AJ: An allometric comparison of the mitochondria of mammalian and reptilian tissue: the implications for the evolution of endothermy, *J Comp Physiol* 156:3-11, 1985.
22. Timm KI, Picton JS, Tylman B: Surface area to volume relationships of snakes support the use of allometric scaling for calculating dosages of pharmaceuticals, *Lab Anim Sci* 44:60-62, 1994.
23. Downes H: Relative metabolic rate as a basis for extrapolation of drug-elimination times from mammals to frogs, *J Herp Med Surg* 12:4-11, 2002.
24. Boxenbaum H: Comparative pharmacokinetics of benzodiazepines in dog and man, *J Pharmacokinet Biopharm* 10:411-426, 1982.
25. Boxenbaum H: Interspecies scaling, allometry, physiological time, and the ground plan of pharmacokinetics, *J Pharmacokinet Biopharm* 10:201-227, 1982.
26. Riviere JE, Martin-Jimenez T, Sundlof SF, Craigmill AL: Interspecies allometric analysis of the comparative pharmacokinetics of 44 drugs across veterinary and laboratory animal species, *J Vet Pharmacol Ther* 20:453-463, 1997.
27. Hu TM, Hayton W: Allometric scaling of xenobiotic clearance: uncertainty versus universality, *AAPS PharmSci* 3:29, 2001.
28. Kaufman GE, Seymour RE, Bonner BB, Court MH, Karas AZ: Use of rocuronium for endotracheal intubation in North American Gulf Coast box turtles, *J Am Vet Med Assoc* 222:1111-1115, 2003.
29. Boxenbaum H, DiLea C: First-time-in-human dose selection: allometric thoughts and perspectives, *J Clin Pharmacol* 35:957-966, 1995.
30. Mordenti J: Pharmacokinetic scale-up: accurate prediction of human pharmacokinetic profiles from animal data, *J Pharm Sci* 74:1097-1099, 1985.
31. McGovren JP, Williams MG, Stewart JC: Interspecies comparison of acivicin pharmacokinetics, *Drug Metab Disp* 16:18-22, 1988.
32. Sawada Y, Hanano M, Sugiyama Y, Iga T: Prediction of disposition of weakly acidic and six weakly basic drugs in humans from pharmacokinetic parameters in rats, *J Pharmacokin Biopharm* 13:477-492, 1985.
33. Swabb EA, Bonner DP: Prediction of aztreonam pharmacokinetics in humans based on data from animals, *J Pharmacokin Biopharm* 11:215-223, 1983.
34. Pahlman I, Edholm M, Kankaanranta S, Odell M-L: Pharmacokinetics of susalimod, a highly biliary-excreted sulphasalazine analogue, in various species: nonpredictable human clearance by allometric scaling, *J Pharm Pharmacol* 49:494-498, 1998.
35. Lave T, Portmann R, Schenker G, Gianni A, Guenzi A, Girometta, MA, et al: Interspecies pharmacokinetic comparisons and allometric scaling of napsagatran, a low molecular weight thrombin inhibitor, *J Pharm Pharmacol* 51:85-91, 1999.

36. Damuth J: Scaling of growth: plants and animals are not so different, *Proc Natl Acad Sci U S A* 98:2113-2114, 2001.
37. Beuchat CA, Braun EJ: Allometry of the kidney: implications for the ontogeny of osmoregulation, *Am J Physiol* 255:R760-767, 1988.
38. Hays GC, Adams CR, Broderick AC, Godley BJ, Lucas DJ, Metcalfe JD, et al: The diving behaviour of green turtles at Ascension Island, *Anim Behav* 3:577-586, 2000.
39. Enquist BJ, Niklas KJ: Invariant scaling relations across tree-dominated communities, *Nature* 410:655-660, 2001.
40. Kirkwood JK: Influence of body size in animals on health and disease, *Vet Rec* 113:287-290, 1983.
41. Else PL, Hulbert AJ: Evolution of mammalian endothermic metabolism: "leaky" membranes as a source of heat, *Am J Physiol* 253:R1-7, 1987.
42. Else PL, Windmill DJ, Markus V: Molecular activity of sodium pumps in endotherms and ectotherms, *Am J Physiol* 271:R1287-1294, 1996.
43. Mahmood I, Balian JD: Interspecies scaling: predicting clearance of drugs in humans: three different approaches, *Xenobiotica* 26:887-895, 1996.
44. Nagy, KA: Energy requirement of free living iguanid lizards. In Burghardt GM, Rand SA, editors: *Iguanas of the world: their behavior, ecology and conservation*, Park Ridge, NJ, 1982, Noyes Publications.
45. Kirkwood JK, Gili C: Food consumption in relation to body-weight in captive snakes, *Res Vet Sci* 57:35-38, 1994.
46. Hartley and Kirkwood: Lecture notes for MSc course in Wild Animal Health, Royal Veterinary College, London, UK, 1999, unpublished.
47. Blakey CSG, Kirwood JK: Body mass to length relationship in chelonia, *Vet Rec* 136:566-568, 1995.
48. Turner FB, Jennrich RI, Weintraub JD: Home range and body size of lizards, *Ecology* 50:1076-1081, 1969.
49. Lawrence K, Muggleton PW, Needham JR: Preliminary study on the use of ceftazadime, a broad spectrum cephalosporin antibiotic, in snakes, *Res Vet Sci* 36:16-20, 1984.
50. Kaufman, GE: Pharmacology, pharmacodynamics, and drug dosing. In Ackerman L, editor: *The biology, husbandry and health care of reptiles and amphibians*, vol 2. Neptune City, NJ, 1997, TFH Publications.
51. Bonner BB: Chelonian therapeutics, *Vet Clin North Am Exot Anim Pract* 3:257-332, 2000.
52. Arrington KA, Legendre AM, Tabeling GS, Frazier DL: Comparison of body surface area-based and weight-based dosage protocols for doxorubicin administration in dogs, *Am J Vet Res* 55:1587-1592, 1994.

26
ALTERNATIVE AND COMPLEMENTARY VETERINARY THERAPIES

BRUCE FERGUSON and NANCY O'LEARY

A number of medical and surgical advances continue to be made in reptile health care. Still, many diseases and conditions exist for which conventional medicine is inadequate, impractical, unsafe, or simply not efficacious. In addition, some clients are reluctant to subject their pets to the perceived or real risks of unapproved drugs or anesthesia and surgery. Might there be other methods that we can use to help these animals?

Complementary therapies, often referred to as alternative therapy (or complementary and alternative veterinary medicine [CAVM]) or, less accurately, holistic medicine, are therapies not generally taught in mainstream veterinary education. Some of these methods have a few thousand years of empirical and clinical trials, and others have been developed more recently and have less empirical or anecdotal evidence for efficacy with few strictly controlled clinical trials. Traditional Chinese veterinary medicine (TCVM), for example, which incorporates several different methods including acupuncture, herbal medicine, nutrition, massage, and meditation, dates back at least 2500 years, while homeopathy has a history of about 200 years.[1] What almost all complementary therapies have in common is that they are targeted to work with the individual animal's natural healing capabilities. They treat the whole individual (thus the term holistic) and the individual body's healing processes. Much criticism has been aimed at these therapies as being nonscientific and lacking in research, controlled, double-blind studies, or other perceived scientific validation. One need only to visit the National Institutes of Health's (NIH) web site to realize the tremendous amount of ongoing research and the already proven benefits of CAVM for many human diseases. Funding for CAVM research is not a federal mandate and sources of private funding are sparse. Nonetheless, clinical work is being undertaken worldwide and empirical results are accumulating.

Many modern diseases and conditions are without safe and effective treatment, at least by mainstream medicine. This is particularly true of chronic problems like arthritis, asthma, allergies, and dermatologic conditions, to name several. Available treatments often carry serious side effects, or merely mask symptoms while the disease or condition progresses. An obvious example is the long-term use of steroids to treat arthritis. Complementary therapies are often more effective without the side effects and may be particularly useful in treating species that cannot tolerate many of the drugs used in human or veterinary medicine. In the future, the term "Integrative Medicine" will hopefully be in common use, melding all the science and therapeutic modalities into one for the benefit of all.

Veterinarians are almost by nature holistic practitioners. We tend to take the entire animal's symptoms and systems into consideration in making a diagnosis. Our examinations must be thorough and complete, and we must take detailed histories that include nutrition and husbandry (particularly when treating reptiles and exotic patients) to diagnose and treat appropriately. This is especially true for exotic veterinarians who must use medications, dosages, and regimens that are based entirely on anecdotal or empirical evidence of efficacy. CAVM may offer treatments that are less toxic and invasive and work to enhance the animal's own healing abilities.

Because of the pervasive constraints of time and funding, few of these technologies have been explicitly studied in reptile patients. Consequently, little data are available for the use of these methods in reptiles. An April 2001 Medline search under the headings Acupuncture, Herbal Medicine, Homeopathy, Chiropractic, Physiotherapies, and Nutraceuticals yielded more than 24,000 citations for humans, almost 500 citations for veterinary medicine, and none for reptiles. Therefore, most of the following extrapolates from mammalian data or uses clinical cases from practicing veterinarians.

This chapter is meant to stimulate thought in this therapeutic area rather than answer all the questions it raises. Our hope is that the ensuing discussion leads to future applications of the following methods with attendant clinical research. In this fashion, as with all incipient medical systems, a database will begin to accumulate that will enlighten us and benefit our reptile patients.

This chapter briefly introduces some of the more common complementary and alternative therapies found to be helpful by clinical veterinarians. Table 26-1 provides definitions for some of the terms used in the chapter. Some of these therapies are immediately applicable to most practicing veterinarians (nutraceuticals and some herbs), and others require more specialized training (e.g., acupuncture, chiropractic, homeopathy). Readers will find a list of resources for further information, organizations, and, most importantly, further education and training at the end of the chapter. We want the reader to view this introduction to CAVM with the knowledge that this area of reptile medicine is in its infancy.

NATURAL HISTORY CONSIDERATIONS

What is the current status of our knowledge of the natural history of reptiles and amphibians in our practice? We are commonly unaware of important details of the environment in which the animals naturally exist. Empirical and experimental data on husbandry for a few popular species have begun to accumulate, yet for most we are still uncertain of the captive conditions that maintain and promote good health.

Ideally, we want to know the precursors of disease in a reptile's natural environment and the normal biologic

Table 26-1	Definitions of Traditional Chinese Medical Terms*
Term	**Definition**
Yin	Nurturing, moist, condensing, soft, internal influences
Yang	Energetic, dry, expansive, hard, external influences
Qi	Life Energy, the impulsive energy of normal organ function
Blood	Western blood plus moist, nutritive influences
Shu	Refers to acupuncture points on dorsum related to internal organ function
Mu	Refers to acupuncture points on ventrum related to internal organ function

*Chinese language is written in derived pictograms, and medical philosophy is metaphorical, though pragmatic. These definitions are very rough translations of Chinese characters.

response to those diseases. For example, do animals with gastrointestinal (GI) parasites significantly vary their ingestive behavior, either quantitatively or qualitatively? Are there items such as herbs that an animal safely ingests in its natural environment that either expel GI parasites or modify gut mucosal immunity to facilitate coexistence? Or are some reptiles susceptible to moderate GI infestation that significantly increases morbidity and mortality, even when in good health otherwise? In such cases, natural or synthetic antiparasitics may be necessary to restore health. Are we aware of the biologically appropriate diets and environments for many of the reptiles with which we work? Prior authors have implicated malnutrition in poor performance, disease, and high mortality.[2] Without such knowledge, our ability to offer veterinary care is only sufficient for acute crises. Chronic health conditions are more likely to be caused by best guess husbandry and nutrition mistakes. We know that ethical and careful owners attempt to address these issues and create a seminatural environment for the animals. But without an appreciation for details of the natural history for each species, correct husbandry advice may be difficult to offer.

Practitioners of CAVM believe that an animal's behavioral and nutritional repertoire in the wild may suggest approaches to healing in captivity. Although we do not claim that an attempt by an animal to heal in the wild is always superior to our intention (e.g., laceration repair), we believe that their behavior in the wild is fertile for ideas to help them heal. We all know that the exact conditions under which most reptiles evolved cannot be replicated. With regard to our daily practice as veterinarians, are we aware of the behavior of healing in the wild? Mechanisms that are possibly important include ingesta (e.g., herbs, foods), thermal gradients, fasting, and immune system automodulation.[3] If we deem any or all of these to be important in the reptile's natural environment, how is it best accomplished in captivity?

A classic example is nutrition (see also Chapter 18). Although we may not be able to completely replicate an animal's biologically appropriate diet, we can choose items that are similar to those in the wild. Much of our shared information on the use of vitamin A, vitamin D, and nonrancid fish oils evolved from close observation in daily clinical practice.

Case Example: Gecko

Signalment: 2-year-old Mediterranean Gecko of unknown gender.

History: Patient was seen with gastric impaction and anorexia. Its diet consisted only of crickets. The adult crickets have a high chitin (lightweight, low moisture) content. In TCVM theory this type of diet is too consistently Yang (dry, light) and eventually consumed Stomach Yin (moisture, cooling).

Diagnosis and Treatment: What is the treatment principle? In this case, a relatively Yang-deficient animal (obligate poikilotherm) was given excess Yang in its diet and the Yin was injured. Dry or Yin deficiency is treated with moisture and Yin. Aloe vera gel was administered orally, and acupuncture was used to stimulate the Q6H and back Shu (Association) points (BL 20 Spleen/Pancreas Pi-Shu, BL 21 Stomach Guan Yuan Shu).

What data do we have on the biologically appropriate diets of many of the unique species with which we work? How might those needs change in an artificial or seminatural environment? In fact, can we speak with any certainty of a reliable shared body of knowledge in the field of reptile nutrition?

We should be alert to any information that may lead us to healthful conclusions in the field of nutrition. As an example that is detailed in another section, antioxidants in human and other mammalian species (vertebrate systems) are important for free radical control in various tissues.[4] Some of the complex phytochemicals are now known to be essential for tissue integrity.[5] Though less well researched in reptiles, a high likelihood exists that similar cellular systems use similar molecules. Evolutionary solutions commonly converge on parsimonous principles. Various fresh food components that may be said to be high in antioxidants and bioflavonoids are commonly ingested in nature by both herbivorous and omnivorous lizards. Carnivores such as snakes eat other creatures that have eaten plant substrates. Are these components necessary to prevent chronic degenerative disorders? Can we be certain that we meet the needs of each reptile?

In summary, we suggest further research into biologically appropriate diets for each species. Further, close scrutiny of natural history events that may be involved in successful health and healing in the wild may become techniques for tomorrow in our daily practice.

HERBAL MEDICINE

Herbal medicine encompasses a broad category of uses and applications from various cultures, including Traditional Chinese Medicine, Western herbal medicine, which includes Native American plants, and Ayurvedic medicine from India. Herbs used in these disciplines may include whole plants or parts of plants and minerals and even animal parts as the Chinese use all three in their herbal formulas.[6] A practitioner may prescribe a single herb or a combination of herbs (an herbal formula) when treating a patient and has several options for the form used. Herbs can be ordered from professional suppliers as bulk herbs, dried extracts, and liquid extracts (usually extracted in alcohol) and therefore can be administered in several ways including capsules, drops, teas, and soups. Many Chinese herbal formulas come conveniently concentrated into a pill form as well. When prescribing an herb as compared with a drug, one prescribes a whole plant or substance where the active constituents may be tempered or enhanced by other parts of the herb. Thus, what may be toxic when isolated becomes safer, or absorption may be increased, or effects may otherwise be altered. Some 25% or

Table 26-2 Common Plant Constituents and Their Actions

Constituent	Actions
Mucilage	Hydrophilic and soothing polysaccharides
Phenols	Broad group of aromatic compounds, astringents (e.g., salicylic acid)
Tannins	Coagulate proteins
Coumarins	Anticoagulants, muscle relaxants
Anthraquinoines	Irritant or cathartic laxatives
Flavonoids	Complex antiinflammatory, antioxidant aromatics
Anthocyanins	Plant pigments that benefit connective tissue
Glucosilinates	Topical counterirritants
Volatile oils	Ketones, esters, and aldehydes with many effects
Saponins	Steroidal and triterpenoidal compounds
Cardiac glycosides	Digitalis, positive inotrope
Cyanogenic glycosides	Cardiac and pulmonary support
Vitamins	Benefit most metabolic processes in body
Bitters	Broad class, stimulates digestion and bile flow
Alkaloids	Broad class (e.g., vincristine, atropine)
Minerals	Support normal metabolic processes (e.g., potassium)

more of the pharmaceuticals used today are derived from specific substances found in medicinal herbs.[7]

Herbal medicines generally work somewhere between nutritional therapy and conventional drug therapy; that is, their actions are generally slower to effect than a pharmaceutical but much faster than nutritional changes or therapies. All of the animals with which we work have coevolved with the plants in their natural habitat. They readily consume many plant types, some of which we cannot commonly duplicate for exotic species. Even the carnivorous reptiles consume herbivores who themselves contain ingested plant materials. Such plants have both nutritional components and other molecules that may have important functions in the body.[8]

Pharmacognosy has revealed a large number of important biologically active compounds in plants, and one can use this knowledge in prescribing herbal products and incorporating historic uses for dispensing herbal medicines. For example, foxglove (digitalis) was discovered by "wisewomen" practitioners to be effective for dropsy (ascites) of congestive heart failure. Hawthorn (various flavonoids) has been and is still used in the European medical community for broad cardiac support. Milk thistle (silymarin) is the primary "drug" used in human medicine in Germany for any hepatopathy and toxic mushroom poisonings.

Active Constituents and Actions

Some of the more common chemical constituents of herbs and their actions may be seen in Table 26-2. So, with use of active constituents and actions, one might prescribe a soothing demulcent such as Marsh Mallow root (*Althea officinalis*) for such diverse conditions as enteritis, colitis, cystitis, and urethritis—all common conditions in veterinary medicine.

Herbal Energetics

Most indigenous herbal medical systems are based on the belief that herbs have specific energies or broad categories of effects in the body. They may, for example, "clear heat," "drain damp," "warm," "cool," or "nourish Yin." Although these categories of herbal energetics may at first sound strange, empirical evidence of these effects can be found.

As an example, a hot pepper is considered to have "Heat" and be "Warming" and is used to "dispel cold and clear the exterior." Yet, when you touch the pepper it is ambient temperature, not "warm." When you eat the pepper, however, you soon begin to sweat and your face and tissues that touched the pepper become red. Detailed experiments have suggested that these physiologic changes are from peripheral vasodilation and increased tissue perfusion, and the flavonoids in the pepper increase neutrophil killing function and generally increase immune system function.[8] Sweating itself has been shown to have a positive influence on the body's ability to deal with pathogens. These are at least a few of the factors that lead an herbal practitioner to give a "warming" herb during the acute phase of viral or bacterial infection (for "wind-cold" in TCVM).

Particularly in Chinese medicine, herbs are prescribed based on the individual's TCVM diagnosis and not the specific symptoms. For example, two patients are seen with chronic diarrhea. One patient has the problem most often in the morning and has weak and slow pulses, a wet tongue, and frequent fatigue, and the other has frequent foul-smelling diarrhea, a fast pulse, and a red dry tongue. One patient is diagnosed with "deficient, cold type," and the other has "heat symptoms." The herbal prescriptions for these patients is heteropathic and as different as the patients themselves!

The art of healing comes from nature, not from the physician, therefore the physician must start from nature with an open mind.
Parcelsus

General Use of Herbs in Veterinary Practice

Primary differences between humans and exotic animals are related to the dietary substrate of these creatures compared with human omnivores. For example, omnivores eat a higher proportion of their diet as plant matter than do carnivores, who are less able to fully use plant nutrients. This is especially true for whole plant parts that are not pulverized before ingestion. Note that carnivores do not have grinding molars to rupture plant cell walls and make the contents bioavailable as do humans and herbivores. If you eat corn on the cob rapidly without chewing the material well and look at your feces the following day, you see whole kernels of corn "off the cob." This should help you realize that all of us, and especially carnivores, need the plant walls ruptured to increase digestion and absorption. Herbivorous animals have done this work for a carnivore and thus contain well-masticated plant matter in their bowels that is beneficial for the carnivores that ingest them.

Metabolic studies conclude that smaller and lighter animals generally have need for relatively higher amounts of herbs than similar larger and heavier individuals. This is based on the relatively higher basal metabolic rate of smaller animals compared with heavier animals. Herbal components are absorbed, used, and excreted more rapidly, on average, by animals of smaller body size. Our broad recommendation is to calculate herb amounts based on mathematic reduction due to smaller body size and increase that amount to account for increased metabolic rates (metabolic scaling, see Chapter 25). That said, our reptile patients differ drastically in metabolism compared with our small animal patients and even more from the avian patients we treat. Dosing should take the reptile's slower metabolic rate into consideration, which can generally be accomplished by less frequent dosing as is often the case with pharmaceuticals we prescribe.

For example, if an adult human dosage of peppermint in an infusion (tea) is 1 tbsp of herb in a pint of water, then the dosage for a 75-lb dog is the same because one increases the amount of peppermint for carnivore inefficiency in using herbal materials. In other words, a 75-lb dog should take one half of the adult human dose by weight, but this is then increased (doubled) because of the canine gut inefficiency. As another example, a 10-lb cat dosage is about $1/15$ that of a human (proportion reduced for body size) and is then increased because of the cat's inefficient use of herbs and its small body size to about $1/2$ tsp. Note that this increase attempts to take into account both body size and dietary preference. These differences may be significant when dealing with herbivorous, omnivorous, or carnivorous reptile patients.

No one knows exactly how much of each herb to use in assorted species of animals of dissimilar sizes and metabolism. When we add to the equation the variability of herbs due to differing growing, harvesting, and storage conditions, more uncertainty may be seen. But these "medicines" are herbs. Most of them lack the dangerous potencies of derived pharmaceutical agents, and we can relax a bit in our calculations of dosages.

A low dosage of any new substance is best to start with. If vomiting, diarrhea, or other possible side effects are seen, discontinue use immediately and restart at a lower dosage or frequency. If your animal patient has no problems, gradually increase the dosage and monitor efficacy over time.

Most herbs and herbal supplements are given over periods of at least weeks and often months. More often than not, the conditions we treat with herbs and other complementary therapies are chronic problems for which conventional medicine has not been effective.

Dosage calculation may seem difficult, but it is one of the simpler aspects of giving herbs to companion animals. Most species we treat are particular about additions to their meals. This is significant because most herbal substances and formulas have distinct and often unpleasant tastes. This is nothing new to veterinarians, but the sheer amount of some herbal powders needed to achieve dosage recommendations can increase the difficulty of our task.

When herbs are not available as pills, and teas and soups are not a viable option, putting the concentrated powdered herb into capsules (usually $1/2$ mg to 2 mg in size) works well. Alternatively, extracts are fairly easy to administer and are believed to have the most rapid GI absorption rate.[9] Alcohol extracts seem to taste terrible to animal patients, but generally only very small amounts are needed. Glycerin extracts are also available and may taste a little better but usually are not as concentrated.

Milk Thistle, for example, is available in health food stores in pill, capsule, and both alcohol and glycerin extract forms. We commonly use it for avian hepatic lipidois, hepatitis, and feline liver diseases and have used it in a common Green Iguana with chronic hepatitis. We use the extract form and find that cats, particularly, salivate profusely with the alcohol extract but take the glycerin extract without problems. We usually administer the dose in lactulose, particularly with hepatic lipidosis cases.

One of the more controversial areas of veterinary medicine is treating behavior disorders with psychotropic drugs. Many behavior problems are such because they are unacceptable in our homes but natural for the animal in its own habitat. Marking and aggression are frequently seen, and treatment is often sought and administered in spite of undesirable side effects. Herbal medicine may offer an effective option for calming anxiety while avoiding the downside of pharmaceuticals like Depo-Provera, Amitriptylline, Buspirone HCL, and others commonly used.

HOMEOPATHY

Homeopathic medicine predates modern medicine by a century or so. At the turn of the 20th century, 22 homeopathic medical schools and 100 homeopathic hospitals existed, and approximately 15% of American physicians considered themselves homeopaths.[11] Samuel Hahnemann, a German physician, first explored homeopathy in the late 1700s and based his theories and practice on the observation of the body's attempts to heal itself. He recognized that symptoms such as fever or pain may represent the body's attempt to deal with infection or trauma. Because the concept of the immune system was unknown, Hahnemann called this innate healing ability and the indication that it was at work (through symptoms of disease) the "vital force."[12]

Homeopathic practitioners believe that conventional medical thought has a fundamental flaw. That is, the assumption

Case Example: Green Iguana

Signalment: Osiris, 6-year-old, female spayed Green Iguana (*Iguana iguana*)

History: Excellent husbandry and diet; annual laboratory, fecal, and physical examinations; egg bound in March 1998; spayed without complications; exhibiting increased restlessness and aggression since February 2001 when placed in new, much larger enclosure; rostral self-trauma when owner walks nearby; aggressive when owner attempts to handle.

Diagnosis and Treatment: A thorough work-up (radiographs, complete blood count, chemistry profile, electrophoresis) had all unremarkable results. Tried inverting the enclosure to resemble the original, increasing humidity, and giving time to adjust to the change. TCVM diagnosis: Shen disturbed. Shen refers to the organizing force of the self, reflected in the mental, emotional, and expressive life of an individual.[10] The patient was prescribed Shen Calmer, an herbal formula designed specifically for animals by Dr Shen Xie, Chi Institute. Shen Calmer uses a number of Chinese herbs in the formula.

Within 2 weeks, the owner reported a return to normal behavior (i.e., no longer aggressive or restless, eating well, tolerant of owner's handling, no further self-trauma). When the owner finished the first 30 days of formula and discontinued treatment, the problem returned. The patient was placed back on herbs for 90 days, and the owner is experimenting with the dose. The patient does well on 1 g every 24 hours, but symptoms return when decreased to $1/2$ g.

that symptoms represent the disease itself, signifying an abnormality with the animal's health, and that these symptoms need to be controlled, managed, or eliminated.[13] Symptoms may in fact be adaptive responses to an organism's physiologic stress. If symptoms are an inherent part of the body's defense mechanisms, eliminating them without addressing the source of the problem may suppress the body's ability to heal. Instead of treating, controlling, or suppressing symptoms, therapies that augment the body's own defenses may make more sense. In modern times, Darwinian Medicine is the label given to the concept that each organism's adaptive response to trauma and disease should be taken into consideration before initiating treatment.

Homeopaths view disease as an imbalance or disturbance in the vital force and, most importantly, believe that these disturbances or symptoms of disease are unique to each patient. This is not dissimilar to the previously discussed TCVM philosophy where two patients with diarrhea may have a different diagnosis, one due to "cold" factors and the other from "damp heat." For example, two iguanas may have enteritis from a bacterial infection such as enteric salmonellosis. One iguana may be anorexic, the other has diarrhea. The conventional diagnosis and treatment are the same. The homeopath views these different manifestations as individual differences in the state of the patients' vital force, and each lizard receives an entirely different prescription.

Homeopathy is said to treat the patient, not the disease, and works on what is called "the law of similars," that is "like treats like." It is here that homeopathic medicine becomes controversial, as the medicines used are extremely dilute, so much that there should be no original material left in the solution. Substances such as herbs or minerals are serially diluted and agitated for a set number of times until, theoretically at least, there is no original solute. What remains is what is used to treat the patient and is considered to be still efficacious. Many theories are put forth for the mechanisms of action, including an immunologic basis similar to vaccines, an electromagnetic "memory" on the water used for diluting, and hypersensitivity to a minute substance, to name a few. Although research is in its infancy, controlled clinical studies have proven that some homeopathic remedies do work, though mechanisms of action are not yet understood.[12,14]

MANUAL THERAPIES

Manual therapies encompass a number of treatment methods that may be subsumed under the heading of physical medicine. These therapies include, but are not limited to, Acupuncture, Chiropractic, Physical Therapy, Massage Therapy, Veterinary Orthopedic Manipulation, and Tellington Touch. Most medical traditions use manual therapies such as massage and body manipulation. These healthful technologies are generally safe and effective, and most are delivered by practitioners to individuals with little medical infrastructure. Manual therapies have the added advantage of being based on human touch. Touch has been shown to increase somatotropin levels and increase immune system function.[15] Another fundamental benefit of manual therapy is that both the giver and the receiver share feelings of appreciation, care, and love. All human cultures likely evolved touch and massage therapies to some degree as healing systems. We limit our discussion to three of these areas—Acupuncture, Chiropractic, and Massage, and we refer you to the end of the chapter for resources to investigate other manual therapies.

Acupuncture

The basis and usage of acupuncture may be viewed in either a conventional scientific or TCVM framework. The placement of small needles (usually 30-gauge to 36-gauge) into exact locations in a subject's body may have a number of positive benefits. Western scientific analyses indicate local, immunologic, neuroreflexive, and central nervous system responses to acupuncture.[16] These effects may include shortened healing time in injured tissues and nervous system activation in neurologic trauma. Increased immune surveillance and heightened immune system function along with reflexive changes in organ system function and pain control are also reported as effects of acupuncture. Studies have shown acupuncture results in an increase in endogenous substances such as enkephalins and endorphins, and the analgesic effects of acupuncture can be reversed with naloxone.[17] Other research has shown that after acupuncture, serotonin concentrations increase 40% in the systemic circulation and beta endorphins and cortisol levels have been found to rise in horses.[18]

Analgesia is not the only measurable effect of acupuncture. Both parasympathetic and sympathetic components of visceral nerves may be stimulated,[19] as well as local changes in cells, nerves, and vessels where the needles are inserted, including mast cell release, vasodilation, and stimulation of neural terminals.[20] Acupuncture can enhance immunity by increasing levels of white blood cells, interferon, antibodies, and immunoglobulins.[21] Hormonal changes including the release of growth hormone, luteinizing hormone, and thyroid hormones have also been measured.[22]

Case Example: American Alligator

Signalment: A 1.5-meter, "hit by car" American Alligator (*Alligator mississippiensis*), age and gender unknown

History: Patient was seen in Florida in early autumn with oral and forelimb tissue avulsion.

Diagnosis and Treatment: Strong Yang-introducing (warm) treatments were avoided because this creature was soon entering a winter estivation. Aloe vera gel was used topically every 8 hours for 6 days, and the animal was left in a quiet environment. Because the GI and metabolic function was decreasing in this animal, no acupuncture points were used that might have awakened the body. Healing to rough granulation tissue led us to release the sluggish creature near its geographic point of origin.

Case Example: Green Iguana

Signalment: Max, 3-ft-long, 3-year-old, Green Iguana (*Iguana iguana*)

History: Housed under average husbandry conditions. Presented with chronic oral abscesses. Treated by the referring DVM with daily intramuscular injections of an antibiotic.

Diagnosis and Treatment: Treated by classical homeopathic analysis with Hekla Lava, 1 M PO every 48 hours. Abscesses reduced in size over the next 2 weeks and have not recurred for more than 1 year.

Alternative and Complementary Veterinary Therapies

In TCVM, the concept of Qi (pronounced chee), and Chinese medicine's perspective on what constitutes health and disease provide the framework for the traditional use and benefits of acupuncture. In TCVM, health is defined as a state of harmony or balance between the body and its internal and external environment. Illness occurs when the homeostatic mechanisms of the body malfunction, becoming overloaded or inefficient.

The Chinese describe this harmony as the theory of Yin and Yang, where all of nature is grouped in pairs or opposites, such as day-night, male-female, hot-cold, which can be applied to all the phenomena in nature. The philosophy is one of opposing forces that are maintained by both mutual antagonism and mutual dependence.

When Yin and Yang become imbalanced, disease occurs. Qi is the life force; where there is life, there is Qi. Qi flows through the body and can be accessed through a system of channels or meridians on which we find our acupuncture points. Qi is energy and involves the energetic functions of the body, which is the focus of acupuncture. In TCVM, when Qi flows freely, there is balance, health, and the absence of pain. When Qi becomes trapped, obstructed, or stagnant, there is pain; if decreased, there may be weakness and disease. Acupuncture restores the free flow of Qi and in TCVM may be used to tonify, strengthen, and balance the body's systems.

One using acupuncture for therapy from a strictly Western viewpoint would likely choose to treat pain (from trauma, for example) based on local points near the injured area along with a-shi points (Figure 26-1). A-shi points are points of pain or sensitivity and do not necessarily correspond to known meridian points.[23] For example, a partial cranial cruciate ligament tear may be treated with rest, a knee brace, a nonsteroidal antiinflammatory drug (NSAID), and acupuncturing points on and around the knee such as ST-36, GB-34, and BL-40. These three points access the Stomach, Gallbladder, and Bladder meridians respectively.

Conversely, a TCVM practitioner might treat an internal medicine case, for example, chronic renal disease, by acupuncturing points that tonify, energize or nourish, and replenish kidney Qi, with points like KI-3 BL-20, 21, and 23 along with ST-36, all considered to be Qi tonification points. Bear in mind, the TCVM practitioner would also likely use herbs and nutrition to hydrate the body, control and replenish electrolyte problems, and treat symptoms related to the underlying imbalance. In TCVM, chronic renal disease is not a diagnosis but certain patterns, Yin deficiency, for example, may result in chronic renal disease symptoms. TCVM treats the pattern.

Most importantly, in modern veterinary medicine, no reason exists why the two cannot be integrated. Chronic renal disease is a common problem in iguanas (Chapter 66). An integrated approach might include fluids or diuresis, correction of electrolyte imbalances via conventional medications, nutritional and husbandry adjustments, and acupuncture to tonify the kidneys, stimulate appetite, and perhaps treat associated problems like constipation. A thorough work-up including a physical examination, rectal examination, blood work, radiography, and possibly celioscopy precedes treatment, along with a detailed history of symptoms, behavior, husbandry, and nutrition, allowing for both a Western and CAVM plan for treatment.

The use of acupuncture on animals transposes traditional Chinese points for humans along 12 major bilaterally distributed meridians, each linked to a specific internal organ, and along 8 extra channels that are not specifically linked to visceral organs. Anatomic differences in various species compared with humans along with uncertain meridian pathways in animals create problems applying the meridian numbering system to animals. Several studies comparing major points between humans and dogs with various electro point finders, or Low Skin Resistant points (LSR), have revealed a fairly high (79% in one study) correlation between human and canine acupuncture points.[20]

Applying acupuncture to reptiles must therefore take anatomic and functional differences into consideration. Meridian points on lizards are easily transposed from canine acupoints, but snakes and turtles are more challenging (Figure 26-2). Meridians found primarily on the extremities are impossible to directly transpose on a limbless animal. It is likely that many of the points found on legs and digits do

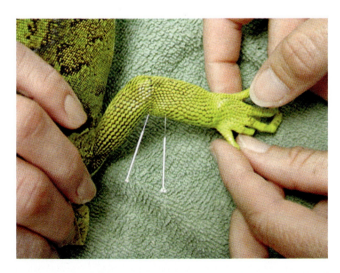

FIGURE 26-1 A-shi acupuncture points are used to treat pain based on local points near the injured area. A-shi points are points of pain or sensitivity and do not necessarily correspond to known meridian points. (*Photograph courtesy D. Mader.*)

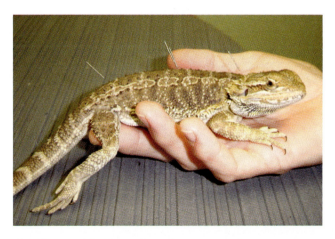

FIGURE 26-2 Meridian points on lizards are easily transposed from canine acupoints; snakes and turtles are more challenging. (*Photograph courtesy D. Mader.*)

exist in some area of the snake's body but have not been discovered or described. Many of the Bladder and Gall Bladder meridians and points on the Spleen, Liver, Kidney, and Stomach meridians are inaccessible on a turtle (Figure 26-3). Some species, particularly amphibians, and more delicate lizards like geckos may have easily identifiable or accessible points, but handling and stress must be conscientiously addressed if one is to attempt needling these species.

Because many of the benefits of acupuncture rely on release of humoral substances like serotonins and endorphins, a highly stressed animal may not receive as much benefit from acupuncture as corticosteroid and epinephrine release may antagonize many of its positive effects.

Numerous animal patients have been successfully treated with acupuncture for a wide range of maladies including, but not limited to, anorexia, GI problems (constipation, decreased GI motility, diarrhea), egg laying, cloacal prolapse, renal failure, respiratory infections, oral inflammation and infection, behavior problems (aggression), musculoskeletal problems, and intervertebral disk disease with resulting neuropathies. Acupuncture does require some basic training, and we strongly recommend interested veterinarians take a formal course before applying acupuncture to their patients. Figures 26-4 and 26-5 show typical acupuncture points used in lizards and turtle patients.

Note that electroacupuncture is a valuable tool for recovery of neural damage. Veterinarians should remember this lesson when considering steroids or euthanasia and hopefully refer these animals to a qualified veterinarian-acupuncturist.[24]

Chiropractic

Chiropractic comes from the Greek words "cheir," meaning hand, and "praxis," meaning practice or done by hand. Chiropractic is based on manual spinal manipulation and is focused on the interactions between neurologic mechanisms and the biomechanics of the spine (Figure 26-8). Treatment is directed at "adjusting" the spine, treating abnormal positional relationships in the contiguous vertebrae, which are described by the chiropractic profession as subluxations. This term should not be confused as a partial dislocation close to a complete luxation as commonly defined in veterinary medicine. Rather, these subluxations may refer to slight changes in the articular surface, which may result in symptoms such as soreness, muscle spasm, tingling, or hard hyperirritable nodular structures called trigger points.[25]

Case Example: Green Iguana

Signalment: Iggy, 5-year-old, intact male Green Iguana (*Iguana iguana*)

History: Adopted at the age of 3 years, previous owners did not feed properly, former husbandry inadequate. Past 2 years had excellent diet and care. Proper temperature, lighting, substrates, humidity, etc., provided. Examined at our clinic about 6 weeks earlier, full laboratory analysis (complete blood count, chemistry profile, electrophoresis) and survey radiographs were performed and all found to be within normal limits.

Iggy was seen with acute onset of posterior paresis and inability to defecate or urinate. Four days before he had done a "back flip" off of the couch. His appetite was normal; he was active, alert, and hydrated. A neurologic examination revealed marked decreased motor bilaterally, conscious proprioceptive deficits but deep pain response remained. Iggy was painful over his caudal thoracic and cranial lumbar vertebrae.

Diagnosis and Treatment: Radiographs showed lesions at T-13/L-1 and L-1/L-2. High-dose dexamethasone was administered, followed by reduced doses 12 and 24 hours later. Strict cage rest was imposed and a (productive) enema given along with subcuticular fluids. Intracoelomic fluids were given after the enema. An herbal formula was prescribed for pain. Several follow-up examinations over a 2-week period revealed a marked reduction in back pain but only minute progress in resolving the paresis and no defecation or urination without enemas. After discussion of a similar case where acupuncture had restored normal eliminations and hindend mobility, the owners agreed to try acupuncture.

The first four sessions used **aquapuncture**, a variance from dry needling where, in this case, vitamin B_{12} was injected into acupoints to treat both constipation and paralysis (Figure 26-6). ST-36, a master point, for spasmolytic effect on the intestines and for the hindend paralysis, BL-40 and BL-60 for analgesia and back pain, BL-20, 21, 23 and Bai Hui for thoracolumbar lesions and pain, BL-11 for bones, GV-14 for spondylosis, and GV-1 for intestinal paralysis.

Iggy's back pain continued to resolve, and hindlimb motor function dramatically improved. Still Iggy could not defecate on his own, although the enema tube now would barely be inserted before a productive bowel movement resulted. Acupuncture therapy was switched to electroacupuncture, where dry needles are inserted into specific points and an electrical current provided via an electronic device designed for this purpose (Figure 26-7). Points used included the previous and the Hua-Tuo-Jia-Ji points (i.e., points just lateral and ventral to the area of spinal trauma as identified on radiographs).

One week later, Iggy's mobility was nearly normal on the left side and continued to improve on the right. He passed some urates on his own the day after his last enema but had still not defecated on his own 3 days after that at the time of his appointment. A Chinese herb was then prescribed to help with defecation in addition to the electroacupuncture.

After the fifth electroacupuncture treatment, Iggy had his first bowel movement, and the following week his owner reported normal defecations occurring every 3 days. After 3 additional weeks of electroacupuncture, the prescribed Chinese herb was discontinued and Iggy's bowel movements increased in frequency to every other day. Iggy is now being treated just once a month as a maintenance therapy, has normal mobility, and appears pain free.

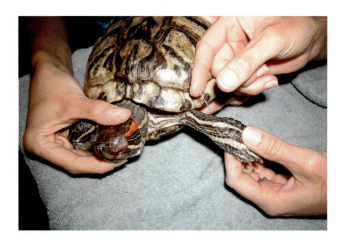

FIGURE 26-3 Most of the bladder and gallbladder meridians and points on spleen, liver, kidney, and stomach meridians are inaccessible on the turtle. Acupuncture is limited to the skin of the legs and neck. (*Photograph courtesy D. Mader.*)

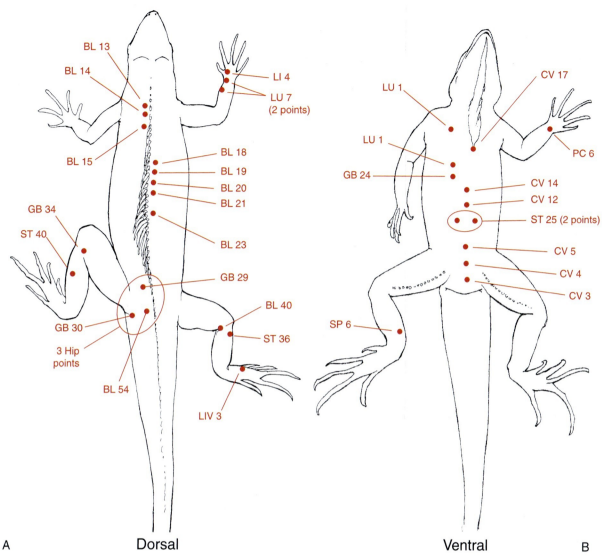

FIGURE 26-4 **A** and **B,** Typical acupuncture points for a lizard patient.

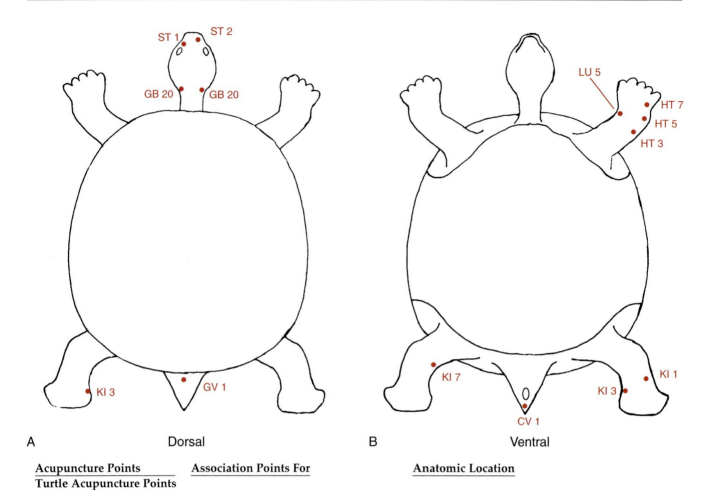

FIGURE 26-5 **A** and **B**, Typical acupuncture points for a turtle patient.

A number of hypotheses have been generated to explain the pathophysiology of subluxations, including nerve compression, facilitation hypothesis, somatoautonomic dysfunction, compressive myelopathy, fixation, vertebrobasilar arterial insufficiency, axoplasmic aberration, and the neurodystrophic hypothesis.[25]

Chiropractic therapy does not try to treat all the varied health problems and disease processes encountered by our profession. Nevertheless, all body functions are innervated and controlled by nerves and the benefits of chiropractic apply to any vertebrate. When neurologic function in the spine is disrupted, disease occurs, and the goal of chiropractic is restoration of normal vertebral function.

Currently, few veterinary chiropractors treat exotic pets, although therapy for equine patients is becoming commonplace, as are applications in canine and feline medicine. However, the potential for application to exotic animals is huge and could potentially treat many conditions commonly

Alternative and Complementary Veterinary Therapies

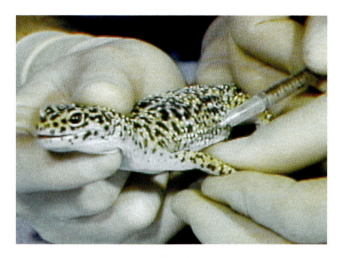

FIGURE 26-6 Small or easily agitated lizards that do not tolerate needling may benefit from aquapuncture. Aquapuncture is a variance from dry needling where, in this case, vitamin B_{12}, diluted with normal saline solution, is injected into acupoints instead of using needles. *(Photograph courtesy D. Mader.)*

Case Example: Uromastix Lizard

Signalment: 3-year-old Uromastyx lizard (*Uromastyx* sp.).

History: Seen with chronic anorexia and lethargy.

Diagnosis and Treatment: The tongue was pale and dry (arid origin lizard). Surrogate pulse indicated a Kidney Yang and Spleen Qi deficiency.

Note that this animal's tongue did not match the pulse diagnosis. Natural "Blood deficiency" seems to be the case in reptiles. Acupuncture was done at BL-21, Guan Yuan Shu and BL-23, Shen Shu (which is probably multiple adjacent back Shu points because of the elongate renal tissues). The animal began to eat with greater vigor, and dietary changes were made. The animal was treated when anorectic twice over the next 3 months and lived uneventfully for another 3 years.

In the last 2 years, the authors have had three cases involving adult male Green Iguanas that had fallen from high ceilings onto cement floors. These are three separate cases, three separate animals and owners, but all of the owners made the same mistake; they kept adult males in mating season together. In this situation, males might fight if not separated, and in our specific cases, the dominant animal chased the weak one to the ceiling and caused the weak one to fall. In nature, the weak one might fall into water or on soft ground, but in captivity, they all fell on cement floors. In all three cases, there was paralysis of one or both hind legs, no fractures or luxations (as none were seen on radiographs), just lower neuron lesions in the area of the pelvis. In all cases, electroacupuncture was used, putting needles in specific points (GB-31 and GB-34) and applying 40 to 80 Hz, direct current in mode dense/disperse for 5 minutes. Usually the animals began flexing and extending stifles after the first treatment, crawling after the second treatment, and running (normal motor restored) by their third treatments.

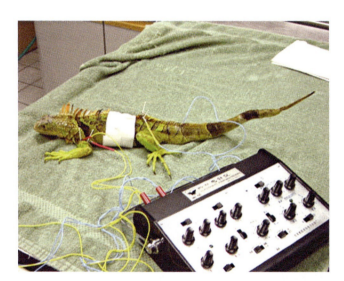

FIGURE 26-7 Electroacupuncture, where dry needles are inserted into specific points and electrical current is applied via an electronic control panel, is a valuable tool for recovery of neural damage. *(Photograph courtesy D. Mader.)*

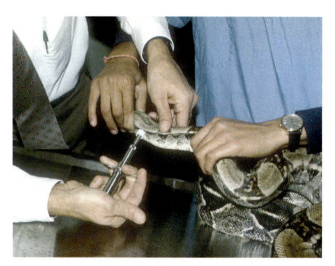

FIGURE 26-8 Chiropractic is based on manual spinal manipulation and is focused on interactions between the neurologic mechanisms and biomechanics of the spine. Here a chiropractor uses an activator to help manipulate a snake's spine. *(Photograph courtesy D. Mader.)*

encountered by avian, reptile, and small animal practitioners. Iguanas and other lizards often have scoliosis from metabolic bone disease of nutritional origin; rabbits and guinea pigs are frequently seen for arthritis, back problems, and lameness; cervical problems may occur in almost any species. Chiropractic (and acupuncture and herbal medicine) can and should be used in wellness or preventive therapy, particularly for the geriatric pet (though beneficial to younger adult animals) that is most prone to deficiencies, imbalances, and subluxations.

Caution must be exercised in treating less flexible creatures (like some lizard species), where disks are fragile, small, or thin and when bone integrity is compromised, as they are in a hypocalcemic iguana. Chiropractic should be applied after corrections have been made (e.g., reestablishing normal calcium homeostasis in a hypocalcemic iguana).

Chiropractic manipulations should only be undertaken by veterinarians with proper training. Unlike humans supporting a vertical column, quadrupeds have less thick and supportive disks. One must be able to visualize the vertebrae in three dimensions with an accurate understanding of articular relationships in the vertebral column and the orientations of joint surfaces. As more veterinarians use Integrated Medicine, manual therapies like acupuncture and chiropractic services will be more readily available and more frequently prescribed for our exotic patients.

Massage

Our best historic records of the origin of massage as a component of an intact medical system come from China. There the indigenous manual therapy system, Tui Na (literally push-pull), was recorded by the physician Bian Que as being used in 2500 BCE. Regardless of its cultural origin, massage therapy has many proponents and styles. These styles may generally be differentiated by the depth and force of touch pressures. Light touch seems more to be correlated with energy transfer between giver and receiver, with receiver receptivity maximally important. Firm touch with deep pressure is more likely to affect local tissue anatomy and physiology, perhaps having reflex activity to deeper body structures as well.

Western massage techniques generally can be classified by overall physical movement involved. Effleurage consists of light gliding movements across the body that do not significantly deviate subcutaneous tissues. Petrissage uses deeper, firmer lifting moves in which superficial and deep tissues are moved together. Connective tissue work involves medium to full depth and pressure moves that slowly push into connective tissue.

Tapotement is a tapping or drumming motion that induces resonant frequency response in the receiver's body. Vibration is now used more commonly with mechanical devices that deliver high-frequency waves to the deepest tissue levels, including into joint capsules. Known effects of massage therapy include both physiologic and psychologic changes.[15] Lymphatic drainage and local vascular function are both benefitted by gentle massage. Muscle relaxation with attendant reduction in myofascial pain and quicker recovery after exercise are facilitated by massage.

Traumatic fibrosis and sprain or strain injuries respond to deep friction massage techniques and range of motion exercises better than to steroids or surgery. Pain relief is probably the most universally reported effect of massage. A sense of well-being is commonly reported by both giver and receiver in human massage. **Contraindications to massage therapy include direct massage of cancerous lesions and no direct massage for sites of recent trauma, inflammation, infection, or fracture.**

Body work is a superb adjunct to many types of surgery, particularly orthopedic. Physiotherapy technologies in human medicine are advanced compared with veterinary medicine. For example, after cranial cruciate ligament surgery, the surgical leg should be manipulated daily. Techniques to use include passive range of motion (gently, never to the point of pain), effleurage, and vibration (5 to 7 days after surgery). If this postsurgical physiotherapy is neglected, cartilage in the greatest weight-bearing area of the joint is lost most rapidly and that same area is then damaged most easily with future return to function. This was emphasized at the North American Veterinary Conference (2001) in multiple lectures and a workshop on physiotherapy techniques. Orthopedic surgeons at the University of Tennessee College of Veterinary Medicine are working with the Health Sciences College program of Physical Therapy to develop innovative approaches to postsurgical physical therapies in small companion animals.[26]

Massage is a valuable addition to acupuncture therapy. Many acupuncture points can be stimulated to good effect with firm finger pressure (acupressure). Clients can extend the effects of acupuncture treatments, with the added benefit that recalcitrant animals may be treated calmly at home rather than stressfully in the office. Manual therapy courses are available to teach veterinarians numerous Tui Na and massage techniques that they can both apply in their office and show to companion animal caretakers so that the caretaker may treat the animal at home.

Massage may also be used instead of surgery. An animal may be a poor surgical candidate or the owner may not want to pursue surgical options. One might even choose to use massage palliatively until an animal or caretaker is mentally or financially prepared for surgery. Massage also can possibly contribute to tissue changes that completely relieve the original problem.

In a paper by Speciale and Fingeroth,[27] the authors conclude, "Persistent use of physical treatment for paralysis that results from conditions affecting the cervical spinal cord may be useful even without concurrent surgical or pharmacologic treatments." In the field of reptile medicine, we may find that soft tissue manipulation techniques can shorten the course of recovery from surgery and trauma.

Relaxation and life extension may be facilitated by massage. Chronic stress is probably one of the major factors that negatively impact human health. For our nonhuman companions, we are uncertain how much stress they perceive. Yet both we and they can benefit from regular massage and body work. The most consistent data on life extension seem to indicate that rest and self-satisfaction are highly correlated with longevity and overall health. When we massage our companion animals, we nourish them and ourselves in both these ways and more. When clients are taught massage techniques to help their companions, they are empowered and included in the healing process. Although unknown, it is likely that such techniques may be of benefit to captive reptiles.

NUTRACEUTICALS AND ORTHOMOLECULAR MEDICINE

Many ingested foods have both nutritional and pharmacologic effects in the body. Sometimes these two cannot be separated. For example, the U.S. Food and Drug Administration (FDA) defines a food as a substance that provides nutrition, taste, or aroma. By FDA definition, a drug is a substance that is a food or nonfood substance that is used to treat, cure, mitigate, or prevent disease (as previous).[28]

Nutraceuticals are mostly foods or food derivatives that have known pharmacologic effects. The North American Veterinary Nutraceutical Council defines a nutraceutical as a nondrug substance that is produced in a purified or extracted form and administered orally to provide agents required for normal body structure and function with the intent of improving the health and well-being of animals.[4]

Nutraceuticals range from macromolecules to simple fatty acids and may act both locally and systemically. For example, numerous species have both quantitative and qualitative fatty acid requirements.[29] Most fats, depending on the natural history and metabolic limits of each reptile, can meet kilocalorie requirements. Some fatty acids may, however, promote inflammation in the body and possibly interfere with normal cytokine production.[30] Further, each bowel segment has an ability to either digest or microbiologically alter fats. Fatty acids that are not biologically appropriate for each species could possibly lead to local bowel inflammation and disharmony and to unbalanced cytokine production and yield less than optimal nutrition to the animal.[5]

Orthomolecular medicine is the use of nutraceuticals and other biologically important molecules, sometimes in supraphysiologic doses, to address various disease conditions. Orthomolecular medicine has become more prevalent with increased research into the role of individual molecules in living creatures. Antioxidant research, for example, has had a few thousand publications in the last 10 years.[4] Generally, the data support the hypothesis of balancing and reducing free radical generation as a key to tissue health. Ocular, vascular, connective tissue, and neuronal and immune system integrity and function have been linked with adequate antioxidant consumption. For example, free radical scavengers were shown to play a role in photoreceptor damage caused by uveitis, and subsequent use of vitamins C and E markedly reduced such damage.[31] A smaller percentage of studies have shown efficacy of supraphysiologic dosages of the antioxidant vitamin E in disease processes such as cardiovascular disease and cancers.[32]

Unfortunately, we are commonly either uncertain of or unable to reproduce the biologically appropriate diet for each species. In such cases, investigation of either diverse fresh foods or food additives with nutraceuticals may be prudent.

Micronutrient imbalances are more difficult to discover and are generally inferred from clinical signs or response to treatment. For example, antioxidants such as vitamin C (most important plasma antioxidant), vitamin E (protects against lipid peroxidation), and beta-carotene and vitamin A (singlet oxygen quencher) deficiencies have been correlated with a number of human degenerative diseases. Some examples include Alzheimer's disease, atherosclerosis, autoimmune disease, cancer, cataracts, and inflammatory diseases. Rarely are all of these important antioxidants added to manufactured diets for captive reptiles.

Most veterinarians have some experience with nutraceuticals in the form of supplements for the hair and coat, multivitamin supplements, and joint supplements, such as chondroitin sulfates and glycosaminoglycans. Geriatric animals in particular may benefit from these substances because of their decreasing ability to absorb and use nutrients. Nutraceuticals may be used to treat more obvious symptoms like arthritis, dry thin skin and coat, impaired vision, and similar problems. For example, we have treated a number of exotics in our practice with joint supplements, including rabbits, guinea pigs, chinchillas, and avian species. One 45-year-old Amazon parrot, barely able to stand on his perch, presented "down on his hocks" and with a decreased appetite and weight loss 3 years ago rapidly improved with diet modification and joint supplementation and continues to do well at this time.

We are left with great uncertainties in the use of nutraceuticals. How to use? When to use? How much to use? Table 26-3

Table 26-3	Trial Dosages for Nutrients and Supplements for Reptile Patients[33]	
Supplement	Daily Dose Range	Possible Adverse Effects
B-complex:		
B_1, B_2, B_6	5-40 mg	Nontoxic
Folic acid, B_{12}	5-100 mg	Nontoxic
Vitamin C*	50-1000 mg	Considered nontoxic
Vitamin E	10-100 IU	Anorexia, increased clotting time?
Vitamin A	500-5000 IU	Anorexia, weight loss
Selenium	5-50 µg	Anorexia, ataxia, weakness
Zinc	5-20 mg	Causes calcium/copper deficiency
Omega-3 fatty acids†	25-250 mg	Dyspepsia, diarrhea

*Should have mixed bioflavonoids in C:bioflavonoid of 1:1 to 1:2.
†Omega-3 fatty acids should be mostly from fish for carnivore supplementation; alpha-lanoline acid from seeds is converted more efficiently to helpful prostaglandins and leukotrienes or eicosanoids in herbivores.

lists some supplements, doses, and possible side effects. We use the previously mentioned joint supplements as recommended on the label but use metabolic scaling where warranted.

RESOURCES FOR FURTHER INFORMATION AND STUDY

We end our chapter with apologies for omitting a number of useful and viable complementary therapies, including, but not limited to Bach Flower Therapy, Aromatherapy, Magnetic Field Therapy and other Bioenergetic Medicines, and Tellington Touch and Physical Therapy. Lack of space, time, and knowledge along with previously mentioned lack of data, especially as regarding the multitude of reptile species, is our excuse. We hope the following resources provide you with opportunities for further education, investigation, and inspiration in applying an integrative approach in your own practices.

Organizations and Training Opportunities in CAVM[9]

Academy of Veterinary Homeopathy
James Schacht, DVM, Corresponding Secretary
6400 E. Independence Boulevard
Charlotte, NC 28212
Phone: 704-535-6688

American Academy of Veterinary Acupuncture
PO Box 419
Hygiene, CO 80433-0419
Phone/fax: 303-722-6726
AAVAoffice@aol.com
www.aava.org

American Holistic Veterinary Medical Association
2218 Old Enmorton Road
Bel Air, MD 21015
Phone: 410-569-0795
Fax: 410-569-2346
AHVMA@compuserve.com

American Veterinarians and Chiropractors Association
623 Main Street
Hillsdale, IL 61257
Phone: 309-658-2920
Fax: 309-658-2622
www.animalchiropractic.org

Chi Institute
9791 NW 160th Street
Reddick, FL 32686
Phone: 352-591-3165
Fax: 352-591-0988
www.chi-institute.com
Acupuncture training; Traditional Chinese Herbalism

Healing Oasis Wellness Center
2555 Wisconsin Street
Sturtevant, WI 53177
Phone: 262-884-9549
Fax: 262-886-6460
www.thehealingoasis.com

International Association for Veterinary Homeopathy
General Secretary: Dr Andreas Schmidt
Sonnhaldenstr. 18
CH-8370 Sirnach
Switzerland
Phone: 41 (73) 26 14 24
Fax: 41 (73) 26 58 14

International Veterinary Acupuncture Society
PO Box 271395
Fort Collins, CO 80527
Phone: 970-266-0666
Fax: 970-266-0777
Ivasoffice@aol.com
www.ivas.org

New Mexico Chinese Herbal Veterinary Medicine Course
1925 Juan Tabo NE, Suite E
Albuquerque, NM 87112
Phone: 505-450-4325
Fax: 505-332-4775

REFERENCES

1. Schoen AM, Wynn SG, editors: *Complementary and alternative veterinary medicine*, Boston, Mass, 1998, Mosby.
2. Donaoghue S, Langenberg J: Nutrition. In Mader D: *Reptile medicine and surgery*, Philadelphia, 1996, WB Saunders.
3. Ober KP: Alterations in fuel metabolism in critical illness. In Ober KP, editor: *Endocrinology of critical disease*, Totowa, NJ, 1997, Humana Press.
4. Bauer JE: Evaluation of nutraceuticals, dietary supplements, and functional food ingredients for companion animals, *J Am Vet Med Assoc* 218(11):1755-1760, 2001.
5. Werbach MR: *Textbook of nutritional medicine*, Tarzana, Calif, 1999, Third Line Press.
6. Xie HS: *Traditional Chinese veterinary medicine*, Beijing, PRC, 1994, Beijing Agricultural University Press.
7. Griffith D: *Herbal medicine*, 1999, Veterinary Information Network Rounds, www.vin.com/Members/SearchDB/Rounds/LC990523.htm.
8. Mills S, Bone K: *Principles and practice of phytotherapy*, Philadelphia, 2000, Churchill Livingstone.
9. Wynn SG: *Organizations and training opportunities in CAVM*, 2001, Veterinary Information Network, www.vin.com/Members/SearchDB/misc/M05000/M00957.htm.
10. Beinfield H, Korngold E: *Between heaven and earth: a guide to Chinese medicine*, New York, 1991, Ballantine.
11. Coulter HC: *Divided legacy: the conflict between homoeopathy and the American Medical Association*, Berkeley, Calif, 1975, North Atlantic.
12. Belavite P: *Homeopathy: a frontier in medical science, experimental studies and theoretical foundations*, Berkeley, Calif, 1995, North Atlantic Books.
13. Ullman D: Homeopathic medicine: principles and research. In Schoen AM, Wynn SG, editors: *Complementary and alternative veterinary medicine*, St Louis, 1998, Mosby.
14. Wynn SG: Animal studies of homeopathy, *J Am Vet Med Assoc* 212(5):719-724, 1998.
15. Yates J: *A physician's guide to therapeutic massage: its physiological effects and their application to treatment*, 1990, Massage Therapists Association of Canada.
16. Hui KKK, et al: Acupuncture modulates the limbic system and subcortical gray structures of the human brain: evidence from MRI studies in normal subjects, *Human Brain Map* 9:13-25, 2000.
17. Cheng RS, Pomeranz BH: Electroacupuncture is mediated by stereospecific opiate receptors and is reversed by antagonists of type 1 receptors, *Life Science*, 26:631, 1980.
18. Bossut DFB, et al: Plasma cortisol and β-endorphins in horses subjected to electroacupuncture for cutaneous analgesia, *Proc Intl Vet Acup Soc* 4:501,1983
19. Altman S: Small animal acupuncture: scientific basis and clinical applications. In Schoen AM, Wynn SG, editors: *Complementary and alternative veterinary medicine*, St Louis, 1988, Mosby.
20. Schoen AM: *Veterinary acupuncture: ancient art to modern medicine*, St Louis, 1994, Mosby.
21. Chao WK, Loh WP: The immunologic responses of acupuncture stimulation, *Acupunct Electrother Res* 12:282, 1987.
22. Xie QW: Endocrinological basis of acupuncture, *Am J Chin Med* 9:298, 1982.
23. Ellis A, et al: *Fundamentals of Chinese acupuncture*, Brookline, Mass, 1991, Paradigm Publications.
24. Sagiv ben-Yakir: *Treatment of three male iguanas with electroacupuncture for spinal trauma*, personal communication, 2001.
25. Leach RA: *The chiropractic theories*, Baltimore, 1986, Williams & Wilkins.
26. Millis D: *Companion animal physiotherapies*, Proceedings from The North American Veterinary Conference, 2001.
27. Speciale J, Fingeroth JM: Use of physiatry as the sole treatment for three paretic or paralyzed dogs with chronic compressive conditions of the caudal portion of the cervical spinal cord, *J Am Vet Med Assoc* 217(1):43-47, 2000.
28. US Food and Drug Administration: FDA's view of dietary supplement legislation, *FDA Vet* 10:5-6, 1995.
29. Harvey RG: Essential fatty acids. In Bonagura JD, editor: *Kirk's current veterinary therapy, XIII*, Philadelphia, 2000, WB Saunders.
30. Messinger LM: Pruritus therapy in the cat. In Bonagura JD, editor: *Kirk's current veterinary therapy, XIII*, Philadelphia, 2000, WB Saunders.
31. van Rooij J: Oral vitamin C and E as additional treatment in patients with acute anterior uveitis: a randomized double masked study in 145 patients, *Br J Ophthalmol* 83(11):1277-1282, 1999.
32. Theriault A: Tocotrienol: a review of its therapeutic potential, *Clin Biochem* 32(5):309-319, 1999.

33. Kendall RV: Basic and preventive nutrition for the cat, dog, and horse. In Schoen AM, Wynn SG, editors: *Complementary and alternative veterinary medicine,* Boston, 1998, Mosby.

ADDITIONAL SUGGESTED READINGS

Bensky D, Gamble A: *Chinese herbal medicine materia medica,* Seattle, 1993, Eastland Press.

Blake SR: Bach flower therapy: a practitioner's perspective. In Schoen AM, Wynn SG, editors: *Complementary and alternative veterinary medicine,* St Louis, 1998, Mosby.

Blumenthal M, Goldberg A, Brinckmann J: *Herbal medicine: expanded commission E mongraphs,* Austin, Tex, 2000, American Botanical Council.

Chuan Y: *Traditional Chinese veterinary acupuncture and moxibustion,* Bejing, PRC, 1995, China Agricultural Press.

Day C, Saxton JGG: Veterinary homeopathy: principles and practice. In Schoen AM, Wynn SG, editors: *Complementary and alternative veterinary medicine,* St Louis, 1998, Mosby.

Harmon D, Ryan M, Kelly A, Bowen M: Acupressure and the prevention of nausea and vomiting during and after spinal anaesthesia for caesarean section, *Br J Anaesth* 84:101-105, 2000.

Holmes P: *The energetics of western herbs,* vols 1 and 2, Boulder, Colo, 1997, Snow Lotus Press.

Maciocia G: *The foundations of Chinese medicine,* London, 1989, Churchill Livingstone.

Mittleman E, Gaynor JS: A brief overview of the analgesic and immunologic effects of acupuncture in domestic animals, *J Am Vet Med Assoc* 217(8):1201-1205, 2000.

Winter WG: *The holistic veterinary handbook,* Lakeville, Minn, 1997, Glade Press.

Wynn SG: *Herb doses for small animal patients,* Veterinary Information Network, 2000, www.vin.com/Members/SearchDB/misc/M05000/M00923.htm.

27
ANESTHESIA AND ANALGESIA

JUERGEN SCHUMACHER and
TRISHA YELEN

Safe and effective anesthesia and analgesia can be challenging in reptiles because of their unique anatomy and physiology and their variable response to anesthetic and analgesic drugs and dosages. Commonly used anesthetic and analgesic agents may also unpredictably compromise homeostasis of the reptilian patient. For successful anesthesia of the variety of reptilian species commonly seen by the practitioner, a thorough knowledge and understanding of their unique anatomy, physiology, and the pathophysiology of diseases is essential. Species and individual differences may be present, and a good understanding of reptile disease processes is recommended for selection and administration of an effective and safe anesthetic protocol for the patient. Reptiles are poikilothermic animals, and all body functions are dependent on the environmental temperature. Reptiles have a species-specific preferred optimal temperature range (POTR) in which all organ systems work most effectively. Consequently, the patient's response to drugs including anesthetic and analgesic agents also depends on the environmental temperature.

Anesthesia and analgesia are important specialties in reptile medicine that need further studies to determine effective drugs and dosage regimen. Few studies have determined the cardiopulmonary effects of anesthetic agents and the pharmacokinetics and effectiveness of analgesic agents in reptiles. Along with the advances of diagnostic and surgical procedures in reptile medicine, safe and effective anesthetic techniques including appropriate analgesic therapy are required. This chapter describes clinical anesthetic and analgesic techniques in reptiles, and comprehensive reviews on reptile anesthesia have been published previously.[1-6]

ANATOMY AND PHYSIOLOGY

The anatomy and physiology of reptiles differs considerably from mammalian and avian species, and knowledge of normal anatomic structures and normal reptilian physiology is essential to successfully anesthetize and monitor the reptilian patient. All anesthetic agents commonly used in reptile anesthesia have profound effects on cardiopulmonary performance, and a detailed understanding of normal respiratory anatomy and function is essential to select a safe and effective anesthetic regimen and facilitate appropriate monitoring of cardiopulmonary function in the preoperative, intraoperative, and postoperative periods.

Respiratory Anatomy and Physiology

The structure and function of the reptilian respiratory system not only differs considerably from mammalian and avian species, but differences are also apparent between orders of reptiles and between species.[7,8] All reptiles lack a functional diaphragm, and the force to move air during inspiration and expiration comes from movement of the intercostal, pectoral, and abdominal musculature, resulting in changes of intrapulmonary pressure.

The glottis of snakes is located rostrally, and air enters through the external nares, the nasal sinuses, and the internal nares.[9] The trachea consists of incomplete cartilagenous rings and bifurcates into short bronchi at the level of the heart. The lungs are elongated sac-like structures lined with respiratory epithelium. Although the left lung is vestigal in most snake species, the right lung extends into a caudal air sac, lined with nonrespiratory epithelium. The glottis of carnivorous lizards is located more rostrally when compared with herbivorous species, where it is commonly found at the base of the tongue (Figure 27-1). Lizards have incomplete tracheal rings, and the trachea bifurcates approximately at the base of the heart. The lungs of most lizard species are single-chambered organs that extend caudally into an air sac. Iguanids have multichambered lungs that consist of an anterior and posterior chamber. In chelonians, the glottis is located at the base of a fleshy tongue. The trachea has complete tracheal rings, is relatively short, and bifurcates into a left and right intrapulmonary bronchus at the level of the thoracic inlet. Turtles and tortoises have paired, multichambered, relatively rigid lungs. In crocodilians, the glottis is located behind the epiglottal flap. The lungs of crocodilians are complex and multichambered, and the bronchi branch into multiple internal lobes.

Reptile respiratory physiology differs considerably between orders and species, especially terrestrial and aquatic species. The lungs are the major organ for gas exchange (oxygen and carbon dioxide); however, some aquatic snake and turtle species feature cutaneous gas exchange, primarily for the elimination of CO_2. Many reptiles, especially aquatic species, are also capable of converting to anaerobic metabolism during long periods of apnea. Reptilian lungs have high compliance values and are relatively easy to inflate. Reptiles increase the minute volume by increasing the respiratory rate. In comparison with mammals, reptiles have larger lung volumes; however, the surface area for gas exchange is

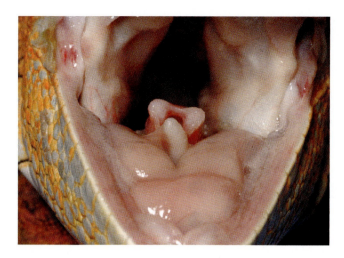

FIGURE 27-1 Glottis of a Green Iguana (*Iguana iguana*).

approximately 20% of that of a mammal of comparative body mass.[7]

Reptilian respiration is controlled by hypoxia and hypercapnia and environmental temperature. Specific receptors increase ventilation during periods of low O_2 and high CO_2. In most reptile species, hypercapnia causes increases in tidal volume and periods of hypoxia increase respiratory rate. In reptiles, the stimulus to breathe comes from low oxygen concentrations. Respiratory rate has been shown in tortoises to increase during hypercapnia but decrease during hypoxia.[8] The higher demand for oxygen during increased temperature or after prolonged dives in aquatic species is met by increasing the tidal volume and not the respiratory rate. In an oxygen-enriched environment, reptiles decrease ventilation, characterized by a decrease in respiratory rate and tidal volume. Intrapulmonary shunts, which represent the portion of pulmonary blood bypassing gas exchange, reduce the efficiency of gas exchange in the lungs and result in a reduction of arterial PO_2 concentrations.[8]

PREANESTHETIC EVALUATION

Reptiles are often seen with chronic disease processes characterized by poor body condition, dehydration, and the presence of secondary bacterial and fungal infections. In many cases, disease is a result of inadequate environmental conditions, and a careful review of husbandry practices and onset of clinical signs of disease is mandatory. For reduction of anesthetic risk and stabilization of the patient's condition, supportive care measures such as fluid therapy and nutritional support should be initiated before anesthesia. In patients with identified infectious bacterial disease processes, treatment should include effective antimicrobial agents, as determined with culture and sensitivity testing. Particular attention should be paid to the cardiopulmonary status and performance of the patient. Rate and depth of respiration should be carefully evaluated for signs of respiratory disease requiring treatment before anesthesia.[10] Baseline respiratory and heart rates and an accurate body weight should be recorded as part of the physical examination.

For assessment of the health status of the reptile, collection of a venous blood sample for hematologic and plasma biochemical parameters is indicated. Minimally, the packed cell volume (PCV), total protein, and glucose levels should be determined. In some patients, however, such as crocodilians, large lizards, and chelonians, sedation or general anesthesia may be necessary to obtain a blood sample and other diagnostic specimen. Additional diagnostic tests should be performed as indicated and should include fecal screens for parasites, collection of biopsy specimen, and aspirates for cytologic and microbiologic evaluation. Imaging procedures such as radiography and ultrasound can be performed in most species with manual restraint alone and are valuable tools in determination of the health status of the patient and identification of organ abnormalities.

Before anesthesia, the patient should be acclimated to temperature and humidity levels appropriate for the species. Fluid therapy should be initiated with indication of volume depletion, on the basis of physical and laboratory findings. The goal of fluid therapy is to restore homeostasis and maintain organ function, and administration of a balanced electrolyte solution is indicated in most patients. Fluid requirements and selection and treatment of disturbances of hydration status have been reported for reptiles.[11] A constant-rate infusion of fluids is preferable over intermittent boluses; therefore, every effort should be made to place an intravenous (IV), or alternatively an intraosseous (IO), catheter. In reptiles with electrolyte imbalances, the underlying problem should be identified and corrected. Normal electrolyte levels in reptiles are species dependent, and a wide range of values has been reported for various species.

In patients in which physical and diagnostic findings indicate that the animal is in pain and discomfort, appropriate analgesic therapy should be initiated before anesthetic induction, as part of a preemptive analgesic regimen.

PREMEDICATION

The type and amount of preanesthetic agents depend on the species of reptile to be anesthetized and the procedure to be performed (Table 27-1). Large crocodilians, large and venomous snakes, and chelonians may need administration of an injectable agent to facilitate handling and induction of anesthesia with an inhalational (e.g., isoflurane) or injectable (e.g., propofol) agent.

Reptiles scheduled to undergo surgical or anticipated painful procedures should be administered a preoperative analgesic agent such as butorphanol or buprenorphine for a balanced anesthetic regimen. Administration of these agents provides intraoperative and postoperative analgesia and often reduces anesthetic maintenance requirements of the inhalational agent. However, a study in Green Iguanas (*Iguana iguana*) determined that butorphanol does not have significant isoflurane-sparing effects.[12] The cardiac anesthetic index of isoflurane in Green Iguanas has been determined to be more than 4.32 and is not affected by the administration of butorphanol.[13] Both butorphanol and buprenorphine, if used alone even at high doses, have minimal to moderate sedative effects in most reptile species. Green Iguanas premedicated with intramuscular (IM) butorphanol (2 mg/kg) showed no changes in heart and respiratory rates 30 minutes after drug administration when compared with baseline values.[14,15] Administered before mask induction, butorphanol or

Table 27-1	Agents Commonly Used for Immobilization and Anesthesia in Reptiles			
Agent	Lizards	Snakes	Chelonians	Comments
Alphaxalone/alphadolone (mg/kg)	6-15 IM, IV	6-15 IM, IV	6-15 IM, IV	Species differences
Diazepam (mg/kg)	0.2-2 IM, IV	0.2-2 IM, IV	0.2-1 IM, IV	All species
Isoflurane (%)	Induction: 4-5 Maintenance: 1.5-3	Induction: 5 Maintenance: 2-3	Induction: 4-5 Maintenance: 2-3	All species
Ketamine (mg/kg)	5-20 IM, IV	10-60 IM	5-50 IM, IV	Rarely used alone
Medetomidine (mg/kg)	0.05-0.1 IM	0.1-0.15 IM	0.03-0.15 IM	Reversible with atipamezole
Midazolam (mg/kg)	1-2 IM, IV	1-2 IM, IV	1-2 IM, IV	All species
Propofol (mg/kg)	3-5 IV, IO	3-5 IV	2-5 IV, IO	Induction agent of choice
Sevoflurane (%)	Induction: 7-8 Maintenance: 2.5-4.5	Induction: 7-8 Maintenance: 2.5-4.5	Induction: 7-8 Maintenance: 2.5-4.5	Species differences
Tiletamine/zolazepam (mg/kg)	2-6 IM, IV	2-6 IM	2-4 IM	Prolonged recoveries, especially in chelonians

IM, Intramuscularly; *IV*, intravenously; *IO*, intraosseously.

buprenorphine results in decreased struggling of the patient, and most animals are less likely to hold their breath during induction of anesthesia.

Benzodiazepines such as diazepam and midazolam if used alone have minimal sedative effects in most reptile species. Midazolam has been reported as a sedative agent in Red-eared Slider Turtles (*Trachemys scripta elegans*) at a dosage of 1.5 mg/kg intramuscularly and resulted in a sedative plane suitable for minor manipulations.[16] In most anesthetic regimens, benzodiazepines are combined with dissociative agents such as ketamine and opioid agents (butorphanol, buprenorphine). Anticholinergic agents such as atropine and glycopyrrolate to reduce respiratory secretions are not routinely used in reptiles.

Hypothermia or deliberate cooling is not an acceptable means for the immobilization of reptiles. Although it causes immobilization, it does not provide analgesia and anesthesia. Hypothermia is painful and associated with decreased metabolism and may also result in necrosis of the brain. Safe and effective injectable and inhalational anesthetic agents are available for reptiles, and hypothermia is an unacceptable inhumane means for immobilization of reptiles.

INJECTABLE ANESTHETIC AGENTS

Many injectable agents have been used and investigated for induction and maintenance of anesthesia in reptiles (see Table 27-1). Most agents, especially when used alone at high dosages, are associated with pronounced cardiopulmonary depressant effects, prolonged induction and recovery times, and poor muscle relaxation and analgesia during maintenance of anesthesia. Species and individual differences are commonly seen in response to parenteral anesthetic agents.

Most commonly, the dissociative anesthetic agent ketamine HCl is used in reptiles to produce immobilization and induce anesthesia. Ketamine has a wide range of safety in most reptiles and can be administered intramuscularly and intravenously. Ketamine alone results in poor muscle relaxation, minimal analgesia, and, if used at high dosages, prolonged recovery times. In snakes, ketamine alone has been shown to produce respiratory depression, hypertension, and tachycardia.[17] Therefore, it is rarely used alone and often combined at lower dosages with synergistic agents such as benzodiazepines (e.g., diazepam, midazolam), opioid agents (e.g., butorphanol, buprenorphine), or alpha$_2$-adrenergic agonists (e.g., medetomidine). The addition of synergistic agents allows for the dose of ketamine to be reduced and results in better quality of anesthesia, characterized by more rapid and smoother induction and recoveries and improved muscle relaxation and analgesia during maintenance. A study of ketamine (60 mg/kg IM) alone or in combination with xylazine (2 mg/kg IM) or midazolam (2 mg/kg IM) in Red-eared Sliders (*Trachemus scripta elegans*) resulted in various degrees of sedation.[18]

Telazol, a combination of tiletamine and zolazepam, has been used for immobilization and induction of anesthesia in reptiles; however, at higher doses (>6 mg/kg IM), it is associated with prolonged recovery times (>48 to 72 hours), especially in chelonians. At a dose of 2 to 4 mg/kg IM, tiletamine/zolazepam is useful to facilitate handling of large chelonians, lizards, and snakes.

The alpha$_2$-agonist medetomidine has been investigated as a sedative agent in reptiles, especially in potentially dangerous species and for short procedures. Similar to use in domestic animals, medetomidine should not be used alone and therefore is commonly combined with a low dose of ketamine and an opioid agent such as butorphanol. Administration of this combination facilitates handling of large reptile species and allows minor procedures to be performed, such as abscess debridement, shell repair, and collection of diagnostic samples. The specific alpha$_2$-antagonist atipamezole should be administered at five times the medetomidine dose to reverse the effects of the alpha$_2$-agonist at the end of the procedure.

Atipamezole administered intravenously to Gopher Tortoises (*Gopherus polyphemus*) immobilized with ketamine-medetomidine resulted in severe hypotension, and the conclusion was that this agent should not be given via the IV route in turtles and tortoises.[19] The sedative effects of medetomidine (150 µg/kg IM) alone have been reported in Desert Tortoises (*Gopherus agassizii*). At the dosage used in this study, all tortoises were sedated; however, pronounced cardiopulmonary depression, including decreases in heart and respiratory rate and hypotension, was present.[20] IV administration of a ketamine (5 mg/kg)–medetomidine (0.1 mg/kg) combination in Gopher Tortoises resulted in effective short-term immobilization adequate for minor procedures. In this study, moderate hypoxemia and hypercapnia and moderate increases in arterial blood pressures were seen. Therefore, recommendation is to provide supplemental oxygen and assist ventilation with this combination.[19]

Propofol an ultra–short-acting induction agent is the injectable agent of choice in reptiles if vascular access is available (Figure 27-2). Propofol has been used in a variety of reptile species for induction and maintenance of anesthesia.[21-23] Propofol has to be administered intravenously or intraosseously and can be used for both induction and maintenance of anesthesia via constant rate infusion (0.3 to 0.5 mg/kg/minute) or with intermittent boluses (0.5 to 1 mg/kg). Propofol does not contain preservatives, and sterile techniques should be used with administration of the agent.

Perivascular injections are not associated with tissue necrosis; however, the potential for infection is present. Although these injections have been shown by some investigators to be effective, the author does not use the intracardiac route for propofol administration for the previous reason.[21] Similar to use of barbiturate induction agents, administration of propofol results in pronounced cardiopulmonary depressant effects in reptiles and therefore should be titrated to effect. Studies in humans and domestic animals have shown that propofol causes systemic hypotension, decreased myocardial contractility, and respiratory depression. Rapid bolus injection of propofol during induction is commonly associated with apnea.[22] The advantage over other induction agents such as barbiturate agents is the shorter duration of action of propofol.

Routes of Drug Administration

In most reptiles, IM administration of anesthetic agents is most effective and practical. Although oral administration of sedative agents has been investigated in domestic and nondomestic species, in reptiles, this route of drug administration is not reliable. Subcutaneous administration of anesthetic agents results in prolonged and unreliable induction times.

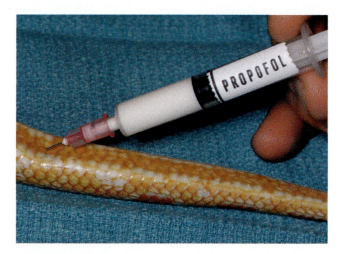

FIGURE 27-2 Administration of propofol into the ventral coccygeal vein of a Cornsnake *(Elaphe guttata)*.

Although a renal portal system has been identified in reptiles, the pharmacokinetics of injectable agents have been shown to be minimally altered if injected into the caudal half of the body.[24,25]

In snakes, IM injections are given into the paravertebral muscles. IV injections can be given into the ventral coccygeal vein or the right jugular vein, after a cutdown procedure. Intracardiac injections should only be given in emergency situations for administration of emergency drugs. In lizards and chelonians, IM injections can be administered into the musculature of the front limbs. In chelonians, the jugular vein can be catheterized for IV access or the coccygeal vein can be used for IV injections. In most lizards, the ventral coccygeal vein is used for IV drug administration. Lizards have a prominent ventral abdominal vein that can be catheterized for administration of anesthetic agents such as propofol and for administration of effective fluid therapy during anesthesia. In patients in which venous access is difficult, an IO catheter can be placed anterograde into the tibia.

LOCAL ANESTHETIC AGENTS

Local anesthetic agents alone are not routinely used in reptiles. However, they can be used for the same indications as in domestic animals.[26] As part of a balanced analgesic regimen, local anesthetic agents such as lidocaine or the longer-acting bupivacaine should be administered concurrently with systemic analgesic agents. Techniques for local and regional anesthesia, including epidural anesthesia, have not been described in reptiles. However, indications for use of local anesthetic techniques are similar to those in domestic animals. Intercostal nerve blocks and interpleural administration of local anesthetic agents are indicated for coeliotomies in reptiles. The most effective local anesthetic agent is bupivacaine at 1 to 2 mg/kg. Administration of bupivacaine should be repeated every 4 to 12 hours if the patient tolerates it. Additional indications for the application of local anesthetic agents in reptiles include orthopedic surgeries in combination with systemic analgesic agents.

INHALATIONAL AGENTS

Most anesthetic regimens in reptiles are based on the administration of inhalational agents either alone or in combination with parenteral agents such as dissociative agents, benzodiazepines, opioid agents, and alpha$_2$-agonists. Inhalational agents can be administered for both induction and maintenance of anesthesia in most reptile species. Inhalational agents should be administered with a precision vaporizer in oxygen, and a nonrebreathing system is indicated in most smaller reptile species (<10 kg body weight). Induction and maintenance requirements of the inhalational agent are determined by the health status of the animal and the amount of preanesthetic agent administered.

At present, the inhalational agent of choice in reptiles is isoflurane because of its rapid induction and recovery times, minimal depressant effects on cardiopulmonary function, and limited hepatic and renal toxicity. For most reptile species, isoflurane concentrations for induction of anesthesia are 5% and maintenance requirements range between 2% and 3%.

In Green Iguanas, the minimum alveolar concentration (MAC) of isoflurane has been determined at 2.1%.[12] Lower concentrations are indicated for severely debilitated patients.

Sevoflurane, commonly used in human and domestic animal anesthesia, has been investigated in several reptile species with various results. Sevoflurane has a low solubility in blood, which results in short induction and recovery times and the ability to rapidly change the depth of anesthesia. During induction with sevoflurane, a rapid increase in alveolar concentration can be seen. In humans and domestic animals, use of premedicants does not change the concentration of sevoflurane necessary for induction of anesthesia. In reptiles, induction times with sevoflurane appear to vary between species, and some species may fail to reach a surgical plane of anesthesia, even at high concentrations.

A study in Desert Tortoises showed minimal cardiopulmonary depressant effects of sevoflurane.[27] A study in Green Iguanas that compared anesthetic and cardiopulmonary effects of sevoflurane and isoflurane after premedication with IM butorphanol (2 mg/kg) showed faster induction and recovery times and improved muscle relaxation with sevoflurane when compared with isoflurane. In sevoflurane-anesthetized iguanas, no significant changes in heart rate were seen over time; however, isoflurane-anesthetized iguanas had significantly lower heart rates approximately 30 minutes after induction of anesthesia. No significant differences between both agents were determined regarding their cardiopulmonary effects.[14,15] If the agent is used alone, most reptile species need sevoflurane concentrations of 7% to 8% for induction and 3.5% to 4.5% for maintenance of a surgical plane of anesthesia.

INDUCTION OF ANESTHESIA

Techniques for induction of anesthesia depend on the species to be anesthetized, the procedure to be performed, and the health status of the patient. For most reptile species, recommendation is administration of a sedative agent (e.g., butorphanol or buprenorphine) before induction to reduce the amount of induction agent necessary and to decrease the likelihood of breath-holding and struggling. In patients in which vascular access has been established, propofol (3 to 5 mg/kg IV/IO) is the induction agent of choice to facilitate endotrachael intubation and maintenance with an inhalational agent. The amount of injectable or inhalational agent necessary for induction of anesthesia depends on the type and dosage of the premedicant, the degree of sedation at the time of induction, and the condition of the reptile and should be adjusted accordingly.

Chelonians

Induction of anesthesia can be challenging in large tortoise species and aquatic species, with the latter often being aggressive and capable of delivering a painful bite. In large tortoises, gaining access to the head and the limbs once retracted into the shell is often difficult. Administration of inhalational agents alone via face mask may result in prolonged induction times, especially in aquatic species capable of prolonged breath-holding. In most species, administration of an injectable anesthetic agent facilitates handling and reduces the amount of induction agent necessary for induction of anesthesia (Figure 27-3). If a peripheral vein is accessible, the author prefers administration of propofol for induction of anesthesia after premedication with IM butorphanol (1 to 2 mg/kg; Figure 27-4). Propofol (3 to 5 mg/kg) can be administered slowly to effect into the jugular vein or the coccygeal vein in most chelonians. In patients where IV access has not been established, IM administration of immobilizing agents is indicated. Ketamine, if given alone for immobilization, requires high dosages, resulting in prolonged recovery times and poor analgesia and muscle relaxation. A combination of ketamine (4 to 10 mg/kg), butorphanol (0.5 to 1 mg/kg), and medetomidine (40 to 150 μg/kg) administered intramuscularly facilitates handling and often allows endotracheal intubation and maintenance of anesthesia with isoflurane or sevoflurane.[28]

Anesthesia was effectively and safely induced in a Loggerhead Seaturtle (*Caretta caretta*) with IV ketamine

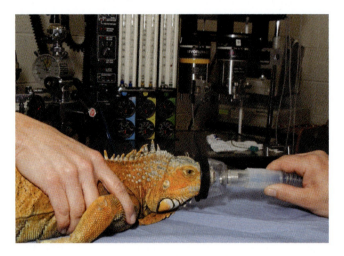

FIGURE 27-3 Mask induction of a Green Iguana (*Iguana iguana*) with sevoflurane after premedication with intramuscular butorphanol (2 mg/kg).

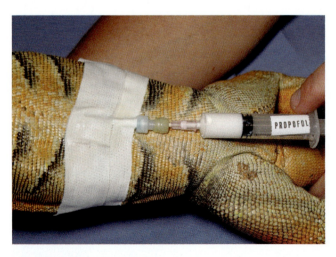

FIGURE 27-4 Induction of a Green Iguana (*Iguana iguana*) with propofol. An intravenous catheter has been placed in the ventral abdominal vein.

(5 mg/kg) and medetomidine (0.05 mg/kg) and maintained with sevoflurane (0.5% to 2.5%).[29] In Snapping Turtles (*Chelydra serpentina*), a combination of ketamine (20 to 40 mg/kg IM) and midazolam (2 mg/kg IM) resulted in good sedation to facilitate handling.[30] A combination of alphaxalon/alphadolon (24 mg/kg) administered intracoelomically resulted in excellent muscle relaxation and a surgical plane of anesthesia in Red-eared Sliders (*Trachemus scripta elegans*).[31]

Rocuronium, a reversible neuromuscular blocking agent, has successfully been investigated in Gulf Coast Box Turtles (*Terrapene Carolina major*) to induce short-term immobilization and facilitate endotracheal intubation. Turtles administered rocuronium at 0.25 to 0.5 mg/kg were effectively immobilized and the trachea was intubated. Reversal of the effects of rocuronium was via administration of neostigmine and glycopyrrolate.[32] Any animal immobilized with a neuromuscular blocking agent is not anesthetized, and no analgesia is provided. Therefore, the length of the procedure should be minimized, and no painful invasive procedures should be performed without prior administration of effective anesthetic and analgesic agents.

Snakes

Most snakes can be premedicated with butorphanol (1 to 4 mg/kg IM) or a low dose of ketamine (5 to 20 mg/kg IM) before induction with an inhalational agent (e.g., 5% isoflurane or 8% sevoflurane). Large snakes such as boid snakes can be premedicated with Telazol (2 to 4 mg/kg IM) to facilitate handling, endotracheal intubation, and induction with an inhalational agent. For IV administration of the induction agent, propofol should be administered into the ventral tail vein. Venomous snakes can be induced in an induction chamber or directly intubated and maintained with an inhalational anesthetic agent. Clear plexiglass tubes are ideal for handling of venomous snakes. They allow safe restraint and visualization of the snake, and tubes are often provided with small holes and slits to allow injections and sample collection. Once the snake is restrained in the tube, an inhalant anesthetic can be administered into the tube to faciliate induction of anesthesia and endotracheal intubation.

Lizards

Most lizards can deliver a painful bite to the inexperienced handler, and one should be aware of the tail and the nails that can inflict injury. The use of leather gloves is recommended for handling large powerful lizard species. Large potentially dangerous lizards can be administered tiletamine-zolazepam (4 to 6 mg/kg IM) to facilitate handling. Butorphanol (1 to 4 mg/kg IM) administered 30 minutes before induction is useful as a preanesthetic and provides preoperative and intraoperative analgesia. Butorphanol alone often does not produce pronounced sedative effects but does reduce the amount of induction agent necessary to induce anesthesia. If venous access is available, propofol (3 to 5 mg/kg IV) administered to effect induces anesthesia to facilitate endotracheal intubation and maintenance with the inhalational anesthetic agents isoflurane or sevoflurane.

The ventral coccygeal vein and the ventral abdominal vein are the preferred venous access sites. Access to the cephalic vein requires a cut-down procedure in most lizards. If inhalational agents are selected for induction of anesthesia, lizards can be induced via facemask with isoflurane (4% to 5%) or sevoflurane (7% to 8%).

Crocodilians

All crocodilians should be considered dangerous and should only be handled by experienced handlers. A variety of injectable agents have been investigated for chemical restraint of crocodilians with variable success.[33-35] Apparent species differences in response to immobilizing agents have been observed in crocodilians. Most anesthetic regimens for crocodilians are based on injectable agents to provide immobilization and safe handling and faciliate induction and maintenance of anesthesia with inhalational agents. Muscle relaxants (e.g., gallamine and succinylcholine) either alone or in combination with other agents (e.g., benzodiazepines, ketamine) have been used in crocodilians to provide immobilization.

Potent opioid agents such as etorphine HCl have been investigated in a variety of crocodilian species. In comparison with mammalian species, crocodilians need higher dosages to induce immobilization, often in excess of 1 mg/kg IM. For small crocodilians that can be manually restrained, propofol (3 to 5 mg/kg IV) is the induction agent of choice and should be given into the ventral coccygeal vein. After induction, the animal should be intubated and maintained on an inhalational agent. Large crocodilians require administration of IM anesthetic agents for safe handling. Tiletamine-zolazepam (5 to 10 mg/kg IM) often provides sufficient immobilization to facilitate handling and endotracheal intubation. However, recovery times after tiletamine-zolazepam administration may be prolonged. A combination of ketamine (5 to 20 mg/kg IM) and medetomidine (80 to 360 μg/kg IM) induced effective and reversible anesthesia in American Alligators (*Alligator mississippiensis*). Reversal with atipamezole was rapid and complete.[36]

Endotracheal Intubation

Endotracheal intubation after induction of anesthesia is relatively easy to perform in most reptile species and is recommended in all patients to maintain a patent airway, prevent aspiration of fluids (e.g., during oral surgery), and allow positive pressure ventilation during maintenance of anesthesia.

The glottis is located rostrally in snakes and in carnivorous lizards. Herbivorous lizards and chelonians have a fleshy tongue, and the glottis is located at the base. For visualization of the tracheal opening, adequate jaw relaxation should be present. A laryngoscope blade and a light source aid in the visualization of the glottis. Chelonians have a relatively short trachea, and care should be taken not to intubate one bronchus. An adequately sized uncuffed endotracheal tube is recommended for most reptiles to avoid damage to the tracheal mucosa that could result in ischemic injury. In oral surgical procedures, cuffed endotracheal tubes can be used, but care should be taken not to overinflate the cuff. Therefore, large-volume low-pressure cuffs are preferable over low-volume high-pressure cuffs. For minimization of the potential for overinflation of the cuff, a small syringe should be used for inflation. In respiratory emergencies, such as obstructive processes in the oral cavity or the trachea (e.g., granulomas, foreign bodies), a tracheostomy can be performed to gain access to the trachea and secure an airway.

MAINTENANCE AND MONITORING

All anesthetic agents have cardiopulmonary depressant effects, and during maintenance of anesthesia, cardiopulmonary performance should be closely monitored. Minimally, rate and depth of respiration and heart rate should be recorded. Supportive care during maintenance of anesthesia includes adequate fluid therapy on the basis of laboratory findings. For correction of major fluid deficits and for maintenance fluid therapy, IV or IO administration of fluids is most effective. In small reptile species, commercially available syringe pumps are mandatory to deliver accurate fluid volumes at a constant rate. The rate of fluid administration depends on the degree of dehydration. In critical cases, a venous blood sample can be collected during anesthesia to monitor success of fluid therapy and initiate corrective measures if indicated. For maintenance fluid requirements, 5 to 10 mL/kg/h of a balanced electrolyte solution is recommended. Also recommended is monitoring of blood parameters such as PCV, hemoglobin, total protein, glucose, and electrolytes during anesthesia and at regular intervals into the recovery period.

During the anesthetic event, the reptile should be maintained within the POTR. Supplemental heat can effectively be provided via heating blankets and heat lamps. During surgery, the reptile should be frequently assessed for effective analgesia. If signs of pain are present during anesthesia and surgery, such as movement or increase in heart and respiratory rate in response to a painful stimulus, the analgesic protocol should be reviewed and additional analgesic agents should be administered during surgery. Critical assessment of the following parameters is recommended for effective anesthetic monitoring of the reptilian patient.

Reflexes

In reptiles, muscular tone and reflexes are evaluated for assessment of anesthetic depth, and the presence or absence of reflexes should be recorded. During a surgical plane of anesthesia, the righting reflex is absent as is the palpebral reflex in chelonians and most lizard species. The corneal reflex should be present; its absence indicates a deep plane of anesthesia. In some lizard species and in all snakes, the palpebral and corneal reflexes cannot be evaluated because of the presence of the spectacle. Additional reflexes to be monitored include the tail, toe, and cloacal reflexes. If no response is found to a surgical stimulus, the anesthetic depth should be critically evaluated to ensure the patient's condition is not too deep. If the reptile is in a surgical plane of anesthesia, slight movement in response to a stimulus is normally not associated with the perception of pain.

Cardiovascular Performance

The most useful monitoring equipment is a Doppler flow device with the probe positioned at the level of the heart (snakes and lizards) or over the carotid artery (chelonians and lizards) to monitor heart rate and rhythm. The probe can also be placed over the coccygeal artery in lizards and snakes. In chelonians, a pencil probe should be placed at the level of the thoracic inlet, close to the heart and the major vessels.

Electrocardiography (ECG) is a useful monitoring tool for detection of changes in heart rate, such as tachycardia and bradycardia and arrhythmias; however, it does not determine mechanical performance of the heart. ECGs can be recorded with leads attached in a conventional manner. ECGs should especially be recorded in reptiles suspected of or diagnosed with cardiac disease or when arrhythmias are detected during routine monitoring.

Direct arterial blood pressure measurements are the most accurate tool for continuous assessment of arterial blood pressure. However, they are impractical in most reptile patients because of the limited access to a peripheral artery. In most cases, a cut-down procedure is necessary to gain access to the femoral or carotid artery. In those lizard and chelonian patients in which arterial catheterization is necessary, the left carotid artery is the most accessible artery. (See Chapter 14 for more information on diagnostic cardiology.)

Respiratory Performance

During a surgical plane of anesthesia, all reptiles exhibit respiratory depression characterized by bradypnea or even apnea. Consequently, **all reptiles need assisted ventilation or intermittent positive pressure ventilation (IPPV) during anesthesia, either manually or via mechanical ventilators** (Figures 27-5 and 27-6). Little work has been published on effective and safe ventilation in anesthetized reptiles. The general principles of IPPV should also be applied in reptilian patients. Manual ventilation can be effectively administered to reptiles, however, it is labor intensive and allows less control of tidal volume and peak airway pressure. Small animal ventilators, pressure driven or volume driven, are commercially available and can be used for reptiles (e.g., Vetronics Small Animal Ventilator VT-9093, BASi Vetronics, West Lafayette, Ind). The tidal volume and respiratory rate determine minute ventilation and in most healthy mammals a tidal volume of 20 mL/kg at a respiratory rate of 10 breaths/minute is adequate to maintain a normal $PaCO_2$.

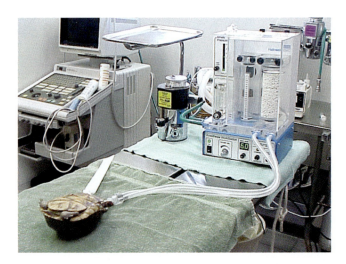

FIGURE 27-5 Box Turtle (*Terrapene carolina*) on a volume-driven mechanical ventilator (Hallowell Anesthesia WorkStation, Hallowell EMC, Pittsfield, Mass, www.hallowell.com), with 2% to 5% isoflurane, 15 to 20 mL/kg, 6 breaths per minute. (*Photograph courtesy D. Mader.*)

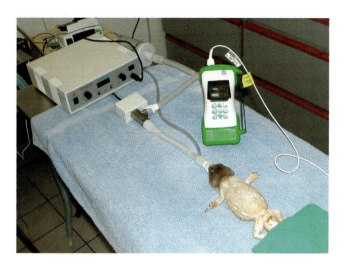

FIGURE 27-6 Bearded Dragon *(Pogona vitticeps)* on a pressure-driven mechanical ventilator (Ventronics, West Lafayette, Ind, www.vetronics.net), with 2% to 5% isoflurane, 10 to 15 cm H_2O, 6 breaths per minute. *(Photograph courtesy D. Mader.)*

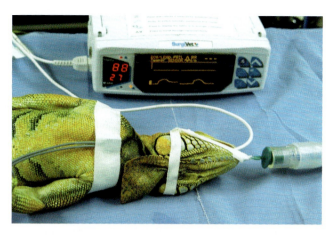

FIGURE 27-7 Monitoring of a Green Iguana *(Iguana iguana)* during maintenance of anesthesia. A reflectance pulse oximeter probe has been placed at the level of the carotid artery to monitor pulse rate and relative arterial oxygen saturation (SpO_2). A Doppler flow probe placed at the level of the heart facilitates audible monitoring of heart rate and rhythm.

However, the tidal volume of reptiles is larger than that of mammals of comparable body mass, and the rate of IPPV is usually set between 4 and 8 breaths/minute. Peak airway pressure should not exceed 10 to 15 cm H_2O and inspiration should not take longer than 1 to 2 seconds. In order to minimize the negative effects of IPPV on cardiovascular performance (e.g., hypotension, decreased cardiac output) the lowest pressure and inspiration time necessary to ensure appropriate ventilation should be used. In reptiles, a useful visual aid for delivery of an adequate tidal volume is also observation of chest expansion during inspiration.

In human and domestic animal anesthesia, pulse oximetry is a useful tool for monitoring heart rate and trends in relative arterial oxygen saturation (SpO_2) and detecting hypoxemia ($SpO_2 < 90\%$). The application of pulse oximetry in reptile anesthesia is limited by the fact that pulse oximeters are calibrated on the basis of the human oxygen hemoglobin dissociation curve, and therefore, values recorded from reptiles should not be interpreted as absolute numbers. One study has found no significant differences in pulse oximeter readings and arterial blood gas analysis between humans and Green Iguanas.[37] In reptiles, pulse oximetry is a useful tool for monitoring trends in arterial oxygen desaturation. Transmission and reflectance probes can be used for reptiles; however, a suitable sampling site is often difficult to find. In most species, an esophageal probe placed at the level of the carotid artery and rectal probes can be used (Figure 27-7). Studies are indicated to further investigate the application and accuracy of pulse oximetry in various reptile species.

Arterial blood gas analysis is impractical in most reptiles, and a cut-down procedure is necessary in most patients to gain arterial access. In addition, the size of the reptile is often the limiting factor in catheterization of a peripheral artery for arterial blood gas determination. Arterial blood gas analyzers directly measure PaO_2, $PaCO_2$, and pH, and these values can be interpreted as absolute numbers. Arterial blood oxygen saturation (SaO_2), however, is calculated on the basis of the human oxygen hemoglobin dissociation curve. Cardiac sampling for blood gas analysis is inaccurate in reptiles because of the mixture of arterial and venous blood within the ventricle. Venous blood gas analysis is of very limited value for assessment of pulmonary function in reptiles.

End-tidal PCO_2 monitoring has become the standard in human anesthesia for determination of respiratory performance and estimation of $PaCO_2$. Capnometry measures CO_2 concentrations in the expired air for determination of adequate ventilation. Analyzers with high sampling rates (>100 mL/minute) are unsuitable for small reptiles; however, analyzers with low sampling rates of 50 mL/minute and less are available and are more suitable for most reptiles. End-tidal CO_2 monitoring in reptiles is limited by the fact that reptiles can develop cardiac shunts. A report in Green Iguanas concluded that no correlation exists between end-tidal CO_2 concentrations and arterial PCO_2 values.[38] However, changes in end-tidal CO_2 may give valuable information on existing complications. A decrease in end-tidal CO_2 may indicate airway leaks, airway obstruction, disconnection of the reptile from the breathing system, or if IPPV is used, malfunction of the ventilator.

RECOVERY AND POSTOPERATIVE CARE

Recovery of the reptilian patient should be in a temperature-controlled and humidity-controlled environment that closely resembles the natural requirements of the species. Small animal incubators are ideal for this purpose, and most offer the ability to provide supplemental oxygen, if indicated (Figure 27-8). The reptile should only be extubated when oral and pharyngeal reflexes have returned and the animal is breathing spontaneously.

Throughout the recovery period, cardiopulmonary parameters, including heart rate and respiratory rate and pattern, should be frequently monitored and recorded. If indicated, respiratory support such as IPPV with room air should be

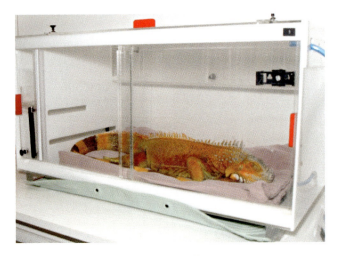

FIGURE 27-8 Recovery of a Green Iguana *(Iguana iguana)* in an incubator.

administered. In reptiles, low oxygen concentrations are the stimulus to breath and high oxygen concentrations in the inspired air may prolong return to spontaneous respiration.[37] In a study with Green Iguanas, patients were found to recover twice as quickly when breathing only room air as compared with those patients on supplemented with oxygen.[37]

If supplemental oxygen is necessary, facemasks are most useful and the flow rate of oxygen should be 2 to 5 L/minute, depending on the size of the patient. Insufflation of oxygen can be achieved with several techniques. For nasal insufflation with oxygen, a rubber catheter is inserted into the nares and then sutured or glued to the scales. Oxygen at a rate of 0.5 to 3 L/minute should be delivered through a humidifier to prevent drying of the airways. In reptiles with obstructive processes in the nasal passageways or the oral cavity, the trachea can be insufflated with oxygen. With this technique, a catheter is inserted percutaneously into the trachea with the tip advanced to the bifurcation.

Throughout the recovery period, the absence or presence of reflexes, such as palpebral, corneal, foot, and tail withdrawal reflexes, should be recorded in regular intervals for assessment of the degree of recovery and return to a preanesthetic state. Adequate fluid therapy should be continued into the recovery period to ensure normovolemia of the patient. Balanced electrolyte solutions are recommended for most species, and if indicated, determination of hematologic and plasma biochemical parameters facilitates accurate assessment of effective fluid therapy. For reduction of recovery time, increase in environmental temperature during the recovery period above the POTR for the species is not recommended. Increases in environmental temperature result in increased metabolism and consequently an increased demand for oxygen by the tissues. During recovery, most reptiles have respiratory depression and may not be able to meet the increased oxygen demand.

Reptiles recovering from anesthesia should be monitored closely for any evidence of postoperative distress or pain. The analgesic regimen should be reevaluated in reptiles with signs of discomfort or pain. If indicated, additional analgesic agents should be administered in the postoperative period.

Only fully recovered animals should be returned to their enclosure, especially if they are housed in groups, to avoid potential injuries from cage mates. Aquatic species should only be returned back to their aquatic environment completely recovered to prevent accidental drowning.

ANALGESIA

Current knowledge of effective analgesic drugs and therapy in reptiles is scant (Table 27-2). Few studies have evaluated effective pain management in common reptile species. Unfortunately, lack of knowledge of effective drugs and dosage regimen often results in neglecting the management of pain in reptilian patients. A recent study concluded that provision of analgesia for the reptilian patient is uncommon.[39] However, all vertebrates experience pain, and the major difference between reptiles and mammalian species may be different pain pathways and receptors. Reptiles possess an endogenous opioid system, and nociceptive neurons in crotaline snakes are similar to those identified in monkeys.[40]

In some cases, lack of recognition of pain in reptiles and unfamiliarity with analgesic agents may result in improper pain management. Conditions such as trauma, neoplasia, surgical procedures, and chronic disease processes commonly associated with pain in humans and mammals also cause pain and discomfort in reptiles.

Before treatment, familiarity with the reptile species is mandatory, including knowledge of normal behavior and signs that indicate discomfort and pain, such as restlessness, increased respiratory rate, anorexia, and aggressiveness. Assessment of pain and the required analgesic regimen is mandatory before treatment. The physiology and pathophysiology of pain have been described in detail elsewere.[41]

Pain, stress, and discomfort are closely related, and effective pain management greatly reduces stress and discomfort of the reptile, thus reducing or eliminating the effects of acute and chronic pain on the animal's metabolism, such as compromised immune function, hematologic and biochemical imbalances, and metabolic changes.[42] Although most veterinary practitioners are familiar with "normal" behavior in domestic animals such as dogs and cats, recognition of normal and abnormal behavior is often challenging in reptiles. Although the reptilian patient does not show obvious well-recognized signs of pain such as vocalization it does not mean the animal does not experience pain and discomfort. However, familiarity with normal behavior and normal body position may help in the diagnosis of pain. Abnormal body position in reptiles, such as hunched-up abdomen or resting in an abnormal position, reluctance to lie down in lizards and tortoises, and abnormal movement such as abnormal gait and restlessness may indicate discomfort. Additional signs in reptiles include anorexia, increased aggressiveness, depression, trembling, and increased respiratory rate.[43]

Analgesic regimens in reptiles are often adjusted from the pharmacokinetic and pharmacodynamic principles known from domestic animals. For effective analgesia and comfort for the reptile, acute pain needs to be differentiated from chronic pain. Acute pain is the result of trauma, surgery, or an infectious event and is of relatively short duration; chronic pain persists beyond an acute injury and has severe effects on metabolic status. Chronic pain such as cancer pain and arthritis serves no biologic function and often results in severe impairment and distress of the animal.

Table 27-2	Analgesic and Local Anesthetic Agents Used for Treatment of Acute and Chronic Pain in Reptiles			
Agent	**Dosage (mg/kg)**	**Route**	**Frequency**	**Comments**
Bupivacaine	1-2	Local infiltration	4-12 h	Maximum dose: 4 mg/kg
Buprenorphine	0.02-0.2	SC, IM	12-24 h	All species
Butorphanol	0.4-2.0	SC, IM, IV	12-24 h	All species
Carprofen	1-4	PO, SC, IM, IV	24 h	All species
Flunixin meglumine	0.5-2	IM	12-24 h	All species
Ketoprofen	2	SC, IM	24 h	All species
Lidocaine	2-5	Topical and local infiltration	—	Maximum dose: 10 mg/kg
Meloxicam	0.1-0.2	PO	24 h	All species
Morphine	0.4-2.0	SC, IM	12 h	Species variability
Oxymorphone	0.1-0.2	SC, IM	12-24 h	Species variability

SC, Subcutaneously; *IM*, intramuscularly; *IV*, intravenously; *PO*, orally.

Prevention of pain is the most effective method of pain management. Therefore, preemptive analgesic techniques are recommended in cases in which the animal undergoes elective surgical procedures. Similar to domestic animals, balanced analgesic techniques are most effective in the treatment of intraoperative and postoperative pain in reptiles. Often this includes administration of systemic analgesic agents (opioid agents) in combination with long-acting local anesthetic agents (e.g., bupivacaine).

Acute Pain Management

Opioid agents such as butorphanol and buprenorphine are most often used for the management of acute pain in reptiles. Indications for the treatment of acute pain include traumatic events such as shell fractures in chelonians; fractures of the long bones in lizards; bite wounds; thermal burns from default heating devices, especially in snakes and lizards; and surgical procedures such as coeliotomies. The latter are commonly performed in reptiles for removal of masses, such as granulomas and neoplasia; reproductive surgeries; and removal of bladder stones. Although effective drugs and dosage intervals are poorly understood in reptiles, the patient should be frequently assessed for evidence of pain, especially in the postoperative period. Recognition of signs of pain and discomfort often facilitates effective analgesic therapy.

Local Anesthetic Agents

In reptiles, local anesthetics are often used for local procedures, such as surgical debridement of abscesses.[26] For invasive procedures, administration of local anesthetic agents should be accompanied by concurrent administration of systemic analgesic agents such as opioid agents as part of a preemptive analgesic regimen. Both lidocaine and bupivacaine can be used in reptiles; the former has a fast onset of action, and the latter is more effective in controlling postoperative pain because of its long duration of action. Many techniques have described in domestic animals the use of local anesthetics to provide topical and regional anesthesia and local infiltration techniques and field blocks. These techniques are often directly applicable to reptiles. Local anesthetics can be directly applied to surgical wounds (e.g., abscess debridement) or injected into coeliotomy incisions in the reptiles. Although toxic doses of both drugs have not been determined in reptiles, one should not exceed 4 mg/kg bupivacaine and 10 mg/kg lidocaine in reptiles to avoid potential side effects such as arrhythmias and seizures.

Chronic Pain Management

Chronic pain management in reptiles is often neglected because of a poor understanding of the effects of drugs used for the management of chronic pain in domestic animals, especially nonsteroidal antiinflammatory agents (NSAIDs). Various metabolic bone diseases, gout, renal disease, and a variety of neoplastic diseases are a few examples of conditions associated with chronic pain in reptiles. NSAIDs can be used for the management of chronic pain in reptiles, although little information is available regarding effective treatment regimens and potential side effects in reptiles. NSAIDs offer the advantage of a long duration of action, and both ketoprofen and carprofen are useful analgesic agents for the reptilian patient diagnosed with chronic pain. Before administration of these agents, every effort should be made to determine the renal status of the patient because both drugs should not be used in patients with severe renal and gastrointestinal disease.

REFERENCES

1. Bennett RA: A review of anesthesia and chemical restraint in reptiles, *J Zoo Wildl Med* 22(3):282-303, 1991.
2. Bennett RA: Anesthesia. In Mader DR, editor: *Reptile medicine and surgery*, Philadelphia, 1996, WB Saunders.
3. Heard DJ: Principles and techniques of anesthesia and analgesia for exotic practice, *Vet Clin North Am Sm Anim Pract* 1301-1327, 1993.
4. Heard DJ: Reptile anesthesia, *Vet Clin North Am Exotic Anim Pract* 83-117, 2001.
5. Page CD: Current reptilian anesthesia procedures. In Fowler ME, editor: *Zoo and wild animal medicine current therapy 3*, Philadelphia, 1993, WB Saunders.
6. Schumacher J: Reptiles and amphibians. In Thurmon JC, Tranquilli, Benson GJ, editors: *Lumb and Jones' veterinary anesthesia*, ed 3, Baltimore, 1996, Williams & Wilkins.
7. Perry SF: Lungs: comparative anatomy, functional morphology, and evolution. In Gans C, Gaunt AS, editors: *Biology of the reptilia, vol 19, morphology G visceral organs*, St Louis, 1998, Society for the Study of Amphibians and Reptiles.
8. Wang T, Smits AW, Burggren WW: Pulmonary function in reptiles. In Gans C, Gaunt AS, editors: *Biology of the reptilia. vol 19, morphology G visceral organs*, St Louis, 1998, Society for the Study of Amphibians and Reptiles.

9. Wallach V: The lungs of snakes. In Gans C, Gaunt AS, editors: *Biology of the reptilia, vol 19, morphology visceral organs*, St. Louis, 1998, Society for the Study of Amphibians and Reptiles.
10. Schumacher J: Reptile respiratory medicine, *Vet Clin North Am Exotic Anim Pract* 6:213-231, 2003.
11. Schumacher J: Fluid therapy in reptiles. In Bonagura JD, editor: *Kirk's current veterinary therapy XIII small animal practice*, Philadelphia, 2000, WB Saunders.
12. Mosley CA, Dyson D, Smith DA: Minimum alveolar concentration of isoflurane in Green Iguanas and the effect of butorphanol on minimum alveolar concentration, *J Am Vet Med Assoc* 222(11):1559-1564, 2003.
13. Mosley CA, Dyson D, Smith DA: The cardiac anesthetic index of isoflurane in Green Iguanas, *J Am Vet Med Assoc* 222(11): 1565-1568, 2003.
14. Hernandez-Divers S, Schumacher J, Read MR, et al: Comparison of isoflurane and sevoflurane following premedication with butorphanol for induction and maintenance of anesthesia in the Green Iguana *(Iguana iguana)*, *Proc Am Assoc Zoo Vet Annual Meeting* 2003.
15. Hernandez-Divers SM, Schumacher J, Stahl S, et al: Comparison of isoflurane and sevoflurane following premedication with butorphanol in the Green Iguana *(Iguana iguana)*, *J Zoo Wildl Med* 36(2), 2005.
16. Oppenheim YC, Moon PF: Sedative effects of midazolam in red-eared slider turtles *(Trachemys scripta elegans)*, *J Zoo Wildl Med* 26(3):409-413, 1995.
17. Schumacher J, Lillywhite HB, Norman WM, et al: Effects of ketamine HCl on cardiopulmonary function in snakes, *Copeia* 2:395, 1997.
18. Holz P, Holz RM: Evaluation of ketamine, ketamine/xylazine and ketamine/midazolam anesthesia in red-eared sliders *(Trachemys scripta elegans)*, *J Zoo Wildl Med* 25(4): 531-537, 1994.
19. Dennis PM, Heard DJ: Cardiopulmonary effects of a medetomidine-ketamine combination administered intravenously in gopher tortoises, *J Am Vet Med Assoc* 220(10):1516-1519, 2002.
20. Sleeman JM, Gaynor J: Sedative and cardiopulmonary effects of medetomidine and reversal with atipamezole in desert tortoises *(Gopherus agassizii)*, *J Zoo Wildl Med* 31(1): 28-35, 2000.
21. Anderson NL, Wack RF, Calloway L, et al: Cardiopulmonary effects and efficacy of propofol as an anesthetic agent in brown tree snakes *(Boiga irregularis)*, *Bull Assoc Reptile Amphib Vet* 9(2):9-15, 1999.
22. Bennett RA, Schumacher J, Hedjazi-Haring K, et al: Cardiopulmonary and anesthetic effects of propofol administered intraosseously to Green Iguanas, *J Am Vet Med Assoc* 212:93-98, 1998.
23. Nevarez JG, Mitchell MA, Wilkelski M: Evaluating the clinical effects of propofol on marine iguanas *(Amblyrhynchus cristatus)*, *Proc Assoc Reptilian Amphib Vet* 48-49, 2003.
24. Benson KG, Forrest L: Characterization of the renal portal system of the common Green Iguana *(Iguana iguana)* by digital subtraction imaging, *J Zoo Wildl Med* 30(2):235-241, 1999.
25. Holz P, Barker IK, Burger JP, et al: The effect of the renal portal system on pharmacokinetic parameters in the red-eared slider *(Trachemys scripta elegans)*, *J Zoo Wildl Med* 28(4): 386-393, 1997.
26. Mader DR: Understanding local analgesics: practical use in the Green Iguana *(Iguana iguana)*, *Proc Assoc Amphib Rept Vet* 7-10, 1998.
27. Rooney MB, Levine G, Gaynor J, et al: Sevoflurane anesthesia in desert tortoises *(Gopherus agassizii)*, *J Zoo Wildl Med* 30(1): 64-69, 1999.
28. Lock BA, Heard DJ, Dennis P: Preliminary evaluation of medetomidine/ketamine combinations for immobilization and reversal with atipamezole in three tortoise species, *Bull Assoc Reptil Amphib Vet* 8(4):6-9, 1998.
29. Chittick EJ, Stamper MA, Beasley JF, et al: Medetomidine, ketamine, and sevoflurane for anesthesia of injured loggerhead sea turtles: 13 cases (1996-2000), *J Am Vet Med Assoc* 221(7):1019-1025, 2002.
30. Bienzle D, Boyd CJ: Sedative effects of ketamine and midazolam in snapping turtles *(Chelydra serpentina)*, *J Zoo Wildl Med* 23(2):201-204, 1992.
31. Hackenbroich C: *Alphaxalon/Alphadolon-Anaesthesie bei der Rotwangen-Schmuckschildkroete (Trachemys scripta elegans)*, Doctoral thesis, Germany, 1999, Justus-Liebig-Universitaet Giessen.
32. Kaufman GE, Seymour RE, Bonner BB, et al: Use of rocuronium for endotracheal intubation of North American Gulf Coast box turtles, *J Am Vet Med Assoc* 222(8):1111-1115, 2003.
33. Clyde VL, Cardeilhac PT, Jacobson ER: Chemical restraint of American alligators *(Alligator mississippiensis)* with atracurium or tiletamine-zolazepam, *J Zoo Wildl Med* 25(4):525-530, 1994.
34. Fleming GJ: Crocodilian anesthesia, *Vet Clin North Am Exotic Anim Pract* 199-145, 2001.
35. Lloyd ML: Crocodilian anesthesia. In Fowler ME, Miller RE, editors: *Zoo and wild animal medicine current therapy 4*, Philadelphia, 1999, WB Saunders.
36. Heaton-Jones TG, Ko JCH, Heaton-Jones DL: Evaluation of medetomidine-ketamine anesthesia with atipamezole reversal in American alligators *(Alligator mississippiensis)*, *J Zoo Wildl Med* 33(1):36-44, 2002.
37. Diethelm G: *The effect of oxygen content of inspiratory air (FIO_2) on recovery times in the Green Iguana (Iguana iguana)*, Doctoral thesis, Germany, 2001, Universitaet Zuerich.
38. Hernandez-Divers SM, Schumacher J, Hernandez-Divers SJ: Blood gas evaluation in the Green Iguana *(Iguana iguana)*, *Proc Assoc Reptil Amphib Vet* 45-46, 2004.
39. Read MR: Evaluation of the use of anesthesia and analgesia in reptiles, *J Am Vet Med Assoc* 224(4):547-552, 2004.
40. Machin KL: Fish, amphibian and reptile analgesia, *Vet Clin North Am Exotic Anim Pract* 19-33, 2001.
41. Muir WW: Physiology and pathophysiology of pain. In Gaynor JS, Muir WW, editors:. *Handbook of veterinary pain management*, St Louis, 2002, Mosby.
42. Muir WW: Pain and stress. In Gaynor JS, Muir WW, editors: *Handbook of veterinary pain management*, St. Louis, 2002, Mosby.
43. Bradley T: Pain management considerations and pain-associated behaviors in reptiles and amphibians, *Proc Assoc Reptil Amphib Vet* 45-49, 2001.

28
CLINICAL PATHOLOGY OF REPTILES

TERRY W. CAMPBELL

REPTILE HEMATOLOGY

The blood of reptiles contains nucleated erythrocytes, nucleated thrombocytes, heterophils, eosinophils, basophils, lymphocytes, and monocytes. Hematology is used to detect conditions that affect these cells, such as anemia, inflammatory diseases, parasitemias, hematopoietic disorders, and hemostatic alterations. The normal hematologic values for reptiles determined by different laboratories can vary significantly. This variation is likely caused by differences in blood sampling, handling, and analytic techniques. Other factors that are likely to contribute to the variation in the normal hematologic values of reptiles include variations in the environmental conditions of the reptiles' habitat, physiologic status of the reptile, age, gender, nutrition, and use of anesthetics. Published hematologic reference values for reptiles often fail to include information that may influence the hemogram, especially the environment of the population of reptiles used as normal controls. For these reasons, the published normal reference values of reptiles vary greatly compared with those of domestic mammals.

Routine evaluation of the reptilian hemogram includes determination of the packed cell volume (PCV), the total erythrocyte and leukocyte counts, and a leukocyte differential and examination of the blood cell morphology on a stained blood film. The microhematocrit method is the quickest and most practical and reproducible method for determination of the PCV and status of the reptilian erythron. The total erythrocyte and leukocyte counts are determined with either manual methods or automated methods (erythrocytes only). The two commonly use methods for the determination of the total leukocyte count in reptilian blood are the semidirect method with phloxine B solution or the direct method with Natt and Herrick's solution. The limitations for the semidirect method include increased error in samples with low heterophil counts and the need for an accurate leukocyte differential. The limitations for the direct method include use of manual diluting pipettes, the need to prepare the diluting solution, and the difficulty in distinguishing between small lymphocytes and thrombocytes. Both methods require training and experience for consistent results.

Because of the limitations on obtaining total cell counts in reptilian blood, especially leukocyte counts; the evaluation of the cell morphology is an important part of the assessment of the reptilian hemogram. Microscope slides containing reptilian blood films are commonly stained with Wright's, Giemsa, or Wright's/Giemsa for evaluation of the blood cells. Quick stains, such as Diff-Quik, can be used but have a tendency to damage some of the cell types (e.g., lymphocytes) and understain immature erythrocytes and lymphocytes.

Whenever possible, examination of blood films obtained from fresh nonanticoagulated blood is best. Ethylenediaminetetraacetic acid (EDTA) may cause the blood to lyse in some species of reptiles (especially chelonians). Therefore, lithium heparin is typically used as an anticoagulant when collecting blood from reptiles. However, heparin often imparts a blue tinge to the overall staining of the blood film and causes clumping of leukocytes and thrombocytes, affecting cell counts. If heparin is used as an anticoagulant for reptilian hematology studies, the sample should be processed immediately to minimize the effects of heparin on the cells.

Reptilian Erythrocytes

Mature erythrocytes of reptiles are permanently nucleated, blunt-ended ellipsoids, which are larger than erythrocytes of birds and mammals. The erythrocyte size for most reptiles range from a length × width of 14 × 8 µm to 23 × 14 µm.[1] The length to width ratio of most reptile erythrocytes is 1.7 to 1.8. Reptile erythrocytes that are round (length to width ratio, ≤1.5) rather than oval are rare and likely to occur in chelonians and some snakes.[1] The mean cellular volume (MCV) of most reptilian mature red blood cells ranges between 200 and 1200 fl. The reptilian erythrocyte has a centrally positioned oval to round (especially chelonians) nucleus that is oriented along the cell's long axis. The nuclei often have irregular margins and contain dense purple chromatin. The cytoplasm stains orange-pink with Romanowsky stains such as Wright's stain. Polychromatophilic erythrocytes have nuclear chromatin that is less dense and cytoplasm that is more basophilic than mature erythrocytes.

Reptiles have lower total erythrocyte counts (300,000 to 2,500,000 erythrocytes/µL) compared with mammals and birds.[2,3] An inverse relationship appears to exist between the total red blood count (TRBC) and the size of the erythrocytes.[2] Lizards tend to have smaller erythrocytes (MCV less than 300 fl) than other reptiles; therefore, they have higher total erythrocyte counts (1,000,000 to 1,500,000 erythrocytes/µL).[2,3] Snakes have lower TRBC values (700,000 to 1,600,000 erythrocytes/µL) than lizards but greater numbers than chelonians. Chelonians have the largest of the reptilian erythrocytes (MCV greater than 500 fl) and the lower TRBC values (≤500,000 erythrocytes/µL). The TRBC, hemoglobin (Hb), and PCV values vary with a number of factors, such as environment (TRBC values are highest before hibernation and lowest immediately after hibernation), nutritional status; and gender (males tend to have higher TRBC values than females).[1-7]

The mean cellular hemoglobin concentration (MCHC) is the red blood cell index denoting the proportion of an average erythrocyte that is comprised of hemoglobin in grams per 100 red blood cells (gHb/100 RBC). The average MCHC for reptiles is 30% (range, 22% to 41%).[1,8,9] The hemoglobin concentration of reptilian blood generally ranges between 6 and 10 g/dL.[10] Most reptiles have multiple hemoglobins, and considerable variation is seen in oxygen affinity between individual red blood cells.[11]

Immature erythrocytes are occasionally seen in the peripheral blood of reptiles, especially very young animals or those undergoing ecdysis. Immature erythrocytes are round to irregular cells with large round nuclei and basophilic cytoplasm (Figure 28-1). The nucleus lacks the dense chromatin clumping of the mature cell and has a characteristic checker board–like pattern. Immature erythrocytes frequently appear smaller than mature erythrocytes, probably because the final stage of erythrocyte maturation involves changing from a spherical cell, which appears small to a flattened ellipsoid and larger. Also, the larger mature cell may contain more hemoglobin. Mitotic activity associated with erythrocytes is common in the peripheral blood of reptiles.

Reticulocytes are detected by staining cells with a supravital stain, such as new methylene blue. They are a normal constituent of reptilian blood, representing 1.5% to 2.5% of the red blood cell population.[12,13] Reptilian reticulocytes that have a distinct ring of aggregated reticulum that encircles the red cell nucleus are probably the cells recently released from erythropoietic tissues. Polychromatic erythrocytes account for less than 1% of the red blood cell population of most clinically healthy reptiles.

Round to irregular basophilic inclusions are frequently seen in the cytoplasm of erythrocytes in peripheral blood films from many species of reptiles. These inclusions most likely represent an artifact of slide preparation because blood films made repeatedly from the same blood sample often reveal varying degrees of these inclusions. Electron microscopy suggests these inclusions are degenerate organelles.[14] Other artifacts found in the erythrocyte cytoplasm include vacuoles and refractile clear areas. These can be minimized with careful blood film preparation.

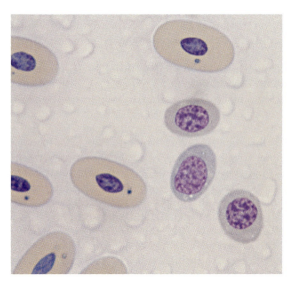

FIGURE 28-1 Immature erythrocytes. Blood film from a Burmese Python (*Python molurus bivittatus*) stained with Wright's stain. The blood was collected in heparin, resulting in an overall blue cast to the blood film.

Erythrocyte Responses in Disease

The normal PCV of most reptiles is approximately 30% (range, 20% to 40%).[4,15,16] Therefore, a PCV less than 20% is suggestive of anemia and values greater than 40% suggest either hemoconcentration or erythrocytosis (polycythemia).

The etiologies of anemia in reptiles are similar to those described for birds and mammals. The anemia can be classified as hemorrhagic (blood loss), hemolytic (increased red cell destruction), or depression anemia (decreased red cell production). Hemorrhagic anemias are usually caused by traumatic injuries or blood-sucking parasites; however, other causes, such as a coagulopathy or an ulcerative lesion, should also be considered. Hemolytic anemia can result from septicemia, parasitemia, or toxemia. Depression anemias are usually associated with chronic inflammatory diseases, especially those associated with infectious agents. Other causes that should be considered as a cause for depression anemia in reptiles include chronic renal or hepatic disease, neoplasia, chemicals, or possibly hypothyroidism.

The degree of polychromasia or reticulocytosis in blood films of normal reptiles is generally low and represents less than 1% of the erythrocyte population. This may be associated with the long erythrocyte life span (i.e., 600 to 800 days in some species) and therefore slow turn over rate of reptilian erythrocytes compared with those of birds and mammals.[2,4] The relatively low metabolic rate of reptiles may also be a factor. Young reptiles tend to have a greater degree of polychromasia than adults.

Slight anisocytosis and poikilocytosis are considered normal for most reptile erythrocytes. Moderate to marked anisocytosis and poikilocytosis are associated with erythrocytic regenerative responses and, less commonly, erythrocyte disorders. An increase in polychromasia and the number of immature erythrocytes is seen in reptiles responding to anemic conditions. The erythrocyte regenerative response in reptiles is slower than in birds and mammals, which respond within 1 week to stimulus. The slow reptilian response (e.g., red cell numbers may return to normal in 4 months after repeated phlebotomy) may be related in part to the long transit time from the rubriblast stage to the mature erythrocyte stage and the long lifespan of the reptilian red blood cell.[17] Young reptiles or those undergoing ecdysis may also exhibit an increase in polychromasia and immature erythrocyte concentration. Erythrocytes exhibiting binucleation, abnormal nuclear shapes (anisokaryosis), or mitotic activity can be associated with marked regenerative responses. However, these nuclear findings may also occur in reptiles awakening from hibernation or in association with severe inflammatory disease, malnutrition, and starvation.[18] Basophilic stippling usually suggests a regenerative response but is also seen in patients with iron deficiency and possibly lead toxicosis. Hypochromatic erythrocytes are associated with iron deficiency or chronic inflammatory disease (presumably in association with iron sequestration). Erythroplastids (anucleated erythrocytes) are an incidental finding (<0.5% of the erythrocytes) in reptilian blood and are most commonly observed in the blood film of snakes.[19-21]

Reptilian Leukocytes

The granulocytes of reptiles can be classified into two groups, acidophils and basophils, on the basis of their appearance in blood films stained with Romanowsky stains. The acidophils are further divided into heterophils and eosinophils. Reptilian heterophils are generally round cells with eosinophilic (bright orange) fusiform cytoplasmic granules (Figures 28-2 and 28-3). The cytoplasm of normal heterophils is colorless. The mature heterophil nucleus is typically round to oval and eccentrically positioned in the cell, with densely clumped nuclear chromatin.[14,18,22-27] Some species of lizards have heterophils with lobed nuclei (Figure 28-4).[1,7] Heterophils range between 10 and 23 μm in size but vary between species and the individual blood sample.[1]

The cytoplasmic granules of reptilian heterophils are usually peroxidase negative, except for a few species of snakes and lizards.[2,14,25,27,28] The heterophils from Green Iguanas *(Iguana iguana)* are similar to mammalian neutrophils because they stain strongly positive with benzidine peroxidase.[7] In addition, reptilian heterophils do not stain for alkaline phosphatase.[14] Therefore, reptilian heterophils are functionally equivalent to mammalian neutrophils but most likely behave like avian heterophils in that they rely more heavily on oxygen-independent mechanisms to destroy phagocytized microorganisms. The peroxidase positive heterophils of Green Iguanas suggest that these cells may possess bactericidal and oxidative properties similar to mammalian neutrophils.[7]

Eosinophils in most reptilian blood films are large round cells with spherical eosinophilic cytoplasmic granules (Figures 28-5 and 28-6). The granules of some species of reptiles, such as iguanas, stain pale blue with Romanowsky stains (Figure 28-7). The cytoplasmic granules of eosinophils stain positive for peroxidase in some species of reptiles, allowing easy differentiation between eosinophils and heterophils in those species with peroxidase-negative heterophils.[14]

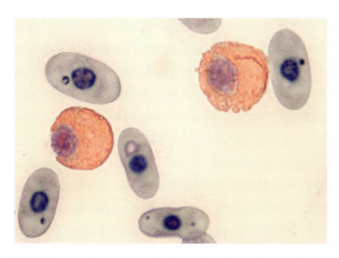

FIGURE 28-2 Two heterophils. Blood film from a Desert Tortoise *(Gopherus agassizii)* stained with Wright's stain. Note the dark inclusions and vacuoles in the cytoplasm of the erythrocytes are artifacts.

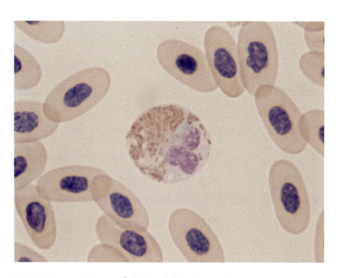

FIGURE 28-4 Heterophil. Blood film from a Green Iguana *(Iguana iguana)* stained with Wright's stain.

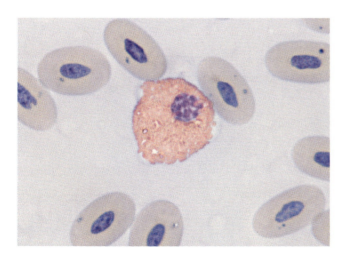

FIGURE 28-3 Heterophil. Blood film from a Burmese Python *(Python molurus bivittatus)* stained with Wright's stain. The blood was collected in heparin, resulting in an overall blue cast to the blood film. Note the dark inclusions in the cytoplasm of the erythrocytes are artifacts.

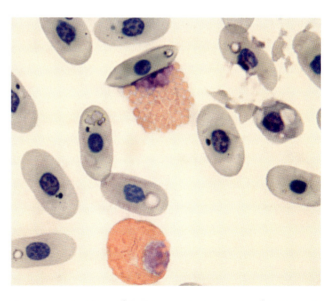

FIGURE 28-5 Heterophil *(bottom cell)* and eosinophil *(top cell)*. Blood film from a Desert Tortoise *(Gopherus agassizii)* stained with Wright's stain. Note the dark inclusions and vacuoles in the cytoplasm of the erythrocytes are artifacts.

The granules of Green Iguana eosinophils do not stain with peroxidase or other common cytochemical stains.[7] Like heterophils, the size of eosinophils varies with the species. For example, snakes have the largest eosinophils, and lizards have the smallest.[1] The nucleus is typically central in its cellular position and is variable in shape, ranging from slightly elongated to lobed.

Basophils are usually small round cells that contain basophilic metachromatic cytoplasmic granules, which often obscure the nucleus (Figures 28-8, 28-9, and 28-10). When visible, the cell nucleus is slightly eccentric in position and nonlobed. Basophil granules are frequently affected by water-based stains, which cause them to partially dissolve. Therefore, alcohol fixation and use of Romanowsky stains provide the best staining for reptilian basophils. Like acidophils,

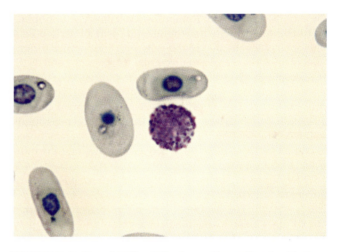

FIGURE 28-8 Basophil. Blood film from a Desert Tortoise (*Gopherus agassizii*) stained with Wright's stain. Note the dark inclusions and vacuoles in the cytoplasm of the erythrocytes are artifacts.

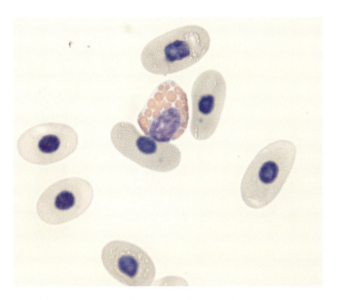

FIGURE 28-6 Eosinophil. Blood film from a Slider (*Trachemys scripta elegans*) stained with Wright's stain.

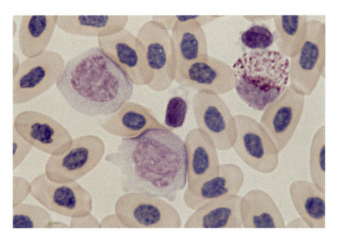

FIGURE 28-9 Basophil (*cell with dark granules*), two monocytes (*large cells*), two thrombocytes, and lymphocyte. Blood film from a Green Iguana (*Iguana iguana*) stained with Wright's stain.

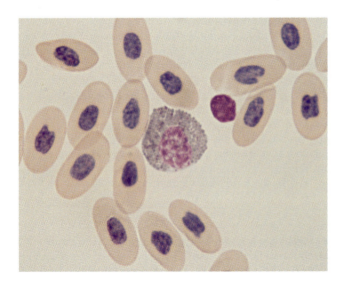

FIGURE 28-7 Eosinophil. Blood film from a Green Iguana (*Iguana iguana*) stained with Wright's stain. Note the blue-staining granules.

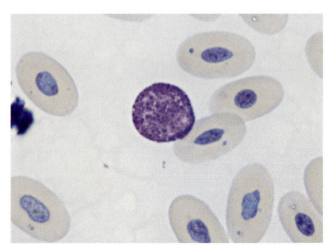

FIGURE 28-10 Basophil. Blood film from a Burmese Python (*Python molurus bivittatus*) stained with Wright's stain. Blood was collected in heparin, resulting in an overall blue cast to blood film. Note the dark inclusions in the cytoplasm of the erythrocytes are artifacts.

basophils vary in size according to the species of reptile but generally range between 7 and 20 µm.[1] Lizards tend to have small basophils, whereas turtles and crocodiles have large basophils.[1]

Reptilian lymphocytes resemble those of birds and mammals (Figures 28-11, 28-12, and 28-13). They vary in size from small (5 to 10 µm) to large (15 µm).[1,2] Lymphocytes are round cells that exhibit irregularity when they mold around adjacent cells in the blood film or fold at their cytoplasmic margin. They have a round or slightly indented nucleus that is centrally or slightly eccentrically positioned in the cell; nuclear chromatin is heavily clumped in mature lymphocytes. Lymphocytes typically have a large nucleus to cytoplasm ratio (N:C). The typical small mature lymphocyte has scant slightly basophilic (pale blue) cytoplasm. Large lymphocytes have more cytoplasmic volume compared with small lymphocytes, and the nucleus is often pale staining. The cytoplasm of a normal lymphocyte appears homogenous and lacks vacuoles and granules.

Monocytes are generally the largest leukocytes in the peripheral blood of reptiles and often resemble those of birds and mammals (Figures 28-14, 28-15, and 28-16). They vary in shape from round to ameboid. The nucleus is variable in shape, ranging between round to oval to lobed. The nuclear chromatin of monocytes is less condensed and stains relatively pale compared with the nuclei of lymphocytes. The abundant cytoplasm of monocytes stains blue-gray, may appear slightly opaque, and may contain vacuoles or fine dust-like eosinophilic or azurophilic granules. The monocyte of snakes often has a round to oval nucleus and contains abundant dust-like azurophilic granules. Although monocytes that have an azurophilic appearance to the cytoplasm are often

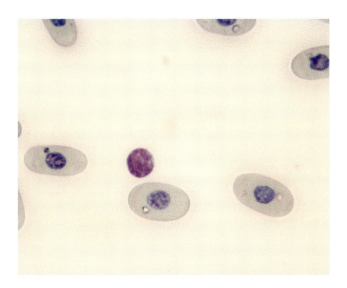

FIGURE 28-11 Small lymphocyte. Blood film from a Desert Tortoise (*Gopherus agassizii*) stained with Wright's stain. Note the dark inclusions and the vacuoles in the cytoplasm of erythrocytes are artifacts.

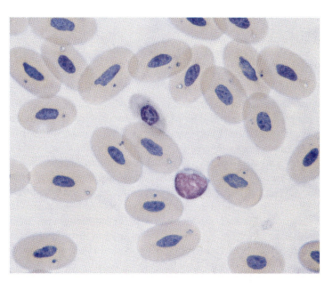

FIGURE 28-13 Lymphocyte. Blood film from a Burmese Python (*Python molurus bivittatus*) stained with Wright's stain. The blood was collected in heparin, resulting in an overall blue cast to the blood film. Note the dark inclusions in the cytoplasm of the erythrocytes are artifacts.

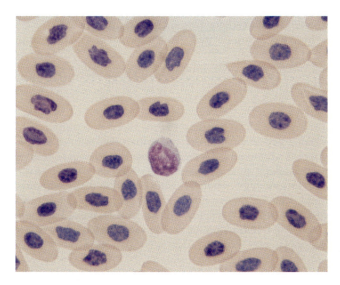

FIGURE 28-12 Lymphocyte. Blood film from a Green Iguana (*Iguana iguana*) stained with Wright's stain.

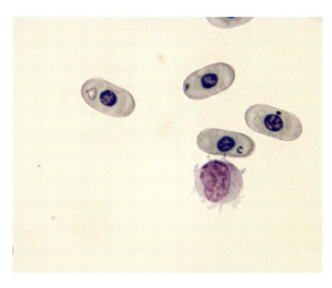

FIGURE 28-14 Monocyte. Blood film from a Desert Tortoise (*Gopherus agassizii*) stained with Wright's stain. Note the dark inclusions and the vacuoles in the cytoplasm of the erythrocytes are artifacts.

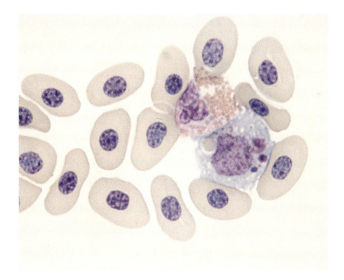

FIGURE 28-15 Monocyte and heterophil. Blood film from a Green Iguana *(Iguana iguana)* stained with Wright's stain. Note the erythrophagocytosis in monocyte.

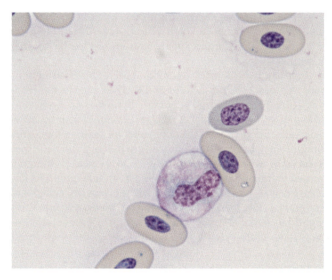

FIGURE 28-16 Monocyte (azurophil). Blood film from a Burmese Python *(Python molurus bivittatus)* stained with Wright's stain. The blood was collected in heparin, resulting in an overall blue cast to the blood film.

referred to as azurophils in the literature, their cytochemical and ultrastructural characteristics are often similar to monocytes and therefore should be reported as monocytes rather than as a separate cell type.[2,7,18,25] The term azurophilic monocyte can be used for these cells.[28] The monocytes of Green Iguanas stain positive with acid phosphatase, alpha-Naphthyl butyrate esterase, and periodic acid-Schiff (PAS) and negative with Sudan black B and peroxidase.[7] Snake monocytes with distinct azurophilic cytoplasmic granules (azurophils) stain positive for peroxidase, Sudan black B, and PAS.[7]

Leukocyte Responses in Disease

The percentage of heterophils in the leukocyte differential of normal reptiles varies with species. Heterophils can represent up to 40% of the leukocytes in some normal reptilian species.[2,3,15,29-32] Heterophil concentration in reptiles is also influenced by seasonal factors. For example, heterophil concentration is highest during the summer and lowest during brumation (hibernation).[3] Because the primary function of heterophils is phagocytosis, significant increases in the heterophil count of reptiles are usually associated with inflammatory disease, especially microbial and parasitic infections or tissue injury. The lack of peroxidase activity in most reptilian heterophils suggests little, if any, oxidative response to stimuli. Noninflammatory conditions that may result in heterophilia include stress (glucocorticosteroid excess), neoplasia, and heterophilic leukemia.

Heterophils may appear abnormal in reptiles with a variety of diseases. For example, heterophils may exhibit varying degrees of toxicity with inflammatory diseases, especially those involving infectious agents such as bacteria. Toxic heterophils exhibit an increase in cytoplasmic basophilia, abnormal granulation (i.e., dark blue to purple granules or granules with abnormal shapes and staining), and cytoplasmic vacuolation (Figures 28-17 and 28-18). Degranulated heterophils may be associated with artifacts of blood film preparation or represent toxic changes. Nuclear lobation in species that normally do not lobate their heterophil nucleus is also an abnormal finding suggestive of severe inflammation.

The number of circulating eosinophils in normal reptiles is variable. In general, lizards tend to have low numbers of eosinophils compared with some species of turtles that can have up to 20% eosinophils.[2,3,15,29-32] Like heterophils, the number of eosinophils present in the peripheral blood is influenced by environmental factors, such as seasonal changes. The number of eosinophils is generally lower during the summer and highest during hibernation in some species.[3] Eosinophilia may be associated with parasitic infections and stimulation of the immune system.[33]

The percent of basophils in the differential leukocyte count of normal reptiles can range between 0 and 40%.[2,3,15,29-32] Seasonal variation in basophil concentration is minimal unlike acidophil concentration, which varies with season.[1] Some species of reptiles normally have high numbers of circulating basophils. For example, some species of turtles typically have circulating basophil numbers that represent up to 40% of the leukocyte differential, although the reason for this is unknown.[34,35]

Reptilian basophils most likely function in a manner similar to that of mammalian basophils based on cytochemical and ultrastructural studies. They appear to process surface immunoglobulins and release histamine on degranulation.[2,34,35] Basophilias have been associated with parasitic and viral infections.[2]

Lymphocyte concentration in the blood of reptiles is also variable and can represent more than 80% of the normal leukocyte differential in some species.[2] Lymphocyte numbers are influenced by a number of environmental and physiologic factors. Like heterophils and eosinophils, lymphocytes are also influenced by seasonal change; lymphocyte counts tend to be lowest during the winter and highest during the summer.[2,3,31] Temperate reptiles have a decrease or absence of lymphocytes during hibernation, and after hibernation, lymphocyte concentration increases.[36-39] Tropical reptiles also show a decrease in circulating lymphocytes during the winter despite lack of hibernate.[2] Lymphocyte numbers are also affected by gender, with the females of some species having significantly higher lymphocyte concentrations than males of the same species.[2,3]

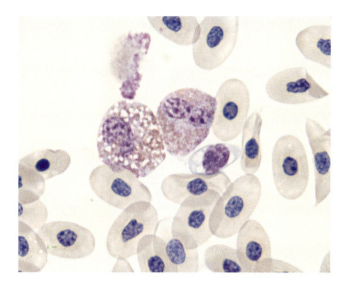

FIGURE 28-17 Toxic heterophils and a thrombocyte. Blood film from a Green Iguana *(Iguana iguana)* stained with Wright's stain. The iguana later died of renal failure and severe necrotic inflammation involving the base of the tail.

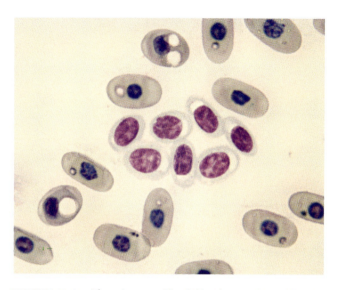

FIGURE 28-19 Thrombocytes. Blood film from a Desert Tortoise *(Gopherus agassizii)* stained with Wright's stain. Note the dark inclusions and the vacuoles in the cytoplasm of the erythrocytes are artifacts.

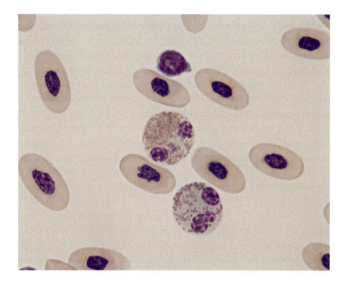

FIGURE 28-18 Normal heterophil, toxic heterophil *(blue cytoplasm)*, and lymphocyte. Blood film from a Green Iguana *(Iguana iguana)* stained with Wright's stain.

Lymphocytosis occurs during wound healing, inflammatory disease, parasitic infection (e.g., anasakiasis and spirorchidiasis), and viral infections. Lymphocytosis also occurs during ecdysis.[16] The presence of reactive lymphocytes and, less commonly, plasma cells suggests stimulation of the immune system. These cells resemble those of birds and mammals. Reactive lymphocytes have more abundant deeply basophilic cytoplasm compared with normal lymphocytes, and the nuclear chromatin may appear less condensed. Plasma cells have abundant intensely basophilic cytoplasm that contains a distinct Golgi zone and eccentrically positioned nucleus.

Monocytes generally occur in low numbers in the blood films of normal reptiles, ranging between 0 and 10% of the leukocyte differential.[2,3,15,29-32,43,44] Snakes typically have monocytes with an azurophilic appearance to the cytoplasm (frequently referred to as azurophils in the literature).[18] Monocyte concentration changes little with seasonal variation.[3] Monocytosis is suggestive of inflammatory diseases, especially granulomatous inflammation.

Although considered to be rare, some cases of leukemia have been reported in reptiles.[45-50] The myeloproliferative diseases of reptiles can be classified in the same manner as in mammals. Special cytochemical studies may be necessary to identify the abnormal cells.

Thrombocytes and Hemostasis

Morphology

Thrombocytes of reptiles appear as elliptical to fusiform nucleated cells (Figures 28-19, 28-20, and 28-21). The centrally positioned nucleus has dense nuclear chromatin that stains purple, and the cytoplasm is typically colorless and may contain a few azurophilic granules. Activated thrombocytes are common and appear as clusters of cells with irregular cytoplasmic margins and vacuoles. Thrombocytes appear devoid of cytoplasm when aggregated. Reptilian thrombocytes often stain PAS-positive, which aids in distinguishing them from the PAS-negative lymphocytes.[7]

Reptilian lymphocytes function in a manner similar to those of birds and mammals. They have the same major classes of lymphocytes, B-lymphocytes and T-lymphocytes that are involved with a variety of immunological functions.[40] However, unlike birds and mammals, the immunologic responses of the ectothermic reptiles are influenced greatly by the environment.[41] For example, low temperatures may suppress or inhibit the immune response in reptiles.

Lymphopenia is often associated with malnutrition or secondary to a number of diseases caused by stress and immunosuppression. A single hydrocortisone acetate dose (1 mg/g body weight) resulted in a 40% to 50% reduction of peripheral blood lymphocytes from lympholysis of lizards that lasted for approximately 4 weeks in one study.[42]

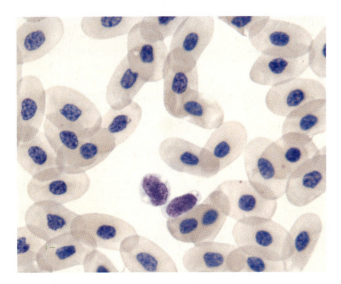

FIGURE 28-20 Thrombocytes. Blood film from a Green Iguana (*Iguana iguana*) stained with Wright's stain.

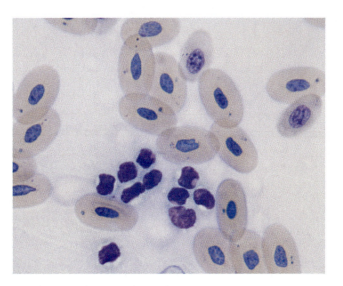

FIGURE 28-21 Thrombocytes. Blood film from a Burmese Python (*Python molurus bivittatus*) stained with Wright's stain. The blood was collected in heparin, resulting in an overall blue cast to blood film. Note the dark inclusions in the cytoplasm of the erythrocytes are artifacts.

Laboratory Evaluation

The actual thrombocyte concentration may be difficult to determine because thrombocytes tend to clump in vitro and when exposed to heparin, a commonly used anticoagulant in reptile hematology. The thrombocyte concentration can be obtained with Natt and Herrick's method for obtaining erythrocyte and leukocyte counts. After preparing the 1:200 dilution of the blood with Natt and Herrick's solution and charging a Neubauer-ruled hemocytometer, the number of thrombocytes in the entire central ruled area (central large square) are counted on both sides of the hemocytometer. The number of thrombocytes per µL of blood is obtained by multiplying that number by 1000. A subjective thrombocyte concentration can be determined based on the number of thrombocytes that appear in a stained blood film and reported as reduced, normal, or increased. Thrombocytes typically occur in numbers that range between 25 and 350 thrombocytes per 100 leukocytes in the blood film of normal reptiles.[2]

Responses to Disease

Reptilian thrombocytes have a significant role in thrombus formation and function similarly to avian thrombocytes and mammalian platelets. The ultrastructural features of activated reptile thrombocytes include pseudopodia with fine granular material and many fibrin-like filaments radiating between and around the cells.[2,36] Immature thrombocytes of reptiles resemble the immature thrombocytes of birds and, when present in blood films, represent a regenerative response. Thrombocytopenias of reptiles most likely occur as a result of excessive peripheral utilization of thrombocytes or a decrease in thrombocyte production. Thrombocytes with polymorphic nuclei are considered abnormal and may be associated with severe inflammatory disease.[18]

Considerations in the Interpretation of the Reptilian Hemogram

When evaluating the hematologic responses of reptiles, external factors such as environmental conditions that may enhance or inhibit the animal's response to disease should not be overlooked. The cellular responses in reptilian blood are less predictable than those of the endothermic mammals and birds whose cellular microenvironments are more stable. A number of intrinsic factors, such as age and gender, also affect the hematologic data from reptiles. In addition, a number of sample handling factors, such as blood collection site, type of anticoagulant used, method of cell counting, and type of stain used, add to the variability of reptilian hemogram values. These factors complicate the establishment of normal reference values in reptiles. Therefore, total and differential leukocyte counts must differ greatly (i.e., two-fold or greater increase or decrease) from normal reference values to be considered significant.

Hematology is most valuable as a tool to assess the response of the reptilian patient to disease or therapy. A favorable response in the leukogram is a shift from a leukocytosis or leukopenia to a normal leukocyte concentration. A normal heterophil, eosinophil, or monocyte count after a heterophilia, eosinophilia, or monocytosis, respectively, usually indicates an improved status of the patient. Disappearance of toxic heterophils, reactive lymphocytes, and plasma cells from the blood film indicates improvement and a favorable response to therapy.

Anemic reptiles with an erythrocytic regenerative response have a better prognosis compared with those with little or no response. Similarly, normal thrombocyte concentration after thrombocytopenia indicates a favorable response. Therefore, hematology can be a valuable tool in the assessment of the reptilian patient.

CLINICAL CHEMISTRIES OF REPTILES

Blood biochemistry profiles are often used to assess the physiologic status of reptilian patients; however, a general lack of controlled studies designed to clarify the meaning of changes in the blood chemistries of reptiles compared with those of domestic mammals exists. Therefore, reptilian clinical chemistry has not achieved the same degree of critical evaluation as seen in domestic mammalian medicine. Currently, interpretations of reptilian blood biochemistries are considered the same as for domestic mammals with the consideration that external factors, such as environmental conditions, have a greater influence on the normal physiology and health of ectothermic vertebrates compared with endotherms. Species, age, gender, nutritional status, season, and physiologic status influence blood biochemistries of reptiles.[10,51,52] This makes interpretation of blood biochemistry results in reptiles challenging.

Normal reference values for specific blood biochemical tests for a few species of reptiles have been reported.[15,16,31,32,53-60] Environmental conditions and physiologic parameters such as nutritional status, gender, and age often have not been taken into consideration when establishing reference intervals, making them less meaningful. Methods of sample collection, handling, and biochemical analysis are additional sources of variation in the published reference values.[61-63] Therefore, published references are generally used as a broad guide to interpretation of blood biochemical results in reptiles. **Because of the difficulty in obtaining meaningful reference intervals for each species of reptile seen in clinical practice, most clinicians use decision levels when assessing reptilian patients. Decision levels are threshold values above or below which a decision is made to respond to a value of an analyte**. The response may vary from repeating the test or ordering additional tests to treatment of the patient. Decision levels may be obtained by using published reference intervals and applying the values to those obtained in the laboratory used by the reptilian hospital. Decision levels may vary to some degree among reptilian clinicians, depending on laboratory results and experience. Values suggested in this text are general guidelines that can be used as decision levels when evaluating each analyte in the reptilian blood biochemical profile. The process of evaluating the blood chemistries of a reptilian patient can be refined by obtaining a set of normal values from that patient housed under a given set of environmental and nutritional parameters. Therefore, when that patient becomes ill, a more meaningful set of reference values specific for that patient can be used to evaluate the chemistry results.

Sample Collection and Handling

Blood samples for biochemical studies can be collected from reptiles with a variety of methods depending on the species, volume needed, size of the reptile, physiologic condition of the patient, and preference of the collector.[64] Depending on the site of blood collection, blood samples collected from reptiles are often contaminated with lymphatic fluid. Most of the analytes such as glucose, calcium, phosphorus, sodium, urea, and enzymes in lymph are comparable with that of plasma or serum in reptiles; however, a significantly lower concentration of total protein and potassium is found in lymph as compared with blood.[61,62] Therefore, the amount of lymph contamination of the blood sample should be considered when interpreting blood biochemical parameters of reptiles. Many clinicians prefer to collect blood with an anticoagulant, such as lithium heparin, for blood biochemical testing of reptiles, primarily because a greater sample volume can be achieved for plasma compared with serum. Collection of blood into lithium heparin also allows for the evaluation of the hemogram and blood biochemistries with one sample. Plasma is preferred over serum because clot formation in reptilian blood is unpredictable and often prolonged, resulting in significant changes in some of the chemistries such as serum electrolytes. Reptilian blood clots slowly because of low intrinsic thromboplastin activity and a strong natural circulating antithrombin factor, which compensates for sluggish blood flow.

Often, the sample size collected from small reptiles is sufficient enough for only a few tests rather than a complete panel. Therefore, the clinician must decide which tests are most beneficial in the evaluation of the reptile patient. **Blood biochemical tests that appear to be most useful in reptilian diagnostics include total protein, albumin, glucose, uric acid, aspartate aminotransferase (AST), creatine kinase (CK), calcium, and phosphorus.** Other tests that may also be helpful include creatine, lactate dehydrogenase (LD), sodium, potassium, chloride, total CO_2, and protein electrophoresis. Many modern blood chemistry analyzers require a small sample size (10 to 30 μL) to perform many of these tests. Commercial veterinary laboratories often offer chemistry profiles that require a minimal amount of serum or plasma (0.5 mL). Blood chemistry analyzers that use dry reagents and reflectance photometry for in-house testing may be used for reptile samples.

The plasma of most reptiles is colorless; however, it may be orange to yellow from carotenoid pigments in the diets of herbivores such as Green Iguanas.[65] The plasma of some snakes such as pythons may be a greenish yellow from carotenoids and riboflavin. Some lizards normally have green plasma because of high plasma concentrations of biliverdin.[65]

Laboratory Evaluation of Reptilian Kidneys

The reptilian renal cortex contains only simple nephrons (cortical nephrons) that have a tubular system devoid of loops of Henle; therefore, reptiles are unable to concentrate their urine. Nitrogenous wastes excreted by the reptilian kidney include variable amounts of uric acid, urea, and ammonia, depending on the animal's natural environment. Freshwater turtles that spend much of their life in water excrete equal amounts of ammonia and urea, whereas those with amphibious habits excrete more urea.[66] Seaturtles excrete uric acid, ammonia, and urea, and alligators excrete ammonia and uric acid.[66] Terrestrial reptiles such as tortoises must conserve water. Ammonia, urea, and other soluble urinary nitrogenous wastes require large amounts of water for excretion; therefore, to conserve water, terrestrial reptiles produce more insoluble nitrogenous waste in the form of uric acid and urate salts, which are eliminated in a semisolid state.

Blood biochemical detection of renal disease in reptiles is more difficult than that of mammals because of the physiologic differences in their kidneys; for example, blood urea nitrogen (BUN) and creatinine concentrations are generally poor indicators of renal disease in reptiles. The normal BUN value of most reptiles is low (<10 mg/dL).[15,16,31,32,53-60] Plasma urea nitrogen may be more useful in the evaluation of renal disease in aquatic reptiles that excrete primarily urea. Because terrestrial reptiles are primarily uricotelic, normal urea nitrogen concentration in these species is less than 15 mg/dL, with the exception of terrestrial chelonians, especially desert species, that typically have plasma urea nitrogen concentrations that can normally vary from 30 to 100 mg/dL.[53,55,57,59] This is considered to be a mechanism to elevate the plasma osmolarity to reduce water loss from the body.[31] The plasma osmolarity of freshwater turtles and crocodilians is approximately the same as that of common domestic mammals but is higher in terrestrial reptiles. An increase in plasma urea nitrogen concentration may be suggestive of severe renal disease, prerenal azotemia, or high dietary urea intake in reptiles. However, BUN does not reliably increase under these conditions in reptiles.

Creatinine is a normal constituent of the urine of mammals, but the amount formed in most reptiles is negligible (<1 mg/dL).[16,31,55,63] **Blood creatinine concentration is generally considered to be of poor diagnostic value in the detection of renal disease in reptiles.** Although blood creatine concentration may be of diagnostic value in the detection of renal disease in some species of reptiles, the test is unavailable from most veterinary laboratories.

Uric acid is the primary catabolic end product of protein, nonprotein nitrogen, and purines in terrestrial reptiles and represents 80% to 90% of the total nitrogen excreted by the kidneys.[67] The normal blood uric acid concentration for most reptiles is less than 10 mg/dL.

Hyperuricemia is indicated by uric acid values greater than 15 mg/dL and is usually associated with renal disease, such as those caused by severe bacteremia, septicemia, nephrocalcinosis, and nephrotoxicity. Plasma uric acid is neither sensitive nor specific for renal disease in reptiles. **Hyperuricemia associated with renal disease most likely reflects loss of two thirds or more of the functional renal mass, and hyperuricemia can also be associated with gout or recent ingestion of a high protein diet.** Carnivorous reptiles tend to have higher blood uric acid concentrations than do herbivorous reptiles, and they exhibit a postprandial hyperuricemia that generally peaks the day after a meal, resulting in a 1.5-fold to 2-fold increase in uric acid.[67] Gout can result from an overproduction of uric acid (primary gout) or an acquired disease that interferes with the normal production and excretion of uric acid (secondary gout). Conditions that result in secondary gout in reptiles include starvation, renal disease (especially tubular damage), severe prolonged dehydration, and excessive dietary purines (i.e., herbivorous reptiles fed diets rich in animal proteins). Hyperuricemia associated with renal disease and gout often results in greater than two-fold increases in uric acid concentrations. See Chapter 54 for more information on gout.

The kidney of reptiles has high alanine aminotransferase (ALT) and alkaline phosphatase (AP) activity.[68] However, significant plasma increases in these enzyme activities do not occur with renal disease because most of the enzymes released from damaged renal cells are released in urine and not the blood.[69]

Reptiles rarely exhibit polyuria with renal disease. Therefore, a urinalysis is rarely performed to assess renal disease. However, valuable information can be obtained, and as more urinalyses are performed, the test is becoming more useful (see Chapter 66).

Electrolytes and Acid Base

Water Balance
The species, diet, and environmental conditions, such as temperature and humidity, influence water consumption of reptiles. Desert reptiles need less water than temperate and tropical species. Some reptiles have developed methods for conserving water.[70] For example, tortoises and some lizards store water in the urinary bladder. Many reptiles can achieve water uptake through the cloaca by soaking.[66] Water is also conserved in reptiles by the elimination of nitrogenous waste in the form of uric acid and urate salts, which are excreted in a semisolid state.

Sodium and Chloride
Dietary sodium is absorbed in the intestines and transported to the kidneys where it is excreted or resorbed depending on the reptile's need for sodium. Reptilian sodium and potassium metabolism involves an active renin-angiotensin system with direct action on osmoregulation.[71] Some reptiles have nasal salt glands that participate in the regulation of sodium, potassium, and chloride in the blood. Therefore, disorders of the salt gland may affect electrolyte balance.

The normal serum or plasma sodium concentration ranges between 120 and 170 mEq/L. Normal plasma sodium concentrations of tortoises and freshwater turtles range between 120 and 150 mEq/L.[72] Seaturtles tend to have higher normal sodium plasma concentrations that range between 150 and 170 mEq/L.[63] The normal plasma sodium concentrations of lizards range between 140 and 170 mEq/L, and those of snakes, such as boas and pythons, range between 130 and 160 mEq/L.[72]

Hyponatremia can result from excessive sodium loss associated with disorders of the gastrointestinal tract (i.e., diarrhea), kidneys, or possibly the salt gland. Iatrogenic hyponatremia can occur with overhydration of the reptilian patient with intravenous or intracoelomic fluids that are low in sodium. Hypernatremia results from dehydration, either from excessive water loss or inadequate water intake, and excessive dietary salt intake.

Chloride is the principle anion in the blood and, along with sodium, represents the primary osmotically active component of plasma in most reptiles. Normal serum or plasma chloride concentration of reptiles varies among species but generally ranges between 100 and 130 mEq/L.[73] Plasma chloride concentrations of turtles tend to range between 100 and 110 mEq/L, whereas those of most lizards and snakes range between 100 and 130 mEq/L.[72] **Blood chloride concentration provides the least clinically useful information of the electrolytes.**

Hypochloremia in reptiles is rare and suggests excessive loss of chloride ions or overhydration with fluids low in chloride ions. Hyperchloremia is associated with dehydration and possibly renal tubular disease or disorders of the salt glands.

Potassium
Normal serum or plasma potassium concentrations also vary with species of reptiles but generally range between 2 and 6 mEq/L. The normal plasma potassium concentrations of most turtles, lizards, and snakes range between 2 and 6, 3 and 5, and 3 and 6 mEq/L, respectively.[72] Common imbalances of serum or plasma potassium include inadequate dietary potassium intake or excessive gastrointestinal potassium loss (hypokalemia) or decreased renal secretion of potassium (hyperkalemia). Hypokalemia can also be associated with severe alkalosis. Hyperkalemia can also result from excessive dietary potassium intake or severe acidosis.

Hyperkalemia in the face of hyperphosphatemia usually indicates erythrocyte lysis (hemolysis) or an otherwise damaged blood sample.

Acid/Base

The normal blood pH of turtles and most other reptiles ranges between 7.5 and 7.7 at 23°C to 25°C.[66,73] The normal blood pH of some snakes and lizards may fall below 7.4. The blood pH of reptiles is labile and changes with temperature fluctuations. An increase in temperature or excitement can cause blood pH to decrease. The blood pH of reptiles may increase during anesthesia from a normal pH of 7.5 to 7.6 to a pH of 7.7 to 7.8. As in mammals, the oxygen dissociation curve for reptilian hemoglobin shifts to the left as the pH increases, resulting in an increase in the affinity of hemoglobin for oxygen but decrease in release to tissues.

The buffering systems that regulate the blood pH in mammals are most likely the same in reptiles, with the bicarbonate/carbonic acid buffer system being the most important because of the rapid rate of CO_2 elimination by the lungs after the conversion from H_2CO_3. Total plasma CO_2 or bicarbonate concentrations are rarely reported in reptiles. However, normal total CO_2 values for most reptiles are expected to range between 20 and 30 mmol/L.[72]

A marked fasting physiologic metabolic alkalosis occurs in postprandial alligators because of an anion shift with bicarbonate replacing chloride in the blood, as chloride is lost as HCl in gastric secretions.[58] Therefore, a postprandial decrease of chloride and increase of bicarbonate concentrations is seen in alligators.[58]

Calcium and Phosphorus

Blood calcium metabolism and the amount of ionized calcium in the plasma of reptiles is mediated by parathormone (PTH), calcitonin (CT), and activated vitamin D_3 (1,25 dihydrocholecalciferol).[74] Other hormones, such as estrogen, thyroxin, and glucagon, may also influence calcium metabolism in reptiles. The primary function of PTH is to maintain normal blood calcium levels by its action on bone, kidneys, and intestinal mucosa. Low blood ionized calcium stimulates the release of PTH, which results in the calcium mobilization from bone, increased calcium absorption from the intestines, and increased calcium reabsorption from the kidneys.

The exact role of calcitonin in reptiles is unknown, but it most likely has a physiologic role opposite that of PTH. Increases in blood calcium stimulate the release of calcitonin from the ultimobranchial gland, which inhibits calcium reabsorption from bone.

The active form of vitamin D_3 stimulates calcium and phosphorus absorption by the intestinal mucosa. Photochemical production of the active form of vitamin D_3 with exposure to ultraviolet (UV) radiation (290 to 320 nm wavelength) is believed to be essential for normal calcium metabolism in reptiles, especially basking species.

Female reptiles exhibit features of calcium metabolism similar to those of birds during egg production. During egg development, female reptiles have hypercalcemia in response to estrogen and reproductive activity.[56] **The increase in the total plasma calcium is associated with an increase in protein-bound calcium during follicular development before ovulation and may increase two to four fold.**

The normal plasma concentration of calcium for most reptiles ranges between 8 and 11 mg/dL.[72] The normal plasma calcium concentration varies with species and physiologic status of the reptile. For example, some species of tortoises have low blood calcium concentrations (i.e., less than 8 mg/dL).[59]

Because of all the factors that affect total calcium measurements in reptilian plasma, measurement of ionized calcium levels may be best. In one study with the Green Iguana, mean ionized calcium concentration measured in blood was 1.47 ± 0.105 mmol/L. Ionized calcium concentration provides a clinical measurement of the physiologically active calcium in circulation. Evaluation of physiologically active calcium in reptiles with suspected calcium imbalance that have total plasma calcium concentrations within reference range or in gravid animals with considerably increased total plasma calcium concentrations is vital for determining a therapeutic plan. A precise evaluation of calcium status provides assistance in the diagnosis of renal disease and seizures and allows for better evaluation of the health status of gravid female iguanas.[75]

Hypocalcemia in most reptiles occurs when plasma calcium concentration is less than 8 mg/dL. Hypocalcemia can occur with dietary calcium and vitamin D_3 deficiencies, excessive dietary phosphorus, alkalosis, hypoalbuminemia, or hypoparathyroidism. Secondary nutritional hyperparathyroidism is a common disorder of herbivorous reptiles, such as Green Iguanas.[76,77] Herbivorous diets are often deficient in calcium and contain excessive amounts of phosphorus. Also, dietary deficiency in vitamin D_3 or lack of proper exposure to ultraviolet light predisposes reptiles to hypocalcemia. Juvenile reptiles (especially Green Iguanas) with secondary nutritional hyperparathyroidism commonly have metabolic bone disease of nutritional origin (NMBD) develop that manifests with fibrous osteodystrophy and pathologic bone fractures.

Adult reptiles often have muscle tremors, paresis, and seizures develop with hypocalcemia. Carnivorous reptiles fed all meat calcium-deficient diets also have hypocalcemia develop associated with nutritional imbalances in calcium and phosphorus. Secondary renal hyperparathyroidism may also result in hypocalcemia in reptiles. See Chapter 61 for more details.

Hypercalcemia in reptiles is indicated by a plasma calcium concentration greater than 20 mg/dL, which occurs with excessive dietary or parenteral vitamin D_3 and calcium. This is typically an iatrogenic condition associated with oversupplementation of calcium and vitamin D_3.[78] Other differentials for hypercalcemia include primary hyperparathyroidism, pseudohyperparathyroidism, and osteolytic bone disease; however, these disorders are rarely reported in reptiles.

The Indigo Snake (*Drymarchon* spp.) has a normal physiologic hypercalcemia, with average plasma calcium level of 159 g/dL (range, 30 to 337 g/dL). Phosphorus levels, likewise, also are high by normal standards with an average of 35 mg/dL (range, 8 to 69 g/dL).[79]

Normal plasma phosphorus concentration for most reptiles ranges between 1 and 5 mg/dL.[72] Hypophosphatemia may result from starvation or nutritional deficiency of phosphorus. Hyperphosphatemia is indicated by a plasma phosphorus concentration greater than 5 mg/dL. Disorders resulting in hyperphosphatemia include excessive dietary phosphorus, hypervitaminosis D_3, and renal disease. Rare causes of hyperphosphatemia include severe tissue trauma and osteolytic bone disease. A factitious hyperphosphatemia can occur when the serum or plasma is not promptly separated from the clot, allowing phosphorus to be released from erythrocytes.

Laboratory Evaluation of the Reptilian Liver

Liver enzymes in reptiles appear to be similar to those of birds and mammals. The LD and AST activities are high in liver tissue of reptiles, and although few critical studies have been applied to the biochemical testing of reptilian blood to evaluate hepatic disease, increases in these enzyme activities in plasma may suggest hepatocellular disease.[69] Plasma AST is not considered to be organ specific because its activity can be found in many tissues. In general, normal plasma AST activity for reptiles is less than 250 IU/L. Increased plasma AST activity suggests hepatic or muscle injury. However, generalized diseases, such as septicemia or toxemia, may damage these tissues, resulting in increased plasma AST activity.

Plasma LD is also considered to have a wide tissue distribution in reptiles. Therefore, increases in plasma LD (activity greater than 1000 IU/L) may be associated with damage to the liver, skeletal muscle, or cardiac muscle. Hemolysis may also result in increased plasma LD activity.

Like AST, plasma ALT is not considered to be organ specific in reptiles. Normal plasma ALT activity for reptiles is usually less than 20 IU/L. Although ALT activity occurs in the liver of reptiles, increases in plasma ALT activity may not be as reliable in the detection of hepatocellular disease as increases in plasma AST or LD activity.

Alkaline phosphatase is also widely distributed in the body of reptiles, and plasma activity of this enzyme is not considered to be organ specific. Little information is found concerning the interpretation of increased plasma AP activity in reptiles; however, increased activity may reflect an increase in osteoblastic activity.

Biliverdin, a green bile pigment, is generally considered to be the primary end product of hemoglobin catabolism in reptiles.[80] Green plasma results from the accumulation of biliverdin in reptilian blood and is usually a pathologic finding suggestive of hepatobiliary disease in these animals. However, a nonpathologic accumulation of biliverdin in the blood of some species of reptiles that are rarely presented for clinical evaluation can occur.[65] The physiologic advantage of this is not known. Biliverdin appears to be less toxic to tissues compared with bilirubin, and the normal biliverdin concentration in the plasma of some species of lizards can be greater than 1000 µmol/L.[65]

Laboratory Evaluation of Plasma and Serum Proteins

The plasma total protein concentration of normal reptiles generally ranges between 3 and 7 g/dL.[72] Female reptiles show marked increases in plasma total protein concentration during active folliculogenesis. This estrogen-induced hyperproteinemia is associated with an increase in proteins, primarily globulins (vitellogenins), necessary for yolk production.[56] The plasma total protein concentration returns to normal after ovulation.

The biuret method is the most accurate method for determination of plasma or serum total protein concentration, although the refractometer method is commonly used to rapidly estimate plasma protein concentration in reptilian blood (the latter measurement being more accurately referred to as total solids).

Protein electrophoresis provides an accurate assessment of serum or plasma albumin concentration in reptilian blood. Absolute concentrations of the various plasma proteins are obtained with determination of the total protein with the biuret method in conjunction with electrophoretic separation of the proteins.

Hyperproteinemia is indicated by total protein values greater than 7 g/dL in most reptiles and occurs with dehydration or hyperglobulinemia associated with chronic inflammatory diseases. The alpha, beta, and gamma globulins may increase with infectious diseases. Normal values, however, have not been established for all the various species. Therefore, interpreting an electrophoresis as a diagnostic tool as yet has no real significance.

Hypoproteinemia, as indicated by a total protein value less than 3 g/dL, is commonly associated with chronic malnutrition in reptiles. However, other causes, such as malabsorption, maldigestion, protein-losing enteropathies (e.g., parasitism), severe blood loss, and chronic hepatic or renal disease, should also be considered.

Laboratory Evaluation of Glucose Metabolism

Normal blood glucose concentration of most reptiles ranges between 60 and 100 mg/dL but is subject to marked physiologic variation.[72,81] The blood glucose concentration of normal reptiles varies with species, nutritional status, and environmental conditions. For example, an increase in temperature results in hypoglycemia in turtles but hyperglycemia in alligators.[81] Normal oral glucose tolerance curves in reptiles differ among the species and with temperature. Reptiles have pancreatic beta and alpha cell types as a source of insulin and glucagon, respectively, similar to mammals and other vertebrates.[82] The action of these hormones is affected by temperature.

Common causes of hypoglycemia in reptiles include starvation and malnutrition, severe hepatobiliary disease, and septicemia. Clinical signs associated with hypoglycemia in reptiles include tremors, loss of righting reflex, torpor, and dilated nonresponsive pupils.

Hyperglycemia in reptiles is often a result of iatrogenic delivery of excessive glucose. A persistent marked hyperglycemia and glucosuria is suggestive of diabetes mellitus, a rarely reported disorder of reptiles. Hyperglycemia may also occur with glucocorticosteroid excess. See Chapter 58 for a thorough discussion of glucose metabolism in reptiles.

Laboratory Detection of Muscle Injury

Creatinine kinase is considered to be a muscle-specific enzyme and is used to test for muscle cell damage. Increases in plasma CK activity can result from muscle cell injury or exertion. Elevations in plasma CK are frequently observed in reptiles that are struggling to resist restraint during blood collection or are exhibiting seizure activity. Increased plasma CK activity resulting from muscle cell damage occurs with traumatic injury, intramuscular injections of irritating drugs (e.g., enrofloxacin) or fluids, and systemic infections that affect skeletal or cardiac muscle. Brain tissue generally has high CK activity; however, whether brain lesions contribute significantly to plasma CK is not known.

Muscle injury also results in mild to moderate increases in plasma AST and LD activities. However, these enzymes are not organ specific for muscle and could increase with hepatobiliary disease. When plasma CK activity is not increased in the face of increased AST and LD activity, hepatobiliary disease should be suspected. Damage to both liver and skeletal muscle can occur simultaneously such as occurs with trauma and septicemia, which results in elevations of plasma AST, LD, and CK.

Laboratory Evaluation of Endocrine Disorders

Laboratory evaluation of the thyroid and adrenal function of reptiles is uncommon. Because of the ectothermic nature of reptiles, their physiologic status, which includes endocrine physiology, is highly dependent on the external environment. For example, the thyroid activity of reptiles is temperature dependent and, even at higher temperatures, is still less active than mammals.[83] Therefore, correction of environmental and nutritional deficits usually results in the restoration of the normal physiologic health of reptiles.

EVALUATION OF THE REPTILIAN CYTOLOGIC SAMPLE

Cytology is a simple, rapid diagnostic procedure that requires little in terms of equipment and cost to the veterinarian. The basic equipment needed includes a microscope with good resolution (especially at 20×, 40×, and 100× oil immersion), clean microscope slides, coverslips, and cytologic stains (i.e., Wright's and stat stains). The basic equipment needed for collection of cytologic samples includes syringes (6 to 12 mL), fine-gauge needles (i.e., 23 to 20 gauge, 1 to 1½ inch), sterile cotton swabs, sterile rubber or soft plastic tubes (i.e., feeding tubes), and sterile physiologic saline solution. A variety of methods can be used to concentrate cells from poorly cellular fluids and washes onto a microscope slide. A simple method is marginating the cells with the spreader slide technique.

Another method is the use of the sedimentation after centrifugation (as used in mammalian urine cytology) or use of a commercial cytocentrifuge. Cells can also be concentrated by allowing them to fall onto the slide via gravity with a sample column and filter paper firmly attached to a microscope slide.

Once the cytologic sample has been collected and stained, it is ready for microscopic evaluation. The primary goal of the cytologist is to evaluate the cellular response, classifying it as either representative of inflammation, tissue hyperplasia (or benign neoplasia), malignant neoplasia, a mixed cellular response (inflammatory and noninflammatory), or normal cellularity. Identification of an etiologic agent, if present, should also be made.

The inflammatory response of reptiles can be classified as either heterophilic, eosinophilic, mixed cell, or macrophagic. The type of inflammatory response may suggest a possible etiology and pathogenesis. Inflammatory responses of reptiles are similar to those described for mammals, except the reptilian heterophil replaces the mammalian neutrophil. The inflammatory cells of reptiles include heterophils, eosinophils, lymphocytes, plasma cells, and macrophages. Heterophil granules in cytologic specimens tend to lose their normal rod-shaped appearance and either appear more rounded or degranulated. Degenerate heterophils have similar characteristics to degenerate mammalian neutrophils (i.e., nuclear hyalinization, swelling, karyorrhexis, and karyolysis and cytoplasmic basophilia and vacuolization) and show varying degrees of degranulation. Degenerate heterophils suggest the presence of toxins, such as bacterial toxins, in the microenvironment.

Heterophilic inflammation is represented by a predominance of heterophils (>80% of the inflammatory cells) in the cytologic sample (Figures 28-22, 28-23, 28-24, and 28-25). Heterophilic inflammation usually indicates an acute phase of the inflammatory response in reptiles. Heterophilic inflammation has shown the ability to develop into a granuloma

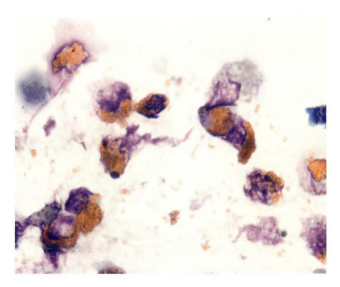

FIGURE 28-22 Heterophilic inflammation. Tracheal/lung wash cytology from a Leopard Tortoise *(Geochelone paradalis)* with noisy respiratory sounds and bubbling nasal discharge. Note the nondegenerate heterophils and lack of an etiologic agent. Radiographic evaluation results were normal. Cytodiagnosis of heterophilic tracheitis and possible pneumonia, suggestive of acute inflammatory response. Diff-Quik stain.

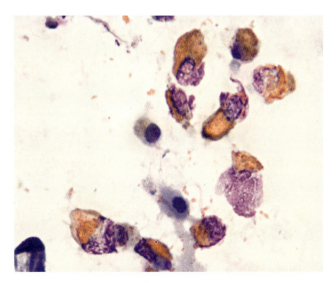

FIGURE 28-23 Heterophilic inflammation. Cytology from the nasal discharge from a Leopard Tortoise *(Geochelone paradalis)* with noisy respiratory sounds and bubbling nasal discharge. Note the nondegenerate heterophils and lack of an etiologic agent. Radiographic evaluation results were normal. Cytodiagnosis of heterophilic rhinitis and possible sinusitis, suggestive of acute inflammatory response. Diff-Quik stain.

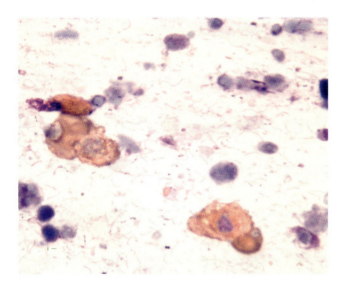

FIGURE 28-24 Heterophilic inflammation. Tracheal/lung wash cytology from a Burmese Python *(Python molurus bivittatus)* with marked dyspnea. Radiographic evaluation results were normal. Note the nondegenerate heterophils. The background contains numerous filamentous structures that resemble shed cilia from respiratory epithelial cells. Cytodiagnosis of heterophilic tracheitis and pneumonia suggests acute inflammatory response. Wright's stain.

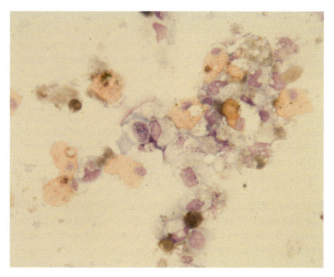

FIGURE 28-26 Mixed-cell inflammation. Tracheal/lung wash cytology from a Red-tailed Boa *(Boa constrictor)* with bubbling nasal discharge and open-mouth breathing. Note the mix of heterophils and macrophages. Cytodiagnosis of chronic active tracheitis and pneumonia. Wright's stain.

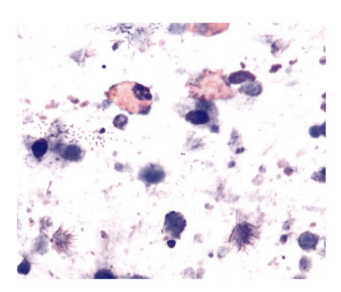

FIGURE 28-25 Heterophilic inflammation. Tracheal/lung wash cytology from a Burmese Python *(Python molurus bivittatus)* with marked dyspnea. Radiographic evaluation results were normal. Note the nondegenerate heterophils. The background contains numerous filamentous structures that resemble shed cilia from respiratory epithelial cells. Note the tags of cytoplasm containing clumps of cilia. The respiratory epithelium in the lung apparently has become degenerate, resulting in lysis of cells. Cytodiagnosis of heterophilic tracheitis and pneumonia suggests acute inflammatory response. Wright's stain.

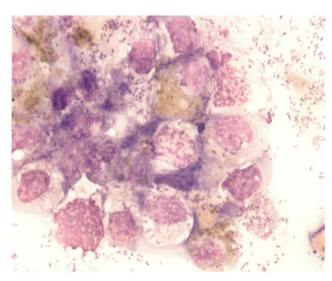

FIGURE 28-27 Mixed-cell inflammation. Oral swab cytology from a Ratsnake *(Elaphe guttata)* with caseous material in the mouth. Note the mixture of heterophils and macrophages indicating chronic active inflammation. The background contains many bacteria; however, unless one can find bacterial phagocytosis, the term *septic inflammation* cannot be used. Wright's stain.

within 1 week.[25,84-86] Apparently, the necrotic center of heterophilic inflammatory lesions produces necrotoxins that are chemotactic to macrophages and a granuloma quickly develops. Therefore, a granuloma formation in reptiles may be in response to necrotic tissue rather than an infectious organism.

Because of the rapid influx of macrophages and lymphocytes into inflammatory lesions, mixed cell inflammation is common to reptiles. Mixed cell inflammation is typically represented by a predominance of heterophils (>50% of the inflammatory cells) with an increased number of mononuclear leukocytes (Figures 28-26 and 28-27). Lymphocytes and plasma cells can be associated with acute heterophilic granulomas, whereas the presence of epithelioid cells (macrophages that contain no vacuoles or phagocytized material) and connective tissue cells (i.e., fibroblasts) suggest chronic granulomas. Frequently, the epithelial and mesenchymal cells adjacent to inflammatory lesions proliferate resulting in the presence of these types of cells showing features of tissue hyperplasia. Heterophilic and mixed cell inflammation are associated with

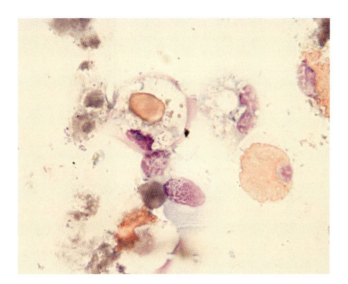

FIGURE 28-28 Septic inflammation. Tracheal/lung wash cytology from a Red-tailed Boa *(Boa constrictor)* with bubbling nasal discharge and open-mouth breathing. Note the degenerate heterophil containing phagocytized bacteria. Cytodiagnosis of septic tracheitis and pneumonia. Wright's stain.

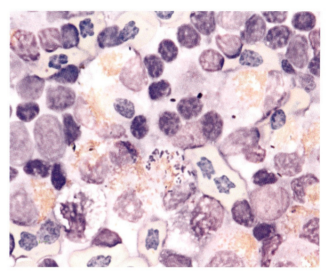

FIGURE 28-29 Septic heterophilic inflammation. Splenic imprint from a Veiled Chameleon *(Chamaeleo calyptratus)*. Cytology indicates fatal septicemia. Wright's stain.

a variety of infectious (i.e., bacterial and fungal) and noninfectious (i.e., traumatic and foreign body) etiologies in reptiles (Figures 28-28 and 28-29)

Macrophagic inflammation may have a different pathogenesis than heterophilic and mixed cell inflammation in reptiles. Macrophagic inflammation is indicated by a predominance of macrophages (>50% of the inflammatory cells) in the cytologic sample. Large vacuolated macrophages that later develop into multinucleated giant cells, apparently responding to necrotic tissue, are a feature of this type of inflammation. Macrophagic inflammation is common in certain reptilian diseases, such as mycobacterial and fungal infections. Areas of macrophagic inflammation and heterophilic inflammation can occur together as macrophages respond to necrotic materials. Therefore, depending on where the sample is obtained from the inflammatory lesion, a macrophagic inflammatory response may predominate the cytology.

Eosinophilic inflammation appears to be rare in reptiles. This may be either the result of the difficulty in differentiating eosinophils from heterophils in cytologic samples with routine cytologic stains or because reptilian eosinophils may behave differently from mammalian eosinophils. Based on cytomorphology, tissue hyperplasia and benign neoplasia are indistinguishable. Tissue hyperplasia is a proliferative process of tissues responding to cellular injury or chronic stimulation (i.e., glandular hyperplasia). Cells representative of tissue hyperplasia or benign neoplasia have increased cytoplasmic basophilia and pale vesicular nuclei. They have a uniform appearance with a uniform nucleus to cytoplasmic ratio (N:C). Cells suggestive of hyperplasia of epithelial and connective tissue often occur in cytologic specimens of chronic inflammation. Other examples of tissue hyperplasia or benign neoplasia that are frequently identified with cytodiagnosis in reptiles include squamous cell hyperplasia or metaplasia associated with hypovitaminosis A and lymphoid hyperplasia.

The cytologic criteria for the diagnosis of malignant neoplasia in domestic mammals also apply to reptilian cytodiagnosis. The criteria for the cytologic diagnosis of malignant neoplasia can be divided into general cellular, nuclear, cytoplasmic, and structural features. General cellular features include the presence on noninflammatory cells with an apparent common origin showing pleomorphism, increased cellularity in samples from tissues that normally provide low cellular samples, and the appearance of cells that are foreign to the tissue being sampled. The more frequently observed nuclear criteria for malignant neoplasia include anisokaryosis, variable N:C ratios, nuclear pleomorphism, abnormal mitoses, abnormal chromatin patterns, and large pleomorphic or multiple (>4) nucleoli. The two important cytoplasmic features of malignant neoplasia include increased basophilia and vacuolation. Increased cytoplasmic basophilia is suggestive of increased RNA activity typical of young, active cells. Increased cytoplasmic vacuolation could suggest cellular degeneration, especially if the vacuoles are small. Cells originating from secretory tissue, such as adenocarcinomas, produce large secretory vacuoles. Finally, structural features of malignant neoplasia refer to those features that may suggest a possible origin of the neoplasm, such as epithelial neoplasia (carcinomas), mesenchymal neoplasia (sarcomas), or discrete cell neoplasia (round cell neoplasms). Epithelial cell neoplasms tend to provide highly cellular samples that contain round to polygonal cells with distinct cell margins and occurring in sheets or clusters. Mesenchymal cell neoplasms usually produce poorly cellular samples that contain spindle-shaped cells with indistinct cytoplasmic margins and generally do not occur in aggregates (Figure 28-30). Discrete cell neoplasms are composed of round to oval cells that exfoliate well as individual cells. A common discrete cell neoplasm of reptiles is lymphoid neoplasia.

The coelomic cavity of normal reptiles contains little, if any, fluid. Therefore, fluid aspirated from the coelomic cavity should be examined for specific gravity, protein content, and cellularity. Fluids can be classified as transudates, modified transudates, exudates, hemorrhagic effusions, or malignant effusions.

Transudative effusions are characterized by low specific gravity (<1.020), low cellularity (<1,000 cells/µL), and low

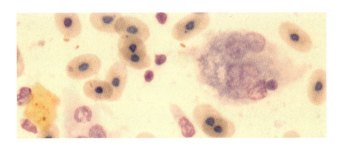

FIGURE 28-30 Multinucleated mesenchymal cells. Imprint from an excised mass on the tongue of a Blanding's Turtle *(Emydoidea blandingi)*. The cytology indicates numerous pleomorphic spindle-shaped cells, some multinucleated, which with lack of inflammatory response is supportive of mesenchymal cell neoplasm. Diff-Quik stain.

total protein (<3 g/dL). Transudates are clear to straw color on gross inspection. The cells found in transudates are primarily macrophages with occasional mesothelial cells, lymphocytes, and nondegenerate heterophils. Transudative effusions in reptiles most likely occur for the same reasons as those for mammals, such as oncotic pressure changes and other circulatory disorders.

Modified transudates resemble transudative effusions grossly but have higher protein content (3 to 3.5 g/dL) and cellularity (1,000 to 5,000 cells/µL). The cells found in modified transudates are primarily macrophages and reactive mesothelial cells. Reactive mesothelial cells are round to oval cells that often have scalloped or villus-like eosinophilic margins, cytoplasmic vacuoles, multiple nuclei, and mitotic activity. Modified transudates occur from long-standing transudative effusions or as a result of hydrostatic pressure changes.

Exudative effusions result from inflammatory processes in the coelomic cavity. They are characterized by a high cellularity (>5000 cells/µL), protein content (>3 g/dL), and specific gravity (>1.020). Exudative effusions vary in color and turbidity, may have a foul odor, and often clot during sample collection. Therefore, use of an anticoagulant (e.g., EDTA) is indicated with coelomic fluids suspected of clotting.

The cellular content of exudates varies with etiology, host response, and duration of time. Exudates that show a heterophilic inflammation suggest an acute inflammatory response. Septic exudates may show intracellular bacteria and degenerate heterophils. Mononuclear leukocytes are characteristic of mild irritation to the coelomic cavity and nonseptic conditions.

Hemorrhagic effusions in the coelomic cavity of reptiles often result from trauma or injury. Hemorrhagic effusions show a variable number of erythrocytes in the fluid sample. Hemorrhagic effusions must be differentiated from peripheral blood contamination of the sample during collection. Because thrombocytes disappear quickly in hemorrhagic effusions, their presence usually suggests peripheral blood contamination of the sample. Chronic and resolving hemorrhagic effusions exhibit varying degrees of erythrophagocytosis that is indicated by leukocytic (usually macrophages) phagocytosis of intact erythrocytes or macrophages containing remnants of erythrocytes, such as red cell fragments and iron pigment. Iron pigment appears as blue-black to gray pigment in the cytoplasm of macrophages with Wright's stain.

Malignant effusions can have features of modified transudates, hemorrhagic effusions, or exudates and may have cells with features of malignant neoplasia. The cytologic features of the malignant cells may allow the cytologist to classify the malignancy involved, such as sarcoma, carcinoma, or lymphoid neoplasia.

REFERENCES

1. Saint Girons MC: Morphology of the circulating blood cell. In Gans C, Parsons TC, editors: *Biology of the reptilia*, vol 3, New York, 1970, Academic Press.
2. Sypik J, Borysenko M: Reptiles. In Rowley AF, Ratcliffe NA, editors: *Vertebrate blood cells*, Cambridge, 1988, Cambridge University Press.
3. Duguy R: Numbers of blood cells and their variations. In Gans C, Parsons TC, editors: *Biology of the reptilia*, vol 3, New York, 1970, Academic Press.
4. Frye FL: Hematology as applied to clinical reptile medicine. In Frye FL: *Biomedical and surgical aspects of captive reptile husbandry*, ed 2, vol 1, Malabar, Fla, 1991, Krieger Publishing.
5. Mussachia XJ, Sievers ML: Effects of induced cold torpor on blood of *Chrysemys picta*, *Am J Physiol* 187:99-102, 1956.
6. Wojtaszek JS: Haematology of the grass snake *Natrix natrix natrix* L, *Comp Biochem Physiol A* 100:805-812, 1991.
7. Harr KE, Alleman AR, Dennis PM, et al: Morphologic and cytochemical characteristics of blood cells and hematologic and plasma biochemical reference ranges in Green Iguanas, *JAVMA* 218:915-921, 2001.
8. Ruiz G, Rosenmann M, Nunez H: Blood values in South American lizards from high and low altitudes, *Comp Biochem Physiol* 106A:713-718, 1993.
9. Pough FH: Blood oxygen transport and delivery in reptiles, *Am Zool* 20:173-185, 1980.
10. Dessauer HC: Blood chemistry of reptiles: physiological and evolutionary aspects. In: Gans C, Parsons TS, editors: *Biology of the reptilia*, vol 3, New York, 1970, Academic Press.
11. Frische S, Bruno S, Fago A, Weber RE, Mozzarelli A: Oxygen binding by single red blood cells from the red-eared turtle *Trachemys scripta*, *J Appl Physiol* 90:1679-1684, 2001.
12. Altland PD, Parker M: Effects of hypoxia upon the box turtle, *Am J Physiol* 180:421-427, 1955.
13. Sheeler P, Barber AA: Reticulocytosis and iron incorporation in the rabbit and turtle: a comparative study, *Comp Biochem Physiol* 16:63-76, 1965.
14. Alleman AR, Jacobson ER, Raskin RE: Morphologic and cytochemical characteristics of blood cells from the desert tortoise *(Gopherus agassizii)*, *Am J Vet Res* 53:1645-1651, 1992.
15. Marks SK, Citino SB: Hematology and serum chemistry of the Radiated tortoise *(Testudo radiata)*, *J Zoo Wildl Med* 21: 342-344, 1990.
16. Wallach JD, Boever WJ: *Diseases of exotic animals, medical and surgical management*, Philadelphia, 1983, WB Saunders.
17. Altland PD, Thompson EC: Some factors affecting blood formation in turtles, *Proc Soc Exp Biol Med* 99:456-459, 1958.
18. Hawkey CM, Dennett TB: Normal and abnormal red cells, granulocytes, lymphocytes, monocytes, and azurophils. In Hawkey CM, Dennett TB, editors: *Color atlas of comparative veterinary hematology*, Ames, Iowa, 1989, Iowa State University Press.
19. Verma GK, Banerjee V: Intergeneric haematological studies in three selected reptiles: erythrocytes, *Indian J Anim Res* 16: 49-53, 1982.
20. Desser SS: Morphological, cytochemical, and biochemical observations on the blood of the tuatara, *Sphenodon punctatus*, *N Z J Zool* 5:503-508, 1978.

21. Desser SS: Haematological observations on a hibernating tuatara, Sphenodon punctatus, N Z J Zool 6:77-78, 1979.
22. Alleman AR, Jacobson ER, Raskin RE: Morphological, cytochemical staining, and ultrastructural characteristics of blood cells from eastern diamondback rattlesnakes (Crotalus adamaneus), Am J Vet Res 60:507-514, 1999.
23. Work TM, Raskin RE, Balazs GH, et al: Morphological and cytochemical characteristics of blood cells from Hawaiian green turtles, Am J Vet Res 59:1252-1257, 1998.
24. Dotson TK, Ramsay EC, Bounous DI: A color atlas of the blood cells of the yellow rat snake, Comp Contin Edu Pract Vet 17:1013-1016, 1995.
25. Montali RK: Comparative pathology of inflammation in higher vertebrates (reptiles, birds, and mammals), J Comp Path 99:1-26, 1988.
26. Campbell, TW: Clinical pathology. In Mader DR, editor: Reptile medicine and surgery, Philadelphia, 1996, WB Saunders.
27. Mateo MR, Roberts ED, Enright FM: Morphological, cytochemical, and functional studies of peripheral blood cells in young healthy American alligators (Alligator mississippiensis), Am J Vet Res 45:1046-1053, 1984.
28. Caxton-Martins AE, Nganwuchu AM: A cytochemical study of the blood of the rainbow lizard (Agama agama), J Anat 125:477-480, 1978.
29. Taylor K, Kaplan HM: Light microscopy of the blood cells of Pseudemyd turtles, Herpetologica 17:186-192, 1961.
30. Wood FE, Ebanks GK: Blood cytology and hematology of the green sea turtle, Chelonia mydas, Herpetologica 40:331-336, 1984.
31. Jacobson ER, Gaskin JM, Brown MB, et al: Chronic upper respiratory tract disease of free-ranging desert tortoises, Xerobates agassizii, J Wild Dis 27:296-316, 1990.
32. Wright KM, Skeba S: Hematology and plasma chemistries of captive prehensile-tailed skinks (Corucia zebrata), J Zoo Wildl Med 23:429-432, 1992.
33. Mead KF, Borysenko M: Surface immunoglobulins on granular and agranular leukocytes in the thymus and spleen of the snapping turtle, Chelydra serpentina, Dev Comp Immunol 8:109-120, 1984.
34. Mead KF, Borysenko M, Findlay SR: Naturally abundant basophils in the snapping turtle, Chelydra serpentina, possess cytophilic surface antibodies with reaginic function, J Immunol 130:384-340, 1983.
35. Sypek JP, Borysenko M, Findlay SR: Anti-immunoglobulin induced histamine release from naturally abundant basophils in the snapping turtle, Chelydra serpentina, Dev Comp Immunol 8:358-366, 1984.
36. Wright RK, Cooper EL: Temperature effects on ectothermic immune responses, Dev Comp Immunol 5, Suppl 1:117-122, 1981.
37. Hussein MF, et al: Effect of seasonal variation on the immune system of the lizard, Scinus scinus, J Exp Zool 209:91-96, 1979.
38. Hussein MF, et al: Lymphoid tissue of the snake, Spalerosophis diadema, in the different seasons, Dev Comp Immunol 3:77-88, 1979.
39. Hussein MF, et al: Differential effect of seasonal variation on lymphoid tissue of the lizard, Chalecides ocellatus, Dev Comp Immunol 2:297-310, 1978.
40. Mansour MH, el Ridi R, Badir N: Surface markers of lymphocytes in the snake, Spalerosophis diadema. L. Investigation of lymphocyte surface markers, Immunology 40:605-611, 1980.
41. Munoz FJ, Galvan A, Lerma M, De la Fuente M: Seasonal changes in peripheral blood leukocyte functions of the turtle Mauremys caspica and their relationship with corticosterone, 17-beta-estradiol and testosterone serum levels, J Vet Immunol Immunopathol 77:27-42, 2000.
42. Saad AH, el Ridi R, el Deeb S, et al: Effect of hydrocortisone on immune system of the lizard, Chalcides ocellatus. III. Effect on cellular and humoral immune responses, J Dev Comp Immunol 10:235-245, 2000.
43. Taylor KW, Kaplan HM, Hirano T: Electron microscope study of turtle blood cells, Cytologia 28:248-256, 1963.
44. Otis VS: Hemocytological and serum chemistry parameters of the African puff adder, Bitis arietans, Herpetologica 29:110-116, 1973.
45. Goldberg SR, Holshuh HJ: A case of leukemia in the desert spiny lizard (sceloporus magister), J Wildl Dis 27:521-525, 1991.
46. Langenberg JA, et al: Hematopoietic and lymphoreticular tumors in zoo animals, Lab Invest 48:48A, 1983.
47. Frey FL, Carney J: Acute lymphocytic leukemia in a boa constrictor, JAVMA 163:653-654, 1973.
48. Frey FL, Carney J: Myeloproliferative disease in a turtle, JAVMA 161:595-599, 1972.
49. Schultze AE, Mason GL, Clyde VL: Lymphosarcoma with leukemic blood profile in a Savannah monitor lizard (Varanus exanthematicus), J Zoo Wildl Med 30:158-164, 1999.
50. Goldberg SR, Holshuh HJ: A case of leukemia in the desert spiny lizard (Sceloporus magister), J Wildl Dis 27:521-525, 1991.
51. Lawrence K: Seasonal variation in blood biochemistry of long term captive Mediterranean tortoises (Testudo graeca and T. hermanni), Res Vet Sci 42:379, 1987.
52. Samour JH, Hawkey CM, Pulger, et al: Clinical and pathologic findings related to malnutrition and husbandry in captive giant tortoises (Geochelone spp.), Vet Rec 118:299, 1986.
53. Rosskopf WJ: Normal hemogram and blood chemistry values for California desert tortoises, VM SAC 77:85, 1982.
54. Chiodini RJ, Sunberg JP: Blood chemical values of the common boa constrictor, Am J Vet Res 43:1701, 1982.
55. Taylor RW Jr, Jacobson ER: Hematology and serum chemistry of the gopher tortoise, Gopherus polyphemus, Comp Biochem Physiol 72A:425, 1982.
56. Dessauer HC: Blood chemistry of reptiles. In Gans C, Parsons TS, editors: Biology of the reptilia, vol 3, New York, 1970, Academic Press.
57. Lawrence K: Seasonal variation in blood biochemistry of long term captive Mediterranean tortoises (Testudo graeca and T. hermanni), Res Vet Sci 43:379, 1987.
58. Dawson WR: Physiological responses to temperature in the lizard Eumeces obsoletus, Physiol Zool 33:87, 1960.
59. Samour JH, Hawkey CM, Pugsley S, Ball D: Clinical and pathologic findings related to malnutrition and husbandry in captive giant tortoises (Geochelone spp.), Vet Rec 118:299, 1986.
60. Mader DR, Horvath CC, Paul-Murphy J: The packed cell volume and serum chemistry of the gopher snake (Pituophis melanoleucus catenifer), J Zoo Anim Med 16:139, 1985.
61. Gottdenker NL, Jacobson ER: Effect of venipuncture sites on hematologic and clinical biochemical values in desert tortoises (Gopherus agassizii), Am J Res 56:19-21, 1995.
62. Crawshaw GJ: Comparison of plasma biochemical values in blood and blood-lymph mixtures from Red-eared slider, Trachemys scripta elegans, Bull Assoc Rept Amphib Vet 6:7-9, 1996.
63. Holz P, Holz RM: Evaluation of ketamine, ketamine/xylazine, and ketamine/medazolam anesthesia in red-eared sliders (Trachemys scripta elegans), J Zoo Wildl Med 25:531-537, 1994.
64. Jacobson ER: Blood collection techniques in reptiles: laboratory investigations. In Fowler ME, editor: Zoo and wild animal medicine: current therapy 3, Philadelphia, 1993, WB Saunders.
65. Austin CC, Jessing KW: Green-blood pigmentation in lizards, Comp Biochem Physiol 109A:619-626, 1994.
66. Davies PMC: Anatomy and physiology. In Cooper JE, Jackson OF, editors: Diseases of the reptilia, vol I, San Diego, 1981, Academic Press.
67. Frye FL: Biomedical and surgical aspects of captive reptile husbandry, ed 2, vol 1, Melbourne, Fla, 1991, Krieger Publishing.

68. Ramsay EC, Dotson TK: Tissue and serum enzyme activities in the yellow rat snake *(Elaphe obsoleta quadrivitatta)*, *Am J Vet Res* 56:423-428, 1995.
69. Boyd JW: Serum enzymes in the diagnosis of diseases in man and animals, *J Comp Pathol* 98:381-404, 1988.
70. Braysher ML: The excretion of hyperosmotic urine and other aspects of the electrolyte balance of the lizard *Amphibolurus maculosus*, *J Comp Biochem Physiol* A 54:341-345, 1976.
71. Uva B, Vallarino M: Reinin-angiotensin system and osmoregulation in the terrestrial chelonian *Testudo hermanni* Gmelin, *J Comp Biochem Physiol* A 71:449-451, 1982.
72. Stein G: Hematologic and blood chemistry values in reptiles. In Mader DR, editor: *Reptile medicine and surgery*, Philadelphia, 1996, WB Saunders.
73. Coulson RA, Henandez T: Reptiles as research models for comparative biochemistry and endocrinology, *JAVMA* 159:1672-1677, 1971.
74. Dubewar D: Effect of hypocalcemic and hypercalcemic substances on the parathyroid histology of the lizard, *Uromastix hardwickii* (Gray), *J Z Mikrosk Anat Forsch* 93:315-320, 1979.
75. Dennis PM, Bennett RA, Harr KE, Lock BA: Plasma concentration of ionized calcium in healthy iguanas, *J Am Vet Med Assoc* 219(3):326-328, 2001; Erratum in *J Am Vet Med Assoc* 219(8):1093, 2001.
76. Boyer TH: Metabolic bone disease. In Mader DR, editor: *Reptile medicine and surgery*, Philadelphia, 1996, WB Saunders.
77. Donoghue S, Langenberg J: Nutrition. In Mader DR, editor: *Reptile medicine and surgery*, Philadelphia, 1996, WB Saunders.
78. Frye FL, Centofanti BV: Successful treatment of iatrogenic (diet-related) hypervitaminosis D and hypercalcemia in an iguana *(Iguana iguana)*, *Proceedings of the Fourth International Colloquium on the Pathology and Therapeutics of Reptiles and Amphibians*, 1991, Bad Nauheim, Germany.
79. Drew ML: Hypercalcemia and hyperphosphatemia in indigo snakes *(Drymarchon corais)* and serum biochemical reference values, *J Zoo Wildl Med* 25:48-52, 1994.
80. Bissell DM: Heme catabolism and bilirubin formation. In Ostrow JD, editor: *Bile pigments and jaundice: molecular, metabolic, and medical aspects*, New York, 1986, Marcel Dekker.
81. Coulson RA, Hernandez T: *Biochemistry of the alligator*, Baton Rouge, 1964, Louisiana State University Press.
82. Kumar S, Khanna SS: Response of the blood glucose and the pancreatic islets of the lizard, *Uromastix hardwicki* (Gray), to exogenous insulin, *J Z Mikrosk Anat Forsch* 91:131-143, 1977.
83. Hulbert AJ, Williams CA: Thyroid function in a lizard, tortoise, and a crocodile, compared with mammals, *J Comp Biochem Physiol* A 90:41-48, 1988.
84. Mateo MR, Roberts ED, Enright FM: Inflammation induced by subcutaneous turpentine in young American alligators *(Alligator mississippiensis)*, *Am J Vet Res* 45:1870, 1984.
85. Ryan ME, Magno G: Acute inflammation, *Am J Pathol* 86:185, 1977.
86. Glassman AB, Bennett CE: Responses of the alligator to infection and thermal stress. In Thorp JH, Gibbons JW, editors: *DOE symposium series, energy and environmental stress in aquatic systems*, Springfield, Va, 1978, National Technical Information Service.

29
DIAGNOSTIC IMAGING
SAM SILVERMAN

This chapter describes techniques for production of radiographs of reptiles, illustrates the normal reptile radiographic anatomy, proposes guidelines for the efficacy of radiographic examination, discusses the principles of radiographic interpretation, and reviews the indications and interpretation of alternative imaging methods, including ultrasound, computed tomography (CT), nuclear medicine, and magnetic resonance imaging (MRI).

Diagnostic imaging, although generally underused in reptile medicine, can contribute significantly to the medical and surgical management of reptiles. Factors that lead to this underutilization include: the relatively small amount of information published regarding imaging techniques and interpretation, a paucity of veterinary radiologists skilled in the interpretation of reptile radiographs, inherent poor radiographic tissue contrast of these species, and the lack of clear guidelines for normal and abnormal radiographic parameters of these species. Fortunately, these conditions are improving: the volume of published information on imaging of reptiles is increasing, and the alternative modalities are providing information not attainable from radiographic studies. Newer film screen systems are capable of producing high detail images at relatively low exposure settings.

Radiographs of reptiles are often characterized by poor image contrast (Figure 29-1). This is caused by the close anatomic proximity of internal organs, a paucity of internal fat, the lack of a clearly demarcated thorax and abdomen, and the image degradation that results from the superimposed exoskeleton or cutaneous scales. Radiology is, nevertheless, an important diagnostic method for evaluation of skeletal and soft tissue structures of reptiles. Because of anatomic and physiologic characteristics of reptiles, the accepted principles used to interpret mammalian (human and domestic animal) radiographs must be modified in interpretation of radiographs of reptiles. A typical example of this is the pattern approach to pulmonary radiographs. The classic alveolar, pleural, and bronchial patterns used in mammalian radiographic interpretation are not present in reptile radiographs, and vascular structures are often indistinct.

Important internal and external anatomic variations between mammals, lizards, snakes, and chelonians are also present. These variations often dictate how the radiographic examination is performed, which radiographic projection provides optimal information, and how the study is interpreted. An example of this is the respiratory tract in chelonians and snakes. The chelonian lung contains muscular bands of tissue, whereas the snake lung is a thin-walled sac-like structure. The lungs are best evaluated in the craniocaudal projection in chelonians and on the lateral projection in snakes. Both of these studies use a horizontally directed radiograph beam.

Even though respiratory movements are less prominent in reptiles than in mammals or birds, the radiographic techniques necessary to produce optimal image detail and contrast use short exposure times and low kilovolt peak (40 to 60 kilovolt peak). Radiographic generators should, therefore, be capable of producing at least 300 milliamperes and exposure times of $1/60$ (0.017) second or shorter with a kilovolt peak range of 45 to 100 kilovolt peak, adjustable in 2 kilovolt peak increments. Diagnostic radiology tubes have two focal spots from which the electrons used to produce the radiographs originate. The smaller focal spot produces a higher quality electron beam but has a lower capacity than the large focal spot. A focal spot size of less than 0.3 mm is optimal for the smaller focal spot. High detail magnification studies require a focal spot sized less than 0.2 mm. Whenever possible, the smaller focal spot should be selected if its use does not result in long exposure times. The exposure time should be less than $1/60$ second if patient motion is present; it can be appreciably longer if motion is not present.

The tube stand and design of the radiology area are important. Because horizontal radiograph beam projections are commonly used, the radiograph tube stand must have the capability to allow 90-degree rotation of the radiograph tube

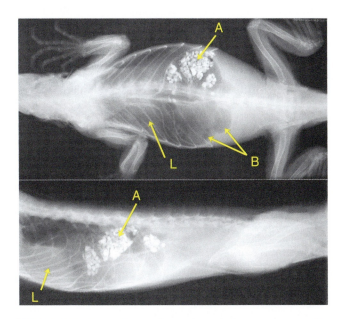

FIGURE 29-1 Green Iguana (*Iguana iguana*). Poor tissue contrast is present. The radiopaque gravel fragments (*A*) are in the stomach, and a moderate amount of intestinal gas (*B*) is seen, but serosal detail is poor. This is a normal finding. The liver (*L*) is visualized, but its borders are indistinct.

471

so that the radiograph beam can be directed parallel to the table top. The horizontal radiograph beam projections require a cassette stand or other device to stabilize the radiograph cassette in the vertical position. Wall-mounted and table-mounted cassette holders are available. The cassette can be supported in the vertical position with tape and rectangular objects such as cardboard boxes if a cassette holder is not available. Sufficient distance also should exist between the radiograph tube and the end of the radiology table or an adjacent wall to make radiographic exposures with a focal film distance of 30 to 40 inches.

High detail film screen systems are recommended. Various film screen combinations are available that result in a 100 to 200 speed system.[1] Dental film can be used for high detail images of selected small areas such as the skull or extremities, but dental film should be used to supplement the standard diagnostic film, not replace it. Although dental film produces high detail high contrast images of bone, soft tissue contrast and resolution may be less than with screen film. Mammography film can also be used for smaller patients; it is slower than screen film and, therefore, requires higher radiograph exposure factors, which may entail long exposure time, but it does produce radiographs with excellent soft tissue detail and is available in larger size than dental film.

RADIOLOGY

Patient Restraint, Positioning, and Exposure Factors: General Comments

The recommended radiographic projections for evaluation of the major organ systems are listed in Table 29-1.

Radiographic studies ideally should not be performed in close proximity to feeding. Distention of the digestive tract often compromises pulmonary inflation, and the radiopacity of the ingesta may obscure detail of superimposed structures.

In positioning of lizards for horizontal radiograph beam studies, the body wall being in direct contact with the radiograph cassette is often not possible because of the laterally protruding legs. The laterally protruding legs may produce a region of intense radiopacity (Figure 29-2). Although the carapace edge of chelonians can be placed against the cassette, the rounded body results in most internal structures being a considerable distance from the cassette. This increased object-film distance detracts from radiographic detail, and right and left lateral studies may be helpful. Use of the small focal spot setting to enhance detail is also advantageous if it does not necessitate a long exposure time. The phase of the respiratory cycle at which the radiographic exposure is made is critical. It should coincide with the peak of inspiration. If an endotracheal tube is in place, the lungs should be inflated with positive pressure of 10 to 15 centimeters of water for radiography (Figure 29-3).

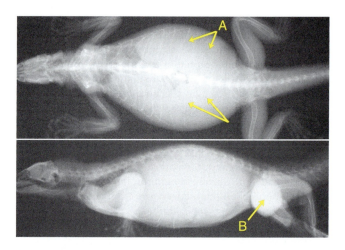

FIGURE 29-2 Gravid Green Iguana (*Iguana iguana*). The round ill-defined soft tissue opacities in the central abdomen are ova (*A*). The intense radiopacity superimposed on the pelvic region is the summated opacity caused by the laterally protruding legs (*B*).

Table 29-1	Recommended Radiographic Exposures for Reptiles		
	Dorso-ventral*	Cranio-caudal†	Lateral†
Chelonians			
Respiratory tract		♦	♦
Digestive tract	♦		
Genitourinary systems	♦		
Carapace and plastron	♦	♦	♦
Skeleton	♦		
Snakes			
Respiratory tract			♦
Digestive tract	♦		♦
Genitourinary systems	♦		♦
Skeleton	♦		♦
Lizards			
Respiratory tract			♦
Digestive tract	♦		♦
Genitourinary systems	♦		♦
Spine	♦		♦
Extremities	♦		

*Vertical radiograph beam.
†Horizontal radiograph beam.

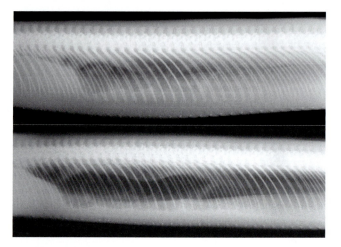

FIGURE 29-3 Boa Constrictor (*Boa constrictor*). The radiograph (horizontal radiograph beam, lateral view) was made with the patient during expiration (*top*) and at peak inspiration (*bottom*). The lungs are more lucent and larger on the inspiratory radiograph. The cardiac silhouette on the *left* of the images serves as a point of reference.

Chelonians

Chelonians are relatively easy to restrain and position for radiographic examinations. If possible, the head and extremities should not be retracted inside the carapace. The exoskeleton and internal anatomy necessitate horizontal radiographic beam lateral and cranial caudal projections for some studies. The selection of patient position (i.e., prone, erect, or lateral recumbent) and direction of the radiograph beam (i.e., horizontal or vertical) is determined by the organ system of primary interest, the pathology present, the volume of coelomic fluid, the degree of digestive tract distention, and the contents of the female reproductive tract. Determination of the optimal radiographic projection and radiograph beam orientation image detail is made with minimizing superimposition of other organs or fluid on the area of interest. For example, if the patient is positioned in sternal recumbency for a horizontal radiograph beam study, the coelomic contents gravitate ventrally away from the dorsally located lungs. For horizontal radiograph studies, the patient is placed in a radiolucent container such as a cardboard box or acrylic tank to minimize movement and, if necessary, it can also be immobilized with tape (Figure 29-4).

Radiopacity and radiographic detail of coelomic contents are affected by the position of the extremities. If the head and neck or legs are retracted into the shell, the radiopacity of the internal organs is increased and image quality of the head, neck, and extremities is degraded. Radiographs should be made with legs and head extending out of the shell. For nonanesthetized studies, this is accomplished with placement of a piece of paper masking tape or bandage tape on the caudal aspect of the carapace and attachment of it to the table restraint device or cassette. The patient attempts to move in a forward direction against the resistance of the tape, and the extremities are, therefore, extended from the exoskeleton. An alternative technique is placement of a small radiolucent object under the patient so that the extremities cannot make full contact with the radiographic cassette. The patient usually attempts to extend its legs and skull. The disadvantage of this technique is that it does produce image unsharpness because of increased object-film distance. The thickness of the separating material should, therefore, be minimized. If the patient is anesthetized, the extremities can be manually extended from the shell.

Evaluation of lungs and the estimation of coelomic fluid volume are best performed with horizontal radiograph beam studies. These studies are made with the patient in the prone, erect, or lateral recumbent position; the craniocaudal prone view is usually preferred for lung evaluation. Erect studies with a horizontal radiograph beam are useful also for estimation of coelomic fluid volume (Figure 29-5). The position of the gas-fluid interface is affected by gravity and other coelomic contents, especially the digestive tract and urinary bladder.

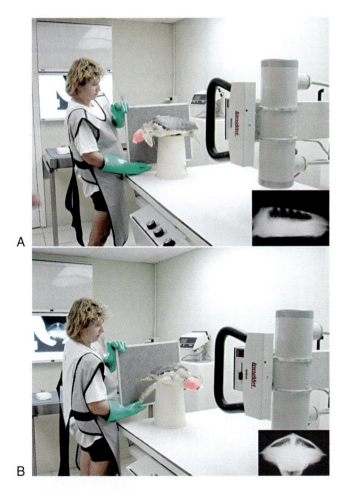

FIGURE 29-4 Chelonian restraint for horizontal radiograph beam, lateral view **(A)** and craniocaudal view **(B)**. For horizontal beam studies, the patient can be placed in a small cardboard box or elevated with placement on a bucket, with the feet kept off the table surface.

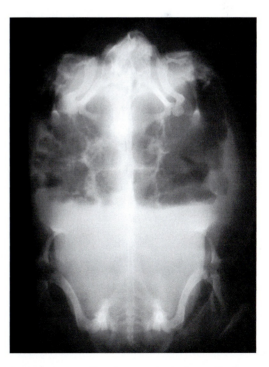

FIGURE 29-5 Cooter (*Pseudemys* sp.). Coelomic fluid is present from coelomitis and pneumonia. The ventrodorsal radiograph was made with the patient in the erect position with a horizontally directed radiograph beam. The straight gas-fluid interface level is helpful to evaluate the volume of coelomic fluid.

Digestive tract or urinary bladder distention affects the appearance and level of the coelomic fluid-gas interface.

The digestive tract, urinary bladder, and skeleton are best evaluated with dorsal ventral projections with a vertical radiograph beam (Figures 29-6 and 29-7). For vertical radiograph beam dorsoventral studies, chelonians can be placed directly on the radiograph cassette or radiograph table.

Evaluation of exoskeleton injuries often requires both horizontal and vertical radiograph beam studies. The patient can be rotated or obliqued in reference to the radiograph beam to optimize visualization of a specific portion of the exoskeleton (Figure 29-8).

Snakes

Radiographs are not recommended to be made with the patient in the coiled position because the internal organs are distorted and symmetry of the spine and ribs is compromised.

General anesthesia is strongly recommended for radiographic studies of snakes. The relaxed state of the patient makes positioning of the patient easier, and it eliminates spinal curvatures associated with normal muscular contractions.

If the patient is not anesthetized, it can be taped to a padded board or placed inside an acrylic tube. An increase in the kilovolt peak slightly to compensate for the acrylic's filtration of the radiograph beam may be necessary. The diameter and wall thickness of the tube should be as small as possible to minimize the object-film distance and to immobilize the patient most effectively. The acrylic tube should not have perforations or other openings over the area radiographed because they produce image artifacts.

Radiographs of larger snakes are often limited to the region of interest (e.g., the respiratory tract or externally abnormal body regions). Familiarity with internal anatomy is essential for localization of the radiograph beam. Localization of the cardiac apex motion on the ventral abdominal wall can be used as a reference point for the beginning of the lung tissue (see Figure 5-15).

If the radiograph beam is well collimated, several exposures can be made on a single piece of film (Figure 29-9). Radiopaque markers are taped to the skin to assist in correlation of radiographic findings with the location on the patient. Metallic number markers are ideal for this purpose. The numbers are attached to the skin in a sequential manner so that the contiguous segments can be identified on the multiple images.

Lizards

Lizards are the most challenging reptiles to position for radiography, and anesthesia is recommended because of their higher activity levels and the difficulty encountered in positioning their extremities. Restraint devices such as those designed for avian radiographic positioning can be used on nonanesthetized lizards. They are best suited for the dorsoventral projection. The guillotine component used to restrain the neck of the avian patient is placed immediately caudal to the pectoral limbs on the lizard. The restraints have limitations for the horizontal radiograph lateral view because the radiograph cassette cannot usually be positioned in apposition to the patient, which results in a lack of image clarity.

Anesthetized or sedated patients can be placed directly on the radiograph cassette for the dorsoventral view and

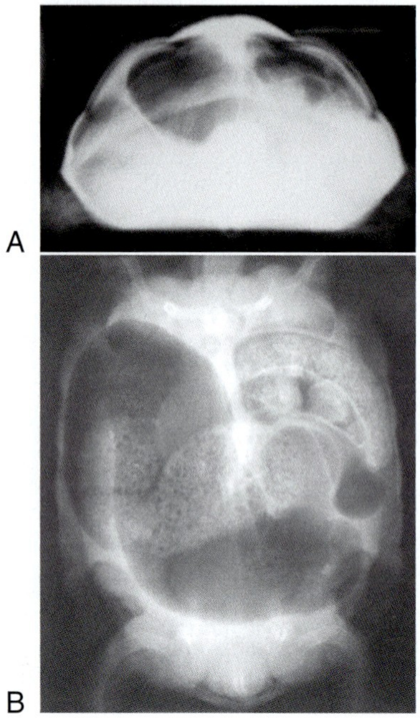

FIGURE 29-6 Desert Tortoise (*Gopherus agassizii*). Intestinal obstruction from corn cob impaction is present. The intestines are severely gas dilated and the foreign bodies are evident on the dorsoventral view *(bottom)*, but the diagnosis cannot be made on the craniocaudal view *(top)* because of superimposition of the internal structures.

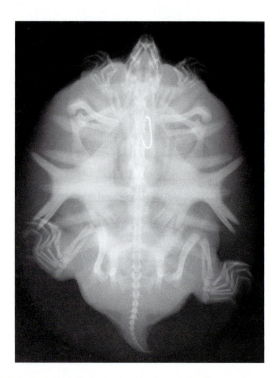

FIGURE 29-7 Softshell Turtle (*Apalone* sp.). The exoskeleton has a unique pattern in this species that is best visualized on the dorsal ventral projection. The fish hook foreign body is in the esophagus.

positioned with the assistance of paper tape or radiolucent bandage tape. The horizontal radiograph beam lateral projection is essential for evaluation of the spine and respiratory tract. The laterally protruding extremities make positioning the body wall in close apposition to the radiograph cassette difficult. Right and left lateral views are recommended for respiratory tract evaluation of larger patients. The pectoral limbs should be positioned as cranial as possible to minimize superimposition on the heart and lungs. The pelvic limbs are usually not a factor in respiratory tract studies, but they can degrade image quality of the caudal abdominal region. They should be extended caudally to minimize their superimposition on the caudal abdominal region.

Radiographic Interpretation

Skeletal System

Skeletal diseases are common indications for radiographic examination of reptiles (Figure 29-10). "Metabolic bone disease" is a term that is extensively used and misused. It includes skeletal diseases caused by nutritional, hormonal, and dietary causes (see Chapter 61). The radiographic manifestations of

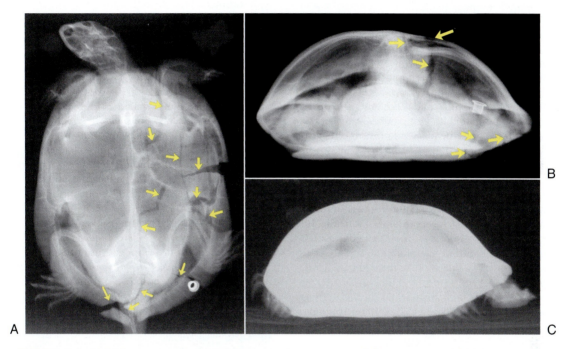

FIGURE 29-8 Multiple carapace fractures (*yellow arrows*) are present, and the true extent of the injuries requires multiple projections. **A,** Dorsal ventral; **B,** craniocaudal. The lateral view **(C)** is underexposed, and fractures are barely visualized.

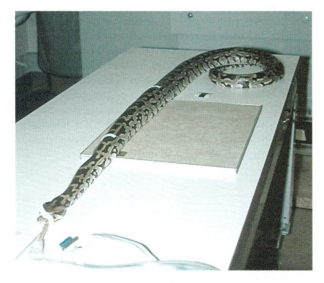

FIGURE 29-9 Several exposures can be made on the same radiographic plate with close columnation. The metallic markers are taped to the patient's skin to assist in correlation of radiographic findings with their location on the patient.

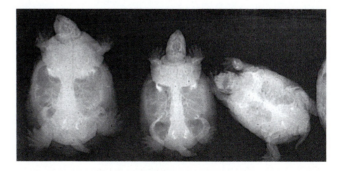

FIGURE 29-10 Metabolic bone disease of nutritional origin (NMBD). Severe decreased bone opacity and soft tissue swelling in the forelimbs and neck were present in these turtles maintained on a vitamin A–deficient and vitamin D–deficient diet. Pelvic and pectoral bone radiopacity is used to assess ossification.

many metabolic bone diseases caused by dietary deficiencies of calcium or vitamin D, insufficient exposure to ultraviolet light, calcium/phosphorus imbalances, and renal or parathyroid disease have similarities but are not identical (see Figure 61-18). The magnitude of the changes is dependent on the age of the patient, when the patient was affected, the duration of the disease, and its severity. Almost all of these diseases result in generalized decreased skeletal opacity, cortical thinning of long bones, pathologic fractures, and angular long bone deformities (Figure 29-11).

In mammals, a 30% decrease in bone calcium is necessary before changes in radiographic bone opacity are recognized. This has not been substantiated in reptiles, but it does emphasize the magnitude of disease necessary to produce radiographic changes. Evaluation of bone radiopacity is based on different criteria in chelonians, snakes, and lizards. In chelonians, the opacity of the pectoral girdle is used as a reference point. The bones of the pectoral girdle should be clearly visualized as radiopaque structures, and they should have crisp outlines, a small medullary canal, and a homogeneous cortical radiopacity. In snakes, the reference point is the radiopacity of ribs, and in lizards, the radiopacity and contrast of long bones and skull are used as references. The normal appendicular skeleton of lizards and chelonians has less distinct medullary borders than mammals, and the reptile trabecular pattern is also less prominent than in mammals. Larger reptiles also tend to have relatively thicker cortices and a higher cortex-to-medullary ratio than mammals. All of these can make diagnosis of early stages of metabolic bone disease difficult, especially if the clinician is unfamiliar with normal appearances of the patient's skeleton. As the decreased bone opacity becomes more severe, cortical thinning of the extremities becomes evident. Subtle changes in the trabecular pattern are sometimes difficult to appreciate without previous radiographs of the same patient or comparison normals of age-matched patients. Jaw and skull opacity are not accurate reference areas of bone opacity in lizards and chelonians because positioning the head in close apposition to the film is difficult. This increased air gap results in decreased detail and radiopacity.

Angular deformities of the long bones are more common in lizards than in chelonians. Progressive bone distortion of the extremities does occur, especially in lizards, in the form of bulbous enlargement of the long bones. The soft tissues adjacent to the mass may also enlarge. The femurs are most commonly affected. The angular deformities and bulbous enlargements are late occurrences in the disease process (Figure 29-12). Rib deformities are seen in lizards and snakes with various metabolic bone diseases.

Pathologic fractures occur latest in the course of the disease and are most common in the ribs of lizards and snakes. Folding fractures, as are common in birds with neonatal metabolic bone disease, are rare in reptiles.

The angular deformities and bulbous distortion of long bones persist throughout life (Figure 29-13). Differentiation of active metabolic bone disease from prior disease is difficult.

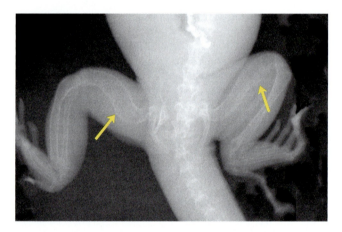

FIGURE 29-12 Green Iguana *(Iguana iguana)*. Severe chronic nutritional metabolic bone disease (NMBD) has resulted in cortical thinning, poor bone opacity, and bulbous distortion of the femur *(yellow arrows)*.

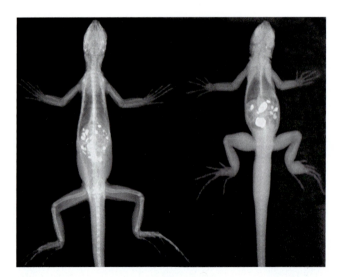

FIGURE 29-11 Green Iguana *(Iguana iguana)*. Severe nutritional metabolic bone disease (NMBD) causes the skeleton to have decreased radiopacity. The animal on the right has severe demineralization. The skeleton, especially the limbs and pelvis, is barely distinguishable from the surrounding soft tissues. Notice the lack of detail in the skull compared with the animal on the *left*.

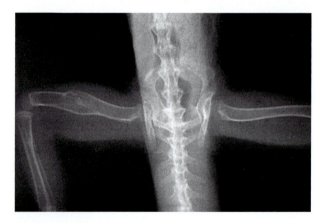

FIGURE 29-13 Green Iguana *(Iguana iguana)*. Healed femoral fracture. Cortical remodeling and mild overriding of the mid-shaft femoral fracture are present. A soft tissue callus is present around the fracture, and minimal periosteal reaction is seen. This is typical of fracture healing in reptiles, where fibrous callus is relatively more important than in mammals.

After correction of the inciting cause, an increase in bone opacity and cortical thickness occurs, but the bones often have a decreased trabecular pattern and indistinct cortical borders as compared with normal.

Soft tissue calcification, especially of vascular structures, is a common abnormal finding in lizards, is occasionally seen in chelonians, and is rare but does occur in snakes (Figure 29-14). Many of these patients have been chronically oversupplemented with vitamin D. These changes can also be associated with atherosclerotic disease of nondietary origin, especially in lizards. Abdominal, thoracic, and peripheral blood vessels become radiopaque. Occasionally, myocardial calcification is identified (see Figure 14-6).

Appendicular skeletal fractures are the most common type of skeletal injury seen in lizards. Digital luxations occur in lizards and, less commonly, in chelonians but are difficult to identify on physical examination. They are relatively rare because of the surrounding soft tissues, and they may often go undiagnosed on physical examination. Radiography is necessary for full diagnosis.

The radiographic characteristics of bone response to fractures in reptiles differ significantly from the changes in mammals. Initially, the fracture fragment edges have distinct margination, but the fracture fragments are not usually severely displaced, although overriding of fracture fragments does occur (Figure 29-15). This relative lack of fracture fragment movement is the result of the fibrous nature of the surrounding tissues. Clinical fracture stability often occurs far earlier than radiographic healing, and radiographic confirmation of complete bony fracture healing in reptiles may not be evident for more than 6 months. Initial radiographs intended to document fracture healing are recommended at 12 to 16 weeks after the injury if no clinical complications occur and healing is thought to be occurring normally. These radiographs are useful in documenting apposition and alignment of the fracture fragments and in ruling out osteolytic disease, which indicates that infection is present. A second set of radiographs is made at 30 weeks. As the healing progresses, the fracture fragment edges become less distinct and often remodeling of the cortical bone occurs. Periosteal new bone formation is evident radiographically; however, it is less prominent than in mammals (Figure 29-16). Prolonged and sometimes lifelong visualization of the radiolucent fracture line is not uncommon because many of the appendicular fractures heal with a combination of a radiopaque callus and fibrous tissue.

Pseudoarthrosis formation, a sign of malunion or nonunion, with the typical "elephant foot" appearance, is not common in reptiles, even with fibrous union.

Rib fractures are common in snakes. Displaced rib fractures with no sign of radiopaque callus are common but are usually incidental findings. The edges of the fracture fragments may be slightly rounded but are often similar in appearance to a recent fracture. Distortion of the fracture end is a sign of chronicity. Distortion of the ribs can also be the result of osteomyelitis (see Figure 29-16).

In lizards, more active rib periosteal response to trauma tends to be seen than in snakes. Another pattern of healed fib fractures is the expansile variant where the fracture line is not visible but the diameter of the rib is increased, its cortex is widened and thinned, and the medullary portion of the rib is widened and slightly more radiolucent than normal.

The response of the vertebrae to insults can be exuberant in snakes and lizards, more so than in mammals. This is in contradiction to the poor response seen in the reptile extremities.

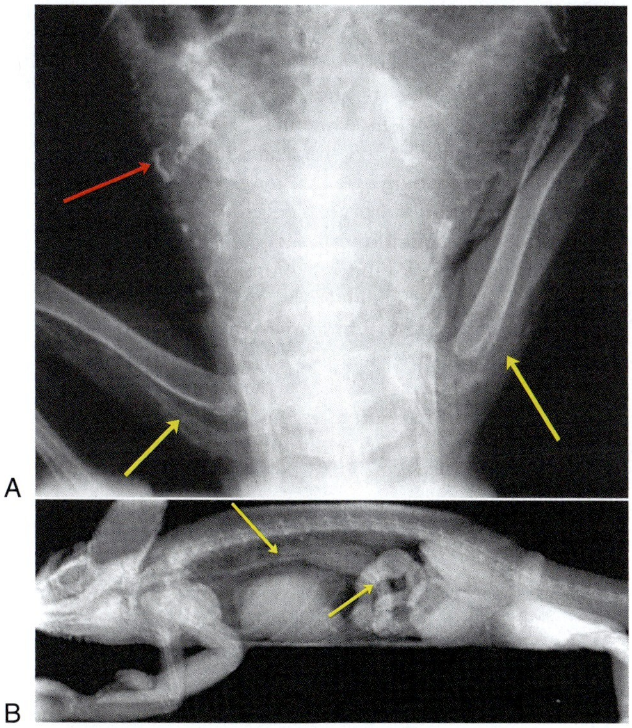

FIGURE 29-14 **A,** Severe mineralization of the major vessels in this Green Iguana *(Iguana iguana);* cause undetermined. The *yellow arrows* point to the femoral veins. The *red arrow* points to calcification in the normally radiolucent fat bodies. *(Photograph courtesy S. Barten.)* **B,** This Veiled Chameleon *(Chamaeleo calyptratus)* had chronic renal failure and dystrophic mineralization of the major vessels *(yellow arrows)*. *(Photograph courtesy D. Mader.)*

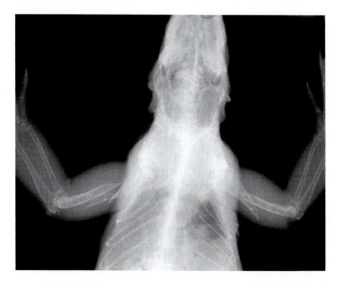

FIGURE 29-15 Green Iguana *(Iguana iguana)*. Acute bilateral humeral fractures occurred after trauma. Bone opacity is normal. The fractures have sharp margins and are comminuted. Moderate overriding of fracture fragments is present.

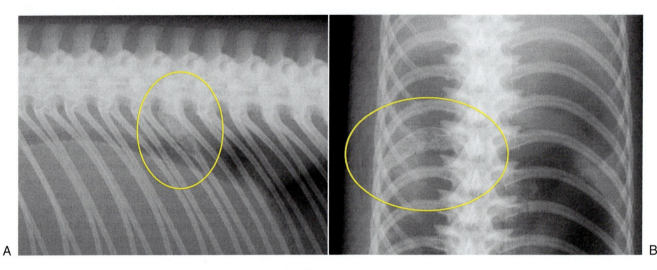

FIGURE 29-16 Close up of patient in Figure 29-3. The proximal portion of the rib is distorted and has an irregular radiopacity. The distortion in the rib may have been the location of a previous fracture or osteomyelitis. Adjacent ribs are normal.

Focal or diffuse regions of spinal deformity or rigidity may be identified clinically, but the radiographic changes are often more dramatic than the clinical signs. The vertebral hyperostosis in lizards may secondarily occlude blood vessels, and some cases of tail necrosis from vascular occlusion caused by the hyperostosis may occur.

The vertebral end plates, bodies, and disc spaces can be involved with lytic and productive changes (Figure 29-17). The etiologies of these changes are diverse. Bacteria have been cultured from some, but not all, cases; histologically, many cases have inflammatory changes. Suggestions have been made that this is similar to Paget's disease in people, but it is not usually associated with abnormal osteoclasts. The skull is not involved in reptiles, but it is frequently involved in people with Paget's disease. See Chapter 69 for a thorough discussion of spinal osteopathy in reptiles.

Computed tomography studies are useful for documentation of the morphology of the vertebral changes, especially spinal canal involvement. Nuclear medical studies are helpful in documentation of areas of new bone production and increased bone blood flow, and early in the course of the disease, they may be more sensitive than radiology.

Appendicular osteomyelitis and infectious arthritis are slowly progressive lytic processes in reptiles (Figure 29-18). The exuberant productive changes described in the vertebrae of lizards and snakes do not occur in the extremities. The secondary periosteal and cortical response to infection is much less prominent in reptiles than it is in mammals. A persistent lytic defect in the bone is often seen after resolution of osteomyelitis in reptiles. In mammals, this is strong evidence for active infection, sequestration, or neoplasia, but in reptiles, this can be a focus of inflammation or nonossified fibrous tissue without contained infection or sequestration. Soft tissue calcification can also be a chronic change as a result of infection (Figures 29-19 and 29-20).

Mandibular and maxillary osteomyelitis is a progressively lytic process. Periosteal new bone production can occur but is less common than in appendicular osteomyelitis. Expansile deformities of the mandible may occur, and teeth are frequently lost (Figure 29-21).

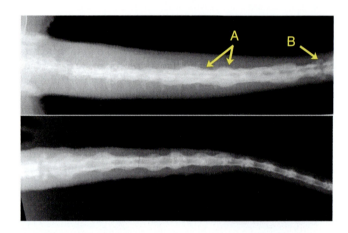

FIGURE 29-17 A 16-year-old Green Iguana (*Iguana iguana*). The tail is rigid and enlarged. Near complete fusion of multiple vertebrae with periosteal bone is present (*A*). Osteolysis can be identified at intervertebral spaces (*B*). Inflammation was identified on histopathology, but organisms were not identified.

Injuries to the exoskeleton of chelonians are common; radiography can be used to document the degree of displacement and soft tissue abnormalities associated with the injuries, especially pulmonary consolidation or hemorrhage adjacent to carapace injuries (see Figure 29-8). CT three-dimensional reconstruction studies are extremely helpful in documentation of the injuries. If CT is not available, appropriate oblique or angulated radiograph beam views highlighting the injury are recommended in addition to the standard dorsal ventral and lateral views.

Digestive System

The dorsal ventral view provides the best visualization of the digestive tract in lizards and chelonians, and the lateral view is usually superior in snakes; however, orthogonal projections are recommended in all cases. The anatomy and physiology of the reptilian and mammalian tracts have major differences. The reptile digestive tract is short compared with

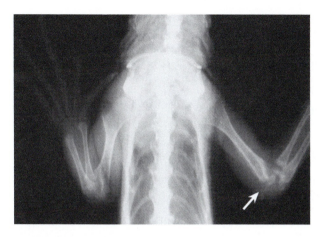

FIGURE 29-18 Green Iguana *(Iguana iguana)*. Septic arthritis. Soft tissue swelling is present around the left pectoral limb, and osteolysis is present in the distal humeral epiphysis, the proximal radius, and the proximal ulna *(arrow)*. Minimal secondary new bone production is present in the early and intermediate stages of osteomyelitis in reptiles. The periosteal and endosteal reactions in mammals are much more prominent than in reptiles.

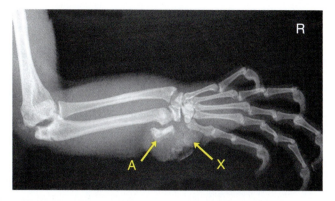

FIGURE 29-20 Same patient as in Figure 29-19. Soft tissue calcification *(X)* of the right carpus from chronic cellulitis, and osteomyelitis are present. The accessory carpal bone *(A)* is partially destroyed.

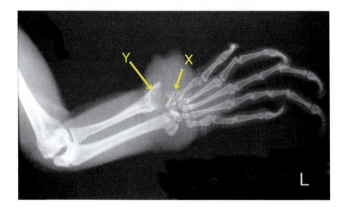

FIGURE 29-19 Green Iguana *(Iguana iguana)*. Chronic bilateral draining carpal wounds are present. The distal radius of the left limb has an expansile lytic region *(X)* with mild periosteal reaction *(Y)*.

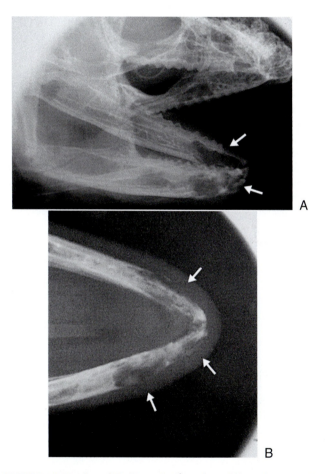

FIGURE 29-21 A and **B,** Parson's Chameleon *(Chamaeleo parsoni)*. High detail dental radiographs show osteolysis in the rostral portions of both mandibular rami without secondary new bone production. Although this is typical of osteomyelitis in reptiles, it is more indicative of neoplasia in mammals.

the mammalian digestive tract, but the transit time of ingesta is generally much longer. Intervals between feedings are much longer in snakes than in other reptiles and mammals.

The digestive tract of reptiles and the accessory digestive organs (i.e., liver and pancreas) are poorly visualized on survey radiographs. Very low inherent tissue contrast is seen because of the close apposition of internal organs and the paucity of internal fat. The stomach can sometimes be identified in the left mid portion of the chelonian coelom on survey radiographs, and the large intestinal contents often have a fibrous appearance. In snakes and lizards, the stomach can usually not be identified unless it is gas filled (usually from aerophagia) or radiopaque food was recently ingested. The appearance of the digestive tract is significantly affected by the time of previous feeding, the nature of the ingesta, and the species of the patient. In snakes, ingesta can often be identified as a bolus of material that produces a regional enlargement of the digestive tract. As the ingesta becomes more digested, the bolus becomes less distinct and is more diffusely distributed.

Relatively more gas is found in the digestive tract in lizards than in snakes or chelonians, but digestive tract gas is usually not prominent unless aerophagia is present. Chelonians tend to have a more granular appearance to their intestinal contents than do other reptiles. The intestinal serosal detail is usually indistinct in all reptiles.

Chelonians and lizards often normally have rocks, gravel, or sand in their digestive tract, but large volumes of these materials can result in constipation or obstruction (Figure 29-22). Intestinal obstruction is characterized by enlargement of the diameter of the digestive tract, but a prominent obstructive gas pattern is not always seen. The hallmark sign for focal intestinal obstruction is the accumulation of luminal contents in a dilated segment of intestines. Lizards frequently ingest foreign objects such as coins or other metallic items. The foreign bodies can remain in the stomach or obstruct the intestines. They can traverse the intestines but become permanently lodged in the cloaca and produce signs of intermittent obstruction (Figure 29-23).

Digestive tract radiographic contrast procedures are often necessary for documentation of intestinal obstruction, foreign bodies, and obstruction (Figure 29-24). These procedures are relatively simple to perform in snakes and lizards but can also be performed on chelonians. The normal appearance and transit times of the contrast media have been described in very few species. If the site of obstruction is the proximal portion of the digestive tract, an upper gastrointestinal study is performed, with 25% barium sulfate or a nonionic iodinated contrast medium. The contrast medium should be warmed to the approximate body temperature of the patient before administration. Barium sulfate appears to be well tolerated if it is extravasated from the digestive tract. Dose rates have not been determined for all species, but the volume of contrast medium administered should be similar to the volume used to tube feed the patient. The noniodinated agents can produce exquisite mucosal detail and do not cause constipation or obstipation. Omnipaque (Iohexal) 240 mg/mL (Nycomed Inc, Princeton, NJ) is the recommended iodinated contrast medium for this study. The agents do not persist in the digestive tract as long as barium sulfate does. Barium sulfate can become desiccated in the digestive tract and result in intestinal obstruction, especially if a large volume of contrast medium is used and remains in the digestive tract for a long time. This situation is not common but should be considered in patients with preexisting ileus or dehydration. If a large volume of contrast medium is present in the distal digestive tract after completion of the study, the contrast medium is recommended to be evacuated after completion of the study with insertion of a catheter into the colon through the cloaca and massaging of the caudal abdomen. In chelonians, evacuation of the digestive tract may be stimulated with placement of the patient in warm water. In snakes, it can be gently milked from the colon with external digital pressure.

Double contrast upper gastrointestinal radiographic contrast procedures can also be performed to document

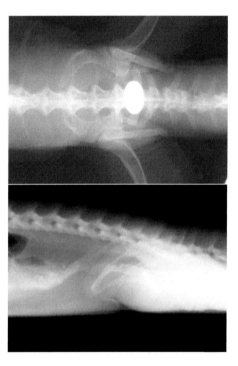

FIGURE 29-23 Green Iguana *(Iguana iguana)*. Intermittent signs of intestinal obstruction had been present for several months. A foreign body (penny) is present in the cloaca on the lateral projection *(bottom)*. It is seen on edge and is more obvious on the dorsal ventral projection *(top)*.

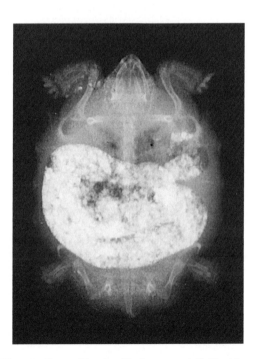

FIGURE 29-22 Desert Tortoise *(Gopherus agassizii)*. Sand impaction. Several immature Desert Tortoises housed on a sand substrate had severe sand impaction of the gastrointestinal tract develop. The impactions were relieved with enemas, and the tortoises were placed on gravel instead of sand.

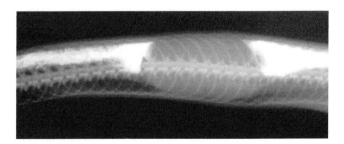

FIGURE 29-24 Gopher Snake *(Pituophis melanoleucas)*. A radiolucent foreign body partially obstructs the intestines. A meniscus effect is proximal and distal to the mass, which was an accumulation of plant material.

mucosal disease, foreign bodies, and strictures or partial obstruction, etc., in the esophagus, stomach, and intestines. They may entail sedation or anesthesia, but double contrast procedure uses a smaller volume of positive contrast medium than the single contrast procedure and allows for a more rapid evaluation of the digestive tract because the gas used propels the contrast positive medium rather than relying on peristalsis. Double contrast studies usually produce superior radiographic mucosal detail than do single contrast studies. A flexible catheter is passed into the stomach. The purpose of the double contrast study is to uniformly coat the digestive tract mucosal surface and produce normal or slightly exaggerated distention of the digestive tract.

The technique recommended for an antegrade double contrast digestive tract examination is as follows. A tube is passed into the stomach, and 100% barium sulfate or nonionic iodinated contrast can be used. Contrast medium is infused into the stomach at a volume estimated to be one third to one half of the gastric volume. Room air is then infused into the stomach in an amount equal to the normal gastric volume. Contrast medium equal to one fourth of the gastric volume is infused into the esophagus as the tube slowly is retracted. When the distal tip of the catheter is in the cranial esophagus, an equal volume of air is infused into the esophagus (one fourth the gastric volume) and the catheter is removed. Radiographs are then made.

If the intestines are the primary region to be evaluated, a retrograde study is performed. These procedures usually require anesthesia because the intestinal distention stimulates peristalsis. A flexible catheter, such as a pediatric nasogastric tube, is introduced into the cloaca and advanced into the distal colon. Contrast medium (barium sulfate or the nonionic iodinated agents) is administered until resistance is encountered. Radiographs can be taken to document the passage of contrast medium and to determine the volume of contrast medium necessary. A potential but infrequently encountered complication of the retrograde studies is accidental introduction of the contrast medium into the ureters and subsequently the kidneys. This could represent a problem with barium sulfate if ureteral or renal concretions develop, especially in dehydrated patients. The double contrast technique is useful in demonstrating distal colonic partial obstruction (Figure 29-25).

The mucosal pattern of the digestive tract varies with location and species and is beyond the scope of this chapter to fully describe. These changes in the esophagus of snake's prominent mucosal folds are common (Figure 29-26). The stomach has a subtle rugal pattern in all species.

Although double contrast radiographic studies are considered optimal for documentation of mucosal disease, ultrasound can be useful in the diagnosis of digestive tract disease, especially if mural thickness is present and the intestines are not filled with gas or fecal material, particularly rocks or sand. This is discussed more fully in the following ultrasound section.

Genitourary System

Urinary bladder calculi are seen most commonly in chelonians but do occur in lizards (Figures 29-27 and 29-28). In chelonians, the urinary bladder is expansive in volume and bilobed in shape. Therefore, the calculi can vary in position and may be located laterally. Typically, calculi are located more cranially than in mammals. The calculi occur with greater frequency in the left lobe of the bladder. They have an irregularly lamellated appearance and an irregularly rounded shape. Renal calcification is not commonly seen, but cloacal calculi are occasionally seen in lizards and chelonians. Cloacal calculi may be radiolucent and, therefore, not visible on survey radiographs. Direct evaluation of the cloaca, or a radiographic contrast study, or ultrasound is necessary for visualization. These methods can result in increased intestinal diameter because of partial intestinal obstruction; this may be visualized without contrast radiography.

After gentle irrigation and evacuation of the cloaca with warm saline solution, a radiographic double contrast cloacogram can be performed to identify masses, foreign bodies, strictures, and perforations. The nonionic iodinated contrast media are preferred. Contrast medium in a volume equal to 50% of the estimated cloacal volume is first infused, followed by infusion of room air in a volume equal to 100% to 200% of the estimated cloacal volume. Sometimes introduction of additional volumes of air between radiographic studies is necessary.

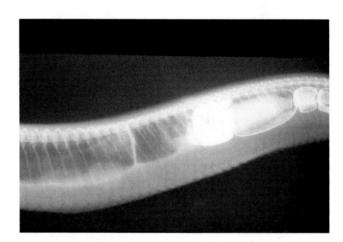

FIGURE 29-25 Emerald Tree Boa (*Corallus caninus*). Chronic abdominal distention was present. The retrograde double contrast study shows an angular constriction caused by an intestinal adenocarcinoma.

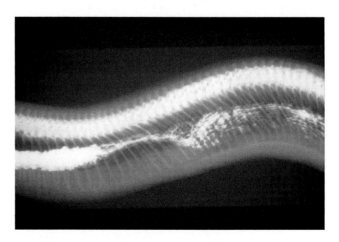

FIGURE 29-26 Red-tailed Boa (*Boa constrictor*). The esophagram shows normal prominent mucosal folds.

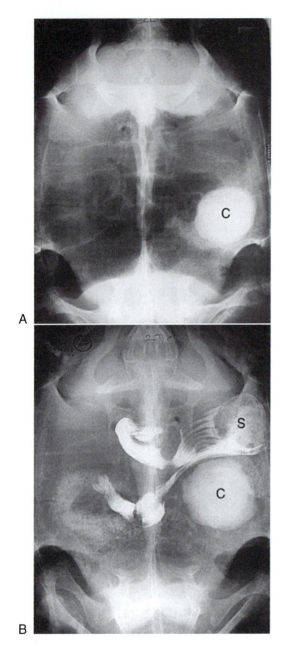

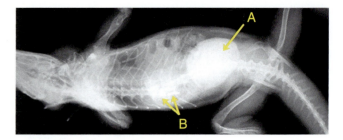

FIGURE 29-28 Green Iguana *(Iguana iguana)*. The urinary bladder calculus *(A)* is radiopaque but has a lamellar pattern. Intestinal foreign bodies (rocks) are also present *(B)*.

FIGURE 29-27 Desert Tortoise *(Gopherus agassizii)*. Urinary calculus. **A,** On day 1, a 5.8-cm-diameter radiopaque urinary bladder calculus is present in the left mid coelomic region. Urinary calculi in turtles and tortoises typically have a high radiopacity and a roughened lamellar architecture. Their borders are often irregular. **B,** Four years later, the calculus is slightly larger. Radiopaque contrast medium was administered to rule out the possibility of a gastrointestinal foreign body. *C*, Calculus; *S*, stomach.

Cloacal soft tissue masses may be difficult to fully evaluate with endoscopic imaging equipment; a double contrast cloacogram is recommended.

Ultrasound may be helpful in the identification of focal mass lesions, including polyp-like masses within the cloaca. The cloaca is irrigated with warm saline solution before the procedure, and the residual cloacal contents are completely flushed from it. The cloaca is then distended with saline solution, the catheter is removed, and the area is imaged with a high detail transducer, 7.5 mHz or higher frequency. The cloaca is scanned when it is fluid distended. Soft tissue equivalent standoff pads may enhance ultrasonographic detail.

Radiographically, pregnancy in lizards and snakes is diagnosed with the identification of rounded, soft tissue opacity structures in the caudal abdomen that are arranged in a linear overlapping pattern that resembles a clumped string of pearls. They are bilateral in location. The ova are well visualized radiographically and may have poorly mineralized calcified shells (Figure 29-29). As the eggs develop, they enlarge and fill the coelom, displacing the intestines cranially. In chelonians, the shells of the ova may be radiopaque (Figure 29-30).

Ultrasound is helpful in documentation of pregnancy and identification of the viability of pregnancy. In chelonians, the probe is placed just craniad to the pelvic limbs; in lizards and snakes, the ventral and lateral abdominal walls are used as the acoustic window. Ultrasound is also effective in documentation of free coelomic fluid or other complications.

The viability of external incubation of ova can be evaluated with ultrasound. Ultrasound coupling gel should not be used because it can affect the permeability of the shell. The egg is cupped in the palm of an assistant, and a water filled surgical glove can be placed on top of the shell to be used as an acoustic stand off. Fetal viability can be imaged through all except the most densely calcified shells. The normal egg has a homogeneous hypoechoic appearance with a central hyperechoic echogenicity.

Cardiopulmonary Systems

The heart may be visualized as a soft tissue opacity in the ventral portion of the body adjacent to the tracheal termination on survey radiographs of chelonians. The cardiac borders are not distinctly visualized, but the approximate size of the heart can be estimated. Evaluation of cardiac size, chamber volume, and contractility are best performed with ultrasound. The lungs are obscured by the coelomic contents on the dorsoventral radiographs but are well visualized on the horizontal radiograph beam studies.

The heart and lungs are not usually well visualized on dorsoventral (Figure 29-31) radiographs of lizards and snakes but are on the lateral view (see Figure 29-3). The location varies between species of lizards but is usually cranial in the thorax. The cardiac silhouette normally does not have discrete borders. If a discrete border is seen, it may indicate pericardial fluid or cardiomegaly is present. The horizontal radiograph beam lateral view is the preferred radiographic

Diagnostic Imaging 483

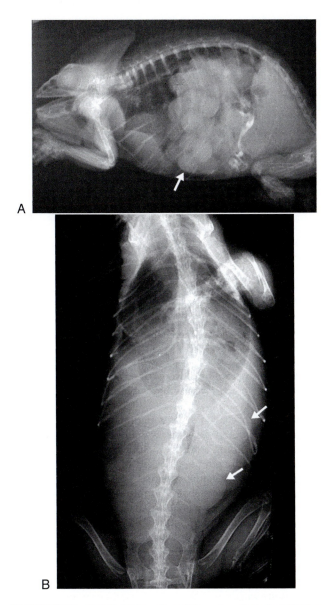

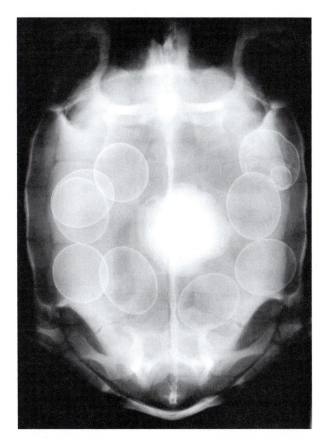

FIGURE 29-30 Desert Tortoise *(Gopherus agassizii)*. Multiple eggs with calcified shells are present, and a urinary bladder calculus is present in the mid abdomen.

FIGURE 29-29 A, Veiled Chameleon *(Chamaeleo calyptratus)*. **B,** Green Iguana *(Iguana iguana)*. Gravid ova in lizards have a soft tissue opacity and do not have radiographically calcified shells *(arrows)*. The ova are usually multiple and appear as overlapping concentric soft tissue opacities. They can displace or compress the viscera. The horizontal radiograph projections of the Veiled Chameleon show the large portion of the coelomic cavity that can be occupied by the ova. In turtles and tortoises, the eggs can have radiopaque shells.

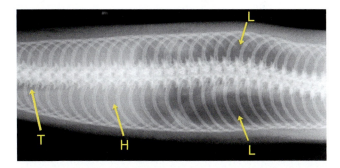

FIGURE 29-31 Red-tailed Boa *(Boa constrictor)*. The region of the lungs *(L)* can be visualized on the dorsal ventral projection, but vascular detail is indistinct. The trachea *(T)* and heart *(H)* are partially visualized.

projection of choice for evaluation of the heart and lungs in snakes. In snakes, the dorsoventral view with the vertical radiograph beam has limited value for respiratory tract evaluation, but it is helpful in evaluation of lizards with cardiomegaly. If severe cardiomegaly or pericardial fluid is present, it may be identified on the dorsal ventral projection.

Craniocaudal and lateral projections with a horizontal radiograph beam are recommended for pulmonary evaluation of chelonians (Figure 29-32). The expansibility of the respiratory tract is affected by the digestive tract and coelomic contents and the depth of respiration. Positive pressure ventilation does influence the radiographic appearance of the lungs, most prominently in snakes and lizards, less so in turtles. The volume of the lungs can be increased with positive pressure ventilation far in excess to what is present with spontaneous respiration in snakes. Also, a subsequent diffuse decrease in pulmonary radiopacity is seen on the positive pressure studies (see Figure 29-3). The effect of positioning devices on lung opacity and detail must be considered (Figure 29-33).

Because the structure of the reptilian lung differs greatly from the mammalian lung, the standard radiographic patterns (i.e., alveolar, interstitial, bronchial, and pleural) used to describe the radiographic appearance of the mammalian lung

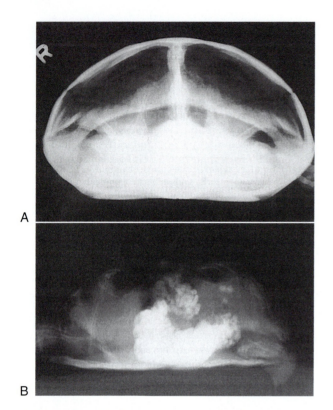

FIGURE 29-32 **A,** Turtle. Normal craniocaudal pulmonary examination. The craniocaudal view with a horizontally directed radiograph allows the viscera to fall ventrally, and the lungs are visualized without the superimposed viscera. The dorsal region occupied by the lungs should be radiolucent. **B,** Desert Tortoise *(Gopherus agassizii)*. Lateral view pulmonary examination. If the digestive tract is filled with contents, it may partially obscure the lung fields, even on a horizontal radiograph beam projection.

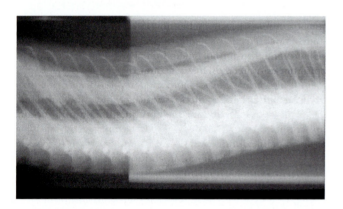

FIGURE 29-33 Acrylic positioning devices *(right side)* can increase radiopacity and decrease image detail.

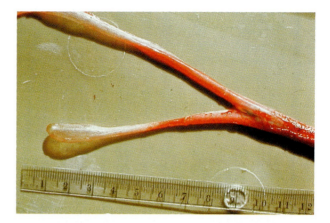

FIGURE 29-34 Snake lung. The left lung *(lower structure)* is variably reduced in size in most snakes.

are not applicable to reptiles. The lungs of snakes and most lizards (except for the New World Chameleons) have a relatively homogeneous radiopacity with more prominence to the pulmonary vasculature in the cranial portions of the lungs. Airway markings are indistinct to indistinguishable throughout. In chelonians, the lungs are composed of irregularly shaped areas of respiratory tissue and interspersed muscular bands. The lungs are closely adhered to the carapace and are not highly expansile. In snakes and most lizards (except for the New World Chameleons), the lungs are more sac-like. Most snakes have only a single functioning lung (the right), with the left side either absent or vestigial (Figure 29-34).

The radiographic manifestation of consolidative pulmonary disease (e.g., pneumonia) is increased pulmonary opacity. In snakes, this is usually a diffuse increase in pulmonary opacity; focal lesions are rarely identified. Focal ill-defined areas of pulmonary consolidation are most commonly identified in chelonians and occasionally in lizards.

The cranial caudal projection is usually most diagnostic for evaluation of pulmonary disease in chelonians. Laterality of lesions can be identified, and the symmetry of opacity and pulmonary markings are used to identify pathology (Figure 29-35). Head and neck position are important factors to consider: the head should be positioned on the mid line and be extended from the shell for optimal pulmonary detail.

In lizards and snakes, the lateral views are usually most diagnostic for respiratory tract evaluation; if the patient's lateral measurement exceeds 6 centimeters, right and left lateral views are recommended. Endotracheal intubation and positive pressure inflation of the lungs for radiography are highly recommended in lizards and snakes. The hyperinflation of the lungs results in decreased pulmonary radiopacity. This can be easily misinterpreted as a positive response to therapy.

Pulmonary parasitism can be documented in snakes with positive contrast bronchography if fiber optic instrumentation is not available. Tantalum powder is used as the contrast medium (Figure 29-36). It is aerosolized and infused into the lungs through an endotracheal catheter. The procedure requires general anesthesia.

Computed tomographic studies are the optimal diagnostic technique for respiratory tract evaluation of reptiles and are discussed subsequently (also see Chapter 86).

ANCILLARY DIAGNOSTIC TECHNIQUES

Computed Tomography

Advances in technology have vastly improved image quality and decreased imaging time for CT studies (Figures 29-37 and 29-38). In addition to rapid production of high-detail

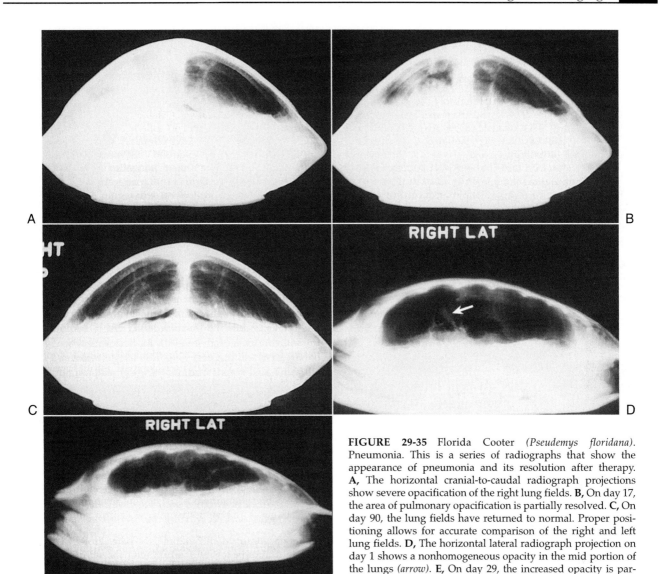

FIGURE 29-35 Florida Cooter *(Pseudemys floridana)*. Pneumonia. This is a series of radiographs that show the appearance of pneumonia and its resolution after therapy. **A,** The horizontal cranial-to-caudal radiograph projections show severe opacification of the right lung fields. **B,** On day 17, the area of pulmonary opacification is partially resolved. **C,** On day 90, the lung fields have returned to normal. Proper positioning allows for accurate comparison of the right and left lung fields. **D,** The horizontal lateral radiograph projection on day 1 shows a nonhomogeneous opacity in the mid portion of the lungs *(arrow)*. **E,** On day 29, the increased opacity is partially resolved.

images, new-generation CT units are also capable of creation of three-dimensional reconstructions of the images. This is especially helpful for evaluation of complex fractures and evaluation of the extent of osteomyelitis and neoplasia, especially in the skull. CT can also be used to quantify bone opacity and, therefore, calcium content. It is an excellent method to monitor patients with various metabolic bone diseases.

Computed tomographic studies are the most accurate imaging technique for evaluation of pulmonary disease in reptiles. The high speed scanners have made it much more practical to image these patients. CT detail is enhanced if respiratory motion can be frozen in complete inspiration with anesthesia and positive pressure ventilation during the study. This is the most important in lizards because of their more rapid respiratory rate.

The liver and digestive tract are in close proximity to each other and have similar tissue opacity. CT is, therefore, not the optimal modality for their evaluation; ultrasound and MRI are preferred.

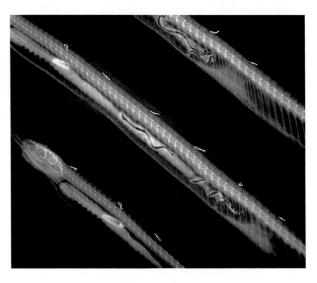

FIGURE 29-36 Ratsnake *(Elaphe* sp.). Pulmonary parasitism (pentastomids) are outlined with the tantalum powder infused through a tracheal catheter.

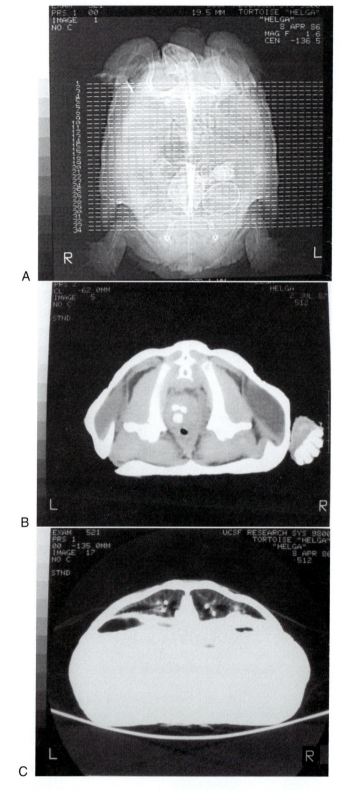

FIGURE 29-37 Desert Tortoise (*Gopherus agassizii*). The computed tomography settings can be manipulated to show soft tissue and skeletal structures. **A,** Scout study shows computed tomographic slice locations. **B,** Soft tissue window at the level of the pectoral girdle. **C,** Lung window.

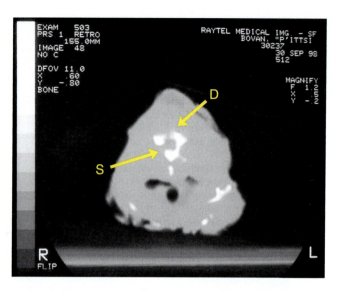

FIGURE 29-38 Sailfin Dragon (*Hydrosaurus* sp.). Vertebral osteomyelitis has partially destroyed the dorsal spinous process (*D*) and lateral portion of the spinal canal (*S*).

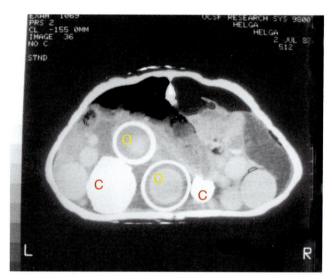

FIGURE 29-39 Desert Tortoise (*Gopherus agassizii*) magnetic resonance imaging. Ova (*O*) and a urinary bladder calculus (*C*) are identified.

See Chapter 86 for a review of normal CT and MRI anatomy of reptiles.

Magnetic Resonance

Magnetic resonance (MR) provides exquisite soft tissue detail, but it is technically limited by the long image acquisition times (Figure 29-39). Several minutes are necessary for each examination. Although information regarding its application to reptiles is minimal, potential areas of utilization include brain, renal, reproductive, and liver disease. If the patient can be immobilized either mechanically or chemically, MRI is an exquisite method of evaluation of the brain and coelomic organs for mass lesions, hemorrhage, inflammation, and congenital or traumatic disease.

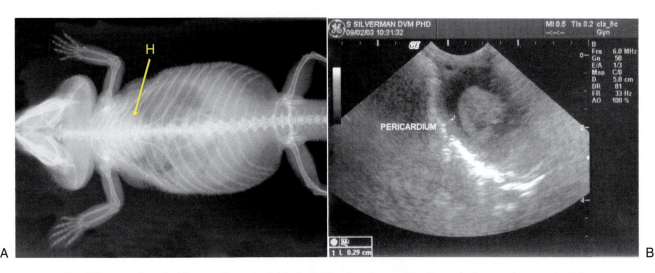

FIGURE 29-40 Bearded Dragon *(Pogona vitticeps)*. **A,** The dorsal ventral radiograph shows enlargement of the cardiac silhouette *(H)*. The ultrasound examination **(B)** showed pericardial fluid to be present. The fluid was aspirated (3 mL of cloudy yellow fluid) and was found to be inflammatory in nature, but infectious agents were not identified.

Before MR examinations are performed on any patient, scout radiographs should be performed to rule out the presence of ferrous metals because these can be dislodged under the influence of the MR unit's magnet and can result in injury to personnel and the patient.

Ultrasonography

Ultrasonography is extensively used in reptile diagnostics.

The examination techniques are not complex but do rely on the use of high resolution equipment. For almost all reptiles, except the larger chelonians, 7.5-mHz transducers with small footprints are recommended. Large chelonians are best imaged with 5-mHz or 3-mHz transducers with a small footprint. Linear array ultrasound transducers designed for human abdominal studies are usually not ideal for use on chelonians because the transducers are too large to fit in the cervical, axillary, or inguinal areas, but these transducers can be used on snakes and larger lizards.

Two methods are used for obtaining ultrasound images of reptiles. Acoustic coupling gel can be liberally applied to the skin before application of the transducer. Copious amounts of gel are necessary to minimize trapped air on the irregular skin and under the scales. Rarely is use of a soft tissue equivalent standoff pad necessary. The second method is water immersion of the patient. This method can be used on more docile or anesthetized patients. The patient is partially submerged in a warm water bath, and transducer-skin contact is not necessary. In chelonians, the transducer can be placed against the skin in the axillary, cervical, and inguinal regions after a generous application of acoustic coupling gel. The patients can also be partially submerged in water, but this may stimulate defecation. Care must be exercised when the transducer is placed next to the skin in the pectoral or inguinal regions because the patient can damage the transducer by wedging it between the shell and the limb. Care must also be used in all patients because the transducer can be damaged with rubbing the transducer against the grain of the skin and scales.

Cardiac evaluation is practical in lizards and snakes (Figure 29-40). The heart can be imaged from lateral and ventral windows in these patients. Cardiac imaging is more difficult in chelonians but is possible via the axillary window. Generalized cardiomegaly, endocarditis, pericardial fluid, and cardiac tumors have been identified with ultrasound. The extracardiac signs of heart failure (e.g., hepatic venous congestion, pericardial effusion, and ascites) can also be identified. Ultrasound is far more useful than radiology for evaluation of cardiovascular disease in reptiles.

Cardiac contractility and internal anatomy are significantly different from mammals. Ventricular contractility in reptiles has a more peristaltic motion as compared with the concentric contraction in mammals. The ventricular myocardium is relatively thick and irregular in contour internally, and reproducible measurement locations are difficult to obtain. We have, therefore, not relied on M-mode measurements or calculations such as fractional shortening.

Intracardiac blood flow velocities are slower in reptiles than in mammals, and atrial swirling flow patterns are normal. These are commonly manifested as "smoke" patterns, which are considered abnormal in mammals. We are currently evaluating the use of caudal venal cave flow patterns and velocities obtained with Doppler interrogation as indices of heart function.

A ventral acoustic window adjacent to the liver is used for hepatic studies. Ultrasound is helpful for evaluation of liver disease in lizards and snakes. Criteria for diagnosis of focal and diffuse disease are similar to those described for mammals. The most common ultrasonographic hepatic abnormality seen in clinical practice is increased hepatic echogenicity, which is usually the result of vacuolar hepatopathy. Irregular areas of echogenicity are more typical of inflammatory disease.

Ultrasound is used to obtain hepatic aspirates for cytologic and microbiologic examinations. The needle is introduced between scales and directed to the appropriate area with ultrasound guidance. A 1.5-inch 27-gauge needle is used for the aspirates. This enables the clinician to obtain the most diagnostic sample while avoiding major vascular structures.

Cholecystocentesis can be performed for microbiologic studies. The gall bladder is visible on ultrasound studies and is accessible for aspiration. The potential for leakage of bile must be considered.

A relatively new area for ultrasound interrogation of reptiles is the digestive tract, especially for the evaluation of paralytic and obstructive ileus. As ileus progresses, the intestinal diameter increases (Figure 29-41). Although normal intestinal peristalsis is sluggish in reptiles, the pressure of atonic dilated fluid-filled intestines in a patient that has not recently eaten should be considered suspicious for ileus. Obstructive soft tissue masses can be identified adjacent to the dilated segments. Intraluminal foreign bodies are usually hyperechoic and exhibit distal acoustic shadowing.

Ultrasound is superior to conventional radiology for evaluation of the reproductive tract, especially in snakes and lizards. Ova have a hyperechoic shell and hypoechoic center. This is in contrast to the diffuse increased echogenicity of urinary bladder calculi. Ova usually produce less distant acoustic shadowing than calculi. Reproductive tract masses can be identified on ultrasound, but the masses are often amorphous in shape and MRI provides a superior documentation of their size and origin.

Ultrasound evaluation of the urinary tract can be performed, but image quality of the urinary bladder can be degraded by the hyperechoic urinary bladder contents. Urinary calculi are hyperechoic and produce distant acoustic shadowing. Considerable experience is required to image and identify the kidneys. To this date, we have not identified any typical ultrasonographic pattern of renal disease.

Nuclear Medicine

Recent studies have shown the efficacy of technetium bone scans in lizards and snakes affected with vertebral hyperostosis (see Figure 69-9). The technetium scans are more sensitive than conventional radiology for identification of abnormal bone blood flow and osteoblastic or osteoclastic activity. Although bone scans are sensitive in identifying "hot spots"

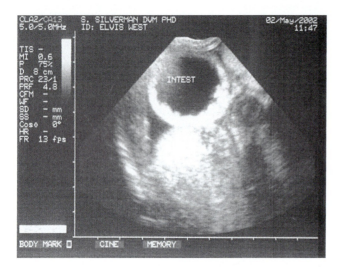

FIGURE 29-41 Water Dragon *(Physignathus cocincinus)*. Chronic ileus has resulted in dilated fluid-filled segments of intestine with poor contractility.

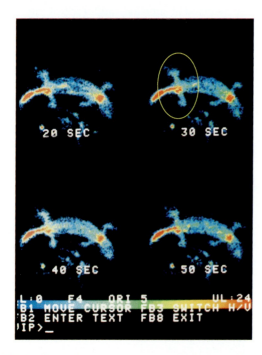

FIGURE 29-42 Technetium scan in a Prehensile-tailed Skink *(Corucia zebrata)*. The scan was performed to evaluate renal perfusion. This series of images represents the "vascular" phase of the scan. Note the area in the *yellow circle*: perfusion to the patient's right kidney is seen, but no contrast is taken up by the left kidney. *(Photograph courtesy D. Mader.)*

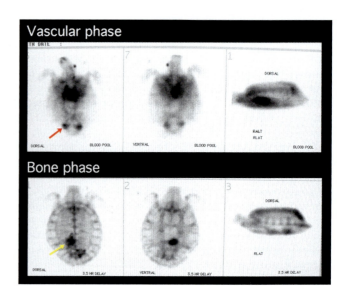

FIGURE 29-43 Bone scan in a Green Seaturtle *(Chelonia mydas)*. The patient has multiple fibropapillomas, with several growing from the surface of the shell. The vascular phase *(top)* shows normal distribution of the isotope in the kidneys *(red arrow)* and heart *(obscured)*. During the bone phase, the isotope scan shows areas of abnormal bone blood flow *(yellow arrow)* specifically regions with increased osteoblast/osteoclast activity. This indicates papilloma growth within the carapacial bone. *(Photograph courtesy D. Mader.)*

of bone activity, the specificity of the examination is poor. The study is, however, invaluable in identification of the extent of polyostotic disease and polyarthropathies.

Nuclear medicine has not been shown to be efficacious for hepatic, renal, and brain scan, as it is in mammals, but is beginning to be used more often (Figure 29-42). Currently, interrogation of these diseases is better understood with MRI or ultrasound. As with many aspects in reptile medicine, as more information is collected, these techniques will gain in usefulness.

Nuclear medicine is also helpful in evaluation of carapace injuries because the vertebral column is encased in the carapace (Figure 29-43).

CONCLUSION

Although conventional radiography and ultrasound remain the mainstay of diagnostic imaging, the ancillary methods are becoming increasingly more important. The high speed spinal CT units and high resolution ultrasound machines are changing the approach to diagnostic imaging and its efficacy for evaluation of diseases in reptiles.

30
DIAGNOSTIC TECHNIQUES

STEPHEN J. HERNANDEZ-DIVERS

The successful diagnosis and treatment of reptile disease require an ability to properly restrain and perform a variety of clinical techniques. The principles of such techniques are similar to those used in domestic companion animal medicine. In particular, the ability to perform a thorough physical examination, which depends on adequate restraint, is considered the cornerstone of clinical reptile practice.[1] Nevertheless, a number of reptile-specific peculiarities must be appreciated in the reptile clinic if potentially serious errors are to be avoided. The following descriptions include clinical techniques that the author has used for the purposes of diagnosis in reptile pets, zoo animals, and wildlife. Some descriptions are general and apply to most if not all species within a group, and others may be more specific. The species of reptile must be identified before clinical interaction so that potential dangers can be appreciated and avoided. Strikes, bites, scratches, crushing injuries, envenomation, and zoonoses are some of the common dangers that face reptile clinicians and their employees.

PHYSICAL RESTRAINT AND EXAMINATION

Reptiles as a group are relatively easy to evaluate, and the standard examination techniques used for domestic companion animals can be used. Clinical evaluation starts with a detailed history, and inexperienced clinicians are advised to consult a history form to ensure that no items are overlooked (Table 30-1). The aim of the physical examination is localization of any lesions or clinical signs to an organ system or systems and formulation of a list of differential diagnoses (Table 30-2). Calm specimens may possibly be observed unrestrained, which permits an assessment of demeanor, locomotion, and obvious neurologic disorders such as lameness, paralysis, paresis, and head tilt. Although seldom possible, observation of reptiles within the usual environment is particularly valuable and should be performed whenever possible. Nervous or aggressive species are best restrained at all times with appropriate techniques, including towels, snake hooks, clear plastic containers, and restraint tubes.[1-8] Gauntlets severely reduce the clinician's tactile sensation but may be necessary with large pugnacious lizards or small to medium aggressive crocodilians. Careful consideration should be given to the safety of veterinary staff, zoo keepers, and private owners with large or venomous reptiles. In many cases, the judicious use of chemical agents can expedite procedures and considerably reduce risks to both reptile and human. Given the improvements in reptile anesthesia, even the more manageable "pet" reptiles may be preferentially sedated or anesthetized for clinical procedures that would otherwise take longer to accomplish and cause unnecessary stress or discomfort to the animal.[3,4,9] Sedatives and anesthetics may affect clinical pathologic results, especially hematology.

A systematic examination from rostrum to tail tip is always indicated, whether the reptile is seen for a postpurchase examination, a yearly health examination, a presurgical assessment, or because it is clinically unwell. The clinician's senses of sight, sound, smell, and touch are all used to examine all accessible areas for abnormalities. With the first tentative steps into reptile medicine, seeking the help of individuals from a local herpetological society for the examination of clinically healthy animals can be invaluable.

A common stress response of many species to handling is the voiding of feces, urine, and urates during the clinical examination (Figure 30-1). In many cases, material is deposited on the table or on the clinician. Any veterinarian blessed with an abundance of clinically valuable material should consider immediate collection for possible laboratory investigation, including urine dipstick, fecal wet preparation, and flotation. Microbiologic results must be interpreted with caution when dealing with material collected in such an unsterile manner.

SPECIAL CONSIDERATIONS

Reptiles are not mammals, and a variety of considerations should be appreciated in examination of this taxonomic class as a whole.[1]

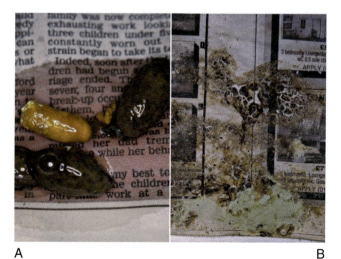

FIGURE 30-1 Feces, urates, and urine that are voided during physical examination should be retained for laboratory investigations. **A,** Normal feces, urates, and urine from a snake. **B,** Diarrhea and abnormal green urates from a tortoise with severe liver disease.

Table 30-1 History Form

Reptile name or ID:
Species, subspecies:
Date of birth, age:
Gender:
Duration in owner's care/captivity:
Origin (captive bred, wild import):
Source (breeder, pet shop):

Enclosure/vivarium specifications:	Type (arboreal, terrestrial, aquatic)
	Size
	Construction (materials, fittings)
	Décor and furnishings
	Ventilation (mesh, grills)
	Cleaning routine (agents used)
Environment:	Heating equipment
	Heating control
	Daytime temperature gradient
	Nighttime temperature gradient
	Water temperature
	Lighting equipment (type, position, age)
	Photoperiod
	Humidity
Diet:	Type and quantities
	Frequency of feeding
	Time when food is offered
	Changes of appetite
Water:	Method of provision (spray, bowl)
	Frequency of water changes; water quality
	Changes in drinking behavior
Supplements in water or food:	Type and frequency of use

Breeding details:
Other specimens in same vivarium:
Other specimens in same room or air space:
Disease history of presented animal:
Details of any diseased in-contact animals:
Quarantine protocol:
Other details of relevance:

From Divers SJ: Clinical evaluation of reptiles, *Vet Clin North Am Exotic Anim Pract* 2(2):291-331, 1999.

Legislation

Many species of reptiles are considered dangerous and may be covered by legislation that restricts their ownership. In particular, venomous snakes (especially front-fanged species), venomous lizards (*Heloderma* spp.), and crocodilians may be covered by national, state, or local legislation. The decision to examine a dangerous reptile should be made by experienced veterinarians with due regard to legislative and safety requirements. In the United Kingdom, no species of chelonia is considered dangerous under the Dangerous Wild Animals Act (1976), and a similar consensus of opinion appears to exist elsewhere (see Chapter 80). Nevertheless, several species (e.g., Snapping Turtles, *Chelydra spp.*) have a ferocious bite that makes them a formidable opponent.

Zoonoses

Reptiles, like all other animal groups, can be a source of disease in humans. The risks of reptile-borne zoonoses are probably no greater than for other animal groups, and basic personal hygiene after the handling of patients reduces these risks to an acceptable minimal level. The major zoonoses of interest include *Salmonella* sp., *Pseudomonas* sp., *Mycobacteria* sp., *Cryptosporidia* sp., *Rickettsia* sp., and pentastomids (arachnid lung parasites) (see Chapter 79). Major public concern centers on the commensal reptile salmonellas, and clinicians are advised to obtain a copy of the statement policy and client brochure on this subject produced by the Association of Reptile and Amphibian Veterinarians (see Chapter 68).[10]

Weight and Length

Every reptile must be accurately weighed because deaths associated with drug overdose, particularly anesthetics and aminoglycosides, are avoidable. In addition, serial weight measurements permit an appraisal of growth and captive management, response to treatment, and disease progression. Relation of body weight to length for an assessment of body condition is a valuable technique that takes practice and experience to master. The ability to discern between the acutely sick reptile and the terminal presentation of chronic disease is a judgment that can be largely determined from body condition. Weight gain and loss are usually most obvious along the tail and around the pelvis and hindlimb areas in the lizards and crocodilians. Some species, such as the Leopard Gecko (*Eublepharis macularius*), store most of their fat reserves within a bulbous tail, and therefore, tail size and shape in this

Table 30-2 Common Differential Diagnoses by Symptoms

Body System	Clinical Sign	Differential Diagnosis
Gastrointestinal	Anorexia	Poor captive husbandry (e.g., inappropriate temperature)
		Captive stress (e.g., maladaption, interspecific/intraspecific aggression)
		Inappropriate food offered
		Food fermentation and colic
		Seasonal (winter) anorexia
		Parasitism (helminth, protozoan)
		Foreign body or impaction
		Ecdysis or dysecdysis
		Normal gravidity
		Dystocia
		Stomatitis, esophagitis, gastritis, enteritis
		Tongue trauma or infection
		Secondary to other localized (e.g., hepatitis, nephritis) or systemic (e.g., metabolic, septicemia, toxemia) disease
	Constipation	Poor captive husbandry (e.g., inappropriate temperature)
		Helminth parasitism
		Dehydration
		Inactivity
		Inappropriate food item (e.g., heavily furred rodents, guinea pigs)
		Cloacolith, fecalith
		Cloacitis
		Intussusception
		Renal disease in iguanas
	Diarrhea	Parasitism (protozoan, helminth)
		Food intolerance (e.g., rotten prey)
		Enteritis, colitis
		Intussusception
		Iatrogenic (e.g., yeast overgrowth caused by antibiotic use, excess oral fluid therapy)
		Secondary to systemic disease
	Prolapsed cloaca or colon	Any cause of increased coelomic pressure/straining (e.g., dyspnea, constipation, and so forth)
		Cloacitis, colitis
		Parasitism
		Renal disease in iguanas
	Regurgitation	Esophagitis, gastritis
		Parasitism (*Cryptosporidium*, helminthiasis)
		Inappropriate or rotten food item
		Postprandial handling
		Inadequate environmental temperature or lack of basking area
		Partial or complete gastrointestinal blockage caused by constipation, abscessation, intussusception, parasites, retained eggs, neoplasia, and so forth
		Boid inclusion body disease
		Septicemia, toxemia
	Stomatitis	Infectious—bacterial, fungal, viral, parasitic
		Exposure gingivitis
		Visceral gout and associated inflammation
		Secondary to esophagitis
		Husbandry predispositions to poor immune status (inadequate nutrition, hygiene, temperature)
		Dental disease (e.g., trauma, abscessation, mandibular/maxillary osteomyelitis)
	Mucous membranes	Pale to black pigmentation—normal coloration
		Yellow—jaundice, biliverdinuria
		Cyanotic—severe cardiovascular or respiratory disease
		Injected—septicemia, toxemia
Respiratory	Dyspnea (open-mouth breathing)	Pneumonia (bacterial, fungal, viral, parasitic)
		Airway obstruction (e.g., foreign body, hemorrhage)
		Heat stress
		Threat or aggressive display
	Glottal discharge	Lower respiratory tract disease
	Nasal discharge	Rhinitis
		Stomatitis
		Pneumonia

Table 30-2	Common Differential Diagnoses by Symptoms—cont'd	
Body System	**Clinical Sign**	**Differential Diagnosis**
Musculoskeletal	Spinal deformities	Normal salt excretion in some lizards
		Predisposition by hypovitaminosis A
		Fractures (pathologic and traumatic)
		Osteomyelitis and abscessation
		Metabolic bone diseases (e.g., secondary nutritional hyperparathyroidism, hypervitaminosis D_3)
		Osteitis deformans, scoliosis, kyphosis
		Congenital anomalies
		Neoplasia
	Lameness	Trauma—fractures, dislocations, soft-tissue injury
		Metabolic bone diseases (e.g., secondary nutritional hyperparathyroidism)
		Degenerative joint disease (age-related)
		Osteomyelitis, septic arthritis, cellulitis, abscessation
		Gout—articular, periarticular, pseudogout
Urogenital	Renomegaly	Renal gout, abscessation, tubulonephrosis, nephritis, neoplasia
	Prolapse	Bladder—urolithiasis
		Shell gland—egg retention, salpingitis
		Hemipenal—trauma or infection
	Infertile mating, laying unfertilized ova	Infertile male or female
		Incompatible pair or grouping
		Unsuccessful copulation
		Inappropriate prebreeding conditioning or poor seasonal stimulation
		Immature breeding
		Reproductive organ disease
	Stillbirths	Poor management of gravid female
		Poor egg incubation, incubator malfunction
		Reproductive tract, fetal, or egg disease
	Dystocia	Stress—interference from owner, other animals
		Competition for nesting sites
		Obesity
		Inappropriate environment
		Infertile eggs, dead fetus
		Grossly malformed egg or fetus
		Reproductive tract disease
		Systemic or metabolic disease (e.g., secondary nutritional hyperparathyroidism)
Circulatory	True anemia	Regenerative—posthemorrhage, excess blood sampling
		Nonregenerative—neoplasia, chronic disease, starvation
	Iatrogenic	Lymph contamination of blood during collection
		Excessive parenteral fluid therapy
	Petechiae	Septicemia, toxemia
	Blood parasites	Usually nonpathogenic
	Circulatory RBC mitosis	Replication of circulating RBC is normal
	Cardiomegaly	Cardiomyopathy
		Illusion caused by starvation and cachexia
		Noncardiac mass
Ophthalmic	Intraocular	Panophthalmitis (often caused by hematogenous spread or penetration)
		Cataract—age-related, hibernation frost damage
		Retinal degeneration—hibernation frost damage
	Cornea	Focal opacity—foreign body, scarring, ulceration, corneal lipidosis
		Keratitis
	Spectacle (snakes and some lizards)	Subspectacular abscess (snakes, some lizards)—ascending infection via nasolacrimal duct from buccal cavity (stomatitis, respiratory disease)
		Diffuse blue haze to spectacle—imminent normal ecdysis
		Wrinkled spectacle—retained spectacle (often caused by low humidity, inappropriate temperature)
	Palpebral swelling, exophthalmos	Ocular venous sinus engorgement
		Trauma—hematoma
		Retrobulbar abscess
		Cellulitis
		Hypovitaminosis A
	Ocular discharge	Conjunctivitis
		Normal tear production and overflow caused by lack of nasolacrimal duct in some species

Continued

Table 30-2	Common Differential Diagnoses by Symptoms—cont'd	
Body System	**Clinical Sign**	**Differential Diagnosis**
Neurologic and behavioral	Lethargy	Poor captive husbandry (e.g., inappropriate temperature, poor lighting, inter/intraspecific stress)
		Gravidity
		Ecdysis
		Visceral gout
		Secondary to any debilitating disease
	Aggression	Normal character of species (e.g., many terrapins and turtles)
		Acquired at sexual maturity or onset of breeding season (e.g., Green Iguana)
		Exposure to natural sunlight
	Tetany	Hypocalcemia—renal disease or severe secondary nutritional hyperparathyroidism
	Convulsions	Septicemia, toxemia
		Head trauma
		Meningitis (bacterial, viral, fungal, parasitic)
		Hepatic encephalopathy
		Renal encephalopathy (hyperphosphatemia)
		Intoxication (e.g., organophosphates, ivermectin)
	Ataxia/paresis	Hypoglycemia
		Hypovitaminosis B_1 (excess thiaminase in fish-eating reptiles)
		Secondary to any debilitating disease
		Ivermectin intoxication, especially in chelonia
	Head tilt, circling	Head trauma
		Ear abcessation
		Hibernation frost damage
	Asymmetrical swimming of chelonia	Unilateral pneumonia
		Unilateral soft-tissue mass
		Unilateral gas production (e.g., gastric bloat)
Integument and shell	Dysecdysis	Parasites (mites, ticks, flies)
		Inappropriate temperature and humidity
		Secondary to generalized debilitation, starvation
	Beak and nails	Overgrowth caused by lack of exercise and soft, easily prehended food material
		Trauma
	Shell	Soft shell—normal in particular species because of secondary nutritional hyperparathyroidism, shell infection
		Deformities—fractures, congenital, metabolic bone diseases, nutritional factors
		Scute loss—trauma, infection, systemic disease
	Skin trauma	Bites from cage mates, prey items
		Damage from poorly designed vivaria (e.g., rostral abrasions caused by repeated escape attempts)
	Abscesses	Subcutaneous abscesses common in most species
	Dermatitis	Bacterial—most common
		Fungal—common secondary to prolonged antibiotic use and in high-humidity environments
		Viral (e.g., papillomavirus of green wall lizards, grey-patch disease of Green Seaturtles)
		Hypovitaminosis A
		Hypervitaminosis A
		Ectoparasites—mites, ticks, flies
		Helminths—transcutaneous hookworm infection, subcutaneous parasitic cysts
	Burns	Chemical—after hypochlorite use
		Thermal—from unscreened heaters
	Blister disease	Noninfectious dermatitis caused by high humidity and mild thermal insult, leading to subcutaneous vesicle formation
	Color	Mutant color selection
		Normal chameleons
		Seasonal (breeding) changes
		Dull coloration caused by systemic or metabolic disease
		Dermatitis, scars, and so forth
Miscellaneous	Weight loss	Inadequate food intake
		Inadequate digestion caused by poor husbandry (especially inappropriate temperature) or intestinal disease
	Submandibular or cephalic swelling	Cellulitis—acute bacterial infection

Table 30-2	Common Differential Diagnoses by Symptoms—cont'd	
Body System	Clinical Sign	Differential Diagnosis
	Hemorrhage—trauma, aneurysm	
	Gross coelomic swelling	Gravid
		Ascites—hypoproteinemia, severe hepatopathy or nephropathy, coelomitis, cardiac disease
		Abscess
		Granuloma
		Neoplasia
		Gastric hypertrophy in snakes caused by *Cryptosporidium*
		Pronounced organ enlargement (e.g., hepatomegaly, intestinal obstipation, enlarged fat bodies and obesity)

From Divers SJ: Clinical evaluation of reptiles, *Vet Clin North Am Exotic Anim Pract* 2(2):291-331, 1999.
RBC, Red blood cell.

species is a particularly good means for assessment of general body condition. In snakes, the fat reserves tend to be more diffuse throughout the elongated coelomic fat reserves; nevertheless, weight loss leads to loose skin folds ("poverty lines"), with pronounced spine and ribs. The snout-vent length (SVL) of lizards, but especially snakes, is well worth noting because organ position and growth can be calculated as a result.

Chelonians present more of a problem. The musculature of the limbs can be assessed, but the best estimation of body condition relies on the relation of total weight to carapace length or body volume. Published charts are available for several common species.[3,11-13] (See Figure 7-20 and Chapter 18.)

Cloacal Temperature

The recommendation for taking a cloacal temperature from an ectotherm may seem a paradox, but in certain situations, the results can be rewarding. Obviously, small reptiles or reptiles maintained out of their enclosure for prolonged periods of time experience changes in core temperature. However, larger reptiles (especially large tortoises, crocodilians, and snakes) that are examined in their home environment or soon after leaving their normal enclosure do not show dramatic changes in their core temperature if they are transported in an insulated container. As a result, a cloacal temperature may provide an indication of the thermal environment in which the reptile resides (see Figure 31-2).

Transillumination

Transillumination of the coelom with a cold light source can be beneficial for visualization of the internal structures of small lizards and snakes and is particularly useful for confirmation of suspected impactions and foreign bodies in the examination room. Care must be exercised with a hot light source (e.g., incandescent spotlight) because of the possibility of thermal damage. A halogen or xenon endoscope light source is ideal. The light can be held against the body of small reptiles or lubricated and inserted into the esophagus or cloaca and colon. Transillumination enables coelomic masses to be identified, and the cardiac shadow can be located for cardiocentesis in small sedated lizards.

Auscultation

Auscultation is certainly possible and can be useful, but the use of a standard diaphragm stethoscope does require a silent consulting room. The adventitious sounds produced between the shell or scales and the stethoscope diaphragm can be reduced with placement of a dampened swab or towel between the stethoscope and the reptilian integument. More recently, the use of electronic stethoscopes has improved the appreciation of heart and respiratory sounds.

SNAKES

Several reviews deal specifically, or in part, with the physical restraint and examination of snakes.[1-4,6-8] The head of an aggressive snake or a snake of unknown disposition should be identified and restrained before the transportation bag is opened and the animal removed. Venomous snakes should be placed in clear plastic tubes or anesthetic induction chambers and anesthetized with isoflurane or sevoflurane before examination (Figure 30-2). In general, the head of the snake is held behind the occiput with the thumb and middle finger supporting the lateral aspects of the cranium. The index finger is placed on top of the head. The other hand is used to support the serpentine body (Figure 30-3). With the snake's head restrained in this manner, greater support can be given to the cranium-cervical junction, which, with only a single occiput, is more prone to dislocation from rough or inappropriate handling. The larger pythons and anacondas can exceed 6 meters and 100 kilograms and are powerful and potentially very dangerous. With large, even docile, boids, a second, third, or even fourth handler is necessary to support the body during the examination. Sedation of a large pugnacious snake is usually safer and more convenient than struggling on and risking injury to the snake, client, or staff.

Nervous or aggressive snakes can be restrained with Plexiglas tubes or sedated before examination (Figures 30-4 and 30-5). Nonvenomous species should be removed from the cloth bag and supported with one or two hands, depending on size. An assessment of demeanor quickly becomes obvious. The snake should be permitted to roam over the hands and arms, thereby enabling the clinician

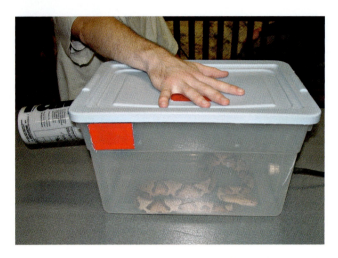

FIGURE 30-2 Venomous Copperhead *(Agkistrodon contortrix)* anesthetized with an induction chamber.

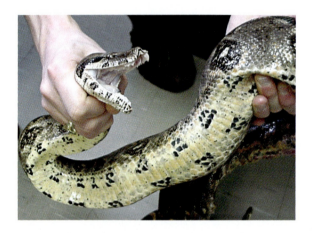

FIGURE 30-3 Restrained snakes must have their head and body supported. Aggressive snakes like the Boa Constrictor *(Boa constrictor)* cannot harm the handler when the heads have been securely grasped and controlled.

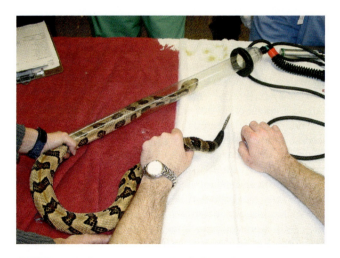

FIGURE 30-4 Restraining a Timber Rattlesnake *(Crotalus horridus)* within a Plexiglas restraint tube permits close observation of dangerous or aggressive snakes and facilitates anesthetic induction for diagnostic procedures.

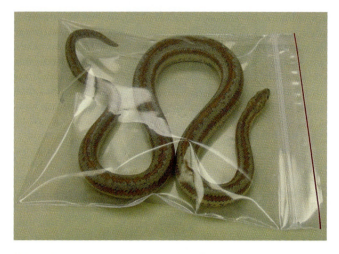

FIGURE 30-5 Nonvenomous snakes that are too nervous to be examined properly can be sedated with placement in a clear or semi-transparent plastic bag with 5% isoflurane or 8% sevoflurane in oxygen. Once righting reflexes have been lost (typically 5 to 15 minutes), the snake can be removed for examination and minor diagnostic procedures.

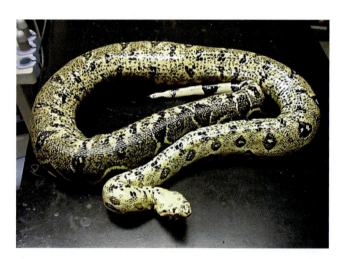

FIGURE 30-6 Complete lack of righting reflexes in *Boa constrictor* with boid inclusion body disease (IBD). *(From Divers SJ: Clinical evaluation of reptiles, Vet Clin North Am Exotic Anim Pract 2[2]: 291-331, 1999.)*

to gauge muscle tone, proprioception, and mobility. Proprioception can be assessed with placing the snake in dorsal recumbency and monitoring the effort and ability of the snake to right itself. Systemically ill serpents often are limp, lack strength, and are less mobile. The healthy serpent imparts a sense of strength and is active during handling. A healthy individual that is permitted to wrap a coil around the handler's wrist while the head is allowed to hang down should be able to raise the head to the level of the tail. Head carriage, body posture, cloacal tone, proprioception, skin pinch, withdrawal, and ocular and righting reflexes can be used to assess neurologic function (Figures 30-6 and 30-7).

The entire integument, particularly the head and ventral scales, should be thoroughly examined for evidence of

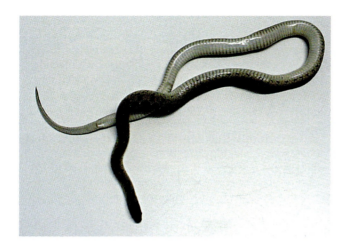

FIGURE 30-7 Poor neurologic function in a Gartersnake (*Thamnophis* sp.) with thiamine deficiency.

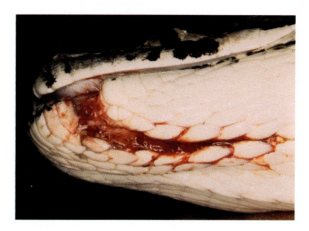

FIGURE 30-9 A submandibular skin laceration caused by another python. Such injuries are common when two snakes strike at the same prey item.

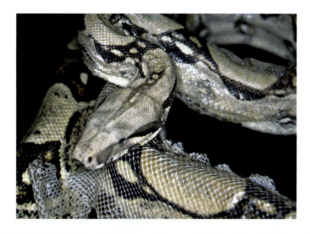

FIGURE 30-8 Dysecdysis in a *Boa constrictor*. (From Divers SJ: Clinical evaluation of reptiles, Vet Clin North Am Exotic Anim Pract 2[2]:291-331, 1999.)

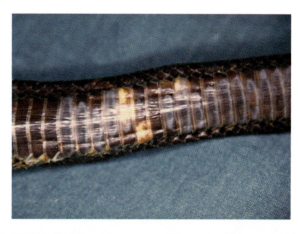

FIGURE 30-10 Blister disease caused by constant dampness within the vivarium.

dysecdysis (poor shedding), trauma, parasitism (especially the common snake mite, *Ophionyssus natricis*, and ticks), and microbiologic infection (Figures 30-8 to 30-15). If available, the recently shed skin should also be examined for evidence of retained spectacles (Figure 30-16). Skin tenting and ridges may indicate cachexia (poverty lines) or dehydration, and ticks and mites may congregate in skin folds, infraorbital pits, nostrils, and corneal rims (Figure 30-17). The infraorbital pits (where present) and the nostrils should be free from discharge or retained skin. The eyes should be clear, unless ecdysis is imminent. In preparation for shedding, snakes produce a lymph-like fluid that creates a white to bluish haze to the eyes. This fluid creates the cleavage zone and facilitates the lifting of the old skin. The spectacles that cover the eyes should be smooth because any wrinkles usually indicate the presence of a retained spectacle (Figure 30-18). The spectacle represents the transparent fused eyelids, and therefore, the cornea is not normally exposed. The subspectacular fluid drains through a duct to the cranial roof of the maxilla. When blocked, the buildup of fluid causes a subspectacular swelling that often becomes infected, resulting in a subspectacular

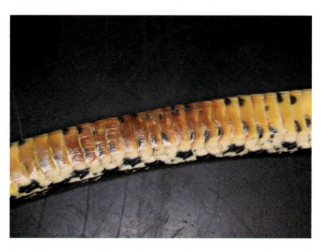

FIGURE 30-11 A thermal burn on the ventrum of a Kingsnake (*Lampropeltis* sp.) caused by a poorly controlled heat mat.

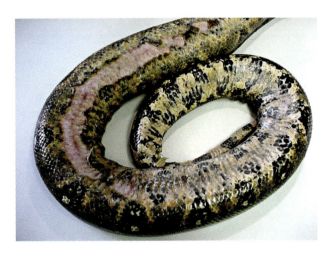

FIGURE 30-12 A *Boa constrictor* with severe bacterial dermatitis and skin necrosis from a burn from an unscreened heater.

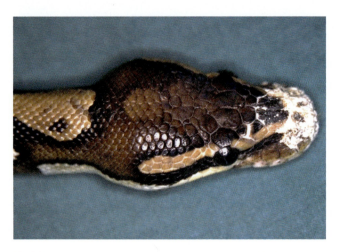

FIGURE 30-15 Mycotic dermatitis in a Royal or Ball Python *(Python regius)*.

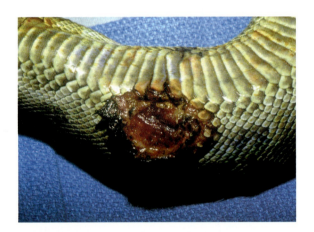

FIGURE 30-13 A focal wound in a Cuban Boa *(Epicrates angulifer)* that involves the skin, subcutis, and underlying musculature.

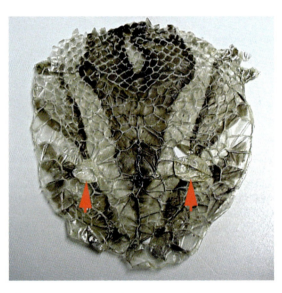

FIGURE 30-16 The dorsal head section of slough from a python. Note the two spectacles *(arrows)*.

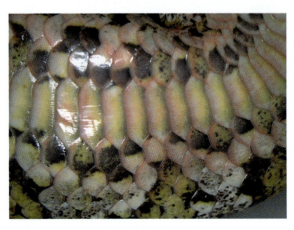

FIGURE 30-14 Subcutaneous hemorrhages can be a sign of generalized infection or toxemia in snakes.

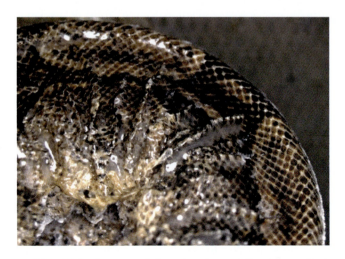

FIGURE 30-17 Pronounced skin ridges (poverty lines) in a cachexic snake.

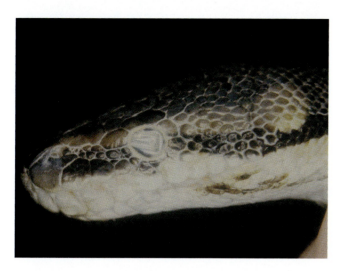

FIGURE 30-18 Retained spectacle in a Royal or Ball Python *(Python regius)*. (From Divers SJ: Clinical evaluation of reptiles, Vet Clin North Am Exotic Anim Pract 2[2]:291-331, 1999.)

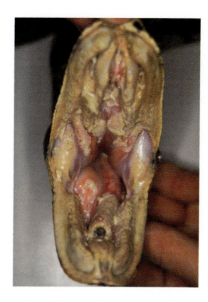

FIGURE 30-20 Severe bacterial stomatitis in a *Boa constrictor*. (From Divers SJ: Clinical evaluation of reptiles, Vet Clin North Am Exotic Anim Pract 2[2]:291-331, 1999.)

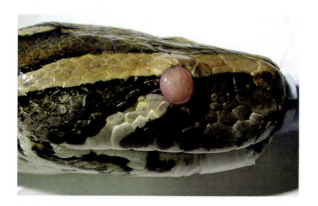

FIGURE 30-19 Subspectacular abscess in a Burmese Python *(Python m. bivittatus)*.

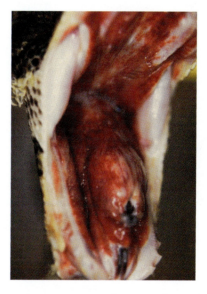

FIGURE 30-21 Severe buccal erythema and hemorrhages associated with viral stomatitis in a *Boa constrictor*.

abscess (Figure 30-19). Damage to the underlying cornea can result in panophthalmitis and ocular swelling, and retrobulbar abscessation results in protrusion of a normal-sized globe. Other ocular pathologies can include uveitis, corneal lipidosis, and spectacular foreign bodies, including slivers of wood chip or other vivarium materials.

Examination of the oral cavity is often left until the end of the examination because many snakes object to such manipulation. However, even before the mouth is opened, the tongue should be seen flicking in and out of the philtrum with regularity. The mouth can be gently opened with a plastic or wooden spatula to permit an assessment of mucous membrane color and buccal examination for evidence of mucosal edema, ptyalism, hemorrhage, necrosis, and inspissated exudates (Figures 30-20 and 30-21). The presence of white deposits may indicate uric acid deposition from visceral gout. The pharynx and glottis should be examined for hemorrhage, foreign bodies, and discharges. Observation of the glottis during respiration is important to attempt to differentiate between discharges originating from the respiratory and gastrointestinal tracts. Unfortunately, because of the stresses of examination, respiratory rates are often elevated in normal reptiles, and therefore, tachypnea may not be considered a definitive indicator of respiratory disease unless observed in the undisturbed snake. However, open mouth breathing is a reliable indicator of respiratory compromise (Figure 30-22). During the oral examination, the patency of the internal nares and the state of the polyphyodontic teeth should be noted.

From cranial to caudal, the head and body are palpated for abnormal swellings, wounds, and other abnormalities (Figures 30-23 and 30-24). The position of any internal anomalies, noted as a distance from the snout and interpreted as a percentage of SVL, enables an assessment of possible organ involvement (Figure 30-25).[14] Depending on the musculature,

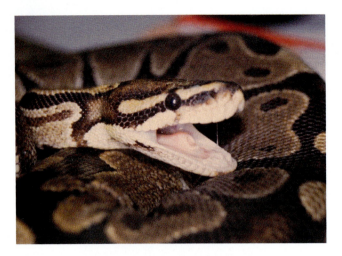

FIGURE 30-22 Dyspnea and open-mouth breathing in a Royal or Ball Python *(Python regius)* with severe pneumonia.

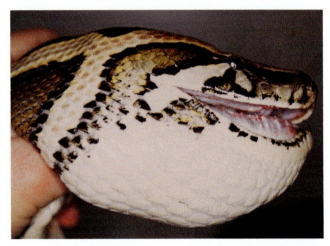

FIGURE 30-24 Submandibular bacterial cellulitis in a Burmese Python *(Python m. bivittatus)*.

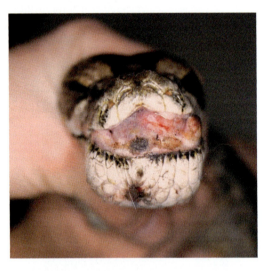

FIGURE 30-23 Mandibular swelling from a lymphosarcoma in a Burmese Python *(Python m. bivittatus)*.

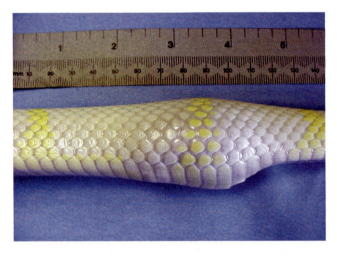

FIGURE 30-25 Intracoelomic mass in a Kingsnake. The mass, located approximately 85% from snout-vent, was a renal carcinoma.

feeding habits, and fat reserves of the snake, palpation of the normal heart, stomach, liver, active ovaries, eggs, kidneys, and fecal material may be possible. Recently fed snakes have a mid-body swelling associated with the prey within the stomach, but handling such individuals may well lead to regurgitation. Eggs and preovulatory follicles may also be palpated. The clinical examination should differentiate between coelomic (internal) and extracoelomic (subcutaneous) masses. Most subcutaneous masses are usually abscesses, but parasitic cysts, blisters, and neoplasia are occasionally seen. Internal masses may represent abscesses, neoplasia, granulomas, obstipation, organ hypertrophy, retained eggs, or ova. The cloaca should have muscle tone and not gape open and be free from fecal staining with no discharges. There should be no prolapsed tissue emanating from the vent (Figure 30-26).

Nervous snakes, especially colubrids, often expel the contents of their cloacal glands and cloacae in a defensive reaction to a perceived threat. This foul-smelling material does not represent infection but merely an annoyance because the

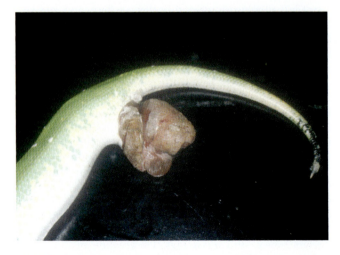

FIGURE 30-26 Cloacocolonic prolapse in a Green Tree Python *(Morelia viridis)*.

Diagnostic Techniques

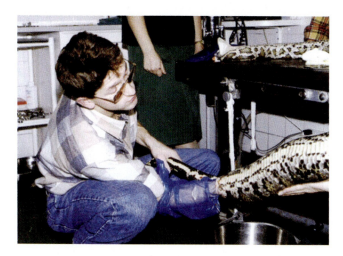

FIGURE 30-27 Cloacocolonic internal examination in a large python using a lubricated, gloved arm.

smell is difficult to eradicate from clothing. Examination of the cloaca can be performed with a dedicated otoscope or, better still, a rigid endoscope. Digital palpation is often overlooked but is a useful technique. In small to medium snakes, a latex-gloved lubricated finger can be passed into the cloaca and may allow palpation of eggs, cloacoliths, fecoliths, or abscesses. In the large constrictors, insertion of a lubricated gloved arm for an internal cloacal and even colonic examination is possible (Figure 30-27). Care is necessary to not force the colonic examination because the lower intestinal wall is thin and prone to perforation. Internal palpation often induces defecation and urination and can be useful to aid the collection of samples. Examination of the tail length or probing of the hemipenes should confirm the gender. The tail length (and the number of subcaudal scales) is always smaller in females than in males, but this method requires access to published information on tail length and scale counts unless both genders are available for simultaneous examination. The hemipenes are entered with a blunt probe, lubricated with a water-soluble material, either side of midline, just inside the caudal vent rim. In males, the probe passes to a depth of 6 to 14 subcaudal scales, whereas in females, the probe enters a cloacal gland to a depth of only 2 to 6 subcaudal scales (Figure 30-28).

LIZARDS

Lizards vary considerably in size, strength, and temperament, and therefore, a variety of handling techniques are necessary to cover most practical situations and permit physical examination.[1-5,7,8] The tegus and monitors are renowned for their powerful bites, and other species, particularly the Green Iguana *(Iguana iguana)*, are much more likely to use their claws and tail to painful effect. The main problem with handling small lizards is restraining them before they flee from an open bag or container. In all cases, the lizard should be transported in a securely tied cloth bag so that the position of the lizard can be identified and held before the bag is even opened. The large lizards are best restrained with the forelimbs held laterally against the thorax and the hindlimbs held laterally against the tail base (Figure 30-29). On no account should the

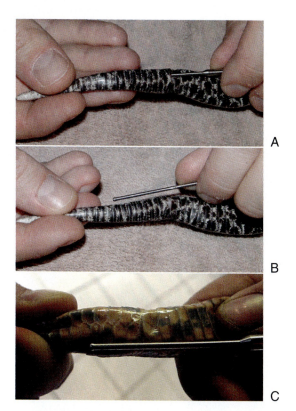

FIGURE 30-28 Gender determination of snakes. **A,** A lubricated blunt sexing probe is inserted into the vent and advanced caudad. **B,** The probe penetrates to a level of 6 to 14 subcaudal scales in males. **C,** The probe penetrates to a level of only 2 to 6 subcaudal scales in females.

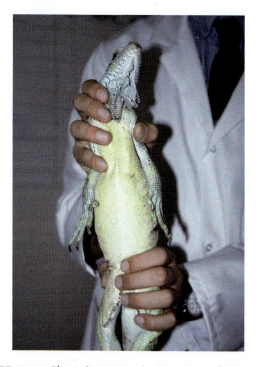

FIGURE 30-29 Physical restraint of a large lizard should include holding the forelimbs against the body and the hindlimbs against the tail base, as shown. If a lizard is prone to whipping its tail, the tail can be secured under the handler's arm.

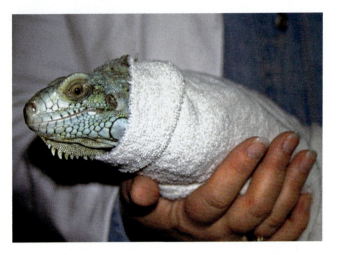

FIGURE 30-30 Restraint of a large lizard with a towel wrap technique.

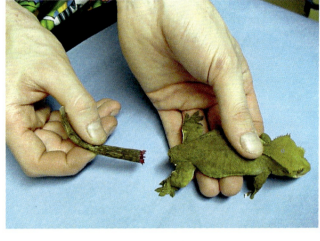

FIGURE 30-32 Many lizards like this Caledonian Lizard (*Rhacodactylus* sp.) can perform autotomy and drop their tails to evade predators. Inappropriate handling by grasping the tail can cause autotomy.

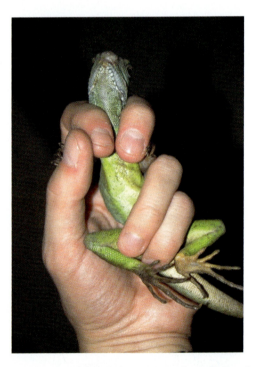

FIGURE 30-31 Single-handed restraint of small lizards must not inhibit coelomic breathing movements.

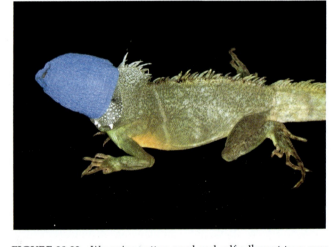

FIGURE 30-33 Wrapping cotton wool and self-adherent tape over the closed eyes of an Asian Water Dragon (*Physignathus cocincinus*) to induce vasovagal response.

limbs be held over the spine because fractures and dislocations are a reported complication. Particularly nervous lizards can be wrapped in a towel to aid restraint (Figure 30-30). Smaller lizards can be restrained around the pectoral girdle with the forelimbs held against the cranial coelom, although care is necessary to not impair respiratory movements (Figure 30-31).

A lizard should never be grasped by the tail because many species can perform autotomy and drop their tails in an attempt to evade a predator (Figure 30-32) (see Chapter 70). Restricting the vision of these animals is often the simplest way to facilitate handling, and a towel placed over the head often facilitates examination of the rest of the body and limbs.

A useful restraint technique for iguanid lizards uses the vasovagal response: gentle digital pressure is applied to both orbits, and in many cases, the lizard enters a state of stupor for up to 45 minutes or until a painful or noisy stimulus is applied (Figure 30-33).[7] This technique can be used to calm nervous iguanids and monitors and enables the mouth to be gently opened without the need for excessive force. If possible, the lizard should be observed unrestrained to appreciate any neurologic problems (Figures 30-34 to 30-37). Calm lizards may be permitted to walk around the examination table or on the floor. However, if in any doubt, the lizard should be placed in a large plastic enclosure to prevent escape during the observation period.

The integument should be examined for parasites, essentially mites and ticks, and evidence of trauma from fighting, mating, and burns (Figures 30-38 to 30-42). Lizards tend to shed their skin in stages, and therefore, retained skin (often

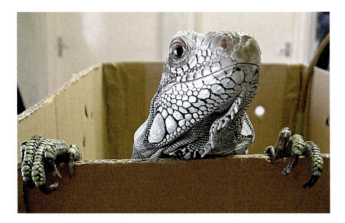

FIGURE 30-34 A healthy alert Green Iguana *(Iguana iguana)*.

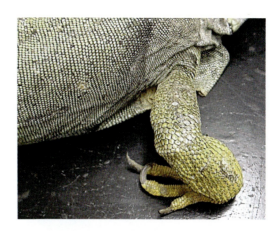

FIGURE 30-37 Propioceptive (placement) deficit in a Green Iguana *(Iguana iguana)* with localized spinal cord compression at T4. Similar presentations can occur with limb fractures.

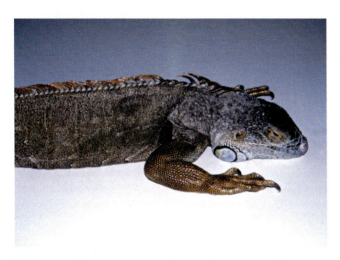

FIGURE 30-35 Moribund Green Iguana *(Iguana iguana)*. Depression is most often associated with severe sepsis or metabolic derangements.

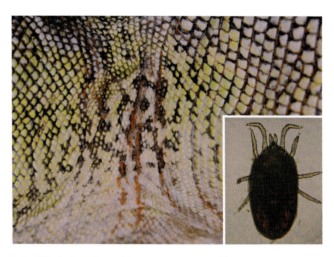

FIGURE 30-38 *Hirstiella* mites are commonly found around area folds in iguanas. *Inset,* Microscopic appearance of the mite.

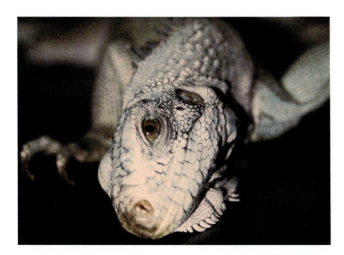

FIGURE 30-36 Right-sided head tilt in a Green Iguana *(Iguana iguana)* after head trauma.

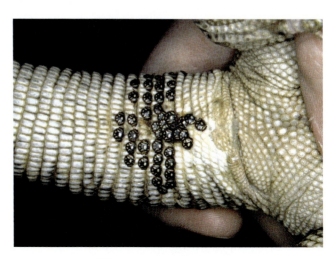

FIGURE 30-39 Ticks located along the ventral tail base of an imported Savannah Monitor *(Varanus exanthematicus)*.

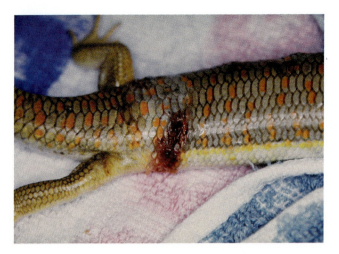

FIGURE 30-40 Infected bite wound in a female Berber Skink *(Eumeces schneideri)* after a mating encounter with an aggressive male.

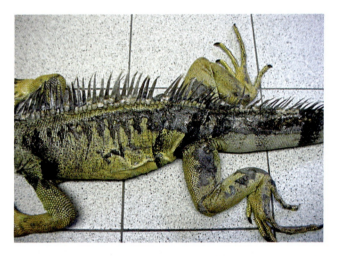

FIGURE 30-41 Severe burns to much of the dorsal surfaces of a Green Iguana *(Iguana iguana)* from an overly powerful radiant heat source within its enclosure.

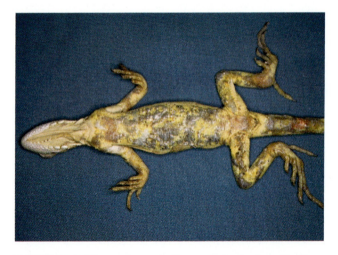

FIGURE 30-42 Severe burns to the ventrum of a juvenile Green Iguana *(Iguana iguana)* that was maintained in a vivarium with a poorly controlled heat mat inside the enclosure.

dry and brown) must be differentiated from normal piecemeal ecdysis (flexible and transparent). Classically, dysecdysis and skin retention occur around the digits and tail, causing ischemic necrosis. Extensive skin folding and tenting are indicators of cachexia and possible dehydration.

The head should be examined for abnormal conformation (Figure 30-43). The mouth can be opened with a blunt spatula or, in iguanids, with gentle pressure to the dewlap (Figure 30-44). Thorough buccal examination for evidence of trauma, infection, neoplasia, and edema, especially pharyngeal edema, and examination of the glottis are considered routine (Figure 30-45). In addition, the internal extent of any rostral abrasions can be evaluated. The nostrils, eyes, and tympanic scales should be clean and free from discharges (Figure 30-46). The presence of white dried material around the nostrils of some iguanid lizards is normal because some species excrete salt through specialized nasal glands. The rostrum should be examined for trauma, often caused by repeated escape attempts from a poorly designed vivarium or by evasion of intraspecific encounters (Figure 30-47). The head, body, and limbs must be palpated for masses or swellings (Figure 30-48). Focal soft tissue masses are usually abscesses, whereas more diffuse swellings around the long bones or mandible are likely to be related to one of a number of possible metabolic bone diseases (Figures 30-49 to 30-51). Lizards with severe hypocalcemia and hyperphosphatemia from secondary nutritional hyperparathyroidism or chronic renal disease exhibit periodic tremors and muscle fasciculations. The coelomic body cavity of most lizards can be gently palpated. In the healthy animal, food and fecal material within the gastrointestinal tract, fat bodies, liver, ova, and eggs are usually appreciable (Figure 30-52). Cystic calculi, fecoliths, enlarged kidneys, impactions, retained eggs or ova, and unusual coelomic masses are considered abnormal (Figure 30-53). An appreciation of species, gender, age, body size, and weight permits an assessment of growth and body condition (Figures 30-54 and 30-55). Auscultation of the heart and lungs is practical with Doppler ultrasound and electronic stethoscopes (Figure 30-56).

The cloaca should be free from fecal staining, with visual and digital examination considered routine (Figures 30-57 and 30-58). In the Green Iguana, renomegaly can be appreciated with digital cloacal palpation. The high incidence rate of dystocia necessitates identification of gender in the examination room. Many species of lizards are sexually dimorphic, although identifying gender in juveniles can be difficult. Adult males tend to be larger and more colorful, exhibit more courting (head bobbing) and territorial behaviors, and possess paired hemipenal bulges at the tail base and more developed femoral or preanal pores (Figure 30-59). Hemipenal eversion and probing are techniques that can be used but are generally more difficult to master than in snakes.

TORTOISES, TURTLES, AND TERRAPINS

There are nearly 300 species of Chelonia within 13 families. Nomenclature varies, largely dependent on which side of the Atlantic the practice is located. In the United States, the term *turtle* is used to refer to both aquatic and terrestrial chelonians, and in Europe, the various species are divided into terrestrial

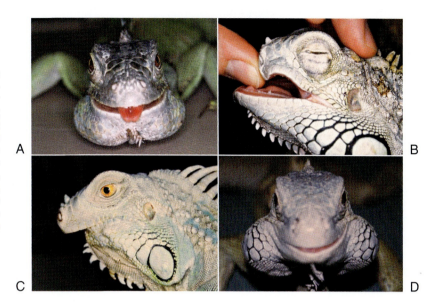

FIGURE 30-43 Abnormal head conformations in Green Iguanas *(Iguana iguana)*. **A**, Bilateral submandibular swelling associated with secondary nutritional hyperparathyroidism. **B**, Softening and compressibility of the maxilla associated with secondary renal hyperparathyroidism. **C**, Acquired agnathia caused by secondary nutritional hyperparathyroidism and continual forces of glossopharyngeal musculature on the softening mandible. **D**, Bilateral submandibular fibromas or osteomas. Biopsies of these pronounced hard swellings indicate that they are not associated with classic secondary nutritional hyperparathyroidism, although their etiology remains unclear.

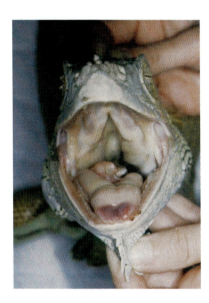

FIGURE 30-44 Gently pulling down on the dewlap of a Green Iguana *(Iguana iguana)* to permit examination of the oral cavity. Note the normal pigmentation at the end of the tongue and the glottis at the base of the tongue.

tortoises, freshwater terrapins, and marine turtles. Aquatic terrapins and turtles have a ferocious bite that may belie an apparently gentle disposition. The major biologic peculiarity of all chelonians is the presence of the shell. The plastron and carapace not only give this group their characteristic structure but also double as a barrier to physical examination. Nevertheless, much can still be achieved in the consulting room before one resorts to imaging techniques.[1-4,8,15]

Small to medium tortoises (e.g., *Testudo* spp.) are not difficult to handle, although their strength and uncooperative nature can hinder the examination and cause frustration. A little patience with the tortoise held head down often persuades a shy individual to protrude the head from the shell, at which time the thumb and middle finger can be placed behind the occipital condyles to prevent retraction of the head. However, in the larger species (e.g., *Geochelone* spp.), keeping a strong individual from pulling free may be physically impossible. In such cases, sedation, anesthesia, or the use of a neuromuscular blocking agent may be necessary.

Steady distractive pressure to the maxilla and mandible can open the mouth, and once the mouth is open, the index finger (in small gentle specimens) or a mouth gag (in larger or aggressive specimens) can be inserted into the mouth to prevent closure (Figure 30-60). This method enables the handler to keep the mouth open with one hand, leaving the other free to examine the head and take samples for laboratory investigation. In aggressive terrapins and turtles, open mouth threat displays provide a good opportunity to examine the buccal cavity with minimal handling. Examination of the head should include the nostrils for any discharges and the beak for damage and overgrowth (Figure 30-61). The eyelids should be open and not obviously distended or inflamed, and the eyes should be clear and bright. Conjunctivitis, corneal ulceration, and opacities are frequent presentations (Figure 30-62). The retina can often have degeneration as a consequence of freezing during hibernation, and ophthalmic examination is warranted in any anorectic animal. The tympanic scales should be examined for signs of swelling associated with aural abscessation (Figure 30-63). Verification of a tympanic abscess can often be made with observation of exudate emanating from the eustachian tubes as they open into the lateral walls of the pharynx. The integument should be free of damage that is often caused by aggressively courting males and subcutaneous swellings that are usually abscesses. Terrapins and turtles appear more susceptible for superficial and deep mycotic dermatitis, especially around the head, neck, and limbs (Figure 30-64). Submandibular swelling and self trauma through forelimb rubbing of the mouth often accompany stomatitis. The buccal cavity must always be examined, particularly for evidence of inflammation, infection, gout, and foreign bodies (Figure 30-65). Stomatitis can quickly lead to a generalized esophagitis, and examination down the pharynx and into the esophagus with a rigid endoscope is advisable. Note should also be made of the mucous membrane

506 Section V CLINICAL TECHNIQUES/PROCEDURES

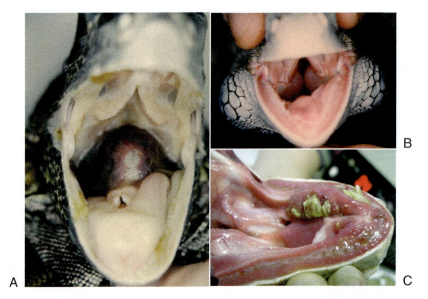

FIGURE 30-45 Oral abnormalities in Green Iguanas *(Iguana iguana)*. **A,** Pharyngeal edema from chronic renal disease. **B,** Intraoral appearance of bilateral fibroma/osteoma as they impinge within the dorsal pharynx. **C,** Oral abscess.

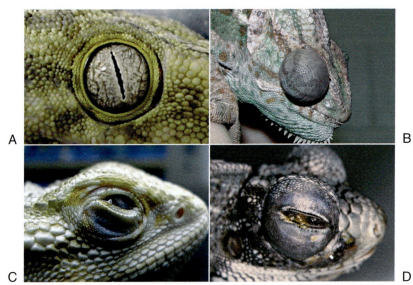

FIGURE 30-46 Lizard eyes. **A,** Normal spectacled (no lids) eye of a *Rhacodactylus* gecko. **B,** Acute swelling associated with trauma and engorgement of retrobulbar venous plexus in a Yemen Chameleon *(Chamaeleo calyptraptus)*. **C,** Blepharospasm and conjunctivitis in a Bearded Dragon associated with corneal ulceration from sand in the eye. **D,** Gross distension of the eye in a Green Iguana *(Iguana iguana)* from panophthalmitis and retrobulbar abscessation.

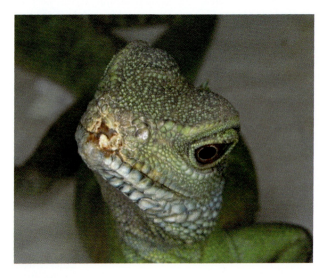

FIGURE 30-47 Rostral abrasions are common in many lizards, like this Asian Water Dragon *(Physignathus cocincinus)*, that fail to recognize and avoid glass barriers.

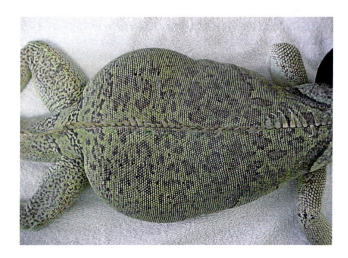

FIGURE 30-48 Coelomic distension in this Green Iguana *(Iguana iguana)* may be from ascites, reproductive activity, organomegaly, neoplasia, or abscess.

Diagnostic Techniques

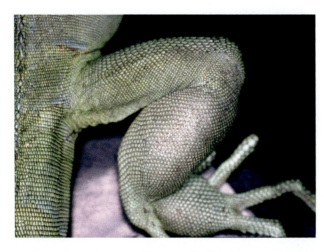

FIGURE 30-49 Firm swelling of the hindlimb in a Green Iguana (*Iguana iguana*) associated with secondary nutritional hyperparathyroidism.

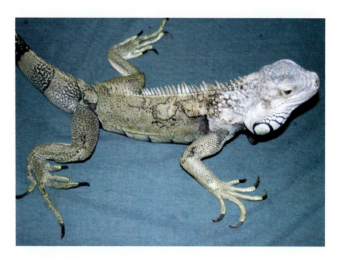

FIGURE 30-52 A green Iguana (*Iguana iguana*) emaciated from chronic renal disease.

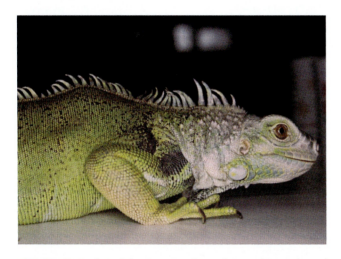

FIGURE 30-50 Spinal fracture in a Green Iguana (*Iguana iguana*) predisposed by secondary nutritional hyperparathyroidism.

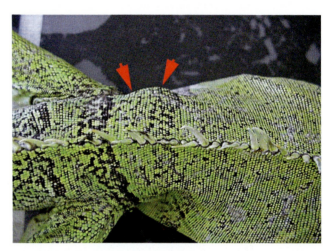

FIGURE 30-53 Enlarged kidney (*arrows*) in a Green Iguana (*Iguana iguana*).

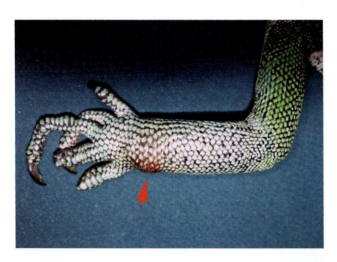

FIGURE 30-51 Swelling of the antebrachium in a Green Iguana (*Iguana iguana*) from localized trauma, abscessation (*arrow*), and subsequent cellulitis.

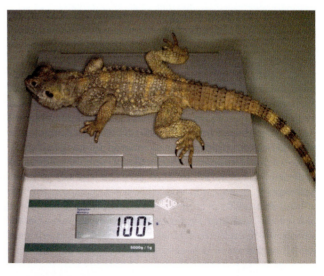

FIGURE 30-54 Accurate weight recording is essential for all reptiles.

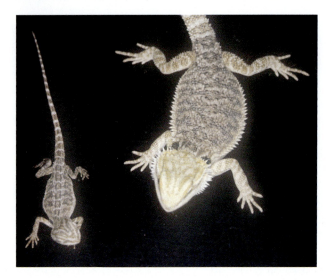

FIGURE 30-55 Sibling Bearded Dragons *(Pogonoa vitticeps)* from the same enclosure. Despite the lack of overt aggression, the sibling on *right* was dominant over the other with regard to food and basking resources and grew much faster.

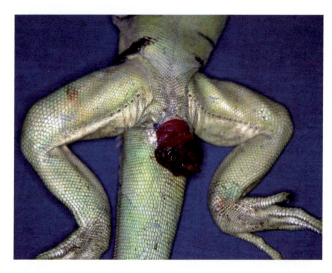

FIGURE 30-57 Cloacal prolapse in a Green Iguana *(Iguana iguana)* with chronic renal disease and secondary renal hyperparathyroidism.

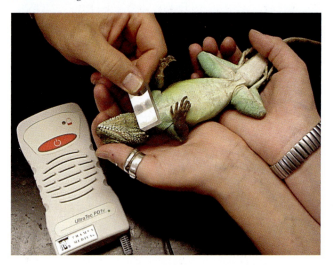

FIGURE 30-56 Doppler ultrasound assessment of the heart of a conscious Asian Water Dragon *(Physignathus cocincinus)*.

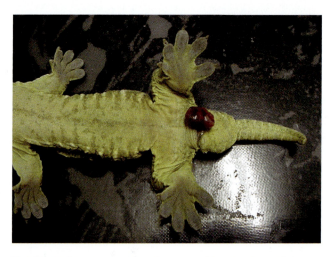

FIGURE 30-58 Hemipenal prolapse in a *Rhacodactylus* gecko.

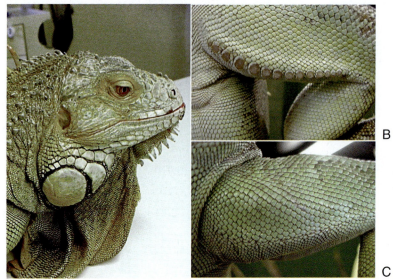

FIGURE 30-59 Sexual characteristics of lizards. **A,** Male Green Iguana. Mature males often have larger, broader heads with more developed crests, dewlaps, and jowls. **B,** Male Green Iguana. Mature males have more developed preanal or femoral pores. **C,** Female Green Iguana. Female lizards tend to have reduced or absent preanal or femoral pores.

Diagnostic Techniques 509

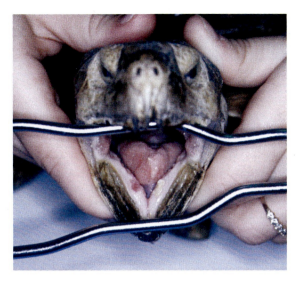

FIGURE 30-60 Use of a metal mouth gag to permit oral examination of an African Spurred Tortoise *(Geochelone sulcata)*.

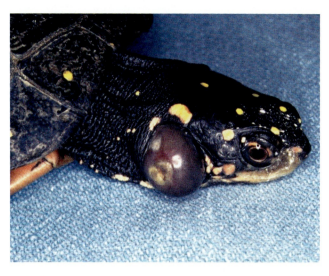

FIGURE 30-63 Aural abscess in a Spotted Turtle *(Clemmys guttata)*.

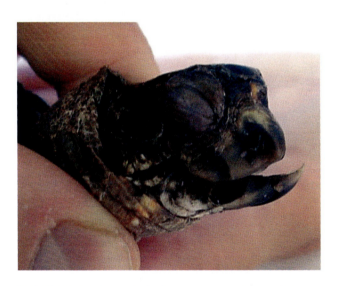

FIGURE 30-61 Overgrown beak of a *(Terrapene* sp.) Box Turtle.

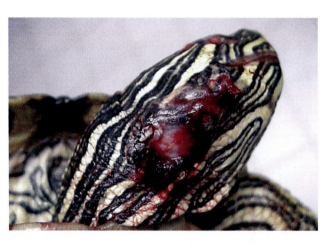

FIGURE 30-64 Mycotic dermatitis and cutaneous ulceration along the ventrolateral border of the mandible in a Red-eared Slider *(Trachemys s. elegans)*.

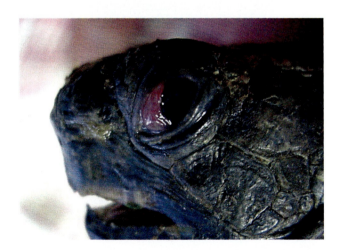

FIGURE 30-62 Protrusion of the nictitating membrane in a Hermann's tortoise *(Testudo hermanni)* with bacterial conjunctivitis.

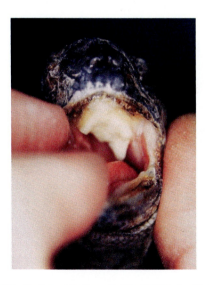

FIGURE 30-65 Oral examination of a Greek Tortoise *(Testudo graeca)* reveals caseous plaque attached to the hard palate.

coloration, which is normally pale pink. Hyperemic membranes may be associated with septicemia or toxemia. Icterus is rare but may occur with biliverdinemia from severe liver disease. Pale membranes are often observed in cases of true anemia. Pale deposits within the oral membranes may represent infection or urate tophi associated with visceral gout. The glottis may be difficult to visualize, being positioned at the back of the fleshy tongue; however, one must check for any inflammation and glottal discharges that may be consistent with respiratory disease (Figure 30-66).

The withdrawn limbs can also be extended from the shell of small to medium chelonians with steady traction. The coelomic space within the shell is restricted, and therefore, gently forcing the hindlimbs into the shell often leads to partial protrusion of the forelimbs and head, and vice versa. The more aggressive species, especially the terrapins and turtles, should be held at the rear of the carapace. Some species (e.g., Alligator Snapping Turtle, *Macroclemys temminckii*) can deliver an extremely powerful bite, and so great care is necessary at all times. Certain species also possess functional hinges at the front or back (or both) of the plastron or carapace, and care should be exercised not to trap a finger when the hinge closes. A wedge or mouth gag can be used to prevent complete closure of a hinge, and no chelonian will close a hinge on its own extended limb. The integument should be examined for parasites, particularly ticks and flies; dysecdysis; trauma; and infection that may arise from rodent, dog, raccoon, or fox attacks (Figures 30-67 and 30-68). Aggressive conflicts and courting trauma must also be considered in the communal environment. Limb fractures are less commonly reported in chelonia than in lizards but are often caused by rough handling, with a greater incidence reported in those individuals with secondary nutritional hyperparathyroidism and road traffic accidents. Focal subcutaneous swellings are usually abscesses, but grossly swollen joints or limbs are more often cases of fracture, osteomyelitis, or septic arthritis (Figure 30-69).

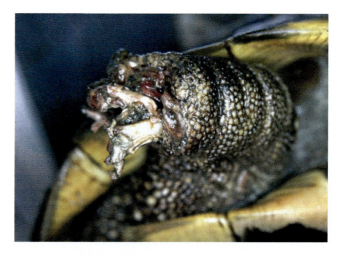

FIGURE 30-68 Severe limb trauma in a tortoise after a fox attack. The tibia and fibula have been exposed.

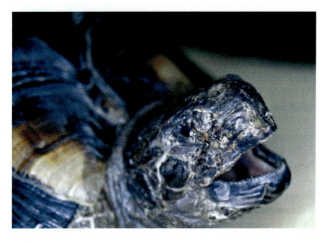

FIGURE 30-66 Dyspnea and open-mouth breathing in a tortoise with severe pneumonia.

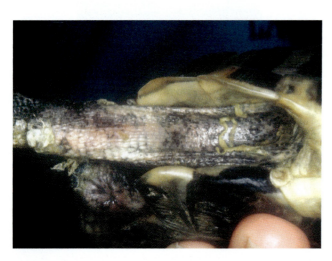

FIGURE 30-67 Skin sloughing and erythema associated with iatrogenic hypervitaminosis A in a tortoise.

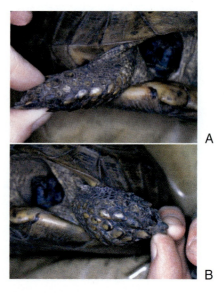

FIGURE 30-69 **A,** Normal forelimb of a *Testudo* tortoise. **B,** Grossly enlarged forelimb of a *Testudo* tortoise from osteomyelitis.

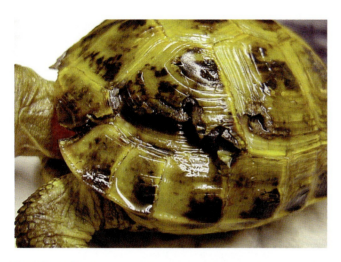

FIGURE 30-70 Fracture of the carapace in a tortoise after a dog attack.

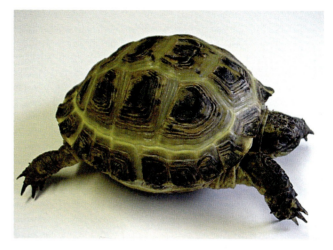

FIGURE 30-72 Excessive growth in this juvenile *Testudo* tortoise is indicated by a broad growth line in the shell.

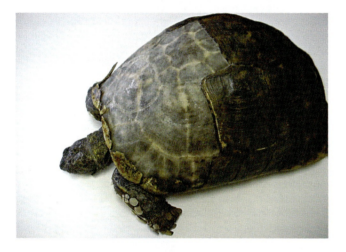

FIGURE 30-71 Sloughing of keratin scutes to reveal the underlying carapacial bones in a tortoise that sustained severe burns in a garage fire.

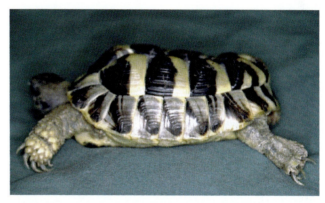

FIGURE 30-73 The deformed shell of a juvenile Greek Tortoise *(Testudo graeca)* from secondary nutritional hyperparathyroidism.

The prefemoral fossae should be palpated with the chelonian held head-up. Gentle rocking of the animal may then enable the clinician to palpate eggs, cystic calculi, or other coelomic masses. The shell should be examined for hardness, poor conformation, trauma, and infection (Figures 30-70 to 30-72). Soft poorly mineralized shells are usually a result of secondary nutritional hyperparathyroidism from dietary deficiencies of calcium, excess phosphorus, or a lack of full spectrum lighting (Figure 30-73). Pyramiding of the shell, historically, has been linked to dietary excesses of protein, although the cause may be multifactorial and include environmental humidity (see Chapter 18). Shell infection may present as loosening and softening of the scutes with erythema, petechiae, purulent or caseous discharges, and a foul odor (Figure 30-74). Deep infections usually involve the bones of the shell and cause osteomyelitis (Figure 30-75).

Prolapses through the vent are obvious, but determination of the structure involved is necessary. Prolapses may include cloacal tissue, shell gland, colon, bladder, or phallus (Figures 30-76 and 30-77). Internal examination with digital palpation and an endoscope is recommended. Male chelonians can be differentiated from females by their longer tails and the

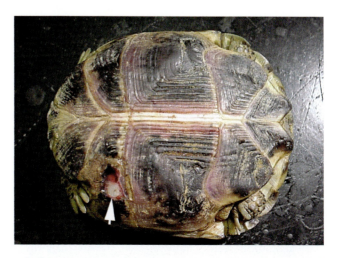

FIGURE 30-74 Hemorrhage and infection between the scutes and the shell of a tortoise. The focal wound *(arrow)* was the presumed portal of entry.

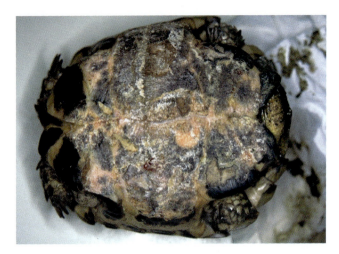

FIGURE 30-75 Generalized plastron infection with osteomyelitis in a tortoise that was maintained in unhygienic conditions on an inappropriate heat mat.

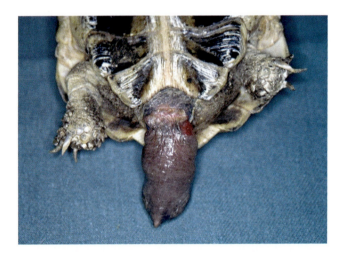

FIGURE 30-76 Phallic prolapse in a *Testudo* tortoise.

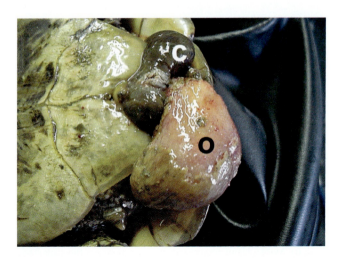

FIGURE 30-77 Prolapse of the cloaca (*c*) and oviduct (*o*) in a *Testudo* tortoise that had been straining and had previously passed several eggs.

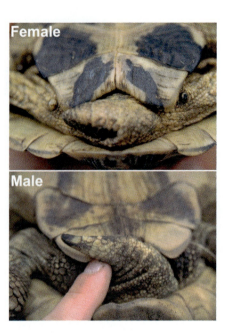

FIGURE 30-78 Gender determination by tail size in a Hermann's Tortoise (*Testudo hermanni*). The female has a smaller tail *(top)* than the male *(bottom)*.

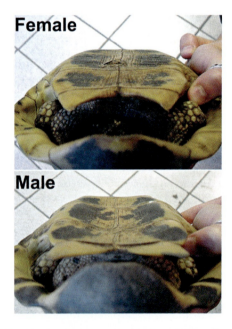

FIGURE 30-79 Gender determination by plastron shape in a Red-footed Tortoise (*Geochelone carbonaria*). The female has a flat plastron *(top)*, whereas the plastron of the male is more concave *(bottom)*.

position of their cloaca caudal to the edge of the carapace (Figure 30-78). Other sexual dimorphism characteristics may also be obvious, including the concavity of the male plastron in many species and the longer forelimb claws of some male terrapins (Figure 30-79).

CROCODILIANS

Individuals of less than 2 meters in total length can often be handled conscious, albeit with extreme caution. Even the small crocodilian can use both tail and jaw to cause injury. The mouth should always be taped and the tail firmly restrained (Figure 30-80).[3] A profound vasovagal induced torpor can be elicited by gently taping the eyes closed (Figure 30-81).[7] Examination of the eyes and mouth is carried out at the end of the examination process, just before the animal is released. Animals may be strapped to a wooden plank to improve physical restraint, but with animals of more than 2 meters in length, serious consideration should be given to the use of chemical restraint.[16] The physical examination of crocodilians follows a similar pattern to that used for large saurians because their body patterns are similar. The clinician should pay particular attention to the extremities and integument, which are often traumatized by conspecifics or poor environment (Figure 30-82).

DIAGNOSTIC SAMPLE COLLECTION

Very few pathognomonic indicators are found in reptile medicine, and therefore, reliance on a variety of diagnostics is usually essential to reach a definitive diagnosis. Ideally, demonstration of a pathologic host reaction is necessary, and of the etiologic agent if one exists. In practice, this often requires a combination of cytologic, histopathologic, microbiologic, toxicologic, hematologic, clinical pathologic, and serologic evaluations on appropriate body fluids or tissues. The advent of various clinical techniques, particularly endoscopy, has enabled far better antemortem diagnoses; previously, necropsy was the common means of achieving a definitive answer.[3,7,17]

Blood and Hemopoietic System

Venipuncture and Blood Collection

The ability to collect quality blood samples is essential in any animal class. Complete or selective hematologic and biochemical evaluations are possible, but the accuracy of results is often adversely affected by poor venipuncture, handling, or laboratory skills. The production of poor-quality blood data can be useless or, even worse, misleading to the clinician.[3,7,18,19] Likewise, the ability to administer intravenous medications, especially anesthetics, or place intravenous catheters also relies on proficient venoclysis technique. Venipuncture in reptiles is generally a blind technique. The jugular vein of certain tortoises may be visible, particularly after temporary caudal occlusion of the vessel, but in any case, anatomic knowledge of the position of veins is vital. Aseptic preparation of the venipuncture site is wise because infection and abscessation after venous access are potential complications. Despite a continuous trickle of published blood ranges, a relative dearth of hematologic or biochemical data still exists for reptiles compared with domesticated animals (see Chapter 88). In addition, blood values can vary dramatically with species, environment,

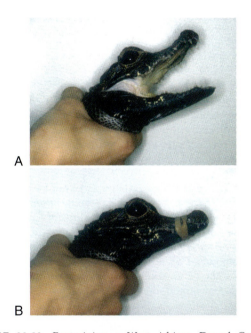

FIGURE 30-80 Restraining a West African Dwarf Crocodile *(Osteolaemus tetraspis)*. **A,** Even small crocodilians have ferocious bites. **B,** Taping the snout closed ameliorates this threat.

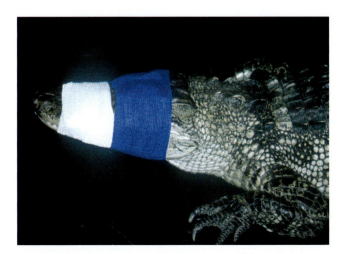

FIGURE 30-81 An adult American Alligator *(Alligator mississippiensis)* with the snout and eyes taped shut to induce vasovagal response and facilitate handling.

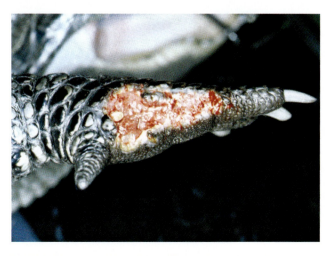

FIGURE 30-82 An infected carpal wound in a juvenile American Alligator *(Alligator mississippiensis)* after trauma from a second alligator.

nutrition, age, breeding status, hibernation, and disease status.[3,7,19] Given this variability, published ranges may be of limited value and should be used with caution. More reliance should be placed on establishment of an individual's observed range and serial sampling to monitor the progress of hematologic and biochemical changes rather than reliance on a single result. The following descriptions indicate the most humane and practical venipuncture sites. Other sites have been indicated for completeness but may have reduced clinical application from increased risk, poor quality sample, or significant welfare and ethical concerns.[18] For example, the use of a toe-nail clip to obtain blood may result in fecal or urate contamination, elevated tissue enzymes, abnormal hemogram and electrolyte changes from the peripheral nature of the sample, and the crushing artifact of collection.[18] Of even greater concern are the ethical and welfare issues that surround a procedure that causes more pain and carries a greater risk of postsampling sepsis.

Snakes. The two common sites for venipuncture in snakes are the caudal (ventral tail) vein and the heart.[3,6,7,19] The caudal (tail) vein is accessed caudal to the cloaca, between 25% and 50% down the tail (Figure 30-83). It is wise to avoid the paired hemipenes of males (that may extend up to 14 to 16 subcaudal scales down the tail) and the paired cloacal musk glands of females (that may extend up to 6 subcaudal scales). The needle is angled at 45 to 60 degrees and positioned in the ventral midline. The needle is advanced in a craniodorsal direction, with a slight negative pressure maintained. If the needle touches a vertebral body, it should be withdrawn slightly and redirected more craniad or caudad. This vessel is most easily entered in larger snakes, and lymphatic contamination is possible.

With the snake preferably sedated and restrained in dorsal recumbency, the heart is located approximately 22% to 33% from snout to vent. The heart is palpated and immobilized. The needle is advanced at 45 degrees in a craniodorsal direction into the apex of the beating ventricle (Figure 30-84). Blood often enters the syringe with each heartbeat. Digital pressure should be maintained for 30 to 60 seconds after this technique. This technique appears to be safe and is less likely to result in lymphatic contamination. It has been used in snakes of all sizes, from 10-g neonates to 150-kg constrictors. Nevertheless, good restraint is essential, and sedation recommended, if significant cardiac trauma is to be avoided. The palatine-pterygoid veins are easily visualized in the dorsal aspect of the oral cavity of large snakes. However, difficulties with physical restraint, appropriate access, and the prevention of a large hematoma make this technique less acceptable.

Lizards. The most clinically useful vessel is the caudal (tail) vein.[3,5,7,19] The needle is positioned in the ventral midline between 20% and 80% down the tail and advanced at 45 to 90 degrees in a craniodorsal direction, with slight negative pressure maintained (Figure 30-85). If a coccygeal vertebra is

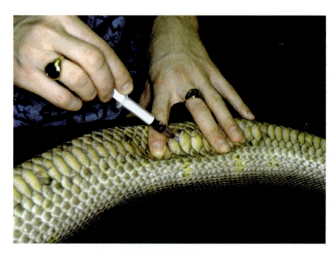

FIGURE 30-84 Blood collection via cardiocentesis in a python. The heart is digitally immobilized before the needle is introduced.

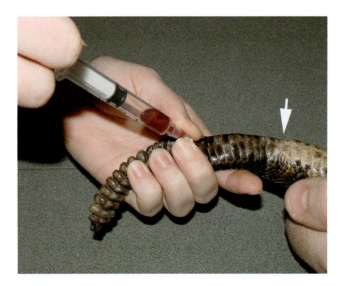

FIGURE 30-83 Blood collection from the caudal (tail) vein of a rattlesnake. Note the position of the needle caudal to cloacal (*arrow*).

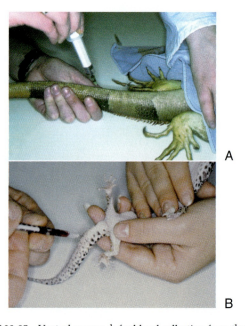

FIGURE 30-85 Ventral approach for blood collection from the caudal (tail) vein of lizards. **A,** Venipuncture in larger lizards, like this Green Iguana (*Iguana iguana*), can be done with the lizard conscious. **B,** Blood collection from small lizards, especially those that perform autotomy, like this Leopard Gecko (*Eublepharis macularius*), is better done with sedation or light anesthesia.

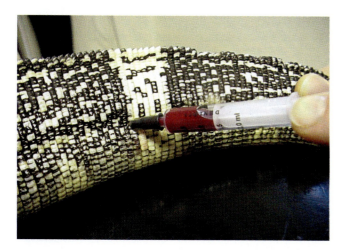

FIGURE 30-86 Lateral approach to the caudal (tail) vein in a large monitor lizard.

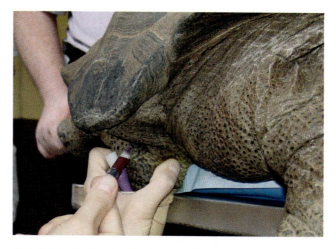

FIGURE 30-87 Blood collection from the dorsal coccygeal vein of an adult Aldabran Tortoise *(Dipsochelys elephantina)*.

encountered, the needle is withdrawn slightly and redirected either further craniad or caudad. An alternative approach that is particularly useful for the larger or more ventrodorsally compressed species is insertion of the needle from the lateral midline (Figure 30-86). The needle is advanced at 45 to 90 degrees in a craniomedial direction, aiming just ventral to the lateral processes of the coccygeal vertebrae. Lymphatic contamination appears more common with the lateral approach.

Lizards possess a large ventral abdominal vein that runs within a suspensory ligament just below the linea alba. This vessel is most easily entered in the caudal coelomic region, cranial to the umbilical scar. The needle is positioned in the ventral midline and advanced in a craniodorsal direction. Apart from the risks of puncture of the gastrointestinal tract or bladder, application of pressure to this vessel is difficult, which makes postvenipuncture hemorrhage a potential complication.

Jugular vein venipuncture is also practical, especially in the larger iguanids and monitor lizards. The jugular veins lie lateral and deep and are seldom visible even when occluded with digital pressure. For most species, the tympanum is a useful anatomic landmark. The lizard is restrained in lateral recumbency, and the clinician inserts the needle in a caudal direction behind the tympanum.

Cardiocentesis in lizards is not as safe as in snakes because the heart cannot be stabilized. Other potential sites include the axillary plexus, orbital sinus, and toe-nail clip, but their use is more problematic, clinically unwarranted, and ethically less acceptable.

Tortoises, Turtles, and Terrapins. The most clinically useful vessels are the jugular, coccygeal, brachial, and subcarapacial veins.[3,7,15,19] Variable species-specific ventral, lateral, and dorsal coccygeal vessels can be used in many chelonia. The dorsal coccygeal vein is probably the most commonly used of the tail veins (Figure 30-87). The needle is angled at 45 to 90 degrees and placed, as craniad as possible, in the dorsal midline of the tail. The needle is advanced in a cranioventral direction, with slight negative pressure maintained. If the needle encounters a vertebra, it is withdrawn slightly and redirected more craniad or caudad. The exact position, size, and even presence of this vessel may vary between species, and a significant risk of lymphatic contamination exists. The left and right jugular veins are preferred because of the greatly reduced

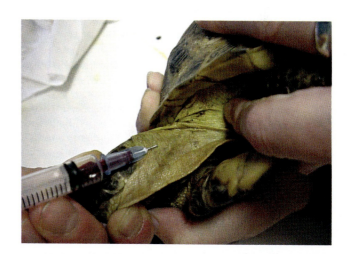

FIGURE 30-88 Blood collection from the jugular vein of a Greek Tortoise *(Testudo graeca)*. Note how the assistant is restraining the forelimbs and occluding the vein at the caudolateral region of the neck.

risk of lymphatic contamination. The regional anatomy varies with species, but the vessel is generally located laterally and may even be visible if temporarily occluded with digital pressure at the base of the neck. The needle is positioned caudal to the tympanum and directed in a caudal direction (Figure 30-88). Postvenipuncture pressure should be applied to prevent hematoma formation.

A subcarapacial site is also available and formed by the venous communication between the most cranial intercostal vessels arising from the paired azygous veins and the caudal cervical anastomosis of the left and right jugular veins. This sinus can be accessed with the chelonian's head either extended or retracted, which makes it useful for uncooperative or aggressive individuals.[20] Depending on the species and conformation of the carapace, the needle may be bent up to 60 degrees and positioned in the midline just caudal to the skin insertion on the ventral aspect of the cranial rim of the carapace (Figure 30-89). The needle is advanced in a caudodorsal direction, with slight negative pressure maintained.

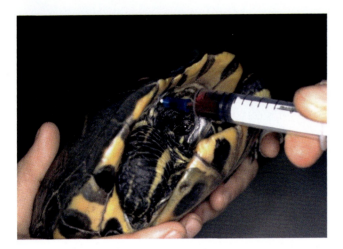

FIGURE 30-89 Blood collection from the subcarapacial site venous sinus (junction of the last caudal anastomosis of the caudal external jugular veins and the cranial intercostal veins) from a Red-eared Slider *(Trachemys scripta elegans)*.

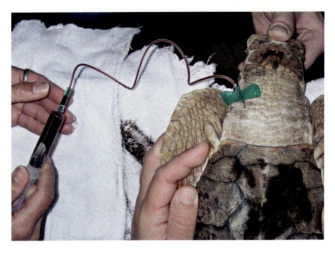

FIGURE 30-90 Blood collection from the dorsal cervical sinus of a juvenile Loggerhead Seaturtle *(Caretta caretta)*.

If a vertebra is encountered, the needle is withdrawn slightly and redirected further craniad or caudad. Lymph contamination appears to be a rare complication.

Cardiocentesis can be achieved in a variety of ways. In those chelonians with soft shells (e.g., Soft-shelled Turtles [*Trionyx* spp.], neonates of most species, and individuals with severe secondary nutritional hyperparathyroidism), a needle can be inserted through the soft plastron directly into the heart. The exact position of the heart varies with species, but it is generally located just dorsal to the plastron, in the midline at the intersection of the abdominal and pectoral scutes. In hard-shelled animals, a temporary osteotomy over the cardiac point of the plastron also permits access to the heart.[15,21] Alternatively, the heart may be approached from a soft tissue approach. The chelonian is held in dorsal recumbency, and on the right side, a point is located midway between the plastron and carapace vertically and between the base of the neck and the shoulder joint horizontally. The needle is inserted at this point and directed toward the junction of the humeral and pectoral scutes.[19]

In seaturtles, the dorsal cervical sinuses are often used (Figure 30-90). Each sinus is located lateral to the cervical vertebrae and is generally easy to access with rare lymphatic contamination.[22] In freshwater turtles the post-occipital sinuses can also be accessed just caudal to the skull. The head should be flexed and the needle inserted just lateral to the dorsal midline.[23] A variety of other venipuncture sites have been discussed, including the brachial and femoral veins and plexuses, orbital sinus, and toe-nail clips. However, they are considered to be of limited or no clinical value.

Crocodilians. The most appropriate venipuncture sites are the caudal (ventral tail) vein in small to medium crocodilians and supravertebral vein in medium to large specimens.[3,7,19] The supravertebral vein is approached with the needle positioned in the dorsal midline, just caudal to the occiput and perpendicular to the surface of the skin (Figure 30-90). The needle is slowly advanced, with slight negative pressure maintained. Excessive penetration may lead to spinal trauma. The technique for caudal (ventral tail) vein access is as

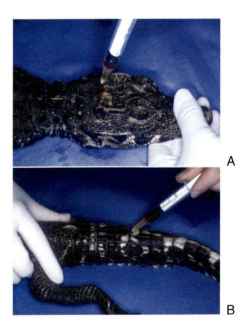

FIGURE 30-91 Venipuncture sites of a West African Dwarf Crocodile *(Osteolaemus tetraspis)*. **A,** Supravertebral venous sinus. **B,** Caudal (ventral tail) vein.

described for lizards (Figure 30-91). The heart is located on the ventral midline, approximately 11 scale rows caudal to the forelimbs. Cardiocentesis in crocodilians is not as safe as in snakes because the heart cannot be stabilized.[19]

Bone Marrow

On occasions bone marrow must be submitted to permit a more detailed hematologic evaluation.[7] The technique for bone marrow collection depends on the size and nature of the reptile. Diagnostic samples can be collected from the femoral or tibial medullary cavities of most lizards, crocodilians, and large chelonians (Figure 30-92). In these reptiles, a suitably sized spinal needle (or hypodermic needle in very small individuals) can be placed into the medullary cavity of the bone

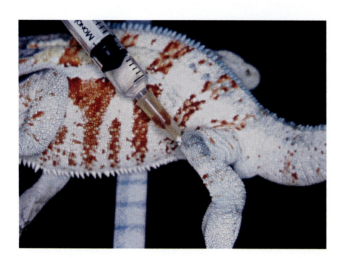

FIGURE 30-92 Bone marrow aspiration from the tibia of a chameleon *(Chamaeleo calyptraptus)* with a hypodermic needle.

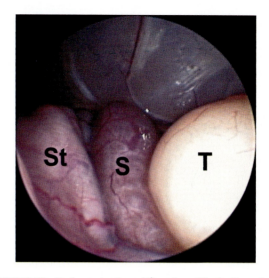

FIGURE 30-94 Endoscopic view of the spleen *(S)* of a Green Iguana *(Iguana iguana)* in preparation for biopsy. Stomach *(St)* and testis *(T)* are also visible.

Hemorrhage has not been a complication, but any damaged intercostal vessels can be sealed with radiosurgery. Depending on the size of the rib and preferences of the histopathologist and hematologist, the entire rib or aspirated marrow may be submitted.

Spleen

The spleen has been cited as an important organ in regards to hemopoietic and lymphopoietic roles, and therefore, biopsies or aspirates may be necessary for further evaluation of hematologic disorders.[24] The spleen varies in size and shape but is usually closely associated with the stomach and pancreas within the dorsal mesentery. In snakes, the spleen and pancreas may be combined into a single splenopancreas organ located approximately 60% to 65% SVL. The spleen can be approached and biopsied in two ways: open surgery and endoscopy. Open surgical biopsy requires a standard coeliotomy approach, whereas endoscopic visualization and biopsy are less invasive and quicker to accomplish (Figure 30-94).[3,7,25] Postbiopsy hemorrhage rarely requires intervention but can be arrested with the use of transendoscopic radiosurgery.

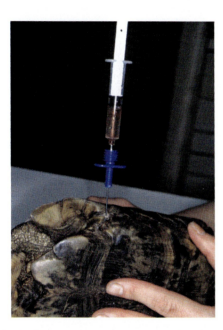

FIGURE 30-93 Bone marrow aspiration from the plastrocarapacial bridge of a tortoise *(Testudo graeca)*.

Cardiovascular Function

There are several means of assessing the cardiovascular system in the examination room, including visual appearance, palpation, and sensitive electrical stethoscopes (Figure 30-95). The detection of abnormal rhythm or rate, and cardiac murmurs, may be appreciated. Further investigation with electrocardiography, diagnostic ultrasound, and radiology is necessary and is dealt with elsewhere (Figure 30-96; see Chapters 14, 29, and 37).

Integument

Dermatologic disease is a frequent presentation, and various levels exist at which the clinician can intervene and collect biologic samples. Shed skin, skin scrapes, impression smears, scale biopsies, and skin biopsies can all be used in the pursuit of a diagnosis.[3,7] The skin and associated structures are perhaps the easiest to sample for laboratory analysis because

and gentle to moderate aspiration used to obtain a sample. An alternative site in chelonia is the plastrocarapacial bridge that laterally connects the plastron and carapace (Figure 30-93). Drilling through the outer layer of keratin and bone to gain access to the medullary cavity and marrow beneath is generally necessary.[7]

In snakes, one must surgically remove and submit a rib for marrow evaluation. A large midbody rib should be selected. A small longitudinal incision is made in the dorsolateral aspect of the body. The rib is palpated and located before cutting the rib as dorsally as possible, close to the epaxial musculature. The lateral muscular attachments are severed in a dorsoventral direction with scissors. The rib is dissected free and elevated through the skin incision.

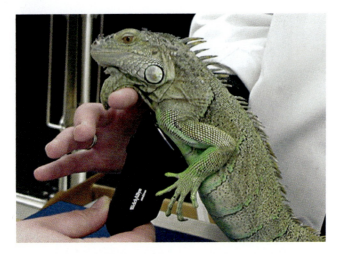

FIGURE 30-95 Auscultation of the heart of a Green Iguana *(Iguana iguana)* with an electronic stethoscope.

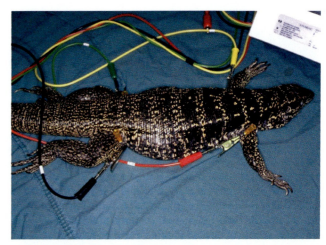

FIGURE 30-96 Electrocardiography of a Tegu Lizard *(Tupinambis teguixin)*. The thick keratinized integument of reptiles often necessitates the use of transcutaneous needles to improve signal strength.

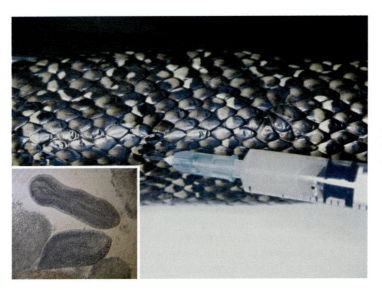

FIGURE 30-97 Fine needle aspiration of a fluctuant cutaneous lesion in a Florida Kingsnake *(Lampropeltis getula)*. *Inset,* Microscopic examination revealed numerous flukes.

of their accessibility (Figure 30-97). However, they can also be the most demanding to interpret because contamination and secondary changes often mask the underlying primary cause. For example, impression smear cytology and bacterial culture may diagnose a severe *Pseudomonas* sp. dermatitis but miss the underlying burn that caused the initial skin damage that facilitated infection. Alternatively, normal and diseased skin often becomes contaminated from fecal Enterobacteriaceae. Therefore, correct sampling and cautious interpretation of microbiologic findings are vital.

Ectoparasites

Various ectoparasites may be clearly seen on the surface of the skin, around nostrils, eyes, and skin folds.[3,7] Mites, ticks, lice, maggots, and flies can often be physically removed and submitted in specimen containers for taxonomic identification.[26] The shed skin of reptiles is also a valuable asset and should be inspected for evidence of parasitism. Suspected mites can be collected directly from the reptile with a wet cotton-tipped applicator and transferred to a microscope slide for closer inspection and identification (Figure 30-98).

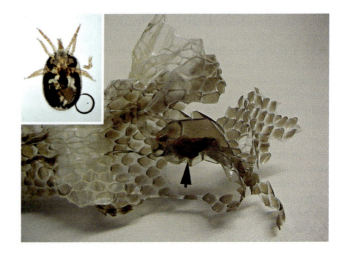

FIGURE 30-98 Shed skin from a snake with severe mite infestation and self-inflicted wounds from intense pruritus. One of these lesions can be appreciated from abnormal slough *(arrow)*. *Inset,* Common snake mite, *Ophionyssus natricis*, recovered from shed skin.

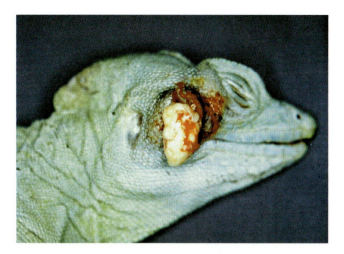

FIGURE 30-99 Facial abscess of a Plumed Basilisk (*Basiliscus plumifrons*). Microbiologic cultures are frequently more rewarding when collected from the peripheral pyogenic capsule rather than from the caseous debris.

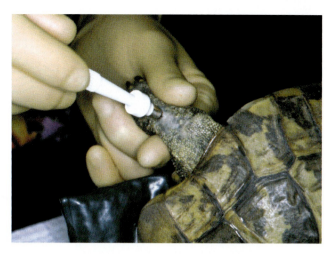

FIGURE 30-101 Skin punch biopsy being taken from the limb of a tortoise.

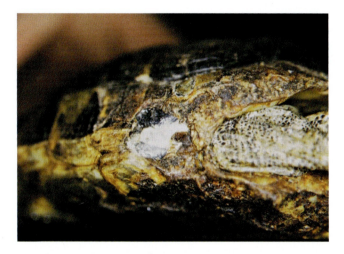

FIGURE 30-100 Scraping a dry skin lesion, such as this mycotic dermatitis of a tortoise, produces material for cytologic and microbiologic investigations.

Skin Scrapes and Impression Smears

Skin lesions are frequently contaminated, and therefore, superficial sampling may not show the primary cause or agent by the time the reptile is presented. Skin lesions are best cleaned and partially debrided with aseptic techniques before the collection of clinical samples.[3,7] Microbiologic swabs should be taken from the periphery of the lesion but deep to any exposed areas (Figure 30-99). Impression smears can be taken after the lesion has been cleaned with sterile saline solution and gently dabbed dry with sterile gauze. Skin scrapes may be useful especially when dealing with drier more proliferative lesions (Figure 30-100). Samples may be prepared for immediate microscopy or submitted to an external laboratory.

Scale and Skin Biopsies

When a skin biopsy is required, the removal of a single scale may be all that is necessary because scales contain both epidermal and dermal elements. A small volume (0.02 to 0.1 mL) of local analgesic (e.g., 2% lidocaine) is injected subcutaneously in the area of interest. With aseptic techniques, a single scale is then elevated and cut close to its insertion with a scalpel blade. If a larger sample is necessary, then a combination of local, regional, or general anesthesia and sharp excision or skin punch biopsy instrument is effective (Figure 30-101).[3,7] A single suture closes the deficit. Biopsy of the chelonian shell requires general anesthesia and cortical biopsy devices (see bone and shell biopsy, musculoskeletal system).

RESPIRATORY SYSTEM

The respiratory system can be conveniently divided into upper and lower respiratory tracts. The upper respiratory tract consists of the nares, buccal cavity, glottis, and trachea, and the lower respiratory tract consists of the bronchi, lung, and, where present, air sac. Very little is found in the way of tubular subdivision into secondary bronchi, bronchioles, and alveoli, as in mammals. The reptilian lung is more reticulated with a large central cavity, although chelonia are an exception because they possess a more three-dimensional, sponge-like lung.[3,27]

Abnormal respiration is a common presentation, and some of these cases are the result of true disease, but many are associated with poor environments that resolve with husbandry improvements. The ability to diagnose pathologic changes within the respiratory system of reptiles is relatively straightforward if reliance is placed on the use of lung lavage for the collection of cytologic and microbiologic samples.[3,7] The collection of tissue biopsies requires anesthesia and surgical or endoscopic techniques and are to be preferred.[24,28,29]

Nares, Glottis, and Cranial Trachea

The upper respiratory tract, including the nares, buccal cavity, glottis, and cranial trachea, can be visualized and often sampled directly without anesthesia. Small-diameter swabs permit the collection of samples, although the greatest concern comes from bacterial contamination by oral commensals,

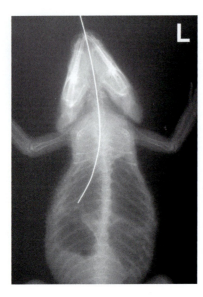

FIGURE 30-102 Radiograph of a Bearded Dragon *(Pogona vitticeps)* shows placement of a lung lavage catheter into the right lung. Note the consolidation and reduction of the right lung field indicating possible disease.

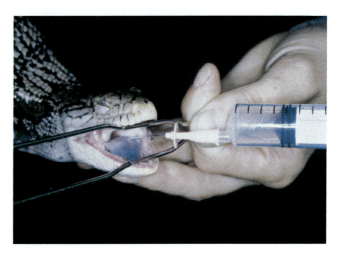

FIGURE 30-103 Lung lavage of a New Guinea Blue-tongued Skink *(Tiliqua gigas)*.

which include gram-negatives and anaerobes. Swabs can be submitted for microbiology or rolled onto glass slides for staining and cytologic evaluation.

Caudal Trachea and Lung Lavage

The simplest method of obtaining a representative sample from the lower respiratory tract is via lavage.[3,7] Although a lung wash or lavage can be performed in the conscious reptile, the discomfort of such a procedure may warrant some degree of sedation or light anesthesia. In addition, general anesthesia and intubation using a sterile endotracheal tube will further reduce the chances of oral contamination of the sample. A sterile catheter of appropriate size is placed through the glottis, with great care taken not to touch the oral membranes. The catheter is advanced down the trachea and into the lung. In snakes, the catheter is advanced caudal to the heart (>30% SVL), but in large specimens, the catheter may not reach the lung and a tracheal lavage is performed. In lizards, the catheter is advanced to a point just caudal to the forelimbs, and in chelonia, a central position appears most appropriate. In lizards and chelonia, the catheter can be preferentially directed into either the left or right lung with insertion of a sterile metal stylet down the catheter before introduction. The catheter and stylet is then given a gentle bend to facilitate introduction into the left or right lung. Proper positioning of the stylet and catheter can be confirmed with radiography (Figure 30-102). Once in place, 0.5 to 1 mL of sterile saline per 100 g of bodyweight can be infused. Sample recovery is often aided with rotation of the animal and repeated aspiration (Figure 30-103). In snakes, lifting of the head and tail also helps accumulate fluid at the dependent area, near the catheter tip.

In chelonia, a unilateral lung wash can also be obtained via a long fine hypodermic needle. The needle is positioned in the dorsocranial area of the prefemoral fossa and directed dorsomedially. Aspiration of air confirms entry into the lung before lavage. Similar techniques are possible in lizards and snakes, but anesthesia and lung inflation are usually necessary. Dependent on the volume and quality of the sample obtained, material should be divided and submitted as requested by the laboratory. The submission of fresh and fixed material, multiple air-dried smears, and a microbiologic swab permits detailed investigation.

Lung Biopsy

Lavage samples do not permit an appreciation of lung architecture. For this, and other histopathologic examinations, tissue biopsies are preferred. Surgical access to the lung can be achieved with a standard coeliotomy because no functional diaphragm exists nor does concern for the maintenance of pleural negative pressure in most squamates.[3,7] In snakes, the respiratory active anterior part of the lung is typically located between 12% and 45% SVL. However, great species variation exists with regards to lung anatomy, including the presence of a tracheal lung in some elapids and viperids, both left and right lungs in boids, and only a right lung in most other snakes.

Biopsy of the anterior lung commonly results in hemorrhage unless appropriate hemostatic measures are taken. Biopsy of the thinner posterior lung (or air sac) is not complicated by hemorrhage, although closing the thin pulmonary membrane without tearing can be challenging. In lizards, the anterior lung is also more highly vascularized than the posterior areas. A cranial coeliotomy, close to the xiphoid process of the sternum, may permit sufficient exposure; otherwise, a lateral approach between ribs may offer better exposure for biopsy of the anterior lung. The Tuatara, some varanids, and crocodilians possess a pseudodiaphragm that should be respected and, if surgically breached, sutured close before closure of the coelom. In chelonia, the lungs are protected by the carapace, which makes surgical access more difficult. Creation of a 4-mm to 5-mm temporary osteotomy in the carapace, over the lung area of interest, does not give sufficient exposure for an excisional biopsy but does permit the collection of a Tru-Cut biopsy (Figures 30-104 and 30-105).[30] The osteotomy can then be closed with acrylic or epoxy.

Diagnostic Techniques

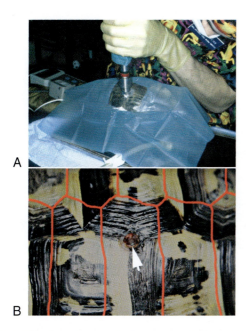

FIGURE 30-104 Lung biopsy of a tortoise. **A,** Drilling a temporary osteotomy in the carapace to gain access to the diseased lung. **B,** The general area of interest is determined with radiography, but the osteotomy site should be through a bone plate at the intersection of the keratin scutes *(arrow)* and not through the peripheral growth plates *(outlined in red)*.

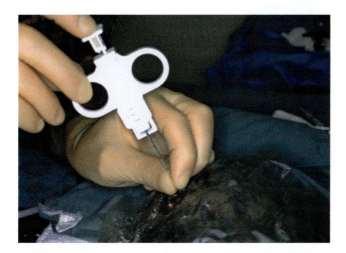

FIGURE 30-105 A Tru-Cut lung biopsy of a tortoise's lung after a temporary osteotomy.

Alternatively, an intrapneumonic catheter can be secured in the osteotomy site to permit continued local therapy.[29] A ventral coeliotomy is not recommended in some chelonians because the septum horizontale (the membrane that divides the lungs from the remaining viscera) is deep to the coelomic viscera and again should be repaired if surgically incised or penetrated in any way.

Endoscopic Biopsy

The use of small rigid telescopes and fine flexible fiberscopes permits endoscopic access to, and biopsy of, lung tissue in most reptiles (Figure 30-106).[28,29] The use of 3F to 5F biopsy

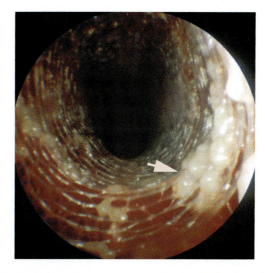

FIGURE 30-106 Endoscopic view of a Royal or Ball Python *(Python regius)* with granulomatous pneumonia *(arrow)*. The diagnosis of pulmonary mycobacteriosis was made after a biopsy as lung lavage proved unrewarding.

instruments permits the collection of tissue samples from reptiles as small as 100 g without deleterious effects. Small biopsies are best submitted in histology filters to avoid loss during transportation and processing. The submission of (digitally captured endoscopy) images of the lesion with the biopsies greatly assists the pathologist in histologic interpretation.

A variety of other sampling devices are also available, including brush biopsy instruments and remote aspiration needles that can also be used deep within the respiratory system to obtain diagnostic material.

The lung of most snakes can be accessed via a tracheal approach. In large constrictors of more than 3 m, reaching the lung via an oral approach may be impossible. In these cases, surgical access to the lung (as described for snake excisional lung biopsy) permits the entry of the endoscope for examination and biopsy both cranial and caudal to the entry point (see Chapter 32). In some lizards, the lungs can be reached via the trachea because the bronchi are often short and easily negotiated. However, with the exception of large seaturtles, the short trachea and long narrow bronchi make entry into the chelonian lung extremely difficult via an oral approach. Endoscopic entry to the lungs can be achieved via a carapacial osteotomy (as described for chelonian lung biopsy) or a prefemoral approach.[29] The prefemoral approach to the lung requires a small incision in the craniodorsal aspect of the prefemoral fossa and identification of the septum horizontale. Retaining sutures are placed through this membrane to elevate it close to the skin incision. A small incision in this membrane permits the entry of the scope and examination of the lung as far craniad as the bronchial opening. Closure of the septum horizontale after biopsy is important to prevent pneumocoelom.

GASTROINTESTINAL SYSTEM

In cases of severe diarrhea or regurgitation, material for laboratory submission is usually available and may be collected

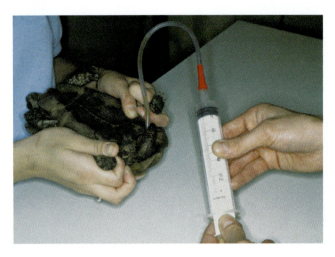

FIGURE 30-107 Cloacocolonic lavage of a conscious *Testudo* tortoise with a flexible catheter.

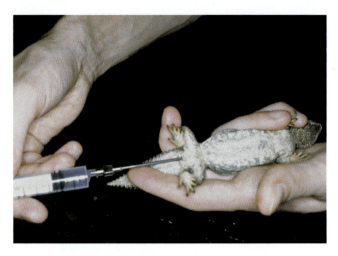

FIGURE 30-108 Cloacocolonic lavage of a small *Uromastyx* lizard with a metal ball-tipped needle.

and presented along with the animal by well-educated owners or keepers. In addition, many reptiles spontaneously defecate and urinate when handled during the examination process. It is important to appreciate that, like birds, the stools of reptiles are composed of fecal, urate, and urine components and that the cloaca is a common chamber for the gastrointestinal, urinary, and reproductive systems.

For example, watery stools from polyuria must be differentiated from true diarrhea, and cloacal bleeding may be intestinal, reproductive, or urinary in origin. Fecal material can be submitted for a variety of parasitologic, cytologic, and microbiologic tests.[3,7,19] The submission of only fecal material in appropriate sterile containers prevents further mixing and contamination by urates and urine during transportation and processing. Microbiologic results from deposited feces should be interpreted with caution because contamination from other organ systems can occur in the cloacal proctodeum before elimination and environmental contamination invariably occurs after elimination.[19] The fresher the material, the more meaningful the laboratory results, although some parasitologic investigations (e.g., helminth egg examination) can be performed on refrigerated material up to 4 weeks or more after elimination.[30]

Cloacocolonic Lavage

Unfortunately, the slow intestinal transit times of most reptiles often necessitate a more direct approach to obtaining material, especially if the animal has been anorectic for several weeks and the intestinal tract is largely empty. A cloacocolonic lavage can be performed on most conscious reptiles and provides the clinician with a diagnostic sample (Figures 30-107 and 30-108). A sterile lubricated round-tipped catheter is inserted into the cloaca and directed craniad toward the colon. A relatively large catheter should be used because this helps prevent kinking of the tube and reduces the risks of perforating the thin intestinal wall. On no account should the catheter be forced. Once in place, 0.5 to 1 mL of sterile saline solution per 100 g of body weight should be gently infused through the catheter and repeatedly aspirated until a sample is obtained. Infusion of an additional 1 mL/100 g is possible if no sample is forthcoming.

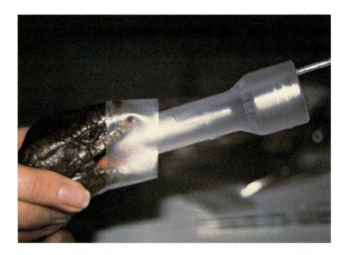

FIGURE 30-109 Gastric lavage of a conscious Solomon Island Skink (*Corucia zebrata*). The cut-off syringe casing acts as a mouth gag and protects the lavage catheter.

The direct collection of fecal material from the distal colon with a lubricated gloved hand offers another practical option in large reptiles (see Figure 30-27).

Gastric Lavage

A similar technique to cloacocolonic lavage can be used to collect samples from the stomach. A relatively large, round-tipped catheter can be inserted into the stomach of most conscious reptiles. In crocodilians, lizards, and chelonia, use of a mouth gag is wise to prevent damage to the tube (Figure 30-109). The catheter should pass to the midcoelomic region before instillation of 0.5 to 1 mL of sterile saline solution per 100 g of body weight.[3] In large snakes, reaching the stomach may not be possible, in which case esophageal lavage is a more appropriate term. Such samples can be examined as a fresh wet preparation for parasites or stained to show microorganisms.[7] Microbiologic cultures are often worthy, but care is necessary in their interpretation because

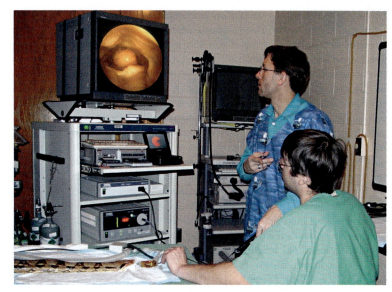

FIGURE 30-110 Gastroscopy of a Boa Constrictor *(Boa constrictor)*.

contamination from the respiratory system and oral cavity is possible.

Gastroscopy and Biopsy

For the collection of gastric or intestinal biopsy specimens, standard coeliotomy and excisional biopsies can be undertaken, but endoscopy is less invasive and preferred (Figure 30-110).[3,7,25] In lizards and chelonians, endoscopic access to the stomach is straightforward, but negotiation of the pylorus and entering of the duodenum can be more difficult. In snakes, the small intestine can be readily entered via the gastric pylorus. Endoscopic biopsy of the large bowel is unwise because the intestinal wall is often thin and easily perforated. Even excisional biopsies of the large intestine can be challenging to ensure adequate closure and prevent leakage (see Chapter 35).

Liver Biopsy

Blood biochemistry, radiography, ultrasonography, and endoscopy may indicate the existence of hepatopathy, but they seldom provide the definitive diagnosis. Liver biopsy remains a most powerful tool for conclusively reaching a diagnosis, indicating specific therapies, and providing a more accurate prognosis. Biopsies may be collected for histopathology and microbiology. Liver samples may be collected percutaneously (with or without ultrasound guidance), surgically, or endoscopically.[31-33] Surgical approaches generally rely on a standard coeliotomy approach to the liver, which in snakes usually results in only a small part of the organ being visible and available for biopsy. Biopsies are best collected with ligation or wedge techniques to avoid postbiopsy hemorrhage. Endoscopic techniques are typically less invasive, permit closer examination of more of the organ, and enable the collection of multiple biopsies (Figure 30-111). Correlations between biochemical tests and histopathology are generally lacking, but serial blood sampling and biopsy currently offer the best diagnostic and monitoring approach to hepatic disease.

Pancreatic Biopsy

The identification of diabetes mellitus should not rely solely on blood glucose values because blood glucose can vary dramatically from stress and handling (see Chapter 58). Therefore, the diagnosis should also rely on the histopathologic demonstration of disease after endoscopic pancreatic biopsy. Likewise, elevations of blood amylase levels should also be viewed cautiously unless histologic confirmation is obtained.

MUSCULOSKELETAL SYSTEM

Despite clinical emphasis on osteomyelitis and secondary nutritional hyperparathyroidism, a variety of other skeletal abnormalities can affect reptiles.[7] The ability to obtain bone material for histologic and microbiologic interpretation greatly aids our understanding and ability to advise on appropriate treatments for these conditions.

Bone and Shell Biopsy

Proliferative and lytic lesions that affect the axial and appendicular skeleton of lizards and snakes are not uncommon.[3,7,34] The radiographic interpretation seldom provides a definitive pathologic diagnosis. The use of cortical bone biopsy instruments designed for humans (e.g., Jamshidi) can also be used for reptiles (Figure 30-112). Care is required not to cause excessive damage and risk fracture, but generally, excellent samples can be obtained with only minor surgical exposure. In very small specimens, a hypodermic needle can be used to obtain a core of bone. This bone core can then be expelled from the needle with insertion of wire through the needle hub. Shell disease of chelonians is also common, and these same cortical biopsy instruments or a Michelle trephine can be used (Figure 30-113).[3,7,15] Care is required to ensure that only a small length of the instrument is exposed so that overly deep penetration into the coelom does not occur.

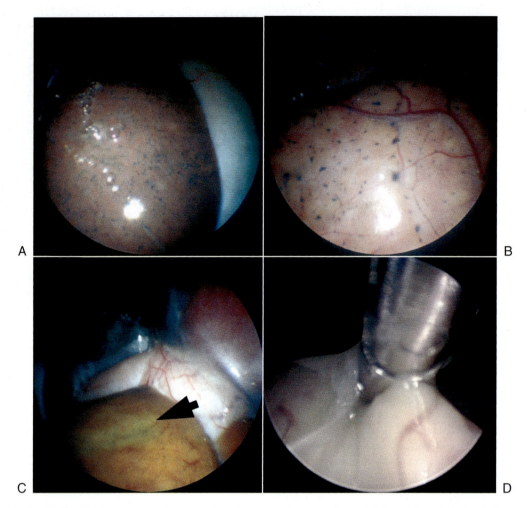

FIGURE 30-111 Endoscopic examination and biopsy of the chelonian liver. **A,** Normal liver in a Greek Tortoise *(Testudo graeca)* shows multifocal pigmentated areas of melanomacrophage aggregation. **B,** Diffusely pale liver in a male Hermann's Tortoise *(Testudo hermanni)* from hepatic lipidosis. **C,** Pale area in the liver of a Leopard Tortoise *(Geochelone pardalis)* from focal bacterial hepatitis *(arrow)*. **D,** Liver biopsy of a juvenile Loggerhead Seaturtle *(Caretta caretta)*.

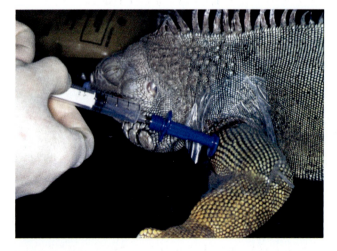

FIGURE 30-112 Cortical bone biopsy in a Green Iguana *(Iguana iguana)*.

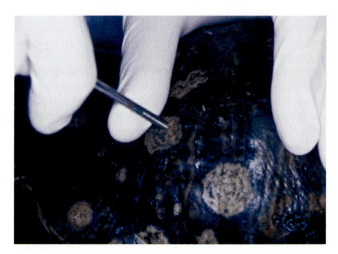

FIGURE 30-113 Full-thickness shell biopsy of the carapace of a *Testudo* tortoise.

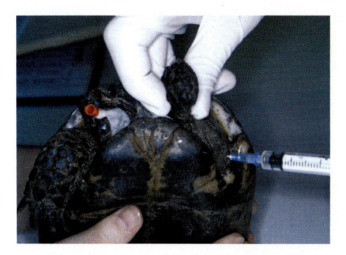

FIGURE 30-114 Scapulohumeral joint aspiration of a *Testudo* tortoise.

Acrylic or epoxy can be used to seal the biopsy site unless obvious infection is present. Septic arthritis is commonly reported after bite wounds to the joints of lizards and tortoises. After aseptic preparation of the area, fine needle aspiration permits the collection of samples for microbiologic and cytologic diagnosis (Figure 30-114).

Muscle Biopsy

Most cases of muscle wastage or weakness are related to nutrition or debilitating disease, but if warranted, muscle biopsies may be collected for histopathologic investigations.[35] The largest affected muscle masses should be selected because many reptiles, especially chameleons and other small lizards, have limited musculature. Surgical exposure of the muscle and longitudinal separation of a number of fibers permit ligation with fine absorbable material at the proximal and distal margins of the biopsy. Sharp excision permits removal of the biopsy. Hemostasis with ligation is preferred over radiosurgery or laser because of the coagulation artifacts that are produced.

URINARY SYSTEM

Diseases of the urinary system can include the kidneys, ureters, urethra, cloaca, and, if present, the bladder.[3,7] In addition to the kidneys, the bladder, cloaca, posterior colon, and remote salt glands can all play important roles in osmoregulation and should be considered part of the osmoregulatory system of reptiles.[36-38] The clinician may assess the osmoregulatory system of reptiles with sampling urine and biopsies from the kidney, bladder, and cloaca.[3,7,39] Ancillary structures such as salt glands are seldom biopsied, although their secretions can often be collected from the reptile's nares or the glass surfaces of enclosures.

Urine

Urinalysis is less helpful in reptiles than in mammals. The reptilian kidney cannot concentrate urine, and so urine specific gravity is of limited use in the assessment of renal function (see Chapter 66).[36] Furthermore, renal urine passes through the urodeum of the cloaca before entering the bladder (or posterior colon in those species that lack a bladder). Bladder urine is therefore not necessarily sterile. The clinical picture is further complicated by the fact that electrolyte and water changes can occur across the bladder or cloacocolonic mucosa.[36] Despite these biochemical drawbacks, urine samples are useful for cytologic assessments of inflammation and infection and for the identification of renal casts.[39-41]

Voided Urine

The urinary, genital, and intestinal tracts empty into a common cloaca, and therefore, any samples voided from the cloaca may represent material derived from, or contaminated by, any of these systems. Voided urine and urates, although useful for cytology, must be critically evaluated whenever a culture is obtained. Urine microbiology must be even more critically judged if the sample was collected from the floor of the enclosure or the examination table. Fresh urine and urate samples can be collected as a free catch. Many reptiles spontaneously void urine and urates (often with fecal material) when handled. More stoic individuals may be encouraged to urinate with gentle digital stimulation of the cloaca.

Cystocentesis

A more representative and less contaminated sample may be collected using cystocentesis in chelonians and those lizards that possess a bladder. However, given the thin fragile nature of the reptilian bladder, the potential danger of postsampling leakage of unsterile urine into the coelom exists. Given the passage of urine through the cloaca and the electrolyte and water changes that can occur in the bladder, urine collected by cystocentesis may not be representative of renal urine with respect to electrolyte composition and osmolarity. Such samples are often unsterile, although a heavy pure microbiologic growth should alert the clinician to potential infection.

Catheterization

One means of obtaining bladder urine without puncturing the bladder is with the placement of a urethral catheter, blind or with the assistance of an endoscope. This procedure has been used in anesthetized tortoises and lizards. Care must be taken not to damage the thin bladder wall. The indwelling catheter can be used to collect fresh urine and empty the bladder.

Renal Biopsy

A variety of infectious, degenerative, and neoplastic renal diseases have been reported in reptiles.[7,42] The poor regenerative capabilities of the kidney make early diagnosis of paramount importance. The relatively poor diagnostic value of urinalysis and the late detection of renal disease using blood biochemistry further exemplify the importance of renal biopsy early in the diagnostic process. The cranial tail cutdown and minimally invasive coeliotomy biopsy techniques permit unilateral access to a single kidney. In these cases, cloacal and coelomic palpation, radiography (including intravenous urography), and ultrasonography can be used to determine whether a left or right approach is most appropriate. Major coeliotomy, ultrasound-guided, and endoscopic

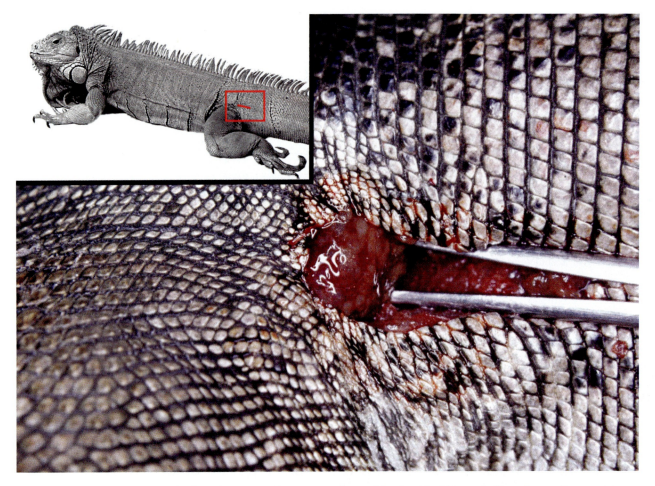

FIGURE 30-115 Cranial tail cut-down procedure to expose the caudal pole of the kidney of a Green Iguana (*Iguana iguana*). *Inset*, Anatomic orientation to the surgical approach.

biopsy procedures can be used to examine and biopsy either or both kidneys.

Cranial Tail Cut-Down Biopsy

A relatively simple technique for biopsy of the intrapelvic kidneys of iguanas requires a cranial tail cut-down with local or general anesthesia.[43] A small longitudinal incision is made in the lateral midline just below the lateral processes of the coccygeal vertebrae. The incision extends for 1 to 3 cm caudad, starting just behind the hindlimb. Blunt dissection between the dorsal and ventral coccygeal muscles permits exposure of the caudolateral aspect of the kidney that can then be sampled (Figure 30-115). Hemorrhage depends on the size of the biopsy, but the temporary application of hemostatic dressings or radiosurgery is effective. This technique is particularly valuable with diffuse renal disease where the kidneys are not enlarged and coelomic approaches to the intrapelvic kidneys are more difficult. It is limited to unilateral biopsy unless bilateral cut-down procedures are undertaken. Furthermore, because only a small area of kidney can be visualized and sampled from, multifocal renal diseases may be missed.

Coeliotomy Biopsy

Where renomegaly is obvious, a coelomic entry and biopsy can be undertaken.[3,39] A standard midline or paramedian coeliotomy enables both kidneys to be assessed in lizards, and excisional or Tru-Cut biopsies can be collected (Figure 30-116). In snakes, the elongated left and right kidneys overlap for a short distance, and coeliotomy and renal biopsy are readily

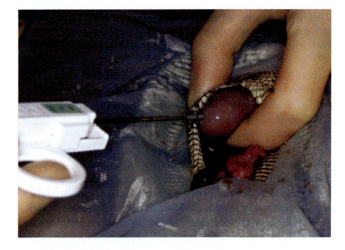

FIGURE 30-116 A Tru-Cut renal biopsy during a standard coeliotomy of a Green Iguana (*Iguana iguana*).

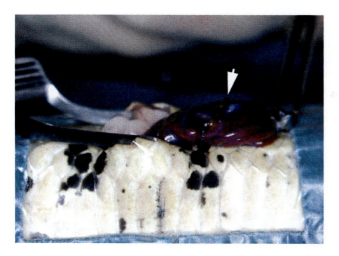

FIGURE 30-117 Renal biopsy of a *Boa constrictor* after a standard coeliotomy. In this case, vascular Hemoclips *(arrow)* have been used to isolate a small kidney lobule before sharp excision.

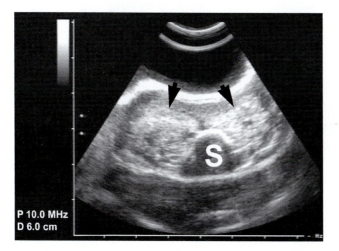

FIGURE 30-118 Ultrasound examination of a Savannah Monitor Lizard *(Varanus exanthematicus)* in preparation for a renal biopsy. Note the two kidneys *(arrows)* separated by the spine *(S)*.

accomplished (Figure 30-117). If an enlarged kidney can be palpated, it can usually be immobilized just under the skin, permitting the use of a Tru-Cut needle biopsy or minimally invasive coeliotomy incision directly over the organ. This technique is suited to the detection of diffuse renal diseases because multifocal diseases may be missed.

Ultrasound-Guided Biopsy

Ultrasound-guided biopsies are useful for coelomic kidneys but are difficult to obtain from intrapelvic tissue.[38] Although ultrasound imaging may permit the identification of gross lesions and aid biopsy needle guidance, dangers are still associated with a technique that does not provide direct three-dimensional visual control (Figure 30-118). In particular, the voluminous bladder, gastrointestinal tract, dorsal aorta, eight to 12 paired renal arteries, efferent renal veins, afferent renal veins, and paired renal veins must be appreciated and avoided. Depending on the quality of the equipment and skill of the ultrasonographer, multifocal or focal lesions may be missed.

Endoscopic Biopsy

The endoscope permits evaluation of the size, color, and shape of both coelomic kidneys via a single surgical entry. The use of endoscopic scissors and biopsy forceps with direct visual control permits the incision of the renal capsule and collection of quality samples with less risk to surrounding structures (Figure 30-119).[44] The excellent optics of the telescope also facilitates an assessment of focal and multifocal disease and the selection of appropriate biopsy sites that may be difficult to ascertain without a real-life, color, magnified image.[24,38]

Bladder Biopsy

The bladder performs important osmoregulatory functions in many reptiles, and biopsy may be necessary for an overall assessment of osmoregulatory function. Proliferative masses of the bladder can also be biopsied to aid identification and direct treatment plans.

Endoscopic Biopsy

Endoscopic entry into the bladder of larger lizards and chelonia has been accomplished with practice. However, endoscopic biopsy of the bladder is not recommended for anything other than grossly proliferative lesions because major dangers are associated with cystic perforation and leakage of unsterile urine and urates into the coelom.

Excisional Biopsy

Surgical excisional biopsy is preferred in most cases because of the importance of preventing postbiopsy leakage. No ureteral connections exist to the bladder, and so bladder biopsies can be collected from almost any site. However, care should be taken to maintain the neural and vascular supplies and avoid the urethra. The technique is similar to that used in mammals, although a double layer enclosure is more difficult because of the very thin nature of the bladder wall. To ensure a waterproof seal, the incision should be closed with an approximating continuous or simple interrupted pattern, followed by a second inverting pattern.

Cloacocolonic Biopsy

Biopsies of the cloacocolonic region may be necessary for a complete assessment of osmoregulatory function, especially in those species that lack a bladder. Because of the intrapelvic position of the coprodeum and urodeum in most reptiles, endoscopic examination and mucosa biopsy are preferred. The cloacal wall tends to be relatively thick, and perforation is unlikely. Nevertheless, care must be taken to identify and avoid the urogenital papillae and oviductal openings within the urodeum. Endoscopic biopsy of the colon is not recommended because the intestinal wall is often thin and prone to perforation.

Renal Function Evaluation

Recently, the use of iohexol excretion studies has been validated in the Green Iguana as a means of measuring

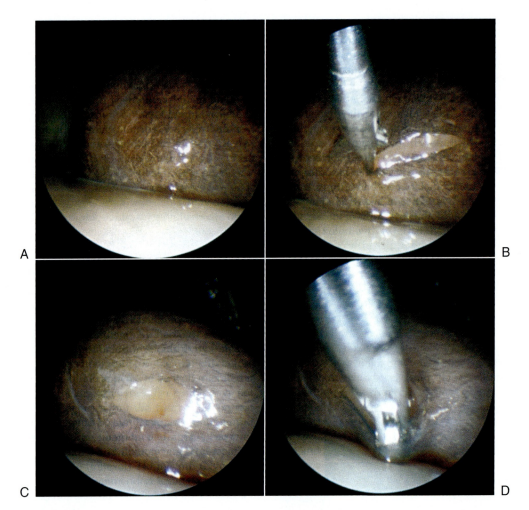

FIGURE 30-119 Endoscopic evaluation and biopsy of an iguanid kidney. **A,** Endoscopic view of an iguanid kidney. **B,** Endoscopic scissors inserted down the instrument channel of the endoscopic sheath into the field of view and used to incise the renal capsule. **C,** The scissors are withdrawn, and the incised capsule reveals renal parenchyma below. **D,** Biopsy forceps inserted into view and through the capsular incision to collect a tissue sample.

glomerular filtration rate and hence renal function (see Chapter 66).[17] A recent study validated this methodology in reptiles where the glomerular filtration rate of healthy iguanas was reported as 16.56 ± 3.90 ml/kg/hr, with a 95% confidence interval of 14.78–18.34 ml/kg/hr. In addition, iguanas with renal disease exhibited significant reductions in GFR even in the absence of other clinical or biochemical signs. A suggested protocol for measuring GFR in iguanas (and potentially other reptiles) is as follows:

1. Contact the Diagnostic Center for Population and Animal Health (Michigan State University, East Lansing, Mich, 48824, USA; Tel 517-353-1683, www.ahdl.msu.edu) to check for any changes to the blood collection and submission requirements for iohexol assay and GFR calculation.
2. Ensure the reptile is hydrated and fasted for 24 hr.
3. Weigh accurately and inject 75 mg/kg iohexol intravenously (intravenous catheterization reduces the risks of perivascular injection that would invalidate the results) at time 0.
4. Collect three 0.5 mL blood samples at 4 hr, 8 hr, and 24 hr post-injection. Record the exact times of blood collection, and send these details with the three separated plasma samples on ice to the Diagnostic Center for Population and Animal Health for iohexol assays and GFR calculation.

Unlike most other clearance techniques, iohexol excretion does not require bladder or ureteral catheterization and, unlike scintigraphy, it does not require expensive equipment or radioisotopes to perform. Given that iohexol assays are commercially available, this technique for renal function evaluation in reptiles can be easily undertaken in private practice.

REPRODUCTIVE SYSTEM

Antemortem pathologic assessment of the reproductive system has not been undertaken to a large degree. However, the advent of minimally invasive endoscopic techniques has brought about an increase in genital evaluation and sampling.

Phallus and Hemipenes

The phallus of chelonians and crocodilians and the hemipenes of squamates may become infected or traumatized

Diagnostic Techniques

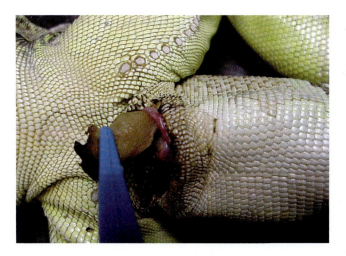

FIGURE 30-120 Removal of a hemipenal plug from a mature male Green Iguana (*Iguana iguana*).

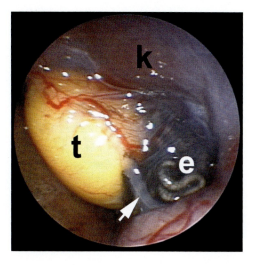

FIGURE 30-121 Endoscopic view of the kidney (*k*), testis (*t*), epididymis (*e*), and vas deferens (*arrow*) of a male tortoise in preparation for gonadal biopsy.

(see Figure 30-76).[3,7] Phallic prolapse is not uncommon, and impression smear cytology and culture may indicate primary or secondary infectious causes that need to be addressed once the organ has been replaced. Where the hemipenes are retracted, a small sterile lubricated catheter can be inserted into the hemipenal sulcus and aspiration or lavage procedures can provide material for cytology and cultures.

In some cases, such an accumulation of cellular debris can exist that a hemipenal "plug" forms that can be removed from the sulcus with forceps (Figure 30-120). The cytologic evaluation of hemipenal material may aid the investigation of male infertility by examining for the presence of spermatozoa and petroleum-based spermicidal lubricants, which may have been previously used for gender determination by probing.

Cloacal (Musk) Glands

The cloacal or musk glands of snakes connect to the cloaca and may on occasions become impacted and infected. Material can often be expressed from these areas manually in the conscious snake, or swabs and lavage techniques can be used for the collection of diagnostic samples.

Oviducts and Vas Deferens

A detailed knowledge of cloacal anatomy and proficiency in endoscopic techniques can facilitate examination of the oviduct. Catheterization of the vas deferens may also be possible and may aid the investigation of male infertility.

Gonads

The gonads of reptiles can be approached using traditional surgery or via endoscopy. The endoscopic identification of gonads has been used as an aid to controlled reproduction and breeding.[25] Testicular biopsy has been used as an aid in the assessment of male infertility in lizards and chelonia (Figure 30-121). Biopsy of the active ovary is not recommended because of the dangers of yolk leakage and coelomitis. Biopsies have been taken from inactive and diseased ovaries without incident.

NERVOUS SYSTEM AND SPECIAL SENSES

The increasing interest in neurologic diseases has led to the pursuit of improvements in neurologic assessment and antemortem sampling techniques.[3] Previously, cytologic or histopathologic assessment of the nervous system was only possible with necropsy, although investigations in the live reptile are still quite limited.

Cerebrospinal Fluid

Some debate exists concerning the anatomy of the reptilian spine and spinal cord. Arguments have been made that reptiles lack a subarachnoid space and therefore cerebrospinal fluid (CSF) collection (and the reptilian equivalent of mammalian myelography) is not possible.[3] Nevertheless, others have used various cervical and lumbar tap techniques in snakes and lizards to obtain CSF samples (and perform spinal contrast studies) in a limited number of cases.[45-47] Obviously awareness of the potential misidentification and misinterpretation of lymph as CSF is important.

The technique is essentially similar to that used in mammals, with emphasis on proper positioning and accurate anatomical knowledge (Figure 30-122). The anesthetized lizard is placed in sternal recumbency with the head and neck maximally flexed. After aseptic preparation of the dorsal neck and lateral retraction of the dorsal crest, the spinal processes of the cervical vertebrae can be palpated. Careful advancement of the needle between C1 and C2 permits the collection of a small volume of CSF. CSF has been collected from the cervical region of lizards, snakes, and chelonians and from the lumbar region of lizards (Figure 30-123).

Strict asepsis is essential, and it is important that either the fluid is permitted to flow from the needle or only minor negative pressure is applied. The greatest complication with this technique is blood contamination, and concurrent hematologic assessment of blood samples can be helpful in assessment

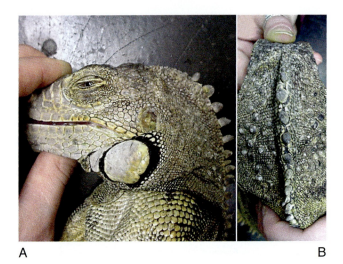

FIGURE 30-122 Positioning for a cerebrospinal fluid tap in a Green Iguana *(Iguana iguana)*. **A,** The head and neck are maximally flexed to improve dorsal access to the spinal canal. **B,** The needle is advanced in the dorsal midline; retracting the crest laterally and palpating the dorsal spinal processes aid proper needle placement.

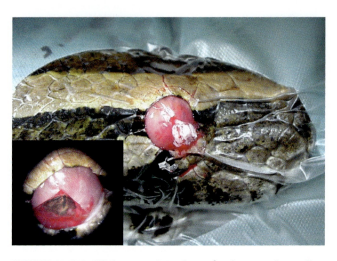

FIGURE 30-124 Wedge resection of a python's spectacle to allow drainage and collection of subspectacular exudates for cytologic and microbiologic investigations. *Inset,* Postoperative view shows a normal cornea below wedge resection.

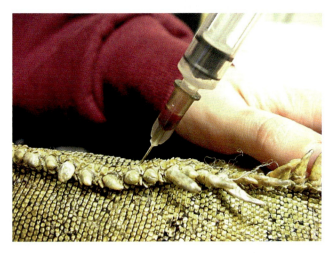

FIGURE 30-123 Lumbosacral cerebrospinal fluid tap in a Green Iguana *(Iguana iguana)*. Cerebrospinal fluid should not be aspirated; it should be allowed to flow slowly. In this case, a syringe is attached because contrast material has been injected for the spinal contrast study.

of CSF blood contamination and artifact.[44] Cytologic and microbiologic evaluations of CSF may be of value in the assessment of central nervous system disease.

Eyes

Subspectacular infections in snakes and some lizards occur with some frequency. Surgical wedge resection of the spectacle permits the collection of exudate for cytologic and microbiologic tests (Figure 30-124).[3,7] Likewise, proliferative corneal lesions can be carefully scraped and retrobulbar swellings aspirated for further investigation (Figure 30-125). Occasionally, eyelid lesions may be seen that can be biopsied using magnification and fine biopsy forceps.

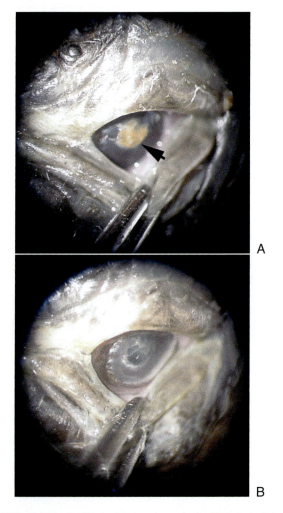

FIGURE 30-125 A, Corneal lesion *(arrow)* of a *Testudo* tortoise as seen at 10× magnification. **B,** The lesion has been carefully removed from the cornea for cytology, leaving the debrided ulcer for further medical therapy.

Ears

Tympanic abscessation in chelonians is common, and surgical access to evacuate the inspissated contents also allows the collection of appropriate samples.[3,7] In lizards, tympanic disease appears to be less common, but a variety of infectious causes, including *Cryptosporidium* sp., have been identified that may not be appreciated without the collection of aspirates or biopsies. The removal of 25% to 50% of the tympanum facilitates both collection of samples and evacuation of exudates. This procedure does not damage the ear, and the tympanum heals by second intention and is renewed during ecdysis (see Chapter 45).

Peripheral Nerve Biopsy

Peripheral neuropathies are seldom encountered, but similar techniques to those in mammals can be used.[34] In most cases, gastrointestinal or muscle biopsies often contain neural tissue.

ACKNOWLEDGMENTS

Sections of this chapter are from the following publications and have been reproduced with permission of the publishers:

Divers SJ: Reptilian renal and reproductive disease diagnosis. In Fudge AM, editor: *Laboratory medicine avian and exotic pets*, Philadelphia, 2000, WB Saunders.

Divers SJ: Reptilian liver and gastro-intestinal testing. In Fudge AM, editor: *Laboratory medicine avian and exotic pets*, Philadelphia, 2000, WB Saunders.

Divers SJ: Clinical evaluation of reptiles, *Vet Clin North Am Exotic Anim Pract* 2(2):291-331, 1999.

REFERENCES

1. Divers SJ: Clinical evaluation of reptiles, *Vet Clin North Am Exotic Anim Pract* 2(2):291-331, 1999.
2. Divers SJ: Basic reptile husbandry, history taking and clinical examination, *J Vet Postgrad Clin Study (In Pract)* 18(2):51-65, 1996.
3. Mader DR: *Reptile medicine and surgery*, ed 1, Philadelphia, 1996, WB Saunders.
4. Beynon PH, Lawton MPC, Cooper JE: *Manual of reptiles*, Cheltenham, England, 1992, BSAVA.
5. Barten SL: The medical care of iguanas and other common pet lizards, *Vet Clin North Am Small Anim Pract* 23(6):1213-1249, 1993.
6. Jacobson ER: Snakes, *Vet Clin North Am Small Anim Pract* 23(6):1179-1212, 1993.
7. Frye FL: *Biomedical and surgical aspects of captive reptile husbandry*, ed 2, Malabar, Fla, 1991, Krieger Publishing.
8. Barnard S: *The reptile keepers handbook*, Malabar, Fla, 1996, Krieger Publishing.
9. Divers SJ, Lafortune M: Prescribing for reptiles. In Bishop Y, editor: *The veterinary formulary*, ed 5, London, 2000, Royal Pharmaceutical Society of London.
10. Bradley T, Angulo FJ, Raiti P: Association of reptilian and amphibian veterinarians guidelines for reducing risk of transmission of *Salmonella* spp from reptiles to humans, *J Am Vet Med Assoc* 213(1):51-52.
11. Jackson OF: Weight and measurement data on tortoises (*Testudo graeca* and *T. hermanni*) and their relationship to health, *J Small Anim Pract* 21:409, 1980.
12. Blakey CS, Kirkwood JK: Body mass to length relationships in chelonia, *Vet Rec* 137:28, 1995.
13. Mader DR, Stoutenberg G: Assessing the body condition of the California Desert Tortoise, *Gopherus agassizii*, using morphometric analysis, *Proceedings of the 5th Association of Reptilian and Amphibian Veterinarians Conference*, 1998.
14. McCracken HE: Organ location in snakes for diagnostic and surgical evaluation. In Fowler ME, Miller RE, editors: *Zoo & wild animal medicine current therapy 4*, Philadelphia, 1999, WB Saunders.
15. Mautino M, Page CD: Biology and medicine of turtles and tortoises, *Vet Clin North Am Small Anim Pract* 23(6):1251-1270, 1993.
16. Lloyd ML: Crocodilian anesthesia. In Fowler ME, Miller RE, editors: *Zoo & wild animal medicine current therapy 4*, Philadelphia, 1999, WB Saunders.
17. Hernandez-Divers SJ, Hernandez-Divers SM, Wilson GM, Srahl SJ: A review of reptile diagnostic celioscopy, *J Herp Med Surg* 15, 2005 (in press).
18. Mader DR. Laboratory sampling in reptile patients: do's and don'ts, *Proceedings of 5th Association of Reptilian and Amphibian Veterinarians Conference*, 1998.
19. Fudge AM: *Laboratory medicine avian and exotic pets*, Philadelphia, 2000, WB Saunders.
20. Divers SJ: Diagnostic techniques in reptiles, *Proc North Am Vet Conf Small Anim Exotics Ed* 14:932-935, 2000.
21. Johnson JD, Mangone B, Wimsatt J: Placement of cardiac access ports for repeated blood sampling in chelonians. *Proceedings of 5th Association of Reptilian and Amphibian Veterinarians Conference*, 1998.
22. Whitaker BR, Krum H: Medical management of sea turtles in aquaria. In Fowler ME, Miller RE, editors: *Zoo & wild animal medicine current therapy 4*, Philadelphia, 1999, WB Saunders.
23. Martinez-Silvestre A, Perpinan D, Marco I, Lavin S: Venipuncture technique of the occipital venous sinus in freshwater aquatic turtles, *JHMS* 12:31-32, 2002.
24. Tanaka Y: Structure of the reptilian spleen. In Gans C, Gaunt AS, editors: *Biology of the reptilia, vol 19, morphology G, visceral organs*, Ithaca, 1998, Society for the Study of Amphibians and Reptiles.
25. Divers SJ: Endoscopy of reptiles, *Proc North Am Vet Conf Small Anim Exotics Ed* 14:937-940, 2000.
26. Barnard SM, Durden LA: *A veterinary guide to the parasites of reptiles, vol 2 arthropods*, Malabar, Fla, 2000, Krieger Publishing.
27. Perry SF: Lungs: comparative anatomy, functional morphology, and evolution. In Gans C, Gaunt AS, editors: *Biology of the reptilia, vol 19, morphology G, visceral organs*, Ithaca, 1998, Society for the Study of Amphibians and Reptiles.
28. Divers SJ: Endoscopic evaluation of the reptile respiratory tract, *Proc Eur Assoc Zoo Wildlife Vet* 303-306, 2000.
29. Divers SJ, Lawton MPC: Two techniques for the endoscopic evaluation of the chelonian lung, *Proceeding of 7th Association of Reptilian and Amphibian Veterinarians Conference*, 2000.
30. Divers SJ: The prevalence of gastro-intestinal parasites in a small population of captive boas and pythons (family Boidae), *Br Herpetol Soc Bull* 50:6-13, 1994.
31. Divers SJ: The diagnosis and treatment of lower respiratory tract disease in tortoises with particular regard to intrapneumonic therapy, *Proceedings of 5th Association of Reptilian and Amphibian Veterinarians Conference*, 1998.
32. Divers SJ: A clinician's approach to liver disease in tortoises. *Proceedings of 4th Association of Reptilian and Amphibian Veterinarians Conference*, 1997.

33. Isaza R, Ackerman N, Schumacher J: Ultrasound guided percutaneous liver biopsy in snakes, *Vet Radiol Ultrasound* 34:452-454, 1993.
34. Klingenberg R: A fast and efficient liver biopsy technique in snakes. Proceedings of the International Conference on Exotics, *Exotic DVM* 3(3):89-93, 2001.
35. Isaza R, Garner M, Jacobson E: Proliferative osteoarthritis and osteoarthrosis in 15 snakes, *J Zoo Wildl Med* 31:20-27, 2000.
36. Bojrab MJ: *Current techniques in small animal surgery*, ed 3, Philadelphia, 1990, Lea & Febiger.
37. Gans C, Dawson WR: *Biology of the Reptilia, vol 5, physiology A*, London, 1976, Academic Press.
38. Gans C, Parsons TS: *Biology of the Reptilia, vol 6, morphology E*, London, 1977, Academic Press.
39. Gans C, Pough FH: *Biology of the Reptilia, vol 12, physiology C*, London, 1982, Academic Press.
40. Divers SJ: Clinician's approach to renal disease in lizards, *Proceedings of 5th Association of Reptilian and Amphibian Veterinarians Conference*, 1998.
41. Innis C: Observations on urinalysis of clinically normal captive tortoises, *Proceedings of 7th Association of Reptilian and Amphibian Veterinarians Conference*, 1997.
42. Hernandez-Divers SJ: Endoscopic evaluation and renal biopsy in 69 chelonians, *Vet Rec* 154:73-80, 2004.
43. Gibbons PM: Urinalysis in box turtles, *Terrapene* spp, *Proceedings of 7th Association of Reptilian and Amphibian Veterinarians Conference*, 1998.
44. Hernandez-Divers SJ, Stahl S, Stedman NL, et al: Renal evaluation in the green iguana (*Iguana iguana*): assessment of plasma biochemistry, glomerular filtration rate, and endoscopic biopsy. *J Zoo Wildl Med*, in press, 2005.
45. Mader DR: A minimally invasive procedure for renal biopsies in the green iguana, *Iguana iguana*, Proceedings of 5th Association of Reptilian and Amphibian Veterinarians Conference, 1998.
46. Divers SJ, Lawton MPC: Spinal osteomyelitis in a green iguana, *Iguana iguana*: cerebrospinal fluid and myelogram diagnosis, *Proceedings of 8th Association of Reptilian and Amphibian Veterinarians Conference*, 2000.
47. Schilliger L: Diseases of the central nervous system in ophidians (snakes), part 2, clinical diagnosis, *Le Point Veterinaire* 30(201):469-476, 1999.

31
EMERGENCY AND CRITICAL CARE

DOUGLAS R. MADER and ELKE RUDLOFF

Few true emergencies are found in reptile medicine. Reptiles do everything slowly; they get sick slowly, and they get well slowly. Most health problems seen in reptiles, with perhaps the exception of trauma (Figure 31-1, *A*), are the result of improper husbandry and nutrition (Figure 31-1, *B*). These key factors, which are essential in successful captive maintenance, exhibit their deleterious effects in an insidious fashion, often taking months to manifest. **The emergency veterinarian is most commonly presented with acute manifestations of these chronic conditions.** The ability to recognize the signs, and familiarity with the pathogenesis of these diseases, better prepares the emergency department staff to diagnose and treat the critical patient.

The single most important principle of emergency care for the reptile patient can best be summarized by one word: heat. Reptiles are ectotherms, which means that they derive their body temperature from the environment. They exhibit a behavior, called thermoregulation, with which they can control their core body temperature through behavioral means rather than endogenous thermoregulation under the influence of the hypothalamus.

Several studies have documented a "behavioral fever" in various species of reptiles in response to endogenous pyrogens (see Chapter 36 for more details). Maintenance of a reptile's core body temperature at or above the species' preferred optimal temperature zone (POTZ) has many beneficial effects: increasing immune response, decreasing healing time, augmenting leukocyte function, and more.

From the perspective of emergent care, it is the rare reptile case that cannot wait 24 hours for the initiation of antibiotic treatment while the patient is properly warmed. Medications, fluids, enterals, and so on have little effect in the cold patient.

Every effort should be made to evaluate the patient's body temperature on initial examination (Figure 31-2). Once determined, adjust either up or down as needed. Emergency facilities that "receive" reptile emergency patients should have appropriate housing/warming cages or devices. Many methods exist for application of heat to reptile patients, but as in mammals, radiant heat is easy and effective (Figure 31-3).

EMERGENCY DIAGNOSTICS

Physical Examination

Chapter 30 reviews examination techniques in all reptile groups. The examination of an emergent reptile patient requires a thorough understanding of the species and a knowledge of the "normal" animal.

Blood Collection

Blood collection is necessary whenever diagnostics are required. No better way is found to assess a patient's internal status than a thorough laboratory evaluation.

The most important credo in medicine is "above all, do not harm." If collection of a laboratory sample will cause more stress or harm to the patient, symptomatic treatment may be more prudent, on the basis of physical examination, history, and other less-diagnostic modalities. As mentioned, it is the rare reptile patient that cannot wait 24 hours to allow for proper warming and rehydration before invasive procedures are initiated.

Chapter 30 reviews venipuncture techniques in all of the common reptile groups. All blood should be collected in lithium heparinized tubes because ethylenediamine tetraacetic acid (EDTA) may cause red cell lysis. In addition, blood should be collected in plastic rather than glass containers. Slides should be available for fresh (nonanticoagulated) whole blood smears.

Blood volumes in reptiles vary from 5% to 8% of total body weight. Of this amount, up to 10% of this volume in a *healthy* patient can be safely collected for analysis without harm. As a rough approximation, the sample size should never be larger than 1% of the animal's total body weight. For example, in a 450-g Green Iguana (*Iguana iguana*), one can safely remove 4.5 mL of blood, which is far more than necessary with even the most antiquated autoanalyzers.

The standard capillary tube holds 70 µL, which means that the volume of a single capillary tube is the maximum amount of blood that can be collected from any patient weighing a minimum of 7 g. Although this is a small sample, enough is collected to yield some valuable diagnostic information.

Capillary tubes are useful for quick assessment of packed cell volume (PCV) and total solids. A tremendous amount of information can be obtained from just a small quantity of blood—enough to help with both diagnostics and the formulation of a therapeutic plan (Table 31-1).

In reality, with the very small patients, only a single drop of blood may be safely collected. A thin, well-prepared blood smear always is of value as a diagnostic aid (see Chapter 28).

Even if reptilian samples are sent to a commercial laboratory, saving one hematocrit tube for in-house analysis is recommended.

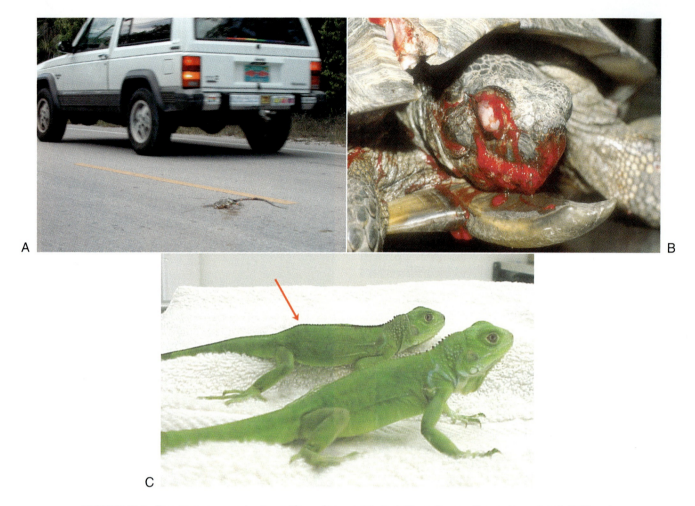

FIGURE 31-1 Few true emergencies in reptile medicine exist. **A,** A Green Iguana *(Iguana iguana)* and, **B,** Desert Tortoise *(Gopherus agassizii)* hit by automobiles usually require immediate attention. Most "emergency" presentations are actually acute manifestations of chronic disease. **C,** A Juvenile Green Iguana *(Iguana iguana)* with a spinal fracture *(red arrow)* as a result of nutritional secondary hyperparathyroidism.

Chapter 88 lists clinical pathologic values for many of the common species.

Diagnostic Imaging

Radiography, ultrasound, and other imaging modalities are important for assessment of emergent reptiles. The accurate diagnosis of trauma, reproductive abnormalities, gastrointestinal impactions, and other internal pathologies benefits from some form of imaging. Techniques are described elsewhere in this book (see Chapters 29, 37, 86, and 87). No special concerns relate directly to the critical reptile patient other than one should be careful not to allow the patient to cool during the procedures.

Microbiologic Sampling

Samples for microbiologic analysis, such as fungal and bacterial culture and sensitivity testing, should always be collected before antimicrobial therapy is initiated. Collecting samples and "holding" them is best, with disposal of the samples if the owner wishes not to pursue the diagnostics, rather than collecting samples that may not be representative once therapeutics have already been started. Chapter 16 reviews proper microbiological sampling protocols.

THERAPEUTICS FOR THE CRITICAL REPTILE PATIENT

Antibiotic Selection

Several antibiotics can be used in the ill reptile. Obvious choices include those antibiotics effective against gram-negative bacteria, but considerations for atypical organisms (such as *Mycoplasma, Chlamydophila, Mycobacterium,* etc.) must be considered. Anticipation of need and consideration for the patient's immediate physiologic state (hydration, hypothermia, anemia) influence choice. See Chapter 36 for guidance and selection. Chapter 89 lists drugs and dosages commonly used in reptilian patients.

Nutritional Support

Reptile patients frequently have a history of anorexia (see subsequent). Plasma blood glucose concentrations in the

Emergency and Critical Care 535

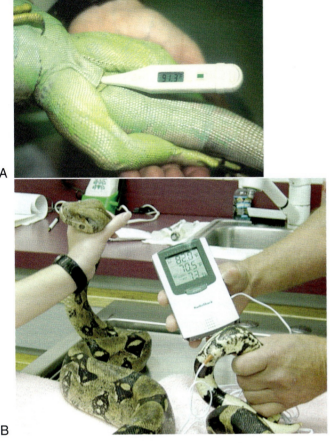

FIGURE 31-2 Essential to proper reptile diagnostics is that core body temperatures are evaluated during the physical examination. **A,** Standard electronic thermometers do not read low enough for most reptile patients. **B,** Inexpensive digital thermometers are available through most electronics stores and are capable of reading low temperatures. These have outdoor thermoprobes made of soft plastic, are readily disinfected, and read in both Celsius and Fahrenheit.

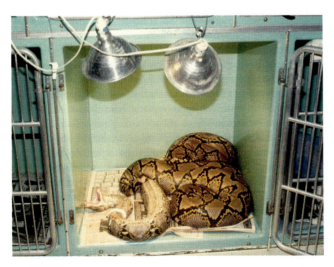

FIGURE 31-3 Supplemental heat is mandatory for hospitalized reptiles. Heating cages, incubators, and radiant lamps should be available for all sizes of reptile patients. Repeated monitoring is essential to prevent burning.

range of 10 to 20 mg/dL are not uncommon, especially in some of the reptiles that infrequently feed (such as the large snakes).

A common practice for exotic veterinarians is to immediately provide caloric or nutritional support. This may not always be necessary, and in some instances (such as animals in a catabolic state or those on potentially nephrotoxic medications), this may even be contraindicated.

A common term used for providing calories to reptile patients is "force feeding." The authors prefer the term "assist feeding" because it implies a more sophisticated, calculated, and gentle approach (Figure 31-4). Refer to Chapter 18 for assist-feeding protocols, placement of feeding tubes, and proper use of nutritional supplements.

FLUID THERAPY

The old adage "if the mouth works, use it" certainly holds true in reptile medicine. However, reptile patients that are not properly warmed do not efficiently absorb enteral fluids. Subcutaneous and intracoelomic fluids are also not well absorbed when the patient is cold. For that reason, whenever possible, intravenous (IV), and rarely, intraosseous (IO) fluids should be administered if the patient is not properly warmed.

Intravenous Catheter Placement

Only one peripheral vessel is visible in reptile patients—the dorsal buccal vein in snakes. Because of its location (inside of the mouth, medial to several dozen sharp teeth), it is not a practical place for indwelling catheter placement in a conscious patient. This vein can be used if the patient is moribund, obtunded, or anesthetized.

Because of this, all IV catheters require a cut down and a minor amount of experience to perform the procedure (see also Chapter 36). Because these procedures are more complicated than simple mammalian IV catheter placement, an additional cost should be charged to the client, and some clients may object to this.

Familiarity with the vascular anatomy of the patient is necessary. The cut-down site should be prepared aseptically with appropriate antiseptics. In all but the most compromised patients, some form of anesthesia or analgesia should be provided (see Chapter 27).

The size of the IV catheter is determined by the size of the patient and the vein being catheterized. Injection ports are needed to cap the catheter once it has been inserted. Tissue glue or monofilament suture is needed to secure the catheter to the cut-down site. A #11 scalpel blade or the fresh tip of an 18-gauge hypodermic needle can be used for the cut-down procedure. Sterile mosquito forceps, a needle driver, and a pair of small-toothed forceps are useful in manipulation of the vessel.

The risk versus benefit must be assessed whenever a marginal patient is anesthetized. If possible, the cut down should be performed with a local rather than a general anesthetic (see Chapter 27).

Severely dehydrated patients can present a challenge. Reptiles have the ability to shunt blood away from the periphery during periods of hypothermia and dehydration. Whenever possible, the patient should be adequately warmed before the cut down is performed.

Table 31-1	Evaluating the Reptilian Hematocrit*
Packed Cell Volume (PCV)[†]: Mechanical estimation of red blood cell (RBC) concentration. Expressed as a %. **Plasma Protein:** A more appropriate term with use of a refractometer is **Total Solids**. This measurement is beneficial in interpretation of the PCV (blood loss versus dehydration). In addition, it is a valuable measurement in monitoring fluid therapy and response to treatment. **Icterus Index:** For reptile patients to have a yellow tinge to their plasma is not uncommon. All color changes should be noted. Green plasma, from hyperbiliverdinemia, is seen in catabolic states (such as in starvation, toxemia, heat stress). Lipemic plasma is also readily detected in plasma samples. **Microfilariae:** Circulating microfilariae found in the area of the buffy coat in wild-caught animals are not uncommon. Although the presence of microfilariae does not necessarily mean clinical disease, it is often an indication of the state of health of the animal. The blood parasites are readily seen with the 10× objective. **Thrombocytes:** In mammals, the platelets collect at the top of the buffy coat layer, appearing as a cream-colored layer as opposed to the light gray of the white blood cells (WBCs).	The visible presence of this layer suggests adequate numbers of platelets. Thrombocyte estimates and morphology can be confirmed with evaluation of the blood smear. **Buffy Coat (BC):** Although no direct correlation exists between the size of the BC and the absolute WBC (this varies by species),[21] in general, the larger the BC, the greater the WBC. Most BC are in the range of 1% to 1.5%. **Buffy Coat Smears:** If the hematocrit tube is snapped at the BC, the concentrated WBCs can be easily smeared and evaluated for the presence of parasites, inclusions, toxic changes, or degranulation. **RBC Health/O_2 Saturation:** The color of the RBC in the hematocrit tube reflects the RBC health, age, oxygen saturation, and toxicity. A patient with respiratory signs that has red blood has less pulmonary compromise than a similar patient with dark purple blood. Likewise, brown coloration may suggest toxicity. **Blood Smear:** If a single drop of blood is used to make a fresh smear before the hematocrit tube is centrifuged, a differential can be performed. In addition, overall cellular morphology can be assessed and a more thorough estimated WBC can be determined.

*Lithium heparin hematocrit tubes.
[†]Note: After the cells have been spun down, the remaining plasma can be used for a limited number of specific chemistries (e.g., uric acid, calcium, phosphorus).

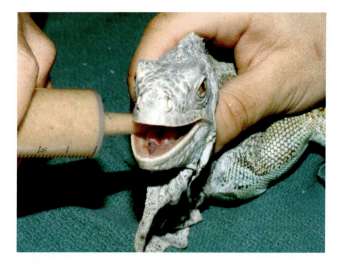

FIGURE 31-4 "Assist feeding," as opposed to "force feeding," may be needed in hospitalized reptile patients. Chapter 18 covers nutritional support.

Important to point out is that even in the face of complete shunting and a completely collapsed vessel, performance of the catheterization is still possible, just with patience and a steady hand.

INTRAVENOUS CUT-DOWN TECHNIQUES

Lizards

The best vessel to catheterize in lizards is the cephalic vein (Figure 31-5). It is located anatomically in the same position as in dogs and cats, running medial to laterally in a proximal to distal direction across the antebrachium.

The vein is found with a transverse cut down starting from the midmedial antebrachium, then progressing 90 degrees in a cranial direction. The vein is superficial and easily damaged with an aggressive skin incision. Just a "nick" to the skin and then gentle blunt dissection to expose the vessel is best.

Once identified, an appropriately sized catheter is placed retrograde into the vessel. The catheter is capped and then sutured or glued in place. A topical antibiotic is applied over the insertion, and a clean dressing is placed around the limb to protect the catheter. Catheter care is performed as in any species.

Turtles

The best place for IV catheter placement is the jugular vein. The right side is usually larger than the left; however, both vessels can be used.

The vein is found with gentle extension of the patient's neck. Once the tympanic membrane is located, an imaginary horizontal line is drawn through the circular membrane extending caudally (Figure 31-6). The jugular vein follows this path. In most species, unless the patient is dehydrated, the "bulge" of the vein is usually visible under the skin.

A small cut down is made over the area of the vessel approximately one third of the way back from the ear toward the body wall. The vein is located with gentle blunt dissection. An appropriately sized catheter is placed in the neck. A standard Teflon catheter can be used. The length of the catheter should be slightly longer than half the length of the turtle's neck. These catheters flex with the patient when it retracts its neck back under the shell (Figure 31-7).

Once the catheter is in place, an injection cap is affixed, and the entire unit is then sutured or glued in place. Wraps or dressings are not necessary and usually are cumbersome to the patient. IV fluids can be administered via a standard

Emergency and Critical Care

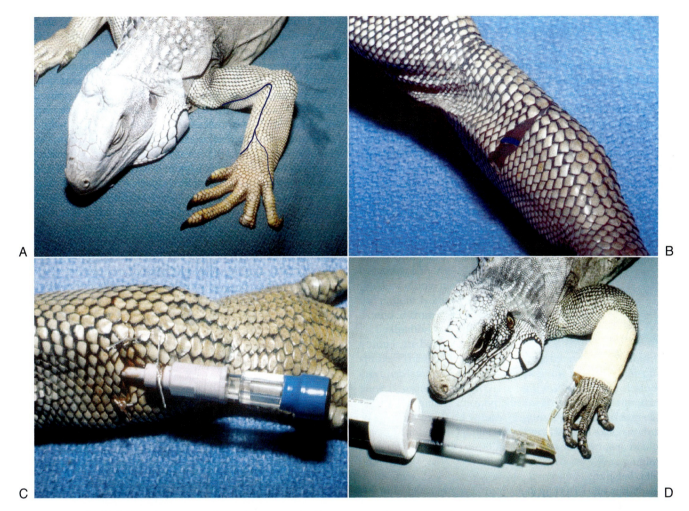

FIGURE 31-5 Intravenous (IV) catheters are the best way to replace fluids and administer medications in a critically ill reptile. **A,** The cephalic vein courses the front limb in a pattern similar to that seen in dogs and cats. **B,** With anesthesia or analgesia, a small cut down is made in the midantebrachial region to expose the cephalic vein. **C,** A standard IV catheter is inserted into the vein and either glued or sutured into place. **D,** The patient can then be placed on IV fluids or administered IV medications as needed.

drip set; however, when the tortoise patient retracts its neck into the shell, the curvature may "kink" the catheter and occlude the flow. A standard infusion pump helps overcome this problem. Mila International makes a small, lightweight, pressure-driven infusion pump system (Flow Line, www.milaint.com) that can be affixed directly to the patient, providing untethered movement within the cage (Figure 31-8).

Snakes

Jugular Catheters

As in the turtle, the right jugular vein is the best location to place an indwelling catheter (Figure 31-9) in a snake. The patient is placed in dorsal recumbency, and the location of the heart is identified by watching for the beating ventral scutes. Once the heart is localized, one should count forward approximately 10 scutes. One should surgically prepare the area and then make a small incision at the margin of the scutes and the lateral body scales. The incision should be two to three scutes long. Now, with blunt dissection, one gently separates the fascia until the jugular vein is exposed. It is superficial and runs medial and parallel to the free margin of the ribs.

When the jugular vein is exposed, then an appropriately sized catheter is carefully inserted, directed toward the heart. Sutures are not needed around the jugular vein but are necessary to affix the catheter to the skin. The catheter hub can be incorporated into the skin closure, and an injection port can be affixed to the end for infusion or sampling. A pledget of antimicrobial ointment should be placed over the incision, and a clean dressing placed around the snake's body at the exit site of the catheter so it is not pulled out.

The catheter is removed by cutting the sutures and removing the catheter. Opening the incision or ligating the jugular vein is not necessary. Pressure should be applied to the site momentarily after the catheter is removed to ensure hemostasis.

Intracardiac Catheters

In an emergency situation, especially one in which owner finances are limited and an IV cut down is not feasible, an intracardiac (IC) catheter is an effective way to get warmed fluids to a dehydrated snake patient (Figure 31-10).

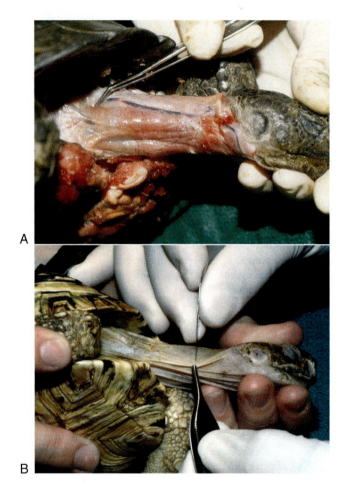

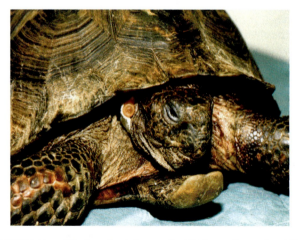

FIGURE 31-6 **A,** The skin has been removed from the neck of this deceased Desert Tortoise *(Gopherus agassizii)* to expose the location of the jugular vein. **B,** A simple cut down approximately one third of the distance between the ear and the body wall (with appropriate anesthesia or analgesia) provides access to the vein, allowing easy insertion of a standard intravenous (IV) catheter.

FIGURE 31-7 The length of the standard Teflon catheter should be slightly longer than half the length of the turtle's neck. These catheters flex with the patient when it retracts its neck back under the shell.

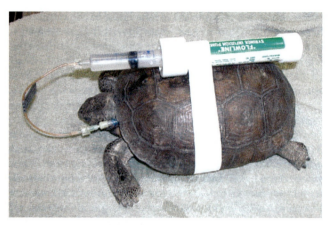

FIGURE 31-8 This tortoise is hooked up to a small, lightweight, portable intravenous (IV) infusion pump. The animal is free to roam about its cage without the restriction of an IV line.

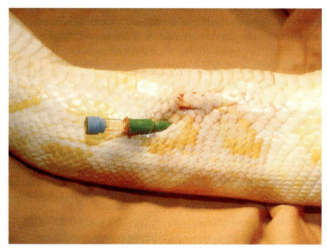

FIGURE 31-9 Jugular catheters in snakes are not difficult to place but require either general anesthesia or local analgesia in a sedate patient to insert. A light dressing protects the catheter port while the snake moves about its cage.

The patient is placed in dorsal recumbency in the usual fashion to identify the cardiac beat. Once the heart is located, the area is aseptically prepared. An appropriately sized standard IV catheter is selected and directed through the ventral skin (between the scutes) directly into the region of the single ventricle. Once a "flash" is seen through the catheter, the metal stylet is removed and the catheter is advanced as far as it goes. An infusion adapter is placed on the end of the catheter, and the entire unit is then taped to the ventrum. The heart beats against the flexible catheter. Because of the normally thick ventricle, the low blood pressure, and slow heart beat, leakage and tamponade are generally not a problem. The benefits of the warm fluid therapy far outweigh any risks involved in this emergency procedure.

Intraosseous Catheters

In practicality, IO catheters are only useful in lizards, although they can be used in small crocodilians and turtles. They can also be placed in the marrow bone of the chelonian shell, but the procedure is difficult and usually requires

Emergency and Critical Care

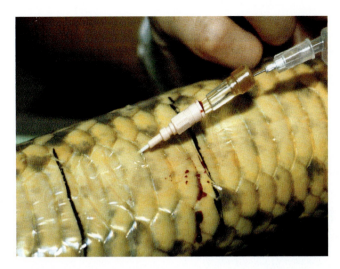

FIGURE 31-10 Intracardiac (IC) catheters are an effective way to provide warm fluids in moribund snakes in emergency situations.

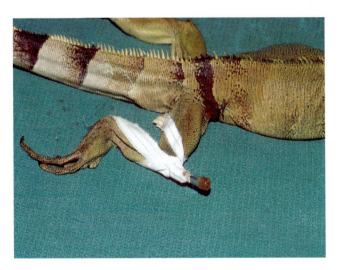

FIGURE 31-11 Intraosseous (IO) catheters are best placed anterograde in tibia of lizards. The insertion point is the tibial crest. Both aseptic technique and some form of analgesia must be used.

an orthopedic drill to accomplish the feat. The long bones of the turtles can also be used, but because they have thick cortices and small marrow spaces and retract their limbs into the shell, placement of IO catheters in turtles is generally not practical. Jugular catheters are so easy that IO catheter placement in turtles is rarely necessary.

In lizards, the preferred site for IO catheter placement is the tibial crest (Figure 31-11). With the leg flexed, the tibial crest region is aseptically prepared. A spinal needle or commercially available IO catheter (both of these have stylets) is inserted anterograde from the tibial crest into the shaft of the tibia. The needle should go no further than the midshaft region of the tibia. Placement should be confirmed with radiography (Figure 31-12).

The marrow space is extremely limited in reptiles (unlike birds). As a result, it is not possible to bolus large volumes of fluids. IO catheters work best if the patient is placed on an infusion pump capable of delivering small continuous volumes (Figure 31-13).

The benefits versus risks of the IO catheters should be evaluated. The authors have seen patients permanently disabled as a result of poorly placed IO catheters and osteomyelitis that developed after placement. In addition, as anyone who has ever donated bone marrow can relate, insertion of a needle into the bone of a patient is painful (Figure 31-14). Aseptic technique and applying a local anesthetic at the periosteum will limit this complication.

ORAL GAVAGE

As previously mentioned, "if the mouth works, use it" holds true with reptile patients and their mammalian counterparts. Clinicians are too hasty to place IO or IV catheters in exotic animal patients, and all too often forget to use the obvious portal for sustenance.

In general, if the patient is less than 5% dehydrated, oral supplementation suffices. If the patient is greater than 5% dehydrated, a combination of oral and parenteral fluids is needed.

Administration of oral preparations in reptiles is not difficult. In reptiles, the glottis is always closed except during breathing, which is the opposite of mammals. In gavaging a reptile, this makes passing a stomach tube easier. When tube feeding the patient, having the preparation prewarmed is prudent.

Placement of feeding tubes has been covered in Chapters 18 and 36. Especially in chelonians, feeding tubes help increase owner compliance with administration of nutritional support and necessary medications (Figure 31-15). Providing an easy means for an owner to help with treatments at home fosters the team approach to health care.

FLUID CHOICES

The fact that reptiles exist on all continents, except Antarctica, is a tribute to the versatility of their water balance capabilities. Water balance is necessary for a number of essential body functions. In the *cell*, water provides a medium for housing organelles and establishing cellular structure. Water provides *interstitial* integrity, allowing unrestricted movement of solutes and waste products between the capillary and the cell. In the *vessel*, water is the transport medium that brings oxygen, solutes, and hormones to the interstitium and waste products from the interstitium to the sanitizing organs (lung, kidney, liver, and spleen). Water also provides a method for heat removal from the body through evaporation from the *skin*.

As a result of their slower metabolic rate, reptiles synthesize water much more slowly than mammals and birds. Reptiles are incapable of producing water in excess of their evaporative water loss, a fact that makes them much more susceptible to a negative water balance when they cease to consume water.[1] In addition, regulation of osmolality is highly dependent on the availability of water to drink, reabsorption of water from the urinary bladder and cloaca,

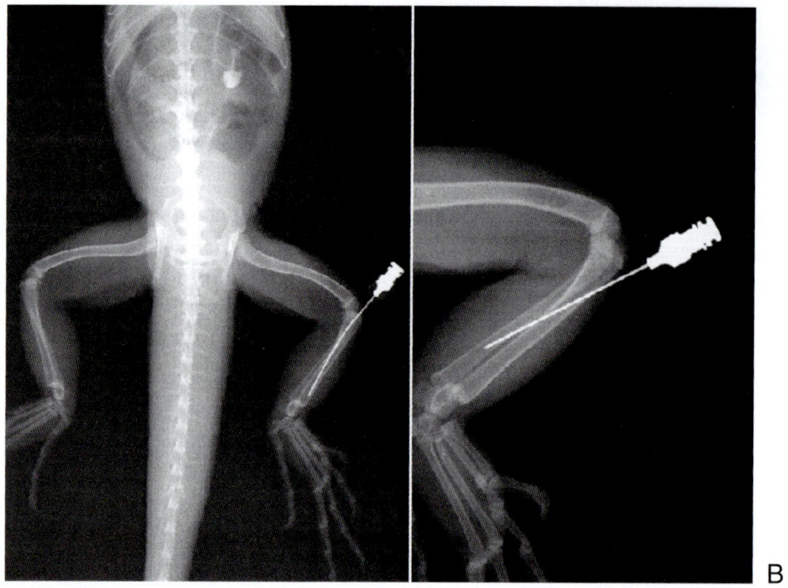

FIGURE 31-12 Placement of the intraosseous (IO) catheter should be confirmed radiographically *(left)*. Misdirection is easy; note the IO needle through the cortex *(right)*.

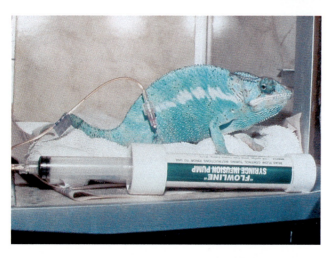

FIGURE 31-13 A chameleon has an intraosseous (IO) catheter placed in the tibia and is hooked up to a small intravenous (IV) infusion pump. These pumps can deliver fluids in a controlled fashion even for small patients.

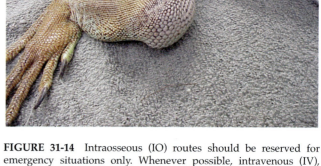

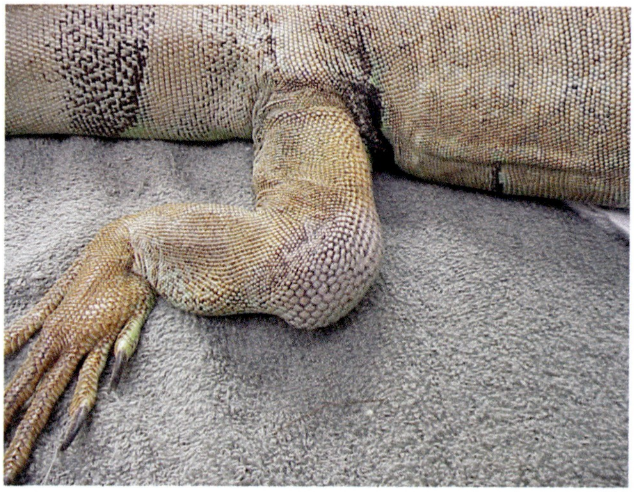

FIGURE 31-14 Intraosseous (IO) routes should be reserved for emergency situations only. Whenever possible, intravenous (IV), oral, or intracoelomic fluids should be attempted first. This Green Iguana *(Iguana iguana)* has a severe osteomyelitis of the stifle that resulted from an IO catheter.

and loss of salts via the salt glands, rather than renal water reabsorption.[2] When a negative water balance occurs, all body systems are adversely affected. Fluid therapy becomes an integral part of reestablishing and maintaining cellular homeostasis.

The principles of fluid therapy are universal across species lines. A basic understanding of body water distribution, forces governing water movement between fluid compartments, fluid pharmacology, and patient assessment are necessary to determine the fluid type, dose, and rate of fluid to be administered.

Body Water Distribution

The physiologic properties of water in normally hydrated reptiles are comparable with those of other vertebrates.[3] Approximately 75% of body weight is water, except in turtles where the presence of the carapace reduces the value closer to that found in mammals, approximately 66%.[1,4] The distribution of total body water (TBW) between the intracellular and extracellular (intravascular and interstitial) fluid compartments in reptiles is slightly different than in mammals. In most reptiles, TBW is equally distributed between the intracellular and extracellular fluid compartments. Of the extracellular fluid volume, approximately 70% exists in the interstitial space and 30% in the intravascular space (Figure 31-16).

Movement of Water

Water movement between the water compartments is regulated by the principles of osmosis and Starling's forces. The cellular and endothelial membranes that separate the

Emergency and Critical Care

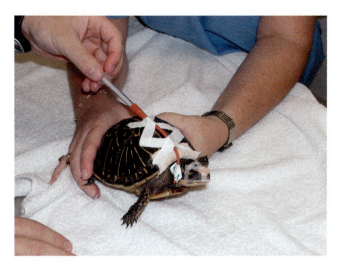

FIGURE 31-15 Feeding tubes help increase owner compliance with administration of nutritional support and necessary medications. This Box Turtle *(Terrapene carolina bauri)* was hit by an automobile and had the rhinotheca fractured. The pharyngostomy tube allows the owner to administer the medications and nutrition without interfering with the healing of the jaws.

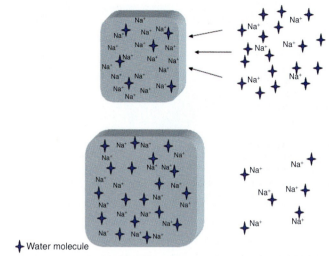

FIGURE 31-17 Osmotic forces across the cell membrane. Water passes from the compartment containing the smaller ion concentration into the compartment containing the greater ion concentration until the ion concentration becomes equal and the osmotic force is eliminated.

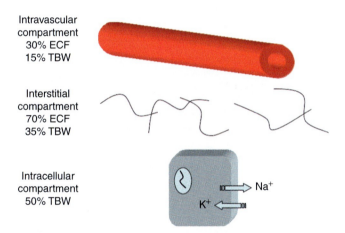

FIGURE 31-16 Distribution of total body water (TBW). The intracellular compartment and extracellular compartment (EC) each contain 50% of the TBW. The EC is divided into the intravascular compartment, which contains 15% of the TBW or 30% of the extracellular fluid (ECF), and the interstitial compartment, which contains 35% of the TBW and 70% of the extracellular fluid.

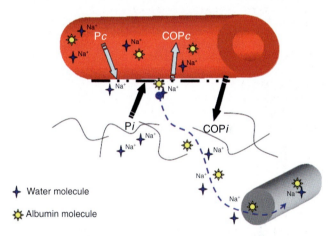

FIGURE 31-18 Starling's Law is the equation that defines the forces that affect the volume of fluid (v) that filters between the capillary (c) and interstitium (i) across the capillary wall. Interendothelial pore size (σ), the pore reflection coefficient (kf), and transcapillary forces of hydrostatic (P) and colloid osmotic (π) pressures work against lymph removal (Q) of fluid.
$$v = [kf(P_c - P_{is} - \sigma(\pi_c - \pi_{is})] - Qlymph$$

fluid compartments are selectively permeable to certain solutes. The cell membrane is impermeable to most ions, and the ion concentration difference between the interstitium and the intracellular compartment produces an osmotic force (Figure 31-17). In addition to osmotic forces, Starling's forces act at the vascular membrane, with the net effect keeping water in the vessel (Figure 31-18). Colloid osmotic pressure is produced by impermeable solutes (plasma proteins) that hold water within a compartment. Plasma proteins are a more heterogenous population in the reptile, compared with mammals; however, their physiologic effects are the same.[5] A negative charge on the protein molecules provides an additional osmotic effect (Gibbs-Donnan effect) by attracting sodium cations (and water) to their vicinity.

Fluid Pharmacology

Both crystalloid and colloid fluids are used for fluid therapy (Figure 31-19). A crystalloid is a water-based solution with small molecules that are osmotically active in the body fluids and permeable to the capillary membrane. A colloid is a water-based solution with both permeable small ions and nonpermeable molecules. The pharmacologic properties of crystalloids and colloids dictate which fluid compartment they enter.

Crystalloids

The amount of crystalloid fluid that remains in the intravascular compartment depends on the osmolality of the fluid

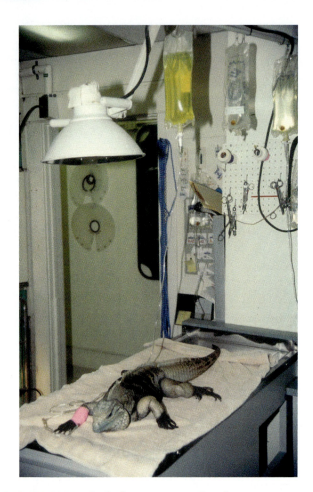

FIGURE 31-19 Fluid therapy in reptiles does require some thought. Many different types of fluids exist, and just as in dog and cat patients, no one single fluid choice is suitable for all conditions.

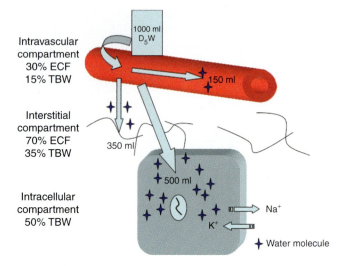

FIGURE 31-20 Distribution of solute-free water, 5% dextrose in water. The dextrose molecules make the fluid isotonic at initial administration; however, the glucose is rapidly metabolized, leaving water to be distributed according the total body water distribution (50% intracellular, 35% interstitial, and only 15% intravascular).

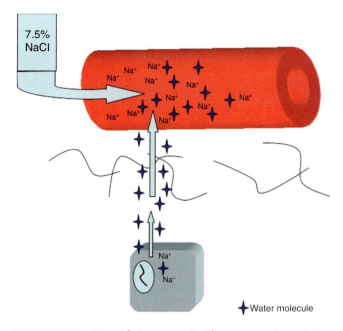

FIGURE 31-21 Water shifts as a result of hypertonic saline solution injection. When hypertonic saline solution is administered into the intravascular compartment, water flows via osmosis from the interstitium and intracellular compartment. The intravascular compartment becomes volume expanded, and the interstitial and cellular compartments are contracted.

compared with the osmolality of the intravascular and interstitial compartments. The sodium concentration in crystalloid fluid is the greatest contributor to fluid osmolality because it is the dominant extracellular ion. Therefore, the amount of crystalloid fluid that remains in the extracellular compartment depends on the sodium concentration of the administered fluid compared with the body fluid compartments.

With regard to crystalloid fluids, convention has defined an *isotonic* fluid as one that has an osmolality equal to that of erythrocytes and therefore does not affect the exchange of fluid across the erythrocyte membrane. A *hypertonic* fluid decreases erythrocyte volume, and a *hypotonic* fluid increases erythrocyte volume.

A hypotonic fluid has an osmolality less than intracellular fluid. The crystalloid 5% dextrose in water (D_5W) is such a fluid (Figure 31-20). Ideal for replacement of intracellular fluid deficits and used as a carrier fluid for drugs, D_5W is not used for intravascular or interstitial fluid replacement. Hypotonic fluid administration should be performed with extreme caution in the chronically dehydrated animal because rapid fluid shifts into the cell can produce cell swelling and membrane disruption.

Hypertonic fluids such as 7% and 23% saline solution have significantly more osmotically active particles per unit volume compared with intracellular fluid (Figure 31-21). After intravenous administration, water moves from the interstitial and intracellular compartments into the intravascular compartment, rapidly increasing intravascular volume. Interstitial sodium concentration (and tonicity) increases, promoting additional movement of intracellular water into the interstitial compartment and intracellular dehydration.

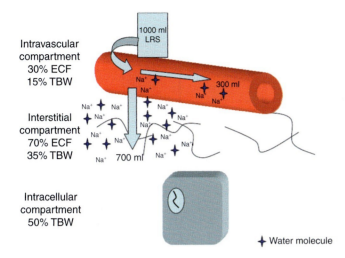

FIGURE 31-22 Water shifts as a result of isotonic replacement crystalloid (LRS) administration. When an isotonic crystalloid is administered containing a similar sodium concentration to the extracellular space, it is distributed according to extracellular distribution volumes. Seventy percent of the fluid administered crosses the capillary membrane into the interstitium within an hour, and only 30% remains in the intravascular compartment.

Sodium and water eventually return to the interstitial compartment as Starling's forces reach equilibrium.

Administration of hypertonic saline solution during hypovolemic resuscitation in mammals is well documented; however, its use in reptiles has not yet been examined. Use of hypertonic saline solution is contraindicated in patients that are dehydrated, hypernatremic, hyperchloremic, or hyperosmolar and that have little tolerance for rapid intravascular volume increases (e.g., active hemorrhage or cardiac or neurologic dysfunction).

Isotonic crystalloids have the same effective osmolality as cells and therefore expand the extracellular space. *Maintenance* isotonic crystalloids (e.g., ½-strength lactated Ringer's solution and 2.5% dextrose) contain half the sodium concentration as plasma and are used to replace daily sensible and insensible water and electrolyte losses in the normovolemic rehydrated animal. Dextrose is added as a 2.5% concentration to make the maintenance fluid isotonic. *Replacement* isotonic crystalloids contain a sodium concentration similar to that of the extracellular space, making them the most useful crystalloid in replacing interstitial and intravascular volume deficits. When isotonic replacement crystalloids are administered intravenously, 70% of the volume administered passes into the interstitial fluid compartment within 1 hour (Figure 31-22). Isotonic crystalloids vary in concentration of potassium, magnesium, and calcium. They also vary in buffer additives (Table 31-2).

In most situations of intravascular volume depletion from reduced water intake, vomiting/reflux, diarrhea, or increased water losses, a crystalloid fluid is part of the fluid plan. The crystalloid chosen should be isotonic, have a comparable sodium composition with that of normal plasma, and contain a buffer when a significant acidemia is present. Because most active snakes and lizards have a sodium concentration between 142 and 165 mmol/L at room temperature[3] and their blood pH varies between 7.3 and 7.5,[3] the replacement isotonic crystalloids that contain comparable sodium and pH include Plasmalyte pH 7.4 (Plasmalyte and LRS, Baxter, North Chicago, Ill), Normosol-R (Normosol, Abbott, New Providence, NJ), and lactated Ringer's solution. Plasmalyte and Normosol-R have a sodium concentration of 140 mmol/L, contain potassium and magnesium, and contain no calcium. Acetate and gluconate, buffers contained in Normosol and Plasmalyte, are metabolized to bicarbonate by the muscle tissue and all cells, respectively. Buffered isotonic replacement crystalloids are expected to correct acidemia in a shorter period of time than buffer-free solutions such as 0.9% sodium chloride, which has a pH of 5.4.

Because land turtles tend to have lower plasma sodium concentration (Na = 113 to 140 mmol/L) and a higher pH (pH = 7.4-8) than other reptiles,[1] lactated Ringer's solution may be considered a more appropriate fluid to administer during extracellular fluid replacement. Lactated Ringer's solution has a slightly lower sodium concentration of 130 mmol/L, contains potassium and calcium, and contains no magnesium. Its buffer, lactate (salt), is metabolized by the liver to bicarbonate. Because land turtles also have a relatively higher blood pH, a buffered solution may be more important for avoiding dramatic reductions in pH.

Some controversy surrounds the administration of lactated Ringer's solution to the reptile: that the buffer may exacerbate hyperlactatemia.[6] Reptiles use anaerobic metabolism for adenosine triphosphate (ATP) production during bursts of activity and can tolerate a high increase of lactate production.[7] By the same mechanism, blood lactate levels increase when inadequate tissue perfusion and oxygen delivery exist.

Lactate salts infused in lactated Ringer's solution do not affect plasma lactate levels unless end-stage liver failure is present or the liver remains persistently hypoperfused.[8-10] Persistent hyperlactatemia exacerbated by lactated Ringer's solution in animals is a phenomenon that has been reported in dogs with lymphoma.[11] Hyperlactatemia is a condition that can occur not only in hypoxic tissue but also in hypermetabolic cells with increased Na^+-K^+-ATPase activity (e.g., neoplastic cells, muscle cells stimulated by epinephrine).[12] Elevated blood lactate levels can be multifactorial, and one should not assume that lactated Ringer's solution administration is the sole cause of hyperlactatemia. Nevertheless, a number of alternative buffered isotonic replacement crystalloids can be safely used during replacement fluid therapy (e.g., Plasmalyte-A, Normosol-R) if there is cause for concern.

Because 0.9% sodium chloride solution is an isotonic crystalloid solution that does not contain additional electrolytes, it is an ideal isotonic crystalloid to use during fluid resuscitation of animals with hyperkalemia (e.g., oliguric renal failure), hypercalcemia, or hypochloremic metabolic alkalosis. Supplemental electrolytes can be added to isotonic fluids according to patient requirements. As a safeguard against acute hyperkalemia, the rate of potassium administration added to resuscitation fluids should not exceed 0.5 mEq/kg/h unless serum electrolytes are frequently monitored.

When the cause of volume depletion is rapidly corrected and the interstitial compartment is capable of handling the added fluid, isotonic replacement crystalloids are an effective means for restoring perfusion after intravascular volume depletion. However, high-volume crystalloid infusion can significantly reduce intravascular colloid osmotic pressure (COP) or exacerbate an existing increased hydrostatic pressure, causing increased movement of fluid into the

Table 31-2 Characteristics of Various Fluid Compositions

Name	Fluid Compartment	Osmolarity (mOsm/L)	pH	Na+ (mEq/L)	Cl− (mEq/L)	K+ (mEq/L)	Mg++ (mEq/L)	Ca++ (mEq/L)	Dextrose (g/L)	Buffer	COP (mm Hg)
Crystalloid											
Replacement											
0.9% Saline solution	Extracellular	308 (isotonic)	5	154	154	0	0	0	0	None	0
Lactated Ringer's	Extracellular	275 (isotonic)	6.5	130	109	4	0	3	0	Lactate	0
Plasmalyte-A	Extracellular	294 (isotonic)	7.4	140	98	5	3	0	0	Acetate, gluconate	0
Normosol-R	Extracellular	295 (isotonic)	5.5-7	140	98	5	3	0	0	Acetate, gluconate	0
7% Saline solution	Extracellular	2396 (hypertonic)		1197	1197	0	0	0	0	None	0
5% Dextrose in water	Intracellular	252 (hypotonic)	4	0	0	0	0	0	50	None	0
Maintenance											
2.5% Dextrose in ½-strength lactated Ringer's	Extracellular	264 (isotonic)	4.5-7.5	65.5	55	2	0	1.5	25	Lactate	0
Jarchow's solution*	Extracellular	(hypotonic)	6	94.3	87.3	1.7	0	1	18	Lactate	0
Colloid											
Natural											
Whole blood	Extracellular	300 (isotonic)	Variable	140	100	4	0	0	0-4	None	20
Frozen plasma	Extracellular	300 (isotonic)	Variable	140	110	4	0	0	0-4	None	20
Synthetic											
6% Hetastarch	Extracellular	310 (isotonic)	5.5	154	154	0	0	0	0	None	30
10% Pentastarch	Extracellular	326 (isotonic)	5	154	154	0	0	0	0	None	25
Dextran 40	Extracellular	311 (isotonic)	3.5-7	154	154	0	0	0	0	None	40
Dextran 70	Extracellular	310 (isotonic)	3-7	154	154	0	0	0	0	None	60

From Jarchow J: Hospital care of the reptile patient. In Jacobson ER, Kollias GV, editors: *Exotic animals*, New York, 1988, Churchill Livingstone.
*Two parts 2.5% dextrose in 0.45% NaCl to one part lactated Ringer's solution.
COP, Colloid oncotic pressure.

interstitial compartment. The local increase in interstitial hydrostatic pressure can result in a physical compression of the lymphatic vessels, reducing lymphatic drainage from the overhydrated interstitium. The detrimental effects of rapid large-volume crystalloid administration increase when moderate to severe anemia is occurring, when increased capillary permeability exists, or when states of reduced fluid tolerance exist (pulmonary disease, neurologic disease, cardiac disease). The addition of colloid fluids during intravascular volume replacement in these situations becomes important.

Colloids

Colloid fluids are isotonic and contain a significant concentration of large molecules that contribute to osmotic pressure. Whole blood, plasma, and concentrated albumin contain natural colloids in the form of proteins. Hydroxyethyl starches (hetastarch and pentastarch) and dextrans (dextran-40 and dextran-70) are synthetically derived colloids that have been administered to reptiles.[13]

Synthetic Colloids

Synthetic colloid fluids contain large molecular weight particles that effectively increase COP beyond what can be obtained with blood product infusion alone. They provide osmotic pressure as a result of their large molecular size, and their negative charge attracts sodium and water. Synthetic colloids provide an extended effect on intravascular volume with less total volume infused as compared with crystalloids. Because they replenish intravascular volume only, synthetic colloids are administered only via intravenous and intraosseous routes and in conjunction with crystalloids to prevent interstitial dehydration. The dose of crystalloid is reduced by 40% to 60%. Synthetic colloid fluids do not provide plasma proteins or hemoglobin.

Hydroxyethyl starches (HES) and dextrans are the most commonly used synthetic colloids during acute intravascular volume replacement, and they have independent characteristics that make them unique.[14] Both are effective at rapid intravascular volume resuscitation. In general, HES have a longer half-life and therefore provide a longer duration of effect. This characteristic is desirable when sustained intravascular volume support is needed for treating diseases causing increased capillary permeability and with less tolerance for large volume infusion (e.g., brain and pulmonary disease or cardiac insufficiency).

Dextran-40 has a greater concentration of smaller molecular weight particles per unit volume than dextran-70 and HES and therefore has a greater initial osmotic effect. However, it is eliminated more rapidly than dextran-70 and HES. Elimination of synthetic colloids occurs via several processes. Smaller molecular weight particles are filtered through the glomerulus and voided in the urine. Larger particles are eliminated in bile, stored in tissue, or broken down into smaller particles by the monocyte-macrophage system.

The potential detrimental effects of synthetic colloid administration become more significant with larger doses. When hetastarch is administered in volumes exceeding 40 mg/kg/day in mammals, an increase in incisional bleeding is reported.[15] This can be attributed to an increase in microcirculatory flow and blood pressure and a dilutional and direct effect of hetastarch on coagulation. On the basis of the author's experience, hetastarch can be expected to increase activated clotting time in mammals by 50% without clinical bleeding. Direct application to reptile patients is unknown.

Whole Blood Transfusion

Random anecdotal reports in the literature and in online chat or message boards are found regarding blood transfusions in reptile patients.[16] Whole blood transfusions are certainly possible and not difficult to perform (Figure 31-23). Little scientific data are available to support definitive protocols. Most transfusions reported involve collecting whole blood (not to exceed 1% of the body weight of the donor) from a healthy conspecific and administering it directly to the recipient. One report recommended NOT using a standard Millipore filter, stating that the large reptilian erythrocytes would not pass through. Strict attention should be paid to aseptic technique. A slide agglutination test can be performed on patients with a history of previous transfusions.

Patient Assessment, Dose Administration, and Monitoring Response to Treatment

The transport of fluid and oxygen through the blood vessels to the capillaries is called *perfusion*. Tissue perfusion is directly dependent on adequate intravascular volume and a normally functioning cardiovascular system. Interstitial *hydration* is the presence of fluid in the interstitial space. Adequate hydration provides support for the cells, transport media for molecules, and shape to the tissue or organ. No single test accurately measures fluid compartment volumes in the clinical setting. A reasonable estimate must be made from historical, clinical, and laboratory information. Perfusion is evaluated and restored before evaluation of hydration parameters and correction of dehydration are performed.

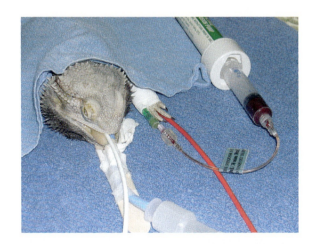

FIGURE 31-23 This Bearded Dragon (*Pogona vitticeps*) is receiving a whole blood transfusion from a healthy conspecific. In addition, it is being maintained after surgery on a pressure-driven ventilator, with its core body temperature recorded with a digital thermometer inserted into the cloaca (red wire) and with its vital signs monitored using a pulse oximeter and a reflectance probe inserted into the esophagus (white wire).

Intravascular Volume Depletion

In mammals, intravascular volume depletion leads to hypovolemia and induces a baroreceptor response that results in sympathetic stimulation causing an elevated heart rate, increase in myocardial contractility, and increased systemic vascular resistance. The same is expected to occur in reptiles; however, because reptiles are ectotherms, their ability to mount an appropriate catecholamine response to hypovolemia requires a warm environment. The degree of hypovolemia may be misjudged if patient assessment relies on heart rate alone.

In addition to clinical judgment on the basis of historical information, clinical parameters such as PCV and total solids (TS) can be useful in assessment of subacute and chronic intravascular plasma water changes. PCV in the reptile is lower than in mammals, ranging from 20% to 40%, and TS are 4 to 6 mg/dL. These values vary between species. When plasma water depletion occurs in the absence of loss of red cell mass (e.g., reduced water intake or increased losses), the PCV and TS increase. Plasma water depletion resulting from acute hemorrhage manifests with a normal to reduced PCV and a reduced TS.

Intravascular volume replacement is best performed via intravascular or intraosseous fluid administration. Isotonic crystalloids alone can be effective in restoring tissue perfusion; however, less volume may be required with concomitant synthetic colloid administration. The reptile and fluids to be administered should always be warmed before and during fluid administration.

Fluids can be kept warm in an incubator or warmed in a microwave (heating times vary between ovens, and testing should be individually performed to determine the best times or intervals for reaching the optimum temperature). The fluid lines can also be placed under heating pads or in warm water baths during administration. Optimal fluid temperatures range between 30°C and 35°C (85°F to 95°F).

Interstitial Hydration

Once perfusion and body temperature have been restored, hydration parameters can be more accurately assessed. The common clinical parameters evaluated during assessment of interstitial hydration in mammals include mucous membrane moisture, position of the ocular globe, and skin elasticity. The latter, skin turgor, is of little value in reptile patients. Factors that can alter these parameters in the absence of interstitial fluid shifts include hypersalivation from oral disease or pain, advanced age, and reduced body fat content. When dehydration is estimated to be greater than 8%, an intravascular volume deficit is expected to occur from osmotic fluid shifts.

Many species of reptiles have a high tolerance for dehydration and increases in plasma sodium and osmolality. The thirst mechanism is highly developed in lizards, and increases in plasma osmolality cause them to drink significant amounts of water and excrete sodium from the salt glands to restore osmolality.[17] Since renal resorptive processes are limited for water retention during acute volume depletion, fluid administration may be necessary in the debilitated reptile. Use of an isotonic replacement crystalloid, with a sodium level comparable with normal plasma, produces less of an osmotic gradient than a maintenance crystalloid.

Interstitial fluid replacement is best performed via an intravascular or intraosseous route in the debilitated reptile. When a rapid recovery is expected, and the patient is properly warmed, fluids can be administered via an intracoelomic or subcutaneous route.

Hyaluronidase (an enzyme derived from bovine testicular tissue) administration has been advocated for enhancing subcutaneous fluid absorption in reptiles. Hyaluronic acid, part of the ground substance that binds the interstitium, is lysed by hyaluronidase. In humans, hyaluronidase is indicated for facilitating fluid and drug absorption from the subcutaneous space and reducing pain during chronic fluid administration. However, no comparable difference between the duration of fluid at the administration site or the presence of pain seems to exist between cancer patients who received hyaluronidase during chronic subcutaneous fluid administration and those who did not.[18,19] No studies have been performed to advocate its use for fluid replacement in the reptile.

Intracellular Hydration

Intracellular hydration is estimated with evaluation of the serum sodium after perfusion and interstitial hydration have been restored. An increase in serum sodium implies a loss in intracellular water as a result of osmotic shifts from the cell into the interstitial and intravascular compartments. Perfusion and hydration parameters must be restored *before* accurate assessment of the intracellular volume status can be made. Cellular swelling caused by rapid shifts of water after inappropriate fluid administration may not be clinically evident until significant loss of cell function has already occurred.

When serum sodium values are greater than 160 mEq/L in the presence of altered mentation, replacement of free water with IV or intracoelomic administration of D_5W is indicated. The free water deficit is calculated and replaced over 12 to 24 hours. When chronic dehydration (>48 to 72 hours) is suspected, this deficit is replaced over 24 to 48 hours. The free water deficit can be estimated with the following calculation for most reptiles:

$$\text{Water deficit (L)} = (0.75 \times \text{lean body weight [kg]}) \times 1 - \text{current pNa}/150*$$

Simultaneously, maintenance and replacement fluids are administered to replace ongoing losses. The serum sodium concentration is reevaluated every 4 to 6 hours, and solute-free water dose is adjusted as needed to prevent excessive osmotic shifts.

COMMON REPTILIAN "EMERGENCIES"

Reptiles are susceptible to a myriad of medical problems. As already stated, very few true emergencies exist, with trauma probably being the most serious and immediately life-threatening. Sepsis, impactions, egg-binding, hypocalcemic tetany, and more are all covered elsewhere in

---

*For land turtles: Water deficit (L) = (0.6 × lean body weight [kg]) × 1 − current pNa/135.

Table 31-3	Recommended Equipment List for a Reptile Practice

Vascular clips (small, medium, and large)
Radioscalpel or CO_2 laser or both
Rigid endoscopy system
Operating magnifying loupes
Air pumps
Sexing probes
Radiology unit with a wide range of mA and kVp settings and the capability of taking both vertical and horizontal beam projections
High-detail radiographic film or screens or both
Electronic digital thermometer capable of rapid read-out with a range from freezing to greater than 100°C; infrared temperature guns are useful
Heat lamps or radiant heat panels with thermostats
Ultraviolet B (UVB) light sources in cages
Thermal water blankets
Capture and restraint equipment (snake hooks, tubes, tongs, bags, plastic storage containers with appropriate ventilation, etc.)
Ventilator, Ambu bag, or ability to manually ventilate anesthetized patients
Pulse oximeter, Doppler flow meter, apnea monitor, or similar equipment for anesthetic monitoring
1-mm to 4-mm uncuffed endotracheal tubes
Dremel (Racine, Wis) or similar rotary cutting tool with appropriate bits for grinding beaks and nails
Dremel or similar rotary cutting tool or orthopedic saw for opening chelonian shells
Oral speculums of various sizes and types
Microliter or insulin syringes
Syringe or infusion pumps

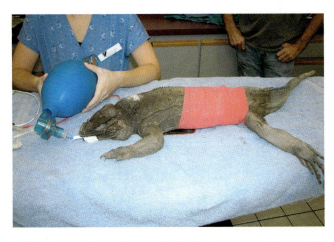

FIGURE 31-24 A ventilator or Ambu bag is a necessity in a reptile practice.

"Exotic Animal Medicine—Standards of Care" symposia.[20] Obviously, a carbon dioxide laser is not absolutely mandatory to be a proficient reptile veterinarian; however, having a mechanical ventilator, or at least an Ambu bag, to manually ventilate a patient is (Figure 31-24).

What constitutes an emergency? No textbook answer is found for that question. What a client considers an emergency (the bump that has been under the skin for the past 2 months) may, in actuality, not be. However, the emergency clinician must be cognizant of the fact that most clients are not trained at assessing the true level of the medical crisis. If they are told that the problem can probably wait until tomorrow ("He seems lethargic, Doc.") and the patient dies, the veterinarian is at fault.

The authors' client credo is: "If it's an emergency to you, it's an emergency to me. Bring it in. If you are not sure, bring it in anyway. It is better to be safe than sorry."

REFERENCES

1. Minnich JE: Reptiles. In Maloiy GMO, editor: *Comparative physiology of osmoregulation in animals,* London, 1979, Academic Press.
2. Fitzsimons JT, Kaufman S: Cellular and extracellular dehydration, and angiotensin as stimuli to drinking in the common iguana *Iguana iguana, J Physiol* 265:443-463, 1977.
3. Minnich JE: The use of water. In Gans C, Pough FH, editors: *Biology of the Reptilia,* vol 12, London, 1982, Academic Press.
4. Smits AW, Kozubowski MM: Partitioning of body fluids and cardiovascular responses to circulatory hypovolaemia in the turtle, Pseudemys scripta elegans; and Thorson TB: Body fluid partitioning in reptilian, *Copeia* 592-601, 1968.
5. Dessauer HC: Blood chemistry of reptiles. In Gans C, editor: *Biology of the Reptilia,* vol 3, London, 1970, Academic Press.
6. Prezant RM, Jarchow JL: Lactated fluid use in reptiles: is there a better solution? *Proc Assoc Reptilian Amphibian Vet* 83-87, 1997.
7. White FN: Circulation. In Gans C, editor: *Biology of the Reptilia,* London, 1976, Academic Press.
8. Trudnowski RL, Goel SB, Lam FT, Evers JT: Effect of Ringer's lactate solution and sodium bicarbonate on surgical acidosis, *Surg Gynecol Obstet* 125:807-814, 1967.
9. Trinkle JK, Rush BF, Eiseman B: Metabolism of lactate following major blood loss, *Surgery* 63:782, 1968.
10. Lowery BP, Clouter CT, Carey LC: Electrolyte solutions in resuscitation in human hemorrhagic shock, *Surg Gynecol Obstet* 133:273, 1971.
11. Vail DM, Ogilvie GK, Fettman MJ, Wheeler SL: Exacerbation of hyperlactatemia by infusion of lactated Ringer's solution in dogs with lymphoma, *JVIM* 4(5):228-232, 1990.
12. McCarter FD, Nierman SR, James JH, Wang L, King JK, Friend LA, et al: Role of skeletal muscle Na^+-K^+-ATPase activity in increased lactate production in sub-acute sepsis, *Life Sci* 70(16):1875-1888, 2002.
13. Wellehan JFX, Gunkel CI: Emergent diseases in reptiles, *Semin Avian Exotic Pet Med* 13(3):160-174, 2004.
14. Rudloff E, Kirby R: The critical need for colloids: administering colloids effectively, *Comp Cont Educ* 20:27-43, 1998.
15. Cheng C, Lerner MA, Lichtewnstein S, et al: Effect of hydroxyethylstarch on hemostasis, *Surg Forum Metab* 48-50, 1998.
16. Wack RF, Anderson NL: Resuscitation of a Hispaiolan slider, Trachemys decorata, using Oxyglobin® and a blood transfusion, *J Herp Med Surg* 14(1):4, 2004.

this book. To review these here is redundant. The more common medical conditions are reviewed, alphabetically, in Chapters 42 to 74.

It would be prudent for regional emergency facilities to be prepared to handle reptile patients. This includes having the appropriate physical plant and necessary equipment to restrain, handle, diagnose, treat, and house these unique patients. Table 31-3 lists recommended equipment for the proper care of reptilian patients. This information was presented at the 2005 North American Veterinary Conference

17. Fitzsimons JT, Kaufman S: Cellular and extracellular dehydration, and angiotensin as stimuli to drinking in the common iguana *Iguana iguana*, *J Physiol* 265:443-463, 1977.
18. Constans T, Dutertre JP, Froge E: Hypodermoclysis in dehydrated elderly patients: local effects with and without hyaluronidase, *J Palliat Care* 7:10-12, 1991.
19. Centeno C, Bruera E: Subcutaneous hydration with no hyaluronidase in patients with advanced cancer [letter], *J Pain Symptom Manag* 17:305-306, 1999.
20. Mader DR, Barten SL: Standards of care: reptile practice, *Proc North Am Vet Conf* 1298-1301, 2005.
21. Lawton MPC, Divers SJ: Comparison of leukocyte counts using two different methods, *Proc Assoc Rept Amphib Vet* 149-152, 1999.

32
ENDOSCOPY
W. MICHAEL TAYLOR

Fine-diameter rigid endoscopes have been used for diagnostic purposes in birds and reptiles since the late 1970s. During the decade of the 1980s, this technology began to be used with greater vigor by veterinarians in zoologic and private practice. The value of a minimally traumatic procedure that allowed excellent visualization of internal structures even in very small patients soon became evident to many avian practitioners. Enhanced diagnostic sampling procedures were slower to develop. Avian medicine has seen spectacular growth in its knowledge base over the past 15 years, including the development of improved endoscopic diagnostic techniques. Reptile medicine is now undergoing many of the exciting growth changes seen in the early 1980s and 1990s in the avian field. Important new applications of endoscopy in reptiles have been developed since the first edition of this book.

EVOLUTION OF THE TECHNIQUE

Bush[1] first described the use of rigid endoscopes for the evaluation of reptiles in the ground-breaking book *Animal Laparoscopy* published in 1980. The first applications of the technology were for gender identification in monomorphic reptiles.[2] Other workers were surprisingly slow to apply the technology to solving clinical problems in reptiles.[3-5] In 1992, Schildger and Wicker[6] described the use of a small-diameter pediatric cystoscope with an integral sheath for examination of the coelom and collection of biopsy specimens from a variety of reptiles and amphibians. This system allowed the insertion of 3-French (1-mm) hand instruments through the channel in the integral sheath. Targeted biopsies could be collected with direct visualization.

Insufflation of the coelom was determined to be necessary in many reptiles and was achieved with connection of a laparoflator or air pump to one of the infusion ports on the sheath. This original cystoscope system is no longer commercially available. Current endoscopic applications for reptiles have arisen from work already completed in avian medicine. The author, working in collaboration with Karl Storz Veterinary Endoscopy, developed a sheath and 2.7-mm endoscope system with 5-French instruments for avian medicine in 1991 (endoscope 64018 BS with sheath 67065 CC, Karl Storz Veterinary Endoscopy, Goleta, Calif; *www.ksvea.com*; Figures 32-1 to 32-3).[7] It soon became evident that this system was applicable to reptiles.

Insufflation is achieved in a manner similar to that described initially by Schildger. Medical carbon dioxide from a manual or electronic laparoflator is infused through one of the lateral stopcocks of the sheath to achieve a pressure of 10 mm of mercury. Room air delivered with a simple pump has also been described as an insufflation source.[8] Effective filtering of the room air can be difficult. The risk of embolism is also greater with room air than with medical-grade carbon dioxide; however, many practitioners have used this technique with no apparent problems. Commercial medical-line filters (e.g., Storz #20400060) are available and can prevent coelomic contamination from fine debris carried by the insufflation gas (Figure 32-4).

Additional regulation of intracoelomic pressure is possible with selective venting of the valve of the opposing stopcock (Figure 32-5). Excess pressure can be released with opening the valve and bleeding off the insufflation gas as necessary.

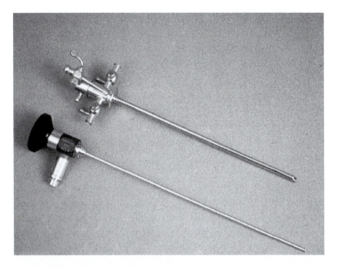

FIGURE 32-1 Storz Avian Sheath system with a 2.7-mm telescope. The telescope is inserted and locked into the sheath. Two side ports are used for infusion of air or water.

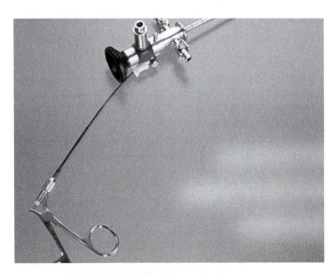

FIGURE 32-2 The top instrument port allows the introduction of semirigid or flexible instruments.

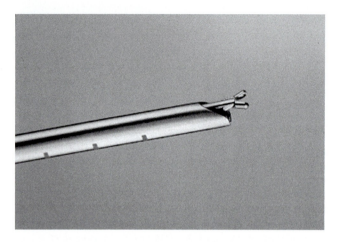

FIGURE 32-3 Instrumentation is visualized as it exits the distal tip of the sheath.

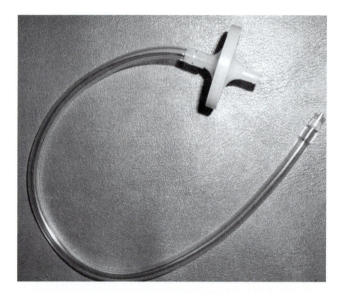

FIGURE 32-4 Insufflation Gas Filter (Storz #20400060).

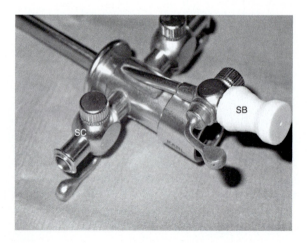

FIGURE 32-5 Close-up of the Storz Sheath. Lateral ports with stopcocks *(SC)* and instrument insertion port with rubber sealing bonnet in place *(SB)*.

A rubber fitting (White rubber sealing bonnet, Storz # 27550 C) placed over the instrument port prevents excessive air or fluid leakage during instrument placement.

The focal directed illumination and magnification achieved with modern rod lens endoscopes are as applicable for work in reptiles as in birds.[9] A thorough coelomic exploratory examination can be performed in many reptiles and most major organs examined. Biopsies may be collected with introduction of a flexible cup biopsy forceps through the rubber fitting and into the instrument channel (see Figure 32-2). Inflammatory debris and fluids may also be collected for cytologic, microbiologic, or molecular biologic testing. As in the bird, the forceps tip may be guided visually to the site of collection with precision, with iatrogenic injury avoided. The Storz equipment is highly recommended because it is the only complete system designed by and for exotic animal practitioners. Attention to detail means that this system has shown tremendous versatility in small and medium-sized reptiles and in birds and small mammals.

RIGID VERSUS FLEXIBLE ENDOSCOPY

The effectiveness of endoscopy as a clinical tool is dependent on several factors (Table 32-1). Of primary importance is optical quality. The endoscope becomes an extension of the clinician's visual system, and in doing so, the resolution, clarity, and magnifying capabilities of the lens system are *crucial to diagnostic decision making.* Modern rod lens designs used in rigid endoscopes have superior optic qualities when compared with similar-diameter flexible endoscopes, especially those with fiberoptic viewing systems. Newer flexible endoscopes with small distal charge coupled device (CCD) viewing systems are the current industry standard in 5-mm and 10-mm diameters. They have revolutionized the practice of human flexible endoscopy but are costly.

The next critical issue becomes diameter of the telescope and the volume of light-carrying bundles that distribute light to the site to be viewed. The greater the number of light-carrying bundles, the greater the focal illumination, but the trade off comes with the necessary increase in endoscope diameter. The third key factor is the length of the instrument. This determines the clinical reach of the endoscope and may become the essential consideration in very large or elongated species.

Table 32-1	Comparison of Rigid Versus Flexible Endoscopes
Rigid	**Flexible**
Rod lenses = gold standard resolution	CCD better than glass fiber imaging systems
Glass fiber illumination system	Same
Length limited by torsional fragility	Long lengths possible
No distal tip deflection, but distal lens angle can be varied	Distal tip deflection in two or four directions
Easier to guide in open cavities	Easier to guide in tubular organs, especially with turns greater than 50 degrees

CCD, Charge coupled device.

Rigid endoscopes are limited in length by the nature of their construction. Torsional rigidity is directly proportional to endoscope diameter and length. Long thin rigid endoscopes are easily damaged.

The last consideration is the distal lens offset (in rigid endoscopes) or planes of control (in flexible endoscopes) available for any given telescope design. Rigid endoscopes do not have the ability to move the distal tip as do flexible endoscopes. The angle of the distal lens in a rigid endoscope can be purchased in a number of variations measured as the degree of offset from the central axis to provide an oblique viewing angle (Figure 32-6). A distal lens offset of 30 degrees proves to be the most useful for standard use. When a 30-degree endoscope is rotated around its long axis, the viewing field is enhanced. Hand instruments can also be more easily viewed entering the operating field.

Differences in species size, shape, and organ morphology determine whether rigid or flexible endoscopy is most appropriate for a given patient. Rigid endoscopes are more useful in the coelomic cavity or cloaca because their rigidity permits better control of placement within open spaces. Flexible endoscopes are most useful in the gastrointestinal tract and airways of reptiles, especially when a longer reach is necessary. Their inherent flexibility is essential with imaging of twisting tubular organs.

GETTING STARTED: THE TOOLS NEEDED

Light Sources

The light necessary to illuminate the endoscopic field may be generated in a number of ways. For routine diagnostic purposes, a halogen reflector lamp of 150 watts is sufficient. A variety of very compact and portable sources in this output range are available. The color temperature of the light produced with a halogen lamp is 3200°K to 3400°K, and although this is perfectly acceptable for viewing with the human eye, it is not suitable for use with "daylight" film emulsions and must be properly white balanced for video use.

Documentation of endoscopic examinations and procedures with film or video often needs more specialized lighting. High-output xenon lamps, although more expensive, produce an intense light with a color temperature similar to daylight (approximately 5500°K). Their continuous intense light output is useful for video recording and certain types of still photography. The highest quality endoscopic still photographs are achieved with specially designed flash generators. These light sources contain some form of constant illumination system, usually halogen, for diagnostic viewing and focusing and a high intensity flash generator for 35-mm still photography. The flash is triggered by the cameras shutter release at the moment an exposure is made, providing an extremely short strobe burst that has the advantage of freezing both patient-produced and operator-produced motion much more successfully than can be achieved with even the most powerful continuously operating xenon lamp. Most current models contain some form of through-the-lens (TTL) flash metering system to ensure consistency of exposure and ease of use and a movable prism to deflect the flash burst down the light cable (Figure 32-7).

Light Guide Cables

Light cables are the flexible tethers that allow rigid endoscopes to be linked to a light source and yet maintain maximum freedom of movement. The cable transmits light produced by the light source via the principle of internal reflection yet transmits very little of the heat. The diameter of the light-transmitting bundle should closely match the diameter of the fiberoptic system of the endoscope to permit the maximum transmission of light from the light source. The size of the internal fiberoptic bundle of the endoscope can

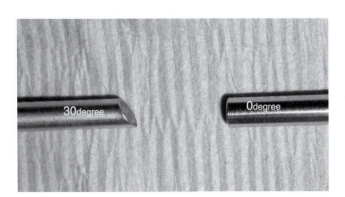

FIGURE 32-6 Comparison view of 0-degree and 30-degree distal lens offsets.

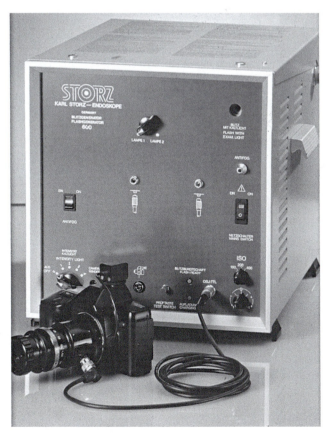

FIGURE 32-7 Storz Model 600 Flash Generator with through-the-lens (TTL) flash measurement.

vary depending on design factors and the overall diameter of the instrument.

Two basic forms of endoscopic light cable are found. The first and most familiar type is the glass fiber optic cable. Constructed of many randomly arranged or "incoherent" specially clad glass fibers of small size (each 10-μm to 25-μm diameter), this cable is very flexible and is therefore most useful for clinical applications. An important principle to remember is that the more a glass fiber cable is flexed the greater the decrease in light transmission from internal reflection losses. This is not a critical problem for diagnostic viewing because the human eye accommodates these changes; however, for critical use (e.g., still photography), keeping the cable as straight as possible is advisable to maximize the transmission of light.

The second type of cable is the liquid or fluid light cable. This device uses an optical liquid to transmit light, and although it is not as flexible as a comparable-diameter glass fiber cable, it offers a greater percentage of light transmission. This can be useful in some applications, but fluid cables transmit a higher proportion of the blue end of the light spectrum that may result in unrealistic blue tones with many daylight film emulsions. Liquid light cables are therefore not recommended for best photographic results.

Endoscopes

The ideal endoscope for reptiles is one with as fine a diameter as possible and with the largest and brightest image that could be achieved, but current design and fabrication limits create important considerations relating to endoscope diameter. As the diameter becomes smaller two practical effects occur. The amount of light that can be transmitted to the viewing field is decreased, and the image circle as viewed at the ocular lens becomes smaller. For diagnostic purposes, this means that 1.9 mm is the smallest diameter endoscope available with high-quality optics. This endoscope is excellent for patients that weigh less than 100 g or in small anatomic sites.

The major disadvantages of these very small endoscopes are their fragility and relatively small field of view. They also transmit less light, which limits their usefulness in larger body cavities. **The 2.7-mm endoscope is most frequently recommended because it provides good light transmission capabilities with an adequate image size at a diameter that may be used in a wide range of reptiles.** This versatility combined with a sheath system means that it is a good choice as the sole or principal endoscope in an exotic animal practice. The author has used the 2.7-mm endoscope in patients that weigh 55 grams to 4 kilograms. Intermediate-sized telescopes (e.g., 2.2 mm) are available and may be preferred by some clinicians. Endoscopes of 4 or 5 mm can also be used in larger patients or when documentation demands. The advantages of the larger optic are greater light transmission and a bigger image circle. Also, most modern 4-mm or 5-mm endoscopes incorporate new distal lens designs that provide a wider field of view. These lens designs are currently unavailable in telescopes with less than 4-mm diameter.

Flexible endoscopes with an instrument channel are available in 2.5-mm, 5-mm, and 10-mm variations. The smaller 2.5-mm flexible endoscopes (e.g., Storz 60003 bronchoscope) do not have CCD imaging but are useful in longer thinner viscera. Standard human flexible endoscopes with CCD imaging are superb and useful in some species, but their purchase cost is high. The clinician must balance the cost of acquisition with the number of clinical procedures that actually require the use of the flexible endoscope on the basis of caseload.

Hand Instrumentation

A variety of hand instruments are available for use with the Storz sheath system. The versatility of the sheath system is enhanced by an assortment of instruments that allow the clinician to perform many procedures. Each is a tool that extends the operator's ability to complete a task in the safest, most efficient manner. Most flexible systems also have biopsy, grasping, and wire baskets available. Having on hand and using the correct instrument is frequently as essential to the success of a procedure for the reptile veterinarian as is having the correct tool for a skilled tradesperson.

Biopsy Forceps

The 5-French elliptical cup forceps (Storz 161Z) is the most important specimen collection tool in the set. It is a versatile biopsy forceps because it can be used in most tissues and collects a deeper longitudinal sample compared with a round cup (Figure 32-8). The 5-French is also useful for sampling exudate and debris. A 5-French round cup forceps (Storz 117Z) is also available. This instrument is the same width as the elliptical but has a round shallow cup suited for collecting smaller samples or when less tissue penetration is desirable. A 3-French forceps is also available and may be used with either the 2.7-mm or 1.9-mm sheath systems.

Grasping and Retrieval

The 5-French grasping forceps (Storz 161T) is the standard for the set and has large serrations. It is particularly useful for retrieving medium to large objects and collecting exudate or debris. The finer 3-French graspers (Storz 071TJ) are most

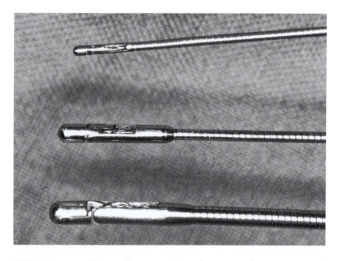

FIGURE 32-8 Biopsy forceps: 3-French, 5-French, and 7-French elliptical cup forceps.

useful for blunt dissection or for grasping smaller objects. This author has had clinical situations in which one or the other size of grasping forceps was essential to the successful outcome of the procedure. As a result, both instruments are recommended to be available.

A wire retrieval basket (Storz 023VK) is also available for use with the sheath system. Many smooth or rounded objects can only be grasped with the use of a retrieval basket such as this.

Incising and Cutting

A superb semirigid 3.5-French scissors (Storz 501EK) with one fixed and one moving blade is an essential part of the operating system. Coelomic and pleural membranes can be easily incised with these miniature scissors. A 22-gauge injection needle with Teflon guide (Storz 071X) has many uses in reptiles. It allows precise injection and aspiration of fluids. The needle may also be connected to a radiosurgical unit (e.g., Ellman Surgitron, Ellman International, Hewlett, NY; *www.ellman.com*) and energized to incise or coagulate structures. The Teflon guide that is designed to promote the easier insertion of the long fine needle within the sheath can also be used alone to aspirate or infuse material where a sharp tip is not necessary.

Documentation Devices

Improvements in video and imaging technologies continue to revolutionize the endoscopic field. Endovideo cameras attach to the ocular of the endoscope and provide superb images when used with an appropriate light source. Examinations can be recorded and reviewed or sent to a consultant. Superb modern endocamera designs (e.g., Storz 202121) fit ergonomically into the hand of the operator, which allows longer procedures and enhanced fine manipulation with lower levels of operator fatigue. The improved ergonomics are attained both by the design of the camera body and by the use of a high-resolution monitor that allows the clinician to sit and view the procedure in a comfortable position with the forearms supported to enable precise movements.

Analog endovideo cameras output a high-quality signal that can be recorded with a standard VHS or, for best results, a super VHS (or equivalent Hi8) recording device. Digital endovideo cameras provide even better images. Medical digital still recording devices are now available and produce good results by capturing the output of the endovideo camera as selected still images. The device converts analog video into a digitized still image that can be recorded onto a data disk for later review or incorporation into digital storage files. The current quality is good and can be expected to improve with the next generation of digital video cameras.

Still photography with 35-mm film has always been a challenge with fine-diameter endoscopes. The small apertures provided by these endoscopes deliver less light to the site to be photographed, which necessitates a high-intensity flash source to enable successful exposure with high-resolution (low ISO speed) film. Superb flash generators such as the Storz Model 600 give excellent exposures and were used to capture the images for this chapter but are relatively costly for clinical practice (see Figure 32-7).

INSTRUMENT CARE AND STERILIZATION

Both rigid and flexible endoscopes are relatively costly precision optic instruments that give excellent long-term performance if maintained properly. Rigid telescopes, especially those of very small diameter, are fragile, and appropriate care must be used during transport, handling, and cleaning to avoid damage to the rod lens elements. Torsional stresses on the long axis of the endoscope must be avoided. This is most important when a fine-diameter telescope is used without a protective sheath as is frequently the case for diagnostic purposes. Particularly important is that the operator be sensitive to the amount of force applied to the telescope during a procedure.

Rigid endoscopes should always be picked up by the ocular (eyepiece) and not by the distal tip. Cleaning the instrument immediately after the procedure is finished is wise. A nonabrasive cleanser may be used to remove fat and debris. In many cases, simply washing the telescope in distilled water is all that is needed. A quality lens paper should be used to clean the lens surfaces. An alcohol wash can be used to chemically dry the endoscope before placement into a padded storage container that meets the manufacturer's recommendations. A simple but effective plastic endoscope sleeve has been manufactured to cover the shaft of the telescope for protection during transport and during soaking (Figure 32-9).

Flexible endoscopes should also be handled with care. They should not be coiled tightly or have objects of any weight placed on the shaft or the glass fiber bundles will be damaged. Instrument channels should be flushed thoroughly with warm soapy water to remove debris after use. Most manufacturers recommend that flexible endoscopes be stored suspended from the ocular end with the flexible shaft allowed to hang vertically. Detailed instructions for endoscope care are provided by most manufacturers to their customers. Technical staff should be properly trained in the handling and cleaning of these sensitive instruments before receiving the responsibility for their care.

Most endoscopic procedures require properly sterilized equipment. Even in examinations of noncritical areas, such as

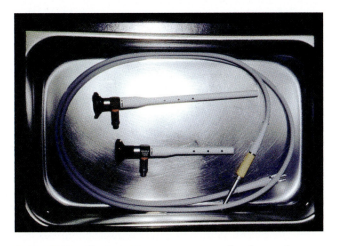

FIGURE 32-9 Plastic endoscope protectors placed on endoscopes in a glutaraldehyde soak tray.

the oral cavity or cloaca, one is prudent to remember that many species may harbor pathogenic organisms that can be physically transferred to another patient without proper handling of the instruments between examinations. Although the stainless steel sheath system can be autoclaved routinely, the sensitive rod lens systems of rigid endoscopes are not generally amenable to this form of sterilization. Expansion and contraction caused by the marked temperature extremes of steam autoclaving damage or severely shorten the life of most telescopes. Some types of recently produced rigid endoscopes are steam autoclavable, although this process may also decrease their working life. One should check with the manufacturer before proceeding and follow their instructions explicitly.

Only two options have been proven safe for sensitive telescopes, hand instruments, and light cables and yet provide consistently reliable sterilization. The first choice is gas sterilization with ethylene oxide. This gas is an extremely effective sterilant, but materials exposed to it must be aerated for a minimum of 8 to 12 hours after the sterilization cycle. Also of note is that ethylene oxide may be a human health hazard and in many jurisdictions must be used under carefully controlled conditions.

Because ethylene oxide is not a practical or safe alternative for the average practitioner, the second choice for office or field sterilization of sensitive endoscopic equipment is soaking in a 2% solution of glutaraldehyde or a peracetic acid solution designed for endoscopes and approved by the manufacturer of the equipment. The solution must be used according to the supplier's directions. One should be aware of the activated life of the product (usually 14 or 28 days) and change solutions accordingly. The equipment manufacturer's instructions should be followed closely regarding the soaking of telescopes, hand instruments, and light cables.

One should avoid the stacking or layering of instruments in the soak tray so that the solution can properly reach all surfaces. Circulating the solution with a syringe is useful to ensure that all surfaces have been contacted. Minimum recommended soaking times in properly prepared glutaraldehyde solutions typically range from 15 to 20 minutes. Greater germicidal effect is achieved the longer the equipment is soaked; however, many manufacturers caution against soaking for longer than 2 hours because damage to glass fibers may occur. Peracetic acid solutions have a slightly shorter soak cycle and may be more likely to cause instrument corrosion. Recommendations should be followed closely.

After the soaking cycle has been completed, the equipment must be rinsed in sterile water to prevent the carryover of irritating solutions to the patient. Glutaraldehyde is extremely irritating to most tissues and may cause local irritation and coelomic reaction. Best results may be achieved with rinsing the equipment in a sterile container of sterile water for 3 to 5 minutes. One should drain and then immerse in a second container of sterile water for 3 to 5 minutes and then wipe dry. A final alcohol wash may be used to chemically dry the equipment if desired. Other types of disinfectant solutions, such as quaternary ammonium compounds, chlorhexidine, and povidone iodine, are not acceptable alternatives to glutaraldehyde or peracetic acid solutions for soaking endoscopic equipment. With the number of resistant viruses and bacteria seen in many reptiles, the endoscopist must ensure that only effective approved products are used or the result may be the unnecessary spread of disease.

ANESTHESIA

Appropriate anesthesia is an essential part of good endoscopic practice. An endoscopic examination is seldom possible to carry out in the physically restrained reptile without the risk of organ contusion or other trauma as a result of patient struggling. Also, one cannot stress strongly enough that consistency in positioning of the patient is essential for anatomic orientation. Maintaining position is neither possible nor humane with physical restraint only. Clinical anesthesia has been thoroughly reviewed in Chapter 27. A variety of parenteral and inhalant anesthetics have been used for endoscopy in reptiles. The anesthetic agent of choice for most endoscopic procedures is isoflurane (AErrane, Anaquest, Madison, Wis).

COELIOSCOPY

One of the most useful applications for rigid endoscopy in reptiles is examination of the coelomic cavity. Knowledge of the variations in reptile coelomic morphology is essential to the endoscopist.[10] The most conserved or "primitive" reptile pleuroperitoneal cavity is simple in layout.[11] The only separate compartment is the pericardium, which is located in the ventral cranial thoracoabdominal cavity at the level of the pectoral girdle (Figure 32-10). This simple form of pleuroperitoneal cavity enables virtually unimpeded endoscopic visualization from the level of the thoracic inlet to the pelvis.

Lizards within the families Iguanidae, Geckonidae, Agamidae, Scinidae, and Helodermatidae are common examples of species with this simple design.[10] In Chelonia (turtles and tortoises), the lungs are located dorsally and are partially adherent to the carapace. They are separated from the coelomic cavity by an oblique postpulmonary septum (septum postpulmonale) that runs from the cranially positioned pericardial sac up to the carapace (Figure 32-11).

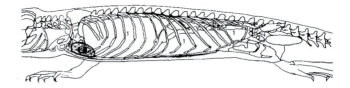

FIGURE 32-10 Schematic representation of the simplest pleuroperitoneal cavity in reptiles (lizard). *1*, Pleuroperitoneal cavity; *2*, pericardial sac.

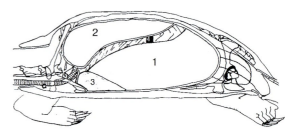

FIGURE 32-11 Schematic representation of the coelomic cavities of the chelonian. *1*, Peritoneal cavity; *2*, pleural cavity; *3*, pericardial sac; *4*, postpulmonary septum.

Monitors (*Varanus* sp.) represent a somewhat more complicated coelomic design, with the separation of the pleural cavities from the peritoneal cavity by a well-developed transverse postpulmonary septum. The lungs are also attached to the dorsal body wall as in Chelonia; however, they completely occupy the cranial portion of the thoracoabdominal cavity. The pericardial sac in monitors is located more caudally, reflecting the transverse position of the postpulmonary septum and the larger lung fields.

Crocodilia have the most complex coelomic design of the reptiles. Like Monitors, they have a prominent transverse postpulmonary septum with large dorsally adherent lungs filling the pleural cavities. The pericardial sac is also situated more caudally. They also have a prominent posthepatic septum (septum horizontale) that separates the liver from the more caudal portions of the peritoneal cavity (Figure 32-12). The posthepatic septum is supplied around its margins with an extensive supply of striated muscle to form the so-called diaphragmatic muscle. Contraction of these striated muscles retracts the posthepatic septum and pulls on the solid liver in a caudal direction. Dunker[11] likens this to the movement of a piston within a cylinder retracting the postpulmonary septum and inflating the lung. This mechanism supports the more traditional respiratory movements produced by the thoracic ribs and their musculature.

In lizards with a simple pleuroperitoneal cavity (e.g., Green Iguana [*Iguana iguana*]), the most frequently used approach for endoscopic examination is made in the lateral region analogous to the mammalian "paralumbar fossa," caudal to the last rib. The skin is incised, and the thin musculature of the body wall may be spread with a fine mosquito forceps. Care should be taken when the thoracoabdominal cavity is first entered to ensure that the lungs are not at full inflation to prevent inadvertent puncture. Insufflation is virtually always necessary in lizards to allow adequate visualization of organs. From this insertion point looking cranially, the operator can view the liver, spleen, stomach, lung, and heart within the large cavity (Figure 32-13).

No diaphragm is present. With the increased intracoelomic pressure from insufflation, the lungs may not inflate well and intermittent positive pressure ventilation (IPPV) is recommended at 2 to 3 breaths per minute. Manual or automated ventilation can be used.

In chelonians, the entry incision is made in the left (or right) prefemoral region after surgical preparation with standard techniques of skin cleansing. The incision is equidistant from the horizontal margins of the carapace and plastron and approximately midway between the femur and the cranial portion of the carapace margin, similar to a surgical approach described previously for laparotomy (Figure 32-14).[12] A fine mosquito forceps is introduced through the body wall in a craniomedial direction. The jaws are opened to gently spread the muscle layers. Insertion of the rigid scope at this site allows visualization of most of the cranial coelomic cavity (Figure 32-15, *A*). Manipulating the scope (repositioning and turning on its axis) also allows visualization of the kidneys and gonads (Figure 32-15, *B*).

Endoscopic examination is indicated whenever the visual inspection of an organ or site may yield additional diagnostic information. Diagnostic endoscopy is usually preceded by the collection of a minimum database, such as a complete blood count, biochemistry profile, or radiology. The patient's history, findings of the physical examination, and the results of laboratory and radiologic studies are frequently inconclusive or may suggest the usefulness of endoscopic examination of a specific site (Table 32-2).

Although conventional radiographic studies are useful, the author's experience has been that endoscopic follow-up

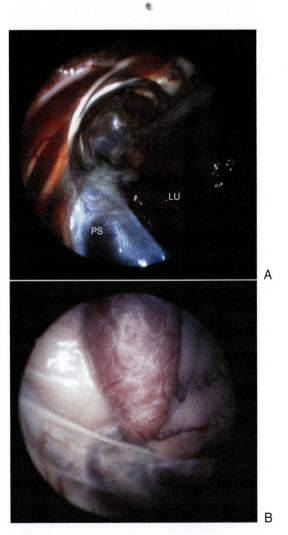

FIGURE 32-13 **A,** View of the cranial pleuroperitoneal cavity of a Green Iguana (*Iguana iguana*). *PS,* Pericardial sac; *LU,* lung. The patient is in right lateral recumbency. Note the lateral body wall and ribs. **B,** Normal Iguana spleen.

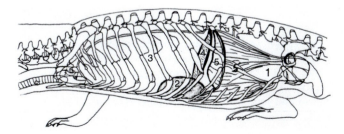

FIGURE 32-12 Schematic representation of the coelomic cavities of the crocodilian. *1,* Peritoneal cavity; *2,* pericardial sac; *3,* pleural cavity; *4,* postpulmonary septum; *5,* posthepatic septum.

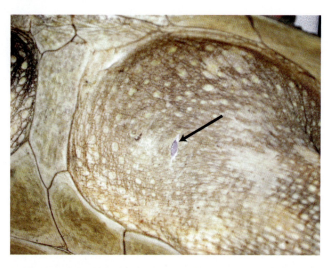

FIGURE 32-14 Incision site *(arrow)* in the midcranial portion of the hind leg fold of Chelonia.

Table 32-2	Indications for Endoscopic Examination

Acute or chronic dyspnea
Sneezing
Abnormal radiographic findings (plain or contrast; e.g., lung organomegaly, gastrointestinal)
Abnormal biochemical studies (e.g., elevated uric acid levels [kidney], elevated bile acids [liver], or enzymology)
Persistent leukocytosis: unexplained or nonresponsive to treatment
Acute or chronic systemic disease
Reproductive system: gender identification in monomorphic species or juveniles, suspected infertility
Polyuria, polydipsia
Follow-up examination to check on lesion resolution ("second look" procedure)

SPECIAL TECHNIQUES

Examination of External Structures

The superb resolution and magnification provided with rigid endoscopes are clinically useful in examination of the external anatomy of reptiles. The Storz 2.7-mm endoscope (Storz #604018 BS) magnifies approximately 20 times at 1 millimeter from the distal lens element. This degree of magnification is useful in examination of external structures such as the integument, nares, tympanic membranes, and ocular and periocular tissues.

Examination of the Respiratory Tract

Examination of the upper respiratory tract is readily accomplished with a rigid endoscope. The external nares, choanal slits, and glottis are magnified and evaluated with gentle manual restraint (Figure 32-16).

Earlier descriptions of examination of the respiratory tract focused on the use of rigid or flexible endoscopes delivered into the lung via the trachea or observations of the lung from the pleuroperitoneal cavity (see Figure 65-14).[6,13] Both techniques provide useful ways to view portions of the reptilian respiratory tract. The anatomy of the species examined has an important effect on the approach or approaches selected. Many *Sauria* have small tracheal diameters compared with their overall body size. This may limit the size of endoscope that can be inserted. The outer surface of the lung can be examined via the coelom. Entrance into the lung from the coelom may cause rents that do not heal because of pressure effects. For this reason, alternative approaches have been developed.

In reptiles with a simple pleuroperitoneal cavity, the lung is also quite simple in design, being single chambered (unicameral). The sac-like unicameral lung is freely movable (Figure 32-17). Divers[8] described a technique to enter the unicameral lung of the Green Iguana (*Iguana iguana*) from a midlateral intercostal approach. The intercostal muscles are carefully separated, and the ribs retracted. The lungs are inflated to full expansion so that the visible lung can be grasped and secured. The endoscope is inserted through the thin wall of the lung for examination. The puncture is closed

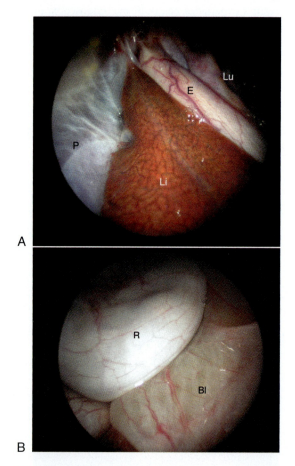

FIGURE 32-15 **A,** Cranial peritoneal cavity of a turtle. *P,* Pericardial sac; *Li,* liver; *E,* esophagus; *Lu,* lung. **B,** Bladder *(Bl)* and rectum *(R)* in an aquatic turtle.

of suspicious findings frequently offers much additional diagnostic information as a result of direct visualization. The minimal invasiveness of fine-diameter rigid endoscopy is particularly useful in Chelonia because of the presence of the restrictive shell and in smaller species where directed illumination and magnification are clinically important.

Endoscopy

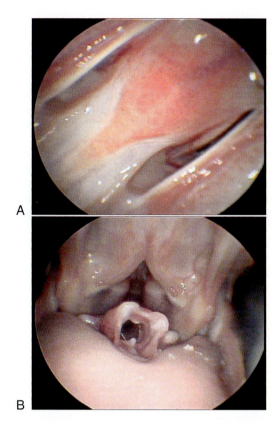

FIGURE 32-16 **A,** Choanal slits (dorsal oral cavity) in a Green Iguana *(Iguana iguana)*. **B,** Glottis during inspiration. Rigid scope allows easy visualization of the inner structures of the oral cavity with minimal restraint. *(Photographs courtesy D. Mader.)*

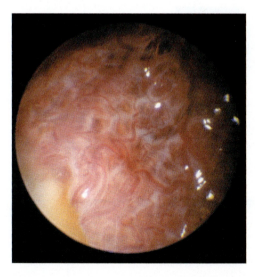

FIGURE 32-17 Collapsed unicameral lung of a Green Iguana *(Iguana iguana).*

with an absorbable suture before return to the pleuroperitoneal cavity.

Access to the lungs of the larger snakes is limited with the smaller rigid telescope. Exploration of the entire lung is possible with flexible endoscopy, although transglottal access may not be possible. Flexible scopes of 100 mm to 150 mm may be needed to access the lungs and air sac tissue in snakes greater than 2 m (6 ft). The diameter of these longer scopes usually exceeds the diameter of the glottis.

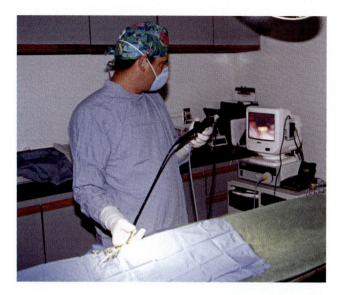

FIGURE 32-18 Flexible endoscopy of a large snake. With general anesthesia, a small stab incision is made approximately mid body. The lung is located and sutured to an opening in the body wall. An incision is made in the lung just large enough to allow insertion of a sterilized endoscope. From this position, exploration of both respiratory and nonrespiratory pulmonary tissue is possible (see Figure 32-19). Note the pulmonary parasites seen on the video monitor. *(Photograph courtesy G. Diethelm.)*

In snakes larger than 2 m (6 ft), access to the entire lung is still possible with a percutaneous approach (D. Mader, personal communication) (Figures 32-18 and 32-19). On average, the junction between the respiratory (vascular) and nonrespiratory (avascular) lung is approximately midway on the snake's body. With anesthesia, the snake is surgically prepped and a small stab incision is made (on the right side in most snakes with a single lung, repeated bilaterally in snakes with two lungs) between the first and second row of scales, just dorsal to the scutes. Blunt dissection is used to penetrate the coelomic cavity and expose the lung. The lung wall is grasped, pierced, and then sutured to the skin incision, thus providing a temporary portal to the lumen of the lung.

A sterile flexible scope is passed into the lung mid body. From this vantage point, caudal deflection allows access and visual inspection to the nonrespiratory (air sac) portion of the lung and cranial deflection allows similar access to the respiratory lung. Object retrieval, biopsies, and cytologic samples are easily collected with this technique (Figure 32-19).

In species in which the lung is adherent to the dorsal body wall (e.g., Chelonia, monitors, and Crocodilia), entering the lung via a dorsal approach is possible. In Chelonia, a transcarapacial technique may be used to access and view the lung. A hole is drilled through the carapace in a region of the appropriate lung.[14] Caution is warranted because removal of the potentially contaminated outer shell first and then a change to a new sterilized burr to make the final entrance to the pleural cavity is necessary. This prevents unnecessary contamination of the insertion site. The endoscope is inserted and can be guided, to a degree, within the parenchyma of the lung near the site, largely dependent on the size of the carapace hole (see Figure 65-13).

In Monitors and crocodiles, the same dorsal approach, lateral to the vertebral column, is used. The more heterogenous lung of these species makes maneuvering somewhat more difficult than in unicameral reptiles; however, a diagnostic examination is possible. Insertion point selection becomes strategically important with a dorsal approach and should be guided with radiography or ultrasonography.

Examination of the Gastrointestinal Tract

The gastrointestinal tract can be entered per os or via the cloaca. Both rigid and flexible endoscopes are of value, depending on the size of the patient and the anatomic location examined.

Flexible gastroscopes have been effectively used to examine and retrieve foreign objects from the stomach of many reptiles in a manner similar to that used with mammals.[15,16] The added length of the flexible systems is particularly useful in snakes, crocodiles, and large monitors. Grasping forceps and wire baskets can be used for object retrieval and may prevent the need for surgical exploration of the stomach. Visualization and mucosal biopsies can also be collected for disease assessment (see Figure 48-2).

Rigid endoscopes allow examination of the oral cavity and associated structures. The philtrum, temporomandibular joint (TMJ), tongue (and sheath), teeth, pharynx, eustachian tubes, and esophagus are readily visualized (Figure 32-20).

In smaller patients, the rigid scopes can also be used to access the stomach. As with the larger flexible endoscopes, air insufflation can be used to distend and improve visualization. When a greater level of mucosal detail is necessary, use of the saline solution infusion is best, as in birds.[17] In this technique **warmed** sterile saline solution is infused into the sheath via one of the lateral ports (see Figure 32-4) with attachment of a standard 1 liter fluid bag with an administration set.

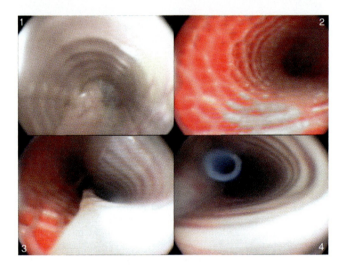

FIGURE 32-19 *1*, Caudal view of the lung (nonrespiratory portion) with a flexible endoscope; *2*, falveolar lining of the respiratory lung; *3*, tracheal lung; note the C-shaped trachea that opens to the respiratory lung; *4*, internal view of the endotracheal tube within the trachea. Note the incomplete tracheal cartilage and dorsal membrane on the left side of the image. *(Photographs courtesy D. Mader.)*

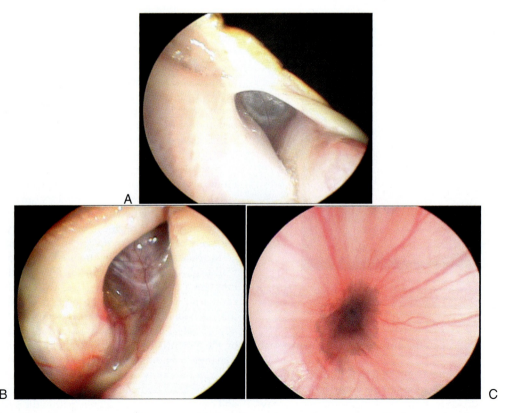

FIGURE 32-20 **A,** Temporomandibular joint (TMJ) of a Green Iguana *(Iguana iguana).* **B,** The eustachian tube in an iguana. **C,** The esophagus and cardia of an iguana. *(Photographs courtesy D. Mader.)*

The bag is suspended at a level above the patient, and the flow rate is controlled with the choice of administration set and with the valve of the lateral port. The trachea and glottis must be protected from aspiration with a tight-fitting endotracheal tube.

Endoscopic Gender Determination

Gender determination is relatively easy because of sexual dimorphism in most species. However, in some species (such as *Heloderma* sp.), differences are not so obvious or require advanced interventive techniques (such as hydrostatic eversion). Endoscopic gender determination can be accomplished much as is done in avian species (Figure 32-21). The standard approaches to the coelomic cavity are used.

Evaluation of breeding soundness or readiness is a more common use of endoscopic inspection of the gonads. Animals evaluated for breeding programs, animals that have failed to produce, or valuable animals needing prepurchase examinations can be safely evaluated with endoscopy. The endoscopist must be familiar with "normals" because the many different patient types may have dramatically different appearances. Unfamiliarity with normal appearance could lead to a misdiagnosis (Figure 32-22).

Cloacoscopy

Coppoolse and Zwart's[3] early yet superb description of cloacoscopy in *Chrysemys scripta* presaged the development of recent advances in avian and reptilian cloacoscopy. The techniques learned in avian cloacoscopy have been applied to reptiles with the Storz diagnostic sheath system and found to be clinically useful.[18,19] The same technique of saline solution infusion described for gastrointestinal examination permits distension of the chambers and provides superb mucosal detail (Figures 32-23, *A, B,* and 32-24, *A*). The bladder and rectum can be entered in many species (Figures 32-23, *C, D,* and 32-24, *B*).

Biopsy

Like the pathologist, the endoscopist must endeavor to become familiar with the normal and pathologic appearance of the tissues to be examined. Every attempt should be made

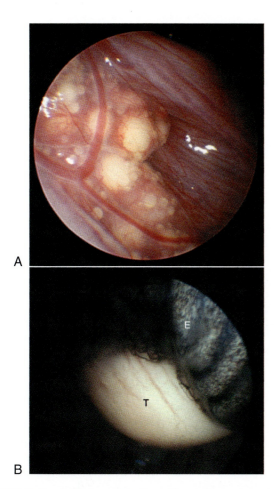

FIGURE 32-21 **A,** The ovary of a Green Iguana *(Iguana iguana).* Very similar in appearance to an avian ovary except that the iguana develops both a right and left ovary. **B,** Testicle (Eastern Painted Turtle) *(Chrysemys picta picta).* Mature testicle *(T)* with well-developed melanin-pigmented epididymis *(E).* Compare with the iguana (see Figure 32-22, *B*).

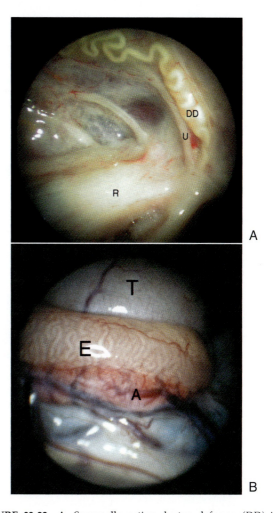

FIGURE 32-22 **A,** Seasonally active ductus deferens *(DD)* in a mature Snapping Turtle *(Chelydra serpentis).* U, Ureter; *R,* rectum. **B,** Seasonally active epididymis *(E)* and testicle *(T)* of a mature Green Iguana *(Iguana iguana).* A, Adrenal.

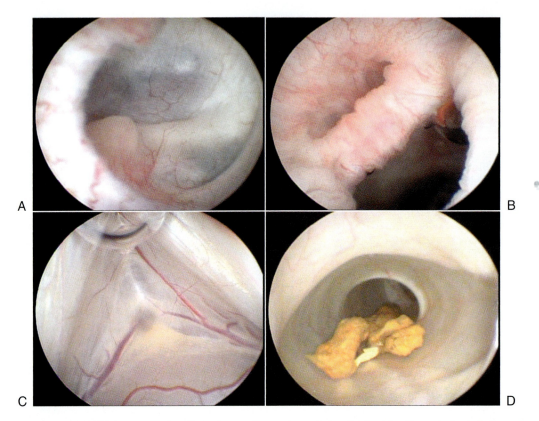

FIGURE 32-23 **A,** Urinary papilla in a Green Iguana *(Iguana iguana)* visualized with saline solution infusion technique. Note the excellent clarity. **B,** Cranial view from within the urodeum. Coprodeum is on the lower right. Urethral opening is on the upper left. **C,** Cystoscopy, view from within the bladder. **D,** Colonoscopy. Distension of the colon is from warm saline solution, not air. *(Photographs courtesy D. Mader.)*

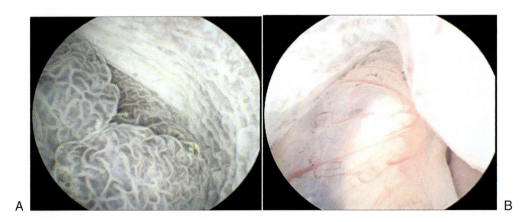

FIGURE 32-24 **A,** Normal proctodeum of a Desert Tortoise *(Gopherus agassizii)*. **B,** Normal bladder in the same animal. Urine in this animal was clear, which is not always the case. In some instances, draining and flushing the bladder, then refilling it with warm saline solution, may be necessary for good visuals. *(Photographs courtesy D. Mader.)*

to describe lesions accurately in terms of their location, color, size, shape, and consistency (Figures 32-25 and 32-26). Photographic or video documentation can be a tremendous aid in this process.

Modern endovideo cameras provide superb imagery at affordable pricing. Clinicians are strongly encouraged to routinely use these tools for data recording during examinations. This technique allows review of procedures in house or via consultants and the sharing of findings with clients. This form of ethical marketing is highly effective and educational. Properly informed and educated clients are better able to understand the procedures proposed for their animal.

Assessment of the appearance of tissue is but the first step in the diagnostic use of endoscopy (Figures 32-27 and 32-28). Improved instrumentation makes routine collection of specimens of suspect or abnormal-appearing tissue and debris for

Endoscopy

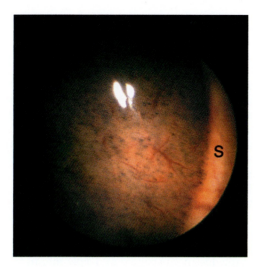

FIGURE 32-25 Liver from a wild Snapping Turtle *(Chelydra serpentina)*. Note the presence of numerous melanomacrophages (black pigment). *S,* Stomach.

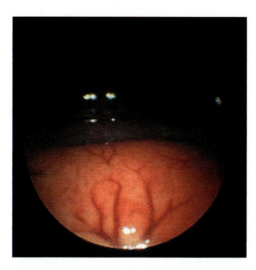

FIGURE 32-26 Liver from a Snapping Turtle *(Chelydra serpentina)* maintained in captivity. Note the hepatic lipidosis (evidenced by yellow appearance).

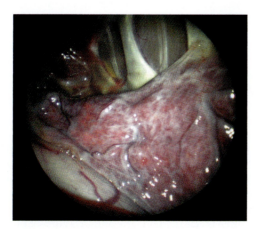

FIGURE 32-27 Lung, collapsed, shows surface edema with some fibrin (Snapping Turtle, *Chelydra serpentina*).

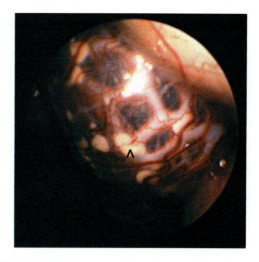

FIGURE 32-28 Lung, inflated, shows granulomatous inflammation *(arrow)* (Red-eared Slider, *Pseudemys scripta*).

histologic, cytologic, and microbiologic examination possible. The use of the Storz system allows a variety of flexible and semirigid instruments to be introduced into the sheath and passed alongside the endoscope and guided to a specific site with greater ease by the operator. Iatrogenic tissue trauma is markedly reduced because instruments are directed to the visual field through the integral sheath, avoiding the blind manipulation necessary to place a second rigid instrument.

Liver

The liver is readily approached in most reptiles from a lateral approach, and biopsies are most easily collected from the lobe margins (Figure 32-29). This technique is useful in generalized hepatic disease, but with focal lesions, the biopsy must be more precisely targeted. In some species, the liver capsule may need to be incised with the semirigid scissors so that the forceps can gain adequate purchase. The 5-French elliptical forceps are usually recommended and are inserted closed through the capsular incision and opened so that a biopsy can be collected (see Figure 30-111). One should avoid opening the forceps to their full extension or crush artifact is created by the packing effect caused by the grasping of too much tissue.

Kidney

In many species, the normal kidneys are located within the pelvic canal and can be difficult to completely visualize, although endoscopy certainly provides one of the few affordable techniques with which to gain clinical information. The kidneys are in a retrocoelomic position. Incision of the coelomic membrane over the kidney is frequently necessary in some species (e.g., Chelonia) to permit access to the renal parenchyma and the collection of biopsy specimens (see Figures 30-119 and 30-121).

The ability to obtain precise target biopsies of specific organs is a natural extension of endoscopic examination and offers a far less traumatic method for obtaining diagnostic specimens in the small reptile than open surgical procedures. Although this is most clinically important in the Chelonia, it is also of value in many other reptile species, especially when renal or hepatic disease is a consideration. Carefully selected

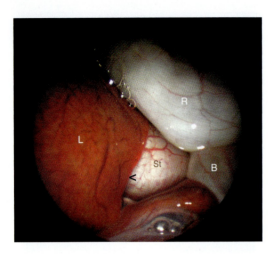

FIGURE 32-29 Left liver lobe of a turtle shows a border ideal for biopsy *(black arrow)*. *L*, Liver; *St*, stomach; *R*, rectum; *B*, bladder.

biopsies of affected organs such as liver, kidney, spleen, pancreas, or gonad are often critical in establishment of an etiologic diagnosis. This allows more precise therapeutic decisions to be made, keeping in mind that reptiles are slow to express outward signs of disease and do so in a limited number of ways. Staging of the lesion as to whether it is acute or chronic is possible. The client can frequently be provided with better prognostic information.

INDICATIONS

Many of the indications for biopsy are similar to those for the visual inspection of tissues and, therefore, endoscopy (see Table 32-2). Abnormal radiographic findings, biochemical parameters that fall outside the reference range, chronic respiratory disease, and polyuria/polydipsia are some of the most common reasons for organ biopsy. The endoscopist is wise to be prepared to collect biopsies during even the most routine examination. Findings of unexpected lesions in patients presented for endoscopic identification of gender are common. Specimens from obvious lesions are easily collected from the border zone where abnormal meets normal tissue. In some cases, gross lesions may not be discerned. This is particularly common in renal disease. If the patient's history, physical examination, or biochemical findings suggest renal or hepatic abnormalities, biopsy of the kidney or liver is recommended, even if they appear normal. Tissues may frequently appear grossly normal even though significant histologic lesions are present.

CONTRAINDICATIONS

The major contraindications for biopsy are related to the blood clotting system of the reptile. Biopsy collection should be delayed in any patient that shows evidence of abnormalities of the hemostatic system. This usually becomes evident at the time of preendoscopic blood collection. Most reptiles should show clot formation in 2 to 5 minutes. Deficiency of vitamin K is the most commonly appreciated coagulation disorder seen in the author's hospital. Vitamin K1 (AquaMephyton, MSD, Rahway, NJ) is administered at the rate of 1 to 2 mg/kg. Blood calcium levels should also be assessed before surgery. As in aves, both calcium and vitamin K appear to play key roles in the primarily extrinsic system-based clotting arcade of reptiles.

A blood film should also be examined for the presence of adequate thrombocyte numbers. Ascites is a relative contraindication. Clot formation is frequently impaired in the presence of ascitic fluid. This is especially important in species with a simple pleuroperitoneal design where fluid accumulates throughout the cavity.

A biopsy cup shape and diameter appropriate to the size of the patient and organ to be biopsied must be chosen. Forceps too large for the purpose may cause excessive organ trauma and hemorrhage. Biopsy cups generally come in only the two shapes, round or elliptical, discussed previously. The round shape does not penetrate as deeply into tissue as the same diameter elliptical cup, which may be indicated for use with certain organs such as the kidney or testes. For general use in reptiles of 200 to 5000 g, an elliptical biopsy cup of 5-French to 7-French (1.7-mm to 2.3-mm) diameter is recommended. In small patients (less than 100 g), a 3-French (1-mm) elliptical or round cup is indicated (see Figure 32-6).

Inexperience with the instrumentation and with approaches to the organ are the two most common causes of iatrogenic biopsy complications. Knowledge of regional anatomic relationships is also essential to good endoscopic technique. A diagnostic evaluation is performed first. If lesions worthy of sampling are discovered, an appropriate biopsy forceps is inserted into the sheath's instrument port. The sheath should be held somewhat away from the expected site of biopsy while the forceps is slowly passed down the instrument channel until it appears in the viewing field. Only then should the entire sheath unit be moved into position for collection of the specimen. One should avoid the temptation to attempt to move the forceps into position without moving the sheath. This can lead to poor control of the instrument tip and unnecessary organ trauma. Repetition and the utilization of good technique reduce the risks of iatrogenic trauma to minimal levels, allowing the clinician to realize the true benefits of minimally invasive procedures.

The techniques of single puncture rigid endoscopy described here are not complicated, but they are associated with a learning curve and do require practice. The clinician is strongly advised to combine a "hands on" wet laboratory experience with work on necropsy specimens to get started. See Chapter 2 for more information on where to attend these valuable training programs.

PREPARATION AND SUBMISSION OF SMALL BIOPSIES

The biopsies obtained with the types of forceps recommended are small. They must be handled with care so that they are not lost or damaged. Various techniques have been recommended in the past to enable the histotechnologist to locate and properly imbed small specimens for processing. Wrapping tiny pieces of tissue in filter paper or a very fine cloth before immersion in the fixative is one method. The author's current preference is to place the specimens into a small stoppered blood collection container without anticoagulant (e.g., Vacutainer red-top

3-mL tube #6381, Becton Dickinson, Rutherford, NJ). This system is simple and effective and allows the technician to clearly visualize the sample. One should avoid placing more than two to three specimens in each clearly labeled container.

Remembering that these small tissue samples require far less time to fix than larger samples, likely less than 2 hours in formalin, is wise. One should always use specifically buffered 10% formalin meant for tissue fixation. Failure to do so leads to precipitates and artifact. If biopsies cannot be processed immediately, storage of the specimens in a solution similar to the first processing solution used by the laboratory (e.g., 97% methyl alcohol) may be recommended to ensure sample quality. One should always refer to the laboratory for specific recommendations.

The last, but arguably most important step in the process of small biopsy submission for the practitioner, is the selection of the pathologist and laboratory. A number of consulting pathologists now have experience and interest in receiving small clinical biopsies from exotic animal practitioners. They must be able to supply rapid turn-around times and have a good working relationship with reptile pathology.

SUMMARY

Rigid endoscopy in reptiles has never offered more potential to the exotic animal practitioner. Improved instrumentation designed to more appropriately meet the needs of the reptile clinician has led to easier implementation of clinical sampling with greater diagnostic return. Improved imaging technologies, especially endovideo cameras, have dramatically altered the way endoscopic techniques can be demonstrated, taught, and reviewed. Participation in intensive 2-day courses for avian and reptilian endoscopy is now possible. These same technologies are making it possible for colleagues to consult on cases in a manner not possible before. The potential for new endosurgical procedures is also great.

REFERENCES

1. Bush M: Laparoscopy in birds and reptiles. In Harrison RM, Wildt DE, editors: *Animal laparoscopy*, Baltimore, 1980, Williams & Wilkins.
2. Schildger BJ: Endoscopic sex determination in reptiles, *Proceedings 1st International Conference on Zoological and Avian Medicine*, Oahu, Hawaii, 1987, AAV/AAZV.
3. Coppoolse KJ, Zwart P: Cloacoscopy in reptiles, *Vet Q* 7(3): 243-245, 1985.
4. Wood JR, Wood FE et al: Laparoscopy of the green sea turtle, *Chelonia mydas*, *Br J Herp* 6:323-327, 1983.
5. Cooper JE, Schildger BJ: Endoscopy in exotic species. In Brearly MJ, Cooper JE, Sullivan M, editors: *Colour atlas of small animal endoscopy*, St Louis, 1991, Mosby.
6. Schildger BJ, Wicker R: Endoscopie bei reptilien und amphibian—indikationen, methoden, befunde, *Der Praktische Tierzart* 6:516-526, 1992.
7. Taylor M. Diagnostic application of a new endoscopic system for birds, *Proc Eur Conf Avian Med Surg*, Utrecht, NL, 1993.
8. Divers SJ: Lizard endoscopic techniques with particular reference to the Green Iguana (*Iguana iguana*), *Semin Avian Exotic Pet Med* 8(3):122-129, 1999.
9. Taylor M: Endoscopic examination and biopsy techniques. In Ritchie BW, Harrison GJ, Harrison LR, editors: *Avian medicine: principles and application*, Lake Worth, Fla, 1994, Wingers Publishing Inc.
10. Schildger BJ, Häfeli W, Kuchling G, Taylor M, Tenhu H, Wicker R: Endoscopic examination of the pleuroperitoneal cavity in reptiles, *Semin Avian Exotic Pet Med* 8(3):130-138, 1999.
11. Dunker HR: Coelom-Gliederung der Wirbeltiere—Funktionelle Aspekte, *Verh Anat Ges* 72:91-112, 1978.
12. Brannian RE: A soft tissue laparotomy technique in turtles, *J Am Vet Med Assoc* 185:1416-1417, 1984.
13. Göbel T, Jurina K: Endoskopie des Respirationstraktes bei Reptilien, *Kleintierpraxis* 39:791-794, 1994.
14. Hernandez-Divers SJ: Endoscopic evaluation of the reptilian respiratory system, *Exotic DVM* 3(3):61-64, 2001.
15. Lumiej JT, Happe RP: Endoscopic diagnosis and removal of gastric foreign bodies in a caiman (*Caiman crocodilus crocodilus*), *Vet Q* 7(3):234-236, 1985.
16. Ackerman J, Carpenter JW: Using endoscopy to remove a gastric foreign body in a python, *Vet Med* 90:761-763, 1995.
17. Murray MJ, Taylor M: Retrieval of proventricular and ventricular foreign bodies with rigid endoscopic equipment, *Proc Assoc Avian Vet* 281-284, 1995.
18. Taylor M, Murray MJ: Endoscopic examination and therapy of the avian gastrointestinal tract, *Sem Avian Exotic Pet Med* 8(3):110-114, 1999.
19. Taylor M: Examining the avian cloaca using saline infusion cloacoscopy, *Exotic DVM* 3(3):77-79, 2001.

33
EUTHANASIA
DOUGLAS R. MADER

Euthanasia: n. 1. An easy and painless death. 2. Act or method of causing death painlessly, to end suffering.
Webster New World Dictionary

Many reasons exist for euthanasia of a reptile. In addition, many different ways exist to accomplish the task. What works for one purpose may not be appropriate for another. All the permutations should be examined to determine what technique is best. The most important point, regardless of the cause and the method, is that the euthanasia is humane.

Euthanasia is an irreversible action. It may be a necessary final step to put an end to suffering from long-term disease or catastrophic injury, or it may be the final end point for an experimental protocol. For some individuals, this act may involve an emotional investment, especially if the animal involved is a companion reptile. For others, the procedure may be more of a mechanical process, especially if the subject is just a data point in an investigation.

One must be cognizant of the ramifications. If the euthanasia involves a companion reptile pet, feelings on the part of the owner/family undoubtedly must be addressed. The bond that forms between a reptile pet and human companion can be just as strong as that seen with dog and cats (see Chapter 3). Considering that many reptiles can far outlive dogs and cats (e.g., tortoises that live in a family for more than 100 years), no wonder multiple generations of a single family may have bonds with a particular reptile pet. Sensitivity to this bond is forever remembered and appreciated.

In many cases, a postmortem examination may be necessary. Cause of death, be it for personal knowledge, academic pursuits, disease monitoring and prevention, or legal purposes, can be compromised if the euthanasia is not performed properly.

Necropsy specimens can either be sent in *toto* to the pathology laboratory or can be evaluated in house and just selected tissues submitted. The author encourages practitioners to perform their own necropsies because the results are immediately available and, oftentimes, complete gross diagnoses can be made without the need for histology.

Owners are encouraged to have their deceased reptiles necropsied, especially if the patient died without a diagnosis. Aside from zoonotic risks, a concern always exists for other reptiles that might be in the same household. One should stress that a great deal can be learned from the dead and that hopefully the information can prevent similar problems in the owner's other animals, especially when contagious diseases are involved.

Not all clients permit a necropsy, and of those that do, few may be willing to pay for the ancillary diagnostic tests needed to complete the proper necropsy examination. Before beginning, the owners should always be informed of the costs involved for the postmortem examination, including necessary ancillary tests such as microbiology, hematology, clinical chemistries, toxicology, and histology. If an owner declines, one should ask permission to perform the necropsy at no cost to the owner and suggest that the owner only pay for the ancillary tests, if necessary. If this fails and it is a case that you feel strongly about, ask permission to perform the postmortem examination only at no cost to the owner. This is usually readily accepted.

The ethical question is whether or not the owners have a right to the information that you discover from the necropsy if they do not pay for the services. The decision is yours. The author usually offers the information to the client. This shows good intent and also educates the client to the necessity of proper diagnostics. If the situation should arise again, insist that the client pay for your services. If the client declines, then do not perform the necropsy. One must convey to the client that the material gathered from a necropsy is invaluable to a diagnosis and, as such, has a value to the client.

Because of a time factor, necropsy of all animals that die in your care may be difficult. A trained technician who does all preliminary procedures for the postmortem, including making an appropriate incision and exposing the internal organs, might be more efficient. You then evaluate the specimen, identify the important structures, and the pathology when applicable, take the necessary photographs, and instruct the technician about the samples to be collected.

This efficient method of postmortem evaluation results in at least the gross examination of most specimens at the author's hospital. Consequently, information is obtained that is otherwise lost.

EUTHANASIA PROTOCOLS

Many methods are available for euthanasia of reptiles. Consideration is important of not only the type and size of the animal being euthanized but also the reason (e.g., culling, alleviating suffering, preparing a specimen for histology). In private veterinary practice, for owners to request euthanasia for a pet and, furthermore, to want to be present during the procedure is not uncommon. This may have a direct effect on the method of euthanasia chosen.

Several protocols for reptile euthanasia have been reviewed in the literature.[1-8] Controversy abounds as to the best, safest, and most humane techniques. Until we have a better understanding of the reptilian nervous system and the reptile's ability to experience pain or discomfort, these controversies may never be settled. In the meantime, to assume that reptiles do feel pain is probably prudent, and when sacrificing these animals, the veterinarian should be cognizant of this point and do all that is necessary to ensure that the procedure is humane.

"Owner present" euthanasias, regardless of the species, are probably one of the most difficult duties that veterinarians are called on to deliver. In reptilian medicine, the procedure is made even more difficult because of the unique anatomy of the patients. Compare how easy injection is of a substance into an obvious cephalic vein in a mammal, perhaps one with a catheter in place, with the stress of being asked to sacrifice a reptile patient that has no visible veins or ready venous access while the emotional owner looks on.

A number of "tricks of the trade" might be useful to a veterinarian in this position. Large, combative, or otherwise active animals benefit from a pre-euthanasia tranquilization, heavy sedation, or anesthetic. This is referred to as **"two-stage" euthanasia.**

The author recommends starting with a sedative such as Telazol (Fort Dodge, Inc, Fort Dodge, Iowa), 25 to 50 mg/kg intramuscularly (IM), or ketamine HCl, 100 mg/kg IM. At these high dosages, approximately 10 to 20 minutes are needed for the drugs to take effect when the patient is at room temperature. Because both of these medications can be administered intramuscularly, delivery to a fractious or dehydrated patient or a patient with inaccessible peripheral veins is facilitated.

After the patient has been administered the medication, it can be tenderly left with the owner with the instructions that the pet will be awake for a few more minutes. This gives the owners a few moments to "say goodbye" if they so desire before the pet loses consciousness.

After the subject/patient has been sedated or anesthetized, the second stage of the euthanasia procedure can proceed. At this time, an intravenous, intracoelomic, intracardiac, or intracranial injection of euthanasia solution can be administered.

One final very important note of warning: sometimes assessment of whether or not a reptile is, in fact, deceased can be difficult. Any practitioner who treats reptiles can share stories of "dead" patients that wake up inside of plastic disposal bags 24 hours later. This is important because occasionally a client takes the remains home for burial, taxidermy, and so forth. It would behoove the practitioner to make absolutely, positively sure that the pet is deceased before it is released to the owner. The situation can be embarrassing if owners call wanting to know why the animal they just paid to have euthanized is walking around. With administration of euthanasia solution to "take home" patients, always give triple the normal dose, or more.

To prevent this type of medicolegal catastrophe, the author has a standing policy that any euthanized reptile patient that is to be taken home with a client either is decapitated (after apparent euthanasia is confirmed) before leaving the premises or, if the owner objects to this, is frozen (after apparent euthanasia is confirmed) for at least 24 hours before the carcass is released to the owner.

Electrocardiogram analysis of postmortem specimens can be misleading because the heart occasionally continues to beat, even hours after the apparent euthanasia. Doppler blood flow analysis may prove useful. However, because a reptile's heart rate can change from beats per minute to minutes per beat with the administration of anesthesia or exposure to cold, definitive determination of death can be enigmatic. This puzzle has no easy answer.

TECHNIQUES AND METHODS

The 2000 American Veterinary Medical Association (AVMA) Panel on Euthanasia has published several guidelines for euthanasia of reptiles.[1] Cooper's monograph on Euthanasia of Amphibians and Reptiles remains the gold standard.[2] Table 33-1 lists recommended procedures for the reptile groups.

The intended use of the carcass (disposal, gross or histologic evaluation, or human consumption [e.g., an alligator]) determines the method of euthanasia. Injection of an overdose of an intravenous barbiturate is the most common method of euthanasia. However, if histopathology is necessary, barbiturates can have an adverse effect on the tissues of the brain, heart, kidneys, and other delicate structures (Mike Garner, personal communication, Northwest ZooPath). As an alternative to a barbiturate overdose if histology of these structures is necessary, an overdose of ketamine HCl, Telazol, or potassium chloride (the latter only acceptable with a surgical plane of anesthesia) may be used.

Another consideration with commercial euthanasia solutions for postmortem examinations is that of microbiologic testing. Most commercial euthanasia solutions are NOT sterile. As a result, when collection bacterial samples form postmortem tissues, the sterility of the sampling is in question and the results may not be valid. This is important, especially in investigation of morbidity and mortality in herd situations or zoonotic outbreaks.

Administration of euthanasia solution or other medications via cardiac puncture is possible in most species. Although this technique is usually easy to perform for trained individuals, in moribund or severely dehydrated animals it may prove difficult. This technique can potentially mechanically and chemically damage heart tissue and may not be ideal

Table 33-1	Recommended Techniques for Reptilian Euthanasia*				
Group	**Deep Freezing†**	**Chemical†**	**Topical**	**Inhalant**	**Physical†‡**
Lizards	<40 g	Yes	No	Yes	Yes
Snakes	<40 g	Yes	No	Yes	Yes
Chelonians	<40 g	Yes	No	No	Yes
Crocodilians	No	Yes	No	No	Yes
Amphibians	<40 g	Yes	Yes	No	Yes

*Sedation or anesthesia is recommended in difficult-to-handle animals.
†Surgical anesthesia is necessary before some forms of euthanasia such as deep freezing, potassium chloride injection, decapitation, or exsanguination.
‡Pithing, concussion, or captive-bolt stun gun or firearm. Exsanguination immediately after brain destruction is recommended before dressing the carcass is commenced.

if accurate cardiac histology is important. If the patient is large, dangerous, or active, sedation as previously described is strongly recommended.

Alternately, the euthanasia solution can be injected directly into the parietal eye (a portal to the brain; Figure 33-1). For the latter technique, the animal must be given a surgical plane of anesthesia.

Euthanasia solutions can also be administered intracoelomically or intramuscularly. These routes are effective but slow. If the patient is dehydrated, cold, or moribund (as they often are when euthanasia is considered), circulation may be poor delaying or even inhibiting absorption.[7]

The patient can be placed in a chamber and exposed to a volatile anesthetic (e.g., halothane, isoflurane, sevoflurane, carbon dioxide, carbon monoxide). Because many reptiles have the capability to breath hold (up to 27 hours for some species), this method may be prolonged. Death in some species may not occur even after prolonged exposure.[9] This method may not be the best for diving and breath-holding species such as crocodilians and turtles. More active species such as the lizards and snakes are better suited for inhalant overdosing. With the myriad of rules concerning employees and exposure to exhaust gases, proper venting of the gas must be performed when the procedure is complete and the container is opened.

External or topical agents, such as Tricaine methane sulfonate (TMS, MS-222) may be used to euthanize amphibians. These agents can be placed in the water (concentrations > 500 mg/L, buffered with to a pH of 7 to 7.5). MS-222 can also be injected directly into the amphibian lymph sac or the coelomic cavity.

Benzocaine hydrochloride can also be used for euthanasia of aquatic amphibians. A concentration exceeding 250 mg/L, used either in a bath or in a recirculating system, is sufficient to kill the animal.

In an emergency situation, aquatic amphibians can be killed with placement in water that contains dissolved carbon dioxide (with the addition of sodium bicarbonate powder or Alka-Seltzer tablets to water).[2]

Rapid freezing, such as dipping in liquid nitrogen, is approved and effective in animals less of than 40 g.[1,4] Larger species may not be rendered unconscious rapidly enough to prevent discomfort.[1]

Reports have stated that placement of a reptile in a conventional freezer is a viable technique for euthanasia.[5] Cooper, Ewebank, and Rosenberg[3] contest that the animals may experience pain as ice crystals form within the tissues and in the skin. This technique is often used by the lay herpetologist and hobbyist. The AVMA Panel on Euthanasia does not consider this an acceptable or humane method for euthanasia, even if prior cooling is performed.

Decapitation (with transection of the cervical spinal cord) may be a useful technique in certain conditions, especially in smaller amphibians and reptiles (Figure 33-2). However, Cooper et al[2] state that in decapitated reptiles the brain may still be able to perceive pain for up to an hour after the spinal cord has been severed. They further recommend immediately pithing the brain. If decapitation is selected, prior surgical plane anesthesia is necessary.

Exsanguination, the removal of the animal's blood while it is still alive, is not approved because it is considered inhumane. Reptiles can tolerate prolonged periods of hypoxia, which is the experience during this procedure. Exsanguination is permitted only in unconscious (anesthetized) reptiles.

Physical means of euthanasia may be the only practical methods in certain situations. Concussion (a crushing blow to the head) either yields the animal unconscious or yields instant death. This is acceptable in certain circumstances but requires training to be performed correctly. This is generally not accepted for pet reptiles.

For the larger reptiles, such as the crocodilians and large chelonians, a captive-bolt stun gun or standard firearm may be necessary. The pistol should be aimed at the brain. The landmark is on the midsagittal line just caudal to the eyes.[3,7] Figure 33-3 shows the locations for "points of aim" for physical techniques for the various amphibian and reptiles.

DISPOSITION OF CARCASS

Always clarify this last point before the euthanasia is performed. Immediately after euthanasia, the owners' emotions

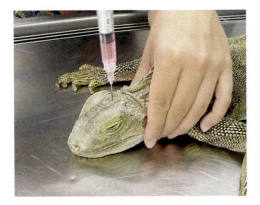

FIGURE 33-1 Pithing, or injection of euthanasia solution directly into the brain, is an approved method for euthanasia. The parietal eye found in many lizard species is a good window or portal directly into the brain. The patient must be anesthetized before the procedure is performed.

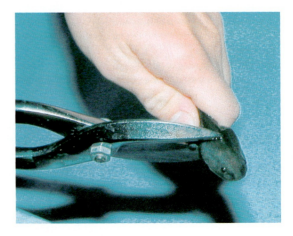

FIGURE 33-2 Physical means of euthanasia such as decapitation are acceptable, providing the animal is anesthetized before the procedure is performed.

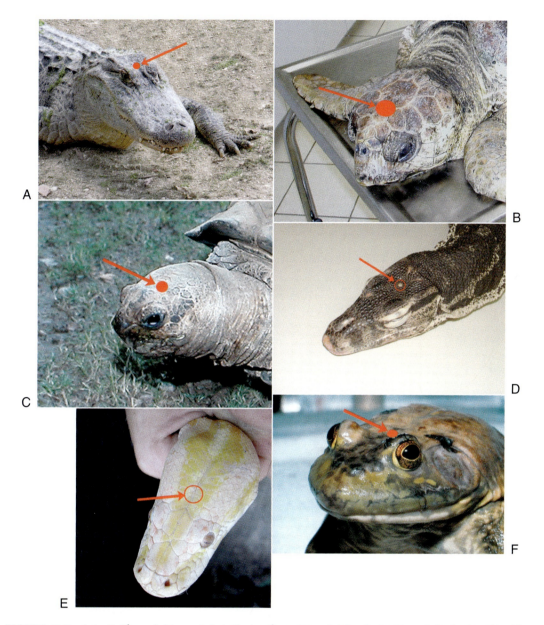

FIGURE 33-3 A to **F**, The *red dot* or *circle* indicates the entry point for destruction of the brain with either a captive-bolt stun gun or a standard firearm. The *angle of the arrow* indicates the recommended direction for the projectile.

may cloud their judgment or make decisions difficult. The best time to discuss disposition of the remains is before the procedure.

One should always receive instructions in writing, and the actual "permission" for the euthanasia. The wording should be clear, concise, and brief. The statement should have the name of the patient, a complete description of the patient (species, age, gender, color, and markings), the name of the owner or authorized agent, the name of the veterinarian performing the procedure, the location, and the date and time. Preprinted forms that are filled out in advance help make an emotional difficult event easier to endure for the veterinary staff and, especially, the owner.

If the owner grants permission for disposal, then one is still wise to retain the carcass until the laboratory verifies that it has received all the samples submitted. In addition, the author recommends saving duplicates of all collected tissues for the occasion when a second opinion may be warranted. One should follow proper disposal guidelines for the carcass as determined by local ordinance.

Some owners are interested in retrieving the remains of deceased pets. Whether for private burial, taxidermy, or salvaging the skin, the ultimate use of the remains is important to know before the postmortem examination is started. A cosmetic postmortem procedure can be accomplished with a single ventral midline incision in most species. The lungs, heart, trachea, and esophagus can be removed through this coelomic incision. The body can be filled with paper towels, and the skin can be closed with a simple interrupted suture. This prevents the body from looking flattened or deflated.

How well the cosmetic procedure is performed might be more important to the owner than what is learned from the procedure. For instance, an accidental scalpel nick can ruin a skin. If a client requests a special procedure, the author recommends that you charge for the extra time; or discussing the options with the client and, if appropriate, returning the eviscerated remains to the owner may be better.

REFERENCES

1. American Veterinary Medical Association: 2000 Report of the AVMA Panel on Euthanasia, *J Am Vet Med Assoc* 218(5): 669-696, 2001.
2. Cooper JE, Ewebank R, Platt E, et al: *Euthanasia of amphibians and reptiles*, Potters Bar, England, 1989, Universities Federation for Animal Welfare.
3. Cooper JE, Ewebank R, Rosenberg ME: Euthanasia of tortoises, *Vet Rec* 114:635, 1984.
4. Hillman H: Humane killing of animals for medical experiments, *World Med J* 25(5):68, 1978.
5. Frye FL: Euthanasia, necropsy techniques and comparative histology of reptiles. In Hoff GL, Frye FL, Jacobson ER, editors: *Diseases of amphibians and reptiles*, New York, 1984, Plenum Press.
6. Frye FL: *Biomedical and surgical aspects of captive reptile husbandry*, ed 2, Melbourne, Fla, 1991, Krieger Publishing.
7. Cooper JE: Humane euthanasia and post-mortem examination. In Girling SJ, Raiti P, editors: *Manual of reptiles,* ed 2, Gloucester, England, 2004, British Small Animal Veterinary Association.
8. *Guidelines for the use of live amphibians and reptiles in field and laboratory research,* ed 2, 2004, revised by the Herpetological Animal Care and Use Committee (HACC) of the American Society of Ichthyologists and Herpetologists. (Committee Chair: Beaupre SJ; Members: Jacobson ER, Lillywhite HB, Zamudio K).
9. Burns R, McMhan B: Euthanasia methods for ectothermic vertebrates. In Bonagura JD, editor: *Continuing veterinary therapy XII,* Philadelphia, 1995, WB Saunders.

34
OVERVIEW OF BIOPSY AND NECROPSY TECHNIQUES

MICHAEL M. GARNER

The contemporary practice of reptile medicine provides the clinician with a vast armament of noninvasive diagnostic tools to aid in the treatment of reptile disease, including radiology, ultrasound, endoscopy, and hematology. Cytology and biopsy procedures are equally important in establishment of a diagnosis in live reptiles. Necropsy is frequently performed in clinical practice to achieve a diagnosis "after the fact" and to apply this information to future treatment protocols or the ongoing health of a collection. Cytology and biopsy techniques are generally performed in-house. Necropsy may be performed at diagnostic laboratories; however, because of the expense, lengthy shipping intervals, and the clinician's own curiosity, necropsies are often performed in-house. This chapter describes techniques to effectively obtain cytology, biopsy, and necropsy specimens for achieving a diagnosis. Clinicians must remember that the most crucial step in obtaining a formal and accurate diagnosis is providing the pathologist with a form that includes the animal's name or number, full signalment, history, and location of the sample (Figure 34-1).

SAMPLE PROCUREMENT

Cytology

Although the level of training received by veterinary students in the procurement and interpretation of cytologic preparations is somewhat variable, many contemporary practitioners are adroit at using this technique as an aid in achieving a rapid in-house diagnosis. In reptiles, as with other animals, many disease processes can be conveniently evaluated with cytologic examination, often without the risk of excessive manual restraint, immobilization, or anesthesia. Ocular, nasal, oral, choanal, cloacal, cutaneous, and fecal specimens are particularly easy to obtain, but aural, intraosseous, intracoelomic, and visceral samples may require more procurement skills, particularly if percutaneous aspiration is used. Interpretation of cytologic specimens is beyond the scope of this chapter, but reviews are available (see Chapter 28). Like anything else, interpretation of cytologic specimens takes practice (and perhaps an affection for microscopy), and clinicians are encouraged to look at the slides before sending them to a pathologist or to save a slide for review after the pathologist's diagnosis is received.

Samples may be obtained with swabs, fine needle aspiration, or tissue imprint. Frosted glass slides are recommended, and the frosted end should be labeled in pencil, not oil-based or water-based markers, which wash off in staining fixatives. Tape should not be used to label slides. The label should include the animal's or owner's name and the site of the sample.

The best method with use of swabs is to lightly roll the swab on the slide, making several lines at the end of the slide opposite the label and preferably extending at least half the length of the slide (Figure 34-2).

With fine needle aspiration, the aspirated specimen can be expressed on the slide at the pole opposite the label. Both smeared and squashed preparations are important to have on multiple slides to circumvent the artifact associated with each of these techniques and to optimize the quality of the material available for examination.

Smear samples are performed with gently lowering another slide onto the sample until it spreads between the glass and then dragging the top slide toward the labeled end of the bottom slide (Figure 34-3). Squash preparations are made in a similar fashion, but after the sample spreads between the glass, the top slide is lifted directly off the bottom slide rather than the slide dragging.

Tissue imprints should be repeatedly blotted on a paper towel until little or no fluid dispersion is noted and then lightly touched onto the surface of the labeled slide in multiple locations (Figure 34-4). At least one slide should be stained in-house with one of the Romanowski-type quick stains, and two to four slides should be left unstained.

The best slide containers for transport or shipping are plastic-shelled rectangular slide holders with snap-cap lids, which usually accommodate four to five slides. A wad of tissue paper should be placed between the slides and the lid to prevent movement of the slides during shipping, and the lid should be taped closed. The slides and submission form with history should then be placed in a padded manila envelope or padded box for shipping. Cardboard slideholders and nonpadded envelopes are a recipe for disaster. These slides often arrive at the diagnostic laboratory fractured into tiny pieces after being run through the stamp machine by the postal service.

When slides are sent in conjunction with formalin-preserved specimens, one must not put the slides and the formalin containers in the same container or bag. Each should be wrapped separately and can then be placed in the same shipping container. Stained and unstained slides exposed to formalin (as with leakage) or formaldehyde fumes can develop artifactual changes that limit their usefulness for diagnostic purposes.

Necropsy Form

Date _____
Referring Veterinarian _____ Clinic Name _____
Address _____
City _____ State _____ Zip Code _____
Phone (_____) _____ Fax _____ E-mail _____
Test Requested
( ) Cytology ( ) Biopsy ( ) Necropsy (call first)
Owner _____
Patient Name or I.D. # _____ Species _____ Breed _____
Age _____ Sex _____ ( ) Captive-bred ( ) Wild-caught
Duration of Illness _____
Manner of Death: ( ) Spontaneous ( ) Euthanasia (agent and route) _____
Carcass Condition: ( ) Fresh ( ) Frozen ( ) Refrigerated _____ hrs
              ( ) Environ. Temp _____ hrs
History, clinical data, description of lesions or necropsy findings

_____
_____
_____
_____
_____
_____
_____
_____
_____
_____

Clinical Diagnosis _____

Tissue Checklist

Skin	Ovary	Kidney	Oral	Brain	Adipose
Pituitary	Oviduct	Liver	Esophagus	Spinal cord	
Adrenal	Testicle	Spleen	Stomach	Vertebrae	
Thyroid	Epididymis	Lung	Intestine	Long bone	
Parathyroid	Urinary bladder	Heart	Colon	Head	
Pancreas	Gall bladder	Muscle	Cloaca	Mesentery	

FIGURE 34-1 Example of the "Necropsy Submission Form" that should accompany all histopathologic submissions to the pathologist. One should be as detailed as possible to help the pathologist with the histopathologic diagnosis.

Biopsies

Table 34-1 summarizes some "dos and don'ts" that apply to procurement and submission of biopsies. The conventional method of biopsy submission is placement of the sample in 10% neutral buffered formalin at approximately 10 parts formalin to 1 part biopsy, immediately after the biopsy is collected. This procedure ensures adequate tissue perfusion by the formalin and limits autolytic artifact (decomposition). If the plan is to prepare cytologic imprints from the biopsy, then obtaining two biopsy specimens is best because the imprint procedure causes significant artifactual change in some cases,

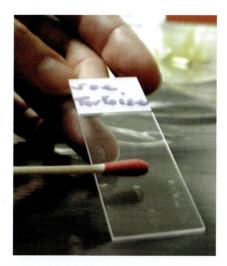

FIGURE 34-2 Swab technique for expression of material onto a glass slide for cytologic interpretation. The swab is rolled from the approximate middle of the slide to the end opposing the label. Two or three lines can be made of varying thickness.

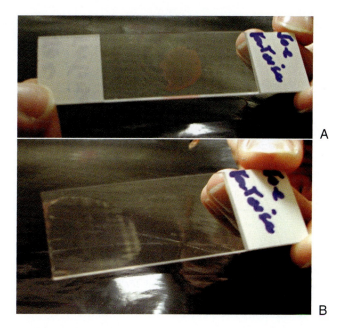

FIGURE 34-3 A and **B,** Smear technique for expression of material onto a glass slide for cytologic interpretation. Material is expressed onto the middle of the glass slide. Another slide is lowered onto the sample slide, and the slides are pulled apart in directions away from labels.

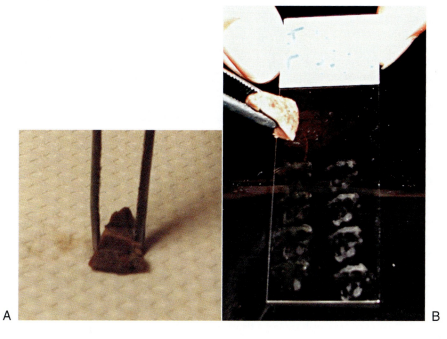

FIGURE 34-4 A and **B,** Imprint technique for expression of material onto a glass slide for cytologic interpretation. A tissue sample is blotted on a paper towel to remove excess fluid, then touched to the bottom half of a glass slide with varying degrees of pressure to obtain a thin film of material.

especially with soft tissue specimens such as kidney, liver, or gut mucosa.

Small biopsy specimens of soft tissue are best obtained with a scalpel or forceps (crush technique). Cautery technique can cause extensive coagulation artifact, which may significantly impede microscopic interpretation. Because some biopsy sites, such as the oral or nasal cavity, bleed profusely, use of cautery may be best to control bleeding after the biopsy is obtained. One should avoid the use of forceps directly on the biopsy specimen because this can cause microscopic crush artifact and impede interpretation.

These principles also apply to core biopsies. An important emphasis is that disease processes are generally dynamic and lesions or parts of lesions may be in different stages of formation or regression. For this reason, obtaining more than one biopsy from different parts of a lesion or from different sites of the same disease process is best. This is particularly applicable for multicentric skin lesions and core biopsies of large or nonresectable masses.

Bone biopsies often pose a significant challenge because the reactive hyperostosis associated with many underlying bone lesions can be more prominent than the actual lesion,

Section V CLINICAL TECHNIQUES/PROCEDURES

Table 34-1 Summary for Proper Handling of Biopsy and Necropsy Specimens

Do	Don't
Use 10% neutral buffered formalin, 10:1 ratio	Overfill container with tissues
Handle biopsy by margins	Grasp body of biopsy with forceps
Obtain more than one biopsy if possible	Use same biopsy for tissue imprints and histopathology
Use scalpel or forceps to collect sample	Cauterize biopsy tissue (cauterize site)
Call laboratory before sending fresh carcass/tissue	Send fresh tissue without calling or on weekend/holiday
Keep extra set of formalin-fixed tissues	Discard tissues until biopsy/necropsy results are known
Culture, freeze tissue and serum	Fix tissues in formalin until all other samples are obtained
Submit head if possible (may cost more)	Tape mouth closed (poor formalin perfusion)
Submit stained and unstained cytology	Expose slides to formalin or formaldehyde fumes
Use plastic slide holders	Use flat cardboard slide holders
Double pack samples, use absorbent liner	Use nonpadded envelopes (boxes are best)

and obtaining representative biopsies becomes difficult, particularly with core biopsy techniques. Importantly, samples should be packaged to ensure that leakage does not occur during shipping because formalin is a hazardous substance that is irritating to skin and mucous membranes.

Necropsy

In most cases, submission of an entire carcass for comprehensive necropsy to a diagnostic laboratory is prearranged after the particulars of the case have been discussed with the pathologist. Consultation with the pathologist before shipping prevents many errors that arise from inadequate communications, particularly regarding legal cases or those cases that may arrive or be waylaid on weekends or holidays. Carcasses are submitted on ice with the most expedient form of transport possible to prevent excessive decomposition of the carcass.

To save on costs and to optimize tissue preservation, most clinicians and field veterinarians or biologists perform their own necropsies. The complexity and gauge of equipment are dependent on the size of the animal.

Most necropsy equipment can be purchased at the local hardware store, but some equipment, such as dissecting scissors, forceps, and T-bars (for chelonians), may be purchased from medical suppliers (Figure 34-5). Generally, the supplies needed are some fairly stout scissors, possibly a scalpel blade, pruning shears, and a hacksaw or a Stryker saw (for chelonians). Sterile culturettes or sterile culture plates may be needed. Ideally, the instruments should be sterile, especially those used to collect tissues for culture, but this is not always practical in field situations. Equipment can be sterilized with dipping the tip in alcohol and then burning off the alcohol with a Bunsen burner or lighter.

Many reptile specimens are small, which makes necropsy an easy procedure. For those animals less than 10 centimeters in length, incision of the coelomic cavity from the thoracic inlet to the pelvis provides enough formalin perfusion and tissue preservation. The carcass can be placed whole in a container of formalin, at approximately 10 parts formalin to 1 part tissue.

Any desired visceral (intracoelomic) bacterial or viral cultures must be obtained at the time the carcass is incised, before placement in formalin. Once placed in formalin, the tissues can no longer be cultured because formalin kills the organisms.

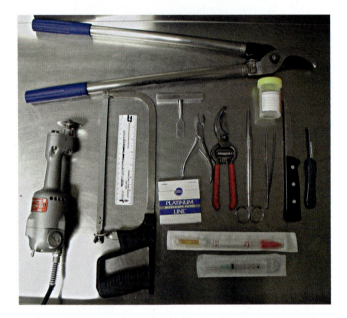

FIGURE 34-5 Some useful instruments and materials for necropsy on a reptile. Tissue forceps and scissors, pruning shears, knife, scalpel, Stryker saw, T-bar, hacksaw, bone rongeur, ruler, frosted glass slides, formalin, syringe, and culturette.

Table 34-2 provides suggested lists of tissues for submission, depending on cost constraints. In the event of cost constraints that may prohibit submission of entire carcasses or a comprehensive set of tissues, maintenance of an in-house log of appropriately labeled frozen and formalin-preserved tissues is often prudent because these tissues can be used for diagnostic purposes at a later date, provided that the original submissions were not diagnostic, or if more specific diagnostic procedures need to be performed.

For those specimens too big to be placed whole in formalin, the following procedures are recommended for the various tissues.

Skin

Skin conditions are common in reptiles, especially trauma, burns, and infectious conditions. The skin should be surveyed closely, with a magnifying glass if necessary. Any abnormalities or asymmetrical discoloration should be noted and collected (and possibly cultured). The distribution and size of the abnormality should be succinctly noted in the history that

Table 34-2 Tissue Collection Protocol for Necropsy Specimens

Procedure	Essentials	Comprehensive	Legal
Histopathology	Lung, liver, kidney, spleen, heart, gut, adrenal, adipose, pancreas (snakes), lesions.	Essentials plus head, trachea, skeletal muscle, skin, long bone, vertebral segment, shell, joint, thyroid, thymus, pancreas, reproductive tissues, urinary, and gallbladder.	As with comprehensive submission, but more sections. Obtain gross photographs of clearly labeled carcass and any lesions.
Additional procedures	Freeze viscera/serum, culture lesions as needed, save duplicate or extra tissues in formalin.	Essentials plus culture lesions and viscera (i.e., liver, lung, gut).	As with comprehensive.

accompanies the necropsy tissues (i.e., "random on the back and legs," "confined to ventral aspects of body [or legs]," "tip of nose [or tail]"). For chelonians, this information also applies to the carapace, plastron, and bridges.

Opening the Body Wall

The animal should be placed in dorsal recumbency (on its back). For squamates (snakes and lizards), scissors are used to cut through the skin and coelomic wall from the tip of the mandibular junction to the cloaca. The skin and body wall are gently parted with fingers, forceps, or scissors, and one should look for obvious abnormalities (lesions). Visceral arrangement and apparent displacement of tissues should be noted. Some lizards, particularly chameleons, normally have extensive melanin pigmentation in the mesentery and inner surfaces of the body wall, and this pigmentation should not be interpreted as a pathologic condition (Figure 34-6). Cultures should be taken of the lung, liver, or kidneys with sterile instruments or swabs before one proceeds with the necropsy.

After cultures are collected, "the pluck" is removed. (See subsequent for opening a chelonian and obtaining the pluck.) This procedure is done with cutting the tongue away from its attachments and pulling it through the ventral intermandibular space. A scissors or fingers is used to carefully dissect soft tissue attachments from the ventral aspect of the dorsal body wall. Caudal traction is applied to the tongue, and the trachea, esophagus, lung, etc., are dissected away back to the cloaca (Figure 34-7).

At this point, the attached viscera can be identified and inspected systematically, with samples collected for histopathology or freezing (for future reference). This procedure may be difficult on large crocodilians and chelonians, and the tissue collection and inspection may need to be done in situ (while still in the carcass). For better exposure, some prosectors prefer to incise around the perimeters of the ventral body wall on large lizards and crocodilians (with pruning shears to cut through the ribs), rather than on the ventral midline, for better exposure.

Shell Removal in Chelonians

A technique for tortoise necropsy is depicted in Figures 34-8 to 34-14. Several methods are used to remove the shell. In young chelonians or those with significant loss of shell bone, the shells can be separated at the bridge with a stout scissors. For larger animals, separation of the shells with a Stryker saw or hacksaw may be necessary.

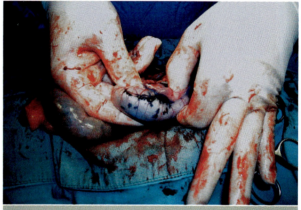
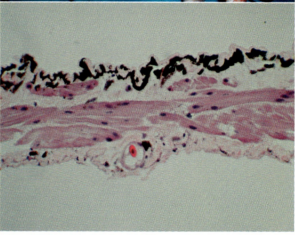

FIGURE 34-6 Normal pigmentation in the coelom of a lizard. A, Gross photograph of the stomach shows black pigmentation. B, Photomicrograph shows accumulation of melanophores in the mesenteric interstitium. *(Photograph courtesy D. Mader.)*

In all cases, the turtle is placed on its back, then tilted laterally to a 45-degree angle. This angle allows gravity to shift the viscera downward, so they are not inadvertently incised during the sawing procedure. This is especially important for obtaining sterile cultures of the viscera and for avoiding a full urinary bladder.

With care taken not to go too deeply with the saw, the shell, and not the underlying soft tissues, is cut. Both bridges are sawed through in this manner.

With the animal still in dorsal recumbency, a scissors is used to cut through the skin at its attachment to the plastron (bottom shell, now facing upwards), both front and rear.

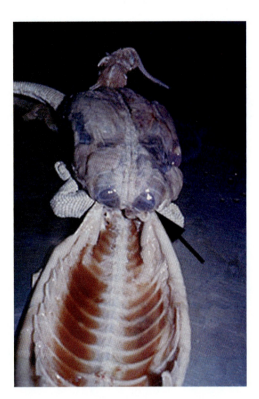

FIGURE 34-7 Savannah Monitor necropsy. Pluck is removed from the carcass with caudal traction. *Arrow* points to the dorsal surface of the kidney. Note the extreme caudal location of the kidney in the coelomic cavity, close to the pelvis. (The tail is at the top.)

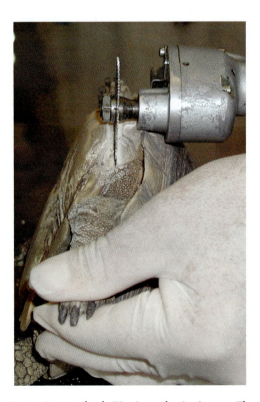

FIGURE 34-8 Incising the shell bridge with a Stryker saw. The carcass is inverted and angled at approximately 45 degrees. The initial cut is at the extreme caudal or cranial bridge junction, and a straight cut is made to opposing end. The opposing bridge is cut in the same manner. Alternatively, a hacksaw may be used if a Stryker saw is not available.

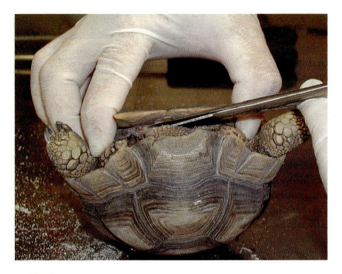

FIGURE 34-9 Removing the carapace. The carcass is inverted, and the carapace rests on the table. With scissors, the skin is dissected from its front and rear attachments to the plastron.

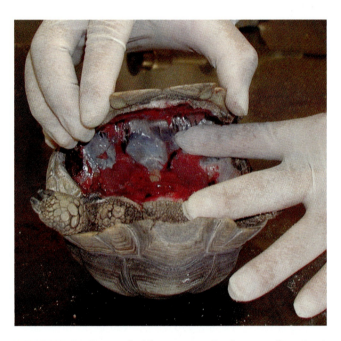

FIGURE 34-10 Removal of the carapace. Gentle upward traction is applied to the plastron for digital dissection of soft tissue attachments.

The soft tissue attachments are bluntly dissected from the top of the plastron, from rear to front. If the procedure is done correctly, the coelomic wall should be intact after removal of the plastron.

For cultures, a small incision can be made in the coelomic wall to allow access to viscera. This provides access to the liver but not the lungs. After cultures are collected, a scissors is used to cut the skin at the junction of the carapace (turtle still in dorsal recumbency), front and rear.

A thick screwdriver, wedge, or T-bar is used to disarticulate the tail vertebrae and the cervical (neck) vertebrae from their attachments to the ventral aspect of the carapace. The turtle is carefully turned over, and gravity is allowed to pull

Overview of Biopsy and Necropsy Techniques 575

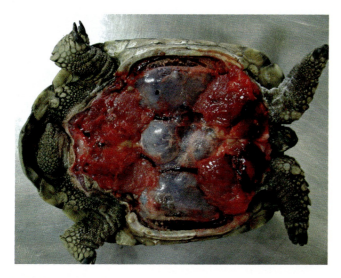

FIGURE 34-11 Plastron removed with body wall intact. The coelomic cavity is still sterile at this point. The pectoral and pelvic musculature is also evident.

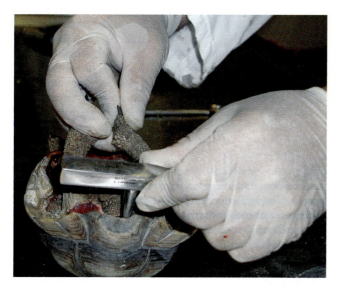

FIGURE 34-12 Disarticulation of the coccygeal vertebrae from the carapace. With the carapace resting on the table, upward traction is applied to the hind legs with one hand and a T-bar is wedged into the junction of the coccygeal vertebrae and carapace. Downward pressure is applied to the T-bar to disarticulate the joint. (The same procedure is used later to disarticulate the cervical vertebrae from the carapace.)

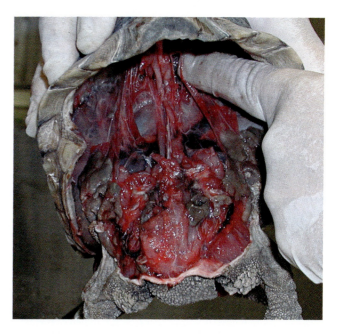

FIGURE 34-13 Removal of the carapace. The carcass is righted, and the carcass is suspended with the carapace held in one hand. With the other hand, the viscera are dissected digitally from the inner surface of the carapace.

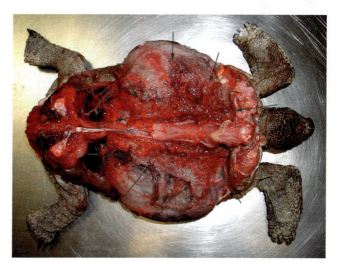

FIGURE 34-14 Carapace removed from the body wall. The coelomic cavity and lungs are still sterile at this point. The lungs (deflated) are apparent on the surface of the rostral half of the body *(arrows)*.

down on the viscera. The tissues are digitally dissected away from the inside aspect of the carapace, starting from the back and moving forward. The large skeletal muscle bundles in the shoulder and pelvic regions may need to be cut with a scissors.

The carcass is placed in sternal recumbency on the necropsy table. If this is done correctly, sterile access is provided to the lung fields and the lung can be cultured with an incision through the wall and swabbing of the inner surfaces (Figure 34-15). This technique is modified for the giant land tortoises and large seaturtles that are too heavy to suspend during dissection of the carcass away from the carapace.

After the shells have been removed (or just the plastron in case of large chelonians) and cultures have been collected, the remaining procedures are similar to the squamates. Most significant anatomy can be seen at this stage of the prosection (Figure 34-16).

Endocrine Tissues

The endocrine glands include the pituitary, pineal, thyroid, parathyroid, ultimobranchial gland, carotid and aortic bodies, pancreas, and adrenal.

Pituitary and Pineal Glands. Recommendation is to submit the entire head of a necropsy specimen. Among other

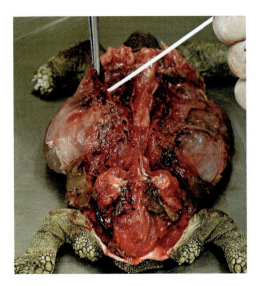

FIGURE 34-15 Culturing of the lung. The lung surface is sterilized with alcohol and incised with a sterile scalpel. The pleura is lifted with sterile tissue forceps to expose the central lumen of the lung, which can then be swabbed with a culturette.

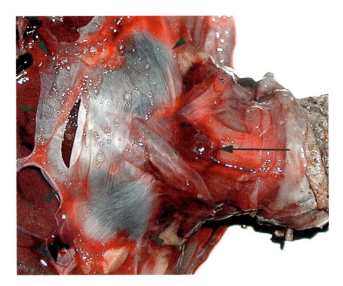

FIGURE 34-17 The pericardial sac and thyroid gland are evident. *Arrowheads* delineate the pericardial sac of this specimen. The thyroid gland *(arrow)* is immediately rostral to the pericardial sac, at the bifurcation of the great vessels exiting the heart.

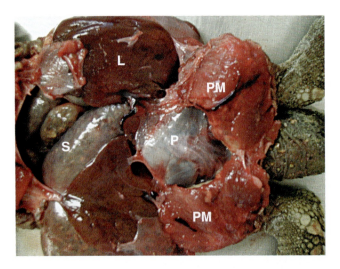

FIGURE 34-16 Ventral view of the viscera with the coelomic wall removed. Liver *(L)*, stomach *(S)*, pericardial sac *(P)*, and pectoral muscles *(PM)* are evident.

reasons, this ensures that both the pituitary and pineal glands are included. In the rare event that these tissues are diseased, the pathologist is able to locate them in sequential sections of the head.

Thyroid, Parathyroid, and Ultimobranchial Body. Examination of the thyroid for evidence of goiter or neoplasia is important. In reptiles, the thyroid is a single structure (not paired, as in mammals and birds) and is located at the bifurcation of the greater vessels (Figure 34-17). It is amber and appears multiloculated on cut surface. It is frequently mistaken for a mass or some form of disease process. Thyroid size may vary from seasonal changes in follicular diameter, so mild "enlargement" may be a physiologic rather than pathologic event. Also in the region of the thyroid are small lobulated structures that represent the thymus, parathyroid, and ultimobranchial bodies. Normally, these can be difficult to see grossly, and sometimes the best method is to submit the soft tissues in this region and "hope for the best."

Carotid and Aortic Bodies. These microscopic glands are located along the greater vessels and are very difficult to find. They are usually detected fortuitously in microscopic sections of the greater vessels and heartbase. Disease involving these structures is rare, and seldom is there a need to submit them for histopathologic evaluation.

Pancreas. The pancreas has both exocrine (digestive) and endocrine functions. Examination of the pancreas is important because it develops microscopic changes indicative of nutritional status. Some infectious disease processes have a tropism for the pancreas, such as paramyxovirus and monocercomoniasis in snakes. Among reptiles, considerable variation is seen in the location of pancreas. In many snakes and some turtles, it is fused with the spleen (splenopancreas) and located in the mesentery next to the gut and gallbladder. In some species, the pancreas is an isolated gland in the mesentery adjacent to the duodenum. Some species have both isolated pancreas and splenopancreas.

Adrenal. The adrenal gland is an important tissue to examine microscopically because it develops microscopic changes that may indicate stress, which can be difficult to evaluate in an otherwise stoic reptile. Neoplasia, degenerative change, necrosis, and neoplasia also are occasionally seen. The adrenal gland is paired in reptiles, but considerable variation in shape and some minor variation in location of the adrenal gland exist. Generally, it is a tubular or ovoid structure in the mesovarium or mesorchium (thin membranes attached to reproductive tract) on the medial aspect of the gonad. In snakes, it is long and can be anterior or posterior to the gonad; careful prosection is necessary to assure both gonad and adrenal are identified before collection of each.

Reproductive Tract

Routine collection of reproductive tissues is important. Common reproductive problems in reptiles and amphibians

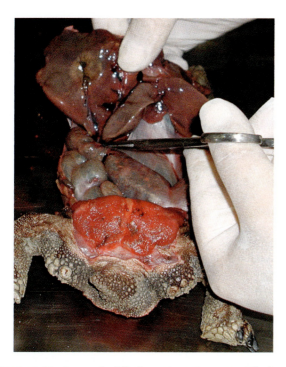

FIGURE 34-18 Removal of the liver. Caudal aspects of the hepatic lobes are lifted, rostral traction is applied, and underlying attachments are incised. The pectoral musculoskeletal system is removed in similar manner.

include bacterial infections; neoplasia; preovulatory and postovulatory follicular stasis; prolapse of the hemipenis, uterus, or cloaca; and mineralization or impaction of the hemipene. The urogenital system is similar in most reptiles. Gonads are paired. Females have a paired oviduct (salpinx), and males have a paired epididymis and vas deferens. Male chelonians and crocodilians have a penis. Lizards and snakes have hemipenes located caudal to the cloaca on both sides of the ventral aspect of the tail.

Urinary Tract

Common disease conditions in reptiles that involve the urinary tract include chronic renal disease (especially iguanas), gout, urolithiasis (stones), nephrocalcinosis, bacterial and parasitic infections, and neoplasia. The kidneys are paired and are generally located in the caudal coelomic cavity. They are especially caudal in the chelonians and some species of lizards (iguanas) and are frequently missed at necropsy. The kidneys are ovoid in most species of reptiles and in the amphibians. In snakes, they are lobulated and cylindrical. Commonly, the gonads are mistaken for kidney. Therefore, identification of the kidneys, gonad, and adrenal in situ is important so that they are not lost or inadvertently overlooked during prosection. Chelonians and some lizards have a urinary bladder. Snakes, crocodilians, and some lizards do not.

Digestive Tract and Liver

Liver and Gallbladder. The liver is generally bilobed in the reptiles, and most species have a gallbladder. The gallbladder is intimately associated with the liver in most lizards and chelonians but considerably caudal to the liver and close to the spleen and pancreas in snakes. Hepatic diseases include infectious processes, neoplasia, toxicosis, lipidosis,

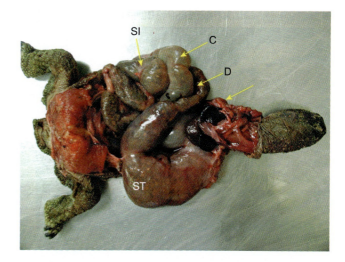

FIGURE 34-19 Ventral view of the viscera. The gut and heart are easily visualized after removal of the liver and front limbs. Note heart (*yellow arrow*), stomach *(ST)*, duodenum *(D)*, small intestine *(SI)*, and colon *(C)*.

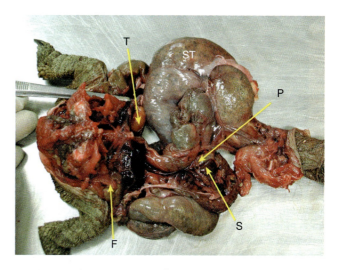

FIGURE 34-20 Dorsal view of the viscera. Evident in this view are the stomach *(ST)*, spleen *(S)*, splenic lobe of the pancreas *(arrow)*, fat bodies *(F)*, and testicle *(T)*.

cirrhosis, and melanosis. Representative sections of liver and gallbladder should be routinely collected at necropsy (Figure 34-18).

Alimentary Tract. Disease conditions of the alimentary tract are especially common in reptiles and amphibians and include a number of bacterial, fungal, viral, and parasitic diseases. Obstruction, plication, or ulceration from luminal passage of foreign bodies, intussusception (telescoping), stasis, and rectal/cloacal prolapse also are occasionally seen. Preferably the pathologist should examine microscopically all segments of the alimentary tract, including the oral cavity (included with the head), esophagus, stomach, small intestine (duodenum, jejunum, and ileum regions), colon, rectum, and cloaca (Figures 34-19 and 34-20).

In some reptiles, difficulty is found with distinguishing microscopically the different segments of small intestine, or the difference between small and large intestine; therefore,

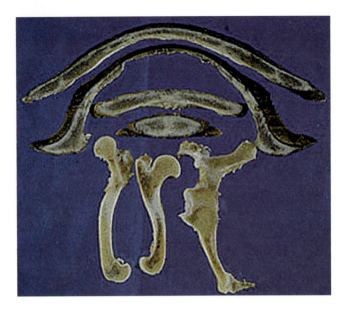

FIGURE 34-21 Sections of bone show the distribution of marrow in a tortoise. The dark shaded areas of bone represent cellular marrow. Note the absence of gelatinous marrow. Note the carapace *(C)*, plastron *(P)*, femur *(F)*, humerus *(H)*, and pelvis *(Pe)*.

labeling the segments of submitted bowel is helpful for interpreting lesion distribution.

Hematopoietic and Lymphoid Tissues (Spleen, Thymus, Bone Marrow, Peripheral Blood)

Examination of these tissues provides clues to immune status, anemia, and various infectious and nutritional problems. Blood films (on slides) can be made from heart blood at necropsy if the blood is not clotted. The spleen is generally a small ovoid brown/red or tan structure located in the mesentery often close to the gallbladder. It can be difficult to find but is important to examine for the presence of infectious disease processes. Evaluation of overall lymphoid cellularity can give a crude estimation of immune status and can also provide evidence of exposure to stress. The thymus is a lobulated structure in the fascia close to the thyroid (see discussion of thyroid) and is responsible for production of lymphocytes. Bone marrow of the long bones is gelatinous in lizards and crocodilians but "trabecular" and difficult to collect separately in snakes and chelonians (Figure 34-21). It is generally examined as part of the microscopic bone examination.

Cardiovascular System

A broad array of disease processes affect the cardiovascular system, such as atherosclerosis, bacterial endocarditis, endocardiosis, degenerative cardiomyopathy, thrombosis of the greater vessels and their main branches, and mineralization of the greater vessels. Visual identification at necropsy of the aorta and major branches and full length examination of the luminal surfaces are recommended, especially if the animal has a history suggestive of thrombosis or vasculitis. For microscopic examination, routine submission of the entire heart (small animals) or full-thickness sections of the ventricle, both atria, and sections of the valves of larger reptiles is recommended.

A short length of cardiac outflow vessels (greater vessels) should routinely be submitted. Opening the heart for formalin perfusion is helpful for adequate fixation and may reveal lesions worthy of culture before formalin submersion. The heart should be prosected with incision of the vena cava with a blunt-tipped scissors at its insertion in the right atrium and with the blade of the scissor to "run" the ventricle down to the right side to the apex, then back up the left side to the aortic outflow. Reflecting the ventricles after this procedure exposes the valves for visual examination.

Respiratory Tract

Numerous disease processes affect the respiratory tract, especially infectious diseases and mineralization from metabolic or nutritional disorders. Submission of the entire head ensures microscopic examination of the nasal cavity and larynx. Representative sections of the trachea and lung should always be submitted. In reptiles, the lung is a hollow sac with a honeycomb appearance on the inner surface. The anterior portion has a thick wall and has respiratory function. The posterior portion is thin-walled and resembles an avian air sac. The anterior portion is generally more useful for diagnostic purposes, but submission of both regions is recommended. In some snakes, the right lung is well developed and the left lung is rudimentary or missing.

Musculoskeletal System

Examination of this system is important because it provides useful information regarding current and past nutritional status. Also, a number of traumatic, degenerative, and infectious conditions affect the musculoskeletal system. When whole carcasses are submitted, microscopic examination of the musculoskeletal system is assured. For carcasses too large to submit whole, an effort should be made to submit the head, a segment of vertebral column, and at least one long bone with articular surface, such as the femur, tibia, humerus, or radius.

Nervous System

Diseases of the nervous system are occasionally seen in reptiles and amphibians and are usually manifestations of other visceral disorders, such as gout, neoplasia, intoxication, or infectious disease. For small reptiles, the brain and cord are easily examined when the entire head and vertebrae are submitted. For those animals too large for submission of an entire vertebra or head, prosection of the spinal cord and brain is necessary.

The mouth should be taped shut so fingers are not impaled on teeth or fangs, and the top of the skull should be removed with a Stryker saw or bone rongeur for exposure to the brain. The top of the vertebral body (dorsal process) can be removed in a similar manner for access to the spinal cord. With submission of the head on venomous reptiles, labeling the containers "venomous" is useful and conscientious so that the technicians trimming the tissue during histologic preparation are aware of the potential danger of handling the tissues. Taping the mouth shut is useful when prosecting the brain but is not recommended when submitting the whole head in formalin because the tape may impede fixation of the tissues.

GROSS PHOTOGRAPHY

The collection of gross photographs of lesions in the live or dead animal is an important and underemphasized procedure. With practice, gross photography can be conveniently and skillfully performed by clinicians. A camera is best kept at the clinic specifically for the purpose of obtaining gross photographs so that it is available as needed.

In live animals, a pretreatment gross photograph is a useful point of reference to measure treatment response and a helpful guide for client communication. Gross photographs can also be included with biopsy submissions and are a useful (and frequently requested) aid in the interpretation of the lesion. In particular, images captured with digital cameras can be rapidly forwarded to a pathologist via the Internet for consultation before biopsy, culture, or treatment. Prints, slides, or images can be stored with the patient records for future reference.

For conventional film cameras, a macro lens is usually needed, especially for small lesions or small patients. Digital cameras have the added flexibility of image enlargement, and color and contrast enhancement after the photograph has been obtained. The lesion should be of a magnification that occupies about 70% to 80% of the field, but an attempt should be made to include a margin of surrounding normal tissue to aid in viewer orientation. Sometimes low and high magnification images are necessary to fully illustrate the location and gross features of the lesion. One should obtain more than one image at each magnification, adjusting for each to obtain the best contrast and focus.

For in situ and ex situ lesion photography, framing the lesion in the center of the image is important. For ex situ photography, a black or dark blue background is best to aid in tissue contrast. One should avoid use of paper towels, wooden cutting boards, cage grates, or tile flooring as backgrounds for tissue photography. A flat, black rubber mat or a piece of clear glass placed over blue or black cloth works particularly well as background. Fluid seepage should be avoided by blotting the tissues before final positioning. A ruler is a useful size guide, especially for ex situ tissue photography; however, the ruler should not occupy more than 10% of the image and should be placed at the bottom or along one side of the tissue. The ruler should not be placed directly on the tissue or in the middle of the slide because this may obscure the lesion or orientation of the lesion in the surrounding tissues. A series of common photographic mistakes are captured in Figures 34-22 to 34-25.

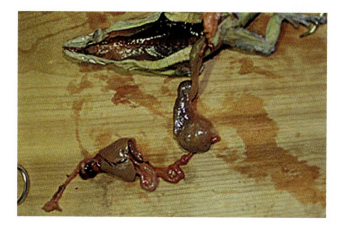

FIGURE 34-23 Poor-quality gross photograph. Carcass of this lizard is not centered in the field and is not entirely in the field, much fluid staining of the background is seen, and the background is absorbent wood. The item of interest is not clear because of the wide spatial arrangement of the tissues. The photograph is about as bad as a gross photograph can be.

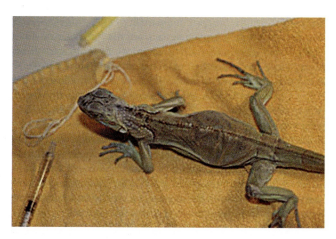

FIGURE 34-22 Poor-quality gross photograph. In this photograph, the entire lizard is not in the field, two different backgrounds are in the field, and much background distraction is seen (e.g., frayed towel and syringe).

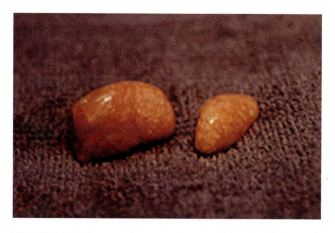

FIGURE 34-24 Poor-quality gross photograph. In this photograph, the subjects (iguana kidneys) are not centered in the field, magnification is too low, and not enough contrast is found between the tissues and background (brown towel).

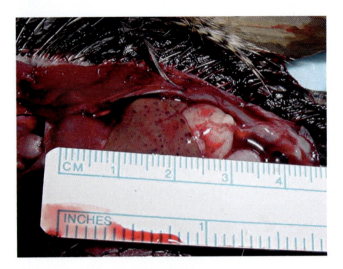

FIGURE 34-25 Poor-quality gross photograph. In this photograph, a ruler is placed directly on tissue, partially obscuring the lesion and markedly obscuring the field of view.

35
SURGERY

DOUGLAS R. MADER, R. AVERY BENNETT,
RICHARD S. FUNK, KEVIN T. FITZGERALD,
REBECCA VERA, and STEPHEN J. HERNANDEZ-DIVERS

SOFT TISSUE, ORTHOPEDICS, AND FRACTURE REPAIR

Douglas R. Mader and R. Avery Bennett

SOFT TISSUE SURGERY

Surgery is a common practice in reptilian medicine. Even with the advent of newer minimally invasive techniques (e.g., endosurgery), the clinician must be able perform a standard set of procedures such as wound repair, exploratory coeliotomy, enterotomy, enucleation, gastrotomy or fracture repair, and amputation. A basic understanding of the unique anatomy and physiology of the particular reptile species is vital before surgery is undertaken.[1] The clinician is referred to the sections of this book that provide information about the body system that needs surgery. Some points of particular relevance to soft tissue or orthopedic surgery are reviewed before discussions concerning specific conditions.

Proper anesthesia and analgesia are paramount. Both subjects are covered in Chapter 27. No excuse exists for not providing some form of pain relief to reptilian patients.

WOUND HEALING

Wound healing in reptiles occurs through phases similar to those observed in mammalian species. This has been studied in snakes.[2] Initially, proteinaceous fluid and fibrin fill the defect to form a scab. A single layer of epithelial cells migrates beneath the scab. This single layer then proliferates to restore the thickness of the normal epithelium. In addition, macrophages and heterophils migrate into the tissue below the scab to clean up bacteria and debris (see Figure 15-19). A transversely arranged fibrous scar is produced by fibroblasts that migrate into the area. Heterophils are present within the scar tissue matrix until maturation has occurred. This is a slow process in reptiles. Consequently, suture removal is generally recommended 4 to 6 weeks after suture placement. The activity of the dermis and epidermis during ecdysis appears to promote healing.[2] If suture removal can be delayed until the subsequent ecdysis, wound strength is likely to be better. In many cases, sutures slough off with the first ecdysis after surgery (Figure 35-1).

Environmental temperature has an effect on wound healing.[2] Maintenance of the patient in the upper end of its optimum range (see Table 4-1) has been shown to promote healing. The orientation of the wound also influences the rate of healing, with cranial to caudal oriented wounds healing faster than transverse wounds. With treatment of open wounds, such as those that occur from lamp burns, good environmental hygiene is important. These wounds do heal well with second intention with a relatively low incidence of secondary infections (see Figure 71-9).

SUTURE MATERIALS

In general, the skin of reptiles is strong and acts as the primary holding layer for maintenance of wound closure. For example, with coelomic surgery, the coelomic membrane and body wall are soft to nonexistent and do not hold sutures well. The success of wound closure relies on strong, well-placed skin sutures. Because the skin is tough, sutures are unlikely to tear through. In addition, most reptiles do not traumatize their incisions, which makes closure with a continuous pattern safe and efficient.

In most situations, steel suture is not necessary and softer materials such as nylon or polypropylene are more comfortable for the patient. Although synthetic absorbable materials are believed to eventually be absorbed by reptilian patients, their absorption appears to be prolonged. If these materials are used for skin closure, removal is required. Chromic catgut does not appear to be an appropriate suture for use in the reptile patient. In a Rhinoceros Viper (*Bitis nasicornis*), the material was still present 12 weeks after placement in both the pleuroperitoneum and the subcutaneous tissues.[3] Other absorbable materials not dependent on proteolysis are recommended for deeper tissue closures.

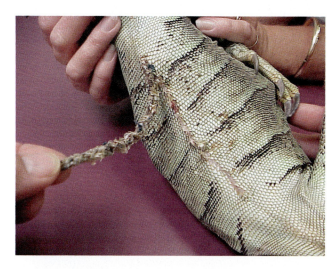

Figure 35-1 If suture removal can be delayed until the subsequent ecdysis, wound strength is likely to be better. In many cases, sutures will slough off with the first ecdysis following surgery. (*Photograph courtesy D. Mader.*)

Govett et al[4] evaluated tissue response to four different absorbable skin sutures in marine turtles. Chromic gut, polyglyconate, polyglactin 910, and poliglecaprone 25 were used in 258 turtles to close a wound produced at the time of laparoscopic gender determination. Gross and histologic tissue reactions to the different suture types were analyzed. Histologically, polyglactin 910 produced a greater tissue reaction than any other suture type. Poliglecaprone 25 and polyglyconate caused the least tissue reaction of the four suture types examined in seaturtle skin.

Suture removal is generally scheduled 4 to 6 weeks after surgery. In squamates, delay of suture removal until after the subsequent ecdysis is often advantageous. If the suture line does not come off with the first ecdysis, the shed skin may stick to the incision site. If this happens, the skin is easily removed with gentle assistance. After suture removal, the skin may stick to the site of the incision for one or two more sheds, but normal ecdysis resumes quickly (Figure 35-2).

Incised reptilian skin has a strong tendency to invert (Figure 35-3). This is most pronounced in squamates, less so in chelonians and crocodilians. If the skin is closed in such a manner that scales oppose scales, the healing is delayed because the cut edges are not in apposition. Skin closure is best accomplished with an everting suture pattern such as horizontal or vertical mattress (Figure 35-4). Skin staples are applicable to reptile patients (Figure 35-5). Not only are they strong, but they also cause eversion of the skin, which allows the incised edges to be maintained in apposition for primary healing. Everting the skin leaves a raw edge exposed. A light dressing can be applied, or alternatively, a liquid bandage can be used to coat the edge and provide a good antiseptic seal (Figure 35-6). Careful placement of sutures and avoidance of overtightening help prevent excessive ridging of the skin.

INSTRUMENTATION

The huge variety in reptile patient size and morphology makes a standard "Reptile" surgery pack impossible. Tiny geckos have thin, delicate skin, whereas others, such as the skinks and of course, the crocodilians, have hard bony osteoderms in the scales. Chelonians, with their shells, add another completely different dimension to the needs of the reptile surgeon.

Some reptile patients necessitate the use of small fine-tipped instruments, such as those used in vascular or ophthalmologic surgery packs. Some form of magnification is recommended for patients that weigh less than 1 kg. Because of the small size and blood volume of many patients, hemostasis is very important. With magnification, vessels are much

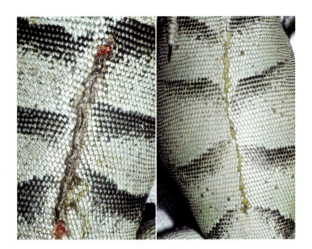

Figure 35-2 Following suture removal, the skin may stick to the site of the incision for one or two more sheds (left) but normal ecdysis resumes quickly (right). *(Photograph courtesy D. Mader.)*

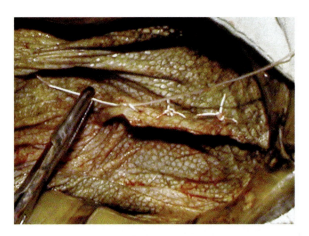

Figure 35-4 Skin closure should be performed with an everting suture pattern, such as a horizontal or vertical mattress. *(Photograph courtesy D. Mader.)*

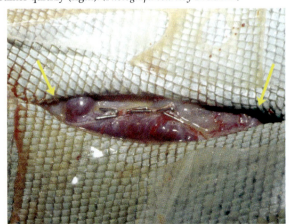

Figure 35-3 Incised reptilian skin has a strong tendency to invert *(yellow arrows)*. *(Photograph courtesy D. Mader.)*

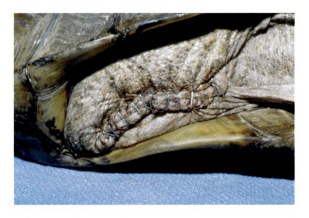

Figure 35-5 Skin staples are strong and also automatically evert the skin, allowing the incised edges to be maintained in apposition for primary healing. *(Photograph courtesy D. Mader.)*

more easily identified for coagulation. Although an operating microscope would be ideal for small patients, binocular magnification loupes of 2.5× to 5× are adequate for most procedures (Surgitel, General Scientific Corp, Ann Arbor, Mich www.surgitel.com; Figure 35-7).

Some ophthalmic instruments are well-suited for magnification surgery. Iris scissors, iris forceps, micromosquito hemostats, iris hooks, eyelid retractors, retinal forceps, jeweler's forceps, spring-handled scissors, and Castroviejo needle holders are particularly useful. Numbers 15 and 11 scalpel blades are most appropriate for reptile surgery. Gauze pads (2 × 2) can be cut from the standard 4 × 4 sponges. Sterile cotton-tipped applicators should also be available. Surgical spears, are small, wedge-shaped, absorbent, synthetic sponges attached to the end of a stick (Weck-Cell Surgical Spears, Research Triangle Park, NC). They are useful for absorbing accumulated blood or fluid in cavities. Surgicel (Johnson & Johnson, Ft. Washington, Pa), a cloth-like product made of an oxidized regenerated cellulose that conforms and adheres to irregular surfaces, and absorbable gelatin sponges (such as Gelfoam, Upjohn, Kansas City, Mo) are used for controlling hemorrhage. Hemostatic clips (Ligaclip, Ethicon, Sommerville, NJ; or Hemoclip, Weck, Research Triangle Park, NC) are available in various sizes and are used to provide hemostasis for vessels in body cavities where application of ligatures is difficult (Figure 35-8). With the applier, the clip is placed across the lumen of the vessel and clamped in place. Several sizes are available that suit the needs of most patients.

Eyelid retractors work well as wound retractors, and the iris hooks can be used to manipulate delicate tissues. A Heiss blunt retractor (Weck) combines quick easy application, small size, good strength, and adequate spread. The blade extends 6.5 mm with a 3.3-mm hook that is less likely to snag sutures. A small Alm retractor with short blunt teeth (Weck) is also effective but slightly larger.

Lonestar Medical Products, Inc. (Stafford, Tex, www.lsmp.com) makes variable-shaped retractors that are ideal for both small and large reptile patients. These retractors can be pre-shaped to fit specific sized patients or unique surgical fields.

Some form of radiosurgery, such as with the Surgitron (Ellman International, Oceanside, NY, www.ellman.com), is also useful in reptile patients. The bipolar ophthalmic forceps have application for abdominal surgery in reptiles because they allow coagulation of vessels deep within the coelomic cavity. Minimization of blood loss is critical in the small patients. The electrosurgical unit may be used for skin incision, body wall incision, organ biopsies, and a variety of other procedures.

Surgical lasers are now readily available and, in many situations, have replaced the scalpel and the radiosurgical units. Lasers allow precise cutting through reptile skin, minimize blood loss, and, in some applications, are useful with endosurgery. Both diode and CO_2 lasers are discussed in detail later in this chapter.

For coelomic surgery in chelonians, some type of bone saw is necessary to cut through the osseous plastron. An oscillating orthopedic saw is ideally suited for this procedure because it can be autoclaved; however, the saw is often prohibitively expensive for the general practitioner. A rotary woodworking or jeweler's tool may be used. The bits are not made of surgical steel and should be autoclaved. In addition, they are not designed to cut through bone and do not last. They must not be overused because a dull blade does not cut

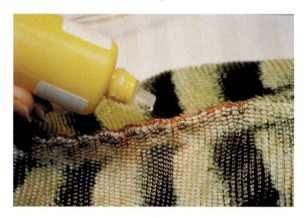

Figure 35-6 Everting the skin leaves a raw edge exposed. A light dressing can be applied, or, alternatively, a liquid bandage or tissue adhesive can be used to coat the edge to provide a good antiseptic seal. *(Photograph courtesy D. Mader.)*

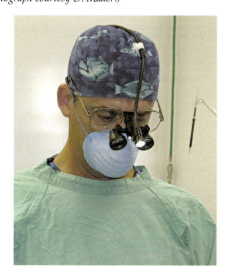

Figure 35-7 Binocular magnification loupes of 2.5× to 5× are adequate for most procedures in small patients (Surgitel, www.surgitel.com). *(Photograph courtesy E. Slomka.)*

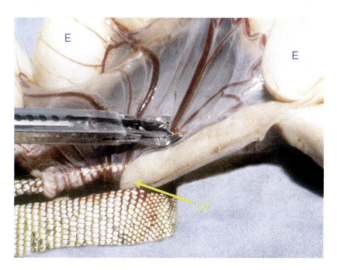

Figure 35-8 Vascular clips are available in various sizes and are used to provide hemostasis for vessels in body cavities where it is difficult to apply ligatures. Using the applicator, the clip is placed across the lumen of the vessel and clamped in place. *(Photograph courtesy D. Mader.)*

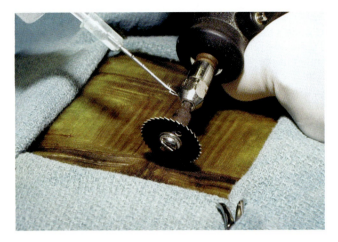

Figure 35-9 Small circular saw blades are available for high-speed rotary tools. A good utility blade for use on most turtles and tortoises is 0.021 inches thick, and has a 7/8-inch diameter and 36 teeth. These blades cut a narrow osteotomy in the plastron, allowing for faster bone healing. Caution should be taken to cool the blade with sterile saline solution during the cut as the blade can overheat, causing thermal damage to the bone. *(Photograph courtesy D. Mader.)*

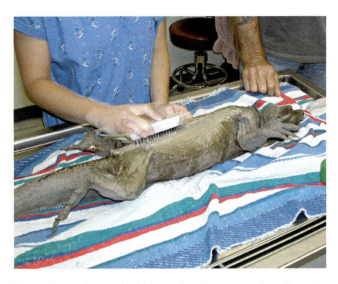

Figure 35-10 The rough, thick, overlapping nature of reptilian skin makes it difficult to effectively aseptically prepare the animal for surgery. Antibacterial preparations, such as betadine or chlorhexidine, with a stiff brush, should be used on all patients. *(Photograph courtesy D. Mader.)*

well and tends to burn the bone, preventing proper healing. Small circular saw blades are available for these high-speed tools. One author (Mader) has found that a good utility blade for cutting through most turtles and tortoises is 0.021-inch thick and has a 7/8-inch diameter and 36 teeth (Micromark, Berkeley Heights, NJ, www.micromark.com) (Figure 35-9). These blades cut a narrow osteotomy in the plastron, allowing for faster bone healing. With careful handling these blades maintain their cutting edge and can be used for two or three patients.

The rotary tools are made of plastic and, as a result, cannot be autoclaved but may be gas sterilized or covered with a sterile stockinette. The bits may be gas or steam sterilized, but steam sterilized bits corrode quickly.

PATIENT PREPARATION

Fasting

Reptiles do not have a problem with regurgitation during anesthesia. Therefore, fasting these animals before surgery is usually not necessary unless a gastrointestinal procedure is planned. Because snakes may go weeks to months between meals, fasting is a nonissue.

Preoperative

All the general principles of anesthesia and preoperative evaluation that apply to mammal patients also apply to reptiles. A thorough preoperative physical examination by the surgeon, appropriate laboratory screening, radiographs, and so on, should all be performed, or at least recommended to the client. Patients should always be classified as to their risk of anesthesia (healthy pet, elective procedure versus patient with major health problems) and the potential surgical risk (simple restraint for laboratory sample collection versus prolonged procedure with potential for major blood loss). Chapters 27, 31, and 36 cover fluids, anesthesia, and analgesia.

Caution should be taken with anemic patients because these animals do not have much blood to start with and even minor hemorrhage can be lethal. Consider preoperative transfusions in those animals at risk, have blood ready for intraoperative transfusions, or, at least, premedicate patients with fluids before procedures.

Because hypothermia is of paramount concern in reptilian patients, the fluids should always be warmed before administration. In weak, emaciated, or severely ill patients, use of a 5% dextrose solution, or a 2.5% dextrose in a balanced electrolyte solution, either before, during, or immediately after surgery, administered either intravenously or intraosseously, may be wise.

Most reptiles have a relatively large surface area to volume ratio (in general, the smaller the patient, the larger the ratio). As mentioned, this larger surface area means that these patients are prone to hypothermia. Some form of supplemental heating is mandatory for these patients: circulating warm water blankets, heated rice bags, warmed anesthetic gases (tube warmers), heated fluids, heated lavage fluids, and for surgical preparation, the use of chlorhexidine rather than alcohol. Bair Hugger (Eden Prairie, Minn) makes a reusable, forced-air warming blanket (model 530 or 555) that is useful for maintaining patient body temperature.

Reptiles, being both ectothermic and breath holders, can be a significant anesthetic challenge. For better control, elimination of temperature as a variable is best. Every reptile group has its own preferred optimal temperature. For instance, the Gartersnake *(Thamnophis* spp.) thrives at temperatures near 27°C (80°F), whereas the Green Iguana *(Iguana iguana)* needs temperatures around 32°C (90°F) or higher to flourish. So, with surgery in these patients, where a Gartersnake may do just fine with a core body temperature of 27°C (80°F), the Green Iguana may be slower to induce, may be more difficult to maintain, and may take much longer to recover.

Reptiles are susceptible to a wide range of microbial infections. Stress from anesthesia and surgery may potentiate natural or iatrogenic infections. In addition, because of the rugous nature of the reptilian skin, an effective sterile preparation may be difficult (Figure 35-10). As a result, perioperative antibiotics are warranted. Chapters 16 and 36 cover common pathogens and antibiotic therapy.

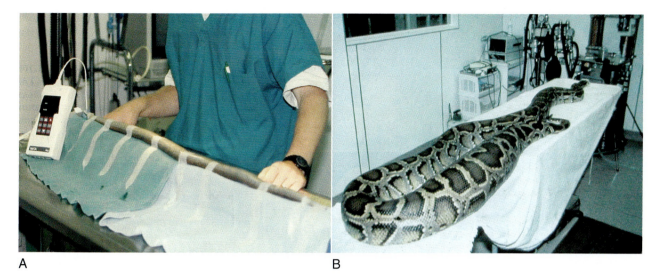

Figure 35-11 **A,** Paper medical tape, or common masking tape, can be used to secure a small snake to a restraint board and does not damage the scales. **B,** Larger snakes can be strapped to a long board, or positioned on tables placed end-to-end. Extremely large animals may have to be doubled back in order to fit on the surgical table(s). *(Photographs courtesy D. Mader.)*

Positioning reptile patients often requires some creativity. Small snakes can be taped to a board for restraint (Figure 35-11, *A*). Paper medical tape or common masking tape works well and does not damage the scales. Larger snakes can also be strapped to a long board or positioned on tables placed end-to-end. Extremely large animals may have to be doubled back to fit on the surgical table or tables (Figure 35-11, *B*).

Turtles and tortoises, when placed in dorsal recumbency, can be balanced in a "V" trough or placed in the middle of a towel rolled into a ring. The feet and legs can either be taped or restrained with surgical ties to prevent motion and stabilize the patient during the procedure.

Lizard morphology varies significantly among species. Most lizards can be positioned in fashions similar to mammalian quadrupeds: dorsal, ventral, or lateral recumbency. Laterally compressed animals, such as the chameleon group, are best positioned in lateral recumbency. From this position, all internal organs can be accessed (Figure 35-12).

A sterile field is as necessary in reptile surgery as in any other species (Figure 35-13, *A*). Clear plastic drapes (VSP, Boca Raton, Fla) provide the necessary sterile field and also allow visual assessment of the patient during surgery (Figure 35-13, *B*). Most clear plastic drapes are of a small size. For creation of a large sterile field, a paper drape with an opening cut large enough to accommodate the patient's size is placed over the clear plastic drape. With this technique, the entire operating table is covered with the sterile paper drape that has a window for observation of the patient. The patient is maintained in an aseptic field covered with the clear plastic drape.

Sterile spray adhesives (Vi-Drape Adhesive, Medical Concepts Development, Inc., Woodbury, Minn) may be used with cloth and paper drapes so that the drapes stick to the patient without the need for towel clamps. This is especially important with chelonians where towel clamps are not applicable. An alternate technique is to gas sterilize a roll of cloth tape and then place a boundary around the surgical site

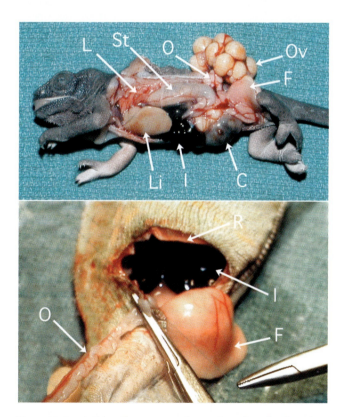

Figure 35-12 **A,** Laterally compressed animals, such as the chameleon group, are best positioned in lateral recumbency. **B,** From this position, all internal organs can be accessed. *L,* Lung, *St;* stomach, *O;* oviduct; *Ov,* ovary; *F,* fat body; *C,* colon; *I,* intestine; *Li,* liver; *R,* rib. *(Photographs courtesy D. Mader.)*

(Figure 35-14). Towel clamps can then be fastened to the sterile cloth tape. The tape is readily removed and discarded after surgery.

Care must be taken when these adhesive-type materials are removed from the patient to avoid damaging the skin.

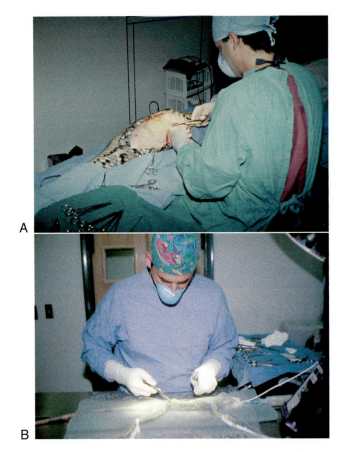

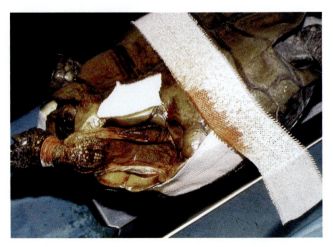

Figure 35-14 In chelonians, where standard towel clamps are not effective, an alternate technique is to gas-sterilize a roll of cloth tape and then place a sterile boundary around the surgical site. Towel clamps can then be fastened to the sterile cloth tape. The tape is readily removed and discarded postoperatively. *(Photograph courtesy D. Mader.)*

Figure 35-13 **A,** A sterile field is as necessary in reptile surgery as in any other species. **B,** Clear plastic drapes provide the necessary sterile field and also allow visual assessment of a small patient intraoperatively. *(Photographs courtesy G. Diethelm.)*

Alcohol or adhesive remover applied to a cotton swab may be used at the skin-adhesive junction to soften the adhesive and aid in removal.

For snakes, draping can be accomplished with a sterile stockinette rolled over the prepared patient. The snake, now inside the stockinette, can be placed over the sterile drape, providing an aseptic field.

Standard patient surgical preparation solutions, such as povidone-iodine and chlorhexidine, are commonly used for reptile patients. Chlorhexidine provides the advantages of a broader spectrum of activity and increased residual activity. When shell repair is necessary for chelonian patients, the surface of the shell must be prepared with cleansing and degreasing the surface so that the restorative material sticks to the shell. Acetone, ether, or trichlorotrifluoroethane (Freon Skin Degreaser, Miller-Stevenson Chemical, Danbury, Conn) may be used for this purpose.

POSTOPERATIVE CARE

The two most important points to address for postoperative reptile patients are warmth and pain control (see Chapter 27). No excuse exists for not providing postoperative analgesia to patients.

During and after anesthetic recovery, the patient should be maintained in a clean, warm, dark, quiet environment. Swimming should be prevented for a period of 7 to 14 days after surgery to allow a scab to form and desiccate. Prevention of brumation (hibernation) for approximately 6 months is best to allow healing to proceed. The nutritional and hydration needs of the patient must be assessed and maintained (see Chapter 18). Fluid therapy is indicated to maintain the hydration status of the patient. Many patients become anorectic after surgery and need tube or assist feeding. In some cases, pharyngostomy tube placement may be necessary to provide long-term alimentation for the patient (see Figure 36-15).

CELIOTOMY

The approach for celiotomy in reptiles varies with the family of reptile.[5] Celiotomy provides access to all the coelomic organs of reptiles and has a wide range of applications. It provides access to thoracic structures, such as the heart and lungs, and abdominal structures, such as the gastrointestinal system and major body organs. Indications include reproductive disorders, gastrointestinal disease, urinary system dysfunction, and exploration for obtaining organ biopsies.

Snakes

Snakes are perhaps the easiest of all reptiles on which to perform surgery. They are essentially one long tube, with all the organs organized in a straight line. Familiarity with normal organ location facilitates the surgical approach. McCracken[6] has published a linear road map, on the basis of relative body positioning with the head as the beginning (0%) and the tip of the tail at 100%. Each organ is expressed, in terms of location along this line, as a percentage somewhere between the head and the tail.[6]

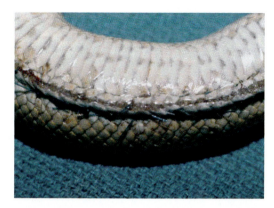

Figure 35-15 The celiotomy incision in snakes should be made next to the lateral margin of the body where the scutes and scales are in apposition. The advantage of making the incision between the first two rows of lateral scales is that when the incision is closed with an everting pattern it does not distort the flat conformation of the ventral scutes. *(Photograph courtesy D. Mader.)*

Alternatively, radiology and ultrasound can be used to identify the location of organs and lesions, and the patient can be labeled with a permanent marker prior to surgical preparation.

In snakes, a celiotomy is best performed at the lateral margin of the body where the scutes and scales are in apposition. The advantage of the incision being made between the first two rows of lateral scales is that when the incision is closed with an everting pattern it does not distort the flat conformation of the ventral scutes (Figure 35-15). The incision should be made between the scales, resulting in a scalloped configuration. This may enhance healing because the incision is made through the softer portion of the skin between the scales. The incision should be made along the body in a position that provides access to the structure being approached. Once the incision has been made through the skin, the body wall must be incised. Keeping in mind that one pair of ribs is associated with each scute to the level of the vent, any trauma to the ends of the ribs is best avoided. Using a #11 blade, cutting edge up, with the incision stroke in an outward direction, helps prevent damage to deeper structures.

Reportedly, no difference exists in exposure gained with a ventral midline incision compared with this lateral approach.[3,7] However, the lateral approach is easier to keep clean because it is not in direct contact with the substrate during the postoperative period and the incision is less stressed by the snake's crawling movements.

Snakes do have a large ventral midline abdominal vein present just inside the body wall in the caudal portion of the body. If a ventral midline approach is used, care must be taken to avoid this vessel. Closure is generally in two layers: one in the body wall (simple continuous) and the second in the skin (an everting pattern).

Lizards and Crocodilians
Ventral Abdominal Vein

For years we were taught that the surgical approach to the coelomic cavity in saurians must be via a paramedian approach

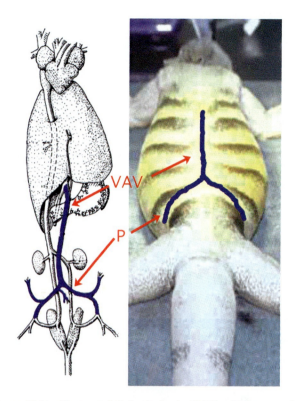

Figure 35-16 The ventral abdominal vein *(VAV)*, which is a confluence of the bilateral pelvic veins *(P)*, which are joined bilaterally by the hypogastric veins and the single ventral pubic vein, can be found roughly along the ventral midline of the patient, deep to the abdominal muscles. *(Photograph courtesy D. Mader.)*

to avoid the large ventral midline vessel that courses down the approximate center of the patient's body.[8]

This school of thought has been dogma simply because no one has thought to evaluate its appropriateness or challenge its viability. As a result, authors and lecturers over the years have promulgated the apparent need to make this surgical approach but at the same time never offered an explanation other than "because a large vein is in the way."

Although the obvious advantage of avoiding such a large vessel (hemorrhage) does exist, several disadvantages far outweigh the single benefit.

An understanding of the anatomy, and of the purpose of this vein, helps clarify its significance from the surgical perspective.

The ventral abdominal vein (VAV), which is a confluence of the bilateral pelvic veins, which are joined bilaterally by the hypogastric veins and the single ventral pubic vein, can be found roughly along the ventral midline of the patient, just axial to the abdominal muscles (Figure 35-16).[9] The origination of the VAV begins just under the abdominal wall as the tributaries conjoin from deeper tissues, cranial to the pubis. The distance from the pubis to the caudal origin of the VAV varies with the species and the size of the patient but is approximately one fourth the distance between the cranial pubic bone and the umbilicus.

The VAV then courses along the inside of the abdominal wall until it reaches the level of the umbilicus, where it takes an approximately 90-degree dorsal turn and confluences with the hepatic vein.

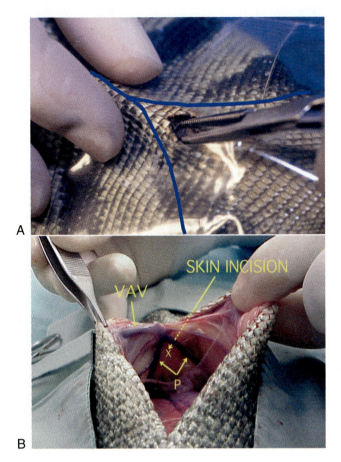

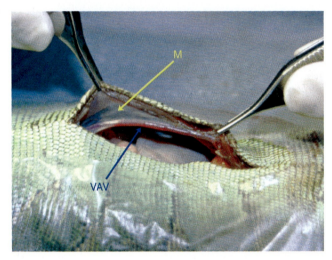

Figure 35-18 The ventral abdominal vein (*VAV*) is supported by a mesovasorum (*M*) that is an extension of the ventral coelomic membrane. (*Photograph courtesy D. Mader.*)

Figure 35-17 **A,** The initial surgical stab is between the pubis and the umbilical scar (*x*) to avoid the ventral abdominal vein (*VAV*) in lizard patients. **B,** By starting the incision at this location, the blade will not contact the ventral abdominal vein. *P*, Pelvic veins. (*Photograph courtesy D. Mader.*)

In summary, between the cranial margin of the pubis extending approximately one fourth of the distance toward the umbilicus and cranial to the umbilicus progressing to the xiphoid, no ventral vessels of any concern are found.

If the initial surgical stab occurs in either of these anatomic locations, the blade will not contact the ventral abdominal vessel (Figure 35-17). From that point onward, the surgeon precedes the incision with a blunt probe or forceps, gently directing the ventral abdominal vein out of harm's way.

The ventral abdominal vein is supported by a mesovasorum that is an extension of the ventral coelomic membrane (Figure 35-18). The mesovasorum varies in overall size from a couple of mm to nearly 1 cm in larger specimens. Whereas anatomically the origin of this mesovasorum does come off the ventral midline, the final resting place of the vein depends on the animal's state of repletion and other space-occupying coelomic structures (e.g., bladder calculi, eggs). In other words, the vessel may rest exactly centerline, or it may be pushed off to either side of the midline by several millimeters in either direction.

The significance here is obvious. When choosing to make a paramedian incision, which side of the sagittal plane to start the cut is a 50:50 guess.

A second, and perhaps more compelling, reason to make a midline incision rather than a paramedian incision involves the concept of minimizing postoperative pain and discomfort. By necessity, with a paramedian incision, the surgeon has to cut through muscle bellies. With a ventral midline approach, no muscles are incised, only skin and fascia of the linea.

We have no way of discerning whether or not this difference in technique makes a difference to reptile patients in terms of pain perception. We know from human patients that the midline approach is less painful than the "bikini cut" laparotomy incisions made to hide scars because the latter involve cutting directly through muscle.

Finally, there is the issue of what would actually happen to the patient if the ventral abdominal vein were accidentally incised during a coeliotomy. This important fact never seems to arise during writings and lectures that advocate the paramedian approach.

Blood coursing through the ventral abdominal vein travels into the hepatic vein, then subsequently the caudal vena cava, and ultimately back to the heart via the right atrium. If the ventral abdominal vein is cut, and ligated, the blood then is redirected back through the pelvic veins into the bilateral renal veins and directly into the vena cava (Figure 35-19).[10]

What is the clinical answer to what happens to the patient if the ventral abdominal vein is accidentally cut and ligated? Both authors have accidentally cut and ligated the VAV several times with no apparent clinical complications.

A ventral coeliotomy approach to both lizards and crocodilians provides access to all major organs. Soft tissue approaches to gastrotomies, enterotomies, cystotomies, and other procedures are no different than in mammals.

Chelonians

In many chelonians, for access to the coelomic cavity, a plastron osteotomy is necessary. With removal of a section of the plastron, one must avoid damaging the pelvic bones, which may be identified on radiographs before surgery (Figure 35-20). In most cases, a trapezoidal incision through the femoral and abdominal shields prevents injury to the pelvic bones (Figure 35-21). The position of the osteotomy should be planned to provide access to the structure being approached,

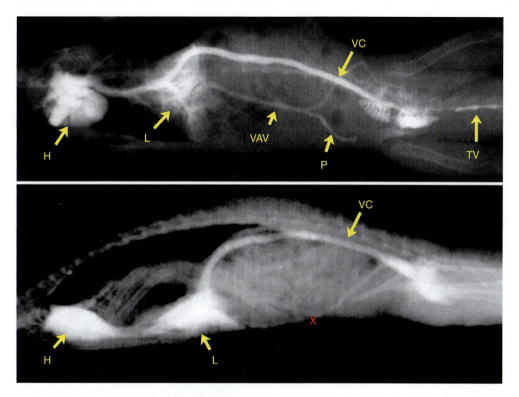

Figure 35-19 Blood from the tail vein *(TV)* courses through the pelvic veins *(P)*, then into the ventral abdominal vein *(VAV)*, where it travels into the hepatic vein to the liver *(L)*, to the vena cava *(VC)*, and ultimately, back to the heart *(H)* via the right atrium. If the ventral abdominal vein is cut, and ligated *(X)*, the blood is redirected through the pelvic veins into the bilateral renal veins and directly into the vena cava. (Photograph courtesy D. Mader.)

and the size of the osteotomy should be appropriate to the procedure to be performed. However, with removal of large calculi, an osteotomy incision large enough to remove the stone intact may not be possible (see Figure 49-9). In that case, the stone can be cut and removed in pieces.

During the osteotomy, fluids should be used to irrigate the osteotomy site to dissipate heat and remove any bone dust that may accumulate (see Figure 35-9). The saw is angled in for each cut, as is done with carving the top out of a pumpkin. This is done for two reasons. First, a wedge-shaped bone flap prevents it from falling back into the coelom when it is replaced. And, more importantly, when the flap is placed back in position, the angled cut provides bone-on-bone contact, thus promoting bone healing.

In some cases, a three-sided osteotomy may be performed with the fourth side along the hinge or a similar location that allows the three-sided osteotomy to be elevated and reflected without completely transecting the fourth side. Where this is not possible, the fourth side (caudal incision) may be made with care taken not to cut the underlying musculature. The flap can be elevated and gently reflected caudally. This provides the advantage of maintaining the blood supply to the section of bone through the fourth side. This theoretically aids in bone healing. However, one should note that removal of the entire flap is possible and it will still heal.

After osteotomy, the section of bone is elevated from the underlying abdominal musculature with the back of the scalpel handle or, more appropriately, a periosteal elevator (Figure 35-22). Once the bone is reflected and the abdominal musculature visualized, two large venous sinuses are identified, one on either side of the midline (Figure 35-23).

One should avoid damaging these sinuses; however, if necessary, they may be ligated.[8] A ventral midline incision should be performed through the easily distensible coelomic membrane to allow access to the coelomic cavity. In many cases, these vessels are large and prominent before incision and manipulation of the ventral coelomic membrane, but by the end of the procedure, they have undergone vasospasm to become almost imperceptible (Figure 35-24). With vasodilation, hemorrhage may occur, making even small leaks in these vessels important to address.

Soft tissue procedures inside the coelomic cavity of a tortoise are performed with protocols similar to those used in mammals. Chromic gut suture should be avoided because it tends to incite an inflammatory response.

In large chelonians, access to the deep recesses of the body cavity can be difficult. The intestinal tract of tortoises is short and attached by a short mesentery to the pleural membrane, which makes exteriorization of the viscera as is done with mammals for the purpose of "running the gut" or performance of a gastrotomy or enterotomy difficult (Figure 35-25). Oftentimes gentle massage of the foreign body either orad or aborad within the intestinal tract to a more accessible portion of the intestine is possible, rather than attempting to perform an enterotomy deep within the coelom where visualization of the site and access are limited.

When the coeliotomy is complete, the cavity should be flushed with warm saline solution to remove any shell debris or other contamination. The warm fluids also serve to provide internal warming to the patient.

The ventral midline should be closed with a simple continuous pattern with an absorbable material (see Figure 35-24).

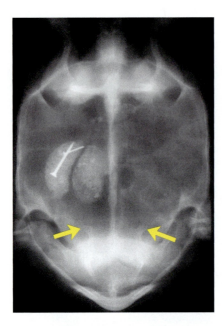

Figure 35-20 When removing a section of the plastron, it is important to avoid damaging the pelvic bones, which may be identified on radiographs preoperatively *(yellow arrows)*. *(Photograph courtesy D. Mader.)*

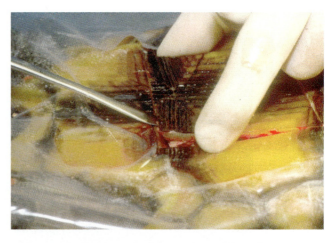

Figure 35-22 The section of bone is elevated from the underlying abdominal musculature after osteotomy. *(Photograph courtesy D. Mader.)*

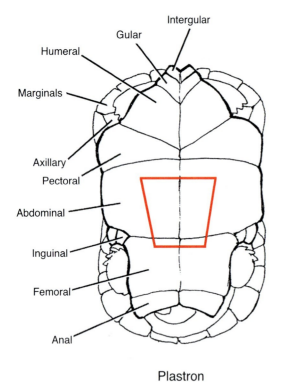

Figure 35-21 A trapezoidal incision, with the largest border along the cranial edge and the lateral incisions crossing through the femoral and abdominal shields, will prevent injury to the pelvic bones. *(Photograph courtesy D. Mader.)*

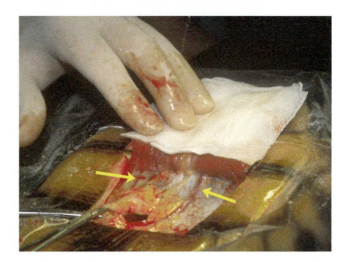

Figure 35-23 Two large venous sinuses will be identified, one on either side of the midline, once the bone is reflected back. *(Photograph courtesy D. Mader.)*

The bone flap is carefully cleaned and placed back into the osteotomy site. Gentle even pressure should be applied to ensure that the edges of the bone are firmly apposed. Any excess blood, saline solution, or tissue fragments should be thoroughly wiped away before the incision is sealed.

Once the flap has been replaced, and the osteotomy site has been cleaned, it should be completely dried.

The flap is sealed in place with a waterproof rapid-setting epoxy resin (Figure 35-26). Some authors advocate placement of bone wax in the incision site to prevent epoxy from dripping into the coelom. If the initial cut was clean, this is not necessary. However, if the cut was irregular and gaps are present, a protective layer of bone wax may be helpful. A thin coat of epoxy is applied to the plastron, covering the flap and extending 1 to 2 cm beyond. A piece of fiberglass mesh (this does *not* have to be sterilized) is then cut and fitted so that it covers the flap and extends at least 1 cm beyond the margins. The mesh is then placed into the epoxy until it is saturated with resin. This layer is allowed to dry, and a second thin coat is then applied over the fiberglass, forming an epoxy-fiberglass-epoxy sandwich.

Thin layers of epoxy are easier to manipulate and harden much faster than thick layers. Although the resin is exothermic as it sets, the heat produced is not enough to cause any damage to underlying bone.

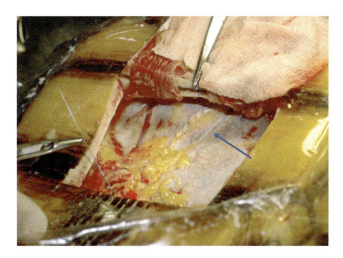

Figure 35-24 The vessels will at first be large and prominent prior to incision and manipulation of the ventral coelomic membrane. However, by the end of the procedure when the coelomic membrane has been sutured closed, the vessels may vasospasm and become almost imperceptible *(blue arrow)*. With vasodilation, hemorrhage may occur, making it important to address even small leaks in these vessels. *(Photograph courtesy D. Mader.)*

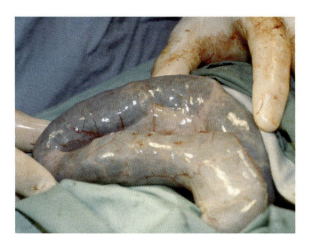

Figure 35-25 The intestinal tract of tortoises is short and attached by a short mesentery to the pleural membrane, making it difficult to exteriorize the viscera as is done with mammals for the purpose of "running the gut" or performing a gastrotomy or enterotomy. *(Photograph courtesy D. Mader.)*

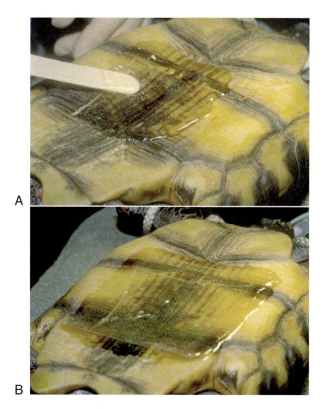

Figure 35-26 **A,** The plastronotomy flap is sealed in place using a waterproof, rapid-setting epoxy resin. **B,** After the first coat is applied, but before it sets, a fiberglass mesh patch is imbedded into the resin. Multiple thin coats are easier to manipulate and will set more efficiently than fewer thick coats of epoxy. *(Photograph courtesy D. Mader.)*

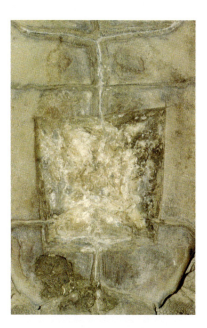

Figure 35-27 A properly performed plastronotomy will heal by primary intention. In the authors' experience, the patch can actually be removed in approximately 1 year, although there is no reason to make this an elective procedure. *(Photograph courtesy D. Mader.)*

In the authors' experience, the patch can be removed in approximately 1 year, although there is no reason to make this an elective procedure (Figure 35-27). Improperly performed osteotomies can lead to thermal necrosis of the bone or osteomyelitis (Figure 35-28), resulting in a patch that has to be removed and the subsequent osteotomy site having to heal as an open wound by second intention. This can be done but is labor intensive, takes months to heal, and carries a guarded-to-grave prognosis.

In young chelonians, cutting through the plastron with a #11 blade is possible with incising over the suture line between the scutes. The plastron can be gently distracted, the coeliotomy performed, and then the shell sutured back together. A light coating of epoxy resin seals the incision site (Figure 35-29). This epoxy will eventually fall off as the patient grows.

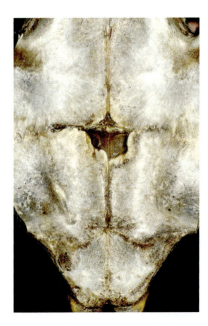

Figure 35-28 Improperly performed plastronotomy incisions can lead to thermal necrosis of the bone or to osteomyelitis. *(Photograph courtesy D. Mader.)*

An alternate approach to a coeliotomy via the plastronotomy is coeliotomy via a soft-tissue prefemoral incision.[11] This is the preferred site for endoscopic access to the coelom (see Chapter 32) and is readily accomplished, even in smaller patients. Surgical access via the soft-tissue approach is limited by patient size, with generally only the larger patients being candidates.

Chelonians with smaller plastrons, such as the snappers and seaturtles, generally have larger prefemoral areas (Figure 35-30 and Figure 76-44). Patients are anesthetized in routine fashion and positioned on an inclined surgical table with the head up. In this position, gravity causes the viscera to rest against the fossa, facilitating access to the various internal organs. The rear limbs are pulled caudally and taped either together or off to the opposite side of the intended incision (see Figure 35-13). A horizontal incision is made midway between the carapace and the plastron, starting at the bridge and extending caudally to the thigh (see Figure 49-17).

The subcutaneous fat is bluntly dissected away, and the underlying abdominal oblique muscles are exposed. These are also incised along the same line as the skin. The next layer of muscle (which may also be obscured by fat) is the transverse abdominis muscle. This is also incised in the same fashion. The coelomic membrane is associated with the deep

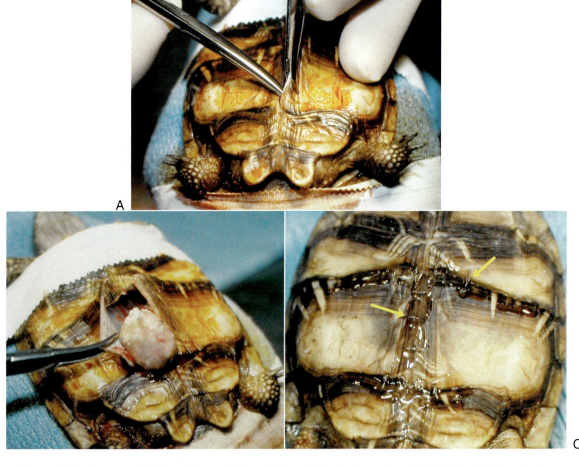

Figure 35-29 In young chelonians it is possible to cut through the plastron using a #11 blade by incising over the suture line between the scutes. The plastron can be gently distracted, the coeliotomy performed, and then the shell sutured back together. A light coating of epoxy resin will seal the incision site. *(Photograph courtesy D. Mader.)*

surface of the transverse abdominis muscle. Incision of the coelomic membrane gains entrance to the coelomic cavity.

Once entrance to the coelomic cavity is attained, visualization may be aided with the use of either a flexible or a rigid endoscope. An ovariohysterectomy hook is useful for gently moving or exteriorizing internal organs.

In the female, the first structures encountered are the ovary and the shell gland. Once these are retracted, the bladder is easily visualized. For cystotomies, the bladder is localized and a portion of it is exteriorized (see Figure 49-17). Stay sutures are placed into the serosa and tacked to the surgical toweling or stabilized by an assistant. The bladder wall is incised, evaluated, and closed in the normal fashion.

After completion of the procedure, the coelomic membrane, abdominal muscles, and fat are all closed with a single, continuous layer of absorbable sutures. The skin is closed with an everting horizontal mattress (see Figures 35-4 and 35-5). The cutaneous sutures are removed in approximately 4 weeks.

This technique allows for complete healing in just 4 weeks, as opposed to 1 to 2 years as in the ventral celiotomy approach through the plastron. One can surmise that considerably less discomfort to the patient occurs with this technique.

Ovariosalpingectomy

Considerable variation exists among reptile species regarding their reproductive physiology (see Chapter 23). The approach to the reproductive system of female reptiles is generally via celiotomy as described previously. Surgery is indicated when noninvasive medical techniques have failed to relieve dystocia or with evidence that natural passage of the eggs or fetuses is not possible (see Chapter 53 for a complete discussion of dystocia).

A decision on when to perform surgery may be difficult to make. In some cases, however, the egg densities are more radiodense than would be expected. Typically, reptilian eggs are not densely calcified and an increase in calcific density indicates that the eggs have been in the oviduct an excessive period of time. This may be the result of infection, resulting in delayed transit. In this situation, surgery is recommended.

In addition, if the eggs are of abnormal size and shape as indicated on a radiograph, precluding passage through the pelvic canal, surgery is indicated.

In general, the oviduct and ovaries of reptiles are fairly mobile within the coelomic cavity. In snakes, the bilateral oviducts are long, approximately 20% to 25% of the length of the animal. For access to this tubular structure, either a single long incision or multiple small sequential incisions are made through the skin and body wall (Figure 35-31).

"Milking" eggs or fetal slugs through the oviduct is not safe. Often, by the time surgical intervention has been elected, the retained eggs or fetuses have begun to deteriorate and are adhered to the oviduct, which is often thin and friable (Figure 35-32 and see Figure 53-5).[3,7,12]

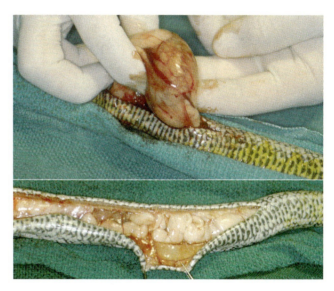

Figure 35-31 The ovaries and oviducts are long in snakes, approximately 20% to 25% of the length of the animal. A single long incision or multiple small, sequential incisions are made through the skin and body wall to access the reproductive structures. *(Photograph courtesy D. Mader.)*

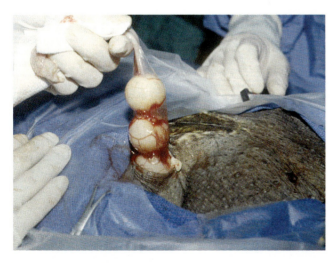

Figure 35-30 An alternate approach to a coeliotomy via the plastronotomy is coeliotomy via a soft-tissue, prefemoral incision, as seen here in a snapper. *(Photograph courtesy K. Rosenthal.)*

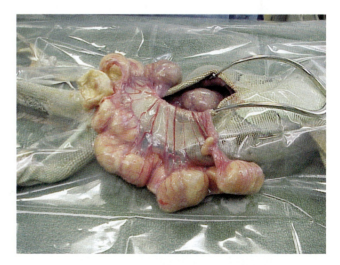

Figure 35-32 It is not safe to "milk" eggs or fetal slugs through the oviduct. Often, by the time surgical intervention has been elected, the retained eggs or fetuses have begun to deteriorate and are adhered to the oviduct, which is often thin and friable. *(Photograph courtesy D. Mader.)*

Salpingotomy (oviduct) incisions are generally repaired with an inverting suture pattern of a light, delicate, absorbable synthetic suture material. Collection of samples for diagnostic evaluation at the time of surgery is always important. In many cases, bacterial infections are causative, and with successful treatment, reproductive viability may be regained.

The reproductive physiology and the feedback loop between the ovary and oviduct of reptiles are not well understood. Both organs do, however, appear to be required for normal reproductive activity. If the ovaries are removed, the oviduct and shell gland appear to begin to atrophy.[13] However, if only the oviduct is removed, the ovaries may remain active. Although no controlled studies have been performed, if only the oviduct and shell gland are removed, the ovaries do appear to release yolks into the coelomic cavity. Whether or not the ovaries develop yolks that are subsequently resorbed remains speculative. **Always take the ovaries whenever attempting to sterilize a reptile patient. Removal of only the oviducts with the ovaries left intact is not acceptable.**

The authors have "respayed" animals that previously had salpingectomies but not ovariectomies. The females exhibited all the signs of normal pregnancy with ultimate clinical signs of what is commonly called "egg binding." During exploratory coeliotomy, free yolks were found in the coelomic cavity. With a lengthy surgery, the ovaries only may be removed.

The physiology and pathology of egg retention in reptiles are covered in Chapters 23 and 53. One must make the distinction between preovulatory and postovulatory in discussion of surgical options (Figure 35-33). In preovulatory conditions, the active ovaries develop mature follicles but do not ovulate (also called follicular stasis). In postovulatory conditions, the ovarian follicles develop as mentioned and the animal ovulates, but the ova do not pass through the oviducts, being stuck in various stages of calcification (Figure 35-34). The former (preovulatory) condition is generally considered to be a surgical condition, whereas the latter (postovulatory) may be treated either medically or surgically. Again, the reader is directed to the previously mentioned chapters for greater detail.

In cases of preovulatory egg binding, the ovaries must be removed. In a healthy lizard patient, the ovaries appear like a cluster of grapes on a short stalk (Figure 35-35); however, if the preovulatory condition has been chronic, the ovaries begin to deteriorate and the ova start to coalesce (Figure 35-36). This structure is extremely friable and readily ruptures during surgical manipulation. The entire ovary should be gently elevated and the vascular attachments ligated with vascular clips (Figure 35-37).

In cases of postovulatory egg binding, where the eggs are within the oviduct, these structures should be removed first, which then allows better access to the underlying ovaries. The oviduct is richly supplied by large blood vessels, especially when reproductively active. These vessels are most easily ligated with hemostatic clips, transecting between two adjacent clips. The process is initiated at the infundibulum, and vessels are ligated and transected, progressing caudally toward the junction of the shell gland with the cloaca (see Figure 35-8). At this location, either two clips or a transfixion ligature is applied to the oviduct, which is then transected and submitted for diagnostic analysis.

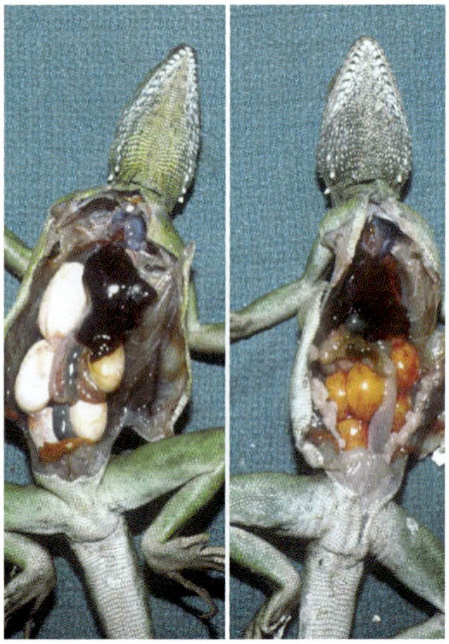

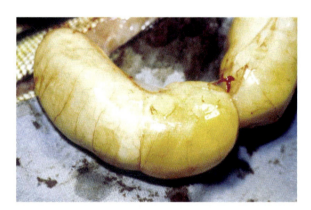

Figure 35-34 In postovulatory conditions, the ovarian follicles develop as mentioned and the animal ovulates, but the ova do not pass through the oviducts, being stuck in various stages of calcification. *(Photograph courtesy D. Mader.)*

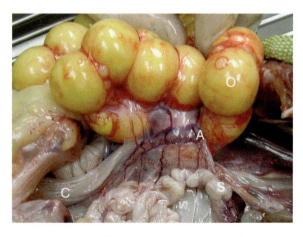

Figure 35-35 In cases of preovulatory egg binding, the ovaries must be removed. In a healthy lizard patient the ovaries appear like a cluster of grapes on a short stalk. *O*, Ovary; *A*, adrenal; *S*, salpinx; *C*, colon. *(Photograph courtesy D. Mader.)*

Figure 35-33 The Water Dragon *(Physignathus cocincinus)* on the left has shelled eggs in the oviducts. This is known as "postovulatory stasis." The animal on the right is showing mature follicles that have not yet ovulated. This is known as "preovulatory stasis." *(Photograph courtesy D. Mader.)*

When performing the ovariectomy, note that the right ovary is very close anatomically to the vena cava (Figure 35-38). Although the left ovary is not anatomically close to the vena cava, the artery and vein that supply it are adhered to the left adrenal gland, and care must be taken to avoid damaging the gland. The hemostatic clips are applied across the vessels where they enter the ovary. The vessels are then transected between the ovary and the clips, allowing removal of the left ovary.

In contrast to the lizards, the chelonians have large fan-shaped mesovaria and an equally long, highly vascular mesosalpinx (Figures 35-39 and 35-40). It is critical that no ovarian tissue be left behind because the animal continues to ovulate, thus predisposing the patient to future problems. Good surgical access to the coelom and the use of vascular clips facilitate the ovariosalpingectomy.

Yolk coelomitis may be the result of yolks being released from the reproductive tract into the coelomic cavity or rupture of follicles while still on the ovary (Figure 35-41 and see Figure 53-4). In some cases, well-formed eggs rupture through the oviduct and may also be found within the coelomic cavity. Another reported cause for egg peritonitis is the presence of cystic calculi, which can traumatize the oviduct and developing eggs within the reproductive tract, allowing them to escape into coelom. The presence of yolk, an egg, or a ruptured egg within the coelomic cavity induces a severe inflammatory reaction, with deposition of fibrin and thickening of the serosal surface of the viscera. Generally, the prognosis for such patients is grave. Treatment consists of removal of the offending material and copious irrigation of the coelomic cavity. Systemic antibiotic therapy, maintenance of hydration, and nutritional balance are also vital.

ORCHIDECTOMY

Male Green Iguanas become very aggressive during the reproductive period. In many cases, this is not acceptable when these animals are maintained as pets. They can cause serious

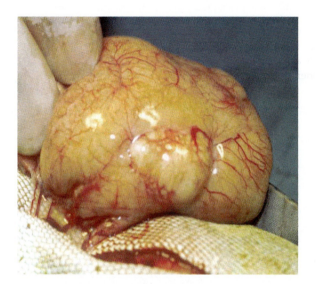

Figure 35-36 If a preovulatory condition has been chronic, the follicles begin to deteriorate and the ova start to coalesce. These structures are extremely friable and rupture easily with even the slightest manipulation. *(Photograph courtesy D. Mader.)*

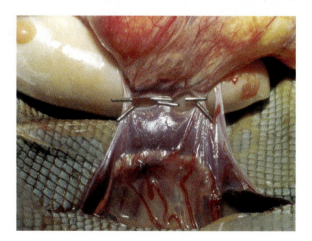

Figure 35-37 The entire ovary should be gently elevated and the vessels double ligated with vascular clips. *(Photograph courtesy D. Mader.)*

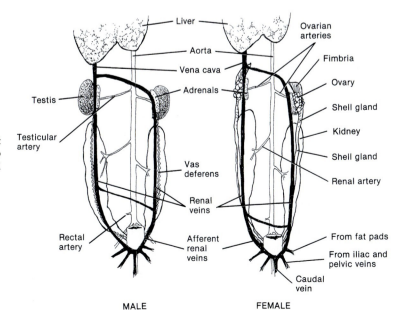

Figure 35-38 When performing a neuter, it is important to note that the right ovary is very close anatomically to the vena cava, and the left gonad is attached to the adrenal gland. *(Photograph courtesy D. Mader.)*

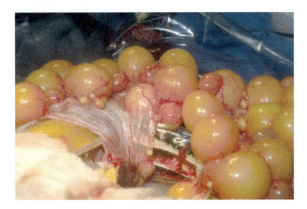

Figure 35-39 In contrast to lizards, the chelonians have large, fan-shaped mesovaria. *(Photograph courtesy D. Mader.)*

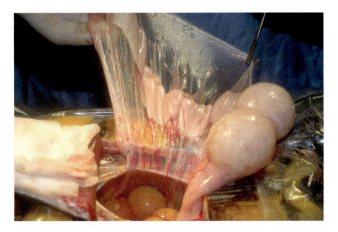

Figure 35-40 A highly vascular mesosalpinx supports the tortoise oviducts. *(Photograph courtesy D. Mader.)*

injury to their owners because such behavior is not expected from the pet. Early clinical evidence suggests that removal of the testicles from these animals may improve behavior during this reproductive period. Chapter 13 discusses aggression in the male iguana in detail.

One should note that castration does not subdue aggressive behaviors immediately after surgery. In almost all cases, a change in temperament is not seen until the animal's subsequent breeding season. The client should be informed of this before the procedure is performed to avoid disappointment.

The approach to castration is identical to that of an ovariectomy. The gonads are tightly adhered in the dorsal coelomic cavity, making surgical access difficult. Exposure is of paramount importance. The coeliotomy incision should extend from a point just caudal to the xiphoid and extend to the pubis.

Each testicle has a rich vascular supply (see Figure 35-38). The right gonad is attached to the vena cava by very short vessels (approximately 1 to 2 mm) (Figure 35-42). The left testicle has its own blood supply—the testicular vein and artery. Interposed between the left testicle and these vessels is the left adrenal gland, an elongated pink granular tissue. It is best not to remove or damage this gland when ligating the testicular vessels. If it is accidentally removed, the patient will survive. The adrenal gland on the right is on the opposite side of the vena cava from the testicle and is unlikely to be damaged during the procedure.

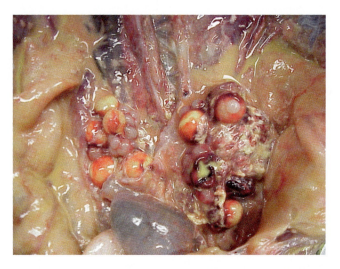

Figure 35-41 Yolk coelomitis may be the result of yolks being released from the reproductive tract into the coelomic cavity or the rupture of follicles while still on the ovary. *(Photograph courtesy D. Mader.)*

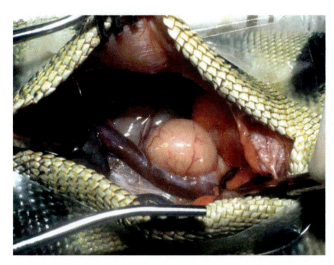

Figure 35-42 Each testicle has a rich vascular supply. The right gonad is attached to the vena cava by very short vessels (approximately 1 to 2 mm), and as is the left ovary, the left testicle is attached to the adrenal gland. *(Photograph courtesy D. Mader.)*

The testes are covered by a capsule, giving them some rigidity, but if aggressively handled, the capsule will rupture. Although bleeding from a ruptured capsule is minute, it makes manipulating the gland during the procedure difficult. Gentle elevation of the testes is necessary to allow visualization and ultimately ligation of the blood supply. To facilitate elevation of the testicle, a suture can be placed through the top of the capsule and gently retracted (Figure 35-43), or if the testicle is small, it can be grasped with Allis tissue forceps. Although manual ligation of these minuscule vessels is possible, the use of vascular clips is highly recommended.

Once the vessels are identified, the vascular clips are gently inserted between the major vessel and the gonad (Figure 35-44). The vascular attachments from the testes to the vena cava or the testicular vein should not be torn. These hemorrhage extensively, and the blood rapidly occludes the surgical field. If either of these major vessels is damaged,

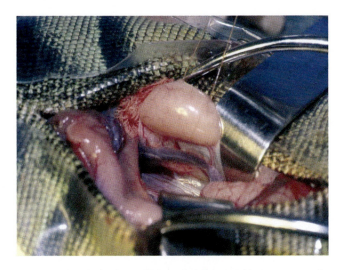

Figure 35-43 To facilitate elevation of the testicle, a suture can be placed through the top of the capsule and then gently retracted. *(Photograph courtesy D. Mader.)*

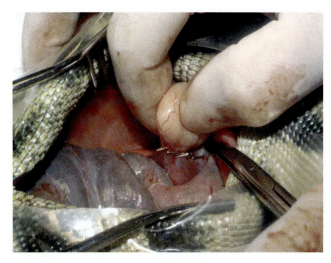

Figure 35-44 Once the vessels are identified, the vascular clips are gently inserted between the major vessel and the gonad. *(Photograph courtesy D. Mader.)*

vascular clips can be applied across the top of the defect, parallel to the vein. This causes changes to the hemodynamics of the blood flow through each of these vessels, but no other choice exists. Depending on the severity of the damage, the patient should heal fine.

If possible, all vessels should be double ligated (clipped). The vessels are then transected adjacent to the capsule and removed. Before the coelomic cavity is closed, the vascular pedicles should be checked for residual hemorrhage.

CYSTOTOMY

Cystic calculi can occur in those species with urinary bladders. Desert Tortoises *(Gopherus agassizii)* and Green Iguanas appear to have an unusually high incidence of calculus formation (see Chapter 49). The formation of cystic calculi has been linked to improper nutrition and also limited access to water, resulting in dehydration. Clinical signs associated with cystic calculi include lethargy, depression, anorexia, constipation, hind limb paresis, and dystocia. Diagnosis is confirmed with palpation or radiography.

Most cystic calculi in reptile patients consist of urate salts. Calcium urate stones are radiodense and easily visualized with radiographs; however, ammonium urate stones are significantly less dense. This type of stone is best diagnosed on palpation.

The urinary bladder of chelonians is usually bilobed, with a left and right section. The right lobe of the liver lies over the right sac of the urinary bladder, preventing large stones from remaining in the right sac. For this reason, most stones in chelonians are visualized on the left side.[14] Small stones may be seen on either the right or the left side.

Techniques for chelonian cystotomy have been described.[15,16] The procedure starts with a coeliotomy as previously described. The bladder is generally readily elevated out of the coelomic cavity (see Figure 49-16). If access is limited or the stone is large, a standard autoclaved kitchen spoon, bent to form an L, can be used as a scoop to gently exteriorize the calculus. The bladder should be isolated with a laparotomy sponge or gauze 4 × 4s, moistened to prevent desiccation. A standard cystotomy is performed as is done in mammals. In normal reptiles, the urinary bladder is thin-walled, almost transparent. Because of the stone and the accompanying cystitis, the bladder wall is usually thickened. A standard two-layer inverting closure is generally recommended. After closure, the coelomic cavity should be copiously irrigated with warmed, sterile saline solution.

Small urinary calculi can be removed through a left flank incision as previously described. If the stone is small, it can be retrieved with a lens loop or small forceps. Larger stones can be grasped with Allis tissue forceps and broken in situ. Most of the stones are layered and can be broken down by chipping away at their masses with the jaws of the forceps. Once the stone is dismantled to a manageable size, its pieces can be exteriorized. Care must be taken not to injure any of the soft tissue within the coelomic cavity during the procedure.

After the stone is out, the exteriorized bladder should be copiously flushed with sterile saline solution. The bladder is then closed with 4-0 monofilament absorbable suture, such as polydioxanone, in a double layered closure, rinsed one final time, and returned to the body cavity. The coelomic membrane, abdominal musculature, and skin closures are routine (see Figures 35-4 and 35-5).

Iguanas and other lizards are also susceptible to urinary calculi. The subject is covered in detail in Chapter 49.

GASTROINTESTINAL PROCEDURES

The basic principles for gastrointestinal surgery in reptile patients are similar to those for mammals. Surgery is indicated for removal of foreign bodies that may cause obstruction, for resolution of intussusception, or for intestinal impaction. Gastrointestinal abnormalities induce clinical signs such as regurgitation, obstipation, weight loss, anorexia, and abdominal distention. Foreign body removal, resection-anastomosis, and anastomosis for colorectal atresia have been successfully performed in reptiles.[8,17-21]

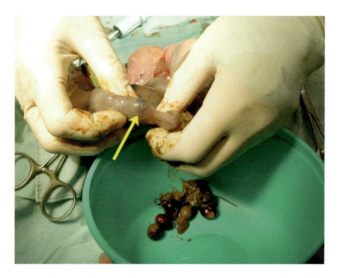

Figure 35-45 In small reptile patients the intestine is thin-walled and tears easily during suturing. A light-gauge, taper-point swedged needle must be used. *(Photograph courtesy D. Mader.)*

In small reptile patients, the intestine is quite thin-walled (Figure 35-45), making the use of fine suture and small atraumatic needles important. The mesentery that suspends the gastrointestinal tract of reptiles is quite variable in length. Exteriorization of the affected section of bowel is preferable to prevent contamination of the coelomic cavity (see Figure 35-25). If this cannot be accomplished, the area to be incised should be isolated with moistened gauze sponges packed within the coelomic cavity of the patient. After closure of the incision in the gastrointestinal tract, copious irrigation should be performed. At this point the surgeon needs to change instrument packs and reglove prior to closing the skin.

CLOACAL PROLAPSE

Cloacal prolapse is covered in detail in Chapter 47. The cause of the prolapse should be determined and corrected before surgical intervention. Several techniques have been described

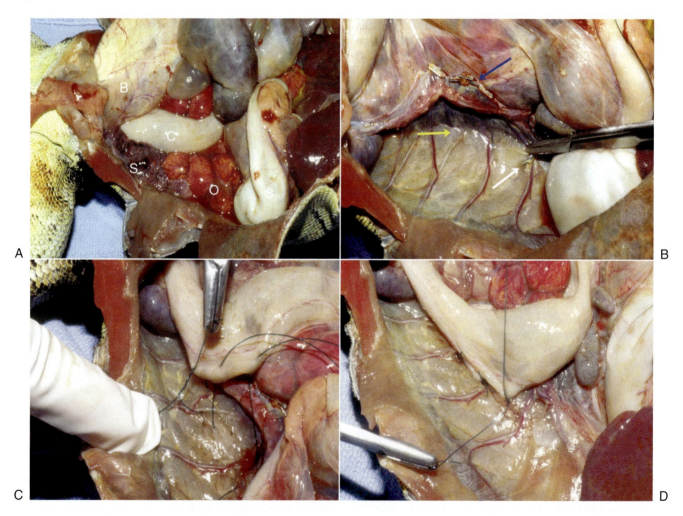

Figure 35-46 A simple, effective colopexy technique involves suturing the colon to the rib cage. **A,** To gain access to the ribs the patient should be spayed or neutered to get the gonad out of the way. *B,* Bladder; *O,* ovary; *S,* salpinx; *C,* colon. **B,** Blue arrow shows the ligated ovarian vessels. The white arrow shows the proper technique used to hook the nonabsorbable suture around the ribs, which are readily identified *(yellow arrow)* adjacent to the spine. **C,** A series of at least three to four preplaced nonabsorbable sutures. **D,** The sutures are tightened, starting at the pelvic canal, and progressing cranially. When the sutures are in place tension on the colon and an inward "pucker" to the cloaca should be seen if the procedure is done correctly. *(Photographs courtesy D. Mader.)*

to correct prolapses, including both intestinal resections and colopexies, with varying degrees of success.[22,23] Each case should be evaluated individually and surgical technique chosen on a case-by-case basis.

Chapter 47 describes several techniques for correcting evolapses. One colopexy technique that is simple and effective involves suturing the colon to the ribs as it courses along the spinal column (Figure 35-46). Because clear access to the ribs is necessary for this procedure, removal of the patient's gonad on the side of the pexy is necessary.

Cloacal prolapses are most common in young growing animals (see Chapter 47 for details). If surgical intervention is necessary to repair a prolapse, it is also an opportune time to discuss neutering the patient.

TRACHEAL RESECTION

Chondromas arising from the tracheal cartilage can cause a gradual onset of dyspnea in snakes.[24,25] Affected snakes present with open-mouth breathing, depression, and anorexia. The lesion is usually visualized on plain radiographs as a soft tissue–dense mass within the air-dense tracheal lumen (Figure 35-47). Endoscopy confirms the presence of a nonmoveable mass within the tracheal lumen.

The trachea is approached as described for celiotomy in snakes on the basis of the radiographic location of the lesion. Snakes do not have a recurrent laryngeal nerve as is seen in mammals. The entire section of affected trachea is removed, and the trachea is anastomosed with a fine monofilament absorbable suture. Suture should encompass one or two tracheal rings on each side of the tracheotomy (Figure 35-48).

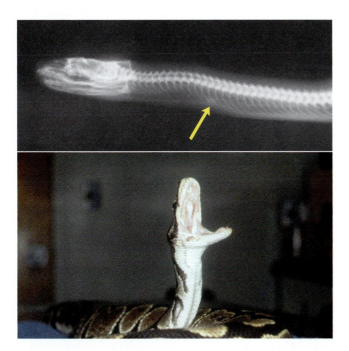

Figure 35-47 Cartilaginous granuloma arising from the tracheal cartilage may cause a gradual onset of dyspnea in snakes. Affected snakes present with open-mouth breathing, depression, and anorexia. The lesion is usually visualized on plain radiographs as a soft tissue–dense mass within the air-dense tracheal lumen (*yellow arrow*). (*Photographs courtesy D. Mader.*)

Remember that snakes have C-shaped tracheal rings and care should be exercised not to damage the dorsal membrane when manipulating the structure. Closure of the surgical site is standard using fine, monofilament sutures in a simple everting pattern. A light wrap or liquid tissue glue is applied over the external surgical site. A broad-spectrum antibiotic and appropriate analgesics are administered perioperatively.

The patient is generally able to breathe without discomfort immediately after surgery. As much as 2.5 cm of trachea has been removed without adverse affect.[24]

ORTHOPEDICS AND FRACTURE REPAIR

Fractures in all reptile groups are not uncommon. Trauma from cagemates, predators, careless handlers, and motor vehicles are the major causes. Pathologic fractures, which may result from any of the various metabolic bone diseases that affect reptiles (see Chapter 61), are the next major cause.

In general, fractures of the extremities in reptiles are rarely open or comminuted. Many fractures, especially pathologic fractures from metabolic bone disease (MBD), are amenable to treatment with external coaptation. In other situations, internal fixation is indicated. Fractures have been successfully stabilized with various forms of internal fixation. In patients with any of the various types of MBD, the CAUSE of the MBD (e.g., nutritional, renal) should be determined and, if possible, corrected before or concurrent with fracture repair. This requires medical management while supporting any pathologic fractures (Figure 35-49). When severe tissue trauma, loss of vascular supply, or granulomatous infection and inflammation exist, amputation may be required. Reptiles generally function well with partial or complete limb amputations.

Most fractures occur as a result of relatively low impact forces, making the incidence rate of comminuted fractures low.[8,26] Most reptiles have tough elastic skin, and fractures are usually not open. Little information is available regarding bone healing in reptiles; however, it appears to occur at a significantly slower rate when compared with birds and mammals. Healing time for traumatic fractures is generally 6 to 18 months. Pathologic fractures that result from one of the MBDs seem to heal more rapidly (6 to 8 wk) if the inciting problem is corrected.

General principles of fracture fixation apply to reptile patients: rigid stabilization and anatomic alignment with minimal disruption of callus and soft tissues. Many factors must be considered when deciding on the method of fixation to be used. **The forces exerted on the fracture (bending, compression, rotation, and shear) must be neutralized to promote healing. Generally, the more forces that must be neutralized by the fixation, the higher the incidence rate of complications and failure** (Figure 35-50). Practical considerations include the patient's functional requirements, cost of the materials, ease of application, availability of equipment, and surgeon's level of experience with various fixation devices. Most closed fractures in reptiles heal without intervention but may have varying degrees of malunion.[26] This resolution may be acceptable for some patients and accepted by their owners. The patient's size and conformation may influence the type of device used and how it is applied.

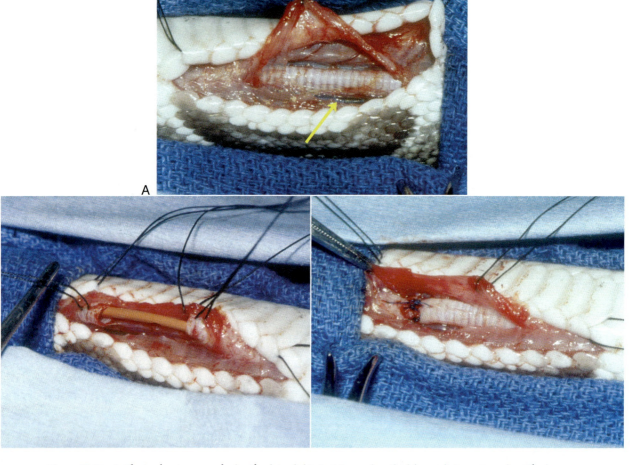

Figure 35-48 **A,** The trachea is approached with a lateral skin incision as described for a celiotomy in snakes. The location of the incision is based on the radiographic location of the lesion. **B,** The entire section of affected trachea is removed, and the trachea is anastomosed using a fine, monofilament absorbable suture. A sterile red-rubber feeding tube is used as a stylet or guide to help align the ends of the trachea during the procedure. The anesthetic gas is passed through this tube. **C,** Suture should encompass one or two tracheal rings on each side of the tracheotomy. *(Photographs courtesy G. Diethelm.)*

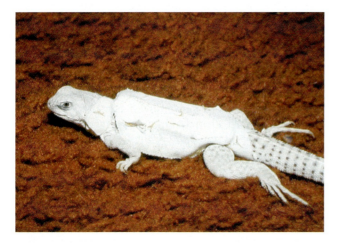

Figure 35-49 This Desert Iguana (*Dipsosaurus dorsalis*) has a pathological spinal fracture that resulted from an NMBD. A rigid, lightweight splint is taped to its back to provide support during healing. It is imperative that the underlying husbandry and nutritional deficiencies be corrected if the patient has a chance to recover. *(Photograph courtesy D. Mader.)*

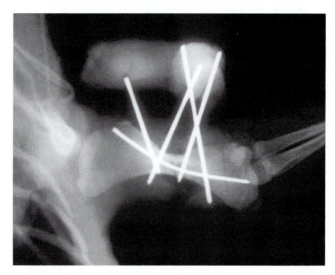

Figure 35-50 The forces exerted on the fracture (bending, compression, rotation, and shear) must be neutralized to promote healing. Generally, the more forces that must be neutralized by the fixation, the higher the incidence of complications and failure. *(Photograph courtesy K. Rosenthal.)*

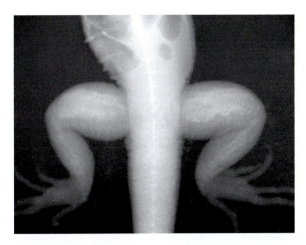

Figure 35-51 Bone is dynamic organ (undergoing constant remodeling); during prolonged hypocalcemia the mineralization process lags behind the deposition of organic bone matrix, resulting in the formation of hypomineralized bone. *(Photograph courtesy D. Mader.)*

The general health and metabolic status of the patient may preclude a surgical procedure for orthopedic repair. Finally, financial concerns must often be considered.

EXTERNAL COAPTATION

External coaptation involves the use of splints, slings, and other bandages to immobilize a fracture. This is probably the most commonly used method of fracture fixation in reptile orthopedics because it is simple, requires little equipment, takes only a short time to apply, requires a brief anesthesia period, and generally is the least expensive. Fractures that are minimally displaced usually heal with minimal support. When dealing with pathologic fractures that result from one of the MBDs, external coaptation is usually the treatment of choice.

Metabolic bone disease is a complex osseous disease that affects reptiles with many causes and factors contributing to its development (see Chapter 61). MBD of nutritional origin (nutritional secondary hyperparathyroidism [NSHP]), also called NMBD, is one of the clinical manifestations of prolonged hypocalcemia and can occur in any captive reptile. Hypocalcemia in reptiles may be the result of improper diet, the presence of organic disease, or failure to provide proper husbandry. Because bone is dynamic (undergoing constant remodeling), during prolonged hypocalcemia, the mineralization process lags behind the deposition of organic bone matrix, resulting in the formation of hypomineralized bone (Figure 35-51).

Orthopedic abnormalities occur when the bone loses approximately one third of its calcium content. Orthopedic problems associated with NMBD include stunted growth, malleable mandibles with loose teeth (rubber jaw), firm fibrous swelling (fibrous osteodystrophy) of the mandible and long bones, bowing of the long bones, and pathologic fractures of the axial and appendicular skeleton (see Chapter 61).

These fractures are difficult to stabilize with internal fixation because the bone is too soft to support implants. If Steinmann pins are inserted, they contact a cortex and penetrate rather than being diverted down the medullary canal.

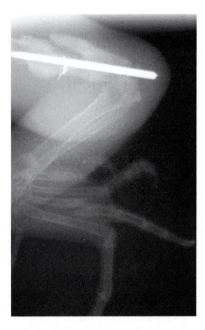

Figure 35-52 Pathologic fractures secondary to NMBD are difficult to stabilize using internal fixation because the bone is too soft to support implants. Cerclage, hemicerclage, and interfragmentary wires tend to collapse the soft bone. *(Photograph courtesy D. Mader.)*

Cerclage, hemicerclage, and interfragmentary wires collapse the soft bone (Figure 35-52). Bone screws have minimal resistance to pulling out when placed in such soft bone. Similarly, external skeletal fixation does not function well because the bone purchase of the fixation pins is minimal. In some cases, intramedullary pins can be carefully inserted to provide axial alignment and some bending stability; however, external coaptation should also be applied because cortical purchase may be minimal.

Fortunately, once the patient's calcium homeostasis has been reestablished, fracture healing progresses rapidly with a fibrous union providing stability as early as 3 to 4 weeks. Medical therapies for hypocalcemia are discussed in Chapter 61.

A wide variety of splinting and casting techniques have been used successfully.[26-29] Anesthesia is recommended during the application of external coaptation to prevent iatrogenic fractures or comminutions and to minimize patient stress and pain. All forms of external coaptation should be monitored closely for evidence of soiling, slippage, creation of vascular compromise, or other problems that may require splint replacement.

Application of external coaptation is an art. Patients tolerate properly fitted, lightweight external splints and casts with minimal stress (Figure 35-53). Soft conforming cast padding (Cast Padding, Johnson & Johnson, http://www.qualitymedicalsupplies.com/page/QMS/CTGY/Johnson-Johnson-Kendall-Wound-Care-Products) and conforming roll gauze (Conform, Kendall Co., http://www.qualitymedical-supplies.com/page/QMS/CTGY/Johnson-Johnson-Kendall-Wound-Care-Products) work well for the initial padding layers. These materials should be cut to an appropriate width for the size of the patient. Use of a roll that is too wide results in a lumpy, cumbersome bandage.

The bandage may be reinforced with a metal paper clip, a wooden applicator stick, a tongue depressor, an aluminum rod, lightweight casting material, or other substance that adds bending stability. Whenever possible, try to stabilize the limb in a slightly flexed position and not fully extended.

Rigid nonmalleable splints do not conform to the normal angles of a reptile's limb, necessitating that the limb be splinted in extension. This can result in a decrease in the range of motion in immobilized joints after splint removal because of periarticular fibrosis (fracture disease). Whenever possible, the limb should be splinted in the normal "walking" position, so that if a limited range of motion results after coaptation, the animal is still able to ambulate (Figure 35-54).

Orthoplast (Johnson & Johnson, New Brunswick, NJ), Hexcelite (Hexcel Medical, Dublin, Calif), and Veterinary Thermoplastic (VTP; IMEX Veterinary, Inc, Longview, Tex) are rigid at room temperature but when heated in water become malleable. This allows the material to conform closely to the configuration of the limb. Orthoplast is a solid sheet, and Hexcelite is a webbing available in roll or sheet form. Hexcelite is much easier to conform but is not as rigid when cool. VTP is available in various sizes and thicknesses. It is a solid sheet with a fibermesh reinforcement within the plastic. It is easily cut to an appropriate size and is more malleable than Orthoplast and more rigid than Hexcelite, making it ideally suited for use as a splint (Figure 35-55).

In lizards, fractures of the humerus or femur can be stabilized with a modified spica splint that crosses over the pelvic

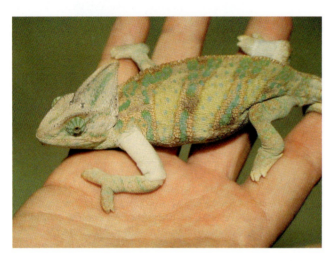

Figure 35-53 Patients will tolerate properly fitted, lightweight external splints and casts with minimal stress. This chameleon has a paper tape splint on both the front and rear legs. *(Photograph courtesy D. Mader.)*

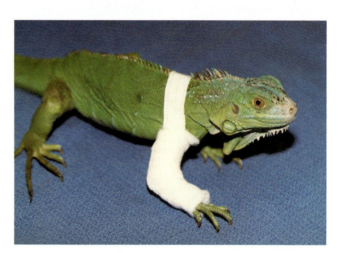

Figure 35-54 Whenever possible the limb should be splinted in the normal "walking" position, so that if a limited range of motion results after postcoaptation, the animal will still be able to ambulate. *(Photograph courtesy D. Mader.)*

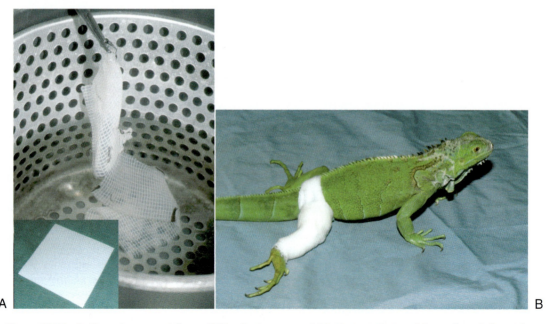

Figure 35-55 **A,** Several commercially available plastics are available that are designed for making lightweight, rigid casts and splints. Vet Thermoplastic comes as a rigid plastic square. When placed in hot water it turns clear, softens, and can be manipulated like a standard cloth tape. The plastic hardens when it cools. **B,** These plastics can be cut off, reheated, and reused. *(Photograph courtesy D. Mader.)*

or pectoral girdle to the opposite limb, thereby stabilizing the hip or shoulder joint and achieving the goal of immobilizing the joints proximal and distal to the fracture. Most lizards stand relatively flat or low with respect to the substrate and use abdominal undulation as an aid to locomotion, allowing them the ability to ambulate even with this type of device. With fractures of the pelvic limb, the splint should cross midline dorsally to allow normal voiding; with fractures of the pectoral limb, it should cross ventrally (see Figures 35-54 and 35-55, *B*).

Tubular traction splints can be used to treat fractures of the crus, antebrachium, distal humerus, and distal femur (Figure 35-56). A tube such as a syringe case of a diameter appropriate to the size of the patient's limb is padded at its proximal end. Tape stirrups are applied to the limb and secured to it. Padding is added to the limb to limit movement within the tube. The tape is then pulled through the tube such that the padded end is forced into the inguinal or axillary region and the limb is maintained in traction. The tape is secured to the outside of the tube maintaining the leg in extension and traction. The disadvantage of this type of splint is that it maintains the limb in complete extension. This can result in a decrease in the range of motion in immobilized joints from periarticular fibrosis (fracture disease).

The bone involved and the conformation of the patient also influence the type of coaptation used. For example, adequate stabilization of a humeral fracture in a chelonian is not possible with a traditional splint because the joint proximal to the fracture is not immobilized. In chelonians with a fractured humerus or femur, the limb can be folded into the cavity created between the plastron and the carapace and taped in place to prevent movement (Figure 35-57). Unfortunately, this does not address fracture alignment; however, the resulting malunion may be acceptable. Radiography of the limb after it is placed into a tape splint is recommended to ensure adequate alignment. If it is not properly apposed, the splint should be removed, the limb set, and the splint then reapplied. Sedation or anesthesia is helpful when trying to align the fracture and also decreases patient pain and stress.

Tortoise fracture splinted in this fashion may take several months to heal. Rechecking the patient, checking the splint, and radiographing the site are recommended every 4 to 6 weeks until union has occurred.

Although not ideal for fracture healing, a fractured limb on an injured lizard may be stabilized by securing it to the body. This is especially applicable in patients with NMBD. For fractures of the femur, the leg is pulled in traction along the tail and secured with adhesive tape. Fractures of the humerus may be stabilized by pulling the leg caudally to apply traction to aid in reduction and securing the limb to the body with adhesive tape (Figure 35-58). The tape must not be applied so tight that it interferes with respiration. With this method, some motion is expected at the fracture site as a result of body movement, but in many cases, the outcome is acceptable.

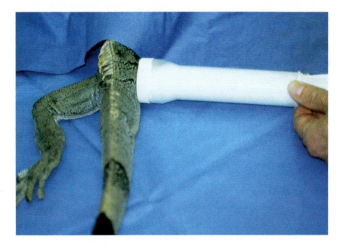

Figure 35-56 Tubular traction splints can be used to treat fractures of the crus, antebrachium, distal humerus, and distal femur. These are easily made from discarded syringe cases. *(Photograph courtesy R. Bennett.)*

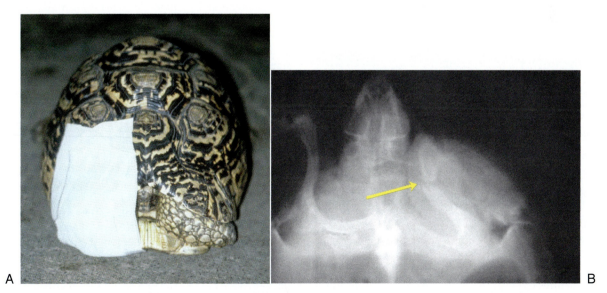

Figure 35-57 **A,** In chelonians with a fractured humerus or femur, the limb can be folded into the cavity created between the plastron and the carapace and taped in place to prevent movement. **B,** It is recommended to radiograph the limb after it is placed into a tape splint to ensure adequate alignment *(arrow).*

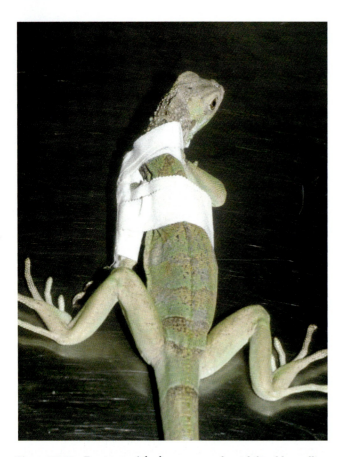

Figure 35-58 Fractures of the humerus can be stabilized by pulling the leg caudally to apply traction to aid in reduction and securing the limb to the body with adhesive tape. Likewise, fractures of the rear leg can be taped securely to the tail base in a similar fashion. *(Photograph courtesy D. Mader.)*

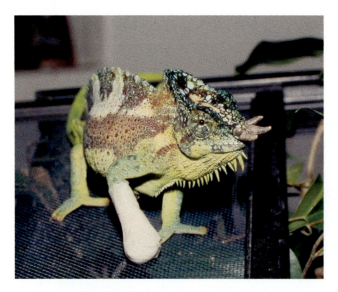

Figure 35-59 With fractures of the digits, manus, or pes, a ball bandage can be used for stabilization. *(Photograph courtesy D. Mader.)*

With fractures of the digits, manus, or pes, a ball bandage can be used for stabilization (Figure 35-59). The affected foot is secured around a ball of cotton in a grasping position. This stabilizes the fracture to allow bone healing.

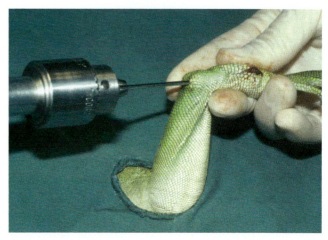

Figure 35-60 Steinmann pins are inexpensive, provide axial alignment and bending stability, and require minimal tissue exposure for insertion. *(Photograph courtesy D. Mader.)*

INTERNAL FIXATION

Internal fixation is indicated for repair of most long bone fractures in reptiles.[26] External coaptation frequently does not provide rigid stabilization and may not be well tolerated by reptile patients. External coaptation is not feasible in aquatic and semiaquatic reptiles. Virtually all methods for internal fracture fixation have been used successfully in reptiles.[28-32] The surgical approach to the long bones and the principles of application of internal fixation in reptiles are similar to those used in mammalian patients.

Most veterinarians are familiar with intramedullary Steinmann pins and orthopedic wires. They are inexpensive, provide axial alignment and bending stability, and require minimal tissue exposure for insertion (Figure 35-60). Kirschner wires can be used as intramedullary pins and are available in sizes as small as 0.028 inches. Spinal needles, which are available as small as 25 gauge × 3.5 inches, can also be used as intramedullary pins in small patients.

External skeletal fixation (ESF) can be used for stabilizing a variety of fractures in reptiles. These devices provide good stability without interfering with joints and may be applied to small patients. In reptiles, they are most often applied parallel to the substrate in a cranial to caudal plane, rather than a medial to lateral plane as in mammals, because of their different method of ambulation (Figure 35-61). Biphasic ESF devices use various size Kirschner wires, Steinmann pins, or hypodermic needles as fixation pins, but the connecting bar and clamps are replaced by acrylic polymer or other rigid material. This modification makes the apparatus less expensive and more lightweight.

In fracture management with ESF, pin loosening occurs for a variety of reasons, and the success of the repair depends on the ability of the bone to heal before the fixation pins loosen and the device fails. Because reptile bones heal slowly, the pins are more likely to loosen before the fracture is stable. Pin purchase can be maximized with threaded pins, preferably with the threads applied onto the pin, not cut into it (Figure 35-62), and inserting the fixation pins in the proper manner as outlined by Egger.[33]

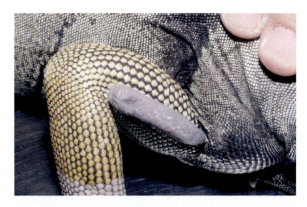

Figure 35-61 External skeletal fixation (ESF) can be used for stabilizing a variety of fractures in reptiles. These devices provide good stability without interfering with joints and may be applied to small patients. In reptiles, they are most often applied parallel to the substrate in a cranial to caudal plane, rather than a medial to lateral plane as in mammals. (*Photograph courtesy D. Mader.*)

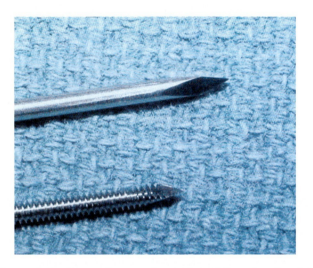

Figure 35-62 Pin purchase can be maximized by using threaded pins, preferably with the threads applied onto the pin, not cut into it. (*Photograph courtesy D. Mader.*)

Bone plating often requires a relatively large patient; however, with the availability of the veterinary cuttable plates (Synthes, Paoli, Pa) with screws as small as 1.5 mm in diameter (1.1 mm core diameter), bones as small as 3 mm in diameter may be plated. Finger plates are also applicable to many long bone fractures in small reptiles. Bone plating is often the treatment of choice for stabilizing femur and humerus fractures in chelonians (Figure 35-63).[27] In some reptiles, especially varanids, long bones are curved. In large patients, 2.7-mm reconstruction plates may be used to allow the plate to be contoured to such bones. Of course, bone plating requires specific expertise.

In most cases, removal of bone plates is not recommended. With intramedullary pins or ESF, the decision to remove implants should be based on radiographic evidence of bone healing. In some cases, a fibrous union may provide adequate stability allowing fracture healing to proceed to completion if the implants fail or must be removed before the development of radiographic union.

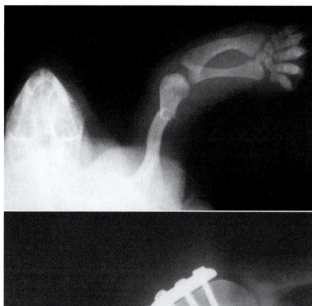
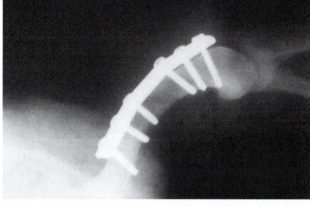

Figure 35-63 Bone plating is often the treatment of choice for stabilizing femur and humerus fractures in chelonians. (*Photograph courtesy D. Mader.*)

BONE GRAFTS AND ADVANCED FRACTURE TREATMENT

Motion at the fracture site is probably the number-one reason for fracture repair failure. Because of the nature of the vast majority of reptilian fractures (trauma, NMBD, hypomineralization, pathologic fractures), rigid fixation is often not possible.

Compression across the fracture site is paramount to ensure primary bone healing. In reptile patients, this may not always be possible. In many cases, external coaptation holds the limb steady with the fracture fragments in approximation but does not provide the same compression as properly applied bone plates.

In complicated fracture repairs, corticocancellous bone grafts may be necessary to perform, just as is done in mammalian patients.[34] In larger reptiles, corticocancellous grafts can be harvested from the proximal humerus or femur. A piece of rib can be collected and morselized for use as a corticocancellous graft. In smaller animals, the wing of the ilium is readily accessible. A small incision is made directly over either wing and a rongeur is used to harvest pieces of bone by taking small bites with the jaws (Figure 35-64). These bone chips can be carefully crushed to increase the surface area of the graft, then packed between and around the fracture site.

Nonunion fracture healing is not uncommon as a result of the aforementioned challenges. Many patients,

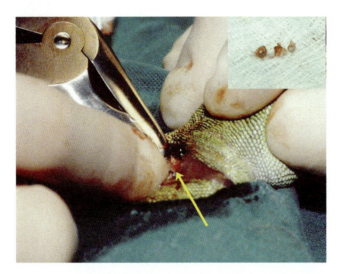

Figure 35-64 Corticocancellous grafts can be harvested from the proximal humerus or femur. A piece of rib can be collected and morselized for use as a graft. In smaller lizards, the wing of the ilium (*yellow arrow*) is readily accessible. (*Photograph courtesy D. Mader.*)

especially those kept as pets, do have an acceptable clinical result even with incomplete fracture healing. Wild animals, those that depend on their limbs for swimming, running, and for fleeing or chasing prey, may not thrive if all of their limbs do not function properly.

Mader and Kerr[35] reported the use of an osteogenic bone stimulator in a Chinese Water Dragon (*Physignathus cocincinus*) to repair a nonunion fracture of the tibia. A 1.5-volt (DC) battery source provided a constant current output (20.5 μA). The IM pin acted as the anode, and a small subcutaneous implant placed directly over the nonunion site served as the cathode. A bone graft was harvested from the ilium and packed around the fracture site to act as a matrix for new bone formation. Finally, an external fixator provided protection against rotation and distraction at the fracture site (Figure 35-65). The bone stimulator was left in place for 3 weeks and then disconnected. The external fixator and IM pin were removed 3 weeks later. At that time, radiographic evidence was seen of callus formation. The patient went on to a complete recovery.

COMPLICATIONS OF INTERNAL AND EXTERNAL FIXATION

As with any orthopedic surgery, complications do occur in reptile patients. Any time implants are used careful attention to aseptic technique is mandatory. Implant loosening and migration, bending of implants, and osteomyelitis are all potential problem areas (Figure 35-66).

Fracture treatment failures should be approached in a fashion similar to that done in mammals. First and foremost, the patient's husbandry must be evaluated and optimized. Implants need to be removed and cultured for pathogens. Antibiotics should be selected on the basis of culture and sensitivity results.

Fistulae should be explored, sequestra removed, and abscesses treated. Once the patient is stabilized and the infection is controlled, attempts to repair the fracture should

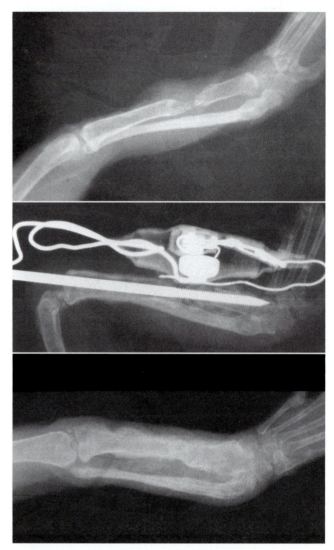

Figure 35-65 The top radiograph shows a nonunion fracture of the tibia in a Chinese Water Dragon (*Physignathus cocincinus*). An osteogenic bone stimulator is applied to the limb to help stimulate healing (middle). The stimulator was removed after 3 weeks. Bottom, the limb 1 year after the successful treatment. (*Photograph courtesy D. Mader.*)

be considered. If owner finance or compliance is a concern, or the limb is not salvageable, amputation is an option that can be discussed.

Implantation of antibiotic-impregnated methylmethacrylate beads has proven successful for the treatment of osteomyelitis.[37] If beads have been placed in a joint, they are removed once the infection is resolved. If the beads are placed in soft tissue or in or around bone, the beads do not need to be recovered.

SKULL AND FACIAL BONE FRACTURES

Although cranial kinesis is common in reptiles, specifically the snakes, fractures still occur even though they have relatively malleable skulls. In those reptiles with a more rigid skull, fractures of the mandible and separation of the symphysis

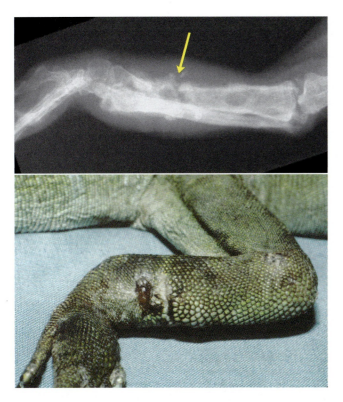

Figure 35-66 Osteomyelitis in the tibia *(yellow arrow)*. A pure culture of *Aeromonas* sp. was cultured from the lesion. After treatment, which included surgical debriding of the wound and antibiotic therapy, the patient made a complete recovery. *(Photograph courtesy D. Mader.)*

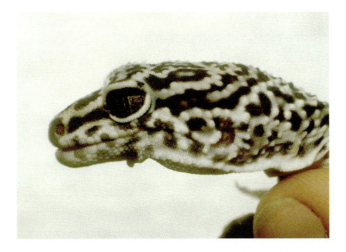

Figure 35-67 Iatrogenic mandibular fractures are not uncommon when opening the mouth of patients with NMBD. *(Photograph courtesy D. Mader.)*

are common. Fractures to the calvarium are seen with high-impact trauma such as encounters with predators (dogs), automobiles, lawnmowers, and boat propellers (see Figure 31-1 and Chapter 76).

Iatrogenic mandibular fractures not uncommonly occur in the veterinary office. Frequently, in an effort to perform a thorough physical examination, when the mouth is opened, the lower jaw fractures (common in cases of NMBD; Figure 35-67).

Snakes in captivity occasionally strike glass while attempting to capture live prey and injure their jaws (Figure 35-68).

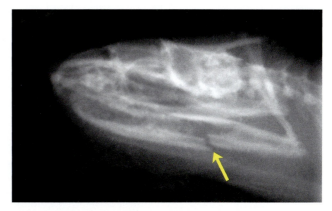

Figure 35-68 Snakes in captivity will occasionally strike glass while attempting to capture live prey and injure their jaws such as the mandibular fracture seen here. *(Photograph courtesy D. Mader.)*

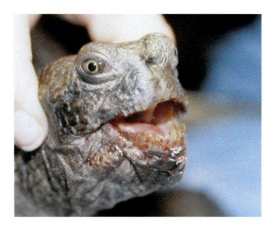

Figure 35-69 Treatment for fractures of the skull should follow standard principles of fracture management used in mammal surgery. In animals with normal bone structure orthopedic wires and bone pins can be used. *(Photograph courtesy D. Mader.)*

Because their skulls are normally distensible, fractures may go unnoticed. Animals may try to eat but are unable to prehend their food.

Treatment for fractures of the skull should follow standard principles of fracture management used in mammal surgery. In animals with normal bone structure, orthopedic wires and bone pins can be used (Figure 35-69).[37] For small patients, hypodermic needles can be used as IM pins in smaller mandibles or for external fixators.

In patients with suboptimal bone health, external coaptation can be applied. Small lightweight paper clips or plastic stays can be affixed to the jaw with tissue glue to position the fractures in place (Figure 35-70). If the appliance loosens, it can be readily reapplied. The process is repeated until the site heals. Alternatively, the jaw can be taped shut and an esophagostomy tube placed in order to provide enterals and medications.

JOINT SURGERY AND ARTHRODESIS

Lameness, although not a common clinical presentation, has been reported in reptile patients. Trauma, luxations, septic arthritis, and idiopathic causes have all been implicated.

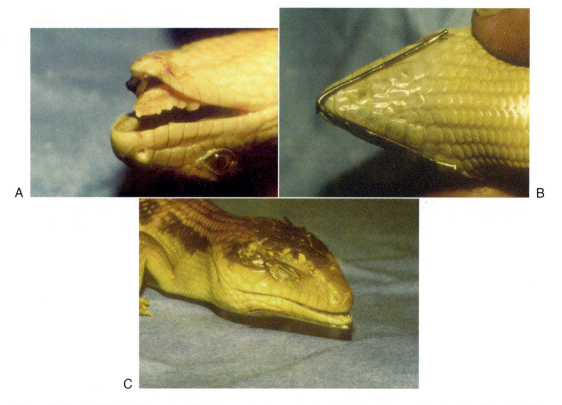

Figure 35-70 **A,** This skink has a mandibular symphysis separation. **B, C,** In patients with suboptimal bone health, external coaptation can be applied. Small, lightweight paperclips or plastic stays can be affixed to the jaw with tissue glue to stabilize the fracture. If the appliance loosens, it can be readily reapplied. The process is repeated until the site heals. *(Photographs courtesy D. Mader.)*

Techniques used in mammalian orthopedics have been attempted with varying degrees of success.[38-40]

Hernandez-Divers[38] reported using an over-the-top (with lateral vastus autograft) technique to repair a damaged stifle in a Spur-thighed Tortoise *(Testudo graeca)*. The technique was similar to that used for cranial cruciate rupture repair in mammals.

Barten[39] attempted a femoral head and neck excision to treat a chronic coxofemoral luxation in a monitor. However, even though the limb function improved, the outcome was less than optimal.

Arthrodesis is necessary in certain situations. Mader (unpublished data) arthrodesed the elbow joint of a Green Iguana that had suffered a severe bite wound from a conspecific. Because of the severity of the soft tissue wounds and the ensuing elbow joint osteomyelitis (Figure 35-71), the limb should have been amputated. However, the opposite front limb had previously been amputated from a similar lesion, so unless this forelimb could be salvaged, the iguana would have had to be euthanized.

An arthrotomy was performed on the elbow joint; what remained of the joint surface was curetted away, and the space was packed with a cancellous bone graft. A type II transarticular external fixator was applied (Figure 35-72). The patient was started on antibiotic therapy (cefadroxil) and kept confined after surgery. Radiographs were made at 6 weeks (Figure 35-73) and 12 weeks (Figure 35-74). At 12 weeks, sufficient callus was found to remove the external fixator. Even with the arthrodesed joint, the patient

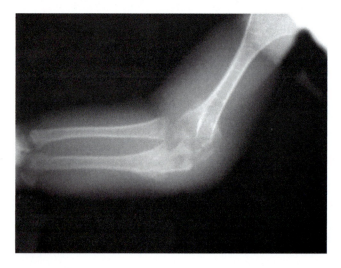

Figure 35-71 Osteomyelitis in the elbow of a Green Iguana *(Iguana iguana). (Photograph courtesy D. Mader.)*

was able to get around and even climb slightly inclined branches.

In a separate unpublished case, Mader described arthrodesing the carpus of a Desert Tortoise after development of radial paralysis that resulted from repeated injections of enrofloxacin in the proximal limb. The animal was dragging its foot in a fashion typical of a mammal with the same pathology. A 20-gauge orthopedic wire was used to force the carpus in permanent extension, allowing the animal to

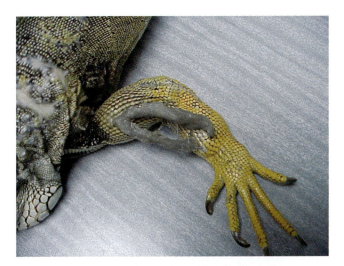

Figure 35-72 An arthrotomy was performed on the elbow joint of the patient in Figure 35-71. The joint surface was curetted away and the space was packed with a corticocancellous bone graft. A biplanar external fixator was applied across the joint for stability. *(Photograph courtesy D. Mader.)*

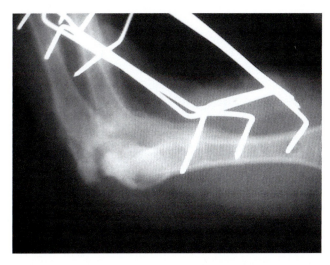

Figure 35-74 Osseous union and arthrodesis were almost complete by 12 weeks postsurgery. The external fixator was removed at this time. *(Photograph courtesy D. Mader.)*

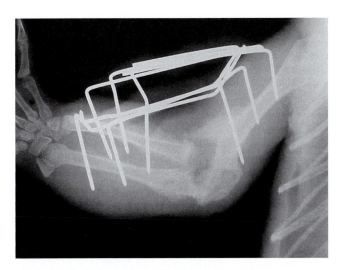

Figure 35-73 Radiographs taken at 6 weeks postsurgery showed initial bridging and callus formation. *(Photograph courtesy D. Mader.)*

walk normally on the foot (Figure 35-75). A hole was drilled through the mid-diaphysis of the radius, encircled ventral to the digits, then connected back to its origin. With tensioning of the wire, the carpus was maintained in permanent extension.

LIMB AMPUTATION

Phalanges or an entire digit may be amputated with good cosmetic result. When a digit is to be amputated, the incision should be planned to allow the skin closure to be flush with the metacarpal or metatarsal portion of the foot, creating a stumpless, cosmetic, functional appendage. Two skin flaps are created with the plantar/palmar flap longer than the dorsal flap. When the two flaps are brought together in apposition, the incision is elevated from the substrate, making it less likely to become severely contaminated or traumatized by the substrate.

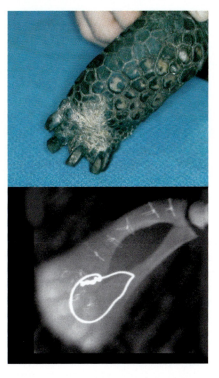

Figure 35-75 *Top,* Radial paralysis in a Desert Tortoise *(Gopherus agassizii)* caused by multiple injections of enrofloxacin in the upper limb. *Bottom,* The carpus was arthrodesed in full dorsoflexion using orthopedic wire. This permitted the animal to walk without dragging the foot. *(Photograph courtesy D. Mader.)*

In most animals in which limb amputation is indicated, amputation is recommended to be performed as proximal as possible to prevent the patient from traumatizing the stump on its substrate (Figure 35-76). This technique has also been recommended for reptiles; however, most reptiles have very tough skin that is resistant to such trauma. Their scar tissue, however, is more delicate and easily abraded. Further, because most lizards stand flat or low to the ground, even a short stump may aid in locomotion. When a limb must be amputated in a lizard and the patient may benefit from the

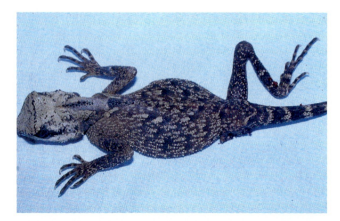

Figure 35-76 In reptiles, amputation should be performed as proximal as possible to prevent the patient from traumatizing the stump. *(Photograph courtesy S. Barten.)*

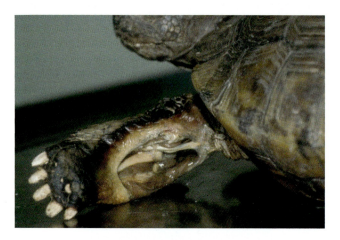

Figure 35-77 Amputation is an appropriate and functional option for patients with end-stage limb disease. *(Photograph courtesy D. Mader.)*

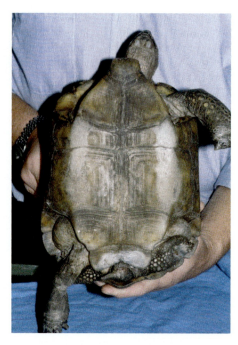

Figure 35-78 In chelonians, it is usually best to amputate as proximal as possible since they stand more upright and are more likely to traumatize the stump. Turtle patients do well, even with double amputations, as long as they have at least one front and one rear leg remaining. *(Photograph courtesy D. Mader.)*

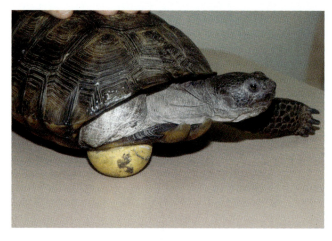

Figure 35-79 A prosthesis may be provided by securing a wood block, furniture coaster, or wheel on the plastron ventral to the shoulder or hip joint using an acrylic cement. *(Photograph courtesy D. Mader.)*

use of a stump, the limb may be amputated in a location that provides a stump that aids in ambulation. The skin should be incised to create a flap on the ventral surface that is placed over the end of the stump and sutured dorsally. This places healthy normal skin in contact with the substrate and the incision/scar tissue dorsal and lateral. The end of the bone should be padded with viable soft tissues before skin closure.

In many cases, because of the nature of the trauma or the presence of infection along fascial planes, the entire limb must be removed (Figure 35-77). This is best performed at the scapulohumeral or the coxofemoral joint. Muscles are transected at their distal insertions to allow for adequate soft tissue coverage of the end of the bone. The muscle bellies are then elevated from the periosteum proximally until the articulation is exposed. Smooth transection of the nerves with a scalpel, or preferably a laser, is recommended.[41] The nerves may be injected with bupivicaine to minimize postoperative pain. The laser "seals" the end of the nerves, theoretically minimizing any chance for neuroma (phantom pain) formation.

In chelonians, amputation as proximal as possible is usually best because they stand more upright and are more likely to traumatize the stump (Figure 35-78). A prosthesis may be provided by securing a wood block, furniture coaster, or wheel on the plastron ventral to the shoulder or hip joint with an acrylic cement (Figure 35-79). This elevates the affected corner of the shell, allowing easier ambulation with the remaining limbs, and prevents erosion of the plastron that could potentially cause injury or pain to the animal.

TAIL AMPUTATIONS

Many lizards and some snakes have the ability to voluntarily break off the tail in a process called autotomy in an effort to escape from a predator (see Figure 70-3). They have the ability to regenerate the lost portion of the tail.[5] The regenerated

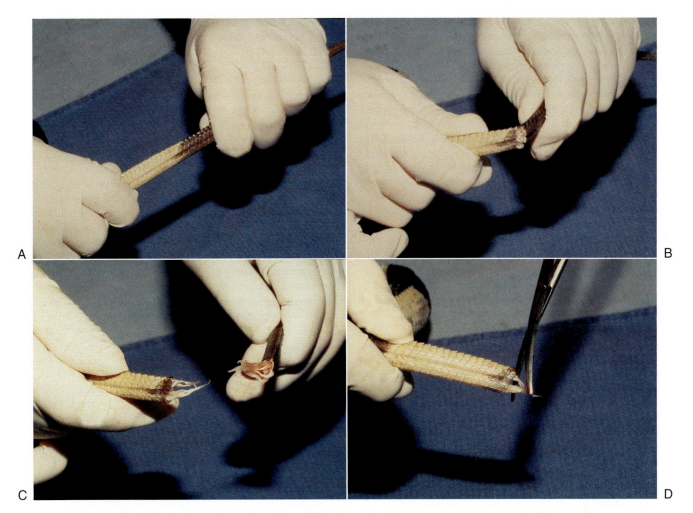

Figure 35-80 **A,** Tail amputation in a Green Iguana *(Iguana iguana)* using the natural fracture plane. Local analgesia should be provided in the form of a ring block proximal to the amputation site. Aseptic techniques should be used. **B,** A quick "snap" is made at the site. **C,** Little hemorrhage occurs as this is a "natural" method of tail loss. **D,** The tendrils of the remaining ligaments can and should be trimmed with scissors for a more aesthetic finished appearance. The amputation site should NOT be sutured. Antibiotics are rarely necessary unless obvious infection is present. *(Photographs courtesy D. Mader.)*

segment contains a cartilaginous rod and a different scale and color pattern. In some instances, only a partial autotomy occurs. Saving these injured tails is possible and worth trying because it yields a more cosmetic result than amputation and regrowth. If the tail fracture is not complete, the distal segment can retain its vascular integrity, allowing the tissue to heal. A padded tubular splint should be applied to prevent progression of the injury during tail movement.[42]

When amputation is necessary, the surgeon can take advantage of the autotomy planes in the caudal vertebrae. The more proximal the tail damage, the less likely the tail will autotomize. No rules dictate exactly how proximal the fracture planes extend in any given patient; however, in general, the older the animal, the fewer proximal fracture planes exist.

When the tail needs to be amputated proximal to the existing damage or disease, the surgeon should transect the tissue in an area where viable tissue is present. If tissue is left in an attempt to salvage as much length of the tail as possible, disease can be left in the surgical field and failure to heal is common.

When the fracture planes are used to amputate a tail, the tail can literally be snapped off at the desired location (Figure 35-80). This is a natural phenomenon and happens routinely in the wild. Some reptile veterinarians advocate doing just that: snapping the tail on an awake patient. The authors do not believe that to be the best method of amputation. Analgesia should be administered, either in the form of general anesthesia or as a local ring block with an injectable analgesic such as lidocaine or bupivicaine.

When the tail is amputated distally, no sutures are needed. In fact, although not proven with controlled studies, many experienced veterinarians believe that suturing an autotomized tail delays healing and tail regrowth.

Surgical autotomy (i.e., when the surgeon manually autotomies the tail) is easily performed in the distal tail region. As the autotomy site progresses proximally, the procedure is complicated by the heavy, strong caudal tail muscles. The controversy arises as to what point anatomically along the tail surgical autotomy should no longer be performed and the tail should be surgically amputated with a scalpel, laser, or radioscalpel, and sutured closed.

In general, if the tail has to be removed with sharp dissection, at that point closure of the skin is recommended. If the tail is amputated in a wedge fashion, with the flaps of the wedge on each side of the coccygeal vertebrae, the tail skin will close in a laterally compressed fashion (a near-normal anatomic apposition). Even animals with these proximal amputations may regrow some of the tail, although it is never as long or as beautiful as the original (Figure 35-81).

If infection is present during the surgery, administration of postoperative antibiotics may be prudent. A broad-spectrum drug should be started and changed on the basis of the results of any bacterial culture and sensitivity performed.

PHYSICAL THERAPY

"Physical therapy" (PT) is the new buzz word in mammal orthopedic surgery. Historically, the practice of PT in reptile patients has been, for the most part, ignored. However, just as postoperative analgesia is critical to patient care, so is postoperative PT.

Martin reported a case involving extensive PT in a Radiated Tortoise (*Geochelone radiata*).[43] A 20-year-old, 7-kg adult male tortoise presented with an injury that involved the left forelimb. It was unable to use the leg and, as a result, could not lift its body off the ground to walk properly. As time progressed, the limb began to atrophy, and even though the initial injury was apparently healing, the limb was not strong enough to support the animal's weight. A "tortoise wheelchair" was designed that allowed the patient to put limited controlled weight on the leg. With time, the weight load increased as did the work load of the limb. Over the course of 1 year, the tortoise eventually regained total use of the leg and no longer had a need for the appliance.

Passive range-of-motion exercises, walking, swimming, and weight training, and appliances can all be applied to reptile patients as to mammals. The imagination is the only limitation.

VENEMOID SURGERY

Richard S. Funk

SNAKES

Venemoid surgery is a surgical technique developed to render a venomous snake functionally nonvenomous by altering the venom production and delivery systems. The first descriptions of this surgery were of an approach to the venom duct through an incision on the side of the snake's face, then transection and double-ligation of the venom duct with the gland left untouched. This technique resulted in facial scars, and a significant number of snakes had a granulomatous response develop at the surgical site, especially in elapids.

The author developed an intraoral technique that leaves no visible facial scars and involves the complete removal of the venom gland and its duct. With isoflurane anesthesia, the snake is draped in dorsal recumbency with the lower jaw opened widely to give a full exposure of the upper jaws. The oral mucosa on each side is aseptically prepared, and an incision is made between the palatine teeth-fang axis and the lip margin with a radiosurgery unit, a CO_2 laser, or a #15 scalpel blade. Careful dissection with small (preferably ophthalmic) instruments exposes the venom gland and its duct. The duct of elapids can be more difficult to handle because of its thickness compared with viperids. Several vessels are associated with both the venom gland and its duct, the largest being encountered dorsomedially; these can be cauterized with a radiosurgery unit or a CO_2 laser, or in the case of large vipers, some can be ligated with absorbable suture. Good hemostasis is important.

The duct is transected at its entrance into the base of the maxillary bone, and the entire duct and venom gland are then elevated out of the incision and cautiously discarded (Figure 35-82). To help preserve the cosmetic postoperative

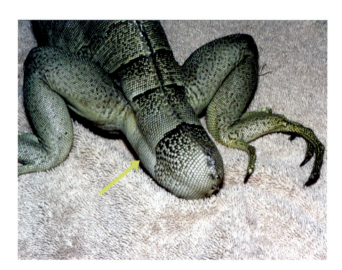

Figure 35-81 High tail amputations should be sutured as hemorrhage is common and more aesthetic healed product results. The tail can be taken as proximal as needed to correct the underlying problem. Caution should be taken in males not to damage the hemipenes (*yellow arrow*). (*Photograph courtesy D. Mader.*)

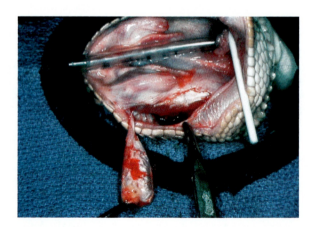

Figure 35-82 Venemoid surgery in an adult Eastern Diamondback Rattlesnake (*Crotalus adamanteus*). The right venom gland has been elevated through an intraoral incision, but the venom duct is still attached to the base of the maxilla. The duct will be separated at its attachment, and the venom gland and duct will thereby be removed. The patient is in dorsal recumbency. (*Photograph courtesy R. Funk.*)

appearance of the head, a sterilized silicone prosthesis is cut to a size slightly smaller than the gland that was removed and then placed into the surgery site. To facilitate future identification, a segment of surgical stainless steel can be inserted into the prosthesis so that it is visible radiographically, or a microchip transponder can be placed into the prosthesis. The mucosal incision is closed with absorbable suture in a simple continuous pattern (Figure 35-83). Because absorbable sutures are used, follow-up suture removal is not necessary.

Perioperative antibiotics are usually given. A broad-spectrum antibiotic is sufficient. If the snake is to be transferred to its owner soon after surgery, the antibiotics may be continued if desired.

After surgery, the snake is not fed for several weeks to help facilitate the healing process and minimize the chances of infection. The cage is kept clean, and the water is changed daily. Thereafter, the snake should be fed only dead prey.

Snakes that this author has rendered venomoid have lived well and even bred subsequently. Legally, most jurisdictions still consider a snake from which the venom glands and ducts have been removed to be a venomous species although it is no longer functionally venomous.

GILA MONSTER VENEMOID SURGERY

Venomoid surgery for Gila Monsters (*Heloderma suspectum*) is performed differently than for venomous snakes because of the anatomic fact that the lizard venom glands are located on the ventral regions of the lower jaws. The Gila is anesthetized, intubated, and maintained on isoflurane gas. The location of each gland is indicated by a prominent swelling or bulge along the anterior and middle region the each lower jaw (Figure 35-84). The skin at each site is surgically prepared, and a ventrolateral linear incision is made over the gland with either a #15 scalpel blade, a CO_2 laser, or a radiosurgery unit. The gland is easily located because little to no subcutaneous tissue overlies it. The slightly pinkish venom gland is carefully elevated from the mandible by a combination of sharp and blunt dissection. No large venom duct is found as in snakes; instead, a number of tiny ducts lead from the gland to several of the teeth. Hemorrhage is minimal. The skin is closed with a nonabsorbable monofilament suture in a simple interrupted (noneverting) pattern. Feeding may be resumed the same week. Sutures are removed in 5 to 6 weeks. A broad-spectrum antibiotic is often used after surgery.

BIOTELEMETRY IN REPTILES

Kevin T. Fitzgerald and Rebecca Vera

Biotelemetry and various forms of remote measurement techniques for biologic data have been applied to various reptilian species for decades.[26,44-47] The last 20 years have witnessed tremendous technologic advances in this area, including miniaturization of electronic components, programmable microcircuitry, and improvement of data transmission systems. These breakthroughs have led to the continued evolution of better remote sensing systems and more consistent performance. Techniques designed for the space program and complex remote physiologic monitoring systems created for humans can now be readily applied to reptiles in the wild. Radiotelemetry for reptiles in the last decade has seen an astounding refinement of attachment techniques, data collection systems, and data storage methods (Table 35-1). Currently, a number of commercial manufacturers are available to supply high-quality advanced telemetry equipment (Table 35-2). Many of these sources have a wealth of information for researchers on the basis of previous telemetry work done in reptiles. As a result, these firms can provide invaluable information concerning design specifications, project needs, and overall practicality of radiotelemetry in herpetofauna.

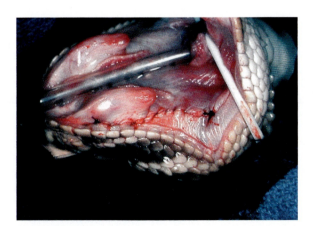

Figure 35-83 Completion of venemoid surgery on the right side of the snake in Figure 35-82. The venom gland and its duct have been removed, a silicone prosthesis has been placed into the space formerly occupied by the gland, and the incision has been closed with absorbable suture in a continuous pattern. *(Photograph courtesy R. Funk.)*

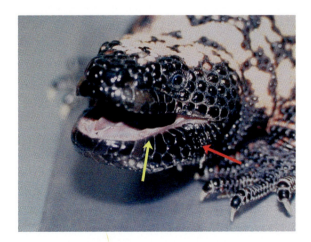

Figure 35-84 The location of the venom gland in the Gila Monster (*Heloderma suspectum*) is noted by a prominent swelling or bulge along the anterior and middle region in each lower jaw *(red arrows)*. There is no large venom duct as is found in snakes; instead, a number of tiny ducts lead from the gland to several of the teeth *(yellow arrow)*.

Table 35-1	Commonly Used Attachment Techniques for Telemetry Units in Reptiles

Subcutaneous implants (surgical)
Coelomic implants (surgical)
Gastric implants (per os; nonsurgical)
Attachment to chelonian carapace (epoxy; nonsurgical)
Sutured to dorsal scales (crocodilians, lizards; surgical)
Backpacks (nonsurgical)
Harnesses (nonsurgical)
Helmets (nonsurgical)

*All surgical implanting *must* be performed aseptically.

Table 35-2	Common Suppliers for Biotelemetry Units for Reptiles

AVM Instrument Company, Ltd
1213 S Auburn Street, PO Box 1898
Colfax, CA 95713
Ph: (530) 346-6300

Advanced Telemetry Systems (ATS)
470 1st Avenue North
Box 398
Isanti, MN 55040
Ph: (612) 444-9267

Custom Telemetry and Consulting
1050 Industrial Drive
Watkinsville, CA 30677
Ph: (404) 769-4067

Telonics
932 East Impala Avenue
Mesa, AZ 85204-6699
Ph: (602) 892-4444

Telinject USA (Biotracks, UK)
9316 Soledad Canyon Road
Saugus, CA 91350
Ph: (805) 268-1105

TRANSMITTERS, POWER SOURCES, ANTENNAS, AND RECEIVERS

Telemetry systems consist of a transmitter, a power supply, an antenna, and the receiver. Special projects may include additional components for other specific data collection. Generally, these are added to either the transmitter or receiver ends of the system. Presently, an astonishing variety of capabilities are available with different systems and configurations, and researchers are limited mainly by their own imagination, experimental design, and financial constraints.

Transmitters

Transmitters are implanted or somehow affixed to the target specimen. The transmitter is the source that is used for locating animals and can also serve to convert collected data into a variety of communication formats. The transmitter and associated sensors can be used to monitor physiologic data such as body temperature, heart rate, blood pressure, body position, movement, or location as determined by geographic positioning systems (GPS). Remote physiologic monitoring has become advanced in humans, and application of this improved technology has been applied to a wide variety of wildlife. Monitoring of reproductive and behavioral patterns has become common in nonhuman species.[48] This type of remote monitoring of biologic data eliminates handling, interactions with humans, and other stressful procedures, which results in a more natural situation in which the animal can be observed and values measured. Signals transmitted can be in any format (e.g., AM, FM, VHF, UHF, M-band). Changes in pulse rate (beeps per minute) are generally used to indicate changes in sensor information.

Transmitters may either continuously send data or store collected data for later transmission. Packages that automatically give a drug injection stored in the transmitter or radio collar have been designed but are generally not available. Relay receivers and transmitters are in use that pick up weak signals and resend them from more distant locations. This is particularly useful for tiny animals and studies done in mountainous or hilly areas.

Power Sources

The power supply of most biotelemetry set-ups has traditionally been batteries. Battery technology and sophistication have improved over the last several decades, but it is still the limiting factor for both transmitter longevity and package size and weight. On account of microcircuitry, sensors and transmitters can be insignificant in size compared with the battery. Reducing the power of the transmitter can significantly prolong the life of the battery. Using the minimum signal wattage necessary for transmission, reducing the length of each pulse (pulse width) and the number of pulses per minute (pulse rate), and designing the transmitter to automatically turn off at regular internals can also enhance battery life. The utilization of such strategies has led to the development of 1.5- to 3-g transmitters that have a 70-day working life. Solar panels have been proposed and designed that could recharge the battery during the day. At present, solar panel attachments have a very limited application for most reptilian species.

Antennas

The transmitter and the receiver require antennas to function. Antenna configuration and radiofrequencies have a tremendous impact on the effectiveness of the system. Antenna size, placement, and configuration are based on the nature of the signal and the physical size and limitations of the animals studied. In general, transmitters are equipped with omnidirectional antennas to optimize signal transmission in all directions, and receivers use directional antennas to determine transmitter locations and maximize reception.

For wildlife applications, frequencies between 140 and 170 MHz (VHF) have traditionally been used. This happened as a result of component design and a compromise of signal transmission and antenna length. For most radio waves, if the length of the antenna is an even multiple of the wavelength used, the transmission of the signal is maximized. The length of antennas of transmitters and receivers is adjusted to match the wavelength selected. One must remember that wavelength is inversely proportional to frequency. Higher frequencies have shorter waves with more waves per second.

Lower frequencies have longer waves. They travel farther and are less attenuated by physical obstruction. However, lower frequencies require longer antennas for successful transmission. Higher frequencies (shorter waves) are more easily attenuated by objects, moisture, and contact, but shorter antennas can be used. Lower frequency (longer wave) transmitters are generally not seen because only very large animals could tolerate the length of the antenna required.

Water and moisture (even high humidity) can affect higher frequencies. Bodily fluids and body contact both dampen transmission by attenuating signals and detuning the antennas, similar to touching a radio or television antenna. Water or contact reduces transmission distance of surgically implanted transmitters. Surgical implants can lose two thirds to three quarters the transmission range present before implantation.[49]

Newer systems that use satellite transmission such as the GPS network operate between 450 to 1600 MHz. Higher frequencies such as these can use extremely short antennas but are easily attenuated. Thick forest cover can greatly interfere with signal transmission of such systems. New technology is being developed that may eliminate such problems.

A variety of factors interfere with the transmission distances available with radiotelemetry. Vegetation type, atmospheric and weather conditions, soil type, and geographic topography can all affect signal transmission. Prediction of the performance of a particular transmitter for a specific site or species is not possible. For the 150- to 170-MHz range used for most wildlife applications, line-of-sight distance for open locations provides a place to start. Signals can usually be detected if distances are in unobstructed, open lines of sight. Systems perform best in flat, open, dry areas, and signals are best detected from an airplane or from the highest point in the local terrain. In suboptimal locales (hills, excessive moisture, dense vegetation, certain soils, etc.), an animal lying behind a hill 100 meters away may not be detectable. Thick, wet vegetation diminishes signal transmission, and rocky surfaces may reflect radio signals, resulting in a false second location transmission.

Receivers

Biotelemetry receivers may be created that satisfy most needs, and they can vary with application requirements and system used. The most commonly used are VHF receivers available commercially. These can be obtained right off the shelf and run the gamut from simple units that can process 12 transmitters to advanced units with programmable scanning, data storage, and computer downloading capacity.

Only one receiver is required to receive data. However, to establish the location of transmitters, triangulation is required if a GPS unit is not integrated in the transmitter package. For triangulation, directional bearings must be obtained from two locations separated by an angle of greater than 30 degrees. Some systems store data in the unit or collar, and information can be downloaded once the animal is recaptured and the unit recovered. These types of systems may save many observation hours and reduce costs necessary to fund such studies.

Satellite receivers are likewise available. The Argos system uses three circumpolar orbiting satellites to retrieve data. It can also calculate location with Doppler shifts of the signal as the satellite crosses the horizon. GPS receivers use geosynchronous orbiting satellites and transmit data with VHF radio communication configurations or through the Argos system. GPS units achieve accurate location readings. Like transmitters, the complexity of receivers and data collection systems is only limited by financial constraints and the breadth of the imagination of the investigator.

Complicating Factors

Placement of external transmitter attachment, implanted transmitters, and even the recovery from anesthesia and surgical procedures can all dramatically affect the physiology and behavior of study species. Collars, tags, and power packs placed on animals provide a novel and unique new stimulus to the animal studies, to conspecifics during social interactions, and to both predator and prey species. Transmitters mounted either externally or internally can affect balance, mobility, hydrodynamics, aerodynamics, and overall energy expenditure.[50-52] Changes in energy budgets as a result of inappropriate transmitter size or placement can affect reproductive success and individual survival. In general, telemetry units should not exceed 2% of the study animal's body weight.[47] Newer, more advanced units are even more conservative and use 1% of the body weight as their guideline.

Ideally, transmitter packages should be removed at the end of the study or designed to fall off the subject in the not-too-distant future. Surgically implanted internal transmitters must not experience instrument corrosion or battery leakage within the animal and optimally are removed at the termination of the study.[47]

Safe and effective placement of transmitters, data storage units, and behavioral or physiologic monitors is essential for success of the study. For surgically implanted units, proper anesthesia, aseptic surgical technique, and appropriate pain management must be observed both for the success of the study and to honor the responsibilities researchers have to their study animals.[53] Biotelemetry raises several ethical, legal, and moral issues. For all such studies, the impact on the animals observed must be the determining factor as to whether the study is undertaken. The short-term and long-term effects of such studies on the animals examined must be determined. Furthermore, the scientific validity of studies that use telemetry units in terms of the experimental design, the interference of observers, and the interference of the implant on the natural behavior, physiology, and anatomy of the animal must all be evaluated. Next we examine surgical placement of telemetry units in reptiles and the associated anesthesia at our practice.

SURGICAL IMPLANTATION

The authors have implanted a variety of transmitter packages in both Bullsnakes (*Pituophis catenifer*) and Prairie Rattlesnakes (*Crotalus viridis viridis*). Our transmitter implants and receivers were obtained through AVM Instrument Company (Colfax, Calif), a supplier traditionally used by herpetologists. To activate the transmitting battery, the magnet taped to the exterior of the module must be removed. To turn the transmitter off, replace the magnet to the unit, securing it back in place with tape. All units should be tested on receipt to ensure they are operational. The preferred means of transmitter sterilization before implantation is gas sterilization.

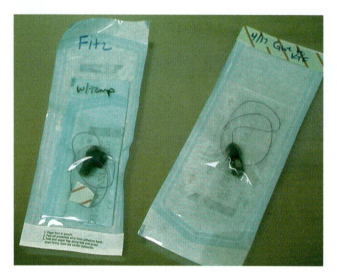

Figure 35-85 The transmitters and antennas implanted in the snakes ranged in weight from 5 to 5.5 g. These must be gas sterilized prior to implantation. *(Photograph courtesy K. Fitzgerald.)*

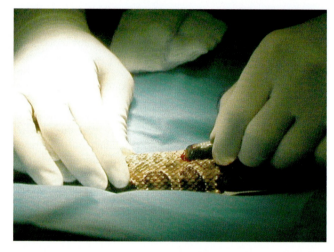

Figure 35-87 Transmitters were implanted below the epidermis and dermis but above the underlying epaxial muscles. The coelom was not entered. The transmitter unit was anchored to the fascia and the deep layer closed using 4-0 nonabsorbable suture. *(Photograph courtesy K. Fitzgerald.)*

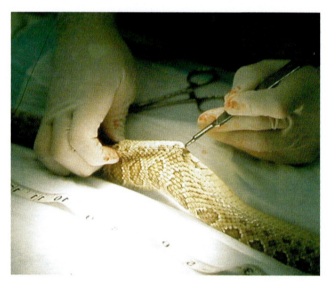

Figure 35-86 The implant site was located approximately one quarter of the body length caudal to the head on the left side. The surgical site was aseptically prepared and a small stab incision was made between the scutes and the lateral scales on the left side. *(Photograph courtesy K. Fitzgerald.)*

To determine the theoretical life in days of each individual transmitter, the battery capacity (given by the supplier) is divided by the individual current drain (also given by the supplier). For our study, transmitters had a life of roughly 8 months (240 days) after activation. Also, our transmitters and antennas implanted in the snakes ranged in weight from 5 to 5.5 g (Figure 35-85).

The day after all implants were gas sterilized, our study snakes were pretreated 20 minutes before surgery with Buprenorphine (Abbott Labs, North Chicago, Ill) at a dosage of 0.01 mg/kg SQ and Telezol (Fort Dodge, Fort Dodge, Iowa) at a dosage of 20 mg/kg IM. Once anesthetized, snakes were maintained with sevoflurone (Abbott Labs) administered through a custom-fitted mask attached to the acrylic snake tube they were pretreated in. The mask was made by cutting a 60-mL syringe case to fit the snake tube on one end and then attaching the other end to the anesthesia machine.

The implant site was located approximately one quarter of the body length caudal to the head on the left side. The surgical site was aseptically prepared, and a small stab incision was made between the scutes and the lateral scales on the left side (Figure 35-86). Transmitters were implanted below the epidermis and dermis but above the underlying epaxial muscles (Figure 35-87). The coelom is not entered. The transmitter unit was anchored to the fascia, and the deep layer closed with 4-0 Novafil (Sherwood, Dams and Geck, Chicago, Ill), a nonabsorbable suture. The subcutaneous tissue was closed with a subcuticular pattern of 3-0 PDS (Ethicon, Pearl River, NY), an absorbable suture. Good apposition of the skin was obtained with this technique, but nevertheless, the skin was closed with surgical glue (Figure 35-88).

The implanted antennas in the transmitter modules were 13.5 in long and were advanced subcutaneously toward the tail (Figure 35-89). A series of small stab incisions was made laterally along the side of the subject, caudal to the transmitter. A long, delicate, straight hemostat was used to tunnel under the skin, with gentle advancing of the antenna to its full length (Figure 35-90).

Larger antennas were selected for our study in an attempt to maximize the distance the signal could be detected. For our study, no snakes smaller than 300 g or less than 36 in (91 cm) were implanted with transmitters. Selection of snakes at least this size ensured that our transmitters (about 5.5 g) were less than the 2% body weight recommendation commonly made for implants. Our implants did not appear to interfere with locomotion or eating and provided a strong signal even when a snake was coiled.

All snakes received lactated Ringer's solution (LRS) at 5 mL/kg SQ after anesthetic recovery. Snakes were held for 3 days after surgery to ensure that they recovered completely and then were released at their point of capture (GPS-validated). All transmitters were determined to be operating before the animals were released.

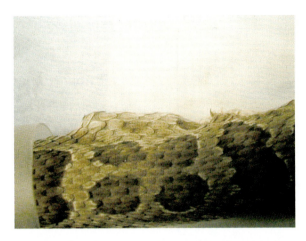

Figure 35-88 The subcutaneous tissue was closed with a subcuticular pattern of 3-0 absorbable suture. Good apposition of the skin was obtained using this technique but, nevertheless, the skin was closed using surgical glue. *(Photograph courtesy K. Fitzgerald.)*

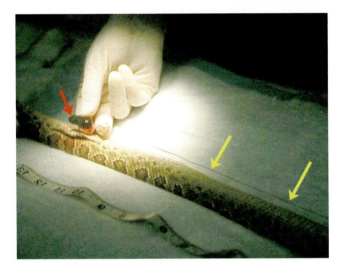

Figure 35-89 The implanted antennas *(yellow arrows)* in the transmitter modules *(red arrows)* were 13.5 in long and were advanced subcutaneously toward the tail. *(Photograph courtesy K. Fitzgerald.)*

The health of the subjects should be monitored as closely as possible without interfering with the study. At the termination of the research or at the end of the useful life of the transmitters, the units should be removed. This surgical removal of the package must also be performed with aseptic technique. In this manner, no subjects are exposed to long-term corrosive effects of the implant, leakage of the battery contents, migration of the unit, or loss of mobility through scarring in the vicinity of the transmitter or the surgical site.

SUMMARY

Biotelemetry units have been implanted in reptiles for many years. Presently, telemetry units are smaller and less expensive and have greater and longer transmitting powers than previous implants. Likewise, receiver modules are less bulky, easier to use, less expensive, and much more sensitive than ever before. A number of competent commercial suppliers are available to provide telemetry units, to supply advice about which unit to use, to examine experimental design, and to offer insights regarding biotelemetry in specific species.

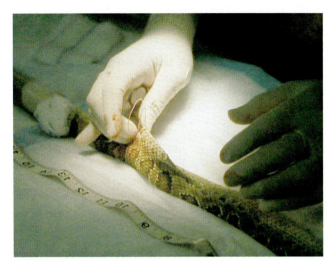

Figure 35-90 A series of small stab incisions were made laterally along the side of the subject, caudal to the transmitter. A long, delicate, straight hemostat was used to tunnel under the skin, gently advancing the antenna to its full length. *(Photograph courtesy K. Fitzgerald.)*

Many significant ethical questions surround biotelemetry studies in animals. The most obvious concern is what effect studies of this type have on the animals observed. One must always remember to "first do no harm." Nevertheless, the short-term and long-term effects of biotelemetry on the animals studied can have far-reaching effects. Potential for risks must be thoroughly considered before such research is undertaken. The information collected from telemetry studies must be so valuable concerning the species studied that the net result far outweighs the risk to the animals. Hopefully such studies add much to our knowledge and understanding of a species and aid in our attempts to protect them. Biotelemetry units must have the well being of the animal at their center, possess a sound experimental design, and ensure that the data obtained are scientifically valid and not tainted by the actions or biases of the researchers. If done correctly, biotelemetry is a powerful tool with which much information can be obtained about the physiology, behavior, and natural history of a species.

ACKNOWLEDGMENTS

We thank Mr Bryan Shipley of the Denver Zoo for including us in his study, for taking us into the field, and for his admirable work ethic. We also thank Dr Robert A. Taylor and the staff at Alameda East Veterinary Hospital for providing us with such a wonderful place to study and treat reptiles.

LASER AND RADIOSURGERY

Stephen J. Hernandez-Divers and Douglas R. Mader

Reptile medicine, as a discipline, has many inherent unique challenges unrealized in more traditional veterinary practice. The obvious, the wide variety of species, is subtly surmounted by the even wider disparity in patient size. Patients may range from a 10-g gecko to a 200-kg tortoise. Blood loss is usually not a problem with the latter but is a critical concern with the former.

Traditional medicine has taught the use of the surgical scalpel, which has always been considered the gold standard for surgical incisions. As with anything, the scalpel has its limitations. Cold steel surgery, even with the best technique, has the risk of excessive hemorrhage.

During the past 20 years, radiosurgery and cryosurgery have become available and, in some situations, have replaced the scalpel blade. Each has its own advantages and disadvantages.

Recent times have seen the introduction of the surgical laser to general veterinary practice. No longer is this sophisticated equipment limited to veterinary institutions and the multimillion-dollar referral practices. Recent graduates are entering the work force with advanced training. Printed media, animal programs on cable television, and the Internet are educating reptile owners on the advances in veterinary medicine, and as a result, newer techniques including laser and radiosurgery are now in demand.

LASER PHYSICS

Since Albert Einstein theorized the concept of lasers in 1916, considerable development has resulted in an array of equipment available to the human surgeon and subsequently, the veterinarian.[54] Practical applications for lasers in veterinary medicine, and particularly in the field of zoologic medicine, have also gained pace.[55-61] The term **LASER** stands for **L**ight **A**mplification by the **S**timulated **E**mission of **R**adiation and relies on the production of electromagnetic radiation in response to photon emission by the lasing medium.[54,55]

A standard light bulb and a laser share one thing in common—they both generate electromagnetic energy, commonly called "light." The electromagnetic spectrum extends from very short wavelengths (gamma radiation at 10^{-11} m) to radio waves (10^{-1} m). The laser wavelengths fall between infrared and ultraviolet, which include the invisible and visible (400 to 700 nm) light spectrum. The wavelengths of medical lasers range from 193 nm (UV-excimer lasers) to 10,600 nm (far-infrared lasers). Only lasers in the wavelengths of 400 to 700 nm are visible to the human eye.

The power behind a laser comes from its ability to store energy in atoms, concentrating the energy and releasing it in the form of powerful waves of light energy. Specifically, an atom in its resting ground state in a given medium (e.g., solid crystal, liquid, or gas) becomes excited to a higher energy state by absorbing thermal, electrical, or optical energy. After the energy is absorbed, the atom spontaneously returns to its resting state by releasing that energy as a photon; this is called stimulated emission.

This released photon resonates between mirrored ends of the laser chamber, further exciting other atoms in the laser medium. The momentum of the particles grows until finally a highly concentrated beam of light passes through a partially transmissive mirror at one end of the laser chamber (Figure 35-91).

Just as sound passes through air, or a ripple in the water, light travels in waves. Frequency is the term for the number of waves that pass a point in time. The frequency of light

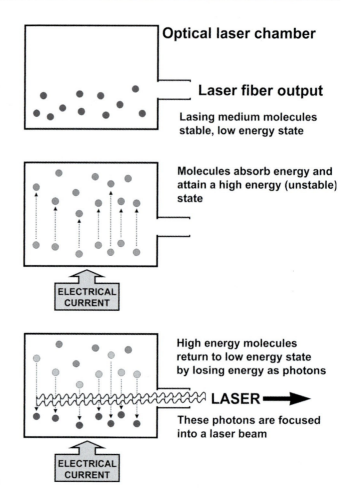

Figure 35-91 Diagrammatic representation of the production of laser. The top diagram demonstrates the resting lasing medium molecules within the optical laser chamber. As energy in the form of electrical current is applied, these molecules attain a higher energy level and become unstable (middle). There is a constant effort to return to a more stable state and the molecules achieve this by losing energy in the form of photons (bottom). These photons leave the optical chamber via the laser fiber output as a laser beam. (*Illustration courtesy S.J. Hernandez-Divers.*)

(known as the number of oscillations per second) combined with its wavelength (the distance between one peak to the next) determines the color of light. Normal white light is *incoherent*, which means it contains many wavelengths radiating in all directions. For example, if light passes through a prism, the beam is broken down into its different colors.

Laser light, in comparison with normal light, is *coherent* and consists of only one color, known as *monochromatic*. The last distinguishing feature of laser light is that it is *collimated* or nonradiating, as is white light. Laser light travels in parallel beams, each reinforcing the beam next to it.

A variety of lasers are available, but carbon dioxide (CO_2) and diode models are the most common in veterinary medicine today (Figure 35-92). Both lasers produce an immediate area of tissue vaporization, surrounded by a zone of irreversible photothermal necrosis, and a further outermost zone of reversible edema (Figure 35-93). With proper technique and a small laser tip, the cellular destruction is limited to a region only three to four cells away from the target area, minimizing tissue devitalization. As a result, the laser

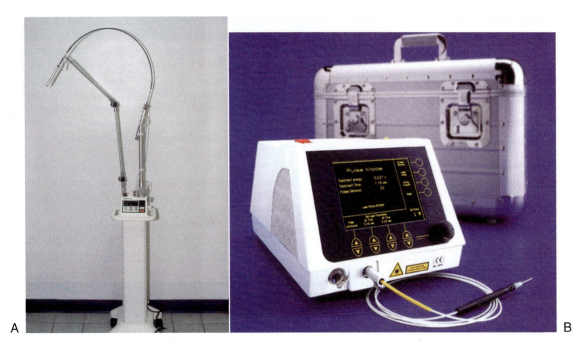

Figure 35-92 **A,** The AccuVet CO_2, 20-W, superpulse laser. CO_2 lasers have an attached wave guide connecting the laser to the hand piece. Wave guides can be fiber optic (shown here) or articulated. **B,** Diode laser. Note the delicate, flexible wave guide that is readily inserted into either a rigid or flexible endoscope. A hand piece can also be attached and used in a fashion similar to the CO_2 laser. (*A, photograph courtesy D. Mader; B, photograph courtesy AccuVet Lasers.*)

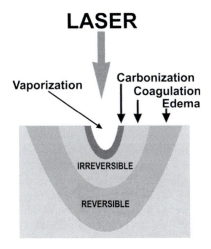

Figure 35-93 The effects of laser on biological tissue. The primary area of vaporized tissue is surrounded by a thin layer of carbonization (char) and then by a zone of thermal necrosis caused by coagulation. The outer-most layer is edema, and is reversible. (*Illustration courtesy Diomed Ltd.*)

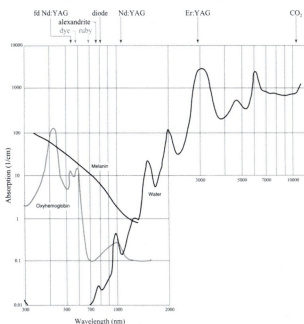

Figure 35-94 The absorption coefficients of hemoglobin, melanin, and water, are shown in relation to diode (810 and 980 nm) and CO_2 (10,600 nm) lasers. The diode is more selective for hemoglobin and melanin (pigmentation), whereas the CO_2 has a far greater affinity for water. (*Illustration courtesy AccuVet Lasers.*)

incision has less lateral tissue damage than either cryosurgery or electrosurgery.

Currently more CO_2 lasers are found in veterinary practices than any other type, and they offer the advantages of accurate noncontact surgery with minimal tissue penetration and a reduced collateral thermal injury of only 0.05 to 0.2 mm, compared with 0.3 to 0.6 mm with diode lasers. This effect is primarily a result of the CO_2 laser's preference for intracellular water (Figure 35-94). Nevertheless, despite these

Table 35-3	Comparison Between CO_2 and Diode Lasers		
Laser	**Advantages**		**Disadvantages**
CO_2 10,600 nm wavelength Highly absorbed by water Ideal for cutting (focused beam) Tissue vaporization (defocused beam) Most common laser in veterinary medicine	Minimal lateral thermal insult Decreased edema (seals lymphatics) Seals nerves (less postoperative pain) No tissue contact (sterilizes as it cuts) Minimizes hemorrhage (seals vessels <0.6-mm diameter)		Cannot pass through endoscope Perceived high cost
Diode 635-980 nm wavelength Ophthalmologic use since 1984	Used with fiberoptic systems Chromophore enhanced tissue ablation Laser welding Photodynamic therapy Ability to function in fluid environments Superior hemostasis (seals blood vessels ≤2 mm in diameter)		Deeper penetration (than CO_2) Less precision Tissue contact

differences, the diode compares well with both CO_2 and neodymium-yttrium aluminium garnet (YAG) lasers, as a comparative study of their effectiveness in human inferior turbinate reduction surgery failed to indicate any significant benefit of one laser over another.[62]

The diode laser has certain advantages over CO_2, specifically: 1, the ability to function in fluid environments (e.g., intestinal tract, fluid-filled abdomen or coelom, and bladder); 2, improved hemostasis (i.e., able to seal blood vessels up to 2 mm in diameter, compared with 0.6 mm with a CO_2 laser); and 3, fiberoptic capability for use with a variety of endoscopes.[63-65] Table 35-3 compares the disadvantages and advantages of both the CO_2 and diode lasers.

CO_2 LASER EQUIPMENT

Several companies sell CO_2 lasers. The CO_2 laser comes in a variety of sizes and power capacities. AccuVet (AccuVet Lasers, Division of Lumenis Inc, Santa Clara, Calif) sells 12-watt, 20-watt, and 20-watt superpulse units. All of the CO_2 lasers are class IV. The invisible 10,600-nanometer beam is beyond the visible wavelength.

When laser light is absorbed by a cell, the water within the cell is boiled and the cell essentially explodes. The cell denatures into smoke and the cell remnant, called char. This smoke, which has been documented to contain DNA, bacteria, and viruses, should always be evacuated with a filtered vacuum.

When the laser is used for cutting, cellular destruction is limited to a region only three to four cells away from the target area, thus minimizing tissue devitalization. In contrast, tissue destruction can be deliberately maximized for purposes of tissue ablation. Tissue cutting versus ablation can be controlled either by tip size or by "defocusing" the laser's beam.

"Focusing" the beam allows the surgeon to use the laser's intensified light beam to "cut" tissue, whereas "defocusing" the beam allows the laser to "ablate" the tissue (Figure 35-95).

A simple analogy can be made with a magnifying glass in the sunlight. The convex glass collects the sun's beams or rays and focuses them to a pinpoint. The light rays can be focused to a fine point by moving the magnifying glass closer or farther away from the surface being imaged. The beam is at its peak intensity when the point of light is at its smallest diameter. This correspondingly is also when the beam of light is at its maximum cutting power, which can be easily demonstrated by focusing the sun beam on a piece of paper and watching it burn with exacting precision.

The laser works in a similar fashion. It actually cuts tissue by searing through it with a highly intense focused beam of generated light. Just like the magnifying glass, the laser has to be positioned so that it is focused on the target tissue (e.g., a growth or abscess).

"Ablation" is especially useful for removal of small growths or tumors. In some situations, "ablating" the tumor is preferable to cutting it off. What this means is that the laser beam is defocused on the tumor, and instead of cutting it away, the laser literally disintegrates it. Of course, this is an important consideration if histopathology is anticipated.

Three factors determine the tissue impact of the delivered laser beam: spot size, power, and exposure.

Spot size refers to the diameter of the aperture that contains 86% of the laser's beam. Several tips permit precise control of spot (cutting) size (Figure 35-96). The tip sizes range anywhere from 0.3 to 3 mm (Figure 35-97), with the most commonly used tips being 0.4 to 0.8 mm. With focused beam tips, the distance of the tip from the target tissue determines the actual spot size at the target. For most tips, the focal distance is typically 1 to 3 mm.

Power is measured in watts, which is defined by the amount of energy applied over time (defined as Joules/second). Power is adjusted on the laser by adjusting the wattage. The greater the wattage, the higher the power.

Power density is affected by the size of the target area. If the spot size is small, the power is concentrated. If the spot size is large, the power is spread out over a larger area and the power density is decreased, thus producing a lesser tissue effect.

Exposure is also a user-controlled variable. Exposure is determined by the duration of the applied laser. The greater the exposure, the greater the tissue impact. Exposure can be delivered as continuous, repeat, or single pulse. Surgical precision is increased respectively.

DIODE LASER EQUIPMENT

Two main types of diode lasers are commercially available for veterinarians: the 15-watt, 30-watt, and 60-watt surgical Diomed lasers (Universal Medical Systems Inc, Bedford Hills, NY) and the 15-watt, 25-watt, and 50-watt AccuVet 980 Lasers (AccuVet Lasers, Division of Lumenis Inc, Santa Clara, Calif). Both the Diomed and AccuVet are class IV

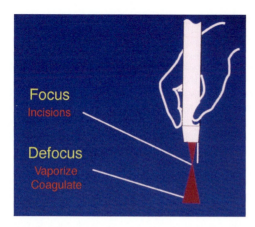

Figure 35-95 The CO_2 laser can be used with a focused beam for cutting or a defocused beam for tissue ablation. *(Photograph courtesy AccuVet Lasers.)*

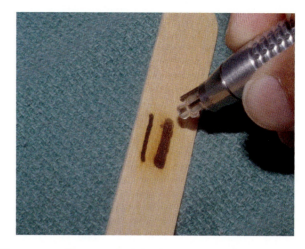

Figure 35-97 The cut on the left is from a 0.4 mm ceramic tip. On the right is a 3-mm scanner tip, used for ablating large tissue areas such as granulomas and surface infections. *(Photograph courtesy D. Mader.)*

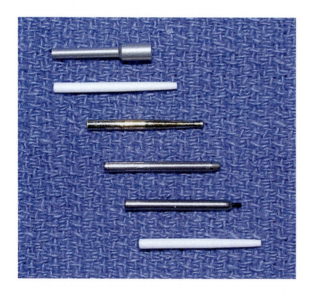

Figure 35-96 A variety of tips can be used with the CO_2 laser. Tip size affects spot size, which affects the laser-tissue interaction and power density. The smaller the tip, the more precise the cut. Shown here, top to bottom, are steel 1.4 mm, ceramic 0.8 mm, gold 0.4 mm, steel 0.4 mm, steel 0.3 mm, and ceramic 0.25 mm. *(Photograph courtesy D. Mader.)*

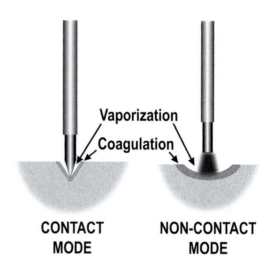

Figure 35-98 Diagrammatic comparison between contact and non-contact modes for the diode laser. Note that the areas of vaporization and coagulation are greatly limited in contact mode. *(Illustration courtesy Diomed Ltd.)*

gallium-aluminum-arsenide diode lasers. The Diomed laser creates a wavelength in the range of 810 nm, and the AccuVet uses 980 nm.

The laser beam is transmitted from the base unit to the surgical site by a solid quartz-core fiberoptic cable. A visible light beam is combined with the invisible laser beam to facilitate aiming. Laser fibers come in a variety of sizes (400 to 1000 µm) and shapes, including flat, conical, orb tips, and air/water cooled. The fibers may be used through the instrument channel of a variety of rigid and flexible endoscopes or in hand-pieces for open surgical use. Unlike the CO_2 fiber, a damaged diode fiber can be trimmed and reused.

The diode laser can be used in direct contact with tissue (contact mode) or at a distance from tissue (noncontact mode; Figure 35-98). In contact mode, the fiber tip is coated with a thin layer of carbon. This is most easily achieved by lightly burning a sterile wooden tongue depressor with the tip of the laser fiber at 10 watts. The carbonized tip absorbs virtually 100% of the laser beam, which causes the tip to instantly heat up to ablative tissue temperatures at relatively low power settings, usually just a few watts.[65] The heated tip can then be used to incise, excise, and coagulate tissue, and a 0.3-mm to 0.6-mm zone of thermocoagulation provides excellent hemostasis of vessels up to 2 mm in diameter. The advantages of carbonized fiber tips are minimized collateral damage and reduced tissue penetration (more comparable with those of CO_2 lasers). This is possible because of the dramatic reduction in both laser power and duration required to achieve a given superficial effect.

This carbonized-tip technique was developed by human neuroendosurgeons who, although keen to use laser technology, were concerned about the potential risks of using high-energy laser in close proximity to vital structures such as the basilar artery in third ventriculostomies.[65] Such concerns are equally applicable to exotic animal surgeons who often find themselves working inside small delicate patients. Furthermore, human neuroendosurgeons reported 100% procedural success with diode lasers with precarbonized tips.[65] For general tissue ablation, the 1000 μm orb fibers can be used, but for microsurgery or endosurgery, the 400 to 600 μm fibers with carbonized microconical tips provide much greater accuracy and finer control.

In noncontact mode, the laser is aimed at the tissue from a short distance. The degree of tissue penetration, coagulation, and vaporization depends on laser type and power setting, duration of exposure, and tissue characteristics (e.g., water content, hemoglobin content, and pigmentation; see Figure 35-94 and Figure 35-99). Generally, the diode lasers can penetrate tissue to a greater degree than other lasers (up to 4 mm in nonpigmented tissue) in noncontact mode. Penetration is greatly reduced to around 0.3 mm when carbonized tips are used in contact mode. The higher wavelength of the 980-nm diode laser may provide an advantage of being less affected by tissue pigmentation and more selective for water and hemoglobin. In practice, contact mode is more accurate and controllable, and noncontact mode is more diffuse with deeper penetration.

For open surgery, the laser fiber is usually housed within a hand-piece that is held much like a pen. The fiber tip is gently stroked across the tissue, either in contact or noncontact modes, until the desired incision or ablative effect is obtained. When used down the operating channel of an endoscope, the fiber is used in contact mode and the entire scope-fiber unit is moved as one. Gentle stroking movements of the scope-fiber unit are used to produce the desired effect, and always under direct visual control.

Power settings tend to vary: 2 to 4 watts for endoscopic surgery, 4 to 8 watts for general surgery, and 5 to 10 watts for tissue ablation. For general surgery, the power is usually continuous, but with very delicate structures, a pulsed output is preferred. Pulsing gives time for the tissue to cool during the interpulse periods and helps reduce collateral thermal damage. The pulse duration and interpulse interval can both be varied to give complete control.

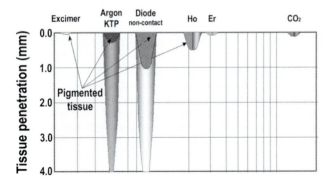

Figure 35-99 Diagrammatic representation of the different tissue penetrations of various lasers in pigmented and nonpigmented tissue. Note that the penetration of the diode laser in noncontact mode is more affected by pigmentation than is the CO_2 laser. *(Illustration courtesy AccuVet Lasers.)*

RADIOSURGERY EQUIPMENT

Electrical current has been used in medical equipment for more than a century. Traditional electrocautery consists of a platinum wire heated with an electric current and has the ability to both cut and coagulate tissues. Further development led to the advent of alternating current and transformer circuitry, which could produce high-electric currents that were used in medicine to coagulate, cut, and destroy tissues. In 1978, Maness showed that 3.8 MHz was a preferred frequency for cutting soft tissues. This frequency served as the starting point for modern radiosurgery units but has been recently surpassed with the development of 4-MHz units.

Surgery performed with a modern radiosurgical unit should not be confused with the results obtained with electrocautery, medical diathermy, spark gap generators, or partially rectified devices that do not provide surgical cutting waveforms. Radiowave surgery is an atraumatic method of cutting and coagulating soft tissue, without the postoperative pain and tissue destruction reported after electrocautery. The cutting effect, known as electrosection, is performed without manual pressure or crushing tissue cells. It results from heat generated by the resistance the tissues offer to the passage of a radiofrequency wave, which is applied with a fine wire called a surgical electrode. The heat vaporizes intracellular water and destroys the cells in the path of the waves. Electrocoagulation is the nonvolatilizing destruction of tissue cells by a radiofrequency wave.

The minimally traumatic nature of electrosection provides a noteworthy advantage over traditional electrical devices. The reduced trauma results in reduced swelling, scar formation, and postoperative discomfort. The other advantage is that the electrodes are also self-sterilizing in use. Unlike electrocautery, radiosurgery offers superior accuracy and reduced collateral damage, similar to CO_2 laser incisions. Histologic studies involving human skin peel grafts concluded that radiosurgery produces less epidermal loss, reduced zone of thermal damage, and reduced dermal fibrosis than the CO_2 laser.[66] In other comparative studies including turbinate ablation and resection, biopsy collection, and effects on oviductal tissue, radiosurgery was comparable with or superior to laser.[67-69]

The two main models available are the 3.8-MHz and the 4.0-MHz dual radiofrequency Surgitron (Ellman International Inc), both of which offer monopolar/bipolar applications with foot-pedal/finger switch control for several waveforms (Figure 35-100):

1. A pure filtered wave form (pure microsmooth cutting; Figure 35-101, *A*). This is used for skin incisions and wire loop excisions where hemostasis is not expected to be a problem. This waveform gives the least lateral heat and is comparable with or better than CO_2 laser incisions.[69]
2. A fully rectified waveform (blended cutting and coagulation; Figure 35-101, *B*). This is used where slight bleeding might be expected. It cuts and coagulates small blood vessels and gives slight lateral heat to the tissues.
3. A partially rectified waveform (Figure 35-101, *C*). This is primarily for hemostasis; it cannot be used for cutting but is excellent for coagulation.

4. A fulgurating current (spark-gap tissue destruction; Figure 35-101, *D*). This is very similar to the unipolar diathermy and gives superficial tissue damage by holding the needle electrode close to the tissue and allowing a stream of sparks to burn the tissues. It is suitable for superficial hemostasis and destruction of cysts and superficial neoplasms.
5. Bipolar coagulation (Figure 35-101, *E*). Very precise hemostasis may be obtained with bipolar forceps. Each blade is connected to the radiosurgical unit so that the current passes between the points of the forceps.

All the previous selections are effected through buttons and displays that give the operator feedback of status. Power level for each mode is indicated by front panel digital displays, which also show the status of self-test and monitoring. The final output power control is made through foot or hand switches. An internal memory provides a special feature for the storage of all the front settings, mode, and power output levels.

Monopolar cutting needles are typically used for dissection, wire loops for tissue biopsies, and bipolar forceps for sealing blood vessels (see Figure 35-100). In addition, a wide variety of standard, microsurgical, and endoscopic instruments are available for use with radiosurgery, which makes it a more versatile technology for veterinary practice.

TISSUE EFFECTS AND HEALING

Very few scientific studies in exotic animal species have assessed either the effects of laser or radiosurgery on tissues or the healing process after surgery. The effects of YAG and CO_2 laser tenotomies of flexor digitorum profundus muscles in rabbits were used to evaluate the effects of laser on collagen tissue.[70] The most consistent observation was variable carbonization (charring) in most cases. Studies on the morphologic consequences of thermosurgery and carbonization in human tissue biopsies and rat organs have shown areas of necrosis, coagulation, and edema, with cellular granulation predominantly by giant cells.

Laser surgery on the buccal mucosa of rats was performed to assess the effects on lymphatic vessels and whether laser tumor resection may lead to iatrogenic metastases via the lymphatics.[71] This study showed that lymphatic vessels are absent from the area of carbonization, occluded by coagulation in the zone of necrosis, and dilated within the zone of edema. The authors concluded that laser resection of tumors was unlikely to result in lymphatic spread. The regeneration of lymphatics was correlated to overall wound healing, being delayed

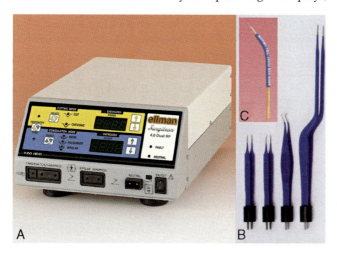

Figure 35-100 A, The 4-MHz dual-frequency Surgitron unit. **B,** Bipolar forceps and, **C,** monopolar cutting electrode. *(Photographs courtesy Ellman International Inc.)*

Figure 35-101 Different radiosurgery waveforms and their surgical uses. *(Illustration courtesy Ellman International Inc.)*

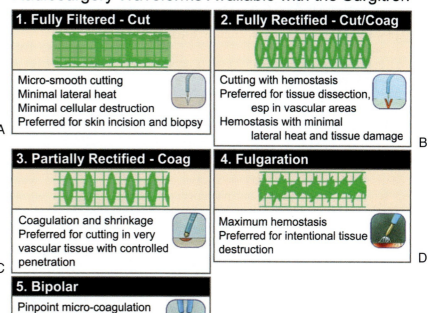

with laser (CO_2 more so than YAG) compared with conventional surgery.

Other studies have confirmed this delayed primary intention wound healing after laser surgery. This delay is primarily from temporary postponement of inflammation, phagocytic resorption, collagen production, and reepithelialization in the early stages of wound healing.[72,73] Later stages of healing compensate, and **laser incisions typically have less scarring than scalpel incisions.**

Healing in rats after hepatectomy with scalpel, electrical diathermy, and laser was followed both at the macroscopic and molecular level.[74] Tissue damage, inflammation, infection, and delayed healing were more common with diathermy, less so with laser, and least after scalpel surgery. Liver regeneration and restoration of function, as determined by protein biosynthesis, started 1 day after scalpel surgery and 2 days after laser or diathermy surgery.

In contrast, the improved healing after laser welding of tissues, compared with conventional surgery, has also been reliably reported, at least in the laboratory rabbit and rat. Clinical and histologic evaluations of small bowel and uterine horn anastomoses with laser welding have resulted in excellent recoveries and primary intention healing with reduced necrosis and inflammation.[75,76] In conclusion, tissue-cooling techniques with moistened gauze during laser surgery combined with low power or pulsed modes of laser delivery and the gentle removal of char result in more rapid favorable healing.[72] Wounds sutured after laser surgery typically heal at a similar pace to those created by sharp incision (i.e., 5 to 10 days in birds, 7 to 14 days in mammals, and 4 to 8 weeks in reptiles).

Several human clinical studies have compared radiosurgery with laser surgery. A study that compared the radiosurgical and CO_2 laser resection of turbinates in humans revealed that although both methodologies were equally effective at completing the procedure and resolving nasal obstruction, CO_2 laser resulted in significantly greater disturbance of mucociliary function.[66] Another comparative study that involved surgery of human oviducts revealed that radiosurgery was the least traumatic instrument used, with CO_2 laser second.[69]

Even fewer studies have compared postoperative pain and complications. However, two independent studies evaluated pain after soft palate resection in humans; both concluded that radiosurgery produced less postoperative pain than CO_2 laser.[77,78] Radiosurgery patients typically had discomfort for 2.6 days after surgery, and 9% needed narcotic analgesics, whereas laser patients experienced pain for 13.8 days, and 100% needed narcotic analgesics.[77] In addition, postoperative side effects (trouble with smell and taste, pharyngeal dryness, globus sensation, voice change, and pharyngonasal reflux) and complications (wound infection, dehiscence, and posterior pillar narrowing) were more common after laser surgery than radiosurgery.[78]

LASER AND RADIOFREQUENCY SAFETY

To prevent retinal damage to personnel in the operating room, protective glasses must be worn at all times that lasers are in use. The safety glasses need to be appropriate for the

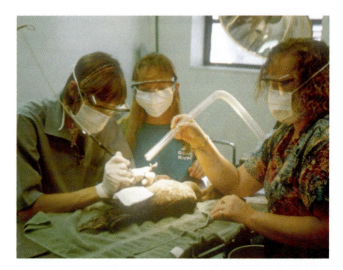

Figure 35-102 Protective glasses and facemasks should be worn by all personal to avoid laser-induced retinal damage and the aspiration of laser smoke. A smoke evacuator with a viral filter is required whenever the laser is in use. *(Photograph courtesy D. Mader.)*

wavelength of the laser used. For instance, safety glasses safe for a diode laser do NOT protect eyes against damage from a CO_2 laser. Likewise, the patient's eyes should be protected by gauze or drapes, unless one is specifically operating on the ocular tissues. No such human health issues occur with the use of radiosurgery.

The use of laser or radiosurgery on tissue produces a smoke plume that may contain pyrolysis products that are known to be cytotoxic.[79] This smoke, which has been documented to contain DNA, bacteria, and viruses, should always be evacuated with a filtered vacuum. In addition, viral-safe facemasks are also strongly recommended (Figure 35-102).

LASERS IN HERPETOLOGIC SURGERY

The diode laser has been successfully used for various procedures in reptiles including coeliotomy, ovariosalpingectomy, ovariectomy, orchidectomy, cystotomy, enterotomy, enterectomy, abscess/neoplasm excision, tail/limb/digit amputation, oral surgery, enucleation, and transendoscopic ablation of lesions within the respiratory tract and coelom. The ability to incise skin with the 810-nm laser is more problematic because of variable skin pigmentation and keratinization, and charring is more obvious. However, incisions through muscle, bladder, oviduct, and intestine are straightforward with no bleeding or clinically apparent delay in wound healing (Figure 35-103).

The CO_2 laser effectively cuts through reptile skin unless osteoderms (bones in the scales) are present because the laser does not cut through bone (Figure 35-104). If bone is present, the bone heats up and burns. In general, if one is uncertain whether or not osteoderms are present, if bones can be seen on a radiograph, the laser should not be used (see Figure 15-4).

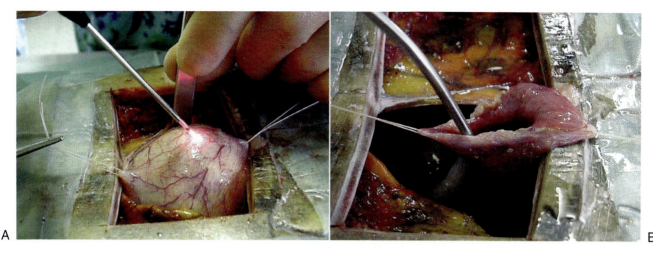

Figure 35-103 **A,** Laser cystotomy (contact mode) in an African Spurred Tortoise *(Geochelone sulcata).* **B,** The cystotomy site after laser incision; note the minimal char associated with the appropriate use of the laser. *(Photographs courtesy S.J. Hernandez-Divers.)*

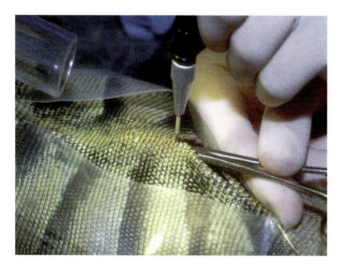

Figure 35-104 Ventral midline incision in a Green Iguana *(Iguana iguana)* using a CO_2 laser. A cutting tip is used, which easily penetrates reptilian skin. A nonreflective hemostat is used as a backstop under the skin to prevent internal damage from the laser's beam as it makes the cut. *(Photograph courtesy D. Mader.)*

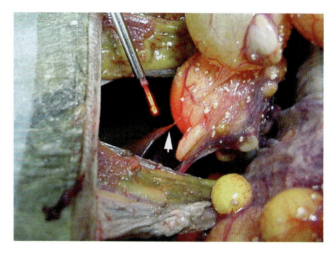

Figure 35-105 Using the laser (contact mode) to separate adhesions between the liver and ovary in a Hermann's Tortoise *(Testudo hermanni)* with postovulatory egg stasis and oophoritis. *(Photograph courtesy S.J. Hernandez-Divers.)*

The laser has also been particularly useful for dissection of abscesses and large granulomas free from adherent tissues (see Chapter 42) and for breaking down adhesions between coelomic viscera, particularly between the liver and ovaries in tortoises (Figure 35-105). Laser coagulation of large vessels such as those that supply the oviducts of larger reptiles, particularly iguanas, is best achieved with the diode laser in noncontact mode because contact tends to result in rupture and bleeding (Figure 35-106). Care is required to mask off surroundings areas with damp gauze to prevent deeper penetration and avoid increased thermal damage (Figure 35-107).

The diode laser has also been used endoscopically (in contact mode) to effect hemostasis after endoscopic surgery and splenic biopsies and to endoscopically ablate small granulomas within the coelom or lung.

Both the diode and CO_2 lasers have been used in amphibians to remove cutaneous lesions and neoplasms. In cases in which dermatologic lesions were removed and the surgical sites were permitted to heal with second intention, subjective assessments indicated that postoperative infections were reduced compared with either radiosurgery or sharp excision.

Incising through the thin amphibian integument for coeliotomy is not as difficult as in reptiles, and charring is reduced (Figure 35-108). Laser incisions through the coelomic structures are uncomplicated, and enterotomy procedures are rapidly performed with minimal charring.

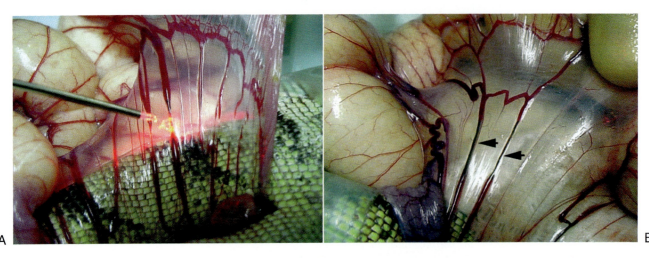

Figure 35-106 **A,** Coagulating the large oviductal blood vessels in a Green Iguana *(Iguana iguana)* using a flat fiber in noncontact mode. **B,** After noncontact laser treatment the blood vessels are contracted and darkened from hemoglobin coagulation *(arrows)*, and can be safely cut without fear of hemorrhage. *(Photographs courtesy S.J. Hernandez-Divers.)*

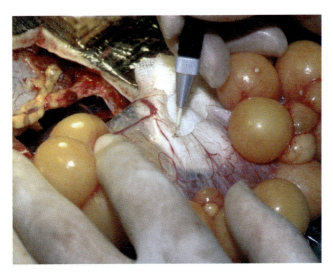

Figure 35-107 A CO_2 laser is being used to photo-coagulate ovarian vessels in a tortoise. Note the moistened gauze placed behind the mesovarium to protect adjacent tissues from laser penetration. *(Photograph courtesy D. Mader.)*

RADIOFREQUENCY IN HERPETOLOGIC SURGERY

Monopolar radiosurgery cutting electrodes can cut through most reptile skin, with the exception of large scales, scutes, and osteoderms. The modern handles can be preprogrammed so that the surgeon can select cutting, cut and coagulation, and fulgurate modes from the hand-piece without changing the settings on the machine (Figure 35-109). Similar cutting electrodes or bipolar forceps can be used to incise coelomic muscles and membranes. With use of bipolar forceps like the Harrison tips, one tip is introduced through a small incision below the tissue and the other is opposed from above. Bipolar activation during withdrawal of the forceps results in the tissue being incised without any risk of penetration deeper into the coelom (Figure 35-110). The 4-MHz Surgitron enables both monopolar and bipolar use simultaneously, making easy the move from one hand-piece to the next without engaging the technical support. Bipolar forceps are used most commonly to arrest hemorrhage from individual vessels but can also be used to stop capillary bed bleeding (Figure 35-111). However, both monopolar and bipolar are useful for dissecting neoplasms, abscesses, and granulomas and transecting or resecting tissues (Figure 35-112).

Radiosurgery has also been used during endoscopic surgery in reptiles and amphibians. The ability to achieve accurate hemostasis is essential during minimally invasive surgery, and radiosurgery units are readily accepted by most endoscopic instruments, turning them into monopolar radiosurgical instruments, or dedicated bipolar forceps (Figure 35-113).

SUMMARY

Laser and radiosurgery are emerging disciplines within zoo and exotic animal surgery. The current list of indications is certain to grow as this technology is further utilized. In the future, those procedures already developed in areas of human medicine, including ophthalmology, gastroenterology, urology, neurology, and gynecology, will continue to filter into the veterinary profession. In addition, the small and delicate nature of many of our exotic species will drive further developments in endoscopic and other minimally invasive procedures.

ACKNOWLEDGMENTS

The authors thank Diomed Ltd and Universal Medical Systems Inc, for the loan of the Diomed 60 Surgical Laser, and Ellman International.

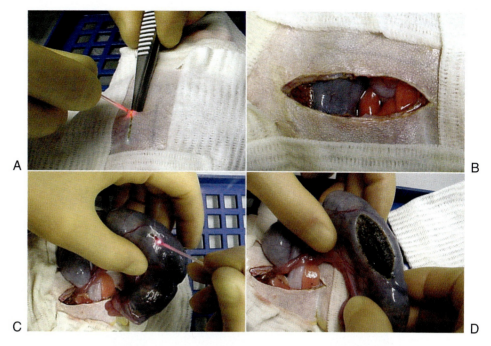

Figure 35-108 Laser coeliotomy and enterotomy in an Argentine Horned Frog *(Ceratophrys ornata)*. **A,** Laser coeliotomy using the diode laser in contact mode; **B,** the coeliotomy incision is essentially bloodless with little carbonization of the wound edges; **C,** laser enterotomy using contact mode; **D,** the enterotomy incision is bloodless with no evidence of char. *(Photographs courtesy S.J. Hernandez-Divers.)*

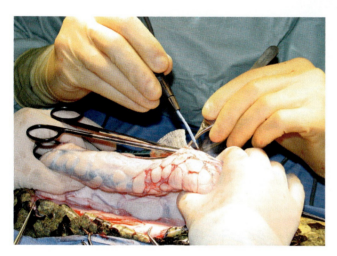

Figure 35-109 Incising through the thickened oviduct of an Anaconda *(Eunectes murinus)* using a monopolar cutting electrode. *(Photograph courtesy S.J. Hernandez-Divers.)*

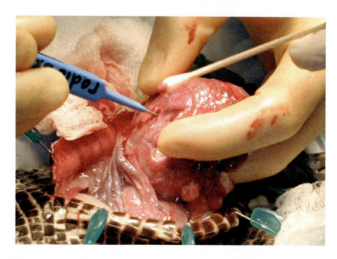

Figure 35-111 Pinpoint coagulation of an oviductal blood vessel using bipolar forceps. *(Photograph courtesy S.J. Hernandez-Divers.)*

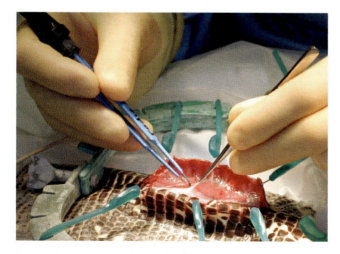

Figure 35-110 Bipolar incision through the coelomic musculature of a Beaded Lizard *(Heloderma horridum)* using bipolar Harrison tips. *(Photograph courtesy S.J. Hernandez-Divers.)*

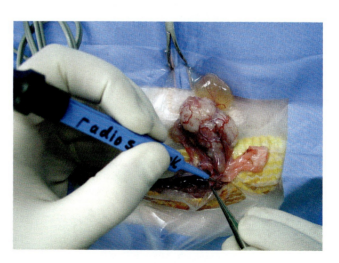

Figure 35-112 Bipolar coagulation and dissection of a granulosa cell tumor from a Cornsnake *(Elaphe guttata)*. *(Photograph courtesy S.J. Hernandez-Divers.)*

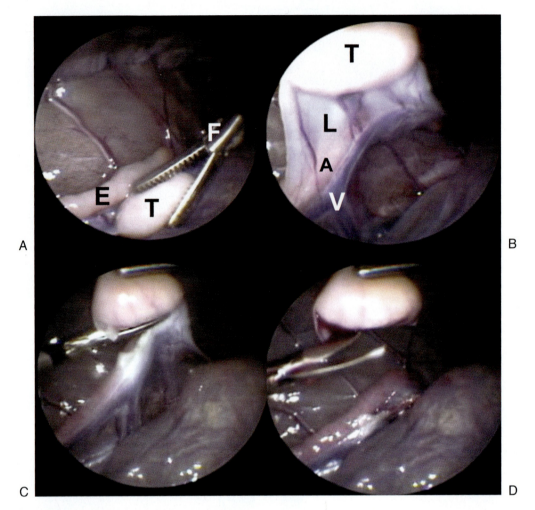

Figure 35-113 A Male Green Iguana *(Iguana iguana)* undergoing endoscopic orchidectomy using monopolar radiosurgery to ensure hemostasis. **A,** The grasping forceps *(F)* are used to grasp the ventral edge of the testis *(T)* as it lies adjacent to the epididymis *(E)*. **B,** The testis *(T)* is elevated revealing the testicular ligament *(L)* and associated blood vessels, the adrenal gland *(A)*, and the renal vein *(V)*. **C,** Scissors with monopolar radiosurgery are used to dissect the testis free. **D,** The testis is removed through the trocar hole. Note the lack of bleeding from the surgical site. *(Photographs courtesy S.J. Hernandez-Divers.)*

REFERENCES

1. Bennett RA: Reptilian surgery: part I: basic principles, *Compend Cont Ed Pract Vet* 11:10, 1989.
2. Smith DA, Barker IA, Allen OB: The effect of ambient temperature and type of wound on the healing of cutaneous wounds in the common garter snake *(Thamnophis sirtalis)*, *Can J Vet Res* 52:120-128, 1988.
3. Millichamp NJ, Lawrence K, Jacobson ER, et al: Egg retention in snakes, *J Am Vet Med Assoc* 183:1213, 1983.
4. Govett PD, Harms CA, Linder KE, Marsh JC, Wyneken J: Effect of four different suture materials on the surgical wound healing of Loggerhead Sea Turtles, *Caretta caretta*, *J Herp Med Surg* 14(4):6-11, 2004.
5. Bennett RA: Reptilian surgery: part II: management of surgical diseases, *Compend Cont Ed Pract Vet* 11:122, 1989.
6. McCracken HE: Organ location in snakes for diagnostic and surgical evaluation. In Miller RE, editor: *Zoo and wildlife medicine, current therapy 4*, Philadelphia, 1999, WB Saunders.
7. Patterson RW, Smith A: Surgical intervention to relieve dystocia in a python, *Vet Rec* 104(24):551, 1979.
8. Frye FL: *Biomedical and surgical aspects of captive reptile husbandry*, Edwardsville, Kan, 1981, Veterinary Medicine Publishing.
9. Oldham JC, Smith HM: *Laboratory anatomy of the iguana*, Dubuque, Iowa, 1975, Wm. C. Brown.
10. Mader DR, Wyneken J: The anatomy and clinical significance of the renal portal vein and ventral abdominal vein in reptiles, *Proc Assoc Rept Amphib Vet* 183-186, 2002.
11. Mangone B, Johnson JD. Surgical removal of a cystic calculi via the inguinal fossa and other techniques applicable to the approach in the Desert Tortoise, *Gopherus agzzizii*, *Proc Assoc Amphib Rept Ann Conf* 87-88, 1998.
12. Peters AR, Coote J: Dystocia in a snake, *Vet Rec* 100(20):423, 1977.
13. Backus KA, Ramsey EC: Ovariectomy for treatment of follicular stress in lizards, *J Zoo Wildl Med* 25:111, 1994.
14. Mader DR, Ling GV, Ruby AL: Cystic calculi in the California Desert Tortoise *(Gopherus agassizii)*: evaluation of 100 cases, *Proc Assoc Amphib Rept Ann Conf* 81-82, 1999.
15. Frye FL. Surgical removal of a cystic calculus from a desert tortoise, *J Am Vet Med Assoc* 15:161(6):600-602, 1972.

16. Mangone B, Johnson JD: Surgical removal of a cystic calculi via the inguinal fossa and other techniques applicable to the approach in the Desert Tortoise, *Gopherus agzzizii*, Proc Assoc Amphib Rept Annual Conf 87-88, 1998.
17. Frye FL: Colo-rectal atresia and its surgical repair in a juvenile amelanistic Burmese python, *J Sm Exotic Anim Med* 2(4):149, 1994.
18. Gould WJ, Yaeger AE, Glenn JC: Surgical correction of an intestinal obstruction in a turtle, *J Am Vet Med Assoc* 200:705, 1992.
19. Isenbugel E, Barandum G: Surgical removal of a foreign body in a bastard turtle, *VM SAC* 76(12):1766, 1981.
20. Jacobson ER, Ingling AL: Pyloroduodenal resection in a Burmese python, *J Am Vet Med Assoc* 169(9):985, 1976.
21. Rosskoph WJ, Woerpel RW, Pitts BJ, et al: Abdominal surgery in turtles and tortoises, *Anim Health Tech* 4(6):326, 1983.
22. Bennett RA, Mader DR: Soft tissue surgery. In Mader DR, editor: *Reptile medicine and surgery*, Philadelphia, 1996, WB Saunders.
23. Bodri MS, Sandanage KK: Circumcostal colopexy in a Python, *JAVMA* 198(2):297, 1991.
24. Diethelm G, Stauber E, Tillson M, Ridgley S: Tracheal resection and anastomosis for an intratracheal chondroma in a ball python, *JAVMA* 209:786-788, 1996.
25. Drew ML, Phalen DN, Berridge BR, Johnson TL, Weeks BR, Miller HA, et al: Partial tracheal obstruction due to tracheal chondromas in Ball Pythons (*Python regius*), *J Zoo Wildl Med* 30:151-157, 1999.
26. Frye FL: *Biomedical and surgical aspect of captive reptile husbandry*, ed 2, Melbourne, Fla, 1991, Kreiger Publishing.
27. Bennett RA: Fracture management. In Mader DR, editor: *Reptile medicine and surgery*, Philadelphia, 1996, WB Saunders.
28. Crane S, Curtis M, Jacobson ER, et al: Neutralization bone plating repair of a fractured humerus in an Aldabra tortoise, *J Am Vet Med Assoc* 177(9):945, 1980.
29. Robinson PT, Sedgwick CJ, Meier JE, et al: Internal fixation of a humerus fracture in a Komodo dragon lizard, *VM SAC* 73(5):645, 1978.
30. Redisch RI: Management of leg fractures in the iguana, *VM SAC* 72(9):1487, 1977.
31. Hartman RA: Use of an intramedullary pin in repair of a midshaft humeral fracture in a green iguana, *VM SAC* 71(11):1634, 1976.
32. Redisch RI: Repair of a fractured femur in an iguana, *VM SAC* 73(12):1547, 1978.
33. Egger EL: External skeletal fixation: general principles. In Slatter D, editor: *Textbook of small animal surgery*, vol 2, ed 2, Philadelphia, 1993, WB Saunders.
34. Brinker WO, Piermatti DL, Flo GL: Bone grafting. In *Handbook of small animal orthopedics and fracture treatment*, Philadelphia, 1997, WB Saunders.
35. Mader DR, Kerr L: Treatment of a non-union fracture of the tibia in a chinese water dragon, including stimulation of osteogenesis with a direct electric current, *JAVMA Wildlife Issue* 189:1141-1142, 1986.
36. Kuehn G: Bilateral transverse mandibular fractures in a turtle, *Proc Am Assoc Zoo Vet* 243, 1973.
37. Divers SJ, Lawton MPC: Antibiotic impregnated methylmethacrylate beads as a treatment for osteomyelitis in reptiles, *Proc Assoc Rept Amphib Vet* 145-147, 1999.
38. Hernandez-Divers SJ: Diagnosis and repair of a stifle luxation in a spur-thighed tortoise (*Testudo graeca*), *J Zoo Wildl Med* 33:125-130, 2002.
39. Barten SL: Treatment of a chronic coxofemoral luxation by femoral head and neck excision arthroplasty in a white-throated monitor (*Varanus albigularis*), *Bull Assoc Rept Amphib Vet* 6:10-13, 1996.
40. Coke RL: External skeletal fixation of bilateral sacroiliac luxations in a savannah monitor, *Varanus exanthematicus*, *Bull Assoc Rept Amphib Vet* 9:4-7, 1999.
41. Weigel JP: Amputations. In Slatter D, editor: *Textbook of small animal surgery*, ed 2, Philadelphia, 1993, WB Saunders.
42. Lutz ME: Surgical and conservative tail repair in iguanas, *J Sm Exotic Anim Med* 1(3):128, 1992.
43. Martin JC. Successful use of physical therapy in resolving a chronic lameness in a large radiated tortoise (*Geochelone radiata*), *Proc Assoc Rept Amphib Vets* 25-26, 2005.
44. Amlaner CJ, McDonald DW, editors: *A handbook on biotelemetry and radio tracking*. Oxford, 1979, Pergamon.
45. Mech D: *Handbook of animal radio-tracking*, Minneapolis, 1980, University of Minnesota Press.
46. Amlaner CJ, editor: *Biotelemetry X*, Fayetteville, 1989, University of Arkansas Press.
47. Karesh WB: Applications of biotelemetry in wildlife medicine. In Fowler ME, Miller RE, editors: *Zoo and wildlife medicine: current therapy 4*, Philadelphia, 1989, WB Saunders.
48. Thompson SP: Biotelemetric studies on mammalian thermoregulation. In Asa C, editor: *Biotelemetry applications to captive animal care and research*, Bethesda, Md, 1991, American Association of Zoological Parks and Aquariums.
49. Korschagen CE, Maxson SJ, Luechle VB: Evaluation of implanted transmitters in ducks, *J Wildl Manage* 48:982-987, 1984.
50. Perry MC: Abnormal behavior of canvasbacks equipped with radio transmitters, *J Wildl Manage* 45:786-789, 1981.
51. Sorenson MD: Effects of neck collar radio on female redheads, *J Field Ornith* 60:523-528, 1989.
52. Foster CC, et al: Survival and reproduction of radio-marked adult spotted owls, *J Wildl Manage* 56: 91-95, 1992.
53. Reynolds PS: White blood cell profiles as a means of evaluating transmitter implant surgery in small mammals, *J Mamm* 73:178-185, 1992.
54. Polanyi TG: Physics of the surgical laser, *Adv Surg Oncol* 1:205-215, 1978.
55. Klause SE, Roberts SM: Lasers and veterinary surgery, *Compend Contin Educ Pract Vet* 12:1565-1571, 1574-1576, 1990.
56. Mader DR: Use of laser in exotic animal medicine, *Vet Pract News* 12:1, 2000.
57. Dvoral L, Bennett RA, Cranor K: Cloacotomy for excision of cloacal papillomas in Catalina Macaw, *J Avian Med Surg* 12:11-15, 1998.
58. Parrott T: Using the CO_2 laser in avian practice, *Proc Conf Assoc Avian Vet* 21, 1998.
59. Hernandez-Divers SJ: Endoscopic diode laser surgery in birds, *Exotic DVM* 3(3):73-74, 2001.
60. Mader DR: The use of lasers in exotic animal surgery, *Exotic DVM* 3(3):70-72, 2001.
61. Mader DR: The use of lasers in reptile medicine, *Proc 7th Assoc Reptil Amphib Vet Conf* 123-125, 2000.
62. DeRowe A, Landsberg R, Leonov Y, Katzir A, Ophir D: Subjective comparison of Nd:YAG, diode, and CO_2 lasers for endoscopically guided inferior turbinate reduction surgery, *Am J Rhinol* 12:209-212, 1998.
63. Morita T, Okamura Y, Ookubo K, Tanaka K, Hirayama R, Daikuzono N: A new instrument for hemostatic vascular management in endoscopic surgery: diode laser (STATLase-SDL) and its hand-piece (dual hook), *J Clin Laser Med Surg* 17:57-61, 1999.
64. Nagatani T, Saito K, Yoshida J: Experimental use of semiconductor diode laser for neuroendoscopic surgery, *Minim Invasive Neurosurg* 40:98-100, 1997.
65. Vandertop WP, Verdaasdonk RM, van Swol CF: Laser-assisted neuroendoscopy using a neodymium-yttrium aluminium garnet or diode contact laser with pretreated fiber tips, *J Neurosurgery* 88:82-92, 1998.

66. Acland KM, Calonje E, Seed PT, Stat C, Barlow RJ: A clinical and histologic comparison of electrosurgical and carbon dioxide laser peels, *J Am Acad Dermatol* 44:492-496, 2001.
67. Sapci T, Sahin B, Karavus A, Akbulut UG: Comparison of the effects of radiofrequency tissue ablation, CO_2 laser ablation, and partial turbinectomy applications on nasal mucociliary functions, *Laryngoscope* 113:514-519, 2003.
68. Turner RJ, Cohen RA, Voet RL, Stephens SR, Weinstein SA: Analysis of tissue margins of cone biopsy specimens obtained with "cold knife," CO_2 and Nd:YAG lasers and a radiofrequency surgical unit, *J Reprod Med* 37:607-610, 1992.
69. Olivar AC, Forouhar FA, Gillies CG, Servanski DR: Transmission electron microscopy: evaluation of damage in human oviducts caused by different surgical instruments, *Ann Clin Lab Sci* 29:281-285, 1999.
70. Gebauer D, Constantinescu MA: Effect of surgical laser on collagen-rich tissue (article in German), *Handchir Mikrochir Plast Chir* 32:38-43, 2000.
71. Werner JA, Lippert BM, Schunke M, Rudert H: Animal experiment studies of laser effects on lymphatic vessels. a contribution to the discussion of laser surgery segmental resection of carcinomas [article in German], *Laryngorhinootologie* 74:748-755, 1995.
72. Hendrick DA, Meyers A: Wound healing after laser surgery, *Otolaryngol Clin North Am* 28:969-986, 1995.
73. Nevorotin AL, Kull' MM: Electron histochemical characteristics of laser necrosis [article in Russian], *Arkh Patol* 7:63-70, 1989.
74. Chinali G, Ferulano GP, Vanni L, et al: Liver regeneration after atypical hepatectomy in the rat. a comparison of CO_2 laser with scalpel and electrical diathermy, *Eur Surg Res* 15:284-288, 1983.
75. Sauer JS, Hinshaw JR, McGuire KP: The first sutureless, laser-welded, end-to-end bowel anastomosis, *Lasers Surg Med* 9:70-73, 1989.
76. Shapiro AG, Carter M, Ahmed A, Sielszak MW: Conventional reanastomosis versus laser welding of rat uterine horns, *Am J Obstet Gynecol* 156:1006-1009, 1987.
77. Troell RJ, Powell NB, Riley RW, Li KK, Guilleminault C: Comparison of postoperative pain between laser-assisted uvulopalatoplasty, uvulopalatopharyngoplasty, and radiofrequency volumetric tissue reduction of the palate, *Otolaryngol Head Neck Surg* 122:402-409, 2000.
78. Rombaux P, Hamoir M, Bertrand B, Aubert G, Liistro G, Rodenstein D: Postoperative pain and side effects after uvulopalatopharyngoplasty, laser-assisted uvulopalatoplasty, and radiofrequency tissue volume reduction in primary snoring, *Laryngoscope* 113:2169-2173, 2003.
79. Plappert UG, Stocker B, Helbig R, Fliedner TM, Seidel HJ: Laser pyrolysis products—genotoxic, clastogenic and mutagenic effects of the particulate aerosol fractions, *Mutat Res* 441:29-41, 1999.

36
THERAPEUTICS

MARK A. MITCHELL

The class Reptilia is composed of more than 7510 species and is divided into four orders: Squamata (Serpentes, 2900 sp.; Lacertilia, 4300 sp.), Chelonia (285 sp.), Crocodylia (23 sp.), and Sphenodontida (2 sp.).[1] Although on the surface the grouping of these four orders into one class suggests similarities among the 7510 species, in fact a high degree of variability exists between the orders and even within genera. This variation is evident not only in the behavior of these animals but also in their physiology. For the veterinarian attempting to develop a therapeutic plan to manage a captive reptile, these differences can prove overwhelming.

A paucity of rigorous scientific studies to determine the specific medical requirements for reptiles further limits the veterinary clinician. Although the management of reptile cases generally follows those guidelines established for birds and mammals, those guidelines can also prove disastrous in other cases. Unlike the higher vertebrates, reptiles are ectotherms and are intimately tied to the environment. Metabolic rate and immune response can vary with environmental conditions. In consideration of therapeutic options for the reptile, including fluid therapy and chemotherapeutics, the veterinarian must optimize the environmental conditions for the reptile to ensure the overall success of a case.

Veterinarians who work with reptiles should develop an understanding of the specific requirements of the reptiles to ensure that they can make informed decisions regarding the care of their patients.

DEVELOPMENT OF A THERAPEUTIC PLAN

Environmental Considerations

Reptiles are ectotherms and depend on environmental temperatures to regulate core body temperature. A number of physiologic factors are affected by the reptile's body temperature, including metabolic rate, heart rate, immune function, embryologic development, and reproductive activity.[2,3] Although a reptile generally maintains a body temperature similar to that of its environment, exceptions do occur. Strel'nikov[4] found *Lacerta agilis* in a montane environment (13,100 feet) to have body temperatures 29.2°C above the environmental temperature. Whereas the body temperature of domestic pet mammals is not generally an important consideration in selection and prescription of a therapeutic for these animals, it is an important consideration for veterinarians who work with reptiles.

Body temperatures for reptiles are highly variable. In a combination of reports of reptilian body temperatures from the literature and data he collected, Brattsstrom[5] published a report of cloacal and deep groin (chelonians) temperatures for 161 species of reptiles.

The range of body temperatures compiled for 13 species of chelonians was 8°C to 37.8°C, with a mean of 28.4°C. The temperature range compiled for 89 species of lizards was 11°C to 46°C (mean, 29.1°C), and the range for 57 species of snakes was 9°C to 38°C (mean, 29.1°C). The lowest body temperatures were recorded for the Tuatara *Sphenodon* sp. (range, 6.2°C to 18°C; mean, 12.5°C), and the American Alligator (*Alligator mississipiensis*) had the highest range of body temperatures (range, 26°C to 37°C; mean, 32°C to 35°C). This high degree of variability in body temperatures between reptilian groups and within species reinforces the amazing physiologic changes that can occur in these animals on a daily basis and the reptile's need for an environmental gradient of temperature.

Although reptiles lack the thermoregulatory function associated with the hypothalamus in higher vertebrates, they have been found to self-regulate body temperature and stimulate a fever response to control a pathogen. Vaughn[6] found that when a reptile was provided a choice between two different environmental temperatures, the reptile chose the warmer temperature in an attempt to stimulate the immune system and eradicate pathogens. Desert Iguanas (*Dipsosaurus dorsalis*) experimentally inoculated with *Aeromonas hydrophila* sought warmer areas within their habitat, whereas no alteration was seen in the behavior of the Desert Iguanas that were given a saline placebo.[7]

The provision of environmental heat or solar radiation for the captive reptile is necessary for a reptile to thermoregulate. However, exposure to excessive temperatures, or no area provided in which a reptile can lower its body temperature, can lead to a fatal hyperthermia. Baldwin[8] showed that *Chrysemys picta* exposed to lethal environmental temperatures (42.2°C) die suddenly. Once the animals achieved core temperatures greater than 27°C, they were found to be in obvious discomfort with tachypnea and frothing at the mouth. A similar series of mortalities was reported in a control group of Desert Iguanas exposed to elevated environmental temperatures for a prolonged period of time.[9]

In contrast to those studies that reported behavioral fever responses in reptiles, Warwick[10] has suggested that some reptiles in an advanced state of disease may select lower environmental temperatures rather than higher environmental temperatures. He theorized that these reptiles may undergo a "biological shut down" to reduce the activity level of an inciting pathogen. The theory was based on anecdotal experience with diseased reptiles and was not rigorously tested. However, the author has had similar experiences with reptiles with advanced disease. Bacterial pathogens are capable of activity at a wide range of temperatures. The author has successfully cultured *Salmonella* spp. from reptiles at a range of temperatures (22.2°C to 37°C). Although pathogens may remain active, other reasons may exist for why reptiles do not use more optimal temperatures, such as a general weakness. To ensure the greatest success with these cases, a thermal gradient must be provided that allows the reptile to self-regulate. In addition, clients should be made aware of the inherent dangers of hyperthermia for the pet reptile and provided assistance from the veterinarian with determination of the most appropriate environmental temperature range for the pet.

Reptile Immune Response

The immune system of the reptile is composed of humoral, cell-mediated, and innate components. Although the components of the reptile immune system are similar to those of higher vertebrates, the reptile immune system is more primitive than that described in higher vertebrates. Because the reptile is ectothermic, the reptile immune system is also dependent on the ability of the reptile to maintain an appropriate core body temperature. In the wild, diurnal reptiles bask during the early morning hours and late afternoon to increase core body temperature. In captivity, reptiles that are not provided an appropriate environmental temperature range may become hypothermic, which can affect immune function.

The humoral component of the reptile immune system functions to produce both specific immunoglobulins (IgY) and nonspecific immunoglobulins (IgM) that interact with foreign antigens and stimulate the cell-mediated immune response. Macrophages phagocitize pathogens or foreign material, process it with a cascade of enzymatic pathways, and present specific antigens to the B-cell lymphocytes for globulin production. IgM is produced first and is a large nonspecific antibody; IgY is a smaller antigen-specific antibody that may appear weeks after the initial encounter. Hyperglobulinemia is a common finding in a reptile with an inflammatory leukogram. Antibody production can be influenced by temperature, the antigen type and concentration, and the route of inoculation.[11] The cell-mediated component of the immune system uses T-cell lymphocytes to seek out and phagocytose foreign antigens. Killer T-cells probably function to eliminate viruses. Our current understanding of this component of the immune system is limited.

Lymphocyte production can be affected by stress, temperature, and season, generally decreasing during the fall and winter.[12] This could reduce the number of active T-lymphocytes that monitor the body for pathogens and the number of B-lymphocytes, which could affect antibody production. Desert Iguanas inoculated with typhoid antigen produced higher concentrations of antibodies when moved from 25°C to 35°C, and lower concentrations of antibodies were recorded when Desert Iguanas were moved from 35°C to 25°C.[12] Antibody production is not only reduced in the face of low environmental temperatures but can also be affected by prolonged high temperatures.[13]

The innate component of the reptile immune system includes the physical barriers that are found in the integument, gastrointestinal, ophthalmic, respiratory, and urogenital systems. Mucous and ciliated epithelial cells can trap pathogens before invading the host body. Disease and traumatic injuries associated with these systems can affect the reptile's ability to prevent the invasion of pathogens. Reptiles with traumatic injuries to the integument are more susceptible to infections and lose valuable moisture and body heat. In management of these cases, one must consider the physiologic and immunologic effects these injuries have on the reptile host.

A number of factors can affect the operation of the immune system in the reptile, including age, environmental temperature, stress, reproductive status, and nutritional status. Young reptiles may have a diminished humoral response because of their naïve immune system, and others may receive persistent maternal antibodies.[14] The production of sex steroids in reptiles has been associated with an inverse decline in circulating antibodies.[15-17] Environmental temperature can affect both antibody production and circulating peripheral white blood cells.

Nutritional Status

The nutritional status of the reptile is an important consideration in development of a therapeutic plan. Reptiles that are fed an inappropriate diet or provided insufficient calories may become dehydrated and have muscle wasting and necrosis, hepatic disease (lipidosis), and renal compromise. Dehydration and alterations to the major organ systems can result in variable responses to therapeutics. The pharmacokinetics of chemotherapeutics that are metabolized by the liver and excreted by the kidneys could be severely affected by alterations to these organ systems. Hypoproteinemia as a result of parasitism, nutritional deficiencies, or loss could be expected to diminish the colloidal affects in the blood and thus chemotherapeutic carrying capacities and immunoglobulin production.

Reptiles in a negative energy balance can be expected to have physiologic disturbances that can affect the management of a case. Severely malnourished reptiles that are hypokalemic and hypophosphatemic may be susceptible to refeeding syndrome, which is characterized by a rapidly fatal cardiac dysfunction.[18] Veterinarians should familiarize themselves with the specific dietary requirements for those species routinely in their care. Reptiles with a negative energy balance should be rehydrated and provided caloric replacement. See Chapter 18 for a complete discussion of reptilian nutrition.

Fluid Therapy

Most reptiles presented to veterinarians have some degree of dehydration. A number of factors can affect the hydration status of a reptile. Dehydration can occur as a result of maintaining a reptile at a low environmental temperature, and thus limiting its metabolism and desire to eat and drink, or as a result of offering an inappropriate food source, especially for those species that acquire much of their moisture through their diet. Not providing reptiles an appropriate water source can also lead to dehydration.

Characterizing the hydration status of a reptile is more difficult than in traditional pets, such as the dog or cat, because the number of physical characteristics used to assess hydration in mammals is greater than those available for reptiles. In addition, reference values for hematologic data used to assess the hydration status, such as total protein (TP; total solids on a refractometer), sodium, chloride, and hematocrit (or packed cell volume [PCV]) values, for different species of reptiles is limited. Characterization of the level of dehydration in a reptile patient is essential to establishment of an appropriate therapeutic regimen.

Dehydration can occur as a result of environmental inadequacies or as a sequela to a specific disease process.

Reptiles that are not provided water in an appropriate receptacle can quickly become dehydrated. Arboreal lizards, such as the Old World Chameleons, rarely leave the protection of the tree foliage and do not climb down to the substrate to drink from a water receptacle. To ensure adequate hydration in these species, water should be sprayed onto the foliage or allowed to pool on arboreal surfaces.

Dehydration can also occur as a result of offering animals an inappropriate diet. Many species of herbivorous reptiles acquire moisture through the vegetation that they consume. Commercial extruded pellet diets generally direct pet owners to feed the diet exclusively to the animal. Unfortunately, these diets are low in moisture and can exacerbate chronic dehydration. Likewise, insectivorous reptiles that are offered a diet composed of freeze-dried insects may also have chronic dehydration develop. Veterinarians should familiarize themselves with the dietary requirements of the reptiles presented to their hospital so that they can make specific dietary recommendations to their clients. See Chapters 4, 18, and 91 for some general guidelines.

Anecdotally, some herpetoculturists recommend limiting water access to certain tortoise species. Although wild tortoises can acquire significant moisture through their diet, in captivity, the selection of feedstuffs is limited and the moisture content may not be sufficient to meet the animal's needs. Visceral gout is a common sequella to chronic dehydration, and the author has observed this in several Sulcata Tortoises (Geochelone sulcata) that were provided limited/restricted access to water.

Low environmental humidity can also lead to dehydration in reptiles as a result of evaporative loss. Maintaining an appropriate environmental humidity in a captive enclosure can be difficult. Wood-base substrates can complicate the situation by absorbing moisture from within the environment. Several different techniques can be used to elevate the environmental humidity, including using live plants, aerating water within the enclosure with an aquarium pump and airstone, or spraying the environment with water several times per day. In general, desert environments should have humidity levels between 25% and 50%, subtropical levels between 60% and 90%, and tropical environments between 70% and 95%.

Reptiles primarily lose moisture through the gastrointestinal and respiratory tracts, although the integument and eye (nonspectacle) are also sites where moisture is lost. Diseases associated with the gastrointestinal tract (e.g., diarrhea) or traumatic injuries to the integument (e.g., thermal burns) can increase the amount of moisture lost in a reptilian patient. Herbivorous species can lose significant amounts of moisture through the gastrointestinal tract because of nondigestible plant products.[19]

The kidneys also play an important role in osmoregulation. Reptiles are metanephric, although their concentration of nephrons is significantly lower than that described in birds and mammals. Crocodilians, squamates, rhynchocephalians, and most testudines excrete uric acid as the primary end product of protein catabolism.[20] Reptiles lack a loop of Henle and therefore do not concentrate their urine. Instead, many reptiles excrete salts through extrarenal sources.[21]

Before a reptile is rehydrated, one must characterize the type of dehydration the animal has: hypertonic, isotonic, or hypotonic. Hypertonic dehydration is common in reptiles that have limited access to water or do not drink. Isotonic dehydration generally occurs as a result of hemorrhage, diarrhea, and short-term anorexia. Hypotonic dehydration is a common sequella to prolonged anorexia. Characterization of the state of dehydration is important to ensure that the reptile is rehydrated correctly.

Fluid Balance in Reptiles

In consideration of the hydration status of the reptile and development of a therapeutic plan to correct any deficiencies, a basic understanding of fluid balance in the reptile is important. Reptile total body water content is generally similar to slightly higher than that found in mammals.[22,23] However, reptiles have higher intracellular (48% to 80%) and lower extracellular (20% to 52%) fluid volumes than mammals.[23] Terrestrial species generally have a higher percentage of extracellular fluid compared with aquatic species.[23] Plasma accounts for approximately 3.3% to 7.0% of the total body weight.[19,23] A high degree of variability exists in the electrolytes important to osmoregulation in reptiles. Terrestrial species generally have higher sodium levels in the extracellular space than aquatic reptiles.[22]

Selection of an Appropriate Replacement Fluid

Historically, isotonic balanced fluids for mammals, such as lactated Ringer's solution (LRS; 273 mosm/L pH, 6.6; Abbott Laboratories, North Chicago, Ill) and Normosol (294 mosm/L pH, 6.6; Abbott Laboratories), have been used to manage dehydration in reptiles. These fluids generally expand the extracellular space without a significant shift into the intracellular space. Prolonged usage of these fluids can lead to hypokalemia. In mammals, physiologic saline solution (0.9%; 308 mosm/L pH, 5.6) is preferred for a need for a rapid expansion of the circulatory volume or for correction of hyponatremia or alkalosis. Other solutions, such as 5% dextrose (252 mosm/L pH, 4.3), are used when fluids are necessary to expand both the intracellular and the extracellular spaces. The caloric input from the glucose is probably negligible, and veterinarians should use appropriate enteral sources of nutrition to provide essential calories and nutrition. Combination fluids, such as 0.45% saline solution and 2.5% dextrose (280 mosm/L pH, 4.3), are also commercially available.

Reptiles can withstand large variation in fluid base, which enables them to survive extreme dehydration.[24] In replenishment of fluid deficiencies in a reptile, rapid expansion of the extracellular space is not necessarily followed by rapid expansion of the intracellular space. Thus, the time necessary to rehydrate a reptile is generally protracted when compared with mammals. When rehydrating a reptile, fluid replacement should focus on delivering the fluids where they are most needed. Reptiles with hypertonic or isotonic dehydration should be provided electrolyte-reduced and hypotonic fluids.[25] The administra-tion of hypertonic fluids limits the diffusion of fluid into the intracellular space, where it is generally needed.

For isotonic/hypertonic dehydration, Jarchow[25] and Prezant and Jarchow[26] recommend an initial solution composed of 2 parts 0.45% saline solution and 2.5% dextrose and one part LRS or Normosol or a 50/50 combination of 5% dextrose and a nonlactated isotonic solution (e.g., Normosol or Plasma Lyte, Baxter Health Care, Deerfield, Ill), followed by balanced fluid replacement.

Although balanced fluids, such as LRS and Normosol, may appear hypertonic for reptiles, they are frequently used with positive results. Plasma biochemistries and venous or arterial blood gases should be measured to determine the most appropriate fluid replenishment plan.

Prezant and Jarchow[26] have suggested the lactate buffered fluids may not be appropriate for reptiles. Reptiles can generate moderate to high concentrations of lactate after moderate to vigorous activity.[27,28] Increased lactate concentrations can lead to an acidemia, which can potentiate an anaerobic cycle. Reptiles in this physiologic condition are also likely to have electrolyte imbalances develop.[29] Prezant and Jarchow[26] suggest that the additional lactate (LRS) may overwhelm the already saturated liver, resulting in prolonged recovery. Instead, they suggest the non–lactate buffered solutions, such as Normosol or Plasma Lyte. Because acetate and gluconate are not dependent on the liver, they are not hindered by the lactic acidosis and buffer the pH to a more appropriate level. This in turn increase hemoglobin's affinity for oxygen and allows the reptile to resume an aerobic metabolism.

Although on the surface this discussion seems to make sense, in reality, reptiles have a large buffer system that allows them to handle any excess production of lactate. Because the lactate in LRS is metabolized to sodium bicarbonate in the liver (an excellent buffer), only a few instances exist in which LRS is not recommended. For general purposes, any balanced crystalloid suffices for rehydration in reptiles. If hepatic disease is suspected, than a nonlactated fluid should be used. See Chapter 31 for a thorough discussion of fluid choices and replacement therapy.

Empiric recommendations for fluid rates for reptiles are between 1% and 3% of the total body weight and are based on the relative volume of plasma in the reptile.[25,30] Overhydration of a reptile with hypertonic solutions could place an enormous strain on the circulatory system and should be avoided. In development of a fluid replacement plan, the volume of fluids administered should include both the maintenance and deficit requirements. Because of the limited extracellular space in reptiles, deficit fluids should be replenished over 72 to 96 hours. The daily fluid replacement plan should include both the daily maintenance (1% to 3% body weight) and 25% to 33% of the deficit. During the rehydration process, the reptile should be examined daily to ensure that the therapy is working. Additional losses may need to be accounted for when a patient has ongoing diseases associated with the gastrointestinal or respiratory tract or integument.

A thorough physical examination is necessary to determine the hydration status of a reptile. In evaluation of the hydration status of a reptile, evaluation of the skin elasticity and mucous membranes is generally recommended. Although skin turgor is generally used in mammals to assess hydration status, it is not as useful in reptiles. Many reptiles, whether they are hydrated or dehydrated, have limited skin elasticity. Dysecdysis is a common sequela to dehydration in reptiles. Dehydrated reptiles generally have thick ropey mucus in the oral cavity. The appearance of the feces and urine should also be recorded. Reptiles that are dehydrated produce dry fecal material and a small volume of urine. As the degree of dehydration increases, generally more than 8% to 10%, the eyes of a reptile appear sunken from the loss of moisture associated with the retroorbital fat pads.

Hematology can play an important role in evaluation of the hydration status of a reptile. The parameters that are generally used to assess a reptile's hydration status include the PCV, TP (total solids on a refractometer), sodium, and chloride. Veterinarians should identify appropriate reference resources to determine appropriate levels for each of these parameters.

The PCV of a dehydrated reptile generally is greater than 45%. However, PCVs between reptiles can vary, and collection of serial samples to fully evaluate the animal's changing status is important. A reptile with a PCV of 33% could be both anemic and dehydrated, presenting a paradoxic clinical picture. In general, the TP of a reptile is less than 8 gram/dL, sodium is less than 160 mg/dL, and chloride is less than 120 mg/dL. Again, this information should be used in combination with the PCV and physical examination findings to determine the animal's hydration status.

Routes of Fluid Administration

The primary methods of fluid replacement in reptiles include the following routes: per os (PO), subcutaneous (SC or SQ), intracoelomic (ICe), intraosseous (IO), and intravenous (IV). The route of administration is generally based on the species and the reptile's health status. In general, parenteral routes should be used for moderate (7%) to severely (>10%) dehydrated patients. The core body temperature of a reptile should be corrected before fluid administration to maximize the absorption of the fluids.

The per os route should be used when an animal is mildly dehydrated (<5%) and has a functional gastrointestinal tract. This route of administration is often underused in veterinary medicine because of our desire to administer fluids via the parenteral routes. Because the gastrointestinal tract is the normal route of fluid absorption in reptiles, this route is appropriate to use when an animal needs mild replenishment. The advantages of administering fluids per os include that the technique is noninvasive, that it stimulates gastrointestinal tract motility, and that reptile owners can be easily trained to administer fluids via this route. Per os fluids should not be administered when a reptile is vomiting or has diarrhea or ileus.

The supplementation of fluids, especially hypertonic fluids, could exacerbate an osmotic diarrhea. Administration of a large volume of fluids could lead to regurgitation and aspiration, so care should be taken to limit the volume administered at a single treatment. In general, the maximum fluid volume that the stomach can hold is 5% to 8% of the reptile's body weight. The author does not recommend administration of more than 2% to 3% of the animals body weight per os at a single time to prevent gastric atony and regurgitation.

Per os fluids can either be administered via a syringe directly into the mouth or with an esophageal or stomach tube. The author prefers to administer fluids via an esophageal or stomach tube because a large bolus can be administered quickly. The tube should be premeasured from the mouth to the midpoint of the reptile, which is the approximate location of the stomach in most species (Figure 36-1).

A soft pliable speculum, such as a rubber spatula or exposed radiograph film, can be used to open the mouth and visualize the glottis and pharynx (Figure 36-2). Aggressive manipulation with the speculum can lead to broken teeth, so care should be taken to gently pry open the mouth. Before the

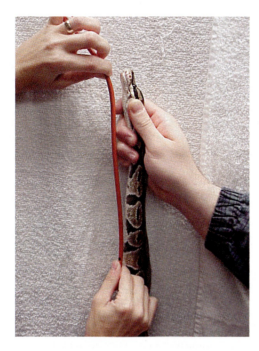

FIGURE 36-1 Always premeasure the feeding tube to ensure proper placement into the distal esophagus or stomach. In this example, a red-rubber feeding tube is premeasured to ensure that a medication is delivered into the esophagus of this Ball Python *(Python regius)*.

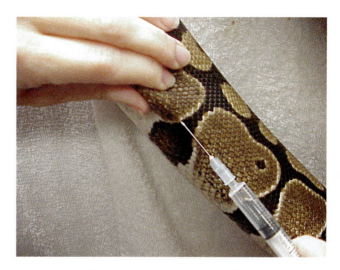

FIGURE 36-3 The subcutaneous space under the lateral body wall of a snake can be used to deliver medications or fluids.

to highly variable absorption rates between reptiles depending on physiologic state. Fluid replacement with the subcutaneous space may be used for reptiles but should be limited to those cases where the reptile is less than 5% to 6% dehydrated. Critically dehydrated reptiles should be rehydrated with the intracoelomic, intravenous, or intraosseous routes.

The primary subcutaneous site for fluid administration in squamates is the lateral body wall (Figure 36-3). The subcutaneous site between and over the scapulae is another site routinely used for lizards. Subcutaneous fluids should be used on a limited basis in those species with high skin tension (e.g., chameleons) because of the likelihood of skin depigmentation and in those with fragile skin (e.g., geckos) because of the likelihood of skin tearing. Chelonians may be given subcutaneous injections in either the axillary or inguinal regions (Figure 36-4). Subcutaneous injections in crocodilians are rare.

Administration of subcutaneous injections to reptiles can be done in a manner used for mammals. Tenting the skin provides a site for injection. The volume of fluids that can be administered at a site varies from reptile to reptile on the basis of its size and health. In general, the veterinarian must make a subjective decision regarding the volume to administer, and the author makes his decision on the basis of the tension on the skin.

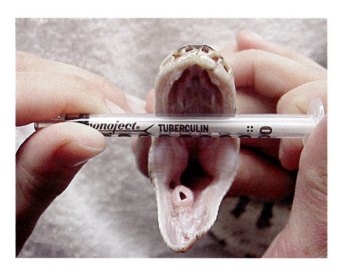

FIGURE 36-2 Opening the oral cavity of a Ball Python *(Python regius)* with a syringe. Note the glottis on the floor of the oral cavity.

Fluid replacement should be provided at body temperature. In mammals, subcutaneous administration of fluids at temperatures lower than body temperature is painful and delays absorption. Care should be taken to avoid administration of irritating compounds. Fluids and injectables with extremes in pH or irritating adjuvants can cause localized inflammatory responses, tissue necrosis, and depigmentation. Hyperosmotic solutions, such as 5% dextrose, should not be administered subcutaneously because they induce sterile abscesses.

tube is passed into the oral cavity, the glottis should be identified. The tube should be passed around the glottis and into the pharynx. The tube can be lubricated with a sterile lubricating jelly, but care should be taken not to introduce the jelly into the glottis.

Subcutaneous fluids are routinely used to replenish fluids in mildly dehydrated mammals. The subcutaneous space in reptiles is limited in comparison with mammals. In addition, the subcutaneous space of reptiles is poorly vascularized. The limited blood supply to the subcutaneous space can lead

The intracoelomic route of fluid administration is a rapid technique to provide large volumes of fluids to a reptile. The coelomic cavity is a large space and is lined with a highly absorptive coelomic membrane. In addition to the coelomic membrane, the serosal surfaces of the viscera are also highly absorptive. Squamates and chelonians do not have a

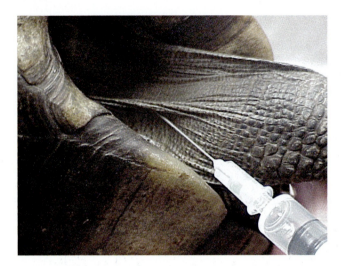

FIGURE 36-4 The subcutaneous space in the inguinal region of this Burmese Mountain Tortoise *(Manouria emys emys)* can be used to deliver medications and fluids.

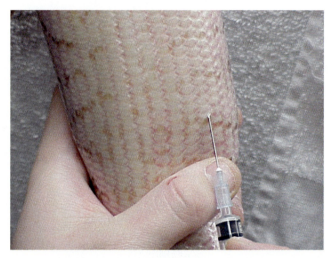

FIGURE 36-5 Intracoelomic fluids should be delivered in the ventrocaudal coelomic cavity of the lizard to avoid the lungs. Note that this Blue-tongued Skink *(Tiliqua scincoides)* has been placed in dorsal recumbency and the needle inserted off the midline to avoid the ventral abdominal vein.

diaphragm, and crocodilians have a pseudodiaphragm. Because reptiles lack a diaphragm, it is important to limit the quantity of fluids placed into the coelomic cavity. That said, the volume of fluids used to replenish losses and provide maintenance requirements does not overload the coelomic cavity.

Intracoelomic fluids should be administered in the caudal third of the coelomic cavity to avoid the lungs or air sac. The lungs of the lizards are located in the dorsal coelomic cavity and can extend the length of the coelomic cavity. Placement of the lizard in dorsal recumbency allows gravity to pull the viscera away from the injection site. The injection site should be disinfected with a topical antiseptic. The hypodermic needle (22 to 25 gauge) or butterfly catheter (22 to 25 gauge) should be inserted off the midline, to avoid the ventral abdominal vein, and slightly off parallel to the skin (Figure 36-5). Once inserted, the syringe should be aspirated to ensure that the needle was not inserted into a lung or air sac. If air is aspirated into the syringe, then the needle/catheter should be removed and reinserted. The same technique can be used to administer fluids to a snake.

For chelonians, the author prefers to administer intracoelomic fluids where the skin folds attach to the bridge of the shell (Figure 36-6). With placement of the chelonian in lateral recumbency, gravity can be used to draw the viscera away from the needle.

Intraosseous fluid administration can be used in those cases in which rapid absorption of the fluids is required but intravenous access is limited or not possible. Intraosseous catheters provide a stable route to administer fluids to a debilitated reptile. The distal femur and proximal tibia are the preferred intraosseous sites for lizards (Figure 36-7). Because the catheter is placed through the periosteum, a local anesthetic should be used. Spinal needles with a stylet should be used to prevent bone coring in the needle. The tibial crest should be used as the primary landmark for the tibial intraosseous catheter. The stifle should be flexed and the needle inserted on the tibial plateau anterior to the joint capsule. A gentle twisting force should be applied to the needle to

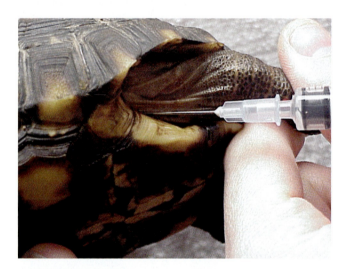

FIGURE 36-6 Intracoelomic fluids should be delivered into the ventrocaudal coelomic cavity of the chelonian to avoid the lungs. Note that this Red-foot Tortoise *(Geochelone carbonaria)* has been placed in lateral recumbency and the needle inserted along the bridge to ensure that the fluids are not delivered into the lungs.

ensure proper purchase into the medullary cavity. The catheter can be secured with suture or tape. Radiography of the limb is recommended to confirm placement (Figure 36-8).

Catheter insertion is similar for the distal femur, although the point of entry is the anterior surface of the metaphysis. Because of the small medullary cavity associated with both the tibia and the femur, large boluses of fluids are difficult. Instead, fluids should be administered slowly over a period of 10 to 15 minutes or via an automatic infusion pump.

Intraosseous catheters are difficult to place in the femur of chelonians because of the sigmoid shape of the femur (Figure 36-9). Although the author has placed intraosseous

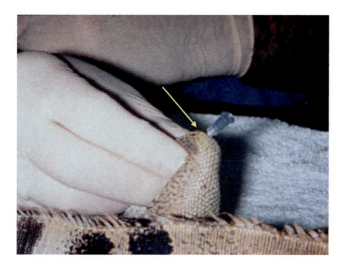

FIGURE 36-7 Final placement of an intraosseous catheter into the tibia of a Green Iguana *(Iguana iguana)*.

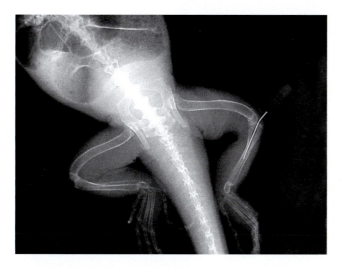

FIGURE 36-8 Dorsoventral survey radiograph of a Green Iguana *(Iguana iguana)* to confirm the placement of an intraosseous catheter.

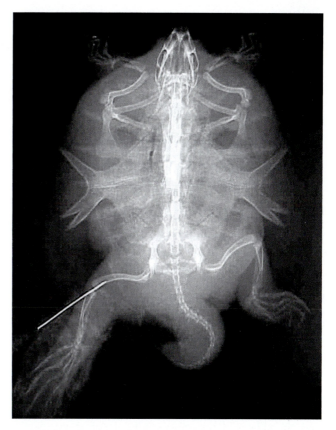

FIGURE 36-9 Attempted placement of an intraosseous femoral catheter in a Spiny Softshell Turtle *(Apalone spinifera)*. Note the sigmoid curvature of the femur. The catheter was used to administer emergency drugs.

catheters in both the femur and the tibia of chelonians, the volume of fluids that could be administered via these routes was negligible unless the catheter was connected to an automatic infusion pump. In addition, if the patient withdraws into its shell, the intraosseous catheter may interfere or be displaced.

The cranial and caudal limits of the bony bridge between the carapace and plastron of chelonians has been suggested as a site for fluid administration. This site is considered analogous to the placement of an intraosseous catheter in other species. However, this site can only be accessed via drilling a hole into the shell. Because of the invasiveness of the procedure, special considerations regarding pain management should be taken. Attempts by the author to locate this site in several species of North American chelonians have been of limited value. Because of the limited accessibility of this site and the invasiveness of the procedure, this site should only be used in rare instances in which other routes of parenteral fluid administration are not possible.

Intravenous fluid therapy is the most effective method for rapid delivery of fluids to the circulatory system. Unfortunately, the intravenous route is rarely used in reptiles because in most cases it requires a surgical (cutdown) approach. In debilitated reptiles that are severely dehydrated (>8% to 10%), the intravenous route provides the best method for rehydrating the patient and should be attempted.

The jugular vein in the lizard is a large vessel located in the lateral cervical area. The vessel can be located with connecting an imaginary line from the point of the shoulder to the middle of the external tympanum (Figure 36-10). Placement of a jugular catheter in lizards requires a surgical incision. This procedure should be performed with a local anesthetic, such as 2% lidocaine HCl, or with an anesthetic agent that provides somatic analgesia, such as Telazol (3 to 5 mg/kg IM; Fort Dodge Laboratories, Inc, Fort Dodge, Iowa) or propofol (10 to 15 mg/kg IV).

The jugular vein of the Green Iguana *(Iguana iguana)* generally courses along the episternocleidomastoieus and constrictor coli muscles. In some cases, the vessel is apparent after the initial incision; however, blunt dissection may be necessary to isolate the jugular vein in other cases. Catheter selection varies from animal to animal on the basis of the size of the animal. In general, an 18- to 22-gauge catheter can be inserted into the jugular vein of an adult Green Iguana or monitor. Before catheter placement, the catheter should be flushed with sodium heparin to prevent clot formation. Once the catheter is placed, it should be sutured into the skin.

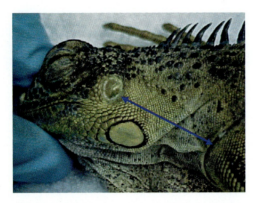

FIGURE 36-10 The jugular vein in most species of lizards is located in the lateral cervical region. This figure shows the approximate location of the jugular vein in the Green Iguana (*Iguana iguana*).

The jugular catheter allows the veterinary clinician to deliver a constant rate of fluids to the reptile patient. If a constant fluid rate is not used, then the catheter should be flushed four times a day to prevent clot formation at the site of the catheter. The catheter site should be attended daily, and the entire catheter should be removed/replaced after 48 to 96 hours of use.

A jugular catheter can generally be placed in chelonians without a skin incision, although certain species have thick scales in the lateral cervical region that require an incision to place the catheter. Although the right jugular vein is usually regarded as larger than the left jugular vein, either vein can be catheterized. To avoid a large incision with a scalpel, a large-gauge hypodermic needle (18- to 20-gauge) can be used to create a small incision or "nick" in the skin in the general area of the jugular vein. This small incision enables the clinician to pass the catheter without damage to the catheter.

The jugular vein is generally found in the area of the latissimus coli muscle. Topical anesthetics may be used to minimize the pain associated with this procedure. Again, once the catheter is situated, it should be sutured into place and flushed with sodium heparin as needed. Even if the neck is withdrawn into the shell, the catheters work, providing the fluids are administered via an infusion pump.

Placement of a jugular catheter in a snake also requires a surgical incision. Most snakes that receive a jugular catheter in the author's practice are moribund, and a catheter can be placed with a local anesthetic alone. In more active specimens, a general anesthetic, such as Telazol (3 to 5 mg/kg IM; Fort Dodge Laboratories, Inc) or propofol (10 to 15 mg/kg IV), is required. The snake should be placed in dorsal recumbency for the procedure. The heart serves as the primary landmark for the procedure and is located approximately one fourth to one third the distance from the head. Either jugular vein can be used, but the author prefers the left side.

The site for the incision should be nine to 10 ventral scales cranial to the location of the heart (Figure 36-11, *A*). The incision should be made between the first and second dorsal scales. The incision site can be manipulated ventrally to expose the medial aspect of the ribs and the rectus abdominis muscle (Figure 36-11, *B*). The jugular vein courses medial to the ribs, and blunt dissection of the surrounding muscles may be necessary to visualize the jugular vein (Figure 36-11, *C*). In consideration of the size of the catheter, one should always

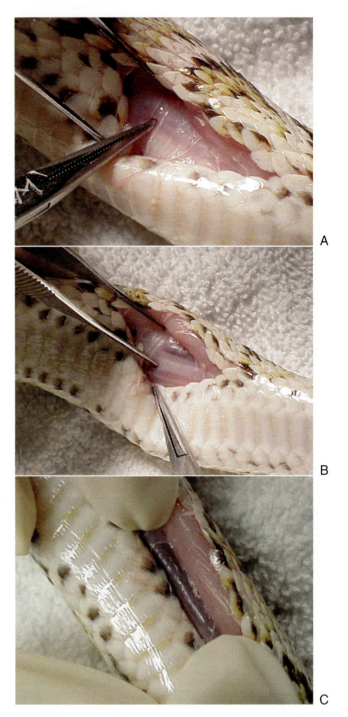

FIGURE 36-11 **A,** The jugular vein of the snake can be located approximately nine scales cranial to the heart. The initial incision should be made between the first and second rows of dorsal scales. **B,** Blunt dissection of the rectus abdominis is necessary to identify the jugular vein. **C,** The jugular vein is a sizeable vessel in the snake. Here is an example of a right jugular vein in a Reticulated Python (*Python reticulatus*).

use the largest bore-catheter. The catheter should be flushed with sodium heparin and sutured into place.

The cephalic vein can be used to deliver fluids in large lizards. The cephalic vein of lizards generally courses along the medial aspect of the antebrachium. An incision that is perpendicular to the direction of the cephalic vein is necessary to find the vein (Figure 36-12). Care must be taken with the incision to prevent laceration of the vessel. The cephalic vein generally can be found in the vicinity of the palmaris longus and flexor carpi ulnaris muscles. When the peripheral circulation is compromised during a hypovolemic crisis, access to the cephalic vein may be limited.

Chemotherapeutics

For the most part, the drugs used to treat reptiles are used off-label. One exception to this is enrofloxacin (Bayer Corp., Shawnee Mission, Kan), which is approved for use in exotics in the United Kingdom. Veterinarians should inform their clients that the drugs used to treat their pets are used off-label. One may be wise to have the owners sign a consent form, which is kept as part of the permanent medical record, whenever a patient is started on medication.

One of the problems that face veterinarians is determination of an appropriate drug dose for a reptile patient. Unfortunately, general drug pharmacokinetic studies are lacking in reptiles, and much of the literature is based on empiric dosing, limited studies, and broad extrapolation.

Drug dosages based on research with mammalian and avian species are routinely used in reptiles. Physiologic differences between reptiles and higher vertebrates should be accounted for in calculation of drug dosages. Because of the slower metabolic rate of reptiles, drugs may have longer half-lives. For those species in which research on the pharmacokinetics of a drug has been done, the drug dose for one reptile species is not necessarily appropriate for another.

Mathematic extrapolations may be more accurate than simple dosing or guesswork. Chapter 25 discusses allometric/metabolic scaling of drug dosages and the physiologic parameters that affect them.

Administration of Therapeutics

In reptiles, the parenteral administration of drugs is generally preferred over the per os route. However, administration of drugs per os does have some advantages. Drugs that are irritating or cause tissue damage should not be administered parenterally. Variability in the gastrointestinal tract anatomy and motility potentially affects the absorption and delivery of drugs in the reptile.[31]

For reptiles that are difficult to medicate orally, the best technique for administration of oral medications is via the food. Gel diets can be prepared to meet the specific nutritional requirements of the reptile patient and also to be combined with a enteral medications. A gel diet can be offered as an exclusive diet during treatment or can be combined with a reptile's primary diet. With medications combined with the diet, limiting the amount of food offered to the reptile is important to ensure that the full dose of the drug is consumed.

Although reptiles have relatively few taste buds, they do avoid a distasteful medication if a large quantity of food is offered. Flavored medications are another method of delivering drugs to reptiles. Herbivorous reptiles, such as Green Iguanas and tortoises, generally readily accept fruit-flavored medications. Many compounding pharmacies have the ability to mimic a variety of flavors for drugs, from cherry fruit to liver and other meat flavors.

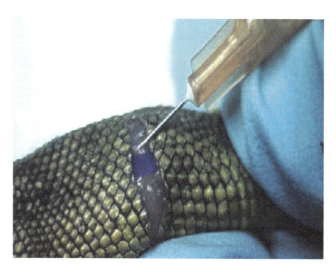

FIGURE 36-12 The cephalic vein of the lizard is generally located on the medial aspect of the antebranchium. To access the vessel, an incision that is perpendicular to the vessel is necessary. Care should be taken to avoid incising the vessel. In this photograph, the cephalic vein has been highlighted in blue.

The chelonians are the most difficult species of reptiles to medicate via the oral route. Once a chelonian has withdrawn it head, access to the oral cavity can be difficult. Attempts to extract the head of a chelonian should be done with caution. The cervical vertebrae of a chelonian are fused to the carapace, and aggressive manipulation of the head and neck can result in a cervical spinal injury. Sedation or anesthesia may be necessary to fully withdraw the head and neck of a chelonian.

A soft pliable speculum, such as a rubber spatula, or a plastic-coated paper clip may be used to gently pry open the beak of a chelonian. Aggressive manipulation of the oral cavity can lead to fractures of the tomia. Either a soft pliable feeding tube or rigid stainless steel ball-tipped feeding tube can be used to deliver a medication (Figure 36-13). These tubes are preferred over placing the drug into the back of the oral cavity because the tubes ensure proper dosing with a decreased likelihood of regurgitation. The dosing tube should be premeasured to deliver the drug directly into the stomach. The stomach of the chelonian is located at approximately the midbody or one third of the distance from the head, to the left of the center line. When passing a stomach tube, the glottis must be avoided. The glottis of the chelonian is located at the base of the tongue. Passage of the stomach tube may be simplified with lubrication of the tube. However, care should be taken to avoid introducing lubricant into the glottis. Chelonians that need frequent oral treatments should have an esophagostomy tube placed to simplify treatment.

An esophagostomy tube can be easily placed in a chelonian. For moribund chelonians, a local anesthetic can be used to provide analgesia, whereas more active chelonians need general anesthesia. A combination of ketamine (2.5 to 10 mg/kg IM; Ketaset, Fort Dodge Laboratories) and medetomidine (0.75 to 0.15 mg/kg IM; Dormitor, Pfizer Animal Health, New York) may be used to provide somatic and visceral analgesia for the procedure. Because the drugs affect cardiopulmonary function, the chelonian should be intubated and ventilated two to four times per minute. The esophagostomy tube should be premeasured before placement. The tube length should be measured

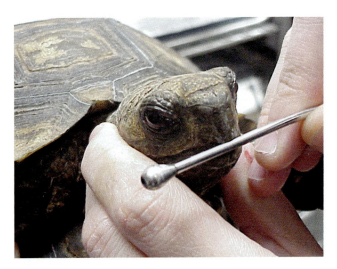

FIGURE 36-13 The oral cavity of a chelonian can be difficult to access. Here a stainless steel, ball-tipped feeding tube was used to gently manipulate the tomia of a Burmese Mountain Tortoise *(Manouria emys emys)*. Once the tube was inserted, it was redirected to deliver the medications.

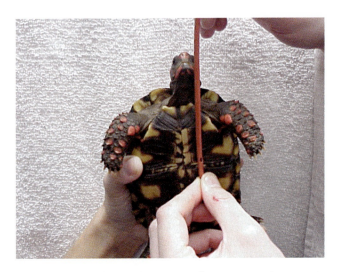

FIGURE 36-14 Always premeasure a pharyngostomy feeding tube to ensure proper placement into the stomach of a chelonian. In this example, a red rubber feeding tube is premeasured for placement into a Cherry-head Red-foot Tortoise *(Geochelone carbonaria)*.

from the lateral surface of the neck to the midbody of the chelonian (Figure 36-14). A permanent marker should be used to mark the distance of the tube as a landmark. The esophagostomy can be made on either the left or right lateral cervical region. Chelonians have paired carotid arteries and jugular veins that are located on the lateral surface of the neck and should be avoided. To avoid accidental incision of an artery or vein, a hemostat can be used as a guard. The hemostat should be inserted through the oral cavity and into the esophagus and displaced laterally. This causes the skin to tent and the major vessels to slip dorsally or ventrally. A small incision should be made through the skin and esophagus with a #15 blade scalpel (Figure 36-15, *A*). The incision should be made as caudal as possible on the neck to limit the opportunity for the chelonian to extract the tube with its forelimbs. The hemostats should be manipulated through the incision, so that they can be used to grasp the feeding tube (Figure 36-15, *B*). The hemostats and the feeding tube should be withdrawn through the oral cavity. The tube should only be withdrawn to the point of the landmark (Figure 36-15, *C*). Once withdrawn, the feeding tube should be redirected down the alimentary canal into the stomach. The tube should be sutured to the skin at the level of the incision with nonabsorbable sutures, and the extended length of the tube secured to the carapace with tape or cyanoacrylic glue (Figure 36-15, *D*). The feeding tube facilitates both administration of medications and supplemental feedings. As the patient convalesces, it is still able to eat even with the feeding tube in place. The tube should be kept in place for at least 1 to 2 weeks after appetite has returned to normal.

Squamates are generally easy to medicate via the oral route, although oral medications for venomous snakes and the *Heloderma* spp. should be avoided or only done by those individuals with extensive experience. For snakes, a dosing syringe or feeding tube can be gently manipulated into the commissure of the mouth to gain access to the oral cavity (Figure 36-16). A soft-pliable rubber spatula can also be used to open the oral cavity. Wooden tongue depressors or rigid speculums should be avoided because they can damage the mucous membranes and teeth.

Alternatively, a large-bore rubber feeding tube can be inserted blind through the philtrum. Use of a large-bore tube prevents any possibility of accidentally passing the tube into the glottis. The feeding tube should be premeasured to a length of approximately one half the length of the patient's body to ensure the placement of the drugs directly into the stomach in small patients.

Because the stomach of the snake is generally located at the midbody, administration of the drugs directly into the stomach is difficult in larger animals. In most cases, the medications are placed into the mid esophagus or distal esophagus. The dosing syringe of tube should be inserted to the back of the pharynx, with care taken to avoid the glottis. Placement of a lubricant on a dosing tube may help facilitate passage, although the esophagus of the snake is lined with numerous mucous glands. After infusing the medication into the esophagus, support the patient's head and neck straight up, and, with the help of gravity, gently "milk" the medication down into the stomach.

Lizards can be medicated with similar techniques, although a speculum is generally necessary. Special care should be taken when manipulating the speculum into the mouth of the lizards to avoid fracturing teeth. Pleurodontic species, such as the Green Iguana regenerate teeth, whereas acrodontic species, such as the Bearded Dragon *(Pogona vitticeps)*, do not. Opening the mouth of those species with a large dewlap is possible without the use of a speculum. In these species, the index finger and thumb of one hand can be placed on the maxillae and the index finger and thumb of the second hand can be used to gently draw on the dewlap to open the mouth. Some species of reptiles, such as the geckos, have an innate ability to lock their jaws. When these species have locked their jaws, attempting to force them open is ill advised because mandibular fractures may occur. Because many species of

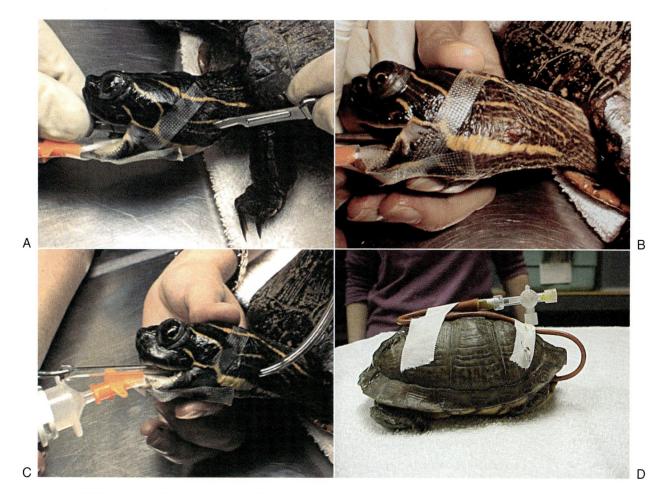

FIGURE 36-15 **A,** The hemostat should be introduced into the oral cavity and directed laterally within the pharynx. This serves as the site for the incision. **B,** The hemostats should be gently forced through the incision and used to grasp the feeding tube. **C,** The feeding tube should be withdrawn through the mouth and redirected back through the oral cavity. This prevents misdirecting the tube into the subcutaneous tissues. **D,** The feeding tube can be affixed to the carapace and a stopcock used to control delivery of fluids, enterals, and medications.

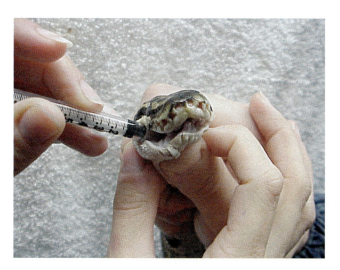

FIGURE 36-16 Gentle insertion of a dosing syringe, such as this tuberculin syringe, into the commissure of the oral cavity can provide access to the oral cavity of a snake.

lizards use their tongue as a chemosensory structure to "taste" products in their environment, they can be trained to readily accept oral drugs.

Lizards readily lap flavored medications that are placed on the tip of the mouth, reducing the need to forcefully open the mouth to deliver the drugs. Special care should be taken when manipulating the mouth of a lizard with suspect secondary nutritional hyperparathyroidism. Fibrous osteodystrophy, a common finding in these patients, could lead to pathologic fractures of the mandible or maxillae.

The preferred method for providing oral medications to crocodilians is through the diet. Commercially prepared extruded pellets can have heat-stable medications added during the milling process to medicate large populations of crocodilians, whereas individually prepared gel diets may be used to medicate individual crocodilians. Because crocodilians can inflict a severe bite injury, only experienced individuals should attempt to tube feed these animals. The crocodilian should be manually restrained, and a speculum (e.g., polyvinyl chloride tube) should be inserted into the mouth to facilitate the passage of the tube. Once the speculum is in place, the jaws of the crocodilian should be taped (e.g., electrical tape or rubber bands) closed. A feeding tube should be used to deliver the medications into the stomach. The tube should be premeasured from the mouth to the midbody to ensure delivery of the drugs into the stomach.

The anatomy of the crocodilian oral cavity is very different than the other reptiles. The velum palati, an extension of the soft palate, and the basihyal valve, a muscular structure located at the base of the tongue, are used to seal the pharynx of these species. With oral dosing of the crocodilian, the tube must be passed over the basihyal valve to ensure passage into the esophagus. An esophagostomy tube should be placed for those cases that need long-term oral medications.

Parenteral Routes

Most chemotherapeutics used to treat reptiles are administered via a parenteral route. The intramuscular route is used most commonly, although the subcutaneous, intracoelomic, intravenous, and intraosseous routes may also be used. The route of administration should be determined on the basis of the reptile's size and general health, the known pharmacokinetics of the drug, and the potential side effects associated with the route of administration.

Subcutaneous

The subcutaneous space in reptiles is limited in comparison with mammals. In addition, the subcutaneous space of reptiles is poorly vascularized. The limited blood supply to the subcutaneous space can lead to highly variable absorption rates between reptiles depending on the physiologic state. The primary subcutaneous site for injection in squamates is the lateral body wall. The subcutaneous site between and over the scapulae is another site routinely used for lizards. Chelonians may be given subcutaneous injections in the axillary and inguinal regions. Subcutaneous injections in crocodilians are rare. Care should be taken to avoid administration of irritating compounds. Compounds with extreme pH levels or irritating adjuvants can cause localized inflammatory responses, tissue necrosis, and skin depigmentation.

Intracoelomic

Although the coelomic cavity is routinely used to administer fluids for reptiles, it is not used as frequently for the administration of drugs. In ornamental fish, the coelomic cavity is routinely used to administer various drugs. The serosa of the viscera and the coelomic membrane are highly absorptive surfaces. Irritating compounds should not be administered intracoelomically. However, irritating compounds, such as enrofloxacin (Baytril, Bayer) are routinely administered intracoelomically to ornamental fish with no apparent ill effects. The technique for intracoelomic administration of a drug is similar to that described for replenishing fluids. One must position the animal in dorsal or lateral recumbency and must insert the needle parallel to the body wall to avoid the viscera.

Intramuscular and Intravenous

Intramuscular and intravenous injections are the most common technique used to administer drugs for reptiles because of access, rapid uptake, and distribution. In general, for life-threatening gram-negative sepsis, the intravenous route is preferred. Unfortunately, this is not always possible because of limited or difficult access. Whenever possible, when an intravenous route is needed, every attempt should be made to acquire one.

Dehydration and hypothermia do not affect drug uptake via the intravenous route as they do with the intramuscular route and other routes of administration. **In general, it is the rare reptile patient that cannot wait 12 to 24 hours for the hydration and thermal status to return to normal before administration of antibiotics or other chemotherapeutics.**

Intramuscular injections are often used when they may not be appropriate, especially for irritating compounds or for reptiles with limited muscle mass. In these cases, intravenous injections may be preferred because they are rapidly diluted. Intramuscular injections should only be given when the manufacturer states on the label that it is appropriate. Certain irritating compounds, such as Baytril (Bayer Corp), recommend a single loading intramuscular injection and additional doses via the oral route. Unfortunately, reports in the literature reinforce the use of multiple intramuscular injections of this compound, which can cause muscle necrosis, skin depigmentation, and sloughing (Figure 36-17).

Intramuscular injections should be avoided in small species of reptiles, such as geckos and chameleons, if possible. Multiple intramuscular injections into a limited muscle mass can cause changes in the reptile's ability to ambulate or cause a temporary paresis. Over an extended period of treatment, this could affect a reptile's ability to acquire food and water, resulting in additional problems.

Egg Treatment

Attempts to reduce or eliminate *Salmonella* in chelonians with antimicrobials were initiated after the US Food and Drug Administration (FDA) ban was implemented in 1975. Treatment of hatchlings with oxytetracycline in the tank water for up to 14 days alleviated shedding in treated turtles but did not affect systemic infection.[38] Treatment of the freshly laid eggs with oxytetracycline or chloramphenicol with a temperature differential egg dip method was successful at eliminating *Salmonella* in eggs less than 1 day old but did not clear eggs greater than 2 days old.[38] Large-scale experimentation on commercial chelonian farms with surface decontamination and pressure or temperature differential treatment of eggs with gentamicin dip solutions for eggs greater than 2 days old, followed by hatching the eggs on *Salmonella*-free bedding, substantially reduced *Salmonella* infections and shedding rates in hatchling turtles.[39] Forty percent of the eggs not treated with the gentamicin were found to harbor *Salmonella*, whereas only 0.15% of the treated eggs were positive.

Legislative implementation of this concurrent method of surface decontamination and gentamicin treatment by the Louisiana Department of Agriculture in 1985 was hailed as victory by chelonian farmers. Unfortunately, use of gentamicin and the other antimicrobials has led to an even greater

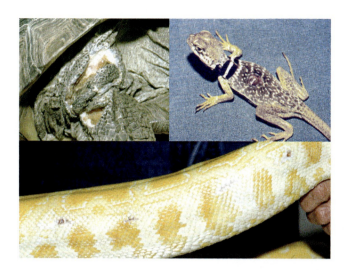

FIGURE 36-17 This series of photographs shows some lesions associated with administration of enrofloxacin intramuscularly. *Upper left*, Desert Tortoise (*Gopherus agassizii*); *upper right*, Collard Lizard (*Crotaphytus collaris*); *bottom*, Burmese Python (*Python molurus bivittatus*). (Photographs courtesy D. Mader.)

concern because of the development and persistence of antimicrobial resistant strains of *Salmonella*.

The occurrence of *Salmonella* in Red-eared Slider (*Pseudemys scripta elegans*) eggs imported to Canada from four different Louisiana turtle farms in 1988 was examined, and of the 28 lots tested, six lots (21%) from three of four exporters were *Salmonella* positive.[40] Of the 37 *Salmonella* strains isolated, 30 (81%) were gentamicin resistant.[40] Similar results have been reported from samples collected directly from the farms in Louisiana.

Shane, Gilbert, and Harrington[41] collected environmental samples and live hatchlings directly from two Louisiana chelonian farms. Isolates of *S. arizonae* and *S. poona* collected from turtles at one of the farms were resistant to erythromycin, gentamicin, tetracycline, and triple sulfa. Pond water samples from both farms showed similar antimicrobial resistant patterns to erythromycin. In 1988, 115 batches of turtle hatchlings were submitted from 28 farms to the Louisiana Department of Agriculture and Forestry for analysis.[41] Five *Salmonella* isolates (4.3%) were obtained. Four of the organisms were submitted for serotyping: three were *S. arizona* and one was *S. poona*. All four isolates were resistant to erythromycin, gentamicin, tetracycline, and triple sulfa. These findings suggest that washing chelonian eggs with antimicrobials is an inconsistent method to control *Salmonella* and that additional techniques that are not susceptible to resistance should be pursued.

The Renal Portal System

The renal portal system is a unique component of the circulatory system of lower vertebrates. Historically, parenteral drug administration into the tail or caudal extremities was not recommended because of the potential side effect (nephrotoxicosis) associated with drug passage through the renal portal system. Although reports exist of nephrotoxicosis associated with the administration of aminoglycosides in reptiles, a review of these cases suggests that the toxicosis were attributed to high doses of gentamicin rather than the route of administration.[32,33] Because aminoglycosides are excreted relatively unchanged, extreme doses could lead to nephrotoxicosis.

Recent work has suggested that parenteral administration of drugs into the caudal extremities may not pose as great a risk as once thought. Holz et al[34] evaluated renal perfusion in Red-eared Sliders (*Trachemys scripta elegans*) with radioangiography. The research suggested that intravenous injections of a radiopaque dye into the dorsal coccygeal vein or femoral vein do not necessarily perfuse the kidneys via the renal portal system.

The renal portal system most likely serves to perfuse the kidneys, more specifically the tubules, during times of water conservation. During times of water conservation, arginine vasotocin increases water resorption at the level of the tubules, while reducing glomerular filtration.[42] Prolactin is the antagonist for this system.[43] Holz et al[34] proposed that a valve located between the abdominal and femoral veins might regulate blood flow through the kidneys. At times of water conservation, a valve in the abdominal vein closes, redirecting blood through the iliac veins and into the kidneys.

Holz et al[37] tested the practicality of this concept by performing two antibiotic pharmacokinetic studies in the Red-eared Slider. Gentamicin and carbenicillin were selected for the study because they are excreted via glomerular filtration and tubular secretion, respectively. A total of 20 Red-eared Sliders were used in the study. Ten Red-eared Sliders received an injection of gentamicin (10 mg/kg) in the musculature of the forelimb or hind limb and, after a 4-week washout period, were given another injection of gentamicin at the site not used for the first injection. Carbenicillin (200 mg/kg) was given to the remaining 10 Red-eared Sliders with the same protocol.

The bioavailability of gentamicin was not affected by injection site. However, this was not unexpected because the renal portal system provides blood to the tubules and should not affect glomerular filtration.[34] The area under the curve for carbenicillin plasma concentrations was significantly lower for the hind limb injections at 1, 4, and 8 hours after injection. Although the plasma concentrations were lower for the hind limb injections, the levels recorded remained above the minimum inhibitory concentration (MIC) required for susceptible bacterial pathogens.

The renal portal system of the iguana may behave differently than that described in chelonians. When three Green Iguanas were given a radiopaque dye intravenously into the ventral caudal vein, the contrast entered the caudal renal parenchyma and moved cranially into the caudal vena cavae.[35] When the radiopaque dye was intraosseously delivered into the femur of three Green Iguanas, the dye entered the common iliac, pelvic, and ventral abdominal veins. The contrast eventually extended into the renal parenchyma. Variation, however, did exist in the movement of the dye in the iguanas, which may be attributed to individual variation or the small sample size.

To determine whether the renal portal system has any affect on drug pharmacokinetics in snakes, Holz et al[44] evaluated injection site on the pharmacokinetics of carbenicillin in Carpet Pythons (*Morelia spilotes variegata*). Seven Carpet Pythons were used for the study, and each received a 200-mg/kg intramuscular dose of carbenicillin in either the cranial or caudal epaxial musculature. Five months after the injection, the snakes again received a 200-mg/kg intramuscular injection of carbenicillin; however, the site of the injection was reversed from the previous example. No significant difference was seen in the pharmacokinetics between injection sites. Although the concentrations of drug given in the cranial half of the snakes were higher over the first 6 to 8 hours, the difference was not significant. However, the range of concentrations was quite varied for each time point, suggesting variability within the sample population. A larger sample population may have led to different results. Regardless of the difference, Holz et al[44] found that the plasma concentrations were sufficient to control susceptible bacterial pathogens.

Research to investigate the pharmacokinetics and the pathologic effects of drugs given in the caudal extremities is limited to a few species, and generalization of these results to all 7500+ species of reptiles could be dangerous. Additional research to elaborate the effects of different drugs on the renal portal system in reptiles should be pursued. See Chapters 10 and 11 for more information on the renal portal system and hemodynamics.

Antimicrobials

Antimicrobial usage in captive reptiles is widespread. Unfortunately, few antibiotic pharmacokinetic studies have been done for reptiles. Because of this limitation, few published drug dosages exist for reptiles. One technique that may be used to estimate a drug dose for a reptile, in the absence of a rigorous study, was described by Lawrence.[45] A mammalian antibiotic dose may last up to 10 times longer in a reptile of similar density and maintained at an appropriate environmental temperature range. Lawrence applied this theory to a study that evaluated carbenicillin in snakes and found that the dose selected, 400 mg/kg, was 10 times greater than that recommended for dogs.[46]

Drug pharmacokinetics in reptiles vary with the physiologic and metabolic condition of the patient. Because reptiles are ectotherms, their metabolic rate, immune function, and general well being are dictated by the ability to thermoregulate. The metabolic rate of reptiles is significantly lower than in endothermic higher vertebrates. Snakes maintained at 37°C have a metabolic rate nearly 80% lower than mammals of the same size.[47] Body temperature can also affect the half-life of a drug, with the half-life increasing with decreasing body temperature. Although the metabolic rate is significantly lower in reptiles than mammals and birds, veterinarians routinely rely on drug dosages reported for higher vertebrates. See Chapter 25, Allometric Scaling, regarding the effects of metabolism and environmental factors on drug dosing in reptiles.

Future research to evaluate the pharmacokinetics of the different classes of drugs used in reptilian medicine should be pursued. In addition, these studies should focus on the interspecific differences between different orders and families of reptiles.

The distribution of drugs in an animal can be altered by various physiologic conditions. Fluctuations in proteins can affect protein binding and drug availability. Alteration in pH can affect the ionization of a drug and chelating agents and a series of other physiologic effects. Unfortunately, measurement of arterial pH is difficult, if not impossible, in most reptiles without surgical catheterization. However, the Rosenthal effect, which suggests that blood pH decreases with increased core body temperature (0.02/1°C), can be used to guide the veterinary clinician in general terms.[48] Many of the drugs used to treat reptiles are active and ionized at a lower pH, reinforcing the importance of maximizing the environmental temperature for the patient.

With some drugs, such as the aminoglycosides, a lower pH could increase the likelihood of a toxic episode. Rats with a metabolic acidosis were more likely to have nephrotoxicosis develop from gentamicin, and the Watersnake (*Nerodia fasciata*) had increased nephrotoxicosis when housed at higher temperatures.[49,50]

Antimicrobial Selection

Several factors should be considered in the selection of an antimicrobial for a case, including antimicrobial sensitivity assay results, antimicrobial spectrum, drug distribution, side effects of the drug, metabolic and excretory pathways, and frequency and ease of dosing. In most cases, a specific isolate is sensitive to several antibiotics. Antimicrobials with a spectrum specific to the isolated pathogen should be selected. When multiple drugs can be used, the drug with the narrowest spectrum should be used to limit the collateral damage to the indigenous microflora. That a drug is distributed to the specific tissue that is affected is vital. Unfortunately, a general lack of information exists regarding the distribution of antimicrobials in reptiles. Although this information is readily available in the domestic animal literature and may be extrapolated for reptiles, anatomic and physiologic differences between species of reptiles and these species may provide varying results.

The specific metabolic and excretory pathways for a drug are important to consider in the selection of an antimicrobial. In a reptile with hepatitis or chronic liver disease, a drug that must be metabolized by the liver may not be appropriate. Because aminoglycosides are excreted unchanged by the kidneys, one must not give one of these compounds to a reptile with a reduced glomerular filtration rate. To minimize the secondary effects of stress on the reptile's immune response, drugs that can be administered with ease and infrequency should be given strong consideration.

If a microbiologic culture and an antimicrobial sensitivity assay cannot be done, then the veterinarian must select an antibiotic on the basis of past experience or generally accepted practices. Most bacterial pathogens isolated from reptiles are gram-negative bacteria. However, gram-positive bacterial infections can also occur.

In cases in which a culture cannot be done, a cytologic examination from a sample of a lesion should be done to determine the predominant bacterial flora (gram-positive versus gram-negative). Drug selection should be made on the basis of general effectiveness of a drug.

Many of the natural penicillins, early cephalosporins, and macrolides have minimal effect against gram-negative bacteria because of intrinsic resistance factors. Microbes can develop resistance either naturally through mutation (intrinsic) or as a result to exposure from the environment.

The widespread use of antibiotics has led to an increased number of reports of antimicrobial resistant pathogens. In the United States, currently more than 100,000 deaths per year are associated with antimicrobial resistant bacteria. Veterinarians should limit antibiotic treatment to those cases in which it is warranted.

Concerns About the Indiscriminant Use of Antibiotics

Salmonella spp., which are generally considered to be a component of the indigenous microflora of reptiles, rarely cause overt clinical disease in reptiles. When reptiles are seen with salmonellosis, antimicrobial treatment is not recommended because of the supposed risk of creating antimicrobial-resistant *Salmonella* pathogens. This therapeutic approach, and the theory that reptiles naturally harbor *Salmonella* spp., suggests that reptiles should not be treated with antibiotics at any time because of the risk of antimicrobial resistance in indigenous flora. However, this is obviously not practiced. An important consideration is that indiscriminant antibiotic use can be dangerous, and until techniques are found to deliver a treatment that does not affect the commensal flora, the risk of creating antimicrobial resistant organisms will exist.

Antibacterials Used in Reptile Medicine

Aminoglycosides

Aminoglycosides are polycations that are minimally bound to protein, are poorly absorbed from the gastrointestinal tract, and are excreted unchanged via the kidneys.[51] Aminoglycosides are bactericidal. These compounds permanently bind to the bacterial 30S ribosome. Antimicrobial resistance to the aminoglycosides is generally associated with the development of inactivating enzymes in the periplasmic space. The aminoglycosides have a narrow therapeutic index and therefore should be used cautiously. The primary side effects associated with aminoglycosides in mammals are ototoxicity and nephrotoxicity. Aminoglycoside toxicity can vary with the specific drug, peak concentration, and hydration and renal status of the patient.

Gentamicin is more nephrotoxic than amikacin.[52] Nephrotoxicity has been reported in snakes given 5 mg/kg of gentamicin for 14 days.[33] Veterinarians should consider evaluating a snake's renal function and hydration status before prescribing aminoglycosides. In mammals, blood urea nitrogen, creatinine, and a urine specific gravity are generally evaluated before aminoglycoside therapy.[51] However, because reptiles are primarily uricotelic and lack a loop of Henle, these parameters are of limited value to the clinician. Instead, the calcium, phosphorus, potassium, TP (total solids on a refractometer), and uric acid can be measured to provide some initial insight. An inverse calcium:phosphorus ratio may be suggestive of reduced renal function and warrants further evaluation, or at least the selection of a nonaminoglycoside antibiotic.

Aminoglycosides are considered the gold standard for gram-negative sepsis and are generally indicated for gram-negative bacterial infections, including *E. coli*, *Klebsiella* spp., *Enterobacter* spp., *Pseudomonas* spp., *Proteus* spp., *Providencia* spp., *Salmonella* spp., and *Serratia* spp.

The aminoglycosides can be used in combination with penicillins to treat gram-positive infections. The MIC required to control gram-negative aerobes with aminoglycosides is dependent on the drug used (gentamicin, 3 to 5 μm/mL amikacin, 5 to 10 μg/mL).[51] In general, up to three to five times the MIC may be necessary to eradicate certain pathogens.[53]

The aminoglycosides were one of the first antibiotics to be used extensively to treat bacterial infections in reptiles. They were also the first class of antibiotics to have pharmacokinetic data that could be used to determine appropriate dosing intervals.

Bush et al[54] were the first to evaluate an aminoglycoside in a chelonian. In the study, 15 Western Painted Turtles (*Chrysemys picta bellii*) and nine Red-eared Sliders were used. The turtles were maintained at 25°C to 27°C for the study. Three different dosing intervals were evaluated, including 10 mg/kg IM every 48 hours, 15 mg/kg IM every 48 hours, and 10 mg/kg IM every 96 hours. The average biologic half-life for gentamicin was 32 hours ± 15 hours, with a range of 8 to 76 hours. The large variation in the half-lives can be attributed to the small sample size. The serum concentrations of gentamicin for the turtles receiving 10 mg/kg every 96 hours provided appropriate serum levels for the first 24 to 48 hours but dropped to subtherapeutic levels thereafter.

The dose of 15 mg/kg every 48 hours achieved serum levels that are considered harmful in mammals. Because of the high levels achieved at this dose, the authors believed it was inappropriate. A dose of 10 mg/kg every 48 hours achieved therapeutic levels deemed appropriate for mammals but could result in toxic doses if used for an extended period (>15 days). On the basis of the results of the study, the authors concluded that 10 mg/kg every 48 hours for less than 14 days was an appropriate dose.

Bush et al[55] were also the first to evaluate these compounds in a snake species, the Gopher Snake (*Pituophis melanoleucas catenifer*). Twenty-one Gopher Snakes were used for the study, and the animals were housed at 24°C. Initially, five snakes received a dose of 2.5 mg/kg IM and an additional five snakes received 5 mg/kg IM. The average biologic half-life of gentamicin for snakes in both groups was 82 hours. No difference was found in biologic half-life between the two dosing regimens.

The half-lives reported in the chelonian and snake studies were 10 to 40 times longer than those reported for mammalian species.[56] A second study was performed to evaluate serial doses of gentamicin over approximately 14 days, including 2.5 mg/kg every 72 hours (n = 4), 2.5 mg/kg every 24 hours (n = 2), 5 mg/kg every 72 hours (n = 2), and 5 mg/kg every 24 hours (n = 3). A stairstep increase in serum concentrations of gentamicin was recorded for all groups. The highest concentrations occurred in the groups receiving daily injections. The authors suggested that this might have occurred because the snakes could not excrete the drug in a timely manner. Although serum concentrations were not as high in the groups receiving the antibiotic every 72 hours, they did achieve therapeutic levels and are less likely to produce negative side effects.

Hilf et al[57] also evaluated gentamicin disposition kinetics in two species of snakes, a Burmese Python (*Python molurus bivittatus*) and Blood Pythons (*Python curtus*). The snakes received a single dose of gentamicin (2.5 mg/kg IM). On the basis of the results from the pilot study, and the authors' desire to achieve peak serum concentrations between 6 and 8 μg/mL, the Blood Pythons (n = 4) were given one of four dosing regimens: 2.5 mg/kg IM followed by 1.5 mg/kg after 72 hours, 2.5 mg/kg IM followed by 1.5 mg/kg after 96 hours, 3 mg/kg IM followed by 1.5 mg/kg after 72 hours, and 3 mg/kg IM followed by 1.5 mg/kg after 96 hours.

Peak serum concentration was achieved within 10 hours. The biologic half-life varied between 32 and 110 hours.

No apparent side effects were seen, although the author used blood uric acid levels to evaluate renal function. Uric acid is not a sensitive assay for renal function in reptiles, and renal biopsy and microscopic review of the tissues would have been more appropriate.

Gentamicin accumulation was observed in these snakes and suggests that multiple dosing could lead to negative side effects. To avoid these potential side effects, the authors suggested medicating Indian Pythons (*Python molurus molurus*) with a loading dose of 2.5 to 3 mg/kg and 1.5 mg/kg every 96 hours thereafter.

Raphael, Clark, and Hudson[58] determined the pharmacokinetics of gentamicin in Red-eared Sliders. Twenty-one turtles were used for the study. The Red-eared Sliders were maintained at approximately 24°C during the study. Two different dosing regimens were tested: 6 mg/kg IM and 10 mg/kg IM. The 6 mg/kg dosing regimen was determined by subtracting approximately 40% of the 10-mg/kg dose to account for the weight of the shell. The plasma half-lives for the 10-mg/kg and 6-mg/kg doses were 56.8 and 31.3 hours, respectively.

Differences in the pharmacokinetics of gentamicin between the turtles studied in the Raphael, Clark, and Hudson[58] and Bush et al[54] papers may have been attributed to injection site or temperature variation. The turtles in Raphael, Clark, and Hudson[58] were housed at cooler temperatures than those in Bush et al.[54] In addition, the Red-eared Sliders in Raphael, Clark, and Hudson[58] were given the injection in the musculature of the forelimb.[58] This information was not provided by Bush et al,[54] and injection site may have led to alterations in the disposition of gentamicin in these chelonians.[54] On the basis of MIC values for susceptible species, the 6-mg/kg IM dose every 48 to 72 hours is appropriate for treatment of susceptible pathogens.

Beck et al[59] determined the pharmacokinetics for gentamicin in the Box Turtle (*Terrapene carolina carolina*). In addition, the authors also evaluated the role of injection site, forelimb versus hind limb, on the pharmacokinetics of the drug. Four turtles received 3 mL/kg of gentamicin in the forelimb, and an additional four animals received the same dose in the rear leg. Uric acid levels were evaluated in all of the test subjects before the antibiotics were given. Although uric acid was used to assess renal function, it does not appear to be a sensitive indicator of renal disease in reptiles. No difference was seen in the plasma concentrations of gentamicin between the two treatment groups. The half-life of gentamicin was 43.9 hours when administered in the rear limb and 40.3 hours when administered in the forelimb. Plasma concentrations remained above 2 μg/mL throughout the study, which should be adequate to achieve MIC for most pathogens. However, it may be insufficient to achieve the levels suggested by Hoperich.[53]

Because gentamicin is excreted via glomerular filtration, these findings were not unexpected. Evaluation of an antibiotic that is excreted via tubular secretion, such as a synthetic penicillin, may be more appropriate for evaluation of the role of the renal portal system in drug pharmacokinetics.

Side effects associated with gentamicin have been well documented. The first report in a lizard was associated with the toxic effects on the basilar papilla of *Calotes versicolor*.[60]

Gentamicin toxicity was also reported in two boid snakes that received 2 mg/lb twice a day for 2 days and then the same dose once a day for 5 additional days.[31] Both snakes had visceral gout develop, which was attributed to gentamicin-induced renal failure.

Many of the problems encountered with this class of antibiotics have been associated with the use of mammalian drug dosages. Montali, Bush, and Smeller[33] evaluated the pathologic effects of administration of a mammalian dose of gentamicin to two snakes. In the study, two Bull Snakes (*Pituophis [melanoleucas] catenifer*) were given gentamicin at 5 mg/kg once every 72 hours, and another two Bull Snakes were given 5 mg/kg once a day for 14 days. Renal biopsy results from the second group of snakes revealed mild to moderate swelling in the proximal tubular cells.

One snake from each of the two treatment groups was given an additional dose of 50 mg/kg once a day for 14 days. Again, swelling was noted in the proximal tubules and advanced to tubular necrosis. Variability in the pharmacokinetics of aminoglycosides in reptiles suggests that veterinarians should be cautious and use lower doses when working with an untested species.

With the advent of newer generation aminoglycosides, and their excellent spectrum against the gram-negative bacteria isolated from reptiles, that additional studies would be done to determine their disposition kinetics in reptiles was not surprising.

Mader, Conzelman, and Baggot[61] determined the pharmacokinetics of a single dose of amikacin (5 mg/kg IM) in Gopher Snakes (*Pituophis [melanoleucus] catenifer cantenifer*) housed at two different temperatures (25°C and 37°C). Because reptiles are ectothermic, the absorption, metabolism, and excretion of an antibiotic might be expected to differ when a reptile is maintained at different temperatures. However, no difference was seen in the absorption and elimination rates of amikacin in the snakes housed at different temperatures. The plasma half-lives for snakes housed at 25°C and 37°C were 71.9 hours and 75.4 hours, respectively.[61]

Snakes housed at the higher temperature did have an increased volume of distribution and body clearance compared to those housed at the cooler temperature. In addition, bacterial isolates were more susceptible to amikacin at higher temperatures. The authors concluded that a single dose of 5 mg/kg IM once, and a 2.5-mg/kg maintenance dose IM every 72 hours, could be used to control susceptible infections.

Although all 4700+ species of snakes are found in the suborder Serpentes, a high degree of variation exists between genera. Unfortunately, few research studies have been pursued to evaluate these differences. In an attempt to discern differences between colubrids and pythons, Johnson et al[62] performed a pharmacokinetic study with Ball Pythons (*Python regius*). They evaluated the effects of ambient temperature on the pharmacokinetics of amikacin in Ball Pythons.

Twelve adult Ball Pythons were used for the study, and the snakes were either housed at 25°C or 37°C. The dose for each snake was determined with metabolic scaling with a canine dose (11 mg/kg twice a day). The drug was delivered either intracardiac (IC) or intramuscularly. After a 4-week washout period, the snakes were treated again; however, the environmental temperature and route of delivery were switched. The elimination half-lives for the 25°C and 37°C treatment groups were 126 and 110 hours, respectively. These half-lives were substantially higher than those reported in the Gopher Snakes. Increased environmental temperature did not affect the rate of elimination in these snakes, which is different from that observed in other reptile species.[61,63]

Drug bioavailability, which is rarely recorded in reptile pharmacokinetic studies, was 74% to 77%. This is substantially less than that reported in mammals (>90%).[64] In comparison of serum concentration with MIC, the authors concluded that a single dose of 3.5 mg/kg is appropriate for susceptible infections in Ball Pythons. A higher dose (12 mg/kg) may be necessary for less sensitive pathogens, such as *Pseudomonas aeruginosa*, but the potential for side effects (e.g., renal pathology) could not be addressed by the authors.

A similar study was done to evaluate the effects of environmental temperature on the pharmacokinetics of amikacin in Gopher Tortoises (*Gopherus polyphemus*).[63] First, a pilot study (n = 3) was done to determine baseline serum concentrations for three different doses: 2.5 mg/kg, 5 mg/kg, and 10 mg/kg IM. The tortoises were maintained at approximately 30°C. The 5-mg/kg dose provided the most consistent results and therapeutic levels. The next component of the study evaluated a single and serial dose of 5 mg/kg IM in a group of six tortoises held at 30°C and an additional six tortoises held at 20°C. Clearance rates, mean residence times, and area under the curve were significantly different between the two treatment groups. The results of the study strongly suggested that environmental temperature could affect metabolic rate in this species, which in turn can affect drug pharmacokinetics in a reptile.

Although crocodilians are an important aquaculture species and display animal at zoologic institutions, clinical research with these species are limited. Jacobson et al[65] were the first to determine the disposition kinetics of gentamicin and amikacin in juvenile American Alligators. Twenty-four alligators were used for the study. The alligators were housed at an ambient temperature of 25°C to 27°C and a water temperature of 21°C to 23°C. Six alligators were allocated to each treatment group, which included dosing intervals of gentamicin at 1.25 mg/kg IM and 1.75 mg/kg IM and amikacin doses of 1.75 mg/kg IM and 2.25 mg/kg IM. A second amikacin dose was given to the amikacin treatment groups 96 hours after the first injection. Gentamicin and amikacin were both rapidly absorbed in the alligators. The distribution of both compounds was biphasic. Serum half-lives for the 1.25-mg/kg and 1.75-mg/kg gentamicin doses and the 1.75-mg/kg IM and 2.25-mg/kg IM amikacin doses were 37.8 hours, 75.4 hours, 49.4 hours, and 52.8 hours, respectively. On the basis of MIC values for pathogenic microbes in crocodilians, such as *Aeromonas hydrophila*, the higher doses used in this study were considered appropriate.

Cephalosporins

The cephalosporins are an important broad-spectrum antibiotic used in veterinary medicine. The cephalosporins, like the penicillins, were originally derived from a microbe (*Cephalosporium acremonium*). These drugs are bactericidal and act to inhibit mucopeptide synthesis in the cell wall. The cephalosporins are generally represented by four classes or generations. In veterinary medicine, classes 1-3 are routinely used, and class 4 is generally cost prohibitive and used in human medicine. The first class of cephalosporins has the narrowest spectrum of activity, generally covering gram-positive aerobes and anaerobes. The second class of cephalosporins has increased activity against gram-negative microbes. The third class of cephalosporins has the greatest spectrum against gram-negative microbes.

Cephalosporins are generally administered parenterally. However, cefadroxil (class 1), cephalexin (class 1), cephradine (class 1), cefaclor (class 2), cefuroxime (class 2), and cefixime (class 3) can be given per os.

The cephalosporins are widely distributed through the tissues in mammals. These compounds are especially useful for treatment of bone infections. Third class cephalosporins can enter the central nervous system (CNS) when the meninges are inflamed. The cephalosporins may be metabolized by the liver and are excreted via the kidneys. Side effects associated with this class of drugs are rare and are generally associated with hypersensitivity reactions. Cephalothin has been associated with renal disease in individuals with compromised renal function but is not generally a concern in those individuals with functional kidneys.[64]

Although these drugs are routinely used in veterinary medicine, few studies evaluate the pharmacokinetics of these drugs in reptiles. Lawrence, Muggleton, and Needham[66] were the first to evaluate the effects of a cephalosporin (ceftazidime) in a reptile. Ceftazidime, a third class cephalosporin, was selected because of its enhanced activity against Gram-negative microbes. This compound also has excellent spectrum against *Pseudomonas aeruginosa*, although the author has observed increased resistance with the continued use of this drug in veterinary medicine.

Eight different snakes, representing five different species, were used for the study. The snakes were maintained at 30°C during the study. Seven of the snakes received one 20-mg/kg dose IM, and one Yellow Ratsnake (*Elaphe obsolete quadrivittata*) received one 35-mg/kg dose IM. The snakes were divided into three groups to facilitate blood collection at different times. Blood samples were collected from one group at 1, 8, and 24 hours; from a second group at 24, 48, and 72 hours; and from a third group at 24, 48, 72, and 96 hours. Peak plasma levels for ceftazidime were variable (26 to 70 μg/mL) and occurred between 1 and 8 hours.

The high degree of variability may have been associated with species differences but could not be evaluated because of a limited sample size. The half-life of the drug was 24 hours, which is almost 12 times longer than that reported in humans.[67] No negative side effects were reported in any of the snakes. From this study, the authors concluded that a dose of 20 mg/kg IM administered every 72 hours is appropriate for sensitive bacterial pathogens isolated from snakes maintained at 30°C. The dose administered might be expected to vary with a different environmental temperature.

A study has also been performed to determine the pharmacokinetics of ceftazidime in Loggerhead Seaturtles (*Caretta caretta*).[68] Eight yearling turtles were used for the study, and the animals were maintained at 24°C ± 2°C. The turtles received a 20-mg/kg dose either IM or IV. Blood samples were collected at 0.5, 1.5, 3, 6, 12, 24, 48, 96, and 120 hours, and the samples were assayed for ceftazidime. The serum half-life for the intravenous route (20.2 hours) was similar to the intramuscular route (19 hours). The plasma concentrations were also similar for both routes and were above 4 μg/mL for 72 hours. The bioavailability of the drug after intramuscular injection was greater than 89%. From this study, the authors concluded that a dose of 20 mg/kg IM every 72 hours is sufficient to treat susceptible infections.

Cefoperazone, another third generation cephalosporin, has also been evaluated in reptiles. Although cephalosporins within the same class have similar mechanisms of action, activity, and distributions within the vertebrate hosts, some differences do exist. For instance, cefoperazome is more liposoluble than ceftazidime, which can increase its distribution to certain tissues. In addition, cefoperazome is excreted primarily via hepatic pathways, unlike most other cephalosporins, which are excreted via glomerular filtration or tubular secretion. Therefore, removal of this drug or negative side effects might be expected in vertebrates with hepatic dysfunction. This may also make it a more appropriate antibiotic than ceftazidime in treatment of a reptile with renal disease.

Speroni, Giambeluca, and Errecalde[69,70] determined the pharmacokinetics of cefoperazome in one snake *(Hydrodynastes gigas)* and one lizard *(Tupinambis teguixin)* after a single dose of 100 mg/kg IM. The reptiles were maintained at 24°C for the study. Peak levels of cefoperazome were achieved much faster in the Tegu (4 hours) than the colubrid (8 hours). In addition, therapeutic levels remained high in the snake much longer (96 hours) than in the lizard (<24 hours). From these results, the authors concluded that the snake should be given a dose of 100 mg/kg every 96 hours and the lizard should be given a dose of 125 mg/kg every 24 hours. The absence of additional reptiles limits the interpretation of these results. The differences found in these animals possibly could be as a result of individual variation (n = 1), but the difference between the Tegu and the colubrid is large enough that the findings more likely are real, which illustrates the differences in the pharmacokinetics between different orders of reptiles.

Chloramphenicol

Chloramphenicol is a broad-spectrum bacteriostatic to bacteriocidal drug (depending on concentration and bacterial susceptibility) that was originally isolated from *Streptomyces venezuelae*.[64] This antibiotic has been found to have activity against aerobic and anaerobic gram-positive and gram-negative bacteria. Chloramphenicol has also been found to be effective against anaerobes isolated from reptiles. Stewart[71] found that 18 anaerobic isolates from reptiles, representing 95% of the anaerobes isolated from clinical samples, were sensitive to chloramphenicol.

Chloramphenicol inhibits protein synthesis by binding to the 50S ribosomal subunit of the bacteria and possibly mammalian cells. The binding to mammalian cells is the cause of the aplastic anemia reported in humans. Chloramphenicol is widely distributed throughout the tissues in mammals. The drug is primarily excreted via the liver, and a small quantity is excreted unchanged via the kidneys. Clients should be made aware of the potential side effects associated with handling chloramphenicol, and humans with hepatic disease and nonregenerative anemias should never handle the drug.

Chloramphenicol, in combination with ampicillin, has been found to eliminate *Salmonella* spp. in both lizards and chelonians.[72] Although only 87% of the reptiles were considered *Salmonella*-free after a 5-day course of the two antibiotics, the remaining animals were "cleared" of *Salmonella* after an additional 5 days of treatment. One should be cautious with interpretation of these results because these animals could have become latent and not actively shed *Salmonella* or the microbes were shed in such low numbers they were below the sensitivity threshold of the assay.

Pharmacokinetic studies for chloramphenicol for reptiles are limited to snakes. Bush et al[55] determined the plasma concentrations of chloramphenicol sodium succinate in Gopher Snakes housed at an environmental temperature of 29°C. Peak concentrations (26 µg/mL) were achieved in 3.5 hours, and the half-life from the subcutaneous injection was approximately 5.5 hours. From these results, the authors concluded that a single 40 mg/kg SC dose of chloramphenicol is sufficient to deliver therapeutic levels in these Gopher Snakes.

An oral dose of chloramphenicol palmitate (12 mg/kg) only achieved peak plasma levels of 10 µg/mL at approximately 12 hours. The oral dose was not considered sufficient to provide therapeutic levels against reptilian pathogens. However, the oral dose was considerably less than that given parenterally.

Clark, Rogers, and Milton[73] determined the plasma concentrations of chloramphenicol in 16 different species of snakes. Two different dosing regimens were evaluated, including 25 and 50 mg/kg SC. The 25-mg/kg SC dose was found to produce low plasma concentrations and was discontinued. The plasma concentrations from the 50-mg/kg dose were found to be highly variable between species. For example, Watersnakes (*Nerodia* spp.) maintained plasma concentrations near 5 µg/mL for 48 to 72 hours, the crotalids maintained concentrations of more than 5 µg/mL for 48 hours, and most of the colubrids eliminated the drug within 24 hours.

Differences in plasma concentrations were also observed between different injectable preparations, with Tevcocin (International Multifoods, Minneapolis, Minn) maintaining higher concentrations than Mychel-Vet (Rachelle Laboratories, Long Beach, Calif). This difference was attributed to an edematous reaction at the site of injection, which was more common with the Mychel-Vet preparation. One Midland Watersnake (*Nerodia sipedon*) had an anemia develop after receiving six injections of chloramphenicol every 72 hours, but no further investigation, such as evaluating the marrow of a rib, was pursued to determine whether the chloramphenicol had a direct effect on blood cell production.

Because of the large variation in plasma concentration between species, the authors concluded that chloramphenicol could be given at 50 mg/kg SC every 12 to 72 hours depending on the species. The dosing frequency should also be based on the environmental temperature because it could affect the metabolism of the chloramphenicol.

Florfenicol

Florfenicol, a fluorinated analog of thiamphenicol, is a relatively recent addition to the veterinarian's antibiotic arsenal. This compound is structurally similar to chloramphenicol, although it lacks the paranitro group that is associated with aplastic anemia in humans.[74] This compound is only approved for cattle, although it has also been used to treat domestic and nontraditional species.

Florfenicol is a broad-spectrum bacteriocidal antibiotic that acts against the 50S ribosome of bacteria. In cattle, the drug is moderately bioavailable (79%) after intramuscular injection.[64] The drug has good distribution into various tissues, including the CNS. Relatively few side effects have been reported in mammalian hosts and are primarily associated with the gastrointestinal tract. However, these side effects can be significant in horses, and the drug is not generally recommended for equids. Similar considerations may need to be taken into account for reptiles that use hindgut fermentation, such as iguanids.

A single published study has been performed to determine the pharmacokinetics of florfenicol in a reptile.[75] Eight yearling Loggerhead Seaturtles were used for the study, and the animals were maintained at 24°C ± 2°C. The turtles received a 30-mg/kg dose either IM or IV. Blood samples were collected at 0.5, 1.5, 3, 6, 12, 24, and 48 hours, and the samples were assayed for florfenicol. An additional two turtles were given 30 mg/kg IV, and blood was collected at 0, 3, 5, 10, 20, 30, and 60 minutes after drug administration.

The serum half-lives for both the intravenous and intramuscular routes were very short. Florfenicol could not be measured in any of the turtles more than 12 hours after receiving the drug. The plasma concentrations in both groups were lower than the acceptable MIC for most reptilian pathogens. From this study, the authors concluded that 30 mg/kg florfenicol either IM or IV in Loggerhead Seaturtles was insufficient to manage bacterial infections.

Fluoroquinolones

Fluoroquinolones are one of the most commonly used groups of antibiotics in human and veterinary medicine. The fluoroquinolones are bactericidal compounds with activity against both gram-positive and gram-negative pathogens.[76,77] These compounds have limited spectrum against anaerobes. Modification of the 4-quinolone ring has enhanced the antimicrobial activity. Oral bioavailability of enrofloxacin is excellent in monogastric mammals and preruminant calves, with up to 80% of the ingested dose absorbed into systemic circulation.[78] Oral absorption of fluoroquinolones is rapid, with peak serum concentrations achieved 1 to 2 hours after administration.[79]

Fluoroquinolones do not readily complex with plasma proteins, which enables metabolites to cross cell membranes readily. In humans, approximately 10% to 40% of the fluoroquinolones are bound to plasma proteins.[78] The fluoroquinolones are widely distributed throughout the body, including the kidneys, liver, bile, prostate, uterus and fallopian tubes, bone, and inflammatory tissues.[80] Excretion of the fluoroquinolones is primarily through the kidneys, with secondary excretion through the liver.[78,80]

Fluoroquinolones alter the action of bacterial DNA gyrase, a type II topoisomerase.[78] This enzyme is involved in unwinding, cutting, and resealing DNA. The two subunits to DNA gyrase are subunit A and subunit B, and fluoroquinolones act on the nalidixic acid locus of the subunit A. Inhibition of the gyrase leads to rapid cell death in bacteria. The concentration of fluoroquinolones necessary to alter the DNA of mammalian cells is two orders of magnitude higher than the concentration against bacterial DNA.[81,82]

Enrofloxacin is a member of the family of 6-fluoro-7-piperazinyl-4-quinolones.[76] Enrofloxacin is highly lipophilic, and the addition of a carboxic acid and a tertiary amine contributes to the amphoteric properties of enrofloxacin.[78] The metabolism of enrofloxacin varies among species. Although enrofloxacin is an active antibiotic, biotransformation to ciprofloxacin may also occur. Biotransformation of enrofloxacin includes N-dealkylation, glucuronide conjugation to the nitrogen in the paraposition of the piperazinyl ring, oxidation in the orthoposition to substituted amine, and opening of the piperazinyl ring.[78]

The elimination half-life of enrofloxacin varies among species. Chickens have a prolonged half-life (7.3 hours) in comparison with mammals, including canines (2.1 hours), calves (1.2 hours), and horses (3.3 hours).[78] The elimination half-life of enrofloxacin is much longer in ectotherms, such as reptiles. Enrofloxacin has a biphasic concentration-response curve.[83] In the first phase, the proportion of bacteria killed increases as the concentration of enrofloxacin is increased. In the second phase, bacteria are killed at a lower rate as the concentration of enrofloxacin is increased.

Selection for resistance to the fluoroquinolones occurs from chromosomal mutations, creation of gyrase modifications, or alterations in permeability.[84,85] No plasmid resistance has been shown. Mutants develop resistance to other fluoroquinolones and other antimicrobials, including cephalosporins, chloramphenicol, and tetracyclines.[86,87]

The adverse effects associated with fluoroquinolones are primarily associated with immature cartilage, the urinary and gastrointestinal tracts, and the CNS. Arthropathies have been reported in immature rats, beagles, guinea pigs, and foals.[88-91] The cartilaginous surfaces of the femur, the humerus, and the tibia are the primary sites where quinolone-induced arthropathies occurred in beagle pups.[89] The most common histologic findings in quinolone-induced arthropathies are erosions of the articular cartilage.[88-90] Histologic lesions may be detected 2 days after treatment.

Fluoroquinolones can achieve a high concentration in the urine because the kidneys are the primary route of excretion for fluoroquinolones. Because the fluoroquinolones have low solubility in water, they crystallize in acidic urine.[78] Crystalluria could be a problem in carnivorous animals fed a high-protein diet. The adverse gastrointestinal effects associated with the fluoroquinolones include nausea, vomiting, and abdominal cramping.[92] The descriptions of adverse effects associated with the CNS have been documented in human patients.[93] Changes in behavior, including psychosis, headaches, hallucinations, and seizures, have been reported after treatment with 250 to 500 mg ciprofloxacin. No adverse effects from enrofloxacin treatment have been reported in reptiles other than the sterile abscesses reported after intramuscular injections already discussed (see Figure 36-17).

Fluoroquinolones are highly effective bacteriocides with relatively low MICs. Clinical *Salmonella arizonae* isolates evaluated at the University of California showed MIC values in 90% of the isolates ranging between 0.128 μg/mL to 1 μg/mL.[78] Berg[91] reported that MICs demonstrated by 96% of Salmonella isolates from clinical samples were less than 0.125 μg/mL. *Salmonella* isolates from urinary tract infections also yielded low MIC levels for ciprofloxacin (0.06 μg/mL).[78] The systemic distributions of enrofloxacin and ciprofloxacin, in combination with the low MIC levels necessary to eradicate *Salmonella* and the levels of enrofloxacin achieved in the serum and tissues, suggest that these compounds are beneficial for treatment of a prospective patient with a *Salmonella* infection.

Enrofloxacin has been evaluated as a method to eliminate *Salmonella* infections in cattle, poultry, and Green Iguanas. Enrofloxacin administered to cattle at 5 mg/kg/day for

10 days eliminated *Salmonella* in more than half the subjects.[94] The *Salmonella* isolates from the cattle that remained infected after treatment were still sensitive to enrofloxacin. Calves experimentally infected with *Salmonella typhimurium* were cleared of the infection after treatment with enrofloxacin at a dose of 5 mg/kg/day for 6 days.[95]

Enrofloxacin administered to poultry in drinking water at 50 parts per million for 5 to 10 days was effective against experimental *Salmonella typhimurium* infection in broilers and turkeys.[95] Broilers reinfected with *Salmonella typhimurium* 14 days after discontinuation of treatment of 100 to 200 parts per million enrofloxacin were reinfected at a similar rate.[95] Enrofloxacin, when administered under controlled conditions, was effective at eliminating *Salmonella* from domestic livestock and poultry.

Salmonella was eliminated from most Green Iguanas treated with enrofloxacin (10 mg/kg PO every 24 hours for 10 days).[96] Enrofloxacin was used to eliminate *Salmonella* from iguanas that were sensitive to the drug to create a *Salmonella* clearance model. The enrofloxacin clearance models were conducted in sterile environments with food and water that were known to be *Salmonella*-free. An interesting side note to the research was that enrofloxacin suppressed shedding of *Salmonella* for up to 70 days. Resistance to the enrofloxacin was not found in any of the isolates recovered from the iguanas.

Veterinarians should not consider using enrofloxacin to eliminate *Salmonella* from apparently normal pet iguanas because enrofloxacin does not provide long-term protection against reinfection with *Salmonella*, which is ubiquitous in the environment.

Enrofloxacin has been used to treat bacterial infection in reptiles because it is active against most of the gram-positive and gram-negative bacteria that affect these species. Enrofloxacin administered at a dose of 10 mg/kg IM or PO at 5 mg/kg in Savannah Monitors (*Varanus exanthematicus*) resulted in minimal conversion to ciprofloxacin.[97] The terminal elimination half-life was 40 hours for the IM and PO routes at 5 mg/kg and 36 and 24 hours for IM and PO routes at 10 mg/kg. The peak plasma concentrations for the IM and oral routes at 10 mg/kg were 10.5 µg/mL and 3.6 µg/mL, respectively. The peak serum concentrations recorded in the monitor lizard are adequate to treat susceptible bacteria.

Maxwell and Jacobson[98] determined the pharmacokinetics of single-dose oral and intramuscular enrofloxacin in Green Iguanas. Six adult Green Iguanas were given 5-mg/kg enrofloxacin PO, and an additional three iguanas were given the same dose IM. The peak plasma concentrations for the oral and IM doses were 1.16 µg/mL and 2 µg/mL, respectively. Therapeutic levels (>0.2 µg/mL) for the PO and IM treatments were maintained for approximately 32 and 16 hours after injection. A high degree of variability was found in the plasma concentrations in the iguanas receiving the oral dose, leading the authors to suggest the parenteral route for critical cases. Because ciprofloxacin was not readily detected, the authors suggested that it is not created in appreciable amounts from the metabolism of enrofloxacin in the Green Iguana.

Pharmacokinetic studies for fluoroquinolones in snakes are limited. Young et al[99] were the first to determine the disposition of enrofloxacin in a species of snake (*Python molurus bivittatus*). Eleven young (1 to 2 years old) Burmese Pythons were used for the study. The snakes were maintained at 30°C for the study and fasted for the week before receiving the antibiotic. Six of the snakes received a single enrofloxacin injection intramuscularly in the cranial half of the body, and the remaining five animals received an enrofloxacin injection intramuscularly once a day for 5 days. A single dose of enrofloxacin resulted in a significant conversion to ciprofloxacin; however, the half-life of ciprofloxacin could not be determined. The peak serum concentration of enrofloxacin in the python was 1.66 µg/mL, and the mean terminal half-life was 6.37 hours.

The multiple dose study revealed that the plasma half-life for ciprofloxacin might be longer than enrofloxacin as a result of the regular conversion of enrofloxacin to ciprofloxacin. On the basis of MIC data for bacterial pathogens isolated from Burmese Pythons, the authors recommended a dose of 10 mg/kg IM every 48 hours for *Pseudomonas* infections and an initial dose of 10 mg/kg with follow-up doses of 5 mg/kg every 48 hours for other susceptible pathogens.

The pharmacokinetic of enrofloxacin have been evaluated in several species of chelonians. Sporle, Gobel, and Schildger[100] evaluated the drug in Hermann's Tortoises (*Testudo hermanni*). A dose of 10 mg/kg IM every 24 hours was sufficient to control susceptible bacterial pathogens.

Prezant, Isaza, and Jacobson[101] evaluated the drug in Gopher Tortoises at a lower dose, 5 mg/kg IM, and found it could be given every 24 to 48 hours to achieve MIC levels for common pathogens. The terminal half-life for enrofloxacin in the Gopher Tortoise (23.1 hours) was significantly longer than other mammal, avian, and reptile species.

Raphael, Papich, and Cook[102] evaluated a similar dose of 5 mg/kg IM in Indian Star Tortoises (*Geochelone elegans*).[102] In the Star Tortoises, peak plasma levels were approximately 3.6 µg/mL, and the plasma half-life was 5.1 hours. Ciprofloxacin was identified after injection, suggesting that these tortoises can convert enrofloxacin to ciprofloxacin. The half-life of ciprofloxacin was 4.8 hours. On the basis of MIC values for pathogens isolated from these tortoises, the authors concluded that a dose of 5 mg/kg IM every 12 to 24 hours should be used to control bacterial infections.

A single study has evaluated the pharmacokinetics of enrofloxacin in an aquatic chelonian (*Trachemys scripta elegans*).[103] In the study, both intramuscular (5 mg/kg) and oral (10 mg/kg) doses of enrofloxacin were evaluated. Peak plasma levels for the IM dose (6.3 µg/mL) and oral dose (3.4 µg/mL) were achieved 2 and 5 hours after injection, respectively. Ciprofloxacin was measured in these Red-eared Sliders, confirming that they can convert enrofloxacin to ciprofloxacin. The average half-life for enrofloxacin was almost 18 and 33 hours for the IM and PO routes. No negative side effects were detected in these turtles. Enrofloxacin at 5 mg/kg IM or 10 mg/kg PO is appropriate for Red-eared Sliders.

The emergence of a pathogenic mycoplasmosis in alligators led Helmick et al[104] to evaluate the pharmacokinetics of enrofloxacin in these reptiles. Seven subadult captive alligators housed at 27°C were used for the study. Five of the alligators received 5-mg/kg enrofloxacin IV once. The peak plasma concentration of enrofloxacin in these alligators was 6 µg/mL, which was much higher than the MIC (1 µg/mL) determined for the *Mycoplasma lacerti* isolated from the alligators. The plasma concentrations measured in these reptiles actually remained above this MIC for an average of 31 hours. On the basis of these data, a dose of 5 mg/kg every 72 hours was suggested to be sufficient to control susceptible infections.

Although negative side effects have been associated with enrofloxacin administration in mammals, they are rare in reptiles. The most common side effect associated with this antibiotic is pain and inflammation at the injection site. Affected reptiles may withdraw the limb where an injection is given, attempt to escape, or experience skin twitching at the site of injection. One report of a more severe reaction was recorded in a Galapagos Tortoise (*Geochelone elephantopus nigra*).[106] The tortoise was empirically treated with 1000 mg of enrofloxacin (Baytril, 10% solution, Bayer AG, Leverkusen, Germany) for a suspected pneumonia. The tortoise became hyperexcitable and uncoordinated and had a profuse diarrhea develop approximately 1 hour after injection. A second lower dose (500 mg, 5% solution) was given approximately 48 hours later. The tortoise again had a negative reaction approximately 1 hour after injection. Because of the similarity in side effects recorded after the enrofloxacin injection, the authors concluded that the tortoise had a hypersensitivity reaction to the enrofloxacin. The side effect associated with this case may have been a direct hypersensitivity to the enrofloxacin or could have been the result of a reaction to the carrier associated with the antibiotic.

The author has used the 2.27% small animal injectable in a number of tortoises, including Giant Tortoises, without negative side effects.

Macrolides

Macrolides were one of the original groups of antibiotics available in veterinary medicine, as were the tetracyclines, and were also originally isolated from a bacteria (erythromycin: *Streptomyces erythreus*). Macrolides are bacteriostatic; however, high doses can be bacteriocidal in susceptible bacteria. Although they are not generally considered to have broad control over anaerobes, Stewart[71] found that 18 anaerobic isolates from snakes, representing 95% of the anaerobes isolated from clinical samples, were sensitive to clindamycin.

By inhibiting the 50S ribosomes, the macrolides restrict protein formation by the bacteria. Macrolides can be excreted unchanged via the bile or partially metabolized by the liver. A limited quantity may also be excreted via the kidneys. In mammals, both food and gastric pH can affect absorption of the macrolides.[64] Macrolides are moderately to significantly bound to protein and have good distribution to most tissues in the body. Although these compounds are generally broad spectrum, widespread use of these compounds in human and veterinary medicine have led to increased resistance.

The first study to determine the pharmacokinetics of a macrolide in a reptile was done by Wimsatt et al[107] when they evaluated clarithromycin in the Desert Tortoise (*Gopherus agassizii*). This drug was evaluated because of its apparent efficacy against mycoplasmosis, which is suspected as the primary etiology responsible for upper respiratory disease syndrome in the *Gopherus* genus.

Male Desert Tortoises were used for the study, and the animals were maintained between 30°C and 33.3°C. Multiple dosing strategies were evaluated in the study. First, a 7.5-mg/kg PO dose given once was evaluated. A second trial evaluated a 15-mg/kg dose PO once. Finally, a series of 15-mg/kg PO doses were given once a day for 9 days.

The 7.5-mg/kg dose was not considered to be appropriate. The 15-mg/kg PO single dose achieved a maximum concentration of 1.37 μg/mL and had a plasma half-life of 11.69 hours. These findings might suggest that a single dose every 24 hours is appropriate; however, in evaluation of the multiple dose study, the authors found that the drug can accumulate. The study suggested that a dose of 15 mg/kg PO every 48 to 72 hours is appropriate to manage susceptible infections.

With the advent of newer more broad-spectrum macrolides, interest has been seen in the veterinary community to evaluate these compounds in reptiles. Coke et al[108] determined the pharmacokinetics of a single dose of azithromycin in Ball Pythons. Azithromycin was selected not only because of its spectrum but also because of the potential for persistent tissue concentrations. Both IV (10 mg/kg) and PO (10 mg/kg) dosing regimens were evaluated. The plasma half-lives for IV and PO were 17 and 51 hours, respectively. Bioavailability after oral dosing was considered good at 77% (± 27%). The authors concluded that a 10-mg/kg dose PO every 2 to 7 days is appropriate to control susceptible infections, depending on site of infection.

Metronidazole

Metronidazole is the most commonly used antimicrobial to manage protozoal and anaerobic bacterial infections. This drug is bactericidal and amebicidal. The cidal mechanism of this compound is not known, although it is thought to inhibit DNA and nucleic acid synthesis.[64] Absorption of metronidazole varies between species. In general, 50% to 100% of the drug is absorbed.[64] Absorption can also vary with gastric contents, with increased absorption reported in canines when fed food and decreased absorption in humans offered food.[64]

Metronidazole is metabolized by the liver and excreted via urine and feces. Because this drug is primarily metabolized via the liver, veterinarians should use caution when giving this drug to a reptile with hepatic dysfunction. In mammals, metronidazole is well distributed in the tissues, including the bones and CNS. In mammals, the half-life of metronidazole ranges from 3 to 8 hours.

Metronidazole toxicity primarily affects the CNS, liver, and gastrointestinal tract. The author has observed three referral reptile cases with severe neurologic disease after treatment with high doses (>200 mg/kg) of metronidazole. In addition, hepatic dysfunction might be expected. In the cases the author has observed, aspartate transferase (AST) levels were significantly increased in the face of mild creatine kinase (CK) elevations. Gastrointestinal disease, including regurgitation and diarrhea, may also occur with metronidazole toxicity.

The presumed toxic cases observed by the author responded to supportive care and the discontinuation of the drug. Funk[109] reported that deaths may occur in Indigo Snakes (*Drymarchon coraes*), California Mountain Kingsnakes (*Lampropeltis zonata*), and Arizona Mountain Kingsnakes (*L. pyromelena*) when doses of more than 100 mg/kg are used. In addition, Jacobson[31] has reported that side effects in Uracoan Rattlesnakes may occur with doses of more than 40 mg/kg.

Metronidazole is available in tablet and injectable forms. Because metronidazole has poor solubility in water, it can be difficult to make into a suspension. Commercial suspensions are available outside of the United States, and many compounding pharmacies in the United States can now make suspensions on special order. Metronidazole is bitter and can cause significant hypersalivation. Flavored medications can be compounded to reduce this effect, or the drug can be administered via a feeding tube.

Metronidazole has been used to treat a variety of clinical problems, from protozoal enteritis to bacterial sepsis to anorexia, with an equally wide range of doses, anywhere from from 20 to 250 mg/kg.[110] Antibacterial doses generally range from 20 to 50 mg/kg, and higher doses are recommended for protozoal infections. Unfortunately, many of these dosages are anecdotal. Appetite stimulant dosages range in the higher end of the range, the latter being anecdotal.

Anaerobic cultures are not routinely collected from clinical specimens because of the difficulty in collecting, transporting, processing, and characterizing anaerobic bacteria. Anaerobes are an important component of the microflora of reptiles and occasionally cause disease. The most common sites from which anaerobic pathogens are isolated are the respiratory tract, coelomic cavity, and integument.[71]

Stewart[71] characterized 21 anaerobes, including *Bacteroides* sp., *Fusobacterium* sp., *Peptostreptococcus* sp., and *Clostridium* sp., from 39 different clinical reptile specimens. All of the isolates were sensitive to metronidazole.

The widespread use of metronidazole as a prophylaxis and antiprotozoal could lead to the development of resistant anaerobic microbes. Veterinarians should use this drug, like other antimicrobials, judiciously to minimize the likelihood of generating metronidazole resistant microbes.

The first study to determine the pharmacokinetics of metronidazole in a reptile was done by Kolmstetter et al[111] with the Green Iguana. The authors evaluated two dosing regimens, 20 mg/kg PO after a single dose and the same dose for 10 days. The iguanas were fed daily during the study. A PCV and plasma chemistry profile, including TP, glucose, albumin, calcium, phosphorus, uric acid, creatinine phosphokinase (CPK), alanine transferase (ALT), lactate dehydrogenase (LDH), AST, and alkaline phosphotase (ALP), was performed on each iguana after the first and last dose of metronidazole.

No negative behavioral side effects or hematologic variations were noted in the iguanas. The half-life (12.7 hours) of metronidazole in the iguana was longer than in mammals, and the peak plasma concentration (7.6 µg/mL) was achieved within 4 hours of dosing. Research evaluating the MICs for metronidazole against common anaerobes suggests that the concentration achieved in these iguanas was sufficient to manage susceptible infections.[112] Variability was noted in the plasma concentrations in these iguanas, suggesting that a 48-hour dosing schedule may not be sufficient in some iguanas. In those cases in which the response to treatment is not sufficient, a 20-mg/kg dose can be given every 24 hours.

Kolmstetter, Cox, and Ramsay[113] also determined the pharmacokinetics of metronidazole in Yellow Ratsnakes after single and multiple oral doses of the drug. The authors evaluated single oral doses of 20 mg/kg and 100 mg/kg and a 6-day course of 20 mg/kg. The snakes were fasted for 10 days before receiving metronidazole. Therefore, determination of whether gastric filling affected absorption in these reptiles was not possible. A PCV and plasma chemistry profile, including TP, glucose, albumin, calcium, phosphorus, uric acid, CPK, ALT, LDH, AST, and ALP, was performed on each snake after the first and last dose of metronidazole. No negative behavioral side effects were reported in these snakes, and they all ate at the end of the study.

The PCV, TP, albumin, glucose, and ALT were significantly lower after the sixth dose, and the CK and LDH were significantly higher after the last dose. The half-life (14 to 15 hours) of metronidazole in the Ratsnakes was also longer than in mammals but similar to the Iguanas. The peak plasma concentration (14 µg/mL) was achieved within 2 hours of dosing. Research evaluating the MICs for metronidazole against common anaerobes suggests that the concentrations achieved in these snakes were sufficient to manage susceptible infections.[112] From the multiple dose study, the authors concluded that a dose of 20 mg/kg every 48 hours is sufficient to manage anaerobic infections in these snakes.

Bodri et al[114] determined the pharmacokinetics of metronidazole in Cornsnakes (*Elaphe guttata*). In this study, higher doses, 50-mg/kg PO and 150-mg/kg PO, were evaluated. The half-life of metronidazole in these snakes was 11.1 hours, and plasma concentrations exceeded MIC values for susceptible microbes for 48 hours. The authors concluded that a 50 mg/kg dose every 48 hours was safe and should be sufficient to control susceptible microbes.

Semisynthetic Penicillins

Carbenicillin and piperacillin are semisynthetic penicillins with extended spectrum against gram-negative bacteria. These drugs were originally found to have antipseudomonal activity; however, increased resistance is reported with increased usage. Lawrence et al[46] reported pseudomonal resistance to carbenicillin in multiple beta-lactamase–producing pseudomonal species in the early 1980s. The semisynthetic penicillins also have some effect against anaerobes.

The primary action of the semisynthetic penicillins is against cell wall synthesis. This class of drugs is susceptible to beta-lactamase. Variable amounts of the semisynthetic penicillins are bound to protein. Distribution of these drugs is greater via the parenteral route. The drugs are excreted primarily via tubular secretion and glomerular filtration. Semisynthetic penicillins cross the placenta in mammals but are not known to have teratogenic effects. Whether these drugs could affect embryos in reptiles is not known.

Studies that evaluate the efficacy of the semisynthetic penicillins are limited in reptiles. Hilf et al[115] determined the pharmacokinetics of piperacillin in Blood Pythons. The half-life of piperacillin between the snakes used in the study was similar. However, the distribution of the drug was variable after intramuscular injection.

The authors also determined the MICs necessary to eliminate several gram-negative bacterial species in vitro. The serum concentration of piperacillin (142.6 to 274 µg/mL) obtained 4 hours after intramuscular injection was sufficient to eliminate the bacterial pathogen (0.25 to 4 µg/kg) isolated for the study. In the case of the blood pythons, a dose of 100 mg/kg IM every 48 hours should be sufficient to eliminate susceptible bacterial infections.

Lawrence et al[46] determined plasma concentrations of a single intramuscular injection of carbenicillin in four different species of snakes. Blood samples were collected on two different time schedules from the snake subjects, limiting the authors' ability to perform a pharmacokinetic study.

Peak plasma levels (177 to 270 µg/mL) were achieved 1 hour after injection. Therapeutic levels (50 to 60 µg/mL) were maintained for 12 hours in the three of the snakes. Although Lawrence et al[46] did not collect sufficient blood volumes to perform a pharmacokinetic study, their recommendation was that 400 mg/kg IM every 24 hours provides therapeutic levels of carbenicillin for snakes. Holtz et al[44] reported that 200 mg/kg IM every 24 hours was appropriate for Carpet Pythons.

Lawrence, Palmer, and Needham et al[116] also evaluated the disposition kinetics of carbenicillin in two species of chelonians, *Testudo graeca* and *T. hermanni*. A total of 11 tortoises were used for the study, and they were divided into three groups on the basis of postinjection blood collection. Carbenicillin was administered in the quadriceps at 400 mg/kg, and blood samples were either collected at 1, 8, and 12 hours after injection (group 1); 1, 4 and 17 hours (group 2); or 37, 44, and 72 hours (group 3). Peak plasma levels were achieved at different times for these two species of tortoise, with *T. graeca* peaking at 1 hour and *T. hermanni* at 8 hours. In addition, a second peak in carbenicillin concentration was recorded at 37 (*T. graeca*) and 72 (*T. hermanni*) hours.

Therapeutic levels were recorded for approximately 12 hours in *T. graeca* and were found throughout the study for *T. hermanni*. Because chelonians, especially tortoises, use their urinary bladders as a site of fluid and electrolyte resorption, resorption of excreted carbenicillin was suggested to possibly also occur. Although limited by the numbers of tortoises used in this study, the authors did report that the tortoises that evacuated urine during the study did have lower carbenicillin concentrations than those that did not micturate, suggesting that the bladder could serve in some capacity in the resorption of ionized drugs. The authors concluded that 400 mg/kg every 48 hours is likely sufficient to provide therapeutic levels in these tortoises.

Tetracyclines

The tetracyclines represent one of the oldest classes of antibiotics available in human or veterinary medicine. Tetracycline was originally isolated from *Streptomyces aureofaciens*. Tetracyclines are bacteriostatic and act by inhibiting protein synthesis by reversibly binding to the 30S ribosome. At high doses, these compounds can also affect eukaryotic cells. Although these compounds are generally reserved for aerobic bacteria, they have been found (in vitro) to be effective against anaerobes isolated from reptiles. Stewart[71] found that 18 anaerobic isolates, representing 95% of the anaerobes isolated from clinical samples in snakes, were sensitive to tetracyclines.

Tetracyclines are variably bound to protein and have good distribution to most tissues in the body. Tetacyclines are not metabolized but are excreted primarily through the gastrointestinal tract or kidneys. These compounds can be chelated by fecal material, thus reducing their effectiveness. In mammals, food can also diminish the absorption by chelating tetracyclines.[64] Because these compounds are excreted via glomerular filtration, reptiles with renal dysfunction may accumulate the compound over time.

Although these compounds are generally broad spectrum, widespread use of these compounds in human and veterinary medicine has led to increased resistance. These compounds, especially doxycycline, have excellent spectrum against *Chamydiophila* spp., *Mycoplasma* spp., and rickettsial organisms. Recent reports of reptilian chlamydiophyllosis and mycoplasmosis suggest that these compounds remain important in reptilian medicine.

Sporle, Gobel, and Schildger[100] determined a therapeutic regimen for doxycycline for treatment of sensitive microbes in the Hermann's Tortoise. In the study, Sporle isolated *Staphylococcus* sp. and *Klebsiella* sp. with MIC values of 8.9 µg/mL and 5.6 µg/mL, respectively. Other microbes, including a *Salmonella* sp. and a *Pseudomonas aeruginosa*, were found to be resistant. The finding of resistance in these microbes should not be considered unusual because they are highly adapted to the tetracyclines. In the study, Sporle determined that a loading dose of 50 mg/kg IM once, followed by 25 mg/kg IM every 72 hours, is appropriate to manage sensitive pathogens in this chelonian.

The emergence of mycoplasmosis in captive crocodilians has led to research to determine the pharmacokinetics of oxytetracycline in American Alligators.[104] Two subadult captive alligators housed at 27°C were used for the study. The alligators received 10 mg/kg oxytetracycline IV once in the supravertebral vein. The peak plasma concentration of oxytetracycline in these alligators was 98 µg/mL, which was much higher than the MIC (1 µg/mL) determined for the *Mycoplasma lacerti* isolated from the alligators. The plasma concentrations measured in these reptiles actually remained above this MIC for an average of 96 hours. The authors concluded that additional samples need to be collected beyond 96 hours to determine the most appropriate dose of oxytetracycline.

Harms et al[105] studied the pharmacokinetics of oxytetracycline in Loggerhead Seaturtles. The recommended IM doses were 41 mg/kg as a loading dose followed by 21 mg/kg every 72 hours or 82 mg/kg first dose then 42 mg/kg every 72 hours.

Potentiated Sulfas: Trimethoprim Sulfadimethoxine

The potentiated sulfas (e.g., trimethoprim sulfadimethoxine) are broad-spectrum antibiotics that are routinely used to treat bacterial and protozoal pathogens in reptiles. Sulfa drugs are generally bacteriostatic; however, the synergism with trimethoprim creates a bactericidal compound. These compounds affect folic acid synthesis. Oral doses are well absorbed in monogastric mammals. This compound has widespread tissue distribution, including the CNS when the meninges are inflamed. Potentiated sulfas are metabolized by the liver and excreted by the kidneys, via both glomerular filtration and tubular secretion.[64] The primary side effects associated with this drug are attributed to hypersensitivity and the potential for crystallization in the urine. The author does not recommend this antibiotic in cases with cystic calculi or severe dehydration.

These compounds are generally delivered via an oral suspension, although compounding pharmacies can create parenteral forms. To date, no pharmacokinetic studies have been performed to determine an appropriate dosing schedule. However, Vree and Vree[117] have determined that Red-eared Slider Turtles can acetylate sulphamethoxazole. Current dosing recommendations are varied, including 15 to 25 mg/kg every 24 hours, 20 to 30 mg/kg every 24 to 48 hours, and 30 mg/kg once a day for 2 days than 30 mg/kg every 48 hours.[31,118] One should remember that these doses are anecdotal and that the veterinarian should consider the general health status of the patient before selecting a dose. Before use of potentiated sulfas, the author always ensures that the patient is hydrated.

Antivirals

Many of the newly documented or emerging diseases reported in captive reptiles are attributed to viruses. Our current understanding of viruses is limited because we do not have the diagnostic assays to isolate or confirm the presence of these pathogens. Until we have described the epidemiology of these viruses, effective treatment and management of reptilian viruses will be difficult. Culling virus-positive reptiles from collections is probably the safest strategy to use in development of a management plan.

A single in vitro study has evaluated the efficacy of antiviral drugs against a virus isolated from a reptile. Marschang, Gravendyck, and Kaleta[119] evaluated the efficacy of acyclovir and ganciclovir (Cymeven; Hoffmann-LaRoche AG, Grenzach-Wyhlen, Germany) in vitro against a herpes virus isolated from a *Testudo hermanni*. Acyclovir at 50 μg/mL and ganciclovir at 25 and 50 μg/mL were sufficient to reduce the virus content of the culture to levels that were not measurable. Acyclovir at 25 μg/mL also inhibited the virus, but some sporadic replication did still occur.

The in vivo use of antiviral drugs in reptiles is limited to anecdotal reports. Cooper, Gschmeissner, and Bone[120] identified herpes-like viral particles in the oral lesions of two Greek tortoises *(Testudo graeca)* with electron microscopy. A topical 5% acyclovir ointment (Zovirax, GlaxoWellcome, Inc, Research Triangle, NC) was used to treat the remaining tortoises in the collection with some success.[120] Klingenberg[118] reported that D.R. Mader recommends the use of oral acyclovir (80 mg/kg PO every 24 hours for 10 days) to treat Desert Tortoises with clinical and histopathologic lesions attributed to herpes virus. The use of antiviral drugs should be limited to those cases in which a confirmed viral diagnosis is made. Widespread use of these compounds could lead to the development of resistant organisms. In addition, antiviral drugs may only induce latent states of infection.

Antifungals

Fungal diseases are reported with an increased frequency in captive reptiles. Although it might appear that these microbes are recent introductions or emerging pathogens, the increased number of cases could be attributed to our improved diagnostic capabilities and the fact that veterinarians are looking for pathogens other than bacteria.

With the increased number of fungal infections reported in reptiles, veterinarians are interested in finding appropriate antifungals to manage these cases.

A variety of topical antiseptics have been used to manage superficial mycoses in reptiles. Farm-raised Green Iguanas frequently have superficial mycoses develop during the wet season in Central America. Wissman and Parsons[121] diagnosed *Geotrichum candidum* in a group of these animals and found that it responded to a topical application of 2% chlorhexidine. A mucormycosis associated with the epidermis of juvenile Florida Soft-shelled Turtles *(Apalone ferox)* responded to malachite green (0.15 mg/L) water baths.[122] Frye et al[123] eliminated *Penicillium* sp. dermatitis in a group of captive American Alligators by improving the water conditions and using a 10-day application of povidone iodine. Jacobson[124] had similar results in treatment of a mycotic dermatitis in a Burmese Python with twice daily soaks of a dilute organic iodine solution. Both an adult and juvenile Eastern Kingsnake *(Lampropeltis getulus getulus)* with necrotizing mycotic dermatitis responded to improved environmental temperatures and a 2-week course of topical 1% tolnaftate.[123] Not all of the cases with topical antifungals are successful, as in the cases of a pair of Royal Pythons that did not respond to the topical application of 1% tolnaftate or systemic griseofulvin (20 mg/kg every 72 hours for five treatments).[124] Although no formal studies have evaluated the efficacy of topical antifungals for superficial mycoses, these reports suggest that they have value in clinical reptile medicine.

The most common systemic antifungals used in reptile medicine are ketoconazole (Janssen Pharmaceutica, Piscataway, NJ), fluconazole (Pfizer), and itraconazole (Ortho Biotech, Raritan, NJ). A review of the literature reveals a combination of empiric and pharmacokinetic reports regarding the specific use of these antifungals in herpetologic medicine. Because of the limited number of pharmacokinetic studies associated with antifungal chemotherapeutics, veterinarians should use caution when determining dosages for untested species.

Ketoconazole is an imidazole antifungal that can be fungistatic to fungicidal depending on fungal sensitivity and serum levels of the drug. Ketoconazole is thought to affect fungal cell membrane permeability by interfering with ergosterol synthesis.[64] Ketoconazole is metabolized by the liver and primarily excreted in the feces.[64] The drug is highly protein bound. Ketaconazole is a teratogen in mammals and should not be given to pregnant placental animals. What effect ketoconazole has on developing reptile embryos is not known. Other side effects associated with ketoconazole include gastrointestinal upset and hepatic toxicity.[64]

Page et al[125] determined the pharmacokinetics of a single oral dose of ketoconazole (30 mg/kg) in Gopher Tortoises. Peak plasma concentrations (3.39 μg/mL) were achieved 10.57 hours after dosing, and the biologic half-life of the drug was 11.57 hours.[125] Therapeutic levels persisted for approximately 32 hours. The only side effect associated with the single dose of ketoconazole was elevated plasma enzymes, including CK, AST, and lactic dehydrogenase. However, the authors attributed the enzymatic changes to the anesthesia (succinylcholine) they used to immobilize the tortoises for catheter placement and the frequent blood sampling (10 samples) necessary to monitor the blood levels of the drug. The authors concluded that a single daily dose of ketoconazole (30 mg/kg PO) should provide sufficient therapeutic levels of ketoconazole for a Gopher Tortoise.

Page et al[126] performed a second study to determine the pharmacokinetics of multiple doses and different concentrations of ketoconazole in Gopher Tortoises. The peak plasma concentration for the 15-mg/kg dose was 2.2 μg/mL, and the peak concentration for the 30-mg/kg dose was 4.4 μg/mL.[126] In mammals, plasma concentrations of more than 1 μg/mL have been found to be approximately 80% effective against mycoses.[127] On the basis of the results of the second study, the authors suggested that a single oral dose of 15 mg/kg/day is sufficient to manage most mycoses encountered in chelonians. Because the effectiveness of ketoconazole may be dose dependent, higher doses (30 mg/kg) may be necessary for more resilient fungal infections.

Similar changes in the plasma enzymes, including elevated CK, AST, and lactic dehydrogenase, were reported in this study. The authors again suggested that the succinylcholine and the frequent blood sampling were responsible for the enzymatic changes.

Fluconazole and itraconazole are triazole compounds that are used extensively in veterinary medicine to manage mycoses. The triazoles, like the imidazoles, are thought to affect fungal cell membrane permeability and limit the absorption of purine and pyrimidines precursors.[64] Although itraconazole is highly protein bound, fluconazole has reduced affinity for proteins. These compounds are metabolized by the liver.[64] Absorption of fluconazole is not affected by gastric pH or the presences of food in the stomach, but these factors do affect the absorption of itraconazole. Both triazole compounds are well distributed throughout the tissues. Because of the long half-life of the triazoles, steady state plasma levels may not be achieved until 6 days after dosing.[64] Itraconazole, like ketaconazole, is a teratogen in mammals. Both triazole compounds have been associated with gastrointestinal upset and mild hepatic toxicity in mammal; however, the incidence rate of toxicity is lower than that for imidazoles because the triazoles are more specific for fungal cytochromes.[64]

Research to investigate the triazoles is limited. Gamble, Alvarado, and Bennett[128] determined the pharmacokinetics of itraconazole in the Spiny Lizard (*Scleropus* sp.). Thirty-five animals were used for the study and divided into 10 groups. Because of the small size of the lizards, blood and tissue samples from the reptiles were pooled to determine the pharmacokinetics. The reptiles were dosed with approximately 23.5 mg/kg (PO every 24 hours) in food for 3 days. Blood and tissue samples were collected at time 0 and 1, 2, 3, 4, 6, 9, 12, and 18 days after treatment. The drug appeared well absorbed from the gastrointestinal tract and has a terminal plasma half-life of approximately 48 hours. The peak concentration was approximately 2.5 µg/mL and was achieved at approximately 99 hours. The dose (23.5 mg/kg) used in this study was considered sufficient to control fungal pathogens for 6 days beyond the peak concentrations.

Fungal diseases are a common finding in seaturtles that experience cold shock or trauma. With the increased number of seaturtles presented to rehabilitation facilities with mycotic disease, research to determine the drug pharmacokinetics for potential antifungal chemotherapeutics is needed.

Mallo et al[129] determined the pharmacokinetics of fluconazole in juvenile Loggerhead Seaturtles. The authors evaluated multiple dosing methods, including single intravenous injection, single subcutaneous injection, and multiple subcutaneous injections. At a dose of 2.5 mg/kg IV, the terminal half-life was approximately 140 hours, and the half-life for a single subcutaneous injection was 133 hours. A second component of the study evaluated multiple dosing regimens over time. Four juvenile turtles were given a loading dose of 21 mg/kg, followed by 10 mg/kg every 5 days. The terminal half-life after the final dose was 143 hours, and the plasma concentration remained above 8 µg/mL throughout the trial. The results suggested that a loading dose of 21 mg/kg, followed by additional 10 mg/kg doses every 5 days, is sufficient to treat mycotic infections in these reptiles.

Empiric use of the triazoles has been met with mixed results. A Panther Chameleon (*Furcifer pardalis*) with a fungal periodontal osteomyelitis given itraconazole (5 mg/kg PO every 24 hours) responded to treatment,[130] whereas a similar dose (5 mg/kg PO every 24 hours) given to a Kemp's Ridley Seaturtle (*Lepidochelys kempi*) was not found to be effective at eliminating *Colletotrichum acutatum*.[131] Differences in physiology between the terrestrial lizard and the seaturtle might account for the difference in response, or the difference may have been associated with limited contact with the drug because of granuloma formation. However, the study by Mallo et al[129] suggests that a higher dose may have been necessary in the seaturtle. Variability in treatment response between different orders might be expected on the basis of our understanding of antibiotic pharmacokinetics in reptiles.

To further evaluate itraconazole in seaturtles, Manire et al[132] determined steady state plasma concentrations of itraconazole in Kemp's Ridley Seaturtles. Juvenile seaturtles undergoing rehabilitation for cold stunning were used for the study. Two different study groups were used, with atotal of 14 turtles. The turtles were on itraconazole, and in some cases antibiotics, for a minimum of 30 days before evaluation of plasma concentrations. Different dosing regimens were evaluated. In the first study (n = 5), doses of 5 and 22 to 25 mg/kg PO every 24 hours were evaluated. In the second study (n = 9), three different doses were evaluated: 5, 10, and 15 mg/kg PO every 72 hours. The plasma levels of itraconazole and its primary metabolite, hydroxyitraconazole, were comparable, whereas in humans, the plasma concentrations are often twice the concentration of itraconazole.[133] This difference may be attributed to the slower metabolism in reptiles. The itraconazole was well tolerated by these turtles, with no ill effects reported. A dose of 5 mg/kg PO every 24 hours or 15 mg/kg PO every 72 hours should provide the steady-state concentrations in these seaturtles to control susceptible fungal pathogens.

Additional Techniques Used to Administer Antimicrobials

Topical Wound Management

Topical dressings are routinely used to manage reptile wounds by limiting opportunistic infections and facilitating the healing response. When wounds become contaminated with bacteria, they stimulate a natural host immune response. This response is generally characterized by the invasion of inflammatory cells, such as the heterophil and macrophage. The release of enzymes and cytokines by the host cells alter the wound microenvironment, leading to indiscriminate destruction of host tissues and thus lengthening healing times. Topical dressings that are antibacterial can limit the destructive nature of the host immune response by restricting bacterial colonization. Topical dressings can also serve as a protective barrier that entraps moisture and prevents the desiccation of viable tissues.[134] In addition, because these products are nonadhering, they reduce the likelihood of incorporating the dermis into the architecture of the scab.[135] Unfortunately, not all topical dressings are beneficial. Application of an excessive quantity of these products to a wound can lead to the development of anoxic conditions that starve damaged tissues, resulting in further tissue necrosis.

A study by Smith, Barker, and Allen[136] to evaluate the effects of various topical dressings on experimental wounds on snakes showed a high degree of variation between the different products. Four different treatments were evaluated in the study, including an occlusive polyurethane film (Op-Site Spray Bandage, Smith and Nephew Inc, Lachine, Quebec,

Canada), an ointment with scarlet red (Dermagen, Hoechst Pharmaceuticals, Montreal, Quebec, Canada), an antimicrobial ointment (Alphadol, Ayerst, Montreal, Quebec, Canada), and an antibiotic powder (Topazone, Austin Laboratories, Joliette, Quebec, Canada). The dressings were applied to experimentally induced wounds, and the wounds were examined for the presence or absence of 17 different characteristics associated with wound healing. In addition to characterizing the wound, the authors evaluated the heterophil and macrophage response to the surgically induced injuries. Overall, the occlusive polyurethane film produced the best results, and the topical antibiotic powder and ointment appeared to slow the healing response.

The use of topical antimicrobial ointments is widespread in our society because they can be used without prescription. A more severe response was observed with the ointment-based materials, too. The results of the study suggested that the value of antibiotic ointments in noncontaminated reptile wounds might be limited.

Nebulization

The respiratory tract of reptiles is primitive. Whereas mammals have a well-developed ciliated epithelial lining and mucociliary escalator in their respiratory tract, the epithelium of the reptile's respiratory tract have few cilia. The absence of cilia diminishes the reptile's ability to remove foreign material from the respiratory tract, leading to the accumulation of mucous and microbes. Infections that occur in the respiratory tract can be difficult to manage in reptiles. Systemic antimicrobials that are well distributed to the respiratory system can be used to manage infections, although systemic antimicrobials alone may not be sufficient.

The nebulization of antimicrobials to treat respiratory tract infections has been used in mammals and birds with a high degree of clinical success. No clinical trials to evaluate the efficacy of antimicrobials in reptiles have been performed, but anecdotal reports suggest that nebulization is beneficial. Success with nebulization is based on the particle size (<5 μm) and the chemotherapeutics. Larger particles might not penetrate the tertiary faveoli in the reptile lung. The duration of treatment is also an important consideration. The author generally nebulizes patients for 15 to 20 minutes twice a day.

Reptiles can be nebulized with a specific antimicrobial or antifungal and sterile water or in combination with a mucolytic agent. Acetylcysteine 20% (200 mg/9 mL Roxane Laboratories, Inc., Columbus, Ohio) can be used to facilitate the breakdown of mucous, increasing the likelihood that the therapeutic is distributed throughout the respiratory tract and maximizing epithelial contact. Because acetylcysteine can be irritating to tissues, exposure times should be limited to 15 to 30 minutes. A sterile ophthalmic ointment may be used to protect the corneas of lizards and chelonians during the nebulization procedure.

Aminophylline (25 g/9 mL sterile saline solution), a bronchodilator, is routinely used to nebulize birds and mammals; however, the author has not used the drug to treat reptiles. A number of different antibiotics and antifungals can be used to nebulize a reptile. However, the ultimate decision should be based on an antimicrobial or antifungal sensitivity assay. Amikacin and gentamicin are excellent first choice antimicrobials when a gram-negative bacterial infection is suspected.

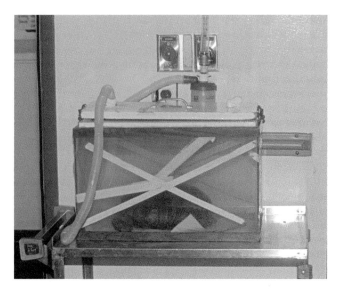

IGURE 36-18 Desert Tortoise (*Gopherus agassizii*) in nebulization chamber. *(Photograph courtesy of D. Mader.)*

A combination of amikacin (50 mg) and sterile saline solution (10 mL) or amikacin (50 mg), sterile saline solution (8 mL) and acetylcysteine 20% (1 mL) can be used to nebulize a reptile for 15 to 30 minutes twice a day. Gentamicin (50 mg) can be substituted for amikacin. Piperacillin (100 mg/10 mL sterile saline solution, 15 to 30 minutes) has been used to treat gram-positive bacterial infections.[137] Additional broad-spectrum antibiotics that may be useful as nebulizing agents include enrofloxacin (10 mg/1 mL sterile saline solution), chloramphenicol (13 mg/1 mL sterile saline solution), and doxycycline (200 mg/15 mL sterile saline solution).[138,139] Amphotercin B (1 mg/1 mL sterile saline solution) can be used to manage fungal infections of the lower respiratory tract. Amphotercin can be used in combination with amikacin, but the reptile must be well hydrated.

The nebulization chamber should only be used for the specific purpose of nebulization to minimize contamination. A large plastic container or aquarium with a secure lid can serve as the nebulization chamber (Figure 36-18). The chamber should be semitransparent to transparent to ensure that the reptiles can be observed during the procedure. A hole should be drilled into the chamber so that the silastic tubing connected to the pump can be inserted into the chamber. Any of a number of aerators can be used for the procedure, although the author prefers the SportNeb model 3050 (Medical Industries America, Inc, Adel, Iowa).

Intrapulmonic

Delivery of an antimicrobial directly into the lung tissue via an external catheter may also be used to deliver a drug directly into the lower respiratory tract. Divers[140] reported treating lesions in the lower respiratory tract by drilling a hole into the carapace over the desired location in the lung and inserting a catheter directly into the pulmonary tissue. Because this procedure requires drilling of an osteoderm and penetration of the coelomic membrane, a general anesthetic, such as propofol (10 to 15 mg/kg IV) or a combination of ketamine HCl (5 to 10 mg/kg IM; Fort Dodge Laboratories, Inc) and medetomidine (100 to 150 mg/kg IM; Pfizer), should be used. The veterinary clinician should adhere to strict surgical disinfection before performing this technique to prevent the introduction of additional opportunistic pathogens. Delivery of an appropriate antimicrobial directly into the pulmonary tissue ensures direct exposure to the compound. Unfortunately, delivery of these compounds with other parenteral techniques may be affected by reduced perfusion and tissue necrosis. This technique does not affect respiration in a chelonian because they do not possess a diaphragm or depend on negative pressure. One must avoid the use of irritating compounds with this technique because of the risk of tissue necrosis. Although aminoglycosides have a low pH (3.3 to 5.5) and can cause tissue irritation, Divers[140] reported no pathologic effects from the treatment.

The catheter site can be closed with inserting gel foam into the deficit and covering it with dental acrylic. The author prefers the use of dental acrylic to epoxy because a risk of tissue necrosis exists if the epoxy comes into contact with the pulmonary tissue. The same techniques can be used in squamates, with the catheter sutured to the skin during the treatment period. After the antimicrobial treatment has been completed, the catheter can be removed and a two-layer closure (body wall and skin) performed.

Antimicrobial Beads

Reptiles respond differently to foreign material than do mammals. In the mammalian cell-mediated response, neutrophils produce myeloperoxidase and other enzymes that liquefy the material surrounding the degranulating cell. Because reptile heterophils lack these enzymatic pathways, abscesses in reptiles are generally caseous in nature. These abscesses can be difficult to treat with systemic antibiotics because the nidus of infection is walled off. For effective treatment of these abscesses, the caseous abscess must be removed and all necrotic tissue debrided. See Chapter 42 for more information regarding the reptilian abscess.

In most cases, this leads to reduced circulation to an affected area, again minimizing the effectiveness of systemic antibiotics. When circulation is compromised or the treatment of an antibiotic must be focused at a local level, antibiotic-impregnated polymethylmethacrylate (PMMA) beads or plaster of Paris can be used.

A variety of heat-stabile compounds can be used to impregnate PMMA. The aminoglycosides and cephalosporins are the most commonly used antibiotics. The author has used amikacin, cefazolin, gentamicin, and clindamycin PMMA beads with excellent results. Divers and Lawton[141] recommend mixing 2 grams of the antibiotic (amikacin, neomycin, clindamycin, gentamicin) to 20 grams of the PMMA.

No studies have been performed to determine whether these concentrations cause negative side effects in reptiles and whether they should therefore be used with caution. In addition, no studies have been done on reptiles to measure antibiotic levels within the general range of the antibiotic beads. If MIC levels are maintained at low levels for extended periods, antimicrobial resistant pathogens possibly could develop. Weisman, Olmstead, and Kowalski[142] did find that at appropriate concentrations MIC values remain effective in vitro for 7 to 10 days.

In creation of antibiotic PMMA beads, several facts must be considered. First, smaller beads generally elute compound faster than larger beads. Antibiotic elution is generally fast over the first 7 to 10 days of bead placement and then can decrease substantially.[141] Finally, the beads elute the antibiotic over a short distance and therefore must be placed directly within the affected area.

One of the first reports of antibiotic PMMA beads was by Bennett.[143] He used antibiotic-impregnated beads to treat a septic arthritis in a Green Iguana. Initial survey radiographs of the iguana revealed significant lysis of the distal femur and proximal tibia. A series of radiographs during the treatment and recovery process revealed substantial bone remodeling. The author has used aminoglycoside-impregnated beads on several occasions to treat lizards with septic arthritis, chelonians with shell fractures, and raptors with pododermatitis with excellent results. Survey radiographs and complete blood counts can be used to monitor the progress of a wound. The beads should remain at the site until appropriate bone sclerosis has occurred. If the beads are not removed, they can initiate a negative immune response by the host.

Nontraditional Therapeutic Methods

Vaccines

Vaccines are widely used in veterinary medicine to reduce or eliminate bacterial and viral diseases in domestic species. The value of vaccines for nontraditional species has only recently been recognized. Canine distemper and rabies vaccines are considered mandatory for captive ferrets (*Mustelus putorious*), and polyoma virus vaccines have been found to protect psittacines against this highly contagious virus. In reptile medicine, vaccines are generally used to control pathogens associated with species raised for aquaculture.

Crocodilians

Mycoplasma crocodyli is an important pathogen in captive crocodiles and has been associated with significant morbidity. Because the introduction of this disease to a farm can be devastating, researchers contend that a successful vaccination program is needed. Mohan et al[144] evaluated an inactivated aluminum adjuvanted *M. crocodyli* vaccine in captive Nile Crocodiles (*Crocodylus niloticus*). The vaccination was administered intramuscularly either once, twice (0 and 7 days), or three times (0, 7, 21 days). The crocodiles were challenged with a homologous strain of *Mycoplasma crocodyli* and monitored for 16 weeks. The vaccine was not found to be pathogenic to the crocodiles or mice, which were also subsequently injected with the vaccine. All of the control crocodiles developed disease, whereas 75% (6/8) of the animals given boosters did not have clinical signs develop. Mohan et al[145] later evaluated an autogenous *M. crocodyli* vaccine to control an outbreak on a farm and found it to be more effective than antimicrobial therapy in alleviating the signs associated with the disease. These finding suggest that management of disease in large populations of reptiles, like in domestic species, may be best managed with preventive methods (e.g., vaccination programs).

Poxvirus is another pathogen that can affect commercial crocodilian aquaculture.[146] Because the crocodile's hide is the most valuable commercial product from the animal, any lesions that affect the hide can reduce the value of the product. Poxvirus in crocodiles can cause wart-like lesions that can occur anywhere on the body but are most frequently found around the head and neck. Horner[147] managed an outbreak of poxvirus in 9-month-old Nile Crocodiles with an autogenous vaccine produced from the tissues of affected crocodiles. The tissues were characterized by eosinophilic intracytoplasmic inclusion bodies in the epithelial cells, and the poxvirus was confirmed with transmission electron microscopy.[147] The crocodiles that received the vaccine healed more quickly than those that were not vaccinated.

Chelonians

Softshelled Turtles *(Apalone sinensis)* are an important commercial species in China. Because of intense farming, these animals are subject to bacterial infections, especially *Aeromonas* spp. Vaccination has been evaluated as a method to reduce the incidence rate of bacterial diseases in cultured Softshelled Turtles. An aluminum hydroxide adjuvanted inactivated *Aeromonas sobria* vaccine was prepared to evaluate the immune response in turtles and mice and to evaluate mortality in the field.[148] No mortalities were found in the turtles or mice in the experimental trial after 30 days, and the mortality rate in the field test was 50% less in the vaccinated turtles.[148] Vaccination against the pathogens most frequently isolated from these turtle farms could significantly reduce the financial losses associated with disease and reduce the overall number of turtles required to ensure quotas are met.

Vaccination has also been used to manage diseases at smaller population levels. Herpesvirus has been associated with significant mortality in captive chelonians. Because no effective treatment method exists for this virus, the development of new control methods, such as vaccines, should be pursued. Marschang, Milde, and Bellavista[149] isolated a virulent herpes virus from a group of tortoises from Italy. The virus was inactivated with formalin and used to create an aluminum-hydroxide adjuvanted vaccine and a nonadjuvanted vaccine. Fifty-seven *Testudo* spp. were used in the study, and the tortoises were vaccinated three times at 45-day intervals. Serial blood samples were collected from the tortoises to measure antibody titers. During the study, no rise in the antibody titers was measured in the vaccinated tortoises, suggesting the vaccine does not stimulate a humoral response.

Snakes

Paramyxovirus is a significant pathogen in captive snakes. The first report of paramyxovirus was from a collection of Fer-de-lance *(Bothrops atrax)* from Switzerland.[150] Since that time, paramyxovirus has been isolated from both viperids and nonviperids, and all snake species should be considered susceptible to the virus. Jacobson et al[151] evaluated the efficacy of three different inactivated paramyxovirus vaccines in Western Diamondback Rattlesnakes *(Crotalus atrox)*. The paramyxovirus used for the study was isolated from a Black Mamba *(Dendroaspis polylepsis)*, inactivated, and used to generate a nonadjuvanted vaccine, aluminum hydroxide vaccine, and oil-emulsion vaccine. Snakes were given one of the three vaccines or a control vaccine. Serconversion was recorded in 50% of the snakes (3/6) given the oil-emulsion vaccine, 33% of the snakes (2/6) given the nonadjuvanted paramyxovirus vaccine, and none of the snakes (0/6) given the aluminum hydroxide paramyxovirus vaccine. The low seroconversion rate suggests the responses to the vaccine were variable and that prediction of protection is hard in these animals challenged by a paramyxovirus.

Autogenous bacterins have also been used to control bacterial infections in captive snakes.[152,153] Addison and Jacobson[152] used an autogenous *Pseudomonas aeruginosa* bacterin to treat a chronic stomatitis in a Reticulated Python *(Python reticulatus)*. The python had a recurrent stomatitis, and *Pseudomonas aeruginosa* was consistently isolated from the lesions. The snake was injected six times with the bacterin (6×10^6 cells/mL) over a 16-day period, and the response was favorable. The infection reoccurred less than a month later and was treated with five bacterin injections over 9 days. The snake did not experience a relapse after the second bacterin treatment. Jacobson, Millichamp, and Gaskin[153] also used a polyvalent autogenous bacterin to treat a mixed *Pseudomonas* sp., *E. coli*, and *Proteus* sp. osteomyelitis in a Rhinoceros Viper *(Bitis nasicornis)*. The snake showed minimal response to antimicrobial therapy, including ceftazidime, carbenicillin, and gentamicin sulfate, but a dramatic response to the polyvalent bacterin. Although not frequently used in reptile medicine, autogenous bacterins should be considered for those cases in which no response is observed with antibiotics.

Lizards

One of the dilemmas facing herpetoculture in the United States is the public health concern over reptile-associated salmonellosis. The concern was significant enough in the 1970s that the US FDA restricted the interstate and intrastate sale of all chelonians under 4 inches in length. Recent reports from the Centers for Disease Control and Prevention suggest that the incidence rate of reptile-associated salmonellosis cases is on the rise again. Will future regulations be imposed on the industry in an attempt to protect public health? Vaccination might be used to counter the risk associated with pet reptile ownership. *Salmonella* vaccines are currently undergoing evaluation as control measures to eliminate salmonellae in domestic animals. Both inactivated and live attenuated vaccines are currently marketed.

Attempts to suppress or eliminate *Salmonella* spp. in Green Iguanas with a commercial poultry double-deletion mutant *S. typhimurium* vaccine (MeganVac1, Megan Health, Inc, St Louis, Mo) were unsuccessful.[154] No difference was found in the prevalence of *Salmonella* between vaccinated and nonvaccinated groups. The poultry variant may have failed to elicit a significant immune response in the iguana. Future research to evaluate reptile-associated serotypes should be pursued.

Competitive Exclusion Products

Competitive microbial exclusion is a phenomena that allows specific microbial constituents of the intestinal flora to inhibit the multiplication of other bacteria, including pathogens, and to inhibit colonization by competing for receptor sites on enterocytes.[155] The concept of competitive exclusion (CE) was documented by Metchnikoff[156] who proposed that beneficial organisms, such as *Lactobacillus*, could displace pathogens, improve intestinal health, and prolong life. Since then, studies on CE have been evaluated with single and mixed populations, and defined and undefined cultures, to control enteropathogens in humans and animals.

Food-borne illness in humans attributed to consumption of *Salmonella*-contaminated poultry has increased since the 1970s, prompting studies to evaluate techniques to reduce salmonellae colonization in poultry.[157] The CE technique has been researched extensively in the poultry industry as a method to prevent colonization of the intestinal tract of chicks and poults with salmonellae. Nurmi and Rantala[158] and Rantala and Nurmi[159] applied this technique to poultry to control an outbreak of *Salmonella infantis* in broiler flocks responsible for food-borne outbreaks in Finland. That chicks are most susceptible to *Salmonella* colonization during the first week after hatch, before establishment of a stable indigenous microflora, was determined. In these naïve birds, as few as one to 10 *Salmonella* organisms in the crop led to colonization. Attempts to exclude *Salmonella* with *Lactobacillus* were unsuccessful. An undefined *Salmonella*-free mixed culture derived from adult birds was administered orally to the chicks and provided protection against *Salmonella infantis*.

The mechanisms used by bacteria to exclude or reduce the growth of an enteropathogen are poorly understood. Rolfe[160] suggested four possible mechanisms, including: (1) creation of a microecology that is hostile to other bacterial species; (2) elimination of available bacterial receptor sites; (3) synthesis of antibacterial compounds; and (4) depletion of essential nutrients. An acidic pH in the intestinal tract can reduce survival of *Salmonella* and other Enterobacteriaceae, and microbes that synthesize volatile fatty acids can reduce intestinal pH levels and inhibit colonization by enteropathogens.[161] Microbes that block receptor sites on enterocytes can effectively reduce the rate of adhesion of pathogens and the invasion of host cells. Antimicrobial substances, such as reuterin, are natural compounds produced by indigenous microbes that can destroy pathogens. Microbial competition for available nutrients may inhibit the establishment and subsequent multiplication of a pathogen, although many organisms can use alternative metabolic pathways to avoid these limiting factors.

Defined CE cultures consist of organisms classified by the US FDA in the category of "generally regarded as safe" (GRAS). Currently, 42 GRAS organisms, principally species of *Lactobacillus*, may be used in defined CE cultures.[162] The mechanism of action used by defined organisms to reduce or control *Salmonella* is poorly understood. Most defined cultures that consist of a single or limited number (<14) of organisms afford limited or negligible protection.[163] A recent study with *Lactobacillus reuteri* reduced colonization of *Salmonella* and *E. coli* in chicks and turkey poults.[164] *Lactobacillus reuteri* produces reuterin, a broad-spectrum antimicrobial, and has been shown to inhibit at least 25 genera of microbial enteropathogens found in mammalian and avian intestines.[165] Reuterin concentrations as low as 10 to 30 µg/mL can destroy *Salmonella*, *E. coli*, and *Campylobacter* within 30 to 40 minutes.[164] Defined cultures consisting of large numbers of organisms (>14) and representing different genera have been shown to provide protection against experimental *Salmonella* colonization.[166-168]

Undefined cultures are routinely prepared from the intestinal microflora of apparently healthy animals. Continuous-flow culture systems have been used to maintain indigenous chicken flora in a steady-state culture system.[169] A characterized continuous flow culture (CF3) of cecal anaerobes that consisted of 29 bacterial isolates comprising 15 facultative anaerobes and of 14 obligate anaerobes representing 10 different genera was patented and licensed for commercial manufacture (BioScience Division, Milk Specialties, Dundee, Ill).[170] This product is effective against experimental *Salmonella typhimurium* colonization and challenge with environmental *Salmonella* in commercially reared broilers.[171,172]

The use of undefined CE cultures has raised concerns regarding the potential transmission of animal or human pathogens. Although undefined cultures contain unidentified organisms, they can be shown to be free of specific animal and human pathogens.[173] The safety of these products has been confirmed in both laboratory and field trials.[174]

Dietary Supplements

The administration of fructooligosaccharides to control bacterial pathogens, such as *Salmonella*, has been studied extensively, with generally inconclusive results.[174] Most salmonellae do not use lactose, in contrast to indigenous intestinal microbes, which metabolize lactose as a primary carbon source. In theory, the addition of dietary lactose should provide a nutrient source for the indigenous flora to compete with salmonellae. The metabolism of lactose produces an acid, which can reduce the intestinal pH and further affect the survival of salmonellae. The addition of mannose or lactose to drinking water of chicks for 10 days reduced colonization of salmonellae, although dextrose, maltose, and sucrose exerted no effect.[175] The administration of lactose to market-age broilers was associated with an increased prevalence of *Salmonella*.[176] More consistent results have been reported when a fructooligosaccharide is combined with a CE culture. The addition of lactose at 5% to the diet (weight/weight) of Leghorn chicks in combination with an undefined CE culture, enhanced resistance to colonization with *S. enteritidis* to a greater extent than CE culture or dietary lactose alone.[162] A subsequent study further supported these findings.[176] A defined CE culture that consisted of 11 indigenous strains of cecal bacteria was maintained in a continuous flow culture with lactose as a primary carbon source. The culture was administered by crop gavage to Leghorn chicks on the day of hatch. Controls received either lactose or the defined CE culture without lactose. Chicks were challenged with *S. enteritidis* PT13 on the following day. When either dietary lactose or the defined CE culture was administered separately, a reduction in salmonellae colonization was determined, but the treatments were not consistently protective. The combination of the two products was effective in prevention of colonization.

Research to elucidate the mechanisms of CE cultures in providing protection and identifying "determinant factors" in inhibition requires further study.[168] For CE-based control to be effective, it must be integrated into a comprehensive preventive health program. The CE culture may be a valuable method to reduce or prevent pathogens from colonizing the gastrointestinal tract of reptiles.

Euthanasia

Although we do not routinely consider euthanasia as a therapeutic option, cases do exist in which euthanasia is the most humane treatment. Barbituate overdose is the most common method of euthanasia for mammals and birds. Unfortunately, establishment of intravenous access to administer a thick barbituate euthanasia solution to a reptile can be difficult, if not impossible. Several different euthanasia methods have been described for reptiles. Historically, placement of a reptile into a freezer was considered an appropriate form of euthanasia. However, this technique is not considered humane because the pain from the crystallization of cells is considered extreme. Carbon dioxide is an acceptable method of euthanasia for laboratory rodents. This technique can also be used to euthanize reptiles, but the time to perform the procedure is generally longer than for mammals because reptiles can hold their breath for extended periods and survive with anaerobic metabolism for an extended period of time. Decapitation has also been suggested as a method of euthanasia; however, Warwick[177] has suggested that the technique is not humane and that the reptiles, functioning on a diminished metabolic rate, could survive extended periods beyond the decapitation. The use of an electroencephalogram might be useful in determination of brain function after decapitation.

Anesthetic overdose is considered the most human method, but the administration of a barbituate intracardiac or into the intracoelomic cavity can create pathologic artifact. The author prefers to overdose the reptile with a dissociative agent or propofol followed by carbon dioxide overdose, decapitation, or a barbituate overdose if a necropsy will not be performed. See Chapter 33 for an in-depth discussion of reptilian euthanasia.

REFERENCES

1. Zug GR, Vitt LJ, Caldwell JP: Classification and diversity. In Zug GR, Vitt LJ, Caldwell JP, editors: *Herpetology*, ed 2, San Diego, 2001, Academic Press.
2. Dawson WR, Bartholomew GA: Relation of oxygen consumption to body weight, temperature, and temperature acclimation in lizards *Uta stansburiana* and *Sceloporus occidentalis*, *Physiol Zool* 29:40-51, 1956.
3. Dawson WR, Bartholomew GA: Metabolic and cardiac responses to temperature in the lizard, *Dipsosaurus dorsalis*, *Physiol Zool* 31:100-111, 1958.
4. Strel'nikov ID: Znachenie solnechnoĭ radiatsiĭ v ékologii vysokogornykh reptiliĭ, *Zool Zh (SSSR)* 23:250-257, 1944.
5. Brattsstrom BH: Body temperatures of reptiles, *Am Midl Nat* 73(2):376-422, 1965.
6. Vaughn EE: Comparative immunology: antibody response in *Dipsosaurus dorsalis* at different temperatures, *Proc Soc Exp Biol* 112:531, 1963.
7. Vaughn LK, Bernheim HA, Kluger M: Fever in the lizard (*Dipsosaurus dorsalis*), *Nature* 252:473, 1974.
8. Baldwin FM: Body temperature changes in turtles and their physiological interpretation, *Am J Physiol* 72:210-218, 1925.
9. Kluger MJ, Ringler DH, Anver MR: Fever and survival, *Science* 188:166, 1975.
10. Warwick C: Observations on disease-associated preferred body temperatures in reptiles, *Appl Anim Behav Sci* 28:375-380, 1991.
11. Cooper EL, Klempau AE, Zapata AG: Reptilian immunity. In Gans C, editor: *Biology of the reptilia*, vol 14, Chicago, 1985, University Chicago Press.
12. Evans EE: Comparative immunology: antibody response in *Dipsosaurus dorsalis* at different temperatures, *Proc Soc Exp Biol Med* 112:531-533, 1963.
13. Evans EE, Cwls RB: Effect of temperature on antibody synthesis in the reptile, *Dipsosaurus dorsalis*, *Proc Soc Exp Biol Med* 101:482-483, 1959.
14. Schumacher IM, Rostal DC, Yates R, et al: Persistence of maternal antibodies against *Mycoplasma agassizii* in Desert Tortoise hatchlings, *Am J Vet Res* 60:826-831, 1999.
15. Leceta J, Zapata A: Seasonal variation in the immune response of the tortoise, *Mauremys caspica*, *Immunology* 57:483-487, 1986.
16. Saad AH, El Deeb S: Immunological changes during pregnancy in the viviparous lizard, *Chalcides ocellatus*, *Vet Immunol Immunopath* 25:279-286, 1990.
17. Zapata AG, Varas A, Torroba M: Seasonal variations in the immune system of lower vertebrates, *Immunol Today* 13:142-147, 1992.
18. Donoghue S, Langenberg J: Nutrition. In Mader D, editor: *Reptile medicine and surgery*, Philadelphia, 1996, WB Saunders.
19. Nagy KA: Water and electrolyte budgets of a free-living desert lizard, *Sauromalas obesus*, *J Comp Physiol* 79:39-62, 1972.
20. Dantzler WH: Renal function: with special emphasis on nitrogen excretion. In Gans C, Dawson WR, editors: *Biology of the reptilia*, New York, 1976, Academic Press.
21. Dunson WA: Salt glands in reptiles. In Gans C, Dawson WR, editors: *Biology of the reptilia*, New York, 1976, Academic Press.
22. Bentley PJ: Osmoregulation. In Gans C, Dawson WR, editors: *Biology of the reptilia*, New York, 1976, Academic Press.
23. Thorson TB: Body fluid partitioning in Reptilia, *Copeia* 592-601, 1968.
24. Munsey LD: Water loss in five species of lizards, *Comp Biochem Physiol* 43A:781-794, 1972.
25. Jarchow J: Hospital care of the reptile patient. In Jacobson ER, Kollias GV, editors: *Exotic animals: contemporary issues in small animal practice*, New York, 1988, Churchill Livingstone.
26. Prezant RM, Jarchow J: *Lactated fluid use in reptiles: is there a better solution?* Houston, 1997, Proc Assoc Rept Amphib Vet.
27. Bennet AF: The energetics of reptilian activity. In Gans C, Pough FH, editors: *Biology of the reptilia*, vol 13, London, 1982, Academic Press.
28. Gotten RR: The use of anaerobiasis by amphibians and reptiles, *Am Zool* 25:945-954, 1985.
29. Dantzlen WH: Renal function. In Gans C, Pough FH, editors: *Biology of reptila*, vol 13, London, 1982, Academic Press.
30. Frye FL: Infectious disease. In Frye FL, editor: *Biomedical and surgical aspects of captive reptile husbandry*, ed 2, vol 1, Melbourne, Fla, 1991, Krieger Publishing.
31. Jacobson ER: Use of chemotherapeutics in reptile medicine. In Jacobson ER, Kollias GV, editors: *Exotic animals: contemporary issues in small animal practice*, New York, 1988, Churchill Livingstone.
32. Jacobson ER: Gentamicin related visceral gout in two boid snakes, *Vet Med Small Anim Clin* 71:361-363, 1976.
33. Montali RJ, Bush M, Smeller JM: The pathology of nephrotoxicity of gentamicin in snakes: a model for reptilian gout, *Vet Pathol* 16:108-115, 1979.
34. Holz P, Barker IK, Crawshaw GJ, Dobson H: The anatomy and perfusion of the renal portal system in the Red-eared Slider (*Trachemys scripta elegans*), *J Zoo Wildl Med* 28(4):378-385, 1997.
35. Benson KG, Forrest L: Characterization of the renal portal system of the common Green Iguana (*Iguana iguana*) by digital subtraction imaging, *J Zoo Wildl Med* 30(2):235-241, 1999.
36. Holz PH: The reptilian renal-portal system: influence on therapy. In Fowler ME, Miller RE, editors: *Zoo and wild animal medicine: current therapy 4*, Philadelphia, 1999, WB Saunders.
37. Holz P, Barker IK, Burger JP, Crawshaw GJ, Conlon PD: The effect of the renal portal system on pharmacokinetic parameters in the Red-eared Slider (*Trachemys scripta elegans*), *J Zoo Wildl Med* 28(4):386-393, 1997.
38. Siebling RJ, Neal PM, Granberry WD: Evaluation of methods for the isolation of *Salmonella* and *Arizona* organisms from pet turtles treated with antimicrobial agents, *Appl Microbiol* 29:240-245, 1975.
39. Siebling RJ, Caruso D, Neuman S: Eradication of *Salmonella* and *Arizona* species from turtle hatchlings produced from

eggs treated on commercial turtle farms, *Appl Environ Microbiol* 47:658-662, 1984.
40. D'Aoust JY, Daley E, Crozier M, Sewell AM: Pet turtles: a continuing international threat to public health, *Am J Epidemiol* 132(2):233-238, 1990.
41. Shane SM, Gilbert R, Harrington KS: *Salmonella* colonization in commercial pet turtles *(Pseudemys scripta elegans), Epidemiol Infect* 105:307-315, 1990.
42. Dantzler WH, Schmidt-Nielson B: Excretion in a fresh-water turtle *(Pseudemys scripta)* and Desert Tortoise *(Gopherus agassizi), Am J Physiol* 210:198-210, 1966.
43. Brewer KJ, Ensor DM: Hormonal control of osmoregulation in the chelonian. I. The effects of prolactin and interregnal steroids in freshwater chelonians, *Gen Comp Endocrinol* 42:304-309, 1980.
44. Holz PH, Burger JP, Pasloske K, Baker R, Young S: Effect of injection site on carbenicillin pharmacokinetics in the carpet python, *Morelia spilota, J Herp Med Surg* 12(4):12-16, 2002.
45. Lawrence K: Drug dosages for chelonians, *Vet Rec* 114: 50-151, 1984.
46. Lawrence K, Needham JR, Palmer GH, Lewis JC: A preliminary study on the use of carbenicillin in snakes, *J Vet Pharmacol Ther* 7:119-124, 1984.
47. Benedict FG: *The physiology of large reptiles*, Washington, 1932, Carnegie Institute.
48. Malan A, Wilson TL, Reeves RB: Intracellular pH in cold-blooded vertebrates as a function of body temperature, *Resp Physiol* 28:29-47, 1976.
49. Hsu CH, Kurtz TW, Easterling RE, et al: Potentiation of gentamicin nephrotoxicity by metabolic acidosis, *Proc Soc Exp Biol Med* 146:894-897, 1974.
50. Hodge MK: The effects of acclimation temperature on gentamicin toxicity in the broad banded water snake *(Natrix fasciata), Proc Am Assoc Zoo Vet* 226-237, 1978.
51. Conzelman GM: Pharmacotherapeutics of aminoglycoside antibiotics, *JAVMA* 176(10):2,1078-1080, 1980.
52. Luft FC, Block R, Sloan RS, et al: Comparative nephrotoxicity of aminoglycosides in rats, *J Infect Dis* 138:541-545, 1978.
53. Hoperich PD, editor: *Infectious diseases,* ed 2, Hagerstown, Md, 1977, Harper & Row.
54. Bush M, Custer R, Smeller JM, Charache P: *Preliminary study of gentamicin in turtles,* Honolulu, 1977, Proc AAZV.
55. Bush M, Smeller JM, Charache P, Arthur R: Biologic half-life of gentamicin in Gopher Snakes, *AJVR* 39:171-173, 1978.
56. Kunin C: Diagnosis and treatment, a guide to use antibiotics in patients with renal diseases, *Ann Int Med* 67:151-157, 1967.
57. Hilf M, Swanson D, Wagner R, Yu VL: A new dosing schedule for gentamicin in blood pythons *(Python curtus)*: a pharmacokinetic study, *Res Vet Sci* 50:127-130, 1991.
58. Raphael B, Clark CH, Hudson R: Plasma concentrations of gentamicin in turtles, *J Zoo Wildl Med* 16:136-139, 1985.
59. Beck K, Loomis M, Lewbart G, Spelman C, Papich M: Preliminary comparison of plasma concentrations of gentamicin injected into the cranial and caudal limb musculature of the eastern box turtle *(Terrapene carolina carolina), J Zoo Wildl Med* 26(5):265-268, 1995.
60. Bagger-Sjoback D, Wersall J: Toxic effects of gentamicin on the basilar papilla in the lizard *(Calotes versicolor), Acta Otolaryngoal* 81:57-65, 1976.
61. Mader DR, Conzelman GM, Baggot JD: Effects of ambient temperature on the half-life and dosage regimen of amikacin in the Gopher Snake, *JAVMA* 187(11):1134-1136, 1985.
62. Johnson JH, Jensen JM, Brumbaugh GW, Boothe DM: Amikacin pharmacokinetics and the effects of ambient temperature on the dosage regimen in Ball Pythons *(Python regius), J Zoo Wildl Med* 28(1):80-88, 1997.
63. Caligiuri K, Kollias GV, Jacobson ER, McNab B, Clark CH, Wilson RC: The effects of ambient temperature on amikacin pharmacokinetics in gopher tortoises, *J Vet Pharmacol Ther* 13:287-291, 1990.
64. Plumb DC: *Veterinary drug handbook,* ed 4, Ames, 2002, Iowa State Press.
65. Jacobson ER, Brown MP, Chung M, Vliet K, Swift R: Serum concentration and disposition kinetics of gentamicin and amikacin in juvenile American alligators, *J Zoo Wildl Med* 19(4):188-197, 1988.
66. Lawrence K, Muggleton PW, Needham JR: Preliminary study on the use of ceftazidime, a broad spectrum cephalosporin antibiotic, in snakes, *Res Vet Sci* 36:16-20, 1984.
67. Harding SM, Ayrton J, Thorton JE, Munro AJ, Hogg MIJ: Pharmacokinetics of ceftazimime in normal subjects, *J Antimicrob Chemother* 8B:261, 1981.
68. Stamper MA, Papich MG, Lewbart GA, May SB, Plummer DD, Stoskopf MK: Pharmacokinetics of ceftazidime in loggerhead seaturtles *(Caretta caretta)* after single intravenous and intramuscular injections, *J Zoo Wild Med* 30(1):32-35, 1999.
69. Speroni JA, Giambeluca L, Errecalde EO: Farmacocinetica de cefoperazona tras su administracion intramuscular a Hydrodynastes gigas *(Ophidia, Colubridae)*, Buenos Aires, Argentina, 1989, AHA Communications meeting.
70. Speroni JA, Giambeluca L, Errecalde EO: Farmacocinetica de cefoperazona tras su administracion intramuscular a Tupinambis teguixin *(Sauria, Teidae)*, Buenos Aires, Argentina, 1989, AHA Communications meeting.
71. Stewart JS: Anaerobic bacterial infections in reptiles, *J Zoo Wildl Med* 21:180-184, 1990.
72. Koopman JP, Kennis HM: Occurrence and treatment of *Salmonella* carriers in tegus *(Tupinambus teguixin)* and tortoise *(Testudo hermanni), Tijdschr diergenesskd* 101:957-961, 1976.
73. Clark CH, Rogers ED, Milton JL: Plasma concentrations of chloramphenicol in snakes, *Am J Vet Res* 46(12):2654-2657, 1985.
74. Manyan DR, Arimura GK, Yunis AA: Comparative metabolic effects of chloramphenicol analogues, *Mol Pharmacol* 11: 520-527, 1975.
75. Stamper MA, Papich MG, Lewbart GA, May SB, Plummer DD, Stoskopf MK: Pharmacokinetics of florfenicol in loggerhead seaturtles *(Caretta caretta)* after single intravenous and intramuscular injections, *J Zoo Wildl Med* 34(1):38, 2003.
76. Hooper D, Wolfson J: The fluoroquinolones: structures, mechanisms of action and resistance and spectra of activity in vitro, *Antimicrob Agents Chemother* 28:581-586, 1985.
77. Scheer M: Studies on the antibacterial activity of Baytril, *Vet Med Rev* 2:90-98, 1987.
78. Vancutsem PM, Babish JG, Schwark WS: The fluoroquinolone antimicrobials: structure, antimicrobial activity, pharmacokinetics, clinical use in domestic animals and toxicity, *Cornell Vet* 80(2):173-186, 1990.
79. Parpia S, Nix D, Hejmanowski H, Goldstein H, Wilton J, Schentag J: Sucralfate reduces the gastrointestinal absorption of norfloxacin, *Antimicrob Agents Chemother* 33(1):99-102, 1989.
80. Montay G, Goueffon Y, Roquet F: Absorption, distribution, metabolic fate, and elimination of pefloxacin mesylate in mice, rats, dogs, monkeys, and humans, *Antimicrob Agents Chemother* 25(4):463-472, 1984.
81. Oomori Y, Yasue T, Aoyama H, Hirai K, Suzue S, Yokota T: Effects of fleroxacin on HeLa cell functions and topoisomerase II, *J Antimicrob Chemother* 22(Supplement D):91-97, 1988.
82. Hussy P, Maass G, Tummler B, Grosse F, Schomburg U: Effect of 4-quinolones and novobiocin on calf thymus DNA polymerase alpha primase complex, topoisomerases I and II, and growth of mammalian lymphoblasts, *Antimicrob Agents Chemother* 29(6):1073-1078, 1986.

83. Diver JM, Wise R: Morphological and biochemical changes in *Escherichia coli* after exposure to ciprofloxacin, *J Antimicrob Chemother* 18(supplement D):31-41, 1986.
84. Easom CSF, Crane JP: Uptake of ciprofloxacin by human neutrophils, *J Antimicrob Chemother* 23:284-288, 1983.
85. Piddock LJV, Wise R: Mechanisms of resistance to quinolones and clinical perspectives, *J Antimicrob Ther* 23:475-481, 1989.
86. Neu HC: Bacterial resistance to fluoroquinolones, *Rev Infect Dis* 10(Supplement D):57-63, 1988.
87. Bellido F, Pechere JC: Laboratory survey of fluoroquinolone activity, *Rev Infect Dis* 11(Supplement 5):917-924, 1989.
88. Kato M, Onodera T: Morphological investigation of cavity formation in articular cartilage induced by ofloxacin in rats, *Fundamental Appl Toxicol* 11:110-119, 1988.
89. Burkhardt JE, Hill MA, Carlton WW, Kesterson JW: Histologic and histochemical changes in articular cartilages of immature beagle dogs dosed with difloxacin, a fluoroquinolone, *Vet Path* 27:162-170, 1990.
90. Bendele AM, Hulman JF, Harvey AK, Hrubey PS, Chandrasekhar S: Passive role of articular chondrocytes in quinolone induced arthropathy in guinea pigs, *Toxicol Pathol* 18(2):304-312, 1990.
91. Berg J: Clinical indications for enrofloxacin in domestic animals and poultry. In: *Quinolones: a symposium: a new class of antimicrobial agents for use in veterinary medicine*, Shawnee, Kan, 1988, Mobay Corporation.
92. Schluter G: Ciprofloxacin: review of potential toxicologic effects, *Am J Med* 82(supplement 4A):91-93, 1987.
93. Ball P: Ciprofloxacin: an overview of adverse experiments, *J Antimicrob Chemother* 18(supplement D):197-193, 1986.
94. Spiecker R: *Untersuchungen zur Wirksamkeit des Chinoloncarbonsaure derivats. Bay Vp 2674 bei der Behandlung der latenten Salmonellen Infektion des Rindes*, dissertation, Hannover, West-Germany, 1986, Tierarztliche Hochschule.
95. Bauditz R: Results of clinical studies with Baytril in calves and pigs, *Vet Med Rev* 2:122-129, 1987.
96. Mitchell MA, Shane SM, Nevarez J, Pesti D, Sanchez S, Wooley RE, et al: Establishing a *Salmonella* free iguana, *Iguana iguana*, model using enrofloxacin, Orlando, Fla, 2001, Proc ARAV.
97. Hungerford C, Spelman L, Papich MG: Pharmacokinetics of enrofloxacin after oral and intramuscular administration in Savannah monitors *(Varanus exanthematicus)*, Houston, 1997, Proc AAZV.
98. Maxwell L, Jacobson ER: Preliminary single-dose pharmacokinetics of enrofloxacin after oral and intramuscular administration in Green Iguanas *(Iguana iguana)*, Houston, 1997, Proc AAZV.
99. Young LA, Schumacher J, Papich MG, Jacobson ER: Disposition of enrofloxacin and its metabolite ciprofloxacin after intramuscular injection in juvenile Burmese Pythons *(Python molurus bivittatus)*, *J Zoo Wild Med* 28(1):71-79, 1997.
100. Sporle H, Gobel T, Schildger B: Blood levels of some anti-infectives in the Hermann's tortoise *(Testudo hermanni)*, Bad Nauheim, Germany, 1991, 4th International Colloqium on Pathology on Medicine of Reptiles and Amphibians.
101. Prezant RM, Isaza R, Jacobson ER: Plasma concentrations and disposition kinetics of enrofloxacin in gopher tortoises *(Gopherus polyphemus)*, *J Zoo Wildl Med* 25: 82-87, 1994.
102. Raphael BL, Papich M, Cook RA: Pharmacokinetics of enrofloxacin after a single intramuscular injection in Indian star tortoises *(Geochelone elegans)*, *J Zoo Wildl Med* 25(1):88-94, 1994.
103. James SB, Calle PP, Raphael BL, Papich M, Breheny J, Cook RA: Comparison of injectable versus oral enrofloxacin pharmacokinetics in Red-eared Slider turtles, *Trachemys scripta elegans*, *J Herp Med Surg* 13(1):5-10, 2003.
104. Helmick KE, Papich MG, Vliet KA, Bennett A, Brown MR, Jacobson ER: Preliminary kinetics of single-dose intravenously administered enrofloxacin and oxytetracycline in the American alligator, Houston, 1997, Proc AAZV.
105. Harms CA, Papich MG, Stamper MA, et al: Pharmacokinetics of oxytetracycline in Loggerhead Seaturtles *(Caretta caretta)* after single intravenous and intramuscular injections, *JZWM* 35(4):477-488, 2004.
106. Casares M, Enders F: Enrofloxacin side effects in a Galapagos tortoise *(Geochelone elephantopus nigra)*, *Proc AAZV* 446-448, 1996.
107. Wimsatt J, Johnson J, Mangone B, Tothill A, Childs JM, Peloquin CA: Clarithromycin pharmacokinetics in the Desert Tortoise *(Gopherus agassizii)*, *J Zoo Wildl Med* 30(1):36-43, 1999.
108. Coke RL, Hunter RP, Isaza R, Koch D, Goatley M, Carpenter JW: Pharmacokinetics and tissue concentrations azithromycin in Ball Pythons *(Python regius)*, *AJVR* 64(2):225-228, 2003.
109. Funk RS: Herp health hints and husbandry: parasiticide dosages for captive amphibians and reptiles, *Chicago Herp Soc Newsletter* 23(2):30, 1988.
110. Carpenter JW, Mashima TY, Rupiper DJ: *Exotic animal formulary*, Philadelphia, 2001, WB Saunders.
111. Kolmstetter CM, Frazier D, Cox S, Ramsay EC: Pharmacokinetics of metronidazole in the Green Iguana *(Iguana iguana)*, *Bull Assoc Rep Amphib Vet* 8:4-7, 1998.
112. Prescott JF, Baggott JD: *Antimicrobial therapy in veterinary medicine*, Boston, 1993, Blackwell Scientific Publishing.
113. Kolmstetter CM, Cox S, Ramsay EC: Pharmacokinetics of metronidazole in the yellow rat snake *(Elaphe obsolete quadrivittata)*, *J Herp Med Surg* 11(2):4-8, 2001.
114. Bodri MS, Rambo TM, Wagner RA, Venkataramanan R: Pharmacokinetics of metronidazole administered as a single oral bolus to corn snakes, *Elaphe guttata*, Orlando, Fla, 2001, Proc ARAV.
115. Hilf M, Swanson D, Wagner R, Yu VL: Pharmacokinetics of piperacillin in blood pythons *(Python curtus)* and in vitro evaluation of efficacy against aerobic gram-negative bacteria, *J Zoo Wildl Med* 22(2):199-203, 1991.
116. Lawrence K, Palmer GH, Needham JR: Use of carbenicllin in two species of tortoise *(Testudo graeca* and *T. hermanni)*, *Res Vet Sci* 40:413-415, 1986.
117. Vree TB, Vree JB: Acetylation of sulphamethoxazole by fresh water turtles, *Pseudemys scripta elegans*, *J Vet Pharmacol Ther* 6:237-240, 1983.
118. Klingenberg RJ: Therapeutics. In Mader DR, editor: *Reptile medicine and surgery*, Philadelphia, 1996, WB Saunders.
119. Marschang RE, Gravendyck M, Kaleta EF: Herpesvirus in tortoises: investigations into virus isolation and the treatment of viral stomatitis in *Testudo hermanni* and *T. graeca*, *J Vet Med* 44:385-394, 1997.
120. Cooper JE, Gschmeissner S, Bone RD: Herpes-like virus particles in necrotic stomatitis of tortoises, *Vet Rec* 123:544, 1988.
121. Wissman MA, Parsons B: Dermatophytosis of Green Iguana *(Iguana iguana)*, *J Small Exotic Anim Med* 2(3):133-136, 1993.
122. Jacobson ER, Calderwood MV, Clubb S: Mucormycosis in hatchling soft-shelled turtles, *JAVMA* 177:835, 1980.
123. Frye FL, Gabrisch K, Schildger B, Zwart P: Penicillium dermatitis in three American alligators *(Alligator mississipiensis)*, Giessen/Lahn, Germany, 1991, Int Cooloq Pathol Ther Reptil Amphib.
124. Jacobson ER: Necrotizing dermatitis in snakes: clinical and pathological features, *JAVMA* 177:838, 1980.
125. Page CD, Mautino M, Meyer JR, Mechlinski W: Preliminary pharmacokinetics of ketoconazole in gopher tortoises *(Gopherus polyphemus)*, *J Vet Pharmacol Ther* 11:397-401, 1988.

126. Page CD, Mautino M, Derendorf H, Mechlinski W: Multiple-dose pharmacokinetics of ketoconazole administered orally to gopher tortoises (Gopherus polyphemus), J Zoo Wildl Med 22(2):191-198, 1991.
127. Levine HB: *Ketoconazole in management of fungal diseases,* New York, 1982, ADIS Press.
128. Gamble KC, Alvarado TP, Bennett CL: Itraconazole plasma and tissue concentrations in the spiny lizard (*Scleropus* sp.) following once daily dosing, J Zoo Wildl Med 28(1):89-93, 1997.
129. Mallo KM, Harms CA, Lewbart GA, Papich MG: Pharmacokinetics of fluconazole in loggerhead sea turtles, *Caretta caretta,* after single intravenous and subcutaneous injections, and multiple subcutaneous injections, J Zoo Wildl Med 33(1):29-35, 2002.
130. Heatley JJ, Mitchell MA, Williams J, Smith JA, Tully TN: Fungal periodontal osteomyelitis in a chameleon (*Furcifer pardalis*), J Herp Med Surg 11(4):7-12, 2001.
131. Manire CA, Rhinehart HL, Sutton DA, Thompson EH, Rinaldi MG, Buck JD, et al: Disseminated mycotic infection caused by *Colletotrichum acutatum* in a Kemp's Ridley sea turtle (*Lepidochelys kempi*), J Clin Microbiol 40(11):4273-4280, 2002.
132. Manire CA, Rhinehart HL, Pennick GJ, Sutton DA, Hunter RP, Rinaldi MG: Steady-state plasma concentrations of itraconazole after oral administration in Kemp's Ridley sea turtles, *Lepidochelys kempi,* J Zoo Wildl Med 34(2):171-178, 2003.
133. Heykants J, van Peer A, van de Velde V, Van Rooy P, Meuldermans W, Lavrijsen K, et al: The clinical pharmacokinetics of itraconazole: an overview, *Mycoses* 32(Supp 1):67-87, 1989.
134. Alvearez OM, Mertz PM, Eaglstein WH: The effect of occlusive dressings on collagen synthesis and re-epithelialization in superficial wounds, J Surg Res 35:142-148, 1983.
135. Winter GD, Scales JY: Effect of air-drying and dressings on the surface of a wound, Nature 197:91-92, 1963.
136. Smith DA, Barker IK, Allen BO: The effect of certain topical medications on healing of cutaneous wounds in the common garter snake (*Thamnophis sirtalis*), Can J Vet Res 52:129-133, 1988.
137. Rupley AE: Emergency procedures; recovering from disaster, Proc Annu Conf Assoc Avi Vet 249-257, 1997.
138. Clippinger TL: Diseases of the lower respiratory tract of companion birds, Semin Avian Exotic Pet Med 6:201-208, 1997.
139. Forbes NA: Respiratory problems. In Benyon PH, Forbes NA, Lawton MPC, editors: *BSAVA manual of psittacine birds,* Ames, 1996, Iowa State University Press.
140. Divers SJ: The diagnosis and treatment of lower respiratory tract disease in tortoises with particular regard to intrapneumonic therapy, Kansas City, Mo, 1998, Proc Assoc Reptil Amphib Vet.
141. Divers SJ, Lawton MPC: Antibiotic-impregnated polymethylmethacrylate beads as a treatment for osteomyelitis in reptiles, Columbus, Ohio, 1999, Proc ARAV.
142. Weisman DL, Olmstead ML, Kowalski JJ: In vitro evaluation of antibiotic elution from polymethylmethacrylate (PMMA) and mechanical assessment of antibiotic-PMMA composites, Vet Surg 29:245-251, 2000.
143. Bennett RA: Antibiotic PMMA beads for septic arthritis in a Green Iguana, Proc ICE 1.3:27-28, 1999.
144. Mohan K, Foggin CM, Muvavarirwa P, Honywill J: Vaccination of farmed crocodiles (*Crocodylus niloticus*) against *Mycoplasma crocodyli* infection, Vet Rec 141(18):476, 1997.
145. Mohan K, Foggin CM, Dziva F, Muvavarirwa P: Vaccination to control an outbreak of *Mycoplasma crocdyli* infection, Onder J Vet Res 68(2):149-150, 2001.
146. Huchzermeyer FW, Huchzermeyer KDA, Putterill JF: Observations of a field outbreak of pox virus infection in young Nile crocodiles (*Crocodylus niloticus*), J S Afr Vet Assoc 62(1):27-29, 1991.
147. Horner RF: Poxvirus in farmed Nile crocodiles, Vet Rec 122(19):458-462, 1988.
148. Shen JY, Yin WL, Qian D, Cao Z, Shen ZH: Bacterin immunization of cultivated soft-shelled turtles against bacterial diseases, J Zhejiang Univ Agric Life Sci 26(3):325-328, 2000.
149. Marschang RE, Milde K, Bellavista M: Virus isolation and vaccination of Mediterranian tortoises against chelonid herpes virus in a chronically infected population in Italy, Deutsche Tierarztliche Wochenschrift 108(9):376-379, 2001.
150. Foelsch DW, Leloup P: Fatale endemische infection in einem serpentarium, Tierrztliche Praxis 4:527, 1976.
151. Jacobson ER, Gaskin JM, Flanagan JP, Odum RA: Antibody responses of western diamondback rattlesnakes (*Crotalus atrox*) to inactivated ophidian paramyxovirus vaccines, J Zoo Wildl Med 22(2):184-190, 1991.
152. Addison JB, Jacobson ER: Use of an autogenous bacterin to treat a chronic mouth infection in a reticulated python, J Zoo Anim Med 5(1):10-11, 1974.
153. Jacobson ER, Millichamp NJ, Gaskin JM: Use of a polyvalent autogenous bacterin for treatment of mixed gram-negative bacterial osteomyelitis in a rhinoceros viper (*Bitis nasicornis*), JAVMA 187(11):1224-1225, 1985.
154. Mitchell MA, Shane SM, Pesti D, Sanchez S, Wooley RE, Ritchie B, et al: Effect of an avirulent *Salmonella* vaccine on *Salmonella* colonization of hatchling Green Iguanas, Orlando, Fla, 2001, Proc ARAV.
155. Greenberg B: Suppression of known populations of bacteria by flies, J Bact 99:629-635, 1969.
156. Metchnikoff E: *Prolongation of life,* New York, 1908, GP Putnam & Sons.
157. O'Brien JDP: Aspects of *Salmonella enteritidis* control in poultry, World Poultry Sci J 46:119-124, 1990.
158. Nurmi E, Rantala M: New aspects of *Salmonella* infection in broiler production, Nature 241:210-211, 1973.
159. Rantala M, Nurmi E: Prevention of the growth of *Salmonella infantis* in chicks by the flora of the alimentary tract of chickens, Br Poultry Sci 14:627-632, 1973.
160. Rolfe RD: Population dynamics of the intestinal tract. In Blakenship LC, editor: *Colonization control of human bacterial enteropathogens in poultry,* San Diego, 1991, Academic Press.
161. Meynell GC: Antibacterial mechanisms of the mouse gut: II: the role of pH and volatile fatty acids in the normal gut, Br J Exp Path 44:209-219, 1963.
162. Corrier DE, Nisbet DJ: Competitive exclusion in the control of *Salmonella enterica* serovar Enteritidis infection in laying poultry. In Saeed AM, editor: *Salmonella Enterica serovar Enteritidis in humans and animals: epidemiology, pathogenesis, and control,* Ames, 1991, Iowa State University Press.
163. Stavric S, Gleeson TM, Buchanan B, Blanchfield B: Experience on the use of probiotics for *Salmonella* control in poultry, Lett Appl Microb 14:69-71, 1992.
164. Edens FW, Parkhurst CR, Casas A, Dobrogos ZWJ: Principles of ex ovo competitive exclusion and in ovo administration of *Lactobacillus reuteri,* Poultry Sci 76(1):179-196, 1997.
165. Chung TC, Axelsson L, Lindgreen SE, Dobrogosz WJ: In vitro studies on reuterin by *Lactobacillus reuteri,* Microb Ecol Health Dis 2:137-144, 1989.
166. Hudault SH, Brewa C, Bridonneau C, Ribaud P: Efficiency of various bacterial suspensions derived from cecal flora of conventional chickens in reducing the population level of *Salmonella typhimurium* in gnotobiotic mice and chicken intestines, Can J Microb 31:832-838, 1985.
167. Impey CS, Mead GC, George SM : Competitive exclusion of salmonellosis from the chick caecum using a defined mixture of bacterial isolates from the caecal microflora of an adult bird, J Hyg 479-490, 1982.

168. Stavric S, Gleeson TM, Blanchfield B, Pivnick H: Competitive exclusion of *Salmonella* from newly hatched chicks by mixtures of pure bacterial cultures isolated from fecal and cecal contents of adult birds, *J Food Protec* 48:778-783, 1985.
169. Nisbet DJ, Ricke SC, Scanlon CM, Corrier DE, Hollister AG, DeLoach JR: Inoculation of broiler chicks with a continuous-flow derived bacterial culture facilitates early cecal bacterial colonization and increases resistance to *Salmonella typhimurium*, *J Food Protec* 75(1):12-15, 1994.
170. Nisbet DJ, Corrier DE, DeLoach JR: *Probiotic for control of Salmonella*, US Patent 5,478,557, 1995.
171. Corrier DE, Nisbet DJ, Scanlan DM, Hollister AG, Cladwell DJ, Thomas LA, et al: Treatment of commercial broiler chickens with a characterized culture of cecal bacteria to reduce *Salmonella* colonization, *Poultry Sci* 74:1093-1101, 1995.
172. Corrier DE, Nisbet DJ, Scanlan DM, Hollister AG, DeLoach JR: Control of *Salmonella typhimurium* colonization in broiler chicks with a continuous-flow characterized mixed culture of cecal bacteria, *Poultry Sci* 74:916-924, 1995.
173. Blakenship LC, Bailey JS, Cox NA, Stern NJ, Brewer R, Williams O: Two-step mucosal competitive exclusion flora treatment to diminish salmonellae in commercial broiler chickens, *Poultry Sci* 72:1667-1672, 1993.
174. Stavric S, D'Aoust JY: Undefined and defined bacterial preparations for the competitive exclusion of *Salmonella* in poultry: a review, *J Food Protec* 56(2):173-180, 1993.
175. Oyofo BA, DeLoach JR, Corrier DE, Norman JO, Ziprin RL, Mollenhauer HH: Effect of carbohydrates on *Salmonella typhimurium* colonization in broiler chickens, *Avian Dis* 33:531-534, 1989.
176. Waldroup AL, Yamaguchi W, Skinner JT, Waldroup PW: Effects of dietary lactose on incidence and levels of salmonellae on carcasses of broiler chickens grown to market age, *Poultry Sci* 71:288-295, 1992.
177. Corrier DE, Nisbet DJ, Hollister AG, Beier RC, Scanlan CM, Hargis BM, et al: Resistance against *Salmonella enteritidis* cecal colonization in leghorn chicks by vent lip application of cecal bacteria culture, *Poultry Sci* 73:648-652, 1994.
178. Warwick C: Euthanasia of reptiles, *N Z Vet J* 1:12, 1986.

37
ULTRASONOGRAPHY

MARK D. STETTER

Ultrasonography is a critical diagnostic tool in veterinary medicine and has many potential uses in reptile medicine. It provides a noninvasive method for peering inside a patient and evaluating anatomic size, location, and architecture.[1-4] Because radiographs of reptiles often provide limited soft tissue information, ultrasonography is an excellent complement to radiography.[5] The organs best viewed with ultrasonography include the heart, liver, gallbladder, urinary bladder, colon, and female reproductive organs.[2,4] In some animals, ultrasonography can also be useful for the evaluation of the stomach, small intestine, spleen, pancreas, kidneys and testes.[2,4]

Ultrasound waves are not transmitted through air or bones, and thus, ultrasound imaging of pulmonary or skeletal structures is not useful. In those reptile species with thick scales or osteoderms (bones in the scales), image quality is often reduced because of the poor penetration of the scales. Placement of the transducer between these thick scales, copious use of ultrasound coupling gel that is given 30 minutes to absorb into the scales, or ultrasound of the patient that is submerged under water may help with image quality.[6] Image quality is also reduced during ecdysis, and patient examination should be postponed until after the animal has shed.[2]

The primary limitation in ultrasonography is the practitioner's experience in performing the scan and in interpretation of these images. Inherent artifacts to the normal ultrasound process, coupled with the additional artifacts associated with the reptile's skin, can make ultrasound evaluation a challenge. The veterinarian is encouraged to use surgical and postmortem procedures to correlate the ultrasound findings and become familiar with image interpretation (Figure 37-1).

ULTRASOUND EQUIPMENT

A rapidly growing range of ultrasound equipment is currently available to the veterinary practitioner. The primary considerations in purchase of equipment should include: size and species of the patients, requirements for a stationary unit versus a portable machine, and financial limitations.

The size of the patients dictates the transducer probes that are needed. Smaller animals (snakes, most lizards) require the use of a 7.5-megahertz (MHz) or 10-MHz transducer. In general, a linear array transducer with a small "footprint" is best suited for small animals.[7] A 5-MHz or 7.5-MHz transducer is used for medium size patients (20 to 50 kg). For large reptiles (i.e., giant tortoises, seaturtles, adult crocodilians), a 2.5-MHz or 3.5-MHz probe may be warranted (Figure 37-2).[8,9]

Prices of ultrasound machines have come down dramatically over the last 10 years, and many high-quality units are now affordable to the veterinary practitioner. In addition to the ultrasound unit and transducers, the clinician should also purchase a digital recording device. Digital images can be recorded as a still picture or can record the patient examination with a digital video unit. Not only is this documentation important for medical record storage and retrieval, but it also is critical as an easy method to acquire consultation from

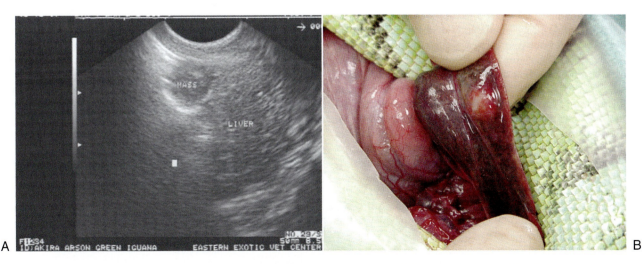

FIGURE 37-1 **A,** Interpretation of ultrasound images in reptiles can be challenging. Aside from the inherent artifacts associated with ultrasound imaging, learning the anatomy and image distortion seen with the thick scales can be difficult. **B,** The hepatic abscess seen in the ultrasound in **A**. Whenever possible, comparison of ultrasound images with gross pathology is recommended. (*Photographs courtesy S. Stahl.*)

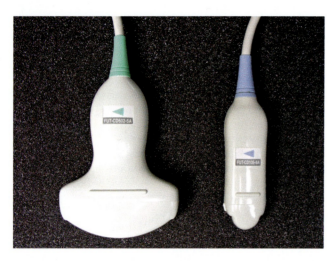

FIGURE 37-2 Transducer frequency directly affects image quality. Lower frequency transducers, such as the 5-MHz convex probe on *left*, give deeper penetration than the higher frequency 8-MHz probe on *right*. The trade-off is that lower frequencies lose resolution and detail. *(Photograph courtesy D. Mader.)*

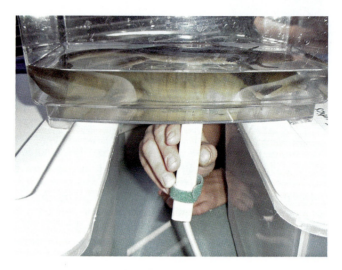

FIGURE 37-3 This axolotol is examined through both the plastic container and water. Ample gel is applied to the transducer, allowing the image to pass through plastic. *(Photograph courtesy S. Stahl.)*

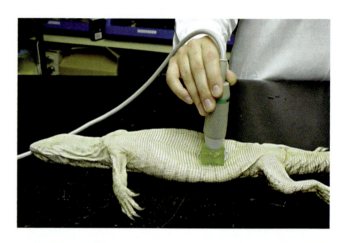

FIGURE 37-4 This lizard is imaged with a gel stand-off pad. The extra thickness of the pad allows the area of interest to be placed in the best focal plane of the transducer. Ample gel is used between both the transducer and the pad, and the pad and the scales on the patient. *(Photograph courtesy S. Divers.)*

other veterinary experts. These digital images can rapidly be sent via e-mail for consultation and interpretation.

ANIMAL RESTRAINT

Survey ultrasonography is a painless procedure, and thus, animal restraint is based more on the patient's size, temperament, and mobility than on the need for analgesia and sedation. Many lizard and crocodilian species can be imaged with manual restraint.[2,6,10-14] Imaging chelonians without sedation is variable and directly dependent on the ability to extend the animal's limbs.[2,8,9,15,16] For those species that tightly retract their limbs, sedation may be necessary (see Chapter 27). Imaging snakes can often be done without sedation, although very active or aggressive animals may need sedation.[17-19]

For small patients, the use of a water bath may provide some distance between the transducer and the patient.[7] This is particularly important with a small animal and only a 7.5-MHz or 5-MHz probe available. The animal can be submerged in a water bath, and the transducer can be placed either directly in the water, or with acoustic gel, the transducer can be pressed against the plastic container itself (Figure 37-3). Alternately, a "stand-off pad," a homogenous gelatinous wafer, can be used to distance the probe from the patient, thus placing the object to be imaged in the focal zone of the transducer (Figure 37-4).

PATIENT POSITIONING

Unless the patient has been sedated, most reptiles require less manual restraint if maintained in sternal recumbency. With the exception of chelonians, the best window for visceral organ imaging is created with placement of the transducer on the ventral surface. Two methods can be used to facilitate this transducer placement while the patient is kept in sternal recumbency. For smaller animals, the patient is simply elevated off the table and the transducer is then placed on the animal's ventrum (Figure 37-5). With larger animals, the animal can be placed on a surface that is fenestrated, allowing for transducer placement (Figure 37-6). For large snakes and crocodilians, this can be accomplished with two tables moved together and a small gap left between them. Many smaller snakes can be manually restrained and placed in dorsal recumbency for ultrasound examination (Figure 37-7).

Chelonians can be imaged in a variety of positions depending on the animal's size and the area of interest.[2,8,9,15,16] Smaller animals can be held off the table for examination, with the area of interest exposed for transducer placement (Figure 37-8). Medium and large chelonians can either be positioned in dorsal recumbency or placed sternally, with their plastron resting on a bucket or table to elevate the feet off the ground (Figure 37-9).[8,9]

PATIENT EXAMINATION

For consistency and thoroughness, a systematic evaluation of all visceral organ systems is best performed. The author

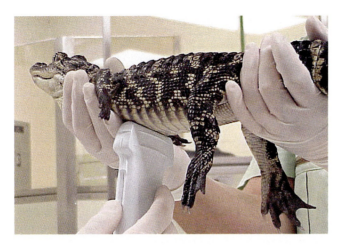

FIGURE 37-5 Ultrasound examination of an American Alligator (*Alligator mississippiensis*). The transducer is placed ventrally with the animal's body elevated off the table. Coupling gel is used to eliminate air between the transducer and the animal's skin. In thick-scaled reptiles, image quality can be improved by applying gel to the scales 15 to 30 minutes before the procedure and allowing the scales to absorb this material.

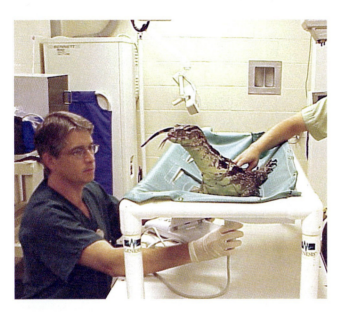

FIGURE 37-6 A monitor lizard (*Varanus* sp.) given an ultrasound examination with minimal manual restraint used. The ultrasound table has several holes in it for transducer placement.

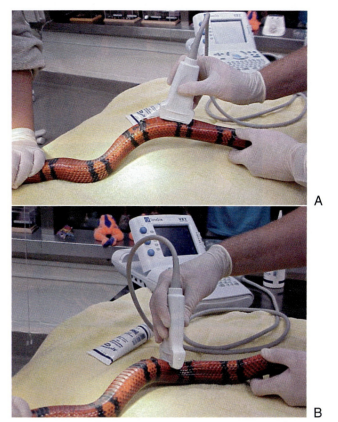

FIGURE 37-7 **A** and **B**, Ultrasound examination of a Honduran Milksnake (*Lampropeltis triangulum hondurensis*). The snake is manually restrained for the procedure. Note that the transducer must be used in two directions to provide a full image of the patient's structures.

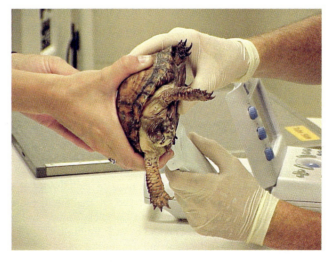

FIGURE 37-8 An ultrasound examination of an Eastern Box Turtle (*Terrapene carolina carolina*). The organs of chelonians are relatively mobile within the shell, and placement of the transducer in the dependent inguinal area provides the best image.

prefers to start at the heart and work caudally to the liver, stomach, gallbladder, intestines, and urogenital systems.

The **heart** provides an ideal landmark for initial orientation and allows the operator to fine-tune the various ultrasound settings: gain, depth, magnification, etc. In most lizards, the heart can be easily located on the ventral midline in the area of the front limbs.[2,10,13,14] In monitor lizards and crocodilians, the heart is often located more caudally than in other lizard species.[2,13] In snakes, the heart is generally located between 20% and 33% of the distance between the nose and the cloaca. Initially, the heart can be located grossly with placement of the animal in dorsal recumbency and visualization of cardiac contractility in that region of the body. Even if the heart cannot be seen grossly, placement of the transducer over this section of the snake rapidly allows identification of the heart (Figure 37-10).

The author commonly uses ultrasound as a method of monitoring anesthesia in reptiles. The transducer can be

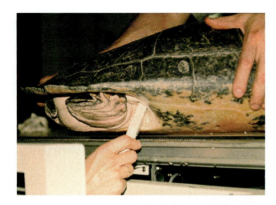

FIGURE 37-9 Ultrasound examination of an Asian Pond Turtle (*Mauremys mutica*). The transducer is placed on the soft skin just in front of the rear legs. This window allows good visualization of the reproductive organs, gastrointestinal tract, and urinary bladder.

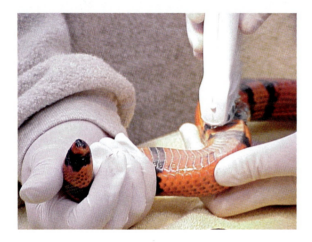

FIGURE 37-10 Cardiac ultrasonography in a Honduran Milksnake (*Lampropeltis triangulum hondurensis*). The transducer is placed on the ventral surface, directly over the heart.

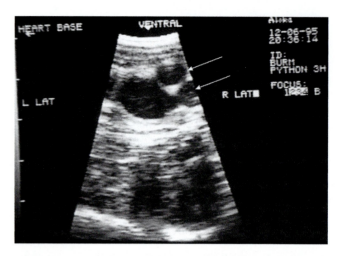

FIGURE 37-11 Ultrasound image of the heart in a Burmese Python (*Python molurus bivittatus*). The prominent paired aortic arches are easily visualized and unique to reptiles (*arrows*).

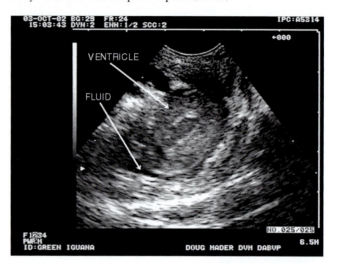

FIGURE 37-12 Reptiles normally have a single muscular ventricle. To the inexperienced clinician, this may look like hypertrophic cardiomyopathy. Finding a small amount of pericardial fluid around a normal reptile heart is not uncommon. (*Photograph courtesy D. Mader.*)

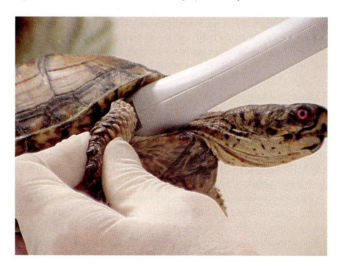

FIGURE 37-13 Ultrasound examination of an Eastern Box Turtle (*Terrapene carolina carolina*). The transducer is placed in the mediastinal window for imaging the heart and liver.

placed over the heart to monitor heart rate and contractility throughout a procedure.

With imaging of reptile hearts, one must remember that, with the exception of crocodilians, reptiles have a single muscular ventricle and that all reptiles have paired aortic arches (Figure 37-11; also Figures 14-22 and 14-23). The finding of a small amount of pericardial fluid in the normal reptile patient is not uncommon (Figure 37-12). See Chapter 14 for a comprehensive discussion on cardiac ultrasound.

With imaging of the heart and liver in chelonians, the transducer placement is recommended in the mediastinal window, between the front limb and the neck (Figure 37-13) or in the axillary region just caudal to each forelimb.[2,16]

In chelonians, the **intestinal** and **urogenital** tracts are best viewed from the inguinal area, with the transducer placed in the soft tissue of the prefemoral fossa (Figure 37-14).[2,16]

As compared with mammals, the relative size of the reptile **liver** is significantly larger. In lizards and chelonians, the liver lies immediately adjacent to the heart.[2] In chelonians, the liver can also be visualized through a window in the right prefemoral fossa. The large bladder is usually juxtaposed between the soft tissue and the liver, providing an excellent unobstructed view of the organ.

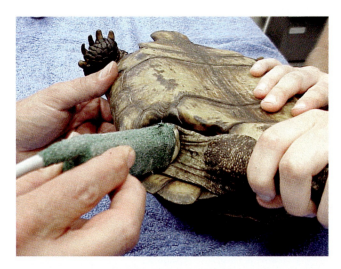

FIGURE 37-14 Ultrasound examination of a Desert Tortoise (*Gopherus agassizii*). The transducer is placed in the inguinal window for imaging of the urinary bladder, intestines, colon, and reproductive tract. The inguinal space between the rear leg and the shell must be completely filled with acoustic gel. (*Photograph courtesy D. Mader.*)

In lizards, the liver is usually visualized from a ventral approach. No specific window exists; rather, the transducer should be manipulated across the midcoelomic region just caudal to the xiphoid until the best image is obtained (Figure 37-15).

In snakes, the liver is separated from the heart by the lungs.[2] The lungs start to diminish in size and the liver gradually enlarges as the transducer moves from the snake's first quarter to the mid body. Snakes have a characteristic large central hepatic vein that helps differentiate the liver from fat bodies (Figure 37-16).

In most species, the **gallbladder** is easily recognized as a large round anechoic structure. In chelonians, the gallbladder is embedded in the liver to the right of midline. In lizards, the gallbladder is attached to the right caudal pole of the liver (Figure 37-17), and in snakes, the gallbladder does not directly contact the liver but can be found at the mid body, caudal to the end of the stomach (Figure 37-18).

If the **stomach** is empty, filled with digesta or fluid, it can be visualized adjacent to the liver (Figure 37-19). If the stomach is filled with gas, it is difficult to visualize.

The female **reproductive tract** of most reptiles can be visualized and often provides valuable information about the reproductive status of the animal. Determination of gender can be difficult in some lizard species, and ultrasonography has proven useful in confirming the gender of these species.[6,11-13] **Testes** may not always be recognized on ultrasound examination. During the nonbreeding season, the testes often regress. At the beginning of the breeding season, the gonads recrudesce, becoming more apparent. Regardless of the season, the **ovaries** are usually readily identified (Figure 37-20).

Gravid animals are usually readily imaged. Ovaries are staged as either "previtellogenic" or "vitellogenic." In previtellogenic females, the ova are round and anechoic and usually arranged in clusters. The ova are small, ranging from 1 to just a few millimeters in diameter.

In preovulatory vitellogenic follicles, the diameter is larger, but they are still round and in clusters. These are more echogenic than previtellogenic follicles.

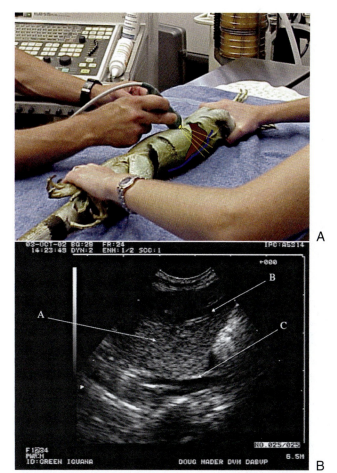

FIGURE 37-15 A, Normal transducer position for evaluating the liver in a Green Iguana (*Iguana iguana*), just caudal to the xiphoid. **B,** Liver (*A*), portal vein (*B*), and hepatic vein (*C*). (*Photograph courtesy D. Mader.*)

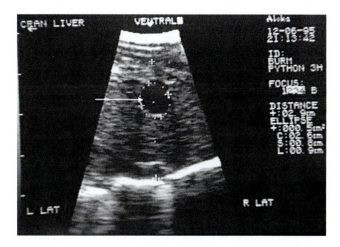

FIGURE 37-16 Ultrasound image of the liver in a Burmese Python (*Python molurus bivittatus*). The transducer has been placed on the ventral midline approximately one third of the distance from the head. The characteristic large central hepatic vein is easily recognized (*arrow*).

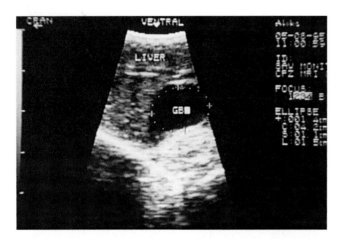

FIGURE 37-17 Ultrasound image of the liver and gallbladder in a Savannah Monitor *(Varanus exanthematicus)*. In lizards, these structures are adjacent to each other. The transducer has been placed on the ventral aspect of the lizard, approximately halfway between the fore and rear legs.

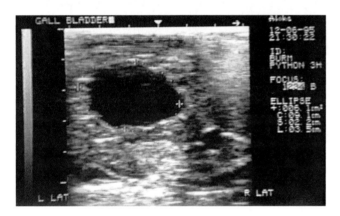

FIGURE 37-18 Ultrasound image of the gallbladder in a Burmese Python *(Python molurus bivittatus)*. In snakes, the gallbladder is recognized as a round hypoechoic structure just caudal to the stomach.

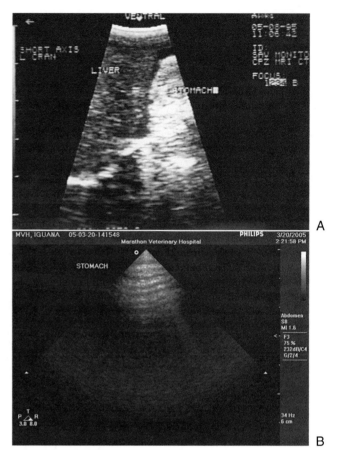

FIGURE 37-19 **A,** Ultrasound image of the liver and stomach in a Savannah Monitor *(Varanus exanthematicus)*. Note the marked difference in echogenicity between the two tissue densities. Image characteristics of the stomach in reptiles vary greatly, dependent on when and what the animal has recently consumed. **B,** Stomach of a Green Iguana *(Iguana iguana)*. Note the normal rugal folds typically associated with an empty stomach. *(Photograph courtesy D. Mader.)*

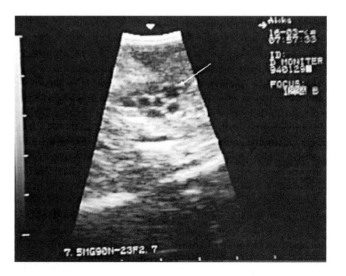

FIGURE 37-20 Ultrasound image of the ovary in a Desert Monitor *(Varanus griseus)*. Note the numerous round, anechoic, ovarian, previtellogenic follicles *(arrow)*. Externally, determination of gender in many species of monitors can be difficult. Ultrasound can be used to identify the gonads in these animals.

In postovulatory follicles the eggs are more oblong and usually in a line rather than a cluster. Postovulatory follicles have a more variable echogenicity with a hypoechoic center and hyperechoic outer line (shell).

Imaging is best when approached from the prefemoral region bilaterally. The bladder provides a clear window to the ovaries and shell glands (Figure 37-21).

In addition to gender determination, ultrasonography is useful for documenting and monitoring the status of the female reproductive tract.[8,9,14,15,17,18] Ovarian activity, ovulation, condition of the ovarian follicles, and presence of ova within the oviduct can be determined (Figures 37-22 and 37-23). In viviparous animals, fetal presence and viability can also be determined with ultrasound (Figure 37-24).

The **kidneys** of many species of reptiles are difficult to image. In those lizards that have renomegaly, and in some chelonian species, the kidneys can be identified in the caudal-most aspect of the dorsal coelom.[2,13]

In iguanas, a large portion of the kidney is located within the base of the tail. In these animals, the kidneys can be visualized with placement of the transducer laterally on either

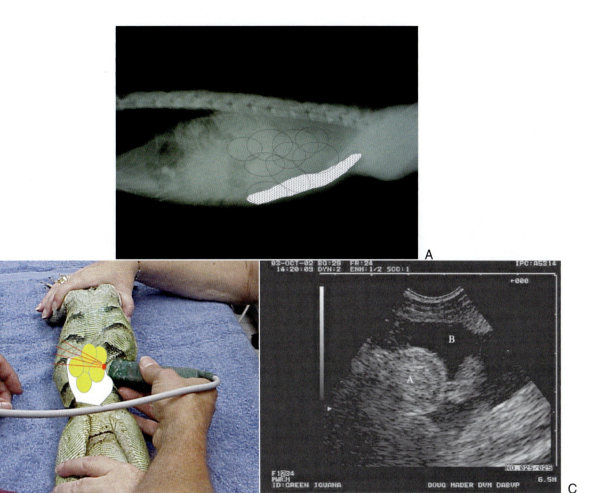

FIGURE 37-21 **A,** Lateral radiograph of a gravid Green Iguana *(Iguana iguana).* The vitellogenic ova are highlighted. The bladder is highlighted in white. **B,** Normal transducer position for evaluation of the reproductive tract. The urine-filled bladder makes an excellent window for clear imaging of the ovaries. **C,** Vitellogenic follicle *(A)* highlighted by urine *(B)* in the bladder. *(Photographs courtesy D. Mader.)*

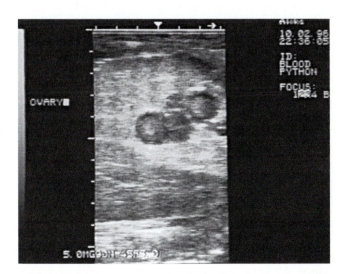

FIGURE 37-22 Ultrasound image of the ovary in a Blood Python *(Python curtis).* Note the numerous round, previtellogenic, ovarian follicles. These structures and their stage of development can be measured with ultrasound.

side of the tail base (Figure 37-25). This can be useful for ultrasound-guided renal biopsies in iguanas.

In snakes, the paired kidneys are generally located in the caudal 75% of the body. The right is cranial to the left and situated on either side of the spine. The best image is acquired from either side of the ventral scutes (Figure 37-26).

Many lizard and chelonian species have a large **urinary bladder** (see Table 11-1). These can be visualized as thin-walled anechoic structures that occupy the caudal coelom. A fluid-filled colon can appear similar to the urinary bladder (Figure 37-27). With a turn of the transducer 90 degrees, the clinician should be able to determine whether the organ is completely round (bladder) or is tubular in a long axis view.

The presence of the urinary bladder or colon should be distinguished from animals that have a significant amount of coelomic transudate (ascites). Differentiation of coelomic fluid from a large urinary bladder or colon is important. The clinician should attempt to identify the wall of the bladder or colon that contains within it the anechoic fluid. With the presence of ascites, significant fluid can be seen between the

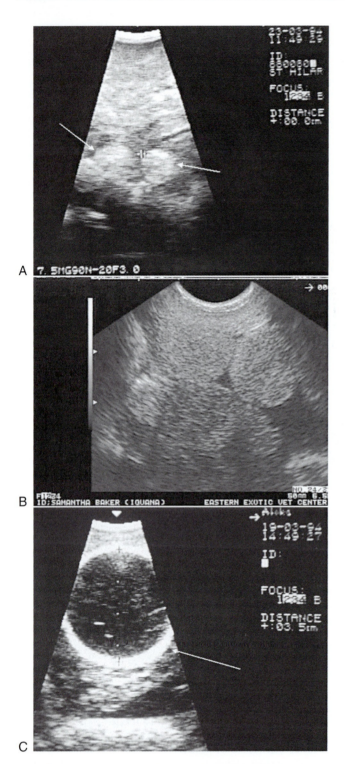

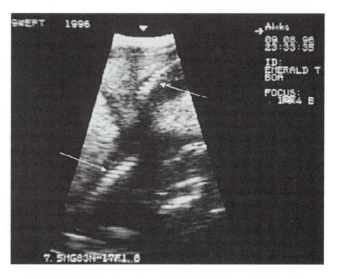

FIGURE 37-24 Ultrasound image of several fetuses in a gravid Emerald Tree Boa *(Corallus caninus)*. The calcified vertebrae of the fetuses can be seen as hyperechoic lines within the uterus *(arrows)*.

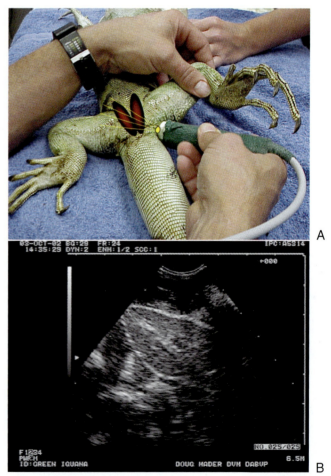

FIGURE 37-23 **A,** Ultrasound image of the ovary in an Asian Pond Turtle *(Mauremys mutica)*. Note the round, hyperechoic, vitellogenic follicles *(arrows)*. **B,** Mature, vitellogenic, postovulatory ova in a Green Iguana *(Iguana iguana)*. Note the hyperechoic nature of the ova. *(Photograph courtesy S. Stahl.)* **C,** Ultrasound image of a calcified egg within the oviduct of an Asian Pond Turtle *(Mauremys mutica)*. The circular hyperechoic line is the outline of a partially calcified eggshell *(arrow)*.

FIGURE 37-25 **A,** Ultrasound probe position for evaluation of the kidneys in a Green Iguana *(Iguana iguana)*. Kidneys (location highlighted in brown) are intrapelvic in iguanas. **B,** Image of normal iguana kidneys from the caudal pelvic window. The hyperechoic capsule around the teardrop-shaped kidneys is the normal appearance. *(Photograph courtesy D. Mader.)*

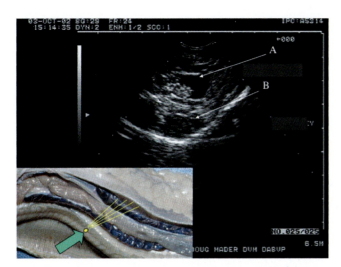

FIGURE 37-26 Normal ultrasound appearance of healthy kidneys in a snake. Fluid-filled colon *(A)*. Kidneys *(B)*—cross-section appearance. *(Photograph courtesy D. Mader.)*

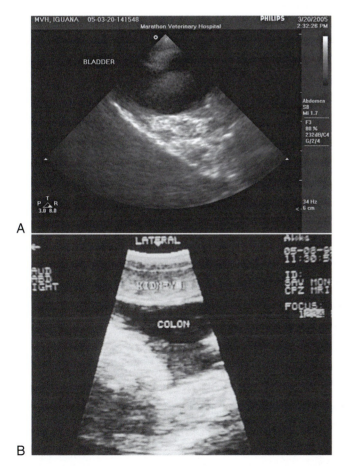

FIGURE 37-27 **A,** Urinary bladder (hypoechoic) adjacent to the body wall (hyperechoic line) in a Green Iguana *(Iguana iguana)*. Adjacent to the bladder are several previtellogenic ova. *(Photograph courtesy D. Mader.)* **B,** Ultrasound image of the colon and kidney in a Savannah Monitor *(Varanus exanthematicus)*. The colon is often seen as a large anechoic structure in the caudal coelom and can easily be confused with the bladder.

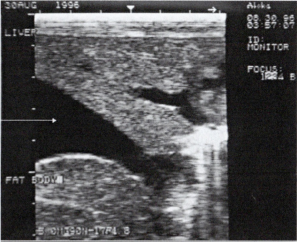

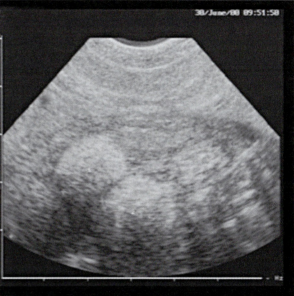

FIGURE 37-28 **A,** Ultrasound image of free coelomic fluid, the liver, and fat bodies in a Savannah Monitor *(Varanus exanthematicus)*. Free coelomic fluid *(arrow)* should be differentiated from other fluid-filled structures, such as the gallbladder and large intestine. Note the prominent vasculature in the liver, which helps differentiate it from lobulated fat bodies in **B**. *(Photograph courtesy of S. Stahl.)*

visceral organs, and in severe cases, the liver, fat bodies, and intestines can be seen floating. In the author's experience, lizards and chelonians normally have a small amount of free coelomic fluid without any evidence of disease.

Fat bodies are common in many reptile species and often can be confused with the liver on ultrasound examination. The fat bodies are paired structures in lizards and often occupy a large portion of the caudal to mid coelom. Remembering that the liver has prominent vasculature within its tissue can help differentiate these structures. In addition, fat bodies may have a thin hyperechoic capsule on their surface and can appear in clumps of round masses versus the tapered edge of a normal liver lobe (Figure 37-28).

REFERENCES

1. Hildebrandt TB, Göritz F, Stetter MD, Hermes R: Applications of sonography in vertebrates, *Zoology* 101:200-209, 1998.
2. Schildger B, Casares M, Kramer M, et al: Technique of ultrasonography in lizards, snakes, and chelonians, *Semin Amian Exot Pet Med* 3:147-155, 1994.
3. Silverman S: Advances in avian and reptilian imaging. In Kirk R, editor: *Current veterinary therapy X: small animal practice*, Philadelphia, 1989, WB Saunders.
4. Stetter M: Diagnostic imaging of reptiles. In Kirk R, editor: *Current veterinary therapy XIII: small animal practice*, Orlando, Fla, 2000, WB Saunders.
5. Stetter M, Raphael B, Cook R, Haramati N, Currie B: Comparison of magnetic resonance imaging, computerized axial tomography, ultrasonography and radiology for reptilian diagnostic imaging, *Proceedings of the American Association of Zoo Veterinarians*, Puerto Vallarta, Mexico, 1996.
6. Wright K, Pugh C, Walker L: Ultrasonographic sexing of helodermatid lizards, *Proceedings of the American Association of Zoo Veterinarians*, East Lansing, Mich, 1995.
7. Silverman S, Janssen D: Diagnostic imaging. In Mader R, editor: *Reptile medicine and surgery*, Philadelphia, 1996, WB Saunders.
8. Robeck T, Rostal D, Burchfield P, Owens D, Kraemer D: Ultrasound imaging of reproductive organs and eggs in Galapagos tortoises (*Geochelone elephantopus* spp.), *Zoo Biol* 9:349-359, 1990.
9. Rostal D, Robeck T, Owens D, Kraemer D: Ultrasound imaging of ovaries and eggs in Kemp's Ridley sea turtles (*Lepidochelys kempi*), *J Zoo Wildl Med* 21(1):27-35, 1990.
10. Fritsch G, Göritz F, Hermes R, Jaroffke D, Gildebrandt T: Anatomic study by means of ultrasonography in tuatara (*Sphenodon punctatus*), *Proc Assoc Reptilian Amphibian Vet*, Orlando, Fla, 2001.
11. Hildebrandt TB, Göritz F, Pitra C, Spelman LH, Walsh TA, Rosscoe R, et al: Sonomorphological sex determination in subadult komodo dragon, *Proc Annu Meet Am Assoc Zoo Vet*, Puerto Vallarta, Mexico, 1996.
12. Morris PJ, Alberts AC: Determination of sex in white-throated monitors (*Varanus albigularis*), gila monster (*Heloderma suspectum*), and bearded lizards (*Heloderma horridum*) using two-dimensional ultrasound imaging, *J Zoo Wildl Med* 27:371-377, 1996.
13. Sainsbury A, Gili C: Ultrasonographic anatomy and scanning technique of the coelomic organs of the bosc monitor (*Varanus exanthematicus*), *J Zoo Wildl Med* 22:421-433, 1991.
14. Schildiger B, Kramer M, Spörle H, Gerwing M, Wicker R: Comparative diagnostic images of the ovary in two saurians: common chuckwalla (*Sauromalus obesus*) and ocellated monitor (*Varanus panoptes*), *Salamandra* 29:240-247, 1993.
15. Kuchling G: Assessment of ovarian follicles and oviductal eggs by ultrasound scanning in live freshwater turtles, *Chelodina oblonga*, *Herpetologica* 45(1):89-94, 1989.
16. Penninck, D, Steward J, Paul-Murphy J, et al: Ultrasonography of the California desert tortoise (*Xerobtes agassizi*): anatomy and application, *Vet Radiol* 32(3):112-116, 1991.
17. Sauer A, Sauer H: Use of ultrasound to evaluate intrauterine findings using the example of the smooth snake (*Coronella austriaca*), *Salamandra* 28:92-94, 1992.
18. Smith CR, Cartee RE, Heathcock JT, Speake DW: Radiographic and ultrasonographic scanning of gravid eastern indigo snakes, *J Herpetol* 23:426-429, 1989.
19. Starck JM, Burann AK: Noninvasive imaging of the gastrointestinal track of snakes: a comparison of normal anatomy, radiography, magnetic resonance imaging, and ultrasonography, *Zoology* 101:210-223, 1998.

Section VI
DIFFERENTIAL DIAGNOSES BY SYMPTOMS

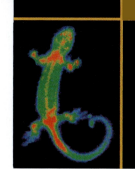

38
SNAKES
RICHARD S. FUNK

SIGNS RELATING TO THE GASTROINTESTINAL TRACT

Anorexia

Anorexia is a nonspecific sign and could be related to disease, husbandry, biology, or a combination of these factors (see Chapter 44). Husbandry-related issues include the temperature being kept too low or, less frequently, too high. Stresses such as constant exposure to view or the cage-tapping public or close proximity to a loudly vibrating home entertainment system can contribute to anorexia. An insecure snake with too small, or too few, hiding places may not feed, neither may a snake offered food during the wrong time of day. Lighting left on for prolonged periods of time, or never turned off, can stress a captive snake and contribute to anorexia, as can overcrowding.

Reproductive conditions can also be associated with anorexia. Some males during the breeding season are more interested in mating than in food. Many gravid females go off feed during all or part of gestation. For instance, the Burmese Python *(Python molurus bivitattus)* normally goes off food toward the end of gestation, which is often mistaken by inexperienced herpetologic veterinarians as a trouble sign, such as "egg-binding."

Temperate zone snakes may enter a fall anorexia in preparation for brumation, and some anorectic hatchlings may first feed after brumation. Freshly imported snakes may take a while to acclimate to captive conditions before commencing to feed. A snake may not eat if the wrong food is offered or if food is offered incorrectly (e.g., on the ground for an arboreal snake or during the day for a nocturnal snake, or a rodent crawls all over the snake all day long). Juvenile snakes of species with ontogenetic dietary shifts may be problem feeders during the transition, for example, from ectothermic to endothermic prey. Snakes nearing shedding ("in the blue") typically do not eat until after ecdysis.

Disease conditions associated with anorexia include gastrointestinal parasitism (helminths, coccidia including *Cryptosporidium*, amebas, cestodes, possibly flagellated protozoans) and gastroenteritis from bacterial, fungal, or viral infections. Gastrointestinal foreign bodies and impactions that include pieces of the cage substrate (bark, wood chips, gravel, towels) can be associated with anorexia.

Oral abscesses, necrotic stomatitis, or an injured or missing or abscessed tongue can also lead to anorexia (see Chapter 72; Figures 38-1 and 72-10). Anorexia may also be associated with gastrointestinal masses; internal space-occupying masses such as abscesses, granulomas, or tumors; or septicemia. Pneumonia, occluded nares, and tracheal ring granulomas can lead to anorexia.

Emesis (Vomiting or Regurgitation)

Vomition and regurgitation are generally not easily differentiated in reptiles; the problem usually is vomition (see Chapter 74). Too large a meal, or too many food items, can cause vomiting, as can housing the snake at inappropriate temperatures. The wrong diet, or an iatrogenically inappropriate or too large a meal, can result in vomiting. Postprandial handling, especially of a nervous snake, can result in vomiting. A stressed insecure snake with no hiding place or too many cage mates may vomit. Rule-outs for vomiting must also include

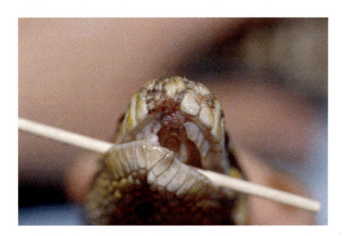

FIGURE 38-1 Infectious stomatitis, or mouth rot, is a common cause of anorexia. Note that infectious stomatitis is *not* disease but rather a symptom of other more serious problems. Patients need a thorough physical evaluation, including a discussion of husbandry and management. *(Photograph courtesy D. Mader.)*

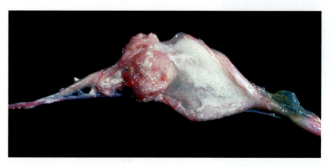

FIGURE 38-2 This mass originated in the gastric mucosa of a Cornsnake *(Elaphe gutatta)*. This severe gastric hypertrophy resulted from an infection with *Cryptosporidium serpentis*.

gastrointestinal stasis such as a foreign body or too frequent feedings so that prior meals have not yet been fully digested and voided. Gastrointestinal parasitism, gastroenteritis, or masses such as neoplasia, granulomas, and abscesses can also cause vomiting. Vomition can be confused with diarrhea in some cases when the act was not actually observed.

Diarrhea

Diarrhea is a nonspecific sign and not a disease entity (see Chapter 50). First, one should ascertain that the feces are truly abnormal: some species have more runny stools than others, and in some species, the stool quality can vary with the meal.

Probably the most common causes of diarrhea in captive snakes are inappropriate (especially too low) environmental temperatures and gastrointestinal parasitism. But foreign bodies, too large a meal, and iatrogenic meals that are inappropriate (such as dairy products) can also result in diarrhea. Bacterial, fungal, or viral gastroenteritis can lead to diarrhea.

Oral Cavity

A good oral examination may reveal necrotic stomatitis (lay term, mouth rot), abscessation, foreign bodies, increased mucus or discharges, petechiation, icterus, parasites, masses, edema, or other problems (see Chapter 72). Masses may be embedded foreign objects, for example, a piece of substrate from the snake's enclosure. Other masses may be bacterial or fungal granulomas, neoplasms, or abscesses. A mass, a broken jaw, or stomatitis can cause a deviation in the opening of the mouth, exposing the gums and leading to an exposure gingivitis.

An inactive tongue can be the result of a tongue sheath abscess or a tongue injury, or rarely the tongue may have been bitten off or necrosed off from an injury. Oral petechiation can be associated with stomatitis, sepsis, hyperthermia, intoxication (as from cedar or organophosphates), or a diffuse intravascular coagulopathy. The oral membranes may also be inflamed from infection. Edema of the oral membranes has been seen with bacterial cellulitis and renal failure, and the author has seen several snakes with head or intermandibular edema associated with having the head stuck partly through a hole in a cage or snake bag. An intraoral discharge or mucus may be the result of an oral infection, a gastrointestinal infection, or a respiratory infection. Dental disease may be seen with stomatitis and with osteomyelitis.

Esophagus and Stomach

Emesis (regurgitation or vomition) may occur with stomatitis, which can extend posteriorly down into the esophagus and stomach. (See the previous section on emesis and Chapter 74.) Esophageal tonsils may enlarge with so-called inclusion body disease of boas and pythons. A mass in the precardiac region may be in the esophagus but may also be in the respiratory system or the rib cage. Cryptosporidiosis, which can cause marked gastric hypertrophy, is often characterized by obvious midbody swelling (Figure 38-2).

Intestines

A mass in the coelomic cavity could be a granuloma, neoplasm, abscess, foreign body, meal, or cryptosporidiosis or may not be intestinal (Figure 38-3). A retained egg or fetus (dystocia) may be mistaken for an intestinal mass. Constipation can be caused by too large a meal, too frequent meals, or dystocia (food unable to pass by the retained conceptus). Obstructive intestinal disease may be caused by helminthiasis, foreign body including bedding material, dystocia, neoplasm, abscess, or granuloma. (See the previous section on diarrhea.) Loose stool may not be diarrhea but may in fact be normal for the species.

A prolapse that protrudes from the cloaca may be the cloacal membranes but could also be the oviduct (in a female) or a hemipenis (in a male; see Chapter 47).

Abdominal Distension

Gastrointestinal problems can lead to distension of the abdomen. Knowledge of the topography of the snake's body helps rule out other causes, including reproductive problems or organomegaly.

In the gastrointestinal system, abdominal distension can be the result of parasitism, including cryptosporidiosis (see Figure 38-3); a blockage, such as a foreign body or fecal impaction; a tumor or granuloma or abscess; or gastrointestinal

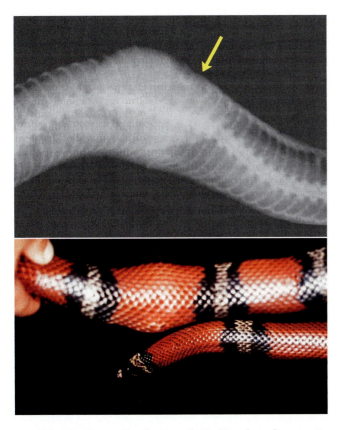

FIGURE 38-3 Externally, all masses look alike; thus, the necessity for biopsies before a prognosis is given. This mass was a chondroma. *(Photograph courtesy D. Mader.)*

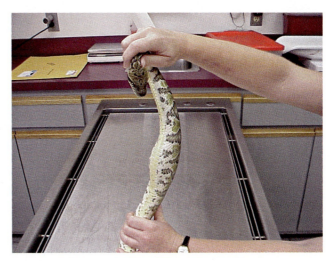

FIGURE 38-4 The midbody swelling seen here is an enlarged heart. On careful observation, rhythmic beating can be seen. *(Photograph courtesy D. Mader.)*

stasis and putrefaction of ingesta in response to suboptimal temperatures. A huge meal may also distend the body. Retention of large solid urate "stones" may enlarge the caudal body, possibly with associated palpable fluid around and anterior to the stones.

Ascites can distend a good portion of a snake's body. Steatitis or hepatic inflammation or neoplasia can also distend the body. An abscess, granuloma, or neoplasm outside of the gastrointestinal system may distend the body (e.g., a renal adenocarcinoma).

Any organomegaly could potentially cause a distension of the body.

Cardiomegaly may appear as an enlargement in the anterior fourth to third of the snake's body, and generally, on inspection, this "mass" may be seen to be beating (Figure 38-4). Renomegaly may occur in the posterior fourth of the body.

Reproductive events may cause abdominal distension: ovulation in boas and pythons, normally enlarging fetuses or eggs, or a dystocia.

INTEGUMENTARY SIGNS

Masses and swellings are most often abscesses, which are usually bacterial infections but can be mycotic or mixed. But tumors and granulomas must be ruled out also. Myiasis is rare in snakes. Sparganosis may appear as subcutaneous masses, particularly in tropical snakes. A generalized cellulitis may accompany dermatitis or even septicemia.

Abrasions, ulcers, and sores may appear on snake skin. Snout-rubbing injuries may appear on snakes that need a more secure hiding place or on those that continually push against a weak or loose area of a cage. Abrasions can become infected but, if the inciting cause is eliminated, may heal after several sheds, although a permanent cellulitis and fibrosis can occur on the snout.

Acanthocephalans may exit the skin of a snake and leave small ulcerated wounds.

Chemical and thermal burns may leave lesions of varying severity, perhaps with associated fluid-filled vesicles in the affected scales, and these may become infected with bacteria and sometimes fungi. So-called "blister disease," with a similar bacterial infection and a vesicular dermatitis, may be seen with thermal burns and with a filthy cage syndrome where a snake literally lies in urine-contaminated and fecal-contaminated substrate or is kept too wet (see Figure 15-16).

Petechiation in the skin may be associated with a generalized or local dermatitis, thermal burns, septicemia, obesity, or osteomyelitis. Wrinkling of the skin can be seen with inanition or dehydration, with dysecdysis, or with postpartum conditions of a female. When snakes have been stuck in tape and the tape is removed, the outer keratin layer of the scales may be removed adherent to the tape, causing a dry nonshiny appearance to the skin, and small wrinkles or even tears in the skin may be found. Similarly, when snakes have become stuck under doors, or escape through a narrow opening in a cage, they may bruise or damage the skin as they do so or as their owners remove them.

Ectoparasites may be found, usually mites but occasionally also ticks. Manual removal of ticks is usually possible, but treatments for both, including the use of ivermectin and various acaricides, are discussed in Chapter 43. The presence of mites can be suspected if a fine whitish powder is found on the snake's skin, with dysecdysis, or if the snake is soaking in its water bowl excessively.

Rodent bite trauma may occur when a snake is offered a live rodent and for whatever reason does not feed. The rodent, left alive in the cage with the snake, may begin chewing on the snake, and the damage done to the snake may range from minor bites needing little veterinary intervention, to wounds that necessitate major surgical repairs, to trauma so severe that humane euthanasia is the only option for treatment (see Chapter 46). Live rodents placed into snake cages must therefore be closely monitored to avoid catastrophe. Rodent bite wounds should be treated as highly infected wounds. Most snakes readily learn to accept dead prey, whether freshly killed or frozen and thawed.

Dysecdysis may occur for a variety of reasons, including ectoparasites, malnutrition, improper humidity, improper substrate or hiding places, systemic disease, dehydration, debilitation, or rough handling when the snake is "blue" (see Chapter 52). The eyecap should normally be shed with the rest of the skin, but if it is not, one should check for mites and husbandry-related problems and carefully manually remove it. Overzealous owners or pet shop personnel may actually remove the normal (functional) spectacle, leading to an exposure keratopathy of the cornea. A snake that stays "blue" too long, or that increases its shedding frequency, may be ill. Snakes with skin lesions, including surgical wounds, may increase this shedding frequency as part of a normal healing process. A reduction in shedding frequency may indicate a lack of feeding, or insufficient feeding, or a normal reduction with maturity as growth slows.

Scars may heal and be depigmented, or hyperpigmented, and large scars may heal with an abnormal scalation.

A wide variety of captive-bred "morphs" or phenotypes (cultivars) are now available in the commercial marketplace for a growing number of snake species. These include many with patterns and coloration that may differ from the normal wild types in a particular species, including those lacking melanocytes (amelanistic partial albinos), those lacking reds and yellows (anerythristic partial albinos), those homozygous recessive for both alleles ("snows" and "blizzards"), leucistics (white with blue eyes), and many other mutations that collectors prize. Occasionally, scaleless snakes are seen—the epidermis is keratinized but not fully formed into scales. The author has seen several Western Diamondback Rattlesnakes (*Crotalus atrox*) and Freckled Pythons (*Liasis fuscus mackloti*) with patches of the skin rotated nearly 180 degrees and the tips pointing anteriorly.

MUSCULOSKELETAL SIGNS

Paresis and paralysis can be from musculoskeletal signs but can also result from neurologic abnormalities (see Chapter 62). Spinal column lesions are the likely cause of paralysis or paresis in a snake, especially from trauma to the vertebral column but also from spinal abscessation, ossifying spondylosis, or even a spinal tumor. Fecal impactions can present as a caudal paresis and usually resolve with treatment. Neurologically related postural abnormalities may be mistaken for musculoskeletal signs.

Fractures can be caused by trauma, such as a bite wound, closure in a cage door or lid, fall from a perch or branch, or rarely, a prey animal. Family pets, mainly dogs and also cats, may injure a pet snake and cause fractures. Osteomyelitis or abscessation can weaken a bony area and contribute to a fracture. Fractures of ribs generally need not be treated unless they are protruding or they penetrate another body organ. In fact, rib fractures, often healed, are common incidental findings during routine radiography.

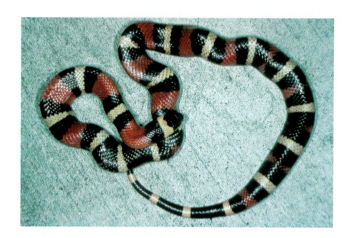

FIGURE 38-5 A captive-bred subadult Pueblan Milksnake (*Lampropeltis triangulum campbelli*) with a series of kinks in the body. Radiographs showed normal skeletal structures. When sedated, the snake relaxed and the scoliosis disappeared. No history of trauma or toxic exposure was the seen, and no lesions were found on necropsy.

Head fractures may be difficult to detect unless one knows the skull anatomy; one should look for asymmetry on skull radiographs, or pain and swelling or palpable abnormalities. Lower jaw fractures may heal if they are closed, the jaw can be realigned closely, and the snake is not fed for a period of time to allow some callus formation; external fixators can be ingeniously constructed, but the cage must be kept quite bare so the fixators do not get caught on cage furniture or bedding.

Musculoskeletal deformities in snakes are rarely attributable to malnutrition because most captive snakes are fed on whole rodents that generally are viewed as being nutritionally complete. Exceptions may be found among snakes that eat invertebrates, when the invertebrates are not fed nutritiously.

Curvatures, kinks, or external lumps or swellings of the body may be the result of musculoskeletal problems such as abscessation, ossifying spondylosis, osteomyelitis, trauma, fractures, congenital defects, or neurologic disorders (Figure 38-5; see also Chapter 69). Cases of so-called Paget's syndrome when fully investigated are most often associated with a septic condition of the spine.

Many deformities are seen in captive-produced snakes, including shortened jaws or snouts, restricted orbits, domed cranial vaults, arched necks or spines, and various types of spinal kinks and bends, and at least some of these may be congenital abnormalities associated with improper incubation or gestation temperatures. A possible role of inbreeding is often invoked but rarely well-documented. One category of congenital defects elicits considerable interest in zoos and from private collectors, including high commercial prices: two-headed snakes exhibiting what has been called axial bifurcation. Sometimes in these two-headed snakes one head seems to be more dominant, but often they can both eat.

Tail tips may be damaged by parasites, such as *Alaria* flukes or ticks; by prey or predator animals; by rodent bites in cages; by the tail being tied in the knot of the collecting or transport bag; by the tail being shut or caught in a cage lid or door; or by injury from a human. Wild rattlesnakes are occasionally found with healed rattleless tails, having had their rattles cut off previously.

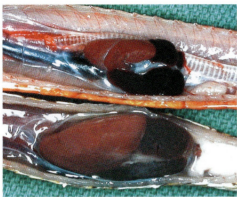

FIGURE 38-6 Two similar-sized adult Cornsnakes *(Elaphe gutatta)* are prosected to show a comparison of the heart sizes. The animal on the bottom had cardiomegaly from an unidentified cause.

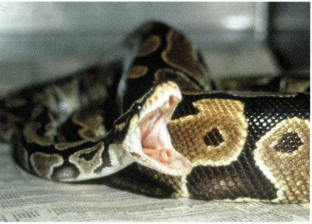

FIGURE 38-7 Open-mouth breathing is *never* normal in snakes. Snakes yawn on occasion and show a "gaping" response after injection with anesthetics such as ketamine or tiletamine, but constant open-mouth breathing is a serious sign. This Ball Python *(Python regius)* had a tracheal chondroma. *(Photograph courtesy G. Diethelm.)*

CARDIOVASCULAR SIGNS

Anemia, if truly present, may originate from blood loss, from neoplasia such as lymphosarcoma, laboratory or clinician error (including lymphatic fluid contamination and dilution), septicemia, or possibly hemic parasites (although the latter are generally considered to be asymptomatic incidental findings; see Chapter 55).

Oral petechiation may be associated with stomatitis, septicemia, diffuse intravascular coagulopathy, hyperthermia, or intoxication and rarely with anemia.

Avascular necrosis of the tail tip has been seen with parasitism, including *Alaria* flukes and microfilariae, or after trauma to the tail. Ischemic necrosis has been documented in the tails of breeding female Burmese Pythons in association with thromboembolic disease.

A snake that is hypovolemic, shocky, anemic, dehydrated, or cold may have a bradycardia or a weak heart beat.

Apparent enlargement of the heart (or radiographically the cardiac silhouette) may be caused by cardiomyopathy or pericardial effusion (cardiac tamponade; Figure 38-6). Starvation with extreme weight loss gives the illusion of an enlarged heart. A noncardiac mass such as an abscess, granuloma, or neoplasm may be mistaken for the heart (but is not contracting).

The presence of mitotic figures in peripheral blood is a normal finding in snakes, although unusually high numbers are suspicious of a disease condition such as lymphosarcoma or hemangiosarcoma. Other clinical pathology abnormalities are addressed in Chapter 28.

RESPIRATORY SIGNS

Respiratory signs in snakes may include nasal discharge; oral discharge; open-mouth breathing (Figure 38-7); crusted external nares; puffy throat; abnormal posturing, including holding the head and neck elevated; bubble blowing; sneezing; and increased respiratory sounds. Many snakes with respiratory illness are anorectic and lethargic; sometimes owners may be unaware of the respiratory component to the snake's illness.

Oral and nasal discharges need to be carefully evaluated to ensure their origin is the respiratory system because gastroenteritis and stomatitis can have confusing discharges. Indeed, stomatitis can occur simultaneously with a respiratory infection. A bacterial, mycoplasma, mycotic, viral, or parasitic pneumonia may present with dyspnea or with oral or nasal discharges. Snakes have difficulty getting rid of excessive pulmonary and tracheal mucus. An aspiration pneumonia can be a sequela of vomition of food or vomition after iatrogenic force feeding of liquid food.

Dyspnea in snakes can be caused by occluded nostrils; a choana full of caseous material or pieces of the cage substrate; a tongue sheath abscess; an intraoral abscess or granuloma; granulomas of the tracheal cartilages (Figure 38-7); hyperthermia; exposure to toxins, such as cedar or excessive ammonia buildup in the cage; an increase in tracheal or pulmonary mucus (occasionally with a relatively large firm mucinous tracheal plug); or near-drowning accidents. Any of these conditions can present as open-mouth breathing, whether constant or intermittent. Tobacco and incense smoke can be a respiratory irritant for some snakes.

Respiratory sounds of snakes can be audible. Abnormal gurgling or wheezing on inspiration, or especially on expiration, should alert one to examine a snake's respiratory system. But some snakes may seem to increase their (normal) respiratory sounds when becoming alert. Some snakes also appear to make slightly increased breathing sounds when nearing shedding, as the skin lining the external nares thickens in preparation for ecdysis and forces the airway to be slightly constricted. These sounds must be evaluated in comparison with the normal for each particular species because defensive hissing may be confused with a respiratory problem.

NERVOUS SYSTEM SIGNS

Lethargy and depression can be difficult to appreciate and evaluate. A client may state that the snake is lethargic, and one may not be able to detect this in the examination room. One should rule out non–nervous system causes such as gravidity, preecdysis, too low an environmental temperature, malnutrition, or illness (e.g., respiratory or gastrointestinal disease, renal disease, or sepsis). In fact, a wide variety of illnesses can also cause a snake to be lethargic.

Depression in snakes can be the result of head trauma, housing at too cool a temperature, a drug reaction, or intoxication (as from organophosphates, etc). Some boas and pythons certainly recognize their individual owners and may appear at least inactive while their owners are away for a period of time, resuming normal activity on the return of their owners; this may not be a true depression.

Paresis and paralysis must be differentiated from musculoskeletal system problems (refer to that previous section). Ataxia may occur from exposure to toxins such as cedar shavings or phenolic cleansers; acaricides and insecticides; head or body trauma; ossifying osteomyelitis; inclusion body disease (viral) of boas, pythons, and colubrids; and thiamine deficiency in snakes fed frozen-thawed fish. Ataxia and incoordination have also been attributed to hypoglycemia (although the author has seen snakes with a blood glucose level of less than 10 mg/dL that were not ataxic), starvation, general debilitation, hepatic encephalopathy, trauma, meningitis, drug intoxication (such as ivermectin and streptomycin), paramyxoviral infection, and the so-called inclusion body disease.

Inclusion body disease, mostly known from boas and pythons but now also known in a few colubrid snakes (including *Lampropeltis*), can cause a head tilt, opisthotonus, flaccid paralysis, disorientation, an inability to right itself, an inability to prehense food or inability to completely ingest food, and death (see Chapter 60).

Nutritional deficiencies rarely contribute to neurologic problems in snakes because most of the popularly kept species are fed rodents, which generally precludes the development of deficiencies in these species. Snakes that are fed invertebrates might be more susceptible to such problems as hypocalcemia if the prey are not properly fed.

Thiamine and biotin deficiencies have been linked to convulsions.

Dehydration or iatrogenic overdosage of gentamicin can lead to renal disease and gout, which can cause incoordination and even seizures and death in snakes.

Hyperactivity in a snake may mistakenly be presented as a neurologic problem and may be the result of insecurity (inadequate hiding places), too high an environmental temperature, thirst or hunger, crowding, or mate-seeking behavior, or it may be a normally very active species. Although these appear to be neurologic disorders, the symptoms are not neural in origin.

Central nervous system tumors are quite rare but can cause lessened activity, incoordination, convulsions, anorexia, and even death.

Hepatic encephalopathy can be associated with lethargy, inappetence, ataxia, and weakness and more rarely with opisthotonus.

Head tilts are uncommonly seen in snakes but can be the result of head trauma, metabolic disease, a unilateral ocular disease, and even sepsis. Central origins include encephalitis, a brain tumor, or inclusion body disease. Head trauma may be the most common cause of a head tilt, such as being shut

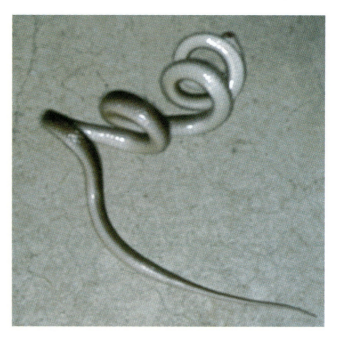

FIGURE 38-8 An adult long-term captive-bred African House Snake (*Lamprophis fuliginosus*) shows bizarre neurologic behavior. The snake crawled normally, then when stimulated, coiled into a series of loops and rolled across the substrate for 1 to 3 minutes. Afterwards, it would lie still, then if undisturbed, would uncoil and act normal. No history of trauma or toxic exposure was seen, and no lesions were found on necropsy.

in the cage door or lid, being hit with an object by a human, being run over by an automobile, falling off a branch or perch, or being dropped by the handler.

Seizures and convulsions can occur from such varied causes as septicemia, including central nervous system abscessation; encephalitis (bacterial; viral, including paramyxovirus; and inclusion body virus); parasite migration; head trauma; toxicity (including cedar, organophosphates, dichlorvos pest strips, insecticides, ivermectin overdosage, streptomycin, paint solvents); metabolic disease (hepatic encephalopathy, renal gout); and very rarely, nutritional deficiencies (thiamin, biotin, hypoglycemia). Unfortunately, many neurologic cases remain undiagnosed (Figure 38-8). See Chapter 62 for more information.

EYES

Retention of eyecaps may be caused by mites in the periorbital space, trauma to the spectacle (and perhaps to the eye as well), ocular abscessation, and husbandry issues, such as inadequate humidity or lack of cage furniture for proper shedding (see Chapter 52).

An apparently bulging eye may be the result of an intraocular mass, such as an abscess or granuloma; a retrobulbar mass; subspectacular abscessation; or increased subspectacular fluid from a blockage of the lacrimal duct. An association with stomatitis or a respiratory infection must be considered (see Chapter 20).

A decrease in eye size may be the result of an infected eye that is becoming phthisical, a congenital microphthalmia, or a reduced palpebral fissure partially covering a normal-sized globe. Anophthalmia may be seen as a congenital abnormality either unilaterally or bilaterally.

Cloudy eyes may be normal and indicative of an impending shed. Or they may be the result of a retained eyecap, injured eyecap, missing spectacle with corneal edema and exposure keratopathy, subspectacular abscess, inflammation of the subspectacular space or cornea, panophthalmitis, or a penetrating wound from a bite or a foreign object. The presence of a subspectacular abscess may make evaluation of the globe underneath impossible.

Cataracts have rarely been seen in snakes but are known in some older animals (the author's 28-year-old Corn Snake has bilateral cataracts) and as a sequela to brumation temperatures that were too cold.

REPRODUCTIVE SIGNS

Infertility is difficult to document. The failure of a snake to breed or be bred necessitates an examination to ascertain that the snake's sexual identity has been accurately determined. If the snake was inadequately nourished or improperly cycled, it may not breed. If the keeper places snakes together during the breeding season but is not present to observe them continuously, whether or not courtship and mating took place may be unknown. If copulation did not occur, infertility may not be the problem. The author once examined a Short-tailed Python (*Python curtus*) that seemingly bred two females, both of which laid infertile eggs; this male had no hemipenes (sex confirmed with endoscopic examination of the testes). A large female Burmese Python that was mated in successive seasons with three adult males always produced a clutch of eggs only about half of which were fertile, as if a problem may have existed with sperm transport or storage in one oviduct.

An infection or blockage of the female reproductive tract could lead to a failure to produce offspring. The author has seen several snakes that had retained one ovum from a prior season and that fed and then bred the next season without producing a clutch. A failure to oviposit may be from a female never actually cycling or breeding or, again, by her not actually being a female.

A dystocia, in which a gravid female does not deliver her brood or clutch or retains part of it, can be the result of a number of factors including: obesity in the female; improper plane of nutrition in the female before breeding; the female's first clutch; "power-feeding" for fast growth but marginal size to carry and deliver a normal clutch; improper gestation temperatures or no thermal gradient; inactivity of the female (restricted cage size); lack of security for the gravid female; lack of a suitable oviposition or birthing site; uterine infection; death of a conceptus; or a prolapse of the oviduct during delivery. Medical and surgical treatments for dystocia are addressed in Chapter 53.

Occasionally a female snake cycles, with palpable follicles present, but she does not produce a clutch and resorbs the unshelled follicles. Shelled follicles, eggs, must be removed if the female cannot pass them.

Birth of stillborn young may be the result of early fetal death or almost any of those factors that contribute to a dystocia. Large livebearing snakes kept confined to relatively tiny cages may have a normal delivery but accidentally crush some neonates because of a lack of cage floor space.

A prolapse at the cloacal opening must be carefully evaluated to ascertain whether it is the cloaca, the oviduct (in a female), or the hemipenis (of a male). The oviduct may prolapse with a retained egg in it. Surgical treatments for prolapses are covered in Chapters 35 and 47.

BEHAVIORAL CHANGES

An increase in a snake's activity can be related to a variety of causes including: the snake being kept too warm; insufficient hiding places for the snake; the snake getting ready to shed within a few hours; mate-seeking behavior; a gravid snake seeking a laying or birthing site; hunger; thirst; mites; an improper substrate (such as no branches for an arboreal species, or nothing into which a fossorial snake can burrow); odors in the room, such as rodents, cats, or incense; or an improper photoperiod (lights are on 24 hours or on an irregular variable cycle).

By contrast, a snake that has become lethargic may be ill, or may be gravid, or digesting food, being kept too cool, or getting ready to shed.

A snake that is spending increasing amounts of time in its water bowl may be too dry, may be nearing shedding, may be too hot, or may have mites.

A snake may spend more time in the warmer end of its cage if the ambient temperature has dropped, if it is gravid, if it is digesting food, or if it is ill.

Some snakes may exhibit unusual defensive postures that must be differentiated from disease conditions (e.g., death-feigning in Hognosed Snakes [see Figure 13-2] and inflated throats in some colubrids [see Chapter 13]).

LUMPS AND BUMPS

"Lumps and bumps," or masses, in snakes are usually abscesses until proven otherwise. But granulomas and tumors cause lumps also. Blisters or vesicles on the skin form from integumentary infections and may (or may not) progress to small abscesses; causes can include too high humidity or too much moisture in the cage, a fecal-contaminated cage (filthy cage syndrome), prey bites, parasitism, and thermal burns. Rib fractures can present as small lumps, as can osteomyelitis and congenital skeletal deformities. Cardiomegaly, internal abscesses and granulomas, tumors, and organomegaly can cause the appearance of an internal mass or lump. Fecal impactions or retained uroliths can present as caudal abdominal masses. Some snakes nearing shedding may hold feces and urates and pass these at the time of shedding. Multiple intraabdominal masses could be the result of a normally cycling female, or gravid female with follicles or concepti, or a dystocia. Impacted or abscessed anal glands, or hemipenes in a male, may cause tail base masses.

WEIGHT LOSS

Weight loss most often occurs if the snake is not eating or is not being fed enough food (lack of calories). If the snake is growing, it may need more food now than previously. A constrictor may start feeding on pinky or fuzzy mice, progress to adult mice, then rats, and then rabbits or larger prey as it grows.

Some species take amphibians or lizards as neonates, then shift to rodents as they mature. Acute weight loss in a female may be the result of just having delivered her brood or clutch.

Systemic illness may lead to weight loss through inappetence (review various previous sections, such as anorexia). But poor husbandry conditions are most likely to be involved and need to be reviewed before other causes for the weight loss.

Cachexia (appearance of general ill health and malnutrition) can result from neoplasia even in the face of an apparently normal appetite. Unthriftiness and weight loss mandates a complete and thorough physical examination and laboratory evaluation.

SUGGESTED READING

Bechtel HB: *Reptile and amphibian variants—colors, patterns, and scales*, Malabar, Fla, 1995, Krieger Publishing.

Girling SJ, Raiti P, editors: *BSAVA manual of reptiles*, ed 2, Gloucestershire, Great Britain, 2004, British Small Animal Vet Association.

Cooper JE, Jackson OF, editors: *Diseases of the Reptilia*, vol 2, San Diego, 1981, Academic Press.

Cunningham B: *Axial bifurcation in serpents: an historical survey of serpent monsters having part of the axial skeleton duplicated*, Durham, NC, 1937, Duke University Press.

Frye FL: *Biomedical and surgical aspects of captive reptile husbandry*, Melbourne, Fla, 1991, Krieger Publishing.

Hoff GL, Frye FL, Jacobson ER, editors: *Diseases of amphibians and reptiles*, New York, 1984, Plenum Press.

Jacobson ER: Snakes, *Vet Clin North Am Small Anim Pract* 23: 1179, 1993.

Marcus LC: *Veterinary biology and medicine of captive amphibians and reptiles*, Philadelphia, 1981, Lea & Febiger.

Wozniak EJ, DeNardo D, Burridge MJ, Walker DH, Funk RS: Roundtable: ectoparasites, *J Herpetol Med Surg* 10(3+4):15-21, 2000.

39
LIZARDS

STEPHEN L. BARTEN

MUSCULOSKELETAL SIGNS

Lameness, Skeletal, and Spinal Abnormalities

Metabolic bone diseases (MBDs), of various origins, are the most common causes of lameness, skeletal, and spinal abnormalities in lizard patients. MBDs can manifest with a range of pathology, including fibrous osteodystrophy, osteomalacia, osteoporosis, osteopetrosis, pathologic fractures, and more (see Chapter 61). Swollen or misshapen mandibles, limbs, or vertebral column are common, and lesions may be symmetric or asymmetric. Other causes of lameness include fractures or soft tissue injuries from trauma, bites from cage mates, neoplasia, and cellulitis and abscesses (Figure 39-1). Joint abnormalities may result in lameness. The affected joints often are swollen and have a limited range of motion. Joint problems may be caused by septic arthritis or degenerative joint disease related to trauma or aging. Articular and periarticular gout and pseudogout have been reported in the Green Iguana (*Iguana iguana*) and Egyptian Spiny-tailed Lizard (*Uromastyx* sp.), respectively.[1,2] Gout consists of radiolucent uric acid deposits in the joints. Pseudogout consists of radiopaque calcium deposits.[2,3] (See Chapter 54 for more information.)

Ossifying spondylosis related to age, osteomyelitis, or metabolic abnormalities can cause a lizard's spine and tail to be stiff and unyielding, resulting in an altered gait.

Hypertrophic osteopathy that results in profound periosteal proliferation of the long bones (see Figure 61-15) has been reported in two Green Iguanas (*Iguana iguana*) with coelomic abscesses and renal gout.[4,5]

Tail

Most iguanid lizards undergo tail autotomy, or loss of the tail, as a defensive strategy. When a predator grabs the tail, it breaks off and wiggles violently for a few minutes. Each caudal vertebra has a cartilaginous fracture plane through the vertebral body and neural arch. Fracture planes are absent in the cranial part of the tail to protect the hemipenes and fat deposits. In iguanas, the fracture planes are replaced by bone as the lizards grow, so the tail breaks off less easily in adults. The lost tail is regenerated with a cartilaginous rod for support and is covered with smaller darker scales in an irregular pattern compared with the original tail. Tail autotomy generally does not occur in agamid lizards, monitors, or true chameleons, and these species do not regenerate tails that are lost from trauma or amputation.

In cases of autotomy, if the tail does not break off cleanly, the regenerated tail can be deformed, resulting in a forked tail or a blunt knob.

Avascular necrosis of the tail is relatively common in Green Iguanas (*Iguana iguana*) and is occasionally seen in other species. The distal tail becomes hard, dry, stiff, and discolored. A zone of devitalized tissue characterized by swelling, erythema, and occasional serous discharge often exists between necrotic and healthy tissue. More than one etiology can cause this symptom. When the symptom occurs within 2 weeks of venipuncture of the ventral caudal vein, iatrogenic vascular damage may be a factor.[6] Likewise, trauma and hematogenous routes of infection can be involved.

Swelling of the ventral tail base, adjacent and caudal to the cloacal opening, in male lizards usually involves the hemipenes. Some male lizards such as Green Iguanas (*Iguana iguana*) and various species of chameleons undergo dramatic enlargement of the hemipenes with sexual maturity. Naive keepers occasionally present young adult male lizards to have these normal but newly enlarged hemipenes evaluated.

Swelling of the ventral tail base is also caused by seminal plugs. These consist of caseous debris that collects within the inverted hemipenes and most often are bilateral and symmetrical. The brown dry tips of the seminal plugs can be seen protruding from the opening of each hemipenis in the caudolateral cloaca (Figure 39-2). Seminal plugs have been suggested to consist of dried semen and desquamated epithelial cells and to occur most often during the breeding season.[7] Seminal plugs have been associated with iatrogenic hypovitaminosis A in chameleons.[8]

Deformities

Axial bifurcation, or conjoined (incomplete) twinning, has occasionally been reported in embryonic or neonate lizards,

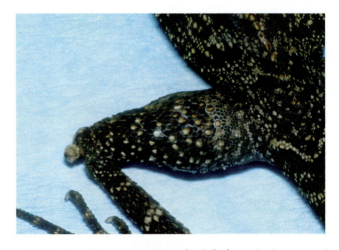

FIGURE 39-1 Fibrous osteodystrophy (which results from any of several different metabolic bone diseases) is the most common cause of swollen limbs in reptile patients. However, the swelling in the thigh of this Horn-headed Lizard (*Acanthosaurus crucigera*) was caused by cellulitis associated with osteomyelitis of the femur. The bone exhibited marked lysis on radiography.

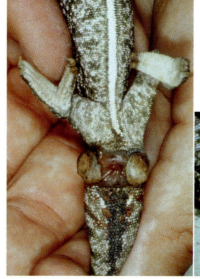
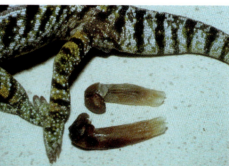

FIGURE 39-2 **A,** A ventral view of the cloacal region in a male chameleon (*Chamaeleo* sp.) shows bilateral seminal plugs. The base of tail is swollen, and the dried tips of the plugs protrude from the hemipenal openings in the caudolateral cloaca. **B,** Seminal plugs after removal in the same lizard.

including the Slow Worm (*Anguis fragilis*), the Sand Lizard (*Lacerta agilis*),[9] and the Blue-tongued Skink (*Tiliqua scincoides*) (Figure 39-3).[2] Congenital malformations of the head may include foreshortening of the upper jaw, cleft palate, and microphthalmia. Short, absent, or kinked tails may also be seen.[9]

Kyphosis and scoliosis of the spine is occasionally seen in Green Iguanas and other lizards. This condition can result from genetic defects, malnutrition, and pathology of the epaxial muscles. In a Green Iguana, disease of the epaxial muscles can be caused by overheating from a heat lamp.[2] Multiple cartilaginous exostoses have been reported in monitor lizards.[2]

Congenital defects may be a result of genetic defects or improper environmental conditions during incubation, primarily temperature levels that are too high or too low for some or all of the incubation. Gravid ovoviviparous or viviparous females subjected to improper temperatures might also produce dead or deformed young. Defects that appear later in life may be genetic or the result of external factors including infection, trauma, neoplasia, and malnutrition (see Chapter 22 for more information).

INTEGUMENT

Dermatitis, Abrasions, Ulcerations, and Open Sores

Rostral abrasions are common in active lizards such as Water Dragons (*Physignathus* spp.) and Basilisks (*Basiliscus* spp.) and result from repeated trauma with glass cage walls during flight responses to stimuli. Rostral abrasions also occur from escape attempts in lizards kept in undersized cages or cages with rough screen wire surfaces. Abrasions on the palmar and plantar surfaces of the feet also occur in lizards kept in cages with rough or wire surfaces. Bite wounds from cage mates or live rodent prey or other trauma may result in defects in the skin. Thermal burns result from direct contact with a heat source or fire and usually involve the ventral or dorsal surface. Chemical burns result from contact with cage disinfectants, such as sodium hypochlorite that has not been

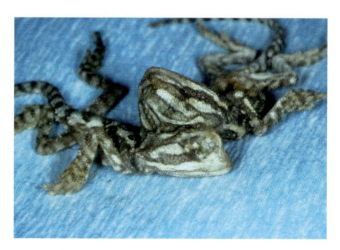

FIGURE 39-3 Conjoined twin Bearded Dragons (*Pogona brevis*). Fully formed but dead twins, joined at the crown of the head, were discovered when the egg was opened after it failed to hatch with the other eggs in the same clutch.

rinsed away adequately. A thorough patient history reveals the cause of the lesion in these cases.

Dermatitis may be ulcerative or necrotizing and result from gram-negative, gram-positive, or anaerobic bacteria and from various fungi and algae (Figure 39-4).[1,2,10,11] Dermatitis may also result from mites (*Ophionyssus* and *Hirstiella*) (Figure 39-5).

Myiasis may cause one or more open holes in the skin, and the fly larvae are usually visible moving within the hole (see Chapter 15).

Crusts, Scabs, Flakes, and Dysecdysis

Crusts and scabs may be seen as a result of bacterial dermatitis or burns. Flakes of skin may represent normal shedding. Most lizards shed in pieces, but in some species (e.g., geckos), the old skin comes off in one piece. In addition, some lizards eat their shed skin. Dysecdysis, or difficult shedding, may result in dry, flaking adherent patches of dead skin. The most common cause of dysecdysis is a lack of humidity. Retained skin surrounding the digits, dorsal spines, or tail tips shrinks

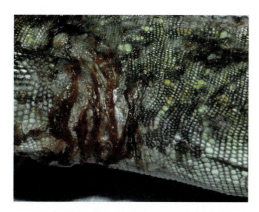

FIGURE 39-4 Generalized moist dermatitis in a Sailfin Lizard (*Hydrosaurus pustulatus*) characterized by inflammation, ulceration, crusts, and foul odor. Numerous yeasts were found on impression smears, and the lizard responded to topical and systemic antifungal drugs.

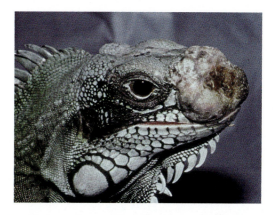

FIGURE 39-6 Most lumps and bumps in reptiles are abscesses. Chronic ones can become quite large, like this rostral abscess in a Green Iguana (*Iguana iguana*).

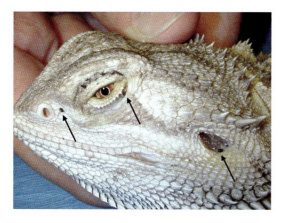

FIGURE 39-5 Snake mites (*Ophionyssus natricis*) infesting a Bearded Dragon (*Pogona vitticeps*). The lizard was housed in a cage that formerly held a Ball Python (*Python regius*) infested with mites.

as it dries, which compromises the blood flow. This results in necrosis and sloughing of the affected part.

Dysecdysis has been associated with iatrogenic hypovitaminosis A in chameleons.[8]

Recently imported Green Iguanas may have widespread focal black raised lesions 1 to 5 mm in diameter that cover the entire surface and resemble a multitude of tiny scabs. The etiology has been reported to be *Geotrichum candidum*,[12] but this is an ubiquitous fungal organism that may be acting as an opportunist in newly imported, overcrowded, stressed, and immunocompromised specimens (see Chapters 16 and 52).

Swellings, Nodules, and Blisters

Most lumps and bumps in reptiles are caused by abscesses, which usually manifest as encapsulated inspissated pockets of caseous debris. Rarely, reptile abscesses contain mucoid or liquid discharge instead. Abscesses often are subcutaneous (Figure 39–6), but they may occur within the coelomic cavity or middle ear or under the ocular spectacle. Abscesses usually occur after bacteria, including anaerobes, or fungi enter through a penetrating wound. Cellulitis often precedes the formation of a pocket of debris (see Chapter 42).

Dermatophilosis has been reported in a number of lizards and results in nodular hyperkeratosis and subcutaneous abscessation.[2,10] This disease is diagnosed with culture or histopathology and has zoonotic potential.

Cryptococcus neoformans was isolated from a subcutaneous mass in a skink.[11]

The protozoan *Trichomonas* sp. caused subcutaneous abscesses in a Leopard Gecko (*Eublepharis macularius*).[13]

Fluid-filled blisters commonly result from conditions of excessive humidity or thermal burns. Cytology should always be done to differentiate between sterile and septic blisters regardless of cause.

Sebaceous cysts have been reported in lizards, primarily in the tails of Green Iguanas. These resemble dry abscesses.[2]

A variety of neoplasms has been reported in lizards, and these may result in dermal, subcutaneous, oral, or coelomic masses. Viral papillomas have been reported in European Green Lizards (*Lacerta viridis*).[10]

Subcutaneous nematodes and filarid parasites may cause subcutaneous masses. These are especially common in chameleons.[14]

Various MBDs and arthritis may cause swelling of the affected limbs and joints (see Lameness). Edema causes swelling of the limbs, pharynx, or coelom (see Distended Coelom).

Cases of pseudoaneurysm or dissecting aneurysm have been observed in the dorsolateral cervical region of captive Bearded Dragons (*Pogona vitticeps*). The condition, seen to date only in adult lizards, presents with a large fluctuant to firm swelling up to 5 cm in diameter on the dorsolateral neck just caudal to the skull (Figure 39-7). Affected animals behave normally and continue to eat unless the aneurysm becomes so large as to interfere with prehension and mastication. Attempts to aspirate the fluid-filled mass generally yield several mL of whole blood. After fluid evacuation, the mass immediately refills with blood, indicating communication with a large or high-pressure blood vessel.

In more chronic cases, the contents of the lesion coagulate and cannot be aspirated. In two cases that were investigated with MR and CT imaging and anatomical dissection respectively, the aneurysm or pseudoaneurysm arose from the internal carotid artery near where it branched off the aorta or from the aorta itself (Wyneken J, personal communication). The aneurysm in the first case was surgically repaired.

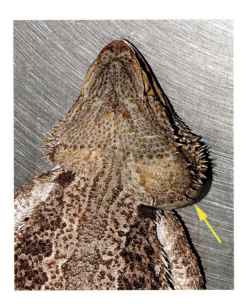

FIGURE 39-7 The yellow arrow points to a large fluid-filled mass on the dorsolateral cervical region of this adult Bearded Dragon (*Pogona vitticeps*). The lesion turned out to be an aneurysm arising from the internal carotid artery.

Intraoperative blood loss required a transfusion from a donor Bearded Dragon (Mader D, personal communication). This patient was still alive and well with no recurrence of the aneurysm 1 year after surgery. In a second case, the affected lizard lived 8 months without treatment, then died acutely.

The etiology of this syndrome is unknown. These vessels are somewhat exposed in the dorsolateral pharynx as they course over the ventral aspect of the neck and skull and might be exposed to trauma or tension. Hypertension cannot be ruled out.

Abnormalities in Color and Color Change

Abnormalities in color commonly occur in reptiles and are often selected for in captive breeding programs. Red, yellow, and white skin pigments are present in addition to melanin. Albinism involving one or more of these pigments produces varying color patterns. Amelanosis, hypomelanosis, anerythrism, and melanosis may be seen. The latter is common in the Mexican Beaded Lizard (*Heloderma horridum*). Pattern abnormalities are more common in snakes than in lizards but may include lack of pattern in normally patterned individuals or stripes where spots or bars should be present or vice versa. Ontogenetic pattern changes occur in some lizards, for example, the Leopard Gecko (*Eublepharis macularius*). In this species, the young are banded but become spotted as they mature.

Rapid color change is highly developed in a number of lizards but most notably among the chameleons (*Chamaeleo* spp.) and anoles (*Anolis* spp.). Control of the chromatophores may be hormonal or neurologic or both.[10] Male chameleons confronted with conspecific males or even their own mirror image quickly assume bright "threat" colors as they attack their rival. Chromatophores may react to stimulation from light or changes in temperature; lizards that are cold or in bright sunlight often become noticeably darker. Age, gender, and season may influence color change. Some male Green Iguanas have a pronounced orange hue develop during the breeding season as a normal condition, but this must be differentiated from the orange discoloration that is occasionally seen with systemic illness. The Ground Iguana (*Cyclura nubila lewisii*) often takes on a bluish tint as it matures. Lizards with systemic disease or malnutrition often become duller or darker than normal in color. Lizards about to shed their skin also appear dull.

Mite infestation may result in color changes. Prostigmatid mites such as *Hirstiella trombidiiformis*, which infests lizards in the deserts of southwestern North America, are red in color. In the lizard, groups of mites appear as focal red patches caudal to the ear opening and in the skin folds adjacent to the limbs. In Green Iguanas, slightly raised, well-demarcated patches of black discoloration often accompany red mite infestations. These lesions are usually confined to the ventral abdomen and the limbs (see Chapter 43).

Scars

Scars from wounds, burns, and other trauma initially are white to pale pink and smooth and lack scales. With each successive shed, the scaleless area becomes smaller as new scales are produced around the periphery of the lesion. The scar does not change appreciably in appearance between sheds but is noticeably smaller immediately after a shed. Once the scarred area is completely filled in, the new scales may be noted to be smaller and darker than the original scales. Also, they usually are arranged haphazardly rather than in neat even rows (see Chapter 71).

ORAL CAVITY

Petechiae

Petechiae are uncommon in lizards. Causes include trauma associated with rostral abrasions, running into cage walls during escape attempts, and the forceful use of oral speculums. Focal, early stomatitis can result in petechiae, but this also is rare in lizards. Coagulation disorders are poorly documented in reptiles, but these could result in petechiae. Disseminated intravascular coagulation has been reported in an iguana with hyperthermia in a locked automobile.[2] Coagulopathy might also result from the ingestion of warfarin-type rodenticides or prey animals that had ingested rodenticides.

Stomatitis, Ulcerations, and Exudates

Stomatitis, which should never be referred to by the archaic and unprofessional term "mouth rot," is common in snakes and chelonians but rare in lizards. It usually occurs as a result of poor husbandry conditions, including suboptimal temperatures, malnutrition, and overcrowding. Stomatitis may be caused by a variety of bacteria, viruses, or fungi. Inflammation, ulceration, abscessation, and caseous deposits often develop. Pneumonia and septicemia are often present in association with stomatitis.

Exposure gingivitis often is mistaken for stomatitis. Lizards that have or have had MBD commonly have deformed mandibles and maxillae, resulting in the exposure of gingival tissue. This condition also is seen in cases with traumatic defects in the lips. The affected gingiva produces a dry reddish-brown scab-like material. This condition does not respond to antibiotic therapy. The exposed gingiva should be kept moist with petrolatum jelly, and the discharge periodically removed.

Oral neoplasia has been seen in lizards and may appear as an ulcerated mass. Chemical or thermal burns, in theory, could result in oral ulcerations. Lizards with renal failure do not typically have oral ulcers develop. Visceral gout can result in inflammation of the oral cavity.

Oral exudates usually result from inflammation of the oral cavity, respiratory tract, or gastrointestinal tract. Stomatitis usually involves exudation. White or mucoid foam may be coughed up in cases of pneumonia. Less commonly, stomach contents may be regurgitated and be present in the oral cavity in cases of gastritis or gastrointestinal obstruction. Septicemia is often present in cases of stomatitis, pneumonia, and gastroenteritis. Inflammation of any tissues is caused by bacterial, viral, fungal, and parasitic agents. Appropriate diagnostic sampling is necessary to differentiate the causative agent.

Chameleons (*Chamaeleo* spp.) have temporal glands dorsolateral to the corners of their mouths that sometimes become infected and distended with caseous debris (Figure 39-8).[14] (See Chapter 72.)

Oral Discharge and Ptyalism

Excessive white foam in the oral cavity is occasionally seen in lizards and is associated with septicemia and pneumonia. Affected lizards are usually moribund. Improper husbandry techniques, such as chilling, malnutrition, lack of parasite control, and overcrowding, are often part of the history.

Pharyngeal Edema

Pharyngeal edema has been associated with renal disease in Green Iguanas. Some chameleon species have an accessory lung lobe attached to the trachea in the ventral neck. Swelling in this area can be caused by infection and cellulitis of this structure.

Mucous Membrane Color

Adult Bearded Dragons and many chameleons have yellow-orange mucous membranes that resemble icterus as a normal condition. Many lizards, including various species of chameleons, geckos, and monitors, have melanotic oral cavities (Figure 39-9). These can vary from jet black to dark purple in color, and the latter must be differentiated from cyanosis.

Icterus may be prehepatic or hepatic and result in jaundiced mucous membranes.[2] Cyanosis may result from respiratory or cardiac compromise but is rare in reptiles. Erythema and congested mucous membranes may be seen in stomatitis.

Reptile mucous membranes are normally pale pink to white in color and are significantly more pale than those of a typical mammal because normal packed cell volumes of reptiles are significantly lower than those of mammals.

Tongue

Chameleons (*Chamaeleo* spp.) and monitors (*Varanus* spp.) have long protrusible tongues that retract inside a sheath rostral to

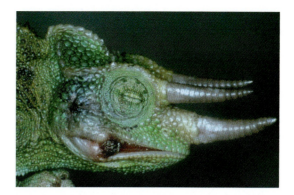

FIGURE 39-8 Abscessation of the temporal gland dorsolateral to the corner of the mouth in a Jackson's Chameleon (*Chamaeleo jacksonii*).

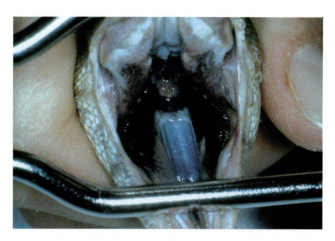

FIGURE 39-9 Mucous membranes in the oral cavity of a subadult Savannah Monitor (*Varanus exanthematicus*). Melanin (dark) pigment is normal and should not be mistaken for disease.

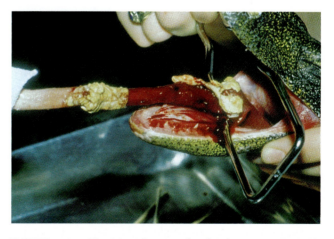

FIGURE 39-10 Glossitis and tongue sheath infection in a Crocodile Monitor (*Varanus salvadorii*). The tongue was adhered to the sheath and could not be protruded. Here adhesions are broken down with sedation. Severe inflammation and copious caseous debris are seen.

the glottis when not in use. Bacterial infection sometimes develops within that sheath.[14] Symptoms include inflammation, discharge, and an inability to protrude the tongue because of adhesions between the tongue and sheath (Figure 39-10).

In chameleons, hypocalcemia commonly results from malnutrition, lack of ultraviolet B light, or renal disease. One of the first symptoms of hypocalcemia in this group is poor muscle tone manifested as flaccid paralysis of the tongue. The affected chameleons either cannot shoot their tongue at prey in a normal fashion or, if they do, are unable to retract it so that it hangs from their mouth.

The tip of the tongue in the Green Iguana is darker than the rest of the tongue, which may be mistaken for glossitis.

Dental Disease

The teeth of lizards are generally pleurodont (attached to the sides of the mandible without sockets), but in some families, the Agamidae and Chamaeleontidae, they are acrodont (attached to the biting edges of the jaws without sockets). Pleurodont teeth are regularly shed and replaced, and dental disease in these species is rare. Acrodont teeth are not replaced except in very young specimens, although new teeth may be added to the posterior end of the tooth row as the lizard grows. Many Agamids have pleurodont teeth in the rostral portion of the dental arcade. Periodontal disease has been reported in captive acrodont lizards, including Bearded Dragons, Water Dragons (*Physignathus lesueurii*), Frilled Lizards (*Chlamydosaurus kingii*), Sailfin Lizards (*Hydrosaurus pustulatus*), and Jackson's Chameleons (*Chamaeleo jacksonii*). Symptoms include gingival erythema, gingival recession, calculus formation, and, in severe cases, osteomyelitis and abscess formation.[15]

Teeth may fracture as a result of biting or chewing on objects, such as oral speculums. Infected gingiva can result. Teeth may become loosened as a result of MBD.

GASTROINTESTINAL SIGNS

Anorexia

Anorexia is a common symptom among captive reptiles. Causes may be environmental or medical.

Environmental causes of anorexia include low temperature, low humidity, excessive handling of shy specimens, stress from overcrowding (this may be seen when only two lizards share a cage or when one lizard confronts its image in a mirror), lack of a hide box for visual security, lack of ultraviolet light sources, and presentation of inappropriate or inadequate diets (e.g., carnivorous lizards such as monitors do not accept vegetarian diets). Determination of both the environmental conditions that *have* been provided and those that *should* be provided is important.[16,17]

In a few cases anorexia is normal in lizards. Gravid females usually eat less than normal, if at all, because the developing eggs or fetuses fill a large percentage of the coelomic cavity and there simply is no room for food. Assist feeding in this instance is extremely stressful. Likewise, many male lizards become so obsessed with territoriality, fighting with rivals, and searching for a mate during their breeding season that eating takes on a low priority. Species that normally brumate (hibernate), especially wild-caught specimens, may have decreased appetites with decreasing photoperiod in the fall even when environmental temperatures are kept high.

Medical causes of anorexia are varied. One of the most common symptoms of virtually any and every disease is a decreased appetite. Anorexia is common with bacterial or viral infections, parasites, nutritional disorders, foreign body (Figure 39-11) or impaction, stomatitis and gastroenteritis. Renal disease, liver disease, metabolic disorders, neoplasia and toxemia, and so on, all result in anorexia. MBD often causes soft flexible mandibles and loosened teeth, which can preclude eating, and ileus of the gastrointestinal tract related to hypocalcemia. Tongue lesions or infection can prevent food prehension. A complete history, physical examination, and appropriate laboratory sampling are necessary to establish a diagnosis (see Chapter 44).

Vomition and Regurgitation

Lizards have a more highly developed cardiac sphincter than snakes and as a result rarely regurgitate. Lizards with regurgitation and vomition usually are in serious condition and often near death.[18] Causes include septicemia, toxemia, gastroenteritis, parasite burdens, gastrointestinal foreign bodies, and gastrointestinal obstruction caused by intussusception or constipation. Extramural causes of gastrointestinal obstruction include nephritis with renal enlargement, uroliths, the presence of eggs or fetuses, abscesses, neoplasia, and a narrowed pelvic canal from trauma or one of the MBDs. Spoiled food or inappropriate temperatures that prevent normal digestion and postprandial handling can cause regurgitation.

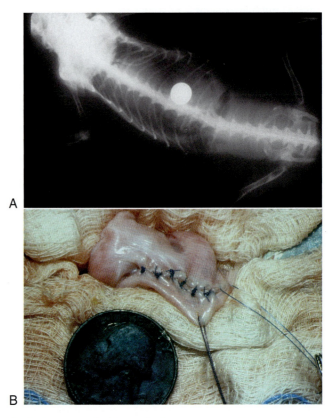

FIGURE 39-11 A, Radiograph shows an ingested coin in a Green Iguana (*Iguana iguana*) with anorexia but no vomition. **B,** Same coin after surgical removal from the stomach.

Vomition may be seen during agonal struggles in terminal cases (see Chapter 74).

Diarrhea

Environmental conditions can result in diarrhea. Low environmental temperatures can cause incomplete digestion, bacterial overgrowth, and diarrhea. Sudden changes in the diet may cause diarrhea in herbivorous lizards, especially when fruits with a high water content are offered. Likewise, lack of fiber in the diet of these lizards can contribute to the formation of loose stools. Feeding chicks, dog food, chicken parts, or other meat products to carnivorous lizards results in looser, more foul-smelling stools than when whole rodents are used.

Diarrhea is caused by a variety of infectious and parasitic agents. Enteritis results from a number of bacteria, including *Salmonella* spp. Fungal enteritis was reported in a Jackson's Chameleon (*Chamaeleo jacksonii*).[1] Viral diseases are poorly documented in lizards. Parasites that can cause diarrhea include hookworms (*Kalicephalus* sp.), ascarids, strongyles (*Rhabdias* sp. and *Strongyloides* sp.), *Entamoeba*, coccidia (*Eimeria* and *Isopora*), flagellates (*Trichomonas* sp., *Monocercomonas* sp., and others), and, less commonly, ciliates (*Nyctotherus* sp.).[1,18] Cryptosporidium is more common in snakes than in lizards, but it has been reported in Leopard Geckos and Gila Monsters.[19,20] The geckos exhibited diarrhea, anorexia, weight loss, and death (see Chapter 50).

Constipation

Lack of bowel movements has many potential causes. Associated husbandry issues include inappropriate temperatures, inappropriate or insufficient water sources, lack of activity from a too-small cage, inappropriate food items (long-haired rodent prey, hard-shelled insect prey), and ingestion of indigestible cage substrates such as gravel, rocks, sand, and bark.

Diseases that cause constipation include parasitism and dehydration. Intussusception and cloacitis can cause physical obstruction of the gastrointestinal tract. Extramural causes of gastrointestinal obstruction include nephritis with renal enlargement, uroliths, the presence of eggs or fetuses, abscesses, neoplasia, and a narrowed pelvic canal from trauma or MBD.

Prolapse from the Cloaca

Several organs can be prolapsed from the cloacal opening. These include the cloaca itself, the bladder when present, and the colon. Female reptiles can prolapse the shell gland, and males one or both hemipenes. Seminal plugs in males can be mistaken for a prolapsed organ.

A prolapse can occur as a result of anything that causes straining. The most common cause of a prolapsed cloaca in juvenile iguanas is poor muscle tone associated with hypocalcemia, a consequence of nutritional secondary hyperparathyroidism (NSHP), a metabolic bone disease of nutritional origin (NMBD). Straining may be caused by any cause of gastroenteritis, including bacterial, fungal, or parasitic enteritis, cloacitis, impactions or ingested foreign objects, intussusception, or constipation. Uroliths, bacterial cystitis, or dystocia can result in excessive straining. Extraluminal gastrointestinal blockage caused by renal enlargement, neoplasia, abscesses, or a narrowed pelvic canal from trauma or MBD all result in straining. Dyspnea can cause straining (see Chapter 47).

REPRODUCTIVE SIGNS

Infertility

Males and females may fail to produce sperm and eggs, respectively, if they are kept at inappropriate temperatures, humidity levels, or photoperiods. Many species need a period of brumation (hibernation) to mate successfully. The specific requirements of specific species must be researched because excessive cooling can result in illness. Social cues play a role, and some species require social groups or male-to-male combat, rather than just a lone male and female, to stimulate successful mating. Some individual pairs seem incompatible with each other. In some cases the keeper has misdiagnosed the gender of one or both of the mated pair. In other cases the animals are too young to breed. Localized illness, such as infection of the reproductive tract, the presence of seminal plugs, or cloacitis, can prevent breeding, as can systemic illness such as septicemia, malnutrition, or renal failure.

Stillbirths and Hatch Failure

Improper environmental conditions for the gravid female or incubating eggs commonly result in stillbirths or failure of eggs to hatch. Low or high environmental temperatures, low or high humidity levels, poor hygiene with mold or fungal contamination of the incubation media, and incubator failure are potential causes. Infection of the cloaca or oviduct, genetic abnormalities, and fetal or egg disease also may be involved.

Dystocia

The presence of eggs or fetuses does not indicate the diagnosis of dystocia. Normal gravid females have distended coelomic cavities develop and become anorectic. Green Iguanas usually refuse food for 4 weeks before they lay eggs.[21] However, they remain bright, alert, and responsive. Gravid lizards with dystocia quickly become depressed and unresponsive and without prompt treatment can die in a short time.

Nonobstructive causes of dystocia may include husbandry issues. Lack of a suitable egg-laying site is one of the most common causes. Iguanas need an enclosed egg-laying chamber, and chameleons often lay eggs in the soil of potted plants within their cage, as long as a climbing branch reaches into the pot. Cool temperatures, malnutrition, dehydration, and poor physical condition from lack of exercise can contribute to dystocia. Infection of the reproductive tract is sometimes seen, but whether this is a cause or a result of the dystocia can be unclear.

Obstructive causes of dystocia include anatomic defects that prevent the passage of eggs or young. Oversized or deformed eggs may be too big to pass through the pelvic canal. The shell gland may have a stricture or torsion. Abscesses, enlarged kidneys, neoplasia, or uroliths may compress and obstruct the oviducts. A narrowed pelvic canal caused by one of the MBDs or trauma may prevent passage of eggs. Fractured or malpositioned eggs can fail to pass.

Preovulatory egg retention occurs when a lizard undergoes vitellogenesis but not ovulation. The enlarged ova remain on the ovaries but fill the coelomic cavity and cause anorexia. In some cases they are resorbed; in others an ovariectomy is necessary (see Chapter 53).

RESPIRATORY SIGNS

Dyspnea

Dyspnea may result from upper or lower airway disease. The nostrils can become plugged with unshed skin, normal discharge from the salt excretion glands, or inflammatory discharge from rhinitis and pneumonia. Both the external and internal nares must be examined for discharge, which may be serous, mucoid, or purulent. Pneumonia may be present at the same time as rhinitis. Plugged nostrils result in open-mouth breathing.

Lower respiratory disease with respiratory embarrassment results in dyspnea as the lizard attempts to obtain more oxygen. Pneumonia is caused by a variety of aerobic and anaerobic bacteria. Viral pneumonia has been reported in snakes and chelonians but not yet in lizards.[22,23] Mycotic pneumonia has been seen in a number of reptiles, including lizards, but is often considered a secondary invader.[2,23,24] Verminous pneumonia is usually accompanied by bacterial pneumonia. *Entomelas*, a helminth similar in appearance to *Rhabdias* of snakes, is the common lungworm in lizards.[2] Pentastomes, trematodes, and migrating nematode larvae also may cause verminous pneumonia in reptiles. Among lizards, parasites are most common in chameleons and monitors. Aspiration pneumonia may be a sequela of assist feeding and the oral administration of medication by inexperienced persons. Appropriate samples must be submitted for cytology and bacterial culture.

Untreated chronic respiratory tract disease often spreads to other areas, resulting in abscess formation in the oral cavity, periorbital space, and parenchymatous coelomic organs, notably the liver. Any lesion that compromises the opening of the glottis, such as abscesses or neoplasia of the oral cavity, can cause severe dyspnea (Figure 39-12).[24]

Respiratory distress in two Green Iguanas was caused by human hair wrapped around the epiglottis and trachea. Normal respiration resumed immediately on removal of the hair, with sedation to facilitate working in the back of the oropharynx (personal observation). Other foreign objects may cause similar signs.

A drowning fatality was observed in a juvenile Green Iguana left unattended in a lukewarm bath (personal observation). Drowning and near-drowning injuries are more common in aquatic chelonians but may occur in lizards or any reptile left soaking unattended.[23]

Primary neoplasms of the respiratory tract are rare in reptiles, but metastasis to the lungs is possible.[2,25] Widespread pulmonary metastasis was noted in a Cornsnake (*Elaphe guttata*) with renal adenocarcinoma, although clinical signs were related to renal failure and renal space–occupying lesions.[26]

Pulmonary edema from cardiac or hepatic disease can result in respiratory signs. Space-occupying coelomic lesions, such as ascites or neoplasia, prevent normal lung expansion and cause dyspnea.[24]

Agonal respiration in terminal patients resembles dyspnea.

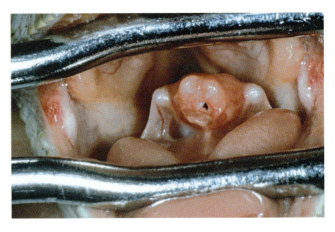

FIGURE 39-12 Idiopathic stenosis of the glottis in a Green Iguana (*Iguana iguana*). The lizard showed exertional dyspnea that resolved when the glottis was surgically enlarged. The glottis is depicted at its widest opening.

Open-mouth panting occurs in some lizards as a cooling mechanism during overheating.

Nasal Discharge

Some lizards, most notably the Green Iguana, have sodium-secreting, potassium-secreting, and chloride-secreting nasal salt glands. These allow the lizard to excrete excess salts without losing significant amounts of water. This results in a clear nasal discharge that dries to a fine white powder, which may be observed around the nares or on the sides of the cage.[2,16]

Sinusitis and rhinitis can produce nasal discharge as well. This material varies from clear with bubbles to thick and mucoid. Because of the position of the internal nares anterior in the oropharynx, stomatitis and pneumonia might also result in nasal discharge. Thorough physical examination helps differentiate between the two groups.

Epistaxis and hemoptysis most commonly occur from metastatic mineralization in Green Iguanas. Iatrogenic hypervitaminosis D and idiopathic causes are associated with marked hypercalcemia. The resulting mineral deposits commonly occur in the smooth muscle of blood vessels, making them abnormally rigid and prone to fracture with minor trauma such as a short fall or vigorous restraint. When a mineralized vessel in the lungs fractures, marked epistaxis and hemoptysis result, often with fatal results. Metastatic mineralization is easily shown on radiographs. Other causes of epistaxis are rare in lizards but might include necrotizing rhinitis and sinusitis caused by bacteria, mycoplasma, or fungi, acquired coagulopathy from septicemia, nutritional deficiency or liver insufficiency, rodenticide toxicity, neoplasia, and foreign bodies.

Causes of discharges in the oropharynx are discussed under Stomatitis, Ulcerations, and Exudates and under Oral Discharge and Ptyalism (see Chapters 65, 67, and 73).

Abnormal Vocalizations

Respiratory sounds may result from any fluids within the respiratory tract as a result of pneumonia, aspiration, or near-drowning. These must be differentiated from hissing and snorting as a defensive gesture in response to a perceived threat. Conversely, a lack of sound might be noted in a fully consolidated lung.

EYES

Palpebral and Spectacle Abnormalities

Reversible, temporary, bilateral periorbital swelling is occasionally seen when a Green Iguana is restrained behind the head and struggles violently. Venous sinuses capable of engorgement exist in this area, presumably to help loosen dead skin during periods of ecdysis, because the skin of the head is tightly adhered to the skull. More permanent venous congestion occurs with systemic and localized infection.

Subcutaneous cellulitis and abscesses are common around the eye and usually result from penetrating wounds or hematogenous sources. These cause asymmetrical swelling and are most common on the ocular turrets of chameleons (Figure 39-13).

Trauma to the palpebrae can result from escape attempts in unsturdy cages, fights with cage mates, and burns from heat lamps. Blepharoplasty to repair severe burn damage in a Green Iguana has been reported.[2]

In species with a spectacle, distention of the subspectacular space with clear lacrimal fluid results when the nasolacrimal duct is occluded. Nasolacrimal occlusion can result from infection, pressure, fibrosis, or congenital malformation.[27,28] The subspectacular space also can become distended with caseous debris from bacterial infection ascending up the nasolacrimal duct or spreading hematogenously.[28] The protozoan *Trichomonas* sp. caused subspectacular abscesses in geckoes.[13] Panophthalmitis must be differentiated from subspectacular abscessation. In the latter condition, the entire globe swells as the interior structures are destroyed by infection originating from wounds or hematogenous spread.[2]

Blepharospasm may result from foreign bodies in the eye, such as sand and other particulate bedding materials. Corneal ulcers also cause blepharospasm and may result from foreign bodies, trauma, or infection with bacteria or viruses.

Eye problems have been associated with iatrogenic hypovitaminosis A in chameleons.[8]

Mites and ticks are commonly found in the ocular adnexa.

Viral papillomas have been reported around the eyes in Green Lizards (*Lacerta* sp.).[27] (See Chapter 20.)

Corneal Abnormalities

Keratitis occurs in reptiles as a result of bacterial or fungal infection. Corneal ulcers may result from trauma, foreign bodies, or infection.

In those species with spectacles, exposure keratitis results from iatrogenic avulsion of the spectacle from improper treatment, perhaps related to misdiagnosis, of retained spectacles.

Leopard Geckos (*Eublepharis macularius*) occasionally have a plug of caseous debris covering the cornea develop. Bacterial conjunctivitis and foreign objects such as sand substrate may result in this presentation. The plug can usually be removed in a single piece with flushing and gentle manipulation. Because the inner surface conforms to the round surface of the cornea, the plug is commonly mistaken for a retained

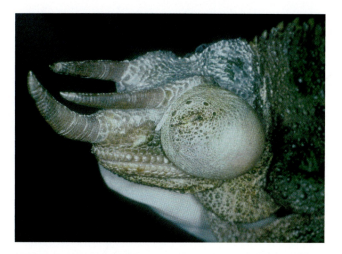

FIGURE 39-13 An abscess involving the ocular turret in a Jackson's Chameleon *(Chamaeleo jacksonii).*

spectacle, but of course this species ("*Eublepharis*" means "true eyelids") lacks a spectacle.

Arcus lipoides corneae is a white band of material that may partially or completely surround the cornea near the limbus. This condition is associated with aging and requires no treatment. It has been observed in monitor lizards (*Varanus* sp.).[2]

Lens Abnormalities

Juvenile cataracts with a postulated genetic etiology have been reported in monitor lizards.[2] Senile cataracts may occur in adult animals. Cataracts in brumating (hibernating) reptiles may sometimes be associated with damage from freezing.[27]

NERVOUS SYSTEM AND BEHAVIORS

Convulsions, Twitching, Coma, Ataxia, and Head Tilts

Neurologic symptoms in reptiles usually overlap (see Chapters 20 and 62). A condition that causes ataxia frequently progresses through muscle weakness, twitching, convulsions, coma, and death. Muscle fasciculations, tetany, and convulsions sometimes are difficult to separate. Head tilts occasionally accompany other neurologic signs (Figure 39-14).

One of the most common pathologic conditions in captive lizards is hypocalcemia. The hypocalcemia results from unbalanced diets, lack of ultraviolet light sources, and inadequate environmental temperatures. Chronic NMBD cases may develop hypocalcemia with symptoms of tetany, muscle fasciculations, and eventually coma and death.[2,16,29]

Another dietary cause of neurologic symptoms is vitamin B complex deficiencies. This condition may be seen in carnivorous reptiles that are fed large amounts of frozen fish or in herbivorous lizards fed large amounts of frozen vegetables. Freezing decreases vitamin levels and increases thiaminase activity, resulting in thiamine (B_1) deficiency. Biotin deficiency has been reported in monitors (*Varanus* spp.) fed raw eggs, which contain avidin, a substance with antibiotic activity.[2,29] Symptoms vary with severity but range from weakness and

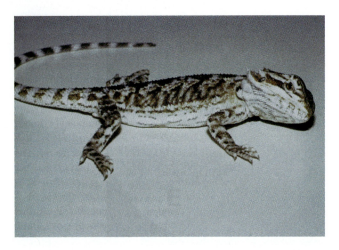

FIGURE 39-14 Idiopathic head tilt in a Bearded Dragon (*Pogona vitticeps*).

incoordination, through twitching and torticollis, and finally to convulsions and death. The diagnosis is confirmed with response to supplementation with B complex vitamins or histopathology.

Vitamin E and selenium deficiencies are occasionally seen in herbivorous lizards with symptoms of muscle weakness, fasciculations, and convulsions. This condition is diagnosed with clinical improvement after the injection of vitamin E and selenium or muscle biopsy.[2,16]

Dehydration and renal pathology can result in gout, causing incoordination and convulsions.[29] Hypoglycemia may result in convulsions, but this condition is rare in reptiles. A heavy parasite burden can result in weakness, lethargy, coma, and death.

Lizards with septicemia may have brain abscesses and neurologic symptoms develop, including convulsions. Viral encephalitis caused by retro-like virus in boid snakes results in disorientation, head tilt, opisthotonos, flaccid paralysis, and death.[22] Similar viruses have not yet been documented in lizards. A chameleon with esophagitis associated with adeno-like virus showed neurologic signs.[30] Acanthamoeba have been isolated from the brain of an iguana with brain lesions.[2] Tumors involving the central nervous system of reptiles are extremely rare.[2,25]

Neurologic lesions may result from physical trauma, such as a blow to the head or damage from freezing.[29]

Toxicity from a variety of substances may result in convulsions. Possible toxins include insecticides, pharmaceuticals such as metronidazole, ivermectin, and aminoglycoside antibiotics, bufotoxins from consumption of a toad of the genus *Bufo*, and various chemicals such as paint solvents.[29] Cedar wood shavings contain aromatic resins, and when used as bedding, these can cause neurologic symptoms in small specimens.[31] Nicotine salts on smokers' fingers also can prove toxic to small reptiles.[29] Toxic plants are occasionally ingested by herbivorous species, the symptoms of which vary with the species of plant. Convulsions, coma, and death followed the consumption of azalea by two Green Iguanas (personal observation). Reptiles also can show alcohol intoxication after the consumption of rotting overripe fruit.[2]

Head tilts are rarely seen in lizards. These may be the result of a lesion in the vestibular system, but documentation of these lesions has not been found.

Paralysis and Paresis

By far the most common cause of paralysis or paresis is spinal cord lesions from the collapse of one or more vertebrae as a sequela to one of the MBDs. Depending on the site of the lesion, paraplegia or quadriplegia may be present. The onset usually is sudden, and a history of trauma may or may not be present. If the lizard is able to defecate and urinate, the prognosis is fair; if not, the prognosis for recovery is poor. These signs must be differentiated from, but may accompany, muscle weakness, twitching, and fasciculations (see Nervous System). Other causes of paralysis and paresis are rare but include spinal cord lesions from trauma such as vertebral fractures, spinal abscesses, and neoplasia.

Behavior Changes

Aggression

Aggression is sometimes divided into offensive and defensive aggression. The former involves unprovoked attacks, and the latter is in response to a real or perceived threat or the defense of territory. Some species of lizards are naturally aggressive and pugnacious, for example, monitor lizards, Tegus (*Tupinambis* spp.), and the Veiled Chameleon (*Chamaeleo calyptratus*). Acquired aggression can coincide with sexual maturation, the onset of breeding season (especially in male Green Iguanas), stimulation by the presence of conspecifics or mirror images, exposure to unfiltered sunlight (especially in monitor lizards and Gila Monsters [*Heloderma* sp.]), and display of throat fans, beards, and dewlaps.[2]

Reproduction

Gravid females often exhibit behavior changes before egg laying that may be mistaken for disease. They often become anorectic and lethargic with distended abdomens. Other individuals become hyperactive, pacing and digging frantically as oviposition nears.

SYSTEMIC SIGNS

Weight Loss

A common cause of weight loss in captive reptiles is an inadequate intake of calories. Some keepers mistakenly offer meals that are too small or too infrequent for the specimen in question. This part of the history must be investigated thoroughly.

Low environmental temperatures can hinder digestion even when adequate diets are eaten. This is especially true in folivorous iguanid lizards that rely on microbial fermentation in their hindgut to break down the cellulose in their high-fiber diet.

Intestinal parasites, renal failure, neoplasia, or any systemic disease can result in rapid weight loss.

Anorexia results in weight loss (see Anorexia; Figure 39-15).

Distended Coelom

Lizards store fat in paired symmetrical fat bodies in their caudal coelomic cavity. In obese animals, these may be huge and cause a distended abdomen. They appear as fat density

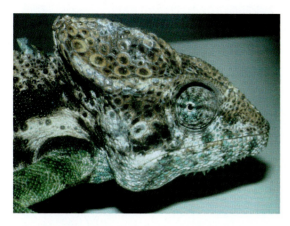

FIGURE 39-15 Sunken eyes in an emaciated Chameleon (*Chamaeleo verrucosus*) with a heavy parasite burden and poor husbandry conditions.

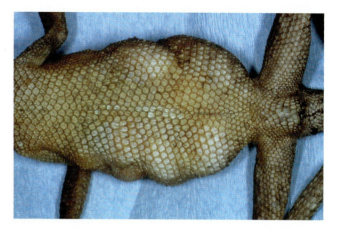

FIGURE 39-17 Distended coelom in a gravid Horn-headed Lizard (*Acanthosaurus crucigera*). Individual eggs can be seen through the skin.

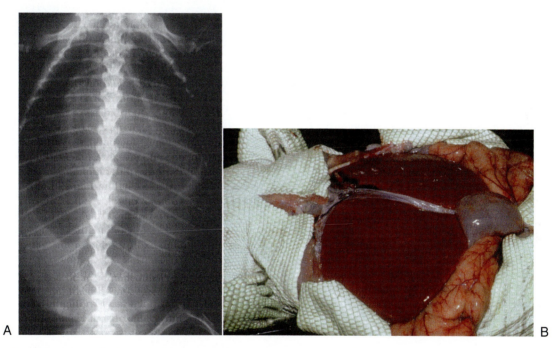

FIGURE 39-16 **A,** Radiograph shows marked hepatomegaly in a Savannah Monitor (*Varanus exanthematicus*). Note the soft-tissue-density liver with prominent blood vessels superimposed over the more radiolucent lungs. **B,** The same lizard at necropsy. The diagnosis was lymphosarcoma, with an antemortem white blood cell count of 100,000/mm^3 and 97% lymphocytes including many blast forms. On histopathology, virtually every organ, including the liver, was massively infiltrated with neoplastic lymphocytes.

on radiographs and often are palpable. Fat bodies may be mistaken for mass lesions.

An apparent distended coelom can result from an enlargement of any of the coelomic viscera. The liver and kidneys may become exaggerated with hepatic lipidosis, granulomatous inflammation, or neoplasia (Figure 39-16). The gastrointestinal tract can become distended with constipation, foreign objects (notably gravel, sand, or other bedding), obstruction, intussusception, or ileus from a spinal cord lesion or profound hypocalcemia. The bladder often becomes grossly distended with urine when denervated by spinal cord lesions, which can be caused by trauma or one of the MBDs.

Ascites is caused by similar mechanisms in reptiles as in mammals. Hypoproteinemia, liver failure, renal failure, cardiac disease, septicemia, and neoplasia may cause ascites. Coelomic neoplasia can result in massive enlargement of the abdomen. Uroliths are occasionally seen in herbivorous lizards with dehydration or unbalanced diets. These tend to be singular and stratified and may be large enough to distend the abdomen.[2]

Female lizards that are gravid or have egg retention have enlarged abdomens. The ova can be palpated, visualized with an ultrasound examination, or shown on radiographs (Figure 39-17).

Lethargy

Environmental conditions such as low temperatures, lack of ultraviolet light, lack of a hiding place, and social stress can cause a lizard to be less active than normal. Lizards that are gravid or about to shed normally have decreased activity. MBDs, nutritional deficiencies, iguana hypercalcemia syndrome, egg retention, renal failure, infections, septicemia, parasite burdens, and just about any illness may result in depression and lack of activity.

A renal failure syndrome in 3-year-old to 5-year-old captive-raised Green Iguanas presents with vague symptoms of anorexia and lethargy in the absence of polyuria and polydipsia. The kidneys are usually enlarged and protrude anterior to the pelvic canal on palpation. Enlarged kidneys also may be shown with digital cloacal palpation and radiographs. Serum blood urea nitrogen (BUN) and creatinine levels are unrewarding in the assessment of renal function in lizards, and uric acid levels only rise in massive end-stage renal failure. The most consistent changes in clinical pathology are the elevation of serum phosphorus levels and a calcium-to-phosphorus ratio of less than one. Affected lizards are usually mildly hypocalcemic, but occasional individuals are profoundly hypercalcemic and sometimes exhibit widespread metastatic mineralization. Ultrasound, the examination of urine sediment for the presence of casts, and kidney biopsy may be used to further evaluate the kidneys. The etiology of this syndrome has not been scientifically documented but may be multifactorial. The use of animal-based protein sources in the diet, lack of exposure to unfiltered sunlight, and chronic dehydration may play a role.[3,16]

One iguana with nonspecific lethargy and illness was diagnosed with lead poisoning. Blood lead levels were measured at 600 µg/dL (N < 40 µg/dL in dogs and cats). The lizard showed response to chelation therapy with CaNa2 ethylenediaminetetraacetic acid (EDTA; personal observation; Figure 39-18).

Often the owners of lizards with lethargy misdiagnose the etiology as attempted brumation (hibernation), even in cases involving tropical species and the presence of high temperatures. Overly cool temperatures and short photoperiods must be corrected, but other causes should be investigated.

Polydipsia and Polyurea

Polydipsia and polyurea are uncommon signs in reptiles. Chronic renal failure may cause these signs. Causes of renal failure include bacterial infection, granulomatous inflammation, and excessive use of aminoglycoside antibiotics. Diabetes mellitus has been reported in a handful of reptiles, none of which were successfully controlled with insulin therapy.[2] Diabetes may be associated with overwhelming septicemia, pancreatitis, and metabolic imbalances but has not been documented as a primary disease.

Sudden Death

Symptoms of disease in reptiles often are subtle, and owners commonly miss them. Thus, many chronic diseases such as septicemia, malnutrition, renal failure, neoplasia, gastrointestinal obstruction, and so on may present as sudden death when in fact they were chronic in nature.

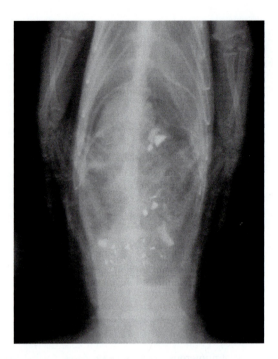

FIGURE 39-18 Radiograph shows metallic densities in a Green Iguana *(Iguana iguana)* with lead poisoning. Blood lead levels were measured at 600 µg/dL (N < 40 µg/dL in dogs and cats). The source of lead was never determined.

Heat stroke from exposure to direct sunlight while a reptile is in an enclosed container or thermostatic malfunction in a heating device can result in sudden death. Victims usually are warm to the touch. Drowning causes sudden death, but the history leaves little doubt as to the cause. Ingestion of certain toxic plants results in relatively rapid death. Several reported cases have been seen where the ingestion of a single firefly caused sudden death in Bearded Dragons.[32] Adenovirus causes sudden death with few or no symptoms in juvenile Bearded Dragons and other species.[33] The protozoan parasite microsporidia caused death with few symptoms in Bearded Dragons.[34]

Epizootics in collections are not uncommon, and various pathogens including bacteria, viruses, fungi, and parasites have been implicated. Microsporidiosis was observed in a colony of Pink-tongued Skinks *(Hemisphaeriodon gerrardi)*.[35] A paramyxo-like virus caused three separate epidemics in colonies of imported Caiman Lizards *(Dracena guianensis)*.[36]

REFERENCES

1. Cooper JE, Jackson OF, editors: *Diseases of the Reptilia,* vol 1 and 2, San Diego, 1981, Academic Press.
2. Frye FL: *Biomedical and surgical aspects of captive reptile husbandry,* ed 2, Melbourne, Fla, 1991, Krieger.
3. Zwart P: Urogenital system. In Beynon PH, Lawton MPC, Cooper JE, editors: *Manual of reptiles,* Gloucestershire, England, 1992, British Small Animal Veterinary Association.
4. Barten SL: What's your diagnosis? Distal leg necrosis in a Green Iguana, *Iguana iguana, J Herpetol Med Surg* 10:48, 2000.
5. Ball RL, Dumonceaux G, MacDonald C: Hypertrophic osteopathy associated with renal gout in a Green Iguana, *Iguana iguana, Proc Assoc Reptil Amphib Vet* 49-50, 1999.

6. Prezant RM, Jarchow JL: Indications and applications of clinical techniques in the Green Iguana, *Semin Avian Exotic Pet Med* 6: 63, 1997.
7. Raiti P: Reproductive problems of reptiles, *Proc Assoc Reptil Amphib Vet* 101-105, 1995.
8. Stahl SJ: Captive management, breeding and common medical problems of the veiled chameleon *(Chamaeleo calyptratus)*, *Proc Assoc Reptil Amphib Vet* 29-40, 1997.
9. Bellairs Ad'A: Congenital and developmental diseases. In Cooper JE, Jackson OF, editors: *Diseases of the Reptilia*, vol 2, San Diego, 1981, Academic Press.
10. Cooper JE: Integument. In Beynon PH, Lawton MPC, Cooper JE, editors: *Manual of reptiles*, Gloucestershire, England, 1992, British Small Animal Veterinary Association.
11. Jacobson ER, Cheatwood JL, Maxwell LK: Mycotic diseases of reptiles, *Vet Clin North Am Exotic Anim Pract* 9:94, 2000.
12. Wissman MA, Parsons B: Dermatophytosis of Green Iguanas *(Iguana iguana)*, *J Small Exotic Anim Med* 2:133, 1993.
13. Miller HA, Frye FL, Graig, TM: Trichomonas associated with ocular and subcutaneous lesions in geckos, *Proc Assoc Reptil Amphib Vet* 102-107, 1994.
14. de Vosjoli P: *The general care and maintenance of true chameleons*, parts I and II, Lakeside, Calif, 1990, Advanced Vivarium Systems.
15. McCracken H, Birch CA: Periodontal disease in lizards—a review of numerous cases, *Proc Am Assoc Zoo Vet* 108-114, 1994.
16. Barten SL: The medical care of iguanas and other common pet lizards, *Vet Clin North Am Small Anim Pract* 23:1213, 1993.
17. de Vosjoli P: Designing environments for captive amphibians and reptiles, *Vet Clin North Am Exotic Anim Pract* 2:43, 1999.
18. Bone RD: Gastrointestinal system. In Beynon PH, Lawton MPC, Cooper JE, editors: *Manual of reptiles*, Gloucestershire, England, 1992, British Small Animal Veterinary Association.
19. Coke RL, Tristan TE: Cryptosporidium infection in a colony of leopard geckos, *Eublepharis macularius*, *Proc Assoc Reptil Amphib Vet* 157-165, 1998.
20. Pare JA, Crawshaw GJ, Barta JR: Treatment of cryptosporidiosis in Gila monsters *(Heloderma suspectum)* with paromomycin, *Proc Assoc Reptil Amphib Vet* 23, 1997.
21. Barten SL: Egg laying problems in Green Iguanas *(Iguana iguana)*. In Bonagura JD, editor: *Kirk's current veterinary therapy XIII: small animal practice*, Philadelphia, 2000, WB Saunders.
22. Jacobson ER: Snakes, *Vet Clin North Am Small Anim Pract* 23:1179, 1993.
23. Stoakes LC: Respiratory system. In Beynon PH, Lawton MPC, Cooper JE, editors: *Manual of reptiles*, Gloucestershire, England, 1992, British Small Animal Veterinary Association.
24. Schumacher J: Respiratory diseases of reptiles, *Vet Clin North Am Exotic Anim Pract* 6:209, 1997.
25. Jacobson ER: Neoplastic diseases. In Cooper JE, Jackson OF, editors: *Diseases of the Reptilia*, vol 2, San Diego, 1981, Academic Press.
26. Barten SL, Davis K, Harris RK, et al: Renal cell carcinoma with metastasis in a corn snake *(Elaphe guttata)*, *J Zoo Wildl Med* 25(1):123, 1994.
27. Lawton MPC: Ophthalmology. In Beynon PH, Lawton MPC, Cooper JE, editors: *Manual of reptiles*, Gloucestershire, England, 1992, British Small Animal Veterinary Association.
28. Millichamp NJ, Jacobson ER, Wolf ED: Diseases of the eye and ocular adnexae in reptiles, *J Am Vet Med Assoc* 183:1205, 1983.
29. Lawton MPC: Neurological diseases. In Beynon PH, Lawton MPC, Cooper JE, editors: *Manual of reptiles*, Gloucestershire, England, 1992, British Small Animal Veterinary Association.
30. Benson KG: Reptilian gastrointestinal diseases, *Semin Avian Exotic Pet Med* 8:90, 1999.
31. Jacobson ER: Evaluation of the reptile patient. In Jacobson ER, Kollias GV, editors: *Contemporary issues in small animal practice: exotic animals*, New York, 1988, Churchill Livingstone.
32. Glor R, Means C, Weintraub MJH, Knight M, Adler K: Two cases of firefly toxicosis in bearded dragons, *Pogona vitticeps*, *Proc Assoc Reptil Amphib Vet* 27-30, 1999.
33. Cranfield M: Adenovirus in the bearded dragon, *Pogona vitticeps*, *Proc Assoc Reptil Amphib Vet* 131-132, 1996.
34. Jacobson ER, Green DE, Undeen AH, Cranfield M, Vaughn KL: Systemic microsporidiosis in inland bearded dragons *(Pogona vitticeps)*, *Proc Assoc Reptil Amphib Vet* 13, 1997.
35. Garner M, Collins D, Joslin J, Didier E, Nordhausen R: Microsporidiosis in a closed colony of pink-tongued skinks, *Hemisphaeriodon gerrardi*, *Proc Assoc Reptil Amphib Vet* 57, 2000.
36. Jacobson ER, Origgi F, Pessier AP, Lamirande EW, Walker I, Whitiker B, et al: Paramyxo-like virus infection in caiman lizards, *Draecena guianensis*, *Proc Assoc Reptil Amphib Vet* 59, 2000.

40

TURTLES, TORTOISES, AND TERRAPINS

THOMAS H. BOYER

CUTANEOUS SIGNS

Cutaneous or Subcutaneous Swelling

Box Turtles (*Terrapene* spp.) and occasionally tortoises and aquatic turtles have myiasis caused by *Cistudinomyia (Sarcophaga) cistudinis*.[1-3] Maggots encyst subcutaneously and breathe through small black-rimmed holes prevalent on the neck and base of the legs, into the axillary and inguinal fossae, and sometimes around the perineum (Figure 40-1). Lesions at the skin-shell interface are easily overlooked. Swelling associated with joints can indicate articular or periarticular gout or pseudogout,[4] joint or bone infection, foreign bodies, parasites, fracture, or luxation. Middle ear abscesses are common in Box Turtles (Figure 40-2). Tumors, such as epidermal squamous papillomas, are a rare cause of skin lesions on the feet of aquatic turtles.[4] Bacterial or fungal infections are more common. Fibropapillomas, common on Green Seaturtles (*Chelonia mydas*), have also been seen on the other species of seaturtles. Gas bubble disease caused large, cutaneous, air-filled, sterile blebs in Malaysian Painted Terrapins, *Callagur borneoensis*, in a large outdoor pool.[5] Gas bubble disease remains rare in turtles; unusual circumstances led to this sole reported case. Mycobacterial and fungal infections can cause nodular skin lesions that fail to respond to antibiotics; the former may be missed without special staining. Spirochid blood fluke eggs can cause intense granulomatous tissue reactions in many organs, including the skin, and can be difficult to diagnose antemortem.[6]

Petechia, Erythema, and Foul Odor

Normally, chelonians have little odor, especially aquatic turtles. However, freshly caught aquatic turtles, such as the Musk Turtle, *Kinosternon odoratus*, and the Mata Mata, *Chelus fimbriatus*, may produce a foul odor from musk glands when under duress. In other turtles, odor often indicates necrosis or infection of the skin or shell, heavy parasitism, poor husbandry, or feces stuck to the animal.

Skin

This condition usually indicates septicemia (endotoxins or exotoxins that may be causing vascular damage), a burn, or hypervitaminosis A, but one should also consider etiologies similar to those of other animals, such as thrombocytopenia, chemical intoxication, and nutritional coagulopathies.[4] Hemoprotozoans are reported to cause similar lesions.[4] One should be aware that many turtles have reddish coloration that may be mistaken for erythema, such as with the juvenile Mata Mata (Figure 40-3).

Shell

Petechia or erythema of the shell usually indicates a bacterial or fungal shell infection, in which case the underlying lesion feels soft (Figure 40-4).[7] Shell infections result from bite wounds, trauma, or, most commonly, poor husbandry, such as unclean water, lack of basking areas, abrasive substrates, or inadequate environmental temperatures. More diffuse shell erythema can also occur with septicemia or starvation or may be normal coloration for some species (see Figure 40-3).[8] Spirochid blood fluke eggs or granulomas may occlude blood vessels in aquatic turtles and manifest as ulcerative ecchmyotic lesions of the plastron or carapace.[6]

Swelling of the Middle Ear Cavity (Tympanic Membranes)

Normally the skin overlying the middle ear should be slightly concave. Middle ear abscesses cause the skin to bulge outward (see Figure 40-2 and Chapter 45).

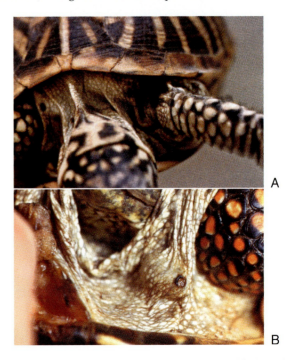

FIGURE 40-1 **A** and **B**, Several botfly pores are visible around the base of the neck in an Ornate Box Turtle, *Terrapene ornata ornata*. Multiple larvae usually share one portal.

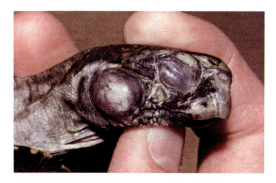

FIGURE 40-2 Swelling over the tympanic membrane is generally a sign of a middle ear abscess; normally the tympanic membrane is slightly concave.

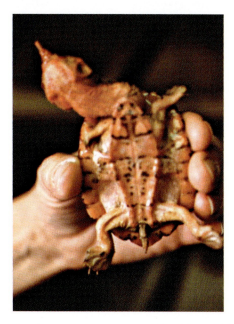

FIGURE 40-3 The underside of a young Mata Mata *(Chelus fimbriatus)* may be normally bright red or orange but should not be confused with erythema.

Whitish Growth on Skin

This condition can be normal incompletely shed skin or a fungal, viral, or parasitic infection. Scar tissue is commonly depigmented.

Whitish Areas on Shell

White areas on the shell represent healed shell lesions, exposed healed bone, mineral deposits, or ongoing shell infection (see Figure 40-4, *B*, versus Figure 40-5, *A, B, C*). One should keep in mind that turtle shell is capable of regrowth such that old areas of exposed bone may be pushed off by underlying newly formed scutes. White areas may also be seen in the seams between scutes in rapidly growing juvenile turtles and tend to darken with age. Texas Tortoises, *Gopherus berlandieri,* from south Texas have been observed to have whitish blemishes in the scutes that may coalesce and eat away the scutes. New growth in the seams is not affected. This necrotizing scute disease is caused by *Fusarium semitectum*.[9]

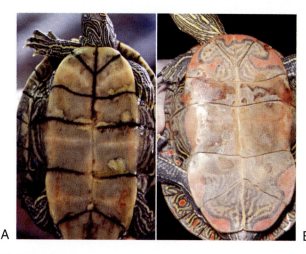

FIGURE 40-4 **A** and **B,** Bacterial infection of bone can cause fluid and cellular debris to accumulate under the scutes; normally no fluid, odor, or discoloration should be present under the scutes.

Box Turtles, *Terrapene ornata*, were resistant to experimental infection.[9]

Algae Growth on Shell

Green algae often colonize the shell of aquatic turtles. As long as husbandry conditions are adequate, simple periodic scrubbing keeps algae under control. Concern is not necessary.

Sloughing

Skin

Chelonians normally shed their skin in a much more piecemeal fashion than squamates, but they still regularly shed. Full-thickness skin sloughing is abnormal and may be associated with iatrogenic hypervitaminosis A (see Chapter 59).[4] Bacterial infection, especially anaerobic bacteria; trauma; starvation; and chemical or thermal burns can also cause skin sloughing. Desert Tortoises *(Gopherus agassizii)* kept too damp during brumation (hibernation) may have an ulcerative dermatitis develop from *Aeromonas hydrophila* along the ventral skin margins of the plastron in the axillary and inguinal regions and in the carpal and tarsal folds.[10]

Scutes

Terrestrial chelonians may slough scutes as a result of bacterial (see Figure 40-4, *A, B*) or fungal infections brought on by a moist environment or from chronic renal failure (Figure 40-6).[4] If renal failure is present, bone plates may loosen and ooze azotemic fluid. Ascites may also be present.[4] In tortoises, nutritional deficiencies may cause flaking and sloughing scutes that are secondarily infected with bacteria or fungi.[3] Aquatic species normally flake off portions of scutes if their shell dries out while out of water, and they periodically shed entire scutes as part of normal growth.

Shell Ulceration or Shell Rot

Traumatic injuries such as bites from other turtles or predators can penetrate the outer keratin layer of the shell. Burns and bacterial (see Figure 40-4) or fungal infections can also lead to

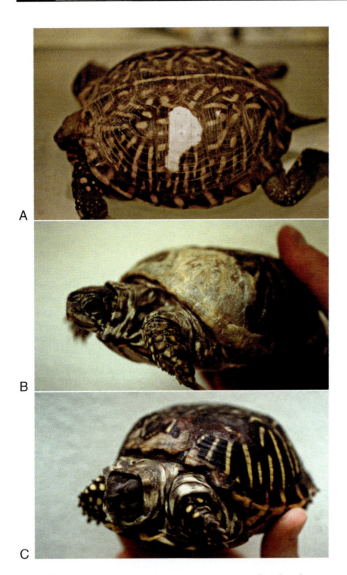

FIGURE 40-5 A, B, and C, Scutes are missing over the whitish areas on the carapaces of these Ornate Box Turtles, *Terrapene ornata ornata*, exposing the underlying bone. New scutes may form under this bone, and eventually the bone will flake off. Unless ongoing disease is present, treatment is not indicated.

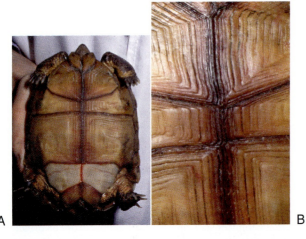

FIGURE 40-6 Note the erythema at the seams between scutes (A) and sloughing of scutes (B) in this Desert Tortoise, *Gopherus agassizii*, with renal failure.

ulcers on the shell. In terrestrial chelonians, wet shell rot tends to be bacterial and dry shell rot tends to be fungal.[8] Ulcerative shell disease or shell rot is a chronic contagious disease that causes pitting of the shell of aquatic turtles.[11] *Beneckeia chitonovora*, a bacteria from shellfish, was thought to be the causative agent.[12,13] Septicemic cutaneous ulcerative disease (SCUD) causes irregular caseated crateriform ulcers, especially on the ventral surfaces of aquatic turtles such as the Softshell Turtles (*Apalone* spp.).[4] As the lesions progress, the patient becomes septicemic. Hepatic necrosis, paralysis, and death may ensue.[4] The etiologic agent was once thought to be *Citrobacter freundii*,[14] yet poor husbandry and other gram-negative bacteria are undoubtedly involved with this condition and with ulcerative shell disease.[4,11]

Box Turtles often have healed pits in the shell from unknown causes, perhaps as a result of invertebrate or vertebrate predation during brumation (hibernation).[4] Free-ranging Desert Tortoises from Riverside County, California, have cutaneous dyskeratosis with a high mortality rate.[15] Lesions commence at the seams and spread toward the middle of the scutes. Lesions are gray-white, sometimes orange, and have a roughened flaky appearance. The plastron is most heavily affected; deficiency or toxicity of some sort is suspected.

Fractures of the Shell

Usually fractures are the result of trauma from dogs, other vertebrate predators, large hoof stock, falls, automobiles, and lawnmowers. Nutritional secondary hyperparathyroidism can cause shell fractures, but other signs of a soft or distorted shell should be present (see Chapter 61).

Overgrown Rhamphotheca (Beak) and Toenails

Overgrowth of the rhamphotheca and toenails may indicate an underlying nutritional deficiency such as nutritional secondary hyperparathyroidism (Figure 40-7). Lack of wear in captivity has been suggested as a cause, yet overgrowth is generally not a problem in captive turtles on balanced diets.[4] Elongated nails (but not rhamphotheca) on the front or rear feet (not both) is a normal secondary sex characteristic in some chelonians (see Sexual Dimorphism, under Clinical Anatomy and Physiology, Chapter 7, Turtles, Tortoises, and Terrapins). Overgrown front and rear nails with a normal rhamphotheca may reflect lack of wear.

Soft Shell

A soft shell may indicate nutritional secondary hyperparathyroidism (see Chapter 61), unless evidence of trauma or bacterial or fungal disease is present. Hatchling chelonians on an adequate ration should have a firm shell develop within the first year. Shell should feel like solid bone, with the exceptions of a few species that normally have soft shells or carapacial fenestrae. These include Pancake Tortoises (*Malacochersus tornieri*), male and immature female giant Asian River Turtles (*Batagur baska*, *Kachuga kachuga*, and *K. dhongoka*),[16] and Softshell Turtles (*Apalone* spp.). Other species have shell kinesis that should not be confused with a soft shell. These include platronal hinges in *Terrapene*, *Cuora*, *Pyxix*, and *Kinosternon*; a caudal carapacial hinge in *Kinixys*; and slight caudal plastron mobility in female *Testudo*.

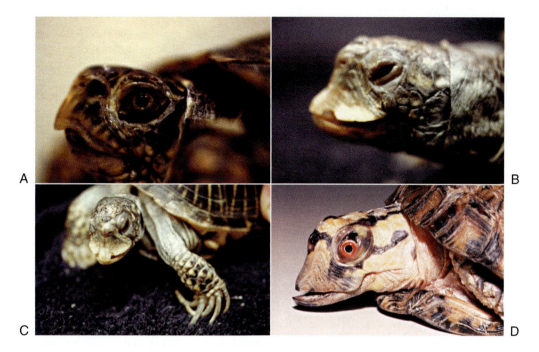

FIGURE 40-7 Normal beak or rhamphotheca (**A**) compared with overgrown rhamphotheca and nails (**B, C,** and **D**). Severely overgrown and misshapen rhamphotheca or nails may represent an underlying nutritional deficiency. (*D, Courtesy S. Barten.*)

Distorted Shell

A distorted shell is common with nutritional secondary hyperparathyroidism or previous trauma. Scute abnormalities can be congenital or the result of various metabolic bone diseases (see also Shell Ulceration or Shell Rot; Figures 40-8 and 40-9).

Pyramidal Shell Growth

The etiology of pyramidal shell growth remains unknown. Tortoises are most often affected (Figure 40-10). Suggested etiologies include excess dietary protein, too rapid growth, vitamin or mineral excess or deficiency, nutritional secondary hyperparathyroidism, low humidity, and species predisposition.[17,18] For a more detailed discussion, see Chapter 18, Nutrition.

Dermal fistulas

Trauma or myiasis can cause holes in the skin (see Cutaneous and Subcutaneous Swelling; see Figure 40-1).

Edema or Ascites

Edema can result from liver, kidney, or cardiopulmonary disease and from vascular or lymphatic obstruction and hypoproteinemia.[4] Myxedema has been observed in tortoises and a Red-eared Slider (*Trachemys scripta elegans*) with goiters.[4,19]

GASTROINTESTINAL SIGNS

Anorexia

Anorexia is a nonspecific sign of almost all chelonian illnesses. Winter anorexia is frequent in species that normally brumate (hibernate).[7]

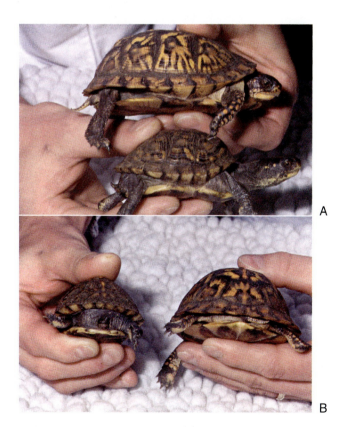

FIGURE 40-8 **A** and **B,** Note abnormal shell growth and increased space between the carapace and plastron in the smaller long-term captive Eastern Box Turtle, *Terrapene carolina carolina*, compared with the larger wild-caught turtle. Abnormal new shell growth indicates underlying deficiency, in this case nutritional secondary hyperparathyroidism.

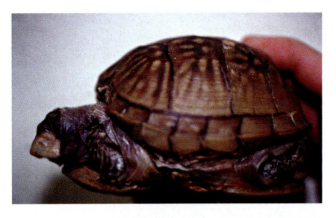

FIGURE 40-9 Note the distorted rhamphothecal and seam growth in the bridge area of this Three-toed Box Turtle, *Terrapene carolina triunguis*, arising from a calcium-deficient diet.

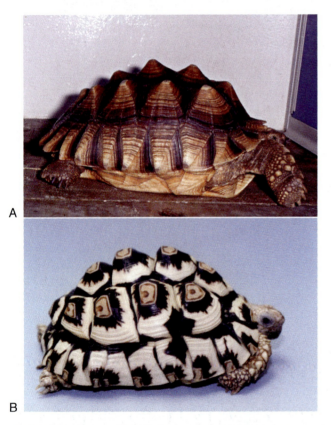

FIGURE 40-10 Pyramidal shell growth in a Spurred Tortoise, *Geochelone sulcata* (**A**), and a Leopard Tortoise, *Geochelone pardalis* (**B**). The causes of pyramidal shell growth are multifactorial. See Chapter 18 for more details.

Emaciation

Emaciation generally indicates starvation from disease, poor husbandry, neoplasia, or any other debilitating conditions.

Pale Tongue and Mucous Membranes

The oral cavity should normally be pale pink, with the tongue even pinker. Pale mucous membranes are often the result of anemia or poor peripheral circulation in severely debilitated animals.[20]

Infectious Stomatitis

Herpesvirus causes necrotic caseous stomatitis (especially involving the palate and internal nares), glossitis, pharnygitis, and tracheitis and is often observable at the back of the oral cavity as coalescing white plaques (see Chapter 57). Herpesvirus is especially common in *Testudo*[21,22] and has been reported in a variety of other turtles; all tortoises are considered susceptible. Other than Herpesvirus infections, infectious stomatitis is rare in chelonians.

Moisture or Dried Mucus on Rhamphotheca (Beak)

Any accumulation of material on the beak is abnormal and may signify oral infection, ulceration, or irritation from a foreign body,[23] broken jaw, or a cracked, overgrown, or misshapen rhamphotheca (see Overgrown Rhamphotheca and Toenails under Cutaneous Signs).

Constipation

Constipation can arise from gastrointestinal impactions as a result of dehydration.[4] Foreign bodies, such as sand, gravel, rocks, cage litter, or other material, can also cause impaction. Fine sand and crushed gravel are particularly worrisome. One should note that tortoises often have a few stones in the gastrointestinal tract that pass uneventfully.[24] Cystic calculi and parasites are less common causes of constipation.

Emesis/Regurgitation

Parasites, foreign bodies, septicemia, and adverse drug reactions can cause regurgitation.[8,24] The author has seen several Box Turtles (*Terrapene* spp.) that vomited within 30 minutes of administration of enrofloxacin and vitamin A at normal dosages. Differential diagnoses should include causes of vomiting typical for other animals. Ptyalism and fluid regurgitation are commonly found in tortoises with intestinal impactions.[25] Tortoises may also present for acute and repeated emesis after ingestion of toadstools (species not determined).[26]

Bloating

Excessive intestinal gas production can result from fermentation of food within the gastrointestinal tract. This condition can result from an abrupt change to protein-rich or carbohydrate-rich foods; force-feeding sick chelonians inappropriate foods (such as dairy products), especially with suboptimal temperatures; or gastrointestinal obstruction or hypomotility.[4,24]

Diarrhea

Loose, watery stools can result from various parasites, bacterial or fungal infections, foreign bodies, or food. Foods with a high water content, such as fruits, can cause diarrhea. For tortoises, lack of roughage, especially with indoor housing, seems to make for more watery stools, which is not necessarily abnormal.

Mass Protruding from Cloaca

The penis is the most common mass observed protruding from the cloaca (Figure 40-11). The penis is a large pink, purple, or

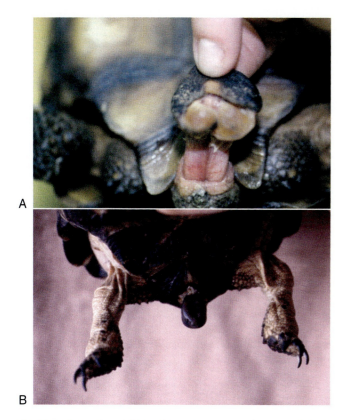

FIGURE 40-11 A and B, Penile prolapse is a common malady in chelonians.

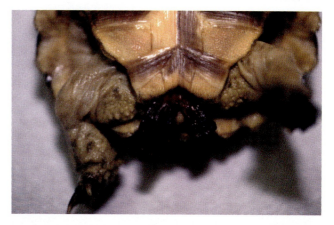

FIGURE 40-12 Not all that prolapses from the cloaca is a penis, such as this prolapsed urinary bladder in a young Desert Tortoise, *Gopherus agassizii*.

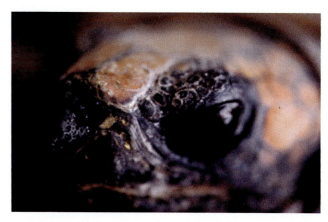

FIGURE 40-13 Nasal discharge should always be considered abnormal in chelonians.

tan mass with a spade-shaped tip. Males periodically have an erection develop that should be no cause for immediate concern unless necrotic or if it does not retract within several hours. See Chapter 64 for more details.

Differential diagnosis for masses protruding from the cloaca include prolapse of the urinary bladder (Figure 40-12), cloaca, colon, or oviduct.[4] Prolapse of the penis can be from nutritional secondary hyperparathyroidism; constipation; impaction of the cloaca with urates; cystic calculi; neurologic defects in the penis rectractor apparatus, cloacal vent, or anal sphincter muscles; bacterial, parasitic, or fungal infections; irritation or desiccation of the penis from substrates during attempts at breeding; or trauma from cagemates or attempts to copulate.

Bleeding from Cloacal Vent

Blood passing from the cloaca often indicates a penis laceration. Differential diagnosis includes gastrointestinal, urogenital, or cloacal bleeding or parasites. Cloacaliths have been seen in several tortoise species (see Figure 49-4).

RESPIRATORY SIGNS

Nasal Discharge

Any nasal discharge, wet or dried, is abnormal in chelonians unless associated with drinking or eating watery foods.

Dorsal pressure on the gular area should not elicit any nasal discharge. *Mycoplasma agassizii* causes upper respiratory tract disease in a variety of tortoises, especially Desert (*Gopherus agassizii*) and Gopher Tortoises (*G. polyphemus*),[27,28] and Box Turtles (*Terrapene carolina bauri*; see Chapter 73). All tortoises should be considered susceptible. Clinical signs include clear to colored discharge or bubbling from the nares (Figure 40-13), rhinitis, ocular discharge, conjunctivitis, palpebral edema, sunken eyes, decreased to no appetite, lethargy, dull coloration, and weight loss without lesions in the mouth.

Herpesvirus can also produce nasal discharge but almost always also has whitish plaques in the oral cavity (see Infectious Stomatitis; see Chapters 57 and 72). Hypovitaminosis A can predispose chelonians to secondary nasal sinus infections and nasal discharge but is probably overdiagnosed, especially in tortoises (Chapter 59).[4] Dietary history is important to rule out vitamin deficiency.[4] Excess salivation[29] and inhaled irritants such as pollen[4] or foreign bodies, such as foxtails or grass awns,[8] can also lead to nasal discharge.

Erosion or Depigmentation of the Nares

Chronic upper respiratory tract disease may erode or depigment the nares (see Nasal Discharge) (Figure 40-14).[23] See also Chapter 73.

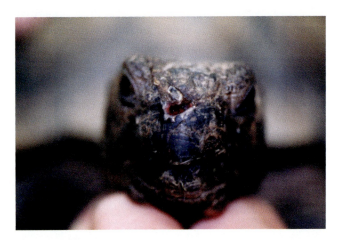

FIGURE 40-14 Erosion of the nares in a Desert Tortoise, *Gopherus agassizii*, with chronic upper respiratory tract disease.

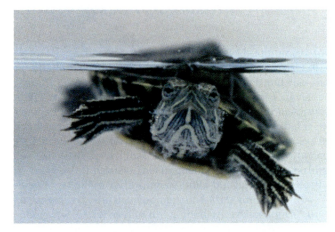

FIGURE 40-16 Although uneven floating in a dorsal plane is typically a sign of pneumonia in aquatic turtles, any unilateral mass or gas production can also cause turtles to list.

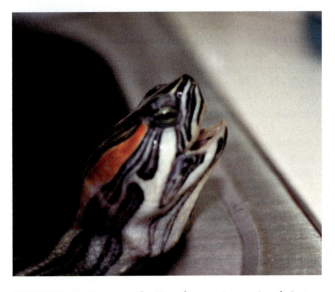

FIGURE 40-15 Open-mouthed breathing is abnormal in chelonians and generally suggests pathology deep to the glottis.

Distortion of Tissue Around Nares

Chronic upper respiratory tract disease or nutritional secondary hyperparathyroidism in young growing tortoises may cause the area around the nares to bulge asymmetrically, much like atrophic rhinitis in swine.[30]

Dyspnea and Abnormal Breath Sounds

Dyspneic turtles may stretch the neck and gape the mouth with obvious labored breathing (Figure 40-15) or pump the head and legs. Movement of the head and limbs is a normal part of breathing in most chelonians but becomes more pronounced with dyspnea. Gular pumping is associated with olfaction and is not a sign of dyspnea. Dyspnea or abnormal breath sounds, such as a click or slight whistle, usually indicate a lower respiratory tract infection. Bacteria, particularly gram-negative bacteria, are the most common culprit.

Mycoplasma spp. have been implicated in tortoises.[28] Other causes include fungal, viral, or parasitic disease or aspirated foreign bodies.

Uneven Floating

Aquatic turtles normally float levelly from side-to-side but not front-to-back. As material accumulates in a pneumonic lung, the lung becomes heavier and the turtle does not float levelly in a lateral plane (Figure 40-16).[4] Any unilateral mass, such as an abscess, tumor, or asymmetric gas production, as with bloating, can cause similar signs.

Inability to Submerge

With emaciation, pneumonia, tumors, and gas accumulation within the coelom or gastrointestinal tract (from infection, trauma, or obstruction)[20] may cause aquatic turtles to lose the ability to submerge. This is a common problem in seaturtles (Chapter 76).

REPRODUCTIVE SIGNS

Penile Prolapse or Mass Protruding from Cloaca

See Mass Protruding from Cloaca under Gastrointestinal Signs (Chapter 47).

Failure to Lay Eggs

Nutritional factors or stress from improper husbandry should be considered primary to all reproductive failures (Chapter 23).

Chelonians often fail to lay eggs because of metabolic bone disease of nutritional origin (NMBD), hypovitaminosis A, hypocalcemia, dehydration, or lack of an appropriate nesting area.[7] Females housed outdoors may be reluctant to continue laying eggs indoors if the substrate is not deep enough (inadequate nesting site). A ruptured, large, or anomalous egg; oviductal rupture; infection; or any mass impinging on the oviduct, such as a urolith, fecalith, or gastrointestinal foreign body, can also lead to egg retention.[4] Eggs may also become ectopically located in the urinary bladder, coelom, or colon or lodged in the pelvis.

Mass in Coelom

The differential diagnoses for coelomic masses include ova, eggs, cystic calculi, gastrointestinal foreign bodies, neoplasia, and abscesses.

MUSCULOSKELETAL SIGNS

Lameness

Lameness can result from fractures, luxations, trauma, foreign bodies, gout, or sepsis and, in females, as a short-term sequela to egg laying and imbalances in calcium homeostasis. Egg retention or cystic calculi can contribute to lameness.[30] One should always consider nutritional or renal secondary hyperparathyroidism as a potential cause of lameness. Large breeding males often traumatize a limb from falling off female's carapace.

Asymmetric Toenail Wear

Uneven wear of the toenails may be associated with lameness in terrestrial species.[23] One should keep in mind normal secondary sex characteristics (see Sexual Dimorphism, under Clinical Anatomy and Physiology, Chapter 7, Turtles, Tortoises, and Terrapins). Some females often have longer nails on the hind limbs for nest excavation, and male aquatic turtles may have longer nails on the forelimbs for courtship.

Swollen Joints

Joint swelling can result from nutritional disorders, infection, luxation, fracture, articular or periarticular gout, or pseudogout (Figure 40-17) (Chapter 54).[4]

Swollen Long Bones

Long bone swelling can result from healed or healing fractures, neoplasia, osteomyelitis, or fibrous osteodystrophy.

Temporal Muscle Atrophy

The temporal muscles are normally prominent with no visible occipital crest. Starvation, emaciation, or extreme dehydration may cause noticeable atrophy of the temporal muscles (Figure 40-18).[23]

NEUROLOGIC SIGNS

Ataxia/Hypermetric Gait

Severe ataxia and a hypermetic gait have been observed in Desert Tortoises after episodes of hyperthermia, near-drowning, or joint luxation. Cerebellar injury may be present perhaps as a result of hypoxia or cerebral edema.[26]

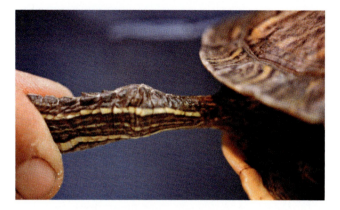

FIGURE 40-17 Joint swelling can result from infection, luxation, fracture, articular or periarticular gout, or pseudogout.

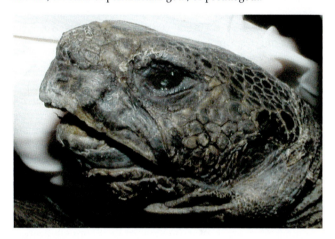

FIGURE 40-18 Note the sunken eyes and temporal muscle atrophy in this cachectic Desert Tortoise, *Gopherus agassizii*. (Photograph courtesy D. Mader.)

Circling

Circling can be a sequela to freezing during brumation (hibernation) (see Blindness), toxemia, septicemia, central nervous system damage, or liver disease.[31]

Flaccid Paresis, Paralysis, or Coma

A comatose turtle could have severe systemic illness, such as septicemia, organ failure, or end-stage starvation, which dictates a poor prognosis. Other less common causes include toxicity to ivermectin or other substances, shock, drowning, hyperthermia, or bloat.[4,30]

Hindlimb Paresis

Chelonians can present with hindlimb paresis from egg retention, oviposition, cystic calculi, spinal cord damage, or orthopedic problems.[30]

OPHTHALMOLOGIC SIGNS

Blindness

Blindness has been reported in *Testudo* spp. after freezing during brumation (hibernation) and may be associated with hyphema, vitreal haze, lenticular opacities, and retinal damage.[31] Additional symptoms include anorexia, head tilt, circling, or holding the head high. Patients improved slowly with time and vitamin A supplementation.[31] Blindness from other causes is possible but not commonly seen (Chapter 20).

Eyelids Swollen Shut

Palpebra edema may indicate hypovitaminosis A (see Figure 59-1, A, B). Emaciated or dehydrated turtles also tend to keep their eyes shut, but the globe is more sunken. The differential diagnosis can include trauma, foreign bodies, bacterial or viral infection, parasites, or metabolic disturbances.[4] Hypovitaminosis A remains rare in tortoises; infectious causes such as mycoplasmosis and herpesvirus are more likely. Box Turtles may hold one eye shut with middle ear abscesses that may, or may not, be advanced enough to cause tympanic swelling.[20] Ulcers or panophthalmitis can also cause blepharospasm.

Exophthalmia

Unilateral exophthalmia may result from retrobulbar abscess, tumor, or injury. Bilateral exophthalmia may result from vascular obstruction or generalized edema.[23] See Eyes Swollen Shut in this section as well.

Sunken Eyes or Enophthalmia

Bilateral enophthalmia can indicate microphthalmia; thiamine deficiency, especially with a diet of frozen fish rich in thiaminases[4]; or emaciation (see Figure 40-18) or dehydration from other disease or poor husbandry or both. Sunken eyes may also indicate severe dehydration or circulatory collapse in septic debilitated chelonians. The eyes often sink way into the orbit just before death.[20] Unilateral enophthalmia may result from orbital injury (particularly automobile trauma) or phthisis bulbi.[23]

Ocular Discharge

Discharge from the eyes can accompany upper respiratory tract disease (see Nasal Discharge under Respiratory Signs), ocular irritants, and hypovitaminosis A (see Figure 40-18).[4] Red-footed (*Geochelone carbonaria*) and Yellow-footed (*G. denticulata*) Tortoises normally have a clear ocular discharge, especially when maintained in conditions of inadequate humidity.

REFERENCES

1. Aldrich JM: *Sarcophaga and allies in North America*, Lafayette, Ind, 1916, Thomas Say Foundation.
2. Townsend CH: New genera and species of American muscoid diptera, *Proc Biol Sci Wash* 30:43, 1917.
3. Jacobson ER: Causes of mortality and diseases in tortoises: a review, *J Zoo Wildl Dis* 25(1):2, 1994.
4. Frye FL: *Biomedical and surgical aspects of captive reptile husbandry*, ed 2, vol 2, Melbourne, Fla, 1991, Kreiger Publishing.
5. Lung NP, Garner M: Gas bubble disease in Malaysian painted terrapins, *Callagar borneoensis*, Proc Assoc Rept Amphib Vets, Reno, Nev, 2000.
6. Conboy GA, Laursen JR, Averbeck GA, Stromberg BE: Diagnostic guide to some of the helminth parasites of aquatic turtles, *Comp Cont Ed Practicing Vet* 15(9):1217-1221, 1993.
7. Boyer TH: Common problems of Box Turtles (*Terrapene* spp.) in captivity, *Bull Assoc Reptil Amphib Vet* 2(1):9, 1992.
8. Highfield AC: *Keeping and breeding tortoises in captivity*, Bristol, Great Britain, 1990, Longdunn Press, Ltd.
9. Rose FL, Koke J, Koehn R, Smith DL: Identification of the etiologic agent for necrotising scute disease in the Texas tortoise, *J Wildl Dis* 37(2):223-228, 2001.
10. Jarchow JL: Cenozoic environments and the evolution of the gopher tortoises (Genus *Gopherus*). In VanDevender TR, editor: *The Sonoran Desert Tortoise: natural history, biology, and conservation*, Univ of AZ Press, Tucson, Ariz. In press.
11. Marcus LC: *Veterinary biology and medicine of captive amphibians and reptiles*, Philadelphia, 1981, Lea & Febiger.
12. Wallach JD: The pathogenesis and etiology of ulcerative shell disease in turtles, *Aquatic Mammals* 4:1, 1976.
13. Wallach JD: Ulcerative shell disease in turtles: identification, prophylaxis and treatment, *Intl Zoo Yb* 17:170, 1977.
14. Kaplan HM: Septicemic cutaneous ulcerative disease of turtles, *Proc Anim Care Panel* 7:273, 1957.
15. Jacobson ER, Wronski TJ, Scumacher J, Reggiardo C, Berry KH: Cutaneous dyskeratosis in free-ranging desert tortoises, *Gopherus agassizii*, in the Colorado desert of southern California, *J Zoo Wildl Med* 25(1):68-81, 1994.
16. Rapheal BL, Behler JL: Clinical challenge, *J Zoo Wildl Med* 25(1):181, 1994.
17. Innis C: Considerations in formulating captive tortoise diets, *Bull Assoc Reptil Amphib Vet* 4(1):8, 1994.
18. Stearns B: The captive status of the African spurred tortoise (*Geocehelone sulcata*); recent developments, *Intl Zoo Yb* 25:87, 1989.
19. Frye FL, Dutra F: Hypothyroidism in turtles and tortoises, *Vet Med Small Anim Clin* 69:990, 1974.
20. Innis CJ: Personal communication, Westboro, Mass, 2001, VCA Westboro Animal Hospital.
21. Cooper JE, Gschmeissner S, Bone RD: Herpes-like virus particles in necrotic stomatitis of tortoises, *Vet Rec* 123:544, 1988.
22. Origgi F, Jacobson ER, Romero CH, Klein PA: Diagnostic tools for Herpesvirus detection in chelonians, *Proc Assoc Reptil Amphib Vet* 2000.
23. Jacobson ER, Behler JL, Jarchow, JL: Health assessment of chelonians and release into the wild. In Fowler ME, Miller RE, editors: *Zoo and wild animal medicine: current therapy 4*, Philadelphia, 1999, WB Saunders.
24. Bone RD: Gastrointestinal system. In Beynon PH, Lawton MPC, Cooper JE, editors: *Manual of reptiles*, Gloucestershire, England, 1992, British Small Animal Veterinary Association.
25. Jarchow JL, Lawler HE, VanDevender TR, Ivanyi CS: Care and diet of captive Sonoran desert tortoises. In VanDevender TR, editor: *The Sonoran Desert Tortoise: natural history, biology, and conservation*, Univ of AZ Press, Tucson, Ariz. In press.
26. Jarchow JL: Personal communication, Tucson, Ariz, 2001, Sonoran Animal Hospital.
27. Jacobson ER, Gaskin JM, Brown MB, Harris RK, Gardiner CH, LaPointe JL, et al: Chronic upper respiratory tract disease of free-ranging desert tortoises (*Xerobates agassizii*), *J Wildl Dis* 27:296-316, 1991.
28. Jacobson ER: The desert tortoise and upper respiratory tract disease, *Bull Assoc Reptil Amphib Vet* 4(1):6, 1994.
29. Stoakes LC: Respiratory system. In Beynon PH, Lawton MPC, Cooper JE, editors: *Manual of reptiles*, Gloucestershire, England, 1992, British Small Animal Veterinary Association.
30. Mader DR: Personal communication, Marathon, Fla, 1999, Marathon Veterinary Hospital.
31. Lawton MPC: Neurological diseases. Ophthalmology. In Beynon PH, Lawton MPC, Cooper JE, editors: *Manual of reptiles*, Gloucestershire, England, 1992, British Small Animal Veterinary Association.

41
CROCODILIAN DIFFERENTIAL DIAGNOSIS

JAVIER NEVAREZ

Crocodilians as a group have a worldwide distribution and have been able to survive for millions of years. Through time, society has integrated crocodilians species into conservation efforts as a natural resource. Countries such as Australia, India, Mexico, Papua New Guinea, South Africa, and the United States maintain intensive production operations for various species. Alligators, crocodiles, and caimans are all found in farm or ranch scenarios where they are raised for skin and meat. Crocodilian farms maintain their own breeding stock of animals from which they collect eggs every year for hatching. On the other hand, a crocodilian ranch is characterized by the harvest of eggs from the wild. A percentage of the eggs collected is then returned to the wild to maintain the population. Most American Alligators (*Alligator mississippiensis*) are raised in a ranch scenario. Regardless of the methodology, this industry has played an integral role in the conservation of crocodilian species around the world. People now view this species as a natural resource that must be protected for future generations.

Like any other intense production animal system, crocodilian species are affected by an array of diseases in captivity. Some of these diseases may also be observed in wild animals. Stress plays a major role in the occurrence of diseases in captive populations. In this section, we concentrate mostly on diseases found in captive-reared crocodilians, but some also apply to the wild populations. Of all the species, the concentration is on the American Alligator, which is the species harvested in the United States. For purposes of this section, we refer to the group containing all species as crocodilians and then refer to each species by common (crocodiles, caimans, alligators, gharials) and scientific names to avoid confusion.

CAPTIVE HUSBANDRY

Captive husbandry of crocodilians varies with species and country of location. In the United States, the American Alligator industry is also varied between and even within states. In Louisiana, most of the operations are ranches. In Florida, both ranches and farm operations are found. In a ranch operation, buildings are either circular (Figure 41-1) or rectangular with some divisions on the inside to create a number of individual pens. The buildings are completely enclosed with one or two entrances and no source of light. The pens usually allow communication of water and are lined with rubber, fiberglass, or other nonporous material. Heating elements may also be contained within the concrete slab to aid in temperature control. Water heaters are used to maintain temperature when refilling the pens. Water sources can be city water, well water, or bayou water. Most operations do not use a filtration system. Temperature is the only water parameter routinely monitored. The frequency of cleaning the pens can range from three to six times a week depending on the ranch and the size of the animals. A commercial pelleted diet is readily available, and some diets are supplemented with chicken, fish, or nutria. Vitamin supplements are sometimes mixed with the feed. Feed is typically placed on a suspended wooden table in the middle of the pen. Feeding frequency is five to six times per week. A complete history is essential in diagnosis of diseases in a crocodilian operation.

STRESS AND IMMUNOSUPPRESSION

Many diseases of crocodilians are considered to be caused by stress. Stress has been defined as "a physiological answer to a perceived threat that includes, but is not restricted to, increased adrenal secretion."[1] Stress is also thought of as any event that challenges homeostasis, and likely the response to that challenge involves more than an adrenal response. The autonomic nervous system, the hypothalamic adrenal axis, neuropeptides, neurotransmitters, and neuroimmunologic mediators all have a role in the response of the immune system to stress.[2] How stress and immunosuppression are measured is still a subject of controversy in veterinary medicine. No one test can be used to measure stress, but rather physiologic changes are combined to give an idea of what is

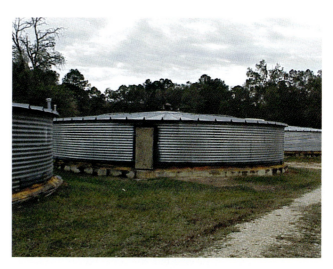

FIGURE 41-1 Circular building for raising captive *Alligator mississippiensis*.

involved in a stress response. A number of research studies have examined the stress response in crocodilians. These studies have looked at the stress associated with restraint, long-term corticosterone implants, cold shock, and stocking densities.[3-6] Lance, Morici, and Elsey[7] provide an overview of the physiology and endocrinology of stress in crocodilians. Catecholamines, glucocorticoids, glucose, and lactate have been implicated in the stress response of crocodilians. In addition, an argument is made for immunosuppression on the basis of changes observed in the white blood cells.[3-5,7] The factors that influence stress in crocodilian and reptile species are reviewed by Rooney and Guillette.[1] Enough evidence exists to suggest that stress plays an important role in the physiology of crocodilians, and it may indeed predispose them to illness. Overcrowding, handling, excessive noise, diet changes, temperature irregularities, etc., should all be considered as predisposing or confounding factors of disease. These need to be a consideration with diagnostics and recommendation of treatment for these species.

NONSPECIFIC CLINICAL SIGNS: ANOREXIA, LETHARGY, AND DEATH

The first signs of illness in captive crocodilians are usually nonspecific in nature. These include anorexia, lethargy, and death. The workers notice excess food remaining on the tables from the day before, which is sometimes followed by a perceived change in the behavior of the animals. One should not underestimate these observations because most workers are well tuned to the daily routine and behavior of the animals. A visit to the ranch or farm should be performed during feeding time to avoid additional stress to the animals. This also allows observation of the feeding and water change practices. At this time, a thorough history and a collection of animals for diagnostics and necropsy can be obtained. In addition to routine samples, tissues should be frozen for possible bacterial, fungal, or viral cultures.

The list of differentials for nonspecific clinical signs must be narrowed after diagnostic samples are obtained. However, one must remember that husbandry and disease go hand in hand. Most systemic diseases of captive crocodilians are thought to be secondary in nature. This is especially true for bacterial and fungal diseases because of the environment in which they are maintained. A number of bacterial infections have been diagnosed in crocodilians. The most data available are from *A. mississippiensis* as presented in Table 41-1. This table presents a large number of isolates from diseased and nondiseased animals. Huchzermeyer et al[8] also have extensive data on enteric bacterial and fungal isolates from African Dwarf Crocodiles (*Osteolaemus tetraspis*).

One bacterium that has been widely studied in reptiles is *Salmonella* sp., in part because of its zoonosis and association with the pet trade. Only a few reports exist of *Mycobacterium* sp. affecting crocodilian species, perhaps because of the difficulties associated with the culture techniques. However, in the author's experience, multiple clinical cases have revealed acid-fast organisms consistent with *Mycobacterium* sp. Their true identity can only be ensured with positive cultures.

More recently, new species of *Mycoplasma, Mycoplasma alligatoris* and *Mycoplasma crocodyli,* have been identified.[9,10]

Chlamydiosis has also been reported in crocodilian species.[21] Fungal infections occur with some frequency in captive crocodilians. Many of these are opportunistic invaders that affect the integument and respiratory system.

Viral diseases are likely underdiagnosed in reptile medicine because of the challenges in diagnostic techniques and the scarce information about them. Poxvirus and most recently West Nile virus (WNV) have been reported as pathogens in crocodilians. An adenovirus-like infection in captive Nile Crocodiles (*Crocodylus niloticus*) was first identified by Jacobson, Gardiner, and Foggin[12] in 1984. Clinical signs are nonspecific, lethargy and anorexia, although conjunctivitis and blepharitis were observed in one of two crocodiles.[11,12] Hepatitis is thought to be the main effect of adenoviral infection. Intestine, pancreas, and lung are also affected on rare occasions.[11] Horizontal transmission is believed to be more common, but vertical transmission has been postulated.[11] Diagnosis is obtained postmortem, and no treatment regimens have been established.

Coronavirus, influenza C virus, and paramyxovirus have been identified with transmission electron microscope in the feces of crocodilians, but their significance remains to be determined. Finally, evidence exists of seroconversion to paramyxovirus and eastern equine encephalitis virus in crocodilians.[11]

Toxicities are not common in captive crocodilian. However, cases have been found of lead toxicity in alligators fed lead-shot nutria. Clinical signs include weakness, lethargy, anorexia, and death. Alligator ranchers and farmers are now more diligent in inquiring about the source and kill method of nutria before feeding the animals. Another phenomenon seen in captive crocodilian operations is runting. This describes the lack of growth and failure to thrive of some animals within a group. In some operations, animals are separated by size and some buildings contain only the runts. A clear size difference is observed in same-age animals between the runts and the otherwise healthy ones. These animals are not as hardy in the captive environment and are potentially more susceptible to disease. Dominance by other animals, environment, and even incubation factors[13] contribute to the presence of runts.

INTEGUMENTARY DISEASE

Integumentary disease is likely the most important process that affects captive crocodilians. The environment in which they are raised predisposes them to it, and the economic impact can be devastating. Most integumentary lesions in crocodilians usually arise from fighting. Lacerations, abscesses, and draining tracts can all be observed in captive and wild crocodilians (Figure 41-2). Consequently, these open wounds can serve as a nidus for microorganisms, especially fungi and bacteria. An additional factor in captive operations is the accumulation of fatty material in the form of slime on the surface of the water. This occurs when meat supplements are fed in addition to a commercial diet. This slime attaches to the skin of the animals and the enclosure, creating an environment for bacterial and fungal growth. A surfactant disinfectant can be used to reduce the amount of slime on the enclosure. Bacterial dermatitis can lead to septicemia and death; therefore, skin lesions must be recognized early for appropriate therapy. Fungal dermatitis is also common because many fungi thrive in the water column and environment of

Table 41-1 Bacteria Isolated from *Alligator mississippiensis* with and without Signs of Disease

Isolate	Tissue	Clinical Signs/Lesions	Reference
Aeromonas hydrophila	Blood	Yes	29
	Lungs, heart, liver, kidneys, intestines, oral cavity	Yes, no	36
	Lungs, blood	Yes	37
	Eye	Yes	38,39
	Oral cavity, water	No	40
Aeromonas sp.	Lungs	Yes	9
Acinetobacter calcoaceticus	Oral cavity	No	40
Aerobacter radiobacter	Oral cavity	No	40
Bacteroides asaccharolyticus	Oral cavity	No	40
Bacteroides bivius	Oral cavity, water	No	40
Bacteroides loescheii/denticola	Oral cavity, water	No	40
Bacteroides oralis	Oral cavity	No	40
Bacteroides sordellii	Oral cavity	No	40
Bacteroides thetaiotamicron	Oral cavity	No	40
Bacteroides vulgatus	Oral cavity	No	40
Bacteroides sp.	Water	No	40
Citrobacter freundii	Blood	Yes	42
	Oral cavity	No	40
Clostridium bifermentans	Oral cavity, water	No	40
	Lungs	Yes	9
Clostridium clostridioforme	Oral cavity	No	40
Clostridium innoculum	Water	No	40
Clostridium limosum	Oral cavity	No	40
Clostridium sordellii	Oral cavity, water	No	40
Clostridium sporogenes	Blood	Yes	9
Clostridium tetani	Oral cavity	No	40
Clostridium sp.	Blood	Yes	9
Corynebacterium sp.	Tail abscess	Yes	37
Diphtheroid sp.	Oral cavity	No	40
Edwardsiella tarda	Kidney, feces	Yes	41
	Fat body, pericardial fluid	Yes	9
Enterobacter aggiomerans	Blood	Yes	42
Enterobacter cloacae	Oral cavity, water	No	40
Enterobacillus sp.	Lungs	Yes	37
Fusobacterium nucleatum	Oral cavity	No	40
Fusobacterium varium	Oral cavity	No	40
Klebsiella oxytoca	Skin	Yes	42
	Oral cavity	No	40
Klebsiella sp.	Lungs	Yes	25
Micrococcus kristinae	Blood	Yes	29
Moraxella sp.	Oral cavity, water	No	40
Morganella morganii	Blood	Yes	42
	Oral cavity	No	40
	Lung	Yes	9
Mycoplasma alligatoris	Multiple tissues	Yes	29
Pasteurella haemolytica	Oral cavity	No	40
Pasteurella multocida	Lungs	Yes	43
Pasteurella sp.	Oral cavity, water	No	40
Peptococcus magnus	Oral cavity	No	40
Peptococcus prevotii	Oral cavity	No	40
Proteus mirabilis	Blood	Yes	29
Proteus vulgaris	Oral cavity	No	40
	Oviduct	Yes	41
	Blood	Yes	29
	Lung	Yes	9
Proteus sp.	Blood	Yes	42
Pseudomonas cepacia	Oral cavity	No	40
Pseudomonas diminuta	Water	No	40
Pseudomonas fluorescens	Water	No	40
Pseudomonas pickettii	Oral cavity	No	40
Pseudomonas vesicularis	Water	No	40

Continued

Table 41-1	Bacteria Isolated from *Alligator mississippiensis* with and without Signs of Disease—cont'd		
Isolate	Tissue	Clinical Signs/Lesions	Reference
Pseudomonas sp.	Lungs, pharynx	Yes	37
	Water	No	40
Salmonella typhimurium	Gastrointestinal tract	Yes	37
Salmonella braenderup, anatum	Cloaca	No	37
Arizona spp.			
Salmonella sp. (subgroup III)	Lung	Yes	44
Serratia marcescens	Skin	Yes	42
Serratia odorifera	Oral cavity	No	40
Staphylococcus aureus	Lungs	Yes	43
Staphylococcus cohnii	Blood	Yes	29
Streptococcus sp., hemolytic	Lungs	Yes	9
Vibrio parahaemolyticus	Blood	Yes	29

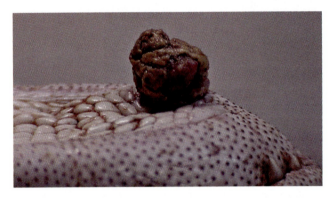

FIGURE 41-2 Mandibular lesion on a captive-reared American Alligator *(A. mississippiensis)*. This lesion involved only skin and did not affect bone.

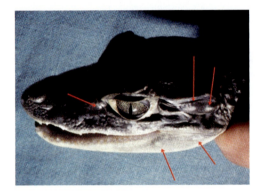

FIGURE 41-3 This caiman *(Caiman sp.)* has pox viral infection. Note the gray patches around the face and eye *(red arrows)*. (Photograph courtesy F. Frye.)

captive alligators. In most instances, both bacteria and fungi are present in skin lesions. Culture and sensitivity testing can be frustrating in these cases because of the mixed flora found in the lesions. Nonetheless, antimicrobial therapy should be instituted. Medications can be mixed in the feed to provide adequate dosage. The use of systemic antifungal medications is cost prohibitive in treatment of a large number of animals; therefore, a combination of good hygiene and water treatments with disinfectants is recommended in these situations.

A number of parasites are known to affect crocodilians. *Paratrichosoma* spp. are capillaroid parasites that cause a zigzag lesion on the skin. These lesions are cosmetic, and no evidence has been found of further pathology in affected animals. This parasite is known to affect various crocodile species in the wild and is believed to have a stage of its lifecycle dependent on soil; therefore, it is not observed in captive scenarios where animals are kept on concrete.[11] Finally, pox virus has been reported in various crocodilian species. Regardless of the etiology, good hygiene is essential in the prevention and treatment of integumentary disease in crocodilians. The etiology itself is at times not as important as what conditions predisposed them to the disease.

Dermatophilosis (Brown Spot Disease)

Dermatophilosis or "brown spot disease" causes brown to red lesions usually located between scales. These can be accompanied by ulcerative lesions and are mostly found on the ventral skin. *Dermatophilus* spp. have been implicated with these lesions. Most of the cultures appear to resemble *Dermatophilus congolensis*.[14,15] This condition has occurred in both alligator and crocodile operations. These filamentous bacteria do not respond well to antibiotic therapy in crocodilian operations; therefore, intensive hygiene practices are necessary to prevent and control outbreaks.

Pox Virus

Parapoxvirus or pox-like viruses have been identified in five different crocodilian species: Spectacled Caiman *(Caiman crocodilus fuscus)*,[16,17] Brazilian Caiman *(Caiman crocodilus yacare)*,[18] Nile Crocodile,[19,20] Saltwater Crocodile *(Crocodylus porosus)*,[21] and Freshwater Crocodile *(Crocodylus johnstoni)*.[21] In caimans, pox virus is characterized by 1- to 3-mm–diameter, gray to white, coalescing to macular skin lesions (Figure 41-3). These can be found on the head, palpebrae, maxilla, mandible, limbs, palate, tongue, and gingiva.[16-18] Other signs observed include palpebral and generalized edema. Resolution of clinical signs was observed 6 weeks after improvement of husbandry in one case[17] and after 5 months in another case with no changes in husbandry.[18]

On the other hand, lesions in crocodiles have been described as 2- to 8-mm–diameter, yellow to brown, wart-like, sometimes firm, and unraised to raised nodules with occasional shallow ulcers. These lesions can be found on the head,

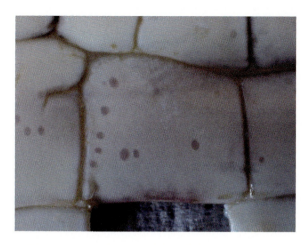

FIGURE 41-4 Gross lesions of lymphohistiocytic proliferative syndrome of alligators. These lesions are sometimes difficult to differentiate from scars and tooth marks.

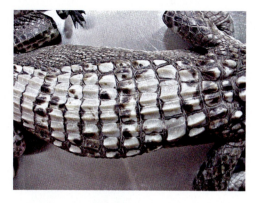

FIGURE 41-5 Skin depigmentation of a captive-reared alligator. This animal was born with normal pigmentation but started to lose pigment after 1 to 2 weeks of age.

palpebrae, nostrils, sides of the mouth, oral cavity, limbs, ventral neck, and coelom and at the root of the tail.[19,20] Resolution of lesions was reported to occur as early as 3 to 4 weeks.[19] Light microscopy reveals epithelial hyperplasia, acanthosis, hyperkeratosis, and necrosis, and at times, Borrel and Bollinger's bodies are also visible.[16-20] Secondary bacterial and fungal infections may also be present at the time of diagnosis. Horner[19] reported the use of an autogenous vaccine to treat pox virus in Nile Crocodiles. No specific treatment recommendations exist. Maintaining appropriate husbandry is essential in the prevention and resolution of pox virus in crocodilian farms.

Lymphohistiocytic Proliferative Syndrome of Alligators (PIX Disease)

Lymphohistiocytic proliferative syndrome of alligators (LPSA), also known as PIX disease, has been recently studied in captive-reared alligators from Florida and Louisiana.[22] This production problem mostly affects the quality of the hide and consequently decreases profit for farmers and ranchers. Gross lesions can be seen as multifocal, 1-mm to 2-mm, gray to red foci on the ventral mandibular, abdominal, and sometimes tail scales (Figure 41-4). They can be found on any section of a scale and do not appear concave or convex with respect to the scale's surface. Routine microscopic examination reveals dermal nodular lymphoid proliferation with perivascular cuffing. Similar lesions have also been observed in other tissues besides the skin. One of the problems with identification of the lesions is that they are sometimes not seen until the hides are removed from the animal. Therefore, antemortem identification is not very accurate at this time. The etiology of this syndrome is unknown, but various research projects are examining the possibilities.

Besides the infectious lesions observed on the integument, other potential noninfectious causes exist. A nutritional deficiency or genetics is suspected in the depigmentation of captive alligators. Some farms in Louisiana have animals that are born with normal pigmentation but start becoming white after a few weeks of life (Figure 41-5). These animals thrive well otherwise and do not appear to be runts. No erosions are associated with the lack of pigment. On palpation of the skin, it appears thinner and has a flakier nature, similar to that observed in leucystic alligators. The processing of the hides is not affected by the pigment deficit. Anecdotal reports of improvement of the condition after vitamin supplementation are found, but this has not been documented.

NEUROLOGIC DISEASE

Neurologic deficits are not commonly seen in crocodilians and deserve special attention if encountered. The most common neurologic presentation relates to the inability to swim properly. This may include swimming in circles, swimming on one side of the body, or any other abnormal swimming behavior. Out of the water, one may observe lethargy, ataxia, head tilt, and muscle tremors. However, animals may still attempt to bite so one must be cautious when handling them. Anorexia often accompanies the neurologic signs. Any infection that affects the nervous system can lead to similar presentation.

Thiamin deficiencies should be considered in animals fed a frozen fish diet. Signs typically include severe lethargy that leads to coma.

Hypoglycemia has also been reported as a cause of neurologic signs in alligators.[23] These animals have muscle tremors, loss of the righting reflex, and mydriasis. Stress seems to be the main contributing factor.

The most recent etiology to cause neurologic signs in crocodilian species is WNV.

West Nile Virus

West Nile virus is a flavivirus that was found to affect American Alligators during 2001 to 2002.[24] It has also been reported in a Nile Crocodile from Israel.[25] Alligators are believed to first contract WNV after being bitten by a mosquito. However, the current thought is that alligators can have high viremias develop and shed the virus in the feces, leading to horizontal transmission of the virus. This represents an opportunity for zoonosis in captive operations. Some suspect cases exist of alligator to human transmission. A strict building quarantine and hygiene strategies should be implemented to prevent spread to other animals in the facility and to the workers. This is now a reportable disease, and one should contact the state veterinarian and the state office of

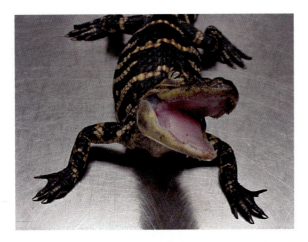

FIGURE 41-6 Young Alligator *(Alligator mississippiensis)* with the head tilt typical of those affected with West Nile virus. Notice that it still maintains an aggressive stand with the mouth open.

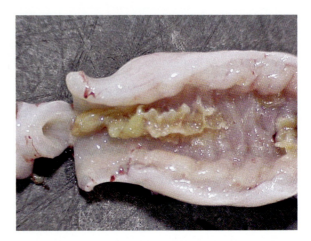

FIGURE 41-7 Enterocolitis from an alligator diagnosed with West Nile virus. This lesion appeared to cause bloating of the colon and caused difficulties for the alligator to submerge.

public health (see Chapter 79). Thoroughly cooked alligator meat should not represent a source of WNV.

Clinical signs include swimming in circles, head tilt (Figure 41-6), muscle tremors, weakness, lethargy, and anorexia. On necropsy, one may also observe evidence of aspiration and pneumonia. Proliferative enteritis has been diagnosed in a group of alligators with positive results for WNV. The colon lesions tested positive for WNV[26] (Figure 41-7). Clinically, these animals appeared bloated and were unable to submerge in the water. This was likely the result of a blockage caused by the fibrous membrane in the colon. Affected animals in captive operations have ranged in age from 1 month to more than 12 months old. In younger animals, infection is usually severe and acute with as much as a 50% mortality rate. The pattern of deaths is usually seen as a sudden onset of mortalities followed by a peak and subsequent decline in the number of deaths. However, sporadic mortalities may also be seen, especially in older animals. No proposed treatments exist for WNV other than increasing hygiene to prevent the accumulation of feces. Once the infection runs its course, the surviving animals continue to thrive. Definitive diagnosis is best accomplished with reverse transcriptase polymerase chain reaction (RT-PCR) and viral culture of brain and spinal cord. Veterinarians should take additional precautions with necropsies of suspect animals.

Respiratory Disease

This is probably one of the most common presentations of captive crocodilians, second only to integumentary disease. In a review of articles on crocodilian diseases, a fair number show lung lesions on necropsy. Respiratory signs can often be confused with neurologic signs, and a clear distinction must be established. On the other hand, respiratory disease may accompany neurologic disease as a consequence of weakness that leads to aspiration. Clinical signs associated with respiratory disease in crocodilians may include abnormal swimming (either in circles or on one side of the body), dyspnea, tachypnea, excessive basking, nasal discharge, and anorexia, among others. As these animals become weak, the basihyoid valve does not function properly and they can aspirate food or water. Because of the pharyngeal anatomy of crocodilians,

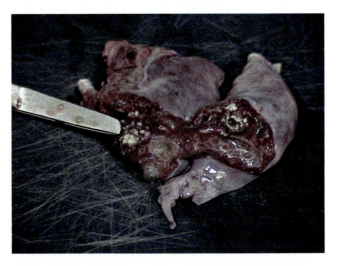

FIGURE 41-8 Caseous material within the bronchi of alligators with respiratory signs. *Klebsiella* sp. susceptible to potentiated sulfa drug was cultured from these lesions, and the animals responded to antibiotic therapy administered with feed.

aspiration is an unlikely event in healthy animals. Therefore, any evidence of it should be indicative of animals with an underlying illness. Most respiratory infections are either bacterial (Figure 41-8) or fungal in origin. A number of rhinitis and pharyngitis syndromes have also been described in some crocodilian species.[11] Fungal infections are perhaps not as commonly diagnosed but still need to be a consideration, especially for captive crocodilians. An early report showed a fungal pneumonia associated with *Beauveria bassiana* in two alligators,[27] and *Fusarium moniliforme* was found in another case.[28] Bacterial and fungal cultures should be obtained from the lungs in cases where respiratory disease is suspected. This allows a choice of appropriate treatment on the basis of sensitivity testing.

Mycoplasmosis

One well-documented respiratory pathogen is *Mycoplasma alligatoris*. Clinical signs are nonspecific and include lethargy,

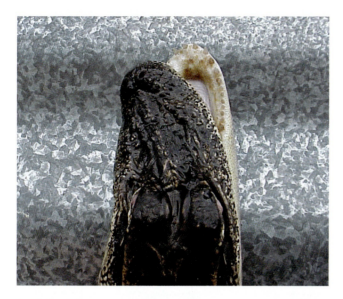

FIGURE 41-9 Congenital abnormality in an American Alligator (*Alligator mississippiensis*). This animal was hatched with this deformity and is able to eat and thrive among others in the group.

weakness, anorexia, white ocular discharge, paresis, and edema (facial, periocular, cervical, limbs).[9] Pneumonia, pericarditis, and polyarthritis can be diagnosed on necropsy. Pathogenicity of *M. alligatoris* has been documented for *A. mississippiensis* and for the Broad-nosed Caiman (*Caiman latirostris*).[29,30] Other crocodilian species closely related to alligators are also potentially susceptible. Treatment should include antimicrobial therapy. Helmick et al.[31] reviewed antimicrobial susceptibility for *M. alligatoris*. A second *Mycoplasma* species, *M. crocodyli*, is known to affect Nile Crocodiles.[10] Lesions are similar to those observed with *M. alligatoris*. Some studies have examined the use of an autogenous vaccine for *M. crocodyli*, but work is still needed to determine its true efficacy.[32,33]

Mycobacteriosis

Another bacterium of interest is *Mycobacterium* sp. Although it is not commonly diagnosed in reptiles, a number of unpublished clinical cases from alligators have shown acid-fast organisms consistent with *Mycobacterium* sp. These animals had evidence of pneumonia on necropsy as shown by multiple white foci, 1 to 4 mm in diameter, on the lung parenchyma.[26] Other cases of pulmonary and enteric mycobacterial infections are mentioned by Youngprapakorn, Ousavaplangchai, and Kanchanapangka.[34] Difficulties of growing *Mycobacterium* sp. make its definitive diagnosis a challenge.

MUSCULOSKELETAL DISEASE

Musculoskeletal disease of crocodilians is commonly seen in captive operations. Many of these are attributed to alterations in the incubation temperature or environment (Figure 41-9). The rest of the musculoskeletal disorders are likely the result of trauma from fighting (Figures 41-10 and 41-11), transport, or restraint. Limb fractures and partial amputations can be seen after altercations. In some farms, observation is possible

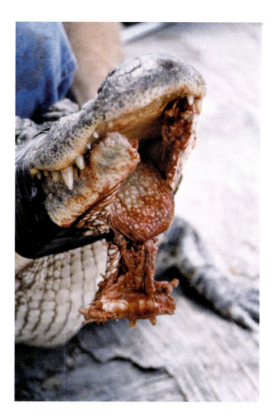

FIGURE 41-10 Mandibular fracture in a wild *A. mississippiensis*. This type of lesion is not uncommon in wild animals.

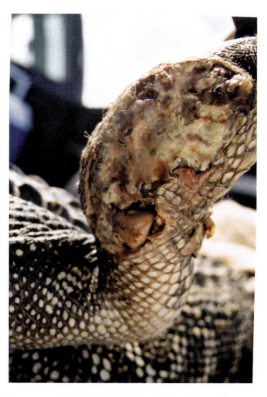

FIGURE 41-11 Rear limb lesion on a wild alligator. Tissue necrosis and part of the bone protruding through skin are seen. Wild animals can recover from these types of lesions, but they can lead to severe septicemia in captive ones.

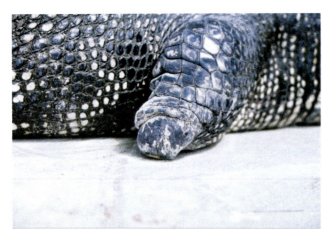

FIGURE 41-12 Wild alligator with a healed lesion that caused amputation of the distal rear limb.

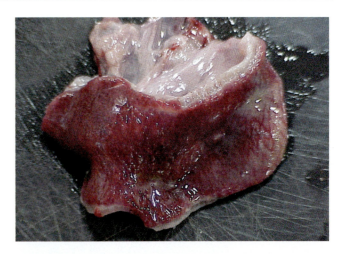

FIGURE 41-13 Enteritis in a captive-reared alligator. Notice the red mucosa.

of animals that have lost limbs after a fight and survived to the point of complete healing. Similar lesions can also be observed in wild alligators (Figure 41-12). These may also lead to nerve or muscle damage and consequent paresis or paralysis. As mentioned in the Respiratory Disease section, *M. alligatoris* and *M. crocodyli* cause polyarthritis, which can be evident antemortem.

Various metabolic bone diseases are seen in young crocodilians and may manifest in different ways depending on the cause (e.g., nutritional, renal). Weakness, lethargy, kyphosis, scoliosis, paresis, tooth decalcification, and other skeletal abnormalities can be observed in crocodilians as well. Only a small number of these abnormalities are observed in most captive operations. Those affected may be runts of the group and have other concurrent disease. This is seen less often as better and improved diets are offered to captive crocodilians. Nonetheless, some operations still may offer no source of calcium in the diet. The innate requirement of ultraviolet B light as a source of vitamin D_3 in crocodilians is not known. They appear to be able to obtain appropriate levels from their diet, but research in this area needs to be performed. The author has seen adult alligators raised in enclosed buildings and offered a pelleted diet with some meat supplement that show no evidence of metabolic disease. However, anecdotal comments from various ranchers indicate that the animals appear to thrive better if exposed to sunlight.

Gout also occurs in crocodilians as either the articular or visceral form. High protein diets, dehydration, and stress are contributing factors to its development. Clinical signs can be nonspecific in nature, but limb paresis/paralysis and joint enlargement may be observed. Ariel, Ladds, and Buenviaje[35] reported a case of gout with concurrent hypovitaminosis A in crocodile hatchlings.

Deficiencies of vitamins A, B, C, or E can also lead to a variety of musculoskeletal disorders. These are not commonly seen when commercial diets are fed in addition to meat products.

GASTROINTESTINAL DISEASE

Anorexia is likely the most common clinical sign associated with gastrointestinal disease in captive crocodilians.

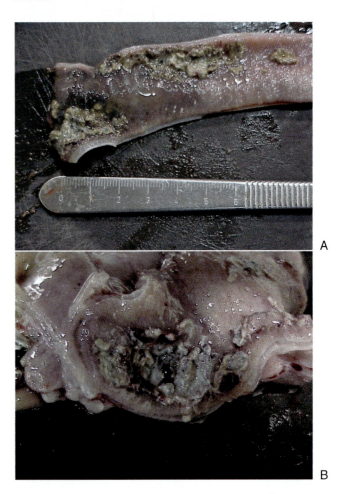

FIGURE 41-14 **A** and **B**, Fibrotic membrane on the intestinal mucosa of a captive-reared alligator. This was an incidental finding for this animal.

Foreign body ingestion, gastric ulcers, enteritis (Figure 41-13), and trauma to the oral cavity can be observed in crocodilians. Ingestion of foreign bodies is more common in wild crocodilians. However, it must also be a differential in captive specimens. Malfunction of water pumps, water filters, or construction can lead to the presence of foreign bodies in the enclosures. These can then be ingested by the animals and cause severe problems in the case of nails and other sharp objects. A more common process is likely associated with infectious enteritis or septicemia. This is difficult to assess grossly because crocodilians have very thick intestines normally. However, crocodilians appear to have a characteristic response to insult of the gastrointestinal tract. Accumulation of fibrous material or necrotizing lesions is commonly seen on necropsy (Figure 41-14). This reaction is aggressive and can even lead to obstructions caused by the fibrous material itself. Obstruction can also occur with fecal impactions and torsions. Gastric ulcerations and abnormalities of the gastric mucosa are also routinely observed on necropsy and may be associated with stress and diet. Finally, the intestinal tract contains a large amount of Peyer's patches and likely represents a site of aggressive inflammatory response to infectious agents.

REFERENCES

1. Rooney AA, Guillette LJJ: Biotic and abiotic factors in crocodilian stress: the challenge of a modern environment. In Grigg GC, Seebacher F, Franklin CE, editors: *Crocodilian biology and evolution*, Chipping Norton, 2001, Surrey Beatty and Sons.
2. Dohms JE, Metz A: Stress-mechanisms of immunosuppression, *Vet Immunol Immunopathol* 30:89-109, 1991.
3. Lance VA, Elsey RM: Plasma catecholamines and plasma corticosterone following restraint stress in juvenile alligators, *J Exp Zool* 283(6):559-565, 1999.
4. Morici LA, Elsey RM, Lance VA: Effects of long-term corticosterone implants on growth and immune function in juvenile alligators, *Alligator mississippiensis*, *J Exp Zool* 279(2): 156-162, 1997.
5. Lance VA, Elsey RM: Hormonal and metabolic response of juvenile alligators to cold shock, *J Exp Zool* 283:566-572, 1999.
6. Elsey RM, et al: Growth rate and plasma corticosterone levels in juvenile alligators maintained at different stocking densities, *J Exp Zool* 255:30-36, 1990.
7. Lance VA, Morici LA, Elsey RM: Physiology and endocrinology of stress in crocodilians. In Grigg GC, Seebacher F, Franklin CE, editors: *Crocodilian biology and evolution*, Chipping Norton, 2001, Surrey Beatty and Sons.
8. Huchzermeyer FW, et al: Aerobic intestinal flora of wild-caught African dwarf crocodiles *Osteolaemus tetraspis*, *Onderstepoort J Vet Res* 67(3):201-204, 2000.
9. Clippinger TL, et al: Morbidity and mortality associated with a new *Mycoplasma* species from captive American alligators *(Alligator mississippiensis)*, *J Zoo Wildl Med* 31(3):303-314, 2000.
10. Mohan K, et al: *Mycoplasma*-associated polyarthritis in farmed crocodiles *(Crocodylus niloticus)* in Zimbabwe, *Onderstepoort J Vet Res* 62(1):45-49, 1995.
11. Huchzermeyer FW: *Crocodiles: biology, husbandry and diseases*, Cambridge, 2003, CABI Publishing.
12. Jacobson ER, Gardiner CH, Foggin CM: Adenovirus-like infection in two Nile crocodiles, *J Am Vet Med Assoc* 185(11):1421-1422, 1984.
13. Allsteadt J, Lang JW: Incubation temperature affects body size and energy reserves of hatchling American Alligators *(Alligator mississippiensis)*, *Physiol Zoo* 68(1):76-97, 1995.
14. Buenviaje GN, et al: Isolation of *Dermatophilus* sp from skin lesions in farmed saltwater crocodiles *(Crocodylus porosus)*, *Aust Vet J* 75(5):365-367, 1997.
15. Buenviaje GN, Ladds PW, Martin Y: Pathology of skin diseases in crocodiles, *Aust Vet J* 76(5):357-363, 1998.
16. Jacobson ER, et al: Poxlike skin lesions in captive caimans, *J Am Vet Med Assoc* 175(9):937-940, 1979.
17. Penrith ML, Nesbit JW, Huchzermeyer FW: Pox virus infection in captive juvenile caimans *(Caiman crocodilus fuscus)* in South Africa, *J S Afr Vet Assoc* 62(3):137-139, 1991.
18. Ramos MC, et al: Poxvirus dermatitis outbreak in farmed Brazilian caimans *(Caiman crocodilus yacare)*, *Aust Vet J* 80(6):371-372, 2002.
19. Horner RF: Poxvirus in farmed Nile crocodiles, *Vet Rec* 122(19):459-462, 1990.
20. Pandey GS, et al: Poxvirus infection in Nile crocodiles *(Crocodylus niloticus)*, *Res Vet Sci* 49(2):171-176, 1990.
21. Buenviaje GN, Ladds PW, Melville L: Poxvirus infection in two crocodiles, *Aust Vet J* 69(1):15-16, 1992
22. Nevarez JG, et al: Lymphohistiocytic proliferative syndrome of captive reared American Alligators *(Alligator mississippiensis)* from Louisiana, *Proc Tenth Ann Conf Assoc Rept Amphib Vet* Minneapolis, Minn, 2003.
23. Wallach JD, Hoessle C, Bennett J: Hypoglycemic shock in captive alligators, *J Am Vet Med Assoc* 151(7):893-896, 1967.
24. Miller DL, et al: West Nile virus in farmed alligators, *Emerg Infect Dis* 9(7):794-799, 2003.
25. Steinman A, et al: West Nile virus infection in crocodiles, *Emerg Infect Dis* 9(7):887-889, 2003.
26. Nevarez JG: *Case series*. Louisiana, 2002-03, unpublished data.
27. Fromtling RA, et al: Fatal *Beauveria bassiana* infection in a captive American alligator, *J Am Vet Med Assoc* 175(9):934-936, 1979.
28. Frelier PF, Sigler L, Nelson PE: Mycotic pneumonia caused by *Fusarium moniliforme* in an alligator, *Sabouraudia* 23(6):399-402, 1985.
29. Brown DR, et al: Pathology of experimental mycoplasmosis in American alligators, *J Wildl Dis* 37(4):671-679, 2001.
30. Pye GW, et al: Experimental inoculation of Broad-Nosed Caimans *(Caiman latirostris)* and Siamese Crocodiles *(Crocodylus siamensis)* with *Mycoplasma alligatoris*, *J Zoo Wildl Med* 32(2):196-201, 2001.
31. Helmick KE, et al: In vitro susceptibility pattern of *Mycoplasma alligatoris* from symptomatic American Alligators *(Alligator mississippiensis)*, *J Zoo Wildl Med* 33(2):108-111, 2002.
32. Mohan K, et al: Vaccination of farmed crocodiles *(Crocodylus niloticus)* against *Mycoplasma crocodyli* infection, *Vet Rec* 141(18):476, 1997.
33. Mohan K, et al: Vaccination to control an outbreak of *Mycoplasma crocodyli* infection, *Onderstepoort J Vet Res* 68(2):149-150, 2001.
34. Youngprapakorn P, Ousavaplangchai L, Kanchanapangka S: *A color atlas of diseases of the crocodile*, Thailand, Style Creative House.
35. Ariel E, Ladds PW, Buenviaje GN: Concurrent gout and suspected hypovitaminosis A in crocodile hatchlings, *Aust Vet J* 75(4):247-249, 1997.
36. Gorden RW, et al: Isolation of *Aeromonas hydrophila* from the American alligator, *Alligator mississippiensis*, *J Wildl Dis* 15(2):239-243, 1979.
37. Shotts EB Jr, et al: *Aeromonas*-induced deaths among fish and reptiles in an eutrophic inland lake, *J Am Vet Med Assoc* 161(6):603-607, 1972.
38. Millichamp NJ, Jacobson ER, Wolf ED: Diseases of the eye and ocular adnexae in reptiles, *J Am Vet Med Assoc* 183(11):1205-1212, 1983.
39. Jacobson ER: Immobilization, blood sampling, necropsy techniques and diseases of crocodilians: a review, *J Zoo An Med* 15:38-45, 1984.
40. Flandry F, et al: Initial antibiotic therapy for alligator bites: characterization of the oral flora of *Alligator mississippiensis*, *South Med J* 82(2):262-266, 1989.

41. Wallace LJ, Gore WFH: Isolation of *Edwardsiella tarda* from a sea lion and two alligators, *J Am Vet Med Assoc* 149(7):881-883, 1966.
42. Novak SS, Seigel RA: Gram-negative septicemia in American alligators *(Alligator mississippiensis)*, *J Wildl Dis* 22(4):484-487, 1986.
43. Mainster ME, et al: Treatment of multiple cases of *Pasteurella multocida* and staphylococcal pneumonia in *Alligator mississippiensis* on a herd basis, *Proc Am Assoc Zoo Vet* 33-36, 1972.
44. Brown DR, et al: *Mycoplasma alligatoris* sp. nov., from American alligators, *Int J Syst Evol Microbiol* 51(Pt 2):419-424, 2001.

Section VII
SPECIFIC DISEASES AND CLINICAL CONDITIONS

42
ABSCESSES

DOUGLAS R. MADER

Abscesses are found in all species, although their presentation may vary. In mammals, the result of abscessation is usually a purulent liquefied exudate. In reptiles, however, abscesses take on an entirely different form.

An abscess is defined as a localized collection of purulent material (pus) in a confined cavity formed by the disintegration of tissues. In mammals, this pus is often a milky, variably colored exudates composed of primarily degenerate or toxic neutrophils, macrophages, lymphocytes, serum, and liquefied necrotic tissue. In reptiles, the heterophils possess a different killing mechanism than that seen in mammals. The exact pathway is not known, but the oxidative pathways seen in the mammalian neutrophil do not exist. As a result, the reptilian abscess is usually not liquefied (Figure 42-1). Reptilian pus is caseous, forming hard, "cheese-like" plugs that are nearly impenetrable to antimicrobial therapy. Typical presentation of a reptilian abscess is lamellar, similar in appearance to a cross-sectional cut through an onion (Figure 42-2). Most reptilian abscesses not only are solid but also are well encapsulated (see Figure 42-2).

INCITING CAUSES

Many causes are found for abscesses. Pyogenic organisms (bacteria, fungi, parasites) or foreign bodies embedded in tissue can lead to the formation of the exudates. If the organisms are not cleared or removed from the body, accumulation of the exudates stimulates the formation of a fibrinous capsule. In mammals, the increase in pressure from accumulation of the purulent exudate may ultimately result in the abscess rupturing, either externally (skin) or internally (intestinal, peritoneal). If a prolonged abscess is present, rather than rupture, a rigid fibrous wall forms around the abscess. If this occurs, eventual healing of the lesion requires filling of the evacuated cavity with granulation tissue. If the inciting cause (organism, foreign body) is not totally removed, a chronic or intermittent discharge or abscess recurrence is likely.

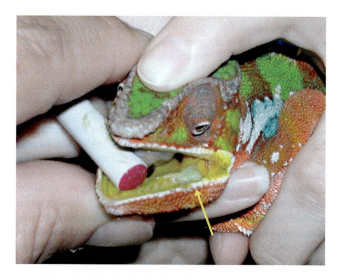

FIGURE 42-1 This Panther Chameleon (*Chamaeleo pardalis*), as is commonly seen in chameleons, has an abscess in the gland at the commissure of its mouth. In this case, the greenish purulent exudate is paste-like, rather than the more common caseous material normally seen in reptiles.

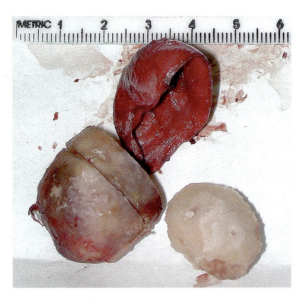

FIGURE 42-2 Most reptilian abscesses are hard, wax-like masses *(bottom two objects)*. On cut surface, they have a lamellar appearance. They are typically surrounded by a thick fibrous capsule *(top)*.

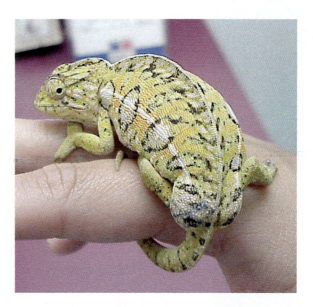

FIGURE 42-3 Abscesses most often occur as a result of trauma, as in this chameleon. Two large bilateral abscesses are seen over the pelvis of this animal as a result of the bite of a cage mate.

Abscesses can be found throughout the body. The portal for entry of the pathogenic organisms can be the skin, the gastrointestinal tract, or the lungs. Once inside the body, hematogenous spread can disseminate the pathogens to the internal organs, tissues, retrobulbar regions, and the brain.

Reptiles are exposed to pathogens on a regular basis. Bites, scratches, and environmental trauma can all predispose these animals to abscess formation (Figure 42-3). Healthy animals can withstand minor insults with no prolonged effects. However, as is often the case with captive reptiles, an immunocompromised individual is more prone to disease development.

Foreign bodies such as plant material (thorns, bark) and other manmade products (plastics, metals) can all lead to abscess formation.

Pyogenic organisms can vary, and bacteria (aerobic and anaerobic), fungi, and parasites (protozoan and metazoan) may all be involved. Bites from prey are a frequent source for anaerobic infections. *Nocardia*, *Clostridium*, and mycobacteria have also been isolated.

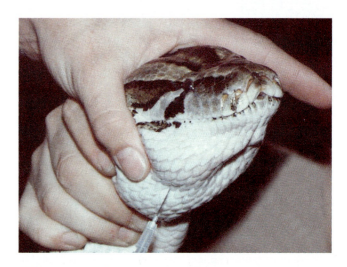

FIGURE 42-4 Cellulitis is a deep diffuse suppurative infection in areas of low oxygen tension that can have a similar presentation to large abscesses but does not have the solid core center. An attempt is being made to aspirate the core contents in this Burmese Python *(Python molurus bivitattus)* with "cephalic cellulitis."

CLINICAL SIGNS

All reptiles are susceptible to abscess formation. No age or sex predilections exist. Husbandry factors seem to play a significant role in the development of abscesses. Poor lighting, inadequate temperature regulation, nutritional deficiencies, and overcrowding are common factors.

Swelling is the hallmark of abscess formation. Unlike what is noted in mammals, heat and erythema are *not* associated with the development of an abscess in the reptile patient. Fever, as seen in mammals, also is not a part of the reptilian clinical disease. Behavioral fever may be involved but is beyond the scope of this discussion (see Chapter 36).

Depending on the organ system involved, the clinical signs may vary. Cutaneous or subcutaneous abscesses manifest as obvious, generally localized, swellings. Cellulitis, a deep diffuse suppurative infection in areas of low oxygen tension, can have a similar presentation to large abscesses but does not have the solid core center (Figure 42-4).

Internal abscesses can have varying clinical signs depending on the organ system involved. Intestinal and hepatic abscess may have gradual wasting, brain abscess with neurologic signs, pulmonary abscesses with evidence of respiratory difficulty, etc. (Figure 42-5).

DIAGNOSIS

The differential diagnoses include any "mass lesions," such as tumors, hematomas, scar tissue, and parasitic cysts. Pain on palpation (not always obvious), internal structure (fluid-filled versus solid), and previous history help with the determination.

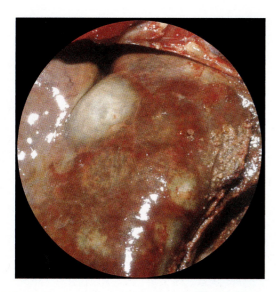

FIGURE 42-5 Abscesses can be internal, such as the lesions seen here on this liver. Animals that are "poor doers" benefit from endoscopy, the best way to diagnose internal abscessation.

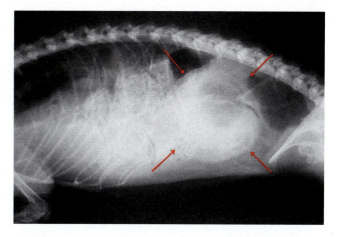

FIGURE 42-6 Radiographs are helpful in diagnosis of internal abscesses. Note the typical lamellar appearance of this coelomic abscess (*between the red arrows*).

Laboratory analysis has limited use in the diagnosis of an abscess. A complete blood count (CBC) and a serum chemistry analysis are usually unremarkable. Animals with generalized abscessation may have normal values, whereas apparently normal animals may have a leukocytosis.

Aspiration of the mass, including cytology and bacterial culture/sensitivity testing, again may have questionable results. Cytology usually reveals amorphous debris. Because of the solid nature of the abscesses, exfoliative cytology is usually nonproductive. Stains should include Gram, Wright's-Giemsa, acid-fast (mycobacteria and *Nocardia*), and periodic acid shift (fungal).

Culture results are usually negative, especially if routine culture techniques are used. Culture submissions can be enhanced with anaerobic and fungal evaluations. Sample collection should be from the inner lining of the fibrous capsule, not the center of the lesion, because the center has often outgrown any blood supply and rarely produces positive culture results.

Radiography, ultrasonography, and advanced imaging, such as magnetic resonance imaging (MRI) or computed tomography (CT), can all be used to help evaluate the presence of internal abscesses (Figure 42-6).

TREATMENT

The key to successful treatment of the reptilian abscess is complete removal of the abscess cavity and surrounding fibrous capsule. Simple lancing and curettage, or removal of the internal caseous material, is not enough to prevent recurrence. Once the abscess capsule has been removed, the wound is left open to heal by secondary intention and granulation. Healing times vary depending on many factors but in general can take anywhere from 4 to 6 weeks. Scar tissue ensues but usually shrinks over time, leaving minimal changes to the skin. See the series in Figure 42-7, *A-L*, to follow excision and healing of a typical large reptilian abscess.

Unlike mammals, in which lancing, and in some cases, placement of a drain, is enough to facilitate healing, the reptilian abscess needs thorough debridement. In most cases, this may mean general anesthesia. A small abscess can be potentially treated with local analgesia (lidocaine, bupivacaine). Caution must be taken not to accidentally overdose small patients with the analgesic (for example, local infiltration should not exceed 10 mg/kg of lidocaine).

Laser ablation of the abscess bed helps sterilize any material left behind after the debridement. Daily topical debridement and application with an iodine-based solution chemically cauterizes any bacteria that remain on the surface.

Antibiotic therapy, preferably based on bacteriologic culture and sensitivity data, is an essential adjunct to surgical debridement. Antibiotics vary in ability to penetrate abscesses or work in anaerobic or acidic environments. **Amikacin and enrofloxacin, two of the most commonly used antibiotics in reptilian medicine, are generally ineffective in the treatment of abscesses.**

Chloramphenicol, a lipophilic bacteriostatic antibiotic, effectively penetrates tissue that is inaccessible to many other antibiotics. It is effective in both anaerobic and acidic conditions. It has a limited spectrum of activity, so its use should be based on supportive bacterial sensitivity testing. Other medications that may prove useful in the treatment of abscesses include potentiated penicillins (e.g., amoxicillin/clavulanic acid), trimethoprim-sulfa, and metronidazole, and some of the newer generation cephalosporins and flouroquinolones can be considered. Drug dosages for these medications have not been established pharmacokinetically, so their use is empirical. See Chapter 89 for drug dosages.

FOLLOW-UP

Drug therapies should continue for a minimum of 14 days. Recheck evaluations are recommended at that time, and the medication can be continued pending the results of the examination. Owners must keep the abscess site clean and debrided on a daily basis during the treatment period.

Underlying deficiencies in husbandry practices must be corrected to prevent future occurrence of disease. The owner should be given a cautiously optimistic prognosis, with the potential for possible recurrence of the abscess or development of new lesions at different locations.

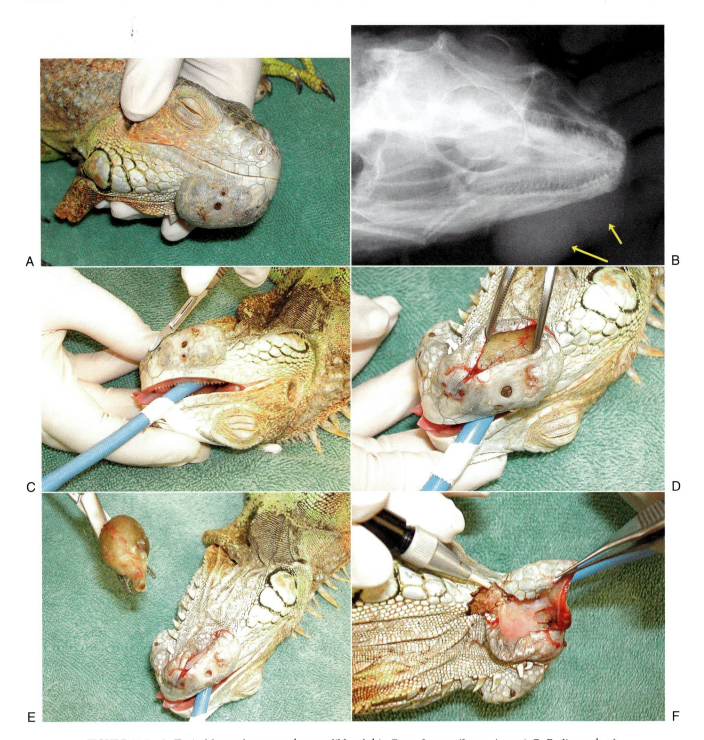

FIGURE 42-7 **A**, Typical large abscess on the mandible of this Green Iguana *(Iguana iguana)*. **B**, Radiograph of patient in **A**. Note the soft tissue swelling *(yellow arrows)*. No involvement is found in the osseous structures of the mandible, which suggests a more favorable prognosis. **C**, The patient is anesthetized, and the area is aseptically prepared. The abscess is incised along the long axis. **D**, The abscess is spread, exposing the caseous plug inside. **E**, As is typical, the abscess "shells out" with little effort. At this point, a bacterial culture should be collected from the inside of the capsule, not the caseous plug. **F**, With a CO_2 laser, the entire wall and capsule of the abscess is excised in toto.

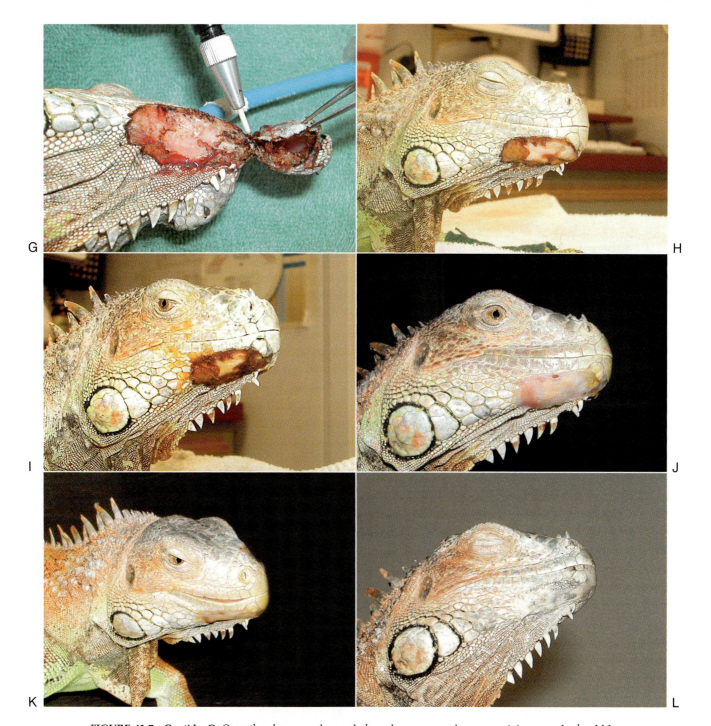

FIGURE 42-7—Cont'd G, Once the abscess and capsule have been removed, any remaining capsule should be peeled off or laser ablated to remove any residual bacteria. **H,** Patient appearance 2 days after surgery. Appropriate analgesics and antibiotics should be administered as long as is needed. **I,** Patient appearance 14 days after surgery. **J,** Near-healed surgical scar 21 days after surgery. **K,** Patient 16 weeks after surgery. Note that the surgical wound has almost completely healed, but minor stricturing is seen of the surrounding tissue, with pulling the lip down and exposing the mandibular gingiva. **L,** Patient 6 months after surgery. The wound has healed, the stricturing has self-corrected, and the pigment has returned. Aggressive surgical debridement is the key to successful management of the reptilian abscess.

43
ACARIASIS
KEVIN T. FITZGERALD and REBECCA VERA

"Ticks gotta eat, too!"

LENNY BRUCE

Life has assumed an awesome variety of forms and strategies. Species interact with an astonishing degree of complexity. *Prey* species provide sustenance and nutrition for *predators*. *Commensal* organisms live together to the obvious overall advantage of neither. For *symbiotic* species, both animals prosper from the relationship. The *parasite* (loosely from the Greek meaning "one who eats at another's table") lives at the expense of *host* animals and can often bring them harm.[1]

Captivity introduces a whole new dimension to parasitism. In captivity, commensal organisms can become pathogenic, and normally relatively harmless parasites can become much more virulent and even cause disease and death.[2] Captive animals may endure a potentially disastrous array of stressors. Neglect, crowding, starvation, unhygienic conditions, low temperatures, and introduction of diseased individuals can all tremendously predispose captive reptiles to the ravages of parasitism. In addition, the captive environment can concentrate parasite numbers to incredible levels by providing conditions and microhabitats powerfully favorable to the parasite and from which the captive reptile cannot escape. Thus, we may see parasite burdens in captive animals that rarely, if ever, are witnessed in wild free-living populations.

Captive reptiles are commonly presented to private practitioners for a variety of ectoparasites. Acarids (ticks and mites) are the parasites most commonly seen.[3-5] Mites and ticks have been reported in both wild and captive reptiles.[6-8] Infestation with ticks and mites is known as *Acariasis*. Parasitism by ticks and mites has been linked to a variety of problems ranging from simple itching and discomfort to dermatitis, anemia, failure to thrive, and the possible transmission of blood-borne pathogens.[9,10] Any level of infestation should be regarded as serious and promptly treated. These parasites can be difficult to eliminate and expensive to treat and have a high incidence rate of recurrence.[11-13] For treatment to be truly successful, the parasites must also be totally eradicated from the environment.[13,14]

This discussion examines the biology, life cycle, and pathogenic nature of the parasites and focuses on the clinical signs, diagnosis, treatment, prevention, and zoonotic potential of acarid parasites of captive reptiles.

PATHOGENESIS AND PARASITE NATURAL HISTORY

Although spiders are the best-known arachnids, ticks and mites are also members of this class. Larval ticks and mites have three pairs of legs, and nymphs and adults have four pairs. The head, thorax, and abdomen of ticks and mites are fused, and antennae and mandibles are absent in these creatures.[15]

Infestation with ticks and mites invariably can be traced to unsanitary conditions, poor husbandry practices, and recent imports of unquarantined diseased animals.[16,17] The snake mite, *Ophionyssus natricis* (Parasitiformes, Macronyssidae), is the most commonly found mite in reptiles. It normally infests snakes but can also be found in captive lizards. *Ophionyssus acertinus*, found on lizards, is usually red and larger than the black snake mite (Figure 43-1). More than 250 other species of mites also can parasitize reptiles. Trombiculid or "chigger" mites can also infect reptiles, but they are only parasitic in the

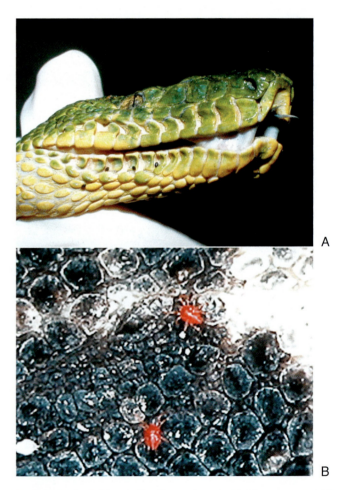

FIGURE 43-1 **A,** This python has snake mites *(Ophionyssus natricis)* in the labial pits. **B,** These red mites *(Ophionyssus acertinus)* are on the skin of a Chuckwalla *(Sauromalus* sp.).

larval form[15,18]; adults are free-living. Also, larval trombiculid mites ingest lymph or dissolved tissue rather than blood. In general, mites that infect reptiles are formidable blood-sucking pests, and infestations may be huge, with hosts supporting up to 10,000 mites.[19]

Seven genera of ticks are able to parasitize reptiles.[7] Both soft and hard ticks are found in snakes, lizards, and turtles.[15] The soft ticks tend to live in nests and burrows where they surreptitiously feed on unsuspecting hosts. Hard ticks live in fields or scrub areas where they lie in wait for passing hosts. Despite these differences in behavior, all ticks are blood-sucking parasites. Nevertheless, ticks rarely occur in numbers large enough to cause serious blood loss and anemia. Hard ticks of the genera *Ixodes, Hyalomma, Haemaphysalis, Amblyomma,* and *Aponomma* have been documented in various reptiles.[15] Many of these hard ticks are host specific. Soft-bodied ticks of two genera *Argasidae* and *Ornithodoros* have been found to infest snakes, lizards, and chelonians. Likewise for the soft ticks, some are host specific and some are not. The soft tick *Ornithodoros talaje* has been reported to transmit the filariid worm *Macdonaldius oschei* to snakes.[20,21] The major concern regarding ticks as parasites is their potential for transmitting a large number of microbial diseases to host animals. In addition, ticks can be responsible for toxicosis associated with their bites, inflict painful bites, result in significant blood loss in certain conditions, and cause a general unthriftiness linked to large tick burdens known as "tick worry."[15] In general, because ticks are considerably larger than mites and as a result are more conspicuous to owners, they are much more likely to be noticed and removed before serious conditions or life-threatening anemias develop. The following information is taken from the seminal work of Camin; recent publications by Wozniak, DeNardo, and others; and the excellent articles by Burridge on eradication of exotic ticks.

The life cycle of the snake mite, *Ophionyssus natricis,* consists of egg, larva, protonymph, deutonymph, and adult stages.[22] One molt occurs between each immature stage. These are blood-feeding mesostigmatid mites. They possess stigmata (respiratory pores) in the middle of their bodies. The life cycle is short (7 to 16 days), which lends itself well to the rapid establishment of dense populations.[22] The mites in the adult and protonymph stages are parasitic and feed on the blood of reptiles. Larva and the deutonymph are nonfeeding, free-living stages. Because of their morphology and behavior, snake mites are believed to have evolved from or share a common lineage with mammalian mites, parasites of the genus *Steatonyssus.*[22] The snake mite has been described as a typical nest parasite. Cages and captive enclosures provide a nearly perfect nest-like environment. These mites thrive on most snakes and many lizards.[13,14]

The eggs of snake mites are frequently laid in sticky clusters on the inner surface of the cage lid, the hide box, or other cage furniture–concealed spots. Eggs are off-white to tan and ovoid and darken at one pole as they mature. They are visible to the naked eye and vary from 300 to 400 µm in length and 200 to 300 µm in width. Unfertilized eggs are somewhat smaller than fertile ones. Embryonic development within the eggs is temperature dependent and doubles with each 5° increase between 20°C and 30°C (68°F to 86°F). At 25°C (77°F), the interval between hatching is only 40 to 50 hours. At temperatures higher than 40°C (104°F), the eggs rapidly desiccate. Eggs hatch into larvae at relative humidities of 85% and higher.

Snake mite larvae are small, fragile, white, nonfeeding, six-legged mites about 400 µm long. Developing fourth legs are visible under the lateral integument caudal to the third leg. Larvae generally remain at the hatch site until they molt into the parasitic protonymphs. Progression to the protonymph stage takes 18 to 24 hours at a temperature of 25°C to 30°C (77°F to 86°F). A relative humidity of at least 75% is necessary. Desiccation, and the resultant ineffective molting, is the major cause of larval mortality.

Protonymphs are similar to larvae in size but have four pairs of legs and well-developed chelicerae. Unfed protonymphs are aggressive blood-feeding mites. Unfed protonymphs often congregate on cage furniture and swarm on any disturbance in the cage, including the reptile occupant, the cleaning utensils, and the hands of the keeper. On contact with a reptile host, they crawl under the scales or around the eyes and commence feeding. The period from attachment to complete engorgement is 3 to 7 days at 25°C (77°F). Engorged protonymphs drop from the host and congregate on dark rough surfaces shielded from light. The period from molting to the deutonymph stage is 12 to 48 hours after engorgement. Protonymphs can persist in the cage environment for up to 31 days without feeding. Molting requires 12 to 48 hours after engorgement and is temperature dependent. Roughly 10% of protonymphs become trapped in the old skin and die.

Deutonymphs are active nonfeeding free-living mites. Usually deutonymphs are found within or on the cage but seldom on the host reptile. The chelicerae of the deutonymph stage are believed to be unable to pierce the skin of host animals. This stage lasts only 24 to 26 hours at 25°C (77°F). Deutonymphs destined to become males are often found riding those destined to become females. Typically they are dark red to black in color and are the same size as engorged protonymphs or unfed adults of either gender. As much as 10% of the deutonymphs become entrapped in the old skin and die even with optimal environmental conditions.

Adult snake mites are active, blood-feeding, and sexually dimorphic. With microscopic visualization, the dorsal and ventral surfaces are covered with a series of scleritized plates and appear hairy. Unfed adults are active mites, can move rapidly, and search incessantly for hosts. Like protonymphs, the adult stage mites feed on the less keratinized skin between and underneath the scales. Engorgement requires 4 to 8 days at 25°C (77°F). Adult males feed but are only slightly wider than unfed males. Engorged females are dark red to black, can exceed 1300 micrometers in length, and are rounded caudally. Variation in color depends on density of ingested erythrocytes and degree of blood meal digestion. Females can ingest up to 1500% of their body weight in host blood with each feeding.

After engorgement, females tend to crawl upward in search of dark moist concealed areas for oviposition. Adult female mites feed two to three times at 1-week to 2-week intervals. After each feeding, the female produces approximately 20 eggs in a sticky cluster. Pairing off and mating take place only before the first adult blood meal and are dependent on the size of the female. Males mate with several females before and after engorgement. Once a female weighs greater than 0.15 mg, males are no longer attracted to her. Blood-fed females reattach and feed once their body weight drops to 0.30 milligrams, so only newly matured females are likely to be bred. Mated females have been shown to lay both fertilized and unfertilized eggs. Fertilized eggs develop into females, and unfertilized eggs become males parthenogenetically. These strategies in egg development result in cyclic shifts in the sex ratios of adult mites. The episodic outbreaks of mites probably represents cycles in which the predominant mites are the more conspicuous, larger, blood-engorged females. With the right temperature and humidity, adult mites can live up to 40 days with or without feeding.

Attached mites try to remain concealed under a scale until engorgement is complete. Blood feeding in snake mites is a diphasic process. A prolonged period of slow ingestion is followed by a brief period, 1 to 2 days, of rapid engorgement at the end of the feeding cycle. Engorgement takes 3 to 7 days in protonymphs and 4 to 8 days in adults.

The mouthpart of ticks and blood-feeding mites consists of a pair of chelicerae on either side of a central peg-like hypostome. The chelicerae create a penetrating wound while the hypostome is inserted into the skin and acts as a hold-fast. Blood and interstitial fluid of the host are absorbed through feeding channels between the chelicerae and hypostome and taken into the stomach-like midgut. Blood is pulled through these channels with capillary action driven by the activity of a pharyngeal pump. This type of feeding by mites (telmophagy) is much different from that used by mosquitoes and other insects that simply penetrate and feed directly from intact blood vessels (solenophagy). Digestion of blood appears to be an intracellular process similar in both mites and ticks.[23] The hypostome of mites lacks the tooth-like denticles of ticks that make feeding mites tremendously vulnerable to mechanical detachment. Mites detached before full engorgement rapidly attempt to reattach and complete feeding, which helps explain the tremendous potential of mites as a mechanical vector for blood-borne pathogens.

The activity and behavior of snake mites depend on a variety of environmental factors. Temperature, relative humidity, odor, gravity, contact, and light all tremendously influence mite behavior. Snake mites stop and congregate in areas of ambient temperatures between 20°C and 23°C (68°F and 73°F). Orthokinesis of mites (rate of locomotion) is directly related to temperature. Higher rates of motion are seen with higher temperatures. Klinokinesis (rate of turning) increases at temperatures either below 20°C (68°F) or higher than 24°C (76°F). Between 20°C and 23°C mites move in a relatively straight line, but after leaving the 20°C to 23°C range, mites rapidly turn and usually come back into the 20°C to 23°C range again. Most stages of mite are akinetic below 10°C (46°F); however, fed females are akinetic at 2°C (35°F), and unfed females become akinetic at 6°C (37°F). Larval stages are akinetic at all temperatures. The thermal death point (where all stages die after a 5-second exposure) is 50°C to 55°C (122°F to 131°F).

Humidity affects hatching success (no hatch if relative humidity is less than 50%), molting success (less than 50% molt if humidity drops to less than 50%), and behavior of snake mites. At 95% humidity, mites become akinetic. Rate of turning (or klinokinesis) increases as mites move away from 95% in an attempt to bring them back to preferred areas of high humidity. Although mites have a marked preference for areas of high relative humidity, they are exceedingly capable of drowning in a drop of water.

Snake mites are able to distinguish between various odors. Snake mites are attracted to a live snake but not to a dead snake, a live mouse, or a human. They are unable, however, to differentiate snake blood from frog blood. Incredibly, snake mites show a preference for snake blood over snake feces, snake skin, or coagulated snake blood. These odor chemosensory receptors are located at the tips of tarsi.

Snake mites are negatively geotactic, meaning they prefer to move upward. They climb rather than go around. When they reach the tops of objects, they typically become akinetic.

For mites to become akinetic and feed, the anterior of the dorsum must be at least partially covered. If snake skin is stretched to remove the overlap of scale over skin, attached mites starve.

Snake mites possess a strong klinokinetic response (rate of turning) to light. Mites move straight in darkness, and when leaving a shaded area, they turn and return to darker areas. Orthokinesis (rate of movement) is unaffected by light intensity. This negative phototactic response is variable and directly correlated to the degree of engorgement. Fully engorged females take a straight path directly away from light, and unfed female avoidance routes can be circuitous. For environmental stimuli in general, snake mites are most akinetic in darkness and in relative humidity of 95%. Intense light stimulates a marked negative phototactic response, gravity provokes a negative geotaxis, and diffuse light and heat are strong influences of activity and behavior.

In summary, the life cycle of the snake mite *Ophionyssus natricis* is as follows. After mating and engorgement with the blood of the host, adult females leave the snake and search for a dark moist concealed site suitable for oviposition. Here they lay their clutch of sticky white eggs. The soft larvae hatch, do not feed, and remain in the hatching area. Larvae molt into the parasitic protonymph stage, and once their skin hardens, they leave the hatching site in search of host animals. Once a host is found, they conceal and attach themselves under the host's scales and commence feeding. If hosts are not found, the nymphs climb onto objects and await passing reptiles. After engorgement, protonymphs leave the host and seek refuges and microhabitats similar to those inhabited by gravid females. Males and females may pair up now until they mature. After another molt, they become nonfeeding deutonymphs. After another molt, they become adults, breed, and once again become more active. The adult mites seek hosts in the environment, conceal themselves under the scales, and begin a blood meal. After dropping off the host, the female can lay 60 to 80 eggs during the next week or two, feeding perhaps two to three times. Females that are unmated produce male eggs parthenogenetically. The duration of snake mite life cycle stages is summarized in Table 43-1.

Larvae of trombiculid mites (chiggers) are parasitic, but nymphs and adults are free-living. These mite larvae (family Trombiculidae) are bright red to orange and six-legged and in other species (cats, dogs, birds, sheep) are intensely pruritic. Chiggers remain on the skin for several days unless dislodged by the actively itching host. The saliva of the mite is injected into the skin, and the cells of the host disintegrate. This resultant necrotic material ("soup") is taken back into the mite as food. Thus, the meal chiggers obtain is not blood but rather dissolved tissue and lymph.

Table 43-1	Duration of Snake Mite Life Cycle Stages at 20°C to 30°C
Egg incubation	28-98 hours
Larval stage (free-living)	18-47 hours
Protonymph stage (parasitic)	3-14 days
Deutonymph stage (free-living)	13-26 hours
Adult stage (parasitic)	10-32 days

Females can lay up to 60-80 eggs after 2-3 feedings.
Unfed nymphs can live for 15-19 days awaiting a meal (perhaps up to 40 days with the right conditions).
Unmated females may parthenogenetically produce male eggs.
Male mites do feed but are much smaller than females.

Understanding the natural history of the snake mite can also help in predicting animals at risk. Although snakes are the most common host for *O. natricis*, some lizards are also vulnerable. On account of the need for mites to have their dorsum in contact with some object for feeding, smooth-scaled lizard species such as Geckos are at low risk for mite infestation. Species with a high requirement for humid environments such as tropical boids are good candidates for mite infestation because the mites thrive at higher relative humidity.

Ticks use a different anatomic strategy than mites to secure their attachment. The anchoring piece or hypostome of ticks is armed with backward projecting teeth, and the chelicerae possess moveable denticles. These structures make dislodging ticks much more difficult than dislodging mites. The soft ticks live in nests, burrows, and sleeping places of their host species. The life stages consist of the egg, larva, two or more nymphal stages, and adult male and female ticks. Unlike hard ticks, which need several days to complete engorgement and feed only once during each stage, adult soft ticks feed to completion in hours or minutes on sleepy hosts and may feed repeatedly. Females lay a clutch after each blood meal. Soft tick larvae feed for several days. Hard tick larvae, nymphs, and adults each feed only once, but several days are necessary for complete engorgement. Eggs are laid in a single clutch and may number in the hundreds. Unlike mites, unfed larvae, nymphs, and adults of many tick species can survive for months without a blood meal. For this reason, treatment of ticks is always necessary. To simply "wait them out" is not advisable. Various ticks parasitize reptiles in North America; among them are *Amblyomma dissimili*, the Iguana tick; *Aponomma elaphensis* for which the Trans-Pecos Ratsnake *(Bogertophis subocularis)* is the sole host; and *Amblyomma tuberculatum*, the Gopher Tortoise tick.[24] The Gopher Tortoise tick is the largest hard tick, with engorged females reaching a length of nearly 25 mm.

CLINICAL SIGNS

Infestations with ticks and mites can cause a variety of health problems in captive reptiles. Anorexia, dermatitis, pruritus, anemia, septicemia, dysecdysis, retained eye caps, failure to thrive, dehydration, and the potential for the transmission of blood-borne pathogens all have been attributed to tick and mite infections in captive animals. Some of the most common clinical signs associated with ectoparasites in these reptiles include behavioral changes. Snakes may remain coiled in

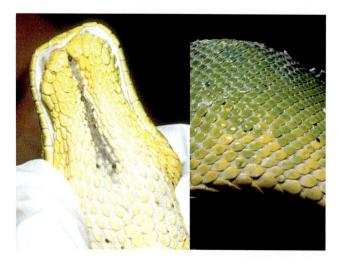

FIGURE 43-2 Snake mites are commonly found between the gular folds, around the eyes, in the labial pits, under the scales, and around the cloaca.

water bowls and soak for inordinate periods in an attempt to rid themselves of pests. Animals also may become hyperactive in cages or frequently rub against cage furniture to try to eradicate the parasites. Persistent or recurrent dysecdysis in snakes may signal mite infestation.[16,17] Typically, frequent ecdysis and shedding problems are not observed in lizards affected by mites. However, even if animals can successfully shed irritated ectoparasite-infected skin, they are quickly reinfested within the confines of the cage.

Although ticks and mites are both hematophagous, only mites in heavy infestations can consume enough host blood to cause life-threatening anemias.

Ticks are capable of inflicting such blood loss, but because they are much larger, owners are likely to notice them long before serious anemia results.

Mite-infested animals have a dull, lackluster, dirty appearance. Mites tend to accumulate on animals where they can best resist desiccation. Skin folds under the chin and under the scutes, the periocular region about the eyes, inside skin folds around the cloaca, and the tympanic recesses in lizards are all commonly affected areas where mites are found (Figure 43-2). Host skin around feeding sites becomes hyperemic, edematous, and infiltrated with heterophils, lymphocytes, and plasma cells. Mites vary in color depending on their species, their gender, and how recently they have fed.

Snake mites (*Ophionyssus* spp.) may be either black or tan depending on the age, gender, and feeding status of the mite (Figures 43-3 and 43-4). Lizard mites (*Hirstiella trombidiiformis*) are red, surface dwellers, and easily seen with the unaided eye (Figure 43-5).

Chigger mites (Trombiculidae) are usually red to orange and are readily visible (Figure 43-6, *A*). Juvenile chiggers are parasitic, have six legs (unlike adult mites with eight legs), and have a distinctive hairy body as seen with the microscope (Figure 43-6, *B*). Chigger mites are commonly found in skin folds behind the rear leg, in the axillary region, and in the tympanic recess. The parasitic larval chigger mites may congregate in clumps large enough to give the appearance of red spots on the skin.[7]

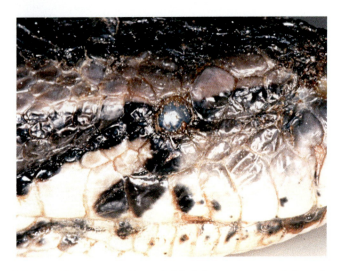

FIGURE 43-3 Snake mites can be black, brown, tan, or red, depending on their life stage and state of repletion. This python is heavily infested with mites around the spectacle and the scales of the face. *(Photo courtesy S. Barten.)*

Ophioptid mites are not surface dwelling and live under the scales of lizards and snakes. Raised telltale skin lesions are highly suggestive of these mites (Figure 43-7).

Mites of the family Cloacaridae live in the cloacal mucosa of aquatic and semiaquatic turtles. Aside from local irritation, they cause little harm. In North America, the two species of Cloacaridae mites found are *Cloacurus beeri* seen in the Painted Turtle and *Cloacurus faini* reported in the Snapping Turtle.[12] Impaction of loreal pits of crotalids and labial pits of boids has been well documented.[25] Two genera of lung mites have been reported in snakes, but their clinical significance and potential pathogenicity are as yet unknown.

With ticks, the typical presentation is one to multiple ticks present without signs of obvious disease. Minor skin irritation may be observed (Figure 43-8). Ticks can be found under the scales of lizards and snakes. They are often similarly colored to the scales of the reptile, can blend in quite well, and can be easily missed on cursory examination (Figure 43-9). They can also be found in the recesses of ears, around the skin folds of the vent in turtles and lizards, and anywhere on the soft skin of turtles. In turtles, ticks commonly can

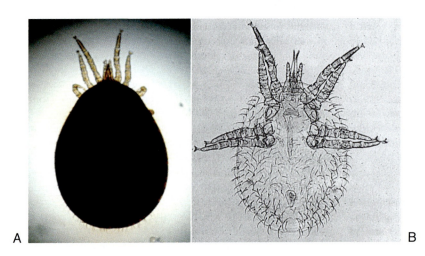

FIGURE 43-4 **A,** The snake mite (*Ophionyssus natricis*) in its typical teardrop appearance under the microscope. **B,** This is a cleared specimen showing the placement of the legs and the fine hairs over the body. *(Photo courtesy R. Houston.)*

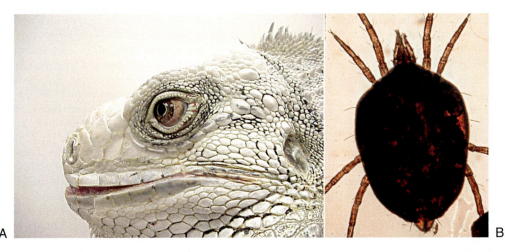

FIGURE 43-5 **A,** The lizard mite (*Hirstiella trombidiiformis*) is easily seen on the surface of the skin. **B,** The shield-shaped body is readily recognizable under the microscope.

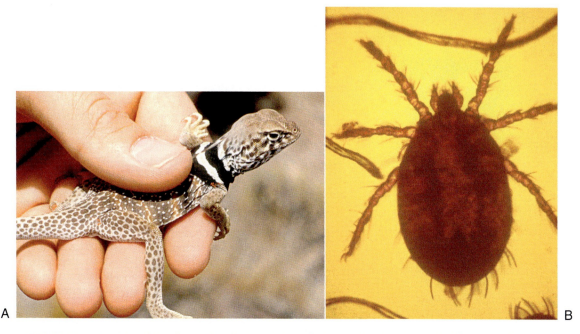

FIGURE 43-6 **A,** This wild Collared Lizard *(Crotophytus collaris)* is infested with trombiculid mites (chiggers). Juvenile chiggers are six legged, and, unlike the adult trombiculids (which have 8 legs), are parasitic. **B,** Typical presentation of a juvenile trombiculid showing the 6 legs and hairy body.

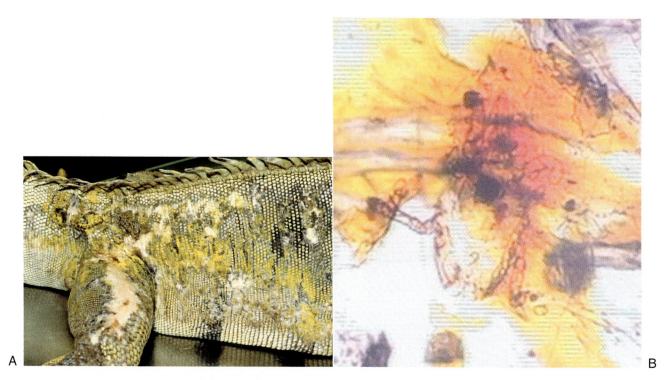

FIGURE 43-7 **A,** This Green Iguana *(Iguana iguana)* is suffering from a generalized mite infestation. Surface mites are not visible; however, the severe dermatitis is typical of parasitism, often complicated with a secondary bacterial or fungal pyoderma. **B,** A deep skin scraping revealed this unidentified subdermal mite.

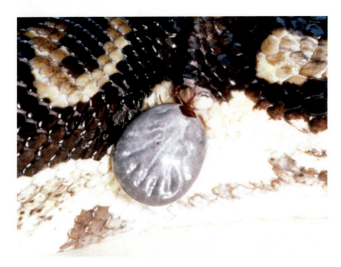

FIGURE 43-8 Ticks may be found solo or in clusters. Note the skin irritation around the site of attachment. *(Photo courtesy S. Barten.)*

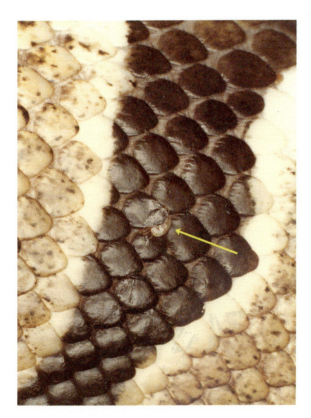

FIGURE 43-9 Both soft- and hard-shelled ticks are found in reptiles. Some ticks can be difficult to see on routine examination *(arrow)*. These smaller parasites can easily be misidentified as scales.

be found up under the shell in the recess in front of the rear legs. Monitor Lizard ticks *Aponomma exornatium* and *Aponomma flavomaculatum* attach inside the nostrils where heavy infestations can cause dyspnea and suffocation.[24] As many as 56 adult *A. exonatum* have been removed from the nostrils of a dyspneic Nile Monitor *(Varanus niloticus)*. Ticks have also been identified in the labial pits of various boids.

Mites have been linked to the transmission of several blood-borne viral, bacterial, and filariid pathogens of snakes. The hematropic protozoan *Hepatozoon* that cycles through hematophagous ticks has been documented in snakes.[20] *Hepatozoon* is not a host-specific organism and can be transferred from one species of reptile to another by fleas, mosquitoes, mites, and ticks.[12] Snake mites are also known carriers of *Aeromonas hydrophilia*, a common bacterium implicated in pneumonia and infectious stomatitis.[3] Blood smears are good inexpensive ways of obtaining diagnostic information and are not done enough. Mites have also been implicated as potential vectors of the boa retrovirus.[26] Ticks may also serve in the transmission of several microbial pathogens.[20] More work is necessary to establish the precise role of acarids in transmission of infectious agents.

Animals infested with acarids can be seen as obviously debilitated or astonishingly still active, feeding, and seemingly unaffected by tremendous parasite burdens. Although not directly a result of the parasite, perhaps the most common clinical presentation associated with mites and ticks is toxicity to host animals from improper and unsafe eradication treatments. These toxicities can be severe, devastating, and often fatal.

DIAGNOSIS

To the vigilant caretaker, mite and tick infestations in captive reptiles are usually quite obvious (Figure 43-10). In the worst cases, animals may have ticks and mites visibly swarming over their bodies. Generally, mites are most readily seen moving on or between scales of the head, the axillary folds, or the trunk of heavily infested lizards. However, casual visual observation is not enough to declare animals or their cages mite free. Too often mites are not noticed until owners find them on their own skin after handling infested reptiles. Captive animals and their environment must be part of a regular inspection program that searches for both free-living and parasitic stages. Frequent inspection of the animals, cages, water bowls, hide boxes, cage furniture, and freshly shed skin is highly recommended. These inspections should be thorough and routinely performed. In examination of water bowls, both the water surface and sediments should be closely examined for drowned parasites.

For the cage itself, the inner surface of the lid and hide boxes should be given particular attention. Here is where resting mites, eggs, digested blood, and fecal material are most likely to be found. Because mites prefer darkness and have a tendency to climb, crevices and corners, particularly those at the top of the cage, must be inspected. In examination of animals, the periocular area, chin shields, and first two rows of scales on the lateral body should receive particular scrutiny. Abnormally reddened areas, the underside of scales, or gaps between scales should be examined with a hand lens. Swabbing the sides of the animal with a gauze sponge or an oil-coated cotton swab and then immediately examining the gauze or cotton for dislodged mites can help detect even low-level infestation. Material recovered from the animal or cage that resembles mites can be fixed in 70% ethyl or isopropyl alcohol, cleared, mounted, and examined microscopically for accurate keying and identification. Full-thickness skin scrapings may be necessary to identify *Ophioptid* mites that live

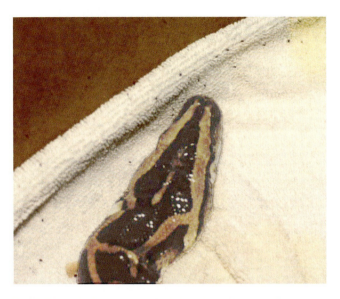

FIGURE 43-10 In severe mite infestations the parasites can be found all over the animal's cage and will readily dislodge, temporarily infesting human hosts.

Table 43-2	Clinical Signs of Mite Infestation

Anorexia
Dermatitis
Pruritus
Restlessness
Extended soaking
Frequent ecdysis
Excessive rubbing
Dehydration
Anemia
Septicemia

Not a direct clinical sign of acariasis, but nevertheless one frequently seen is toxicity as a result of incorrect treatment.

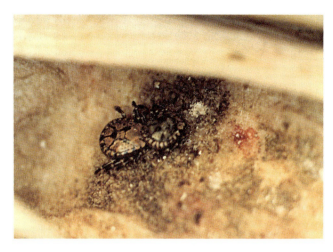

FIGURE 43-11 A common place to find ticks on tortoises is under the shell, just cranial to the thigh in the prefemoral fossa.

Table 43-3	Partial List of Historic Treatments for Reptile Acarids*

Water baths
Oil baths
Pyrethrins
Pyrethroids
Ivermectin
Trichlorfon
Dichlorvos strips
DDT
Diazinon
Bleach
Silica gels and drying agents
Quartenary ammonia
Biologic control

*Many of these therapies are considered dangerous and should not be used. See text for acceptable methods.

under the scales of snakes and lizards (see Figure 43-7, *B*). Dermatitis, pruritus, and frequent ecdysis can indicate the presence of parasites.[16,17] One should not underestimate the aid in diagnosis that magnification with a hand lens can provide. A summary of clinical signs of mite infestation is included in Table 43-2.

Ticks are generally much easier to identify and diagnose than are mites. One should pay particular attention to the skin in front of the rear legs in turtles, the nostrils of certain lizards and snakes, and the labial pits of snakes for the presence of hiding ticks. Other favorite spots for tick attachment in reptiles include: the anterior axillae, on and around the elbow, between digits in larger animals, and around the cloaca and eyes. For tortoises, one should also check the skin around the neck up under the shell (Figure 43-11). Continuous surveillance is the surest aid to early detection and diagnosis of mites and ticks in captive animals.

TREATMENT

A large and often confusing number of therapies have been proposed for the elimination of ticks and mites from captive reptiles and their environments (Tables 43-3 and 43-4). These protocols vary in their ease of application, expense, efficacy, and potential for harming the animals treated. All stages of the mite life cycle spend some time off the lizard or snake. The egg, larvae, and deutonymph spend their entire time off the host and never blood feed. Thus, any treatment plan that only deals with mites on the host and not the surrounding environment is doomed to failure. This section focuses on and compares these various regimens, centers particularly on those we have experience with, and attempts to identify the safest and most effective treatments.

Mites

Treatment protocols for management and eradication of the snake mite *(Ophionyssus natricis)* must address a variety of factors. The condition of the animal to be treated, the number of infested individuals, the budget of the caretaker, and the size of the infested area must all be considered before initiation of any therapy. The complex life cycle of the snake mite

Table 43-4 Treatments Proposed for Acarid Therapy in Captive Reptiles

Drug	Species	Route	Dosage	Interval
Carbaryl powder (5%)	Lizards, snakes	Topical	Lightly dust animal and cage; rinse after 1 hour	Repeat in 7 days
Pyrethrins (Mite & Lice Bird Spray)	Lizards, snakes	Spray	0.03%	Repeat in 14 days
Pyrethroids:				
a) Permethrin (Provent-a-mite)	Tortoises (for ticks)	Spray	0.01%	Repeat in 14 days
b) Permethrin	Lizards, snakes	Spray	0.007%–0.002%	Repeat in 14 days
c) Permectrin	Lizards, snakes	Spray	1%	Repeat in 10 days
Ivermectin	Lizards, snakes (never use in chelonians)	Spray / Injectable (IM/SC)	5 mg ivermectin / 1 quart H_2O / 200 µg/kg IM/SQ	Repeat in 14 days
Fipronil	Lizards, snakes	Spray	0.29% topical spray. Spray animal; wipe with dampened gauze; wash off with H_2O after 5 min	Repeat in 7 days
Dichlorvos strips	Various reptiles	Strips placed in well-ventilated cage; remove after 3 days. Toxicities reported; safer therapies exist. **Use only to treat empty cages**		
Trichlorfon	Lizards, snakes	Spray	0.15% for animals	Repeat in 14 days

It must be remembered that none of these therapies can be successful if only the animal is treated and the cage environment is not also aggressively managed.

(some stages on the animal, some stages free-living in the environment) and its intense wandering ability make this parasite difficult to eradicate and control. Persistent and recurrent infestations are common even for the experienced keepers. Parasites that possess complex life cycles are best managed with treatment programs that target all life stages of the organism. Successful treatment deals concurrently with the parasite species, the host species, and the cage environment. A sensible multifaceted integrated approach for snake mites has recently been described and uses isolation, sanitation, topical and systemic acarides, and habitat-directed pesticide applications to attempt to successfully eradicate the mites.

Isolation or Quarantine

The power of quarantining new reptiles should never be underestimated. New animals are recommended to be isolated a minimum of 3 months before they are placed with resident animals in the same room as the rest of the collection. New additions can be safely treated with 5% Sevin dust (carbaryl) for 6 hours in a ventilated container.

The ability of unfed mites to survive for extended periods makes isolation-quarantine a central part of parasite management. Cages that house infested animals should be kept in separate rooms and animals maintained there for 2 to 4 weeks past the time mites are last detected.

For maximal assurance that mites are detected and for assessment of treatment progress, animals, cages, and rooms should be examined daily. Widely recommended is that cages be isolated with a moat system. In this method, cages are mounted in a shallow water bath. A few drops of dishwashing detergent placed in the water decrease the surface tension enough that any mites in the water sink and drown. One should not underestimate the wandering capability of these mites.

Sanitation and Cleaning

Snake mites thrive in the warmth, filth, and favorable conditions of unwashed neglected cages. In a short time, huge populations of these nest parasites can develop. Housing for mite-infested animals should be kept as simply furnished as possible. Cages should be emptied, totally scrubbed, and refurnished at a minimum of twice weekly. Hide boxes, substrate, and other cage furniture should be disposable, be composed of nonporous material, and minimize the microhabitats sought by the parasites. To be effective, cages (including lids) should be washed in hot water (>50°C [122°F]). Waste products from infected cages should be bagged and sealed, treated with insecticides, incinerated, autoclaved, and totally removed from the facility. During each cleaning, animals can be examined closely, rinsed with water, and wiped with gauze in an attempt to reduce the number of mites and monitor the progress of therapy.

In instances of heavy snake mite infestations, the cage, cage rocks, and room should be thoroughly scrubbed and treated with an insecticide after animals have been removed. A pyrethrin, pyrethroid, carbaryl, or organophosphate-containing insecticide should be used. For this purpose, interiors and caged environments can be sprayed with 0.15% trichlorfon (an organophosphate) or 1% permectin (a pyrethroid). In addition, cages (including cracks), hide boxes, soaking bowls, climbing branches, and any other cage furniture should be thoroughly cleaned with either Roccal D (Pfizer Animal Health, New York, NY), a 3% bleach solution, or another quaternary ammonia compound such as A-33 Dry (Airken Professional Products, Ecolab Inc, St Paul, Minn). Roccal D is formulated in a dilution of 10-mL concentrate in 1 gal of water, and A-33 Dry is made with addition of one 16-g packet to 1 gal of water. These substances should *never* be applied to live animals. Residual disinfectant can be removed with wiping interiors with a clean cloth or wettened sponge, and all treated cages, shelving, and related surfaces must be allowed to adequately dry and air out a minimum of 24 hours before the return of live animals.

Pyrethrins/Pyrethroids

A variety of dilute insecticide products have been recommended for use on live animals to reduce or eliminate mite infestations. Pyrethroids, particularly resmethrin (0.35% active ingredient; Durakyl, DVM Pharmaceuticals, Miami, Fla), have also been reported to be effective.[7] Pyrethrins are naturally derived from chrysanthemum flowers. Pyrethroids are synthetic molecules. In general, pyrethroids are more potent and have a longer half-life than do pyrethrins.[13,27,28] These parasiticides work by disrupting sodium and potassium ion transport and blocking neurotransmission. Because the potential exists for transcutaneous absorption and accidental poisoning, pyrethrin and pyrethroid topical sprays must be thoroughly rinsed from the animal immediately after application. Gentle rinsing in lukewarm running water is usually sufficient. Other compounds that contain insect growth inhibitors, oils, or synergistic parasiticides are *not* recommended and should be avoided because they hasten the rate of transcutaneous absorption or they are toxic in their own right. Dilute pyrethrin (0.03%; Mite & Lice Bird Spray, 8 in 1 Products, Inc, Hauppauge, NY) has been reported to be effective against snake mites. Products used by veterinarians for flea and tick infestations in cats and dogs should *not* be used in reptiles because they can have pyrethrin concentrations of 0.18%. Patients with toxicity typically show signs within 15 minutes of application. Salivation, muscle fasciculations, and ataxia are commonly seen. Treatment with atropine (0.4 mg/kg intramuscularly [IM]), diazepam (0.5 mg/kg IM, as needed for seizures), and fluids can be effective.

Permectrin II (Bio-Ceutic Division, Boehringer Ingelheim Animal Health, Inc, St Joseph, Mo) is a synthetic pyrethroid compound found to be safe for eliminating mites from both hosts and infested housing.[19] The active ingredient is 10% permethrin emulsible insecticide. The permectrin concentrate is diluted to 1% in tap water and applied as a spray. Animals are removed to a well-ventilated clean enclosure. The reptile is lightly sprayed over the whole body including ventral surfaces. Excess solution is carefully blotted off. The animal is confined to this cage without water for 24 hours. The spray should be applied again in 10 days. If mites are still present after the second treatment, a third treatment should be performed in 10 days. Animals should be washed with water 24 hours before repeat treatments to reduce mite numbers. Several species of snake and some lizards have been safely and successfully treated with this technique. Toxic reactions have been seen in animals treated with permectrin after earlier trichlorfon spraying. Pyrethrins, pyrethroids, carbaryl, and organophosphates should not be used on animals concurrently with other cholinesterase-inhibiting compounds.

Although normally considered fairly safe for eliminating mites, pyrethrins and pyrethroids have been implicated in several reported toxicities.[13,14] The occasional toxic encounter with these molecules may be the result of variation in available products, how they are used, the species treated, and the housing conditions in use. The carrier material in commercial pyrethrin and pyrethroid products vary; some are water-based, and some are oil-based. These variations may contribute to fatalities. Pyrethrins and pyrethroids are applied as sprays either to the animal or the environment. Sprays to environments such as cage surfaces are effective but may leave toxic residues. Animals treated with such sprays should be rinsed with water after exposure. Rinsing for oil-based products should also include a gentle soap to help remove residues from the animal. Animals housed in poorly ventilated cages appear especially prone to toxicity. Intoxications are best treated supportively as described, with complete removal of any toxic residuals from the animal or the cage environment and provision of clean air and adequate ventilation. Pyrethrin-containing and pyrethroid-containing products must be used diligently to prevent toxicity. Particular attention must be paid to the nature of the product used, the frequency of the treatment, the duration of each treatment, the species treated, the carrier material in use (water-based versus oil-based), how and to what it is applied, and the specific housing and ventilation conditions that exist. Any toxicities are most likely a miscalculation in one or more of these parameters.

Organophosphates

Trichlorfon (Trichlorfon, Chem-Tronics, Inc, Leavenworth, Kan; or Neguvon, Cutter Animal Health, Mobay Corp, Animal Health Division, Shawnee, Kan), an organophosphate, has also been shown to be effective against the snake mite.[29] Trichlorfon is sprayed both on the animal and on the cage in a 0.15% application and left on for 24 hours. Differing concentrations (0.08%, 0.15%, 1%, and 2%) have been researched, but 0.15% is considered the safest while still efficacious formulation. (To make a 0.15% solution, mix 8 mL of an 8% stock Trichlorfon solution with 400 mL of water. It is not soluble in water, so shake vigorously before use. In this fashion, it can easily be applied with spray bottles.) Cages, hide boxes, and other cage props must all be treated to remove any eggs or mites and allowed to air out and dry for 24 hours. Treated cages should not be completely closed or totally air tight. Snakes and lizards should be lightly but thoroughly sprayed. Include the eyes and labial pits; small amounts accidentally sprayed into the mouth seem to be tolerated. For lizards, eyes should be protected with ophthalmic lubricants before spraying is started. A second treatment should follow in 14 days. Water dishes and bowls should be removed for 24 hours after treatment to avoid accidental ingestion when drinking or soaking.

A large number of species including Boas and Pythons, Kingsnakes, Gartersnakes, Vipers and Pit Vipers, and various Cobras have been successfully treated without incident. However, shedding opaque animals are more likely to display adverse reactions and should not be treated. Several lizard species (iguanas, Collared Lizards, Fence Lizards, and Chuckwallas) have likewise been safely treated. One should note that geckos are reported not to tolerate Trichlorfon, so alternative methods should be used.

Organophosphates like trichlorfon act neurotoxically with inhibition of the enzyme acetylcholinesterase. Rigid paralysis results. Any animals treated with trichlorfon should be watched closely for signs of toxicosis. Signs of organophosphate toxicity in reptiles include salivation, ataxia, muscle tremors and twitching, bizarre postures, and an inability to right themselves.[30] Treatment should be immediately halted in animals that display these signs, and they should be rinsed thoroughly in tepid soapy water. They should be treated with atropine (0.4 mg/kg IM) or fluids (20 mL/kg intravenously [IV], intracoelomically [ICe], intraosseously [IO], or subcutaneously [SC] in that order), and if seizures are occurring, diazepam (0.5 mg/kg IM) has been shown to be effective. Because of the potential for organophosphate toxicity, simultaneous use of trichlorfon and other cholinesterase-inhibiting insecticides (organophosphates or carbamates) is not recommended.

Ivermectin

Ivermectin applied as a topical spray has been advocated as a control for reptilian mites.[7,13,14,31,32] To prepare the spray, 0.5 mL of ivermectin for cattle (10 mg/mL) is added to 1 quart of water and applied to the animals and to the cage. Animals can be safely treated with this spray concentration three times at 2-week intervals. Because ivermectin is not water soluble, the spray solution must be shaken vigorously before each use. All ivermectin formulations must be maintained in opaque containers to retard light degradation. The main advantage of ivermectin is that it can act systemically and has a relatively long biologic half-life (several days in cattle). It can remain in the bloodstream at therapeutic levels for extended periods. Whether ivermectin is absorbed through reptilian skin has not been determined; thus, its effects when applied as a spray may only be local.

Ivermectin is a gamma-aminobutyric acid (GABA) agonist that results in paralysis of arthropod and nematode parasites through binding to the alpha subunit of glutamate gated chloride channels.[27,28] This causes neuronal hyperpolarization and paralysis through the influx of chloride ions. If injected or given orally, ivermectin is systemically absorbed into host tissues. When mites and ticks take a blood meal, the ivermectin is absorbed by the parasites. In addition to use as a spray, ivermectin can be injected (200 µg/kg SC). Although this recommended dosage may be sufficient to kill some mites, experimental work with ivermectin in the closely related fowl mite of birds (*Dermanyssus gallinae*) has shown the dosage necessary to kill adult mites is 400 to 500 µg/kg.[33] Further work on the susceptibility of snake mites to ivermectin, the margin of safety of this drug in snakes, and the potential for cumulative concerns regarding this drug needs to be undertaken before dosages like those used in fowl can be recommended. Remarkably, evidence shows that mites and ticks can recover from paralysis caused by ivermectin.[33] On account of this development, an integrated approach including quarantine, proper sanitation, and concurrent use of other acaricidal sprays for the environment is a highly recommended adjunct to ivermectin therapy alone. One should note that ivermectin should *never* be used on or around chelonians because it can cause paralysis, coma, and death.[34,35] Ivermectin sprays to the environment should be applied weekly for 3 to 4 weeks. Although ivermectin is easily applied and relatively inexpensive, its biggest drawbacks include that it is not 100% effective (some animals and environments seem particularly resistant) and that it is toxic to turtles and tortoises. Interesting to note is that although treatment of the cage environment is undoubtedly beneficial, it may be unnecessary with ivermectin because of the long half-life of the drug.[36] Mites off the host eventually must take a blood meal at which time they are exposed to the ivermectin. Reports of toxicity exist for lizards and snakes; however, lizards appear to be much more sensitive.[24,31]

Fipronil

Recently, fipronil (Frontline Spray Treatment, Merial, Duluth, Ga; active ingredient 0.29% fipronil) has also been recommended as an effective topical spray treatment for mites and ticks.[38] Fipronil is a phenylpyrazole antiparasitic substance. Its mechanism of action in invertebrates is to disrupt the passage of chloride ions in GABA-regulated chloride channels. In this fashion, it interferes with central nervous system activity. Fipronil has been shown to be useful if sprayed on the patient, with the excess wiped off with wettened gauze and then totally washed off with water after 5 minutes. It can be used weekly in this manner. In dogs and cats, no adverse effects have been reported, but it is contraindicated in rabbits. It should not be used in conjunction with other insecticides. Safety and efficacy data for this drug when used on reptiles have not been determined.

Antiparasitic sprays must be applied in thoroughly ventilated areas by persons wearing disposable impermeable latex gloves; aprons; and face shields, goggles, or other protective eyewear. Any skin contact should be avoided, and material sprayed or spilled on the skin must be immediately and thoroughly rinsed off with soap and ample amounts of fresh water. Spills on floors or counters should be quickly cleaned up. Care must be taken to ensure that domestic animals are not allowed in areas where antiparasitic spraying has occurred to protect them from spills, concentrated fumes, or other inadvertent contact.

One must point out that reptiles severely debilitated from mite-related anemia, severe infestations, or any other mite-linked diseases should be stabilized before treatment for mites is initiated. Animals anemic, dehydrated, and weakened from heavy mite infestations must receive fluids, blood transfusions, and support before treatment for acarids. Treat the patient, not the parasite. Antibiotics may be advisable for some patients because mites potentially can carry several serious diseases. Once again, although the spectacles on the eyes of snakes protect their corneas from the application of sprays, eyes of lizards should be pretreated with ophthalmic lubricants before spray therapies are initiated.

Dichlorvos Strips

Dichlorvos (DDVP, Vapona, United Industries, St. Louis, Mo) organophosphate insecticide works through the same mechanism of action as trichlorfon. Historically, dichlorvos therapy has been used in both the host animal and the environment. Dichlorvos-impregnated strips (such as No Pest Strips, United Industries, St Louis, Mo) placed in the cage at 6 mm of strip per 10 cubic feet of cage for 3 hours, three times a week for 2 consecutive weeks, have long been recommended as an effective therapy for mites.[7,13,14]

Dichlorvos is volatile and leaves the strips as a vapor. Inside the cage, this vapor condenses into a thin film that condenses on every surface, including animals. The older literature for reptilian/mite control recommends cut pieces of dog or cat flea collars (containing dichlorvos) be left in cages for varying lengths of time. Make no mistake—this is a hazardous chemical. The strips should be handled only wearing gloves and used in strict accordance with packaging labels.

In laboratory animals, topical application of concentrated liquid formulations has been shown responsible for transcutaneous absorption leading to dermal mutagenesis.[39] Human studies have shown rapid and protracted decreases in plasma and red blood cell cholinesterase activity in people exposed to high dichlorvos levels. People poisoned with organic insecticides such as organophosphates report a spectrum of clinical signs including gastrointestinal problems, acute neurologic signs (such as weakness, paralysis, and seizures), and cardiac arrhythmias. Organophosphate toxicity can range from simple mucous membrane irritation to the aforementioned acute signs.

An insidious chronic form of organophosphate intoxication has also been shown to exist and cause delayed systemic and particularly neurologic signs, thought to be from prolonged exposure. This deterioration may take months, manifest itself as nonspecific signs, and be hard to document even from necropsy findings. Furthermore, these substances pose a potential threat to nontarget species, such as humans and companion animals. Descriptions in reptiles of toxic reaction to this treatment have been reported.[7,13,14,24,30,40] Nevertheless, other studies report no adverse side effects at recommended dosages. Various snake species ranging from Pit Vipers (*Crotalus* and *Agkistrodon* spp.), to Ratsnakes (*Elaphe* spp.), to boids (*Python* spp. and *Boa* spp.), to Gartersnakes (*Thamnophis* spp.) have all been reported to be safely and successfully treated with this method. In a recent study, Rainbow Boas were exposed to strips 10 times the recommended width. No clinical signs were observed in any of the exposed animals, and no differences in plasma or red blood cell cholinesterase activity were shown in high-dosage, normal-dose, or untreated control animals.

Researchers who advocate dichlorvos strip use do recommend suspending the strips in a ventilated container to prevent direct contact with animals, removing water bowls before treatment to minimize ingestion, and not using dichlorvos strips in conjunction with any other acetylcholinesterase-inhibiting pesticide.

Species differences, with some species appearing vulnerable to dichlorvos exposure and others able to be treated both safely and successfully, may account for differing sensitivities to organophosphates. However, no matter what mite control therapy is chosen, animals treated with dichlorvos must be closely observed and monitored for signs of poisoning. Animals that show signs of toxicosis should be taken off therapy and treated as described with atropine, fluids, and, if necessary, diazepam. Methocarbamol (100 mg/kg) may also be useful for muscle tremors. The authors no longer recommend use of "no-pest" strips because both better and safer treatment methods exist; long-term exposure to the vapors are a potential risk to reptiles, to humans, and to other nontarget domestic species; long-term exposure causes chronic, nonspecific, debilitating changes in reptiles; and monitoring, regulating, or preventing the commonly seen overzealous client use of these products, which leads to intoxication in captive reptile species, is impossible.

Alternative Methods

A number of other time-honored (but not necessarily effective) methods for mite control have been suggested. Probably the safest for host animals is to bathe the reptile in lukewarm water for 30 minutes. This drowns most of the mites. However, it does nothing to treat the reptile's environment and does not kill the mites that have accumulated on the host's head. As a result, the method is not 100% effective. If meticulous cleansing and treatment (pyrethroid spray) of the cage, hide boxes, and food and water dishes are not performed; if disposable cage furniture, branches, and substrate are not replaced; and if even one contaminated object is left behind untreated, the mites are back in force within 14 to 21 days.

Although not an efficient treatment if used alone, water can be a successful aid in mite elimination. All stages of mites are vulnerable to drowning and to high temperatures. Soaking cages, cage furniture, hide boxes, lids, etc., in hot water can be an effective nontoxic adjunct treatment in mite control. Severely debilitated animals (dehydrated, anemic, etc.) from heavy mite infestations can have the parasite load reduced considerably with daily water soaks until the general condition of the snake allows appropriate chemical treatment. Remember, soaking reptiles should *never* be left unattended, and animals should *never* be placed in scalding water.

A safe (but messy) method for mite eradication is to cover the entire animal body with a thin film of olive oil, which suffocates the mites. To smother the mites by blocking the spiracles, oil should remain on the infested reptile for about an hour, followed by thorough rinsing. Like bathing, the disadvantage of the olive oil technique is that it only kills mites on the host. Nothing is done about adult or juvenile mite forms present in the reptile's cage environment. Unless the environment also is treated and the non–host-residing mite stages are simultaneously killed, the infestation on the animal quickly reoccurs. Oil treatments should be done in the tub at home; they are messy, and caretakers should wear old clothes. Treatment results in a slimy pet, but the oil does not hurt the reptile. Snakes may shed multiple scales in response to oil therapy, but the skin should return to normal after the next shed. Unless the environment is also treated with thorough cleansing and a pyrethroid spray, oil therapy is not an effective method for mite control.

Dilute bleach solutions (1:20 with water) may be used to clean an infested cage or enclosure (including cage furniture) but should *never* be used on the animals themselves. The bleach solution must be thoroughly rinsed off all surfaces and allowed to air out for 24 hours before animals can be safely reintroduced. Bleach residues can be irritating to skin, mucous membranes, and upper airways.

Most stages of the mite life cycle require a humid environment. Some control can be achieved with manipulation of humidity and drying out the cage environment. Removing animals from infested cages and allowing them to dry out even for a month is not enough because unfed mites can live in excess of 40 days.

The silica gel powder (Dri-Die, Rhone-Poulenc Ag Company, Portland, Ore) abrades the cuticle of mites and thereby decreases their resistance to water loss and results in their desiccation. It is effective at killing mites, but it can also dry out neonatal and small species of lizards and snakes. In addition, the dust can aerosolize and be inhaled by the animal and the caretaker, and the powder can cause quite a severe foreign body reaction. Silica gel powders must be used in such a way that chances for aerosolization are diminished. Silica gel products should be avoided in neonatal animals and in tiny species more susceptible to their dehydrating effects. Dri-Die has little effect on attached protonymphs and adults because it has poor ability to penetrate the protected microhabitat under the host reptile's scales. Furthermore, because mites are natural climbers, contact with the desiccating powder may not always occur. In addition, crystalline silica has been shown to be a potent carcinogen. Caution must be observed with this product. More effective and less dangerous treatments are available than with silica gel powders such as Dri-Die.

In the older literature, chlorinated hydrocarbons such as dichlorodiphenyltrichloroethane (DDT) and diazinon have been listed as possible mite treatments. With the advent of much safer, effective, alternative treatments, these two past therapies should be discontinued because they are just too toxic.

A word about substrate should be noted here. During acarid treatment, paper should be used as substrate. It is inexpensive and can be discarded and replaced easily, and the enclosure can be disinfected readily and frequently. Avoid substrates that provide suitable microhabitats and hiding spots for the parasites.

Growth Regulators

Insect growth regulators such as lufenuron have been examined for use against ectoparasites. These substances impede egg hatching and molting by inhibiting chitin synthesis. Their advantage is their systemic ability and their long biologic half-life. Their disadvantage for clinical cases is they do not kill the mites immediately. This treatment has not been used to any extent in reptiles.

Biologic Control of Mites

Sterile male mites have been postulated as being introduced into the population as done with the screw worm fly (*Cochliomyia hominovorax*). This is a particularly effective strategy in an arthropod that mates only once, such as the snake mite. At present, this therapy is merely theoretic.

In addition, the utilization and effectiveness of so-called "cannibal mites" that would selectively find and destroy the parasitic mites have been investigated and evaluated. Presently, this therapy is neither practical nor widely available to the general public. Recently, a biocontrol computer website was encountered that claimed success in biologic control of snake mites (access at www.biconet.com/biocontrol/hypoaspis.html). This site claimed that female *Hypoaspis* mites lay their eggs in the soil where they hatch in 1 to 3 days. Nymphs and adults feed on other pests. The article states each *Hypoaspis* mite consumes five to 20 prey or eggs per day. Their entire life cycle is 7 to 11 days, and they are said to be effective at ridding pet tarantulas, lizards, and snakes of mites. Presently, we have no experience with these "cannibals." However, this type of natural mite control and "gee-whiz" biology is tremendously exciting. Identification and subsequent application of natural brakes and inhibitors on mite infestations is by far preferable to the often toxic treatments available until now. We must continue to identify therapy regimens more toxic to the parasite and less toxic to the host, humans, associated companion species, and the environment.

Life Cycle–Directed Control Strategies

Specific therapy intended and used to target specific stages of the mite life cycle can be effective. Various combinations of these strategies together with quarantine, thorough cage cleaning and better sanitation, and aggressive treatment of the environment can act to rapidly reduce mite populations.

The free-living stages of egg, larva, and deutonymph are best managed with an active treatment protocol that addresses the cage and housing environment. Moat isolation; bleaches; thorough cleansing; treatment of the environment with ivermectin, a permethrin product, dichlorvos strips, or silica gel dusts (Dri-Die); keeping infested cages empty for 3 to 6 months after cleansing and treatment; and following and using proper quarantine techniques are all therapies aimed at eradication of free-living stages. We find it safest and most effective to disinfect the cage and furniture with hot water and dilute bleaches and then spray it with a permethrin product. The cage is then allowed to air out for 24 to 48 hours before animals are returned. We believe in isolation moats for all cages, in routine monitoring of cages for mites, and in regular replacement of disposable cage furniture, substrate, and hide boxes. As discussed, many of the treatment agents can have adverse reactions. In particular, therapies with dichlorvos strips, ivermectin, organophosphates, and silica gel powders must be closely monitored. We find permethrin treatment of cage environments safe and effective.

The parasitic stages, protonymphs and adult mites, attach to hosts and feed for prolonged periods (3 to 7 days). As a result, these stages of the life cycle are best treated with agents either applied topically or injected directly into the host. Topical agents such as ivermectin spray, topcial agents such as pyrethrin or pyrethroid sprays, and injectable ivermectin are all methods geared directly at killing the parasitic stages.

The overall efficacy and margin of safety of ivermectin in reptiles are open to question. Recent work in birds indicates higher dosages of ivermectin may be necessary to kill mites. Ivermectin given topically or systemically may display adverse reactions (lethargy, depression), and it should never be administered to chelonians. We typically use a pyrethroid spray to host animals followed immediately by a thorough rinsing with tepid water. We also recommend dusting all new acquisitions for 6 hours in a ventilated enclosure with 5% Sevin dust (carbaryl). New reptiles are then quarantined for a minimum of 3 to 6 months before they are admitted to the resident collection.

Therapy for mites in reptiles may involve multiple approaches and a combination of treatments directed at various life cycle stages. However, no one method can ultimately be successful that does not couple host therapy with aggressive treatment of the cage environment and elimination of the nest microhabitats favorable and necessary for completion of the mite life cycle.

Ticks

Ticks should be removed from reptiles with delicate forceps. Ticks should be grabbed under the head on the mouthparts and extracted. Mouthparts left behind may cause abscessation (Figure 43-12). After removal, irritated skin around tick attachment sites may be treated with a topical broad-spectrum antibacterial ointment. Ivermectin has been suggested as a method of tick removal and may be the only effective treatment for ticks hiding in nostrils, labial/loreal pits, or other body recesses. As mentioned, ivermectin must *never* be given to chelonians.

Recently, an effective regimen for the treatment of ticks that infest reptiles has been described.[41,42] A permethrin product (Provent-a-mite, Pro Products, Mahopac, NY) was shown to be both safe and effective at killing ticks at a dilution of 0.01% and 0.5%. Ticks are killed within 4 hours of application. This protocol was effective with the permethrin product sprayed directly on tortoises or directly on the substrate for lizards and snakes. No signs of toxicity have been reported at this dosage in tortoises, snakes, or lizards, and no signs of toxicity were shown by Leopard Tortoises when twice the recommended dosage was used. Likewise, permethrin has been shown to be safe in tortoises, lizards, and snakes when applied at 10 times the recommended dosage.[42] At present, permethrin is the safest acaricide to use in reptiles.

At present, use of the permethrin product on reptiles together with a 0.01% of cyfluthrin (Tempo, Bayer Corporation, Kansas City, Mo) formulated for premise treatment has been shown to be effective in the eradication of ticks from infested tortoise enclosures. One should point out that, unlike pyrethrin, cyfluthrin (although safe for chelonians) has been shown to be toxic to lizards and snakes even in very low dosages. Method of treatment with permethrin differs with reptile groups. In tortoises, the permethrin is sprayed directly onto the animal from a few inches away (10 centimeters), with a 1-second burst of spray into each leg opening of smaller animals. In larger tortoises, two 1-second bursts are used for each opening. In snakes and lizards, the reptiles are removed from their cages and the permethrin is sprayed directly onto the substrate from a distance of 12 to 15 inches (30 to 40 cm). A 1-second burst per 1 foot (30 cm) of surface is used. Snakes and lizards are returned to treated cages only after several hours when the permethrin spray has completely dried and all fumes have totally dispersed.

For tick-infested tortoise premises, this protocol recommends treatment of animals with permethrin and removal to a tick-free area. Then, the empty cages and housings are sprayed with the cyfluthrin product formulated for premises treatment, with hide boxes, cage furniture, and all lid cage surfaces adequately treated. This step is repeated again in 2 weeks. One week after the second treatment, animals are returned and closely monitored for the recurrence of ticks. Another permethrin spray (Preventic Virbac, Ft. Worth, Tex) has been suggested for cage, shelving, and room treatment of ticks. Here too, caution must be used, proper ventilation must be ensured, and animals should not be returned to treated cages for 24 hours.

The permethrin methods developed and effective in tortoises are likewise encouraging in squamates. Nevertheless, to avoid toxicities, many of these treatments are best performed within the veterinary hospital by veterinarians and their staff or applied in the home by licensed pest control companies. Although ticks are more visible than mites, their control and eradication can still be difficult. Ticks spend most of their lives off their vertebrate hosts. Monitoring the captive environment can be difficult, time consuming, and lengthy. Juvenile stages can exist in bedding, in houses, and in outdoor enclosures. These animals wander and can therefore spread readily to other enclosures and to other animals. Like successful mite therapy, the most effective treatment methods for ticks in reptiles include close inspection and quarantine of new animals, treatment of infected animals, aggressive treatment of captive environments, and frequent subsequent monitoring.

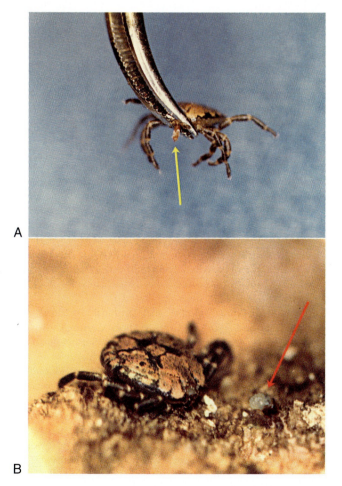

FIGURE 43-12 **A,** Ticks should be removed, individually, with delicate forceps. It is imperative to grasp the mouthparts when removing the tick *(white arrow).* **B,** If left behind in the skin *(red arrow),* an abscess will likely result.

ZOONOTIC POTENTIAL AND IMPLICATIONS FOR OTHER SPECIES

Ticks and mites that parasitize reptiles only temporarily infest humans who are accidental hosts. Snake mite protonymphs swarm on and bite humans who handle infested cages. Bite-associated dermatitis, pruritic papular lesions, and skin puncture and bleeding have been documented in humans.[43,44] Although they cannot complete their life cycle with humans as hosts, acarid parasites of reptiles may function as vectors for a variety of bacterial and viral diseases where the reptile serves as the reservoir. In a parasite like the snake mite that feeds once as a protonymph and multiple times as an adult and in chiggers, snake mites, and ticks that are all easily displaced and able to reattach to different hosts, the mechanical and biologic transmission of infectious agents is definitely possible. The snake mite (*Ophionyssus natricis*) is found worldwide on snakes and lizards, so the potential for the transmission of various agents to humans through temporary association with mites is far reaching. Chigger mites and their parasitic larvae parasitize turtles, snakes, and various lizards. Their cousin the harvest mite (*Neotrombiculi autumnalis*) is found on snakes and lizards in Europe. All of the parasitic larvae of these trombiculid mites have been shown to cause dermatitis in humans.

A variety of ticks potentially attack man (Figure 43-13). The relapsing fever tick (*Ornithodoros turicata*) of the United States and Mexico has been found infesting various native reptile species.[45] This tick transmits relapsing fever, also known as borreliosis and spirochetosis. The tick may also be able to transmit *Leptospira pomona*.

Immature stages of the tick *Haemaphysalis punctata* have been found on lizards and snakes in Europe, Northwest Africa, and Southwest Asia. This tick may transmit Siberian tick typhus (*Rickettsia siberica* or *Dermacentroxenus sibericus*) to humans. The immature stages of *Haemaphysalis concinna*, a tick found in Europe and Northern Asia, have also been found on various reptiles. This tick transmits the Flavivirus responsible for Russian spring-summer encephalitis and Siberian tick typhus.

Immature stages of the California Black-legged Tick (*Ixodes pacificus*) have been found on lizards and snakes in the Pacific Coastal region of the United States. The bite of these common ticks causes irritation and trauma in humans and is implicated in the transmission of tularemia (*Francisella tularensis*). They may also be a vector for Lyme disease (*Borrelia burgdorferi*). The immature European version of this tick (*Ixodes ricinus*) is rarely found on reptiles. However, its bite can cause irritation, pruritus, and paralysis in human beings. This tick may also transmit Lyme disease, central European tick-borne encephalitis, and Boutonneuse fever (*Rickettsia conorii* or *Dermacentroxenus conorii*). Ticks and mites that infest reptiles are themselves only a temporary problem to humans. Nonetheless, acarids are widespread throughout the world and, more insidiously, may serve as vectors in the transmission of several serious infectious agents from reptiles to people.

Heartwater disease is caused by the rickettsia *Ehrlichia ruminantium*. This organism is transmitted by ticks of the genus *Amblyomma*.[24,46-48] Heartwater can affect both wild and domestic ruminants including deer, antelope, cattle, sheep, and goats. It gets its name from the accumulation of fluid found at necropsy in the chest and pericardium of its victims. Clinical signs in ruminants include inappetence, fever, respiratory signs, and often neurological manifestations. Mortality may reach 100%. At present, heartwater is not treatable in a ruminant once clinical signs are present. Currently there is no vaccine available to control the disease.

African ticks of the genus *Amblyomma* that can carry heartwater have been found on imported monitor lizards, tortoises, ostriches, rhinoceros, antelopes, buffalos, giraffes, elephants, and zebras.[49-51] Some of these were *Amblyomma variegatum*, a major vehicle of heartwater disease, and a tick that has been introduced and spread throughout much of the Caribbean where heartwater also has been found. Another African tick, the African tortoise tick (*Amblyomma marmoreum*), was identified in a Florida reptile breeding premise in 1997. This is concerning since it too has been confirmed as a capable vector of heartwater. Furthermore, it has been demonstrated experimentally that at least two ticks native to the United States, the Cayenne Tick (*Amblyomma cajennense*) and the Gulf Coast tick (*Amblyomma maculatum*), are able to transmit heartwater. Obviously, if heartwater were to gain a foothold in the U.S., this would be disastrous for the goat, sheep, and cattle industries.

Although over 500 exotic ticks capable of transmitting heartwater had been discovered on imported reptiles and mammals, it was not until late 1999 that 15 African *Amblyomma sparsum* ticks tested positive for heartwater. These infected exotic ticks were found on Leopard Tortoises (*Geochelone pardalis*) imported from Africa. Since the majority of African *Amblyomma* ticks are found on African Spurred Tortoises (*Geochelone sulcata*) and Leopard Tortoises, the Florida Fish and Wildlife Conservation Commission and Department of Agriculture and Consumer Services prohibited the importation or transportation into the state of any African Spurred Tortoise or Leopard Tortoise in December 1999.[24] It will allow interstate movement of these species if they are accompanied by a special permit issued by the Commission. In early 2000 the USDA followed suit and banned importation into the United States of African Spurred Tortoises, Leopard Tortoises, and Bells Hingeback Tortoises (*Kinxys belliana*). These measures should help prevent the unregulated flow of exotic ticks into the United States. It should be noted, however, that the USDA will allow interstate movement of these three tortoise species if the animals are accompanied by a health certificate signed by a federal or

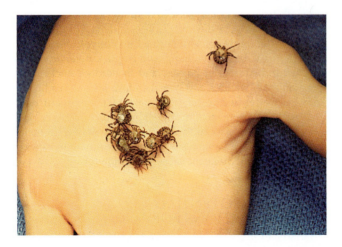

FIGURE 43-13 A variety of ticks have the potential to parasitize man and other mammals. Several of these ticks have been shown to carry communicable diseases such as relapsing fever and heartwater.

accredited veterinarian stating the tortoises have been examined by that veterinarian and have been found free of ticks.

Due to the natural history, behavior, and worldwide distribution of mites and ticks their potential as vectors in the transmission of infectious agents to both humans and to other species is staggering. We must remain constantly vigilant and proactive.

PREVENTION

A well-designed prevention program for ticks and mites in captive reptiles must focus upon quarantine of new individuals (for at least 3 months), aggressive sanitation and regular cage cleansing techniques, moat-isolation strategies, immediate therapy for infested animals, and thorough and effective treatment of infested cage environments. Routine monitoring of animals and enclosures for the presence of these parasites must be regularly performed. Cleaning tools, food and water dishes, cage furniture, caretakers' hands, and any object that has contacted animals or the cages of animals of uncertain mite and tick status should be viewed with suspicion. Proper sanitization of these items must be carried out before their contact with acarid-free animals. Established mite-free and tick-free facilities should not admit anyone who has recently handled reptiles of unknown ectoparasite status until that person has bathed and undergone a change of clothes. Exhibitions of reptiles featuring the indiscriminate handling of both mite-free and infested animals can be a tremendous source of acarid infestations. Any reptiles exhibited in such shows and exposed to other animals of uncertain status should be quarantined all over again and treated no differently than new animal acquisitions.

Snake mites are species specific for reptiles and do not live and reproduce on mice, rats, or other rodents. However, snake mites can temporarily infest mice and rats. Thus, rodents could act as carriers of snake mites if they are indiscriminately transferred among or moved between infested and parasite free reptile cages.[7] This relationship between the mites and the mouse is not parasitism but one of *phoresis*. In addition, mice have their own species of macronyssid mites that resemble snake mites, but these do not infest reptiles.[52] Nevertheless, to avoid problems (and since mice, bedding, and rodent accessories are difficult to sanitize), it is best to obtain feeder rodents from outlets that do not house snakes or other reptiles. An alternative strategy would be to freeze dead food animals or any suspected mite-contaminated objects below –20°C (–4°F, which is standard freezer temperature) for a minimum of five days to kill off any potentially harmful mites or other parasites.

If maintaining a rodent colony as a food source for reptiles, elimination of mites from a rodent population can be almost as challenging as eradication of parasites from a reptile collection. Dusting the rodents with Sevin dust (5% carbaryl) can be fairly effective. Do not forget the dust can be irritating to animals and to humans. Those applying such dust treatments must use well-ventilated areas, wear protective gloves, and wear a mask. Do not dust pinkies or fuzzies. Once dusted with an external parasiticide rodents are toxic as food items. As a result, dusted mice and rats should be rinsed with copious amounts of fresh water. Wait at least 2 weeks before using them as food.

The same methodology in eliminating mites from a reptile collection must be applied in attempting to eliminate mites from a rodent colony. Infested cage material should be removed and discarded or thoroughly disinfected. After rodents are treated, they must be placed into a mite-free environment or they will be almost immediately reinfested. Rodents then represent yet another way that acarid parasites can be transmitted among captive reptiles. Maintaining rodent colonies as food for reptile collections can be rewarding, but vigorous measures must be taken to prevent and eradicate the occurrence of rodent mites within these populations. Furthermore, these rodent populations must be prevented from acting as carriers of reptilian parasites between infested and non-infested herptile enclosures. The successful prevention of acarids in captive reptiles depends upon constant vigilance, early detection, and decisive treatment of outbreaks of infested animals. Maintaining ectoparasite-free animals is a time-consuming, expensive, and never-ending proposition. Still, we owe captive animals healthy, safe, parasite-free conditions. Better treatments now exist so that such environments may be provided.

PROGNOSIS

The outcome of various therapy protocols for management of ectoparasites in captive reptiles is dependent on (1) how successfully they treat the infested host species, (2) how thoroughly they treat and control the affected housing environment, and (3) how effective they are in targeting and eradicating specific life stages of the parasite.

Infestation with ticks and mites can be responsible for anorexia, lethargy, pruritus, anemia, and dehydration and has been implicated in the transmission of several blood-borne infectious agents. Severely debilitated animals must be treated supportively before acarid therapies are initiated. In addition, these parasites possess widespread zoonotic potential and have far-reaching implications for other non-target species. In general, acarids are hematophagous parasite species (with the exception of the Trombiculid "chigger" mites where the parasitic larval stage ingests dissolved tissue and lymph), and they are spectacularly well adapted for infesting captive reptile species. Despite a wide variety of suggested products for parasite control, acarid parasites remain a formidable problem in captive reptiles.

These ectoparasites are easily diagnosed and with selection of the right combination of protocols can be managed and eliminated. However, ticks and mites have an uncanny ability to escape parasiticides and control measures. This is due, at least in part, to their complex life cycle involving both free-living and parasitic stages and their incessant wandering behavior. As a result, the most successful control programs are integrated, combination protocols that safely and effectively target the parasite on the host, the captive environment and cages, and the various stages of the parasite life cycle.

Possible integrated and combinations of control measures include quarantine and barrier procedures, aggressive sanitation and treatment of captive environment, and several neurotoxic compounds that target various parasite neuromuscular pathways and interfere with tick and mite physiology.

Applied together, these techniques incapacitate the parasites, poison them, attack them on and off the host, or provide an inhospitable microhabitat. They interrupt the parasite life cycle and kill them. Treated parasites may dehydrate due to loss of appropriate microhabitat, deposit their eggs in unsuitable locations, and be unable to find suitable hosts, or be poisoned outright. The effect of an integrated, combination therapy approach is a rapid reduction in parasite population density.

Successful prognosis in treatment of ticks and mites in captive reptiles depends upon a combination of control protocols involving rigid quarantine and barrier practices, therapies that target various parasite stages and continuously disrupt the life cycle, and perpetual monitoring and surveillance. Such treatment is time-consuming, difficult, not inexpensive, and, due to its high potential for toxicity, may be beyond the capabilities of the inexperienced or novice caretaker. Many of these treatments should be performed by veterinarians in a controlled environment.

In summary, successful treatment of mite infestations generally includes a combination of several of the following regimens: (1) a rigorous quarantine system, (2) a warm water bath/soak, (3) dilute ivermectin spray or ivermectin 0.2 mg/kg SC (*never* to be used in chelonians), (4) topical application of a pyrethroid spray to the host (immediately followed by a thorough rinsing), (5) disposal of infested bedding, cage furniture, branches, etc., (6) disinfection of non-disposable hide boxes, food and water dishes, and other permanent cage furniture, (7) treatment of the cage, lid, and cage environment, and associated surfaces with a permethrin product, and (8) continued adherence to permanent quarantine system (including moat-isolation) to prevent recurrence. Frequent monitoring and surveillance for parasites must be continually performed. Vigilance must also be maintained for the appearance of adverse reactions in captive animals treated with any of these potentially toxic therapies.

Successful tick therapy involves physical removal of the parasite, application of an antibacterial ointment to the irritated area of attachment, and spray application of a permethrin product (at 0.5% dilution). Ivermectin (0.2 mg/kg SC) may be necessary for severe tick infestations of nostrils and labial pits. Keep in mind ivermectin must never be administered to tortoises and turtles. Veterinarians must be aware of the zoonotic capabilities of ticks and remain vigilant for the potentially devastating implications tick infestations can possess for other non-target species as well.

The future appears promising for the treatment of ticks and mites. Hopefully, we shall see safer compounds utilized, more effective methods for treating and disinfecting the cage environment, and the potential biological control of parasite populations. However, no acarid control method can ever be successful that merely deals with the parasites on the host and does not also actively eliminate the parasites concealed within the countless favorable microhabitats provided by the captive environment.

SUMMARY

Infestations with ticks and mites can cause anorexia, dermatitis, pruritus, anemia, septicemia, dysecdysis, retained eye caps, failure to thrive, dehydration, and the transmission of blood-borne pathogens in captive reptiles.

Infestations with ticks and mites invariably can be traced to unsanitary conditions, poor husbandry practices, and recent imports of unquarantined, diseased animals.

For snake mites, protonymphs and adults are parasitic while eggs, larval stages, and deutonymphs are non-feeding. Only the parasitic stages are found on the host.

Unfed, parasitic protonymph stage snake mites can persist in the cage environment for up to 31 days without eating.

Under the right conditions, adult mites can survive up to 40 days with or without feeding. Treatment protocols must address this fact.

Snake mites lay their eggs on the inner surface of cage lids, hide boxes, and any other concealed spots on cage furniture.

Mated female snake mites lay both fertilized and unfertilized eggs. Fertilized eggs become females while unfertilized eggs parthenogenetically become males.

Due to differences in anchoring pieces, ticks are much more difficult to dislodge than are mites.

Ticks may infest the nostrils of various captive lizards and can cause dyspnea and suffocation. Likewise, ticks have been found infesting the loreal pits of various crotalids and labial pits of the boids.

Sadly, perhaps the most frequent clinical sign of acarid infestation is toxicity due to improper or unsafe therapy.

All stages (including eggs) are visible to the naked eye. However, mites and ticks can be easily overlooked in both animals and cages with casual visual observation alone.

Do not underestimate the aid in diagnosis that magnification with a hand lens provides.

Infestations can often be diagnosed by the presence of dead mites found floating in bath water.

For any treatment to be successful, acarid parasites must also be totally eradicated from the captive environment.

The most successful treatment protocols consider and treat the parasite, the host, *and* the cage environment concurrently.

Selection of any therapy for acarid infestation of captive reptiles must reflect ease of application, number of animals to be treated, expense, efficacy, experience of the caretaker, and relative potential toxicity of the material chosen.

Contact with parasiticides by humans must be avoided. Spills of these toxic substances must be quickly and meticulously cleaned and contact with other non-target species should be minimized.

Bleach solutions used for cleaning cage enclosures should *never* be applied to living animals.

Ivermectin should *never* be administered to chelonians.

The 0.15% solution of Trichlorfon is considered the safest concentration.

Any treated cages, shelving, or related surfaces must be allowed to adequately dry and air out a minimum of 24 hours prior to returning live animals to their enclosure.

The most successful therapies for tick and mite infestation are a combination of quarantine and barrier practices, treatments that target and disrupt the parasite life cycle and provide continuous surveillance to monitor their return.

Mites and ticks that parasitize reptiles only temporarily infest humans who are accidental hosts.

The natural history, behavior, and worldwide distribution of ticks and mites gives them tremendous potential as vectors for zoonotic diseases. In addition to humans, other non-target species can be implicated. We must remain vigilant and proactive in regard to the introduction, distribution, and monitoring of acarid parasites in order to early detect deleterious microbes they may carry and transmit.

Moat isolation to counter the wandering behavior of these parasites is a good addition to any successful control protocol.

Introduction of any persons or animals of unknown parasite status into established parasite-free collections should be discouraged.

New animals should be isolated a minimum of three months in a separate room before they are placed with existing, parasite-free resident reptiles.

Individual animals traveling to shows or exhibitions where animals of unknown status are present should be quarantined again to prevent infestation to resident reptiles.

Cleaning utensils, hide boxes, other cage "furniture," and food and water dishes should never be exchanged between parasite-free and infested cages. Likewise similar items must never be switched between quarantine and resident housing areas. To prevent infestation each cage should have its own items.

A pyrethrin, pyrethroid, carbaryl, or organophosphate should be used to treat infested cage environments. In addition, cages (including cracks), hide boxes, soaking bowls, climbing branches, or other cage props should be thoroughly cleaned with a 3% bleach solution or Roccal D.

If the captive reptile, the cage enclosure and surroundings, and the specific parasite life stages are not *all* successfully treated, reinfestations with ticks and mites are very common.

ACKNOWLEDGMENTS

The authors wish to thank Dr Douglas Mader for his unflagging support, encouragement, and example. We also wish to thank Dr David Chizar for his kind help over the years, teacher Dr Richard E. Jones for his contagious enthusiasm and flare for "gee-whiz biology," and Dr Hobart M. Smith for showing us how to be lifelong students of herpetology. As always we thank Dr Robert A. Taylor and the whole staff at the Alameda East Veterinary Hospital for providing such a wonderful environment in which to treat sick reptiles.

REFERENCES

1. Clayton DH, Moore J: *Host-parasite evolution*, Oxford and New York, 1997, Oxford University Press.
2. Cooper JE: Host-parasite relations in reptiles and amphibians, *ARAV Proceedings Eighth Annual Conference*, 2001.
3. Maxwell L: Infectious and noninfectious diseases. In Jacobson ER, editor: *Biology, husbandry, and medicine of the green iguana*, Malabar, Fla, 2003, Krieger Publishing.
4. Frank W: Ectoparasites. In Cooper JE, Jackson OF, editors, *Diseases of the Reptilia*, vol 1, New York, 1981, Academia Press.
5. Jacobson ER: Parasitic diseases of reptiles. In Fowler M editor: *Zoo and wild animal medicine*, ed 2, Philadelphia, 1986, WB Saunders.
6. Mader DR, Houston R, Frye FL: Hirstiella trombidiiformis infestation in a colony of chuckwallas, *JAVMA* 189(9):1138, 1986.
7. Mader DR: Acariasis. In Mader DR editor: *Reptile medicine and surgery*, Philadelphia, 1996, WB Saunders.
8. Boyer TH: *Reptiles: a guide for practitioners*, Lakewood, Colo, 1998, AAHA Press.
9. Camin JH: Mite transmission of a hemorrhagic septicemia in snakes, *J Parasitol* 34:345, 1948.
10. Chiodini RJ, Holdeman LV, Gandelman AL: Infectious necrotic hepatitis caused by an unclassified anaerobic bacillus in the water snake, *J Comp Path* 63(2):235-242, 1983.
11. Mader DR, Palazzolo C: Common reptile parasites not always easy to treat, *Vet Product News*, 1995 (Jan), pp. 32-33.
12. Lane TJ, Mader DR: Parasitology. In Mader DR editor: *Reptile medicine and surgery*, Philadelphia, 1996, WB Saunders.
13. Denardo D, Wozniak EJ: Understanding the snake mite and current therapies for control, *Proceedings of Assoc Rept Amph Veterin*, 1997.
14. Wozniak EJ, DeNardo DF: The biology, clinical significance and control of the common snake mite, *Ophionyssus natricis*, in captive reptiles, *Jour Herp Med Surg* 10(3):4-10, 2000.
15. Bowman DD: *Georgis' parasitology for veterinarians*, ed 8, Philadelphia, 2003, WB Saunders.
16. Harkewicz KA: Dermatology of reptiles: a clinical approach to diagnosis and treatment, *Vet Clin North Am Exotic Anim Pract*, 4:441-461, 2000.
17. Harkewicz KA: Dermatologic problems of reptiles, *Seminars in Avian and Exotic Pet Medicine* 4(3):151-161, 2002.
18. Hirst AS: On the parasitic mites of the subordae prostigmata (Trombidiodea) found on lizards, *J Linn Soc Lond Zool* 36:173, 1925.
19. Boyer D: Snake mite (*Ophionyssus natricis*) eradication utilizing permectrin spray, *Bull Assoc Reptil Amphib Vet* 5(1):4-5, 1995.
20. Rossi JV: Dermatology. In Mader DR editor: *Reptile medicine and surgery*, Philadelphia, 1996, WB Saunders.
21. Jacobson ER: Reptile dermatology. In Kirk R, Bonagura J, editors: *Current veterinary therapy XI: small animal practice*, Philadelphia, 1992, WB Saunders.
22. Camin, JH: Observations on the life history and sensory behavior of the snake mite *Ophionyssus natricis* (Gervais). Chicago Acad. Science Spec. Pub., 10:1-75, 1953.
23. Coons LB, Rosell-Davis R, Tarnowski BI: Bloodmeal digestion in ticks. In Sauer JR, Hair JA, editors: *Morphology, physiology, and behavioral biology of ticks*, London, 1986, Ellis Harwood.
24. Wosniak EJ et al: Ectoparasites, *Jour Herp Med Surg* 10(3): 15-21, 2000.
25. Garrett CM, Harwell G: Loreal impaction in a black speckled palm viper (*Bothriechis nigroviridis*), *J Zoo Wildl Med* 22: 249-251, 1991.
26. Schumacher J et al: Inclusion body disease in boid snakes, *J Zoo Wildl Med* 25(4):511-524, 1994.
27. Plumb DC: *Veterinary drug handbook*, ed 4, Ames, 2002, Iowa State Press.
28. Papich MG: *Handbook of veterinary drugs*, Philadelphia, 2002, WB Saunders.
29. Boyer D, Boyer T: Trichlorfon spray for snake mites (*Ophionyssus natricis*), *Bull Assoc Reptil Amphib Vet* 1:2-3, 1991.
30. Jamal GA: Neurological syndromes of organophosphorus compounds, *Adv Drug React Toxicol Rev* 16(3):133-170, 1997.
31. Rosskopf WJ: Ivermectin as a treatment for snake mites, *Bull ARAV* 2(1)7, 1992.
32. Abrahams R: Ivermectin as a spray for treatment of snake mites, *Bull ARAV* 2(1):8, 1992.
33. Ash LS, Oliver JH Jr: Susceptibility of *Ornithodoros parkeri* (cooley) (Acari: Argasidae) and *Dermanyssidae gallinae* (Acari:Dermanyssidae) to ivermectin, *J Med Entomol* 26(3): 133-139, 1989.
34. Teare J, Bush M: Toxicity and efficacy of ivermectin in chelonians, *JAVMA* 183(11):1195-1197, 1983.
35. Rosskopf WJ: Ivermectin dangerous in chelonians, *Bull ARAV* 2(1):7, 1992.

36. Guillot FS, Wright FC, Oehler D, et al: Concentration of ivermectin in bovine serum and its effect on the fecundity of psoroptic mange mites, *Am J Vet Res* 47:525-527, 1985.
37. Boyer DM: Adverse ivermectin reaction in the prehensile-tailed skink, *Corucia zebrata, Bull Assoc Rept Amph Vet* 2(2):6, 1992.
38. Funk RS: A formulary for lizards, snakes and crocodilians, *Vet Clin North Am Exotic Anim Pract* 3(1):333-358, 2000.
39. Tungul A et al: Micronuclei induction by dichlorvos in mouse skin, *Mutagenesis* 6(5):405-408, 1991.
40. Nathan R: Further notes on mite eradication "Cold Blooded News," vol 21, no 4, April 1994, Colo. Herp. Soc.
41. Burridge MJ: Control and eradication of exotic tick infestations on reptiles, *Proceedings of Association of Reptilian and Amphibian Reptiles,* 2001.
42. Burridge MJ, Simmons LA, Hofer CC: Clinical study of a permethrin formulation for direct or indirect use in control of ticks on tortoises, snakes and lizards, *J Herp Med Surg* 13(4):16-19, 2003.
43. Schultz H: Human infestation by *Ophionyssus natricis* snake mite, *Br J Dermatol* 93:695, 1975.
44. Beck W: Animal mites as a cause of epizoonoses, *Tierische Milben als Epizoonoseerreger und ihre Bedeutung in der Dermatologie,* 47(10):744-748, 1996.
45. Johnson-Delaney CA: Reptile zoonoses and threats to public health. In Mader DR, editor: *Reptile medicine and surgery,* Philadelphia, 1996, WB Saunders.
46. Burridge MJ, Simmons LA, Simbi BH, et al: Evidence of *Cowdria ruminentium* infection (heartwater) in *Amblyomma sparsum* ticks found on tortoises imported into Florida, *J Parasitol* 86:1135-1136, 2000.
47. Burridge MJ, Simmons LA, Allan SA: Introduction of potential heartwater vectors and other exotic ticks into Florida on imported reptiles, *J Parasitol* 86:700-704, 2000.
48. Peter TF, Burridge MJ, Mohan SM: Competence of the African tortoise tick, *Amblyomma marmoreum* (Acari: Ixodidae) as a vector of the agent of heartwater *(Cowdria ruminantium), J Parasitol* 86:438-441, 2000.
49. Simmons LA, Burridge MJ: Introduction of the exotic ticks *Amblyomma humerale* Koch and *Amblyomma geoemydae* (Cantoa) (Acari: Ixodidae) into the United States on imported reptiles, *Int J Acarol* 26:239-242, 2000.
50. Clark L and Doten E: Ticks on imported reptiles into Miami International Airport: November 1994 through January 1995, *Proc Vet Epidemiology and Economy,* 1995.
51. Burridge MJ: Ticks (Acari: Ixodidae) spread by the international trade in reptiles and their potential roles in dissemination of diseases, *Bull Entomol Res* 91:3-23, 2001.
52. Flynn RJ: Arthropods. In *Parasites of laboratory animals,* Ames, 1973, Iowa State University Press.

44
ANOREXIA
RICHARD S. FUNK

ANOREXIA IS A SYMPTOM, NOT A DISEASE

Anorexia may be defined as the lack of an appetite or the lack of a feeding response. It is a symptom that may accompany a wide variety of infectious and metabolic diseases and husbandry conditions and also may result from behavioral problems.

Anorexia may occur in a recently acquired reptile that never eats or as a result of cessation of feeding in an animal that previously had a good appetite. A good history is critical to evaluation of the presence and etiology of anorexia in a reptile patient. Anorexia may accompany diarrhea, and chronic anorexia may lead to debilitation and ultimately death. A thorough physical examination should accompany the evaluation of an anorectic patient, including positive identification of the reptile down to the species level.

Most often, anorexia is related directly to improper husbandry conditions, frequently without the presence of any disease process (Figure 44-1). Temperate climate reptiles may undergo an "autumn anorexia" as they physiologically ready themselves for the approach of winter and brumation, a seasonal anorexia. Brumation is the proper term for winter dormancy in reptiles.[1,2] The Flat-tailed Horned Lizard, *Phrynosoma mcallii*, undergoes a physiologic brumation in the fall regardless of the temperature at which it is kept in captivity.[1] Reptiles offered food during the wrong time of day may exhibit a client-perceived anorexia; for example, some nocturnal species may not feed if offered food only during daylight hours, but feeding may occur if the food is presented during the animal's normal activity cycle. A proper diel cycle and lighting of sufficient intensity and quality are important. Lights should never remain on for 24 hours a day.

Food offered in the wrong location of the animal's captive environment may not be eaten; for example, a terrestrial reptile may not find food placed in a tree branch and a strictly aquatic reptile may not locate food placed on the shore. Improper food may be offered because of a misidentification of the reptile by the client or insufficient knowledge of what the normal diet is in the wild (Figure 44-2). The client may offer produce to a carnivorous lizard or aquatic turtle or pinky mice to an insectivore. Some insectivorous lizards may not recognize dead insects as prey and need the movement of living prey to elicit a feeding response. Improperly sized food items also may not be eaten. Or the patient may already be sated.

Feeding snakes a diet of obese rats may lead to anorexia,[3] and feeding crocodilians a diet too high in fat may lead to steatitis and anorexia.[4] Nutritional inadequacies in the diet including hypovitaminosis and hypervitaminosis, and improper usage of nutritional supplements, may eventually lead to metabolic disturbances and anorexia. Consult the Nutrition chapter (Chapter 18).

The cage setup should be examined, or the client should be asked to describe the cage in detail. Does an arboreal reptile have appropriate cage furnishings (e.g., tree branches) on which to climb and feel secure? Does an aquatic or semi-aquatic reptile have good quality water? Lack of a secure hiding place or a variety of hiding places (e.g., in warmer and cooler areas of the enclosure) may contribute to anorexia. If the animal is on public display, the constant traffic of patrons past its cage, usually with nearly constant tapping or banging on the enclosure, may create stressful conditions that cause anorexia. Handling of the animal too frequently, particularly if a regular feeding regimen has not yet been established, as with a new pet, can cause anorexia.

Occasionally captives seem to grow "tired" of a repetitious diet. The author has hospitalized a number of chameleons, for example, that had been fed only crickets, with part of the presenting signs that the captive was off feed. In some cases, an offering of another arthropod prey species that they have not had, such as a moth, roach, or spider, elicits a feeding response. After successive days on the same produce, some iguanas and tortoises may appear inappetent or uninterested but if given something different eat a full meal. With some captives, just an available choice may break the anorexia. A variety of foods for wild-caught or newly imported captives is often a good idea. Anorectic Ball Pythons *(Python regius),* which repeatedly refuse rats or mice, may feed on gerbils.

Improper temperatures are a frequent cause of anorexia; a thorough discourse on temperature requirements of captive reptiles is outside the scope of this chapter (see Chapter 4). Briefly, if the reptile cannot reach its selected (or "preferred")

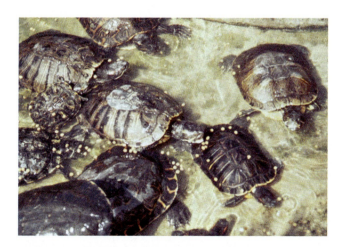

FIGURE 44-1 Most cases of reptilian anorexia are related to improper husbandry. Inappropriate housing, temperature, humidity, diet, and crowding (stress) can all contribute to anorexia. In this pond, larger specimens out-compete and intimidate smaller animals. *(Photograph courtesy D. Mader.)*

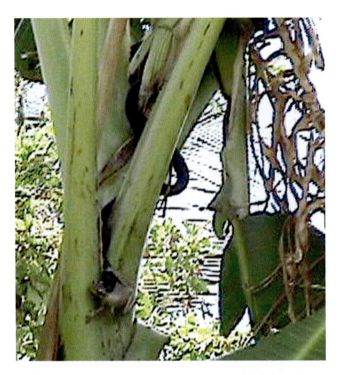

FIGURE 44-2 Many reptiles have specific dietary requirements. This Black Racer (*Coluber constrictor*) is eating a frog high up in a banana tree. Matching natural conditions in the captive setting is extremely difficult. Wild-caught reptiles may have trouble recognizing contrived diets as appropriate. *(Photograph courtesy G. Diethelm.)*

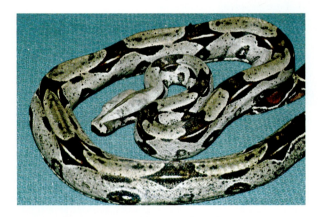

FIGURE 44-3 Although husbandry is often the underlying cause of many reptile problems, medical pathology must be ruled out as the primary cause. A thorough history, physical examination, and minimal database (complete blood cell count, serum chemistry, radiographs, and more) must be performed in all cases of anorexia. *(Photograph courtesy D. Mader.)*

body temperature (T_s or T_p) in a captive environment, it may not feed.[5] Keeping a reptile too cool often leads to anorexia, as can keeping it too hot without an opportunity to cool off or escape the heat. Optimal cages offer the reptile inhabitants the opportunity to thermoregulate, and a thermal gradient improves the long-term well-being of almost any reptile. Clues to a patient's proper temperature requirements are found in its native habitat and geographic origin.

Occasionally some neonate temperate zone snakes appear anorectic after hatching in spite of apparent good husbandry practices. In some cases, these neonates may feed after brumation.

Social and reproductive factors may also lead to anorexia. A dominant individual may inhibit a subordinate from eating or may eat most or all of the available food. Many gravid snakes stop feeding during gestation, and pythons that brood their eggs usually refuse food until after the young have hatched. Some tortoises may be temporarily anorectic at the time of ovulation or oviposition (personal observation). Female reptiles with dystocias often are anorectic. Reproductively active male reptiles may also exhibit a temporary anorexia. Breeding male and postcopulatory (gravid) Green Iguanas (*Iguana iguana*) generally stop feeding in the wild.[6]

A maladaption syndrome has been described in which certain individual reptiles fail to adapt to captive conditions, exhibiting among other symptoms anorexia, even when other individuals of the same species are apparently thriving (Figure 44-3).[7,8]

Gastrointestinal problems may lead to anorexia, including necrotic stomatitis, which may also accompany esophagitis or gastroenteritis; dental disease; abscessation or neoplasms anywhere in the gastrointestinal tract; and rarely an intussusception (usually diagnosed postmortem). Oral abscesses commonly contribute to anorexia in Green Iguanas, chameleons, and snakes.

Gastroenteritis may result from infectious or parasitic causes and lead to anorexia. Parasitic causes may include cestodes, nematodes, acanthocephalans, and protozoans including *Entamoeba* sp. and coccidia (especially *Cryptosporidium* sp.). Yeast or fungal gastrointestinal infections are less commonly encountered. Viral infections are reported to be associated with anorexia in reptiles, including herpesvirus in tortoises,[9] paramyxovirus in snakes,[9] and adenovirus and herpesvirus in Rat Snakes (*Elaphe* spp.).[10]

Mycoplasmosis in Desert Tortoises (*Gopherus agassizii*) also is associated with anorexia.[9] Neoplastic diseases in reptiles may be accompanied by a terminal anorexia.

Gastrointestinal foreign bodies and impactions can lead to anorexia. A good history or examination of the captive environment may be necessary to suspect the presence of a foreign body. For example, bedding materials, such as pebbles, ground corn cob, and wood and bark chips, and plastic cage decorations or towels and pieces of cloth may be ingested and cause intestinal obstruction.

In many snakes, anorexia occurs at the time of shedding. Often no meal is taken during the shedding process, and a failure to feed may only signal the approach of ecdysis in a healthy captive. Many newly acquired snakes may feed for the first time immediately after a shed.

Respiratory disease, including pneumonia, sinusitis, and a secondary aspiration pneumonia, can lead to anorexia (e.g., after vomition or assist-feeding). An iatrogenic bronchoesophageal fistula from overly aggressive assist-feeding may cause anorexia.

DIAGNOSIS

In diagnosing the causes of anorexia, the history and physical examination are critical. Techniques that may aid in determination of underlying etiologies include a complete blood

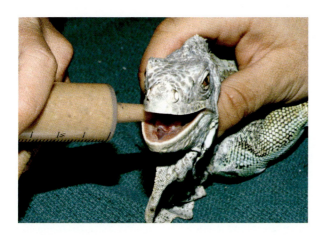

FIGURE 44-4 Regardless of the cause of anorexia, a debilitated patient must be supported with appropriate medical care and nutritional support. This Green Iguana *(Iguana iguana)* is being assist-fed with high-calorie, readily digestible gruel. *(Photograph courtesy D. Mader.)*

count and blood chemistry analysis, a fecal examination for parasites, gastric lavage to check for parasites or infectious agents, fecal culture, radiography, endoscopy, ultrasonography, and biopsy or aspiration of masses for cytologic examination.

Treatment

Anorexia is a symptom, not a disease. Its treatment therefore depends on a determination of the underlying cause or causes. Most often this involves correcting the husbandry techniques and frequently treating the reptile for parasites. If a cause or causes can be identified, the veterinary clinician must guide the client in correcting and treating the problems if possible and owner compliance is essential. A debilitated animal may need to be fed, perhaps via gastric gavage or with assist-feeding, even with the use of a pharyngostomy tube (Figure 44-4).

The client must be willing to make necessary husbandry and nutrition changes if an anorectic patient is to recover, regardless of the cause.

REFERENCES

1. Mayhew WW: Hibernation in the Horned Lizard *(Phrynosoma m'calli), Comp Biochem Physiol* 16:103-119, 1965.
2. Mayhew WW: Biology of desert amphibians and reptiles. In Brown GW, editor: *Desert biology,* vol I, New York, 1968, Academic Press.
3. Frye FL: *Husbandry, medicine, and surgery in captive reptiles,* Bonner Springs, Kan, 1973, Vet Med Publishing.
4. Jackson OF, Cooper JE: Nutritional diseases. In Cooper JE, Jackson OF, editors: *Diseases of the Reptilia,* vol 2, San Diego, 1981, Academic Press.
5. DeNardo DF: Reptile thermal biology: a veterinary perspective, *Proc Assoc Rept Amphib Vet* 157-163, 2004.
6. Rodda GH: The mating behavior of *Iguana iguana, Smithson Contr Zool* 544:1, 1992.
7. Cowan DF: Diseases of captive reptiles, *J Am Vet Med Assoc* 153: 848, 1968.
8. Funk RS: Lizard reproductive medicine and surgery, *Vet Clin No Amer Small Anim Pract* 5:579-613, 2002.
9. Jacobson ER: Viral diseases of reptiles. In Fowler ME, editor: *Zoo & wild animal medicine: current therapy* 3, Philadelphia, 1993, WB Saunders.
10. Heldstab A, Bestetti G: Virus-associated gastrointestinal disease in snakes, *J Zoo Anim Med* 15:118, 1984.

45
AURAL ABSCESSES

MICHAEL J. MURRAY

Aural abscesses or abscessation of the middle ear is a common clinical disease in chelonians, particularly Box Turtles (*Terrapene carolina*), and occasionally lizards (Figure 45-1). The condition is seen in apparently normal individuals. However, it is most commonly associated with reptiles maintained in suboptimal husbandry conditions. This multifactorial aspect of the aural abscess creates the primary challenge to the clinician. Typically, a large number of predisposing factors must be considered in addressing both therapy and prevention.

ANATOMY OF THE REPTILE EAR

The ear of the reptile is often a conspicuous structure located just caudoventral to the eye and covered either by an enlarged cutaneous scale or a transparent to translucent tympanum. Snakes lack an external ear, a factor used in the differentiation of snakes and legless lizards. Species with a well-developed tympanum have a good sense of hearing, and atympanic species have hearing limited to a low-frequency range of 150 to 600 Hz.[1]

The reptilian ear, as is seen in mammals, is divided into three parts: the external ear, which collects sound waves from the environment; the middle ear, which transmits and amplifies these sound waves into vibrations to a chain of bony ossicles; and the inner ear, which transmits these vibrations to a fluid medium that in turn causes movement of cochlear hair cells, movements that are subsequently transmitted to the brain by the vestibulocochlear nerve for interpretation. In most reptile species, the external ear is either absent or significantly diminished. Exceptions to this statement include the geckos, which have a discernible external ear canal, and the crocodilians, which have an earflap that can completely cover the slightly depressed tympanum. Most lizard species have a superficial tympanum and lack an external ear. The chelonian tympanum is flush with the surrounding skin with no external ear. The middle ear consists of the tympanic membrane laterally, the ossicular chain, the tympanic cavity, an air space through which the ossicular chain passes, and the oval window of the cochlea on which the ossicular chain inserts medially (Figure 45-2). The reptilian ossicular chain consists of the columella, an elongated version of the stapes, and the extracolumella, a cartilaginous expansion of the distal portion of the columella. Both the incus and malleus are absent in the reptile.

The tympanic cavity is quite variable in its size and expanse among the reptile orders. In turtles, the large cavity extends caudally into a blind-ended sac (Figure 45-3). The crocodilian species have an extensive tympanic cavity with communication between the left and right sides. The lizard tympanic cavity is situated in such a manner as to appear to be a portion of the pharynx.[2] Despite the absence of a tympanic membrane, snakes do have a tympanic cavity, which is reduced to a narrow fissure.[2] As a result, snakes rarely have aural abscesses develop.

The sole reptilian ossicle, the columella, is a slender osseous structure that spans the tympanic cavity from the tympanum where it connects with the extracolumella to its insertion on the oval window of the cochlea. At this point, the ossicular vibrations are transferred to the fluid medium of the inner ear. The extracolumella has a variable number of processes that extend over the medial aspect of the tympanum. Its function is controversial; however, it appears to stiffen the tympanum and aid in the transfer of vibrations to the columella.[2]

Of particular clinical importance is the presence of eustachian tubes, which connect the middle ear to the oropharynx. Through this structure, pathogens may ascend into the tympanic cavity or inflammatory debris may course into the pharynx (Figure 45-4). The pharyngeal orifice of the eustachian tube is readily identified on the buccal oral mucosa just caudal to the angle of the jaw of the chelonian.

As in mammals, the inner ear has two primary functions: auditory and equilibrium. As expected, the structure and function of the inner ear are quite complex. An extensive description of this aspect of aural anatomy is beyond the scope of this discussion. Surprisingly, vestibular signs and their implication of inner ear involvement are generally not associated with aural abscessation.

ETIOPATHOGENESIS

Although the exact cause of aural abscesses cannot be definitively stated, most appear to be the result of several

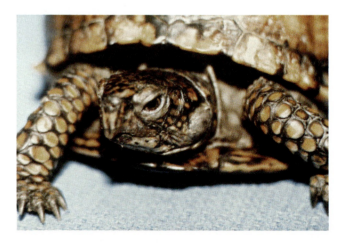

FIGURE 45-1 Typical appearance of an aural abscess in a Box Turtle (*Terrapene carolina*). The tympanum is swollen laterally and is slightly more pale in color. (*Photograph courtesy D. Mader.*)

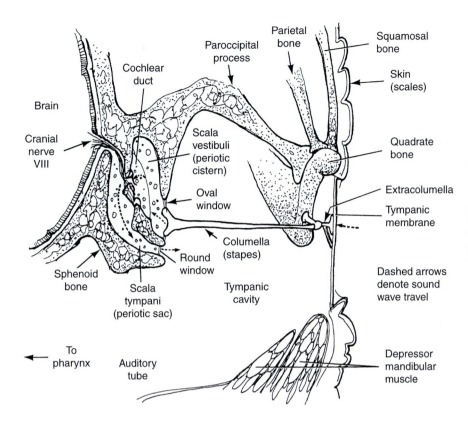

FIGURE 45-2 General relations of the middle and inner ear structures in the lizard *Scleroporus magister*. The right ear is viewed from behind and from the left, so that the inner surface of the tympanic membrane is exposed. (Adapted from Wever EG: *The reptile ear*, Princeton, NJ, 1978, Princeton University Press.)

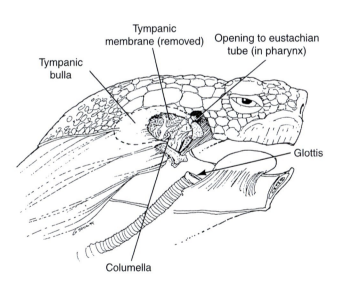

FIGURE 45-3 Head of a Box Turtle (*Terrapene* sp.) with the right lower jaw removed. Note the extent of the middle ear cavity demarcated by the *dashed line*. (Adapted from Boyer TH: Common problems of Box Turtles [*Terrapene* spp.] in captivity, Bull ARAV 2[1]:11, 1992.)

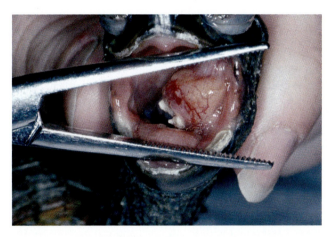

FIGURE 45-4 The eustachian tube connects the middle ear to the oropharynx. Digital pressure on the tympanic membrane may force inflammatory debris through the passage into the pharynx. (*Photograph courtesy S. Barten.*)

predisposing factors. Affected animals are often victims of chronic suboptimal temperatures, improper husbandry, and inadequate nutrition. As a result, the reptile tends to be immunosuppressed with secondary opportunistic infection. The accumulation of potential pathogenic bacteria in an unsanitary cage and dirty water are of particular concern because bacteria tend to flourish in this liquid medium. Ingestion of contaminated water over an extended time period may result in colonization of the oropharynx by pathogenic organisms. Finally, inadequate nutrition, especially hypovitaminosis A, tends to predispose the reptile to aural abscess formation. The squamous metaplasia within the eustachian tube and middle ear, which occurs secondary to hypovitaminosis A, predisposes the animal to colonization and subsequent infection by a variety of bacterial pathogens. In addition, the exfoliating squamous cells tend to accumulate within the tympanic cavity, becoming a constituent of the caseous plug associated with aural abscesses.

Although hematogenous and traumatic etiologies are feasible, most aural abscesses occur as bacterial pathogens that ascend the eustachian tube to enter the tympanic cavity. The cell-mediated immunologic response to these organisms within the middle ear is manifested as an accumulation of granulocytes and histiocytes. As a result of the relative or absolute lack of lysozymes within the reptilian granulocytic leukocytes, the inflammatory exudate tends to be caseous rather than liquid as in mammals. As the disease becomes more chronic, the inflammatory response becomes more mononuclear. Increased chronicity results in the presence of multinucleated giant cells and, in some cases, the formation of a fibrous connective tissue capsule.[3] The abscess center remains avascular throughout the disease process, which tends to prevent the diffusion of parenterally administered antibiotics into the core.

A variety of organisms have been isolated from reptilian aural abscesses. Because most aural abscesses occur from the extension of oropharyngeal bacterial colonization, organisms associated with the disease tend to reflect the normal or commensal flora of the oral cavity. Most tend to be aerobic gram-negative bacteria; however, anaerobic organisms were recovered from an aural abscess in an Eastern Box Turtle (*Terrapene carolina carolina*).[4]

DIAGNOSTIC PLAN

As in the evaluation of mammalian patients, a thorough history is paramount. Specific questions regarding the reptile's water source and frequency of water changes and water bowl disinfection are recommended. In conducting the nutritional review, particular attention should be paid to the vitamin A or beta-carotenoid content of the diet. The clinician must be cautioned to avoid "tunnel vision" and perform a complete and thorough physical examination of the entire patient. Other body systems are often concurrently afflicted as a result of the suboptimal conditions to which the reptile has been subjected. Although the aural abscess itself tends not to be significantly debilitating, the predisposing factors may cause significant systemic illness. Aural abscesses appear as **unilateral** or **bilateral** firm to semifirm swellings of the reptile's tympanum (Figure 45-5). The swelling may appear slightly yellow in color as a result of the accumulation of caseous material within the tympanic cavity. Some degree of discomfort may be noted on opening the mouth, probably as a result of pain associated with the disease, and can account for the patient's discomfort. Gentle digital pressure on the surface of the swelling often expresses small amounts of inflammatory debris from the tympanic cavity through the eustachian tube into the oropharynx (see Figure 45-4).

Ancillary diagnostic testing may seem frivolous but may provide important therapeutic and prognostic data. Fine-needle aspiration of the swelling tends to reveal varying numbers of granulocytes, macrophages, and eosinophilic proteinaceous background material. Samples for culture and sensitivity testing may be collected via centesis; however, a more significant sample is often obtained at the time of surgical debridement. Microorganisms may or may not be identified.

Some level of systemic evaluation of the patient is indicated. Abnormalities of the hemogram, such as leukocytosis, heterophilia with or without toxic changes, monocytosis, or azurophilia, may imply systemic illness and indicate the need for appropriate therapy. Clinical chemistries, with particular attention to renal function, may be indicated. Other ancillary examinations may be warranted, depending on the results of the historic, environmental, nutritional, and physical examinations.

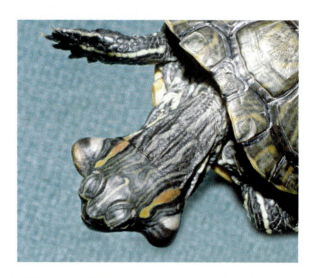

FIGURE 45-5 Aural abscesses may be unilateral or bilateral, as seen in this young Red-eared Slider (*Trachemys scripta elegans*). (*Photograph courtesy D. Mader.*)

THERAPEUTIC PLAN

The nature of the reptilian inflammatory response, the location of the inflammatory exudate, and the relative ease of surgical manipulation mandate a surgical approach to the aural abscess. Cases of long-standing abscesses and those with evidence of systemic disease may benefit from delay of surgical intervention and initiation of systemic antibiotics, fluids, and appropriate supportive care for 3 to 4 days. This approach tends to decrease the local inflammatory response and may decrease local hemorrhage during surgery. In addition, a short delay may enhance the patient's ability to tolerate general anesthesia through correction of fluid and electrolyte imbalances and may elevate the core body temperature to a point within the preferred optimal temperature zone (POTZ).

Surgical manipulation of aural abscesses should occur with appropriate anesthesia. Although a variety of anesthetic agents have been advocated, intravenous propofol is the author's preference. This facilitates adequate debridement of the tympanic cavity and alleviates the pain associated with the disease process. The surgical wound is allowed to heal with secondary intention, but a sterile surgical preparation should be used before surgery and is especially important if collection of specimens for culture and sensitivity is anticipated.

An incision is made through the entire thickness of the tympanum along its ventral border from the 9 o'clock to the 3 o'clock position. The incision is then connected in a horizontal direction across the center of the tympanum.[5] Inflammatory debris may then be removed with small ear loops or curettes (Figure 45-6). An alternative surgical technique in which a cross incision is made, dividing the tympanum into four quadrants, has been described as well.[6] Care must be taken not to damage the columella during debridement. Specimens for culture and sensitivity should be collected at this time. The oral cavity must be examined frequently to prevent the possibility of aspiration because debris

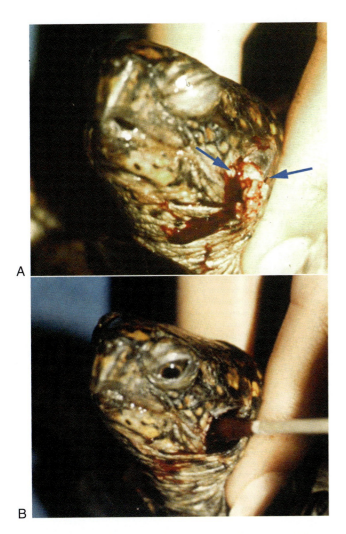

FIGURE 45-6 **A,** This Box Turtle *(Terrapene carolina triunguis)* has an inspissated aural abscess. The first step is to incise through the tympanum from the 3 o'clock to the 9 o'clock position *(blue arrows)*, then continue the incision in an inverted arch to connect both sides. **B,** The caseous inflammatory debris needs to be gently removed. Afterward, the cavity should be flushed with warm saline and treated with Betadyne. *(Photograph courtesy D. Mader.)*

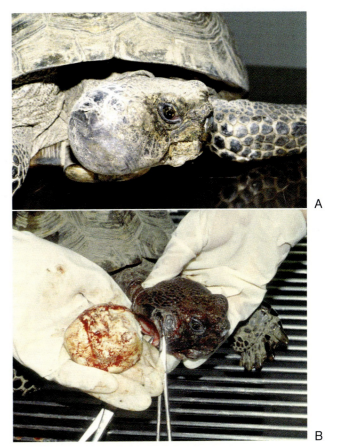

FIGURE 45-7 **A,** Large aural abscess in a California Desert Tortoise *(Gopherus agassizii).* **B,** After removal of the concretion, the area needs to be flushed and examined for extent of damage. The site needs to be cleaned daily and allowed to heal by secondary intention. *(Photograph courtesy D. Mader.)*

may be forced through the eustachian tube into the oropharynx.[7] After removal of the typically large caseous pearl, the surgeon should closely inspect the caudal aspects of the tympanic cavity because debris may extend quite far in the more chronic cases (Figure 45-7). After complete removal of the abscess contents from the tympanic cavity is ensured, the eustachian tube should be gently flushed with saline solution to completely remove all debris. Placement of several cotton-tipped applicators in the caudal oropharynx is generally adequate to prevent aspiration of the flushed material.

After debridement of the abscess, the tympanic cavity should be liberally lavaged with an appropriate antimicrobial agent. Although dilute povidone-iodine (P-I) solution has been advocated, its use remains controversial. In vitro studies have shown that concentrations in excess of 1% P-I solution killed fibroblasts.[8] Free iodine, the active antimicrobial ingredient of P-I, is inactivated in the presence of the proteins of serum, which is often present after surgery within the tympanic cavity. The preferred lavage solution is dilute chlorhexidine (1 part chlorhexidine:30 parts saline) solution. It has a wide spectrum of activity, is relatively nontoxic to tissue, and maintains a sustained residual activity.[8]

After lavage, the wound may be packed with an appropriate antibiotic ointment, such as gentamicin ophthalmic ointment, and allowed to heal with secondary intention. The surgical wound should continue to be lavaged and packed on a daily basis until healed. The decision to place the patient on systemic antibiotics is dependent on several factors. Patients with evidence of systemic illness as determined with physical examination or hematologic changes should benefit from antibiotic therapy.

Concurrent hypovitaminosis A should be investigated, as should continued maintenance of fluid and electrolyte balance. Oral beta-carotenoids, such as those found in orange, yellow, and dark green leafy vegetables, rather than injectable vitamin A, may be indicated in herbivorous reptiles to prevent the possibility of iatrogenic hypervitaminosis A.[9] Until a normal appetite returns, the animal should receive routine assist feedings to maintain a positive calorie balance.

Most aural abscesses respond well to surgical manipulation and heal completely.

Recurrences do occur and are typically the result of inadequate surgical debridement or failure to address the underlying predisposing causes of the disease. Owners should be extensively counseled on appropriate husbandry, sanitation, and nutrition of the species under their care.

To what degree the reptile's auditory capability is compromised by this disease process is, at this time, uncertain. The substantial fibrotic changes that occur during the healing process must certainly affect the ability of the columella to transmit sound to the inner ear. This decreased hearing capability appears to have no long-term effect on the reptiles commonly presented with aural abscesses.

REFERENCES

1. Cooper JE, Jackson OF: *Disease of the Reptilia*, vol I, San Diego, 1981, Academic Press.
2. Wever EG: *The reptile ear*, Princeton, NJ, 1978, Princeton University Press.
3. Frye FL: *Biomedical and surgical aspects of captive reptile husbandry*, ed 2, Melbourne, Fla, 1991, Krieger Publishing.
4. Stewart JS: Anaerobic bacterial infections in reptiles, *J Zoo Wildl Med* 21(2):180, 1990.
5. Mader DR: Turtle and tortoise medicine and surgery, *Proc Calif Vet Med Assoc*, Reno, Nev, 1991.
6. de la Navarre BJS: Diagnosis and treatment of aural abscesses in turtles, *Proc Assoc Reptil Amphib Vet* 9-13, 2000.
7. Boyer TH: Common problems of box turtles (*Terrapene* spp.) in captivity, *Bull Assoc Reptil Amphib Vet* 2(1):9, 1992.
8. Swaim SF, Lee AH: Topical wound medications: a review, *J Am Vet Med Assoc* 190(12):1588, 1987.
9. Palmer DG, Rubel A, Mettler F, et al: Experimentell erzeugte Hautveranderungen bei Landschildkroten durch hohe parenterale Gaben von Vitamin A, *Zbl Vet Med A* 31: 625, 1984.

46
BITES FROM PREY
STEPHEN L. BARTEN

Keepers commonly feed live rodents to carnivorous reptiles and amphibians. This practice is discouraged. Many captive reptiles refuse live food but readily accept prekilled prey items. The use of prekilled food allows more humane euthanasia of the prey. Prekilled prey may be purchased in bulk at lower prices than live prey and stored frozen until used. Finally, prekilled prey cannot injure the reptile to which it is fed.

Captive reptiles occasionally choose not to eat a live rodent as soon as it is offered, which gives the prey a chance to injure the reptile. Husbandry factors may be the reason. These include lack of proper temperatures, lack of a hiding place, sharing the cage with another reptile, excessive handling, and rodents offered to species that normally do not eat them. Many reptiles normally refuse food when they are opaque or about to shed or are gravid, during the breeding season, or during the fall in species that normally brumate (hibernate). Virtually any illness also can cause a reptile to refuse food.

When a live rodent is left in a cage with a reptile that is anorectic for any reason, the rodent often gnaws on the reptile, causing wounds along its sides and back (Figure 46-1). Bite wounds can be superficial and minor or can involve massive tissue destruction (Figure 46-2). Reptiles do not kill rodents to prevent further damage during an attack. Fatalities may result from a bite to the neck just caudal to the occiput. Rodents also may bite in self defense when seized by a hungry reptile in any manner that fails to cause immediate death. This usually results in wounds to the tongue, lips, eyes, or head of the reptile (Figures 46-3 and 46-4). If a rodent must be left unattended in a cage with a reptile, rodent food should be left in the cage as well, although this does not guarantee that the rodent will leave the reptile alone.

The best way to prevent bite wounds from prey is to feed only prekilled prey. Reptiles that refuse prekilled prey may be trained to accept the prey with offering a two-rodent meal that consists of a live rodent followed by a stunned one. The next meal uses a stunned rodent followed by a dead one. After that, a dead rodent is offered. More feeding trials than this may be necessary, but once prekilled food is accepted, live prey never should be offered again. Species that need movement to recognize food items can be trained to accept prekilled rodents with dangling the prey from a long pair of forceps.

Live rodents must never be left unattended in a cage. If a reptile does not seize the prey within 10 to 15 minutes, it probably will not eat that day.

TREATMENT

Bite wounds are contaminated and should be flushed copiously with sterile saline or balanced electrolyte solutions. In all but minor wounds, sedation is recommended during treatment. Anesthesia and basic surgical techniques for reptiles have been discussed in detail elsewhere (see Chapters 27 and 35).[1-7] Necrotic and avascular tissue is removed, and defects should be sutured if possible. Old or obviously infected wounds should not be sutured until infection has been controlled and a healthy bed of granulation tissue established. Reptile skin adheres tightly to the subcutis, especially over the skull, so that sliding full-thickness skin grafts are difficult to construct. Undue tension on suture lines must be avoided and bite wounds from prey often result in large defects; thus, many bite wounds must be allowed to heal by granulation. Severely damaged tail tips and digits may heal faster with amputation than with granulation (Figure 46-5). Wounds around the face may result in gross disfigurement. A ruptured globe should be enucleated. A scarred rostrum may necessitate reconstruction of the nares.[4] If the tongue or lingual sheath is damaged, care must be taken to prevent the formations of adhesions. Application of an antibiotic steroid

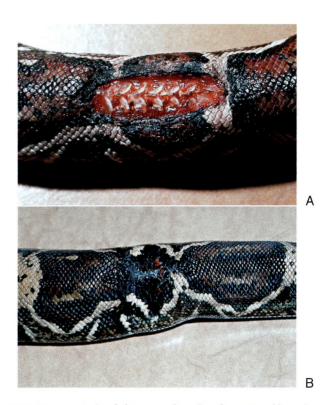

FIGURE 46-1 **A,** Single bite wound in a Boa Constrictor *(Constrictor constrictor)* inflicted by a live mouse left in the cage overnight. The vertebrae have been exposed. Suturing was not possible because of skin tension across the wound. The wound was allowed to heal by granulation, with bandaging and systemic antibiotics. **B,** The same snake after 20 months. Healing is complete with minimal scarring.

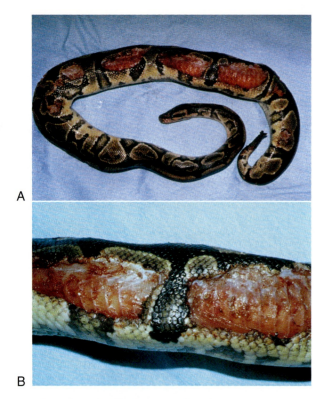

FIGURE 46-2 **A,** Multiple bite wounds with massive tissue loss in a Ball Python *(Python regius)* fed a live rat. Although capable of doing so, the snake did not kill the rat to stop the attack. **B,** Close-up of bite wounds in the same snake.

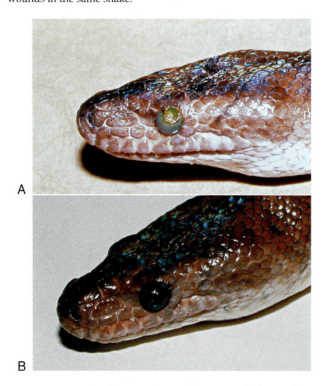

FIGURE 46-3 **A,** Rainbow Boa *(Epicrates cenchria)* with a hole in the left spectacle inflicted by a mouse during feeding. The snake struck the mouse in the hind end, which allowed the mouse to turn and bite the snake in the eye before the snake could apply constriction or the owner could intervene. Note that the cornea was positive for fluorescein stain. Treatment consisted of topical antibiotic ophthalmic ointment. **B,** Same snake seen 2 years later for a different problem; healing is complete.

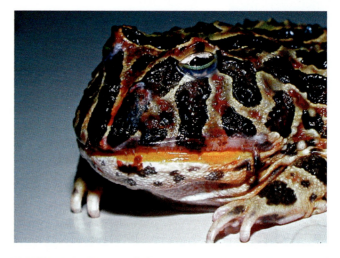

FIGURE 46-4 Bite wounds from prey are not confined to snakes. A live mouse was left in the cage with this Argentine Horned Frog *(Ceratophrys ornata)*. The lips, rostrum, and eyelids were gnawed.

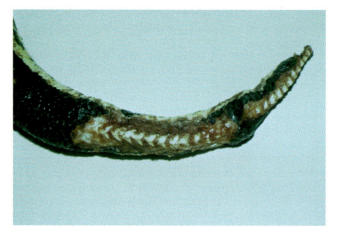

FIGURE 46-5 Rodent bite wounds exposed most of the vertebrae in the tail of this Boa Constrictor *(Constrictor constrictor)*. The tail was amputated back to healthy tissue.

ophthalmic ointment containing steroids to the tongue sheath two to three times a day during the healing process helps avoid this sequela. A single injection of 0.01 to 0.05 mL of methylprednisolone acetate (Depo-Medrol, Pharmacia & Upjohn, Kalamazoo, Mich) or triamcinolone acetonide (Vetalog, Fort Dodge Animal Health, Overland Park, Kan) may be given intralesionally if adhesions develop.[4] Snakes that lose the use of their tongue, either through amputation or adhesions, must be hand-fed for the remainder of their life.

All but the most minor open wounds should be bandaged. Antiseptic liquid bandage (New Skin, Prestige Brands Holdings, Inc., Irvington, NY) can be used to cover superficial wounds. It is not appropriate for deep wounds, should not be used in conjunction with other topical medications, and must be reapplied every 24 to 48 hours. Adhesive tape sticks to reptile skin, but ointment on the skin prevents sticking. Honey or sugar bandages have gained popularity in the treatment of contaminated wounds. Wet-to-dry bandages are useful to promote the development of healthy granulation tissue (Figure 46-6). Biosynthetic absorbent wound dressing (BioDres, DVM Pharmaceuticals, Inc., Miami, Fla) protects

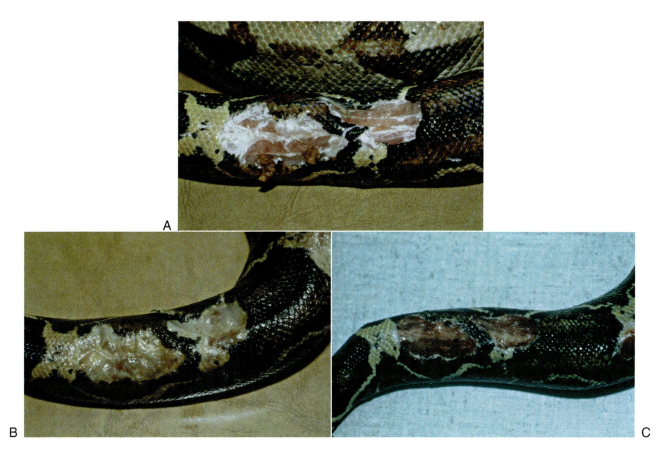

FIGURE 46-6 **A,** Deep bite wounds in a Boa Constrictor *(Constrictor constrictor)* inflicted by a rat. These fresh lesions were contaminated with bedding material. Not enough skin was present for suturing across the lesions. Instead the wounds were treated with wet-to-dry bandages changed every other day along with systemic and topical antibiotics. **B,** The same wounds show copious discharge on day 14. **C,** A healthy granulation bed on day 21. Healing was complete with moderate scarring.

the wound during healing and sticks to areas that otherwise are difficult to bandage, such as the rostrum. All bandage materials should be changed every 1 to 2 days.

Extracellular matrix from porcine intestinal submucosa (VetBioSISt, Global Veterinary Products, Inc., New Buffalo, Mich) is another product that may be used to cover large skin defects.[8] Principles of its use include the control of infection, development of a healthy granulation bed before application, rehydration of the matrix before use, and suturing the matrix in place and bandaging the area to keep the matrix clean, moist, and infection free.

Some reptiles, particularly snakes, are adept at crawling out of bandages. An alternative to bandaging is to house the patient for the first few days in a waterproof container such as a small aquarium, plastic cage, or plastic picnic chest with adequate ventilation. This container is lined with clean toweling soaked in dilute povidone-iodine (Betadine solution, Purdue Pharma L.P., Stamford, Conn) or chlorhexidine (Nolvasan, Fort Dodge Animal Health, Overland Park, Kan) solution.[4] The towels and solutions should be changed daily.

During healing, reptiles with open wounds should be kept in bare cages or in cages lined with clean newspaper, paper towels, or cloth towels. Particulate bedding material may stick to wounds and should be avoided.[4]

Topical and systemic antibiotics are indicated for contaminated bite wounds. One percent silver sulfadiazine cream (various manufacturers) is an excellent topical for *Pseudomonas* spp. and other gram-negative bacteria. Two percent mupirocin ointment (Bactoderm, SmithKline Beecham Inc., Philadelphia, Pa) is another good choice. Antibiotic combination ointments or creams with polymyxin B sulfate, neomycin, and bacitracin (various manufacturers) also are good choices for topical therapy. Systemic, parenteral, bactericidal antibiotics should be used to prevent and treat infection and septicemia (see Chapter 36). Material for bacterial culture and sensitivity should be collected from wounds that are obviously infected.

Healing by granulation can take from as little as a few months to more than a year. Changing bandages and wound cleaning are necessary every day or every other day. Topical enzymatic agents may be used when copious necrotic debris is present. Choices include collagenase ointment, 250 units per gram (Collagenase Santyl, Smith & Nephew, Inc., Largo, Fla), and preparations with combinations of trypsin, papain, balsam of Peru, castor oil, urea, and chlorophyll derivatives (various manufacturers). Defects from bite wounds may appear unchanging between periods of ecdysis, then appear partially epithelialized after a shed. As many as six to 10 shedding cycles may occur before a large defect is completely healed. The area around healing wounds may shed incompletely and necessitate soaking and manual removal of the old skin. Massive scarring with interruption of the normal symmetrical scale pattern often results.

REFERENCES

1. Bennett RA: Reptilian surgery; part I: basic principles, *Compend Contin Educ Pract Vet* 11:10, 1989.
2. Bennett RA: Reptilian surgery; part II: management of surgical diseases, *Compend Contin Educ Pract Vet* 11:122, 1989.
3. Bennett RA: A review of aneshesia and chemical restraint in reptiles, *Zoo Wildl Med* 22:282, 1991.
4. Frye FL: *Biomedical and surgical aspects of captive reptile husbandry*, ed 2, Melbourne, Fla, 1991, Krieger Publishing.
5. Lawton MPC: Anaesthesia. In Beynon PH, Lawton MPC, Cooper JE, editors: *Manual of reptiles*, Gloucestershire, England, 1992, British Small Animal Veterinary Association.
6. Lawton MPC, Stoakes LC: Surgery. In Beynon PH, Lawton MPC, Cooper JE, editors: *Manual of reptiles*, Gloucestershire, England, 1992, British Small Animal Veterinary Association.
7. Millichamp NJ: Surgical techniques in reptiles. In Jacobson ER, Kollias GV, editors: *Contemporary issues in small animal practice: exotic animals*, New York, 1988, Churchill Livingstone.
8. Divers S: Use of VetBioSISt® skin grafting techniques in reptiles, *Exotic DVM Vet Mag* 2:62, 2000.

47
CLOACAL PROLAPSE

R. AVERY BENNETT and
DOUGLAS R. MADER

ANATOMY

Three compartments are located within the cloaca (see Figure 11-1). The coprodeum is the most cranial and is located where the rectum enters the cloaca. Fecal and urinary waste from the terminal colon is deposited into this chamber. The urodeum is in the midsection of the cloaca and contains the openings of the ureters and the reproductive system. The proctodeum is the caudal-most portion of the cloaca and serves as the reservoir for fecal and urinary waste before excretion. The openings of the musk glands are located within this compartment.

When an organ prolapses, it is not always easy to identify, especially for the lay person. Prolapses should always be considered and treated as an emergency. When a client calls and claims that the herp pet has "something coming out of its rear end," instruct them to bring the animal in right away. Have them protect the tissue from further damage by wrapping the cloacal area with a clean damp facial cloth, diaper, or some other cotton fabric (Figure 47-1). Paper and tape that could potentially damage the tissue should be avoided. Also tell the owner *not* to try and reduce the prolapse because further damage may occur or current injuries may be hidden.

CLOACAL ORGAN PROLAPSE

In reptiles, the distal gastrointestinal tract, the urinary bladder, the penis (chelonians, crocodilians) or hemipenes (all other reptiles) of males, and the oviduct of females may prolapse through the cloaca and out through the vent. Cloacal organ prolapse is generally the result of an excessive amount of straining from some inciting cause. For example, enteritis may result in excessive straining and prolapse of the colon. Identification of the underlying cause for the prolapse, in addition to treatment of the prolapse itself, is important. For example, in a female California Desert Tortoise (*Gopherus agassizii*), prolapse of the reproductive tract was the result of a cystic urinary calculus.[1]

Which organ has prolapsed must be determined before a treatment plan is decided on. The urinary bladder is thin walled and translucent (Figure 47-2). Coelomic fluid may collect within the everted bladder, giving the impression of a "urine"-filled, albeit exteriorized, bladder. A penis or hemipenis prolapse presents as a solid tissue mass protruding from the vent (Figure 47-3) (see also Chapter 64). These structures have no lumen (but a central "groove" or "sulcus" may be present) and are therefore unique. With a prolapse of the colon, a lumen should be present (Figure 47-4, *A*). The surface is generally smooth, and in many cases, fecal material can be obtained through the lumen, either passed directly or with aspiration through a small catheter inserted into the lumen (Figure 47-4, *B*) (see also Figure 47-7, *A*). With an oviductal prolapse, the prolapsed structure has a lumen but no feces are identified. Although this structure also has a lumen, longitudinal striations are present on the surface that are not present on the colon (Figure 47-5).

Copulatory Organ Prolapse

Prolapse of the penis or hemipenis is most commonly the result of infection, swelling from sex determination probing, or forced separation during copulation. Other reported causes include constipation and neurologic dysfunction.[2,3]

The protruding tissue should be cleaned, lubricated, and gently replaced into the cloaca. Frequently, a moistened cotton-tipped applicator is helpful in reducing the prolapse.

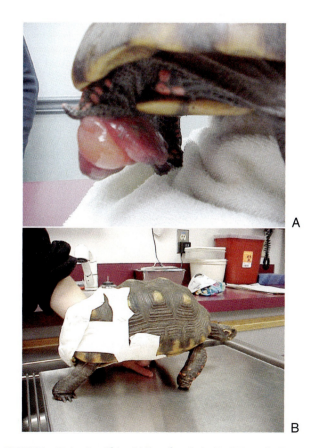

FIGURE 47-1 **A,** This Yellow-headed Red-Footed Tortoise (*Geochelone carbonara*) has a prolapsed oviduct. **B,** The emergency veterinarian wrapped the tissue in saline solution–soaked gauze and then taped the tissue into a makeshift "diaper" to protect the tissue until the patient could be seen by a specialist. (*Photographs courtesy D. Mader.*)

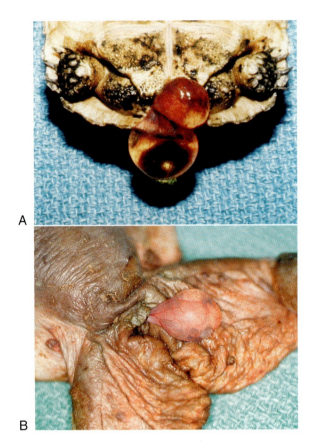

FIGURE 47-2 Prolapsed bladder in a tortoise **(A)** and a frog **(B)**. Note the fluid-filled, thin-walled, membranous urinary bladder. The fluid is not urine. It is coelomic fluid that has been trapped within the everted structure. *(Photographs courtesy D. Mader.)*

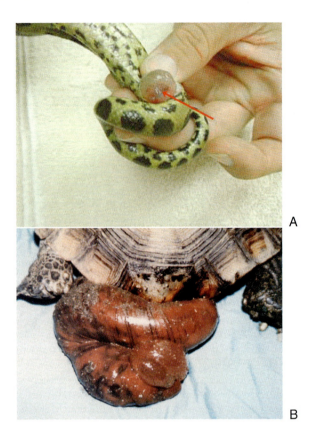

FIGURE 47-4 Prolapsed colon in, **A**, a juvenile Anaconda (*Eunectes* sp.) and, **B**, Desert Tortoise (*Gopherus agassizii*). The tissue is smooth and shiny and may be gas filled. Feces can often be found within the lumen of the prolapsed organ. *(Photographs courtesy D. Mader.)*

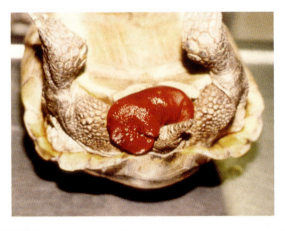

FIGURE 47-3 An engorged prolapsed penis in a tortoise. This reproductive organ is so swollen that it cannot be replaced. A small incision can be made in the lateral cloacal wall to help reduce the tissue. Compare this prolapse with the images in Chapter 64. *(Photograph courtesy D. Mader.)*

Glycerin or concentrated sugar solutions may be helpful in decreasing the tissue edema if the organ is significantly enlarged.

If the prolapse cannot be manually reduced, the vent opening may be enlarged with incision of the vent laterally on one or both sides (see Figure 47-3). This enlarges the vent opening, allowing the swollen gland to be reduced. Once the organ is replaced, a purse-string or transverse cloacal suture may be placed to prevent the organ from prolapsing again (see Chapter 64 for details). The transverse cloacal suture provides the advantage of allowing normal urination and defecation.

If the tissue is badly damaged, severely swollen, or necrotic, amputation may be performed. Because the urinary system does not pass through the penis or hemipenes, no disruption is seen in the flow of urine. Mattress sutures are placed at the base of the prolapsed organ to control hemorrhage, and the tissues are transected distal to the sutures. The stump may then be replaced within the cloaca. In those species with hemipenes, if one organ is amputated, the animal is still considered fertile because the opposite side should still be functional.[3]

Prolapse of the Oviduct

Females may have the oviduct prolapse as a result of egg binding or other conditions that cause tenesmus. In some cases, reduction of the prolapse may be possible; however, the suspensory structures likely have been damaged. This affects the ability of the oviduct to receive yolks ovulated from the ovary in the future. Amputation of the exposed and damaged tissue has been performed in some cases.[4] In most cases, celiotomy for removal of the affected portion of the reproductive tract and its accompanying ovary is recommended.

Cloacal Prolapse

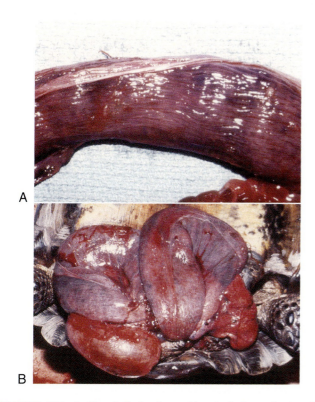

FIGURE 47-5 **A,** The shell gland or oviduct is fleshy and striated. **B,** Both the oviducts *(purple tissue)* and colon *(red tissue)* prolapsed in this Desert Tortoise *(Gopherus agassizii)*. *(Photographs courtesy D. Mader.)*

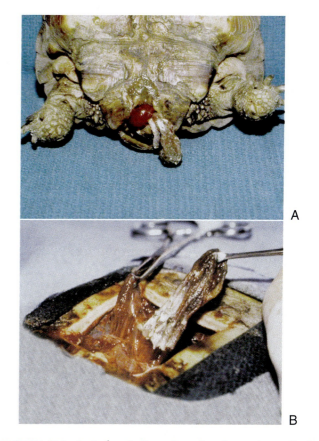

FIGURE 47-6 **A,** A chronically prolapsed, and now traumatized, urinary bladder in a Desert Tortoise *(Gopherus agassizii)*. Note that one lobe of the bladder is necrotic. **B,** The same tortoise as in Figure 47-6, *A.* A ventral celiotomy has been performed to allow enough access to properly excise the diseased tissue. Captive animals can handle subtotal cystectomies provided they are allowed continuous access to fresh water. *(Photographs courtesy D. Mader.)*

Female reptiles have a bicornuate reproductive system and two ovaries. Through celiotomy, if one side of the reproductive tract is involved, the oviduct, and the ovary on the affected side may be removed. With the contralateral side left intact, the patient is still be able to reproduce. In reptiles in which reproduction is not a concern, bilateral ovariohysterectomy should be performed to prevent future occurrence of this condition or other reproductive tract–related abnormalities (see Chapter 35 for surgical procedures).

Urinary Bladder Prolapse

In most cases prolapse of the urinary bladder is the result of cystitis, often associated with cystic calculi (see Chapter 49). Because the ureters empty into the urodeum and do not have a direct connection to the urinary bladder, they are seldom affected or damaged in a simple prolapse of the bladder.

If a small portion of the urinary bladder is prolapsed, it may be successfully reduced with the previously described techniques. If the exposed tissue appears to be nonviable, it needs to be resected (Figure 47-6, *A*). An atraumatic clamp may be placed across the viable section of tissue, allowing the nonviable tissue to be removed distal to the clamp. A double-layer inverting closure is then placed distal to the clamp, sealing the urinary bladder. The remainder is then replaced through the cloaca and into the coelomic cavity. If a large portion of the bladder is damaged, a celiotomy may be performed for better exposure and excision of the diseased tissue (Figure 47-6, *B*). One must keep in mind that the bladder does participate in water and electrolyte reabsorption from the urinary system, and if possible, an attempt should be made to salvage as much of the viable bladder tissue as possible.

Colon Prolapse

Prolapse of the colon is generally the result of tenesmus. Constipation, bacterial enteritis, and parasitic enteritis have been implicated. Constipation may result from environmental factors, such as an enclosure that is excessively small and inhibits sufficient exercise to stimulate normal defecation. Determination of the cause of tenesmus and treatment of this in conjunction with management of the prolapse are important.

In the acute phase, the prolapsed tissue is easily reduced and can be managed with either purse-string or transverse cloacal sutures. The venous return from the prolapsed colon is frequently compromised, resulting in rapid engorgement of the tissue. The tissue becomes edematous and friable. This type of prolapse is often difficult or impossible to reduce. In such cases, a celiotomy allows for traction to be applied to the colon and for external pulsion, resulting in reduction of the prolapse. In addition, through a celiotomy approach, a colopexy may be performed to prevent recurrence of the prolapse (see Chapter 35 for surgical procedures).

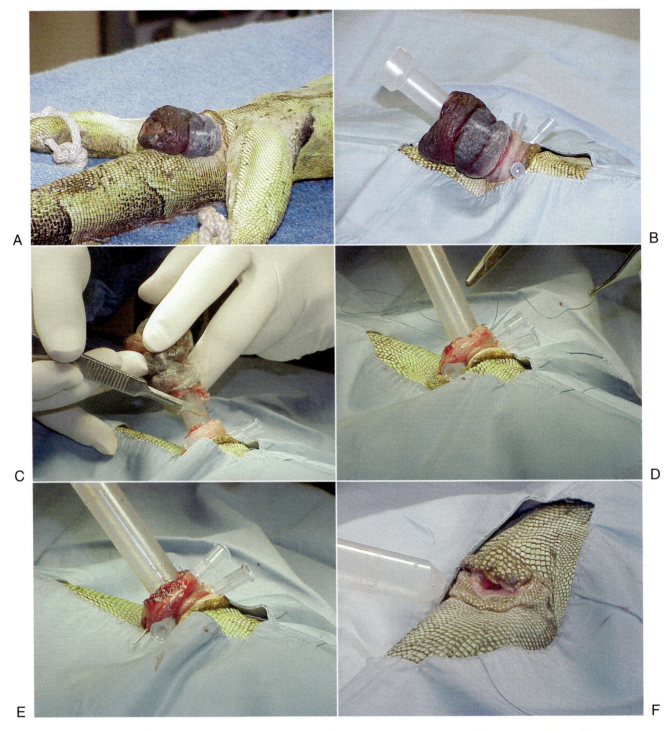

FIGURE 47-7 **A,** Prolapsed colon in a Green Iguana *(Iguana iguana).* **B,** A syringe case is lubricated and placed into the prolapsed lumen. The tissue is cross-pinned through the viable areas. **C,** The necrotic portion is excised. **D** and **E,** The remaining two layers are then anastomosed with a monofilament, synthetic, absorbable suture material. **F,** The dead tissue and syringe case are then removed, allowing the healthy tissue to retract back into the coelomic cavity. *(Photographs courtesy D. Mader.)*

If the primary cause of tenesmus is identified and treated, creation of permanent adhesions between the colon and the body wall is not necessary. However, during the treatment period, internal suturing of the colon is beneficial so that it will not prolapse. The coloplexy should be performed in an area of healthy viable colon tissue.[5] In this location, sutures are placed between the colon and the body wall. A small atraumatic needle should be used to minimize the amount of colon contents that leak through the suture tracks.

Alternatively, the colon may be incorporated into the body wall closure, thus immobilizing the colon. With this technique, the suture is passed through one side of the body wall, through the colon, then through the other side of the body wall, and tied. This technique is used along the length of the body wall incision.

In cases of colon prolapse in which the exposed tissue is devitalized, a resection and anastomosis can be performed.[6] This may be performed without celiotomy with insertion of a smooth, tubular object into the lumen of the colon (Figure 47-7). In many patients, a thermometer or clean syringe case is of an appropriate size to provide support to the lumen. Mattress sutures are placed from the external surface toward the thermometer or stent, bouncing off the stent and exiting to the external surface. These sutures are placed circumferentially around the tubular colon in a healthy portion of tissue. Once these mattress sutures have been placed circumferentially, the tissue may be transected distal to the sutures. When the exposed tissue is returned to the coelomic cavity, an inverting end-to-end intestinal anastomosis is created. Alternatively, a resection and anastomosis may be performed through a celiotomy with standard techniques.

REFERENCES

1. Bennett RA: *Uterine prolapse caused by cystic calculus in a California desert tortoise* (Gopherus agassizii), Orlando, Fla, 1993, Proceedings of the North American Veterinary Conference.
2. Rosskoph WJ, Woerpel RW, Pitts BJ: Paraphimosis in a California desert tortoise, *Calif Vet* 36(1):29, 1982.
3. Frye FL: *Biomedical and surgical aspects of captive reptile husbandry*, Edwardsville, Kan, 1981, Veterinary Medicine Publishing.
4. Frye FL: Clinical obstetric and gynecological disorders in reptiles, *Proc AAHA* 41:497, 1974.
5. Bodri MS, Sadanaga KK: Circumcostal cloacapexy in a python, *JAVMA* 198:297, 1991.
6. Leash AM: Amputation of a prolapsed rectum in an African rock python, *J Am Vet Med Assoc* 171:980, 1977.

48
CRYPTOSPORIDIOSIS

MICHAEL R. CRANFIELD and
THADDEUS K. GRACZYK

The apicomplexan genus *Cryptosporidium* contains about 11 species[1] and has been identified in numerous hosts, including mammals, birds, reptiles, and fishes.[2] This monogenous (life cycle in one host) protozoan inhabits the gastrointestinal tract along with gastric glands[3] and has been reported from the avian respiratory system.[4] *Cryptosporidium* has a worldwide distribution.[5] To date, *Cryptosporidium* infection in amphibians has been reported as an incidental finding.[6] *Cryptosporidium* sp. was seen on fecal examination of an American toad at the Baltimore Zoo and in the feces of Bell's Horned Frog in a zoo in Canada.[7,8]

The first report in the literature of *Cryptosporidium* in reptiles describes infections in 14 snakes belonging to four species and three genera (*Elaphe*, *Crotalus*, and *Sansinia*) at the Baltimore Zoo.[9] More recent reports of cryptosporidiosis concern snakes, lizards, and turtles.[10-15]

Cryptosporidiosis was reported in three species of geckos (*Hemidaxctylus turcicus turcicus*, *Phelsuma madagascariensis grandis*, and *Eublepharis macularius*), and the infection was limited to the cloaca.[16-18] The previously mentioned reports and comparison of the biology of reptilian and mammalian isolates suggest that *Cryptosporidium* recovered from reptilian gastric mucosa represents a different species. Investigation of 528 wild and captive reptiles for cryptosporidial infections suggests that cryptosporidiosis is common in wild and captive populations and that, although not proven, at least four species may exist among the reptiles examined.[11]

The name of *Cryptosporidium* (hidden sporocyst) was given[3] when the endogenous pathogen stages that adhere to the microvillous borders of mouse intestines were found to be covered by the enterocyte-derived membrane. The lack of distinguishable morphologic features on the oocyst wall has generated a lot of confusion[19] in the classification of the genus *Cryptosporidium* since 1907. Small oocyst size, moderate rate of infection, and fluctuation in shedding the oocyst make oocyst detection difficult.

LIFE CYCLE

The life cycle in reptiles has not been delineated but is thought to be similar to the mammalian life cycle described subsequently. The differences in life cycle between human or calf-derived *Cryptosporidium* spp. isolates and other Coccidia (*Eimeria* spp., *Isospora* spp.) concern the site of infection of comparable intracellular stages within the microvillus. *Cryptosporidium* spp. inhabit a parasitophorous (produced by the parasite) vacuole confined to the microvillous region, whereas *Eimeria* spp. or *Isospora* spp. parasitophorous vacuoles occupy deeper regions of the gastric mucosa. *Cryptosporidium* spp. oocysts sporulate within the host cells and are infective immediately after release with the feces.

In the mouse model, approximately 20% of *C. muris* oocysts do not form a thick, two-layered, environmentally resistant wall, but four sporozoites are surrounded by a single membrane.[20] After the sporozoites are released from the oocyst, they penetrate into the enterocyte microvillous region, reinitiating the life cycle. Most (approximately 80%) *C. muris* oocysts develop a thick wall resistant to environmental factors.

The thick-walled oocysts are considered transmission agents, and the thin-walled oocysts are autoinfective and maintain the life cycle within an infested individual. Severity of infection is a result of reinfection with thin-walled oocysts, repeated exposure to the thick-walled oocysts, and the immune status of the infested host.[14,15]

TRANSMISSION

The mode of *Cryptosporidium* transmission in reptiles is the fecal-oral route from one animal to the next by direct contact or through contact with contaminated objects.[14,15] In mammals, it is also considered a water-borne disease, with water sources contaminated by *C. parvum* from cattle or deer.[5] This route is not likely important to reptiles in captivity. In a study at the Baltimore Zoo in which 2000 oocysts were given via stomach tube to healthy snakes, five of nine became fecal-positive between 8 to 28 weeks (average, 14 weeks) after infection.[21] Dexamethasone administration at 1 mg/lb for 5 days before and after dosing the snakes increased the rate of infection.[21]

TRANSMISSION STUDIES AND ZOONOTIC IMPLICATIONS

Cryptosporidium parvum can pass through the digestive tract of birds and lower vertebrates, causing no disease, but defecated oocysts remain infective to mammals (Table 48-1).[8,11,22] Therefore, if a reptile eats a *C. parvum*–infected host, it is not infected, but contact with the reptile's feces could result in a *C. parvum* infection in a handler.[22] *Cryptosporidium* sp. and *C. serpentis* from reptiles did not cause disease in neonatal Bagg Albino/c mutation BALB/c mice (the golden standard for mammal infectivity).[23] Therefore, according to current knowledge, reptiles infected with *Cryptosporidium* are not a zoonotic problem.[14,15] *Cryptosporidium parvum* and *C. muris* do not cause infection in reptiles, and *C. parvum*–positive and *C. muris*–positive food items are not a problem when fed to reptiles.[22]

Species specificity does not appear to exist to *C. serpentis* within reptiles. *Cryptosporidium* oocysts from Bog Turtles (*Clemmys muhlenbegi*), Star Tortoises (*Geochelone elegans*), Mountain Chameleons (*Chamaelo montium*), and Savannah Monitors (*Veranus exanthematicus*) caused severe infections

Table 48-1 Cross-Transmission Studies

Organism	Mammals	Birds	Reptiles	Amphibians	Fish
C. parvum	+	+/−*	−	−	−
C. muris	+	−	−	?	?
Cryptosporidium spp. in reptiles	−	−	+	−	?
C. serpentis	−	−	+	−	?
C. baileyi	−	+	−	?	?
C. meleagridis	−	+	−	?	?

*One study showed *Cryptosporidium* from bovine feces to cause respiratory infections in 1-day-old and 7-day-old ducks.[27]

in young Cornsnakes *(Elaphe obsoleta)* when experimentally transferred.[14,22]

CLINICAL SIGNS

Three manifestations of *Cryptosporidium* appear to exist in reptiles:

Subclinical (Carrier State)

Clinically healthy snakes are able to pass oocysts intermittently for years.[14,15] At the Baltimore Zoo, one death from cryptosporidiosis has occurred in a snake in the last decade.[14] This low mortality rate has occurred despite a high prevalence rate in the collection of snakes that have shed oocysts in their feces for up to 20 years without clinical signs.[14] Most positive snakes are intermittent fecal shedders, oscillating between periods of shedding high numbers of oocysts to periods during which feces are cryptosporidia-negative.[14,24] These cases were undetected unless routine fecal studies by skilled technicians showed the presence of the parasite.[24] Although subclinical carrier states are most frequently found in snakes, the authors have also seen them in turtles and lizards.[13-15,25] The organisms from these carriers were pathogenic to young snakes when experimentally infected.[22]

Clinical

Gastric Hyperplasia of the Mucus-Secreting Cells (Snakes)

The usual history in clinical cases of snakes is weight loss with persistent or periodical postprandial regurgitation of undigested mice 3 to 4 days after ingestion.[15] These clinically affected snakes may live for days to years.[14] Clinically affected snakes have a noticeable swelling in the gastric region, located half the distance between the mouth and the cloaca (Figure 48-1).[14] Barium studies reveal thickened gastric walls with associated constriction of the gastric lumen. Some species such as rattlesnakes and amelanotic snakes appear to be more prone to the overt clinical syndrome, but no set patterns to this rule are found.[14,15] In snakes, the disease differs from that in mammals and birds in that it appears to affect snakes of all ages and is not acute and self-limiting.[14]

Enteritis

A chronic debilitating enteritis without gastric involvement has been seen in lizards, chelonians, and snakes.[14] Although in some cases *Cryptosporidium* was concluded to be the main

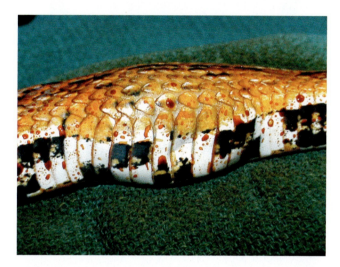

FIGURE 48-1 Firm midbody swellings are common in chronically infected snakes. This patient has been prepared for gastric biopsy. *(Photograph courtesy D. Mader.)*

pathogen responsible for death, it was often associated with other stressors, such as concurrent disease or suboptimal environmental conditions.[13-15]

GROSS PATHOLOGY

The pathologic changes in snakes with cryptosporidiosis are almost always limited to the stomach and vary in severity.[14] Chronic shedders with no clinical signs may have grossly normal gastric mucosa, and clinical cases may have an increase in the diameter of the stomach, with reduction in the gastric luminal diameter.[14,15] The gastric mucosa of affected snakes may be edematous, with mucosal thickening and exaggeration of the normal longitudinal rugae to which copious mucus is adhered (see Figure 48-2).[14,15] Mucosal petechiae (Figure 48-2), brush hemorrhages, and focal necrosis are common. In cases of pathogenic enteritis, inflammation of bowel and loose contents throughout the complete intestinal tract are usually seen.[9,14,15]

HISTOLOGY

In snakes, the lesions vary with the severity of the disease but usually range from mild, with little architectural change and low numbers of organisms on the surface of the brush border, to severe, with loss of brush border, flattening of epithelial

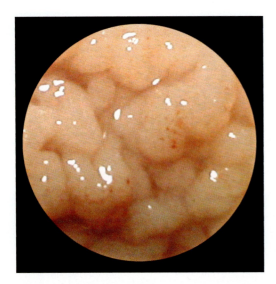

FIGURE 48-2 Endoscopic view of thickened gastric rugae. Note the petechial hemorrhages in the mucosa. *(Photograph courtesy D. Mader.)*

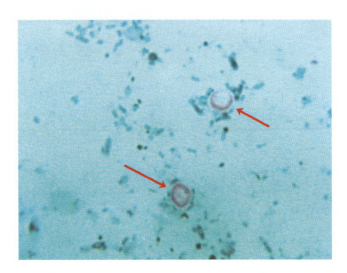

FIGURE 48-4 *Cryptosporidium serpentis* stained with the modified acid-fast stain *(arrows)* in direct wet smear prepared from fecal specimens of subclinically infected Cornsnakes *(Elaphe guttata)*. The mean size of *C. serpentis* oocysts is 6.3 × 5.5 μm.

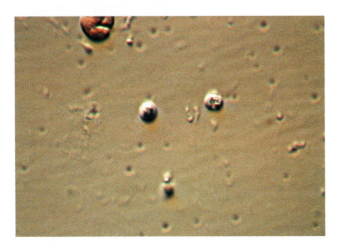

FIGURE 48-3 Wet mount preparation photographed with sheared light illumination. The two circular objects in the center of the image are *Cryptosporidium* sp. The larger circular object on the upper left is an erythrocyte. (Magnification, ×402; *Photograph courtesy F.L. Frye.*)

cells, and proliferation of gastric mucous cells.[9,14,15] Intestinal lesions in lizards, chelonians, and (rarely) snakes consist of heterophil, lymphocyte, and macrophage infiltration and occasionally more than 80% of the cells harboring parasites.[14,15]

DIAGNOSTICS

Noninvasive

Examination of Feces or Mucus from Regurgitated Food Items

Although cryptosporidia can be detected in an unstained smear (Figure 48-3), the sensitivity increases greatly with an acid-fast stain (Figure 48-4; Table 48-2) and is the most sensitive with an immunofluorescent antibody (IFA) stain (Merifluor, Meridian Diagnostic, Cincinnati, Ohio; Figure 48-5).[26,27] Merifluor is 16 times more sensitive in detection of *Cryptosporidium* in the feces than the acid-fast stain.[26,27] Sensitivity increases again when techniques to concentrate the *Cryptosporidium*, such as Sheathers sugar flotation, are used in combination with IFA.[24,26] The concentration of *Cryptosporidium* in the fecal sample increases with volume of feces defecated.[24] This is thought to occur because of postprandial increase in gastric metabolism and associated increase in metabolism of the parasite.[24] As the Merifluor test takes advantage of cross-reactive antigens on the surface of reptilian *Cryptosporidium* to *C. parvum* antibodies, *C. parvum* oocysts from ingestion of a positive food item produce a false-positive reaction.[15]

Gastric Lavage

Gastric lavage is a more sensitive test because mild infections of *Cryptosporidium* can be regional within the stomach and is less invasive than gastric biopsy (which necessitates endoscopy or surgery).[28] The stomach in a snake is half the distance between the mouth and the cloaca.[28] For lavage, a stomach tube is inserted into the stomach, and 0.9% NaCl at a volume equal to 2% of the animal's body weight is introduced into the stomach.[28] The region is mildly massaged externally, and as much of the NaCl and stomach contents as possible is gently aspirated.[28] The resulting volume of aspirated fluid is usually 50% of that introduced.[28] The sample is centrifuged for 15 minutes at 7500 gravity and examined with the IFA or acid-fast stain.[28] Because little debris is usually found in this sample, the sensitivity of IFA and acid-fast are approximately the same. Again, increased sensitivity can be gained if the test is done 3 days after routine feeding (or if the animal is off food, then 3 days after stomach tubing) with a highly digestible protein item, such as beef baby food.[28]

Serum Antibody Titers

Snakes take 6 weeks after infection to develop antibodies to *Cryptosporidium*. The presence of serum antibodies in snakes

Table 48-2	Dimethyl Sulfoxide (DMSO) Acid-Fast Fecal Technique

1. A small amount of fecal material is smeared onto a clean glass slide and allowed to air dry. Slides are prefixed in a Coplin jar of absolute methanol for at least 10 seconds.
2. Slides are stained in carbol fuchsin-DMSO solution in a Coplin jar for at least 5 minutes. Slides are rinsed under gently running tap water until excess solution no longer runs off (approximately 10 to 30 s/slide).
3. Slides are then placed in a Coplin jar of decolorizing counterstain for at least 1 minute. These are then rinsed for about 10 seconds, blotted with paper toweling, and allowed to air dry.
4. With an applicator stick, a thin layer of immersion oil is applied over the stained smear. Slides are examined with a microscope.
5. Slides are scanned with high-dry objective. Suspect particles are checked with 100× oil immersion lens. Oocysts are brilliant pink to fuchsia against pale green background. The cyst is 4 to 5 µm in size, with typical internal vacuole with material clumped to one side. Ghosts, or empty cyst walls, may also be shed. They do not stain well and appear as empty space of the typical size and shape of cyst with no remaining internal structures.
6. Other particles that could be confused with *Cryptosporidium* oocysts do not stain same way. Yeast cells and leukocytes are not acid-fast and stain blue-green. Erythrocytes stain partially acid fast and have brown or black overcast or a distinctive rough geometric shell.

Stain Preparation

A. Carbol fuchsin-DMSO stain

4 g basic fuchsin crystals (Color Index no. 42500, certified, 99% dye content, Fisher Scientific Company, Pittsburgh)
- dissolved in -
25 mL 99% ethyl alcohol
   +
12 g phenol crystals liquified in water bath
or
12 mL liquified phenol (Mallinckrodt, Paris, Ky)
Add together and mix well with glass stirring rod
   - add -
25 mL glycerol, chemically pure
25 mL DMSO (Sigma Chemical Company, St Louis)
75 mL distilled water
Mix well. Allow solution to stand at room temperature for 30 minutes, then filter. Stain may be stored indefinitely at room temperature in amber glass bottle.

B. Decolorizer–counterstain

220 mL 2% aqueous solution malachite green (Color Index no. 42000, certified, 99% dye content, Harleco, Philadelphia)
30 mL glacial acetic acid (99.5%)
50 mL glycerol, chemically pure

Add together and mix well. Filtration is not necessary. Stain keeps indefinitely at room temperature in closed container.

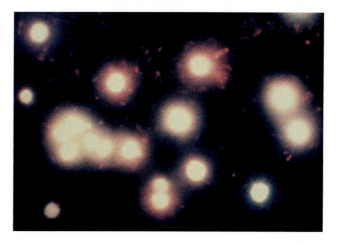

FIGURE 48-5 *Cryptosporidium serpentis* in a direct wet smear prepared from fecal specimens of subclinically infected Cornsnakes (*Elaphe guttata*). The oocysts are detected with Meriflour *Cryptosporidium*/*Giardia* monoclonal antibody (Mab) combination reagent for direct fluorescence detection of the fecal *C. parvum* oocysts and *Giardia* spp. cysts. The mean size of *C. serpentis* oocysts is 6.3 × 5.5 micrometers.

indicates exposure to the organism. Because most infections are long term, a positive serum ELISA test represents either exposure or active infection of *C. serpentis*.[29] The best method is combination of either fecal or gastric lavage with the serum enzyme-linked immunosorbent assay (ELISA) test.[28,29] If both the serum test and the fecal test results are positive, the animal is infected and actively shedding *C. serpentis*. If both results are negative, then the animal is *Cryptosporidium*-negative.[29]

If the fecal sample is positive and the IFA negative, either the animal is passing nonreptilian *Cryptosporidium* oocysts or the infection is new (<6 weeks).[29] If the IFA is positive and the fecal negative, then the animal has *Cryptosporidium* but either is not shedding or is shedding at an undetectable level.[29]

Recently, anti-*Cryptosporidium* immunoglobulins in snakes have been discovered to transfer maternally through the egg yolk and then be detected in newly hatched snakes for approximately 2 months (unpublished). Thus, in certain cases, if the female is *Cryptosporidium*-seropositive, the serum of the hatchlings is also positive because of the maternal antibody titer (unpublished).

Unfortunately, the commercial serum ELISA is no longer available.

Barium Studies

A barium study can differentiate nongastrointestinal masses in the stomach region from the *Cryptosporidium* diagnosis.[14,15,21] If the snake has classical midbody swelling from *Cryptosporidium*, then a narrowing of the lumen or occlusion of the stomach (in advanced cases) is seen with the barium test.[14,15,21]

Gastric Biopsies

Gastric biopsies (endoscopic or surgical) are relatively easy to perform and aid in the prognosis of the disease because histology reveals the extent of gastric mucosal hyperplasia (see Figure 48-2).[14,15] However, because the organism can have a patchy distribution within the stomach, false-negative results are not uncommon.[14,15]

Postmortem Examination

In a postmortem, one should see exaggerated gastric rugae on gross examination (Figure 48-6) and, microscopically, the organisms on the mucosal surface (Figure 48-7).[14,15] Again, false-negative results occur in mild cases.[14,15] To decrease the number of false-negative results, multiple sections should be trimmed in and mucosal scraping should be done of the

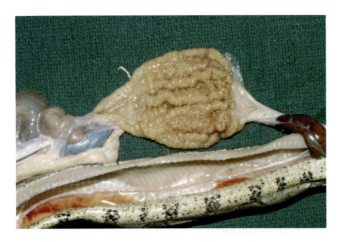

FIGURE 48-6 The gastric mucosa of affected snakes may be edematous, with mucosal thickening and exaggeration of the normal longitudinal rugae to which copious mucus is adhered. *(Photograph courtesy D. Mader.)*

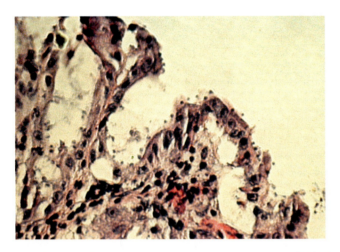

FIGURE 48-7 Histologic section (hematoxylin and eosin [H&E] stain) of gastric mucosa infected with *Cryptosporidium* sp. The organisms line the microvilli or "brush" borders along the luminal surfaces. *(Photograph courtesy F.L. Frye.)*

remaining portion of the organ and washed with 0.9% NaCl, centrifuged, and examined with IFA or acid-fast stain.[14,15]

TREATMENT

In most warm-blooded animals, the infection is usually self-limiting, with transient clinical signs.[20] A great effort, however, has been made to discover an effective treatment for cryptosporidia because of the economic loss in domestic animals and the life-threatening disease in patients with AIDS.[30-32] Approximately 50 anticoccidial or other antiparasitic agents, including sulfonamides, have proven ineffective against cryptosporidia in mammals.[30] Spiramycin (Spirasol, May and Baker, Toronto) and paromomycin (Humatin, Caraco Pharmaceutical Laboratories, Detroit, Mich) have shown limited success at reducing the effects of cryptosporidia in patients and mammals with AIDS.[30,33] Halofuginone (Collgard Biopharmaceuticals, Montreal, Canada) and Arprinocid (Merck and Co, North Bank, NJ) have received limited acclaim as treatments in mice, cattle, and chickens[31] but are toxic in reptiles.[34] Treatment to eliminate the parasite is a high priority in reptiles because cryptosporidia do not appear to be self-limiting and chronic shedding occurs.[14,15] Historically, reptile medication has been based on mammalian treatments in the literature or anticoccidial protocols.

No commercially available effective treatments to eliminate the parasite in reptiles are documented in the literature.[35] Trimethoprin sulfa (SMA-TMP Biocraft Laboratories Elmwood Park, NJ; 30 mg/kg) once a day for 14 days and then one to three times weekly for several months,[34] spiramycin (160 mg/kg) for 7 days and then twice a week for 3 months[34] (author's experience), and paromomycin (100 mg/kg) for 7 days and then twice a week for 3 months[34] were effective at reducing clinical signs and reducing or eliminating oocyte shedding.[34] Although spiramycin and paromomycin treatment produced negative fecal results, postmortem results revealed cryptosporidial organisms still present on gastric mucosa.[34] Necropsies were not done after the other treatment regime, although gastric biopsies collected after trimethoprim sulfa treatment had negative results.[34]

In each of these treatment regimes, the snakes were given extensive supportive treatment, such as high environmental temperatures (≥80°F), subcutaneous fluids, and regular stomach tubing with highly digestible foods. These added treatments may have influenced the course of the disease or been synergistic with treatment.

In patients with AIDS with cryptosporidiosis (which mimics the reptile carrier syndrome), the approach to treatment changed to hyperimmune bovine colostrum, with moderate success.[32] This practice was abandoned when protease inhibitors came into use on humans, boosting the impaired immune system, so that people eliminated the disease without treatment.

Encouraging results occurred with the hyperimmune bovine colostrum in reptiles (Table 48-3).[16,17,36,37] The animals were first diagnosed positive with fecal examination or gastric lavage. They were then treated with the colostrum (1% body weight by volume) via stomach tube once a week for 6 weeks.[16,17,36,37] Animal fecal examinations were followed, as were gastric lavages and postmortem examinations, with histologic sections and scrapings, to confirm a negative status. Positive controls were used in the studies.[16,17,36,37] The product is hoped to be commercially available in the near future.

The *Cryptosporidium* from the geckos with positive acid-fast results, but not IFA-positive results, suggests an antigenically different organism, and therefore, the cross-reactivity to the bovine colostrum may not have occurred.[17,37]

Fifty percent of the snakes cleared the organism during the study.[16] More aggressive (higher doses) or longer therapy might have been more effective.[16,37]

Often cryptosporidiosis is an intestinal condition in turtles, and the colostrum may be altered passing through the gastric region.

Preliminary data indicate that repeated immunization of snakes with *C. serpentis* oocyst wall antigens can elicit high magnitude humoral responses to the pathogens (unpublished). In one trial, as determined on the basis of the oocyst output, such humoral responses were protective against subsequent challenge with *C. serpentis* oocysts (unpublished).

Table 48-3	Results of Hyperimmune Bovine Colostrum Treatment in Reptiles			
Species	Reduced Fecal Concentration	Negative Status	Clinical Improvement	Oocyst Shedding Eliminated
Leopard Gecko	Yes	No	Yes	No
Snake	Yes	Yes (50%)	Yes	Yes
Monitor Lizard	Yes	Yes (100%)	Yes	Yes
Turtle	Yes	No	?	Yes/No

CONTROL

Strict hygiene and good management are essential in the control of cryptosporidiosis.[14,15] Mammalian cryptosporidiosis is self-limiting in immunocompetent people and life-threatening in immunosuppressed individuals.[5] This may hold true for reptiles as well. "Nervous" snakes, such as rattlesnakes and closely inbred amelanotic snakes, seem to have a higher incidence rate of pathology attributable to cryptosporidiosis.[14,15] Elimination of any environmental, nutritional, or concurrent disease problems appears to be as effective as any anticryptosporidial drug at this time.[14,15,37]

Currently, the most effective ways to disrupt the life cycle of *Cryptosporidium* spp. are moist heat, freezing, or thorough desiccation.[14,15] Of seven common disinfectants, only ammonia (5%) and formal saline solution (10%) were effective in eliminating oocyst infectivity after 18 hours of contact at 4°C.[14,38] Ineffective disinfectants included iodophores (1% to 4%), cresylic acid (2.5% and 5%), sodium hypochlorite (3%), benzalkonium chloride (5% and 10%), and sodium hydroxide (0.02 mol/L).[38]

Infectivity of oocysts was neutralized with exposure to moist heat between 45°C and 60°C for 5 to 9 minutes.[14] Because oocysts stored at 4°C remain infective for 2 to 6 months,[28] cleanliness and removal of organic matter should be emphasized.[14,15] Crates, pens, feeding bottles, and utensils should be thoroughly cleaned with an ammonia solution and allowed to dry for a period of at least 3 days.[14,15] Known shedders should be isolated from "clean" animals and should be cared for after care for the rest of the collection is completed.[14,15]

CONCLUSIONS

A need exists to further characterize *Cryptosporidium* infecting reptiles, specifically to see how many species can induce infection and disease in this vertebrate group. *Cryptosporidium serpentis* originally described from snakes can infect other reptiles. So far, *C. saurophilum* described from skinks[39] has been shown to be infectious only for lizards,[39] but the cross-transmission experiments within reptiles were not extensive enough to fully justify this statement. Most of the molecular studies on reptilian *Cryptosporidum* are focused on phylogenetic relationships to human infectious species of *Cryptosporidium*.[40]

The question why only a small percentage of *Cryptosporidium*-exposed snakes become clinically ill needs to be scientifically addressed. Is it because of strain differences of the pathogen or differences in the host immune system that dictate the severity of infection? Perhaps chronically stressed animals, such as "nervous" rattlesnakes, are more susceptible because of higher cortisol levels.[14,15] A concurrent illness (e.g., microsporidial infection) has been postulated to predispose the snakes to the clinical syndrome,[37] and possibly even a snake lentivirus is present.

No efficacious commercially available treatment for cryptosporidiosis in reptiles has been found, although promising results from supportive care and treatment with spiramycin or paromomycin in reptiles have been obtained.[14,15,34,41] Hyperimmune bovine colostrum treatment on the basis of passive immune transfer has been shown to be the best treatment in snakes and certain species of lizards.[16,17,36,37] Hyperimmune bovine colostrum treatment may become commercially available in the near future to treat reptilian cryptosporidiosis.

REFERENCES

1. Levine ND: Taxonomy and review of coccidian genus *Cryptosporidium* (Protozoa, Apicomplexa), *J Protozool* 31(1):94, 1984.
2. Angus WA: Cryptosporidiosis in man, domestic animals, and birds: a review, *J Royal Soc Med* 76:26, 1993.
3. Tyzzer EE: A sporozoan found in the peptic glands of the common mouse, *Proc Soc Exp Biol Med* 5:12, 1907.
4. Goodwin MA, Davis JF: Fatal bronchopneumonia associated with *Cryptosporidium* in a wood duck, *J Assoc Avian Vet* 7(2):77, 1993.
5. Graczyk TK, Fayer R, Cranfield MR: Zoonotic potential of cross-transmission of *Cryptosporidium parvum*: implications for waterborne cryptosporidiosis, *Parasitol Today* 13(9):348, 1997.
6. Arcay L, DeBorgenes EB, Bruzual E: Criptosporidiosis experimental en la escala de vertebrados, I, Infeciones experimentales, II, Estudio histopathologico, *Parasitol al Dia* 19:20-29, 1995.
7. Crawshaw GJ, Mehren KG: Cryptosporidiosis in zoo animals. In Ippen R, Schroeder HD, editors: *Erkrankungen der zootiere*, Berlin, 1987, Academie Verlag.
8. Graczyk TK, Cranfield MR, Geitner A: Multiple *Cryptosporidium serpentis* oocyst isolates from captive snakes are not transmissible to amphibians, *J Parasitol* 84(6):1298, 1998.
9. Brownstein DG, Strandber JD, Montali RJ, et al: *Cryptosporidium* in snakes with hypertrophic gastritis, *Vet Pathol* 14:606, 1977.
10. Godshalk CP, MacCoy DM, Patterson JS, et al: Gastric hypertrophy associated with cryptosporidiosis in a snake, *J Am Vet Med Assoc* 189(9):1126, 1986.
11. Upton SJ, McAllister CT, Freed PS, et al.: *Cryptosporidium* spp. in wild and captive reptiles, *J Wildl* 25(1):20, 1989.
12. Frost DF, Nichols DK, Citino SB: Gastric cryptosporidiosis in two ocellated lacertas (*Lacerta lepida*), *J Zoo Wildl Med* 25(1):138, 1994.
13. Graczyk TK, Cranfield MR, Mann J: Intestinal *Cryptosporidium* sp. infection in Egyptian tortoise (*Testudo kleinmanni*), *Int J Parasitol* 28(12):1885, 1998.

14. Cranfield MR, Graczyk TK, Wright K, et al: Cryptosporidiosis, *Bull Assoc Reptl Amphib Vet* 9(3):15, 1999.
15. Graczyk TK, Cranfield MR: *Cryptosporidium serpentis* oocysts and microsporidian spores in stools of captive snakes, *J Parasitol* 86(2):413, 2000.
16. Upton SJ, Barnard SM: Two new species of coccidia (Apicomplexa, Eimeridae) from Madagascar gekkonids, *J Protozool* 34:452, 1987.
17. Graczyk TK, Cranfield MR, Bostwick EF: Hyperimmune bovine colostrum treatment of moribund Leopard geckos *(Eublepharis macularius)* infected with *Cryptosporidium* sp, *Vet Res* 30(4):377, 1999.
18. Cranfield MR, Graczyk TK: Cryptosporidia in reptiles. In Bonagura JD, editor: *Kirk's current veterinary therapy XIII small animal practice*, London, 2000, WB Saunders.
19. Tzipori S, Angus KW, Campbell I, et al: *Cryptosporidium*: evidence for a single species genus, *Infect Immun* 30(3):884, 1980.
20. Hoffman KA, Sandoval SI: Cryptosporidiosis, *Vet Tech* 10(2):124, 1989.
21. Cranfield MR, Ialeggio DM, Noranbrook R, et al: Cryptosporidiosis, *Proc 7th Avian Exotic Animal Medicine Symposium*, Davis, Calif, 1992.
22. Graczyk TK, Cranfield MR: Experimental transmission of *Cryptosporidium* oocyst isolates from mammals, birds, and reptiles to captive snakes, *Vet Res* 29(2):187, 1998.
23. Fayer R, Graczyk TK, Cranfield MR: Multiple heterogenous isolates of *Cryptosporidium serpentis* from captive snakes are not transmissible to neonatal BALB/c mice *(Mus musculus)*, *J Parasitol* 81(3):482, 1995.
24. Graczyk TK, Cranfield MR: Assessment of the conventional detection of fecal *Cryptosporidium serpentis* oocysts of subclinically infected captive snakes, *Vet Res* 27(2):185, 1996.
25. Frye FL, Garman RH, Graczyk TK, et al: Atypical nonalimentary cryptosporidiosis in three lizards. In Boyer LC, editor: *Proceedings of the Association of Reptilian and Amphibian Veterinarians*, Columbus, Ohio, 1999.
26. Graczyk TK, Cranfield MR, Fayer R: A comparative assessment of direct fluorescence antibody, modified acid fast stain, and sucrose flotation techniques for detection of *Cryptosporidium serpentis* oocysts in snake fecal specimens, *J Zoo Wildl Med* 26(3):396, 1995.
27. Graczyk TK, Cranfield MR, Fayer R: Evaluation of commercial enzyme immunoassay (EIA) and immunofluorescent antibody (IFA) tests kits for detection of *Cryptosporidium* oocysts other than *Cryptosporidium parvum*, *Am J Trop Med Hyg* 54(3):274, 1996.
28. Graczyk TK, Owens R, Cranfield MR: Diagnosis of subclinical cryptosporidiosis in captive snakes based on stomach lavage and cloacal sampling, *Vet Parasitol* 67(3-4):143, 1996.
29. Graczyk TK, Cranfield MR: Detection of *Cryptosporidium*-specific immunoglobulins in captive snakes by a polyclonal antibody in the indirect ELISA, *Vet Res* 28 (2):131, 1997.
30. Fayer R, Ellis W: Paromomycin is effective as prophylaxix for cryptosporidiosis in dairy calves, *J Parasitol* 79(5):771, 1993.
31. Linday DS, Blagburn BL, Sunderman CA, et al: Chemoprophylaxix of cryptosporidiosis in chickens using halofuginone, salinomycin, lasalocid, and nomesin, *Am J Vet Res* 48(3):354, 1987.
32. Nord J, Ma P, DiJohn D, et al: Treatment with bovine hyperimmune colostrum of cryptosporidial diarrhea in AIDS patients, *AIDS* 4(6):581, 1990.
33. Phila AM, Rybak MJ: Spiramycinin the treatment of cryptosporidiosis, *Pharmacology* 7(5):188, 1987.
34. Graczyk TK, Cranfield MR, Hill SL: Therapeutical efficacy of Spiramycin and Halofuginone treatment against *Cryptosporidium serpentis* (Apicomplexa: Cryptosporiidiidae) infections in captive snakes, *Parasitol Res* 82(2):143, 1996.
35. Funk RS: Implications of cryptosporidiosis in emerald tree boas *(Corallus caninus)*, *Proc 11th International Herpetological Symposium*, Chicago, 1987.
36. Graczyk TK, Cranfield MR, Bostwick EF: Therapeutic efficacy of hyperimmune bovine colostrum therapy against *Cryptosporidium* infections in reptiles. In CK Baer, editor: *Proceedings of the American Association of Zoo Veterinarians*, Columbus, Ohio, October 1999.
37. Cranfield MR, Graczyk TK, Bostwick EF: A comparative assessment of therapeutic efficacy of hyperimmune bovine colostrum treatment against *Cryptosporidium* infections in Leopard geckos *(Eublepharis macularius)* and Savanna monitors *(Varanus exanthematicus)*. In MM Willette, editor: *Proceedings of the Association of Reptilian and Amphibian Veterinarians*, Columbus, Ohio, October 1999.
38. Campbell I, Tzipori S: Effects of disinfectants on survival of *Cryptosporidium* oocysts, *Vet Rec* 111:414, 1982.
39. Graczyk TK, Cranfield MR, Bostwick EF: Successful hyperimmune bovine colostrum treatment of Savanna monitors *(Varanus exanthematicus)* infected with *Cryptosporidium* sp, *J Parasitol* 86(3):631, 2000.
40. Morgan UM, Xiao L, Fayer R, et al: Phylogenetic analysis of 18S rDNA sequence data and RAPD analysis of *Cryptosporidium* isolates from captive snakes, *J Parasitol* 85(3):525-530, 1999.
41. Graczyk TK, Fayer R, Cranfield MR: *Cryptosporidium parvum* is not transmissible to fish, amphibia, or reptiles, *J Parasitol* 82(5):748, 1996.

49
CALCULI: URINARY

DOUGLAS MADER

The term *urinary calculi* refers to any macroscopic precipitates, or polycrystalline concretions, found anywhere in the urinary tract. Also called urolithiasis, this is a common finding in reptile patients. Uroliths have been reported in amphibians, lizards, turtles, and snakes (Figure 49-1).[1-6] Although snakes do not have bladders, concretions are not uncommonly found in the distal ureters where urine is frequently stored (Figure 49-2).

When located in the bladder, urinary calculi are also known as cystic calculi or bladder stones. Although the bladder is the most common place for these concretions to form, they have also been reported in the ureters and the cloaca (Figures 49-3 and 49-4).[7,8]

Kidney stones, or renal calculi, have not been reported in reptiles. However, calcified kidneys (which could be misconstrued as a renolith) are not uncommonly seen in the Green Iguana *(Iguana iguana)* in captivity (personal observation; Figure 49-5).

ETIOLOGY OF CALCULI FORMATION

Most of the reports in the literature discuss treatment or pathology findings, not cause of stone formation. Likely many different causes exist for the formation of urinary calculi; however, nutritional links have been suggested most frequently. Causes include deficiencies in vitamins A

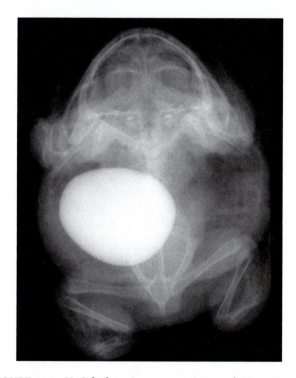

FIGURE 49-1 Uroliths have been reported in amphibians, lizards, turtles, and snakes. This Argentine Horned Frog *(Ceratrophrys ornata)* had a bladder stone, clearly seen as a smooth, elongated radiodense object on the left side of the patient. This was readily removed via cystotomy.

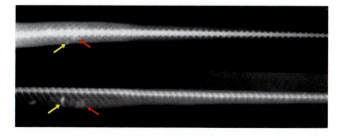

FIGURE 49-2 Although snakes do not have bladders, concretions are not uncommonly found in the distal ureters where urine is frequently stored *(yellow arrows)*. The *red arrow* indicates a fecalith.

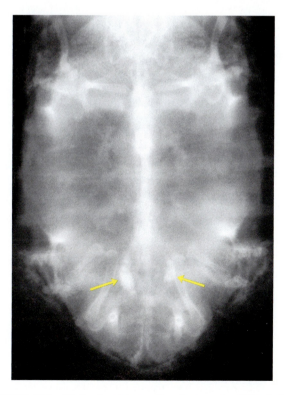

FIGURE 49-3 Bilateral calcium phosphate ureteroliths *(yellow arrows)* in a Red-eared Slider Turtle *(Trachemys scripta elegans)*. (Photograph courtesy C. Innis.)

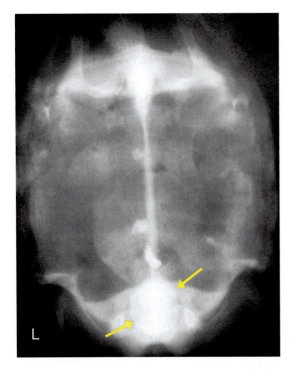

FIGURE 49-4 Cloacalith *(between yellow arrows)* in a Leopard Tortoise *(Geochelone pardalis)*. Because of the location, within the bony pelvis, these stones are easily missed on radiographs.

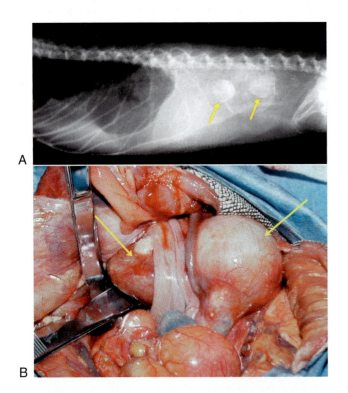

FIGURE 49-5 A, Two round calcified renal abscesses *(yellow arrows)* appear on the radiograph to be either uroliths or fecaliths. **B,** Renoliths have not been reported in reptiles. However, in this Green Iguana *(Iguana iguana)*, the two renal abscesses *(yellow arrows)* calcified within the renal parynchema, giving the appearance of large renal calculi. *(Photograph courtesy S. Barten.)*

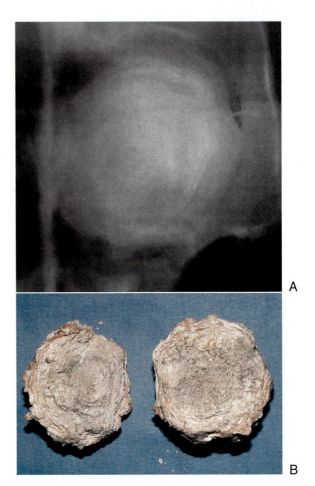

FIGURE 49-6 A, Radiographic appearance of a urolith. Note the obvious lamellar appearance. **B,** Same calculus as in **A,** cut in half. Again, note the lamellar onion-like construction.

and D and the mineral calcium, excesses of dietary protein (as seen when dog or cat food is fed to herbivores), excess oxalates (as seen in spinach), bacterial infection, and suture remnants.[9]

Regardless of the cause, the formation of a urinary stone involves the "seeding" of a supersaturated solution. Some factor acts as a nidus from which the balance of the stone develops. This is readily appreciated with looking at the lamellar nature of the stones, both radiographically and in gross cross section (Figure 49-6).

Almost everybody has grown "crystals" in science class. The easiest way to create or grow crystals is to supersaturate a solution with a substance, such as sugar. The solvent is heated to facilitate the saturation of the solute. For instance, water is heated and sugar is added into the solution until no more dissolves. The solution is then allowed to slowly cool. As this happens, a supersaturation point is reached and crystals begin to form. If no crystals form, either the solution is not properly saturated or a stimulus to form the crystals is needed. Usually dropping a few tiny sugar crystals directly into the solution starts the process.

Multiple small crystals begin to grow and eventually touch. They do not join together to form one large crystal; rather, they remain a jumble of small individual crystals that form a polycrystalline mass. The mass continues to grow unchecked until the concentration of solute decreases to the point that not enough is left to form more crystals.

This is a model for how the urinary calculi form. Obviously, the urine (solution) is not superheated to allow maximum concentration of solute (calculi) in the case of reptiles. Crystals may form even without superheating the solution. Everyone has seen mineral crystals form around a faucet.

In the reptile, a common variable for most calculi formation is dehydration. Regardless of the solute (e.g., urate salts), if the animal is dehydrated, especially captive herps with chronic dehydration, production of the solute continues, thus increasing its concentration, and the volume of solution decreases (from the dehydration). Eventually, supersaturation occurs, or a nidus (such as a coagulum of bacteria and inflammatory cells) develops, and the crystal forms.

Reptiles are uricotelic, excreting nitrogenous waste in the form of uric acid rather than as urea as done in mammals. Uric acid is minimally soluble in water and easily forms urate salts with cations that are normally filtered through the kidneys. These insoluble urates eventually form aggregates in the bladder, which then act as the nidus for further deposition and stone formation.

Pseudocalculi are also seen in tortoises. The short urethra opens into the urodeum, sharing this space with both the distal rectum (via the proctodeum), the paired ureters, and the paired oviducts. Although not common, fully developed eggs are occasionally retropulsed into the bladder. Once inside, they are unable to be passed to the exterior and progressively develop into a calculus (Figure 49-7).

EFFECTS OF URINARY CALCULI

Clients with reptiles that have stones not uncommonly say "My old vet said not to worry about it; they are commonly found in the wild." In fact, that is true. Stones have been found in both wild turtles and tortoises.[5,6] What is important to point out is that most of the bladder calculi that are found are discovered in dead animals.

Small calculi probably do not cause significant problems other than minor irritation to the lining of the bladder and hematuria. This constant irritation usually induces thickening and hypertrophy of the bladder wall. Larger stones, because of their size and weight, can act as a space-occupying lesion, making eating and breathing difficult and inciting internal inflammatory responses in the patient (Figures 49-8 and 49-9). Pressure necrosis to the bladder wall and internal viscera, adhesions, and postrenal azotemia can all develop if stones are not removed.

CLINICAL SIGNS OF CALCULI

No "typical" presenting signs of urolithiasis exist. Human patients frequently report pain as one of the more common signs. Reptile patients cannot articulate that, so, as a result, we have to look for signs that suggest an internal problem.[1]

One hundred cases of urinary calculi were evaluated in California Desert Tortoises (Gopherus agassizii).[3] Ninety-two of the cases were diagnosed during routine annual physical

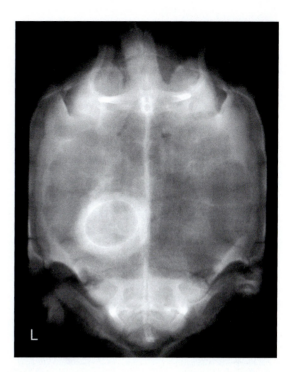

FIGURE 49-7 A "pseudocalculus" in a California Desert Tortoise (Gopherus agassizii). An egg had retropulsed back into the bladder from the cloaca during oviposition and acted like a nidus, forming crystals as does a typical urolith.

examinations. Of the remaining eight cases, one presented for anorexia, one for constipation, three for egg binding (see Figure 29-30), one for dysuria, and two for poor growth.

Other anecdotal reports include rear-limb unilateral or bilateral paralysis, walking like a wheelbarrow (rear legs up, head down), constant straining (to urinate), cloacal prolapse, and passing blood from the cloaca. Owners occasionally report that the pet has been producing "more white stuff" in the excrement than normal. The important clinical point is that the uroliths are generally occult until health problems occur. Clinicians must check for the presence of calculi during every examination.

DIAGNOSIS

Palpation of the abdomen is relatively simple in amphibians and most lizards, with the exception of some of the larger specimens. Even in chelonians, palpation of the bladder is possible with digital palpation of the inguinal fossa with the animal held vertical (Figure 49-10). Gentle rocking of the patient from side to side allows the stones to ballot off the fingertips.

With smaller stones or calculi in large obese animals or animals that have defensively "inflated" themselves, palpation may not be possible. Occasionally, digital cloacal examination permits palpation of either cloacal or urinary calculi in some patients.

The gold standard for detection of urinary calculi is radiography. Generally radiographs are not part of routine annual examinations; however, considering that 92% of the stones reported in the previous study were discovered on

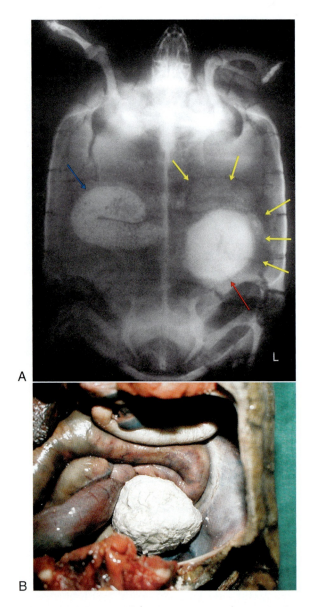

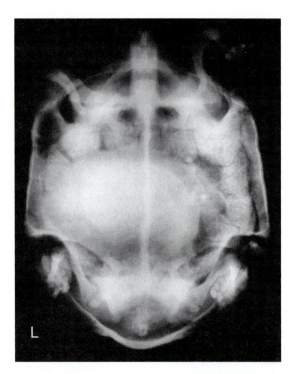

FIGURE 49-9 This radiograph shows an extremely large bladder stone (stone weight greater than 10% of the animal's total body weight). These large stones can produce significant internal pathology such as pressure necrosis to the bladder wall and other internal viscera, adhesions, and postrenal azotemia. A plastronotomy was performed on this patient, and the stone was chiseled into pieces so it could be removed. The tortoise had a complete recovery.

FIGURE 49-8 **A,** Large uroliths can act as a space-occupying lesion. In this radiograph, one can see how the bladder stone has constricted the descending colon *(red arrow).* Note the impacted fecal material proximal to the constriction. **B,** Prosection of a tortoise with a large stone shows the effect seen in **A.** The bladder has been removed in this case, showing just the location of the stone.

a routine physical, making radiography a standard part of the annual examination seems prudent.

In general, cystine and urate stones are radiolucent. Reptile calculi are predominantly urate in origin and are therefore expected to be radiolucent. However, the stones are usually potassium or calcium urate salts, which are radiodense.[10] Because the stones can be variably complexed with different minerals, the radiographic appearance likewise varies greatly (Figures 49-11 and 49-12).

No clinical pathologic changes are pathognomonic for urolithiasis. Uric acid is generally *not* elevated in reptiles with urinary calculi unless primary renal disease is present. A mild inflammatory leukogram may be seen, especially in patients with large calculi.

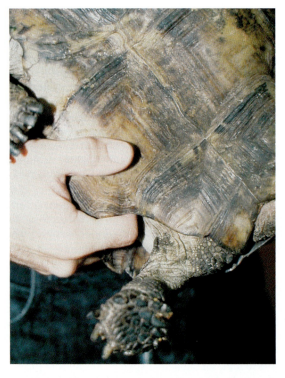

FIGURE 49-10 Digital ballottement is enhanced by holding the tortoise patient vertical, placing the fingers bilaterally in the prefemoral fossa, and gently rocking the animal side to side.

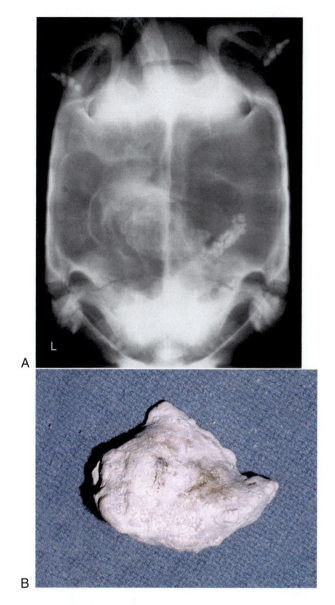

FIGURE 49-11 **A,** All uroliths are some type of urate salt. Urates are generally radiolucent. Radiodensity depends on the minerals, such as calcium or phosphate, which are complexed with the urates. **B,** Gross specimen from **A**.

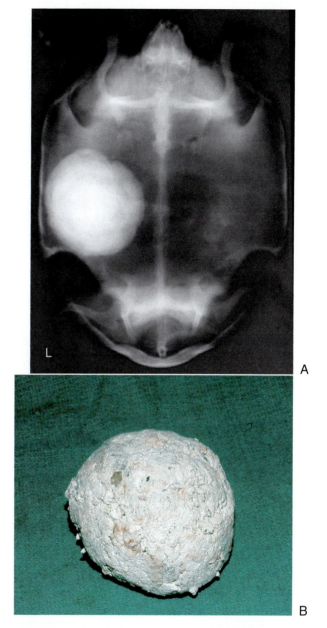

FIGURE 49-12 **A,** Radiograph shows a large, very radiodense urolith in a tortoise (compare with urolith in Figure 49-11, *A*). **B,** Gross specimen from **A**. Note that externally, other than the shape, it looks just as "solid" as the stone in Figure 49-11, *B*.

Microscopic examination of urine is of no value because urate crystals are commonly found in reptilian urine. The presence of white blood cells or red blood cells may indicate an inflammatory response, but because reptile urine commingles with feces, whether the cellular response is from the bladder or the gastrointestinal tract is not possible to tell.

Of the 100 published cases evaluated,[9] males made up the majority of cases (60%). Seventy-three cases had single calculi; of the remaining 27%, 21 had two calculi, five had three calculi, and one had five calculi. No patients had four stones.

The calculi averaged 5.4 cm in diameter in size (range, 0.4 to 14 cm; standard deviation, 2.76 cm; n = 135). Forty-seven percent of the calculi were in the left lobe of the bladder. Thirty percent of the calculi were in the right lobe, and the remaining stones (23%) were considered to be on the midline (Figure 49-13). All of the stones were some form of urate salt.

Several papers have presented cases of urolithiasis in reptile patients. Unfortunately, many only report treatment and not stone analysis.[1,2,11,12]

Kolle et al[4] evaluated 49 "samples" (20 bladder stones and 29 concrements). Fifty-one percent of the samples consisted of single substance, and 49% consisted of two or more substances (Table 49-1).

Mayer[13] reported a single case of a dual urolith in a Uromastyx (*Uromastyx maliensis*). One of the stones was

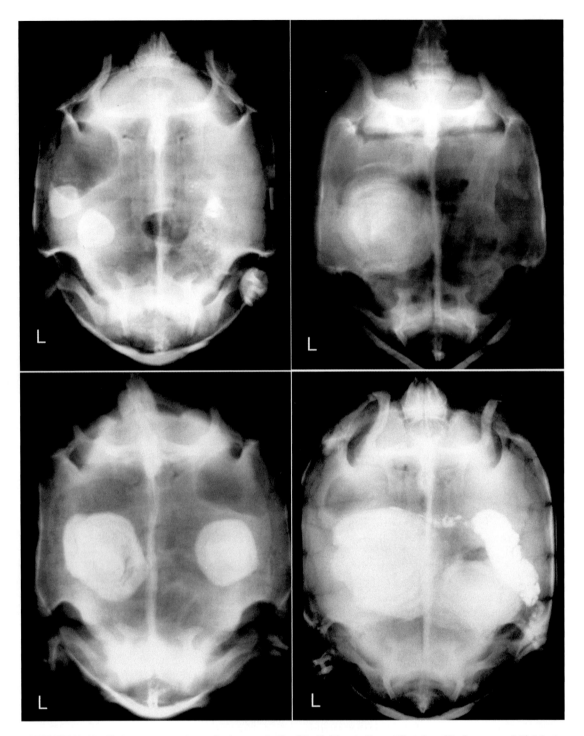

FIGURE 49-13 Various presentations of urinary calculi, all in California Desert Tortoises *(Gopherus agassizii)*. Most of the calculi are found in the left lobe of the bladder. The large liver lobe on the right side tends to push the calculi toward the opposite side. All of these patients recovered and thrived after cystotomy.

subjected to a detailed morphologic and elemental composition analysis with scanning microscopic techniques, energy dispersive radiographic microanalysis, and inductively coupled plasma metal analysis. The sophisticated tests, commonly used in human calculi analysis, revealed a comprehensive description of the stone's composition. The following metals were identified: potassium, 16.79%; calcium, 0.45%; sodium, 0.18%; magnesium, 0.05%; copper, 0.0011%; and iron, 0.00099%. Manganese, lead, and arsenic were not detected. Unknown "others" made up the balance of 72.93%.[13]

Mayer[14] further published a review paper that discussed multiple stone analysis techniques. Standard urolith analysis techniques such as chemical analysis, infrared spectroscopy, and optical crystallography were compared with radiographic microanalysis and scanning electron microscopy.

Table 49-1	Constituents in Reptile Urinary Calculi[4]
Substance	Percent of Samples
Uric acid dihydrate	18.4
Ammonium urate	14.3
Sodium urate	12.2
Calcium urate	6.2
Potassium urate	2
Combination*	16.2

*Struvite, 3 calculi; calcium apatite and calcium phosphate, 1 calculus.

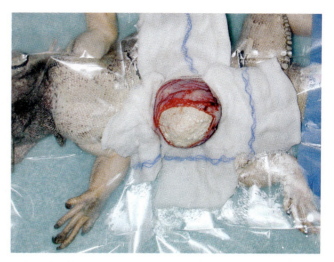

FIGURE 49-15 A standard ventral midline approach was used to remove the large bladder calculi from this Green Iguana *(Iguana iguana)*. The procedure is not much different than that used in mammals. *(Photograph courtesy S. Barten.)*

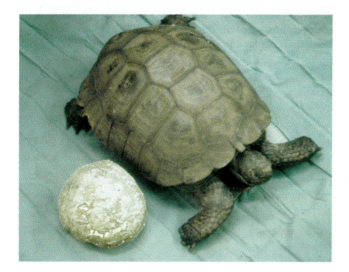

FIGURE 49-14 Bladder stones only get bigger. Surgical removal is easier and fewer complications occur when the calculi are removed while still small. This stone weighed greater than 10% of the patient's total body weight. This tortoise had a complete recovery.

Mayer states that the combination of radiographic microanalysis and scanning electron microscopy provides the best results for many reasons. One major advantage is the simplicity of sample preparation that permits rapid analysis. In addition, the nondestructive nature of the testing allows for both the exterior and interior of the stone to be analyzed separately and independently.[14]

TREATMENT

Regardless of the size of the urinary stone, a proper preoperative evaluation is a must. This author has performed cystotomies on more than 700 tortoise patients. Some of the animals had stones with weights greater than 10% of their body weight (Figure 49-14). These stones are a chronic problem, and surgery is *not* an emergent action. A minimal database of blood analysis and radiographs is a must. If the patient is anorectic, assist feeding and fluid therapy for several days is warranted. In addition, because bladders are *not* sterile, preoperative antibiotic therapy is necessary. The author typically starts patients on oral cefadroxil, 20 mg/kg, orally every 24 hours.

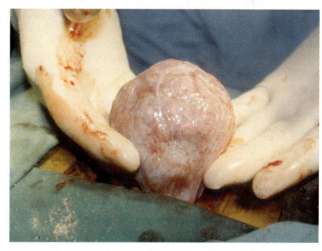

FIGURE 49-16 Plastronotomies are the most common approach used to remove large uroliths from tortoises. The plastronotomy cut should be made large enough to permit removal of the stone (premeasure with the radiograph as a guide). In cases with large stones, it is not possible to make a cut big enough. When that happens, the stone can be cut into pieces with an osteotome while still within the body. The fragments of the urolith can then be removed through the smaller opening.

Historically, the treatment of choice for the removal of urinary calculi has been a coeliotomy with cystotomy. In lizards and frogs, a standard soft-tissue approach through the ventral midline has been the technique of choice (see Chapters 35 and 75 for surgical techniques; Figure 49-15). A plastronotomy approach has been described in tortoises by Frye[11] (Figure 49-16). A soft-tissue approach to the coelom and bladder of tortoises has also been described (Figure 49-17).[15] See Chapter 35 for a thorough description of the surgical techniques.

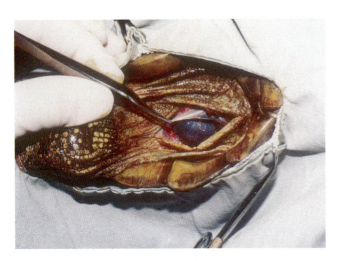

FIGURE 49-17 A prefemoral soft-tissue approach can be used to access the bladder. Radiographs help determine on which side the approach should be made. This is an effective technique for removing small stones and permits rapid healing.

Mangone and Johnson[12] discussed a series of 10 cases of urolithiasis in the Desert Tortoise in which the stones were retrieved with a soft-tissue prefemoral approach. The authors felt that this technique was valuable in patients with a carapace length over 15 cm and with calculi with diameters less than twice the length of the fossa and no laminated radiographic appearance. The surgical site showed good healing by 21 days after surgery. One of the 10 animals died in the postoperative period.

In this author's 100 case series, 90 of the patients had the calculi removed via a plastronotomy. Ten cases, selected on the basis of the size of the urolith, had the calculi removed via a prefemoral approach.[3]

Of the 10 prefemoral surgical cases, a plastronotomy was also performed to assess intraoperative damage after the inguinal approach was completed. Small bladder rents, adhesions, and internal pathology (such as bruising and evidence of pressure necrosis) were missed in each case.

All 100 patients were reported alive and well 1 year after surgery. The conclusion was that, especially with the larger stones (stones with diameters larger than the distance between the plastron and the carapace in the inguinal fossa), the plastronotomy approach was a preferable technique for removal of cystic calculi.[3]

Chapter 35 describes both the plastronotomy and soft tissue techniques. Chapter 27 discusses appropriate anesthesia and analgesia.

Smaller cystic calculi can be readily removed either endoscopically or with long forceps (Figure 49-18).

Advanced techniques such as lithotripsy and laser stone ablation have yet to find use in reptile medicine. Lithotripsy in turtles and tortoises may prove problematic because the sound waves may not effectively penetrate the plastron or carapace. The technique may have some usefulness in lizards.

Nutritional dissolution of stones has also not been reported. The author has tried chemical dissolution of tortoise calculi experimentally in vitro with no success.

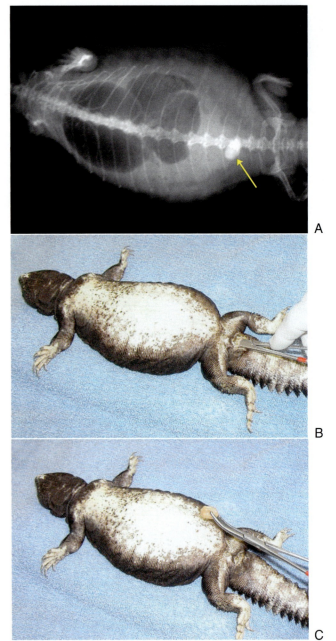

FIGURE 49-18 **A,** Small cystic calculi (*yellow arrow*) in the bladder of a Uromastyx (*Uromastyx* sp.). **B** and **C,** Many of these small uroliths can be removed manually with long forceps. The patient is sedated.

SUMMARY

Urinary calculi are a common problem in both captive and, most likely to a lesser extent, wild reptiles. The cause is likely multifactorial, ranging from improper nutrition to problems with hydration to infectious etiologies.

How long calculi take to form is not known. The author has removed more than 700 calculi from various tortoise species (Figure 49-19). During that time, there was one repeat patient.

A 6-cm–diameter bladder calculus was removed from an adult male Desert Tortoise via a plastronotomy. Ten years

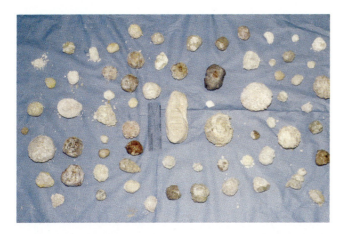

FIGURE 49-19 Cystic calculi come in many shapes, sizes, and colors, depending on the chemical composition, the size of the patient, and the length of time the stone was present before diagnosis. All of these uroliths came from California Desert Tortoises (*Gopherus agassizii*).

later, the same patient once again presented, with similar signs, with a second bladder stone, this one measuring approximately 5 cm in diameter. Of interest to note, the patient had the same owner the entire time, and after the first surgery, the owner made a conscious effort to ensure the pet always had fresh food and ample water available. The owner brought the pet in for annual examinations yearly for the first 4 years after surgery, then moved away and did not take the pet to the veterinarian until it once again showed signs of illness.

Removal should be the goal whenever the diagnosis of urolithiasis is made, regardless of the size of the calculus. Small stones only get larger. Large stones can kill the patient. Obviously, smaller stones are much easier to remove, oftentimes without the need for surgery.

Until more can be learned about the causes, accurate advice for prevention is not possible. With the advent of the more sophisticated calculi analysis techniques, tracking patterns and developing prevention plans may be possible.

In the meantime, early diagnosis via rigorous regular annual physical examinations and prompt treatment is the best recommendation.

REFERENCES

1. Greek TJ: Cystic calculi in the frog *Phyllomedusa sauvagei*, *Proc Assoc Amphib Rept Annual Conf*, 3-5, 2000.
2. Blahak S: Urolithiasis in a green iguana (*Iguana iguana*), *Tierarztl Prax* 22(2):187-190, 1994.
3. Mader DR, Ling GV, Ruby AL: Cyctic calculi in the California Desert Tortoise (*Gopherus agassizii*): evaluation of 100 cases, *Proc Assoc Amphib Rept Annual Conf* 81-82, 1999.
4. Kolle P, Hoffmann R, Wolters M, Hesse A: Cystic calculi in reptiles, *Proc Assoc Amphib Rept Annual Conf* 191-192, 2001.
5. McKown RD: A cystic calculus from a wild Western Spiny Softshell Turtle (*Apalone [Trionyx] spiniferus hartwegi*), *J Zoo Wildl Med* 29(3):347, 1998.
6. Homer BL, Berry KH, Brown MB, Ellis G, Jacobson ER: Pathology of diseases in wild desert tortoises from California, *J Wildl Dis* 34(3):508-523, 1998.
7. Innis CJ, Kincaid AL: Bilateral calcium phosphate ureteroliths and spirorchid trematode infection in a Red-eared Slider Turtle, *Trachemys scripta elegans*, with a review of the pathology of spirorchiasis, *Assoc Reptilian Amphibian Vet* 9(3):32-35, 1999.
8. Raiti P: Endoscopic-assisted retrieval of a cloacal urolith in an African Spurred Tortoise (*Geochelone sulcata*), *Proc Assoc Amphib Rept Annual Conf* 145, 2004.
9. Frye FL: *Biomedical and surgical aspects of captive reptile husbandry*, 1991, Malabar, Fla, Krieger Publishing.
10. Mayer J, Golden E: *Analysis of reptile uroliths using scanning electron microscopy, energy-dispersive x-ray microanalysis, and inductively coupled argon plasma spectrography*, unpublished data.
11. Frye FL: Surgical removal of a cystic calculus from a desert tortoise, *J Am Vet Med Assoc* 161(6):600-602, 1972.
12. Mangone B, Johnson JD: Surgical removal of a cystic calculi via the ingujinal fossa and other techniques applicable to the approach in the Desert Tortoise, *Gopherus agassizii*, *Proc Assoc Amphib Rept Annual Conf* 87-88, 1998.
13. Mayer J: Identification and morphologic analysis of a urolith from a Uromastyx Lizard (*Uromastyx maliensis*) using scanning electron microscopic techniques and energy dispersive x-ray microanalysis, *Proc Assoc Amphib Rept Annual Conf* 43-45, 2003.
14. Mayer J: Comparison of different methods applicable for the reptilian urolith analysis, *J Herp Med Surg* 15(1):31-35, 2005.
15. Bennett RA, Mader DR: Soft tissue surgery. In Mader DR, editor: *Reptile medicine and surgery*, Philadelphia, 1996, WB Saunders.

50
DIARRHEA
RICHARD S. FUNK

Diarrhea may be defined as the production of excessive quantity of soft or liquid feces and results from increased water content in the feces. Diarrhea is a symptom of a variety of disease and husbandry conditions and is not a disease entity itself.

For evaluation of diarrhea in reptiles, one must first determine that the patient indeed has diarrhea; a client may present some material for evaluation without having seen the animal produce it. The material may be abnormal feces or it may be another substance, such as vomitus, urine, or respiratory discharge.

The submitted specimen must be evaluated in light of what a normal stool is for a particular species. For example, boas and pythons usually produce firm stools, but Indigo Snakes (*Drymarchon* spp.) and many cobras normally have much softer stools. "Normal" cobra stool is considered "diarrhea" in a python. The good clinician must know the normal to diagnose the abnormal (Figure 50-1).

Diagnosis of the cause of diarrhea is made on the basis of a good history and physical examination. The following information should be obtained:

1. The duration and mode of onset.
2. The clinical course.
3. Descriptive characterization of the diarrhea.
4. Whether the diarrhea correlates with a change in the animal's diet or stressful events.
5. Whether the diarrhea is associated with any other signs, such as anorexia or vomition.
6. Any prior treatment attempted, whether it was successful, and what was administered.

In canine and feline medicine, diarrhea may be classified on the basis of mechanisms (hypermotility, increased permeability, hypersecretion, malabsorption) or etiology (infection, mechanical, inflammation, dietary, drugs and toxins, metabolic, psychogenic, neoplastic, and others).[1] Sufficient information is not yet available for reptiles to facilitate this degree of classification, but the clinician should attempt to quantify and describe the signs.

Reptile diarrhea should be classified as acute or chronic. Acute diarrhea includes a sudden onset and short duration and may be self-limiting. Chronic diarrhea is more persistent or has periodic recurrence but is uncommon.

Because both the intestines and the cloaca in reptiles are involved in water conservation, chronic diarrhea may be more severe and lead to dehydration and electrolyte imbalances. Acute diarrhea may be associated with vomition.

The differences between small and large bowel diarrhea commonly observed in canine and feline medicine are not well-documented in reptiles, but steatorrhea (fat in the feces) and flatulence may indicate a small bowel problem and hematochezia (frank blood in the feces) and increased mucus may be indicative of a large bowel problem. The transit time for food through the gastrointestinal tract in reptiles is normally much longer that it is in mammals and varies among reptile species.

Causes of diarrhea may include parasites, such as a variety of helminths; protozoans, including coccidia such as *Eimeria* spp.[2] or *Cryptosporidium* spp.; ameba[2]; or *Giardia* (Figure 50-2). Bacterial gastroenteritis caused by *Salmonella* spp., *Shigella* spp., and *Proteus* spp. may be associated with diarrhea. Other causes of diarrhea include viral infections, such as an undescribed parvovirus infection in colubrid snakes (personal observation), adenovirus in ratsnakes (*Elaphe* spp.),[3] chlamydiophylosis in baby Green Iguanas (personal observation), and some poorly documented fungal enteritides.

Iatrogenic diarrhea may result from the use of medications or the administration of certain inappropriate foods such as dairy products. Dystocias can rarely be associated with diarrhea, more often with anorexia.

Husbandry-related causes of diarrhea may relate to temperature, with the animal too cool or too warm (see Chapter 44, Anorexia), the ingestion of too large a meal, a lack of a secure hiding place to facilitate normal digestion, or food items that are partially autolyzed.

Changes in diet may also lead to diarrhea (e.g., feeding baby chicks to a snake that normally eats rodents). Often in zoos, large tortoises are housed outside and permitted to graze on grass during the warmer portion of the year; when they are brought inside for the winter and fed a higher proportion of food with a higher moisture content, such as fruits, diarrhea

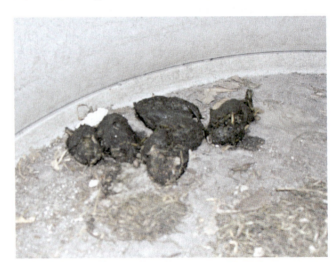

FIGURE 50-1 The clinician must know what is normal for a particular species to recognize the abnormal. Leopard Tortoises (*Geochelone pardalis*) produce voluminous, almost horse-like feces, whereas other species produce a more pasty liquid material. (*Photograph courtesy D. Mader.*)

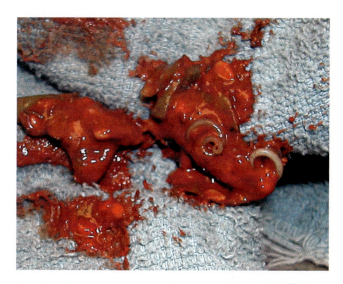

FIGURE 50-2 Parasites are a common cause of diarrhea in reptiles. Speciation of a particular parasite is rarely necessary. However, an attempt should be made to place the parasite into a category such as round worms, tape worms, protozoans, etc. Once the category of parasite is identified, treatment can be started. *(Photograph courtesy D. Mader.)*

may ensue. The presence of a gastrointestinal foreign body may cause diarrhea if the animal is still feeding.

DIAGNOSIS

Diagnostic aids that can be used include fecal parasite examinations and bacterial/fungal cultures, gastric washes and colonic or cloacal washes, plain and contrast radiography, ultrasound, endoscopy, and exploratory surgery and biopsy. Blood work may reveal sepsis, anemia, heterophilia, heteropenia, dehydration, hepatic disease, electrolyte imbalances, or other abnormalities associated with the diarrhea. See Chapter 21 for excellent descriptions on various fecal analysis techniques.

TREATMENT

Treatment is aimed at identification and correction of the underlying problems. Simultaneously, an attempt to eliminate the diarrhea and address any imbalances (such as dehydration) is important.

If parasites are implicated, they should be eliminated with the use of appropriate parasiticides.[4,5] If bacterial or fungal pathogens are present, appropriate chemotherapeutic agents should be used. If the diarrhea is the result of poor husbandry practices, one should work together with the client to improve these conditions (e.g., better attention to cleanliness, diet, and temperature).

Oral or parenteral rehydration should be used as indicated. The use of narcotic or other drugs to slow the passage of ingesta may be worth investigating. Some clinicians believe that the empiric use of aluminum hydroxide, bismuth subsalicylate, or pectin products is beneficial in treatment of acute diarrhea in lizards. If the diarrhea is nonresponsive to therapy, one should reevaluate the diagnostic and therapeutic approach.

SUMMARY

Remember, **diarrhea is a symptom, not a disease.** The cause must be found. Empiric treatment (random treatment with antibiotics) may have detrimental effects. For instance, a *Salmonella*-related diarrhea that is treated with antibiotics may result in antibiotic-resistant strains. This is not only detrimental to the patient but may also have zoonotic implications. Discussion of the risks and benefits of random antibiotic treatment with owners/curators is paramount, as is documentation of all treatment decisions in the patient's medical record.

REFERENCES

1. DiBartola SP: Gastrointestinal problems. In Fenner WR, editor: *Quick reference to veterinary medicine*, Philadelphia, 1982, JB Lippincott.
2. Keymer IF: Protozoa. In Cooper JE, Jackson OF, editors: *Diseases of the Reptilia*, San Diego, 1981, Academic Press.
3. Heldstab A, Bestetti G: Virus-associated gastrointestinal disease in snakes, *J Zoo Anim Med* 15:118, 1984.
4. Funk RS: A formulary for lizards, snakes and crocodilians, *Vet Clin North Am Exotic Anim Pract* 3(1):333-358, 2000.
5. Bonner BB: Chelonian therapeutics, *Vet Clin North Am Exotic Anim Pract* 3(1):257-332, 2000.

51
DIGIT ABNORMALITIES

GERALDINE DIETHELM

Reptiles are often seen with pathology to their digits and feet. This pathology may be the primary reason for the presentation but is often an incidental finding. Abnormalities and deformities in feet and toes should not be disregarded because they commonly provide insight to the overall health of the patient. As with most ailments, problems in the feet are often a reflection of improper husbandry, whether it be incorrect temperature, humidity, inadequate housing, or improper diet.

HISTORY AND PHYSICAL EXAMINATION

A thorough patient history is as critical to the diagnosis of the foot and digit problems as is the physical examination. Questions relating to diseases of the digit must include information related to temperature, humidity, light-dark cycles, cage furniture, diet (frequency and type of food), and types and numbers of cage mates. Important inquiries include when the last shed occurred and the quality of that shed (complete versus partial). One should find out how the supplemental heat is delivered (under-tank heating, "hot rocks," heat lamps, etc.) and whether soaking places exist or water is available only in small drinking bowls.

Although the patient is seen for digit or foot problems, a complete nose-to-tail physical examination must be performed. One should look for evidence of retained spectacles, tags of old skin around the face, ears (if present), and cloaca, and for evidence of sepsis (petechia, ecchymosis), serum oozing from between the scales, etc. Particular attention should be paid to the joints, looking for swelling or disfigurement. See Chapter 30 for a thorough discussion of the physical examination.

Further diagnostic testing is often necessary, such as complete blood counts and chemistry panels, radiographs, cytology, and culture of joint fluid or blood.

MISSING TOES OR TOENAILS

One should ask the owner about housing and shedding of the patient. Retained shed (dysecdysis) around the digits can form strictures and cut off circulation to the appendage, therefore causing sloughing of the toe (Figure 51-1). This condition is seen when humidity in the enclosure is inadequate to promote proper shedding. Carpet fibers or hair can also wrap around the digits with the same effect. Chameleons frequently catch their nails in the mesh of the cage as they climb up the sides, which can lead to an open portal for infections of the toe, digit, and joint abscesses and ultimately sepsis (Figure 51-2).

SWOLLEN TOES OR JOINTS

Swelling of the toes without signs of external trauma requires closer inspection. Fibrous osteodystrophy, trauma, gout, and neoplasia should be considered when the swelling is seen in this region.

Gout is often seen in the metatarsal-phalangeal joints. Lysis and deposition of crystals in or around the joints may

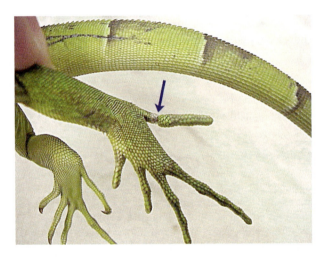

FIGURE 51-1 Retained ringlets of old skin (*blue arrow*) can constrict the digits and result in avascular necrosis and sloughing of the digits and toenails. This is a common sequela of improper husbandry, specifically cool temperatures and low humidity. (*Photograph courtesy D. Mader.*)

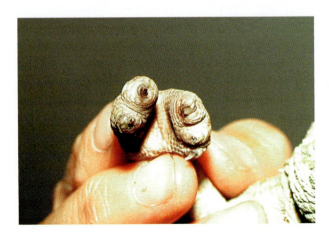

FIGURE 51-2 Screen mesh can be hazardous to arboreal reptiles. The toenails become caught in the screen and are injured. Infections around the nail bed can lead to loss of toes, abscesses, and potentially systemic infections. (*Photograph courtesy D. Mader.*)

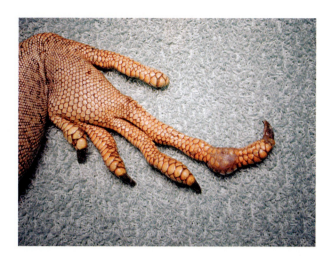

FIGURE 51-3 This Green Iguana (*Iguana iguana*) was seen for a mass on the toe that did not respond to antimicrobial therapy. Eventually the mass was biopsied. The resulting histopathologic analysis revealed a sarcoma. *(Photograph courtesy S. Barten.)*

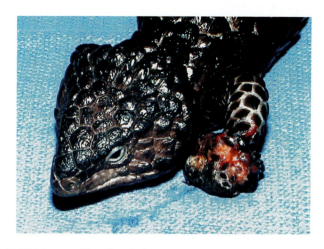

FIGURE 51-4 This Shingle-backed Skink (*Trachydosaurus rugosas*) was seen with an infected foot that had sloughed all the digits. Impression smears of the mass revealed acid-fast organisms suggestive of mycobacteria. Instead of euthanasia, the limb was amputated. *(Photograph courtesy D. Mader.)*

be noted on needle aspirate or radiographic evaluation of the digit and foot (see Chapter 54). Whole body survey radiographs may demonstrate mineralization in other organs and fat bodies. Tophi may also be noted in mucous membranes during the oral examination. Laboratory analysis may reveal an increased uric acid (but not always), indicating possible dehydration or renal impairment.

Nutritional secondary hyperparathyroidism (NSHP) can result in fibrous osteodystrophy. This change results in swelling of the digits and limbs of one or more legs (see Chapter 61). This is radiographically confirmed with lysis of the cortex of the digits and long bones, and hips and vertebrae, and deposition of fibrous tissue. Signs of old pathologic fractures suggest that this patient probably has had NSHP.

Although uncommon, neoplasia has been reported in the digits of reptiles (see Chapter 19). Because neoplasia is so uncommon, it often goes undiagnosed. Frequently, lumps and bumps in the foot/digit that do not respond to traditional antimicrobial therapy are often surgically removed (usually via amputation of the digit/limb). As a result, the neoplasia is often passed off as an antibiotic-unresponsive granuloma (Figure 51-3).

Infection of the toes from external trauma as seen with inadequate housing, where lizards catch their toes in the wire mesh of the enclosure or in the carpeting around the house, is not uncommon. If this is combined with poor husbandry, these local infections can often become systemic. Generalized signs of illness, such as inappetence and lethargy, may result.

Microorganisms such as *Escherichia coli* or *Salmonella* and other coliform bacteria are often found in blood or joint cultures in such cases. Cuts and open wounds caused by improper housing and materials often cause swelling even once the wounds have healed.

Mycobacterium spp. are ubiquitous in the reptile's environment. Potentially pathogenic species in the reptiles include *M. marinum*, *M. chelonei*, and *M. thamnopheos*. These bacteria are commonly isolated or identified from the interdigital lesions. In addition to causing localized dermal infections, mycobacteria can also cause systemic disease that is usually fatal. Treatment is questionable because of the risk of creating antibiotic resistance to a potentially zoonotic organism. If distal portions of an extremity are the only clinical signs associated with the infection, amputation may be a realistic option to euthanasia (Figure 51-4).

Artificial turf is commonly used as an easy-to-clean surface for reptile's cages. The vertical fibers are cut plastic. New carpets may have razor-sharp edges on the surface that can leave microscopic wounds between the toes (Figure 51-5). These cuts can lead to infections that can ascend to joints and surrounding tissue. Treatment involves cleaning of the wounds, appropriate antimicrobial therapy, and removal of the inciting cause.

FRACTURES

Fractured digits can be traumatic, infectious, or metabolic in origin. A thorough examination, radiographs, and blood work help differentiate the three. Trauma from cage mates (bites), crushing injuries, being dropped, and appendages caught in cages is common.

Immobilization of the fracture with splints, provision of analgesia, and correction of the underlying deficiencies speed recovery. Useful lightweight splints can be made from padded paper clips, tongue depressors, and veterinary thermoplastic. Reptiles heal slowly, so the splints may need to stay in place for at least 8 weeks. The splints should be checked regularly to avoid sloughing of distal appendages.

Internal fixation is unrealistic in all but the largest reptile patients, such as some of the larger lizards, chelonians, and crocodilians. Open fractures must be treated with antibiotic therapy and stabilization to avoid local and systemic infection. In the case of comminuted fractures or severe localized infection, amputation of the digit is a viable alternative.

In pathologic fractures that result from NSHP, bone healing is further delayed by the generalized deficiency of calcium. This condition must be corrected before healing can be expected (see Chapter 61).

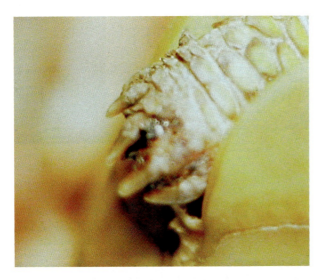

FIGURE 51-5 Small lacerations between the toes are easily infected if the environment is not maintained in a hygienic state. The cuts on this Box Turtle (*Terrapene* sp.) were caused by the sharp edges of the "grass" stems on the artificial turf carpet. *(Photograph courtesy D. Mader.)*

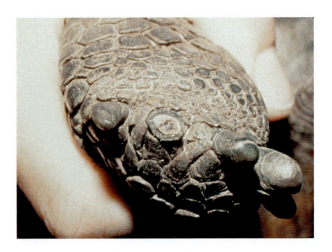

FIGURE 51-6 This Desert Tortoise (*Gopherus agassizii*) was intentionally "short-clipped" to collect a blood sample. This technique is considered inhumane and should not be used as a method of blood collection. *(Photograph courtesy D. Mader.)*

Although only limited studies have been seen on pain control in reptiles, the most common combination drug is the use of a nonsteroidal antiinflammatory such as meloxicam with an analgesic such as butorphanol. See Chapter 89 for drugs and dosages.

TWITCHING TOES

One of the most subtle and common symptoms of NSHP is an uncontrollable tremor in the toes, which is commonly called "playing the piano" by lay herpetologists. The condition is typically intermittent and commences with excitement or movement. As calcium availability decreases, it can become a constant tremor that eventually ends in flaccidity of muscles and an inability to move.

Other toxicities, such as zinc or lead, can also cause neurologic signs. Sepsis, hypoglycemia, and hyperthermia must also be ruled out.

ABNORMAL SKIN

Skin that is necrotic, sloughing, or black may indicate burns, trauma, ectoparasites, and infection beneath the skin. Burns must be treated locally and systemically because the moisture underneath dead skin can predispose to bacterial growth that can spread to other parts of the body. Debridement and topical application of creams such as calendula ointment or silver sulfadiazine cream, and sugar or honey bandages, can decrease healing time and prevent secondary bacterial infections.

Mites look like spots on or under the scales and can cause inflammation or infection with severe infestation, eventually leading to the sloughing of the toenails. They can cause blistering or dullness of scales, with improper shedding around the toes. A scraping of the affected area and microscopic evaluation typically reveal the parasites.

Treatment with ivermectin and antimicrobials may be needed in severe cases. Soaking the feet in antiseptic baths or Epsom salts and decontamination of the environment are crucial in ridding the patient of infection.

Any part of the enclosure that cannot be thoroughly scrubbed and treated is best disposed of because it serves as a source of recontamination when the pet is reintroduced into its habitat.

IATROGENIC

Unfortunately, it has long been a common practice in reptile medicine to collect blood samples by short-clipping toenails (Figure 51-6). This procedure is outdated and considered barbaric. Short-clipping, or "quicking," nails to get blood samples demonstrates a lack of knowledge of proper sampling techniques and suggests that practitioners performing such antiquated procedures should refer their reptile patients to more qualified colleagues.

Short-clipping nails destroys normal keratin, severs vessels, and damages nerves. Anyone who has ever cut their own fingernails or toenails too short can vouch that pain is involved. In addition, leaving the site unprotected opens a portal for potential local or systemic infection.

Nails damaged in such a fashion should be cauterized to seal the open end, and antibiotics and analgesics should be administered as needed.

TREATMENT

Treatment of any digit or foot abnormalities depends on the cause of the pathology. Underlying causes must be identified and corrected if treatment of actual lesions is to be successful.

Antimicrobial selection should be based on cytology (Gram stains), culture and sensitivity data, biopsy and histopathologic analysis, and patient type (oral versus injectable medications). Immobilization, analgesia, and supportive care should be administered as needed. In the case of gout or nutritional or toxic insults, appropriate medical therapy should be initiated.

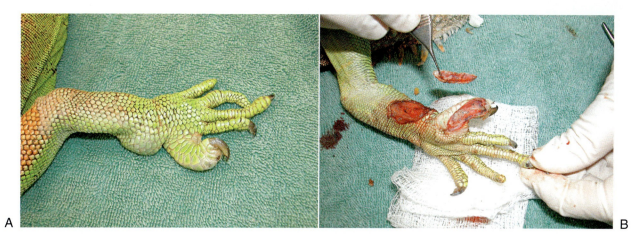

FIGURE 51-7 **A,** A bilobed abscess is seen on the carpus and first digit of this Green Iguana *(Iguana iguana)*. Note the similarity to the sarcoma noted in the toe of the Iguana in Figure 51-3. **B,** Surgical debulking of the abscesses are often necessary to promote healing. This patient had a full recovery after a course of antibiotics and wound care. *(Photograph courtesy D. Mader.)*

Surgical debridement is usually needed in the cases of abscesses because antimicrobials rarely penetrate pus and granulomas (Figure 51-7). Amputation, when necessary, may be a viable alternative to euthanasia in some patients.

SUMMARY

As mentioned, damage to the digits and feet is often an ancillary finding during examinations for other presentations. Many wild and captive reptiles have injuries to their feet. Mild injuries often self-heal. As a result, finding recent imports that are missing one or many digits is not uncommon. The clinically relevant fact is that these animals appear to do fine and the findings are merely incidental.

When a patient has pathology to the digits or feet, a complete physical examination and a thorough history are mandatory on the part of the veterinarian. The pathology usually reflects some underlying deficiencies or problems that may have dire consequences to the patient if not corrected.

52
DYSECDYSIS

KEVIN T. FITZGERALD and REBECCA VERA

"Oh skin—shape of life!"
William Shakespeare

Skin may be the most versatile of all organs. Its many functions include support and protection of internal structures, establishment of a preventative barrier from infectious microbes and parasites, a role in physiologic processes such as heat regulation and respiration, desiccation retardation, housing of the structures necessary for sensory evaluation of the environment, and provision of the basis for pigmentation and coloration. Even more remarkably, along with all these diverse purposes, skin must still permit movement, allow expansion, and accommodate for growth of the animal. The appearance and condition of the skin of a living organism are accurate indicators of its general well being.

Compared with their amphibian ancestors, reptiles have a more desiccation-resistant thicker keratinized layer of epidermis.[1] Healthy reptiles regularly lose this keratinized outer layer of skin. Chelonians, crocodilians, and most lizards continuously slough patches of their skin.[2] However, unlike most vertebrates, the skin of snakes and some geckos is not continuously renewed. For these animals, cell replacement in germinal epidermal layers is cyclic and takes place during limited periods called renewal phases.[3] Unlike other reptiles, shedding in most snakes is a synchronous epidermal mechanism that results in the entire outer skin being lost in one piece out of which the animal crawls. This special shedding or molting adaptation, known as ecdysis, is a complex multifactoral process dependent on such varied environmental cues as temperature, humidity, hydration, and photoperiod. It is also a function of age, gender, and hormonal regulators. Finally, disease processes such as infection (bacterial, viral, and fungal), parasitism, trauma, crowding, malnutrition, and other stressors may likewise influence normal shedding. This discussion examines the shedding process and its normal control (ecdysis), what can cause the process to go wrong (dysecdysis), and the specific treatment, management, and prevention of shedding problems in captive reptiles.

THE SHEDDING COMPLEX

The architecture and function of the epidermis in reptiles, birds, and mammals varies tremendously. The magnificent avian plumage and the diversity of mammalian pelage are widely thought to have evolved from the scales of some ancestral stem reptile. One aspect that the skin of all these groups has in common is the eventual shedding of the most superficial keratinized cells. Although most vertebrate groups display continuous desquamation (slow, irregular, and mainly from wearing), the skin of snakes and a few lizards is characterized by epidermal shedding only during very specific periods.[4,5]

As with any vertebrate, the epidermis of snakes is made up of living and keratinized cells. What sets them apart and defines the characteristic skin sloughing is the evolution of a specialized epidermal fission layer or shedding complex. This structure develops through the formation of an intraepidermal interface that results in an outer generation of older epidermal cells and an inner generation of newer epidermal cells (see Figure 15-8).[6,7] The formation and separation of these layers have no counterpoint in any other vertebrate. Epidermal splitting occurs after the infiltration of lymph and enzymes into a cleavage zone between the old and new layers. The presence of the lymphatic infiltrate contributes to the dull hazy "blueing" of the skin in snakes about to molt. The enzymatic lysis and digestion of the intercellular desmosomal proteins that hold the two generations of layers together, coupled with the friction and shearing forces caused by the snake's movement and behavior, result in a synchronous shedding. Interesting to note is that the laterally placed cellular contact bridges (desmosomes) are not digested by the action of the lymph and enzymes and the two generations separate from each other but remain tight with their own generation. This lateral bonding is strong enough to account for the sloughed outer skin holding together in one piece as the snake crawls out of its own skin.

Keratin layers in reptiles are thickest dorsally and thinnest on ventral surfaces. Younger more rapidly growing reptiles shed more frequently than do older more mature animals.[8] Quickly growing animals may shed as often as once a month. In snake embryos, where growth is especially spectacular, a shedding complex forms before hatching, perhaps in response to water loss from the egg, and the peridermis is lost (in ovo) before hatching.[9] Thus, snakes appear to start shedding before they hatch. The second (postembryonic) shedding may occur within 7 to 10 days after hatching.[9] One explanation for the development of this unique synchronous epidermal shedding mechanism in snakes is the need to accommodate somatic growth, which is seasonal in these animals. The development and appearance of such a system allow for maximal growth when environmental factors are most favorable.

Evidence also exists that the evolution of the shedding complex most likely involved separation of cells capable of synthesizing alpha-keratin from cells that synthesized beta-keratin, resulting in synchronal functional shedding of snakes.[9] However, the single most important evolutionary step that leads to synchronal molting is the appearance and formation of the specialized fission layer, the shedding complex, which uniquely characterizes the epidermis of snakes and is responsible for their distinctive specialized ecdysis.

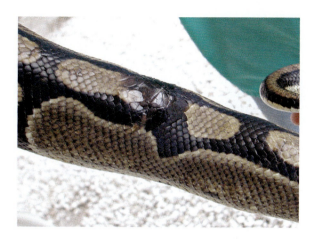

FIGURE 52-1 Old scars can be a source of repeat shedding problems. Trauma, burns, and surgical lesions can disrupt normal congruency of the skin that acts as a nidus for retention of sloughed skin. *(Photograph courtesy D. Mader.)*

CLINICAL SIGNS

The eye may be the window to the soul, but the skin gives the alert clinician a glimpse of how the whole organism is functioning. The outward condition and appearance of the skin of a reptile are a sound yardstick for its overall health. Captive animals must be examined frequently so that potential problems can be dealt with as early as possible. With recognition of the normal, the abnormal can be identified more swiftly and effective therapy regimens initiated sooner. How frequently an animal sheds and when the last molt occurred are questions that should be part of every herpetologic history taking. The entire skin of the reptile must be closely examined. Critically ill animals, those chronically ill, and stressed animals may shed more slowly or not at all. Old injuries, scars, and burns can lead to local areas of retained scales and abnormal sloughing. Scars can become problem areas each time the animal sheds and require the owner's continued vigilance and assistance (Figure 52-1).

Snakes and certain lizards shed their skin in a single synchronous slough (Figure 52-2, *A, B*), and crocodilians, chelonians, and most lizards shed asynchronously in pieces (Figure 52-2, *C*; see Figure 15-30). The skin of giant snakes may tear or break so that they appear to shed in patches rather than in a single piece like other snakes. Younger growing animals shed more frequently than do older mature individuals. Every attempt must be made to identify the species, gender, and age of the patients to better understand their natural history and assist in their shedding habits. Owners should be questioned extensively. As much information as possible should be gathered about the history, environment, diet, and habits of the reptile presented. This information may help to better explain the clinical signs shown. Laboratory results and new technologies can be helpful, but no substitute exists for a complete history and a thorough physical examination. In this section, the clinical signs of dysecdysis are identified and examined.

During normal shedding in snakes, the skin takes on a more hazy appearance. Markings become less distinct, and the skin color seems faded. This starts on the underside of the

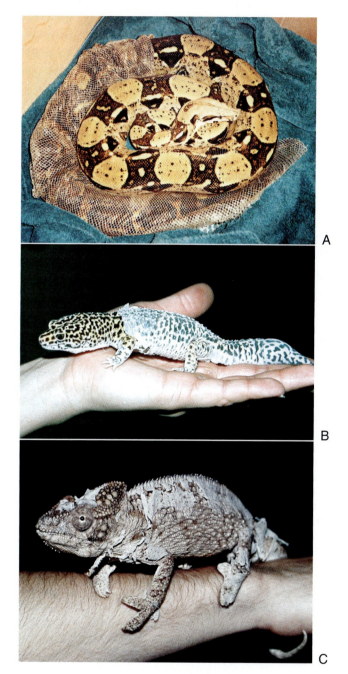

FIGURE 52-2 A, This Boa Constrictor (*Boa constrictor*), like all snakes, normally sheds in one piece. **B,** Some lizards also shed in a single piece, such as this Leopard Gecko (*Eublepharis macularius*). **C,** Most lizards, like this Veiled Chameleon (*Chamaeleo calyptratus*), normally shed in pieces. *(Photographs courtesy D. Mader.)*

tail and spreads anteriorly to the head. When the process reaches the head, the eyes become cloudy and milky blue ("blue-eye"; see Figure 5-22). In this stage, the snake is often called "opaque." The vision of the animal is dramatically impaired during this time, and eating may cease. Animals in this condition are tremendously vulnerable to predation and are often injured by live rodents provided by well-intentioned owners. Snakes in this stage can become quite irritable, and even normally docile animals may strike or bite during shedding.

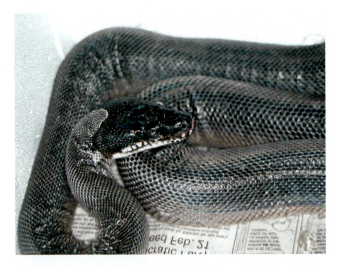

FIGURE 52-3 This D'Albert's Python *(Liasis albertisii)* is having problems shedding. No heavy or rigid objects that can be used to assist with removing old skin are found in the cage. Note the abraded rostrum from constant rubbing on the walls and paper substrate. *(Photograph courtesy D. Mader.)*

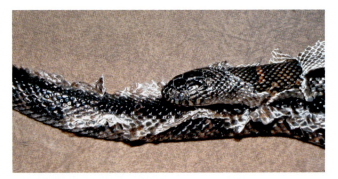

FIGURE 52-4 Regardless of the outward appearance of a patient, prognosis is usually good. One or two shed cycles may be necessary for all old skin to come off and for underlying scales to return to normal. Dysecdysis is not a disease, it is a symptom of other problems; systemic disease, improper husbandry, and ectoparasites are possible causes. *(Photograph courtesy S. Barten.)*

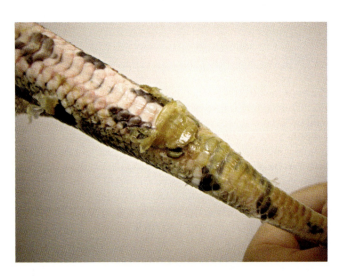

FIGURE 52-5 Retained skin needs to be carefully removed. Skin left in place can act as a nidus for infection, as bacteria and fungus can easily accumulate under old slough. *(Photograph courtesy D. Mader.)*

Under the old outer layers of the eye cap, newer layers of epithelium are forming, and just before shedding, the eye clears. At this point, the skin of snakes becomes shiny and is described as having a metallic appearance. The new skin is extremely fragile at this stage. While in this condition, snakes should not be manipulated. One should resist the temptation to aggressively peel off retained portions of shedding skin. If the older layers are removed prematurely before the newer layers have fully developed, permanent damage and scarring can result. Usually within 3 to 4 days of the eye clearing and this shiny phase, snakes start the shedding process. With rocks, branches, or other various cage "furniture," they begin rubbing the skin on the tip of the nose or the lower jaw (Figure 52-3). As the skin starts to peel, the snake crawls through the remainder of the skin by snagging it on a stationary object and inverting it backward in the opposite direction from which it is moving. The period from the first signs of dull cloudy skin to the actual shedding takes about 14 days. Normal healthy shedding in snakes results in a single piece of inside-out, nonpigmented, transparent skin slough.

For lizards, dysecdysis may present as constricting bands of tissue, particularly around the toes or encircling the tail. These incomplete sloughs can act as a tourniquet, impede local circulation, and result in avascular necrosis and sloughing of distal extremities (toes, tail tips). Constricting bands of tightly adherent encircling skin can also occur on the tail of snakes. Animals with severe cases of dysecdysis usually respond to corrective treatment (Figure 52-4). Any reptile with signs of dysecdysis should be treated because of the potential that retained scales have for infection (bacterial, fungal, ectoparasites, etc.) and other subsequent complications (vascular compromise and dry gangrene; Figure 52-5).

Retained ocular spectacle tissue in snakes and some geckos may result from the accumulation of several incomplete sloughs. Retained eye caps appear dull and dry when compared with normal eyes in the nonshedding animal. Retained spectacles can occur either unilaterally or bilaterally. A wrinkled dull appearance of the eye caps is normal for some species (the Ball Python [*Python regius*] is the most notable example) and is often mistaken for retained spectacles (Figure 52-6). Retained eye caps and their treatment are discussed separately in a later section.

The biggest problem seen in private practice in regard to dysecdysis involves temperature, humidity, age, and overzealous aid of molting reptiles by well-meaning owners. Animals kept for extended periods of time at temperatures suboptimal for their species typically show decreased metabolic activity. Chilling and extended cooling are the underlying culprits for many shedding problems. Cold animals do not eat, and anorexic animals do not grow because they lack the nutritional matrix necessary for new skin growth. Chilled animals are compromised immunologically and are more susceptible to disease and infections of the skin, whether bacterial, viral, fungal, or parasitic. Finally, animals kept too cold are unable to generate the movement necessary to remove the sloughed skin.

Improper humidity brings its own series of problems to shedding. Excessively dry environments result in dehydrated

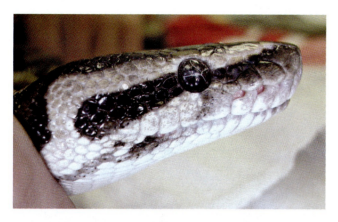

FIGURE 52-6 The Ball Python (*Python regius*) normally has a wrinkled spectacle, which can easily be mistaken for a retained eye cap. *(Photograph courtesy D. Mader.)*

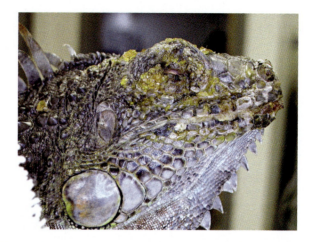

FIGURE 52-7 This Green Iguana (*Iguana iguana*) has severe mite infestation. Mites, combined with secondary pyoderma, can do harm to the skin and affect the shed. *(Photograph courtesy D. Mader.)*

animals and starve the cleavage zone of the fluids necessary for normal segregation and separation of layers and impede normal molts. Aquatic and semiaquatic reptiles likewise can display problem skin sloughs. This can be the result of poor water quality and can lead not only to retained skin but also to secondary infection. One must remember that there is no typical reptile. The natural history and specific temperature and humidity requirements of each of our patients must be recognized and faithfully provided to ensure healthy shedding. Desert dwelling animals have far differing requirements than species from tropical rain forests. Nevertheless, proper husbandry (in terms of correct temperature, humidity, and photoperiod) coupled with proper nutrition goes a long way in countering unhealthy molting.

Age is another important factor where shedding is considered. Young actively growing reptiles shed more frequently than do mature animals. Young snakes shed more often than older snakes, usually about once a month. Starvation and malnutrition of young animals result in a hypoproteinemic state. In this condition, new epidermal layers are not produced and enzymes necessary for the breakdown of the fission layer are not manufactured. Poor nutrition thus leads to incomplete separation of sloughing layers, retained scales, and delayed shedding.

Ecdysis with too rapid a frequency (shedding again in only 10 to 14 days after a cycle is completed) has been linked to hyperthyroidism in some snake species.[3] This condition has been documented in the Rainbow Boa (*Epicrates cenchria cenchria*) and the Red Ratsnake (*Elaphe guttata*). However, results of treatment with methimazole (Tapazole, Eli Lilly and Co, Indianapolis) in these snakes have been equivocal and inconclusive.

Ectoparasites can also cause increased shedding frequency either through secondary infection or by the reptile inducing a shed in an attempt to rid itself of the irritating parasites. In addition, ectoparasites can cause such severe dermatitis that the animal may not shed properly because of the mechanical irritation and subsequent inflammation (Figure 52-7). Animals presented for dysecdysis must be carefully examined for external parasites.

Dysecdysis may be mistaken for respiratory infection. Respiratory sounds generally increase before and during shedding[10] because retained scales in and around the nostrils can cause whistling, wheezing sounds, and even total occlusion of the nares. A thorough physical examination includes establishing whether or not both nostrils are clear and open.

Retained scales can accumulate on and under upper and lower lips. This incompletely shed skin can become secondarily infected and lead to infectious stomatitis. Retained skin can thus result in severe infection of the oral cavity in snakes and lizards. A thorough oral inspection should be a part of any complete reptilian physical examination.

Excessive handling by owners and their misguided attempts at removing retained skin frequently result in seriously damaged tissues. Owners must be counseled in how they can assist shedding reptiles, become well schooled as to what is normal ecdysis, taught to resist overeager efforts in removing retained skin, and advised when to seek professional veterinary assistance.

Dysecdysis itself is not a primary disease. Improper shedding and all its accompanying signs are the hallmark of some other underlying problem. The most prevalent factors associated with dysecdysis are listed in Table 52-1. Generally, once these factors are identified and corrected, shedding returns to normal. Next we investigate specific therapy for dysecdysis.

TREATMENT

The most important factor in successful treatment of shedding problems in captive reptiles is in identification of the underlying cause that led to the dysecdysis. In all reptiles, any patches or areas of skin retained after shedding should always be removed.[11-13] As discussed, failure to do so can lead to a variety of problems, ranging from infection to gangrene.

For snakes, retained skin sloughs are generally readily removed with gentle 20-minute soaks in warm (85°F), shallow tap water. Various agents have been advocated to be added to the bath water to help rehydrate and remove loose skin. Among those recommended are chlorhexidene soaks (Nolvasan Solution, Fort Dodge Laboratories, Fort Dodge, Iowa), tamed iodine (Betadine Solution, Purdue-Frederick, Norwalk, Conn) in a 1:50 dilution with water, resembling weak ice tea), hydrogen peroxide, and various aloe-containing formulations.

Table 52-1	Factors That Contribute to Dysecdysis

Temperature
Humidity
Photoperiod
Nutrition
Hydration
Age
Gender
Infection (bacterial, viral, fungal)
Parasitism
Trauma
Hormonal regulation
Stress (crowding, filthy cage, no hide box, etc.)

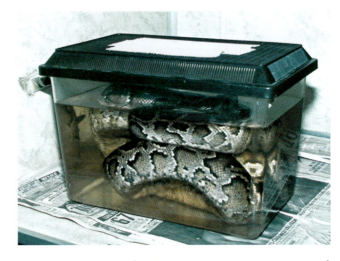

FIGURE 52-8 Soaking the patient may be necessary to assist with rehydrating the skin. After the soak, old skin can be gently peeled off. Snakes should never be left in the soaking chamber unattended because they can potentially drown. *(Photograph courtesy D. Mader.)*

Our experience has been that plain water alone is usually safest and successful. In fact, recent evidence points to potentially toxic situations from overzealous soaks with various agents in the water, particularly with regard to reptiles and chlorhexidine baths.[14] Furthermore, hydrogen peroxide is not only not bactericidal but also potentially cytotoxic to tender new epithelium. Betadine is bactericidal and not cytotoxic; however, a good rule of thumb is production of concentrations dilute enough that newsprint can still be read through the Betadine/water mixture.[15] One should be certain that air temperature is warm enough (24°C to 29°C [75°F to 85°F]) and that no drafts are present that might chill wet reptiles after soaking.

The container should be deep enough to cover the animal's body with water but kept fairly shallow. Too large a container, too deep a bath, or too long an immersion can result in drowned animals. One should never leave reptiles unattended during soaking (Figure 52-8).

In addition, snakes can be wrapped in warm wet cotton towels or terry cloth and allowed to pull themselves out and through the damp rough surface. This process can be repeated over a period of days until all unsloughed skin is gone and is usually quite successful.

Another safe time-honored method is putting the snake into a pillowcase with warm wet heavy towels. The weight of the damp towels assists in helping lift off the shed skin. How long the problem has been occurring and how many cycles of improperly shed skin are present determine how many soaks and warm towel applications are necessary.

Alternatively, spraying both the snake and the environment with a fine mist of lukewarm tap water usually aids in removal of retained skin. Generally, the shed is completed within a day or two of this. Various substances have been suggested to be added to the spray, but we still believe simple tap water is adequate.

The temptation to aggressively peel back shedding skin should be resisted. Rarely is problem shedding ever an emergency situation. Usually providing sprays and soaks, adjusting temperature and humidity, providing proper cage furniture (branches, rocks, rough substrate, etc.) for rubbing against, and providing adequate nutrition remedy ecdysis. If assistance is necessary, start at the head and gently peel skin back posteriorly toward the tail. Avoid removal of large pieces out of sequence. Reptiles may need assistance and have problems around old scars. Scarred areas of previous trauma may not shed normally and may interfere with the shedding of adjacent skin. Owners that keep individuals with signs of old injuries must be taught to aid the animal with soaks, sprays, and warm towels or how to remove retained scales around scars with lotions and gently rolling back the skin with moistened cotton applicators. One is wise to always err in favor of being too gentle. Overaggressive assistance in shedding can damage new underlying skin, often permanently. Sometimes the best method is to continue conservative soaks and wait and see what happens with the next shed cycle.

Lizards housed in too dry an environment (particularly Leopard Geckos [*Eublepharis macularius*]) retain skin around the eyes, toes, feet, and tail. Soaking these areas as in snakes loosens unsloughed skin. If several layers of old dead skin are present, several daily soaks may be necessary to successfully remove the problem area. Sloughing layers can also be lifted with the use of fine iris forceps. Remember that gentleness is essential.

Turtles can be soaked, provided baths are safe with regard to length of time immersed, depth of the soak involved, and composition of the bath water. Retained sloughing scutes on the plastron or carapace can be removed with warm soaks or gently by hand.

For many desert species of lizards and snakes, natural habitats provide areas such as underground burrows, dens with leaf litter or plant debris, or other microhabitats of higher humidity. When animals are ready to shed, humidity boxes with moist sphagnum moss or vermiculite can be placed into the enclosure to attempt to provide more moisture and facilitate normal shedding (Table 52-2). Animals can then seek out this moister environment to help prevent problem skin sheds.

Bacterial infections can commonly result from patches of retained sloughed skin. Gram-negative organisms are the most frequent cause of bacterial infections in reptiles.[16] These infections stem from opportunistic exploitation of normal skin bacteria or invasion by exogenous pathogens. Animals with such infections can become immunocompromised and unable to halt the infection. *Pseudomonas aeruginosa*, *Aeromonas hydrophilia*, *Klebsiella oxytoca*, and *Salmonella arizonae* have all been isolated from the skin of both healthy and diseased reptiles.[16,17] In addition to these gram-negative bacteria,

Table 52-2	How to Make a Humidity Box

Use a pliable plastic container (such as a food container)
Cut an entrance hole in the side or lid
Place a thin layer of moistened sphagnum moss or vermiculite in the bottom of the container

Place a humidity box in the reptile's enclosure at the beginning of each shed as soon as signs of ecdysis are noted. Shedding animals seek out this moist environment. A humidity box also serves to reduce stress by acting as a hide box during molting.

anaerobic agents such as *Bacteroides, Fusobacterium,* and *Clostridium* are commonly cultured and can play a significant role in the development of bacterial skin disease.[18-20] Proper culture and isolation techniques to aid in identification of specific pathogenic organisms combined with antibiotic sensitivity should be undertaken before selection of an antibacterial agent. Because of the nature of these infections in reptiles, a bactericidal antibiotic is preferable to a bacteriostatic agent.[16,21] Topical solutions such as chlorhexidene and Betadine and antibacterial ointments such as 1% silver sulfadiazine (Silvadene Cream, Marion Laboratories, Mansfield, Mass) can be applied to infected areas around or beneath retained skin to combat bacterial skin conditions. Specific selection of antibiotics and reptilian therapeutics is discussed in detail elsewhere in this book. Concurrent medical problems can also predispose the reptile to secondary bacterial infections, so conditions other than dysecdysis must be identified and corrected.

Areas of retained skin can also become prone to fungal infections. The integument is the most common site of mycotic infection.[22] Poor husbandry is the number one cause of fungal skin disease in reptiles. Persistently low environmental temperatures, environments that are too moist, and accumulation of filth and debris in cages predispose animals to cutaneous mycoses. Aspergillosis, candidiasis, phycomycosis, geotrichosis, and fusariosis have all been documented in reptiles.[21] Biopsy of the infected area or proper fungal culture is necessary to confirm mycotic infections. Cutaneous fungal infections can be treated with topical chlorhexidine or tamed iodine solutions, antifungal ointments, and systemic antifungal drugs (see Chapter 89). Polyene macrolides and imidazole derivative drugs are the most common antifungals used in herpetofauna. Specific therapy with reptilian antifungal therapeutics is discussed in detail in another chapter. Unfortunately, if not treated, cutaneous mycotic diseases can become life-threatening systemic fungal infections. Successful treatment centers on early diagnosis.

In addition, ectoparasites such as mites and ticks can invade areas of unsloughed skin (see Chapter 43). They may be present before molting and actually help to induce dysecdysis. Crowded dirty cages can contribute to these infections. The snake mite *(Ophionyssus natricis)* is the most common mite in reptiles.[15] These mites can be present in huge numbers, feed on the host's blood, and cause anemia. Small animals are particularly vulnerable. Pruritus may be present, and mites may be found floating in the water after soaks. Sometimes they can be seen moving on the scales of the head and body of infected animals. Less severely infested reptiles may need skin scrapes or wipes with oil-coated cotton swabs to diagnose the presence. Ticks are much larger and so are more quickly identified. A variety of treatment options are available for ticks and mites, and these are discussed in detail in another chapter. However, one must point out that for effective and successful eradication of ectoparasites both the infected animals and the environment must be treated.

Retained skin under the lips of lizards and snakes should be removed with a moistened cotton applicator for prevention of subsequent infectious stomatitis. If infection is already present, a broad-spectrum antibiotic and regular flushing should be initiated. This condition may be slow to heal and deep seated and must be treated aggressively.

Determination of the exact cause of dysecdysis is crucial in not allowing problems in skin sloughs to occur with each subsequent molt. The natural history of the species we care for must be well understood to prevent dysecdysis and the debilitating complications that stem from problem skin sloughs.

DYSECDYSIS-RETAINED SPECTACLES

The spectacles in snakes function as fused transparent eyelids that protect the corneas from injury. Retention of the spectacles or eye caps can lead to subsequent eye infection. Some species of gecko may also retain ocular and periocular tissue in incomplete sheds. Snake owners should be trained to examine shed skin in an attempt to determine whether the spectacles have successfully sloughed (Figure 52-9). They should also know when the last shed occurred.

Veterinarians must become familiar with the normal ocular anatomy of various reptilian species. The spectacles of certain snakes (Ball Pythons in particular) normally display a wrinkled appearance (see Figure 52-6). Mistaking these for retained spectacles can lead to permanent damage to the eye, avulsed corneas, and even blindness (Figure 52-10).

True retained eye shields may represent several previous incomplete shedding cycles. Eyes with retained spectacles appear dry and dull; they may also involve adjacent periocular skin, and the eye itself may not be visible. Retained eye caps can occur either unilaterally or bilaterally. Snakes with retained eye shields may stop eating. With this condition, even normally docile animals can become quite irritable and may even strike or bite if handled. Retained eye caps in snakes provide a great habitat for parasitism by snake mites.

Retained eye shields can be difficult to successfully remove. If any doubt at all exists as to their successful safe removal, the most prudent path is to wait until the next shed cycle and see whether they slough naturally. Wetting retained spectacles with lukewarm water, artificial tears, or a 10% acetylcysteine solution (Mucomyst, American Regent Laboratories Inc, Shirley, NY) may aid in their removal with a cotton-tipped applicator or gentle lifting with an ocular forceps. A sound technique that ensures maximum safety is gently pressing a piece of cellophane tape onto the retained eye cap and then slowly, gently, and even more carefully lifting the tape off. Barring other complications, retained spectacles should come off with the tape.

Elevation of a retained eye shield off the eye with the blunt tip of a forceps is also a proven method that minimizes potential damage to the cornea or to the rest of the eye (Figure 52-11). However, grabbing the edge of the retained eye cap with a forceps or tweezers is strongly discouraged and can cause severe and permanent damage. Retained spectacles are not

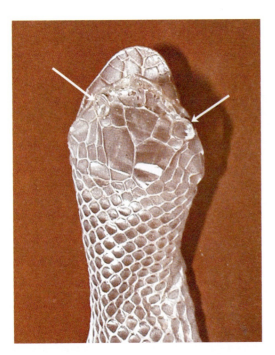

FIGURE 52-9 One should always check shed skin to verify that the eye caps have been sloughed *(yellow arrows)*. *(Photograph courtesy D. Mader.)*

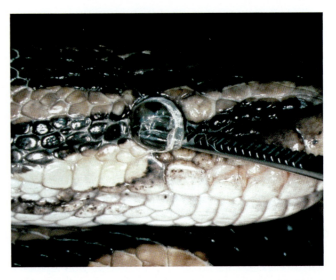

FIGURE 52-11 The best way to remove a retained eye cap is gentle elevation of the scale with a blunt-tip forceps or probe. One should never grab the edge and pull because the eye can be irreversibly damaged (see Figure 52-10). *(Photograph courtesy S. Barten.)*

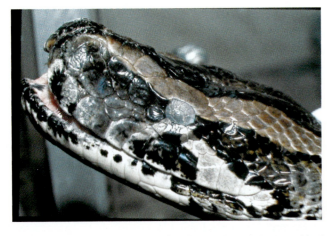

FIGURE 52-10 This Burmese Python *(Python molurus bivitattus)* had a severe corneal injury. In an attempt to remove what was thought to be a retained spectacle, the cornea was damaged. *(Photograph courtesy D. Mader.)*

an emergency situation. Be patient. If eye caps cannot be removed with one or two attempts, the clinician should wait, strive to identify and correct the underlying cause of dysecdysis, and then see if the retained eye shields resolve on their own after the next cycle. Previous trauma and scarring can lead to recurrent retention of ocular spectacles, and these animals may require regular assistance in sloughing the eye caps.

PREVENTION

Poor husbandry is the main cause of dysecdysis in captive reptiles. Within this category, consistently low temperature is the major culprit. One should recognize and provide optimal temperatures so that metabolic pathways are able to function and drive the reactions necessary for normal shedding. The appropriate humidity, neither too dry nor too moist, should be supplied for that particular species. The use of humidity boxes is an excellent way to provide a moist microhabitat for molting and to reduce stress during shedding. Improper photoperiods interfere with hormonal regulation of normal cycles. Malnourished animals and those with substandard hydration cannot fuel the enzymatic machinery necessary for healthy molting. Animals kept at improper temperatures, those housed in incorrect humidity, and those maintained with inhospitable photoperiods all become stressed and are in danger of chronic immunocompromise. Likewise, animals kept from adequate food and water eventually display weakened immune responses. Infections (bacterial, viral, and fungal) and parasitism (internal and external) can both cause dysecdysis themselves and secondarily complicate shedding once it has started. To guarantee successful therapy, infections must be recognized and managed early. One must remember that younger growing animals shed more frequently than older more mature ones. As a result, growing animals must be provided the support necessary to ensure successful growth-related sheds. Gravid and pregnant females may need additional assistance in molting on account of their condition. Energy necessary for effective reproduction may short change that needed for shedding cycles, and dysecdysis can result. The breeding status of all animals must always be ascertained.

Hormonal regulation of reptilian ecdysis is a complex affair that involves the pituitary gland, the thyroid gland, the adrenal gland, and the posterior hypophysis. Animals must be kept in good condition if the hormonal axis is to function. Areas of previous trauma must be watched closely to ensure sloughed skin is not retained around a scar. These retained scales can serve as a nidus for secondary infection. Old scars and burns may require continued vigilance with each successive shed to ensure sloughed skin does not accumulate.

Finally, stress in the form of crowding, filthy cage conditions, insufficient hiding areas, etc., must be minimized to make certain ecdysis may proceed normally. Ecdysis and the formation of new epidermal layers are thought to promote wound healing. Some surgeons recommend waiting for suture removal until after the next subsequent shed because wound strength is most likely elevated from increased mitotic activity.[23] The successful prevention of dysecdysis depends on reptile keepers and veterinarians being aware of the various factors that influence healthy molting in captive reptiles.

PROGNOSIS

As we have seen, dysecdysis is not a primary disease but rather the outward sign of underlying problems. If the actual source of dysecdysis is not determined, captive reptiles are doomed to repeat the problem with each subsequent shed. Once the primary cause of problem shedding has been revealed and treated, normal ecdysis should return within two to three cycles. Do not give up! Even though animals can appear severely debilitated, with persistent support and care, many can make stunning recoveries. If the problem is detected and dealt with early, most animals have an excellent chance of recovery.

Captive reptiles are completely dependent on their keepers for their health and well being. Owners must become educated in the natural history, habits, and requirements of the species they keep. Reptiles share the same life force that we possess and as a result deserve our attention, our respect, and our kindness in the care that we provide.

PEARLS OF PRACTICE

To summarize the diagnosis, treatment, and prognosis of dysecdysis in captive reptiles, the following basic "pearls of practice" should be remembered.

Pearl 1. Dysecdysis is not a primary problem, and for successful management of the condition, the underlying causes must be identified.

Pearl 2. Dysecdysis is rarely an emergency. If any doubt exists that patches of retained skin can be removed safely, one is wise to wait until the next cycle.

Pearl 3. Humidity boxes provided at the start of each cycle can provide microhabitats that aid shedding and an area for hiding during molting to reduce stress.

Pearl 4. Bath water should be routinely checked for mites and the presence of other ectoparasites.

Pearl 5. Soaking animals should **never** be left unattended.

Pearl 6. The spectacle of Ball Pythons is normally wrinkled and dry in appearance. Excessive manipulation of these delicate tissues can permanently damage the eye.

Pearl 7. Retained spectacles can be gently removed with pressing a piece of cellophane tape to the unsloughed eye cap and carefully lifting it.

Pearl 8. Retained unsloughed skin around the nares can rattle, whistle, obstruct the nostrils, and mimic upper respiratory infections. Ensuring that nostrils are open should be a part of the physical examination for every reptile.

Pearl 9. Areas of scarring and old trauma may become problem areas during shedding and require special assistance and vigilance with each successive shed.

Pearl 10. Leave sutures in until after the next subsequent shed to maximize wound strength and wound healing.

Pearl 11. Be patient. With gentle persistent nursing care and support, even the most dramatically affected animals can make full recoveries from dysecdysis.

Pearl 12. Be gentle when manipulating the skin of any reptile. We cannot always help them, but we can sure hurt them. Be gentle!

ACKNOWLEDGMENTS

We acknowledge the guidance and example of Dr Douglas Mader. Dr Richard E. Jones provided valuable advice on the hormonal control of shedding. Finally, we thank Dr Robert A. Taylor and the staff of Alameda East Veterinary Hospital for a wonderful place to treat sick reptiles.

REFERENCES

1. Zug GR, Vitt LJ, Caldwell GP: *Herpetology: an introductory biology of amphibians and reptiles*, ed 2, San Diego, 2001, Academic Press.
2. Weldon PJ, et al: A survey of shed skin-eating (dermatophagy) in amphibians and reptiles, *J Herpetol* 27(2):219-228, 1993.
3. Maderson PFA: *Biology of the Reptilia*, vol 14, New York, 1985, Wiley Interscience.
4. Harkewicz KA: Dermatology of reptiles: a clinical approach to diagnosis and treatment, *Vet Clin North Am Exotic Anim Pract* 4:441-461, 2000.
5. Harkewicz KA: Dermatologic problems of reptiles, *Semin Avian Exotic Pet Med* 11(3):151-161, 2002.
6. Alibardi L: Histidine uptake in the epidermis of lizards and snakes in relation to the formation of the shedding complex, *J Exp* 292:331-344, 2002.
7. Alibardi L: Ultrastructure of the embryonic snake skin and putative role of histidine in the differentiation of the shedding complex, *J Morphol* 251:149-168, 2002.
8. Boyer TH: *Reptiles: a guide for practitioners*, Lakewood, Colo, 1998, AAHA Press.
9. Alibardi L, Thompson MB: Epidermal differentiation during ontogeny and after hatching in the snake *Liasis fuscus* (Pythonidae, Serpentes, Reptilia), with emphasis on the formation of the shedding complex, *J Morphol* 256:29-41, 2003.
10. Boyer TH: Respiratory changes before ecdysis, *Bull Assoc Reptil Amphib Vet* 1(1):2, 1991.
11. Jacobson ER: Reptile dermatology. In Kirk RW, Bonagura JD, editors: *Kirk's current veterinary therapy XI, small animal practice*, Philadelphia, 1992, WB Saunders.
12. Wright K: Dysecdysis in boid snakes with neurologic diseases, *Bull Assoc Reptil Amphib Vet* 2(1):5, 1992.
13. Rossi JV: Dermatology. In Mader DR, editor: *Reptile medicine and surgery*, Philadelphia, 1996, WB Saunders.
14. Lloyd M: Chlorhexidine toxicosis from soaking in Red-Bellied Short-Necked Turtles, *Emydura subglobosa*, *Bull Assoc Reptil Amphib Vet* 6(4):6-7, 1996.

15. Mader DR: Dysecdysis: abnormal shedding and retained eye caps. In Mader DR, editor: *Reptile medicine and surgery,* Philadelphia, 1996, WB Saunders.
16. Maxwell LK, Helmick KE: Drug dosages and chemotherapeutics. In Jacobson ER, editor: *Biology, husbandry, and medicine of the Green Iguana,* Malabar, Fla, 2003, Krieger Publishing.
17. Jacobson ER: Antimicrobial drug use in reptiles. In Prescott JF, Baggot JD, editors: *Antimicrobial therapy in veterinary medicine,* ed 2, Ames, 1988, Iowa State University Press.
18. Stewart JS: Anaerobic bacterial infection in reptiles, *J Zoo Wildl Med* 21:80-184, 1990.
19. Barrett SJ, et al: A new species of *Neisseria* from iguanid lizards, *Neisseria iguanae* sp, *Nov Lett Appl Micro* 18:200-202, 1994.
20. Plowman CA, et al: Septicemia and chronic abscesses in iguanas (*Cyclura cornata* and *Iguana iguana*) associated with a *Neisseria* species, *J Zoo Anim Med* 18:86-93, 1987.
21. Maxwell LK: Infectious and noninfectious diseases. In Jacobson ER, editor: *Biology, husbandry, and medicine of the Green Iguana,* Malabar, Fla, 2003, Krieger Publishing.
22. Migaki G, Jacobson ER, Casey H: Fungal diseases in reptiles. In Hoff G, Frye F, Jacobson ER, editors: *Diseases of reptiles and amphibians,* New York, 1984, Plenum Press.
23. Bennett RA: Reptilian surgery part I and II, basic principles. In Johnston DE, editor: *The compendium collection, exotic animal medicine in practice,* Trenton, NJ, 1991, Veterinary Learning Systems.

53
DYSTOCIAS

DALE DeNARDO

In most species, dystocia refers to difficulty associated with the birthing process. In reptiles, the term is used more broadly as any situation with failure by the female to either complete (e.g., parturition, oviposition) or reverse (e.g., resorption) the reproductive process. As a result, ova remain within the female and cause both local and generalized physiologic changes that can lead to sterility and even death. Dystocia is commonly referred to as egg binding or egg retention.

Dystocia has been rarely reported in wild reptiles.[1-3] Although this deficiency may in part be a result of an inability to detect dystocia before the death of a wild animal, the dearth of reports of dystocia in reproductive studies in which wild reptiles are closely monitored suggests that dystocia is not a common natural occurrence. Unlike conditions in the natural setting, dystocia is relatively common in captive reptiles. In a survey of various facilities housing a total of nearly 1600 reptiles, dystocias occurred in approximately 10% of the captive reptile population annually, with 42% of the dystocias occurring in snakes, 39% in turtles, and 18% in lizards.[4] Because the proportion of snakes, turtles, and lizards in captivity was not determined, no conclusions can be made regarding the relative prevalence of dystocia among the various taxa of reptiles. Regardless, dystocia represents a substantial proportion of clinical presentations. Twenty percent of all Green Iguana *(Iguana iguana)* presentations at one veterinary teaching hospital were diagnosed with dystocia.[5]

As a result of its prevalence and seriousness, dystocia receives considerable attention in the lay literature (e.g., herpetocultural magazines, herpetologic society newsletters)[6-8] and at herpetocultural conferences.[9,10] However, the scientific literature on dystocia is limited, with predominantly clinical case reports that focus on treatment. Therefore, much of the information provided here is based on the author's experience, personal communications with colleagues, and the limited scientific literature.

ETIOLOGY

Dystocia can be caused by a variety of factors. Although determination of the exact cause of a dystocia allows one to correct the underlying problem and decrease the risk of recurrence, the etiology of most cases goes unresolved. Factors that have been attributed to causing dystocia cover a vast gamut of situations, but they can be usefully divided into two broad groups: obstructive and nonobstructive.

Obstructive Dystocias

An obstructive dystocia is a result of an anatomic inability to pass one or more eggs or fetuses through the oviduct and cloaca. The causative defect may be a fetal or maternal abnormality. Fetal abnormalities include oversized and malformed eggs or fetuses (Figure 53-1). Maternal abnormalities include misshapen pelvis, oviductal stricture, or nonreproductive masses including abscesses and cystic calculi (Figure 53-2). In addition, obstructive dystocias may be a result of a complication during oviposition, such as malpositioning of eggs or egg fracture.

Nonobstructive Dystocias

A large number of dystocias occur where no obstructive etiology can be found. In these cases, the eggs or fetuses appear to be of normal size and shape and the female appears anatomically normal. These nonobstructive dystocias have been attributed to several possibilities, mainly based on correlational rather than causal evidence. That is, both the dystocia and suspected etiologic condition are present, but which one leads to the other is unknown. For example, a bacterial culture of retained ova or fetuses often reveals one or more microorganisms, but whether these organisms caused the dystocia or whether they invaded as a result of the dystocia is difficult to determine.

Many dystocias may be a direct result of poor husbandry. Improper nesting site, improper temperature, malnutrition, and dehydration may each lead to dystocia. Therefore, females must be provided with the proper environment for that species during gestation and oviposition/parturition. Environmental requirements of pregnant or gravid females are often different than those of nonreproductive conspecifics.[11,12]

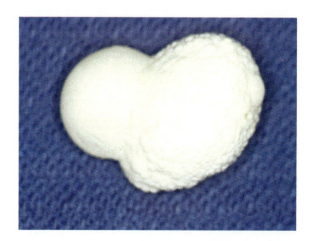

FIGURE 53-1 Malformed, broken, or oversized eggs are often a cause of dystocia. This abnormally shaped egg is from a California Desert Tortoise *(Gopherus agassizii)* and had to be removed via a coeliotomy. *(Photograph courtesy D. Mader.)*

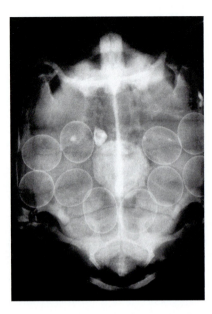

FIGURE 53-2 Anatomic strictures, coelomic masses, old trauma, and cystic calculi can result in an inability for normal eggs to pass during oviposition. This tortoise has a large bladder stone that acts like a ball valve in the pelvis, blocking the passage of eggs. *(Photograph courtesy D. Mader.)*

Another potential cause of dystocia is poor physical condition of the female.[13] Captive reptiles are extremely sedentary compared with their wild counterparts and, as a result, may possess poor muscle tone. Oviposition requires a substantial muscular effort, and if a female is in poor condition because of inactivity, she may fail to complete the task. The predominant presentation of dystocia cases in oviparous snakes supports this theory. Most dystocias in this group of reptiles involve the uneventful oviposition of most of the clutch but retention of the last egg or two without any indication of an obstructive process.

Although definitive determination of an etiology is difficult, effort should be made to identify the cause of a dystocia. Such information can help in assessment of a prognosis for the case and prevention of recurrence or future presentation in other individuals. Regardless of the etiology, the author has anecdotally noted an increased prevalence of dystocia in snakes and lizards that are first-time breeders, have had a previous dystocia, or are carrying a predominantly infertile clutch.

DIAGNOSIS

In diagnosis of dystocia, three questions should be addressed:

- Is a mass present in the coelomic cavity?
- Is the mass an egg or fetus?
- Is there difficulty in passing the egg/fetus, or is the egg/fetus retained beyond what is normal for reproduction?

Although each of these questions must obviously be answered in the affirmative for the case to be a dystocia, diagnoses of dystocia are oftentimes made prematurely. As a result, normal animals or animals with other clinical problems are treated inappropriately or unnecessarily. Differential diagnoses for a coelomic mass include fecal masses, cystic calculi, abscesses, and tumors. However, the location, size, shape, and firmness of the mass can usually differentiate eggs or fetuses from other masses with noninvasive techniques. Distinguishing a dystocia from the normal reproductive process can be simple or challenging. Straining without successful oviposition or parturition is a clear sign of dystocia. Production of one or more eggs or fetuses, but not the entire clutch, is also strongly suggestive of a dystocia. However, diagnosis of dystocia in animals that contain the entire clutch can be challenging. A clear understanding of the reproductive biology of the species, a thorough history, a physical examination, and, in some cases, supplemental diagnostic tests usually provide ample information to ensure a case is a dystocia before initiation of treatment.

Snakes

A history of recent oviposition and the visual presence of a caudally located mass make diagnosis of dystocia simple for most oviparous snakes (Figure 53-3). In pythons, however, large girth often conceals the visual recognition of the retained eggs, making abdominal palpation critical. Behaviorally, snakes with dystocia are usually normal. Dystocia can be more difficult to diagnose in viviparous snakes because the pliability of fetuses makes them less evident. In addition, unlike oviparous species, viviparous species oftentimes retain the entire clutch. Because gestation is quite long and parturition dates are difficult to accurately predict, distinguishing a dystocia from a normal pregnancy can be troublesome. Prolonged straining or cloacal prolapse may indicate unsuccessful attempts to pass fetuses. Ultrasonography can be valuable in assessment of cases in which the diagnosis is uncertain. In addition to simply identifying eggs or fetuses, ultrasonography can detect a fetal heart beat (or lack thereof).

Radiography can also aid in diagnosis of dystocia. However, one must realize that many reptiles (all snakes, most lizards) produce eggshells that have little or no calcium in them, and thus, the shell is not clearly discernible in a radiograph.

Lizards

As with viviparous snakes, distinguishing dystocia from normal pregnancy in lizards may also be quite difficult. Frequently, iguanas are presented as "impacted" with eggs because they are anorectic, show marked weight loss, and have an extremely distended abdomen with obvious outlines of many eggs. However, these signs are indicative of a normal gravid lizard, and the only step warranted is the provision of a structurally and thermally adequate nesting environment. Inadequate nesting sites appear to be a major cause of dystocia in lizards. The best determinant of dystocia in lizards is the animal's attitude. Healthy gravid lizards, although not eating and sometimes ambling awkwardly, are alert and active. Unlike snakes, lizards with retained eggs rapidly become depressed and unresponsive. If such behavioral signs are noted in a gravid lizard, immediate steps should be taken to correct the dystocia. Although snakes can tolerate a dystocia for extended periods of time (with variable local damage occurring), dystocia in lizards often leads to death within several days. That many lizards, including iguanas, can produce a clutch of eggs without the presence of a male is noteworthy.

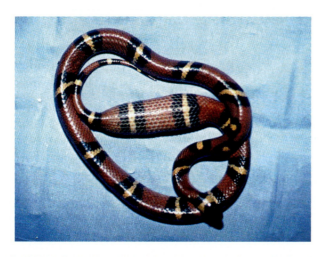

FIGURE 53-3 Prolonged straining, inanition, and poor husbandry can all lead to egg retention. Diagnosis is easy in cases such as this Milksnake (*Lampropeltis triangulum* sp.) in which egg masses are easily seen. *(Photograph courtesy D. Mader.)*

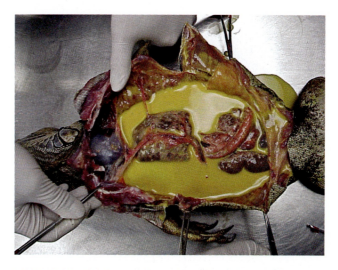

FIGURE 53-4 This Iguana (*Iguana iguana*) died of egg yolk coelomitis. If the condition is caught in time, patients have a good prognosis for recovery with proper supportive care and surgical intervention. *(Photograph courtesy D. Mader.)*

These clutches are usually infertile (although sperm storage is possible) and frequently retained.

Egg yolk coelomitis has been reported in several species of lizards, including the Green Iguana and the Bearded Dragon (*Pogona vitticeps*). Although the condition is dramatic when discovered, these patients often respond well to supportive care and surgical intervention (Figure 53-4).

Chelonians

Egg retention in chelonians is nearly impossible to detect without the benefit of radiographs. Even with radiographs, the decision as to whether the eggs are retained is again a difficult one. If eggs are abnormal (in shape, size, or shell thickness) or if the turtle shows clinical signs such as straining or cloacal swelling, egg removal efforts should be initiated. Generalized symptoms such as depression or respiratory distress can be a result of retained eggs, with cessation of clinical signs after removal of the eggs.[14]

TREATMENT

Although dystocias are usually not emergency situations, except perhaps for lizards, a delayed diagnosis and, therefore, delayed treatment increase the risk of complications that reduce the prognosis for future reproduction and even survival. Contrarily, instigation of treatment on a normal gravid or pregnant female is unnecessary and jeopardizes the survival of the developing clutch. In cases in which the female begins but does not complete delivery, treatment to remove the retained eggs or fetuses should be initiated within 48 hours after cessation of the incomplete oviposition or parturition. The female sometimes naturally completes the delivery during the first 48 hours but rarely does so after this time. Whether to initiate treatment immediately or wait 24 to 48 hours depends on the nature of the dystocia (obstructive versus nonobstructive), the condition of the female, the species, and the relative importance of the female compared with the clutch. During the observational time before treatment, the animal must be maintained in a proper environment that is conducive to oviposition/parturition. The specific treatment to be used is dependent on the species of reptile, the characteristics of the dystocia, and the duration of the dystocia.

Physical Manipulation

One of the more common methods used to attempt removal of retained eggs or fetuses in snakes is manual palpation. Eggs are literally forced out by firmly running a finger down the ventrum of the animal, usually a snake. Although some hobbyists claim reasonable success with this method, the risks are substantial. Common complications associated with manual palpation include oviductal rupture,[15] oviductal prolapse,[16,17] and even death.[17] Consequently, one should never attempt to physically force eggs or fetuses from a female.

If a retained egg can be visualized through the cloaca, attempts can be made to extract the eggs.[16] However, similar procedures used by others have had deleterious outcomes, including egg rupture in a tortoise[18] and death in a snake,[19] so extreme care should be taken (Figure 53-5).

Hormonal Stimulation

Commonly, the first approach to treatment of dystocias is to stimulate oviductal contractions with posterior pituitary hormones. Oxytocin has been routinely used intramuscularly or intracoelomically at doses ranging from 5 to 30 IU/kg.[4] However, doses as low as 1 IU/kg have been effective in turtles.[14] Frequently, a second dose (50% to 100% of the initial dose) is given 20 to 60 minutes after the first. Because temperature influences the effect of oxytocin on oviductal muscles,[20] patients should be maintained at or near their optimal body temperature during treatment. The efficacy of oxytocin in removal of retained eggs or fetuses is variable depending on the species and the duration of the retention. Oxytocin appears to be much more effective when given within the

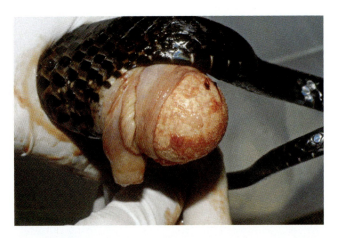

FIGURE 53-5 Snakes can retain eggs for prolonged periods before they show systemic illness. It is not uncommon for eggs that have been retained for prolonged periods to develop a layer of fibrin that surrounds the egg, essentially "sticking" the shell to the inside of the oviduct. With this occurrence, manual extraction of eggs without damage to the patient is usually not possible. *(Photograph courtesy D. Mader.)*

first 48 hours of dystocia. Even at this time, the author has had less than a 50% effectiveness rate in snakes. Lizards respond slightly better, and chelonians respond quite well (>90% effectiveness).

Arginine vasotocin, the natural oxytocin equivalent in reptiles, can also be used to treat dystocias. Reptile oviducts are 10 times more sensitive to arginine vasotocin than to oxytocin.[20] Lloyd[4] reported that arginine vasotocin (at 0.01 to 1 μg/kg, intravenously or intracoelomically) was 73% effective, with 18% of the cases previously unsuccessfully treated with oxytocin.

Although little doubt exists that arginine vasotocin is more effective at stimulating oviductal contraction in reptiles, it does have its drawbacks. Currently, arginine vasotocin is only available as a research drug. In addition, arginine vasotocin is extremely unstable, requiring that it be kept frozen in its powdered form. Once reconstituted in sterile water or saline solution, it must be used within 6 weeks if frozen or 5 days if refrigerated.[4] Aminosuberic arginine vasotocin is less active but more stable, withstanding several freeze-thaw cycles.

One must remember that posterior pituitary hormones merely cause oviductal contraction, not "egg removal." Use of oxytocin or arginine vasotocin on animals that have an obstructive dystocia can have detrimental consequences. Increased pressure on eggs or fetuses that cannot proceed down the oviduct may cause egg fracture, oviduct rupture, or hemorrhage, and each of these can lead to death. These drugs should not be used in individuals that have displayed active contractions but failed to eliminate an egg or fetus.

A multitude of adjunct treatments have been suggested to increase the efficacy of the posterior pituitary hormones, including simultaneous treatment of the patient with calcium or reproductive steroids (e.g., estrogen, progesterone). The efficacy of these adjunct treatments has not been thoroughly studied; however, estrogen and progesterone both failed to have an effect on isolated lizard oviducts treated with oxytocin.[21] Pretreatment with propranolol has experimentally been shown to increase the effectiveness of parturition-inducing drugs.[22] In that study, a dose of 1 μg/g was used in a small lizard species (approximate body weight of 10 g) 15 minutes before anterior pituitary hormone treatment. The clinical value of propranolol in treatment of dystocias remains unknown but warrants further investigation.

Percutaneous Ovocentesis

A second treatment for dystocia used in oviparous snakes is aspiration of the contents of the retained egg(s) with insertion of a sterile needle into the egg through the ventrum of the snake. Caution must be taken not to contaminate the coelomic cavity with egg contents. Removing the yolk from the egg decreases the size of the egg, making it easier for the snake to expel. As with the use of posterior pituitary hormones, aspiration must be performed shortly after the onset of dystocia (usually within 48 hours). With time, the egg contents solidify and become impossible to extract through a needle.

Once the egg's contents have been removed, the snake can be allowed to pass the egg naturally, with oviposition occurring from a few hours to a couple days after aspiration. To assure a more rapid oviposition of the aspirated egg, posterior pituitary hormones can be administered after aspiration.[13,23] If the aspirated egg is not expelled within 48 hours, surgical removal is indicated because of a risk of infection or coelomitis as a result of residual yolk leaking through the newly created hole in the eggshell.

A similar procedure has been used successfully in turtles that produce placid eggs when the egg can be visualized through the cloaca. The egg is aspirated through the cloaca, and the collapsed egg is then removed with forceps.[24]

Surgery

Snakes

Surgery is indicated if retained eggs or fetuses cannot be removed with the use of hormones or aspiration or if the etiology is suspected to be obstructive in nature. After anesthesia, but before surgery, gentle manual palpation may be used to attempt to remove retained eggs or fetuses. The relaxation of the oviductal sphincter from the anesthesia decreases the risk of injury from manual palpation and increases the likelihood of success. Nevertheless, care must be used to avoid prolapse or rupture. In larger species (e.g., large pythons), the oviductal sphincter can be opened with gentle digital palpation through the cloaca.

Depending on the condition of the oviducts and surrounding tissue, a single or multiple salpingotomy, a unilateral or bilateral salpingectomy, or a unilateral or bilateral ovariosalpingectomy may be necessary. Because the condition of the tissue governs the particular procedure performed and the prognosis for survival and future reproduction, clients must be informed of the various possibilities. The species involved and the history of the case can aid in providing the client with a predictive prognosis; however, a more detailed prognosis cannot be made until after surgery.

Most surgeries are simple, with a ventrolateral incision between the first and second scale row of the skin overlying the retained egg or fetus. The oviduct is then incised and the egg/fetus is removed (Figure 53-6). Additional eggs/fetuses may be removed through the same incision, but care should be taken not to traumatize the tissue by attempting to "milk" eggs or fetuses through the oviduct. Additional oviductal incisions over each egg or fetus are usually preferred because such an approach is less traumatic. The oviduct should be

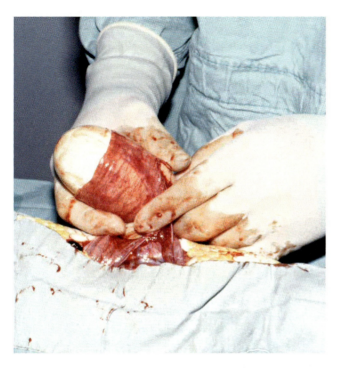

FIGURE 53-6 Reptile oviducts are long and tubular. Usually multiple salpingotomy incisions are required to remove multiple eggs from a single oviduct. Milking of eggs within the oviduct in order to remove eggs through a single incision is possible, but can cause considerable tissue trauma. *(Photograph courtesy D. Mader.)*

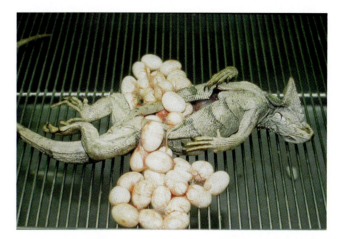

FIGURE 53-7 Dystocia involving 20 to 40 eggs is not uncommon in Green Iguanas *(Iguana iguana)*. Unless the animal is to be used for breeding, a bilateral ovariosalpingectomy is often more efficient than removal of eggs one at a time via multiple salpingotomies. *(Photograph courtesy D. Mader)*

closed with a simple continuous pattern with a fine long-lasting absorbable suture (e.g., 5-0 Vicryl). Some surgeons choose not to close the oviduct, but theoretically this may lead to an increased chance of oviductal scarring and stricture. If excessive adhesions have formed between the retained tissue and the oviduct or if severe tissue damage has occurred, the reproductive tissue may need to be removed. If an oviduct needs to be removed, removal also of the ipsilateral ovary is best. However, the linear alignment of the organs often makes the entire reproductive tract inaccessible through a single skin incision. In such instances, either multiple skin incisions need to be made or a salpingectomy can be performed leaving the ovary intact. Although not common, a salpingectomy can lead to a subsequent dystocia should ovulation from the ipsilateral ovary occur. Salpingectomies (alone or in combination with an ovariectomy) are more likely necessary with dystocias of extended duration, especially in viviparous species. Reptiles that have had all or part of one reproductive tract surgically removed readily reproduce from the other ovary in future seasons.

Lizards

Surgery to remove eggs in lizards can be performed through a single ventral midline incision or through bilateral ventrolateral incisions. Either way, care must be taken to avoid the central vein located on the ventral midline just under the skin. Dystocias involving 20 to 40 retained eggs are common in Green Iguanas, thus making a salpin-gotomy an extended procedure in this species (Figure 53-7). If there is no intention of breeding the lizard in the future, performance of an ovariosalpingectomy rather than multiple salpingotomies is highly recommended. This greatly shortens the surgery time and prevents recurrence of the problem.

Simply isolating an intact female from males does not necessarily prevent recurrence of dystocia because female iguanas often produce eggs regardless of whether a male is present. Because of the extensive surgery that may need to be performed (if multiple salpingotomies are performed) and because many lizards with a dystocia are in poor presurgical condition, the presurgical prognosis for most lizards is usually less optimistic than it is for snakes. Oftentimes, however, successful surgery is rewarded with a dramatic positive change in the lizard's attitude almost immediately after surgery.

Chelonians

Surgery can also be used to remove retained eggs from chelonians.[25] The procedure is usually unnecessary, however, because of the effectiveness of oxytocin in these species. If oxytocin fails or if the eggs are oversized, malformed, or fractured, surgery is necessary. In addition, eggs have been identified in the urinary bladder,[26,27] and such situations require surgical intervention.

The shell of chelonians makes surgical removal of eggs much more complicated than the equivalent procedure in snakes (see Chapter 35 for a detailed description of a plastral surgical approach). Unlike snakes and lizards, recovery from these surgeries is relatively slow, requiring several days before the turtle exhibits normal behavior.

An alternative to a plastral surgical approach is a soft tissue approach through the rear limb fossae, just cranial to the femur.[28,29] Access to the coelomic cavity is limited in this procedure, sometimes making location and removal of the eggs difficult. However, this soft-tissue approach greatly shortens healing time.

VIABILITY OF RETAINED EGGS OR FETUSES

Although countless numbers of retained, and often fertile, eggs have been removed from reptiles, successful incubation of the eggs is rare. However, eggs removed with oxytocin from gravid, but not retaining, female turtles are commonly incubated successfully.[30] Success has been seen with removal of live fetuses from snake dystocia cases via salpingotomy.[31,32]

FUTURE REPRODUCTION AND RECURRENCE

The prognosis for survival is excellent in most cases, provided the female is in good general health. Future reproduction usually carries a good to excellent prognosis provided no complications were noted during the dystocia and at least one of the reproductive tracts was left intact. Successful reproduction the year after a surgical correction of a dystocia is common.[17,33,34] The author has also noted viable second clutches produced within 1 to 2 months of both hormonal and surgical correction of dystocias in snakes.

Although the potential for future reproduction is good, anecdotal evidence suggests that snakes that have retained eggs in the past are more likely to retain eggs in the future. The increased incidence rate of repeat dystocias could be related to failure to correct the causative problem, but further work is needed before any conclusions can be made.

PREVENTION OF FUTURE REPRODUCTION

With the broadening interest in reptiles as personal pets, an increased interest has been seen by owners to prevent their reptiles from becoming reproductively active. This is especially true for species that show dramatic physical and behavioral changes associated with reproduction or a high prevalence rate for dystocia (e.g., iguanas). Social isolation prevents reproduction in many species, but it does not guarantee the cessation of reproductive activity. Many species initiate folliculogenesis in the absence of a male, and some (e.g., iguanas, geckos, cornsnakes) may even lay eggs under these conditions. Currently, the only clinical prevention of reproduction is a bilateral ovariosalpingectomy. Although such a procedure is clearly effective, many owners believe it is excessively expensive or risky. Recently, tamoxifen, an antiestrogen, has been experimentally used to inhibit reproductive activity in Leopard Geckos (*Eublepharis macularius*),[35] but its clinical value remains untested.

REFERENCES

1. Lapasha NA, Parmerlee JS Jr, Powell R, Smith DD: *Nerodia erythrogaster transversa* (blotched water snake), *Reprod Herpetol Rev* 16(3):81, 1985.
2. Plummer MV: *Heterodon platyrhinos* (eastern hognose snake), *Mortal Herpetol Rev* 27(3):146, 1996.
3. Blazquez MC, Diaz-Paniagua C, Mateo JA: Egg retention and mortality of gravid and nesting female chameleons (*Chamaeleo chamaeleon*) in southern Spain, *Herpetol J* 10(3):91-94, 2000.
4. Lloyd ML: Reptilian dystocias review: causes, prevention, management and comments on the synthetic hormone vasotocin, *Proceedings of the American Association of Zoo Veterinarians* 1990.
5. Campbell TW: Clinical laboratory evaluation of dystocia in lizards, *Proc Assoc Reptil Amphib Vet* 6:123-131, 1999.
6. Barten SL: Egg retention in captive snakes, *Bull Chicago Herpetol Soc* 21(3-4):65-71, 1986.
7. Klingenberg RJ: Egg-binding in colubrid snakes, *Vivarium* 3(2):32-35, 1991.
8. Divers SJ, Williams D: Dystocia (egg-binding) in reptiles, *Br Herpetol Soc Bull* 45:14-19, 1993.
9. Opferman RR: Prevention and treatment of dystocia in reptiles, *Ann Reptil Symp Captive Propagation Husbandry Proc* 7:26-30, 1983.
10. Raiti P: Dystocia in colubrid snakes, *Proc Assoc Reptil Amphib Vet* 3:93-95, 1996.
11. Gier PJ, Wallace RL, Ingermann RL: Influence of pregnancy on behavioral thermoregulation in the northern Pacific rattlesnake, *Crotalus viridis oreganus*, *J Exp Biol* 145:465-469, 1989.
12. Tu MC, Hutchison VH: Influence of pregnancy on thermoregulation of water snakes (*Nerodia rhombifera*), *J Therm Biol* 19(4):255-259, 1994.
13. Grain E Jr, Evans JE Jr: Egg retention in four snakes, *J Am Vet Med Assoc* 185(6):679, 1984.
14. Glassford JF, Brown K: Treatment of egg retention in a turtle, *Vet Med Small Anim Clin* 72:1641, 1977.
15. Barten SL: Oviductal rupture in a Burmese python (*Python molurus bivittatus*) treated with oxytocin for egg retention, *J Zoo Anim Med* 16:141, 1985.
16. Wagner E, Foster J: Removing retained eggs from snakes, *Proceedings of the 8th International Herpetological Symposium* 1984.
17. Brown CW, Martin RA: Dystocias in snakes, *Comp Small Anim* 12(3):361, 1990.
18. Jordon RD, Kyzar CT: Intra-abdominal removal of eggs from a gopher tortoise, *Vet Med Small Anim Clin* 73:1051, 1978.
19. Millichamp NJ, Lawrence K, Jacobson ER, et al: Egg retention in snakes, *J Am Vet Med Assoc* 183(11):1213, 1983.
20. LaPointe J: Comparative physiology of neurohypophyseal hormone action on the vertebrate oviduct-uterus, *Am Zool* 17:763-773, 1977.
21. Lapointe J: Effects of ovarian steroids and neurohypophyseal hormones on the oviduct of the viviparous lizard, *Klauberina riversiana*, *J Endocrinol* 43:197, 1969.
22. Gross TS, Guillette LJ, Gross DA, et al: Control of oviposition in reptiles and amphibians, *Proceedings of the Joint Meeting of AAZV/AAWV* 1992.
23. Peters AR, Coote J: Dystocia in a snake, *Vet Rec* 100(20):423, 1977.
24. Rosskopf WJ Jr, Woerpel R: Treatment of an egg-bound turtle, *Mod Vet Prac* August:644, 1982.
25. Frye FL, Schuchman SM: Salpingotomy and cesarian delivery of impacted ova in a tortoise, *Vet Med Sm Anim Clin* 69(4):454, 1974.
26. Frye FL: *Reptile care, an atlas of diseases and treatments*, Neptune City, NJ, 1991, TFH Publications.
27. Thomas HL, Willer CJ, Wosar MA, Spaulding KA, Lewbart GA: Egg-retention in the urinary bladder of a Florida Cooter turtle, *Pseudemys floridana floridana*, *J Herpetol Med Surg* 12(1):4-6, 2002.
28. Brannian RE: A soft tissue laparotomy technique in turtles, *J Am Vet Med Assoc* 185(11):1416, 1984.
29. Page CD: Soft-tissue celiotomy in an Aldabra tortoise, *J Zoo Anim Med* 16:113, 1985.
30. Ewert MA, Legler JM: hormonal induction of oviposition in turtles, *Herpetologica* 34:314, 1978.
31. Vandeventer TL, Schmidt M: Caesarean section on a western Gaboon viper (*Bitis gabonica rhinoceros*), *Int Zoo Yb* 17:140, 1977.
32. DeNardo D: Unpublished data.
33. Loomis M, Smith R: Fertility following caesarean section in an Aruba Island rattlesnake (*Crotalus unicolor*), *Int Zoo Yb* 26:187, 1987.
34. Lichtenhan JB: Caesarean section (CBAC) in an amelanistic corn snake, *Reptil Amphib Mag* 91:16, 1991.
35. DeNardo DF, Helminski G: The use of hormone antagonists to inhibit reproduction in the lizard *Eublepharis macularius*, *J Herpetol Med Surg* 11(3):4-7, 2001.

54
GOUT
DOUGLAS R. MADER

Gout, in any of its forms—visceral, articular, and periarticular—is a common affliction in reptilian patients. Hippocrates, 2500 years ago, wrote of gout as a disease of the big toe, hand, or knee of man and called it Podagra, Cheigagra, or Gonagra, respectively, depending on the joint affected. Little new was added to the description of gout until the late seventeenth century when Anton van Leeuwenhoek described the crystals that we now routinely associate with gouty tophi. Over the last three decades, gout, and other crystal-related joint diseases (e.g., pseudogout), has been thoroughly elucidated in human medicine.

Although gout is frequently seen in humans and primates, it is not a common problem in general veterinary medicine. Other than in the Dalmatian dog, gout is not a topic of much discussion in the veterinary literature.[1] As a result, exotic animal veterinarians, especially those who specialize in avian and reptilian patients, must rely on the human medical literature for information regarding the diagnosis and treatment of this disease.[2-8]

Few studies have been reported that cite the incidence of gout in reptile patients. Kolle and Hoffman[9] reported a retrospective analysis of 280 European Tortoise carcasses that showed an incidence rate of 64.3% of all necropsies had evidence of renal disease. Of those, 16% showed signs typical of gout with tophi in the kidneys.[9]

CAUSES

All reptiles need protein in their diets. Not all protein is the same. For example, there are animal source proteins (meat) and plant source proteins (vegetables). Carnivores, such as snakes and monitor lizards (*Varanus* spp.), need animal source proteins in their diet, whereas vegetarians, such as the Green Iguana (*Iguana iguana*), must have plant source protein in their diet (Figure 54-1). Each type of animal is physiologically adapted to efficiently use a specific type of dietary protein.

Although carnivores can eat plant source proteins, the diet is not complete and they eventually have certain amino acid deficiencies. In comparison, vegetarians can eat animal source proteins, but the differences in the amino acids may overwhelm the animal's ability to efficiently process the nutrients and may lead to serious side effects.

Nucleic acids in the diet are degraded by nucleases to nucleotides (Figure 54-2). These nucleotides undergo further enzymatic hydrolysis to yield free purine and pyrimidine bases. Additional purine and pyrimidine bases are synthesized in the liver from amino acids. If these free bases are not reused by the body, they are further degraded and ultimately excreted. The pyrimidines are catabolized to the end products CO_2 and NH_3.

In some vertebrates, including man, nonhuman primates, the Dalmatian dog, birds, and some reptiles, the end product of purine degradation is uric acid (Figure 54-3).[10] In the remaining mammals and reptiles, the end product is allantoin. In the fishes, the allantoin is further broken down into allantoic acid and urea.

In aquatic invertebrates, the end product of purine metabolism is ammonia. One other notable exception occurs in the pig and the spider where the excretory end product of purine degradation is guanine.[10]

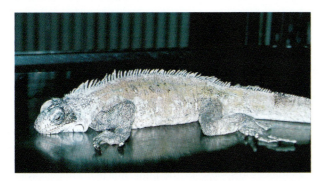

FIGURE 54-1   This gouty Green Iguana (*Iguana iguana*) was fed a diet that consisted mainly of cat food for its entire life. Note the poor condition of the scales, the swollen eyes, and the knobby curled digits.

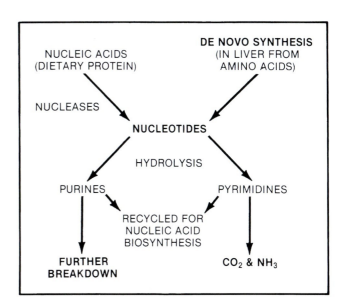

FIGURE 54-2   Nucleic acid breakdown and nucleotide formation.

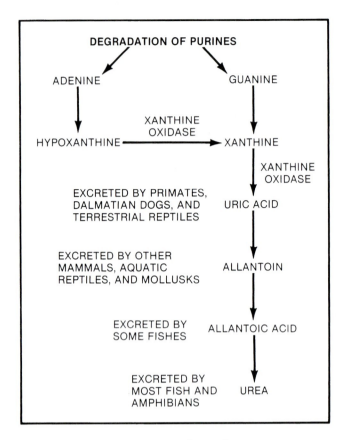

FIGURE 54-3 Degradation of purines.

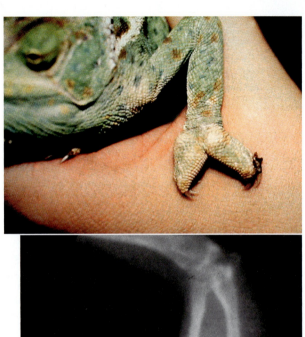

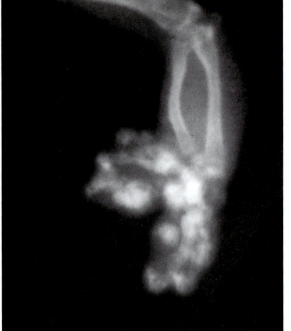

FIGURE 54-4 A, Veiled Chameleon *(Chamaeleo calyptratus)* with whitish-yellow nodules around and over the carpal joints. This patient had difficulty ambulating or grasping with its digits. **B,** Radiograph of the carpal joint. Note the gout-induced lytic damage to the bones.

In humans, the formation of uric acid from the degradation of purines has been extensively studied. Degradation of the major purines, adenine and guanine, starts initially with a conversion to hypoxanthine and then to xanthine for adenine and directly to xanthine for guanine. Both of these pathways require the flavoprotein, xanthine oxidase, to form uric acid (see Figure 54-3).[10]

In vertebrates, this uric acid is derived from both exogenous and endogenous nucleic acids. In man, approximately 0.5 gram of uric acid is excreted daily, even though as much as 5 grams of free purines are formed during the same period.[11]

In reptiles, uric acid is cleared from the blood through the kidney tubules, unlike in mammals, where urea is excreted primarily with filtration. Urates are poorly water soluble and precipitate at low concentrations. In alligators, studies have shown that dehydration does not impair uric acid excretion, but lower ambient temperature does decrease renal tubule function.[12] Dantzler,[13] however, reports that the nephron actively secretes three times more urates when normally hydrated. In the bird, uric acid excretion is regulated with plasma uric acid concentration and renal portal blood flow.[14]

In the blood, uric acid is present predominantly as monosodium urate. Both the free uric acid and the urate salts are relatively insoluble in water. When the concentration of either or both of these forms becomes elevated in the blood (a condition called hyperuricemia) or in other body fluids, such as synovial fluid, the uric acid crystallizes, forming insoluble precipitates that are deposited in various tissues throughout the body.

Crystallization that occurs in the synovial fluid results in an acute painful inflammation of the joint, a condition called gouty arthritis (Figure 54-4). Crystals can also deposit around the joints (periarticular gout) (Figure 54-5) and in other subcutaneous and internal tissues (visceral gout) (Figure 54-6). The uric acid crystals form small white nodules, called tophi, that are clearly visible to the unaided eye.

True gout is caused by the presence of monosodium urate crystals. Pseudogout, which occurs as a result of any crystal other than sodium urate, also causes an acute inflammatory response in the joint affected. Wenker et al[15] reported a case of pseudogout caused by calcium hydroxyapatite $(Ca_{10}[PO_4]_6[OH]_2)$ in two Red-bellied Short-necked Turtles *(Emydura albertisii)*.

Gout

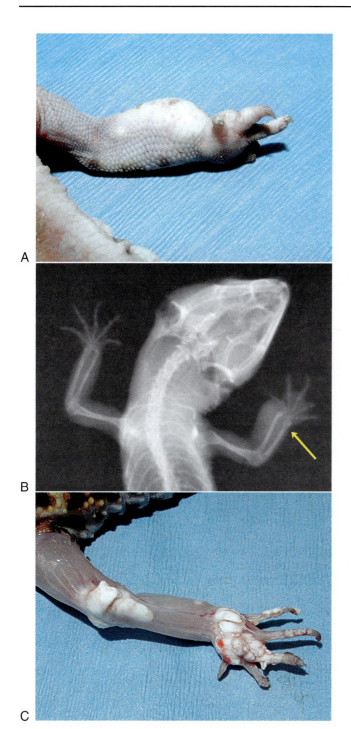

FIGURE 54-5 **A**, Periarticular gout in a gecko. Note the whitish nodules around and over the carpal joints. **B**, Radiograph of the carpal joint. Note the joint itself does not appear to be damaged. **C**, Prosection of the patient in **A** and **B**. Note the periarticular accumulation of tophi around the elbow, carpus, and phalanges. *(Photographs courtesy S. Barten.)*

TYPES

The two classifications of gout are primary and secondary. In primary gout, the hyperuricemia is the result of an overproduction of uric acid. Approximately 95% of the humans affected with gout have the primary form, which is believed to be familial and possibly related to inherited enzyme defects.

Secondary gout occurs when the hyperuricemia results from an acquired chronic disease or a drug that interferes with the normal balance between the production and excretion of uric acid. Diuretics are the drugs most implicated in causing gout. Furosemide, a diuretic frequently used in veterinary medicine, decreases the renal tubular excretion of urates and is contraindicated in dehydration, hyperuricemia, or cases of suspected gout.

Examples of chronic diseases that affect uric acid excretion include renal disease, hypertension, and starvation. Hyperuricemia can also be caused by myeloproliferative disorders (accelerated metabolic processes) and hemolytic disorders (increase in cellular breakdown).

In humans, hyperuricemia is associated with obesity and drug, alcohol, and protein (purine) consumption, which suggests that environmental factors and genetic factors contribute to the development of gout. In reptile medicine, the environmental factors are the most commonly implicated.

Three stages of gout are described in humans. The first is an asymptomatic hyperuricemia. In this stage, tophi, renal stones, and arthritic symptoms are not present. A person may remain asymptomatically hyperuricemic throughout life.

In the second stage, which is an acute gouty arthritis, the symptoms can occur abruptly, with the most common symptom being pain. Arthritic attacks may subside without treatment. On recovery, all symptoms resolve completely. Subsequent attacks may or may not occur. The "intercritical period" between attacks can be days to years.

The third stage is called tophaceous gout. A progressive inability to excrete uric acid results in urate crystal deposits (tophi) in cartilage, synovial membranes, tendons, and soft tissue. Each tophus consists of a complex of urate crystals surrounded by a granuloma. This granuloma consists of macrophages that have developed into epithelial and giant cells. These tophi produce irregular swellings around joints.

In reptilian patients, common sites for tophi deposition include the pericardial sac, kidneys, liver, spleen, lungs, subcutaneous tissue, and other areas of soft tissue.

In humans, renal calculi occur with increasing levels of serum urates. The stones can range in color from pale yellow to reddish brown. Some of the stones consist of 100% monosodium urate, which are radiolucent, and others, which are complexed with calcium oxalate or calcium phosphate, are radiopaque. Cystic, not renal, calculi are a common finding in reptilian patients. However, renal tophi are a common finding in patients with visceral gout (Figure 54-7).

In reptile medicine, various risk factors contribute to the development of gout, such as dehydration, kidney damage (especially tubular disease), and excessive intake of purine-rich meals. This latter condition is common in herbivorous animals fed a diet high in animal protein (e.g., Green Iguanas fed a diet of cat food).[16]

Misuse of potentially nephrotoxic antibiotics, such as the aminoglycosides and the sulfonamides, can cause tubular nephrosis and predispose the patient to hyperuricemia. This is a common sequela in patients being treated, but the state of hydration is ignored (Figure 54-8).

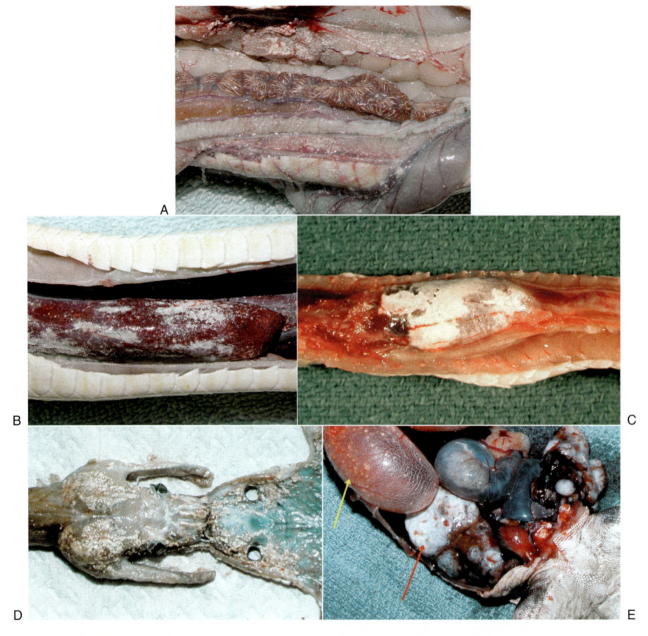

FIGURE 54-6 In reptilian patients, common sites for tophi deposition include **A,** the kidneys (note the powdery tophi crystals scattered throughout the membranes); **B,** the liver; **C,** the pericardial sac; **D,** the muscles of the head and subcutaneous tissue; and **E,** the lungs *(yellow arrow)* and fat pads *(red arrow)*.

DIAGNOSIS

Diagnosis of gout, either articular or visceral, is made on the basis of history and clinical examination. Diet, availability of water, ambient temperature, and humidity all play important roles in development of the disease. Laboratory sampling may or may not show hyperuricemia, depending on the state of health at the time of sampling. Blood urea nitrogen and creatinine are usually of little value in interpretation of renal disease in reptilian species.

Radiographs may reveal lytic lesions in, around, or near the joints. If renal or cystic calculi are composed of monosodium urate stones, they may go unnoticed; but if the calculi are complexed with calcium, the stones are readily apparent.

A definitive diagnosis of gout is made on demonstration of monosodium urate crystals in the joints of affected patients or within tophi of diseased tissue (Figure 54-9). A polarizing filter makes identification of the biorefringent crystals easier.[16,17]

TREATMENT

Treatment of gout in human medicine is threefold: lower the serum uric acid level with antihyperuricemic drugs such as

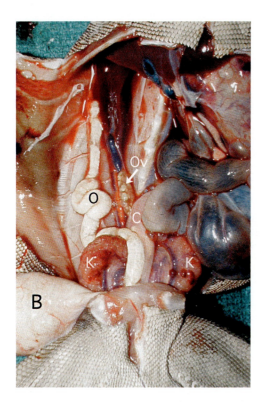

FIGURE 54-7 A Green Iguana *(Iguana iguana)* with severe renomegaly from gout. The kidneys were so enlarged that the pelvis was almost completely obstructed. As a result, urate-laden urine refluxed back into the animal's right oviduct. *O,* Oviduct; *Ov,* ovary; *C,* colon; *K,* kidney; *B,* bladder.

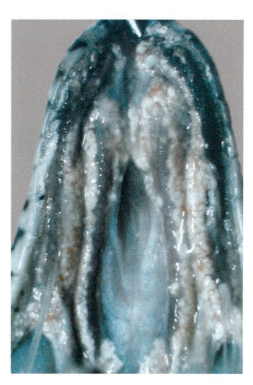

FIGURE 54-8 This python was treated with an aminoglycoside for infectious stomatitis. The veterinarian noticed the whitish lesions in the gingiva. Thinking it was a progression of the infectious stomatitis, he increased the dose. In actuality, the lesions were not infectious in origin but were depositions of gouty tophi. The snake died of extensive visceral gout.

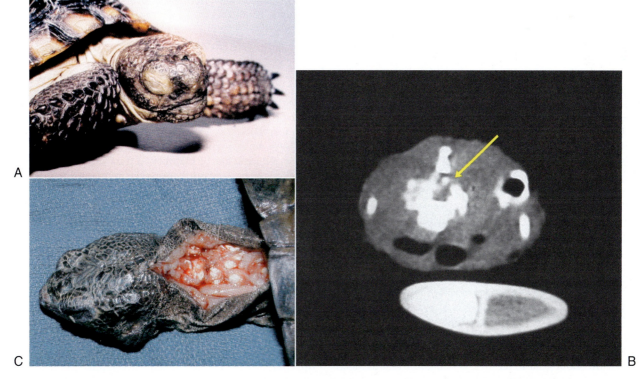

FIGURE 54-9 A, This tortoise presented with a right-sided head tilt. **B,** The computed tomographic cross section through the neck of this patient shows a small area of bone destruction caused by uric acid crystals *(yellow arrow).* **C,** The patient was euthanized, and necropsy was performed. The numerous whitish crystals along the dorsal cervical region were all gouty tophi.

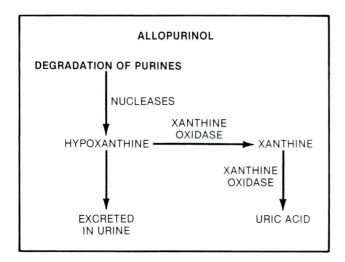

FIGURE 54-10 Allopurinol decreases uric acid production by inhibiting the actions of xanthine oxidase.

allopurinol (Figure 54-10), promote urate excretion with uricosuric drugs such as probenecid, and manage acute gouty arthritis attacks with antiinflammatory drugs such as colchicine and corticosteroids. In humans, the goal of therapy is to keep the serum uric acid levels less than 6 mg/dL. Doing so is believed to prevent future attacks and to dissolve existing tophi.

In theory, the treatment goals for reptiles with gout are similar to those in humans. However, little research has been done surrounding the treatment of gout in reptiles. Recent reports suggest that allopurinol therapy is effective in reptiles (Figure 54-11),[18] with results consistent with goals in human medicine.[19,20]

Many different dosages have been reported in the recent herpetologic literature (Table 54-1). Most dosages used, however, are based on extrapolations from the human dosages (Table 54-2). These drugs are not without side effects, and the clients should be warned when they are used in reptile patients.

If the patient has severe gouty arthritis, surgically entering the affected joint and physically removing the uric acid crystals is possible. However, by the time the crystals have formed, severe joint damage is usually present. Between this damage and the surgical damage done to the joint, even by the best of surgeons, the joint is usually permanently affected. In these cases, treatment may be best attempted with long-term allopurinol therapy.

CONCLUSION

All this points to the fact that gout is a serious problem in reptiles. Because of their primitive physiology and unique, often poorly understood nutritional requirements, they are more prone to this disease. Although we still have a great deal to learn about gout in reptiles, we do know that in most instances it is usually preventable.

Proper diet, correct ambient temperatures, and continuous access to fresh clean water all thwart the development

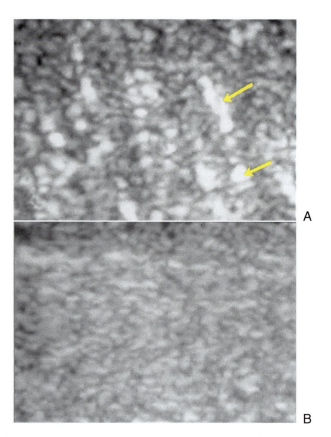

FIGURE 54-11 A, Renal ultrasound from a European Tortoise with severe renal gout. The tophi, which are scattered throughout the renal parynchema, are hyperechoic *(yellow arrows).* **B,** The same patient as in **A**. Note the homogenous-appearing renal parynchema and the absence of hyperechoic tophi. The tophi dissolved after 2 to 4 months of treatment with 50 mg/kg allopurinol, given every third day. *(Photographs courtesy P. Kolle.)*

of gout. In addition, the proper use of medications, especially antibiotics, can ensure against kidney damage and secondary gout formation.

The overall prognosis for patients with severe gout is poor. Advanced cases can be maintained for a short period. Keep in mind, on the basis of our knowledge in human medicine, that acute gouty attacks are painful, and although how reptiles interpret pain is not known for sure, one can only assume that they feel the same discomfort as their human counterparts. As such, patients with gout should be given proper medications to alleviate any pain and suffering that they might experience.

More research needs to be done on reptilian patients with gouty symptoms. Newer drugs are available on the human market that show promise and have potential for use in herpetologic medicine. Xanthine oxidase inhibitors such as oxipurinol and febuxostat are first-line treatments for human patients with renal calculi, renal insufficiency, and hyperuricemia. These are safe and well tolerated with few side effects.[21]

Recombinant urate oxidase is used for the treatment of tumor lysis hyperuricemia in human cancer patients.

Table 54-1 Dosages of Allopurinol Reported in Clinical Reptile Cases

Dose	Frequency	Duration	Comment	no.	Reference
50 mg/kg	q 24 h	30 d	A	73	18
Followed by:					
50 mg/kg	q 72 h	3 y	B		
9.93 mg/kg	q 24 h	30 d	C	1	19
Followed by:					
3.31 mg/g	q 24 h	90 d			
20 mg/kg	q 24 h	90 d	D	1	20
At 21 days into therapy, the following was added:					
Probenecid (250 mg)	q 12 h	45 d	E	1	

All doses were administered orally.
A, 97.3% of all tortoises showed decrease in [uric acid] by day 7. B, Uric acid tophi in kidneys disappeared 2 to 4 months after [uric acid] < 2 mg/dL. C, Joint inflammation disappeared after 5 months of treatment; all clinical signs gone by 7 months later. D, [Uric acid] returned to normal (8 mg/dL) after 75 d of allopurinol, 52 days after the start of probenecid. E, The tortoise had a relapse and died 30 days later, despite reinstatement of treatment.

Table 54-2 Medications Commonly Used for the Treatment of Gout in Humans

Drug	Dose	Comments
Allopurinol	20 mg/kg, PO, q 24 h	Decreases production of uric acid (blocks xanthine oxidase)
Probenecid	250 mg, PO, bid (increase as needed)	Blocks resorption of uric acid by kidney tubules, increasing uric acid excretion
Sulfinpyrazone	100-200 mg, PO, bid (increase as needed)	Blocks resorption of uric acid by kidney tubules, increasing uric acid excretion
Colchicine	0.5-1.2 mg, PO q 2 h; or 2 mg loading dose IV, followed by 0.5 mg IV q 6 h	Reduces inflammatory response to monosodium urate crystals in joint tissues; positive response usually seen within 24 h

PO, Orally; *q*, every; *bid*, twice a day; *IV*, intravenous.

Pegylated urate oxidase shows promise in patients with hyperuricemia and gout.[22]

When diagnosed early, gout can be managed and the patient maintained comfortably. The author has a number of patients on long-term gout medications. As long as the owners remember to administer the drugs, the pets do fine. On the rare occasion when the owner forgets, runs out of the prescription, or for some reason does not give the medication, the patients often have quick relapses.

REFERENCES

1. Lewis LD, Morris ML, Hand MS: *Small animal clinical nutrition III*, Topeka, Kan, 1987, Mark L. Morris Associates.
2. Fam AG: Strategies for treating gout and hyperuricemia, *J Musculoskel Med* 5(3):83, 1988.
3. German DC, Holmes EW: Gout and hyperuricemia: diagnosis and management, *Hosp Pract* 21(11):119, 1986.
4. Lo B: Hyperuricemia and gout (topics in primary care medicine), *West J Med* 142:104, 1985.
5. McCance KL, Huether SE: *Pathophysiology: the biological basis of disease in adults and children*, St Louis, 1990, Mosby.
6. Smyth CJ: Monoarticular arthritis: suspect gout, *Diagnosis* 86, 1987.
7. Vawter RL, Spadaro Antonelli MA: Rational treatment of gout, *Postgrad Med* 91(2):115, 1992.
8. Wolfe F: Gout and hyperuricemia, *AFP* 43(6):2141, 1991.
9. Kolle P, Hoffman R: Incidence of nephropathies in European Tortoises, *Proc Assoc Rept Amphib Vet* 33-35, 2002.
10. Lehninger AL: *Biochemistry*, New York, 1975, Worth Publishers.
11. Ganong WF: *Review of medical physiology*, Los Altos, Calif, 1981, Lange Medical Publications.
12. Dessauer HC: Blood chemistry of reptiles: physiological and evolutionary aspects. In Gans C, editor: *Biology of the Reptilia*, San Diego, 1970, Academic Press.
13. Dantzler WH: Comparative aspects of renal urate transport, *Kidney Int* 49:1549-1551, 1996.
14. Campbell TW, Coles EH: Avian clinical pathology. In Coles EH, editor: *Veterinary clinical pathology*, Philadelphia, 1986, WB Saunders.
15. Wenker CJ, Bart M, Guscetti F, Hatt J, Isenbugal E: Periarticular hydroxyapatite deposition disease in two Red-bellied Short-necked Turtles (*Emydura albertisii*), *Proc Am Assoc Zoo Vet* 23-26, 1999.
16. Frye FL: *Biomedical and surgical aspects of captive reptile husbandry*, Melbourne, Fla, 1991, Krieger Publishing.
17. Casimire-Etzioni AL, Wellehan AFX, Embury JE, Terrell SP, Raskin RE: Synovial fluid from an African Spur-thighed Tortoise (*Geochelone sulcatta*), *Vet Clin Path* 33(1):43-46, 2004.

18. Kolle P: Efficacy of allopurinol in European Tortoises with hyperglycemia, *Proc Assoc Rept Amphib Vet* 185-186, 2001.
19. Figureres JM: Treatment of articular gout in a Mediterranean Pond Turtle *(Mauremys leprosa)*, *Assoc Rept Amphib Vet* 7(4):5-7, 1997.
20. Martin-Silvestre A: Treatment with allopurinol and probenecid for visceral gout in a Greek Tortoise *(Testudo graeca)*, *Assoc Rept Amphib Vet* 7(4):4-5, 1997.
21. Becker MA, Schumacher HR, Wortman RL, et al: Febuxostat, a novel nonpurine selective inhibitor of xanthine oxidase: a twenty-eight-day, multicenter, phase II, randomized, double-blind, placebo-controlled, dose-response clinical trial examining safety and efficacy in patients with gout, *Arthritis Rheum* 52(3):216-223, 2005.
22. Bomalaski JS, Clark MA: Serum uric acid–lowering therapies: where are we heading in management of hyperuricemia and the potential role of uricase, *Curr Rheumatol Rep* 6(3):240-247, 2004.

55
HEMOPARASITES
TERRY W. CAMPBELL

Ectothermic vertebrates, such as reptiles, are hosts for a variety of blood parasites. Intraerythrocytic parasites include protozoa, viruses, and structures of uncertain status. Reptilian parasites, and those of any ectothermic vertebrate, experience host temperature fluctuations, host reproductive strategies, population genetics, host habitat, and migratory behavior that are unlike those of the endothermic mammals and birds.[1] Also, the biology of the reptilian erythrocyte compared with that of the mammalian erythrocyte might influence the nature of the intraerythrocytic parasite behavior. Therefore, most blood parasites of reptiles are relatively harmless to their reptilian hosts and are an incidental finding. This is in contrast to the many blood parasites of mammals and some birds that harm their hosts. However, some reptilian blood parasites are highly pathogenic and have the potential to cause diseases, such as hemolytic anemia and inanition. Pathogenic species often cause disease in both young and geriatric reptiles. Factors that contribute to the pathology associated with parasitic infection in reptiles include nutritional disorders and environmental stresses, such as maintaining reptiles in temperatures outside the reptile's optimal range, overcrowding, and poor sanitation that includes poor control of ectoparasites or other invertebrate vectors. Concern also exists that the practice of grouping reptiles that originate from a variety of global locations together in the same captive environment might create severe parasitic infections in unnatural reptilian hosts.[2-4]

Common hemoprotozoa include the hemogregarines, trypanosomatids, and *Plasmodium* spp. Less commonly encountered hemoprotozoans include *Sauroleishmania*, *Sauroplasma*, *Haemoproteus*, and *Schellackia*. Microfilaria also can be found in the peripheral blood films of reptiles (Table 55-1).

Reptile parasites in the Phylum Apicomplexa and Subclass Coccidiasina are the most common group of blood parasites found in reptiles.[5] Organisms in this phylum possess an apical complex at some stage in their development. The apical complex identified by parasitologists consists of polar rings, rhoptries, micronemes, a conoid, and subpellicular microtubules. These organisms usually reproduce sexually with syngamy and asexually with multiple or binary fission.

HEMOGREGARINES (HAEMOGREGARINIDS)

Hemogregarines (also, Haemogregarinids) are the most common group of sporozoan hemoparasites that affect reptiles. These parasites are in the Phylum Apicomplexa, Subclass Coccidiasina, Suborder Adeleorina, and Family Haemogregorinidae. The Suborder Adeleorina contains coccidia that have macrogametes and microgamonts associated in syzygy during development, and microgamonts usually produce one to four microgametes.[5] Reptile coccidia in the Family Haemogregorinidae have an indirect life cycle, with intermediate hosts that include leeches, ticks, mosquitoes, or mites. Three genera of the Family Haemogregorinidae of parasites that are common in reptiles are *Haemogregarina*, *Hepatozoon*, and *Karyolysus*.[5-9] Genera in this family can only be identified by the appearance of the oocytes in the invertebrate host. Therefore, the hemogregarines are not easily differentiated on the basis of the appearance of their gametocytes within the cytoplasm of erythrocytes or tissue schizonts. The definitive hosts for the genus *Haemogregarina* include freshwater turtles, tortoises of the genera *Geoemyda* and *Testudo*, the Tuatara, some lizards, and most snakes and crocodilians.[5-9] The definitive hosts for the genus *Hepatozoon* are primarily reptiles, especially snakes.[5] The definitive hosts for the genus *Karyolysus* are primarily Old World lizards and, possibly, tree snakes.[6-9] No cases of haemogregariniasis have been reported in seaturtles.[7] Because an accurate classification of the hemogregarines into their appropriate genus cannot be accomplished on the basis of their appearance in the blood film alone, the general terms hemogregarine or haemogregarinids are used in reports of their presence in blood films during hematologic examinations.

Hemogregarines are identified by the presence of intracytoplasmic gametocytes in erythrocytes in stained blood films. The sausage-shaped (or banana-shaped) gametocytes lack the refractile pigment granules found in the gametocytes of *Plasmodium* and *Haemoproteus*, and they often distort the host cell by creating a bulge in the cytoplasm or displacing the nucleus laterally. Typically, only one gametocyte is found per erythrocyte; however, in heavy infections, two gametocytes may be found in one cell (Figures 55-1 to 55-3).

Hemogregarines have a life cycle that involves sexual reproduction (sporogony) in an invertebrate host and asexual multiplication (merogony) in a reptilian host. The parasite infects the reptilian host when the sporozoites are transmitted from the invertebrate host as it feeds on the blood of the reptile or is ingested by the reptile. Several biting invertebrate hosts (i.e., mites, ticks, mosquitoes, flies, and bugs) can transmit the parasite to terrestrial reptiles, whereas leeches appear to be the primary intermediate host for the hemogregarines of aquatic reptiles.[6] Reptilian hemogregarines are well adapted to their natural host and do not typically cause clinical disease; however, heavy infestations can cause anemia and inanition. Because they are relatively non-host-specific, the haemogregarinids can cause significant clinical disease in unnatural or aberrant host species.[3,4] Such infections result in severe inflammatory lesions associated with schizonts in a variety of organs.[3,4,10-12] No reported treatments are effective in the treatment of haemogregariniasis.

Table 55-1 Blood Parasites of Reptiles

Parasite	Stage in Peripheral Blood	Intermediate Host	Blood Location	Description
Trypanosomes (L, S, C, Cr)	Trypanomastigote or trypanosome stage	Dipteran biting flies or leeches	Extracellular	Blade-like shape, single flagellum, undulating membrane
Leishmania (L)	Amastigote or leishmanial stage	Sand flies	Intracytoplasmic in thrombocyte, lymphocyte, monocyte	Round to oval (2 to 4 μm), blue cytoplasm, oval red nucleus
Haemogregarina (aquatic reptiles)	Gametocytes	Ticks, mites, flies, bugs, leeches, mosquitoes	Intracytoplasmic in RBC	Sausage-shaped nonpigmented, gametocytes
Hepatozoon (S)	Gametocytes	Ticks, mites, flies, bugs, leeches, mosquitoes	Intracytoplasmic in RBC and extracellular	Sausage-shaped, nonpigmented, gametocytes
Karyloysus (Old World Lizards)	Gametocytes	Ticks, mites, flies, bugs, leeches, mosquitoes	Intracytoplasmic in RBC and extracellular	Sausage-shaped, nonpigmented, gametocytes
Plasmodium (L, S, C)	Schizonts, gametocytes, trophozoites	Dipteran biting insects	Intracytoplasmic in RBC, WBC, thrombocytes	Trophozoite: small, signet ring–shaped. Schizogony: packets of merozoites. Gametocyte: refractile pigment granules
Haemoproteus (Haemocystidium; L, C)	Gametocytes	Dipteran biting flies	Intracytoplasmic in RBC	Gametocytes that encircle cell nucleus with pigment granules
Saurocytozoon (L)	Gametocytes	Biting insects (mosquitoes)	Intracytoplasmic in WBC	Large, round, nonpigmented gametocytes that grossly distort host cell
Schellackia (L)	Gametocytes	Dipteran biting insects	Intracytoplasmic in RBC, WBC (lymphocytes)	Round to oval inclusions that often deform host cell nucleus
Babesia (L, S, C)	Trophozoites (0.5 to 1 μm) Schizonts (2 to 4 μm)	Ticks	Intracytoplasmic in RBC	Small round to piriform
Aegyptianella (Tunetella)	Trophozoites, schizonts	Biting insects or arthropods	Intracytoplasmic in RBC	Small round to piriform
Sauroplasma (L)	Piroplasma-like	Biting insects	Intracytoplasmic in RBC	Multiple, small, punctate, nonpigmented, signet ring–like vacuoles (1 to 2 μm)
Serpentoplasma (S)	Piroplasma-like	Biting insects	Intracytoplasmic in RBC	Morphologically similar to Sauroplasma

C, Chelonians; Cr, crocodilean; L, lizards; RBC, red blood cell; S, snakes; WBC, white blood cell.

PIROPLASMS

Piroplasms are in the Phylum Apicomplexa, Subclass Coccidiasina, and Suborder Piroplasmorina. Piroplasms are identified by the appearance of asexual stages of the organism in the cytoplasm of erythrocytes and occasionally in other cells. They appear as small (1 to 2 microns in diameter) nonpigmented intracytoplasmic inclusions. These inclusions vary in shape from piriform, spherical, rod-like, or amoeboid (Figure 55-4). Sporogony occurs in invertebrates, which thus far have been shown to be ticks. Piroplasms lack oocytes, sporocysts, cysts, flagella, and a typical conoid.[5] The only piroplasmid to infect reptiles belong to the genus Sauroplasma (also known as Serpentoplasma). Sauroplasma spp. have been reported in chameleons and other lizards (Gymnodactylus, Uroplatus, Lacerta, Cordylus, and Zonurus).[5]

SCHELLACKIA

Schellackia spp. (also called Atoxoplasma, Gordonella, Lainsonia, Lankesterella) belong to the Phylum Apicomplexa, Subclass Coccidiasina, and Suborder Eimeriorina. Most species of this suborder (i.e., Cryptosporidium, Eimeria, Isospora, Sacrocystis, and Toxoplasma) inhabit the intestinal epithelium of reptiles where they are detected microscopically by the presence of oocytes in the feces or histopathology of the intestines.[5] However, the Schellackia spp. are detected by the appearance of intracytoplasmic sporozoites in erythrocytes and mononuclear leukocytes, primarily lymphocytes.[7] These inclusions resemble the intracytoplasmic inclusions of Atoxoplasma in birds. The parasite is identified by the round to oval, pale staining, nonpigmented inclusions in lymphocytes that deform the host-cell nucleus into a crescent shape. The definitive hosts for

Hemoparasites

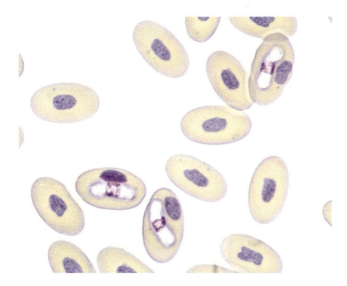

FIGURE 55-1 Hemogregarine, most likely *Hepatozoon*, in the blood film of a snake *(Corallus caninus)*. Modified Wright-Giemsa stain; original photograph, 500×.

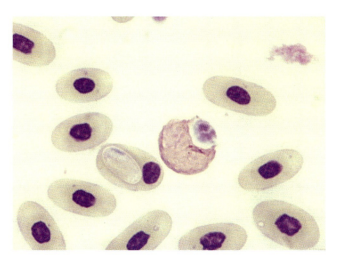

FIGURE 55-2 Erythrocytic inclusion resembling that of hemogregarine in the blood film of a tortoise *(Manouria emys)*. Modified Wright-Giemsa stain; original photograph, 500×.

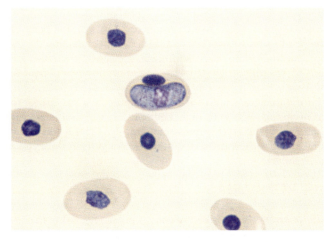

FIGURE 55-3 Hemogregarine in the blood film of a freshwater turtle *(Trachemys scripta elegans)*. Wright stain; original photograph, 500×.

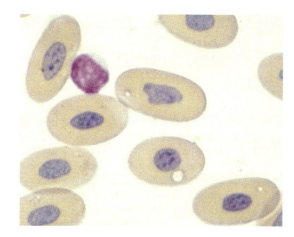

FIGURE 55-4 Erythrocytic cytoplasmic *Sauroplasma (Serpentoplasma)* inclusion in the blood film of a snake *(Corallus canina)*. Modified Wright-Giemsa stain; original photograph, 500×.

this parasite are lizards.[5] *Schellackia* spp. are considered to be an incidental finding because no known disease has been associated with them.

MALARIA-CAUSING PARASITES

The parasites considered to cause malaria in reptiles belong to the Phylum Apicomplexa, Subclass Coccidiasina, and Suborder Haemospororina. These blood parasites have an indirect life cycle where schizogony and gamogony occur in reptiles and fertilization and sporogony occur in arthropods. The arthropod vectors include sandflies, mosquitoes, gnats, and perhaps mites. In general, these parasites are not pathogenic to their reptilian hosts, but they can occasionally cause a hemolytic anemia. No effective chemotherapeutic agents are found to treat infections with these parasites. These parasites are detected by the presence of microscopic intraerythrocytic trophozoites, schizonts, or gametes in stained blood films.

Haemoproteus spp. (also known as *Haemamoeba*, *Haemocystidium*, *Halteridium*, *Parahaemoproteus*, and *Simondis*) are identified by the presence of intracytoplasmic gametocytes within erythrocytes in stained peripheral blood films. The gametocytes contain refractile pigment granules (hemozoin). Only the gametocyte stage of this parasite can be found in the peripheral blood film of reptiles, whereas schizogony occurs only in reticuloendothelial cells in tissues. Birds are considered to be the primary hosts for *Haemoproteus*; however, the parasite has also been reported in lizards and turtles.[5,7,13] Some parasitologists believe *Haemoproteus* of lizards should be placed in the genus *Haemocystidium* and those of turtles should be placed in the genus *Simondia*.[14] No known effective treatment exists for *Haemoproteus*.

More than 60 species of *Plasmodium* have been described in reptiles; most have been identified in lizards and a few snakes.[6,13] *Plasmodium* in reptiles resemble those found in birds. The intracytoplasmic gametocytes have refractile pigment granules (hemozoin) that aid in differentiation between *Plasmodium* and the hemogregarines. Unlike *Haemoproteus*, schizogony of *Plasmodium* can occur in blood cells. The trophozoites are small signet-ring inclusions in the cytoplasm of erythrocytes. The life cycle of *Plasmodium* involves a sporogony stage in an insect host, such as the mosquito, and schizogony and gametogony in a reptile host. Heavy infections with some species of *Plasmodium* can result in a severe hemolytic anemia and death, whereas other species may cause splenomegaly.

Saurocytozoon are identified by large round gametocytes that lack the refractile pigment of *Plasmodium* and *Hemoproteus*. The gametocytes grossly distort the host cell, usually an erythrocyte, that it parasitizes. This parasite is transmitted through the bite of an arthropod vector, such as a mosquito, to the definitive reptilian hosts, which are lizards.[5,7] *Saurocytozoon* is usually considered nonpathogenic to reptiles but may cause anemia in susceptible animals. No known effective treatment is found for saurocytozoonosis.

Fallisia spp. are considered by some parasitologists to be the same as *Saurocytozoon* because of their identical morphologic features. This parasite has been reported in lizards of the genera *Draco, Neusticurus, Plica, Tropidurus,* and *Uranoscodon*.[5]

TRYPANOSOMATIDS

Trypanosoma and *Sauroleishmania* belong to the Phylum Apicomplexa, Subclass Coccidiasina, and Order Kinetoplastida. Members of this order of parasites are flagellate protozoans with one or two flagella, typically with a single long mitochondrion and one or more kinetoplasts.[5] They reproduce by binary fission. Approximately 60 species of *Trypanosoma* parasitize reptiles. All orders of reptiles can be parasitized by trypanosomes. Some species are also pathogenic to humans and other mammals. The trypomastigote form is common in the blood of vertebrates. They are large extracellular flagellate protozoa with a blade-like shape, a single flagellum, and a prominent undulating membrane (Figure 55-5). The body size varies with species. Trypanosomes are digenetic and require a blood-sucking invertebrate host, such as biting flies for terrestrial reptiles or leeches for aquatic reptiles, for transmission. Trypanosomes have a worldwide distribution. However, they rarely cause clinical disease and are often associated with lifelong infections.

Sauroleishmania need more than one host to complete a life cycle and develop as promastigotes (the form with a free anterior flagellum that resembles the typical adult form) or similar forms in phlebotomine sandflies. Until recently, these reptilian parasites were considered to be species of *Leishmania*.[5,7] About 12 species have been reported to be parasitic to reptiles. This rare parasite of lizards and some snakes is identified as a circular to oval (1.5 to 5 microns) amastigote (leishmanial stage) in the blood film. The intracytoplasmic organism is found in thrombocytes or mononuclear leukocytes and has a blue cytoplasm and a prominent oval red nucleus and kinetoplast and no external flagellum. *Sauroleishmania* is considered to be nonpathogenic to reptiles.

PIRHEMOCYTON

Pirhemocytonosis is characterized by the presence of intraerythrocytic inclusions in lizards. The inclusions appear as red punctate to oval bodies that may be associated with vacuoles (albuminoid vacuoles) and irregular pale-staining areas in the cytoplasm of erythrocytes in Giemsa-stained

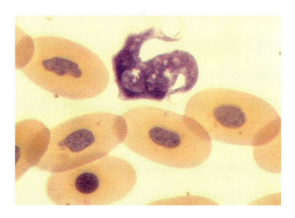

FIGURE 55-5 Trypanosome in the blood film of a snake *(Corallus canina)*. Modified Wright-Giemsa stain; original photograph, 500×.

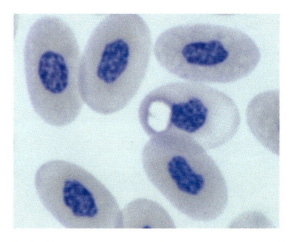

FIGURE 55-6 Rectangular vacuole-like inclusion resembling that of pirhemocyton in the cytoplasm of an erythrocyte in the blood film of a lizard *(Iguana iguana)*. Wright stain; original photograph, 500×.

blood films (Figure 55-6).[15] Similar inclusions have been reported in snakes and turtles.[6] These intraerythrocytic inclusions of reptiles were previously considered to be a piroplasm, referred to as Pirhemocyton, until ultrastructural studies revealed the presence of a virus consistent with members of the Iridoviridae. One report of pirhemocytonosis in snakes was suggestive of an oncornavirus on the basis of the results of ultrastructural studies.[16] As the infection develops, the inclusions increase in size, measuring between 0.5 and 1.5 microns. A single inclusion per erythrocyte is typical; however, two inclusions per cell may occur on occasion. Natural infections with the lizard erythrocyte virus appear to be nonfatal, even with high viremia (i.e., even with greater than 85% of the erythrocytes being infected) that result in the appearance of spindle-shaped or thin elongate erythrocytes.

MICROFILARIA

Microfilaremia in reptiles typically is not associated with clinical signs of illness or changes in the hemogram or blood biochemical profile. The reptile typically survives for years with these parasites, and microfilaria are detected as an incidental

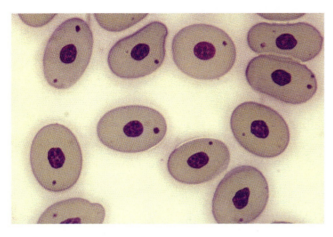

FIGURE 55-7 Artifacts in the cytoplasm of the erythrocytes in a Loggerhead Turtle *(Caretta caretta)*. Wright stain; original photograph, 500×.

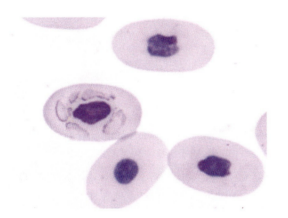

FIGURE 55-8 Artifact in the cytoplasm of a tortoise *(Gopherus polyphemus)*. Wright stain; original photograph, 500×.

finding on examination of routine Romanowsky-stained blood films. Microfilaria are produced by adult female filarid nematodes, which can live in various locations in the body of a reptile. Microfilaria are ingested by a suitable blood-sucking arthropod (i.e., tick or mite) or insect (i.e., mosquito), in which they develop into the infective third-stage larval form. The life cycle is complete when the infective form enters a new reptilian host during intermediate-host feeding.

ARTIFACTS (PSEUDOPARASITES)

Round to irregular basophilic inclusions frequently are seen in the cytoplasm of erythrocytes in the peripheral blood films from many species of reptiles (Figure 55-7). These inclusions most likely represent artifact of slide preparation because blood films made repeatedly from the same sample often reveal varying degrees of these inclusions. For example, the erythrocyte inclusions seen in the blood film of a Loggerhead Seaturtle *(Caretta caretta)* (a species not noted for having blood parasites) in Figure 55-7 appeared in nearly every erythrocyte on the original blood film; however, a second blood film made from the same blood sample revealed very few of these inclusions. Electron-microscopic images suggest that these inclusions are degenerate organelles.[16] Other artifacts found in the erythrocyte cytoplasm include vacuoles and refractile clear areas (Figure 55-8). These later artifacts can be minimized with careful preparation of blood films.

REFERENCES

1. Davies AJ, Johnston MR: The biology of some intraerythrocytic parasites of fishes, amphibia, and reptiles, *Adv Parasitol* 45:1-107, 2000.
2. Wozniak EJ, Kazacos KR, Telford SR, McLaughlin GL: Characterization of the clinical and anatomical pathological changes associated with *Hepatozoon mocassini* infections in unnatural reptilian hosts, *Int J Parasitol* 26(2):141-146, 1996.
3. Wozniak EJ, Telford SR: The fate of possibly two *Hepatozoon* species naturally infecting Florida black racers and water snakes in potential mosquito and soft tick vectors: histological evidence of pathogenicity in unnatural host species, *Int J Parasitol* 21:511-516, 1991.
4. Wozniak EJ, Telford SR, McLaughlin GL: Employment of the polymerase chain reaction in the molecular differentiation of reptilian hemogregarines and its application to preventative zoological medicine, *J Zoo Wildl Med* 25:538-549, 1994.
5. Barnard SM, Upton SJ: *A veterinary guide to the parasites of reptiles, vol 1, protozoa*, Malabar, Fla, 1994, Krieger Publishing.
6. Telford SR: Haemoparasites of reptiles. In Hoff GL, Frye FL, Jacobson ER, editors: *Diseases of amphibians and reptiles*, New York, 1984, Plenum.
7. Keymer IF: Protozoa. In Cooper JE, Jackson OF, editors: *Diseases of the Reptilia*, San Diego, 1981, Academic Press.
8. Lowichik A, Yeager RG: Ecological aspects of snake hemogregarine infections from two habitats in Southern Louisiana, *J Parasitol* 73:1109-1115, 1987.
9. Frye FL: Hemoparasites. In Frye FL, editor: *Biomedical and surgical aspects of captive reptile husbandry*, ed 2, Melbourne, Fla, 1991, Krieger Publishing.
10. Griner LA: *Pathology of zoo animals*, San Diego, 1983, Zoological Society of San Diego.
11. Wozniak EJ, McLaughlin GL, Telford SR: Description of the vertebrate stages of a hemogregarine species naturally infecting Mojave Desert Sidewinder rattlesnakes *(Crotalus cerastes cerastes)*, *J Zoo Wildl Med* 25:103-110, 1994.
12. Jacobson E: Parasitic diseases of reptiles. In Fowler ME, editor: *Zoo and wild animal medicine*, ed 2, Philadelphia, 1986, WB Saunders.
13. Garnham PCC: *Malaria parasites and other haemosporidia*, Oxford, 1966, Blackwell Scientific Publications.
14. Telford SR, Jacobson ER. Lizard erythrocytic virus in East African chameleons, *J Wildl Dis* 29:57-63, 1993.
15. Daly JJ, Mayhue M, Menna JH, Calhon CH: Viruslike particles associated with Pirhemocyton inclusion bodies in the erythrocytes of a water snake, *Nerodia erythrogster flavigaster*, *J Parasitol* 66:82-87, 1980.
16. Alleman AR, Jacobson ER, Raskin RE: Morphologic and cytochemical characteristics of blood cells from the desert tortoise [*Gopherus agassizii*], *Am J Res* 53:1645-1651, 1992.

56
HEPATIC LIPIDOSIS

STEPHEN J. HERNANDEZ-DIVERS and
JOHN E. COOPER

Hepatic lipidosis is a well-recognized condition that is frequently diagnosed postmortem in numerous species of reptiles. Unfortunately, a paucity of information exists concerning the pathogenesis of hepatic lipidosis in reptiles and, until relatively recently, the collection of biopsies for definitive antemortem diagnosis presented a challenge to clinicians. Although many of the difficulties of sample acquisition have now been overcome, the practitioner is still faced with the problems of microscopic (histopathologic and electron microscopic) interpretation. A logical case investigation is described with particular emphasis on histologic interpretation through the grading of microscopic lesions.

Liver disease, and more specifically, hepatic lipidosis, is probably one of the most frequently stated and misunderstood diagnoses made by clinicians and pathologists alike. Metabolic changes that lead to an increase in hepatic fat can lead a pathologist to make a postmortem diagnosis of hepatic lipidosis. Likewise, clinicians may also be forgiven for making a presumptive diagnosis of "fatty liver" when confronted with an obese captive reptile that has been consistently overfed and underexercised. However, the problem is far more complex and extensive than perhaps has been previously appreciated.

THE REPTILE LIVER

Anatomy

The macroscopic appearance of the liver of reptiles is little different from that of other vertebrate animals. Its shape varies according to the morphology of the animal; thus, it is long and thin in most snakes but short and broad in chelonians and most lizards.

The liver comprises 3% to 4% of body weight in most squamate species, generally less in chelonians and crocodilians.[1] However, its size and weight (mass) can fluctuate according to time of year and nutritional or reproductive status.

Different forms of the reptilian liver were first described long ago by comparative anatomists, culminating in the work of Richard Owen (1804-1892). Since then, remarkably little study has taken place, and as a result, we remain ignorant of the specific features of liver anatomy of many reptiles. Some of the variations are discussed by Schaffner.[2]

The liver originates (in most species) from the endodermal gut. Usually it consists of two lobes and varies in color from dark brown to black. A gallbladder is usually present. The blood supply to the liver is from the hepatic portal vein and hepatic artery.

Physiology

The functions of the reptile liver are similar to those of mammals and birds—essentially fat, protein (including globulin) and glycogen metabolism, and the production of uric acid and clotting factors. However, these functions may vary markedly as the animal progresses from egg to juvenile to breeding adult and may also be dramatically affected by seasonal changes, especially brumation (hibernation) and sometimes estivation. A full review of hepatic metabolism of carbohydrates, fats, bile acids and pigments, proteins, and hormones is given by Schaffner.[2]

Mammals and birds tend to store fat in subcutaneous sites, primarily as a means of thermal insulation. Such an adaptation is less helpful and, judged from extant species, has not evolved within the Reptilia. Instead, most reptiles store fat in specific fat bodies; these organs are located within the caudoventral coelom. The main role of these fat stores is to provide lipid for vitellogenesis and to act as an energy store during brumation (hibernation) or estivation and fasting.[3] Hepatic lipid reserves of species studied are highest in females just before brumation (hibernation) and lowest in males in late brumation (hibernation).[4,5] Fats are transported from the intestinal tract and the fat bodies to the liver in the form of unesterified fatty acids. All fat transportation away from the liver is in an esterified form, being protein-bound as lipoproteins. These very low-density lipoproteins are recycled as low-density lipoprotein fragments. The formulation of phospholipids and cholesterol is also under hepatic regulation, again from lipid precursors.

DIAGNOSIS OF HEPATIC LIPIDOSIS

Anamnesis (History) and Physical Examination

One must remember that hepatic lipidosis is a metabolic derangement and not a single clinical disease. A host of factors can predispose to increased hepatic fat. Classically, the high-fat diet (e.g., obese laboratory rats, waxworms) has been implicated in obesity, an increase in the size of coelomic fat bodies, and an increase in hepatic fat. Equally, reduction in activity, which frequently afflicts captive reptiles, must also be considered. Therefore, careful questioning of the keeper or owner with regard to exercise, food items, and feeding frequency is essential. The usual environmental information, particularly with regard to thermal provision, is obviously essential. One other common aspect to this condition is the apparent prevalence in nonbreeding adult to aged females.

Many female reptiles undergo seasonal cycles of lipogenesis in preparation for folliculogenesis. Those females that do not have the opportunity to breed and produce eggs appear more prone to obesity in captivity.

Hepatic disease can be classified as acute or chronic, inflammatory (hepatitis) or degenerative (hepatosis). Hepatic lipidosis is usually chronic, and observant owners and keepers who maintain accurate records may report a gradual reduction in appetite, activity, fecundity and fertility, retarded weight gain or gradual weight loss, brumation (hibernation) problems including postbrumation (posthibernation) anorexia, and changes in fecal character and color. However, the underlying liver disease may become clinically apparent only during episodes of increased physiologic demand (e.g., brumation [hibernation], breeding, concurrent disease, etc.). Unfortunately, many caretakers miss these early signs of disease. As a result, veterinary attention is only sought once the animal has deteriorated to a life-threatening condition. When lipidosis is advanced, most affected reptiles are in poor body condition, flaccid, weak, and cachectic. The bodyweight (mass) is usually below normal, often critically so, although in cases of ascites, weight may be artificially maintained or even increased. Diarrhea is uncommon as most affected animals have been anorectic for a prolonged period of time.

Acute hepatitis (an inflammatory change) is not uncommon in reptiles and is often associated with infectious agents. Acute hepatosis (degenerative liver disease) is much less common. Rare situations exist where toxic insult may cause acute degenerative changes. Ivermectin-induced hepatic lipidosis is a well-documented example.[6] Reptiles with acute liver disease usually are seen in good body condition but with sudden onset depression and anorexia (Figure 56-1). If several animals are affected simultaneously, a common etiology is most likely and infection or intoxication should be primarily considered. Diarrhea is not uncommon, and if the urates are pigmented yellow-green, then the excretion of biliverdin may indicate severe liver compromise and bile stasis. Regurgitation is considered to be a poor sign. Severely affected animals usually are depressed, lethargic, and weak, and mucous membranes may be pale, hyperemic, or icteric. As already stated, the early signs of chronic disease may be missed; this, in conjunction with the rapid onset of severe clinical signs, may confuse and convince the clinician that this is an acute hepatitis rather than the end-stage presentation of a chronic hepatosis.

Laboratory Investigations

A full clinicopathologic investigation is essential to differentiate accurately between acute and chronic liver disease, and pretreatment blood samples must be collected before the instigation of fluid therapy and other supportive measures.[7]

Reptiles with severe hepatopathies may be seen with diarrhea and biliverdinuria (green urine or urates). Hypoalbuminemia can result in the production of an acellular low-protein coelomic transudate. A more complete review of laboratory liver assessment is given by Divers.[7]

Hematologic parameters can vary with species, gender, age, and seasonal status, but marked elevation of packed cell volume usually indicates dehydration (Table 56-1). However, in cases of chronic hepatopathy, anemia may be evident and can mask serious fluid deficits. Acute inflammation or

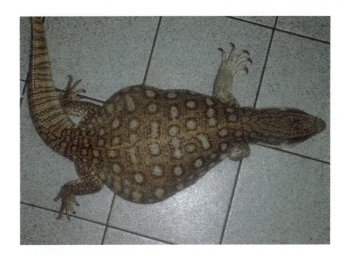

FIGURE 56-1 Obese Savannah Monitor *(Varanus exanthematicus)*. *(Photo courtesy S.J. Hernandez Divers.)*

necrosis of the liver usually results in a dramatic heterophilia and monocytosis (including azurophilia in many species). Chronic bacterial hepatitis usually only causes minor elevations of the total white blood cell count, although shifts in the lymphocyte/monocyte:heterophil ratio often occur. Eosinophilia may be expected in cases of parasitic disease.

Hepatocellular damage as noted in mammals may lead to elevations of several enzymes including aspartate aminotransferase (AST), γ-glutamyltransferase (GGT), alkaline phosphatase (ALP), alanine aminotransferase (ALT), and lactate dehydrogenase (LDH) (Table 56-2). Unfortunately, most of these parameters are widely distributed in other tissues, including muscle and kidney. Assessment of creatinine phosphokinase (CPK) can be helpful in distinguishing between muscle and nonmuscle sources. In mammals, hepatocellular LDH isoenzymes, AST, ALP, ALT, and the biliary tract brushborder enzyme GGT appear to be more useful. However, in reptiles, tissue distribution of many of these enzymes appears more widespread and tissue values of GGT may be very low.[8,9] In the future, isoenzyme analyses may improve the organ specificity of sensitive indicators such as LDH. In hepatic lipidosis, little hepatocellular damage occurs and so enzyme levels may remain normal.

Bile acids are considered to be useful in the assessment of liver function in many birds and mammals, but their application in reptile medicine has yet to be conclusively determined. Unpublished observations by the authors and Greendale Laboratories (Surrey, England) suggest normal values of less than 60 μmol with commercial enzymatic assays for 3α-hydroxy-bile acids. The major bile acid varies with the taxonomic order of the reptile, and therefore, concern must exist as to the universal application of a single assay for all reptiles.[10] Practical protocols for bile acid stimulation tests have not been documented. Assuming specificity and sensitivity, they may offer an accurate assessment of liver function and a means of identifying those cases of severe liver compromise where little or no hepatocellular damage exists.

Biliverdin is the major bile pigment produced by reptiles because they lack the biliverdin reductase enzyme necessary to produce bilirubin. To date, no readily available commercial assays are found for this metabolite.

Table 56-1 Hematologic Parameters Used in Assessment of Liver Disease

Blood Parameter	Observed Range	Diagnostic Use
Total WBC ($\times 10^9$/L)	2-10	Raised during inflammation and infection, may be depressed or low during brumation (hibernation) or after brumation (hibernation)
Heterophils ($\times 10^9$/L)	1.0-4.0	Classic reptile acute inflammatory cell, usually raised in sepsis and necrosis
Lymphocytes ($\times 10^9$/L)	1.0-6.0	Highly variable but may be elevated in cases of viral disease
Azurophils ($\times 10^9$/L)	0.0-0.7	Elevated during bacterial infections and necrosis
Monocytes ($\times 10^9$/L)	0.0-0.5	Elevated in cases of chronic disease and chronic immunogenic stimulation
Eosinophils ($\times 10^9$/L)	0.0-0.8	Variable in number, elevated in protozoal and helminth infections
PCV (L/L)	0.2-0.4	Useful to assess hydration status, anemia
RBC ($\times 10^{12}$/L)	0.12-0.75	Decreased in cases of chronic disease
Hb (g/dL)	3.5-8.6	Decreased in cases of chronic disease

Divers SJ, Cooper JE: Reptile Hepatic Lipidosis. *Semin Avian Exotic Pet Med*, 9(3):153-164, 2000.
Hb, Hemoglobin; *PCV*, packed cell volume; *RBC*, red blood cell; *WBC*, white blood cell.

Table 56-2 Biochemistry Parameters Used in Assessment of Liver Disease

Blood Parameter	Observed Range	Diagnostic Use
ALT (U/L)	5-120	Not always raised in cases of liver disease and not liver-specific because also present in other tissues
ALKP (U/L)	20-150	Widespread tissue distribution, not specific or very sensitive of liver disease
AST (U/L)	5-130	Sensitive indicator of both liver and muscle disease; also elevated in cases of renal disease
GT (U/L)	0.0-3	Liver-specific, but normal tissue values may be low
Bile acids (µmol/L)	<60	May be specific and sensitive for liver function; normal values yet to be documented for most species
Biliverdin	NA	Biliverdin is major bile pigment, but commercial assays remain elusive
Cholesterol (mmol/L)	0.6-6 (23.2-231.7 mg/dL)	Often elevated from triglycerides in cases of hepatic lipidosis, but may be physiologically elevated during normal vitellogenesis and before brumation (hibernation)
Triglycerides (mmol/L)	0.6-6 (53.1-531 mg/dL)	Often elevated in cases of hepatic lipidosis, but may be physiologically elevated during normal vitellogenesis and prebrumation (prehibernation)
Total protein (g/L)	32-66 (3.2-6.6 g/dL)	Decreased with malnutrition, blood loss, intestinal disease, chronic liver and kidney disease; alpha globulins may decrease with hepatic disease
Albumin (g/L)	10-35 (1-3.5 g/dL)	May fall as result of prolonged anorexia, protein-losing enteropathies, or nephropathies or chronic hepatic disease; rises because of dehydration and vitellogenesis
Glucose (mmol/L)	2.5-5.5 (45.5-99.1 mg/dL)	Varies with metabolic state, nutrition, stress, but may be reduced in severe hepatopathies; elevations seen in rare cases of diabetes mellitus
Uric acid (µmol/L)	10-400 (0.17-6.7 mg/dL) (up to 1000 µmol/L [16.8 mg/dL] may be normal in some species and situations)	Raised during severe dehydration, but hepatic production may be reduced in cases of liver disease; normal range highly variable between species but more limited within species
Urea (mmol/L)	0.0-16.7 (0-96.8 mg/dL)	Production low and excretion usually variable; may have some limited use as guide to early dehydration in chelonia but not considered clinically useful

From Divers SJ: Reptilian liver and gastro-intestinal testing. In Fudge AM, editor: *Laboratory medicine, avian and exotic pets*, Philadelphia, 1999, WB Saunders. These values are approximate ranges and vary with species, nutrition, environment, season, and reproductive status.
ALKP, alkaline phosphatase; *ALT*, alanine aminotransferase; *AST*, aspartate aminotransferase; *GT*, glutamyl transferase; *NA*, not applicable.

Diagnostic Imaging

The radiographic hepatic shadow is often appreciable in horizontal beam radiographs of lizards, less so in snakes, and least of all in chelonians because of the superimposition of the shell. Gross hepatomegaly or microhepatica may be discernible in some lizards and snakes. Ultrasound has proven to be useful for the assessment of hepatic size and shape in many reptiles, including chelonians. Detection of macrohepatic changes may even be possible, such as the generalized hyperechoic appearance in cases of severe hepatic lipidosis. Ultrasound also has the advantage of permitting guided biopsies of the liver parenchyma.

The senior author's preferred method of imaging the liver is endoscopically with a rigid 2.7-mm Hopkins telescope (67208B, Karl Storz Endoscopy, Tuttingen, Germany). A minimally invasive technique that requires general anesthesia, endoscopy permits the examination and appreciation of the size, color, shape, and contours of the liver and allows the collection of multiple tissue biopsies with direct visual control (Figures 56-2 to 56-4).

Some researchers have used magnetic resonance imaging (MRI) and computed tomography (CT) because these technologies produce excellent soft tissue resolution. However, such devices are beyond the capabilities of most private practices

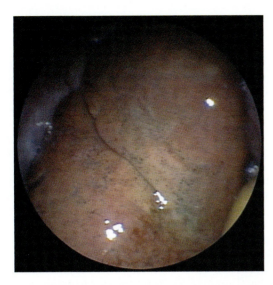

FIGURE 56-2 Coelioscopic view of a normal chelonian liver. Note the dark red coloration that makes identification of melanomacrophage aggregations difficult. *(Photograph courtesy S.J. Hernandez-Divers.)*

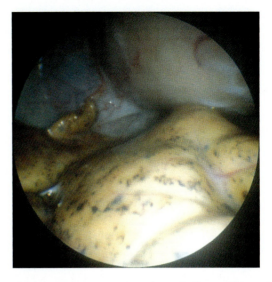

FIGURE 56-3 Coelioscopic view of a pale liver within a Greek Tortoise *(Testudo graeca)*. Note the obvious pale color that often accompanies hepatic lipidosis and accentuates melanomacrophage aggregations. *(Photograph courtesy S.J. Hernandez-Divers.)*

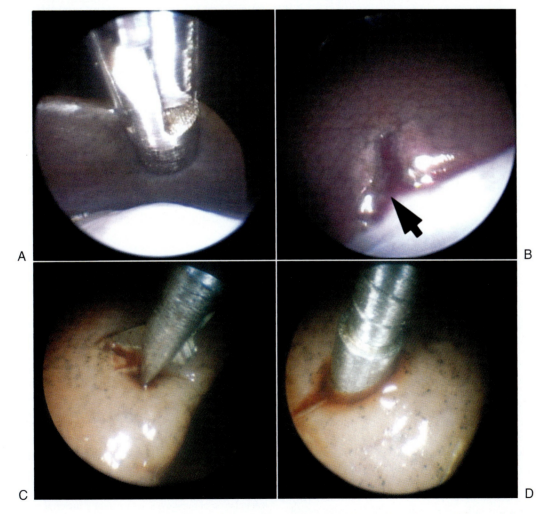

FIGURE 56-4 Endoscopic examination and biopsy techniques. **A,** Caudal edge liver biopsy with 5-French biopsy forceps in a Green Iguana *(Iguana iguana)*. **B,** Minimal hemorrhage from the biopsy site *(arrow)*. **C,** Incision through the hepatic membrane of an Egyptian Tortoise *(Testudo kleinmanni)* in preparation for a liver biopsy. **D,** Insertion of the biopsy forceps into the liver of the same Egyptian Tortoise for collection of a deeper parenchymal biopsy. *(Photograph courtesy S.J. Hernandez-Divers.)*

and zoo departments and do not readily lend themselves to the collection of tissue samples, and little has been done to correlate these images with reptilian histologic structure and pathology.

Liver Biopsy

At present, nothing to appears to surpass the diagnostic value of a hepatic biopsy for both microscopic (histology and transmission electron microscopy [TEM]) interpretation and, where infectious agents may be present, microbiologic culture (see Figure 56-4). In addition to facilitating a definitive diagnosis, serial biopsies offer the best means of monitoring disease progression and response to treatment and are invaluable for providing the client with the most accurate prognosis. Tissue samples can be taken with ultrasound guided Tru-Cut biopsy needles (e.g., Quick-core disposable biopsy needle, Cook Veterinary Products, Queensland, Australia), via the instrument port of the rigid endoscope (e.g., 2.7-mm Hopkins telescope, Karl Storz Endoscopy) (see Figure 56-4) or surgically after a coeliotomy approach to the liver. Small biopsies must be handled with care, and where significant pressure has been applied, this fact should be relayed to the pathologist because it can lead to confusing artifact.

Biopsies should, whenever possible, be handled with atraumatic instruments to minimize damage. Small tissue samples are placed into histology filters before submission in 10% neutral buffered formalin for histopathology, in appropriate fixative for TEM, or in 10% methanol/ethanol for urate tophi demonstration. Tissue samples for microbiology should be sent in appropriate transport media depending on whether fungal, bacterial, or viral investigations are most important.[11]

PATHOLOGIC FEATURES

Postmortem Features

With performance of a necropsy on an animal with suspected hepatic lipidosis, care must be taken to ensure that all other body organs are meticulously examined. In particular, note should be taken of (1) other fat deposits, including the size of fat bodies and presence or absence of adipose tissue under the skin and around the heart,[12] and (2) changes in other organs, such as the pancreas, that may have predisposed to fatty change. In crocodilians, the size of the fat body is carefully assessed as part of the postmortem evaluation of condition, either by weighing or by comparing its size with the animal's ventricles (F.W. Huchzermeyer, personal communication). Similar techniques could prove useful in other reptiles.

In hepatic lipidosis, the color may be pale tan to almost white (see Figures 56-2 to 56-4).[13] The color may also be affected by the natural color of fat in the species, and that in turn can be influenced by diet. A "fatty liver" is usually swollen with rounded nonangular edges and may weigh more than normal; organ weights can be helpful in this respect. Markedly fatty livers have a soft fatty "feel" when held for cutting and are friable (easily torn). Both the surfaces of the scalpel and the touch preparation, even before staining with specific stain (ORO, Sudan), show greasy fat droplets.[14]

Histopathologic Features

Thomson, subsequently cited in Carlton and McGavin,[15] defined hepatic lipidosis as "excessive accumulation of lipid within hepatocytes," and Elkan[16] drew attention to the fact that both normal and pathologic deposition of fat could exist within the liver. These and other references are a reminder of the fact that the presence of some intrahepatic lipid can be quite normal. Schaffner,[2] writing specifically about the reptilian liver, states categorically that "small fat droplets normally may be found in cytoplasm."[2] He goes on to emphasize that the amount of fat can vary depending on such factors as gender and season. Thus, the *presence* of fat in the liver of reptiles is not, per se, indicative of lipidosis. A more accurate description is "fatty change" but not necessarily "lipidosis."

The *detection* of fat in a reptile's liver is not usually difficult. In a standard paraffin-embedded section, the lipid appears as "holes" (vacuoles or vesicles) that usually can be assumed to be fat (Figure 56-5). However, some caution is needed because vacuoles can, on occasion, contain water, glycogen, or other material as opposed to fat.[13] Sometimes light microscopy per se permits a distinction to be made, but often other tests are needed, such as special stains or even TEM.

Once fat has been ascertained to be present in the liver of a reptile on histologic examination, a number of subsidiary questions need to be asked before a diagnosis (tentative or definite) of hepatic lipidosis can be made. These include an appreciation of the precise location, position, and size of the fat vacuoles. Evidence of hepatocellular dysfunction or degeneration and inflammatory changes must also be noted.

It should be mentioned that other techniques could also be used to investigate fatty change in the liver of reptiles. TEM is hardly suitable for routine diagnosis but has an important role to play in working with valuable or endangered species, for instance, where lipidosis is a feature of a disease "outbreak," perhaps linked with other metabolic changes, such as xanthomatosis. In such cases, TEM can provide essential information on pathogenesis, including the presence or

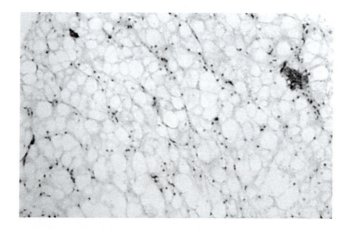

FIGURE 56-5 Histologic section of the liver of a Greek Tortoise (*Testudo graeca*) shows marked, predominantly macrovesicular, vacuolation of hepatocytes. Apparent paucity of nuclei is found, and those that are visible have a dark, pyknotic appearance, which suggests impairment of hepatic function (hematoxylin and eosin; original magnification, ×20). (*From Divers SJ, Cooper JE: Reptile Hepatic Lipidosis.* Semin Avian Exotic Pet Med, **9**(3):153-164, 2000.)

absence of changes in intracellular organelles or the presence of pathogens (Figure 56-6).[17] TEM is also one of the keys to more research on fat metabolism in reptiles.[18]

Even when the presence of what appears to be "excess" fat has been established, a diagnosis of hepatic lipidosis cannot usually be confirmed without taking into account (1) the clinical history and the clinician's assessment of the case (including other laboratory results) and (2) the patient's details and circumstances, for example, species, age, gender, reproductive status, brumation (hibernation), estivation, and diet. These were all previously discussed.

TREATMENT

Although specific therapy for hepatic lipidosis is usually reserved until the diagnosis has been confirmed histologically and the precise etiology has been identified, much can be done in general to support a reptile with hepatic dysfunction, whether infectious or noninfectious. Medical stabilization with fluid therapy is essential, and the provision of the species-specific preferred optimum temperature zone (within which the reptile can select a preferred body temperature) can be instrumental in improvement.

Fluid and Nutritional Support

The route of therapy is directed by the animal's condition at the time of presentation. Mild to moderate cases of hepatic lipidosis are usually anorectic on presentation but in good condition, and in these cases, oral fluids are adequate. Reptiles with severe disease often need intracoelomic, intravenous, or intraosseous infusion. In cases of severe liver pathology, avoidance of solutions that contain lactate may be wise. Other medications may be used at the clinician's discretion, but care should be taken not to invalidate future diagnostic investigations. For example, blood samples should be collected before fluid therapy, and antibiotic medication should be delayed until after liver biopsy and culture.

In many instances, hepatic lipidosis is a chronic disease that may take months, if not years, to reverse. Therefore, a means of providing long-term fluid and nutritional support should be explored. Most lizards and snakes are easily stomach-tubed; however, most chelonians and some squamates are better served by the placement of an esophagostomy tube with local or light general anesthesia (Figure 56-7). A variety of mammalian nasogastric and esophagostomy tubes can be modified, but the senior author prefers silicone tubes because they appear to cause the least reaction. For complete nutrition, estimation of total calorific requirements and total daily food requirements is important.[19] However, care is necessary to avoid gastric overload and stasis that may ensue from the use of a high-volume semisolid diet. In addition to long-term fluid and nutritional support, the esophagostomy tube can be used to deliver oral medication. The importance of nutritional support cannot be overemphasized and, given the available literature in human and veterinary medicine, appears to offer the best therapeutic approach to hepatic lipidosis. When providing nutritional support, one must consider (1) the patient's energy and nutritional requirements, (2) the patient's natural dietary preference (e.g., herbivorous, omnivorous, or carnivorous), and (3) the attempt to use natural foods in preference to artificial substitutes (e.g., whole rodent preferred to Hills a/d).

Carnitine

Carnitine, a derivative of lysine, is necessary for the transportation of acyl-coenzyme A (CoA) across the inner mitochondrial membrane of hepatocytes.[20] In human and more recently in feline medicine, carnitine supplementation to improve the transport of acyl-CoA and hence, the hepatic metabolism of fat has been suggested.[21,22] However, carnitine deficiency could not be shown in cats with hepatic lipidosis, and therefore,

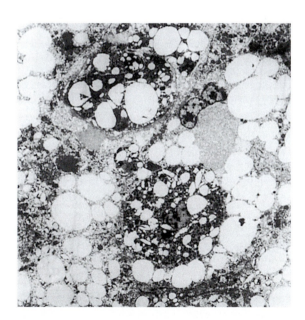

FIGURE 56-6 Transmission electron micrograph (TEM) of the liver of Round Island Gecko (*Phelsuma guentheri*) shows a mixture of macrovesicles and microvesicles. Some lipid has been phagocytosed by granulocytes (magnification, ×3000). (*From Divers SJ, Cooper JE: Reptile Hepatic Lipidosis.* Semin Avian Exotic Pet Med, *9(3):153-164, 2000.*)

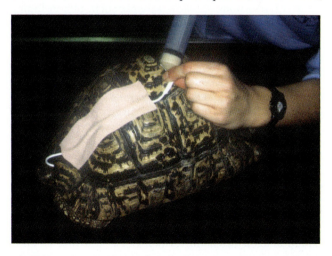

FIGURE 56-7 Assist-feeding a Leopard Tortoise (*Geochelone pardalis*) with an esophagostomy tube. These tubes permit long-term nutritional support and can be maintained for up to 4 months. (*Photograph courtesy S.J. Hernandez-Divers.*)

dietary supplementation with carnitine remains questionable.[23] Nevertheless, a daily dose of 250 mg/kg carnitine mixed with the tube-feeding formula appears to be safe in reptiles.

Choline and Methionine

Choline is lipotropic and is believed to promote the conversion of hepatic fat into phospholipids, which are more rapidly transferred from the liver into blood.[24] In addition, choline is used in the production of membrane phospholipids necessary for lipoprotein synthesis. The requirement for choline in conditions that predispose to hepatic lipidosis, such as diabetes mellitus, malnutrition, and cirrhosis, has been well documented in humans.[24] Methionine, a precursor of choline, may also exert lipotropic effects, but despite the general view that both of these supplements may be of benefit, only anecdotal reports support their use. Indeed, in the rat, choline has been shown to be ineffective in prevention and suppression of hepatic lipidosis.[25] Nevertheless, despite these drawbacks, a daily dose of 40 to 50 mg/kg has been suggested for mammals and appears to be safe in reptiles.[24]

Thyroxine and Anabolic Steroids

On the basis of clinical applications in small animal medicine and the author's clinical experience, thyroxine (20 mg/kg by mouth every 48 hours) and nandrolone (0.5 to 5 mg/kg intramuscularly every 7 to 28 days) have been advocated in an attempt to improve the hepatic metabolism of fat, to reduce catabolism, and to improve appetite.[26,27]

CONCLUSIONS AND RECOMMENDATIONS

Although hepatic lipidosis of reptiles has traditionally been considered to be associated with overfeeding, obesity, and underexercise, now this clearly is not always true.[13,14] As in other animals, including humans, excess lipid deposition in the liver can be from, or follow, a number of insults, including toxins, anoxia, and impaired metabolism of carbohydrate and volatile fatty acids.

In humans and domestic animals, a whole spectrum of diseases that can lead to fatty change are recognized. In *Homo sapiens*, for example, causes include alcoholism, diabetes, congenital metabolic defects of the urea cycle or fatty acid oxidation, side effects of drugs (e.g., corticosteroids), systemic disease (especially with pyrexia), pregnancy, Reye's syndrome, and certain drug toxicities (e.g., tetracycline).[28] In domestic animals, the list is shorter, but a whole range of fatty liver syndromes has been reported in species as diverse as birds of prey, cats, and dairy cows.[29,30]

Although hepatic lipidosis in reptiles shows in its natural history a number of significant differences from its counterpart in mammals and birds, much value can accrue from a certain amount of careful extrapolation. The first of these is in the *description and classification* of fatty change where the medical profession, in particular, has done sterling work in differentiating between conditions on the basis of, for example, size and distribution of vesicles. In this context, medical pathologists have been able to bring a degree of precision to the diagnosis of fatty liver in humans by proposing that the term should be used when lipid accumulation exceeds the normal 5% of body weight. Secondly, the medical profession has been able to bring to its investigations of lipidosis a weight of technical expertise and experience, much of which might, in due course, be applied to reptiles.[31]

Research on domestic mammals and birds can also be relevant. Again, substantial work has been performed that has shed light on the changes that occur in hepatocytes (and elsewhere) when lipid is deposited and why this can predispose to bacterial infections and endotoxemia.

Given the variability of clinical presentation, blood chemistries, and the lack of standardized reference points for ultrasonographic diagnosis compared with mammals, it appears that histopathology and TEM, in combination with the aforementioned, offer the best approach to diagnosis. Indeed, serial tissue samples not only aid prognosis but may well help our understanding of the pathogenesis of both disease progression and recovery. To this end, biopsy appears to be key in the successful diagnosis and monitoring of lipidosis and, indeed, other hepatopathies in reptiles. Despite our improved ability to safely biopsy the reptilian liver, our understanding of hepatic metabolism and the pathogenesis of hepatic disease remains in its infancy.

ACKNOWLEDGMENTS

This text was modified from: Divers SJ, Cooper JE: Reptile hepatic lipidosis, *Semin Avian Exotic Pet Med* 9(3):153-164, 2000. The authors are grateful to the publishers for granting permission for reproduction for this chapter.

REFERENCES

1. Abdul-Raheem K, Okasha S, El-Deib S, et al: Hibernation in reptiles 3; carbohydrate metabolism in *Eryx colubrinus* and *Eumeces schneideri*, *J Thermal Biol* 14:133-137, 1989.
2. Schaffner F: The liver. In Gans C, Gaunt AS, editors: *Biology of the Reptilia*, vol 19, morphology G, visceral organs, *Missouri Soc Study Amphib Reptil* 19:485-531, 1998.
3. Gatten RE: The uses of anaerobiosis by amphibians and reptiles, *Am Zool* 25:945-954, 1985.
4. Ferrer C, Zuasti A, Bellesta J, et al: The liver of *Testudo graeca* (Chelonia), a comparative study of hibernating and non-hibernating animals, *J Submicro Cytol* 19:275-282, 1987.
5. Ji X, Wang PC: Annual cycle of lipid contents and caloric values of carcass and some organs of the gecko (*Gekko japonicus*), *Comp Biochem Physiol* 96A:267-271, 1990.
6. Bush M, Teare JA: Toxicology and efficacy of ivermectin in chelonians, *J Am Vet Med Assoc* 183:1195, 1983.
7. Divers SJ: Reptilian liver and gastro-intestinal testing. In Fudge AM, editor: *Laboratory medicine, avian and exotic pets*, Philadelphia, 1999, WB Saunders.
8. Ramsay EC, Dotson TK: Tissue and serum enzyme activities in the yellow rat snake (*Elaphe obsoleta quadrivittatta*), *Am J Vet Res* 56:423, 1995.
9. Wagner RA, Wetzel R: Tissue and plasma enzyme activities in juvenile green iguanas, *Am J Vet Res* 60(2):201-203, 1999.
10. Skoczylas R: Physiology of the digestive tract. In Gans C, Gans KA, editors: *Biology of the Reptilia*, vol 8, physiology B, London, 1978, Academic Press.

11. Cooper JE: Reptilian microbiology. In Fudge AM, editor: *Laboratory medicine, avian and exotic pets,* Philadelphia, 1999, WB Saunders.
12. Elkan E: Reptilian fat bodies, *Br J Herpetol* 6:75-77, 1981.
13. Frye FL: *Biomedical and surgical aspects of captive reptile husbandry,* ed 2, Melbourne, Fla, 1991, Krieger.
14. Vegad JL: *Textbook of veterinary general pathology,* India, 1995, Vikas, Jabalpur.
15. Carlton WW, McGavin MD: *Thomson's special veterinary pathology,* St Louis, 1995, Mosby.
16. Elkan E: Pathology and histopathological techniques. In Cooper JE, Jackson OF, editors: *Diseases of the Reptilia,* London, 1981, Academic Press.
17. Cooper JE, Bloxam QMC, Tonge SJ: Pathology of Round Island geckos *Phelsuma guentheri*: some unexpected findings, *Dodo J Wildlife Preservation Trusts* 4:153-158, 1999.
18. De Brito Gitirana L: The fine structure of the fat-storing cell (Ito cell) in the liver of some reptiles, *Z Mikrosk anat Forsch* 102:143-149, 1988.
19. Donoghue S, Langenberg J: Nutrition. In Mader DR, editor: *Reptile medicine and surgery,* Philadelphia, 1996, WB Saunders.
20. Stryer L: Fatty acid metabolism. In Stryer L, editor: *Biochemistry,* ed 3, New York, 1988, WH Freeman.
21. Cornelius LM, Jacobs G: Feline hepatic lipidosis. In Kirk RW, editor: *Current veterinary therapy X small animal practice,* Philadelphia, 1989, WB Saunders.
22. Jacobs G, Cornelius L, Allen S, et al: Treatment of idiopathic hepatic lipidosis in cats: 11 cases (1986-1989), *J Am Vet Med Assoc* 195(5):635-638, 1989.
23. Jacobs G, Cornelius L, Keene B, et al: Comparison of plasma, liver, and skeletal muscle carnitine concentrations in cats with idiopathic hepatic lipidosis and in healthy cats, *J Am Vet Res* 51(9):1349-1351, 1990.
24. Jenkins WL: Drugs affecting gastrointestinal functions. In Booth NH, McDonald LE, editors: *Veterinary pharmacology and therapeutics,* ed 6, Ames, 1988, Iowa State University.
25. Leclerc J, Miller ML: Inositol and choline levels in the diet and neutral lipid hepatic content of lactating rat, *Int J Vitam Nutr Res* 59(2):180-183, 1989.
26. Jackson OF: Reptiles part one chelonians. In Beynon PH, Cooper JE, editors: *Manual of exotic pets,* ed 2, Cheltenham, 1991, BSAVA.
27. Divers SJ: A clinician's approach to liver disease in tortoises. *Proceedings of the Association of Reptilian and Amphibian Veterinarians,* Houston, Texas, 1997.
28. McGee J, Isaacson PG, Wright NA: *Oxford textbook of pathology,* Oxford, 1992, Oxford University Press.
29. Forbes NA, Cooper JE: Fatty liver-kidney syndrome of merlins. In Redig PT, Cooper JE, Remple D, Hunter B, editors: *Raptor biomedicine,* Minneapolis, Minne, 1993, University of Minnesota.
30. Dimski DS: Feline hepatic lipidosis, *Semin Vet Med Surg (Small Anim)* 12(1):28-33, 1997.
31. Patrick RS, McGee JOD: *Biopsy pathology of the liver,* London, 1980, Chapman and Hall.

57
HERPESVIRUS IN TORTOISES

FRANCESCO C. ORIGGI

INTRODUCTION

The members of the family Herpesviridae are infectious agents associated with diseases that affect many species of animals, from invertebrates to primates.[1] These double-stranded DNA viruses are divided into three subfamilies named alpha, beta, and gamma Herpesvirinae whose paradigms are considered the herpes simplex virus (HSV1-alpha), the human cytomegalovirus (HCMV-beta), and the Epstein-Barr virus (EBV-gamma), respectively.

Herpesvirus-like particles have been observed in several species of reptiles, including the Green Iguana (*Iguana iguana*),[2] the Green Lizard (*Lacerta viridis*),[3] the Sudan Plated Lizard (*Gerrhosaurus major*),[4] the Green Tree Monitor (*Varanus prasinus*),[5] the Banded Krait (*Bungarus fasciatus*), the Indian Cobra (*Naja naja*),[6] the Siamese Cobra (*Naja naja kaouthia*),[7] and the Saltwater Crocodile (*Crocodylus porosus*).[8] However, most herpesvirus infections of reptiles have been documented in freshwater and seawater turtles and land tortoises.

The first report to call attention to a herpesvirus agent in chelonians was that of Rebell, Rywlin, and Haines[9] that described the gray patch disease (GPD) in Green Seaturtles (*Chelonia mydas*) in an intensive commercial aquaculture facility in the Cayman Islands. The classic skin lesions that gave the name to the disease could be observed only in turtles 2 to 4 months of age and differed in severity. The lesions ranged from nonspreading papules on the neck and the flippers of the turtles that had tendency to regress naturally to severe lesions that consisted of spreading gray patches with superficial epidermal necrosis. The disease seemed to be age dependent, with the most severely affected age group being hatchlings, with mortality rates ranging from 5% and 20% to 100% during natural and experimental infections, respectively. Water temperature was proven to play an important role in the pathogenesis of the disease.[10]

More than 10 years later, Jacobson et al[11] investigated the lung-eye-trachea disease (LETD) in Green Seaturtles characterized by the presence of caseous exudate that covered the eyes and was around the glottis and within the trachea. Most of the affected turtles were 12 months old to 24 months old, and mortality rates varied between 8% and 38%. The turtles either died after several weeks of illness or remained chronically infected with clinical signs that persisted for months. Currently, the LETD herpesvirus is the only seaturtle herpesvirus agent that has been successfully isolated and propagated in cell culture.

A fibropapilloma-associated herpesvirus was described by Jacobson, Buergelt, and Williams[12] in 1991. The affected seaturtles had cutaneous or visceral fibropapillomatous masses. Despite several attempts, the isolation of a herpesviral agent associated with this pathology was unsuccessful, and its role in the pathogenesis of the seaturtle fibropapillomatosis still remains unclear.[13]

Herpesvirus-like particles have also been observed by Frye et al[14] in two Pacific Pond Turtles (*Clemmys marmorata*); by Cox, Rapley, and Barker[15] in a Painted Turtle (*Clemmys picta*); and by Jacobson, Gaskin, and Wahlquist[16] in a False Map Turtle (*Graptemys pseudogeographica*) and a Barbour's Map Turtle (*Graptemys barbouri*).

Among land tortoises, four reports described the detection of herpesvirus particles in ill Desert Tortoises (*Gopherus agassizii*),[17-20] and Jacobson et al[21] described an epidemic associated with herpesvirus infection in a large shipment of Argentine Tortoises (*Geochelone chilensis*) imported into the United States by an animal dealer along with several Red Footed Tortoises (*Geochelone carbonaria*). More recently, herpesvirus-like particles were also detected[22] in Leopard Tortoises (*Geochelone pardalis*) from a breeding colony in Yorkshire in the United Kingdom and in imported Pancake Tortoises (*Malachochersus tornieri*) in Japan.[23] It is generally accepted that most if not all tortoises should be considered susceptible to tortoise herpesvirus infection[24]; however, Mediterranean Tortoises (*Testudo* sp.) seem to be the land tortoise species most targeted by herpesvirus.[22,23,25-32,34]

The first successful isolation attempts of a tortoise herpesvirus agent were those of Biermann and Blaha[25] and Kabish and Frost[34] who isolated herpesviruses from Hermann's and Horsfield's Tortoises (*Testudo hermanni* and *T. horsfieldii*) more than a decade ago. Since then, several new isolates have been obtained and at least two serologically and genetically distinct tortoise herpesviruses known to infect Mediterranean Tortoises have been isolated and identified.[35]

During these years several features of this viral agent have been investigated such as pathogenesis,[36] physical properties,[37] serological reactivity,[35] and sensitivity to antiviral drugs (acyclovir and gancyclovir in vitro)[29] and to environmental agents.[38]

CLINICAL SIGNS

Several terms have been used to name the array of clinical signs that are commonly associated with herpesvirus infection in tortoises; *stomatitis-rhinitis* is the most common term used. The term "stomatitis" refers to the inflammation of the oral cavity. This clinical sign is often associated with and characterized by the presence of diphtheritic plaques (Figure 57-1); the extension and location may vary, but it is generally limited to the tissues of the oral cavity, rarely extending caudally to the cranial portion of the esophagus.[32,33] The diphtheritic plaques may be very large and impair basic physical activity of the animals, such as eating. No clear explanation for the

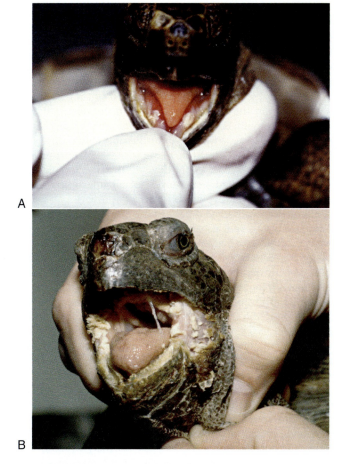

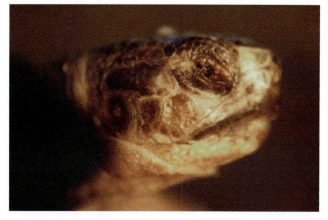

FIGURE 57-1 **A,** Shown are diphteritic plaques in the oral cavity of a Greek Tortoise *(Testudo graeca)*. Observe the presence of hemorrhagic inflammation of the oral mucosa surrounding the plaques. Plaques are in the early stage of formation. Notice the perfect symmetry shown by the lesions. **B,** Herpesvirus in a California Desert Tortoise *(Gopherus agassizii)*. Note the oral plaques and hemorrhagic rhinitis. *(B, Photograph courtesy D. Mader.)*

FIGURE 57-2 Severe conjunctivitis in a Greek Tortoise *(Testudo graeca)*. The presence of thick exudates has sealed the eyelids of the tortoise together, making it impossible for the animal to open its eyes.

cyclic appearance and resolution of the oral plaques exists. The pathogenetic mechanism responsible for these lesions is unknown at the moment. Furthermore, whether the diphtheritic plaques are the consequence of a direct action of the virus or whether they are an indirect by-product of the herpesviral infection is unknown. Some new insights in the pathogenesis of the diphtheritic plaques associated with tortoise herpesvirus infection have been obtained during an experimental infection of Greek Tortoises *(Testudo graeca)* with two different live isolates of serotype 1 tortoise herpesvirus.[36] Four Greek Tortoises were inoculated with one of two different tortoise herpesvirus serotype 1 isolates either intranasally (IN) or intramuscularly (IM) while an additional non-infected control was inoculated with phosphate buffer saline (PBS). The diphtheritic plaques started to develop 11 to 12 days after the viral administration in two of the four infected tortoises (one tortoise infected IN and one tortoise infected IM). Following the maximum extension in size, the plaques started to regress and they disappeared in one of the two tortoises (infected IN), while there was only a partial regression in the other tortoise (infected IM). The entire cycle of appearance and regression that was fully observed only in one tortoise lasted for about 2 weeks. The two tortoises that developed the diphtheritic plaques showed a consistent bilateral and symmetrical location of the lesions, which were preceded in their appearance by a hemorrhagic inflammation.[36] Two experimentally infected tortoises never developed the diphtheritic plaques, suggesting that the absence of diphtheritic plaques in suspected infected tortoises could not rule out an actual tortoise herpesvirus infection. It is not known if the appearance and the regression of the plaques that was observed in experimental conditions follow the same pattern during the occurrence of a natural infection where additional factors could influence the course of the disease.

Rhinitis and "runny nose" are other terms used to name the tortoise herpesvirus–associated disease and to describe other clinical signs associated with the infection. The term refers to a nasal discharge that may vary in intensity and appearance when the disease occurs. Observation is common of the presence of a clear-serous nasal discharge at the beginning of the disease that can become thicker and mucopurulent when the disease progresses and part of the lower respiratory tract is affected.

Conjunctivitis is another clinical sign associated with tortoise herpesvirus infection. Tortoises with monolateral or bilateral conjunctivitis have swollen eyelids often associated with ocular discharge, aqueous or mucoid in appearance. The ocular discharge can be as intermittent as the conjunctivitis itself. The conjunctivitis can last for a few days and reappear a few days or several weeks after the last recrudescence. In the most severe cases, the tortoises cannot open their eyes (Figure 57-2).[39]

Along with the nasal and ocular discharge, observation is possible of an oral discharge in some ill tortoises[36,40] that can leave a white "chalky-like" deposit following the margin of the lower jaw (Figure 57-3).

Along with these local clinical signs, other more systemic signs are possible to observe in the advanced stages of the disease. Heldstab and Bestetti[27] described the presence of central nervous system (CNS) disease in Mediterranean Tortoises infected with herpesvirus. The tortoises may circle around with the head tilted in the same direction of the circling.

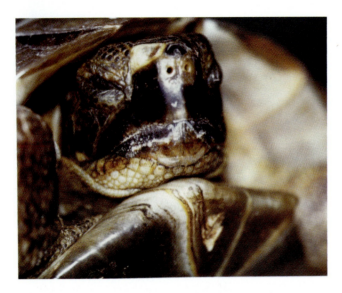

FIGURE 57-3 The whitish line parallel to the rim of the lower jaw of this Greek Tortoise *(Testudo graeca)* is what is left of the oral discharge that occurred 24 hours earlier.

The pathogenic mechanism that accounts for the CNS disease and its related clinical signs is not known. The herpesvirus colonization of the brain[36,41] and its recurrent reactivation from latency[42] (possibly occuring also during tortoise herpesvirus infection) are likely to be pivotal in the explanation of the appearance of the clinical signs reported. In support of this hypothesis, during the experimental infection of Greek Tortoises reported above,[36] it was possible to detect a large amount of herpesviral DNA in the CNS of three out of four infected tortoises, but none of them showed neurological signs. Considering that in the experimentally infected tortoise, no actively replicating virus was detected (possibly indicating a latent status of the virus) it could be reasonable to speculate that the neurological signs could be associated to an active infection (or reactivation) of the virus in the brain of the infected animal and not when the virus is dormant (latent).

Weight loss, cachexia, and difficult breathing have also been reported during the chronic stages of the disease.[27]

Of the two distinct serotypes known to infect tortoise herpesvirus, serotype 1 appears to cause severe disease in naïve susceptible tortoise species. The other serotype (serotype 2) causes significantly lower morbidity and mortality in the affected populations.[43]

DIAGNOSIS

Clinical Diagnosis

As for many other diseases of reptiles, the first diagnostic opportunity is the physical examination. Clinical signs such as stomatitis, monolateral or bilateral conjunctivitis along with ocular and nasal discharge, respiratory signs, and CNS disease could suggest to the clinician the possibility of the involvement of a herpesvirus in the pathogenesis of the disease of the tortoise patient brought into the clinic.

Unfortunately, reliance on just the clinical signs for a diagnosis of tortoise herpesvirus infection is difficult, if not impossible. Conjunctivitis and rhinitis are two clinical signs described also for other respiratory diseases of tortoises and among these, also that known as upper respiratory tract disease (URTD), which is caused by a pathogenic mycoplasma *(M. agassizii)* (see Chapter 73).[44-47] The overlapping of these clinical signs makes the differential diagnosis of tortoise herpesvirus and URTD difficult if not impossible if based only on the physical examination performed by the clinician. Stomatitis, along with the presence of diptheritic plaques, can play a critical role for the differential diagnosis between URTD and tortoise herpesvirus because tortoises with URTD are known to not develop diphtheritic plaques. However, as reported previously, not all infected tortoises develop diphtheritic plaques,[36] and diphtheritic plaques similar to those observed during tortoise herpesvirus infection have been observed also in association with iridovirus and virus x infections,[43] suggesting that the formation of diphtheric plaques in tortoises could be the result of a common pathogenetic pathway that gets activated in the host in response to different etiological insults.

Although examples of mycoplasma-herpesvirus productive interaction in the same host are not reported in the literature, *Mycoplasma hyopneumoniae* is known to potentiate the severity of the pneumonia induced by the porcine reproductive and respiratory syndrome virus (PRRSV) in pigs.[48] However, whether *Mycoplasma agassizii* and tortoise herpesvirus can interact with each other, potentiating one another in URTD or in stomatitis-rhinitis, is not known. Recently,[40] the serologic exposure of a group of Mediterranean Tortoises to both herpesvirus and mycoplasma was proven with serology. However, this investigation has not clarified whether any synergism exists between herpesvirus and mycoplasma in the coinfected tortoises.

The clinical diagnosis of tortoise herpesvirus infection is also complicated by the inconsistent appearance and timing of the array of clinical signs reported previously. Additionally, there is evidence of a viral titer-dependent effect of the clinical signs as observed experimentally.[36,39] When Greek Tortoises were infected with a viral dose of 10^4 tissue culture infectious dose 50 ($TCID_{50}$), the only consistent clinical sign detectable in all the infected tortoises was either a transient unilateral or bilateral recurrent, mild to severe conjunctivitis.[39] Following the administration of an inoculum 10 times higher (10^5 $TCID_{50}$) all of the array of clinical signs described in the literature with the exception of the nasal discharge was observed.[36] If this phenomenon would occur also during the natural infection, it would be another critical confounding factor to consider during the clinical approach. Overall, a conclusive diagnosis of tortoise herpesvirus is difficult, if not impossible, in most of the cases, when it is based only on the general physical examination of the tortoises presented in the clinic.

Laboratory Diagnosis

The experimental data that have been acquired in the last decade on tortoise herpesvirus, thanks to the extensive work that has been performed, set the ground for the development of several serologically or molecular-based diagnostic tests for the laboratory diagnosis of tortoise herpesvirus infection, in both live and dead tortoises.

Serologic tests have been proven useful in detection of the exposure of live tortoises to herpesvirus. The first serologic test used for the diagnosis of herpesvirus infection was the serum neutralization test (SN).[29] The SN test is based on the detection of the presence of serum neutralizing antibodies directed against tortoise herpesvirus. More recently, a new enzyme-linked immunosorbent assay (ELISA) has been developed for herpesvirus exposure detection in tortoises.[39] This new test has been shown to be as statistically reliable as the SN test, and it can be completed in 1 day, differently from the SN test that requires 11 to 14 days to be read. The ELISA test can detect the seroconversion after herpesvirus infection in about 4 to 7 weeks postinfection, 2 to 5 weeks earlier than the SN test in experimental conditions.[39] Both tests have been shown to detect the presence of antiherpesvirus antibodies for more than 10 months after a single exposure to the virus.[39]

Along with these two serological tests, the detection of anti-tortoise herpesvirus antibodies is now possible using an indirect immunoperoxidase-based technique that was recently developed.[37]

The growing knowledge about the genetic information carried by the nucleic acid of tortoise herpesvirus has allowed the development of new molecular-based diagnostic tests. Teifke and his colleagues[41] showed that it was possible to detect the presence of tortoise herpesvirus DNA sequences in formalin-fix, paraffin-embedded tissues. However, the detection of tortoise herpesvirus DNA proved to be more practical using the polymerase chain reaction assay (PCR), a technique that allows the exponential amplification of a specific target DNA sequence.

Currently, three tortoise herpesvirus-specific PCR tests[36,41,49] are available along with a "non-native tortoise herpesvirus" PCR[50] for the detection of tortoise herpesvirus DNA in tissues and biological samples. These assays can detect a very limited amount of DNA and specifically that developed by the author of this chapter has been shown to detect as few as 0.5 femtograms (10^{-15}g) of target viral DNA in ideal conditions.[36] This great sensitivity also allows the diagnosis of tortoise herpesvirus infection when the viral load present in the tissue or in the biological sample is minimal. PCR finds its most useful application during the acute phase of tortoise herpesvirus infection, when the virus is actively shed and can be found in body fluids while the anti-herpesvirus antibodies are still absent in the bloodstream (see above). In contrast, during the chronic (and latent) stage of the infection, serological tests are the diagnostic tools of choice, since the anti-herpesvirus antibodies are now present in the bloodstream while the virus might not be shed any longer at this time, making the use of PCR of limited value in this stage of the disease. Marschang and colleagues[51] compared the ability of the PCR assays developed by Origgi et al,[36] Teifke et al,[41] and Van Devanter et al[50] in detecting tortoise herpesviral DNA from serotype 1 and 2. According to their results, only the PCR assay from Van Devanter (non-native for tortoise herpesvirus) could detect both the serotypes, while the other PCR assays were specific for serotype one.

Recently, an additional molecular-based tool, the reverse transcription PCR (RT-PCR) assay has been applied to differentiate between active and latent tortoise herpesvirus infection.[36] Along with the high-tech diagnostic tools described above, a very simple method was reported by Muller and colleagues[32] for the detection of tortoise herpesvirus infection in live tortoises. It consists in the staining of impression smears of the tongue of the suspected tortoise with Giemsa or hematoxylin and eosin (H&E) stain. The presence of the characteristic intranuclear inclusions in the infected cells would be a very strong evidence of herpesvirus infection.

The array of diagnostic tests described is instrumental for the laboratory diagnosis of herpesvirus infection in tortoises. However, viral isolation from the tissues or samples collected from the infected tortoises remains the most conclusive diagnostic tool for herpesvirus infection diagnosis. Unfortunately, herpesvirus isolation is not always an easy task to perform and requires specialized tools and personnel. Isolation can be performed antemortem from infected animals with oral swabs, nasal washes, and blood and postmortem from a variety of tissues, and it seems to be strongly influenced by the timing of the sampling. Furthermore, all the different steps that are performed, from the sampling to the delivery of the samples to the laboratory, are critical for the successful herpesviral isolation from herpesvirus-infected animals.

Despite several reports that discuss the clinical features of tortoise herpesvirus, little information in the literature concerns the hematologic data of tortoises infected with herpesvirus. In 1998, Muro et al[33] compared a group of herpesvirus-infected Mediterranean Tortoises with a control group of healthy Mediterranean Tortoises. Blood analysis revealed some differences between the ill and the control group of tortoises. The affected tortoises had marked lymphocytosis and heteropenia when compared with the healthy control group of tortoises. Aspartate aminotransferase (AST) and the alpha-globulin fraction were significantly higher in the symptomatic group of tortoises.

Postmortem Diagnosis

Unfortunately, the diagnosis of tortoise herpesvirus infection is frequently made solely on the necropsy table. At gross examination, observation of the presence of the diphtheritic plaques described previously is common. The size and location may vary, but they are generally easily recognizable and limited to the oral cavity, even if an author has described the presence of these plaques extending to the cranial portion of the esophagus and the bifurcation of the trachea.[33]

The presence of disepithelization of the mucosa of the oral cavity where the plaques are located is common. Sometimes, the presence of caseous material is accompanied by cell debris and other necrotic material free in the oral cavity.[17,33] Other major lesions are uncommon on gross examination of a tortoise that died with clinical signs characteristics of the stomatitis-rhinitis. Often other major lesions are caused by secondary pathologies. The poor general conditions of many subjects in the advanced stages of the disease after the heavy loss of weight are a common finding.

Histology

The histologic examination carried out with light and electron microscopy provides critical information for the diagnosis of stomatitis–rhinitis, herpesvirus-associated, when the clinical signs and the gross examination fail to reveal the characteristic signs of the disease. The most important histologic finding is the presence of the characteristic eosinophilic intranuclear inclusions. These inclusion bodies have been detected in the epithelium of many different tissues spanning from the mucosa of the oral cavity to the digestive, urinary, and reproductive tract.[21,27,32,33,41] The presence of some inclusions in the CNS in several reports might be a direct link to the CNS disease observed clinically in some affected tortoises. A mild to severe mononuclear inflammatory cell infiltrate is often observed in the infected tissues with eosinophilic intranuclear inclusions. The multicentric distribution of tortoise herpesvirus in the tortoises has been more recently confirmed by PCR and in situ hybridization,[36,41] showing a prevalent neurotropism of the virus.[36]

The histologic diagnosis of tortoise herpesvirus might be limited either by the absence or by the low number of intranuclear inclusions. How long the inclusions take to appear from the beginning of the viral infection and how long the same inclusions last in the tissues are not known.

Data obtained during an experimental infection of Greek Tortoises with tortoise herpesvirus showed that it was not possible to observe any viral inclusion in the tissue examined (all the main organs including CNS) after 4 weeks from the last viral inoculation,[36] suggesting that the detection of the characteristic viral inclusions might be limited to the acute phase of the disease. When the conventional histological examination of the tissues is not conclusive, it is strongly advised to use complementary tests such as those described above. In situ hybridization has been already described, but other tools are available, such as a new application of a direct immunoperoxidase-staining technique which can be used to detect the presence of herpesvirus protein antigen in formalin-fixed tissues.[37]

The value of an array of diagnostic tests is extremely important especially when facing such a complex disease characterized by different stages and activity of the pathogen. Each of the diagnostic tests discussed gives an answer to each specific diagnostic question. Along with the availability of the test, that the clinician evaluate the appropriate diagnostic test to use to set the appropriate treatment is critical. Table 57-1 lists commercial diagnostic laboratories that offer serologic testing for tortoise herpevirus.

THERAPY, PREVENTION, AND MANAGEMENT

The only study ever conducted on the sensitivity of tortoise herpesvirus to antiherpesviral drugs is that of Marschang, Gravendyck, and Kaleta,[29] who showed that both gancyclovir and acyclovir were able to inhibit the replication of tortoise herpesvirus in vitro. No further investigations have been conducted in this important area of the tortoise herpesvirus research, and more information is needed. An in vivo study to determine the pharmacokinetics of antiherpesvirus drugs and their possible toxicity levels is necessary to establish the best drug treatment and the most appropriate route of administration.

Mader (personal communication) reported that a dose of 80 mg/kg of acyclovir administered once a day is effective for the remission of herpesvirus infection–associated clinical signs in Desert Tortoises. McArthur[52] described variable results with acyclovir at the same dosage reported in *Testudo* sp. The drug therapy needs to be complemented by the supportive care. Stabilization of the patient is imperative, with particular attention paid to the hydration and nutrition status of the tortoise. Appropriate fluid therapy and assist-feeding through an esophagostomy[53] need to be considered on a case-by-case basis.

The prognosis is dependent on many factors. The presence of naïve tortoises, the viral load that infected the animal, the season, the immune status and the immunity make-up of the tortoise, the presence of progressed illnesses, the nature of

Table 57-1 Diagnostic Laboratories That Provide Serologic Testing for Tortoise Herpesvirus

United States
Elliott Jacobson
Veterinary Medical Teaching Hospital
University of Florida
Box J-103, JHMHC
Gainesville, FL 32610

Germany
Rachel Marschang
Institut fur Umwelt- und Tierhygiene (460)
Hohenheim University
Garbenstr 30
70599 Stuttgart
Germany
Phone: +49-(0)711-459-2468
Fax: +49-(0)711-459-2431
E-mail: rachelm@uni-hohenheim.de

Silvia Blahak
Staatliches VetUAmt Detmold
Westernfeld Str 1
32758 Detmold
Germany
Phone: +49-(0)5231-911-640
Fax: +49-(0)5231-911-503
E-mail: silvia.blahak@svua-detmold.nrw.de

Prof E.F. Kaleta
Institut fur Gefluglekrankheiten
Justus Liebig University Giessen
Frankfurter Str 91
35392 Giessen
Germany
Phone: +49-(0)641-99-38430
Fax: +49-(0)641-99-38439
E-mail: Erhard.F.Kaleta@vetmed.uni-giessen.de

Italy
Francesco Origgi
Human Virology Unit
Department of Immunology and Infectious Diseases
San Raffaele Scientific Institute
Via Olgettina 58
20132 Milan, Italy
Phone: +39 02 26434913
Fax: +39 02 26434905
E-mail: (1) origgi.francesco@hsr.it
E-mail: (2) origgif@yahoo.com

England
Michael Waters
Lecturer in Exotic, Zoo and Wildlife Pathology
Department of Pathology and Infectious Diseases
Royal Veterinary College
Hawkshead Lane, North Mymms
Hatfield, Herts AL9 7TA
United Kingdom
E-mail: mwaters@rvc.ac.uk

the infection (primary or secondary), and the care provided by the owner are all important points to be considered by the clinician for a realistic prognosis.

During a tortoise herpesvirus outbreak in a private collection of Mediterranean Tortoises, the author has treated all the infected and suspected infected tortoises with acyclovir at 80 mg/kg along with supportive fluid and antibiotic therapy.[54] Only one tortoise out of 25 that were put under treatment died after the beginning of the therapy. At this time, it is not possible to determine if the success of the therapy was dependent solely on the activity of acyclovir and more studies are need to clarify this aspect.

According to some preliminary data,[36,39] the clinical signs characteristic of tortoise herpesvirus appear to be viral-dose dependent. If so, a tortoise infected with a high viral load is more likely to have a poor prognosis than a mildly infected tortoise. The immune make-up of the tortoise, and probably also the species,[29,33,41,55] appears to play a critical role in the progression of the disease.

In those subjects that survive the primary infection and that are likely to host the virus for life, consideration of the overall health status of the tortoise is important. The presence of serum neutralizing antibodies does not protect from reinfection and does not block the appearance of clinical signs.[36] As known for all the other herpesviruses, it is likely that for tortoise herpesvirus too the pathogen can cycle back from its latent status to its active one, thanks to one or more of several possible stimuli. Among these, immunosuppression and immunodepression, stress, and progressed pathologies can open up the doors to the virus for a recrudescence that can be aggressive if the general conditions of the tortoises have been severely degraded.[42]

Anecdotal reports suggest that seasonality might influence the occurrence of herpesvirus infection in tortoises. The disease is observed often during the beginning of the spring and later on at the beginning of the fall, at the end and at the beginning of the brumation (hibernation), respectively. The appearance of the disease may possibly be influenced by the immune status of the tortoise and by the season of the year.[56]

Great care needs to be adopted not only for the ill animals but also for the apparently healthy tortoises that belong to the same tortoise colony where the outbreak occurred. Despite the presence of few symptomatic animals, many others likely could have been exposed to the pathogen. In these particular scenarios, the serologic testing may be useful. Consideration of the time window for the seroconversion to occur is critical to interpret correctly the result of the test.[39]

Separation of the symptomatic and exposed animals from the unexposed is important. Great care in the disinfection of the facility is necessary. Diluted bleach[57] is considered one of the most effective treatments for the facilities (1/2 cup of bleach for each gallon of water [100 mL bleach to each liter of water]).

No clear evidence is found of a preferential infection route by the virus, but as for many other herpesviruses, the airways and the mucosal openings might be critical. In an experimental infection in Greek Tortoises, both the IN and IM routes proved to be effective for inducing viral infection with comparable clinical signs.[36] The detection of the virus in the epithelia of the genital tract suggests a possible shedding of the virus through the excreta and a sexual transmission of the infection.[32]

Marschang et al[38] reported the virus can persist for months in the soil and still be infective. Replacement of the possibly infected substrate with a new one is appropriate, and if not possible, irradiation of the soil in full sunlight or with ultraviolet lights is recommended. Water bowls, food containers, and other cage or pen furniture need to be thoroughly disinfected or replaced with new ones if possible. For established colonies that are about to host new tortoises, a period of strict quarantine that needs to be as long as possible, and never shorter than 6 months, is extremely important. Simple but effective rules are critical to avoid any opportunity of spreading the infection. The new animals must be fed and taken care of only after the established colony has been cared for. Use of disposable gloves to handle tortoises from the established collection and from the new group is best. If not available, one should always wash hands after handling a tortoise and before handling another one. If entering into the pen is necessary, one should change shoes or wear disposable shoe covers that could prevent the passage of infectious material from one pen to the other.

All tortoises that are considered for purchase or exchange need to be tested serologically for herpesvirus exposure. The serologic testing needs to be repeated two times at an interval of 8 weeks (when the ELISA test is used).[39] Finally, the animal in quarantine needs to be in a separate room, or better in a separate building, with no physical access to the location where the established colony of tortoises is kept.

Prevention is the most effective "treatment" against tortoise herpesvirus to date, since the therapeutic protocols are currently experimental, and our information on the tortoise immune system is still too primitive for designing of an efficacious vaccine.

CONSERVATION

All the tortoise herpesvirus outbreaks that have been documented are those that occurred in captive tortoises or colonies of tortoises. Up to now, only anecdotal reports discuss the presence of herpesvirus in wild tortoises. No herpesvirus isolates have ever been recovered from a wild tortoise. We have only indirect evidence that suggests the presence of herpesvirus in wild tortoises at the moment.[58,59]

An important point to clarify is in which direction, if any, the herpesvirus infection has been moving during these last 30 years. Determination is critical of whether tortoise herpesvirus has always been present in wild tortoises or whether it is just a pathologic feature of captive tortoises where some "captive" herpesvirus strain might have originated from some other host and later on colonized tortoises. Then, understanding how the virus was able to spread from the captive to the wild population is important if this passage is ever to be fully demonstrated. Understanding these aspects of the herpesvirus infection epidemiology in captive and wild tortoises is pivotal to set strategies to control and prevent new infections in captive and wild tortoises.

Overall, much information about tortoise herpesvirus clinical manifestations and pathogenesis is now available. Nevertheless, we are far from understanding the intimate dynamics of the disease and its significance in the ecology of tortoises. We have demonstrated that tortoise herpesvirus is one of the etiologic agents of stomatitis-rhinitis of tortoises,[36] but we do not know whether tortoise herpesvirus is the only etiologic agent responsible for this disease of tortoises, or whether any other pathogen is involved.

Many investigations are needed to unravel some key points in the pathogenesis of the disease, such as the transmission route, the possibility of a vertical transmission, the actual species sensitivity, if any, and the mechanisms of reactivation of the virus.

REFERENCES

1. Murphy FA, Gibbs EPJ, Horzinek MC, Studdert MJ: Herpesviridae. *Veterinary virology*, ed 3, New York, 1999, Academic Press.
2. Clark HF, Karzon DT: Iguana Virus, a herpes-like virus isolated from cultured cells of a lizard, *Iguana iguana*, *Infect Immun* 5:559-569, 1972.
3. Raynaud A, Adrian M: Cutaneous lesions with papillomatous structure associated with viruses in the green lizard (*Lacerta viridis*), *C R Acad Sci Hebd Seances Acad Sci* 283:845-847, 1976.
4. Wellehan JF, Nichols DK, Li LL, Kapur V: Three novel herpesviruses associated with stomatitis in Sudan plated lizards (*Gerrhosaurus major*) and a black-lined plated lizard (*Gerrhosaurus nigrolineatus*), *J Zoo Wildl Med* 35:50-54, 2004.
5. Wellehan JF, Johnson AJ, Latimer KS, Whiteside DP, Crawshaw GJ, Detrisac CG, et al: Varanid herpesvirus 1: a novel herpesvirus associated with proliferative stomatitis in green tree monitors (*Varanus prasinus*), *Vet Microbiol* 105:83-92, 2005.
6. Padgett F, Levine AS: Fine structure of the Rauscher leukemia virus as revealed by incubation in snake venom, *Virology* 30:623-630, 1966.
7. Simpson CF, Jacobson ER, Gaskin JM: Herpesvirus-like infection of the venom gland of Siamese cobras, *J Am Vet Med Assoc* 175:941-943, 1979.
8. McCowan C, Shepherdley C, Slocombe RF: Herpesvirus-like particles in the skin of a saltwater crocodile (*Crocodylus porosus*), *Aust Vet J* 82:375-377, 2004.
9. Rebell H, Rywlin A, Haines H: A herpesvirus-type agent associated with skin lesions of green turtles in aquaculture, *Am J Vet Res* 36:1221-1224, 1975.
10. Haines H, Kleese WC: Effect of water temperature on a herpesvirus infection of sea turtles, *Infect Immun* 15:756-759, 1977.
11. Jacobson ER, Gaskin JM, Roelke M, Greiner EC, Allen J: Conjunctivitis, tracheitis, and pneumonia associated with herpesvirus infection in green sea turtles, *J Am Vet Med Assoc* 189:1220-1223, 1986.
12. Jacobson ER, Buergelt C, Williams B: Herpesvirus in cutaneous fibropapillomas of the green turtle (*Chelonia mydas*), *Dis Aquat Org* 12:1-6, 1991.
13. Herbst HL: *The etiology and pathogenesis of Green Turtle fibropapillomatosis*, Doctoral Dissertation, University of Florida, 1995.
14. Frye FL, Oshiro SL, Dutra FR, Carney JD: Herpesvirus-like infection in two pacific pond turtles, *J Am Vet Med Assoc* 171:882-883, 1977.
15. Cox WR, Rapley WA, Barker IK: Herpesvirus-like infection in a painted turtle (*Chrysemys picta*), *J Wild Dis* 16:445-449, 1980.
16. Jacobson ER, Gaskin JM, Wahlquist H: Herpesvirus-like infection in map turtles, *J Am Vet Med Assoc* 181:1392-1394, 1982.
17. Harper PAW, Hammond DC, Heuschele WP: A herpesvirus-like agent associated with a pharyngeal abscess in a desert tortoise, *J Wild Dis* 18:491-494, 1982.
18. Johnson AJ, Jacobson ER, Origgi FC, Brown R: Herpesvirus infection in a captive desert tortoise (*Gopherus agassizii*), pp. 37-38, *Proceedings of the 10th Association of Reptilian and Amphibian Veterinarians Conference*, Minneapolis, Minn, 2003.
19. Martinez-Silvestre A, Majo N, Ramis A: Caso clinico: herpesvirosis en tortuga de disierto Americana (*Gopherus agassizii*), *Clin Vet Pequ Anim* 19:99-106, 1999.
20. Pettan-Brewer KCB, Drew ME, Ramsey E, Mohr FC, Lowenstine LJ: Herpesvirus particles associated with oral and respiratory lesions in a California Desert tortoise (*Gopherus agassizii*), *J Wild Dis* 32:521-526, 1996.
21. Jacobson ER, Clubb S, Gaskin JM, Gardiner CH: Herpesvirus-like infection in Argentine tortoises, *J Am Vet Med Assoc* 187:1227-1229, 1985.
22. Drury SE, Gough RE, McArthur S, Jessop M: Detection of herpesvirus-like and papillomavirus associated with diseases of tortoises, *Vet Rec* 143:639, 1998.
23. Une Y, Uemura K, Nakano Y, Kamiie J, Ishiabashi T, Nomura Y: Herpesvirus infection in tortoises (*Malacochersus tornieri* and *Testudo horsfieldii*), *Vet Pathol* 36:624-627, 1999.
24. McArthur S, Blahak S, Koelle P, Jacobson ER, Marschang RE, Origgi F: Chelonian Herpesvirus. Roundtable, *J Herp Med Surg* 12:14-31, 2002.
25. Biermann R, Blahak S: First isolation of a herpesvirus from tortoises with diphtheroid-necrotizing stomatitis, *Proceedings of the 2nd World Congress of Herpetology*, Adelaide, Australia, 1993.
26. Cooper JE, Gschmeissner S, Bone RD: Herpes-like virus particles in necrotic stomatitis of tortoises, *Vet Rec* 123:544, 1988.
27. Heldstab A, Bestetti G: Herpesviridae causing glossitis and meningoencephalitis in land tortoises (*Testudo hermanni*), *Herpetopathologia* 1:5-9, 1989.
28. Lange H, Herbst W, Wiechert JM, Schliesser TH: Elektronemmikroskopischer nachweis von herpesviren beieinem massensterben von griechischen landschildkroten (*Testudo hermanni*) und vierzehenschildkroten (*Agrionemys horsfieldii*), *Tierarztl Prax* 17:319-321, 1989.
29. Marschang RE, Gravendyck M, Kaleta EF: Investigation into virus isolation and the treatment of viral stomatitis in *T. hermanni* and *T. graeca*, *J Vet Med Series B* 44:385-394, 1997.
30. Marschang RE, Posthaus H, Gravendyck M, Kaleta EF, Bacciarini LN: Isolation of viruses from land tortoises in Switzerland, p.281-284, *Proceedings of the American Association of Zoo Veterinarians and American Association of Wildlife Veterinarians Joint Conference*, Omaha, Neb, 1998.
31. Marschang RE: Evidence for a new herpesvirus serotype associated with stomatitis in Afghan Tortoises, *Testudo horsfieldii*, p. 77-79, *Proceedings of the 6th Association of Reptilian and Amphibian Veterinarians Conference*, Columbus, Ohio, 1999.
32. Muller M, Sachsse W, Zangger N: Herpesvirus-Epidemie Bei Der Griechischen Landschildkrote (*Testudo graeca*) in der Sweiz, *Schweiz Arch Tierheilk* 132:199-203, 1990.
33. Muro J, Ramis A, Pastor J, Velarde L, Tarres J, Lavin S: Chronic rhinitis associated with herpesviral infection in captive spur-thighed tortoise from Spain, *J Wild Dis* 34:487-495, 1998.
34. Kabish D, Frost JW: Isolation of herpesvirus from *Testudo hermanni* and *Agrionemys horsfieldii*, *Verh Ber Erkrg Zootiere* 36:241-245, 1994.
35. Marschang, RE, Frost JW, Gravendyck M, Kaleta EF: Comparison of 16 chelonid herpesviruses by virus neutralization tests and restriction endonuclease digestion of viral DNA, *J Vet Med B* 48:393-399, 2001.
36. Origgi FC, Romero CH, Bloom DC, Klein PA, Gaskin JM, Tucker SJ, Jacobson ER: Experimental transmission of a herpesvirus in Greek tortoises (*Testudo graeca*) *Vet Pathol* 41:50-61, 2004.
37. Origgi FC, Klein PA, Tucker SJ, Jacobson ER: Application of immunoperoxidase based techniques to detect herpesvirus infection in tortoises, *J Vet Diagn Invest* 15:133-140, 2003.
38. Marschang RE, Reinauer S, Bohm R: Inactivation of tortoise viruses in environment, p. 24, *Proceedings of the 12th Association of Reptilian and Amphibian Veterinarians Conference*, Tucson, Ariz.

39. Origgi FC, Klein PA, Mathes K, Blahak S, Marschang RE, Tucker SJ, et al: An enzyme linked immunosorbent assay (ELISA) for detecting herpesvirus exposure in Mediterranean tortoises [Spur-Thighed tortoise *(Testudo graecai)* and Hermann's tortoise *(Testudo hermanni)*], *J Clin Micro* 39:3156-3163, 2001.
40. Mathes KA, Jacobson ER, Blahak S, Brown DR, Schumacher IM, Fertard B: Mycoplasma and herpesvirus detection in European terrestrial tortoises in France and Morocco, pp. 97-99, *Proceedings of the 8th conference of the Association of Reptilian and Amphibian Veterinarians*, Orlando, Fla, 2001.
41. Teifke JP, Lohr CV, Marschang RE, Osterreider N, Posthaus H: Detection of chelonid herpesvirus DNA by nonradioactive in situ hybridization in tissues from tortoises suffering from stomatitis-rhinitis complex in Europe and North America, *Vet Pathol* 37:377-385, 2000.
42. Wagner EK, Bloom DC: Experimental investigation of herpes simplex virus latency, *Clin Micro Rev* 10:419-443, 1997.
43. Marschang RE, Origgi FC: Diagnosis of herpesvirus infections in tortoises—a review, *Verh Ber Erkrg Zootiere* 41:47-52, 2003.
44. Brown MB, Schumacher IM, Klein PA, Harris K, Correll T, Jacobson ER: *Mycoplasma agassizii* causes upper respiratory tract disease in the desert tortoise, *Infect Immun* 62:4580-4586, 1994.
45. Brown MB, McLaughlin GS, Klein PA, Crenshaw BC, Schumacher IM, Brown DR, et al: Upper respiratory tract disease in the gopher tortoises is caused by *Mycoplasma agassizii*, *J Clin Micro* 37:2262-2269, 1999.
46. Brown MB, Brown DR, Klein PA, McLaughlin GA, Schumacher IM, Jacobson ER, et al: *Mycoplasma agassizii* sp. nov., isolated from the upper respiratory tract of the desert tortoise *(Gopherus agassizii)* and the gopher tortoise *(Gopherus polyphemus)*, *Int J Syst Evol Microbiol* 51:413-418, 2001.
47. Jacobson ER, Gaskin JM, Brown MB, Harris RK, Gardiner CH, LaPointe JL, et al: Chronic upper respiratory tract disease of free-ranging desert tortoises, *Xerobates agassizii*, *J Wild Dis* 27:296-316, 1991.
48. Thacker EL, Halbur PG, Ross RF, Thanawongnuwech R, Thacker BJ: *Mycoplasma hyopneumoniae* potentiation of porcine reproductive and respiratory syndrome virus-induced pneumonia, *J Clin Micro* 37:620-627, 1999.
49. Murakami M, Matsuba C, Une Y, Nomura Y, Fujitani H: Development of species-specific PCR techniques for the detection of tortoise herpesvirus, *J Vet Diagn Invest* 13:513-516, 2001.
50. Van Devanter DR, Warrener P, Bennett L, Schultz ER, Coulter S, Garber RL, Rose TM: Detection and analysis of diverse herpesviral species by consensus primer PCR, *J Clin Microbiol* 34:1666-1671, 1996.
51. Marschang RE, McArtur S, Bohm R: Comparison of 5 different methods for the detection of tortoise herpesvirus infection in a group of *Testudo horsfieldii* in Great Britain, pp. 15-18, *Proceeding of the 10th Association of Reptilian and Amphibian Veterinarians Conference*, Minneapolis, Minn, 2003.
52. McArthur SDJ: An acyclovir trial in *Testudo sp*, *Proceedings of the BVZS, Spring Meeting, Emerging Diseases*, Burford, United Kingdom, 2000.
53. McArthur SDJ: Emerging viral-associated diseases of chelonians in the United Kingdom, pp. 103-116, *Proceedings of the 8th Conference of the Association of Reptilian and Amphibian Veterinarians*, Orlando, Fla, 2001.
54. Origgi FC, Rigoni D: A tortoise herpesvirus outbreak in Italy: history, diagnosis, therapy and follow up, pp. 21-23, *Proceedings of the 10th Conference of the Association of Reptilian and Amphibian Veterinarians*, Minneapolis, Minn, 2003.
55. Frost JW, Schmidt A: Serological evidence of susceptibility of various species of tortoises to infection by herpesviruses, *Verh Ber Erkrg Zootiere* 38:25-27, 1997.
56. Zapata A, Varas A, Torroba M: Seasonal variation in the immune system of the lower vertebrate, *Immunol Today* 13:113-149, 1992.
57. McKeown S: General husbandry and management. In Mader D, editor: *Reptile medicine and surgery*, Philadelphia, 1996, Saunders.
58. Origgi FC, Romero CH, Klein PA, Berry KH, Jacobson ER: Preliminary serological and molecular evidences of tortoise herpesvirus exposure and infection in desert tortoises, *Gopherus agassizii*, from the Mojave and Colorado Desert of California, pp. 27-29, *Proceedings of the 9th Conference of the Association of Reptilian and Amphibian Veterinarians*, Reno, Nev, 2002.
59. Marschang RE, Schneider RM: Detection of antibodies against chelonid viruses in wild-caught spur-thighed tortoises, *Testudo graeca*, in Turkey, pp. 95-97, *Proceedings of the 8th Conference of the Association of Reptilian and Amphibian Veterinarians*, Reno, Nev, 2002.

58
HYPERGLYCEMIA IN REPTILES

SCOTT J. STAHL

Hyperglycemia, an elevation of blood glucose, is an uncommon clinical abnormality in reptiles. Hyperglycemia has not been established as a consistent or specific indicator of pancreatic disease or diabetes mellitus. Elevations in blood glucose are more often related to other metabolic conditions, systemic diseases, and physiologic variables. A better understanding of the reptile endocrine pancreas and continued research are necessary to determine the significance of hyperglycemia and its relationship to clinical disease.

HYPERGLYCEMIA VERSUS DIABETES MELLITUS

Diabetes mellitus has been reported in the reptilian literature. However, in some of the cases, whether diabetes, in fact, was the true diagnosis or whether the patient had hyperglycemia from some other cause, was not clear. A diagnosis of "diabetes mellitus" in the reptile patient should be made with caution. It is an uncommon condition, and metabolic and physiologic factors can have a major influence on blood glucose. These factors must first be considered and ruled out. Persistent hyperglycemia is perhaps a better description for a reptile with elevated blood glucose values until further evaluation can determine possible etiologies.

In mammals, diabetes mellitus results from a lack of or deficiency of insulin or an inability of insulin to transport glucose into cells. Reptile blood glucose appears to be regulated by insulin as it is in mammals. Damage to the reptile pancreas (thus, the pancreatic islet cells) from disease, trauma, or autoimmune disease is expected to elevate blood glucose as is seen in mammals.[1]

Campbell[2] believes that reptiles with a persistent marked hyperglycemia (>200 mg/dL with or without concurrent glucosuria) are potential candidates for diabetes mellitus. A diagnosis of diabetes mellitus in reptiles, according to Frye[3] and Mader,[4] starts with persistent elevated blood glucose values above 300 mg/dL.

For the clinician to approach and assist the hyperglycemic reptile, an understanding of the reptile endocrine pancreas and the influential factors that can affect glucose levels is imperative.

ENDOCRINE PANCREAS

Unlike mammals, most reptilian islet tissue lacks a sharp demarcation from exocrine pancreatic tissue. Islet tissue is usually associated with first-order exocrine ducts and tubules and lacks a capsule. The pancreatic islets of lizards and snakes are larger than those of turtles and crocodilians.[5] The lizard islet is more centrally located than in the snake, where it is more peripheral. Turtle islets are the smallest and are the most diffusely distributed, and crocodilian islets are highly branched.

Alpha and beta cells are equally proportioned in snakes, turtles, and crocodilians, but alpha cells are more abundant in lizards.[5] The high alpha cell predominance in lizards is not understood. A similar observation has been found in ducks, which also have high levels of alpha cells in the pancreas. In ducks and other avian species, the alpha cells and elevated levels of glucagon are thought to play a significant role in the maintenance of blood sugar.[6] However, more research is necessary to better understand the glucagon and insulin balance in reptiles and the significance of alpha cells and glucagon in the lizard pancreas.

Studies on various species of reptiles have shown a great deal of variation in the pancreatic islet morphology between different reptile orders.[7] Generally, four major cell types are present in the reptile endocrine pancreas: insulin (B), glucagon (A), somatostatin (D), and pancreatic polypeptide (PP) cells.[8] Reptile insulin, glucagon, somatostatin, and pancreatic polypeptide appear to cross-react with antisera raised against mammalian insulin, glucagon, somatostatin, and pancreatic polypeptide. Most studies done on the reptile endocrine pancreas used these mammalian-based antisera.[8]

In another report, the comparative morphology of the endocrine pancreas was studied in 11 species of lacertid lizards. The study found that the endocrine islets always contain primarily three cell types: A, B, and D cells, and only occasional F cells. However, F and D cells were found to be much more abundant in the exocrine pancreatic parenchyma then A and B cells. These F and D cells were often associated with blood capillaries. These F and D cells may be influencing pancreatic exocrine function, therefore supporting the hypothesis that, as with other vertebrates, the reptiles' islet hormones may have a local action within the exocrine pancreas along with systemic action.[9] Different species of reptiles may have variation in the actual location of certain endocrine cells within the pancreas itself. Additionally, research has identified endocrine pancreatic islets associated with other organ systems such as the stomach and intestinal mucosa.[10]

Clinically, this information is valuable because it indicates the importance of submitting the entire pancreas, spleen, and perhaps even portions of the gastrointestinal tract for histopathologic analysis to avoid missing the sites of islet

Hyperglycemia in Reptiles

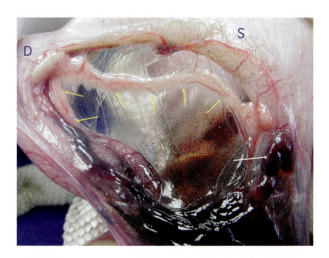

FIGURE 58-1 The normal pancreas of a Bearded Dragon (*Pogona vitticeps*). This was a necropsy specimen. Note the complexity of the pancreas with several arms that move toward other organs. The light-colored pancreas (*yellow arrows*) is suspended in the mesentery between the stomach (S) and duodenum (D). The spleen (*white arrow*) is to the right.

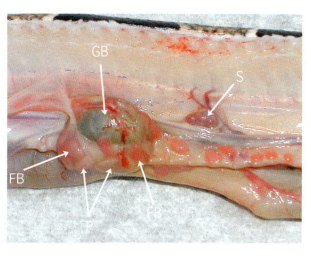

FIGURE 58-3 Normal "triad" in a Ball Python (*Python regius*). The pancreas (P) and spleen (S) are separate in the Boidae. The gallbladder (GB) is on the left. The fat bodies (FB) are easily confused with pancreatic tissue and are frequently submitted for histology as part of the pancreas. (*Photograph courtesy D. Mader.*)

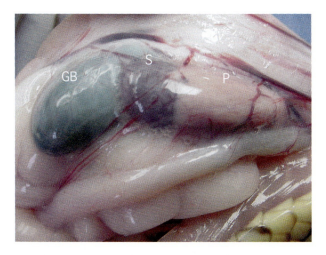

FIGURE 58-2 The normal pancreas (P) of an Eastern Kingsnake (*Lampropeltis getulus getulus*). This was a necropsy specimen. In snakes, the pancreas is often found in close association with the spleen (S) and the more cranially positioned gallbladder (GB). This anatomic association is often referred to as the "triad." In some snakes, the pancreas is just posterior to the spleen (see Figure 58-3), and in some, it may be in contact and actually associated with the spleen (see Figure 58-4).

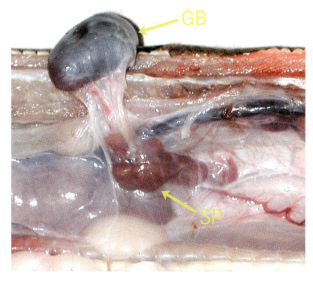

FIGURE 58-4 Typical appearance of a "splenopancreas" (SP) in a colubrid snake. The gallbladder (GB) is retracted dorsally and to the left. The spleen and the pancreas are intermixed and almost impossible to distinguish grossly. In this case, the entire organ should be submitted for histopathologic analysis. (*Photograph courtesy D. Mader.*)

concentration (Figures 58-1 to 58-5). Pancreatic biopsy may not be as useful a tool to evaluate islet presence or activity because the limited tissue available for ante mortem analysis may or may not be representative. In a case report involving a Chinese Water Dragon (*Physignathus cocincinus*) with persistent hyperglycemia, initial submission of pancreatic tissue revealed no endocrine islet tissue present.[11] The gross specimen was reevaluated, and the splenic portion of the pancreas was submitted. Islet tissue was subsequently identified in this portion.

FACTORS THAT AFFECT BLOOD GLUCOSE IN REPTILES

Variations in blood glucose may be more common in reptiles because of variable metabolic rate, environmental influences and adaptations, and relative insulin resistance. Physiologic changes must also be considered because they can seriously impact blood glucose levels. Of particular clinical importance in the reptile patient is stress-associated hyperglycemia,

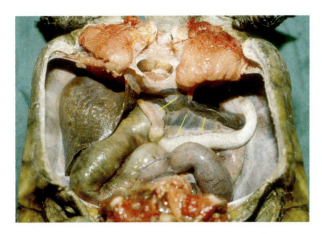

FIGURE 58-5 The pancreas *(yellow arrows)* is seen in this emaciated Desert Tortoise *(Gopherus agassizii)* adjacent to the greater curvature of the stomach and the mesenteric border of the duodenum. *(Photograph courtesy D. Mader.)*

which is the result of glucocorticoid and epinephrine release. Stress-associated hyperglycemia has been reported in a number of reptile species.[5,12-14]

Experimentally, an injection of glucose or epinephrine produces a prolonged increase in the blood glucose of lizards, snakes, tortoises, and caiman. In addition, after these injections, reptiles showed a much slower return to the normal blood glucose levels compared with mammals and birds.[5]

More research is necessary to determine the roles of hormones from the pituitary, thyroid, and adrenal glands in the regulation of blood sugar in lower vertebrates.

A normal seasonal variation in blood glucose levels may occur in many species of reptiles.[15] Temperate reptiles generally have higher blood glucose levels during the breeding season.[16] When the peripheral blood glucose is higher during the breeding season, the liver glycogen and the fat body reserves are low. However, in the fall, when most temperate species are increasing fat-body storage, peripheral blood glucose is low. Tropical reptiles, however, may not show seasonal blood sugar variations.[16]

In a study involving captive Mediterranean Tortoises *(Testudo graeca* and *T. hermanni)*, blood glucose values were found to have a statistically significant peak in April and in May at emergence from brumation (hibernation).[17] This sudden peak of glucose may act as a trigger for arousal and may be associated with a rise in environmental temperature. This elevated blood glucose then provides a readily available energy source for tortoises until they begin to feed again.

In another study involving brumating (hibernating) reptiles, the level of glycemia in the winter is inversely correlated with the amount of glycogen stored in the liver.[18]

Fresh-water turtles were found to show a marked hyperglycemia when diving, which is probably related to increased anaerobic metabolism.[19]

Other studies have been done that indicate reptiles may exhibit hyperglycemia of several days' duration after a meal.[20] In a laboratory setting, 2 months of starvation at approximately 70°F (21°C) was necessary before blood-sugar levels became hypoglycemic.[20]

In contrast, in a study on Savannah Monitors *(Varanus exanthematicus)*, starvation altered B-cell constituents, resulting in a reduction in the biosynthesis of insulin-like material and subsequent hyperglycemia.[21] However, the other endocrine hormones of the pancreas were well conserved and seemingly unaffected. This may be clinically relevant in cases of sick reptiles that have been anorectic for extended periods. The inanition may result in damage to B cells with a subsequent reduction in insulin and possible clinical hyperglycemia.

Total pancreatectomy in the Tegu lizards *Tupinambis teguixin* and *T. rufescens* caused an initial hypoglycemia that lasted approximately 2 weeks and was followed by an intense and permanent diabetic hyperglycemia.[22] In the False Viper Snake *(Xenodon merremii)*, a total pancreatectomy resulted in an initial hypoglycemia that lasted 3 to 4 days followed by a permanent intense hyperglycemia.[23]

Similar to some reptiles, ducks were observed to have a marked hypoglycemia after total pancreatectomy.[6] Hypoglycemia in birds has been attributed to the suppression of glucagon, which typically keeps blood glucose at a normal level. More work needs to be done with reptiles, however, to firmly establish that neutralization of glucagon results in hypoglycemia and neutralization of insulin results in hyperglycemia.

Research indicates that compared with mammals and birds reptiles respond very slowly to the administration of mammalian insulin.[5]

Reptiles, especially lizards, seem to tolerate larger doses of mammalian insulin than mammals and birds. In one study, lizards were treated with insulin at 5 to 10 IU/kg body weight. No deaths occurred at this dose, and only one lizard died after receiving an injection of 100 IU/kg.[22] This insulin resistance in lizards is most likely the result of insulin stimulating the central nervous system, which may have both direct and indirect effects on regulation of carbohydrate metabolism.[5]

In another study, lizards were experimentally pancreatectomized to induce hyperglycemia. Three weeks later, they were injected with 100 IU/kg body weight of insulin. The lizards showed a decrease in blood glucose of 150 mg/dL below the initial diabetic level 3 days after the injection. Recovery of the hyperglycemic level was established on the seventh day.[5]

In another study, experimentally induced hyperglycemic lizards were treated with intracoelomic injections of insulin to determine the effect. As the dose of insulin was increased, it caused a greater reduction in blood glucose; however, the larger dose also caused a more prolonged effect. A dose of insulin of 10 IU/kg body weight resulted in a reduction in the blood glucose of 43 mg/dL below the initial level. This effect lasted for 3 days before the blood glucose returned to the initial elevated value. A dose of insulin of 20 IU/kg body weight caused a decrease in blood glucose of 80 mg/dL below the initial level in 2 days, with a recovery of the initial level on the third day. A dose of insulin of 100 IU/kg body weight caused a decrease of 93 mg/dL below the initial level on the third day after the injection, and the normal level was not recovered until the seventh day. No deaths occurred.[22]

On the basis of published research, turtles and snakes seem to be much more sensitive to insulin than lizards. If 1 to 2 IU/kg body weight of mammalian insulin is administered to turtles or snakes, hypoglycemia of several hours' duration usually occurs.[24]

Alligators tend to be more like lizards and are less sensitive to insulin. In one study, the minimum blood glucose–affecting dose for alligators was approximately 10 IU/kg body weight.[5,25] One unusual finding from use of high insulin doses was an initial increase in glucose followed eventually by the expected decrease.[22]

Although lower doses of insulin in reptiles did not elicit a hyperglycemic phase before the hypoglycemic response, larger doses (10 IU/kg in chelonians,[5] 100 IU/kg in the crocodilians,[25] and more than 100 IU/kg in lizards[5]) consistently did. The exact mechanism for these initial hyperglycemic responses is not well understood. Factors unrelated to the pancreas, such as an adrenal medullary response, direct or indirect nervous system effects, or other endocrine effects, may be responsible.

These research experiments have clinical significance because they show that many variables such as season, body and liver condition, and physiologic variables such as anaerobic metabolism and feeding can affect blood glucose values in reptiles. More research is needed to determine whether feeding effects are related to the type of food, rate of digestion and absorption, variations of temperature at which these processes occur, or basic metabolic differences among reptiles.

APPROACH TO THE HYPERGLYCEMIC REPTILE PATIENT

Because blood glucose values in reptiles can be affected by physiologic and environmental factors, a complete history is important to obtain. Husbandry information obtained should include housing, lighting, heating, diet, vitamin and mineral supplementation, and feeding history. Any recent changes in the environment, previous medical history, and treatment with any drugs should also be reviewed.

Seasonal cycles including brumation (hibernation) and reproduction, both past and present, are important variables that may reflect on blood glucose and thus should be noted.

Reptiles with hyperglycemia are often presented for a variety of nonspecific clinical signs, including anorexia, weight loss, lethargy, and severe depression.[3] Polyuria and polydipsia may be present but are not common clinical signs.[3]

Physical Examination

Physical examination findings may also be nonspecific as described for the previous clinical signs but may include loss of muscle mass, weakness, loss of righting reflex, stupor, and severe depression. Some reptiles may present over-conditioned or obese.

Blood Glucose Sampling

External factors influence the blood biochemistry of reptiles more so than mammals and birds. These factors must be considered with attempts to interpret results of blood sampling. Plasma glucose values for normal reptiles vary among species and by nutritional status, season, age, gender, and environmental conditions.[2] In addition, few controlled studies establish the meaning of specific changes in the biochemical profile of reptiles. Thus, interpretation of reptilian clinical chemistry values has not yet achieved the level of accuracy that is seen in small mammals and avian patients.[2]

Blood glucose can be evaluated on whole blood, plasma, or serum, although most published values are based on plasma, preferably harvested from spun whole blood samples, anticoagulated with lithium heparin. Glucose samples can be evaluated with either bench top chemistry analyzers or hand-held glucometers. Bear in mind, most of the patient-side glucose meters tend to read approximately 20% lower than the actual value. In addition, the hand-held units lose accuracy as the glucose values decrease, meaning a greater margin of error the lower the glucose reading.

In general, blood glucose values for normal reptiles are between 60 and 100 mg/dL.[2-4] In one study, a range of blood glucose values in various species of normal-appearing reptiles was found to be between 30 and 205 mg/dL, with average values usually in the range of 90 to 100 mg/dL.[5]

A single blood sample may reveal an elevation in blood glucose, but because a number of external variables can affect blood glucose values, one elevated value may have limited clinical significance in the sick reptile. However, multiple sampling or serial sampling can be valuable in confirming true hyperglycemia, establishing general trends, and helping to determine the clinical progression of the reptile patient.

In addition, if other reptiles of the same species in the same collection (and kept under similar environmental conditions) are sampled, it helps to establish a baseline for reptiles in this group. These values are more valuable and specific to this patient than published reference ranges.

Glucosuria

Glucosuria may be noted in reptiles with persistent hyperglycemia.[11]

Reptile urine is typically not sterile because it is exposed to contents of the proctodeum and coprodeum and, in many species, it is actually held within the terminal colon before being released. More research is needed to understand the effects of fecal contamination on urine and urate testing for the presence of glucose. See Chapter 66 for more information on evaluating reptile urine.

Blood Insulin

Blood insulin levels may prove to be useful in an attempt to differentiate between diabetes mellitus and other causes of hyperglycemia.

More research is necessary to establish normal values for reptiles and to validate the use of mammalian insulin radioimmunoassays in reptiles. However, reptile insulin appears to have a high affinity for human and other mammalian insulin receptors and may favorably react with mammalian radioimmunoassays. Specifically, one study found that the affinity of python insulin for human insulin receptors was very similar to that of human insulin.[26] Furthermore, a mammalian insulin radioimmunoassay was used with apparent success in a hyperglycemic Bearded Dragon (*Pognia vitticeps*).[27]

Further research has revealed that specific physiologic factors, such as inanition or starvation, may result in a reduction

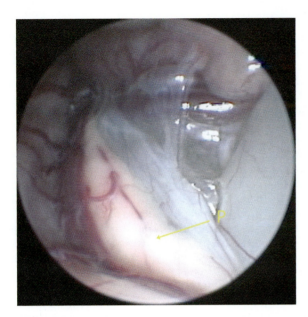

FIGURE 58-6 Endoscopic evaluation of a normal pancreas in the Green Iguana (*Iguana iguana*). The stomach is seen in the upper left, and the lighter-colored pancreas (P) on the bottom. Endoscopic biopsy may have its limitations in diagnosis of specific endocrine disease of the pancreas because the islet tissue tends to be found in focal areas that may not be readily accessible. (*Photograph courtesy S.J. Hernandez-Divers.*)

of immunoreactive insulin content in the pancreas of reptiles. A study in Savannah Monitors found that prolonged starvation resulted in a reduction of immunoreactive insulin content in the pancreas.[21] Whether this decreased immunoreactivity of insulin specifically or directly correlates with hypoinsulinemia and hyperglycemia is not clear, though.

Ketosis

Ketoacidosis is a concurrent clinical condition seen commonly with diabetes mellitus in mammals. This condition may or may not be present in reptiles; however, experimentally total pancreatectomy resulted in an increase in ketone production. One study in lizards found a significant rise in ketone bodies 3 weeks after pancreatectomy that continued to elevate through the eighth week when the experiment ended.[22]

Pancreatic Biopsy

Pancreatic evaluation and biopsy at exploratory surgery or during celioscopy may prove to be a useful tool for diagnosis of pancreatic disease ante mortem (Figure 58-6). Unfortunately, in most cases of persistent hyperglycemia reported, a biopsy was not performed because of the moribund nature of the patient.

An important consideration with a pancreatic biopsy as a diagnostic tool is awareness of the location of the islet tissue in the pancreas. For example, in the Savannah Monitor, all of the islet tissue is concentrated in the splenic portion of the pancreas.[28] This localized concentration of islet tissue in some reptiles may make assessment of islet tissue difficult on an ante mortem biopsy alone.

Necropsy and Histopathology

Because of the severity of the reptile's condition at presentation, most documented cases of persistent hyperglycemia in reptiles have been investigated at necropsy (Table 58-1).

A review of the anatomy of the pancreas and the primary location of islet tissue in reptiles is important to ensure the evaluation of the pancreatic islet tissue on the gross necropsy and histopathology. For example, in the more advanced snake species (family Colubridae), most endocrine cells are actually found within the spleen.[33]

As more reptile species are studied, a great deal of variation will likely be found in the location and abundance of pancreatic islet tissue and specific endocrine cell types. Thus, generalizations should be made with caution. To be clinically thorough, submission of the entire pancreas for histopathologic analysis is imperative.

On histopathology, characteristic lesions are seen in cases of suspected pancreatic insulin deficiency. Typically, the islets of Langerhans may display atrophic characteristics or may be entirely absent. When present, the islets of insulin-producing cells may reveal hydropic degenerative changes, hyalinization, amyloid deposition, and a loss of intracytoplasmic granulation of beta cells.[3,30]

In review of the cases of persistent hyperglycemia described in the literature, some similarities in changes or involvement of other organs is apparent (see Table 58-1). The liver appears to play a significant role in many of these cases. The diagnosis of liver disease is becoming more common in reptiles through the use of improved and more specific diagnostic tools such as ultrasonography and endoscopic biopsy. As more cases of liver disease are documented and described, it may become evident that liver pathology may play a primary role in influencing hyperglycemia.

Liver histopathologic changes associated with persistent hyperglycemia in reptiles include hydropic degeneration, hepatocellular lipidosis, and centrilobular necrosis (see Table 58-1).[3] Hepatic lipidosis is commonly associated with diabetes mellitus in mammals. Hepatic lipidosis is a common condition seen in reptiles and has been associated with persistent hyperglycemia. However, it has not been shown to have a consistent association with persistent hyperglycemia in reptiles.[3,4,11,30,34]

Histopathologic changes associated with hyperglycemia have also been found in the kidneys of reptiles and typically include chronic glomerulonephritis and interstitial nephritis or nephrosclerosis (see Table 58-1).[3,11] The diagnosis of kidney disease is also becoming more common in reptiles with the use of improved and more specific diagnostic tools including ultrasonography and endoscopic biopsy. As more cases of renal disease are described it may become evident that kidney pathology may influence glucose levels in reptiles (Figure 58-7).

MANAGEMENT OF HYPERGLYCEMIA

Because of the multifactorial causes of hyperglycemia, management of the syndrome is both difficult and poorly documented. Anecdotal reports on individual cases exist, but little information on clinical treatment is available. Indeed, no controlled clinical studies have been published,

Hyperglycemia in Reptiles 827

Table 58-1 Cases of Reptile Hyperglycemia Reported in the Literature

Species	History/Presentation	Blood Glucose	Treatment	Case Summary	Reference no.
Red-eared Slider (*Trachemys scripta elegans*)	Anorexic for 3 wk Semistupor	830 mg/dL	NPN Zinc insulin injection(s) 3 days No response	Died Histology of pancreas Granular degeneration Reduction in islet tissue	3
Desert Tortoise (*Gopherus agassizii*)				Died Granulomatous pancreatitis No islet tissue found Primary GI adenocarcinoma	3
Red-eared Slider (*Trachemys scripta elegans*)	Anorexic (2 wk) Progressive lethargy Muscle weakness	610.7 mg/dL		Died Pancreatic islet cell atrophy Hepatic hydropic degeneration Chronic glomerulonephritis	29
Chinese Water Dragon (*Physignathus cocincinus*)	4-y-old male Reduced appetite Weight loss Mandibular osteomyelitis	794 mg/dL	Regular insulin: 5× feline dose 0.097 IU IM No response Glipizide: 0.25 mg PO; then 3 mg PO No response Ocreotide acetate: 6 mg No effect	Died Severe diffuse hepatic lipidosis Renal lipidosis (cortical tubular) Pancreatic islet tissue with random minimal cell pyknosis Human immunohistochemistry stains negative for presence of insulin	11
Western Pond Turtle (*Clemmys m. marmorata*)	Wild caught Acute lethargy Anorexia	842 mg/dL		Died Histology: wide cuff of lymphoplasmacytic leukocytes with occasional large histiocytic macrophages surrounding every pancreatic islet; no normal pancreatic tissue found Immune-mediated disease	30
Exuma Island Iguana (*Cyclura c. figgensi*)	Depression Rear-limb lameness	987 mg/dL	Single dose regular insulin: 1 unit IM No response	Died Histology: round to irregular shaped islets with edges bordered by fibrovascular stroma Immunohistochemical staining with specific antiglucagon reagents from monoclonal antirabbit glucagons Alpha-cell glucagonoma	31
Inland Bearded Dragon (*Pogona vitticeps*)	6-y-old female Lethargy Anorexia	604 mg/dL and 576 mg/dL, weeks apart Plasma insulin: canine/feline Radioimmunoassay		Died Histology: pancreatic hyperplasia with proliferating exocrine acini and fibrovascular stroma No pancreatic neoplasia Hepatocellular carcinoma	27

Continued

Table 58-1 Cases of Reptile Hyperglycemia Reported in the Literature—cont'd

Species	History/Presentation	Blood Glucose	Treatment	Case Summary	Reference no.
Green Iguana (*Iguana iguana*)	5-y-old male Swelling mandible Renomegaly	259 mg/dL initial 700 mg/DL (2 mo later) 594.8 mg/DL (1 d after #2) 384.1 mg/dL (4 d after #2) Plasma insulin: 1 pmol/L (4 d after #2) 1.8 ng/dL this dragon 13.1 ng/dL control		Immunoperoxidase staining positive for insulin, glucagon, and somatostatin in pancreas No stain in hepatic carcinoma Died Enlarged kidneys Histology: pancreatic tissue normal Renal failure Diffuse hydropic change and mild lipidosis in liver and adrenal glands	32

GI, gastrointestinal; *IM*, intramuscularly; *PO*, orally.

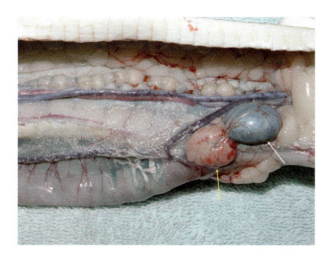

FIGURE 58-7 Splenopancreas (*yellow arrow*) and gallbladder (*white arrow*) in a snake with severe visceral gout (*white speckling* in mesentery). The patient died of a combination of gout and renal disease. The animal was hyperglycemic ante mortem. (*Photograph courtesy S. Barten.*)

and all treatments are empirical at this time. Reported cases and treatment in the literature are summarized, as is academic research. Rough guidelines can be extrapolated from this information to initiate treatment.

Initially, management should focus on a diagnosis of the cause of the persistent hyperglycemia. Is it related to underlying metabolic disease, neoplasia (see Figure 19-5), physiologic circumstances (e.g., gestational diabetes), or true diabetes mellitus?

The clinician must evaluate the entire patient, review all the variables that may affect blood glucose levels, and rule out these influences. Physical examination, biochemical analysis, radiology, ultrasonography, endoscopy, and surgery are all modalities that can be used.

Persistent hyperglycemia should be established with serial sampling, and attempts should be made to rule out underlying diseases and environmental or physiologic influences before the use of insulin or other glucose-regulating drugs.

On the basis of the clinical evaluation, supportive care including hydration, alimentation, liver support, and other appropriate chemotherapeutics as indicated should be initiated.

Even with a review of the clinical cases and published research, much work is still needed to provide clinically relevant information. To date, no clinical trials or even long-term management of individual cases with the use of mammalian insulin or other glucose-regulating agents have been reported in reptiles. Variables such as dosage, frequency of dosing, dramatic physiologic differences among reptiles, and their unique adaptations to the environment (xeric, tropical, aquatic, etc.) make establishment of standardized dosing regimens for reptiles difficult.

If all factors indicate that the patient is truly a strong candidate for diabetes mellitus, an uncommon diagnosis in reptiles, and the clinician feels some glucose-regulating agent must be initiated, then a **starting point** for regular mammalian insulin may be:

Lizards and crocodilians: 5 to 10 IU/kg every 24 to 48 hours

Snakes and chelonians: 1 to 5 IU/kg every 24 to 48 hours

These doses are empirical and should be adjusted on the basis of response to therapy and continued serial sampling of blood glucose. Clinicians must be aware that intracoelomic injections often took 24 to 48 hours before any response was seen. So, a change in dosing regimen should be considered only after looking at serial sampling for several days. Clinicians must continue to document and report cases of persistent hyperglycemia, treatment regimens, and responses to therapy to improve the clinical management of these cases.

SUMMARY

In summary, if a reptile patient presents with hyperglycemia, *do not* think diabetes mellitus. Because true diabetes mellitus is not common, ruling out other causes for the hyperglycemia is prudent.

A great deal of research is still needed to better understand hyperglycemia in reptiles, especially with regard to diagnosis and treatment. However, vigilant clinicians and pathologists have important roles to play in expanding our knowledge base in this field and are encouraged to share their findings through publications and presentations.

REFERENCES

1. Stahl SJ: Diseases of the reptile pancreas, *Vet Clin Exot Anim* 6:191-212, 2003.
2. Campbell TW: Clinical pathology. In Mader DR, editor: *Reptile medicine and surgery*, Philadelphia, 1996, WB Saunders.
3. Frye FL: *Biomedical and surgical aspects of captive reptile husbandry*, ed 2, Malabar, Fla, 1991, Krieger.
4. Mader DR: Reptilian metabolic disorders. In Fudge AM, editor: *Laboratory medicine avian and exotic pets*, Philadelphia, 2000, WB Saunders.
5. Miller MR: Pancreatic islet histology and carbohydrate metabolism in amphibians and reptiles, *Diabetes* 9(4):318-323, 1960.
6. Mialhe P: Glucagon, insuline et regulation endocrine chez le canard, *Acta Endocrinol* 28:9-134, 1958.
7. Miller MR: Observations on the comparative histology of the reptilian pancreatic islet, *Gen Comp Endocrinol* 2:407-414, 1962.
8. El-Salhy M, Grimelius L: Histological and immuno-histochemical studies of the endocrine pancreas of lizards, *Histochemistry* 72:237-247, 1981.
9. Putti R, Della Rossa A, Varano L, Laforgia V, Cavagnuolo A: An immunocytochemical study of the endocrine pancreas in three genera of lacertids, *Gen Comp Endocrinol* 87:249-259, 1992.
10. Perez-Tomas R, Ballesta J, Pastor LM, Madrid JF, Polak JM: Comparative immunohistochemical study of the gastro-enteropancreatic endocrine system of three reptiles, *Gen Comp Endocrinol* 76:171-191, 1989.
11. Heatley JJ, Johnson A, Tully T, Mitchell M: *Persistent hyperglycemia in a Chinese water dragon*, Physignathus cocincinus, Orlando, Fla, 2001, Proc Assoc Reptilian Amphibian Veterinarians.
12. Aguirre AA, Balazs GH, Spraker TR, Gross TS: Adrenal and hematological responses to stress in juvenile green turtles (*Chelonia mydas*) with and without fibropapillomas, *Physiol Zool* 68:831-854, 1995.

13. Britton SW, Klein RF: Emotional hyperglycemia and hyperthermia in tropical mammals and reptiles, *Am J Physiol* 18:221-232, 1939.
14. Gregory LF, Schmid JR: Stress responses and sexing of wild Kemp's Ridley sea turtles (*Lepidochelys kempii*) in the northeastern Gulf of Mexico, *Gen Comp Endocrinol* 124:66-74, 2001.
15. Coulson RA, Hernandez T: *Biochemistry of the alligator*, Baton Rouge, La, 1964, Louisiana State University Press.
16. Prado JL: Glucose tolerance test in Ophidia and the effect of feeding on their glycemia, *Rev Can Biol* 5:564-569, 1946.
17. Lawrence K: Seasonal variation in blood biochemistry of long term captive Mediterranean tortoises (*Testudo graeca* and *T. hermanni*), *Res Vet Sci* 43:379-383, 1987.
18. Gregory PT: Hibernation. In Gans C, Pough FH, editors: *Biology of the Reptilia*, vol 13, London, 1982, Academic Press.
19. Dessauer HC: Blood chemistry of reptiles. In Gans C, Parsons TC, editors: *Biology of the Reptilia*, vol 3, New York, 1970, Academic Press.
20. Miller MR, Wurster DH: Studies on the blood glucose and pancreatic islets of lizards, *Endocrinology* 63:114-120, 1956.
21. Godet R, Mattei X, Dupe-Godet M: Alterations of endocrine pancreas B cells in a Sahelian reptile (*Varanus exanthematicus*) during starvation, *J Morphol* 180:173-180, 1984.
22. Penhos JC, Houssay BA, Lujan MA: Total pancreatectomy in lizards: effects of several hormones, *Endocrinology* 76:989-993, 1965.
23. Houssay BA: Comparative physiology of the endocrine pancreas. In Gorbman A, editor: *Comparative endocrinology*, New York, 1959, John Wiley.
24. Lopes N, Wagner E, Barros M, Marques M: Glucose, insulin and epinephrine tolerance tests in the normal and hypophysectomized turtle *Psuedemys d'Orbignyi*, *Acta Physiol Latinoamer* 4:190-199, 1954.
25. Stevenson OR, Coulson RA, Hernandez T: Effects of hormones on carbohydrate metabolism in the alligator, *Am J Physiol* 191:95-102, 1957.
26. Conlon JM, Secor SM, Adrian TE, Mynarcik DC, Whittaker J: Purification and characterization of islet hormones (insulin, glucagon, pancreatic polypeptide and somatostatin) from the Burmese python, *Python molurus*, *Regul Pept* 71(3):191-198, 1997.
27. Griswold WG: *Hepatocellular carcinoma with associated hyperglycemia in an inland bearded dragon*, Pogona vitticeps, Orlando, Fla, 2001, Proc Assoc Reptilian Amphibian Veterinarians.
28. Moscona AA: Anatomy of the pancreas and Langerhans islets in snakes and lizards, *Anat Rec* 227:232-244, 1990.
29. Frye FL, Dutra FR, Carney JD, Johnson B: Spontaneous diabetes mellitus in a turtle, *Vet Med Small Anim Clin* 71(7):935-939, 1976.
30. Frye FL: *Spontaneous autoimmune pancreatitis and diabetes mellitus in a western pond turtle*, Clemmys m marmorata, Columbus, Ohio, 1999, Proc Assoc Reptilian Amphibian Veterinarians.
31. Frye FL, McNeely HE, Corcoran JH: *Functional pancreatic glucagonoma in the rhinoceros iguana*, Cyclura c. figgensi, *characterized by immunocytochemistry*, Columbus, Ohio, 1999, Proc Assoc Reptilian Amphibian Veterinarians.
32. Crocker C, Miller D: *Persistent elevated blood glucose in the iguana*, Iguana iguana: *a case study*, Reno, Nev, 2002, Proc Assoc Reptilian Amphibian Veterinarians.
33. Miller MR, Lagios M: The pancreas. In Gans C, Parsons TC, editors: *Biology of the Reptilia*, vol 3, New York, 1970, Academic Press.
34. Divers SJ, Cooper JE: Reptile hepatic lipidosis, *Semin Avian Exotic Pet Med* 9(3):153-164, 2000.

59
HYPOVITAMINOSIS A AND HYPERVITAMINOSIS A

THOMAS H. BOYER

HYPOVITAMINOSIS A

Hypovitaminosis A is primarily a disease of chelonians, with Box Turtles (*Terrapene* spp.) currently most commonly affected. Hypovitaminosis A used to be seen in small aquatic turtles before they were banned for sale in the United States but is less commonly seen in aquatic turtles now. Tortoises are generally not affected. Any reptile is theoretically susceptible. Although hypovitaminosis A has been reported in iguanas,[1] it is rarely seen in lizards. It has also been seen in farm-raised crocodiles.[2,3]

Pathogenesis

Vitamin A deficiency arises in reptiles fed an unbalanced diet lacking adequate levels of vitamin A. Elkan and Zwart[4] first detailed the pathology of hypovitaminosis in 1967. The fundamental disorder of vitamin A deficiency is multifocal squamous metaplasia and hyperkeratosis of epithelium.[4-6] Epithelia in the respiratory, ocular, endocrine, gastrointestinal, and genitourinary systems (in respective order) are most often involved.[6] Early changes include epithelial necrosis or atrophy. Cellular debris fills spaces between cells, and eosinophils and heterophils move *en masse*. The normal columnar or cuboidal epithelium is replaced by flattened cells, which continually desquamate. Granulocytes and desquamated material fill multiple retention cysts (keratin pearls). Ducts in the pancreas, kidney, and oculonasal glands become blocked with desquamated debris.[4] The compromised epithelial barriers are susceptible to opportunistic bacterial infections.[6]

In chelonians, two tear-secreting ophthalmic glands, the anteromedial Harderian and the posterolateral lacrimal, merit special mention. Vitamin A deficiency causes these glands to expand outward in the direction of least resistance. This forces the eyelids to gradually swell shut.[4] Cellular debris accumulates underneath the eyelids in the conjunctival sac. In severe chronic cases, the ever-enlarging ophthalmic glands can evert the conjunctiva, giving the superficial impression of a fused eyelid.[4]

Vitamin A deficiency was implicated as a cause of renal tubular squamous metaplasia and hyperkeratosis in young farm-raised saltwater *Crocodylus porosus* and freshwater crocodiles, *C. johnstoni* that had been fed a diet deficient in vitamin A.[3] Tubular damage and subsequent gram-negative bacterial colonization, in conjunction with a high-protein diet, were thought to contribute to renal and visceral gout.[3] On the surface of the crocodiles' tongues were multiple pale brown nodules up to 5 mm in diameter. Microscopically, these tongue lesions consisted of glandular squamous metaplasia and marked hyperkeratosis with secondary bacterial and fungal infection.

Clinical Signs

In chelonians, the most obvious clinical sign is blepharedema, usually with (in chronic cases), or without (in early cases), solid whitish-yellow cellular debris underneath the eyelids (Figure 59-1). Involvement is not always bilaterally uniform; one eye may be affected long before the other.[4] Other symptoms may include lethargy, anorexia, weight loss, and nasal or ocular discharge (Figure 59-2).

Middle ear and respiratory tract infections and egg retention are common in Box Turtles with hypovitaminosis A. Juvenile seaturtles exhibit dermal hyperkeratosis of the external surfaces of the eyelids.[7] Postbrumation (hibernation) blindness in Mediterranean Tortoises (*Testudo graeca* and *T. hermani*) from retinal damage responded to time and vitamin A supplementation.[8] Inguinal and axillary edema can be a sign of kidney failure from vitamin A deficiency and dictates a poor prognosis.[9] Fatty degeneration of the liver was found in several terrapins with hypovitaminosis A.[4]

In the past, vitamin A deficiency and respiratory tract disease were thought to be often concurrent in Desert Tortoises (*Gopherus agassizii*).[5] Most green plants are rich in carotenoids (precursors of vitamin A), and thus, to ever encounter vitamin A deficiency in tortoises that eat greens is extremely unlikely. Because hypovitaminosis A is rare in tortoises, tortoises with clinical signs suggestive of deficiency should be thoroughly evaluated for diseases that cause blepharedema before parenteral vitamin A therapy is started (see Chapters 40, 57, and 73).

External gross lesions of vitamin A deficiency in saltwater and freshwater crocodiles were limited to multiple pale brown nodules, up to 5 mm in diameter, in the dorsal epithelium of the tongue.[3]

The author has diagnosed vitamin A deficiency in one lizard, a Jackson's Chameleon, *Chamaeleo jacksonii*. The lizard had chronically swollen lips (Figure 59-3) that oozed thick clear mucus, reminiscent of saliva, with firm digital pressure. One month of antibiotic therapy had negligible affect on the lips. Biopsies revealed hyperkeratosis and marked squamous metaplasia of salivary duct with chronic fibrosing cheilitis; no bacteria were seen. The changes were suggestive of vitamin A deficiency. A single vitamin A (5000 IU) and D injection returned the lips to normal within 2 weeks. The author suspects swollen lips were the result of blocked ducts within salivary glands of upper and lower jaws.

Diagnosis

Vitamin A assay of liver, or large quantities of blood, are needed for definitive antemortem diagnosis. Two Map Turtles (*Graptemys geographica*) with confirmed hypovitaminosis A

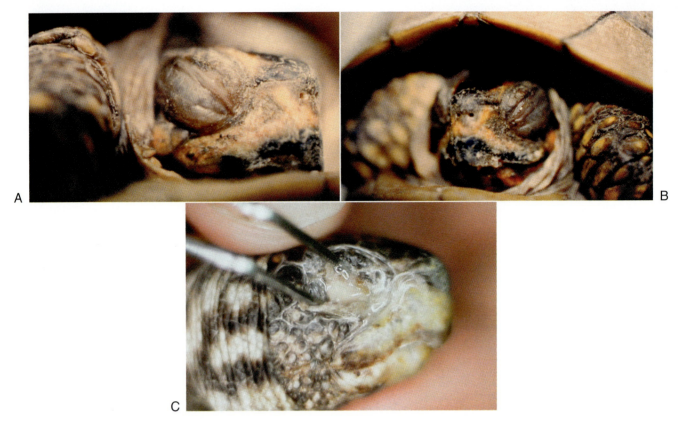

FIGURE 59-1 **A** and **B**, Blepharedema is a classic sign of vitamin A deficiency. **C**, In severe cases, caseous exudate may be found under the palpebrum. (*C, Photograph courtesy D. Mader.*)

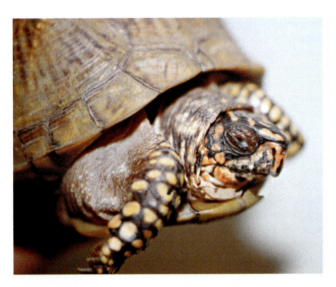

FIGURE 59-2 Mucopurulent ocular discharge and moderate blepharedema in a Three-toed Box Turtle (*Terrapene carolina triunguis*) from hypovitaminosis A.

had 9 and 19 IU vitamin A/g of liver.[4] Normal liver vitamin A levels have been reported to be more than 1000 IU/g in monitors and snakes[4] and 10, 30, and 80 IU/g liver in three *Testudo hermanni*.[10] Concentrations of 500 to 1000 IU/g are not uncommon in most species (other than fish and humans).[11] Liver biopsy is not a difficult procedure in most reptile species; however, it may not be clinically practical in suspected cases of hypovitaminosis A.[12]

Vitamin A status and dietary adequacy cannot be easily determined with blood sampling.[13,14] However, retinol can be used for an assessment of vitamin A.[14] Mean plasma retinol values in 193 turtles from 10 genera ranged from 0.04 to 0.35 μm/mL, and in 345 tortoises from five genera, means ranged from 0.04 to 0.61 μm/mL. No statistically significant differences were found between zoo and wild populations. These values tended to be at the lower end of expected normal ranges (0.2 to 0.8 μm/mL) for domestic livestock species.[14] Interesting to note is that chelonians normally may have levels of retinol below 0.2 μm/mL, which is considered below normal for most other species.[11] If chelonians normally have low levels of vitamin A in liver and retinol in blood, that they should be more sensitive to dietary deficiencies makes sense.

Although measurement of plasma retinol levels is possible, most diagnoses of hypovitaminosis A are currently based on dietary history, clinical signs, and response to treatment.[7,12] Dietary history is especially important because blepharitis can also be caused by trauma, foreign bodies, pollen, and viral, mycotic, bacterial, or nematode infections.[7] Biopsies or exfoliative cytology, which show desquamated keratocytes and granulocytes, may also aid diagnosis in rare cases with dietary history not suggestive of hypovitaminosis A[7,15] or in cases in which hypovitaminosis A is not suspected.

Farm-raised crocodiles had vitamin A deficiency develop when fed thawed frozen diets (75% kangaroo meat,

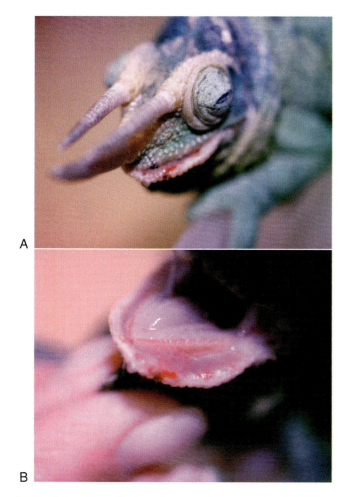

FIGURE 59-3 **A** and **B**, Cheilitis in a Jackson's Chameleon (*Chamaeleo jacksonii*) that failed to respond to antibiotics. Histopathology revealed hyperkeratosis and marked squamous metaplasia of the salivary ducts, suggesting hypovitaminosis A. The cheilitis resolved completely within 2 weeks of a single dose of vitamin A. Vitamin A deficiencies remain rare in lizards.

25% chicken heads, and a multivitamin supplement) that contained 125 IU vitamin A/kg feed.[3]

Treatment

Fat-soluble vitamin A is recommended over water-soluble vitamin A.[10] Subcutaneous injections of 500 to 5000 IU/kg vitamin A for one or two treatments (every 14 days) is an effective treatment for hypovitaminosis A. Symptoms resolve gradually within 2 to 4 weeks, depending on the severity of presenting clinical signs (Figure 59-4); one should be sure to warn owners of this.

Cellular debris under the eyelids can be carefully removed with a blunt probe and digital pressure. Ophthalmic antibiotic ointments or solutions are warranted if secondary infection is present. If nasal discharge or other evidence of respiratory disease (dyspnea, rales, nasal discharge) is present, systemic antibiotics should be given. Nephrotoxic drugs should be avoided because of potential renal compromise.[5,12]

Shallow warm water (24°C to 27°C [75°F to 80°F]) soaks for several hours daily ensure rehydration. Patients do not start eating again until their eyes open. If the patient is

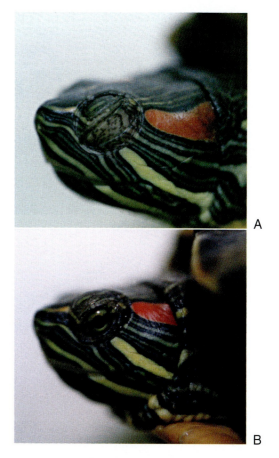

FIGURE 59-4 **A**, Blepharedema in a Red-eared Slider (*Trachemys scripta elegans*) that presented after 2 months of misdiagnosis and treatment with topical and systemic antibiotics. **B**, The same turtle 2 weeks after discontinuation of antibiotics and a single dose of vitamin A subcutaneously.

severely underweight, force-feeding, or placement of an esophagostomy tube, is recommended. Box Turtles generally respond well to treatment, even in severe cases.

Long-term treatment and prevention involves expanding the diet to include foods rich in carotenes, especially the beta-carotenes. For tortoises and Box Turtles, these foods include dark leafy greens (spinach, dandelions, turnip and mustard greens, bok choy, broccoli) and yellow-colored or orange-colored vegetables or fruits (steamed winter squashes, carrots, green peppers, sweet potatoes, cantaloupe). For aquatic turtles, liver in whole mice or fish is a good source of vitamin A, as are algae and pond weeds.[15] Many commercial diets suitable for reptiles (Purina Trout Chow, Tetra Reptomin Floating Food Sticks) are good sources of vitamin A.[7]

IATROGENIC HYPERVITAMINOSIS A

Vitamin A, like other fat-soluble vitamins, has been shown to have toxic effects in most species studied. Reptiles are no exception. Most veterinarians are aware of the propensity of certain chelonians for hypovitaminosis A, such as Box Turtles and aquatic turtles. Before the discovery that mycoplasmal infections in tortoises caused upper respiratory tract disease, vitamin A deficiency was thought to be involved.[5] Vitamin A treatment gradually became part of the standard treatment for many chelonians, often for any symptom. Vitamin A toxicity was not yet appreciated. Unfortunately, a wide range of empiric dosages for vitamin A was found in the reptile veterinary literature. Dosages were often listed simply as IU without regard to weight. Most commercial sources of vitamin A were designed for larger mammals and contained 100,000 to 500,000 IU vitamin A/mL, which made administration of toxic doses easy even with small volumes (less than 0.1 mL). Also, that water-soluble vitamin A was much faster acting than fat-soluble vitamin A, and perhaps more toxic, was not known.[10] Thus, with wide dosage ranges, concentrated and different sources of vitamin A, and small patients, iatrogenic hypervitaminosis became the unknowing mistake of many veterinarians.[16]

Pathogenesis and Clinical Signs

Carotenoids are converted to retinol in the intestines or liver and stored in the liver. Retinol is transported from the liver to tissue with retinol-binding protein. The liver acts as a reservoir to protect against deficiency and excess. Toxicity results when massive doses of vitamin A overwhelm the storage and processing capabilities of the liver and free retinol, not bound to retinol-binding protein, becomes present in tissue.[11] In chelonians, early retinol toxicity primarily affects the epidermis, initially causing dry flaky skin (xeroderma).[7] Within a few days, erythematous areas spread over the skin.

Histologically, early changes in these areas include marked flattening of the stratum corneum and stratum germanitivum.[10,17] The stratum corneum separates from the stratum germanitivum, and subcorneal acantholysis, intercellular edema, and well-differentiated acanthosis are seen.[10] Grossly, blisters typically form on the skin of the neck and legs but may occur on any skin surface.[17] The blisters, or bullae, break open and expose moist, reddened, or gray underlying tissue and eventually slough (Figure 59-5). With increased toxicity, the cells in the upper levels of the stratum corneum become parakeratotic and cells in the upper stratum germinativum become swollen.[10]

Water-soluble vitamin A produces these lesions within 10 to 15 days, yet fat-soluble vitamin A at identical doses did not, even though liver levels of vitamin A were similar.[10] The study by Palmer et al[10] terminated at 15 days, so whether the tortoises would have eventually sloughed their skin or whether fat soluble vitamin A is truly less toxic remains unknown. Cumulative toxic doses for parenteral water-soluble vitamin A are thought to be from 50,000 to 100,000 IU/kg.[10,16] Further confusing the entire issue is the fact that elevated intakes of vitamins D, E, or K may reduce vitamin A toxicity by interfering with vitamin A assimilation or restoring their respective adequacies.[11] Protein deficiency may have a protective effect against hypervitaminosis A. Decreased retinol-binding protein may slow removal of excess vitamin A from liver into tissue and thereby decrease toxicity.[11]

Treatment

Treatment of hypervitaminosis A is essentially identical to that of severe burns (see Chapter 71).[17] Prognosis is dependent on many factors, the most important of which include the dosage of vitamin A, the health status before administration, and the aggressiveness of treatment. Most chelonians survive with treatment, but high dosages can definitely be lethal. Recovery may take 4 to 6 months.

Vitamin A should not be used unless dietary history and clinical signs suggest a deficiency. Vitamin A deficiency in tortoises remains unlikely given their diet.[7] Vitamin A should be dosed carefully in other chelonians. **Until more is known, avoidance of water-soluble vitamin A and use of fat-soluble vitamin A instead seems prudent.**[10]

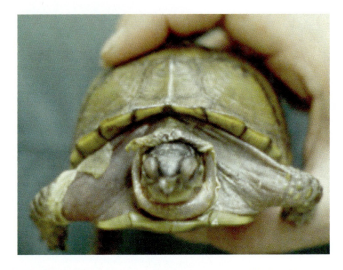

FIGURE 59-5 Epidermal sloughing in a Box Turtle *(Terrapene carolina triunguis)* from hypervitaminosis A.

REFERENCES

1. Anderson NL: Husbandry and clinical evaluation of *Iguana iguana, Compend Cont Ed Pract Vet* 13:1265, 1991.
2. Foggin CM: Diseases and disease control crocodile farms in Zimbabwe. In Webb GJW, Manolis SC, Whitehead PJ, editors: *Wildlife management: crocodiles and alligators,* New South Wales, 1987, Surrey Beatty.
3. Ariel E, Ladds PW, Buenviaje GN: Concurrent gout and suspected hypovitaminosis A in crocodile hatchlings, *Aust Vet J* 75(4):247-249, 1997.
4. Elkan E, Zwart P: The ocular disease of young terrapins caused by vitamin A deficiency, *Pathologia Vet* 4:201, 1967.
5. Fowler ME: Comparison of respiratory infection and hypovitaminosis A in desert tortoises. In Montali RJ, Migaki G, editors: *Comparative pathology of zoo animals,* Washington, DC, 1980, Smithsonian Institute.
6. Frye FL: Nutritional disorders in reptiles. In Hoff GL, Frye FL, Jacobson ER, editors: *Diseases of amphibians and reptiles,* New York, 1984, Plenum Press.
7. Frye FL: *Biomedical and surgical aspects of captive reptile husbandry,* ed 2, Melbourne, Fla, 1991, Kreiger Publishing.
8. Lawton MPC, Stoakes LC: Post-hibernation blindness in tortoises, *Third International Colloquium on the Pathology of Reptiles and Amphibians,* Orlando, Fla, 1989.
9. Lawton MPC: Neurological problems of exotic species. In Wheeler SJ, editor: *Manual of small animal neurology,* Cheltenham, 1989, British Small Animal Veterinary Association.
10. Palmer DG, Rubel A, Mettler F, Volker L: Experimentally induced skin changes in land tortoises by giving high doses

of vitamin A parenterally, *Gaben von Vitamin A Zbl Vet Med A* 31:625, 1984.
11. National Research Council: *Vitamin A: vitamin tolerance of animals, Subcommittee on Vitamin Tolerance, Committee on Animal Nutrition, Board of Agriculture, National Research Council,* Washington, DC, 1987, National Academy Press.
12. Stoakes LC: Respiratory system. In Beynon PH, Lawton MPC, Cooper JC, editors: *Manual of reptiles,* Cheltenham, 1992, British Small Animal Veterinary Association.
13. Gibson RS: *Principles of nutrition assessment,* New York, 1990, Oxford University Press.
14. Dierenfeld ES, Leontyeva OA, Karesh WB, Calle PP: Circulating α-tocopherol and retinol concentrations in free-ranging and zoo turtles and tortoises, *Proc Amer Assoc Zoo Vet,* Columbus, OH, 1999.
15. Williams DL: Opthalmology. In Mader DR, editor: *Reptile medicine and surgery,* Philadelphia, 1996, WB Saunders.
16. Boyer TH: Vitamin A toxicity, *Bull Assoc Amphib Reptil Vet* 1(1):2, 1991.
17. Frye FL: Vitamin A sources, hypovitaminosis A, and iatrogenic hypervitaminosis A in captive chelonians. In Kirk RW, editor: *Current vet therapy,* vol 10, Philadelphia, 1989, WB Saunders.

60
INCLUSION BODY DISEASE VIRUS

JUERGEN SCHUMACHER

Inclusion body disease (IBD) of boid snakes is the most important viral disease that affects captive collections of boas and pythons and has been associated with high morbidity and mortality rates. IBD has been named after the presence of characteristic eosinophilic intracytoplamic inclusions in visceral epithelial cells and neurons of the central nervous system of affected snakes. This disease has been recognized in the United States, Africa, Australia, and Europe since the 1980s,[1-6] and outbreaks have been reported from private and zoologic collections of boid snakes. Although most likely all snakes of the family Boidae are susceptible to this infection, the most common species diagnosed with IBD are Boa Constrictors (*Boa constrictor constrictor*) and Burmese Pythons (*Python molurus bivittatus*), probably because of their high popularity in the pet trade and in breeding facilities. Exclusively members of the family Boidae have been diagnosed with this infection, but evidence exists that other reptile species either may act as carriers of the virus or may show different clinical and pathologic signs than boas and pythons[7,8] and therefore may go undiagnosed. A study of captive-bred and wild-caught Palm Vipers (*Bothriechis marchi*) with clinical signs similar to boid snakes with IBD showed eosinophilic inclusions with ultrastructural features similar to IBD.[8,9]

The etiologic agent of IBD appears to be a retrovirus-like agent that has been detected in tissues of affected snakes, both on electron microscopic examination and on viral isolation.[4,10,11] A distinct possibility also exists that several strains of this virus exist.[7,10] Current and future research focuses on the isolation and identification of the etiologic agent and on the development of a serologic test and transmission studies to identify carriers and susceptible species.[7] An enzyme-linked immunosorbent assay has been developed to determine exposure of Boa Constrictors to specific antigens.[12]

PATHOLOGY

Inclusion body disease is characterized by a unique pathogenesis usually not associated with retrovirus infections, such as the presence of characteristic eosinophilic intracytoplasmic inclusion bodies in epithelial cells of all visceral organs.

Necropsy findings are often limited to gross changes associated with secondary bacterial infections, such as pneumonia, stomatitis, and bacterial granulomas within the liver and kidneys. In some species, such as Boa Constrictors, fibrous changes and atrophy of the spleen may be seen.[4]

Histologically, the most consistent finding is the presence of eosinophilic intracytoplasmic inclusion bodies in hematoxylin and eosin (H&E)–stained epithelial cells of all major organs, including liver, kidney, stomach, pancreas, and brain (Figures 60-1 and 60-2). **In *Boa* spp., inclusions are often found in all visceral organs, and in *Python* spp., inclusions are more abundant within the tissue of the central nervous system.** Inclusions vary in size (1 to 4 µm) and often exceed the size of the nucleus. Affected cells typically exhibit vacuolization and degeneration of the cytoplasm, and affected organs may show multiple areas of necrosis. Histologic evaluation of the brain of infected snakes often reveals a non-suppurative

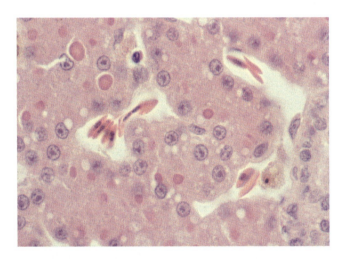

FIGURE 60-1 Section of the liver of a Boa Constrictor (*Boa constrictor constrictor*) with inclusion body disease. Eosinophilic intracytoplasmic inclusions are present within multiple hepatocytes.

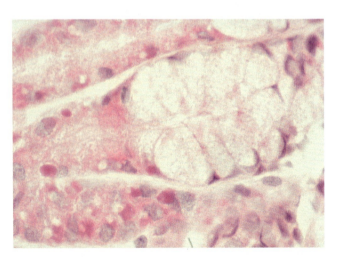

FIGURE 60-2 Section of the stomach of a Boa Constrictor (*Boa constrictor constrictor*) with inclusion body disease. Inclusion bodies are located within the cytoplasm of gastric mucosal cells.

meningoencephalitis that includes neuronal degeneration, gliosis, and demyelinization (Figure 60-3). The inflammatory response is more pronounced in pythons than in boas. In pythons especially, inclusion bodies can often be detected in the cytoplasm of degenerating neurons that are commonly surrounded by mononuclear cell infiltrates.

On electron microscopy, inclusions appear as electron-dense structures that may vary in size and shape (Figure 60-4). Inclusions may either present previral material or some type of storage material of a dysfunctional cell. In one study, an antigenically distinct 68-kilodalton protein was isolated and characterized from nonviral inclusions in IBD-infected Boa Constrictors.[13] A study in Cornsnakes *(Elaphe guttata)* revealed inclusions similar to inclusions of IBD on light microscopy.[14]

Viral agents morphologically compatible with members of the family retroviridae have been detected in tissue (brain, kidney) sections of infected Boa Constrictors and Burmese Pythons. Morphologically, similar particles have also been detected with electron microscopy in primary kidney cell cultures established from infected Boa Constrictors and Burmese Pythons (see Figure 60-4).[4,10] Viral particles measured 90 to 120 nm were enveloped, and the nucleoid was enclosed by a hexagonal nucleocapsid. Viral particles were budding from membranes of the endoplasmic reticulum. Mature particles had an electron-dense core and were located extracellularly. The enzyme reverse transcriptase has been detected in the serum of infected Boa Constrictors and Burmese Pythons and in supernatant fluids of primary kidney cell cultures of infected snakes.[4,10] Several retroviruses have been isolated from boid snakes, but a causal relationship between these isolates and IBD has not yet been confirmed.[11]

CLINICAL SIGNS

No clinical signs are pathognomonic for IBD. Any boid snake with an acute onset of neurologic signs or a history of chronic wasting should be suspected of IBD (Figure 60-5). IBD is characterized by a variety of signs and symptoms that may be slow progressing and difficult to differentiate from other conditions, especially in *Boa* spp. Boas are often presented with a history of regurgitation and progressive weight loss. In most cases, determination of the time of exposure to the agent is impossible; therefore, the term *acute stage* of the disease is clinically more accurately described as a stage of IBD when clinical signs are first noticeable. These can include mild neurologic signs (e.g., head tremor, stargazing, and flaccid

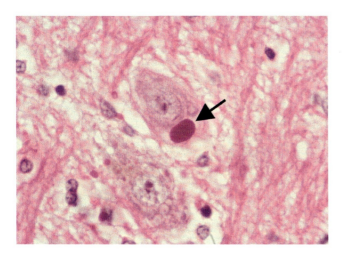

FIGURE 60-3 Nonsuppurative encephalitis and demyelinization in the brain of a Boa Constrictor *(Boa constrictor constrictor)*. Inclusions can be seen within the cytoplasm of degenerating neurons.

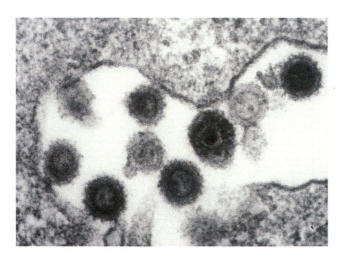

FIGURE 60-4 Electron photomicrograph of immature viral particles within the vacuoles in the cytoplasm of a primary kidney cell culture, established from an infected Boa Constrictor *(Boa constrictor constrictor)*.

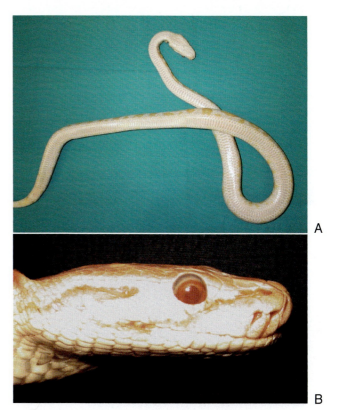

FIGURE 60-5 A, Juvenile Burmese Python *(Python molurus bivittatus)* presented with acute onset of neurologic signs, including loss of the righting reflex and disorientation. **B,** The same snake with dilated pupils.

paralysis of the musculature) or decreased activity levels. In later stages of the infection, secondary bacterial infections often cause respiratory tract disease, stomatitis, and dermatitis. In several instances, cutaneous neoplasia and leukemias have been reported associated with IBD.[7] In the final stages of the disease, affected boas are commonly anorectic and dehydrated and exhibit severe neurologic symptoms, such as incoordination and failure to right themselves when placed in dorsal recumbency. *Python* spp. are most often presented with acute onset of neurologic signs, including loss of righting reflex, disequilibrium, and opisthotonos (Figures 60-6 and 60-7). In pythons, the infection appears to progress faster when compared with *Boa* spp., and clinical signs may be present within a few weeks after exposure to the agent.[4] Remission from IBD has never been observed, and infected snakes do die.

The route of natural transmission is unknown and may be horizontal (e.g., respiratory tract, oral). Arthropods such as the snake mite *Ophionyssus natricis* may also serve as a vector.[4]

DIAGNOSIS

A definite antemortem diagnosis of IBD is often challenging because of the unavailability of a serologic test to identify infected and exposed snakes. Often, a diagnosis of IBD is made on postmortem histologic detection of typical inclusions

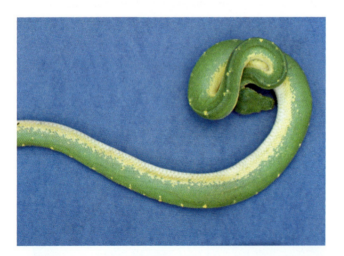

FIGURE 60-6 Green Tree Python *(Morelia [Chondropython] viridis)* with loss of motor function and paralysis of the musculature of the caudal half of the body.

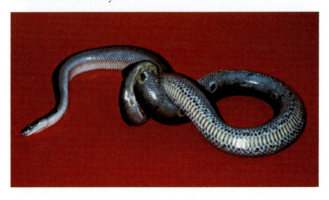

FIGURE 60-7 Papuan Python *(Liasis papuanus)* with signs of incoordination and disorientation.

within epithelial cells of all major organs including the brain. With presentation of a suspected case of IBD, one must first rule out all other causes of regurgitation, respiratory disease, and neurologic disease. The list of differentials should include bacterial and parasitic infections, trauma, and exposure to toxins. A thorough history and collection of a combination of diagnostic samples from a live snake are often necessary to diagnose the disease. However, because of the variety of clinical symptoms especially between boas and pythons and often the lack of inclusions within epithelial cells of major organs in pythons, the disease may go undiagnosed in some cases. Although the detection of inclusions is diagnostic for IBD, absence of inclusions does not rule out infection or exposure to the agent. The following lists antemortem and postmortem diagnostic approaches to workup in suspected cases of IBD.

Antemortem Diagnosis

1. A thorough history detailing the origin of the snake and potential exposure to other boid snakes should be obtained. Any recent additions, including both boid and nonboid snakes, to an existing collection should be noted. The quarantine program if existent should be reviewed.
2. Date of onset and progression of clinical signs and species of snakes affected should be recorded.
3. A complete physical examination, including neurologic examination, should be performed.
4. A venous blood sample for a complete white blood cell count (WBC), including differential count and plasma biochemistries, should be collected. Infected snakes may be seen with a leukocytosis (WBC > 30,000 cells/mL) and a pronounced lymphocytosis. In advanced stages of the disease, snakes may have developed a pronounced leukopenia (WBC < 5000 cells/mL). Plasma biochemistries are indicated to evaluate organ (e.g., kidney, liver) function.
5. A buffy coat can be prepared from a venous blood sample and stained with H&E, Diff-Quik, or Wright's Giemsa. The cytoplasma of white blood cells, especially of circulating lymphocytes, should be examined for the presence of inclusion bodies.
6. Collection of biopsy specimens is the most useful tool for the diagnosis of IBD. Biopsies can be collected from a variety of different organs, fixed in 10% formalin, and submitted for histopathologic evaluation. Most commonly, biopsies of the liver, stomach, esophageal tonsils, and skin are evaluated (Figure 60-8). Biopsies of the stomach and distal esophagus can be collected with fiberoptic equipment, and biopsies of the liver can either be obtained with ultrasound guidance[15] or with surgery. In one study, wedge biopsies of the liver were reported to be the best method for the diagnosis of IBD.[16]

Further diagnostic tests and extended quarantine of the snake are recommended if the previously mentioned tests fail to make a diagnosis. This is especially true for *Python* spp., which commonly lack inclusions in visceral organs.

Postmortem Diagnosis

At present, a definite diagnosis of IBD can only be with histopathology, electron microscopy, and viral isolation and detection of typical inclusions in epithelial cells or demonstration and isolation of the virus.

1. A thorough necropsy and collection of samples of all major organ systems, including brain and spinal cord, should be performed on any snake suspected of IBD. After collection, samples should be placed in 10% neutral buffered formalin (NBF) and submitted for histopathologic evaluation. In addition, sections of all major organs (lung, liver, kidney, pancreas, and spleen) should be frozen at $-70°C$ for future viral isolation attempts.
2. Samples of the brain, liver, kidney, and pancreas can also be processed for electron microscopy and detection of inclusions or viral particles.
3. At present, viral isolation is the most accurate technique for diagnosis of IBD. However, only a few laboratories have the expertise and equipment to process reptilian cell cultures. A qualified laboratory should be contacted before necropsy to verify processing and handling of diagnostic specimen.

CLINICAL MANAGEMENT AND TREATMENT

At present, no known treatment exists for IBD. Supportive therapy of a suspected or confirmed case of IBD should be determined from a management point of view. Although a single pet snake with IBD may receive supportive therapy, every attempt should be made to limit outbreaks in collections of boid snakes. In the latter, every suspected and exposed snake should be isolated from the rest of the collection and diagnostic tests should be performed as described previously. The most important step to prevent introduction of the agent into an established collection is a strict quarantine protocol and strict hygiene. Because nonboid snakes may serve as carriers of the disease, they should be kept separated from boid snakes.

Although infected *Python* spp. are often presented with severe neurologic signs and are diagnosed in earlier stages of the infection, *Boa* spp. represent a major challenge to the clinician because of unspecific clinical signs. Especially, chronically infected Boas may not develop noticeable clinical signs in early stages of the disease and may potentially introduce the agent into the collection. Confirmed cases of boas with IBD have been observed for more than 1 year without development of clinical signs suggestive of IBD. This represents a major problem regarding the recommended length of quarantine. Although a quarantine period of 3 months is recommended for all reptile species, a minimum of 6 months for boas and pythons may be safer and is recommended for large and valuable collections. During quarantine, strict hygiene procedures should be followed to prevent possible spread of the agent through the collection.

No treatment exists for IBD. Supportive care, including adequate fluid therapy for dehydrated patients, nutritional support, and antimicrobial treatment for secondary bacterial infections, does not alter the course of the disease. Infected snakes eventually succumb to the disease, and euthanasia of confirmed cases is recommended to prevent further spread of the infection.[17]

PREVENTION AND CONTROL

Because no known treatment exists for IBD, prevention of introduction of the agent into an established collection of snakes is critical. Once introduced, the agent often spreads rapidly within a collection, especially in *Python* spp. During an outbreak, no snake should be allowed to enter or leave the collection. All incoming snakes, including nonboid snakes, into a collection of boid snakes should be quarantined for at least 6 months. A distinct possibility exists that the agent responsible for IBD may not cause the same clinical and pathologic changes (e.g., formation of eosinophilic inclusions) in nonboid snakes as it does in boid species. Therefore, this disease may go undetected in these animals. Because *Boa* spp. are often unidentified carriers of IBD, they should be kept separate from *Python* spp. and a strict hygiene protocol should be followed.

Before acquisition of a new snake or shipment of snakes, a detailed history of the origin and potential exposure to other snakes should be obtained. In cases in which no such information is available, the potential risk to the existing collection should be considered.

During quarantine, a thorough physical examination should be performed, fecal samples examined, and a venous blood sample collected at the beginning and the end of quarantine for hematologic and plasma biochemistry determinations. Ideally, the quarantine facility should be a separate building from the main collection and footbaths should be used before entering and after leaving the facility. If the main collection and the quarantine facility are in the same building, no exchange of airflow should occur between the two and utensils should not be shared between facilities.

An apparently "poor doing" (chronic weight loss, lethargy, persistent or reoccurring bacterial infections, etc.) snake should never be introduced into the collection, even if diagnostic tests are inconclusive. All snakes that die during quarantine or that are euthanized should be necropsied, and samples from all major organs should be collected for histopathology and future studies. An apparently sick snake should never be introduced into the collection. At the end

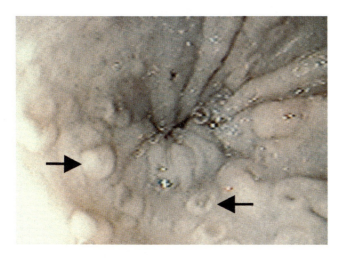

FIGURE 60-8 Endoscopic demonstration of prominent esophageal tonsils in the distal esophagus of a Boa Constrictor (*Boa constrictor* sp.) with inclusion body disease.

of the quarantine period, all cages and equipment should be thoroughly disinfected.

Sick snakes or snakes with unspecific clinical signs should be removed from the collection and kept in isolation for diagnostic workup and treatment. Confirmed carriers of IBD should be euthanized and submitted for histopathology. All cage furniture that has been in contact with infected snakes should be either discarded or disinfected. Effective disinfectants include sodium hypochlorite and chlorhexidine (see Chapter 85).

REFERENCES

1. Axthelm MK: Viral encephalitis of boid snakes, *Proc Int Colloq Pathol Reptil Amphib* 3:25, 1989.
2. Jacobson ER: Viral diseases of reptiles. In Fowler ME, editor: *Zoo & wild animal medicine, current therapy 3*, Philadelphia, 1993, WB Saunders.
3. Konstantinov A, Ippen R: Erythroleukosis with presence of virus particles in two Boa Constrictors, *Proc Int Colloq Pathol Reptil Amphib* 1:123-128, 1982.
4. Schumacher J, Jacobson ER, Homer BL, et al: Inclusion body disease in boid snakes, *J Zoo Wildl Med* 25(4):511-524, 1994.
5. Schumacher J: Viral diseases. In Mader DR, editor: *Reptile medicine and surgery*, Philadelphia, 1996, WB Saunders.
6. Carlisle-Nowak MS, Sullivan N, Carrigan M, et al: Inclusion body disease in two captive Australian pythons (*Morelia spilota variegata* and *Morelia spilota spilota*), *Aust Vet J* 76:98-100, 1998.
7. Jacobson ER, Klingenberg RJ, Homer BL, et al: Inclusion body disease: roundtable discussion, *Bull Assoc Reptil Amphib Vet* 9(2):18-25, 1999.
8. Garner MM, Raymond JT, Nordhausen RW, et al: Inclusion body disease in captive palm vipers, *Bothriechis marchi*, *Proceedings Association of Reptile and Amphibian Veterinarians*, Reno, Nevada, 2000.
9. Raymond JT, Garner MM, Nordhausen RW, et al: A disease resembling inclusion body disease of boid snakes in captive palm vipers (*Bothriechis marchi*), *J Vet Diagn Invest* 13:82-86, 2001.
10. Jacobson ER, Tucker S, Oros J, et al: Studies with retroviruses isolated from Boa Constrictors, *Boa constrictor*, with inclusion body disease, *Proceedings Association of Reptile and Amphibian Veterinarians*, Columbus, Ohio, 1999.
11. Jacobson ER, Oros J, Tucker SJ, et al: Partial characterization of retroviruses from boid snakes with inclusion body disease, *Am J Vet Res* 62:217-224, 2001.
12. Lock BA, Green LG, Jacobson ER, et al: Enzyme-linked immunosorbent assay for detecting the antibody response in Argentine Boa Constrictors (*Boa constrictor occidentalis*), *Am J Vet Res* 64:388-395, 2003.
13. Wozniak E, McBride J, DeNardo D, et al: Isolation and characterization of an antigenically distinct 68-kd protein from nonviral intracytoplasmic inclusions in Boa Constrictors chronically infected with the inclusion body disease virus (IBDV: Retroviridae), *Vet Pathol* 37:449-459, 2000.
14. Fleming GJ, Heard DJ, Jacobson ER, et al: Cytoplasmic inclusions in corn snakes, *Elaphe guttata*, resembling inclusion body disease of boid snakes, *J Herp Med Surg* 13:18-22, 2003.
15. Isaza R, Ackerman N, Schumacher J: Ultrasound-guided percutaneous liver biopsy in snakes, *Vet Rad Ultra* 34(6):452, 1993.
16. Garner MM, Raymond JT: Methods for diagnosing inclusion body disease in snakes, *Proceedings Association of Reptilian and Amphibian Veterinarians*, Naples, Fla, 2004.
17. Schumacher J, Jacobson ER: Inclusion body disease in boid snakes: a review, *American Association of Zoo Veterinarians, infectious disease manual*, 1999.

61
METABOLIC BONE DISEASES

DOUGLAS R. MADER

Metabolic bone diseases are common in captive herpetofauna. In fact, in the author's veterinary practice, this group of diseases accounts for a majority of patient veterinary visits. **The term** *metabolic bone disease (MBD)* **is not actually a single disease entity but rather a term used to describe a collection of medical disorders that affect the integrity and function of bones.** Many different types of metabolic bone diseases (Table 61-1) affect both animals and humans alike. In an effort to maintain purity in medical description, the terms *metabolic bone disease* and *MBD* should NOT be used to describe diseases of herpetofauna unless accompanied by a qualifier such as "nutritional" or "renal" (e.g., the Green Iguana [*Iguana iguana*] had metabolic bone disease of nutritional origin). Hereafter, MBD of nutritional origin is referred to as NMBD and of renal origin as RMBD.

Nutritional secondary hyperparathyroidism (NSHP) is the most common MBD diagnosed in captive herpetofauna. Thus, most of this chapter discusses NMBD; however, RMBD and other documented cases of metabolic bone diseases in reptiles are also reviewed.

NUTRITIONAL SECONDARY HYPERPARATHYROIDISM

"Rubber jaw" is the lay term often used in the pet stores and herpetologic societies. Although this term is not technically correct, the origin of "rubber jaw" comes from the fact that animals with NSHP often have grotesque facial deformities that usually affect and soften the lower jaw (Figure 61-1).

Nutritional secondary hyperparathyroidism occurs as a result of dietary or husbandry mismanagement. The most commonly implicated factors are a prolonged deficiency of dietary calcium or vitamin D_3, an imbalance of the calcium-to-phosphorus ratio in the diet (usually an excess of phosphorus), or inadequate exposure to ultraviolet (UV) radiation in diurnal animals.

Nutritional secondary hyperparathyroidism can potentially affect all reptilian and amphibian species, but it is most commonly described in lizards and aquatic turtles (Figure 61-2).[1] Animals that eat a whole animal diet, such as the snakes, typically are more likely to receive balanced nutrition. NSHP is common in the Green Iguana, and although their diets have been studied in the wild,[2] nutritionally balanced captive diets, coupled with comprehensive applied husbandry in captivity, have yet to be fully elucidated. Chapter 18 discusses recommended diets for the various reptile groups and offers tables that describe nutritive values of various feedstuffs.

Under natural conditions, the body synthesizes its own vitamin D when it is exposed to sunlight. Light from the ultraviolet spectrum (290 to 320 nm) reacts with the body's skin to convert cholesterol to the inactive form of vitamin D. This vitamin D is then converted to a hormone called 1,25 dihydroxycholecalciferol (1,25-DHCC) through pathways involving the liver and kidneys. The active form of 1,25-DHCC is used by the body to facilitate absorption of calcium from the intestinal tract (Figure 61-3).

Table 61-1	Examples of Different Types of Common Metabolic Bone Diseases in Mammals

*Fibrous osteodystrophy
Hypertrophic osteodystrophy
*Hypertrophic osteopathy
*Nutritional secondary hyperparathyroidism
*Osteomalacia
*Osteopetrosis
Osteoporosis
*Paget's disease
Panosteitis
*Renal secondary hyperparathyroidism
Rickets

*Reported in reptiles.

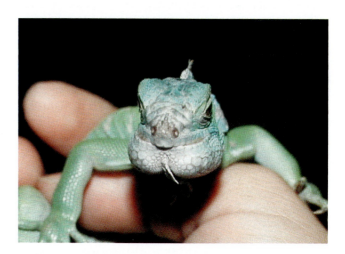

FIGURE 61-1 A Juvenile Green Iguana (*Iguana iguana*) with advanced metabolic bone disease (MBD) from nutritional secondary hyperparathyroidism (NSHP). This image represents the "classic" presentation of nutritional MBD (NMBD). However, what is seen here is actually an advanced state of the disease. Early signs are much more subtle.

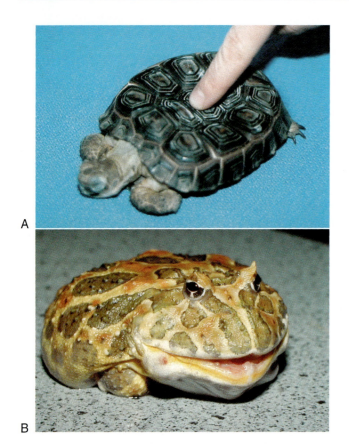

FIGURE 61-2 Nutritional metabolic bone disease (NMBD) affects all herp species, including tortoises **(A)**, such as this juvenile California Desert Tortoise *(Gopherus agassizii)*, and amphibians **(B)**, such as this Argentine Horned Frog *(Ceratophrys ornata)*.

In the wild, exposure to natural sunlight is not a problem for most diurnal animals. Animals in a captive environment do not always get the proper exposure to natural unobstructed sunlight. Important to note is that the part of the spectrum of ultraviolet light that is necessary for vitamin D synthesis in the skin may be filtered out as it passes through ordinary glass. Animals kept in aquaria next to a window that is exposed to sunlight may not get adequate ultraviolet light and as a result are unable to synthesize the needed vitamin D. Fortunately, a type of window glass is now available that permits approximately 80% of the natural UV light to pass through to the animal on the other side.

An alternative to natural sunlight is artificial light that mimics the spectrum of natural light. A number of artificial lighting systems are available that provide an ultraviolet light spectrum that simulates natural sunlight (see Table 18-12 and Chapter 84). Although they are advertised as mimicking natural sunlight, one should note that not all of these lights actually produce the necessary wavelengths required to stimulate vitamin D synthesis in the skin. Several excellent lights are available to reptile and amphibian owners.

Even with the best lights on the market, one should remember that they are NOT a replacement for natural sunlight (Figure 61-4). In addition, when positioning these lights in the animal's cage, placement of the lights close enough that they are still effective is crucial. All ultraviolet light sources should be placed within 16 to 24 inches of the animal for maximum effect (consult the directions on the product). On a final note, these fluorescent lights need to be replaced every 6 to 12 months because the ultraviolet output decreases with use (follow manufacturer's recommendations for set-up details and bulb replacement schedules).

In situations in which the animal cannot be provided with proper exposure to ultraviolet light, vitamin D must be supplemented in the diet. The two major analogues of vitamin D are vitamin D_2 and vitamin D_3. Plants synthesize vitamin D_2, and mammals synthesize vitamin D_3. Most mammals can use both forms of the vitamins. Whether reptiles are able to use vitamin D_2 is not known, and some researchers believe that certain reptiles are not able to use oral vitamin D_3 at all. Therefore, until further research is done, only the vitamin D_3 form should be used as a dietary supplement. See Chapter 18 for a more thorough discussion of vitamin D.

Physiologic Response to Nutritional Secondary Hyperparathyroidism

In NSHP, an excessive production is seen of parathyroid hormone from the parathyroid gland in response to the diet/management-induced hypocalcemia.[3] Calcium is resorbed from the bones to compensate for the deficiency. The resulting osteopenia weakens the integrity of the bones. If this condition occurs in a young growing animal, it is called rickets. If it occurs in an adult, it is referred to as osteomalacia.[3]

Laboratory findings of low normal blood calcium levels are common in NSHP.[4] As the blood calcium levels drop, parathyroid hormone (PTH) is released from the parathyroid glands, which increases blood calcium by increasing bone resorption, increasing renal tubular reabsorption of calcium, and simultaneously increasing phosphate excretion in the urine. PTH also stimulates formation of 1,25 dihydroxycholecalciferol, which increases absorption of intestinal calcium (see Figure 61-3).[4]

Calcium deficits cause partial depolarization of nerves and muscle because of an increase in the threshold potential.[3,4] Resultant symptoms (in humans) include confusion, paresthesias around the mouth and in the digits, carpopedal spasms, and hyperreflexia.[3] Similar (clinical) signs are presumed to occur in reptile patients. "Playing the piano" is a common phrase used to describe the rhythmic twitching of the digits seen in iguanas.

An increase in neuromuscular excitability, caused by hypocalcemia, can account for the reptile's spastic tremors when stimulated with a pinch of a digit. Snakes fed a "pinkie"-only diet (consisting of only neonatal mice) have been reported to exhibit signs of tremors, disorientation, and ataxia (see Chapter 17).

In humans, intestinal cramping and bloating result from the effects of the hypocalcemia on the smooth muscle of the gastrointestinal tract.[3] Cloacal prolapse, from hypocalcemia, is a common finding in the young Iguana (Figure 61-5). See Chapter 47 for a comprehensive review of treatment for cloacal prolapse.

Young animals with active bone growth are the most affected. No typical presentations of the disease are found. Affected animals may show any or all of the following: thickening and swelling of the long bones and mandibles (fibrous osteodystrophy), pathologic fractures of the long bones

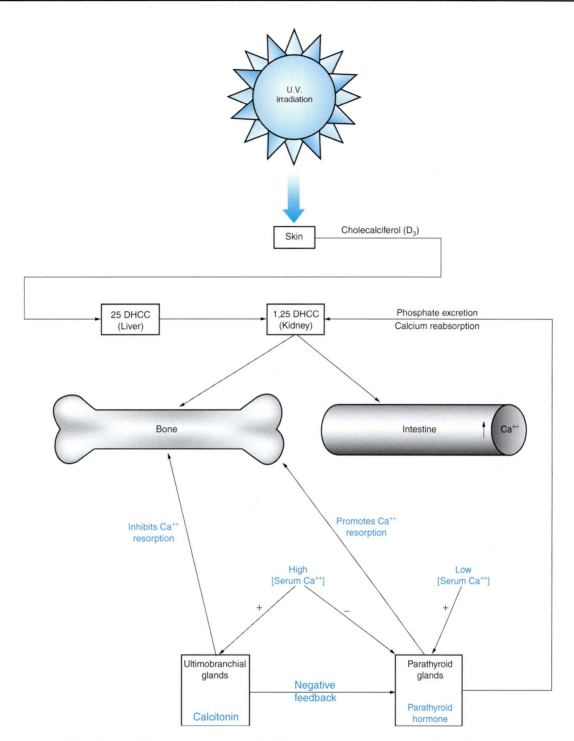

FIGURE 61-3 Physiologic interrelationship between Ca^{++}, calcitonin, and parathyroid hormone.

and spine (generally seen with 40% or greater loss of bone mass), horizontal (rather than the normal vertical) rotation of the scapulae, tetany (clinical hypocalcemia), muscle fasciculations, hyperreflexia, cloacal or rectal prolapse, anorexia, inability to ambulate (carpal walking), and stunted growth (Figures 61-6 to 61-10). The severity of presenting signs depends on a number of factors, including extent of the disease, the age and type of patient, and the experience of the owner at recognizing early signs of trouble.

Clinical differentials for NSHP must include renal secondary hyperparathyroidism, hypertrophic osteopathy, osteomyelitis (bacterial and fungal), and diffuse osteomalacia.

Treatment of Nutritional Secondary Hyperparathyroidism

Numerous reviews and suggested treatments of NSHP have appeared in recent literature.[5] Initial therapy of NSHP

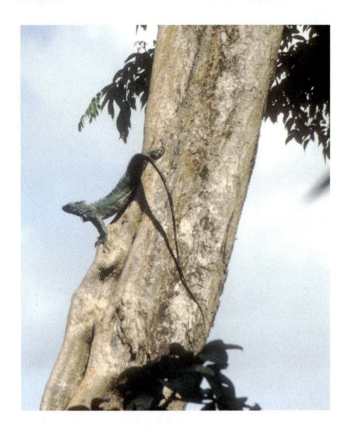

FIGURE 61-4 In the wild, most diurnal animals live for the sunshine. Many excellent artificial lights are on the market, but nothing replaces natural sunlight.

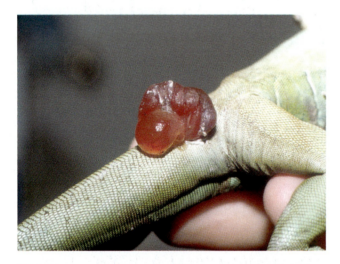

FIGURE 61-5 A common early sign of nutritional metabolic bone disease (NMBD) is cloacal prolapse. Calcium is critical to maintaining normal gastrointestinal peristalsis. In hypocalcemia, intestinal stasis occurs, resulting in bloating, which results in prolapse. These conditions are commonly diagnosed as a prolapse from internal parasites, and the calcium homeostasis is frequently ignored during treatment.

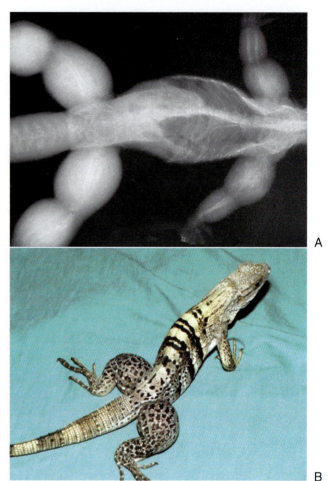

FIGURE 61-6 **A,** Radiograph of a Green Iguana (*Iguana iguana*) with severe nutritional metabolic bone disease (NMBD). Note the productive periosteal changes so typical of advanced fibrous osteodystrophy. **B,** Severe fibrous osteodystrophy in a Spiny-tailed Iguana (*Ctenosaura pectinata*). Note how the thighs appear to be "fat." This is from the fibrous connective tissue that has been deposited around the hypomineralized bones.

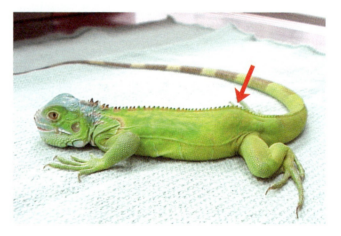

FIGURE 61-7 Pathological spinal fracture (*red arrow*) from nutritional metabolic bone disease (NMBD) in a juvenile Green Iguana (*Iguana iguana*).

generally centers around the treatment of life-threatening disorders (such as hypocalcemic tetany) and splinting or supporting pathologic fractures.

Historically, the main focus on treatment for NSHP has been to correct husbandry and nutritional problems and

Metabolic Bone Disorders 845

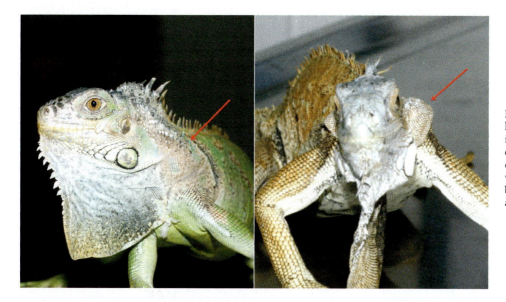

FIGURE 61-8 The scapula on a healthy Green Iguana (*Iguana iguana*) is vertical *(red arrow, left picture)*. In early nutritional metabolic bone disease (NMBD), the bones soften, with a resultant bowing of the flat bone, giving a more horizontal appearance *(red arrow, right picture)*.

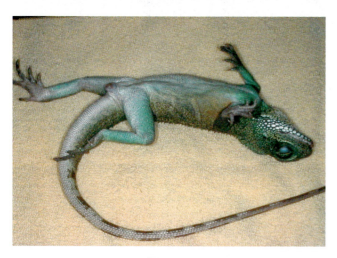

FIGURE 61-9 Hypocalcemic tetany, loss of balance, and inability to right itself are all signs of hypocalcemia, the prelude to nutritional metabolic bone disease (NMBD). *(Photograph courtesy R. Funk.)*

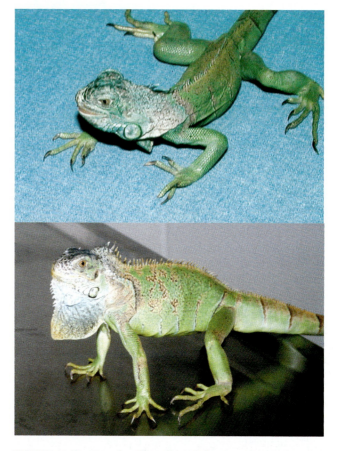

FIGURE 61-10 Carpal walking *(top)* in this juvenile Green Iguana (*Iguana iguana*) is another early sign of nutritional metabolic bone disease (NMBD), seen long before the typical fibrous osteodystrophy of the long bones and jaws as seen in Figures 61-1 and 61-5. Normal Iguanas walk on their toes *(bottom)*.

provide exposure to natural sunlight. However, this is often not enough, especially in severe cases of NSHP.

With chronic NSHP, stimulation of the parathyroid glands causes a compensatory parathyroid hypertrophy.[3] Of particular significance with this parathyroid hypertrophy is the loss of the negative feedback influence by increasing levels of serum calcium on the continued production of parathyroid hormone from the hypertrophied (overactive) parathyroid gland.

Immediate treatment goals for NSHP should focus on reversing the bone loss and promoting new bone production. For this to be accomplished, the deleterious effects of the parathyroid gland must be reversed.

Blood calcium concentration is mediated by a feedback system that involves two hormones. Low blood calcium stimulates PTH secretion. When the blood calcium concentration is above normal, PTH secretion is halted and calcitonin, which is produced from the ultimobranchial bodies, increases.[4]

Calcitonin lowers circulating calcium and phosphorus through negative feedback on the parathyroid gland, thus ceasing the production of parathormone and inhibiting bone resorption. A decrease is seen in osteoclast activity and number, as is a stimulatory effect on osteoblast bone formation.

Table 61-2	Effects of Synthetic Salmon Calcitonin in Mammals

Inhibition of osteoclastic activity (negative feedback on the parathyroid gland to stop production of parathyroid hormone).
Stimulation of osteoblasts.
Decreased blood calcium concentration with increased urinary calcium excretion.
Salmon calcitonin (SCT) is also reported to have an analgesic effect against skeletal pain. This results from SCT's ability to stabilize or augment bone mass, change the skeletal blood flow, stimulate endogenous endorphin production, and directly affect the pain centers in the brain.

Table 61-3	Standard Protocol for Treatment of Nutritional Secondary Hyperparathyroidism (NSHP) in Green Iguanas *(Iguana iguana)* with Salmon Calcitonin (SCT)
Initial visit	Evaluate patient (include radiographs) Determine plasma [calcium] 400 IU/kg, IM, Vitamin D_3 23 mg/kg Calcium glubionate, PO, BID Support patient (tube feeding, etc.) Correct diet, housing, etc.
1-Week follow-up	2nd Vitamin D_3 injection (400 IU/kg, IM) 1st Calcitonin injection (50 IU/kg, IM)* Continue with calcium glubionate Continue with supportive care
2-Week follow-up	2nd Calcitonin injection (50 IU/kg, IM) Supportive care as needed

*Hypocalcemic patients or patients with low normal plasma calcium should not receive calcitonin until their calcium level has been stabilized. Calcitonin can potentially cause acute hypocalcemia and death if administered in patients with marginal plasma calcium values. Never give calcitonin to a patient that has not had its calcium level stabilized.
IM, Intramuscularly; *PO*, orally; *BID*, twice daily.

Calcitonin also decreases blood calcium concentration by increasing urinary calcium excretion (Table 61-2).[4,6]

A synthetic calcitonin, called Salmon Calcitonin (SCT), has been used successfully to treat osteoporosis in women who are postmenopausal.[6,7] Synthetic SCT, which has been approved by the U.S. Food and Drug Administration for the treatment of MBDs in humans since 1975, is modeled after the salmon calcitonin molecule and is 40 to 50 times more potent than human calcitonin.[7]

On the basis of the effectiveness of calcitonin in the therapy for osteoporosis in women and the similarity between human and reptilian calcitonin molecules,[8] similar applications have been used with success in the Green Iguana for the treatment of NSHP.[9]

In humans, the dose of SCT for the treatment of osteoporosis is 100 IU daily to every other day for a minimum of 2 years.[7] The dose of SCT used in the Green Iguana is 50 IU of SCT, given once per week for 2 weeks. On the basis of the clinical and radiographic response to SCT treatment in several hundred patients in a clinical setting, this dose appears to be adequate.[9] Some Iguanas with severe chronic fibrous osteodystrophy may on occasion require a third dose. See Table 61-3 for a guideline for the treatment of NSHP.

The side effects of SCT in humans include anorexia, nausea, vomiting, skin flushing, nonspecific rash, urticaria, polyuria, pruritus, and edema.[7] The amino acid sequence of synthetic SCT is not the same as that in human calcitonin. As a result, an antibody response in humans (as evidenced by a type I hypersensitivity reaction) to SCT after chronic administration lasting longer than 6 months is not uncommon.[7] Because the duration of treatment with SCT for NSHP in iguanas is substantially shorter than it is for osteoporosis, an antibody response is unlikely and to date has not been reported.

The administration of calcitonin does have the potential of causing life-threatening hypocalcemic tetany in reptiles. Because of this, SCT should not be given to a patient with unknown or suspected low blood calcium levels. If owner compliance prevents proper preadministration screening, then one is wise to start the patient on appropriate supplements. Vitamin D_3 and supplemental calcium, preferably oral, should be given for at least 3 days before dosing with SCT (see Table 61-2 for specific instructions).

Patients with hypocalcemic tetany should be treated for the hypocalcemia before the bone pathology is addressed. Animals in tetany should be treated with appropriate fluid therapy, warmth, calorie replacement, and a calcium supplement. If tetany is present, calcium gluconate, 10%, can be administered at 100 mg/kg intramuscularly or intracoelomically every 6 hours until the tetany ceases. Once the tetany stops, the patient should be switched over to oral calcium supplementation with calcium glubionate.

There is never any justification to treat ANY bone pathology with injectable calcium. Aside from being a dangerous practice, calcium injections have been shown to be painful to the patient and most importantly, can cause permanent damage to the patient's kidneys at high dosages. Long-term therapy for NSHP should only be conducted with appropriate oral vitamin and mineral supplementation.

Historically, patients with NSHP typically take 4 to 6 months of intensive supportive care to recover from NSHP. Now, with SCT therapy in conjunction with standard therapies, patients are responding in 4 to 6 weeks.

In addition, in humans, SCT is also reported to have an analgesic effect against skeletal pain. This results from SCT's ability to stabilize or augment bone mass, change the skeletal blood flow, stimulate endogenous endorphin production, and directly affect the pain centers in the brain.[7] This may be an additional benefit with use of SCT in the treatment of MBD in reptiles.

Wagner and Bodri[10] reported that a single dose of SCT (50 IU/kg) had no effect on calcium concentrations on a long-term basis. Unfortunately, the researchers evaluated total plasma calcium concentrations, not ionized calcium. SCT exerts its effects on ionized calcium, not protein-bound calcium (as evidenced by the immediate hypocalcemic tetany seen after injection of SCT in a debilitated patient). Tetanic animals that have been dosed with SCT respond immediately to intravenous calcium supplementation.

In summary, SCT should not be used in cases of hypocalcemia. Its best use is in patients with NSHP that have clinically apparent bone involvement, such as softening or swelling of the long bones or the mandible that results from osteoclastic bone resorption.[11] SCT should not be used alone

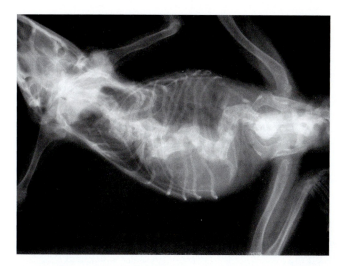

FIGURE 61-11 This radiograph shows a severe scoliosis in an adult female Green Iguana *(Iguana iguana)* with severe nutritional metabolic bone disease (NMBD) as a juvenile. Although these animals can survive, certain behaviors and activities, such as oviposition (with or without breeding), can be a problem at maturity. These females benefit from a salpingectomy while young.

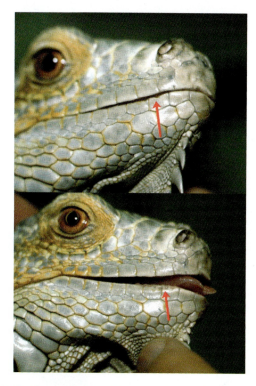

FIGURE 61-12 Mandibular deformities that result from nutritional metabolic bone disease (NMBD) usually never completely resolve. Adult animals with chronic ptyalism as a result of subtle malocclusions that resulted from NMBD while a juvenile are not uncommon. The *red arrows* point to impressions left on the labium from the opposing dental arcade.

but as an adjunct to proper medical care, and most importantly, coinciding with necessary corrections in the animal's husbandry and diet.

Prognosis for Nutritional Secondary Hyperparathyroidism

Depending on the degree of involvement, the prognosis for patients with NSHP varies from good to grave. As mentioned, NSHP starts with the effects of hypocalcemia long before pathologic changes to the bony skeleton occur. Tremors, hyperreflexiveness, ataxia, and cloacal prolapses are all early signs. Fibrous osteodystrophy, pathologic fractures, and paralysis suggest significant disease and carry a much worse prognosis.

Important to note is that reptiles have an amazing ability to heal. Even animals with severe scoliosis (S-shaped spinal deformities) may survive (Figure 61-11). They may be deformed for the rest of their lives, but, as a pet, they do just fine.

A common consequence of NSHP and the resultant mandibular fibrous osteodystrophy of the lower jaw is malocclusion. These animals often have chronic gingivitis and ptyalism (because the jaws and lips do not meet in the normal fashion; Figure 61-12). This condition is not an antibiotic responsive problem but rather a husbandry/maintenance challenge. Daily applications of a quality petrolatum lip balm over the exposed areas usually prevent the continuance of the gingivitis.

The misshapen jaws, so commonly seen with NSHP, usually do not return to normal. All sorts of facial deformities are noted as the animal matures (Figure 61-13). However, once again, in captivity, these deformities are no reason to euthanize a pet. It is prudent to advise the owner that, even with successful treatment, the prognosis for their pet to return to a morphologically normal specimen is unlikely. Documentation of this, including photographs of the deformities, should be made in the medical record.

Female lizards and turtles that have had severe spinal-deforming NSHP as a juvenile may have a second problem facing them as they mature. Once they reach maturity, oftentimes they have difficulty laying eggs because of the damage and deformity of the pelvic canals (the eggs do not pass through; see Figure 61-11). These patients may benefit from elective ovariosalpingectomy.

For paralyzed animals, if a spinal fracture has occurred and if the animal has lost its ability to urinate and defecate, this author recommends that the owners think about euthanasia. Note that in early stages of the disease, an animal can be urinary or fecal incontinent, but as therapy progresses, they may regain the function of the bladder and bowel. Owners are encouraged to give the animal several weeks before they make a decision to euthanize.

Some owners want to try and offer continual nursing care to these paralyzed patients. The owners can be taught to give enemas and pass urinary catheters for some of these chronic spinal animals. These incontinent patients usually have ascending urinary tract infections develop over time and often die of renal failure from pyelonephritis.

METABOLIC BONE DISEASES OF NON-NUTRITIONAL ORIGIN

Renal Secondary Hyperparathyroidism

Hyperphosphatemia is the hallmark of renal secondary hyperparathyroidism (RSHP), a consequence of chronic renal

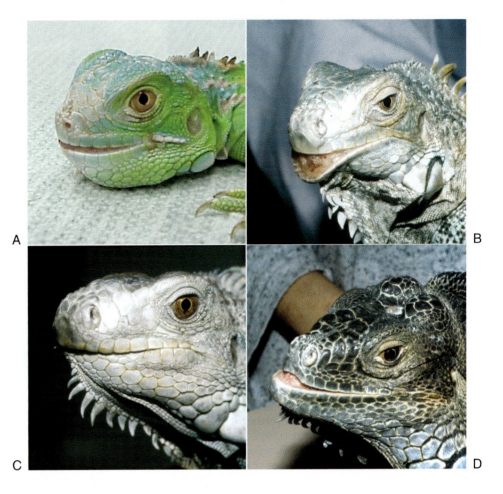

FIGURE 61-13 The many faces of juvenile (A) and adult (B to D) postnutritional metabolic bone disease (NMBD) facial deformities.

disease. The hyperphosphatemia is associated with reduced calcitriol levels, soft tissue calcification, renal osteodystrophy, and hypocalcemia.

Phosphorus is absorbed from the gastrointestinal tract and eliminated via the kidneys. Excretion of phosphorus is a sum of glomerular filtration and tubular resorption. In renal failure, decreasing filtration rate leads to phosphorus retention and hyperphosphatemia.

Calcitriol, the most active form of vitamin D in mammals, is formed by renal hydroxylation of 25-hydroxycholecalciferol. This hydroxylation reaction is promoted by parathyroid hormone. The elevated phosphates have a negative effect on the hydroxylase activity in renal tubular cells. In turn, because elevated calcitriol normally has a negative feedback effect on PTH production, this decreased calcitriol formation, which results from the hyperphosphatemia, promotes RSHP and osteodystrophy (Figure 61-14).

Phosphate retention also decreases extracellular calcium as a result of the mass law equation. In addition, the decreased production of calcitriol further limits absorption of calcium from the intestinal tract. These changes result in low normal or low serum calcium levels.

See Chapter 66 for diagnostics and treatment of renal disease.

Differentials for RSHP must include NSHP, hypertrophic osteopathy (HO), and osteomyelitis (bacterial and fungal).

Hypertrophic Osteopathy

Although not common, HO has been reported in lizards.[12] In mammals, HO, formerly called hypertrophic pulmonary osteoarthropathy or hypertrophic osteoarthropathy, is characterized by lameness, painful limbs, and reluctance to move. Pulmonary pathology has been associated with this condition in greater than 90% of the cases.

Radiographic signs consist of extensive periosteal proliferation beginning in the distal long bones and progressing proximally (digits proximal to the humerus or femur; Figures 61-15 and 61-16). The pathogenesis is unknown, but theories include chronic anoxia, toxins, and complicated neurologic pathways involving the vagus nerve.

In mammals, once HO has been diagnosed, the condition is usually terminal. If an identifiable thoracic mass is found, resection may result in temporary resolution of the clinical signs, which may take several months to regress.

Differentials for HO must include NSHP, RSHP, gout, tumoral calcinosis (pseudogout), and osteomyelitis (bacterial and fungal).

Osteopetrosis

Osteopetrosis (OP) is a rare hereditary disease in humans. Two forms, one an autosomal recessive and the second an autosomal dominant, cause excessive thickening of the

Metabolic Bone Disorders   849

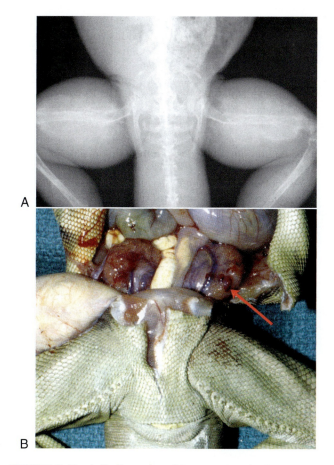

FIGURE 61-14 **A,** Radiograph and **B,** prosection of a Green Iguana *(Iguana iguana)* with severe, advanced, renal metabolic bone disease (RMBD). The *arrow* points to the cranial pole of the massively enlarged kidneys.

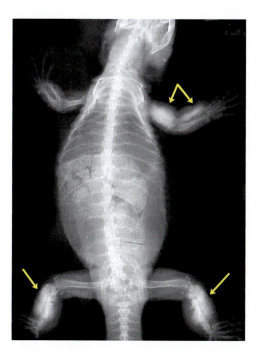

FIGURE 61-15 Hypertrophic osteopathy (HO) in a Black and White Tegu *(Tupinambus teguixin)*. Note the odd distribution of lesions, that they do not include the joints, and their general difference in appearance to the fibrous osteodystrophy seen in nutritional metabolic bone disease (NMBD) or renal MBD (RMBD; see Figures 61-5 and 61-13).

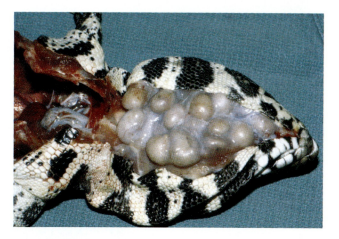

FIGURE 61-16 Lesions (abscesses) in the gular region from the same animal with the hypertrophic osteopathy (HO) lesions in Figure 61-15.

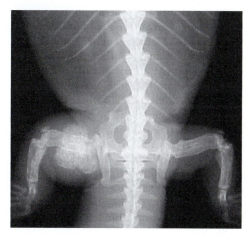

FIGURE 61-17 Osteopetrosis (OP) lesions in a Savannah Monitor *(Varanus exanthematicus)*. Note the solid cortices and medullary cavities. The bones become brittle and fracture easily. A pathologic fracture of the left femur is seen. Note the intense periosteal reaction at the fracture site. *(Radiograph courtesy M. Koob.)*

bones. The bones become radiographically dense, eventually obliterating the marrow cavity (Figure 61-17). The cause is not known but is believed to be an inability to resorb bone in a normal fashion. Because the marrow cavity is destroyed, the patients become anemic. Nerve foramina in the skull become diminished, which leads to blindness and hearing impairments. The bones become brittle and fracture easily.

Cases of osteopetrosis in reptiles in this author's practice (unpublished), with radiologic diagnosis only, have had similar clinical presentations.

In birds, similar signs are seen as a result of avian leukosis virus infection. A parallel situation in reptile patients has not been identified but has been suggested in earlier literature.

Differentials for OP must include NSHP, RSHP, HO, osteomyelitis (bacterial and fungal), excessive dietary supplementation of vitamin D, and calcium and inappropriate nutrition.

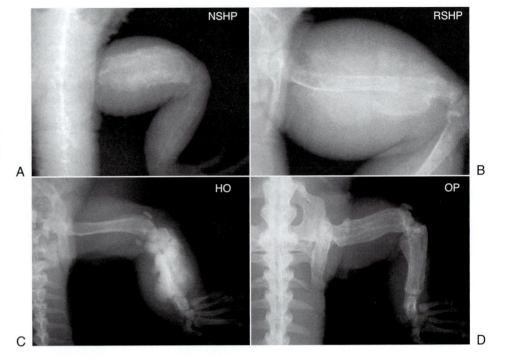

FIGURE 61-18 Radiographic comparison of the femurs of four common reptilian metabolic bone diseases (MBDs).

Paget's Disease

A Paget's disease (PD)–like condition has been reported numerous times in the reptilian literature.[1] In humans, this condition, also known as osteitis deformans, results from repeated cycles of bone resorption and deposition. The bone eventually becomes dense and brittle. Pain and pathologic fractures are common (see Figure 69-5).

In people, many cases are asymptomatic. The diagnosis is made through radiographs, physical examination, and laboratory testing. The cause is not known, but research at the National Institutes of Health (NIH) suggests the possibility of a slow virus being involved. Genetic influence may also play a role.

The primary event in human Paget's disease that is thought to be the cause of the pathology is osteoclastic resorption. Synthetic SCT inhibits this process and has been used extensively in treatment of symptomatic Paget's disease in human patients.[13]

The name *Paget's disease* has been used to described the lesions seen in reptiles for many years. Current opinion and recent studies suggest that this may be an inappropriate term because it is based on the mosaic appearance of the bone changes in humans. In reptiles, this mosaic pattern of bone growth may be a normal feature. In addition, many snakes with this disorder have active inflammatory changes from which bacteria have been isolated, such as *Salmonella, Klebsiella, Morganella*, and *Providencia*, and bacterial osteomyelitis may be a more appropriate term.[14] See Chapter 69 for more information on spinal osteopathy.

Differentials for PD must include gout, fibrous osteodystrophy, trauma, tumors (usually solitary), and tumoral calcinosis. Lesions so noted in reptile patients should be properly evaluated rather than just assumed to be Paget's disease.

CONCLUSION

As mentioned, the term *metabolic bone disease* is not just a single entity but rather a complex assortment of pathology that affects the integrity and function of the bones. Ostensibly, many of the presentations look alike (Figure 61-18). However, they are very different, each with its own etiology and treatment. A treatment for one may be contraindicated for another (e.g., administration of calcium to a patient with RSHP and elevated phosphorus).

The practitioner should collect a thorough history, perform a complete physical examination, and collect appropriate laboratory tests. A thorough understanding of the different causes of bone pathology helps the clinician diagnose and treat the problem where appropriate or at least provide counseling to the owner regarding prognosis.

REFERENCES

1. Frye FL: *Biomedical and surgical aspects of captive reptile husbandry*, ed 2, Malabar, Fla, 1991, Krieger Publishing.
2. Troyer K: Diet selection and digestion in *Iguana iguana*, the importance of age and nutrient requirements, *Oecologia* 61:201, 1984.
3. McCance KL, Huether SE: *Pathophysiology: the biological basis of disease in adults and children*, St Louis, 1990, CV Mosby Company.
4. Ganong WF: *Review of medical physiology*, Los Altos, Calif, 1981, Lange.

5. Boyer TH: Metabolic bone disease. In Mader DR, editor: *Reptile medicine and surgery*, Philadelphia, 1996, WB Saunders.
6. Riggs BL: Overview of osteoporosis, *West J Med* 154:63, 1991.
7. Wallach S: Calcitonin treatment in osteoporosis, *Female Patient* 17:35, 1992.
8. Kline LW, Longmore GA: Determination of calcitonin in reptilian serum by heterologous radioimmunoassay, *Gen Comp Endocrinol* 61(1):1-4, 1986.
9. Mader DR: Nutritional secondary hyperparathyroidism in Green Iguanas. In Bonagura JD, editor: *Kirk's current veterinary therapy XIII*, Philadelphia, 2000, WB Saunders.
10. Wagner RA, Bodri MS: Injectable calcium dynamics and calcitonin response in Green Iguana (*Iguana iguana*), *Proc Assoc Amphib Rept Vet* 117-118, 1996.
11. Rosol TJ, Taylor JL, Fischbach DG, et al: Effects of daily administration of human parathyroid hormone (1-34) or salmon calcitonin in green iguanas (*Iguana iguana*). In Danks J, Dacke C, Flik G, Gay C, editors: *Calcium metabolism: comparative endocrinology*, Bristol, 1999, Bioscientifica Ltd.
12. Barten SL: Distal leg necrosis in a Green Iguana, *Iguana iguana*, *J Herp Med Surg* 10(1):48-50, 2000.
13. Austin LA, Heath H: Medical progress: calcitonin, *N Engl J Med* 304(5):269-278, 1981.
14. Isaza R, Garner MM, Jacobson E: Proliferative osteoarthritis and osteoarthrosis in 15 snakes, *J Zoo Wildl Med* 31(1): 21-27, 2000.

62
NEUROLOGIC DISORDERS

LISA DONE

Neurologic disorders in reptiles manifest in many ways, from hyperexcitability to lethargy to postural abnormalities to generalized tremors to a completely normal clinical appearance. Apparent neurologic abnormalities in reptiles are common and, when present, usually signify serious underlying disease. However obvious the physical signs may be, they typically are not pathognomonic for any specific system or organ pathology. The reptile clinician must be able to formulate a differential for neurologic symptoms. To facilitate this, grouping these observations by clinical presentation is helpful. The cause of problems may be metabolic, neurologic, or musculoskeletal. Etiologies include infectious, toxic, and degenerative causes. In general, a complete evaluation of the client's husbandry practices is a must.

Neurologic disease may mimic musculoskeletal or metabolic disease, and vice versa, which makes diagnosis difficult (Figure 62-1). Whole body weakness, listing to one side, loss of righting reflex, inability to strike prey, and paresis and paralysis are considered generalized signs. These signs are most likely systemic or neurologic in origin but can result from musculoskeletal disorders. If these signs are present in conjunction with ataxia, seizures, walking in circles, or star gazing, the primary etiology is most likely neurologic. The clinician must use a combination of history, physical examination, laboratory tests, and diagnostic imaging to discern neurologic from musculoskeletal and metabolic origins.

In all reptile species, abnormalities of the head are often the first signs noted by both the owners and the veterinarians. In generalized illness, the head is often the first body part affected. The head, and for the sake of this discussion, the neck can be affected in various ways. Signs may range from tilting of the head (roll) to the twisting of the neck and head, with one side of the head held superior to the other (yaw). Other head postural abnormalities include lateral displacement of the head and neck, dorsoflexion or ventroflexion of the head, or cork-screwing of the neck just caudal to the head (wryneck or torticollis).

Head tilt is usually associated with vestibular disease (peripheral or central), and abnormal head positioning can be related to systemic, metabolic, or central neurologic disease. Unfortunately, most references do not distinguish between the two clinical signs. In general, the head tilt is usually toward the side of the lesion. If circling is present, tight circles generally indicate vestibular lesions (circling toward the side of the lesion). However, movement in the opposite direction has been noted with central vestibular lesions (paradoxic vestibular disease).

Nystagmus, commonly seen in mammals with vestibular or central disease, is uncommon in reptiles. However, strabismus is noted in reptilian patients with cephalic abnormalities and may help localize lesions when identified (Figure 62-2).

Although peripheral abnormalities may be seen unilaterally, they can still be the result of systemic disease. For example, hypocalcemic tetany may appear as muscle spasms in only one limb. Although a peripheral postural abnormality is observed, the underlying disease process is a systemic metabolic disease.

In this chapter, neurologic abnormalities in each reptile order are grouped according to signs. This is followed by a list of differential diagnoses for that sign, suggestions for diagnostic tests, and, when appropriate, suggested therapeutics.

CHELONIANS

Aquatic Signs

Body listing during swimming is a common abnormality in aquatic and semiaquatic turtles (see Figure 40-16). The patient

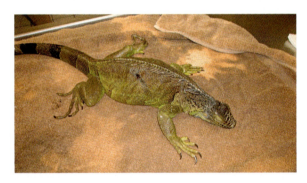

FIGURE 62-1 Neurologic disease can present with many different symptoms. Reptiles are difficult to evaluate neurologically, and as a result, many conditions go undiagnosed, as in the case of this Green Iguana (*Iguana iguana*). The patient had generalized weakness with no apparent cause. (*Photograph courtesy D. Mader.*)

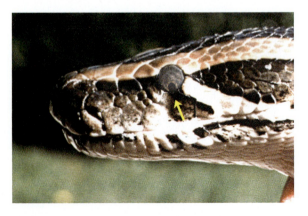

FIGURE 62-2 Strabismus can be a sign of either central nervous system or cranial nerve damage. (*Photograph courtesy D. Mader.*)

typically is seen with an inability to swim or float in a level fashion, usually resulting in a circular swimming pattern. The normal turtle lung acts as an aid in buoyancy. If either lung is compromised, especially if it is consolidated, there is a change in the density of the lung and the turtle lists to the affected side.[1] Bacterial and, less commonly, mycotic pneumonia may be a cause.[2] Radiographs (horizontal beam, craniocaudal, and lateral projections) are the diagnostic test of choice, but hematology, clinical chemistries, lung cytology, and culture are recommended. Treatment is based on the results of sensitivity data, with appropriate antimicrobials. Prognosis for return to normal swimming attitude is guarded because of possible damage from scar tissue in the air spaces, but prognosis for a return to health is good.

Free air in the coelom or intestinal gas can also cause listing in the water. A complete examination is necessary to determine the cause. "Floaters" are a common problem in seaturtles (see Chapter 76). The exact cause often goes undetected.

Whole Body Twitching or Tremors

Muscle tremors or muscle fasciculations are a common condition in many reptiles but are only infrequently seen in chelonians. These can result from systemic disease such as sepsis; central neurologic disease, including cerebral neoplasia; and toxicities. In chelonians, the most common causes of generalized twitching or tremors are nutritional imbalances such as hypocalcemia and thiamin deficiency. The latter occurs in aquatic chelonians that are fed fresh or thawed frozen fish that have significant levels of thiaminase (see Chapter 18). Diagnosis is made on the basis of history and physical signs. Treatment is aimed at correction of the deficiencies.[3-5] Injectable thiamin should be given at 50 to 100 mg/kg daily until resolution of clinical signs. If the thiamin deficiency has caused irreversible damage (e.g., cataracts), the prognosis is guarded at best.

Circling

Circling (in or out of the water) can result from either central or peripheral causes. Lesions associated with the cerebrum usually result in large circles and aimless wandering, whereas brain stem, cerebellar, and vestibular lesions tend to cause tight circling. In general, the animal circles toward the side of the lesion.

Freeze damage (during brumation [hibernation]) can cause toxemia and blindness in chelonians, and as a result, the affected animal may walk in circles.[1,3] Severe inner or middle ear infections have also been implicated in cases of circling.[6] The latter may be accompanied by a head tilt. A thorough history identifies those animals that were brumated (hibernated) in an environment that was too cold. Prognosis depends on the cause and the severity of the condition. For instance, treatment for aural abscesses involves marsupializing the tympanic membrane, curetting and flushing the abscess, and, if indicated, appropriate antibiotic and vitamin therapy (see Chapter 45).

Abnormal Gait or Reluctance to Move

Freeze damage can also cause an abnormal gait or reluctance to move.[3] Trauma, resulting in fractured limbs[4] or compression damage to the carapace with associated injury to the spinal cord, may result in an abnormal gait or reluctance to move.[1,3] Generalized disease, debilitation, and hypothermia should be considered whenever a patient is moribund. Again, a thorough history and physical examination help elucidate the cause of the presenting problems.

Hindlimb-Frontlimb Paresis or Paralysis

Egg binding, constipation, large bladder calculi, and trauma are all potential causes of hindlimb paresis or paralysis in chelonians (Figure 53-2). The paresis or paralysis results when these space-occupying masses put pressure on the internal organs. In addition, conditions such as enlarged kidneys can compress the sciatic nerves and thereby cause hindlimb paresis or the inability to stand.[7] Diagnosis is readily made from radiographs, although a skilled practitioner can usually diagnose these problems with palpation.

Treatment depends on the cause. Egg retention and binding should be managed medically whenever possible (see Chapter 53). Likewise, constipated animals should be properly hydrated and given laxatives, wetting agents, and enemas as needed. If medical treatment is unsuccessful, celiotomy may be necessary (see Chapter 35).

Spinal cord fractures, common manifestations of lawn mower accidents, can cause paralysis.[3,8] Surgical repair of the carapace is possible, but neurologic damage might be so severe that the paralysis may be irreversible. Chelonians are amazing animals. One should not underestimate their ability to recover from seemingly terminal wounds.

Osteomyelitis and osteolysis of the spine and long bones can cause signs that relate to limb paresis or paralysis (Figure 62-3). Diagnosis is from radiographs and, when feasible, from bacterial and fungal cultures of the affected site. If a causal organism can be identified, antibiotics may be effective. Amputation of the affected limb may be necessary in severe cases.[1,3]

Head Tilt and Other Abnormal Head Positions

Head tilts are most commonly associated with vestibular abnormalities. These can be either central (brain stem, cerebellar)

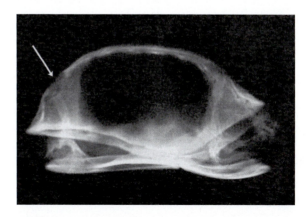

FIGURE 62-3 This Eastern Box Turtle (*Terrapene carolina carolina*) was paralytic in the rear legs. Lateral horizontal beam radiographs showed a lytic lesion in the carapacial bone directly over the spinal cord. This was not apparent on the external physical examination. (*Photograph courtesy D. Mader.*)

or peripheral (inner ear, eighth cranial nerve). In general, the head is tilted toward the side of the lesion (Figure 62-4).

Internal or middle ear infections are common in aquatic and semiaquatic turtles. Although not a common sequela, these infections can cause a head tilt. Usually, aural abscesses are seen as a large swelling on the side of the head, just behind the angle of the jaw (see Chapter 45). Bacterial and mycotic components can be involved.[1,6]

A common site for venipuncture is the jugular vein. Iatrogenic damage to nerves in the vagosympathetic trunk could feasibly cause a head tilt or other abnormal head posture.

A chelonian may hold its head off to the side, without the "tilt," as a result of neurologic damage associated with freezing episodes during hibernation. Sideways head holding may also be the result of toxemia, especially with concurrent liver damage from secondary bacterial infection or fatty liver disease.[3] Diagnosis is made on the basis of a thorough history and physical examination and complete blood analysis. Depending on the cause, treatment is often only supportive.

Freeze damage can also cause blindness from retinal damage that can manifest in the head held back or abnormally high. The retinal damage can show on fundic examination as a general lack of refractivity; the fundus appears dull gray instead of its normal bright red, green, and brown.[3]

Blindness from any cause should be included as a differential diagnosis for abnormal head positions. A thorough ophthalmologic examination should be part of the physical examination (see Chapter 20). Depending on the cause, vision may return but may take as long as 18 months in some cases.[3] Supportive care is usually the mainstay of therapy for these patients.

Miscellaneous causes for abnormal head posturing include respiratory disease, septicemia, and trauma. Again, the key to diagnosis is a thorough history and physical examination.

CROCODILIANS

Muscular Weakness and Locomotion Difficulties

Paresis or paralysis in all four limbs, and in the head and neck, is commonly the result of osteodystrophy. Nutritional osteodystrophy results from imbalances of calcium, phosphorus, and vitamin D_3.[3,9,10] Dietary history, a thorough physical examination, and radiography aid in diagnosis. Typically, crocodilians with nutritional osteodystrophy have generalized osteopenia. Treatment is aimed at correction of nutritional deficiencies and any osseous abnormalities that result from the demineralized bone.

Muscle Twitching and Incoordination

Thiamin deficiency and hypocalcemia can produce muscle twitching and incoordination. The causes and treatments are the same as for chelonians.[4,5] Stress-induced hypoglycemia is a frequent cause of muscle tremors and loss of righting reflex during capture and restraint.[10]

West Nile virus has been found in crocodilians in the United States. Affected animals have an acute onset of loss of leg control, neck spasms, and a "star-gazing" appearance before death. See Chapters 17, 24, and 42 for more details.

LIZARDS

Head Tilt and Other Abnormal Head Positions

Head tilts are most commonly associated with vestibular abnormalities. These can be either central (brain stem, cerebellar) or peripheral (inner ear, eighth cranial nerve). In general, the head is tilted toward the side of the lesion.

Nonvestibular lesions can also occur. Neoplasia, abscesses, and trauma can also account for head tilts. An adult male Panther Chameleon (*Furcifer pardalis*) was seen for a head tilt. The animal was quiet and depressed. No obvious external lesions were seen, and the standard database results of bloodwork and survey radiographs were unremarkable. On computed tomography (CT) examination, an occluded carotid artery was found (Figure 62-5).

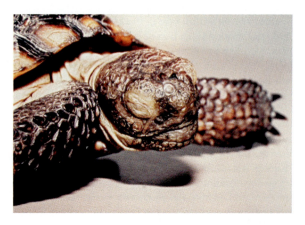

FIGURE 62-4 This California Desert Tortoise (*Gopherus agassizii*) shows a head tilt. In this case, the neurologic manifestation was the result of careless placement of a pharyngostomy feeding tube that damaged the vagosympathetic trunk. (*Photograph courtesy D. Mader.*)

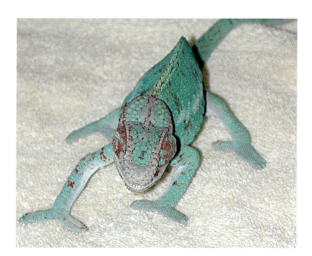

FIGURE 62-5 Head tilt and balance problems in a Panther Chameleon (*Furcifer pardalis*). No obvious external lesions were found, and the standard database results of blood work and survey radiographs were unremarkable. On computed tomographic (CT) examination, an occluded carotid artery was found. (*Photograph courtesy J. Wyneken.*)

Flaccid Paralysis or Muscle Weakness

A vitamin E/selenium deficiency, which causes white muscle disease or myopathy in mammals, has been proposed to result in flaccid paralysis. Supposedly, it can occur in animals fed foliage grown in soil that is deficient in vitamin E and selenium. Anecdotal reports exist that animals with this condition respond to vitamin E/selenium injections or supplementation.[11]

Pathologic fractures with spinal damage, a common sequela to various metabolic bone diseases, are a common cause of hindlimb paresis and paralysis (Figure 62-6). Clinical signs vary depending on the location of the injury, but they usually reflect upper motor neuron lesions. Hyporeflexia to hyperreflexia of the rear limbs, fecal and urinary incontinence, and inability to ambulate are frequent findings. See Chapter 61 for more information regarding diagnosis and treatment.

Monitor lizards fed a diet of raw eggs can have a biotin deficiency as a result of the avidin in the egg white, which can result in muscle weakness.[3,12] Treatment is with supplemental biotin and correction of the diet.

Although uncommon, electrocution has been reported to cause incoordination and flaccid paralysis. Dermal burns may or may not be present. Spontaneous recovery can sometimes occur in 4 to 5 days.[13]

Muscle Twitching

Hypocalcemic tetany, a common sequela to nutritional deficiencies, egg production, and environmental mismanagement, is not always a generalized or bilateral condition.[3,5,9] The most common presentation is usually bilateral or unilateral trembling of the frontlimbs, the hindlimbs, or a single limb. Diagnosis is made on the basis of history, physical examination, and radiography. Blood calcium levels may or may not be decreased. Treatment is aimed at correction of the underlying conditions and calcium and vitamin D therapy as needed.

SNAKES

Incoordination, Ataxia, and Muscle Twitching

Encephalitis from bacterial, mycotic, viral, and parasitic infections is frequently encountered in snakes.[2] Bacterial infections can progress to septicemia and microabscesses in the brain.[2,3] Paramyxovirus, which may initially present as a respiratory infection, may cause central nervous system signs (Chapter 63).[14] Inclusion body disease of boid snakes can also cause central nervous system signs, including disorientation, head tilting, opisthotonos, flaccid paralysis, and progressive loss of motor tone (see Chapter 60). With inclusion body disease, clinical signs are usually more apparent in pythons than in boas. Other signs include chronic pneumonia, regurgitation, and cachexia.[14-16]

Entamoeba invadens, a protozoan parasite considered a commensal in chelonians, can be fatal to snakes. Clinically affected snakes may convulse. This condition is thought to occur as a result of abscesses that form in the brain.[17] Free-living *Acanthamoeba* have been isolated from the brains of neurologically abnormal reptiles. These protozoans are thought to induce a meningoencephalitis.[17]

Diagnosis of encephalitis is with clinical signs, history (e.g., introduction of wild-caught or new snakes that can be carriers of paramyxovirus), clinical pathology, fecal analysis, and viral titers. Cerebrospinal analysis is not practical in reptiles, so antemortem diagnosis of acanthamoebiasis is unlikely. Depending on the cause, treatment may or may not be helpful. Likewise, the prognosis also depends on the etiology. But, regardless of the cause, the prognosis for a snake with any of the mentioned signs is usually guarded at best.

Convulsions can result from generalized septicemia, which may represent a terminal event because sepsis can be lethal. The bacteremia can be nonneurologic in origin, commonly initiating as a respiratory infection.[18]

Additional rule outs for generalized neurologic signs should include toxic reactions. Many disinfectants, common chemicals (iodine, naphthalene, chloroform, and paint solvents), and insecticides (especially organophosphates) can be toxic.[18] Dichlorvos, an organophosphate found in no-pest strips that are used in the treatment of mites, can cause muscle fasciculations, flaccid paralysis, and convulsions.[18,19] Toxic reactions can also result from some poisonous plants and ethylene glycol.[7]

Treatment of toxic reactions is supportive, with fluids, cooling, and atropine (when indicated). Light sedation (e.g., diazepam, 0.5 mg/kg intramuscularly [IM]) or anesthesia may be needed to reduce the severity of neurologic signs.[3,6,20]

Antibiotics, when given or used improperly, have toxic potential. Although no longer in common use, streptomycin can cause vestibular nerve damage in snakes, which manifests as incoordination.[21] Discontinuing the drug, administering fluids, and providing supportive care help correct the situation.

Renal failure and gout can cause convulsions. Tophi formation around the heart and great vessels and in the brain may be responsible. Diagnosis is not always easy. Plasma uric acid, total protein, and calcium:phosphorus ratios may give the clinician some indication of renal function (see Chapters 54 and 66). Treatment attempts should include diuresis, phosphate binders, and allopurinol (20 mg/kg orally [PO]). By the time renal disease or gout has progressed to neurologic signs, the prognosis is guarded to grave.

Thiamin deficiency can also occur in fish-eating snakes fed frozen fish. The freezing causes an increase in the thiaminase activity, which decreases the availability of vitamin B_1; signs

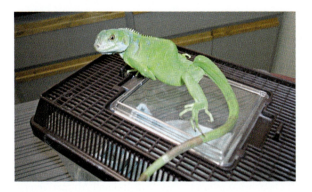

FIGURE 62-6 Healed spinal lesions can leave a patient, such as this juvenile Green Iguana (*Iguana iguana*), with severe postural abnormalities. As long as the patient is still urinary and fecal continent, it makes a good pet. (*Photograph courtesy D. Mader.*)

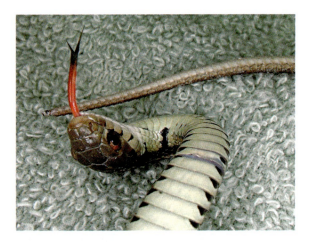

FIGURE 62-7 This Gartersnake (*Thamnophis* sp.) was unable to right itself. These neurologic symptoms are commonly seen in boids with viral encephalitis. This patient had been fed frozen fish and had a thiamin deficiency. When supplemental thiamin was administered, the patient had a full recovery. *(Photograph courtesy S.L. Barten.)*

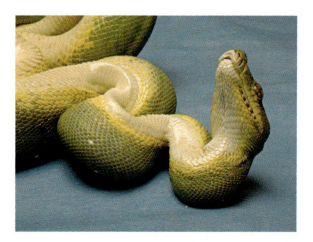

FIGURE 62-8 Head tilts, star gazing, and other neurologic disorders as seen here in this Green Tree Python (*Morelia viridis*) can be associated with any number of diseases such as bacterial, viral, and parasitic meningitis. *(Photograph courtesy S.L. Barten.)*

include incoordination and convulsions (Figure 62-7). Treatment can be accomplished with oral thiamin at 50 to 100 mg/kg daily and encouraging the snake to eat earthworms, guppies, and tadpoles.[3-5]

Paralysis

Fractures and spinal trauma often produce paralysis caudal to the site of the lesion.[4] Lack of dermal sensation, inability to move the body caudal to the lesion, and radiography are used in the diagnosis. Treatment is supportive, including fluids, corticosteroids, assist-feedings, and stabilizing the fracture site with tube splints. The prognosis is usually grave when the fracture is cranial to the cloaca.

Aminoglycoside antibiotics can cause neuromuscular blockade, especially when they are used in conjunction with anesthesia and muscle relaxants.[18]

Electrocution has been documented as a cause of flaccid paralysis or convulsions in snakes.[13]

Loss of Righting Reflex, Abnormal Body Position and Movement, and Inability to Strike at Prey

Some snakes display rolling and lying in dorsal recumbency as normal behaviors. Hog-nosed Snakes (*Heterodon* spp.) feign death, and female pythons carrying eggs frequently rest on their backs (see Chapter 13).

Any condition that causes generalized debilitation such as emaciation, septicemia, and neoplasia or spinal conditions such as myelitis (bacterial or viral), osteomyelitis, osteitis deformans, and spinal cord trauma can cause apparent neurologic disease.

The snake's body distal to the spinal lesion usually displays obvious clinical signs. Swelling, flaccid paralysis, and lack of proprioception are all apparent. The portion of the body cranial to the lesion is usually normal.[4]

Congenital spinal deformities, such as asymmetric changes or kinks of the vertebral column, may manifest as lordosis, kyphosis, or scoliosis.[22]

Osteitis deformans is a syndrome that produces spinal fusion, exotoses along the vertebral column, and remodeling of the vertebrae (see Chapter 69). Subsequent vertebral column fractures occur. Diagnosis is with palpation of the bony proliferations along the backbone and with radiographs that show exotosis along the vertebral bodies, pathologic fractures, and dislocations. Antibiotics are possibly useful, but supportive treatment is usually unrewarding.[23,24]

Osteomyelitis that causes spinal abscesses can also produce abnormal postures.[25] Radiographs along with culture and sensitivity testing are diagnostic. Treatment is with antibiotics and surgical curettage, if indicated.

Opisthotonos and Head Tilt (Star Gazing)

Star gazing results from contracture of cervical musculature (Figure 62-8). Encephalitis is the primary cause of this posture and can be caused by bacterial, mycotic,[2,3] and viral infections. Paramyxovirus, inclusion body disease of boids, and acanthamoebic meningioencephalitis have been implicated. This should be differentiated from posturing seen in respiratory disease.

REFERENCES

1. Jackson OF, Lawrence K: Chelonians. In Cooper JE, Hutchison MF, Jackson OF, et al, editors: *Manual of exotic pets*, revised ed, Cheltenham, England, 1985, British Small Animal Veterinary Association.
2. Frye FL: Infectious diseases. In Frye FL, editor: *Reptile care: an atlas of diseases and treatments*, vol I, Neptune City, NJ, 1991, TFH Publishing.
3. Lawton MPC: Neurological diseases. In Beynon PH, Lawton MP, Cooper JE, editors: *Manual of reptiles*, Cheltenham, England, 1992, British Small Animal Veterinary Association.
4. Frye FL: Nutritional disorders in reptiles. In Hoff GL, Frye FL, Jacobson ER, editors: Disease of amphibians and reptiles, New York, 1984, Plenum Press.

5. Frye FL: Feeding and nutritional disorders. In Fowler ME, editor: *Zoo and wild animal medicine: current therapy 3,* Philadelphia, 1986, WB Saunders.
6. Cooper JE, Jackson OF: Miscellaneous diseases. In Cooper JE, Jackson OF, editors: *Diseases of the Reptilia,* vol 2, San Diego, 1981, Academic Press.
7. Frye FL: Radiology and imaging. In Frye FL, editor: *Reptile care: an atlas of diseases and treatments,* vol I, Neptune City, NJ, 1991, TFH Publishing.
8. Frye FL: Traumatic and physical diseases. In Cooper JE, Jackson OF, editors: *Diseases of the Reptilia,* vol 2, San Diego, 1981, Academic Press.
9. Fowler ME: Metabolic bone disease. In Fowler ME, editor: *Zoo and wild animal medicine,* Philadelphia, 1986, WB Saunders.
10. Jackson OF: Crocodiles. In Cooper JE, Hutchison MF, Jackson OF, et al, editors: *Manual of exotic pets,* revised ed, Cheltenham, 1985, British Small Animal Veterinary Association.
11. Frye FL: Common pathologic lesions and disease processes, miscellaneous myopathies. In Frye FL, editor: *Reptile care: an atlas of diseases and treatments,* vol II, Neptune City, NJ, 1991, TFH Publishing.
12. Lawrence K: Lizards. In Cooper JE, Hutchison MF, Jackson OF, et al, editors: *Manual of exotic pets,* revised ed, Cheltenham, 1985, British Small Animal Veterinary Association.
13. Cooper JE: Physical influences. In Hoff GL, Frye FL, Jacobson ER, editors: *Diseases of amphibians and reptiles,* New York, 1984, Plenum Press.
14. Jacobson ER: Viral disease of reptiles. In Fowler ME, editor: *Zoo and wild animal medicine: current therapy 3,* Philadelphia, 1993, WB Saunders.
15. Schumacher J, Jacobson ER, Gaskin J: *Inclusion-body disease in boid snakes: a retrospective and prospective study,* South Padre Island, Tex, 1990, Proceedings of the American Association of Zoo Veterinarians.
16. Axthelm M: *Viral encephalitis of boid snakes,* Orlando, Fla, 1989, Proceedings Third International Colloquium on the Pathology of Reptiles and Amphibians.
17. Frank W: Non-hemoparasitic protozoans. In Hoff GL, Frye FL, Jacobson ER, editors: *Disease of amphibians and reptiles,* New York, 1984, Plenum Press.
18. Duma R, Ferrell R, Nelson E, et al: Primary amebic meningoencephalitis, *N Engl J Med* 281:1315, 1969.
19. Holt PE: Drugs and dosages. In Cooper JE, Jackson OF, editors: *Diseases of the reptilia,* vol 2, San Diego, 1981, Academic Press.
20. Marcus LC: Specific diseases of herpetofauna. In Marcus LC, editor: *Veterinary biology and medicine of captive amphibians and reptiles,* Philadelphia, 1981, Lea & Febiger.
21. Marcus LC: Principles of husbandry and veterinary care of herpetofauna. In Marcus LC, editor: *Veterinary biology and medicine of captive amphibians and reptiles,* Philadelphia, 1981, Lea & Febiger.
22. Zwart P, Moppes MC: *Congenital deformaties in the vertebral column of snakes,* Orlando, Fla, 1989, Proceedings Third Colloquium International on the Pathology of Reptiles and Amphibians.
23. Kiel J: Spinal osteodystrophy in two southern copperheads, *J Zoo Med* 8(2):21, 1977.
24. Kiel J: *Paget's diseases in snakes,* 1983, Proceedings of the American Association of Zoo Veterinarians.
25. Frye F, Kiel J: *Multifocal granulomatous spondylitis in a rattlesnake,* Scottsdale, Ariz, 1985, Proceedings of the American Association of Zoo Veterinarians.

63
PARAMYXOVIRUS

ELLEN BRONSON and
MICHAEL R. CRANFIELD

Ophidian paramyxovirus (OPMV) was first isolated in 1973 from a Fer-de-lance (Bothrops moojeni) after an outbreak in a Swiss serpentarium that killed 25% of 431 specimens.[1] Since then, numerous documented outbreaks of paramyxovirus have been seen in private and zoologic collections. Paramyxovirus has been isolated from all major snake families, including elapids, boids, colubrids, and viperids. Crotalids appear to be the most susceptible.

Paramyxovirus is an enveloped RNA virus 120 to 150 μm in diameter that reproduces by budding from cell membranes. Two distinct subgroups have been shown to exist with several intermediate isolates. This grouping does not appear to be species specific, although geographic correlations were found.[2,3] Recently, a transmission study was carried out in Aruba Island Rattlesnakes and Koch's postulates were fulfilled.[4]

CLINICAL SIGNS

There are no pathognomonic signs for the diagnosis of paramyxovirus infection. The disease affects primarily the respiratory system but can present with a tremendous variation of signs, which makes diagnosis difficult for the clinician. The symptoms are divided into three categories.

Acute and Peracute

Often minimal to nonexistent promontory signs are noticed by the keeper or owner; the animals are often just found dead. Anorexia and regurgitation are occasionally seen. The most common symptoms include respiratory compromise, blood in the oral cavity, or neurologic involvement such as head tremors, excitement, star gazing, flaccid paralysis, or convulsions (Figure 63-1). The time from exposure to death can range from 6 to more than 10 weeks. Animals often die of secondary bacterial infections. OPMV should be included in the differential diagnosis in boids with neurologic symptoms suspected of inclusion body disease.

The virus may overwhelm the immune system, with death occurring before a detectable antibody response. Improper husbandry and environmental conditions may play a critical role in immunologic incompetence, particularly the absence of a thermal gradient.

Chronic "Poor Doer"

Anorexia, hypophagia, and regurgitation are the earliest signs and have been seen up to 7 months before any other signs of disease. Animals exhibit other general signs of debilitation, such as reluctance to move, increased use of heat plates, emaciation, and poor muscle tone. Respiratory symptoms include variable degrees of stridor and dyspnea, often developing into secondary bacterial pneumonia. Gastrointestinal signs may include gaseous bowel distention, mucoid diarrhea, malodorous stools, and protozoal overgrowth. Directed antiprotozoal and antibacterial treatment increase survival times.

Specimens usually have high titers. However, antibody presence does not prevent viral shedding, as shown by animals able to infect or induce seroconversion in cagemates. These snakes eventually succumb to the disease but actively shed virus and pose the greatest threat to the collection.

Clinically Healthy Animals

Specimens may remain asymptomatic for up to 10 months, although most individuals eventually become chronic "poor doers." Sustained high titers may be indicative of a chronic carrier state and not necessarily immunity. Some specimens have been documented as overcoming a viral encounter and surviving.

In the authors' experience with a paramyxovirus outbreak, the animals with a regular appetite became anorectic, and respiratory compromise developed. They became severely lethargic and died within 1 week of the onset of signs. A few specimens had horizontal head tremors develop that varied from subtle to broad-swinging movements frequently accompanied with star-gazing behavior. One specimen, a Bushmaster (Lactesis mutus), did not show any clinical signs despite a seropositive status for 9 months. A Northern Copperhead (Agkistrodon contortrix) placed in an adjacent

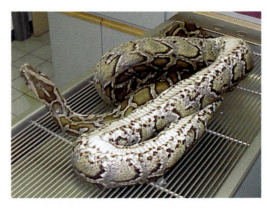

FIGURE 63-1 This Burmese Python (Python molurus bivittatus) exhibited signs of acute OPMV infection, including respiratory compromise and evidence of neurologic involvement. When placed on its back, it was unable to right itself. (Photograph courtesy D. Mader.)

Table 63-1	Laboratories That Test for Ophidian Paramyxovirus with Hemagglutination Inhibition (HI)				
Laboratory*	Sample	Shipping	Turnaround	Price
University of Florida Dr Elliot Jacobson PO Box 100126, HSC 2015 SW 16th Avenue College of Veterinary Medicine Gainesville, FL 32610 (352) 392-4700, ext 5700 www.vetmed.ufl.edu/sacs/wildlife/proto.html	0.5 mL Plasma, frozen until shipped	On dry ice	Batched and tested 1 week per month	$30
University of Tennessee UTCVM Clinical Virology Laboratory Department of Comparative Medicine 2407 River Drive, Room A-239 Knoxville, TN 37996-4543 (865) 974-5643 www.vet.utk.edu/diagnostic	0.25 mL Serum/plasma	On ice	Batched and tested once weekly	$15
Texas Veterinary Medical Diagnostic Laboratory Drawer 3040 College Station, TX 77841-3040 (979) 845-3414 www.tvmdlweb.tamu.edu	0.2 mL Serum/plasma	On ice	Batched and tested once weekly	$12

*Always call the laboratory for current pricing and packaging information before submitting samples.

aquarium did not have a titer or lesions develop after 8 weeks of exposure to the Bushmaster.[5]

DIAGNOSIS

Presumptive diagnosis of paramyxovirus infection may be based on a history of exposure and clinical signs. Ill animals should be closely monitored. A thorough clinical examination should be performed, including pulmonary auscultation and fecal examination. If abnormal lung sounds are detected, transtracheal washes for cytology and bacterial culture should be performed because both secondary bacterial and verminous pneumonia are common.

If OPMV is suspected, serum should be assayed for the presence of antibody with hemagglutination inhibition (HI). Titers only reflect exposure, and a rising titer is necessary for diagnosis of active disease. Seroconversion generally takes more than 8 weeks. The laboratory of Dr Elliott Jacobson at the University of Florida, the University of Tennessee, and the Texas State Diagnostic Laboratory currently perform HI serologic testing for titers to OPMV (Table 63-1). Titers do not necessarily correspond among laboratories because different test antigens are used in each.[6]

Any animal suspected to have died of OPMV should be necropsied as soon as possible. Blood should be collected, centrifuged, and serum frozen pending histologic findings. Three sets of tissue are recommended to be collected. Special attention should be given to include lung (cranial, mid, and caudal sections), liver, kidney, and splenopancreatic tissue in all sets of tissue saved. Garner (Northwest ZooPath, personal communication) also recommends brain and salivary gland.

The first set of tissues should be preserved in 10% neutral buffered formalin for conventional staining and microscopic examination; the second should be placed in formalin for 48 hours, then removed and placed into 70% ethanol. This improves the likelihood of finding lesions with special staining techniques. A third set of tissues should be frozen and kept for virus isolation, should this be indicated by histopathologic findings.

Gross pathologic lesions range from no visible lesions to clear mucus or blood in the oral cavity, slight pulmonary congestion, and a frothy serous or hemorrhagic exudate in the lung and air sacs (Figure 63-2). Severe cases may exhibit caseous exudative pneumonia that results from the secondary infections.

Histologic lesions in the respiratory system include proliferation of epithelial cells and thickening of the pulmonary septa. Macrophages, heterophils, and mononuclear cells often infiltrate the tissue, and moderate amounts of cellular debris, bacterial colonies, and exudate can be found in the primary bronchus and air spaces.[4] Rarely, epithelial cells may contain eosinophilic intracytoplasmic inclusions. If the brain is involved, an encephalitis can be observed, with multifocal areas of gliosis and minimal perivascular cuffing. Moderate ballooning of axon fibers may occur in the brain stem and proximal spinal cord.[7,8] In many snakes with paramyxoviral lesions in the lung, hepatic pathology also consists of diffuse hepatic necrosis or multifocal pyogranulomatous inflammation. Hyperplasia of pancreatic ducts and acinar cells with cystic dilation have also been observed.[9] In the salivary glands, ductular dilatation, flattening and crowding of ductular epithelium, and accumulation of cellular debris and secretory material may be noted in the ductular lumina (Garner, Northwest ZooPath, personal communication; Figure 63-3).

Definitive diagnosis of OPMV infection requires isolation of the virus from tissues. Thus far, this has only been achieved with tissue samples harvested at postmortem examination.

Electron microscopy can be used to show virions budding from the apical membranes of type I and II alveolar cells.

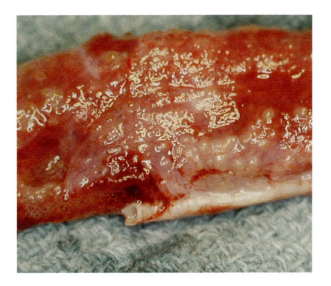

FIGURE 63-2 A resected portion of lung from a Burmese Python (*Python molurus bivitattus*) that died of pneumonia secondary to a chronic paramyxovirus infection. Note the thickened lung tissue along the cut margin on the lower left. The trachea runs along the lower right border of the tissue sample. Also note the frothy exudates typical of chronic paramyxovirus infections. (*Photograph courtesy D. Mader.*)

Occasionally, intracytoplasmic inclusions can be observed in affected cells and consisting of paramyxoviral nucleocapsid material.[4,8]

Immunofluorescence and immunoperoxidase staining techniques have also been developed to show viral antigen in affected tissues.[4,10,11] In situ hybridization has recently been used to identify paramyxoviral nucleic acid.[8]

PREVENTION AND CONTROL

Strict quarantine policies should be followed for all incoming snakes, particularly those that are more susceptible or snakes from questionable origin. The following list applies mainly for zoologic situations but can be modified to suit other scenarios.

Recommended general quarantine protocols:

Quarantine all new animals for a minimum of 60 to 90 days.
Obtain OPMV titers at entrance and exit from quarantine.
Eliminate ectoparasites and endoparasites; obtain a minimum of two negative fecal specimens before quarantine is ended.

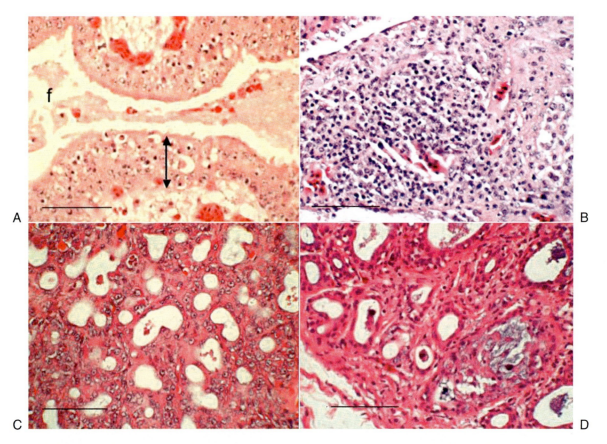

FIGURE 63-3 Paramyxovirus infection, snake tissues. **A**, Lung. Note the zone of marked hyperplasia of the respiratory epithelium (*arrow*) and edema with cellular debris in the lumen of adjacent faveolus (*f*). **B**, Brain. Note the severe nonsuppurative inflammation around the blood vessels in the brain. **C**, Pancreas. Note ductular dilatation, flattening and crowding of the ductular epithelium, and accumulation of cellular debris and secretory material in the ductular lumina. **D**, Salivary gland. Note ductular changes that mirror those of the pancreatic ducts in **C**. All photos, hematoxylin and eosin (H&E); bars, 200 μm. (*Photographs courtesy M. Garner, Northwest ZooPath.*)

House quarantined animals individually to monitor food consumption and fecal output.

Monitor animals closely for abnormal behavior or posturing.

Weigh animals as they enter and exit quarantine.

Animals feed on a regular basis and otherwise appear healthy before quarantine is ended.

Use footbaths when entering or departing the isolation area. Bleach ($1/2$ cup per gallon of water [120mL/L]; changed daily) is recommended for disinfection.

The quarantine room should have a separate set of husbandry tools. These should be disinfected after each use.

No exchange should exist in the air duct systems of the quarantine or isolation room and the main collection.

Disinfect or destroy all cage materials after removal of animals from quarantine.

Euthanize all "poor doers."

Necropsy all quarantined animals that die or are euthanized. Save tissues on all necropsied specimens according to previous recommendations.

The main mode of virus transmission is considered to be airborne, with contaminated utensils and cage furniture playing a contributing role. Medical management of clinical cases should include treatment with metronidazole, amikacin, and a cephalosporin and supportive care. OPMV, like other paramyxoviruses, may cause immune incompetence, and unless careful treated, secondary bacterial infections may result in mortality. Good husbandry practices, particularly the provision of an appropriate thermal gradient, should be integrated into the treatment if they do not already exist.

Cagemates of seropositive animals and those that show clinical signs should be isolated from the collection for at least 3 months from the time of diagnosis or onset of clinical signs. Necessary husbandry for that isolated group should be performed by a separate caretaker or by the same caretaker but at the end of the day after the healthy (nonaffected) animals have been handled. If the remaining animals appear healthy and are seronegative with HI 90 days after the last death, they can be considered a low threat to the collection. Various stressors such as shipment and ambient temperature fluctuations may result in latent infections becoming active. Chronic carriers that are potential shedders of paramyxovirus should be identified and eliminated from the collection.[6]

No vaccine is currently available for OPMV. Vaccine trials have shown that snakes can develop antibody titers to inactivated vaccines, but responses have been variable and transient.[12] Further work is needed in this area.

REFERENCES

1. Foelsch DW, Leloup P: Fatale endemische infection in einem Serpentarium, *Tieraerztl Praxis* 4:527, 1976.
2. Ahne W, Batts WN, Kurath G, Winton JR: Comparative sequence analyses of sixteen reptilian paramyxoviruses, *Vir Res* 63(1-2):65-74, 1999.
3. Franke J, Essbauer S, Ahne W, Blahak S: Identification and molecular characterization of 18 paramyxoviruses isolated from snakes, *Vir Res* 80(1-2):67-74, 2001.
4. Jacobson ER, Adams HP, Geisbert TW, Tucker SJ, Hall BJ, Homer BL: Pulmonary lesions in experimental ophidian paramyxovirus pneumonia of Aruba Island rattlesnakes, *Crotalus unicolor*, *Vet Pathol* 34:450-459, 1997.
5. Cranfield MR, Graczyk TK: Ophidian paramyxovirus. In Mader D, editor: *Reptile medicine and surgery*, Philadelphia, 1996, WB Saunders.
6. Jocobson ER, Flanagan JP, Rideout B, Ramsay EC, Morris P: Roundtable: ophidian paramyxovirus, *Bull ARAV* 9(1):15-22, 1999.
7. Jacobson ER: Paramyxo-like virus infection in a rock rattlesnake, *J Am Vet Med Assoc* 177(9):796, 1980.
8. West G, Garner M, Raymond J, Latimer KS, Nordhausen R: Meningoencephalitis in a Boelen's python (*Morelia boeleni*) associated with paramyxovirus infection, *J Zoo Wildl Med* 32(3):360-365, 2001.
9. Jacobson ER, Gaskin JM, Wells S, Bowler K, Schumacher J: Epizootic of ophidian paramyxovirus in a zoological collection: pathological, microbiological and serological findings, *J Zoo Wildl Med* 23(3):318-327, 1992.
10. Orós J, Sicilia J, Torrent A, Castro P, Déniz S, Casal AB, et al: Immunohistochemical detection of ophidian paramyxovirus in snakes in the Canary Islands, *Vet Rec* 149(1):21-23, 2001.
11. Homer BL, Sundberg JP, Gaskin JM, Schuhmacher J, Jacobson ER: Immunoperoxidase detection of ophidian paramyxovirus in snake lung using a polyclonal antibody, *J Vet Diagn Invest* 7(1):72-77, 1995.
12. Jacobson ER, Gaskin JM, Flanagan JP, Odum RA: Antibody responses of western diamondback rattlesnakes (*Crotalus atrox*) to inactivated ophidian paramyxovirus vaccines, *J Zoo Wildl Med* 22(2):184-190, 1991.

64
PENILE PROLAPSE
STEPHEN L. BARTEN

Male chelonians possess a single copulatory organ, the penis. This is large and fleshy and varies in color from pink to deep purple to black depending on the species. Normally, the penis is retracted within the cloaca and lies on the ventral floor of the proctodeum. Male turtles can be differentiated from females by their longer thicker tails with the cloacal opening well distal to the caudal margin of the carapace. Chelonians may evert the penis briefly when excited. Male snakes and lizards have paired copulatory organs, the hemipenes. Only one hemipenis is used at a time during copulation. The hemipenes are stored in an inverted position in the base of the tail, and male squamates often have longer tails with a broader base than females. Neither penis nor the hemipenes contain a urethra, and these organs are not used for urination.

Penile prolapse is most common in chelonians but also occurs in snakes and lizards. Causes include trauma, such as bite wounds from cage mates, traction during copulation, infection, inflammation, nutritional secondary hyperparathyroidism, neurologic or traumatic deficits involving the retractor penis muscles or cloacal sphincter, and straining from intestinal parasites, impaction of the cloaca with gastrointestinal foreign bodies (ingested substrate such as sand, bark chips, or gravel), or bladder or cloacal uroliths.[1-3]

The prolapsed tissue should be evaluated and identified. Differentials for cloacal prolapses include the phallus, the bladder (in those species that possess bladders), and the distal intestinal tract (in males). Male squamates occasionally form seminal plugs consisting of keratinized material filling one or both hemipenes. The ends of the seminal plugs often protrude from the cloaca and may be confused with a true prolapse. In females, the animal can also prolapse its oviducts. Proper identification is essential to appropriate treatment (see Chapter 47).

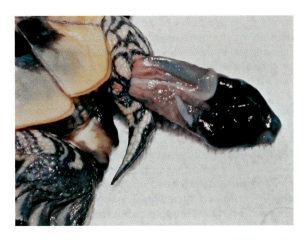

FIGURE 64-1 Penile prolapse in a Red-eared Slider (*Trachemys scripts elegans*). A cage mate was attracted to the prolapsed organ and bit it several times, causing several lacerations that required repair.

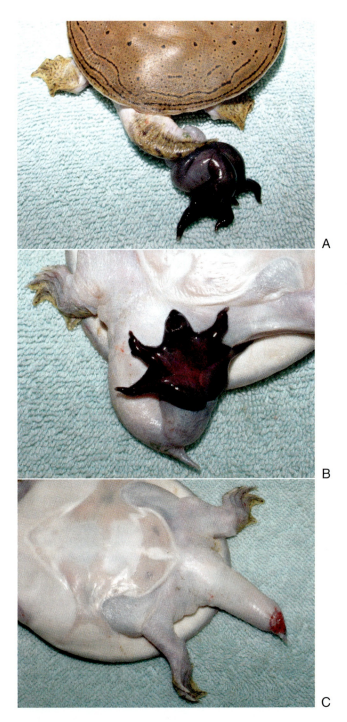

FIGURE 64-2 **A,** Uncomplicated penile prolapse in a Spiny Softshell (*Apalone spinifera*). **B,** Note the dark color and lobulated shape of the penis. **C,** After sedation, the prolapsed penis was replaced and a purse-string suture was used to partially close the cloaca and hold the penis in place. The suture was removed after 2 weeks and the prolapse did not recur.

A prolapsed phallus is often edematous and may have lacerations or bite wounds from cage mates (Figure 64-1) or secondary infections and necrotic tissue from exposure. The exposed tissue is often covered with inflammatory exudate.

Sedation is usually necessary for replacement of the prolapsed organ, especially if the tissue is swollen or damaged or the patient is refractory. The exposed tissue should be cleansed, and any lacerations repaired. A synthetic absorbable suture of appropriate size, with an atraumatic swedged on needle, is preferred.

Edema may be controlled with the application of cold compresses or hygroscopic fluid. The prolapse is reduced and held in place with a cloacal purse-string suture (nonabsorbable, cutting needle). In chelonians, a standard purse-string is effective (Figure 64-2, A-C). In snakes and lizards, the cloacal opening is linear rather than round. Two interrupted sutures in the lateral margins of the cloaca serve to hold it partially closed (Figure 64-3, A-C). The purse-string suture should be tight enough to prevent the prolapse from recurring but loose enough to allow the passage of urates and stool. In larger snakes and lizards, the opening from which the affected hemipenis protrudes may be closed with a purse-string suture within the cloaca after repositioning of the hemipenis. Antibiotics are given if infection is present. An attempt should be made to identify and correct any predisposing factors. The purse-string suture is removed in 2 weeks. The owners or caretakers should monitor the patient carefully on a daily basis to ensure that the patient passes stools and urates. The purse-string suture should be replaced if it is too tight.

If severe neurologic deficit, damage, infection, or necrosis is present, or in cases of a recurring prolapse, the penis or hemipenis may be amputated without compromising the ability to urinate.[1-6] In snakes and lizards, amputation of a

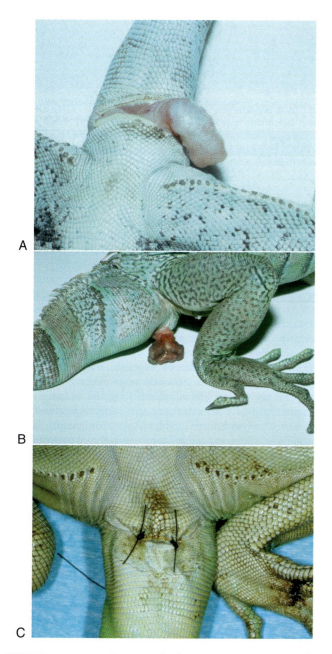

FIGURE 64-3 **A,** Prolapse of the hemipenis in a Green Iguana (*Iguana iguana*). **B,** Another prolapse of the hemipenis in a different Green Iguana (*Iguana iguana*) with incidental scoliosis of the spine. In both cases the tissue was viable and the prolapse was reduced successfully. **C,** Because the cloacal opening of lizards and snakes is linear, traditional, circumferential purse-string sutures are awkward. Rather, two simple interrupted sutures in the lateral margins of the cloaca serve to hold it partially closed.

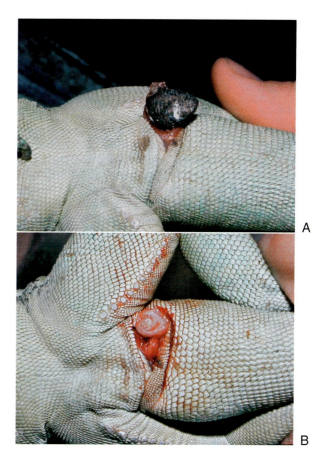

FIGURE 64-4 **A,** Penile prolapse of the left hemipenis in a Green Iguana (*Iguana iguana*). The tissue was necrotic. **B,** After amputation of the necrotic left hemipenis. The iguana was anesthetized and the hemipenis was clamped across its base. It was ligated with synthetic absorbable suture in a through-and-through horizontal mattress pattern. After amputation the mucosa of the stump was closed in a simple continuous pattern and the stump was returned to within the cloaca.

single hemipenis does not prevent future reproduction with the remaining hemipenis. With appropriate anesthesia, gentle traction is used to expose the penis or hemipenis. A ligature is placed proximal to the damaged tissue, and the organ is amputated. In larger chelonians, the blood supply and corpus cavernosa on each side are ligated separately. Through-and-through horizontal mattress sutures work well (Figure 64-4, *A, B*).[2,6] The mucosa of the stump is sutured with a continuous pattern, and the stump is returned to the cloaca.[5] Synthetic, absorbable suture material such as polyglyconate or poliglecaprone 25 is recommended. An antibacterial ointment such as 1% silver sulfadiazine cream (various manufacturers) or 2% mupirocin ointment (Bactoderm, SmithKline Beecham Pharmaceuticals, Philadelphia, Pa) is instilled into the cloaca. Systemic antibiotics are indicated when infection is present.

REFERENCES

1. Frye FL: *Biomedical and surgical aspects of captive reptile husbandry*, ed 2, Melbourne, Fla, 1991, Krieger Publishing.
2. Mautino M, Page CD: Biology and medicine of turtles and tortoises, *Vet Clin North Am Small Anim Pract* 23:1251, 1993.
3. Zwart P: Urogenital system. In Beynon PH, Lawton MPC, Cooper JE, editors: *Manual of reptiles*, Gloucestershire, England, 1992, British Small Animal Veterinary Association.
4. Bennett RA: Reptilian surgery, part I: basic principles, *Compend Contin Educ Pract Vet* 11:10, 1989.
5. Lawton MPC, Stoakes LC: Surgery. In Beynon PH, Lawton MPC, Cooper JE, editors: *Manual of reptiles*, Gloucestershire, England, 1992, British Small Animal Veterinary Association.
6. Millichamp NJ: Surgical techniques in reptiles. In Jacobson ER, Kollias GV, editors: *Contemporary issues in small animal practice: exotic animals*, New York, 1988, Churchill Livingstone.

65
PNEUMONIA AND LOWER RESPIRATORY TRACT DISEASE

MICHAEL J. MURRAY

Pneumonia is a common problem in captive reptiles. Often called "respiratory" by lay herpetologists, pneumonia, with its multiple etiologies, can easily be life-threatening if not aggressively managed. Although a number of infectious agents are capable of causing primary pneumonia, many clinical cases are the result of the intermingling of any of several predisposing deficiencies in husbandry, sanitation, and nutrition. A clinical diagnosis of pneumonia should be made on the basis of the sound principles of clinical medicine, history, physical examination, and a variety of ancillary diagnostic techniques. The sole use of apparent clinical signs often results in erroneous diagnostic and subsequent therapeutic measures (Figure 65-1).

DIAGNOSTIC PLAN

History

The historic data collected from owners of suspected pneumonic reptiles can be quite variable. In most instances, however, significant deficiencies exist in the husbandry of the species presented. Recent transport through the retail pet shop trade, importation, severe endoparasitism and ectoparasitism, malnutrition, and suboptimal temperature are all stressors that predispose the reptile to severe respiratory disease. Collection of a complete and thorough history is critical to the diagnosis, treatment, and prognosis of pneumonia. Of particular interest to the clinician are the origin of the animal, the quarantine procedures used, the presence of other reptiles within the collection, the type and frequency of disinfection of the environment, and the progression of clinical signs.

Maintenance of the reptile within its preferred optimal temperature zone (POTZ) is critically important for normal respiratory function and normal immune system activity. Provision of a temperature gradient allows the captive reptile the opportunity to actively select its desired temperature. Humidity is often an overlooked factor in the development of pneumonia in reptiles. Although most captives do well at relative humidity of 50% to 70%, certain species have peculiar requirements. Housing in cages with excessively high or low humidity may cause changes within the lower respiratory tract that predispose the reptile to pneumonia.

Nutritional imbalances, particularly hypovitaminosis A, are often associated with respiratory disease in the reptile. Inadequate dietary vitamin A results in squamous metaplasia of respiratory epithelial cells and the ducts of the mucus-producing glands. Such changes may either predispose the respiratory tract to opportunistic bacterial infection or cause clinical signs that mimic pneumonia (see Chapter 59).

Inadequate dietary protein may also act as a nutritional predisposing factor to pneumonia.

Proper sanitation of the reptile's environment is critically important in the prevention of pneumonia and lower respiratory tract disease. Because many of the pathogens associated with pneumonia are opportunistic, poor hygiene causes exponential increases in microbial populations that may eventually wear down the most efficient immune systems.

Significant ectoparasite loads are often associated with poor environmental hygiene. Snake mites (*Ophionyssus natricis*) have been implicated as vectors of several infectious causes of pneumonia, such as aeromoniasis.[1]

Physical Examination

Clinical signs of pneumonia often are not apparent to the owner until they are so advanced that they overwhelm the reptile's ability to physiologically compensate. In such situations, affected animals are critically compromised and need aggressive diagnostic and therapeutic measures. Although a complete and thorough physical examination is indicated for any patient, this discussion limits itself to a description of the signs typically associated with the respiratory system and pneumonia.

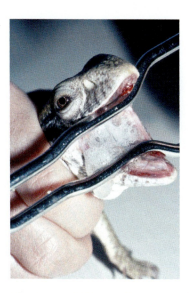

FIGURE 65-1 This Savannah Monitor (*Varanus exanthematicus*) has profound frothy oral discharge. Without a complete work-up, the origin (gastric, respiratory, or sinus) is not possible to tell. (*Photograph courtesy S. Barten.*)

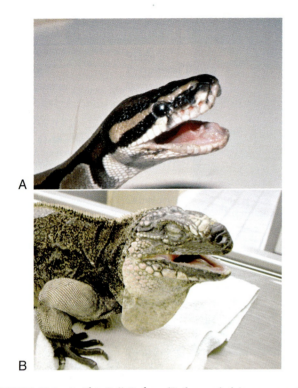

FIGURE 65-2 A, This Ball Python *(Python regius)* is open-mouth breathing. With rare exceptions, this is a sign of severe pathology in snakes. Lizards, crocodilians, and turtles may thermoregulate with an open mouth. **B,** This Cyclura had a large ovarian abscess compromising lung volume. (**A,** *Photograph courtesy G. Diethelm.* **B,** *Photograph courtesy D. Mader.*)

The most dramatic clinical presentation involves dyspnea, generally inspiratory but often inspiratory and expiratory. The respiratory rate is generally elevated with exaggerated respiratory movements of the body. Open-mouth breathing is common, especially after any exertion (Figure 65-2). Snakes and lizards tend to extend the neck, hold up the head, and may breathe with an open mouth (Figure 65-3). Chelonians breathe with the head and neck extended, often oblivious to their surroundings. Aquatic species may spend less time in the water.

Nasal discharge may or may not be associated with pneumonia (Figure 65-4). An upper respiratory component is not unusual in lower respiratory disease; however, the conditions may occur separately. The anatomy of the lower respiratory tract, particularly the bronchi and trachea, and the oftentimes caseous exudates produced in reptilian pneumonias make the movement of respiratory discharges from the lungs to the nares unlikely (Figure 65-5). Therefore, the presence of nasal discharge is not a sign of pneumonia but a reflection of disease within the upper airway or oral cavity.

Varying degrees of pathology may be detectable with auscultation in clinical cases of pneumonia. Rales are often detected as air moves over accumulations of mucus and other inflammatory debris within airways. Use of a moistened gauze sponge over the diaphragm of the stethoscope facilitates auscultation of the lungs. The clinician should pay particular

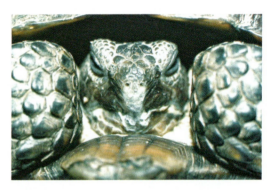

FIGURE 65-4 Nasal discharge does not necessarily mean lower respiratory pathology. Upper respiratory tract disease (URTD) is common in many tortoise species (see Chapter 73). (*Photograph courtesy D. Mader.*)

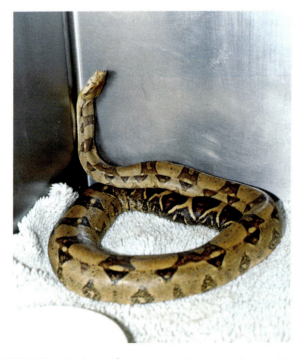

FIGURE 65-3 Snakes with respiratory disease may "posture" in an attempt to facilitate breathing. Resting in a vertical position prevents exudate from blocking the airway. (*Photograph courtesy D. Mader.*)

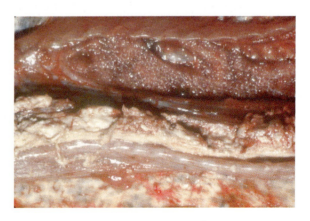

FIGURE 65-5 Most respiratory infections have a caseous component. Lack of a cough reflex and thickness of exudate prevent phlegm from mobilizing up the airway and being expelled. (*Photograph courtesy D. Mader.*)

attention to the presence of abnormal sounds and asymmetry during the auscultation.

Reptilian patients with pneumonia are typically systemically ill. Cyanotic mucous membranes, especially in the oral cavity, imply severe respiratory compromise and warrant a poor to grave prognosis. Clinicians should take note of the animal's mental status because most are depressed and lethargic. In aquatic turtles, unilateral pneumonias often result in asymmetrical swimming, with the affected side carried lower in the water (see Figure 40-16). The state of hydration is a critically important parameter with significant therapeutic ramifications and should be noted.

Radiography

A radiographic examination is necessary for a definitive diagnosis of pneumonia in the reptile. In addition, radiographic examination may prove valuable in evaluation of the patient's response to therapy. The most important factor in use of radiography in lower respiratory tract disease is the selection of radiographic views. The dorsoventral view provides limited information for the clinician regarding the respiratory tract in chelonians but is of use in snakes, lizards, and crocodilians. Complete radiographic evaluation of the lungs requires orthogonal views, specifically either a vertical, or preferably, a horizontal beam lateral.

Use of **horizontal** beam projections of the craniocaudal view (in chelonians) and the lateral view (in all species) is of significant value (see Chapter 29). These horizontal beam projections allow the clinician to examine the lung fields without the confusion of the underlying visceral anatomy present in the dorsoventral vertical beam projection. A disadvantage of the lateral view is the superimposition of the two lung fields because discerning which lung has the pathology is not possible (Figure 65-6).

Quality radiographs permit the clinician to evaluate the trachea and bronchi as they leave the cervical region and enter the lungs near the heart (Figure 65-7). The normal pulmonary parenchyma has a delicate reticular pattern with fine soft tissue septa often observable within the organ.[2] The reticular pattern is lost in snakes as the lung progresses caudally into the air sac–like division.

Increased densities within one or both lungs suggest pathologic changes consistent with pneumonia. Horizontal beam projections may reveal actual fluid lines not detectable in the dorsoventral view (Figure 65-8). Pneumonic changes may be diffuse, with the entire lung involved, or regionalized, with only a portion of the lung affected. Clinicians are recommended to collect a series of "normal" radiographs of a variety of reptile species to aid in the interpretation of the more subtle changes in the lung fields.

Advanced imaging, such as computed tomographic (CT) scans and magnetic resonance imaging (MRI), are the best techniques for localizing pulmonary lesions in the chelonian. The use of orthogonal radiographic views (dorsoventral, lateral, and craniocaudal projections) allows calculation of lesion location. However, CT and MRI images permit precise calculations of lesion location and extent (Figure 65-9).

Newer digital imaging techniques allow the clinician to alter brightness or contrast of the images. Adjusting parameters can help highlight areas that may be missed on an otherwise minimally diagnostic film. In addition, reversing the image (with a negative instead of a positive image) allows the eye to focus on portions of the radiograph that might otherwise go unnoticed (Figure 65-10).

Transtracheal Wash

Transtracheal washes may be indicated in cases of pneumonia or suspected pneumonia. The technique is relatively safe and

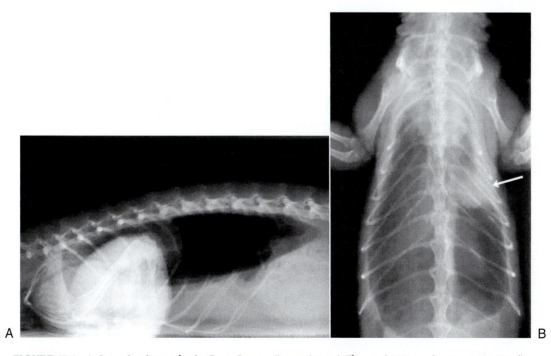

FIGURE 65-6 **A,** Lateral radiograph of a Green Iguana *(Iguana iguana)*. The combination of poor positioning (legs not drawn forward) and superimposition of the lung fields and limbs dramatically limits the diagnostic quality of the film. **B,** Same animal as in **A.** This dorsoventral view clearly shows a pulmonary abscess *(yellow arrow)* in the right lung and shows the importance of orthogonal views. *(Photograph courtesy R. Brown.)*

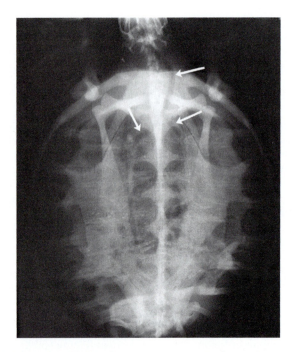

FIGURE 65-7 Reptiles have a prominent trachea and primary bronchi, easily seen on the dorsoventral view of this seaturtle. *(Photograph courtesy D. Mader.)*

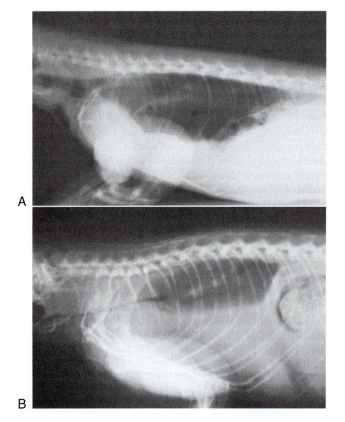

FIGURE 65-8 A, Well-positioned horizontal beam lateral view of the lung fields in a normal Green Iguana *(Iguana iguana)*. **B,** Lateral horizontal beam view clearly shows a fluid line in the cranial coelom of this Iguana patient. *(Photographs courtesy D. Mader.)*

simple; however, chemical restraint may be indicated as an aid in maintaining sterile technique. The glottis is identified, and a sterile red rubber catheter is passed through the glottis into the lung. A volume equal to 0.5% to 1.0% of the animal's body weight of sterile saline solution (not bacteriostatic) is instilled into the lung while the animal is restrained in the horizontal position. The fluid is then immediately aspirated with the body's position altered to a head-down configuration. The syringe and cannula should be withdrawn slowly with gentle negative pressure maintained on the syringe (see Figure 30-103).[3]

In cases of unilateral pathology, directing the catheter into the preferred lung with an internal stylet as determined through radiology may be necessary (Figure 65-11).

A percutaneous lung wash is often advantageous in those species with a glottis protected by a fleshy muscular tongue, such as the chelonians. In the chelonian, the inguinal fold is prepared for an aseptic procedure. The preferential side is typically determined radiographically. Sterile saline solution is then instilled into the lung through a needle of sufficient length to access the organ. Again, the fluid is immediately aspirated with the affected side held in a lower position.

The sample collected from the lung may then be used for several diagnostic procedures. First, a wet mount is prepared for direct visualization of parasite larvae, ova, and protozoal organisms. Several slides of the material should be prepared and held for exfoliative cytology and special stains. Finally, the remainder of the sample should be prepared for submission for microbiologic evaluation, aerobic and anaerobic culture, fungal culture, and viral culture, depending on other test results.

One must use caution in the interpretation of lung wash results, particularly those that contain potentially "normal" oropharangeal flora or those with equivocal or negative results. The potential for specimen contamination is great; therefore, particular attention must be paid to methodology and aseptic technique.

Not surprisingly, many of the infectious causes of pneumonia in the reptile incite a granulomatous response (Figure 65-12). For that reason, the recovered fluid may never truly come into contact with pathogenic organisms, instead washing against granulomata. Unfortunately, many of the cells involved in the granulomatous inflammatory response exfoliate poorly and may not be recoverable. As a result, cytology and microbial culture may be unrevealing.

Endoscopy

Endoscopic examination of the lungs provides the best opportunity for the determination of a definitive diagnosis. This technique facilitates both direct visualization of the trachea and lung and the opportunity for collection of representative tissue specimens for cytology, culture, and histologic examination (see Figure 30-106). Instrument selection is dependent on the size and species involved. Traditional rigid rod-lens telescopes may be introduced through the glottis and into the trachea and even lungs in appropriately sized lizards and snakes. Larger specimens may require the use of flexible bronchoscopes (see Chapter 32).

Introduction of an endoscopic telescope directly into a lung through a surgical approach is also possible. Bearing in mind the location of the heart, the lateral aspect of a lung may

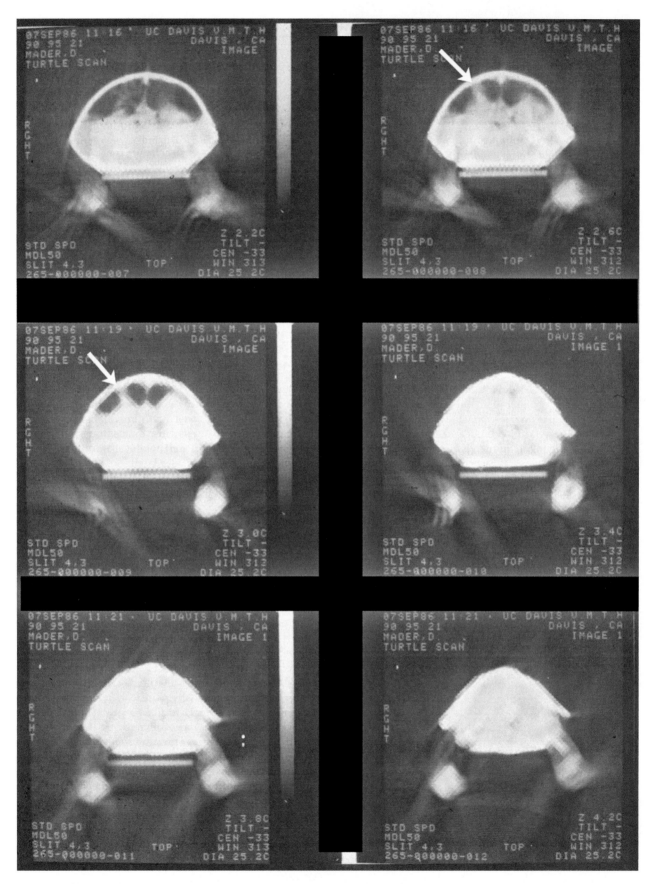

FIGURE 65-9 Computed tomographic series of a Desert Tortoise *(Gopherus agassizii)*. The *yellow arrow* points to a pulmonary abscess that did not image on a standard survey radiograph. *(Photograph courtesy D. Mader.)*

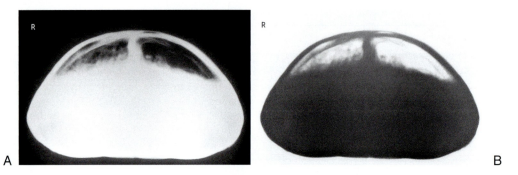

FIGURE 65-10 **A,** Horizontal beam cranial-caudal (anterior-posterior) view of a tortoise with right-sided pneumonia. Digital manipulation of images allows for altering contrast and brightness, thus enhancing an otherwise poor-quality radiograph. **B,** Negative image of **A.** Reversal of colors visually enhances delicate septa and pathology. *(Photographs courtesy D. Mader.)*

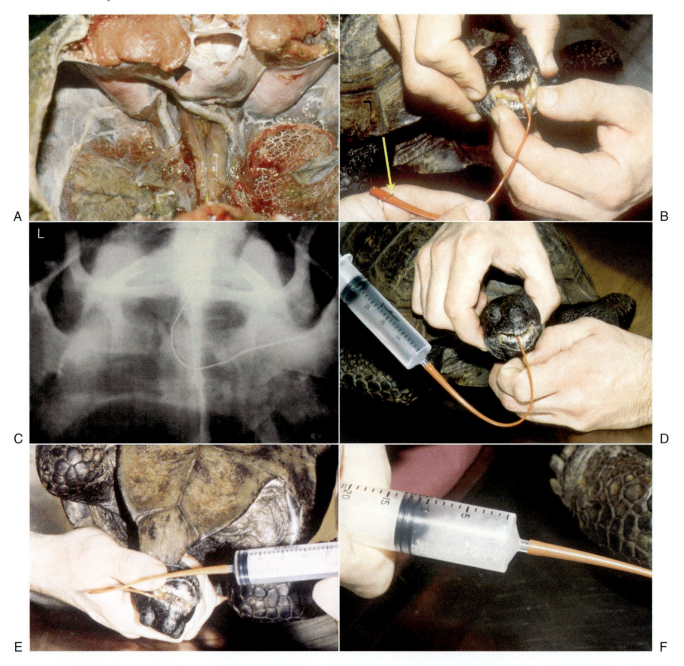

FIGURE 65-11 **A,** Development of unilateral pneumonia (right lung lobe, pictured on *left*) is not uncommon in tortoises. **B,** A catheter is inserted into the trachea with a sterile technique. Sterile cerclage wire *(yellow arrow)* is used as a stylet to "stiffen" the catheter and give it direction during insertion. **C,** On the basis of radiographic findings, the catheter is directed into the affected lung. A dorsoventral radiograph verifies placement. **D,** Sterile nonbacteriostatic saline solution, 0.5% to 1% of patient's body weight, is infused into the affected lung. **E,** The patient is inverted and gently "rocked" back and forth to mix the saline solution with lung fluids. **F,** The aspirate is collected and then submitted for cytologic analysis and bacterial culture and sensitivity testing. *(Photographs courtesy D. Mader.)*

be exposed through an intercostal approach. The pleural surface is then easily sutured closed after examination.

The anatomy of the chelonian patient mandates a different approach to endoscopic examination of the lungs. The proximal location of the tracheal bifurcation coupled with long narrow bronchi interferes with traditional transglottal approaches to pneumonoscopy. Instead, two unique approaches to the chelonian lung have been described—a prefemoral approach and a carapacial approach through a temporary osteotomy (Figure 65-13).[4] Both approaches require complete radiographic work-ups because the bony shell of the chelonian restricts movement of the telescope; therefore, targeting of the pulmonary lesion is necessary.

The prefemoral approach is a soft tissue surgical approach to the more caudal aspects of the lung (Figure 65-14). After identification of the more severely affected lung, the turtle is anesthetized and placed in lateral recumbency, affected side up.

A skin incision is made into the prefemoral skin fold at its most craniodorsal aspect. With the animal maintained in maximum inspiration, the septum horizontale is grasped and secured with stay sutures. A small incision then permits access to the lung. After examination, the incisions are closed routinely.[4]

A temporary osteotomy is necessary for endoscopic examination of the lung via the carapacial approach. As in the prefemoral approach, targeting the site of entry is critically important. With the turtle adequately anesthetized and placed in ventral recumbency, the area of carapace over the site of lung pathology is prepared for aseptic surgery. Assurance that the entry site is lateral to the spine is important.

A 4-mm osteotomy is then created with a short sterile orthopedic drill. The osteotomy is preferably performed with the patient held in expiration (see Figure 30-104). With a trocar or fine hemostats, entry into the lung is accomplished with the animal held in inspiration. One must recognize that the endoscopist's ability to maneuver the telescope within the lung is significantly limited by the rigid carapace. After lung examination and sample collection, the osteotomy site may be closed with an epoxy resin or a catheter instilled to facilitate intrapulmonic drug administration.[4]

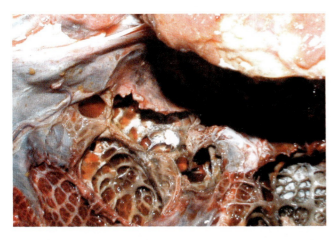

FIGURE 65-12 Many reptile patients form granulomas in their lungs as a consequence of infection. As a result, negative bacterial growth yielded by lung wash is not uncommon. *(Photograph courtesy D. Mader.)*

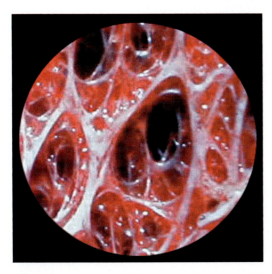

FIGURE 65-13 Transcarapacial approach to the lung parynchema of a tortoise. The endoscopist's ability to maneuver the telescope within the lung is significantly limited by the rigid carapace. *(Photograph courtesy D. Mader.)*

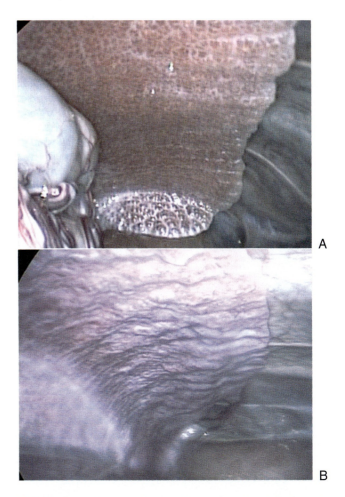

FIGURE 65-14 Prefemoral approach to evaluation of the lungs in a seaturtle. This approach allows excellent visualization of the outside of the lung parenchyma. **A,** Normal lung. **B,** Patient with pneumonia. Note the consolidated opaque appearance of the pulmonary tissue. *(Photographs courtesy D. Mader.)*

Systemic Evaluation

Most reptiles with pneumonia are critically ill. Therefore, secondary effects on a variety of organ systems may be anticipated. Because aggressive antimicrobials are frequently indicated as a component of the therapeutic regimen, evaluation of renal and hepatic function is prudent before the administration of nephrotoxic or hepatotoxic drugs. Collection of blood for a baseline hemogram aids in prognostication and helps to establish an endpoint for therapy.

DIFFERENTIAL DIAGNOSIS

Bacterial

Many cases of pneumonia diagnosed are caused by bacterial infections. As anticipated, many isolates are gram-negative organisms, which may be identified in clinically healthy animals. Bacterial pneumonia may occur as a primary entity, as an extension of another disease process such as infectious stomatitis, or as the establishment of a normal commensal organism in an abnormal location such as the lung. Bacterial pneumonias can be focal, unilateral, or bilateral (Figure 65-15). Many potential pathogens, such as *Escherichia coli, Klebsiella* spp., *Pseudomonas* spp., *Proteus* spp., and *Aeromonas* spp., may be recovered with some frequency from water sources within the reptile's environment.[5]

The bacterial organisms most commonly isolated in healthy snakes, which implies that they are normal airway inhabitants, are *Providencia rettgeri* and coagulase negative *Staphylococcus* spp.[5] The most common pathogenic isolates are aerobic gram-negative bacteria, including *Aeromonas, Pseudomonas, Salmonella, Arizona, Klebsiella,* and *Proteus.*[5] Although these organisms may be identified in the oral cavity of normal individuals, their recovery from the lower respiratory tract is significant. Reports are also found of *Salmonella arizonae* being a primary pathogen, not a secondary invader.[6] *Pasteurella testudinis* has been reported to be associated with pneumonia in Desert Tortoises *(Gopherus agassizii).*

Although one study of the airway flora in healthy and pneumonic snakes failed to identify any anaerobic bacteria,[5] anaerobic organisms associated with pneumonia in several reptile species have been identified.[7] Organisms recovered from the lung included *Bacteroides, Peptostreptococcus, Fusobacterium,* and *Clostridium.*

Atypical bacteria, such as *Mycoplasma* and *Chlamydophila,* have also been associated with pneumonia in reptiles. *Mycoplasma agassizii* has been recovered from Desert Tortoises and Gopher Tortoises *(G. polyphemus)* with pneumonia and appears to be intimately involved in the upper respiratory disease complex of these species.[8,9] Other species of *Mycoplasma* have been associated with pneumonia in a variety of chelonian species, American Alligators *(Alligator mississippiensis),* and Burmese Pythons *(Python molurus bivittatus).*[10-12]

Chlamydial infection in a group of puff adders has been reported.[13] Although the infection was systemic, respiratory signs and pneumonia were a component of the clinical presentation. Acid-fast organisms, such as mycobacteria, may also cause pneumonia. In most cases, the granulomatous mycobacterial infection does not affect the respiratory tract as a primary site of infection but causes pneumonia by extension from another location.[14]

Viral

Although reptilian virology is in its infancy, several viral diseases have been identified that have a respiratory component. Unfortunately, antiviral therapies have not been well documented in reptiles; however, knowledge of a viral etiology may have significant impact on the management and prognosis of a collection of susceptible species.

A paramyxovirus with a combination of respiratory and central nervous signs was initially identified in viperid snakes (see Chapter 63).[15] The virus has since been identified in other common snake families such as elapids, boids, and colubrids.[16] The viral infection has three predominant clinical presentations: (1) acute and peracute; (2) chronic "poor doer"; and (3) asymptomatic carriers.[17]

Acutely affected snakes may be dyspneic with open-mouthed breathing and expel blood-tinged brown mucoid discharge from the oral cavity, pharynx, and trachea. The disease advances quickly with the development of nervous signs including convulsions and loss of the righting reflex. Death may occur within 1 to 3 days of the initiation of respiratory signs. Chronically affected snakes have a number of clinical signs consistent with a reptile that is failing to thrive. Respiratory signs in these cases are typically the result of secondary bacterial invaders and the subsequent pneumonia. The diagnosis of ophidian paramyxovirus (OPMV) infection is typically made on the basis of clinical signs, history, postmortem examination, and serology. A hemagglutination inhibition test for the presence of antibodies to OPMV is available.

An unidentified viral disease of boids, referred to as inclusion body disease, has been recognized for many years. Electron microscopy has tentatively placed the virus within

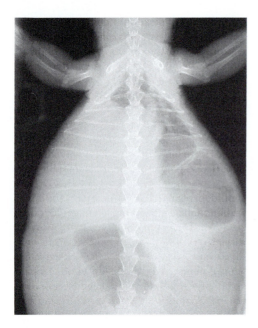

FIGURE 65-15 Unilateral bacterial pneumonia in a monitor. Bacterial culture revealed a pure culture of *Klebsiella pneumoniae.* (Photograph courtesy D. Mader.)

the family Retroviridae.[18] The typical clinical signs are chronic regurgitation and cachexia, although a chronic pneumonia may also exist.

Neurologic signs, progressive loss of motor function, disorientation, and loss of righting reflex are most common in pythons.

Diagnosis is made on the basis of the demonstration of eosinophilic intracytoplasmic inclusion bodies within affected tissues, particularly the kidney and pancreas.

A herpesvirus has been associated with respiratory disease in several species of chelonian (see Chapter 57). Severe necrotizing bronchitis, pneumonitis, and hepatitis have been identified. An enzyme-linked immunosorbent assay (ELISA) has been developed for identification of herpesvirus exposure in tortoises.[19] A herpesvirus appears to be associated with a respiratory disease characterized by conjunctivitis, tracheitis, and pneumonia in Green Seaturtles *(Chelonia mydas)*.[14]

Fungal

Mycotic pneumonia is occasionally, but uncommonly, diagnosed in captive reptiles (Figure 65-16). Because most of the organisms are ubiquitous in nature, abnormal environmental or host situations must exist for infection to occur. Typically, fungal infections occur in a patient that is overexposed to fungal spores or one that is immunocompromised. Cases have been related to the overuse of antibiotics.

Any of the previously described stressors within the captive environment—temperature, humidity, nutrition, and concurrent disease—may be sufficient to suppress the immune system adequately for secondary fungal infection. Excessive environmental humidity coupled with cage substrates, such as ground corncob, walnut shell, and alfalfa pellets, which tend to support fungal growth, may provide large numbers of fungal spores that may overwhelm the reptile's ability to mount an appropriate immune response.

Environmental temperature appears to be critically important in the development of fungal pneumonia. Not only does maintenance of sub-POTZ interfere with normal reptile immunologic activity, but many fungi grow more rapidly at the lower sub-POTZ than at the typical temperature zones required by most captive reptiles.[20] A number of species of fungi have been associated with pneumonia in reptiles, including *Aspergillus, Candida, Mucor, Geotrichum, Penicillium, Cladosporium, Rhizopus, Chrysosporium,* and *Beauveria* (see Chapter 16).[14,20,21]

The systemic deep mycoses occasionally diagnosed in mammals, such as blastomycosis and histoplasmosis, have not been diagnosed in reptiles to date.[22] A case of pneumonia from *Coccidioides immitis* has been reported in a Sonoran Gophersnake *(Pituophis melanoleucus)*.[23]

A single case of cryptococcosis, caused by *Cryptococcus neoformans*, has been reported in a captive Anaconda *(Eunectes murinus)*.[24] This individual presented with signs attributable to the central nervous system; however, pulmonary involvement was identified on postmortem examination.

A diagnosis of fungal pneumonia is often difficult to make antemortem. Recovery of fungal elements, hyphae, or spores,

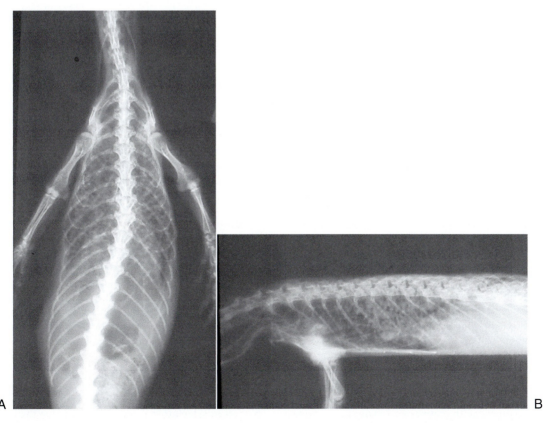

FIGURE 65-16 **A** and **B**, Dorsoventral and lateral views of a monitor with diffuse fungal pneumonia. Orthogonal views help differentiate artifacts caused by overlay of scales from true pathology. *(Photographs courtesy D. Mader.)*

or culture of a fungal agent from a transtracheal wash, is supportive of a diagnosis of fungal pneumonia. Because most pulmonary fungal infections stimulate the formation of focal or diffuse granulomata, radiographic identification of pulmonary nodules is suggestive of mycotic infection. Typically, however, the diagnosis of fungal pneumonia is made on postmortem examination. Gross pathologic changes of mycotic pneumonia include pulmonary granulomata, lung consolidation, and occasionally extension of the disease into adjacent organs.

Unfortunately, most treatment regimens for fungal pneumonia are unsuccessful. Obviously, should a cure be effected, the clinician must educate the reptile owner to correct those husbandry and nutritional deficiencies that probably predisposed the animal to the secondary fungal disease.

Parasitic

A number of parasites encountered in captive reptiles have a portion of their life cycle within the lungs (see Chapter 21). Except in the cases with overwhelming parasite loads, most respiratory parasites cause localized inflammation and irritation, and associated pneumonias tend to be secondary bacterial infections.

Lungworms

These nematode parasites of the genus *Rhabdias* live in the lungs of snakes and lizards. Although most parasite loads are low, heavy infestation may result in secondary bacterial infections. The parthenogenic females lay their eggs within the lung. The eggs are then transported up the trachea, are swallowed, and are passed in the feces. Infective larvae then enter the susceptible host via either ingestion or cutaneous penetration. Infestation is diagnosed with the identification of the eggs in either fecal examinations or transtracheal washes. The currently recommended treatment is ivermectin, 200 µg/kg subcutaneously, repeated in 2 weeks. Levamisole phosphate (Levasole Injection 13.65%, Schering-Plough, Union, NJ) at a dose of 10 mg/kg intracoelomically, repeated in 2 weeks, is also effective. Quarantine of newly acquired individuals and sound hygiene are important preventative measures.

Pentastomids

Annulate metazoan parasites of the lungs, trachea, and nasal passages of snakes, lizards, turtles, and crocodilians, the "tongue worms," are often seen in wild-caught specimens. The adults feed on tissue fluids within the lung and pass the embryonated eggs from the respiratory tract to the oral cavity where they are swallowed and passed through the feces. An intermediate host, often a small mammal, then consumes larvae. Consumption of the intermediate host then infects the reptile. Humans may serve as incidental hosts, so a zoonotic potential exists. Heavy parasite loads may cause significant localized inflammatory disease, subsequent respiratory compromise from obstruction, and occasionally a secondary bacterial pneumonia.[14] No reliable chemotherapeutic treatment is currently described; however, surgical or endoscopic removal is curative (see Figure 21-67). Anecdotal reports exist of successful treatment with ivermectin 200 µg/kg.[25] The use of captive-bred prey species as a food source for carnivorous reptiles is recommended.

Trematodes

Renifers, trematodes of the genera *Dasymetra, Lechriochis, Aeugochis, Ochestosoma,* and *Stomatrema,* are occasionally found in the lower respiratory tract. Although most infestations are asymptomatic, heavy parasite loads may cause enough damage to predispose the animal to a secondary pneumonia. Most renifers use amphibians as their intermediate host. The diagnosis is made on the basis of the identification of the typical fluke eggs on transtracheal wash. Currently, no effective and safe treatment has been advocated.[16]

Infection of aquatic turtles with digenetic spirorchid trematodes of the genera *Spirorchus, Henotosoma, Unicaecum, Vasotrema,* or *Hapalorhynchus* may result in clinical signs suggestive of pneumonia. Although the adult flukes reside in the heart and great vessels, the eggs are released into the circulatory system. The granulomatous inflammatory reaction associated with the eggs as they occlude terminal vascular beds is responsible for the clinical disease associated with the spirorchids. Substantial granulomatous reaction within the lungs may result in an asymmetric appearance in the water, with the affected side floating lower than the contralateral side.

The diagnosis of spirorchid fluke infection is difficult. Typical fluke eggs may be identified in direct saline solution mounts from lung washes or in sedimentation concentration of fecal samples. Often, however, the diagnosis is made at postmortem with the identification of adults within the cardiovascular system or in squash preparations of pulmonary tissue. Treatment is often ineffective; however, the use of praziquantel may be beneficial.[26] In a study performed in the Green Seaturtle (*Chelonia mydas*), praziquantel was safe and effective in eliminating cardiovascular trematodes. In contrast to earlier published reports, the dosage administered was 50 mg/kg orally for a single day at hours 0, 7, and 9.[27] Unfortunately, the granulomatous verminous pneumonia is unlikely to resolve because it is initiated by the presence of the fluke eggs within the pulmonary vasculature.

Others

Other nematode parasites have a visceral larval migrans component within their life cycle. During the pulmonary aspect of the larval migrans, ascarid or hookworm larvae may be associated with pneumonia (Figure 65-17).[16] Typically, their presence is merely irritating; however, sufficient pulmonary pathology may occur in heavy parasite loads, predisposing the reptile to a secondary bacterial pneumonia.

Intranuclear coccidia have been reported in captive tortoises (*Geochelone* spp.).[28] The biology and significance of these coccidia are yet to be determined.

The obligate intracellular parasite, microsporidia, has been identified within pulmonary cells of inland Bearded Dragons (*Pogona vitticeps*) dying of the systemic effects of the disease.[29] Although the primary target organs appear to be the liver and kidney, the significance of pulmonary infection is yet to be determined.

NONINFECTIOUS CAUSES

Not all inflammatory diseases that involve the lower respiratory tract of reptiles are infectious by nature. Aspiration of foreign material, either iatrogenically or by chance, is certain to

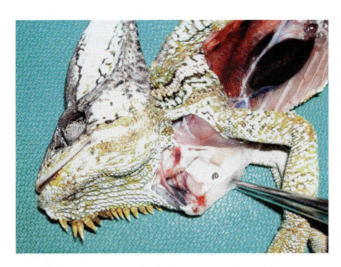

FIGURE 65-17 A nematode in the accessory lung lobe (at tip of forceps) in a chameleon. Small numbers of lung parasites do not usually cause a problem. However, in stressed or immunocompromised patients, parasites can lead to inflammation and pneumonia. *(Photograph courtesy D. Mader.)*

cause a substantial inflammatory reaction within the lungs. Inhalation pneumonia begins as a foreign body reaction; however, if neglected, it progresses rapidly to a secondary bacterial pneumonia.

Diseases that compromise tidal volume may mimic pneumonia because affected reptiles are frequently presented dyspneic. Obesity, ascites, and space-occupying lesions have the potential for respiratory compromise, thereby giving the appearance of pneumonia. Other nonrespiratory causes of dyspnea, such as cardiac or hepatic disease, may similarly mimic pneumonia. Conditions as innocuous as the loosening of skin around the nares immediately before ecdysis may be interpreted as pneumonia. The movement of air over this area often creates an audible respiratory noise similar to that noted in respiratory tract disease. The "problem" is self-resolving after completion of ecdysis.

TREATMENT

Because most cases of lower respiratory tract disease are well advanced at the time of presentation and diagnosis, treatment must be quite aggressive, yet within the limits of the patient. Ideally, antibacterial therapy should be directed against specific pathogens, as dictated by the culture and sensitivity results. Unfortunately, the serious nature of the reptile with pneumonia does not permit the delay necessary for microbiologic testing.

Suspected aerobic bacterial pneumonias are best treated with bactericidal drugs. The author prefers a synergistic combination of aminoglycoside and beta-lactam antibiotics (see Chapters 89 and 90). Because most organisms recovered from affected cases are gram-negative bacteria, selection of agents with an enhanced spectrum of activity is suggested. Cases with a suspected anaerobic bacterial etiology may be treated with metronidazole, 20 mg/kg orally every 24 hours.[30-32]

The unique nature of the mycoplasma species often associated with pneumonia, particularly in chelonians mandates special therapeutic consideration. Antibiotics whose mechanism of action affects the bacterial cell wall, such as the beta-lactams, are obviously ineffective in organisms like *Mycoplasma* or *Chlamydia*, which lack cell walls. Treatment options recommended include the use of one of the following: the fluoroquinolone enrofloxacin (5 mg/kg every 48 to 72 hours) or the macrolides clarithromycin (15 mg/kg orally every 48 to 72 hours)[33] or azithromycin (10 mg/kg orally every 2 to 7 days).

The pharmacokinetics of most antifungal drugs are not well described for reptiles. In addition, the granulomatous inflammatory response and its fibrocollagenous capsule often preclude entry of antifungal agents into the site of infection. For this reason, discrete fungal granulomas are best surgically excised.

On the basis of extrapolation of data from mammalian and avian medicine, combination antifungal therapy appears to have the most promise in eliminating pulmonary fungal disease. Such protocols should be used cautiously with an understanding of the potential for toxicity or other undesired side effects. Nebulization therapy with diluted amphotericin B (Fungizone, Geneva, Broomfield, Colo), a fungicidal drug, 5 mg in 150 mm of saline solution, for 1 hour every 12 hours, has been advocated.[34] Ketoconazole, a fungistatic drug, may also be administered at a dose of 15 to 30 mg/kg orally every 24 hours.[35] Itraconazole may also be used at 23.5 mg/kg orally every 24 hours. After 3 days of treatment, peak levels are attained, and therapeutic levels are maintained for 6 days beyond peak concentration.[36]

The use of aerosol or nebulization therapy may prove beneficial to the patient with pneumonia. The use of such techniques has several therapeutic advantages. First, increasing the humidity of the microenvironment at the level of the respiratory epithelium tends to promote proper hydration of the area and may increase the efficiency of the mucociliary transport mechanism. Nebulization may also aid in the breakup of necrotic and inflammatory debris. When combined with antimicrobials, aerosols may be delivered deeply into the site of infection (Table 65-1). To reach the lungs, aerosolized particle size must not exceed 3 μm. Particles in the 3-μm to 7-μm size tend to be deposited in the trachea and on the mucosal surface of the nasal cavity. Nebulization episodes are typically 10 to 30 minutes in length and are repeated 2 to 4 times per day for 5 to 7 days.

A technique for direct administration of drugs into affected lungs in the chelonian has been reported.[37] As described for transcarapacial endoscopy, effective treatment mandates accurate pinpointing of the lesion within the lung. With the approach previously described, a catheter is secured to the carapace and enters the lung. Therapeutics may then be administered directly to the site of pneumonia. In most cases, standard systemic doses may be used; however, drugs with potentially toxic side effects should have dosages reduced. Of particular interest to the clinician is that drugs such as amphotericin B and gentamicin are poorly absorbed, thereby minimizing potential toxic side effects when given at standard parenteral doses.[37]

The use of mucolytic agents should be approached cautiously. Acetylcysteine has been reported to be irritating in several species of birds and mammals. Although the reports have not included reptiles, the clinician that uses this compound should watch closely for signs of dyspnea, lethargy, edema, and tachycardia. Other techniques for the breakdown

Table 65-1	Antibiotics Commonly Used in Nebulization	
Antibiotic	**Dose**	**Administered**
Amikacin*	5 mg/10 mL saline solution	30 min daily
Cefotaxime	100 mg/10 mL saline solution	30 min daily
Piperacillin	100 mg/10 mL saline solution	30 min daily

*Monitor renal function and administer supplemental fluids.

and elimination of pulmonary exudates have been advocated. The use of cuppage to dislodge inflammatory debris may facilitate a more rapid clearance of the material. Judicious use of transtracheal suction with sterile red rubber tubes may also aid in the direct removal of inflammatory exudates.

The use of atropine cannot be advocated. Parasympatholytic drugs of this type tend to thicken respiratory secretions, thereby inhibiting their removal from the respiratory tract. Extensive supportive care must be provided for reptiles with pneumonia. Patients should be maintained at the upper end of their POTZ to facilitate inherent immunologic function. Generally, the relative humidity is maintained within the species' normal range. Supplemental fluid therapy is mandatory, especially if potentially nephrotoxic drugs are administered. Fluid therapy should be designed to provide both maintenance and replacement fluids. In most cases, the administration of 1% to 2% of the patient's body weight is administered subcutaneously, intracoelomically, or orally on a daily basis. Animals in crisis should be given intravenous fluids if at all possible.

Patients with pneumonia are often anorectic. Patients should be encouraged to voluntarily consume normal food items. The goal is to place the animal in a positive calorie balance. Assist-feedings should be approached with some trepidation because the stress of such a procedure may overwhelm and decompensate a critically ill reptile. Parenteral vitamin supplementation, particularly with water-soluble vitamins, may aid in the recovery process.

Supplemental oxygen therapy may be contraindicated in most pneumonia cases. As previously discussed (see Chapter 10), one of the driving parameters for reptilian respiration is PO_2. Significantly elevated environmental oxygen tensions may inhibit respiration, thereby compromising the reptile's already marginal ability to eliminate inflammatory debris from the lower respiratory tract. If supplemental oxygen is to be provided, levels of 30% to 40% oxygen should suffice, thus providing a 100% increase from atmospheric oxygen concentrations. Supplemental oxygen should be humidified during administration because failure to do so tends to irritate respiratory mucous membranes, compromising already marginal respiratory abilities.

Even the most well-designed therapeutic regimen is doomed for eventual failure should the clinician neglect correction of the underlying etiopathogenesis of the pneumonia. Environmental, hygienic, and nutritional deficiencies should be corrected. Appropriate quarantine and isolation procedures should be instituted in multiple reptile collections. Elimination of both ectoparasite and endoparasite loads appears to be critically important in the resolution and prevention of reptile pneumonia.

One of the most perplexing problems facing the clinician treating a reptile with pneumonia is when to stop therapy. Although no definitive answers to this question exist, several guidelines are offered:

1. Have clinical signs been eliminated? If not, cessation of therapy may be inappropriate. Evaluation of serial hemograms provides the clinician with an impression of the progress of treatment. Most reptilian hemograms remain abnormal in the face of infectious pneumonia.
2. Serial radiographic examination, although not terribly sensitive, does detect significant pulmonary pathology.
3. Repeated transtracheal washes, especially for exfoliative cytology, provide local cellular information concerning the case progression.
4. Repeat endoscopic examinations are often invaluable.
5. The clinician's judgment and intuition should not be overlooked. Does this patient appear to be feeling well? Is it eating? If not, further investigation is warranted.

Pneumonia in the reptile is a significant clinical entity with multifactorial etiologies and a complex etiopathogenesis. The reptile's tolerance for extended anaerobic metabolism facilitates the concealment of clinical signs until the disease is well advanced, thereby complicating the clinician's therapeutic task. Aggressive diagnostic and therapeutic measures are necessary if treatment is to be successful.

REFERENCES

1. Cooper JE: Integument. In Benyon PH, Lawton MP, Cooper JE, editors: *Manual of reptiles*, Gloucestershire, England, 1992, British Small Animal Veterinary Association.
2. Rubel A, Kuoni W, Frye FL: Radiology and imaging. In Frye FL, editor: *Biomedical and surgical aspects of captive reptile husbandry*, ed 2, vol I, Melbourne, Fla, 1992, Krieger Publishing.
3. Jacobson ER: Reptiles: exotic pet medicine, *Vet Clin North Am Small Anim Pract* 17(5):1203, 1987.
4. Divers SJ, Lawton MPC: Two techniques for endoscopic evaluation of the chelonian lung, *Proceedings Association of Reptilian and Amphibian Veterinarians*, 2000.
5. Hilf M, Wagner RA, Yu VL: A prospective study of upper airway flora in healthy boid snakes and snakes with pneumonia, *J Zoo Wildl Med* 21(3):318, 1990.
6. Oros J, et al: Respiratory and digestive lesions caused by *Salmonella arizonae* in two snakes, *J Comp Path* 115:185-189, 1996.
7. Stewart JS: Anaerobic bacterial infections in reptiles, *J Zoo Wildl Med* 21(2):180, 1990.
8. Mader DR: Turtle and tortoise medicine and surgery, *Proceedings of the California Veterinary Medicine Association*, 1991.
9. Jacobson ER, et al: An update on mycoplasmal respiratory disease of tortoises. *Proceedings Association of Reptilian and Amphibian Veterinarians*, 2000.
10. Jacobson ER, McLaughlin GS: Chelonian mycoplasmosis. *Proceedings Association of Reptilian and Amphibian Veterinarians*, 1997.
11. Clippinger TL, et al: Morbidity and mortality associated with a new *Mycoplasma* species from captive American alligators (*Alligator mississippiensis*), *J Zoo Wildl Med* 31(3): 303-314, 2000.
12. Penner JD, et al: A novel *Mycoplasma* sp associated with proliferative tracheitis and pneumonia in a Burmese python, *Python molurus bivittatus*, *J Comp Path* 117:283-288, 1997.

13. Jacobson ER, Gaskin JM, Mansell J: Chlamydial infection in puff adders (*Bitis arietans*), *J Zoo Wildl Med* 20(3):364, 1989.
14. Junge RE, Miller RE: Reptile respiratory diseases. In Kirk RW, Bonagura JD, editors: *Current veterinary therapy XI*, Philadelphia, 1992, WB Saunders.
15. Jacobson ER, Gaskin JM, Page D, et al: Illness associated with paramyxo-like virus infection in a zoologic collection of snakes, *J Am Vet Med Assoc* 179(11):1227, 1981.
16. Stoakes LC: Respiratory system. In Benyon PH, Lawton MP, Cooper JE, editors: *Manual of reptiles*, Gloucestershire, England, 1992, British Small Animal Veterinary Association.
17. Lloyd ML, Flanagan J: Recent developments in ophidian paramyxovirus research and recommendations on control, *Proceedings of the American Association of Zoo Veterinarians*, 1991.
18. Schumacher J, Jacobson ER, Gaskin JM: Inclusion-body disease in boid snakes: a retrospective and prospective study, *Proceedings of the American Association of Zoo Veterinarians*, 1990.
19. Origgi FC, Jacobson ER: Development of an ELISA and an immunoperoxidase based test for herpesvirus exposure detection in tortoises, *Proceedings Association of Reptilian and Amphibian Veterinarians*, 1999.
20. Fromtling RA, Kosanke SD, Jensen JM, et al: Fatal *Beauveria bassiana* infection in a captive American alligator, *J Am Vet Med Assoc* 175(9):934, 1979.
21. Jacobson ER, Cheatwood JL, Maxwell LK: Mycotic diseases of reptiles, *Semin Av Exotic Pet Med* 9(2):94-101, 2000.
22. Zwart P: Infectious diseases of reptiles. In Fowler ME, editor: *Zoo and wild animal medicine*, ed 2, Philadelphia, 1986, WB Saunders.
23. Timm KI, Sonn RJ, Hultgren BD: Coccidioidomycosis in a Sonoran gopher snake, *Pituophis melanoleucus affinis*, *J Med Vet Mycology* 26(2):101-104, 1988.
24. McNamara TS, Cook RA, Behler JL, et al: Cryptococcosis in a common anaconda (*Eunectes murinus*), *J Zoo Wildl Med* 25(1):128, 1994.
25. Driggers T: Respiratory diseases, diagnostics, and therapy in snakes, *Vet Clin North Am Ex Anim Pract* 3(2):519-536, 2000.
26. Conboy GA, Laursen JR, Averbeck GA, et al: Diagnostic guide to some of the helminth parasites of aquatic turtles, *Compend Cont Ed Pract Vet* 15(10):1217, 1993.
27. Adnyana W, Ladds PW, Blair D: Efficacy of praziquantel in the treatment of green sea turtles with spontaneous infection of cardiovascular flukes, *Aust Vet J* 75(6):405-407, 1997.
28. Origgi FC, Jacobson ER: Diseases of the respiratory tract of chelonians, *Vet Clin North Am Ex Anim Pract* 3(2):537-549, 2000.
29. Jacobson ER, et al: Systemic microsporidiosis in inland bearded dragons (*Pogona vitticeps*), *J Zoo Wildl Med* 29(3):315-323, 1998.
30. Jacobson ER: *Use of antimicrobial therapy in reptiles, Antimicrobial therapy in caged birds and exotic pets*, Trenton, NJ, 1995, Veterinary Learning Systems.
31. Kolmstetter CM, et al: Pharmacokinetics of metronidazole in the green iguana, *Iguana iguana*, *Bull Assoc Rept Amph Vet* 8:4-7, 1998.
32. Kolmstetter CM, et al: Metronidazole pharmacokinetics in yellow rat snakes (*Elaphe obsolete quadrivittata*), *Proceedings Association of Zoo Veterinarians*, 1997.
33. Johnson JD, Mangone B, Jarchow JL: A review of mycoplasmosis infections in tortoises and options for treatment, *Proceedings Association of Reptilian and Amphibian Veterinarians*, 1998.
34. Jacobson ER: Use of chemotherapeutics in reptile medicine. In Jacobson ER, Kollias GV Jr, editors: *Exotic animals*, New York, 1988, Churchill Livingstone.
35. Page CD, Mautino M, Meyer JR, et al: Preliminary pharmacokinetics of ketoconazole in gopher tortoises (*Gopherus polyphemus*), *Proceedings of the American Association of Zoo Veterinarians and American Association of Wildlife Veterinarians*, 1988.
36. Gamble KC, Alvarado TP, Bennett CL: Itraconazole plasma and tissue concentrations in the spiny lizard (*Sceloporus* sp.) following once-daily dosing, *J Zoo Wildl Med* 28:89-93, 1997.
37. Divers SJ: The diagnosis and treatment of lower respiratory tract disease in tortoises with particular regard to intrapneumonic therapy, *Proceedings Association of Reptilian and Amphibian Veterinarians*, 1998.

66
RENAL DISEASE IN REPTILES: DIAGNOSIS AND CLINICAL MANAGEMENT

STEPHEN J. HERNANDEZ-DIVERS and CHARLES J. INNIS

Continued strides in captive husbandry and nutrition of reptiles have resulted in many animals surviving to adult and geriatric ages.[1,2] Nevertheless, renal disease remains a major cause of morbidity and mortality, particularly among older iguanas, and continues to be of significant concern to veterinarians and reptile keepers alike.[3-6] Inadequate captive husbandry, poor nutrition, and secondary nutritional hyperparathyroidism are considered to be common predisposing factors to chronic renal disease, and acute renal failure tends to be the result of infectious or toxic causes and more sporadic in nature.[3,5,6] Although most of the information presented here relates to lizards, and especially the Green Iguana (*Iguana iguana*), much has direct relevance to reptiles in general.

RENAL PHYSIOLOGY

For a comprehensive discussion of renal anatomy see Chapter 11.

In some species of snakes (*Storeria* sp. and *Thamnophis* sp.), direct micropuncture techniques have indicated that individual nephron glomerular filtration rates (GFRs) average 2.04 nm/min.[7] Overall GFR has been calculated for several species with clearance methods, and results varied with hydration status.[8] A single study of Green Iguanas (*Iguana iguana*) has determined normal GFR of 14.78-18.34 mL/kg/h, while GFR in another rainforest saurian, the Puerto Rican Gecko (*Hemidactylus* sp.) was calculated at 10.4 ± 0.77 mL/kg/h.[6,9] During dehydration (experimentally studied with the intravenous infusion of hyperosmotic saline solution), GFR tends to decrease, and water-loading (experimentally studied with the intravenous injection of sterile water) increases GFR; however, considerable variation exists between different species from different habitats. As an example, GFR of the Puerto Rican Gecko is 3.33 ± 0.37 mL/kg/h with dehydration and 24.3 mL/kg/h with water-loading.[9] In some species that possess an alternate method for salt excretion (e.g., nasal salt glands of the Sand Monitor, (*Varanus gouldii*), dramatic elevations of plasma osmolarity may not cause the expected decrease in GFR because mechanisms for postrenal reabsorption of water from the cloaca, colon, or bladder are usually well-developed.[10]

Few studies have evaluated the effects of temperature on GFR in reptiles, but in two saurian species (*Trachydosaurus rugosus* and *Sauromalus obesus*), significant increases in GFR have been associated with increasing temperature from 5°C to 25°C, mediated by increases in mean arterial pressure.[11,12] However, these same studies also indicate that within the preferred optimal temperature zone, mean systemic arterial pressure and urine flow appear to be virtually independent of temperature.

The concept that overall GFR is mediated by changes in the number of filtering glomeruli rather than subtle variations in individual nephron filtration rates appears justified because the maximum rate for renal tubular transport of para-amino-hippurate (PAH) has been shown to vary directly with GFR.[13] If changes in GFR resulted from changes in the amount filtered by each glomerulus with all glomeruli continuing to function, the renal tubular transport for PAH would not be expected to change because the mass of tissue transporting PAH would not have changed.[14] In addition, microscopic studies in various reptile species, including the eastern Blue-tongue Skink (*Tiliqua scincoides*), have indicated that the ratio of open-to-closed proximal tubular lumina correlates with GFR.[15] A tubule collapses when the glomerulus ceases filtering, supporting the concept that changes in GFR result from changes in the number of functioning nephrons.[8]

Precise control of GFR and tubular function in lizards is not well understood. Studies in *V. gouldii* have shown a significant reduction in GFR after arginine vasotocin (AVT) administration. The effect appears to be independent of systemic arterial pressure and presumably is the result of constriction of the afferent glomerular arteriole.[10] More recent studies in the agamid lizard (*Ctenophorus ornatus*) have suggested that AVT may also stimulate dilution of urinary fluid in the thin-intermediate segment and facilitate water reabsorption along an osmotic gradient as the urine passes through the final segments of the nephron.[16] Antidiuretic effects and reductions in GFR have been attributed to high doses of oxytocin; however, at least in some species, these effects appear to be mediated by reductions in systemic arterial blood pressure.[8]

Tubular function includes the regulation of water, sodium, potassium, hydrogen ion, calcium, phosphorus, and nitrogenous compounds, predominantly urate in most terrestrial reptiles.[8] Urate is freely filtered by the glomerulus in snakes, and presumably in nonophidian species as well.[7] For those species in which clearance data are available, net tubular secretion of urate occurs in the proximal tubule.[8] Urate secretion requires the active transport of urate against a diffusion gradient from the blood into the proximal tubular cell and passive diffusion into the lumen of the proximal tubule.[8]

In tubules with greatly reduced GFR and tubular flow, the passive diffusion of urate into the lumen ceases as urate concentrations equalize across the luminal membrane.[8] The proximal tubular secretion of urate is dependent on and directly associated with GFR. Urate complexed with various ions, particularly potassium, and urinary proteins forms a colloidal suspension that passes from the nephron into the collecting duct.

In the cloaca, colon, or bladder, the acidification of urine through hydrogen ion secretion or bicarbonate absorption, combined with water reabsorption, leads to the precipitation of uric acid.[8] Failure to adequately excrete urate leads to hyperuricemia, gout, and death.[3] Electrolytes, including sodium and potassium, are freely filtered by the glomerulus. Most of the ultrafiltrate sodium (and water) is reabsorbed from the nephron, collecting duct, colon, cloaca, or bladder. Studies in hydrated Geckos (*Hemidactylus* sp.) and Iguanids (*Phrynosoma* sp. and *Tropidurus* sp.) have indicated that only 15% to 46% of glomerular filtered sodium is actually excreted in urine.[8] Isosmotic sodium reabsorption occurs in the proximal tubule. However, because the osmolarity of ureteral urine is generally lower than plasma, fluid reabsorbed from the distal tubule must vary from isosmotic to hyperosmotic.[8] In many species, colon, cloaca, and bladder are more important sites for the regulation of sodium excretion and water reabsorption than the kidneys. Control of sodium and potassium regulation has been poorly studied in reptiles, but AVT, aldosterone, and temperature have been shown to exert significant effects.[8] Finally, the theoretic ineffectiveness of furosemide in the reptile kidney, lacking a loop of Henle, has not been confirmed experimentally. Indeed, studies in chelonians and lizards have shown that furosemide exerts significant diuretic effects by increasing sodium, chloride, potassium, and water losses from the kidney, colon, cloaca, and bladder.[17-19]

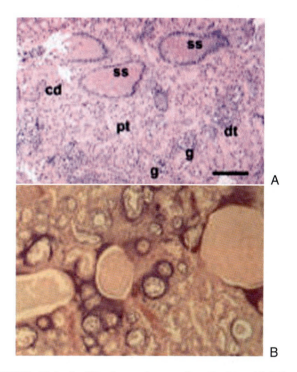

FIGURE 66-1 **A,** Histology of normal male iguanid kidney shows glomeruli (*g*), proximal tubules (*pt*), distal tubules (*dt*), collecting ducts (*cd*), and sexual segments (*ss*). Hematoxylin and eosin, bar = 100 μm. **B,** Histology of severe tubulonephrosis, glomerulonephrosis, and renal mineralization in an iguanid kidney. *(Photographs courtesy S.J. Hernandez-Divers.)*

RENAL DISEASES

A variety of renal diseases have been described in iguanas and other reptiles, including renal cysts, interstitial nephritis, glomerulonephritis, pyelonephritis, glomerulosclerosis, nephrosclerosis, glomerulonephrosis, tubulonephrosis, renal edema, amyloidosis, gout, bacterial nephritis, tubular adenoma, adenocarcinoma, and metastatic adrenal (interrenal) carcinoma (Figure 66-1, *A*).[2,20]

Degenerative nephroses represent the most common diseases encountered and are usually characterized by variable degeneration or necrosis of the glomeruli (glomerulonephrosis) or tubules (tubulonephrosis).[2,3,5,6] In the terminal stages, aberrant calcium metabolism may cause metastatic calcification of the cardiorespiratory and gastrointestinal systems (Figure 66-2, *B*). Calcification of the great vessels and myocardium can lead to congestion of peripheral blood vessels (especially obvious on the sclera of the eye), poor circulation, and ischemic necrosis of the tail. Gastrointestinal effects may include vomiting and passing poorly digested food.

High-protein diets are considered a predisposing cause of hyperuricemia, gout, and nephrosis in herbivorous reptiles, and modern texts now recommend avoidance of such foods.[4,21-23] Blockage of the renal tubules with secreted urate

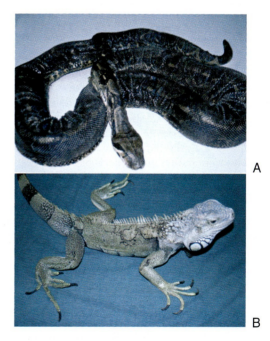

FIGURE 66-2 Physical presentation of reptiles with chronic renal failure. **A,** Boa Constrictor *(Boa constrictor)* with severe nephrosis and renal gout from inclusion body disease. **B,** Green Iguana *(Iguana iguana)* with tubulonephrosis and glomerulonephrosis attributed to high-protein diet, low humidity, and inappropriate water provision. *(Photographs courtesy S.J. Hernandez-Divers.)*

is another process that impairs renal function and has been associated with chronic dehydration in snakes. The maintenance of the high-humidity, rainforest species in dry captive conditions is suggested as a cause of chronic dehydration and nephropathy.

CLINICAL INVESTIGATION

Currently, diagnosis of renal disease in reptiles is made on the basis of history, physical examination, hematology, biochemistry, urinalysis, diagnostic imaging, and ultimately renal histopathology and microbiology.[3] However, the recent advent of measurement of iohexol excretion to determine GFR offers the first practical means for assessment of renal function.[6]

Anamnesis

A detailed history is most important in investigation of any disease; moreover, in cases of suspected renal disease, history can often differentiate between true acute renal disease and chronic renal failure. Usually little history is associated with acute renal disease. In most cases, the lizard presents with acute onset depression, anorexia, and usually cessation of urine and urate output. Such cases often involve individuals that are poorly managed in unhygienic conditions. Recent exposure to nephrotoxins including aminoglycoside antibiotics and high doses of vitamin D_3 may be inferred from a detailed case history and previous medical or owner records. Total water deprivation, severe dehydration, or hemorrhage could also theoretically lead to poor renal perfusion and acute renal failure.

Reptiles with chronic renal disease often have had long-term mismanagement. High-protein diets rich in purines and in particular the use of canned dog or cat foods can lead to abnormal hyperuricemia in herbivores, with increased demands for effective urate excretion. Likewise, persistently inadequate humidity or inappropriate water provision (e.g., water bowl instead of daily spraying) can result in chronic dehydration. The regular use of oral vitamin D_3 as a substitute for broad-spectrum lighting can cause nephrocalcinosis, and reptiles that recover from secondary nutritional hyperparathyroidism may have sustained chronic renal damage from the cytotoxic effects of excess parathyroid hormone.[24] Affected animals tend to have a more protracted history, including deteriorating body condition, capricious appetite, and lethargy that may extend over weeks or months, and as a result, most cases present dehydrated and emaciated. Only occasionally do owners report polydipsia or polyuria.

Physical Examination

A thorough physical examination is always indicated and should include an accurate measurement of weight.[25] Reptiles with severe renal compromise present in a depressed and weakened state (see Figure 66-2). In cases of acute disease, the animal often presents in good body condition, whereas the chronic renal case is likely to be significantly underweight. Dehydration may be inferred from reductions in skin elasticity, salivary, and ocular secretions.

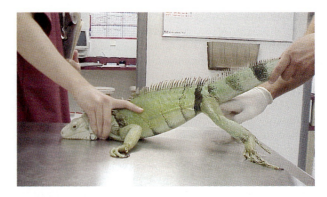

FIGURE 66-3 Digital palpation of the kidneys should be performed on all patients as part of the complete evaluation. The finger is gently inserted into the cloaca, palm down; then, after the pelvic canal is entered, the palm is rotated up to allow palpation of the kidneys. The normal iguana kidney should be completely within the bony pelvis. (*Photograph courtesy D. Mader.*)

Pharyngeal edema is not uncommon, and where digital palpation of the kidneys per cutaneous or per cloaca is possible, the size, shape, and contours of the kidneys can be determined (Figure 66-3) and should be a part of every physical examination. Pronounced renomegaly may cause constipation and cloacal prolapse.

Routine Blood Analysis

Blood collection and analysis is an essential part of the diagnostic investigation. Considerable variation exists in published hematologic and biochemical results derived from different populations of the same species, which often complicates detailed interpretation.[26-28] Many of these differences are probably a reflection of differing husbandry practices, laboratory methodologies, and the inclusion of normal, abnormal, and reproductively active females. Preference should be given to generating normal reference data for each individual animal when healthy (i.e., yearly health examinations with blood screens). When this is not possible, the careful extrapolation of published ranges can be helpful.

Hematology

Pathologic elevations of hematocrit are usually related to dehydration. The clinician must also be aware that chronic renal disease may lead to a nonregenerative anemia that may mask hemoconcentration. Unless immunosuppression is present, acute infection or inflammation usually results in heterophilia or azurophilia. In cases of chronic renal disease, a decreased, normal, or mildly increased total white blood cell count is more common, with monocytosis not an unusual feature. Reptiles constantly exposed to temperatures below the preferred optimum temperature zone may become immunocompromised and fail to show an appropriate leukocyte response, even in the face of overwhelming infection.

Biochemistry

The major nitrogenous waste product of terrestrial reptiles is urate or uric acid; however, many aquatic chelonians excrete significant quantities of urea.[8] Hyperuricemia or uremia seldom ensues before terminal renal failure.[6,28] In clinical practice, urea and creatinine are considered poor indicators of renal disease in most species because of their low production and variable excretion in most reptiles.[3,6,8,28] Only chelonians and rhynchocephalids excrete urea as a consistently significant fraction of urinary nitrogen, although noteworthy bladder urea levels have been reported in certain saurians (*Anolis carolinensis* and *Lacerta viridis*).[9] Low or undetectable levels of urea have been previously reported in the Green Iguana.[6,27] Creatinine and creatine values have been described in a limited number of healthy and renal-diseased iguanas.[24,27] Creatinine production and excretion appear to be too variable for useful clinical interpretation, and creatine, like uric acid, only rises during renal failure.[6,28] In Green Iguanas, calcium:phosphorus ratios may become inverted in many, but not all, cases of renal failure.[6,28,29]

Other electrolytes, including sodium and potassium, have received less attention in the diagnosis of renal disease. Significant regulation of sodium and potassium is possible at extrarenal sites (e.g., nasal salt glands). The ranges for sodium and potassium determined in previous studies may assist in the evaluation of electrolyte changes during disease.[6,26,27] Hyponatremia and hyperkalemia may be expected from dysfunction of the distal tubules, cloaca, colon, bladder, or distal extrarenal salt glands, but more detailed evaluation is necessary in healthy animals and those with renal disease.[3,28]

Other parameters, including aspartate aminotransferase (AST), creatinine phosphokinase (CPK), and lactate dehydrogenase (LDH), may be elevated during renal disease, but their wide tissue distribution makes them poor specific markers of renal damage.[28,30] Tubular disease may be expected to result in increased urinary loss of the brush border enzyme, γ-glutamyl transferase; however, further studies are necessary to confirm this theory. Severe glomerular disease may increase urinary loss of albumin and lead to hypoalbuminemia. Acute renal inflammation is uncommon, but it may result in leukocytosis and elevated fibrinogen.[28] Chronic disease may lead to secondary renal hyperparathyroidism as a result of inadequate hydroxylation of vitamin D_3 by the kidneys or to phosphate retention resulting in hypocalcemia and increased parathyroid hormone secretion.[31-34]

Even within the same species, gender, season, nutrition, and management can significantly affect biochemical values, and therefore, published reference values must be interpreted with caution (Table 66-1). Given these variations, biochemical profiles collected from the healthy individual may prove to be the most useful reference range for that individual.

Urinalysis

Urinalysis is less helpful in reptiles than in mammals. The reptilian kidney cannot concentrate urine, and so urine specific gravity is of limited use in the assessment of renal function. Furthermore, renal urine passes through the urodeum of the cloaca before entering the bladder, and therefore, bladder urine is often nonsterile. The clinical picture is further complicated by electrolyte and water changes that can occur across the bladder membrane.[18] Nevertheless, despite these biochemical drawbacks, reptile urine samples are useful for cytologic assessments of inflammation and infection and for the identification of renal casts.

Voided Urine

The urinary, genital, and intestinal tracts empty into a common cloaca, and therefore, any samples voided from the cloaca may represent material derived from, or contaminated by, any of these systems. Voided urine and urates, although useful for cytology, must be critically evaluated whenever a culture is obtained. Urine microbiology results must be

Table 66-1 Selected Biochemical Parameters Used in the Evaluation of Renal Damage Disease in Captive Green Iguanas (*Iguana iguana*)

Parameter	Published Ranges				
	Divers et al[32,A]	Hernandez-Divers et al[6,B]	Harr et al[31,C]	Fudge[87,D]	ISIS[88,E]
Albumin (g/L)	21-28	23-28	13-30	20-31	10-39
Total protein (g/L)	50-78	55-69	42-76	49-78	41-91
Globulin (g/L)	25-43	31-43	22-52	13-38	24-61
A/G ratio	0.5-1.1	0.5-0.9	0.3-1	1.1-2.9	0.16-1.6
Uric acid (μmol/L)	70-140	122-322	40-390	113-654	0-375
Calcium (mmol/L)	2.2-3.5	2.8-3.2	2.1-5.8	2.2-4	2-3.9
Ionized calcium (mmol/L)	NA	1.37-1.39	NA	NA	NA
Phosphorus (mmol/L)	1.5-3.0	1.04-1.6	0.9-3	NA	1.1-3.8
Sodium (mmol/L)	140-183	145-151	152-172	NA	146-189
Chloride (mmol/L)	110-125	NA	113-129	NA	104-128
Potassium (mmol/L)	1.3-4	2.2-3	2.0-6.1	NA	1-5.7
AST (IU/L)	5-52	NA	7-102	12-84	2-172
GGT (IU/L)	0-3	NA	NA	NA	0-1

[A]Divers et al (1996) include blood from 10 healthy Green Iguanas (including males and nongravid females) kept indoors in artificial conditions.
[B]Hernandez-Divers et al (2005) include blood from 23 recently imported, healthy Green Iguanas kept in laboratory conditions. All lizards were reproductively inactive and had normal kidneys as determined with glomerular filtration rate measurements, necropsy, and histologic examinations.
[C]Harr et al (2001) include blood from 51 healthy iguanas kept outdoors in three separate locations in Florida (gravid females excluded to avoid biochemistry extremes associated with reproduction).
[D]Fudge (2000) includes blood from 886 iguanas submitted through the California Avian Laboratory.
[E]International Species Information System (1999), physiologic reference ranges from 16 institutions (females excluded to avoid biochemistry extremes associated with reproduction).
A/G, Albumin/globulin ratio; *AST*, aspartate transaminase; *GGT*, gamma-glutamyl transferase; *NA*, not applicable.

particularly scrutinized if the sample was collected from the floor of the enclosure or the examination table. Fresh urine and urate samples can be collected as a free catch. Many reptiles spontaneously void urine and urates (often with fecal material) when handled. More stoic individuals may be encouraged to urinate with gentle digital stimulation of the cloaca.

In general, catheterization of the bladder is a "blind-stick," although dilation of the cloaca with a nasal or vaginal speculum or evaluation by cloacoscopy may allow visualization of the urethral opening ventral to the rectum.

Cystocentesis

A more representative and less contaminated sample may be collected with cystocentesis. However, given the thin fragile nature of the reptilian bladder, the potential danger of postsampling leakage of unsterile urine into the coelom exists. Given the passage of urine through the cloaca and the electrolyte and water changes that can occur in the bladder, urine collected with cystocentesis may not be representative of renal urine with respect to electrolyte composition and osmolarity. Such samples are often unsterile, although a heavy pure microbiologic growth should alert the clinician to potential infection.

Cystocentesis is possible but must be performed carefully. The large bladder can be accessed from either side in most lizards (Figure 66-4). Because of the caudal extent of the liver on the right side of the coelom in chelonians, cystocentesis is performed most safely when the needle is introduced into the left prefemoral fossa (Figure 66-5). Rotation of chelonians may allow the bladder to fall toward the prefemoral fossa and increase the chance of success. In lizards, one should approach the bladder laterally or ventrally just anterior to the pelvis, aiming the needle anteromedially. A 22-gauge to 25-gauge needle is appropriate, but the smaller needle sizes may become clogged if the urine is very viscous. In large specimens, ultrasound-guided cystocentesis is possible.

Endoscopic Catheterization

One means of obtaining bladder urine without puncturing the bladder is with the endoscope-guided placement of a urethral catheter. This procedure has been used in anesthetized iguanas. Care must be taken not to damage the thin bladder wall.

Standard urinalysis technique can be used to evaluate reptilian urine. Ideally, urinalysis should be performed immediately on obtaining a sample because changes in pH and bacterial populations, lysis of cells, and precipitation of crystals could occur as the urine ages. However, such changes may occur more slowly in reptilian urine than in mammalian urine, making timing of urinalysis less critical.[35] As in mammalian medicine, a complete urinalysis should include gross observation, biochemical testing, specific gravity measurement, and microscopic sediment analysis.

A gross evaluation of the urine is the appropriate first step. Much can be learned regarding the patient's well-being with evaluation of the appearance of the urine sample. Urine color, while ranging from clear to yellow, may be a good reflection of the animal's energy balance. Starvation and hepatic disease promote the production of biliverdin in the urine, turning it a lime green color (Figure 66-6).

Standard urine chemistry dipsticks appear to be useful, albeit unvalidated, for most assays. Although not all dipstick assays are of value, several assays appear to provide important information. Unless otherwise specified, detection of abnormalities with urinalysis should prompt the clinician to consider any and all causes of the abnormal values as seen in other species. For example, severe proteinuria may be seen with protein-losing nephropathy, and hematuria may be seen with cystic calculi, etc.

URINE DIPSTICK EVALUATION

Urine pH

Initial studies in chelonians indicate that urine pH may have significant diagnostic value. Innis[36] and Koelle[37] independently produced data indicating that the urine pH of several

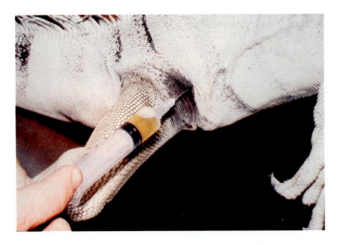

FIGURE 66-4 Cystocentesis in the Green Iguana (*Iguana iguana*). The area just cranial to the thigh is aseptically prepared. The smallest gauge and length needle that will penetrate the body and bladder walls should be chosen. (*Photograph courtesy D. Mader.*)

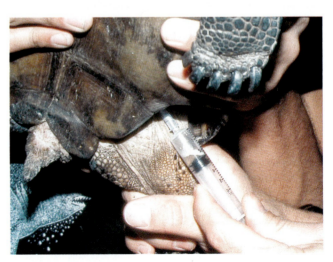

FIGURE 66-5 Cystocentesis in the Desert Tortoise (*Gopherus agassizii*). Because of the large liver lobe on the right side, the bladder tends to rest against the left prefemoral region. Holding the patient vertical permits gravity to settle the bladder adjacent to the fossa. (*Photograph courtesy D. Mader.*)

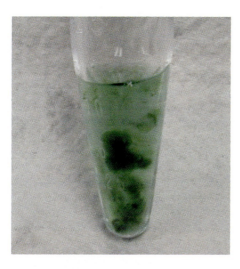

FIGURE 66-6 Urine from a cachectic reptile. The green color is biliverdin pigment. *(Photograph courtesy C. Innis.)*

herbivorous tortoise species is normally alkaline. This is consistent with other herbivorous animals that typically produce alkaline urine. Christopher, Brigmon, and Jacobson[38] showed neutral to slightly alkaline pH in the Desert Tortoise *(Gopherus agassizii)* during periods of abundant forage and rainfall and during early brumation (hibernation). Published reports of the urine pH of other herbivorous reptiles are lacking.

Gibbons, Horton, and Brandl[39] reported the mean urine pH of the omnivorous Box Turtles *Terrapene carolina* and *Terrapene ornata* to be 6.6 and 6.4, respectively. Dantzler and Schmidt-Nielsen[40] reported the urine pH of the Red-eared Turtles *(Pseudemys [Trachemys] scripta)* fed a meat diet to be 6.7. These observations may indicate that, as expected, non-herbivorous reptiles may normally produce acidic urine. Published reports of the urine pH of other omnivorous and carnivorous reptiles are lacking.

Until further data are obtained, suspicion of an abnormality may be appropriate if an herbivorous reptile produces very acidic urine or if a carnivorous reptile produces very alkaline urine. Acidic urine has been observed in herbivorous tortoises under conditions of drought, with high-protein diets, near the end of hibernation, or during prolonged periods of anorexia from illness.[36-38] Although the pathogenesis of acidic urine production in these tortoises is unclear, protein catabolism, and ketogenesis, likely may contribute.[36,38] In most cases, tortoise urine pH has been shown to return to the alkaline range within several weeks of active foraging after hibernation or recovery from illness.[36] As such, monitoring the urine pH of herbivorous reptiles may be a simple means of monitoring recovery from illness and return to positive energy balance. Speculation is interesting that urate cystic calculi commonly found in herbivorous reptiles could form, perhaps, partly from precipitation of urate crystals under conditions of acidic pH and dehydration. If so, attempts to alkalinize the urine through dietary change and medical therapy may be of use in preventing recurrence of such stones after surgical removal.

Although not yet proven in reptiles, alkaline urine in a carnivorous species possibly could indicate the presence of urinary tract infection from a urea-splitting organism. This situation has been well documented in humans and traditional veterinary patients.[41-43]

Protein

Urine dipstick protein assays primarily respond to the presence of albumin. False-positive protein readings may occur with hematuria and pyuria or in the presence of reproductive secretions.[41,42] Initial observations of tortoise and Box Turtle urine indicate that zero to trace protein levels are detected in active healthy specimens. Protein levels of 30 mg/dL or higher have been noted during hibernation or during illness.[36,37,39]

Glucose

Glucosuria is not normally present in significant amounts in those reptiles that have been studied. False-positive results for glucose have been reported in humans after large doses of aspirin, vitamin C, or cephalosporins.[42] Glucosuria was noted by Koelle[37] in 12 of 25 tortoises with renal disease and by Gibbons, Horton, and Brandl[39] in several Box Turtles, including one that was hyperglycemic (plasma glucose = 372 mg/dL). Better documentation of glucosuria and correlation with plasma glucose and organ pathology are needed to ascertain the significance of glucosuria in reptiles.

Blood

Free hemoglobin, myoglobin, or intact erythrocytes may produce a positive reaction for "blood." As expected, Koelle[37] noted hematuria in tortoise urine samples obtained via cystocentesis and bladder expression but not in voided samples. Gibbons, Horton, and Brandl[39] and Innis[36] noted trace to moderate hematuria in a small number of clinically healthy Box Turtles and a tortoise. A positive dipstick reaction for "blood" should be verified with urine sediment evaluation. However, one should note that studies in humans indicate that very dilute urine (specific gravity, <1.008) may result in lysis of erythrocytes, thus producing a false-negative sediment.[42] In light of the generally low specific gravity of reptile urine, this possibility should be considered.

Ketones

The role of ketones in reptile physiology is largely unstudied. Christopher, Brigmon, and Jacobson[38] provide evidence of increased plasma and urine beta-hydroxybutyrate in Desert Tortoises in response to drought but not hibernation, indicating that this may be a clinically important ketone in reptiles. Unfortunately, however, most urine dipstick ketone assays react to acetoacetic acid and sometimes acetones but not to beta-hydroxybutyrate.[41] Further studies on the pathophysiology of reptile ketogenesis and the relative amounts of various ketones produced are needed. Trace ketonuria has been detected with dipstick in the urine of tortoises emerging from brumation (hibernation) but resolved within several weeks of resumed activity and feeding.[36] Abnormal urine color may result in false-positive ketone reaction on dipsticks.[41]

LEUKOCYTES AND NITRITE

The leukocyte test on urine dipsticks reacts to the presence of esterases produced by granulocytes and is considered to be an accurate assay in human medicine.[41,42] However, it has been shown to be poorly sensitive in dogs.[43] Its utility in reptile urinalysis has not been evaluated. Similarly, the nitrite assay, which reacts to the presence of nitrite produced by nitrate-reducing bacteria, is useful in humans but has not been validated for other species.[41,42] The urine nitrite test was reported to be positive in three of 50 healthy tortoises and five of 25 ill tortoises by Koelle.[37] The significance of this finding is unclear because, as discussed subsequently, the presence of bacteria in reptile urine is considered normal.

Urobilinogen and Bilirubin

The role of urobilinogen in reptiles is unclear, and it has not been reported to be present in reptile urine.[36] Because most reptiles (with the exception of some species of snakes) produce very little bilirubin, the bilirubin assay is generally considered to be of no use in reptile medicine.[44] An assay for biliverdin, if developed for routine clinical use, may be more informative.

Urine Specific Gravity

Although dipstick specific gravity assays have been validated for human urine, the test correlates poorly with refractometric results in various domestic animals.[42,43] This assay has not been studied in reptiles; therefore, standard refractometry should be used to evaluate reptilian urine specific gravity.

URINE SEDIMENT EVALUATION

Microscopic evaluation of the urine sediment is an important part of reptile urinalysis. Reptile urine may be centrifuged as in standard mammalian urinalysis procedure, or very low volume samples may be simply placed on a slide with a coverslip. On the basis of the preference of the microscopist, urine sediment stains may or may not be used. In some cases, dried smears of the sediment for examination as a cytologic specimen may be useful in addition to the wet-mounted sample. Erythrocytes, leukocytes, epithelial cells, microorganisms, spermatozoa, crystals, and casts may be identified in reptile urine (Figures 66-7 and 66-8).

Observations of normal tortoise and Box Turtle urine reveal that small numbers of leukocytes and epithelial cells may be seen but that urine is often acellular.[36,39,37] Erythrocytes are not routinely seen unless catheterization or cystocentesis has been performed. Some reptile bladder epithelial cells are ciliated, and finding such cells in the urine sediment in small numbers should not be surprising.[45] The presence of large numbers of leukocytes, erythrocytes, or epithelial cells should prompt consideration of further urinary tract evaluation including plasma biochemical evaluation, radiographs, ultrasound, endoscopy, renal biopsy, and urine culture.

In light of the anatomy of the reptile urinary tract, one should expect that some amount of bacterial contamination

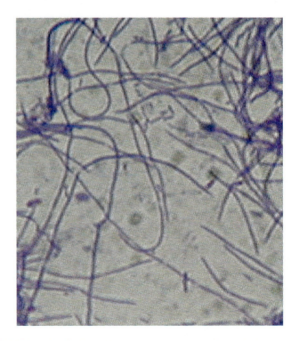

FIGURE 66-7 Rods in the urine of a tortoise collected via cystocentesis. (*Photograph courtesy C. Innis.*)

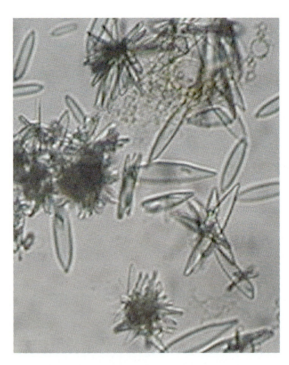

FIGURE 66-8 Urate crystals (normal) as seen in the urine of a Green Iguana (*Iguana iguana*). (*Photograph courtesy C. Innis.*)

of the urine occurs within the cloaca and certainly within the colon in those species that lack a bladder. With experience, however, the microscopist may become comfortable with subjectively assessing the relative numbers and morphology of the urine flora. For example, a mixed population of moderate numbers of rods and cocci may be normal, but huge numbers of a monomorphic bacterial population, or large numbers of budding yeast or fungal hyphae, are generally abnormal. If ancillary testing indicates the possibility of urinary tract disease, culture of reptile urine may be useful. At this time, qualitative and quantitative data on reptile urine flora are lacking. Therefore, clinicians must use their judgement in interpreting culture results. Pure cultures of high concentrations of known reptilian pathogens should be viewed with suspicion.[46] As renal biopsy becomes more common, data correlating renal tissue culture and histopathology with urine culture results should better define the value of urine culture in diagnosing bacterial nephropathies.

Occasionally, protozoan or metazoan parasites may be detected through urinalysis. The flagellated protozoan and renal parasite *Hexamita* has been reported by many authors and is often seen in chelonian urine samples.[36,37,39,47,48] The author (CI) has also observed amoebae (Figure 66-9) in chelonian urine. In snakes and crocodilians where urine is stored in the colon, urine evaluation can often be a useful substitute for fecal testing in an animal that is not producing feces because of anorexia. Koelle[37] reported finding *Hexamita*, ciliates, and helminth eggs in tortoise urine samples.

The presence of casts and crystals in reptile urine may be significant, but much more data are needed before definite statements can be made. Although crystals and casts may be seen, one should be cautious in assuming that these have the same significance as their mammalian counterparts on the basis of appearance alone. For example, biochemical assays to determine the chemical composition of various crystals and histochemical staining to determine the nature of cast components have not been performed for reptile urine. Until such research is done, one may cautiously, subjectively assess the numbers and morphology of casts and crystals in an attempt to differentiate "normal" from "abnormal."

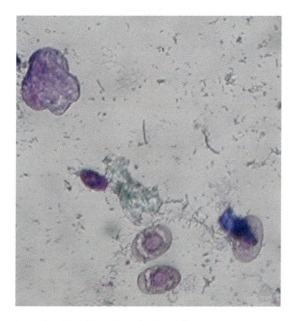

FIGURE 66-9 Amoeba *(upper left)* in the urine from a tortoise. Compare the size with the erythrocytes in the *lower right*. *(Photograph courtesy C. Innis.)*

In many reptilian urine sediment samples, small spherical crystals may be seen. These are likely to be urate crystals as described by Minnich and Piehl.[49] Other crystals that have been noted in reptile urine on the basis of morphology include calcium oxalate, cholesterol, cystine, hippuric acid, leucine, sodium urate, tyrosine, bilirubin, and triple phosphate.[37] Although Koelle[37] found these types of crystals in tortoises with renal disease, but not in healthy tortoises, the significance and pathogenesis of crystal formation have not yet been elucidated.

Casts, or cast-like objects, have been noted in chelonian urine. In some cases, small spherical urate crystals aggregate to form cast-like structures. Unclear, however, is whether these are truly casts that formed in the kidney or whether they are simply aggregates that formed in the bladder. Koelle[37] reported the presence of casts (granular, hyaline, bacterial, and ammonium biurate) in tortoises with renal disease but not in healthy tortoises.

Clearly, worthwhile information can be obtained from traditional urinalysis of reptile urine. Urinalysis is an inexpensive and minimally time-consuming test that can form a valuable piece of the diagnostic puzzle, particularly for the diagnostically challenging reptilian patient. Although initial observations have been made, a need exists for controlled studies of factors that affect chemical and physical properties of reptile urine in health and disease. Clinicians may contribute to this research by carefully accumulating data on urinalysis results of various species and publishing their findings. One obvious area of research is the evaluation of urinalysis for early diagnosis of renal disease in the Green Iguana. Likely, as-yet-unstudied urine chemical parameters will be of importance in the future of reptile clinical pathology.

Diagnostic Imaging

Radiography

The normal kidneys are not always readily appreciable on plain radiographs; however, dorsoventral and lateral (horizontal beam) views are generally the most useful.[50,51] Radiographs can reveal renomegaly, radiopaque uroliths, macroscopic soft tissue mineralization, and severe gout (Figures 66-10 and 66-11). In the iguana, the only organs to occupy the pelvic canal are the kidneys and the lower intestinal tract; therefore, renomegaly often causes extramural obstruction of the colon with resultant constipation. This constipation is often radiographically more obvious than the renomegaly. Negative contrast radiographs can be obtained with an intracoelomic injection of air (5 to 10 mg/kg) and help to differentiate enlarged kidneys from other coelomic soft tissues (e.g., active ovaries). Intravenous urography can be used to highlight the kidneys, identify masses (abscesses, neoplasia, calculi), and show renal or ureteral damage or obstruction. Bolus intravenous injection of 800 to 1000 mg/kg of aqueous iodine contrast media (e.g., iohexol) is followed by serial dorsoventral and lateral radiographs at 0, 0.5, 2, 5, 15, 30, and 60 minutes, with the reptile maintained within the species-specific preferred optimum temperature zone.[51] Cranial intravenous administration results in an excretory urogram; however, caudal vein administration may produce different results as the contrast agent courses through the portal renal system before entering the general circulation and the glomeruli.

Ultrasonography

Ultrasonography, with a 7.5-mHz to 10-mHz sector transducer, permits an appreciation of normal tissue and mineralization, cysts, and other gross pathologic changes (Figure 66-12).[51] Ultrasonography also aids kidney visualization for transcutaneous biopsy. In the iguana, the bony pelvis is a barrier to ultrasound waves, and therefore, the transducer must be angled caudally from a prepelvic location in the ventral midline just cranial to the hindlimbs or cranially from a cloacal position at the ventral tail base. The scaled nature of the integument necessitates the use of copious ultrasound gel or a water bath to reduce air artifacts. In general, a 10-mHz probe is well suited to neonates and juveniles up to 800 g in weight. Animals over 800 g are best examined with a 7.5-mHz transducer, and giant reptiles can be sonographed with 5 mHz.

Scintigraphy

Technetium has been shown to be useful to evaluate renal function in healthy Green Iguanas. Experimental scintigraphy studies involving 10 normal iguanas documented normal renal uptake of technetium-99m dimercaptosuccinic acid (^{99m}Tc-DMSA), and iguanas with reduced functional renal mass have been postulated to exhibit a decrease in technetium uptake.[52] However, the expense of such equipment combined with radiation regulations makes this an impractical method for most private practices.

Endoscopy

The use of fine-diameter rigid endoscopes has revolutionized reptile medicine, permitting the direct visualization of a color magnified image of visceral organs, including the kidneys, through a small surgical entrance into the coelomic cavity (Figure 66-13).[5,6,53,54] The authors prefer a 2.7-mm, 30-degree oblique Hopkins telescope powered by a xenon light source and attached to a video camera and monitor (avian and exotic rigid endoscopy equipment; Karl Storz Veterinary Endoscopy America, Goleta, Calif). Insufflation, preferably with carbon dioxide, is essential. General anesthesia, lateral positioning, aseptic preparation, and paralumbar entry permit examination of the coelomic cavity. In the iguana, the paired kidneys are normally located within the pelvic canal and, being hidden by the terminal colon, fat bodies, and bladder, are difficult to find without insufflation. In cases of generalized renomegaly, the kidneys protrude from the pelvic canal into the coelomic cavity. In most cases, adequate examination of both kidneys from a single entry point is possible. A more midline approach may aid examination of both kidneys, but the midline vein and the associated suspensory ligament can still be a hindrance, and therefore, a second contralateral entry point can be made if necessary. The endoscope entry site requires a single suture for closure. Endoscopy offers an unrivaled appreciation of renal size, surface contours, color, and lesions, which should be documented as focal, multifocal, or diffuse.

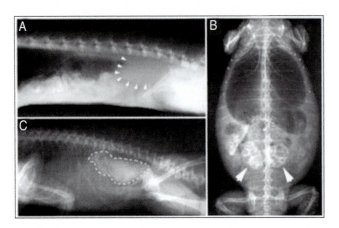

FIGURE 66-10 A, Lateral horizontal beam radiograph of a Green Iguana *(Iguana iguana)* shows renomegaly *(arrows)*. **B,** Dorsoventral radiograph of a Spiny-tailed Lizard *(Uromastyx aegyptius)* shows cystic mineralization of both kidneys *(arrows)*. **C,** Lateral horizontal excretory urogram of a Chinese Water Dragon *(Physignathus cocincinus)* shows irregular renomegaly *(dotted line)*. *(Photographs courtesy S.J. Hernandez-Divers.)*

Renal Biopsy

The relatively poor diagnostic value of urinalysis, the late detection of renal disease with blood biochemistry, and the poor regenerative capabilities of the diseased kidney exemplify the importance of renal biopsy early in the diagnostic process. The cranial tail cut-down and minimally invasive coeliotomy biopsy techniques permit unilateral access to a single kidney. In these cases, palpation and diagnostic imaging can be helpful in determining whether a left or right approach is most appropriate. Major coeliotomy, ultrasound-guided, and endoscopic biopsy procedures can usually be used to examine and biopsy either or both kidneys.

The nasal salt glands, bladder, and colon perform important osmoregulatory functions in many species, and biopsy of these extrarenal sites may, on rare occasions, be useful for an overall assessment of osmoregulation.

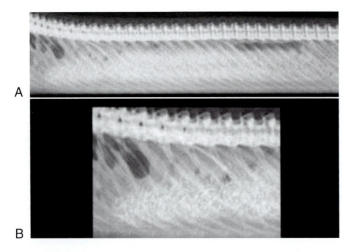

FIGURE 66-11 A, Lateral horizontal radiograph of a Boa Constrictor *(Boa constrictor)* with renal gout and secondary mineralization. **B,** Close-up of the cranial pole of the left kidney shows the radiating pattern of mineralized urate tophi. *(Photographs courtesy S.J. Hernandez-Divers.)*

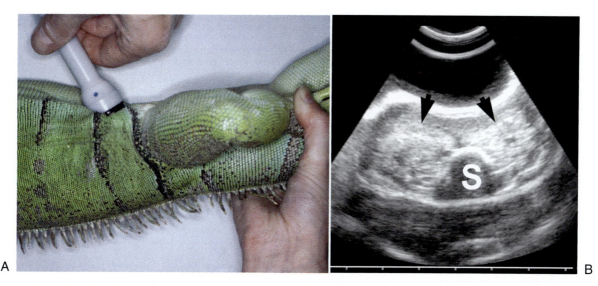

FIGURE 66-12 **A,** Ultrasonography of an iguanid's kidneys with a 7.5-MHz transducer angled caudad to visualize the cranial aspect of the kidneys. **B,** Ultrasonogram of diseased, hyperechoic kidneys in a Green Iguana (*Iguana iguana*). (*Photographs courtesy S.J. Hernandez-Divers.*)

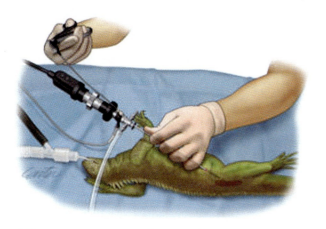

FIGURE 66-13 Endoscopic technique for the coelioscopic examination of the intrapelvic kidneys of the Green Iguana (*Iguana iguana*). Note the one-handed support of the telescope that permits the single surgeon concurrent use of biopsy forceps. (*Photograph courtesy S.J. Hernandez-Divers.*)

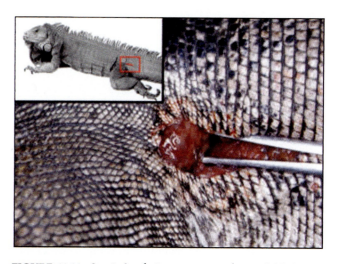

FIGURE 66-14 Surgical technique to expose the caudal kidney at the craniolateral aspect of the iguanid tail for biopsy. (*Photograph courtesy S.J. Hernandez-Divers.*)

Cranial Tail Cut-Down Biopsy

A relatively simple technique to biopsy the intrapelvic kidneys of Iguanas requires a cranial tail cut-down with local or general anesthesia. A small longitudinal incision is made in the lateral midline just below the lateral processes of the coccygeal vertebrae (Figure 66-14). The incision extends for 1 to 3 cm caudad, starting just behind the hindlimb. Blunt dissection between the dorsal and ventral coccygeal muscles permits exposure of the caudolateral aspect of the kidney that can then be sampled. Hemorrhage depends on the size of the biopsy, but the temporary application of hemostatic dressings or radiosurgery is effective. This technique is particularly valuable with diffuse renal disease where the kidneys are not enlarged and coelomic approaches to the intrapelvic kidneys are more difficult. It is limited to unilateral biopsy unless bilateral cut-down procedures are undertaken. Furthermore, because only a small area of the caudal kidney can be visualized and sampled, this technique is best reserved for diffuse or focal diseases of the caudal kidney. Focal or multifocal renal diseases may be missed.

Coeliotomy Biopsy

Where renomegaly is obvious, a standard coeliotomy and renal biopsy can be undertaken (Figure 66-15). A standard midline or paramedian coeliotomy in lizards enables both kidneys to be assessed, and excisional or Tru-Cut biopsies can be collected. In snakes, a standard ventrolateral approach 75% to 95% snout-to-vent provides access to one or both kidneys; however, precise renal position varies with taxonomy, and anatomic references should be consulted before surgery. In chelonians, the kidney is positioned in the caudodorsal retrocoelomic region and, being protected by the carapace,

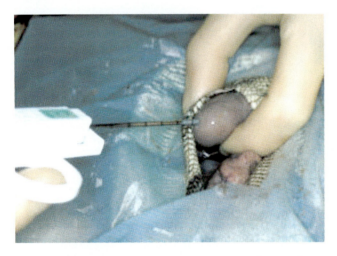

FIGURE 66-15 Standard coeliotomy in a Green Iguana (*Iguana iguana*) and biopsy of an enlarged kidney with a Tru-Cut biopsy device. *(Photograph courtesy S.J. Hernandez-Divers.)*

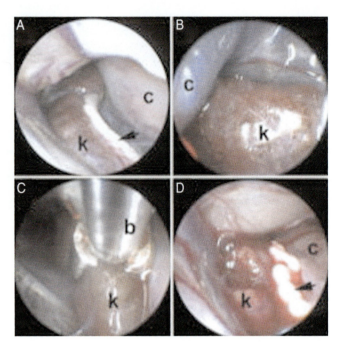

FIGURE 66-16 Endoscopic evaluation and biopsy of the iguanid kidney. **A,** Coelioscopic view of the normal kidney (*k*) protruding from the pelvic inlet, terminal colon (*c*), and vas deferens (*arrow*). **B,** Close-up examination of the left kidney (*k*) reveals normal lobulated pattern and coloration. The terminal colon (*c*) is also visible. **C,** Positioning of biopsy forceps (*b*) at the cranial pole of the kidney (*k*) in preparation for biopsy. **D,** View of the kidney (*k*) immediately after biopsy. Note the minimal hemorrhage and the undamaged colon (*c*) and vas deferens (*arrow*). *(Photographs courtesy S.J. Hernandez-Divers.)*

is difficult to access. If an enlarged kidney can be palpated, it can usually be immobilized just under the skin, permitting the use of a Tru-Cut needle biopsy or minimally invasive coeliotomy incision directly over the organ. This technique is suited to the detection of focal, multifocal, and diffuse renal diseases, but focal disease may be missed.

Ultrasound-Guided Biopsy

Ultrasound-guided biopsies are practical in many species but can be problematic with intrapelvic tissue of iguanids. Even in those species in which ultrasonography permits the identification of gross lesions and aids biopsy needle guidance, dangers are still associated with a technique that does not permit direct, three-dimensional, visual control. In particular, the voluminous bladder, gastrointestinal tract, and several large arteries and veins must be appreciated and avoided. Depending on the quality of the equipment and skill of the ultrasonographer, multifocal or focal lesions may be missed.

Endoscopic Biopsy

The endoscope permits evaluation of the size, color, and shape of both coelomic kidneys via a single surgical entry.[5,6] The use of endoscopic scissors and biopsy forceps with direct visual control permits the incision of the renal capsule and collection of quality samples with less risk to surrounding structures (Figure 66-16). The excellent optics of the telescope also permit an assessment of focal and multifocal disease and the selection of appropriate biopsies that may otherwise be difficult to ascertain without a color, magnified image. The diagnostic quality of endoscopic renal biopsies in Green Iguanas has been found to be excellent.[6]

Assessment of Renal Function

Elevations of nitrogenous metabolites in plasma are poor indicators of renal *function* because they can be affected by hydration status and because pathologic changes tend to occur late in the course of disease. In human and domestic animal medicine, measurement of renal function has been established as an important tool in the diagnosis and surveillance of kidney disease.[55-69] The most advanced techniques use imaging modalities including scintigraphy, computed tomography, and magnetic resonance imaging to measure renal blood flow or renal clearance of radioactive nuclides or contrast agents. Other techniques rely on determination of the plasma clearance of an exogenous compound (e.g., phenolsulfonphthalein, insulin, creatinine), which requires intravenous drug administration, serial blood sampling, and catheterization for urine collection. Because of the postrenal modification of urine in the reptilian cloaca, colon, or bladder, catheterization of the ureters is essential to differentiate the roles of glomerular filtration and tubular transport from those of the cloaca, colon, and bladder.[8] Recently, iohexol clearance studies have proven useful for determination of GFR in mammals without bladder catheterization.[60,70-76]

Iohexol is a nonionic radiographic iodine contrast medium of low osmolarity that is extensively used in clinical radiology and considered essentially free from side effects when used correctly.[77-82] Iohexol is excreted solely by glomerular filtration with negligible extrarenal elimination in mammals.[83] The plasma clearance of iohexol (PCI) can be determined with analysis of plasma iohexol concentration over time after a single intravenous injection (Figure 66-17). The rate of clearance of iohexol from plasma can be used to estimate GFR with dividing the iohexol dose by the area under the curve (AUC) because elimination is solely by

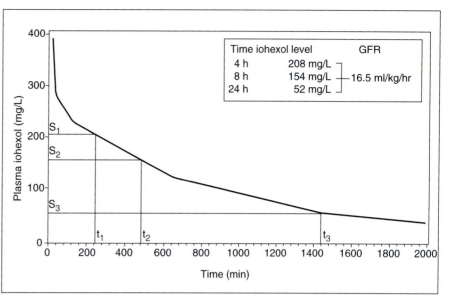

FIGURE 66-17 Example of an iohexol excretion curve against time from a healthy Green Iguana *(Iguana iguana)*. Three samples taken at 4, 8, and 24 hours provide three separate plasma iohexol values that can be used to calculate glomerular filtration rate and, hence, renal function. *(Photograph courtesy S.J. Hernandez-Divers, UGA.)*

glomerular filtration. In addition, this methodology has the distinct advantage of relying on blood collection and not urinary catheterization for the collection of urine. Calculation of GFR by this method has been used and validated in dogs, cats, pigs, rats, humans, and iguanas.[60,70-76,84,85] The established protocol for dogs and cats is 300 mg/kg iohexol intravenously followed by blood collection for iohexol levels at 2 hours, 3 hours, and 4 hours after injection.[86] A recent study validated this methodology in reptiles, and in the healthy Green Iguanas, GFR was reported to be 16.56 ± 3.90 mL/kg/h, with a 95% confidence interval of 14.78 to 18.34 mL/kg/h.[6] In addition, iguanas with renal disease exhibited significant reductions in GFR even in the absence of other clinical or biochemical signs. A suggested protocol for measurement of GFR in iguanas (and potentially other reptiles) is as follows:

- Contact the Diagnostic Center for Population and Animal Health (Michigan State University, East Lansing, MI 48824, [517] 353-1683, www.ahdl.msu.edu) to check for any changes to the blood collection and submission requirements for iohexol assay and GFR calculation.
- Ensure the reptile is hydrated and fasted for 24 hours.
- Weigh accurately, and inject 75 mg/kg iohexol intravenously (intravenous catheterization reduces the risks of perivascular injection that invalidates the results) at time 0.
- Collect three 0.5-mL blood samples at 4 hours, 8 hours, and 24 hours after injection. Record the exact times of blood collection, and send these details with the three separated plasma samples on ice to the Diagnostic Center for Population and Animal Health for iohexol assays and GFR calculation.

Unlike most other clearance techniques, iohexol excretion does not require bladder or ureteral catheterization, and unlike scintigraphy, it does not require expensive equipment or radioisotopes to perform. Given that iohexol assays are commercially available, this technique for renal function evaluation in reptiles can be easily undertaken in private practice.

CONCLUSION

Renal disease remains an important disease process of captive reptiles, especially the Green Iguana. In cases of chronic renal disease, clinical signs and biochemical changes are unlikely to become apparent until late in the course of disease. Iohexol clearance, at least in the iguana, appears to be a safe and practical method for estimation of GFR, and for the first time, *renal function* can be evaluated in practice. Endoscopic evaluation provides a safe and effective means for visualization and biopsy of kidneys, and this technique has again been validated, at least in the iguanas and chelonians. Histopathologic quality of endoscopic renal biopsies is excellent and correlates well with necropsy findings. Endoscopic renal evaluation with biopsy is recommended as an important tool for the accurate diagnosis of renal disease in reptiles.

Much remains to be learned about reptile renal physiology and pathophysiology. In many cases, initiating causes are often inferred from poor husbandry and nutrition or extrapolated from histopathologic interpretations made late in the course of the disease, or most often at postmortem examination. The link between parathyroid hormone and renal disease in humans has been well documented, and given the high prevalence of clinical (and subclinical) secondary nutritional hyperparathyroidism in many captively reared reptiles, this certainly warrants further investigation. Apart from hyperparathyroidism, chronic water deprivation also appears to be a common historic factor in certain rainforest-adapted species. As a folivore originating from the high humidity rainforests of Central and South America, water recovery is not considered to be an adaptive stress response in *Iguana iguana,* and therefore, renal anatomy and physiology are considered to be nonspecialized compared with more arid or aquatic reptiles. In addition, arboreal reptiles do not voluntarily drink from open water but instead imbibe rain or dew droplets from foliage. Maintaining such species in low relative humidity with a water bowl from which to drink is likely to both increase insensible water losses and interfere with normal water intake.

Appropriate therapeutic decisions (including euthanasia) can only be made after an accurate diagnosis. To date, our diagnoses are based largely on the structural evaluations of renal histopathology, and renal biopsy remains our most useful tool for a definitive diagnosis. However, the advent of renal function testing by quantifying GFR offers a new modality for diagnosis and prognosis.

ACKNOWLEDGMENTS

The author thanks WB Saunders and the American Association of Zoo and Wildlife Medicine for granting permission to reproduce sections from the following articles in the preparation of this chapter:

Divers SJ: Reptilian renal and reproductive disease diagnosis. In Fudge AM, editor: *Laboratory medicine: avian and exotic pets,* Philadelphia, 2000, WB Saunders.

Divers SJ: Lizard endoscopic techniques with particular reference to the Green Iguana (*Iguana iguana*), *Semin Avian Exotic Pet Med* 8(3):122-129, 1999.

Hernandez-Divers SJ: Green Iguana nephrology: a review of diagnostic techniques, *Vet Clinics North Am Exotic Anim Pract* 6:233-250, 2002.

Hernandez-Divers SJ, Stahl SJ, Stedman NL, Hernandez-Divers SM, Schumacher J, Hanley CS, et al: Renal evaluation in the Green Iguana (*Iguana iguana*): assessment of plasma biochemistry, glomerular filtration rate, and endoscopic biopsy, *J Zoo Wildl Med* 36:155-168, 2005.

REFERENCES

1. Mader DR: *Reptile medicine and surgery,* Philadelphia, 1996, WB Saunders.
2. Frye FL: *Biomedical and surgical aspects of captive reptile husbandry,* Malabar, Fla, 1992, Krieger Publishing.
3. Hernandez-Divers SJ: Green Iguana nephrology: a review of diagnostic techniques, *Vet Clin North Am Exotic Anim Pract* 6:233-250, 2003.
4. Jacobson E: *Biology, husbandry, and medicine of the Green Iguana,* Malabar, Fla, 2003, Krieger Publishing.
5. Hernandez-Divers SJ: Endoscopic renal evaluation and biopsy in Chelonia, *Vet Rec* 154:73-80, 2004.
6. Hernandez-Divers SJ, Stahl S, Stedman NL, et al: Renal evaluation in the Green Iguana (*Iguana iguana*): assessment of plasma biochemistry, glomerular filtration rate, and endoscopic biopsy, *J Zoo Wildl Med* 36:155-168, 2005.
7. Bordley J, Richards AN: Quantitative studies of the composition of glomerular urine: VII: the concentration of uric acid in glomerular urine of snakes and frogs, determined by an ultramicroadaption of Folin's method, *J Biol Chem* 101:193-221, 1933.
8. Dantzler WH: Renal fucntion (with special emphasis on nitrogen excretion). In Gans C, Dawson WR, editors: *Biology of the Reptilia, physiology A,* London, 1976, Academic Press.
9. Roberts JS, Schmidt-Nielson K: Renal ultrastructure and excretion of salt and water by three terrestrial lizards, *Am J Physiol* 211:476-486, 1969.
10. Green B: Aspects of renal function in the lizard, *Varanus gouldii, Comp Biochem Physiol* 42:747-756, 1972.
11. Shoemaker VH, Licht P, Dawson WR: Effects of temperature on kidney function in the lizard *Tiliqua rugosa, Physiol Zool* 39:244-252, 1966.
12. Templeton JR: Cardiovascular response to temperature in the lizard *Sauromalus obesus, Physiol Zool* 37:300-306, 1964.
13. Dantzler WH, Schmidt-Nielson B: Excretion in freshwater (*Pseudemys scripta*) and the desert tortoise (*Gopherus agassizii*), *Am J Physiol* 210:198-210, 1966.
14. Ranges HA, Chasis H, Goldring W, Smith HW: The functional measurement of a number of active glomeruli and tubules in kidneys of normal and hypertensive subjects, *Am J Physiol* 126:103, 1939.
15. Schmidt-Nielson B, Davies LE: Fluid transport and tubular intercellular spaces in reptilian kidneys, *Science* 159:1105-1108, 1968.
16. Bradshaw SD, Bradshaw FJ: Arginine vasotocin: site and mode of action in the reptilian kidney, *Gen Comp Endocrinol* 126:7-13, 2002.
17. Badia P, Gomez T, Diaz M, Lorenzo A: Mechanisms of transport of Na^+ and Cl^- in the lizard colon, *Comp Biochem Physiol A* 87:883-887, 1987.
18. Ehrenspeck G, Voner C: Effect of furosemide on ion transport in the turtle bladder: evidence for direct inhibition of active acid-base transport, *Biochim Biophys Acta* 817:318-326, 1985.
19. Stephens GA, Robertson FM: Renal responses to diuretics in the turtle, *J Comp Physiol* 155:387-393, 1985.
20. Frye FL: Diagnosis and surgical treatment of reptilian neoplasms with a compilation of cases 1966-1993, *In Vivo* 8:885-892, 1994.
21. Barnard S: *Reptile keeper's handbook,* Malabar, Fla, 1996, Krieger Publishing.
22. McArthur S, Wilkinson R, Meyer J, et al: *Medicine and surgery of tortoises and turtles,* Oxford, 2004, Blackwell Publishing.
23. Raiti P, Girling S: *Manual of reptiles,* Cheltenham, England, 2004, British Small Animal Veterinary Association.
24. Massry SG, Fadda GZ: Chronic renal failure is a state of cellular calcium toxicity, *Am J Kidney Dis* 21:81-86, 1993.
25. Divers SJ: Clinical evaluation of reptiles, *Vet Clin North Am Exot Anim Pract* 2:291-331, 1999.
26. Harr KE, Alleman AR, Dennis PM, et al: Morphologic and cytochemical characteristics of blood cells and hematologic and plasma biochemical reference ranges in Green Iguanas, *J Am Vet Med Assoc* 218:915-921, 2001.
27. Divers SJ, Redmayne G, Aves EK: Haematological and biochemical values of 10 Green Iguanas (*Iguana iguana*), *Vet Rec* 138:203-205, 1996.
28. Divers SJ: Reptilian renal and reproductive disease diagnosis. In Fudge AM, editor: *Laboratory medicine avian and exotic pets,* Philadelphia, 2000, WB Saunders.
29. Innis C, Hawes M, Stone M, Seymour R: What's your diagnosis? Case 2, *Bull Assoc Reptilian Amphibian Vet* 9:50-52, 1999.
30. Suedmeyer K: Hypocalcaemia and hyperphosphataemia in a Green Iguana, Iguana iguana, with concurrent elevation of serum glutamic oxalic transaminase, *Bull Assoc Rept Amph Vets* 5:5-6, 1995.
31. Meints RH, Carver FJ, Gerst JW, McLaughlin DW: Erythropoietic activity in the turtle: the influence of hemolytic anemia, hypoxia and hemorrhage on hemopoietic function, *Comp Biochem Physiol A* 50:419-422, 1975.

32. Elder G: Pathophysiology and recent advances in the management of renal osteodystrophy, *J Bone Miner Res* 17:2094-2105, 2002.
33. Malluche HH, Monier-Faugere MC: Understanding and managing hyperphosphatemia in patients with chronic renal disease, *Clin Nephrol* 52:267-77, 1999.
34. Block GA: The impact of calcimimetics on mineral metabolism and secondary hyperparathyroidism in end-stage renal disease, *Kidney Int Suppl* S131-6, 2003.
35. Lane R. *California avian and exotics laboratory*, personal communication, 2001.
36. Innis CJ: Observations on urinalyses of clinically normal captive tortoises, *Proc ARAV 4th Ann Conf*, 1997.
37. Koelle P: Urinalysis in tortoises, *Proc ARAV 7th Ann Conf*, 2000.
38. Christopher MM, Brigmon R, Jacobson E: Seasonal alterations in plasma β-hydroxybutyrate and related biochemical parameters in the desert tortoise *(Gopherus agassizii)*, *Comp Biochem Physiol* 108A:303, 1994.
39. Gibbons PM, Horton SJ, Brandl SRW: Urinalysis in box turtles, *Terrapene* species, *Proc ARAV 7th Ann Conf*, 2000.
40. Dantzler WH, Schmidt-Nielsen B: Excretion in the freshwater turtle *(Pseudemys scripta)* and desert tortoise *(Gopherus agassizii)*, *Am J Physiol* 210:198, 1965.
41. Lowe F, Brendler C: Evaluation of the urologic patient. In Walsh P, editor: *Campbell's urology*, ed 6, Philadelphia, 1992, WB Saunders.
42. Williams RD, Kreder KJ: Urologic laboratory evaluation. In Tanagho E, McAninch J, editors: *Smith's general urology*, Norwalk, Conn, 1995, Appleton & Lange.
43. Chew DJ, DiBartola SP: Diagnosis and pathophysiology of renal disease. In Ettinger SJ, editor: *Textbook of veterinary internal medicine*, Philadelphia, 1989, WB Saunders.
44. Campbell T: Clinical pathology. In Mader DR, editor: *Reptile medicine and surgery*, Philadelphia, 1996, WB Saunders.
45. Bolton PM, Beuchat CA: Cilia in the urinary bladder of reptiles and amphibians: a correlate of urate production, *Copeia* 3:711-717, 1991.
46. Divers S: Reptilian renal and reproductive disease diagnosis. In Fudge AM, editor: *Laboratory medicine: avian and exotic pets*, Philadelphia, 2000, WB Saunders.
47. Frye FL: *Biomedical and surgical aspects of captive reptile husbandry*, Malabar, Fla, 1991, Krieger Publishing.
48. McArthur S: *Veterinary management of tortoises and turtles*, Oxford, 1996, Blackwell Science.
49. Minnich J, Piehl P: Spherical precipitates in the urine of reptiles, *Comp Biochem Physiol* 41A:551, 1972.
50. Hernandez-Divers SJ, Lafortune M: Radiology. In McArthur S, Wilkinson R, Meyer J, et al, editors: *Medicine and surgery of tortoises and turtles*, London, 2004, Blackwell Scientific Publications.
51. Hernandez-Divers SM, Hernandez-Divers SJ: Diagnostic imaging of reptiles, *In Practice* 23:370-391, 2001.
52. Greer LL, Daniel GB, Shearn-Bochsler VI, Ramsay EC: Evaluation of the use of technetium Tc 99m diethylenetriamine pentaacetic acid and technetium Tc 99m dimercaptosuccinic acid for scintigraphic imaging of the kidneys in Green Iguanas *(Iguana iguana)*, *Am J Vet Res* 66:87-92, 2005.
53. Hernandez-Divers SJ, Stahl S, Hernandez-Divers SM, et al: Coelomic endoscopy of the Green Iguana *(Iguana iguana)*, *J Herp Med Surg* 14:10-18, 2004.
54. Hernandez-Divers SJ: Diagnostic and surgical endoscopy. In Raiti P, Girling S, editors: *Manual of reptiles*, Cheltenham, England, 2004, British Small Animal Veterinary Association.
55. Lora-Michiels M, Anzola K, Amaya G, Solano M: Quantitative and qualitative scintigraphic measurement of renal function in dogs exposed to toxic doses of Gentamicin, *Vet Radiol Ultrasound* 42:553-561, 2001.
56. Tsushima Y, Blomley MJ, Kusano S, Endo K: Use of contrast-enhanced computed tomography to measure clearance per unit renal volume: a novel measurement of renal function and fractional vascular volume, *Am J Kidney Dis* 33:754-760, 1999.
57. Toto RD: Conventional measurement of renal function utilizing serum creatinine, creatinine clearance, inulin and para-aminohippuric acid clearance, *Curr Opin Nephrol Hypertens* 4:503-509, 1995.
58. Fox M, Natarajan V, Trippodo NC: Measurement of cardiovascular and renal function in unrestrained hamsters, *Lab Anim Sci* 43:94-98, 1993.
59. Levey AS: Measurement of renal function in chronic renal disease, *Kidney Int* 38:167-184, 1990.
60. Effersoe H, Rosenkilde P, Groth S, et al: Measurement of renal function with iohexol: a comparison of iohexol, 99mTc-DTPA, and 51Cr-EDTA clearance, *Invest Radiol* 25:778-782, 1990.
61. Russell CD, Dubovsky EV: Measurement of renal function with radionuclides, *J Nucl Med* 30:2053-2057, 1989.
62. Shirley DG, Walter SJ, Zewde T: Measurement of renal function in unrestrained conscious rats, *J Physiol* 408:67-76, 1989.
63. Yamashita M, Inaba T, Kawase Y, et al: Quantitative measurement of renal function using Ga-68-EDTA, *Tohoku J Exp Med* 155:207-208, 1988.
64. Nimmo MJ, Merrick MV, Allan PL: Measurement of relative renal function: a comparison of methods and assessment of reproducibility, *Br J Radiol* 60:861-864, 1987.
65. Chachati A, Meyers A, Godon JP, Rigo P: Rapid method for the measurement of differential renal function: validation, *J Nucl Med* 28:829-836, 1987.
66. Bianchi C, Donadio C, Tramonti G: Noninvasive methods for the measurement of total renal function, *Nephron* 28:53-57, 1981.
67. Buck AC, Macleod MA, Blacklock NJ: The advantages of 99mTc DTPA(Sn) in dynamic renal scintigraphy and measurement of renal function, *Br J Urol* 52:174-186, 1980.
68. Cole BR, Giangiacomo J, Ingelfinger JR, Robson AM: Measurement of renal function without urine collection: a critical evaluation of the constant-infusion technique for determination of inulin and para-aminohippurate, *N Engl J Med* 287:1109-1114, 1972.
69. Gault MH, Dossetor JB: The place of phenosulfonphthalein (PSP) in the measurement of renal function, *Am Heart J* 75:723-727, 1968.
70. Brown SA, Finco DR, Boudinot FD, et al: Evaluation of a single injection method, using iohexol, for estimating glomerular filtration rate in cats and dogs, *Am J Vet Res* 57:105-110, 1996.
71. Finco DR, Braselton WE, Cooper TA: Relationship between plasma iohexol clearance and urinary exogenous creatinine clearance in dogs, *J Vet Intern Med* 15:368-373, 2001.
72. Frennby B, Sterner G, Almen T, et al: Clearance of iohexol, 51Cr-EDTA and endogenous creatinine for determination of glomerular filtration rate in pigs with reduced renal function: a comparison between different clearance techniques, *Scand J Clin Lab Invest* 57:241-252, 1997.
73. Gleadhill A, Michell AR: Evaluation of iohexol as a marker for the clinical measurement of glomerular filtration rate in dogs, *Res Vet Sci* 60:117-121, 1996.
74. Dencausse A, Chambon C, Violas X, Bonnemain B: Comparative study of the dialysability of iobitridol and iohexol in the rat with impaired renal function, *Acta Radiol* 36:545-548, 1995.
75. Nossen JO, Jakobsen JA, Kjaersgaard P, et al: Elimination of the non-ionic X-ray contrast media iodixanol and iohexol in patients with severely impaired renal function, *Scand J Clin Lab Invest* 55:341-350, 1995.

76. Moe L, Heiene R: Estimation of glomerular filtration rate in dogs with 99M-Tc-DTPA and iohexol, *Res Vet Sci* 58:138-143, 1995.
77. Lundqvist S, Holmberg G, Jakobsson G, et al: Assessment of possible nephrotoxicity from iohexol in patients with normal and impaired renal function, *Acta Radiol* 39:362-367, 1998.
78. Thomsen HS, Golman K, Svendsen O: Muscle toxicity of diatrizoate and iohexol in rabbits: a model for local tissue damage, *Acta Radiol* 32:182-183, 1991.
79. Donadio C, Tramonti G, Giordani R, et al: Effects on renal hemodynamics and tubular function of the contrast medium iohexol in renal patients, *Ren Fail* 12:141-146, 1990.
80. Haughton VM: Intrathecal toxicity of iohexol vs. metrizamide: survey and current state, *Invest Radiol* 20:14-17, 1985.
81. Salvesen S: Acute intravenous toxicity of iohexol in the mouse and in the rat, *Acta Radiol Suppl* 362:73-75, 1980.
82. Albrechtsson U, Hultberg B, Larusdottir H, Norgren L: Nephrotoxicity of ionic and non-ionic contrast media in aorto-femoral angiography, *Acta Radiol Diagnosis* 26:615-618, 1985.
83. Nilsson-Ehle P, Grubb A: New markers for the determination of GFR: iohexol clearance and cystatin C serum concentration, *Kidney Int Suppl* 47:17-19, 1994.
84. Frennby B, Sterner G, Almen T, et al: Clearance of iohexol, chromium-51-ethylenediaminetetraacetic acid, and creatinine for determining the glomerular filtration rate in pigs with normal renal function: comparison of different clearance techniques, *Acad Radiol* 3:651-659, 1996.
85. Frennby B, Sterner G, Almen T, et al: The use of iohexol clearance to determine GFR in patients with severe chronic renal failure: a comparison between different clearance techniques, *Clin Nephrol* 43:35-46, 1995.
86. Kruger JM, Braselton WE, Becker T, et al: Putting GFR into practice: clinical applications of iohexol clearance, *Proc 16th ACVIM Forum* 657-658, 1998.
87. Fudge AM: *Laboratory medicine: avian and exotic pets*, Philadelphia, 2000, WB Saunders.
88. Teare JA: *Physiological data reference values CD ROM*, International Species Information System, 1999.

67
SHELL DAMAGE
STEPHEN L. BARTEN

ANATOMY

The chelonian shell consists of an upper carapace and lower plastron, connected by lateral bridges. The shell is composed of plates of dermal bone covered by horny epidermal keratin scutes (see Figure 7-13). The seams between keratin scutes do not align with the sutures between the underlying bony plates, and this arrangement adds strength to the shell.[1,2] In most chelonians, the keratin scutes are not shed regularly, although the older outer ones may show wear. As growth occurs, larger new scutes develop deep to the smaller old scutes so that the exposed edges of the new scutes form a series of growth rings.[1] These rings do not develop annually and cannot be used to accurately estimate the age of a turtle or tortoise. Other species of chelonian, notably aquatic species, shed the outer layer of the keratin scutes at irregular intervals and thus have smooth shells without growth rings.

The bones of the carapace include a row of neural bones along the midline. The anterior midline bone is the nuchal, and the posterior midline one is the pygal. Just anterior to the pygal and caudal to the neurals on the midline are two suprapygal bones. Lateral to the neural bones are the costals. The margin of the carapace between the neural and pygal on each side consists of the peripherals. The corresponding scutes of the carapace include a central row of vertebrals, the most anterior of which is called the cervical. Lateral to these are the pleurals, and the edge of the shell caudal to the cervical on each side is covered by marginals. The bones of the plastron include a single central entoplastron. The other plastral bones are divided into pairs by a central seam. Anterior to the entoplastron are the epiplastrons. Caudal to it are, respectively, the hyoplastrons, hypoplastrons, and xiphiplastrons. The plastral scutes also are paired. They are, from anterior to posterior, the gulars, humerals, pectorals, abdominals, femorals, and anals. These arrangements are typical, but variations exist (see Chapter 7).[2]

The bones of the carapace and plastron in the Softshells (Trionychidae), Leatherback Seaturtle (*Dermochelys coriacea*), Fly River Turtle (*Carettochelys insculpta*), and Pancake Tortoise (*Malacochersus tornieri*) are reduced in number or size, resulting in atypical abbreviated shell structure. The former three have leathery skin that covers the shell in place of the typical keratinized scutes. The latter has a soft flexible carapace and plastron, which allows the tortoise to avoid predators by wedging itself into rocky crevices and inflating its body with air.[1,2] The plastrons of Alligator Snapping Turtles (*Macrochelys temminckii*), Mud Turtles (*Kinosternon* spp.), Musk Turtles (*Sternotherus* spp.), Snapping Turtles (*Chelydra serpentina*), and Softshells are reduced, which allows a soft tissue surgical approach to the coelomic cavity rather than plastronotomy (see Chapter 35).[2]

Box Turtles (*Terrapene* spp.) lack a bridge that connects the carapace and plastron, and Alligator Snapping Turtles possess a row of small supramarginal scutes between the posterior pleural and marginal scutes.[2]

The following turtles have a transverse hinge between the pectoral and abdominal scutes of the plastron, which allows them to more or less close the shell for protection: Box Turtle, Musk Turtle, Blanding's Turtle (*Emydoidea blandingii*), Asian Box Turtle (*Cuora* spp.), Leaf Turtle (*Cyclemys* spp.), Keeled Box Turtle (*Pyxidea mouhotii*), Malayan Flat-shelled Turtle (*Notochelys platynota*), European Pond Turtle (*Emys orbicularis*), African Mud Turtle (*Pelusios* spp.), Mediterranean and Middle Eastern Tortoises (*Testudo* spp.), and Malagasy Spider Tortoise (*Pyxis arachnoides*).[2] Most species of Mud Turtle have two plastral hinges, just anterior and posterior to the abdominal scutes. Hinged-back Tortoises (*Kinixys* spp.) have hinges between the fourth and fifth costal and the seventh and eighth peripheral bones of the caudolateral carapace, which allows them to close the carapace over the hind legs and tail. Some female chelonians such as Desert Tortoises (*Gopherus* spp.), which lack a hinge, nevertheless have a transverse flexible suture between the hypoplastron and xiphiplastron bones of the plastron (just anterior to the seam between the anal and femoral plastral scutes). This allows expansion of the caudal plastron for passage of eggs. This normal suture might be mistaken for a fracture on a radiograph (Figure 67-1). These normal hinges and flexible sutures must be considered in shell repair techniques.

The plastron of several species of turtle is normally pinkish red in color and may be mistaken for infection or inflammation by inexperienced persons. Examples include the Painted Turtle (*Chrysemys picta*), juvenile Mud Turtle, Red-bellied Short-necked Turtle (*Emydura subglobosa*), and juvenile Mata Mata (*Chelus fimbriatus*).

The vertebrae, except for the neck and tail, are fused to the medial aspect of the midline neural bones of the carapace, and a fracture of the midline carapace could result in spinal cord damage. The ribs are fused to the medial aspect of the lateral costal bones of the carapace. The pectoral and pelvic girdles, therefore, are medial to the rib cage, unlike any other group of vertebrates.[1]

SUPERFICIAL SHELL ABSCESSES AND EROSIONS

Superficial abscesses and erosions of the keratin scutes that cover the bony shell are common in aquatic chelonians. Defects or discolorations of the scutes characterize these lesions. Affected areas usually are focal but may be widespread. Discoloration can be dark, pale, or bloody. Part or all of the affected scutes may become loose. Common aspects of the history include poor water quality (lack of a filtration system, infrequent water changes, lack of water conditioners), rough

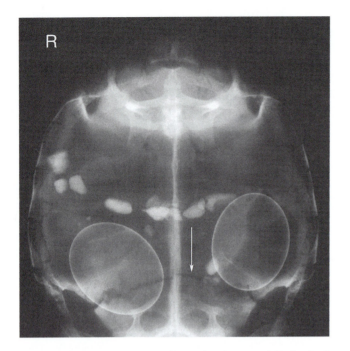

FIGURE 67-1 Dorsoventral radiograph of a gravid Berlandier's Tortoise *(Gopherus berlandieri)*. Two eggs and ingested gravel are visible. Note the radiolucent suture between the hypoplastron and xiphiplastron bones of the plastron (just anterior to the seam between the anal and femoral plastral scutes). This allows expansion of the caudal plastron to allow passage of the eggs. This normal suture might be mistaken for a fracture.

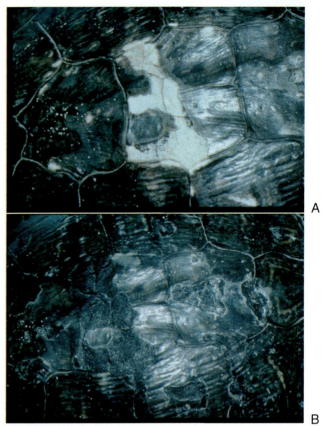

FIGURE 67-2 A, Superficial erosions in the carapace of Red-eared Slider *(Trachemys scripta elegans)*. Thin, bone-white plaque deep to loosened scutes resembles dermal bone but is not. Debridement and topical antibiotic ointments are the only treatment necessary. **B,** Keratin scute material has been exposed after the white plaque has been removed.

substrates, inadequate temperatures, the stress of poor nutrition or overcrowding, the lack of a basking site for complete drying, and insufficient ultraviolet light sources.

Treatment in all cases begins with evaluation and correction of the husbandry conditions. Extensive dry docking has been recommended historically, but is unnecessary for healing and promotes dehydration and inanition.[3] Dry docking in a warm environment is limited to 2 to 4 hours per day for specimens that do not bask voluntarily. All necrotic debris and loosened scutes must be debrided; dental picks are useful for this purpose. Thin, dry, bone-white plaques often lie deep to the loosened scutes, and these are easily removed. In those cases in which the debris and shell underlying the lesion are dry, topical antibiotic ointments applied twice a day are the only therapeutics necessary (Figure 67-2). One percent silver sulfadiazine cream (various manufacturers) is an excellent topical for *Pseudomonas* spp. and other gram-negative bacteria. Two percent mupirocin ointment (Bactoderm, SmithKline Beecham Pharmaceuticals, Philadelphia, Pa) is another good choice. Antibiotic combination ointments or creams that contain polymyxin B sulfate, neomycin, and bacitracin (various manufacturers) also are good choices for topical therapy. Topical enzymatic agents may be used when copious necrotic debris is present. Options include collagenase ointment, 250 units per gram (Collagenase Santyl, Smith & Nephew, Inc., Largo, Fla), and preparations that contain combinations of trypsin, papain, balsam of Peru, castor oil, urea, and chlorophyll derivatives (various manufacturers).

Algae commonly grow on the carapace of aquatic chelonians. This is seen in wild specimens, captives housed outdoors, and, to a lesser degree, those kept indoors. It has been suggested that the algae and the turtle enjoy a commensal or even mutualistic relationship because the turtle is camouflaged and the algae may derive benefit from mobility. At the same time, algae may pit the shell, allowing the entry of opportunistic bacterial pathogens. Likewise, they are unsightly. Wild turtles temporarily lose their algae burden when they shed their keratin scutes. Algae can be removed from captive specimens with scrubbing with a toothbrush and an antiseptic like dilute chlorhexidine or povidone iodine.

DEEP SHELL ABSCESSES

In other cases, shell abscesses are deep, the debris is necrotic and foul smelling, and the underlying shell may be moist or bloody (Figures 67-3 and 67-4). Some abscesses penetrate the full thickness of the shell down to the coelomic membrane. Aggressive surgical debridement is essential, with the goal of a smooth-sided bowl-shaped defect lacking pockets and overlying bone.[3] Anesthesia for pain control and sterile technique are used. Dental picks, bone rongeurs, bone curettes, and rotary power tools (Dremel Tool, Robert Bosch Tool Corporation, Racine, Wis) are used for debridement. Material should be collected for bacterial culture and sensitivity. Fungal cultures should be considered, but fungal infections

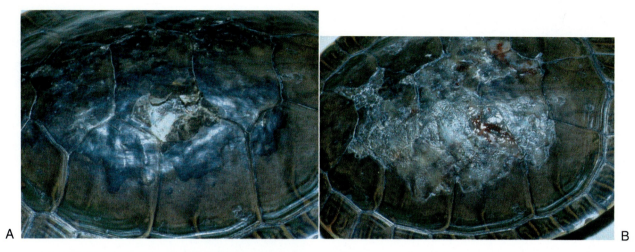

FIGURE 67-3 **A,** Deep shell abscessation in the carapace of a Red-eared Slider *(Trachemys scripta elegans)*. This is a much more serious infection. Sedation, deep debridement, systemic antibiotics based on culture and sensitivity, and supportive care are indicated. **B,** After debridement, raw bloody areas with discharge and foul odor are exposed.

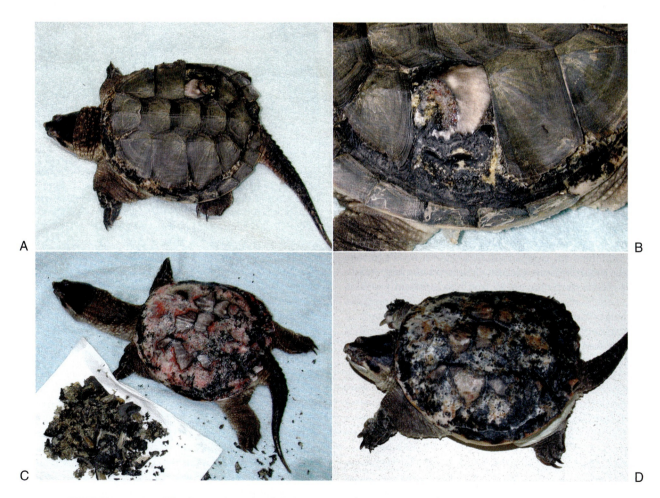

FIGURE 67-4 **A, B,** This Snapping Turtle, *Chelydra serpentina,* had been kept without supplemental heat for 9 years, and had peeling scutes, discharge from the edges of scutes, and foul odor for 2 years. Most of the scutes were loose and easily removed. **C,** Using general anesthesia the shell was aggressively debrided down to healthy tissue. Copious amounts of necrotic tissue, necrotic bone, and caseous debris were removed. Topical and synthetic antibiotics were given, and husbandry improvements in the form of an aquarium heater, basking light, filtration system, and water changes were implemented. **D,** In only 22 days, the lesions had begun to epithelialize and the turtle showed increased activity and appetite.

are less common than bacterial infections and often represent secondary invaders.

Husbandry must be optimized, including temperatures of water, land, and basking sites, diet, UV light sources, and water quality. Treatment with systemic antibiotics on the basis of culture results is important in these cases. The lesions are flushed with sterile saline or electrolyte solutions, coated with topical antibiotic ointments as previously mentioned, and covered with semipermeable, self-adhesive bandages (e.g., Tegaderm, 3M, St. Paul, Minn) daily or every other day. Close monitoring and thorough wound treatment on a regular schedule are essential during the healing period as relapses are common. Treatment may be prolonged and last weeks or months.

Shell repair with epoxy resin is contraindicated in cases of infection because this technique prevents drainage and wound cleaning.

THERAPEUTIC ENDPOINT

In both superficial and deep shell abscesses, the shell is healed when it is smooth, dry, and free from odor and discharge. Deep irregular scars remain in the shell for years, usually for the life of the turtle.

EXPOSED DERMAL BONE

In some cases, infection-damaged or burn-damaged keratin scutes slough, exposing the dermal bone underneath. This results in avascular necrosis of the exposed bone. Nevertheless, turtle shells have a remarkable ability to heal even when lesions are very large. In cases where less than an entire bony plate is exposed, the exposed bone can remain in place and without symptoms for the life of the turtle. When one or more entire bony plates are exposed, the shell membrane deep to the bone generates a layer of scar tissue, a pseudoshell, with the bone acting as a scab. After the pseudoshell forms, which may take more than a year, the bony plates slough off. The result is a heavily scarred but fully functional turtle (Figure 67-5).

Some cases of superficial shell erosions form thin hard bone-white plaques of dried material deep to the affected keratin scutes. These plaques may resemble exposed dermal bone; however, they are easily removed with a dental pick to expose dry rough keratin material. Dermal bone is rarely exposed or involved in these cases.

SEPTICEMIC CUTANEOUS ULCERATIVE DISEASE

Septicemic cutaneous ulcerative disease (SCUD) has been described as a disease syndrome in aquatic turtles. It is most common in Softshells (*Apalone* spp.) and is characterized by cutaneous ulceration, anorexia, lethargy, septicemia, and death. A variety of gram-negative bacteria, including *Citrobacter* spp., have been implicated in this disease.[4] Early detection and treatment are necessary for therapeutic success. SCUD should be treated as for deep shell abscesses, including the use of systemic antibiotics and supportive care.

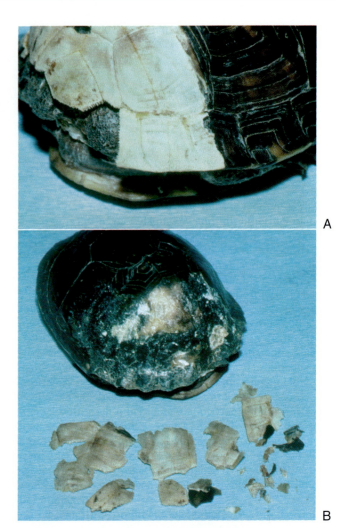

FIGURE 67-5 **A,** Necrosis of the exposed bony plates in the carapace of a Box Turtle *(Terrapene carolina)*. Infection, now resolved, caused the keratin scutes to slough and exposed the bony plates of the caudal third of the carapace. Four years later, several of the exposed peripheral bones fell off and other bones were obviously loose. **B,** The remaining exposed bony plates, consisting of peripheral, costal, pygal, suprapygal, and neural bones, were easily removed with gentle traction and manipulation. A hard irregular pseudoshell had formed deep to the necrotic bone. In spite of the fact that the vertebral column is attached to a deep layer of neural bones, no neurologic deficits occurred in this turtle.

SHELL FRACTURES

Shell fractures result from trauma when the turtle is dropped, stepped on, hit by an automobile or lawn mower, or gnawed on by a dog. The healing ability of the shell is remarkable, and chelonians with completely healed, but noticeably scarred, shell fractures are frequently encountered in wild populations (personal observations; Figures 67-6 and 67-7). Treatment of shell fractures begins with a thorough evaluation of the patient. The trauma involved with shell fracture commonly causes additional damage, including shock, internal hemorrhage, and pulmonary contusions. Some of these patients carry a poor anesthetic risk. Turtles lack a diaphragm, and respiratory movements are accomplished with contraction of intrapulmonary smooth muscle and

Shell Damage

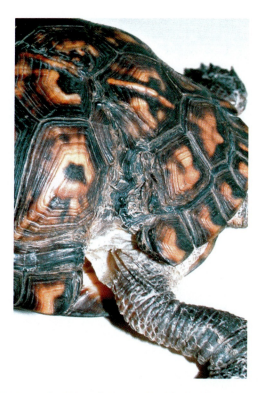

FIGURE 67-6 A wild-caught Eastern Box Turtle *(Terrapene c. carolina)* with a healed fracture of the carapace above the left hind leg.

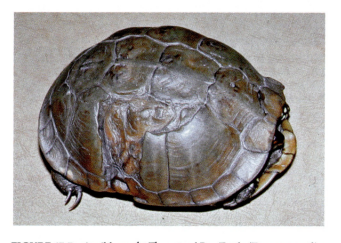

FIGURE 67-7 A wild-caught Three-toed Box Turtle *(Terrapene carolina triunguis)* with a healed fracture of the carapace.

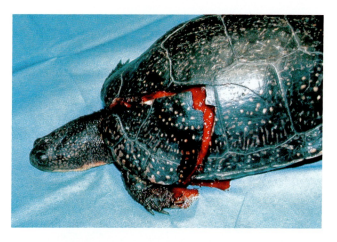

FIGURE 67-8 A Blanding's Turtle *(Emydoidea blandingii)* with a fracture of the carapace as a result of being struck by an automobile. Even though the left lung is visible under the fracture line, respiration continues normally, and negative pressure is not necessary to establish within the shell after repair.

skeletal muscle in the brachial girdle.[4] Thus, respiration continues normally even when the carapace is breached by a fracture, and it is not necessary to establish negative pressure within the shell for respiration (Figure 67-8). Nevertheless, when the lungs are involved, necrotizing pneumonia can develop. This complication responds poorly to therapy and carries a guarded prognosis.[5] Whole body radiographs, including dorsoventral views and horizontal beams of the lateral and anteroposterior views, are useful in evaluation of the extent of the damage to the shell and appendicular skeleton. The vertebrae are fused to the dorsal midline of the shell, and fractures in this area can result in spinal cord lesions, with posterior paresis and paralysis. Assessment of such lesions is difficult because severe spinal cord injury does not always cause complete paralysis. Turtles with a severed spinal cord are able to spinal walk.[5] The prognosis for recovery in these cases is poor, with a slow death months later from bladder atony and colonic obstruction.[2,5]

TREATMENT

Fresh wounds are contaminated but not infected. These should be flushed copiously with sterile saline or electrolyte solutions and repaired immediately. Wounds more than a few hours old are infected, and the infection must be completely controlled before primary repair to prevent abscess formation.[6] These wounds must be treated with topical and systemic antibiotics as discussed previously under Shell Abscesses. Standard bandaging materials stick nicely to the shell, but ointment on the shell prevents sticking. Wet-to-dry bandages or honey or sugar bandages are applied and changed daily until a healthy granulation bed develops, after which primary repair may be accomplished. Semipermeable, self-adhesive bandages (Tegaderm, 3M, St. Paul, Minn) may be used as an outer layer. A bead of cyanoacrylate ester (Superglue, Henkel Loctite Corporation, Rocky Hill, Conn) around the periphery of the bandage causes it to stick for 24 to 48 hours even in totally aquatic seaturtles.[7] This allows swimming during healing. Semiaquatic species should be allowed the opportunity to swim and bask. For individuals that do not bask, 2 to 4 hours of forced dry docking in a warm environment allows complete drying. Extensive dry docking is stressful and promotes dehydration, anorexia, and stress, and is no longer recommended.

Anesthesia is necessary to prevent pain and accomplish restraint in most cases of shell repair, and postoperative pain management must be addressed (see Chapter 27). Devitalized pieces of shell should be removed, and vital fragments returned to their normal position. Dental instruments are useful for elevation of depressed fragments. Fragments may be held in apposition with orthopedic wires inserted through holes drilled through the shell (Figures 67-9 and 67-10),

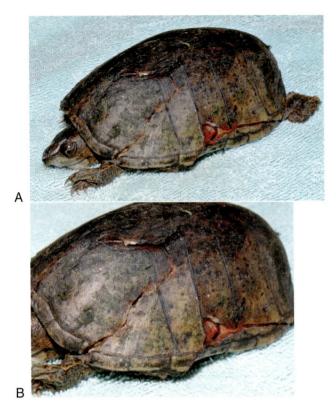

FIGURE 67-9 This Common Musk Turtle or Stinkpot (*Sternotherus odoratus*) was hit by a car and had multiple fractures of the carapace and bridge. The person who brought it in had misidentified it as a protected Blanding's Turtle (*Emydoidea blandingii*).

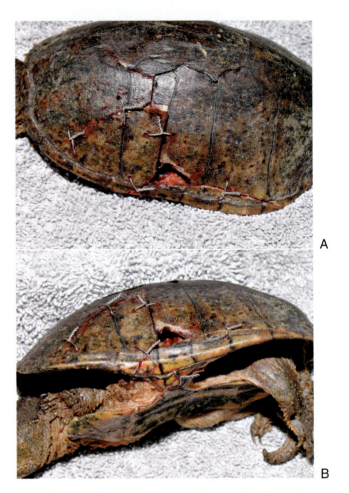

FIGURE 67-10 The fractures were stabilized with orthopedic wires passed through holes drilled in the shell. Upper fracture lines were incomplete and quite stable without additional wires. The hole left by the missing shell fragment was protected with bandages that were changed daily.

with bone plates and screws or with self-tapping orthopedic screws on either side of fracture lines connected by figure-8 wires.[5] These methods allow rigid fixation with compression between fragments and adequate wound drainage.

A simple and inexpensive technique for shell repair is the use of metal bridges affixed across fracture lines with epoxy glue (Devcon 5 Minute Epoxy, ITW Performance Polymers Consumer Division, Riviera Beach, Fla) as external fixators. These are constructed with 16- to 30-gauge aluminum, brass or steel, available from heating contractors, and sterilized by conventional methods. The strips are cut to size with metal shears, a typical size being 0.5 by 3 cm, and bent with pliers to conform to the shell. Strips applied to the carapace may have a high arch to allow wound treatment under the metal bridge, but strips on the plastron must conform more to the shell to allow ambulation.[8]

Practice of shell repair techniques on specimens salvaged from road casualties is beneficial.[9]

Rapid polymerizing 5-minute epoxy resin and fiberglass mesh were once considered the treatment of choice for shell repair.[3,5,9-12] This technique has fallen out of favor and is no longer recommended because most if not all cases followed long term developed osteomyelitis or cellulitis under the epoxy patch from a lack of drainage.[5] Rigid, occlusive, semi-permanent bandages are contraindicated for contaminated wounds. Instead, conventional wound management techniques result in rapid healing and decreased morbidity and mortality rates.[5]

Cases with a shell defect, where a shell fragment is missing or has been discarded, are managed as open wounds. Debris is removed manually and with thorough lavage with sterile saline or balanced electrolyte solutions. The wounds are covered with traditional wet-to-dry bandages or honey or sugar bandages, which are changed regularly until a granulation bed develops. Turtle shell has a remarkable ability to repair even large defects if aggressive supportive care is provided (Figure 67-11).[5]

In cases of severe injury that results in decreased appetite or concomitant head injury that prevents normal feeding, a pharygostomy tube should be inserted. This allows assist feeding and administration of oral medications with minimal stress (see Chapters 18 and 36).

Regardless of the method used, complete shell healing may take 1 to 2 years.[3,10,13,14] Chelonians with healing fractures should not be allowed to brumate or hibernate. Radiographic evidence of healing should be shown before orthopedic devices are removed. Wounds should be healed, orthopedic devices removed, and the shell rigid before wild turtles are released.

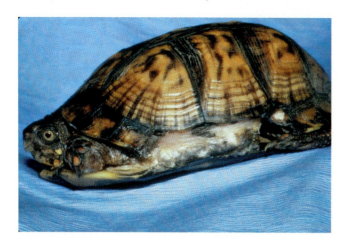

FIGURE 67-11 Fracture of the lateral carapace in a Box Turtle *(Terrapene carolina)*. The wound was contaminated and infected on presentation. It was treated as an open wound with bandaging and both topical and systemic antibiotics. Here injury is resolved with the loss of some lateral peripheral bones and marginal scutes but no residual infection or loss of function.

VACUUM-ASSISTED CLOSURE

Chelonian shell wounds with defects or missing fragments require constant wound management for weeks to months because of the slow healing process. Vacuum-assisted closure is a human technique that has been successfully applied to chelonians to expedite the healing process. Negative pressure suctions fluids continuously and promotes granulation, and an occlusive dressing prevents contamination. Wounds are debrided and packed with a sterile open-cell sponge. They are covered with transparent adhesive dressing (Steri-Drape and Tegaderm, 3M, St. Paul, Minn) and connected to a suction pump set at 10 to 12 cm Hg with plastic tubing placed in the sponge. Bandages are changed daily, and patients are kept dry except for water baths between bandage changes. Treatment may last 1 to 4 weeks or longer.[15,16]

CABLE TIE SHELL REPAIR

A novel approach to shell repair was reported by Forrester and Satta.[17] Carapace fractures are cleaned and aligned (using appropriate anesthesia or analgesia). Once aligned, standard nylon cable ties (used for bundling electrical wiring) are used to stabilize the pieces and prevent movement. Cable tie mounts are glued or epoxied to either side of the fracture(s). A cable tie is then fed through one guide on one side of the fracture, across the fracture line, and into the mount on the other side. The tie is then tightened either manually or with a cable tie gun until there is good compression at the fracture site. This is structurally sound and also allows visualization of the fracture to monitor healing and permit cleaning as needed.

Once the fracture is healed the cable tie mounts are gently elevated off the carapace with the edge of a screwdriver or small chisel. This does not damage the shell or the carapacial bone.

REFERENCES

1. Pough FH, Andrews RM, Cadle JE, Crump ML, Savitzky AH, Wells KD: *Herpetology*, Upper Saddle River, NJ, 1998, Prentice Hall.
2. Ernst CH, Barbour RW: *Turtles of the world*, Washington DC, 1989, Smithsonian Institution Press.
3. Clayton L, Mylniczenko N, Greenwell M: Review of etiology and treatment options for nontraumatic deep shell lesions in freshwater turtles, p 103, *Proceedings of the Association of Reptilian and Amphibian Veterinarians Annual Conference*, 2003.
4. Frye FL: *Biomedical and surgical aspects of captive reptile husbandry*, ed 2, Melbourne, Fla, 1991, Krieger Publishing.
5. Heard DJ: Shell repair in turtles and tortoises: an heretical approach, *Proceedings of the North American Veterinary Conference*, 1999.
6. Mader DR: Shell repair in turtles and tortoises, *Vivarium* 4:9, 1992.
7. Campbell TW: Semi-occlusive bandaging in aquatic turtles, p 823, *Proceedings of the North American Veterinary Conference*, 1996.
8. Richards J: Metal bridges—a new technique of turtle shell repair, *Journ Herp Med Surg* 11:31, 2001.
9. Rosskopf WJ: Shell disease in turtles and tortoises. In Kirk RW, editor: *Current veterinary therapy: a small animal practice*, Philadelphia, 1986, WB Saunders.
10. Mautino M, Page CD: Biology and medicine of turtles and tortoises, *Vet Clin North Am Small Anim Pract* 23:1251, 1993.
11. Bennett RA: Reptilian surgery part II: management of surgical diseases, *Compend Contin Educ Pract Vet* 11:122, 1989.
12. Harwell G: Repair of injuries to the chelonian plastron and carapace. In Kirk RW, editor: *Current veterinary therapy 10: small animal practice*, Philadelphia, 1989, WB Saunders.
13. Lawton MPC, Stoakes LC: Surgery. In Beynon PH, Lawton MPC, Cooper JE, editors: *Manual of reptiles*, Gloucestershire, England, 1992, British Small Animal Veterinary Association.
14. Millichamp NJ: Surgical techniques in reptiles. In Jacobson ER, Kollias GV, editors: *Contemporary issues in small animal practice: exotic animals*, New York, 1988, Churchill Livingstone.
15. Lafortune M, Wellehan JFX, Heard D: Vacuum-assisted closure (VAC) in chelonians, p 28, *Proceedings of the Association of Reptilian and Amphibian Veterinarians Annual Conference*, 2003.
16. Coke RL, Reyes-Fore PA, Finkelstein AD: Treatment of a carapace abscess in an Aldabra Tortoise *(Geochelone gigantea)* with negative pressure wound therapy, p 86, *Proceedings of the Association of Reptilian and Amphibian Veterinarians Annual Conference*, 2005.
17. Forrester H, Satta J: Easy shell repair, *Exotic DVM* 6(6):13, 2005.

68
SALMONELLA: DIAGNOSTIC METHODS FOR REPTILES

MARK A. MITCHELL

SALMONELLA NOMENCLATURE

Salmonella are gram-negative facultative anaerobes with a cosmopolitan distribution. The classification system for *Salmonella* was revised in 1997 to include two species: *Salmonella enterica* and *S. bongori*. Currently, six medically important subspecies of *S. enterica* exist, including *enterica* (subspecies I), *salamae* (subspecies II), *arizonae* (subspecies III), *diarizonae* (subspecies IIIb), *houtenae* (subspecies IV), and *indica* (subspecies V).[1] Subspecies II to V are frequently isolated from poikilotherms and the environment. The *arizonae* and *diarizonae* subspecies, which are generally associated with reptiles and amphibians, have 94 and 321 serotypes, respectively.

More than 2435 *Salmonella* serotypes exist, and most, if not all, of the described serotypes are considered pathogenic.[1] *Salmonella* are serotyped according to their heat stabile somatic (O) antigens, heat labile capsular (Vi) antigens, and flagellar (H) antigens. Serotypes are characterized with the Kauffman-White scheme, which defines the serotypes by their O antigens, Vi antigens (when present), and phase I and phase II (when present) H antigens.[2] Serotyping is an important diagnostic tool used by public health officials to identify a point source of *Salmonella* in human salmonellosis cases.

The nomenclature used to report *Salmonella* isolates has changed. Historically, the genus and serotype of a *Salmonella* isolate were italicized (e.g., *Salmonella typhimurium*). However, the current accepted nomenclature requires the italicization of the genus, while the serotype is capitalized and not italicized (e.g., *Salmonella* Typhimurium).

SALMONELLA DIAGNOSTIC METHODS

A number of different diagnostic methods can be used to determine the *Salmonella* status of a reptile. Although microbiologic culture is the most frequently used diagnostic test, new improved molecular assays, such as enzyme-linked immunosorbent assays (ELISAs) and the polymerase chain reaction (PCR) technique, have gained favor among clinicians. Diagnostic test selection should be based on the veterinary clinician's objective in characterizing the status of a reptile. For example, the PCR technique is extremely sensitive and may be capable of detecting a small number of *Salmonella* organisms (10^2 to 10^4); however, if a specific serotype must be identified, then microbiologic culture is necessary. A review of the current *Salmonella* diagnostic testing methods follows.

MICROBIOLOGIC ISOLATION METHODS

Microbiologic culture is the most common diagnostic method used to isolate *Salmonella* from various tissues and excretions. In general, a highly selective enrichment broth and growth-promoting agar are used to isolate *Salmonella*. The enrichment broth is generally used to provide additional energy to injured *Salmonella* and increase the probability of recovery. The three most common enrichment medias used to isolate *Salmonella* include tetrathionate broth, Rappaport-Vassiliadis, and Selenite broth. The type of enrichment broth can affect the recovery of *Salmonella* serotypes. For example, certain *Salmonella* serotypes may be inhibited in tetrathionate broth if the inoculum is small.[3] Rappaport enrichment broth is frequently used to isolate *Salmonella* from poultry; however, only 27% (3/11) of the strains of subgenus III, which are the most common isolates from reptiles, were subcultured from Rappaport.[4] The author has also experienced difficulty subculturing *Salmonella* from Green Iguanas (*Iguana iguana*) with Rappaport and prefers Selenite enrichment broth. Enrichment broth is generally incubated in aerobic conditions at 37°C for 18 to 24 hours. Because *Salmonella* are facultative anaerobes, they can be incubated in 5% CO_2; however, this is generally not necessary. After enrichment, an aliquot of the enrichment broth is removed with sterile technique and streaked onto a selective medium.

A number of different selective agars are used to isolate *Salmonella*, with some agars more selective than others. Low selective media, such as MacConkey and eosin methylene blue agar, are rarely used to isolate *Salmonella*. *Salmonella* identification on these low selective medias with colony morphology is difficult because the *Salmonella* may or may not ferment lactose and their colonies look similar to other Enterobacteriaceae. Xylose-lysine-desoxycholate (XLD) agar and *Salmonella-Shigella* agar are generally considered intermediate selective agars. Although XLD is only considered to have moderate selectivity for *Salmonella*, the author has used XLD to isolate *Salmonella* from squamates and chelonians with a high degree of success. Bismuth sulfite agar and xylose-lysine tergitol 4 (XLT-4) are considered highly selective. XLT-4 agar is the author's preferred agar for isolating reptile *Salmonella*. Bismuth sulfite, XLD, and XLT-4 contain hydrogen sulfide (H_2S) indicator systems that can detect lactose-fermenting *Salmonella*.

Once bacteria have been isolated on an agar, suspect colonies may be inoculated onto selective screening media. The author generally uses lysine iron agar (LIA), urea, and triple sugar iron agar (TSI) to screen isolates. *Salmonella* decarboxylates lysine and produces H_2S. *Salmonella* does not use urea. On the TSI media, *Salmonella* ferment glucose and produce gas and hydrogen sulfide. Commercial biochemical test kits (API 20E Test Strips, bioMerieux Vitek, Inc, Hazelwood, Mo) can also be used to characterize a *Salmonella* isolate to the group level. The slide agglutination test, which measures antisera for *Salmonella* O groups, may also be used to confirm the presence of *Salmonella*.[5]

Delayed secondary enrichment (DSE) may be used in addition to the standard enrichment method to promote the growth of *Salmonella* organisms that were damaged by antibiotics or required additional time for multiplication because of low numbers. This technique is not frequently used in traditional veterinary medical diagnostic laboratories, as reported by a questionnaire administered to veterinary diagnostic laboratories in the United States where 51% of respondents confirmed the use of a 24-hour enrichment period for culturing *Salmonella*.[6] To determine the value of DSE, the authors of the questionnaire collected 4377 samples from poultry and their environment to evaluate the recovery rates associated with a 24-hour enrichment period and a 5-day DSE.[6] Two hundred sixty-nine *Salmonella* (58%) were isolated after the 24-hour enrichment, and 421 were isolated after the 5-day DSE. Forty-three of the *Salmonella* (9%) were isolated after the 24-hour enrichment and not the DSE, compared with 195 that were only isolated after the DSE. The DSE improved overall recovery of *Salmonella* by approximately 64%. The scientists also evaluated a 3-day DSE and found that the combination of a 24-hour and 5-day DSE provided the most optimal results. The author has not found 3-day or 5-day DSE to significantly improve *Salmonella* recovery in Green Iguanas. However, the prevalence of *Salmonella* in the Green Iguanas evaluated was more than 80%, whereas the prevalence in the poultry samples was much less than that. The DSE technique may be more appropriate when the prevalence of *Salmonella* in a population of reptiles is low.

A number of parameters can affect the reliability of culture, including collection method, quantity or type of sample collected, temporal variation in shedding, and culture method.[7-9] The time necessary to isolate and confirm a microbe is also an impediment. The delay imposed by culture techniques may defer the initiation of appropriate antimicrobial therapy and control procedures.

Microbiologic Culture Techniques to Isolate *Salmonella* from Reptiles

The microbiologic techniques used to isolate *Salmonella* from reptiles are based on those developed for subspecies from mammals and poultry. Because *Salmonella* isolates from reptiles are primarily subspecies III and IIIb, they may use different biochemical pathways than other subspecies and need different enrichment medias and selective agars. Comparative studies to evaluate isolation success for reptile *Salmonella* serotypes with available enrichment broths and selective media are limited.

Fecal samples collected from 20 different species of reptiles at the Bristol Zoological Gardens were used to evaluate the effectiveness of two *Salmonella* enrichment broths, selenite F and Muller-Kauffmann tetrathionate, and three selective agars, brilliant green MacConkey agar, desoxycholate citrate agar, and de Loureiro's three stock solution modification of bismuth sulfite agar.[10] All of the fecal samples were divided equally and placed into either selenite F enrichment broth or Muller-Kauffmann tetrathionate broth. The samples were incubated in aerobic conditions at 43°C for 24 hours. An aliquot from each of the enrichment broths was subcultured onto the three selective agars and incubated at 37°C for 24 hours. *Salmonella* were more consistently isolated from selenite F (81%) than Muller-Kauffmann tetrathionate (63%).

In another study to determine the efficacy of different enrichment broths and selective media, fecal samples were collected from 32 chelonians, comprising nine species, and inoculated into two different enrichment broths, either selenite and tetrathionate, and subcultured onto three selective agars, including Rambach, *Salmonella-Shigella*, or XLT-4.[11] Fecal material was placed in each of the enrichment broths and incubated at 37°C for 24 hours in aerobic conditions. An aliquot from each of the enrichment broths was subcultured onto the three different selective agars and incubated at 37°C for an additional 24 hours. Thirteen of the 32 samples (41%) were *Salmonella*-positive. Thirteen isolates were recovered from selenite broth, compared with 11 with tetrathionate. All 13 isolates grew on Rambach and *Salmonella-Shigella* agar, compared with 12 on XLT-4.

The results of these two studies are similar to those that the author has observed with selenite and tetrathionate broth to recover *Salmonella* from reptiles. These results differ from the poultry industry, which generally prefers the tetrathionate broth to the selenite. Diagnostic laboratories should select enrichment media on the basis of current trends to increase the likelihood of recovering *Salmonella* from different vertebrates.

The method used to collect a sample can also affect the *Salmonella* recovery rate. Wells, McConnell Clark, and Morris[12] compared three methods for isolating *Salmonella* from turtles or their environment, including water samples, specific organs from euthanized turtles, and whole carcasses. Samples were collected from the water of unfed turtles (n = 50); the yolk, bile, liver, spleen, small intestine, colon, and kidney of euthanized turtles (n = 50); and individually blended (whole) turtles (n = 50). The samples were enriched in tetrathionate broth containing brilliant green broth and incubated at 37°C for 48 hours and then subcultured onto brilliant green agar and incubated at 37°C for 48 hours. *Salmonella* was isolated from 17 of the carcasses (34%) and from 24 water samples (48%); however, this difference was not significant. The overall frequency of recovery from individual parts (20%) was significantly lower than the water samples or whole carcasses.

NONCULTURE DIAGNOSTIC METHODS

Enzyme-Linked Immunosorbent Assays

The impact of *Salmonella* on human and animal health has created a need for rapid and accurate detection methods for *Salmonella*. ELISAs combine a specific antiimmunoglobulin with an enzyme to detect a specific microbial antigen. The ELISA has been used extensively in the poultry industry, where labor and economics are important to the business management plan.[13-15] Desmidt, Haesebrouck, and Ducatelle[13] compared a commercial ELISA to microbiologic culture for detection of *Salmonella* from cloacal swabs of poultry and drag swabs of litter. No difference between the two detection methods was found in comparison of cloacal swabs (ELISA, 22/73; culture, 25/73); however, the ELISA (39/42) was more sensitive than culture (22/42) for detection of *Salmonella* in litter samples. The high sensitivity of the ELISA was attributed to the detection of antigen from dead *Salmonella* cells.

Pelton et al[14] compared an antigen capture ELISA with microbiologic culture for detection of *Salmonella* from equine, avian, and reptile fecal samples. Thirty-five culture-negative samples and 35 culture-positive samples were assayed with the ELISA. Of the culture-negative samples, one (3%) was positive with the ELISA in contrast to the culture-positive samples, of which 11 (31%) were positive with the ELISA. Test sensitivity was 69%, and test specificity was 97%. The ELISA used in this study is an acceptable indicator of positive status but only a fair indicator of negative status.

Tan, Gyles, and Wilkie compared a lipopolysaccharide-specific competitive ELISA with motility enrichment culture for detection of *Salmonella* Typhimurium and *S*. Enteritidis in chickens.[15] Of the 3928 samples collected, 1085 (28%) were positive with the ELISA procedure and 1067 (27%) yielded a *Salmonella* isolate on culture. The sensitivity of the ELISA was 93%, and the specificity was 96.7%. The ELISA used in this study is an acceptable indicator of infection.

The ELISA procedure can be used to detect *Salmonella* from various biologic and environmental samples. Benefits of the procedure include speed and low labor requirements compared with culture. Further research on the diagnostic value of the ELISA as a method to detect *Salmonella* in reptiles should be pursued.

Polymerase Chain Reaction Technique

Polymerase chain reaction, once considered only a research technique, is used more frequently in the clinical diagnosis of disease and for epidemiologic investigations. PCR assay is an enzyme-mediated process used to replicate DNA from an organism with specific oligonucleotide primers that are complementary to specific nucleotide sequences of the subject organism. Because the PCR technique can be used to create logarithmic copies of microbial DNA from a limited amount of sample, the technique can identify organisms in clinical or environmental samples at levels too low to detect with culture.

The PCR assay is considered to be more sensitive than culture because it can amplify DNA from a single organism or part of an organism in suitable conditions. Specificity of the PCR assay can also be very high depending on the primers used. PCR assay may be prone to false-positive reactions if processing of the samples is not performed in sterile conditions. A number of biologic inhibitors affect the results of a PCR assay, including blood, blood culture media, urine, sputum, and vitreous humor.[16] Sample processing can influence PCR assay results, yielding false-negative results if the DNA extraction technique does not release microbial DNA or if the quantity of DNA available for the reaction is low.

Another potential advantage of the PCR assay is supposed to be the ability to detect low numbers of organisms in a sample. In a study that evaluated the minimal detection numbers of *Salmonella* in experimentally infected feces from horses with the PCR assay, the minimal detection limit for PCR was 10^3 to 10^4 colony-forming unit (CFU)/gram feces, compared with the minimal detection limit for culture of 10^2 to 10^3 CFU/g feces.[17,18] However, culture results were based on enrichment in selenite broth; in this study, the samples tested with PCR were not enriched. A short enrichment period in selenite may have lowered the minimal detection levels for PCR. PCR diagnosis was more rapid than culture, requiring 10 to 12 hours for PCR versus 2 to 4 days for culture.

Polymerase chain reaction assays may also be used to detect *Salmonella* in the environment.[19] Poultry litter drag swabs collected from 18 poultry houses at nine different broiler farms were tested for *Salmonella* with the PCR assay and culture. Of 50 samples tested, 47 of the PCR samples (94%) and 29 of the culture samples (58%) were positive for *Salmonella*. The PCR was significantly more sensitive than culture for detecting *Salmonella* in poultry litter.

Although laboratory-based comparisons of diagnostic assays are common, relatively few diagnostic tests are compared in natural conditions.[20] Cohen et al[20] compared a PCR assay with standard microbiologic culture for detection of salmonellae from naturally infected equine feces and environmental samples from the teaching hospital at the Texas A&M University, College of Veterinary Medicine. Of the 313 environmental samples collected, eight (3%) were positive based on the PCR assay, but none of the cultures detected *Salmonella*. Fecal samples were collected from an outpatient group without enteric signs and a hospitalized group with gastrointestinal disease. Of the 152 outpatient horses tested, 26 (17%) were positive based on the PCR assay, but none of the cultures yielded an isolate. Of the 110 subjects with gastrointestinal disease, 71 of the samples (65%) were positive with the PCR assay, in contrast to only 11 of the cultured samples (10%). The PCR assay detected all 11 of the cultured isolates. Results indicated that the PCR assay is a useful technique for epidemiologic investigations in evaluation of a population with a low prevalence of *Salmonella*.

ESTIMATING TEST SENSITIVITY AND SPECIFICITY FOR MICROBIOLOGIC CULTURE, ENZYME-LINKED IMMUNOSORBENT ASSAY, AND POLYMERASE CHAIN REACTION ASSAY FOR REPTILES

As previously described, much of the research to evaluate diagnostic methods for *Salmonella* have focused on higher vertebrates. Because the *Salmonella* serotypes isolated from mammals and birds can differ from those isolated from reptiles, these diagnostic methods may be inadequate. Published reports that specifically address the *Salmonella* status of reptiles have primarily been limited to microbiologic culture and ELISA, and no formal studies have estimated the test characteristics for the various diagnostic assays for *Salmonella*.[14,21-23]

As new diagnostic tests become available, a need exists to compare them with other standard tests, preferably a gold standard, to determine their sensitivity and specificity. Clinicians rely on this information in application of specific health programs. Unfortunately, few "true" gold standards are available to make these comparisons. Although microbiologic culture has historically been considered to be the gold standard for detection of bacterial infections in vertebrates, it is susceptible to misclassification.

Latent exact modeling can be used to estimate the sensitivity and specificity of one or more tests in one or more populations in the absence of a gold standard.[24] Although this method does not provide exact measurements of the test parameters and population prevalence, it does increase our understanding of the tests by providing a range of values that incorporate the true value.

A study was performed to determine the test characteristics for a standard microbiologic method, with a selenite enrichment and XLT-4 agar, a commercial ELISA (Salmonella ELISA Test 96/1, Bioline, Polarvej 60, DK-7100 Vejle, Denmark), and a PCR (University of Georgia, College of Veterinary Medicine, Athens, Ga) for samples specifically collected from reptiles.[25] Two populations of Green Iguanas from El Salvador were used for the study, and 119 animals were sampled from each study population.

The estimated sensitivity for PCR was 0.92 (95% credible intervals [CI], 0.87 to 0.95), and the estimated specificity was 0.94 (95% CI, 0.92 to 0.97). The estimated sensitivity for the ELISA was 0.81 (95% CI, 0.77 to 0.85), and the estimated specificity was 0.86 (95% CI, 0.80 to 0.90). Finally, the estimated sensitivity and specificity for microbiologic culture were 0.67 (95% CI, 0.62 to 0.71) and 0.99 (95% CI, 0.98 to 0.99), respectively.

The PCR assay was considerably more sensitive than either the ELISA or microbiologic culture. The specificity of microbiologic culture was higher than the PCR and ELISA assays. The results suggest that the PCR is the preferred assay to identify *Salmonella*-positive reptiles, and culture is the preferred assay for cases in which false-negative results were undesirable. The results of the study also suggest that as many as three to four *Salmonella*-positive iguanas could be misclassified with standard microbiologic culture. Because the PCR assay is both highly sensitive and specific and microbial culture is required for serotyping, parallel testing with both the PCR assay and microbiologic culture could be used to further increase the overall sensitivity and specificity of the testing methods.

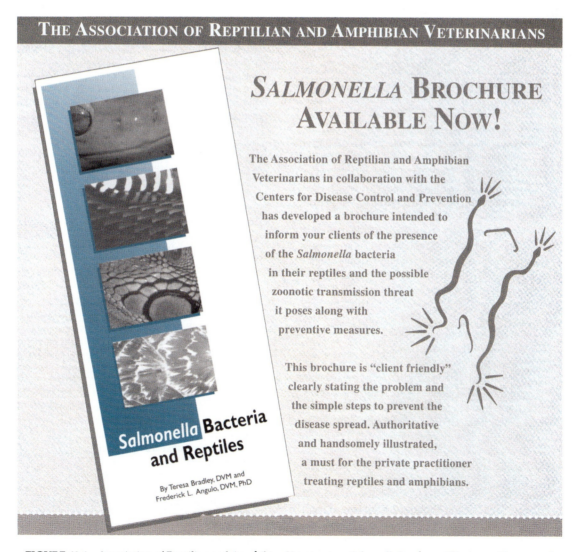

FIGURE 68-1 Association of Reptilian and Amphibian Veterinarians *Salmonella* brochure. Clients must be warned of potential risks of reptile ownership. (Go to www.arav.org to order brochures.)

INTERPRETATION OF TEST RESULTS

Because of the public health risk attributed to pet reptile ownership (reptile-associated salmonellosis), pet owners may ask veterinarians to determine the *Salmonella* status of their pet reptile. From the current literature, obviously a number of different methods can be used to determine the *Salmonella* status of a reptile. However, the difficulty comes with the interpretation of the results.

Because most veterinary clinicians have access only to microbiologic culture, the interpretation of the results should take into account the relative test sensitivity. The moderate test sensitivity of microbiologic culture suggests that it is susceptible to false-negative results that can lead to the misclassification of infected reptiles.

What should a veterinarian tell a client if a single cloacal/fecal culture yielded a negative result? Suggesting that a reptile is *Salmonella*-free based on one cloacal/fecal culture would be malpractice. Clients should be informed of the possibility of false-negative results and of the importance of collecting sequential samples to confirm *Salmonella* status. A minimum of five samples should be collected over a 30-day period to determine the *Salmonella* status of a reptile. Reptiles that have received antibiotics may need to be tested over a longer period of time. Green Iguanas given enrofloxacin (10 mg/kg, per os, every 24 hours) for 14 days did not shed *Salmonella* for 70 days after antibiotic administration, even though at necropsy they were *Salmonella*-positive.[26]

If *Salmonella* is diagnosed, the question exists of what to do with the result. Apparently normal reptiles can harbor *Salmonella*. If the reptile does not have specific clinical signs associated with salmonellosis, then treatment is not justified. The use of antimicrobials in appropriate conditions may eliminate *Salmonella*, but no evidence exists of long-term protection. Antibiotic selection should always be based on the results of culture and sensitivity testing.

Administration of antibiotics to reptiles harboring *Salmonella* bacteria can lead to the development of antibiotic resistant strains. The client should be warned of this potentially significant possibility, and such warning should be documented in the client's medical record.

If the environment of the reptile is not properly sanitized and disinfected, reinfection can occur from the animal's own environment. Contaminated food sources, such as fresh produce, can also serve as a source of infection.

Clients should be made aware of the risks of owning reptiles and should be apprised of appropriate husbandry and sanitation procedures. Hand washing with soap and warm water is an excellent method to eliminate *Salmonella*. Pet owners should be directed to avoid using bathroom basins or kitchen sinks to clean an iguana or any component of its environment. The purchase of a separate washing receptacle, such as a plastic container, is recommended. Dilute bleach solution should be used to clean the environment and food and water bowls (see Chapter 85).

The veterinarian can play an important role as a public health official by providing clients with current literature regarding reptile-associated salmonellosis (Figure 68-1). This enables the client to make informed decisions regarding the pet reptile. Veterinarians can also serve as an important liaison with the pet industry by educating local pet retailers as to the risks of pet reptile ownership. This ensures that important public health information is delivered to prospective pet owners before purchase of a reptile.

REFERENCES

1. Popoff MY, LeMinor L: *Antigenic formulas of the* Salmonella *serovars*, revision 7, Paris, 1997, World Health Organization Collaborating Center for Reference Research on *Salmonella*, Pasteur Institute.
2. McWhorter-Murlin AC, Hickman-Brenner FW: *Identification and serotyping of* Salmonella *and an update of the Kaufmann-White scheme*, Atlanta, 1994, Centers for Disease Control.
3. Van Schothorst M, VanLeusden FM, Jeunink J, deDreu J: Studies on the multiplication of *Salmonellas* in various enrichment media at different incubation temperatures, *J Appl Bacteriology* 42:157, 1977.
4. Vassiliadis P: *Shigella, Salmonella* Cholerae-suis and Arizona in Rappaport's medium, *J Appl Bacteriology* 31:367, 1968.
5. Guthrie RK: Taxonomy and grouping. In Guthrie RK, editor: *Salmonella*, Boca Raton, Fla, 1992, CRC Press.
6. Waltman WD, Horne AM, Pirkle C, Dickson T: Use of delayed secondary enrichment for the isolation of *Salmonella* in poultry and poultry environments, *Avian Dis* 35:88-92, 1991.
7. Hird DW, Pappaioanow M, Smith BP: Case control study of risk factors associated with isolation of *Salmonella* St. Paul in hospitalized horses, *Am J Epidemiol* 120:852-864, 1984.
8. Owens RR, Fullerton J, Barnum DA: Effects of transportation, surgery and antibiotic therapy in ponies infected with *Salmonella, Am J Vet Res* 44:46-50, 1983.
9. Smith BP: Salmonellosis. In Smith BP, editor: *Large animal internal medicine*, St. Louis, 1991, CV Mosby.
10. Harvey RS, Price TH: *Salmonella* isolation from reptilian faeces: a discussion of appropriate techniques, *J Hyg* 91:25-32, 1983.
11. Kodjo A, Villard L, Prave M, Ray S, Grezarl D, Lacheretz A, et al: Isolation and identification of *Salmonella* species from chelonians using combined selective media, serotyping, and ribotyping, *Am Vet Med Series B (Berlin)* 44:625-629, 1997.
12. Wells JG, McConnell Clark G, Morris GK: Evaluation of methods for isolating *Salmonella* and *Arizona* organisms from pet turtles, *Appl Microbiol* 27(1):8-10, 1974.
13. Desmidt M, Haesebrouck F, Ducatelle R: Comparison of *Salmonella*-Tek ELISA to culture methods for detection of *Salmonella* Enteritidis in litter and cloacal swabs of poultry, *Am Vet Med Series B (Berlin)* 41:523-528, 1994.
14. Pelton JA, Dilling GW, Smith BP, Jang S: Comparison of a commercial antigen-capture ELISA with enrichment culture for detection of *Salmonella* from fecal samples, *J Vet Diagn Invest* 6:501-502, 1994.
15. Tan S, Gyles CL, Wilkie BN: Comparison of an LPS-specific competitive ELISA with a motility enrichment culture method for detection of *Salmonella* Typhimurium and *S.* Enteritidis in chickens, *Vet Microbiol* 56:79-86, 1997.
16. Fredricks DN, Relman DA: Application of polymerase chain reaction to the diagnosis of infectious diseases, *Clin Infect Dis* 29:475-488, 1999.
17. Cohen ND, Neibergs HL, McGruder ED, Whitford HW, Behle RW, Ray PM, et al: Genus-specific detection of salmonellae using the polymerase chain reaction, *J Vet Diagn Invest* 5:368-371, 1993.
18. Cohen ND, Neibergs HL, Wallis DE, Simpson RB, McGruder ED, Hargis BM: Genus-specific detection of salmonellae in equine feces by use of the polymerase chain reaction, *Am J Vet Res* 55(8):1049-1054, 1994.

19. Cohen ND, Wallis DE, Neibergs HL, McElroy AP, McGruder ED, DeLoach JR, et al: Comparison of the polymerase chain reaction using genus-specific oligonucleotide primers and microbiologic culture for the detection of *Salmonella* in drag-swabs from poultry houses, *Poultry Sci* 73:1276-1281, 1994.
20. Cohen ND, Martin J, Simpson B, Wallis DE, Neibergs HL: Comparison of polymerase chain reaction and microbiologic culture for detection of salmonellae in equine feces and environmental samples, *Am J Vet Res* 57(6):780-786, 1996.
21. Burnham BR, Atchley DH, DeFusco RP, Ferris KE, Zicarelli JC, Lee JH, et al: Prevalence of fecal shedding of *Salmonella* organisms among captive green iguanas and potential health implications, *J Am Vet Med Assoc* 213(1):48-52, 1998.
22. Cambre RC, Green DE, Smith EE, Montali RJ, Bush M: Salmonellosis and Arizonosis in the reptile collection at the National Zoological Park, *J Am Vet Med Assoc* 177(9):800-803, 1980.
23. Onderka DK, Finlayson MC: Salmonellae and salmonellosis in captive reptiles, *Can J Comp Med* 49:268-270, 1985.
24. Joseph L, Gyorkos TW, Coupal L: Bayesian estimation of disease prevalence and the parameters of diagnostic tests in the absence of a gold standard, *Am J Epidemiol* 141(3):263-272, 1995.
25. Mitchell MA, Shane Nevarez J, Maurer K, Orr K, Scholl D, Pesti SM, et al: Sensitivity and specificity estimation of three diagnostic tests for *Salmonella* in green iguanas. Dissertation.
26. Mitchell MA, Shane SM, Pesti D, Sanchez S, Wooley R, Ritchie B: Establishing a *Salmonella*-clearance model in the green iguana (*Iguana iguana*) using enrofloxacin. Dissertation.

69
SPINAL OSTEOPATHY

KEVIN T. FITZGERALD and
REBECCA VERA

*"The camel's hump is an ugly lump
which well you may see at the zoo;
but uglier yet is the hump we get
from having too little to do."*
                From *How the Camel Got His Hump*, Rudyard Kipling

Vertebrates of several classes have been reported to show anomalous distortions of the vertebral column.[1-11] *Osteoarthritis* is defined as a disorder of moveable joints characterized by deterioration of articular cartilage, osteophyte formation, bone remodeling, changes in periarticular tissues, and a low-grade nonpurulent inflammation of variable degree.[12] This presence or absence of inflammation has spawned considerable debate concerning appropriate terminology. Osteoarthritis can be inflammatory or noninflammatory. Inflammatory arthritis usually implies an influx of inflammatory cells and is most appropriately associated with conditions with immune-mediated or infectious etiologies.

The classic example of an immune-mediated condition is *rheumatoid* arthritis in which immune cell invasion of periarticular tissues occurs, bone is destroyed, and erosive changes develop in articular cartilage. Rheumatoid immune mediated–type arthritis is considered serious, is often swiftly progressive, and is debilitating.

Localized or generalized inflammation and destruction of bone from pyogenic infectious etiologic agents is known as *osteomyelitis*.[13] Osteomyelitis can cause local inflammation, stiffening of joints, destruction of bone, loss of range of motion, septicemia, and death.

Osteoarthrosis has come to imply the absence of inflammation in degenerative disease of the joints. Noninflammatory osteoarthritis is generally a slowly progressive degenerative joint disease. Typically, the highly moveable or diarthrodial joints are involved. The exact etiology of noninflammatory osteoarthritis may be difficult to determine, but usually it is secondary to some type of trauma. This includes application of an abnormal force to a normal joint (trauma) or normal force to an abnormal joint (congenital malformation). Despite these varying causes, the end result to bones and joints is stereotypical. All these syndromes lead to common cellular and molecular pathways that end in disruption of periarticular cartilage, destruction and remodeling of subchondral bone, interruption of the normal synovium, destabilization of the joint capsule, and loss of normal function. Many of the same mediators, including cytokines, prostaglandins, leukotrienes, degradative enzymes, and other destructive agents, are common to immune-mediated, infectious, and noninflammatory osteoarthritis. As a result of these very different processes having a very similar-appearing outcome, determination of the exact nature of the osteopathy that an animal has can be extremely difficult. Furthermore, examples of all these degenerative processes (immune-mediated, infectious, and noninflammatory) are widespread and have been documented for every vertebrate group. Interesting to note is that average or even vigorous and prolonged use of normal joints is not believed to result in osteoarthritis.[14,15] However, similar use of an anatomically abnormal joint, trauma, infection, invasion of immune cells, neoplasia, or inadequate nutrition all hasten the development of osteoarthritis.[9,12,16-19]

Proliferative spinal osteopathy (PSO) has been described in turtles, lizards, and snakes.[3,6,8-11,16] Anomalous displacement of the spinal column in a sagittal plane, especially dorsal and usually thoracic, is termed *kyphosis* (humpback). If the displacement is ventral, usually in the lumbar or cervical area, it is called *lordosis* (swayback). Displacement in a frontal plane, to either side, is known as *scoliosis* (lateral curvature). All three conditions may occur to different extents simultaneously within the same animal. The term *rhoecosis* (from the Greek *rhoikos*, meaning crooked) has been proposed to describe the condition in which all three types of distortion are present together (Figure 69-1).[9]

PATHOGENESIS

A number of cases of reptiles with vertebral osteopathy characterized by proliferative segmented spondylosis have been described.[3,6,8-11,16-18] Snakes appear to be particularly vulnerable (Figure 69-2). However, fairly extensive literature exists even for turtles.[3,8,9,16] The precise cause (or causes) of this condition remains uncertain. Spinal osteopathy has been attributed to trauma (Figure 69-3), unknown viral etiology, dietary deficiency (hypovitaminosis D, hypervitaminosis A), prolonged inactivity because of cage confinement, slow-developing neoplasm, and association with previous soft tissue bacterial infection and septicemia (Table 69-1).[20-24] Speculation exists that the spinal lesions may be caused by an immune-mediated reaction from the septicemia and triggered by bacterial endotoxins. This type of gammopathy involving polyclonal B cells has been shown in several types of bacterial infection. This theory is supported by the fact that these spinal lesions frequently culture positive for bacterial organisms.[25-28] *Salmonella*, long considered a bacteria frequently cultured from reptiles but nonpathogenic to their hosts, has recently been implicated in several cases of vertebral osteomyelitis in snakes.[25,27,28] Reptile-origin *Salmonella* has also been implicated as a cause of osteomyelitis in humans.[29,30] Blood flow in the region of the intervertebral discs has also been suggested to promote seeding of bacteria in this area during bouts of septicemic infection and to predispose to immune-mediated response. An association between spinal disease and previous soft tissue bacterial infections has been suggested in various reptiles.[20-22,24,25] Nevertheless, infection cannot be the whole answer because some animals with similar-appearing

Spinal Osteopathy

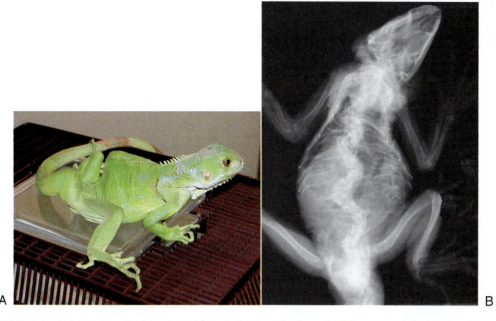

FIGURE 69-1 **A,** Anomalous displacement of the spinal column in the sagittal plane, especially dorsal and usually thoracic, is termed *kyphosis* (humpback). Ventral displacement, usually in the lumbar or cervical area, is called *lordosis* (swayback). Displacement in the frontal plane, to either side, is known as *scoliosis* (lateral curvature). All three conditions may occur to different extents simultaneously within the same animal, as is seen in this Green Iguana (*Iguana iguana*), which is termed "rhoecosis." **B,** Radiograph of a Green Iguana (not the same animal as in **A**) with severe spinal osteopathy that resulted from nutritional secondary hyperparathyroidism. (*Photograph courtesy D. Mader.*)

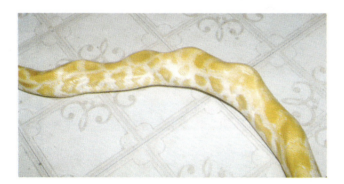

FIGURE 69-2 Proliferative segmented spondylosis (proliferative spinal osteopathy) has been described in turtles, lizards, and snakes, which appear to be particularly vulnerable. This Burmese Python (*Python molurus bivitattus*) presented with multiple "kinks" down the entire length of the spine. (*Photograph courtesy D. Mader.*)

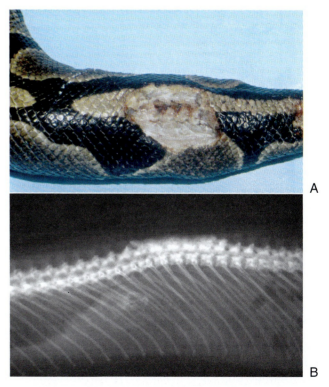

FIGURE 69-3 **A,** Rat bite in a Ball Python (*Python regius*). According to the owner, this bite had occurred only 1 week before presentation. **B,** Radiograph of the lesion from the snake pictured in **A.** Note the extensive spinal involvement. (*Photograph courtesy D. Mader.*)

lesions consistently test negative for bacteria on bone and blood culture.

Recently, the extent of bacterial involvement in PSO has been further investigated.[13,25-28,31,32] In one study, snakes with similar clinical and radiologic signs of spinal osteoarthritis were examined.[24] On radiographs, all snakes had evidence of segmented fusion of adjacent affected vertebra. Adjacent vertebra were fused dorsally, ventrally, or laterally by foci of irregular proliferative bone. Early on, sclerosis of vertebral end plates and varying lysis of the vertebral body were seen, initially sparing the adjacent ribs. In advancing stages, the

Table 69-1	Documented Etiologies for Proliferative Spinal Osteopathy in Vertebrates

Trauma
Dietary deficiency (hypovitaminosis D, hypervitaminosis A)
Prolonged inactivity (captivity)
Metabolic disease
Bacterial infection
Viral etiology
Immune reaction
Neoplasia
Inherited condition (congenital malformation)

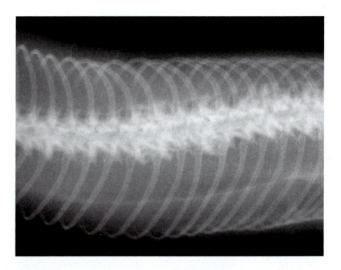

FIGURE 69-4 Snakes with spinal osteopathy have evidence of segmented fusion of adjacent affected vertebra by foci of irregular proliferative bone. Early on, sclerosis is seen of vertebral end plates with or without lysis of the vertebrae. In advanced stages, periarticular bony proliferation involves the dorsolateral articular facets and costovertebral joints. Eventually, osseous metaplasia may bridge adjoining vertebrae (ankylosis). *(Photograph courtesy D. Mader.)*

periarticular bony proliferation noticeably involved the dorsolateral articular facets, the costovertebral joints, and osseous metaplasia, occasionally bridging joint spaces (Figure 69-4). Finally, ribs were seen to be involved, and costovertebral articulations displayed areas of anklyosis. In most of the snakes, the proliferative reactive bone arose from the cortical surface of the vertebral laminae or arches. Proliferative bone occasionally bridged joint spaces of lateral facets and the ventral caudal margins of vertebral condyles (ankylosis). Pathologic fracture was occasionally seen in foci of proliferative reactive bone exostoses (Figure 69-5). As a result of the unique nature of the degenerative progression of this process, it is very different from either ankylosing spondylosis or spondylosis deformans. The proliferative periosteal new bone formation is consistent with a localized attempt at stabilization in response to the degenerative process at work.

Interesting to note is that if bacterial colonies are detected, they are found within joint spaces, around synovial membranes, along superficial surfaces of cortical bone, or at interfaces of subchondral bone and articular cartilage.[25]

Three distinct histologic types of lesions were found in these snakes. The first group had evidence of active bacterial osteoarthritis on histopathology, blood culture, and bone culture. Radiographs were used to confirm spinal disease but could not identify inflammation or identify or distinguish between active or chronic infection. The second group had predominantly noninflammatory lesions with multifocal centers of inflammation. This group had no histopathologic evidence of bacteria but tested positive on bone culture, suggestive of chronic bacterial osteoarthritis. The last group displayed noninflammatory lesions consistent with osteoarthritis, with no evidence of inflammation or bacteria on histopathology or blood or bone culture. The lesions in this last group were said to resemble those in snakes with *osteitis deformans* (Paget's disease). The lesions in the different groups were suggested to represent a continuum from acute to chronic bacterial infection. This study implies that the inflammation and infection caused by active bacterial osteoarthritis may resolve over time and leave behind proliferation of bone as the prominent histologic lesion. Nevertheless, multiple unrelated disease processes could be responsible for the pathologic lesions seen in this study.

As mentioned, some lesions of spinal osteopathy in reptiles have been **compared** with *osteitis deformans* (Paget's disease) in humans.[20,21,23,33] It is a fairly commonly diagnosed human osteopathy. The disease is a localized disorder initially marked by excessive bone resorption followed by

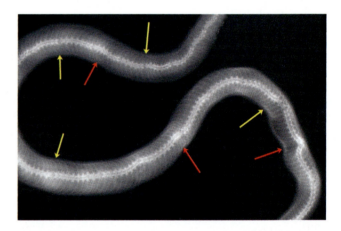

FIGURE 69-5 Ankylosis *(red arrows)* can spread along the spine, involving large segments. Pathologic fractures *(yellow arrows)* can occur in regions of inflexibility. *(Photograph courtesy D. Mader.)*

deformity and then excessive bone formation. Lamellar bone laid down during the osteoblastic phase forms a mosaic pattern. This later sclerotic period is represented by local increased vascularity, fibrosis of adjacent marrow, osteolysis, and collapse of bony architecture.[23] Pathologic fractures may occur in the diseased bone. This condition resembles "ringbone" in horses. Histopathologically, lesions of affected bone reveal marked thickening that extends into the endosteum and marrow spaces and a mosaic pattern created by multiple irregular cement lines of lamellar bone. This is typical of *osteitis deformans* in humans. In general, these lesions show focal masses of neoosseous woven bone, the classic mosaic formed by myriad irregular cement lines, considerable ankylosis, osteolysis, osteoporosis, and later pathologic fractures. These features are consistent with Paget's disease of bone as

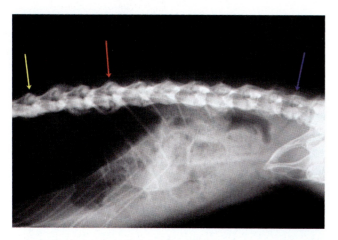

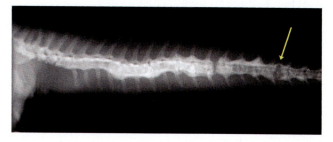

FIGURE 69-7 Ankylosis of the tail vertebrae in a Green Iguana (*Iguana iguana*). Note the area of osteomyelitis (*yellow arrow*). (*Photograph courtesy D. Mader.*)

FIGURE 69-6 Proliferative spinal osteopathy has also been seen in lizards. Causes of spinal osteopathy in lizards include vertebral instability from various metabolic diseases, degenerative joint disease stemming from underlying trauma, periosteal bony response from infection or inflammation, proliferative new bone growth of unknown etiology, and neoplastic processes. (*Photograph courtesy D. Mader.*)

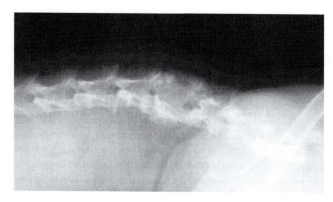

FIGURE 69-8 Osteosarcoma in the lumbar spine of a Green Iguana (*Iguana iguana*). (*Photograph courtesy D. Mader.*)

seen in humans. It was first described in a snake in 1974; subsequently, the condition has been documented in a variety of snake species, and recently, a Paget's disease–like histopathologic description has been reported in lizards. The cause of this condition in humans has not been determined. However, a viral agent as an etiologic agent has been suggested.[22] Paget's disease in reptiles has been postulated to also have an autoimmune etiology stemming from infectious disease.[23]

Many affected reptiles show irregular mosaic patterns in vertebral bones.[23] Some authors believe the mosaic pattern reflects the normal appearance of reptilian bone remodeling.[25] More work is necessary to ascertain the normal progression of bone formation in reptiles to determine the significance of this mosaic pattern in diseased animals.

Proliferative spinal osteopathy has also been seen in lizards (Figure 69-6).[31-33] Causes of spinal osteopathy in lizards include vertebral instability from various metabolic diseases, degenerative joint disease stemming from underlying trauma, periosteal bony response from infection or inflammation, proliferative new bone growth of unknown etiology, and neoplastic processes. Animals with underlying metabolic disease are prone to osteoporosis, pathologic fracture, and subsequent paresis. Animals with a history of trauma may have surface scarring (remnants of focal trauma), vertebral fractures, kinks, osteophyte formation, destruction of articular cartilage, and periosteal new bone formation and ankylosis between adjacent damaged vertebrae (Figure 69-7). Animals with an underlying infectious etiology have spinal osteopathy develop similar to the disease process reported in snakes. However, at the authors' practice, not as many lizards are presented for PSO diseases as are snakes. This could reflect geographic location and what species are most prevalently sold or kept in a region. A number of lizards are presented for spinal osteopathies and periosteal new bone formation from an etiology that is never determined. Finally, at our practice, osteosarcoma, fibrosarcoma, and chondrosarcoma have all been documented in the vertebrae of lizards (Figure 69-8).

Osteoarthritis, osteoarthrosis, and osteomyelitis in reptiles can be difficult to differentiate radiographically.[34,35]

Radiographic signs of osteomyelitis in reptiles are unlike mammalian osteomyelitis lesions.[13] Osteomyelitis in reptiles causes osteolysis (see Figure 69-7). These lytic lesions may persist for prolonged periods after the organisms have been cleared. The periosteal reaction usually present in mammalian osteomyelitis is absent or indistinguishable in reptiles. As a result, lytic areas without evidence of new bone formation are typical of osteomyelitis in reptiles but resemble neoplasia in mammalian bone. Consequently, these lesions can be misinterpreted by inexperienced reptile practitioners with often dire results.

A histologic distinction between spinal osteoarthritis and inflammatory spinal osteomyelitis can be difficult. However, a distinctive feature of osteomyelitis infections in one report was the presence of rib lesions in every confirmed case.[27] In conclusion, a knowledge of the underlying pathophysiology of these conditions aids in a correct diagnosis.

CLINICAL SIGNS

Clinical signs of PSO in reptiles may vary depending on the severity and location of the lesions. Animals with vertebral lesions limited to only a few vertebrae can show minimal deficits. Animals with extensive vertebral lesions can show limited movement or no movement at all in the affected area. Affected vertebral regions can be remarkably extensive, sometimes as much as 30 cm (12 in) long. Clinical signs can include

Table 69-2	Clinical Signs of Proliferative Spinal Osteopathy in Reptiles
Kyphosis	Lower motor neuron signs caudal to lesion
Lordosis	Abnormal posturing
Scoliosis	Loss of righting reflex
Rhoecosis (combination of previous signs)	Constipation
Torsion along long axis	Fecal incontinence
Torticollis	Urinary incontinence
Loss of sensation	Inability to constrict, strike, or eat
Loss of movement	Behavioral changes
Pain	Pathologic fractures
Hyperreflexia	
Upper motor neuron signs cranial to lesion	

vertebral column stiffness and resultant decreased mobility, kyphosis, scoliosis, and occasionally pathologic fractures.

Early on, focal nodular swellings may be visible along the dorsum or bulges on the sides of the body. Palpation of the spine may reveal variably sized segments of ankylosis, kyphosis, scoliosis, or lordosis. Digital pressure may also prove painful, with the animal resenting palpation. Animals may be hyperreflexic cranial to the spinal lesion. Hyperreflexia or upper motor neuron signs are often seen cranial to the lesion, and lower motor neuron signs are seen caudal to the lesion. Motor deficits in somatic musculature, slight or dramatic torsion of the body below the affected area, torticollis, trembling, and subtle or acute spinal kinking may be exhibited. Affected snakes may not be able to balance on a hook, right themselves if placed in dorsal recumbency, or effectively strike at prey objects.

Eventually, affected animals cannot move, constrict, strike, or swallow prey. If severe luxation and rotation of vertebrae are present, animals may display bizarre corkscrew postures. Affected lizards may show proprioceptive deficits, severely distorted postures, and partial to total paresis depending on the site of the lesion. It is interesting to observe that even severely debilitated animals may continue to eat and drink if offered. A summary of clinical signs is included in Table 69-2.

DIAGNOSIS

Radiography is the gold standard of PSO. However, the complete diagnosis depends on clinical history, physical examination, blood culture, bone culture, histopathology, and necropsy findings. Radiographs are useful to confirm the presence of spinal disease but cannot identify active infection or inflammation.[13,34,35] Advanced diagnostics such as computed tomographic (CT) scans or nuclear (bone scan) imaging may help to identify the sites of active disease (Figure 69-9).[36]

Bacterial cultures of bone biopsies or joint swabs are useful for isolating bacteria in cases of bacterial osteoarthritis. However, evidence exists that bony lesions of spinal osteopathy do not develop for as much as 22 to 36 months after the initial episode of local infection or septicemia.[21] In addition, many animals can have noninflammatory osteoarthrosis with no histologic evidence of bacteria.[25] Small foci of inflammation may be present. Inflammation in these cases is suggestive of previous or chronic low-grade osteoarthritis,

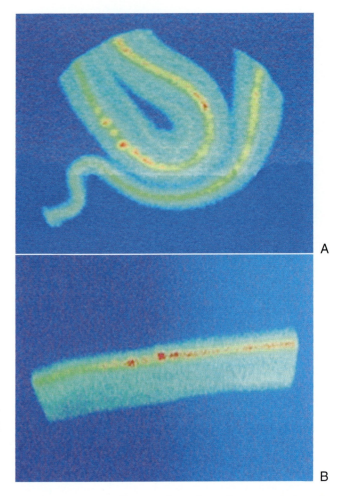

FIGURE 69-9 *A,* Nuclear scan, bone phase, dorsoventral view of a boa with spinal osteopathy. *B,* Lateral view. *Red* foci represent areas of active bone involvement (increased blood flow, infection, proliferation). *(Photograph courtesy D. Mader.)*

supported by isolation of bacteria from blood, bone, and joint lesions.[25] Biopsy of bone in living reptiles is possible (Figure 69-10). The heavy epaxial muscle present over vertebral bodies can make access to the dorsal spinous processes a challenge. Also, antemortem vertebral biopsy has the potential for producing iatrogenic fractures of the spine.

The strong correlation between blood and bone culture results implies that blood culture may be a suitable alternative method of identification of active bacterial osteoarthritis.[25] Animals with radiographic evidence of PSO should also receive blood cultures and local bone aspirates to identify bacteria present either systemically or within bony lesions. Early identification of causative agents may better enable therapeutic success.

TREATMENT

Proliferative spinal osteopathy can be difficult to treat.[25-27] Early diagnosis is essential, identifying a causative agent is crucial, and aggressive appropriate long-term therapy may be necessary. Effective treatment can include appropriate

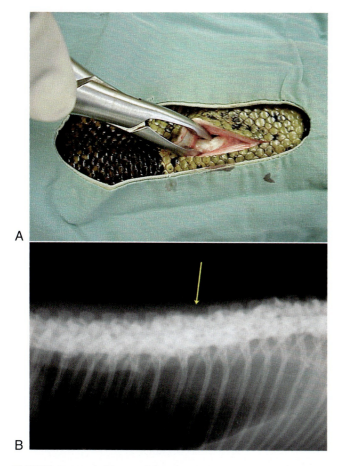

FIGURE 69-10 **A,** Biopsy of dorsal spinous process from the boa in Figure 69-9. **B,** Radiograph of the biopsy site. This is a simple procedure and can be performed with a local block with or without minor sedation. *(Photograph courtesy D. Mader.)*

antimicrobial selection, surgical debridement of granulomatous or lytic areas, use of antiinflammatory medications, and separation of affected and unaffected individuals. Because of the nature of these lesions, medications may not be able to reach the area without intravenous or intraosseous administration or even surgical intervention.[13]

After the initial treatment, intramuscular administration of medications may need to be continued for extended periods of time. If bacterial etiologic agents are suspected, antimicrobials with good penetration of bone must be selected. Therapy regimens have been discouraging. Implantation of antibiotic-impregnated polymethyl methacrylate beads has been used in an attempt to stem deep-seated bony infections in snakes. However, either the antibiotic chosen or the antibiotic dosage of the beads failed in clearing the infection. Perhaps another antibiotic or more antibiotic incorporated into the beads could have been more successful.

Limited data exist to support the effectiveness of nonsteroidal antiinflammatories in reptiles. However, the authors have tried injectable carprofen (1 mg/kg subcutaneously) in affected snakes with seemingly little response to weekly treatments.

At present, most current therapies suggested have been unsuccessful. Nevertheless, effective treatment may depend on early identification of causative agents, aggressive treatment with appropriate antibiotics, and establishment of effective methods of delivering antimicrobials to the affected bony site. Successful treatment depends tremendously on early and aggressive diagnostic techniques such as radiographs, bone biopsy, blood culture, and bone culture.

PROGNOSIS

At present, the prognosis for reptiles with PSO is poor to grave. Most reptiles display advanced lesions at the time of presentation.

Early recognition of this process through implementation of a thorough diagnostic battery and then aggressive long-term antibiotic and analgesic therapy or surgical debridement can make a difference. Every effort must be made to separate affected animals from unaffected animals as early as possible in an attempt to prevent subsequent infection. Further investigation is necessary in every aspect of this debilitating syndrome so that both its true pathogenesis can be understood and effective therapies can be identified and employed. Caretakers of captive reptiles must be more vigilant of their charges and are encouraged to seek earlier more comprehensive treatment for sick individuals. Veterinarians that treat sick reptiles must endeavor to continue to develop effective therapies for frustrating disease processes.

ACKNOWLEDGMENTS

The authors thank Dr Douglas Mader for his patience and help with this chapter. We thank Dr David Chizar and Dr Jeff Baier for their help with the literature search, and we are indebted to Dr Preston Stubbs for discussions regarding osteoarthritis. As always, we thank Dr Robert A. Taylor and the entire staff at Alameda East Veterinary Hospital for such a wonderful place to treat, study, and help sick reptiles. Finally, we thank Dr Hobart M. Smith for providing the initial kyphotic ("rhoecotic") garter snake.

REFERENCES

1. Kroger RL, Guthrie JF: Incidence of crooked vertebral columns in juvenile Atlantic menhaden *Brevoortia tyrannus*, *Chesapeake Sci* 12:276-278, 1971.
2. Dorfman D: Vertebral deformities in an Atlantic silversides, *Underwater Nat* 7:44, 1972.
3. White JB, Murphy GG: A kyphotic eastern spiny soft-shelled turtle, *Trionyx spinifer spinifer*, *J Tenn Acad Sci* 47:61, 1972.
4. Moore CJ, Burton DT: Some skeletal anomalies in Potomac River White perch, *Morone americana*, *Bull Assoc SE Biol* 22:69, 1975.
5. Hadeen SE: Scoliosis and hydrops in a *Rana catesbiana* (Amphibia, Anura, Ranidae) tadpole population, *J Herpetol* 10:261-262, 1976.
6. Grogan WL Jr: Scoliosis in the African lizard, *Agama a. anchietae* (Reptilia, Lacertilia, Agamidae), *J Herpetol* 10:262-263, 1976.
7. Riggins RS, et al: Scoliosis in chickens, *J Bone Surg* 59:1020-1026, 1977.
8. Plymale HH, Jackson CG Jr, Collier G: Kyphosis in *Chrysemys scripta yaguia* (Testudines: Emydidae) and other turtles, *Southwestern Nat* 23:457-462, 1978.

9. Smith HM, Fitzgerald KT: Trauma-induced developmental vertebral displacement (rhoecosis) in a garter snake, *Herp Review* 14(3):69-72, 1983.
10. Chiodini RT, Nielsen SW: Vertebral osteophytes in an iguanid lizard, *Vet Pathol* 20:372-375, 1983.
11. Frye FL, Kiel JL: Multifocal granulomatous spondylitis in a rattlesnake, *Proc Am Assoc Zoo Vet* 60-63, 1985.
12. Johnston SA: Osteoarthritis, *Vet Clin North Am Small Anim Pract* 27(4):699-723, 1997.
13. Antinoff N: Osteomyelitis in reptiles, *Proc Assoc Rept Amph Vet* 149-152, 1997.
14. Lane NE, Buckwalter JA: Exercise: a cause of osteoarthritis, *Rheum Dis Clin North Am* 19:617, 1993.
15. Buckwalter JA: Osteoarthritis and articular cartilate use, disuse, and abuse: experimental studies, *J Rheumatol* 22:13, 1995.
16. Ogden JA, et al: Pathobiology of septic arthritis and contiguous osteomyelitis in a leatherback turtle (*Dermochelys coriacea*), *J Wildl Dis* 17(2):277-287, 1981.
17. Heard DJ, et al: Bacteremia and septic arthritis in a West African dwarf crocodile, *J Am Vet Med Assoc* 192(10):1453-1454, 1988.
18. Russo EA: Anorexia and spinal fracture in a boa constrictor, *Avian Exotic Pract* 2(3):7, 1985.
19. Frye FL: Feeding and nutritional diseases. In Fowler ME, editor: *Zoo and wild animal medicine*, ed 2, Philadelphia, 1986, WB Saunders.
20. Frye FL, Carney J: Osteitis deformans (Paget's disease) in a boa constrictor, *Vet Med Small Anim Clin* 69:186-188, 1974.
21. Kiel JL: Spinal osteoarthropathy in two southern copperheads, *J Zoo Anim Med* 8(2):21-24, 1977.
22. Lewis LD, Morris ML, Hand MS: *Small animal clinical nutrition III*, Topeka, Kan, 1987, Mark Morris Assoc.
23. Kiel JL: Paget's disease in snakes, *Proc Am Assoc Zoo Vet* 201-207, 1983.
24. Frye FL: Viral diseases. In: *Biomedical and surgical aspects of captive reptile husbandry*, ed 2, Malabar, Fla, 1991, Krieger Publishing.
25. Isaza R, Garner M, Jacobson E: Proliferative osteoarthritis and osteoarthrosis in 15 snakes, *J Zoo Wildl Med* 31:20-27, 2000.
26. Jacobson ER, Millichamp NJ, Gaskin NM: Use of a polyvalent autogenous bacterin for treatment of mixed gram-negative bacterial osteomyelitis in a rhinoceros viper, *J Am Vet Med Assoc* 187(11):1224-1225, 1985.
27. Ramsay EC, et al: Osteomyelitis associated with *Salmonella enterica* SS *arizonae* in a colony of ridgenose rattlesnakes (*Crotalus willardi*), *J Zoo Wildl Med* 33:301-310, 2002.
28. Bemis DA, et al: Comparison of phenotypic traits and genetic relatedness of *Salmonella enterica* subspecies *arizonae* isolates from a colony of ridge nose rattlesnakes with osteomyelitis, *J Vet Diagn Invest* 15(4):382-387, 2003.
29. Croop JM, et al: *Arizona hinshawii* osteomyelitis associated with a pet snake, *Pediatr Infect Dis* 3(2):188, 1984.
30. Nowinski RJ: Iguana-transmitted *Salmonella* osteomyelitis, *Orthopedics* 24(7):694, 2001.
31. Divers SJ, Lawton MPC: Spinal osteomyelitis in a green iguana, *Iguana iguana*: cerebrospinal fluid and myelogram diagnosis, *Proc Assoc Rept Amph Vet* 77, 2000.
32. Greek TJ: Osteomyelitis in a green iguana, *Iguana iguana*, *Proc Eighth Ann Conf Assoc Rept Amph Vet* 163-164, 2001.
33. Funk RS: Tail damage. In Mader DR, editor: *Reptile medicine and surgery*, Philadelphia, 1996, WB Saunders.
34. Rubel A, Kuoni W, Frye FL: Radiology and imaging. In Frye FL, editor: *Reptile care: an atlas of diseases and treatments*, Neptune City, NJ, 1991, TFH Publications.
35. Silverman S, Janssen DL: Diagnostic imaging. In Mader DR, editor: *Reptile medicine and surgery*, Philadelphia, 1996, WB Saunders.
36. Blood DC, Studdert VP: *Veterinary dictionary*, ed 2, New York, 1988, WB Saunders.

70
TAIL DAMAGE
RICHARD S. FUNK

Tail damage results from a variety of causes, including mechanical and infectious etiologies. In general, a reptile tail is normally a functional part of its body, often used for social signaling or as a counterbalance or swimming aid, and is a functional caudal extension of the vertebral column. The skin and its scales are resistant to desiccation and abrasion. If the tail is deformed, possible causes include congenital defect, trauma, and infection.

If part of the tail is missing, trauma may have occurred from a cage mate in a display of interspecific or intraspecific aggression; the tail may have been mistaken for food and been bitten off; or the tail may have been bitten off by a predator. Humans may be responsible for the missing portion with an accidental cutting of the tail with a knife, shovel, hoe, or hatchet.

Tail infection of the Gartersnake (Thamnophis sirtalis) by the trematode *Alaria* sp. in the Great Lakes region may result in amputation of a portion of the tail from avascular necrosis (personal observation). An ischemic necrosis of the tail tip of breeding adult female Burmese Pythons (Python molurus bivittatus) has been associated with thromboembolic disease.[3]

Many lizards possess autotomy planes in the tail vertebrae such that when the tail is grasped or bitten by a predator, the portion distal to the insult breaks away by autotomy (see Figure 6-17). When the tail tip regenerates, it is smaller and usually a different color or pattern than the original (Figure 70-1). In addition, the actual tail vertebrae do not regenerate but rather are replaced by a cartilaginous core (Figure 70-2).

The ability to autotomize the tail is widespread among the lizards but is lacking in chameleons, monitors, helodermatids, and a few others. With the understanding that tail autotomy is a natural phenomenon in many lizards, the clinician must be careful in handling these species so as not to cause an iatrogenic tail loss (Figure 70-3). Tail loss has clinical significance in that if a portion of the tail of a species that can autotomize its tail needs amputation, one may be able to "assist" it in autotomizing naturally and then not suture it closed so that regeneration can occur. Conservative treatment, even with a temporary bandage, may be suitable (see Chapter 35 for more details).

Some lizards may have forked tails from an incomplete tail autotomy; the original one "broke" but was not completely separated, and the stimulus occurred for regeneration so a "fork" was produced (Figure 70-4). The few snakes that are known to be capable of autotomy lack a fracture plane and separation occurs between the vertebrae, without subsequent regeneration.

A common cause of tail amputation is trauma from a rodent bite. If a live rodent is left in a reptile cage overnight and the reptile does not feed, the rodent can attack and feed on the reptile, damaging the reptile's body, including the tail.

Paralysis of the tail can be caused by fracture or luxation of one or more caudal vertebrae, a bacterial or protozoal infection that involves the caudal spinal cord, a spinal tumor, or proliferative ossifying spondylosis or osteomyelitis lesions that usually are bacterial and resistant to treatment (Figure 70-5).

A common presentation in Green Iguanas (Iguana iguana) is an ascending avascular necrosis (Figure 70-6). Although the etiology may be multifactorial and often not identified, one of the more common causes results from aggressive (territorial) animals slapping their tails against the cage walls.

Masses and swellings of the tail are common. Many small masses are epidermal or dermal and represent manifestations of a dermatitis. Abscesses are common and must be differentiated from rare granulomas and neoplasms.

Both genders of squamates have scent glands located in the ventral tail base that may enlarge as secretions accumulate. These glands may become inspissated or abscessed.

The hemipenes of male lizards and snakes are also located in the ventral tail base and may also become swollen or abscessed. A careful examination differentiates the scent gland from the hemipenis. Some lizards accumulate a plug of cells and cellular secretions in the hemipenis, termed a hemipenial plug, that may cause swelling and discomfort; this may often be manually removed but may require sedation and sometimes minor surgical intervention (Figure 70-7). In the author's practice, these hemipenial plugs are most often seen in Green Iguanas, Leopard Geckos (Eublepharis macularius), and Bearded Dragons (Pogona vitticeps). A prolapsed hemipenis can become infected or necrotic and lead to tail infection.

An iatrogenic tail swelling/infection very rarely may result from venipuncture. Proper attention to aseptic technique and proper choice of needle size prevent these complications.

Metabolic bone diseases from various causes commonly lead to abnormal curvatures of the tail in lizards (see Chapter 61).

Cloacal problems, including bacterial cloacitis or chronic cloacal prolapse, can lead to lesions on the base of the adjacent tail.

Damage to the tail skin may be from infectious causes such as bacterial or fungal dermatitis, bites from cage mates or rodents (often penetrating through the underlying musculature), contact dermatitis, dysecdysis that necessitates careful removal of the retained skin (Figure 70-8), ectoparasites (e.g., snake mites, tick), or owner-induced trauma such as forcibly pulling from a tight refuge (in or out of a cage) or slamming the cage door on the tail.

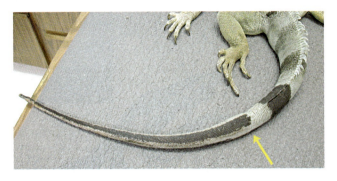

FIGURE 70-1 Avulsed tails usually grow back (*yellow arrow* marks the site of the regrowth). However, the new growth is never the same as the original. The scales are smaller and discolored, and pigment patterns vary. *(Photograph courtesy D. Mader.)*

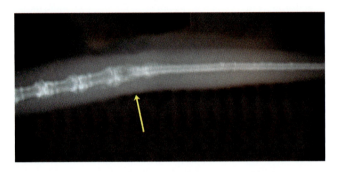

FIGURE 70-2 The regrown tail does not regenerate the vertebrae; rather the bone is replaced with a cartilaginous core (starting at the *yellow arrow*). *(Photograph courtesy D. Mader.)*

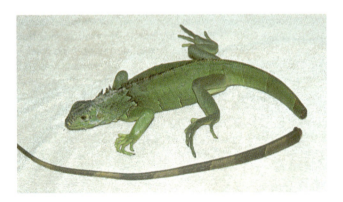

FIGURE 70-3 Lizards that have tail autotomy can avulse their tails when stressed, injured, or caught. Care must be taken not to damage the tails of patients. *(Photograph courtesy D. Mader.)*

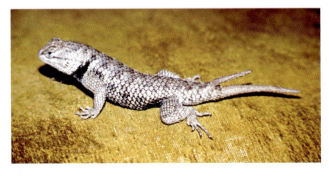

FIGURE 70-4 Partial damage to tails can result in abnormal healing, including the development of "forked tails." *(Photograph courtesy D. Mader.)*

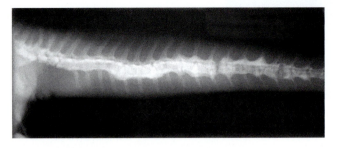

FIGURE 70-5 A form of bridging spondylosis, from various causes such as trauma, nutritional imbalances, or infections, is common in captive lizards, especially the Green Iguana (*Iguana iguana*). These animals frequently "fracture" their ossified tails. *(Photograph courtesy D. Mader.)*

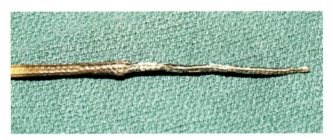

FIGURE 70-6 A common presentation in Green Iguanas (*Iguana iguana*) is an ascending avascular necrosis. The etiology may be multifactorial and oftentimes is not identified. One of the more common causes is aggressive (territorial) animals slapping their tails against the cage walls. *(Photograph courtesy D. Mader.)*

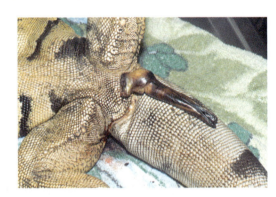

FIGURE 70-7 Mature male Green Iguanas (*Iguana iguana*) commonly masturbate during breeding season. Inspissated impacted seminal plugs can cause infection and pain. These may need to be removed under anesthesia. *(Photograph courtesy D. Mader.)*

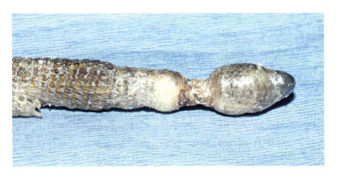

FIGURE 70-8 Improper shedding (dysecdysis), from low environmental humidity, can result in constricting bands of old skin around the tail. As these rings build up and the patient grows, avascular necrosis and sloughing of the distal portion of the tail result. *(Photograph courtesy D. Mader.)*

Occasionally tail skin loss occurs if the tail is stuck to tape. Wild-caught reptiles commonly exhibit scars or wounds on their tails, presumably from predators or occasionally from prey, injuries, or even their human captors. The Trans-Pecos Ratsnake *(Bogertophis subocularis)* is the sole host of a peculiar tick *Aponomma elaphensis*; engorged ticks are found on the tail of the snakes, and wild-caught snakes commonly have tick-damaged tails, with the tip occasionally missing.[5]

These conditions should be treated with chemotherapeutic agents if indicated; amputation if necessary; surgical removal of abscesses, granulomas, or tumors; or even surgical closure of skin defects if possible (see Chapter 35). Delays in treatment may result in a greater likelihood of infection and permanent scarring.

REFERENCES

1. Bellairs A d'A, Bryant SV: Autotomy and regeneration in reptiles. In Gans C, Billett F, editors: *Biology of the Reptilia, development B*, vol 15, New York, 1985, John Wiley & Sons.
2. Frye FL: *Biomedical and surgical aspects of captive reptile husbandry*, Melbourne, Fla, 1991, Krieger Publishing.
3. Heard DJ: Idiopathic chronic pneumonia and thromboembolic disease in captive Burmese Pythons *(Python molurus bivitattus)*, Proc Assoc Rept Amphib Vet 89-91, 1996.
4. Marcus LC: *Veterinary biology and medicine of captive amphibians and reptiles*, Philadelphia, 1981, Lea & Febiger.
5. Shaw CE, Campbell S: *Snakes of the American West*, New York, 1974, AA Knopf.

71
THERMAL BURNS
DOUGLAS R. MADER

Thermal burns in reptiles are one of the most common injuries seen by reptile veterinarians. Exactly why reptiles seem so prone to burns is not understood, but something about their behavior makes them more susceptible to this type of injury than any other captive animal (Figure 71-1).

Because reptiles do everything slowly, for an animal to be burned but not actually show signs of the injury for several days is not uncommon. This is especially true for minor or first-degree burns and is significant because burns, even apparently mild injuries, can have severe consequences if not treated properly. For proper treatment of burns, one must understand the causes of burns and how to recognize them in their early stages.

THERMODYNAMICS

The study of heat and its properties is called thermodynamics. As herpetologists, we are all familiar with the importance of proper temperatures in the cage environment. Over the years, we have seen the evolution of heating devices from the original "hot rocks" to more advanced thermostatically controlled environmental chambers.

Not only do captive reptiles need supplemental heat, but they need supplemental heat provided in the proper fashion. For instance, a 5-m (15-foot) python does not fare well with a single 30-cm (12-inch) hot rock. Likewise, a nocturnal lizard suffers if its cage is heated with a bright heat lamp.

A look at animals in their natural environment assists in the understanding of the principles of thermodynamics from a practical (captive) perspective (Figure 71-2). As an example, we should evaluate the heating strategies of the Green Iguana (*Iguana iguana*) in the rain forest.

These animals live for the sun. On an initial glance, they appear to derive their energy-providing heat from basking in the sunlight. But, on closer inspection, much more is involved than an animal merely perched atop a branch soaking in the sun's rays.

For an object to get warm, or heat up, a transfer of heat must occur from some outside source to the object that is heated. Heat always moves from a warmer area to a cooler area. As the heat leaves the first object and enters the second object, the first object becomes cooler and the second object becomes warmer. Eventually, the temperatures of the two objects become equal, or equilibrate. Heat never continues to leave the first object such that it becomes cooler, resulting in the new object becoming the hotter of the two.

The three ways that an object can gain heat, or become warmed, are via conduction, convection, and radiant heat.

Conduction is the transfer of heat within an object (such as down a long metal pole) or between two objects that are touching each other. A classic example of conduction is a pan on a stove. The burner on the stove heats up. A cold pan is placed on the hot burner, and the heat then transfers from the hot burner directly to the cooler pan, thereby heating up the pan and the contents inside.

A herpetologic analogy here is the use of a hot rock. A hot rock is a solid block-like structure, usually made of brick, concrete, plaster, or heavy molded plastic. Imbedded within the rock is some sort of heating coil. When the heating coil is plugged in, it generates heat. This heat, in turn, heats up the rock.

If a lizard (or any reptile) crawls up on the rock, the heat from the hot rock then transfers, via conduction, to the lizard. The path of the heat transfers from the surface of the hot rock through the feet and belly and tail of the lizard, or whatever parts of the animal are in *direct* contact with the rock's surface.

Convection, on the other hand, involves the motion of large-scale quantities of matter. In plain words, convection usually involves the movement of either gases (such as air) or liquids (such as water). Heat is transferred via movement of this matter (e.g., air or water).

For instance, consider the air over a desert. As the surface of the desert heats up from the sun, it warms the air that touches it (this is conduction). This warm air, which is lighter than cooler air, then rises. As it rises, it pushes (displaces) the air above and on the sides away, forcing the cool air back down to the earth. This cool air warms and then follows the path of the warm air before it, upwards (convection). Hence, you get a warming effect, or a thermal, developing. Birds, hang gliders, and airplanes use these thermals to soar high in the sky with hardly any energy used to stay aloft.

In the iguana example, in the jungle, where it is very hot, the warm air that blows across the animal while it is basking, exposed, on the end of a branch is an example of convective heating.

Radiant heat is the last type of heat transfer. Radiation heat transfer involves the flow of thermal energy by electromagnetic waves. In contrast to conductive heating, where objects must touch, or convective heating, where the matter (gas or water) must touch the object to be heated, radiant heat does not have to have any matter involved (no touching needed for heat transfer).

The classic example here is the fast-food hamburger under the red heat lamp. The lamp does not need to touch the burger to keep it warm, and likewise, a wind current or water flow over the lamp and the burger is not needed to keep the food hot.

The obvious example here is the iguana that basks in the sunlight. It soaks up the electromagnetic radiation produced by the sun's rays. In captivity, this source of electromagnetic radiation is replaced by any number of artificial means, usually a heat lamp or a ceramic bulb.

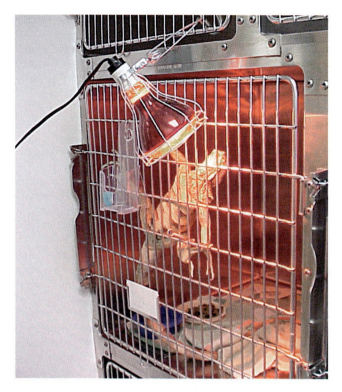

FIGURE 71-1 Burns are a common injury in captive reptiles. No one knows why a reptile does not avoid or withdraw from a noxious stimulus such as a heat lamp. Reptiles not uncommonly fall asleep under a heat lamp or on a hot rock and acquire severe burns.

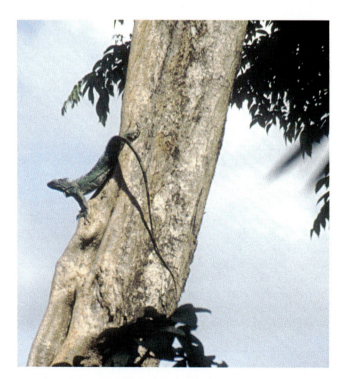

FIGURE 71-2 The transfer of thermal energy in the wild is a complicated process that is not always duplicated in captivity. This wild Green Iguana (*Iguana iguana*) thermoregulates via three different means: conduction, convection, and radiant heat.

So, in review, this apparently simple equation of an iguana sitting on a branch to get warm really is much more complicated than it looks (see Figure 71-2). The iguana in the wild gets its warmth three ways:

1. Radiant heat: The lizard absorbs the electromagnetic radiation from the sun.
2. Convective heat: The warm air that blows across the animal.
3. Conductive heat: From sitting on a branch that has been warmed by the sun. The branch then acts as a conductive heat source, passing the warmth back into the animal resting on it.

The best type of heat source for a captive pet depends on the type of animal caged. As mentioned, a small heat rock is inappropriate for a large snake. These animals do better with convective or radiant heat. Likewise, a big heat lamp is not proper for an arboreal animal that normally gets its heat from either conduction or convection.

Several other variables play important roles in heat transfer and warming. A big factor is humidity. Moist air, or high humidity, tends to hold heat much better than dry heat. When figuring temperatures and thermal gradients, careful attention should be paid to humidity. A hot humid cage is much more stifling than a hot dry cage.

Ventilation is important in any cage design. A well-designed cage has good ventilation. Stagnant air, especially in hot humid cages, leads to build up of pathogens, or disease-causing bacteria and fungi. Proper ventilation dilutes out any potential problem before it reaches concentrations that may be dangerous.

However, for all the good that proper ventilation does, it does have its drawbacks. A well-ventilated cage tends to lose heat and humidity (it gets exhausted outside). Really nothing is wrong with this, except that the heat and humidity need to be replaced, and in the overall scheme of design, it ends up costing more to maintain a steady state of temperature and humidity.

HEAT AND TISSUE INJURY

Of the three types of heat transfer, the two that cause the most injuries are radiant heat and conductive heat. Over the years, the author has seen several hundred burns caused by hot rocks. These crude heating devices have variable heat output, often unevenly distributed over the surface of the rock, and can reach temperatures that sear the flesh off any animal that rests on it.

In addition, the author has personally seen many hot rocks that have "shorted out" (Figure 71-3). In one case in which a hot rock shorted out, it caught fire and set the owner's bedroom ablaze.

Humans have a withdrawal reflex. When we touch something hot, without any cognizant thought, we automatically, immediately, withdraw our hand. Even young children and mammals display this reflex. This author has touched new hot rocks, and their surface has been so hot that the same withdrawal reflex was experienced. They are so hot that the author could not physically keep a hand on the surface.

Why then, when reptiles rest on such a "hot" hot rock, do they not also immediately jump off? How is it that a reptile

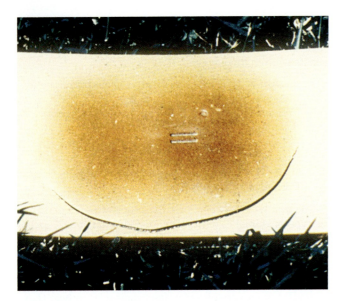

FIGURE 71-3 Hot rocks can pose a severe danger to captive reptiles. This hot rock shorted out. The resultant heat got so extreme that it melted and cracked the plastic.

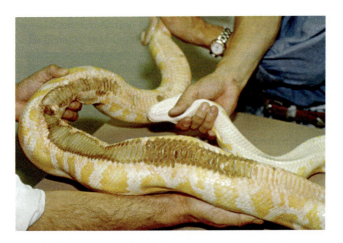

FIGURE 71-4 This Burmese Python *(Python molurus bivitattus)* coiled around a heat lamp. The resulting burn extended over 25% of its ventral scales.

can fall asleep under a heat lamp, acquire a severe burn, and not move away?

Nobody seems to have an easy answer for those questions. For a snake to wrap its coils around a bare light bulb because it is attracted to the warmth that the light emits is not uncommon (Figure 71-4). So, it must feel the warmth; why then, does it not feel the burning heat?

One answer is that the nerve receptors that sense heat and the receptors that sense pain are different. Also possible is that in the wild, such pain receptors have no evolutionary significance (reptiles do not come into contact with intensely hot objects in the wild). Therefore, evolutionarily, a reptile has no reason to have a hot-pain withdrawal reflex.

Other theories put forth suggest that because reptiles do not reason in the same fashion that people do, or other mammals for that matter, even though they may feel pain, they do not associate it with the object that they are touching.

Hence, they do not realize that they need to move for the pain to subside.

Bottom line is, nobody really knows. So, until we understand why these animals are so prone to burns, the best thing to do is make every effort to prevent the burns in the first place.

TYPES OF BURNS

Burns are classified by the type of burn and by the severity of the injury or extent of the body surface area affected. The three basic classifications of burns in mammals are categories that can also be used in reptiles. Understanding the nature of the burn helps one to assess the need for intervention. Is this something that can be handled at home, or should the animal be hospitalized for competent medical care?

The extent and severity of a burn are related to several factors. Obviously the **temperature** of the heat source plays a significant role. Touching a stove burner set on "warm" results in a far less severe burn than touching the same burner set on "high."

Duration of contact also affects the severity of the burn wound. Again, touching a stove burner set on "warm" only briefly may result in a minor burn, whereas holding one's hand on the same burner for several minutes may result in much more severe tissue damage. This is perhaps why we see such intense damage in reptiles that have fallen asleep on what seems like only a mildly hot heating element like a hot rock.

Lastly, the **heat conductance** characteristics of the material touched also play a role in the severity of the burn. For instance, touching a hot piece of metal causes a more severe burn than touching a piece of wood at the same temperature.

Types of burns include thermal, electrical, chemical, and radiation. Thermal burns include all the categories that have been discussed so far, such as burns by hot rocks and heat lamps. An electrical burn, although not common in reptiles, can be seen with direct contact with an electrical current, such as with a short in a wire that has electrical arcing or an animal that bites through an electrical cord that is plugged into a live socket.

Chemical burns are caused by strong acids or alkalis, such as cleaning supplies like pure bleach (an alkali agent). These are also uncommon in reptile patients but do occur, especially when chemicals are spilled or agents are not thoroughly rinsed after a cage is cleaned. (See Figure 15-22.)

Radiation burns in reptiles are extremely uncommon. These are usually related to the use of radiation therapy in treatment of certain types of cancers. Because radiation therapy has been used in reptile patients, this type of burn is possible.

In older terminology, burns used to be classified as first, second, or third degree, depending on the severity of the damage. In more recent classification, the terms partial-thickness and full-thickness burns are more commonly used. "Thickness" refers to the outer layer of skin.

First-degree burns are superficial or partial-thickness injuries that only involve the epidermis (outer skin; Figure 71-5; see also Figures 15-17 and 15-18). These burns are painful. In mammals, damage may occur to the hair or fur (singing). The skin is reddened, and in severe

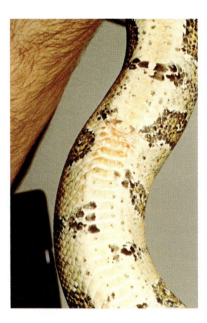

FIGURE 71-5 First-degree burns are superficial or partial-thickness injuries that involve only the epidermis.

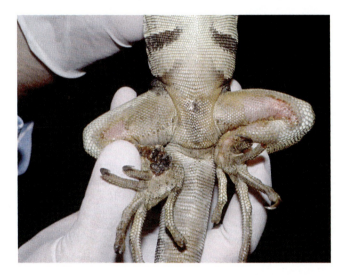

FIGURE 71-6 Second-degree burns are deeper partial-thickness injuries with usually full destruction of the epidermis and variable damage to the underlying dermis. These burns are characterized by intense pain.

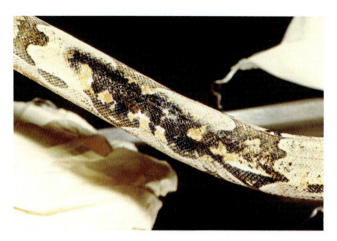

FIGURE 71-7 In third-degree burns, the entire thickness of the skin is destroyed. The burn is actually painless (all the pain-sensing nerves are destroyed), and the tissue takes on either a whitish or charcoal-black appearance.

first-degree burns, blisters may be seen (such as in a severe sunburn).

In reptiles, blisters are rarely seen, although they may occur, and occasionally, one may see singeing of the scales, depending on the type of exposure. Usually, reddening of the skin occurs, and often what looks like "bruises" under the scales, especially in white, pale, or clear scales.

These burns usually heal well and rarely leave a scar. In an otherwise healthy reptile, healing takes about 1 month and a good shed for the burn to completely resolve.

Second-degree burns are deeper partial-thickness injuries with usually full destruction of the epidermis and variable damage to the underlying dermis (inner, deep layer; Figure 71-6). In mammals, although more damage occurs to the dermis, the fur or hair may not necessarily be damaged. The burns are painful, and extensive subcutaneous swelling does occur. In reptiles, blistering and oozing of serum from the burn site are seen. Extensive bruising and discoloration of the tissue are seen. These injuries lead to the formation of a scab-like covering over the burn.

Healing occurs from the margins of the wound inward. In these wounds, especially in burns that cover a large surface area, healing may be prolonged and significant scarring may occur.

In **third-degree** burns, the entire thickness of the skin is destroyed. The burn is actually painless (all the pain-sensing nerves are destroyed), and the tissue takes on either a whitish or charcoal black appearance (Figure 71-7). In mammals, the hair and fur fall out or are destroyed. Third-degree burns are four times as serious as second-degree burns of similar size.

Healing of third-degree or full-thickness burns occurs with contraction of the wound (shrinking) and epithelialization (regrowth and migration of new skin from the margins of the wound toward the center). In some cases of third-degree burns, skin grafting may be necessary. These burns may take many months (4 to 6) to heal completely. Severe scarring is a hallmark of third-degree burns.

The classification of a **fourth-degree** burn is occasionally used to describe a third-degree burn that not only involves the full thickness of the skin but also the underlying tissue such as muscle and bone. These injuries carry a grave prognosis.

BURN TREATMENT

Reptiles have a penchant for healing far greater than mammals. Some of the wounds that have been seen in reptiles would have spelled doom for most other animals. Incredibly, the author has also seen scars on wild reptiles that bore the legacy of previous severe wounds, wounds that healed without the benefit of veterinary intervention. That does not mean that we should ignore wounds in captivity, that they will heal without help, but it does give us hope when we see a bad wound, knowing that with proper care and time, it should heal fine (Table 71-1).

Table 71-1 Treatment of Burns

First-Degree Burns

Brief cool-water rinses, cold compresses.
Do not open blisters; if open, keep clean.
Antibiotics/analgesics usually not necessary if burn is minor.

Second-Degree Burns

Analgesics (butorphenol, nonsteroidal antiinflammatory drugs [NSAIDS]).
Antibiotics (systemic ceftazidime, amikacin, topical silver sulfadiazine; can switch to oral antibiotics for chronic treatment as needed).
Daily debriding and wound care (with or without anesthesia, wet-to-dry, sugar or honey bandages).
Fluid therapy (intravenous [IV], intracoelomic [ICe], oral).
Ensure adequate nutrition (assist-feed as needed).

Third-Degree (and Fourth-Degree) Burns

As in second-degree burns, just more extensive.
Pay close attention to analgesia as the wounds start to heal because pain usually intensifies.

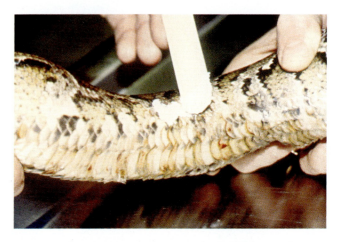

FIGURE 71-8 Silver sulfadiazine burn cream is applied to the damaged skin on this snake. This cream, which is used extensively in humans, is effective against many common bacteria, including *Pseudomonas aeruginosa* and *Candida albicans*, a common fungal pathogen found in chronic burn wounds.

Minor burns often do well with first aid. However, severe burns require medical attention and possible hospitalization for pain relief, infection control, and treatment for shock.

In general, first-degree burns, unless they affect extensive portions of the body, can be treated at home. If the burn is recent, cold-water rinses or cold compresses (not ice) should be applied for no more than 20 minutes to help reduce swelling and pain to the affected area. Application of ice to the tissue can cause frostbite, actually causing freeze damage to the tissue.

If blisters are present, they should NOT be broken. Doing so damages the skin's natural barrier against infection. The blisters should be let to either resolve or break on their own.

Infection is a common, and potentially serious, complication of burns. When the skin is compromised, as with broken blisters, careful attention should be paid to contamination, with the affected area kept as clean as possible. A nonirritating antibacterial soap, such as chlorhexidine, or even a gentle hand soap, such as Ivory or Dove, works well.

If damaged skin exists, then application of a topical burn dressing, after gentle wound cleansing, is appropriate (Figure 71-8). The burn should then be dressed, or covered, with a sterile nonstick bandage. This can be tricky, especially when the burn is on the underside of a snake.

In an animal with extensive burns, the author recommends keeping the animal in a glass or Plexiglas enclosure without substrate. Although this is not a natural way to house a reptile, these cages are easy to clean and disinfect, thus minimizing the risk of infection. Their benefits outweigh the disadvantages of the temporary housing.

Second-degree burns, because of the extensive tissue damage, need veterinary attention. If for no other reason, the veterinarian can provide medications for pain relief as pain is a hallmark of second-degree burns.

If the animal is in shock, therapy must be initiated to counter the effects. Wounds are cleaned and debrided. Topical burn creams, such as silver sulfadiazine, are applied, and the patient is started on antibiotics to prevent infection at the burn site. Injectable ceftazidime and oral cefadroxil (see Chapter 89 for dosages) are the first drugs of choice.

Fluids, either intravenous, oral, or otherwise, must be administered to counter the effects of shock and fluid loss from the burn. Daily cleansing of the wound and sterile bandage changes are needed to effect rapid healing. This process may take several weeks to months to fully heal.

Third-degree, or full thickness burns, require intensive care. Depending on the extent of the burn, the owner of the reptile should be apprised of the potentially grave prognosis and the anticipated prolonged treatment that is required (Figure 71-9).

Treatment of third-degree burns involves all the care involved for the second-degree burn, plus more. As the tissue starts to heal, the pain during healing can be intense. The pain from the daily cleanings and debridements can also intensify as the patient recovers feeling to the burn area.

Antibiotic therapy may be protracted, often lasting for several months. Regular assessment of the patient's renal parameters is prudent. Wound care can become expensive, considering that the bandages may need to be changed daily for many months. **As a veterinarian, consideration of all the costs of return visits, bandage materials, follow-up laboratory sampling, and other miscellaneous costs is important when quoting estimates to the clients.** Even in the face of such odds, many people do elect to treat pets with extensive burns.

Even some of the fourth-degree burns, with the underlying tissue as well as the skin destroyed, have the potential to heal if cared for properly. A Blue Tongue Skink (*Tiliqua scincoides*) had a full-thickness burn through its abdominal wall that left a complete fistula in the coelomic cavity. This animal was taken to surgery after it was stabilized and treated for shock. The devitalized tissue was removed, and the edges of the defect were apposed. So much tissue damage occurred that after the damaged tissue was removed, the patient looked like an hourglass when the sides were pulled together. After extensive wound care, bandage changes, and antibiotic therapy, the patient recovered, nearly 6 months later. Other than the tremendous scar, the animal was back to normal (Figure 71-10).

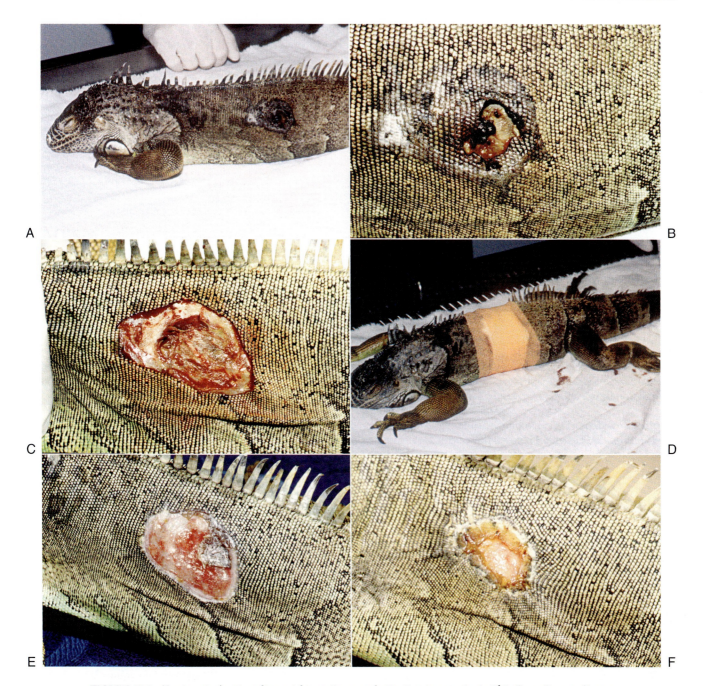

FIGURE 71-9 Treatment of serious burns takes patience and attention to asepsis. **A,** This Green Iguana *(Iguana iguana)* was burned by a heat lamp. **B,** The burn was full thickness (third degree). Note the devitalized tissue (black and depigmented white). The coelomic membrane is visible near the center of the wound. **C,** With anesthesia, and with aseptic technique, the burn is debrided, with removal of all the devitalized tissue back to healthy skin and underlying fascia. Careful attention was made not to penetrate the coelom. **D,** Wet-to-dry sterile bandages were applied daily. No other topical medications were used. The patient was also started on ceftazidime, oral fluids, and butorphenol. **E,** One week after the initial burn, a fungal infection started under the bandage (noted on a cytologic scraping of the wound). A bacterial culture and sensitivity was performed on the wound and revealed a pure growth of *Pseudomonas aeruginosa*, sensitive to amikacin. The patient was then started on daily systemic amikacin combined with topical application of silver sulfadiazine cream. The ceftazidime was discontinued. **F,** By 4 weeks after the burn, reepithelialization of the wound was evident. Note how the wound reepithelializes from the outside in.

Continued

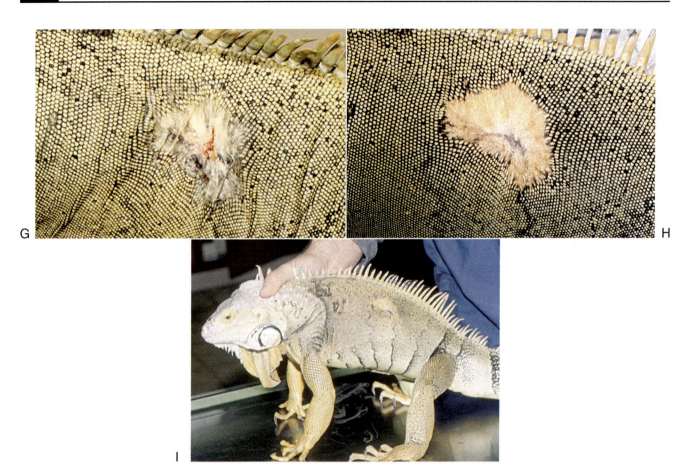

FIGURE 71-9—Cont'd **G,** At 8 weeks after the injury. **H,** At 16 weeks after the injury. The wound has healed, leaving behind only a depigmented scar. **I,** The patient recovered completely. Note the difference in the color of the patient on the day of presentation with the healthy animal.

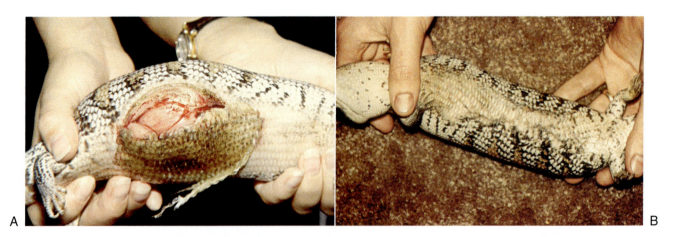

FIGURE 71-10 **A,** This skink had a severe hot-rock burn that penetrated the entire abdominal wall. The wound was resected, and the healthy edges of the skin were apposed. **B,** At 6 months after the initial injury, the patient had made a full recovery. *(Photographs courtesy E. Ivey.)* Clients should be made aware of the usual prolonged recovery times that are necessary for some of these severe burn injuries.

Thermal Burns 923

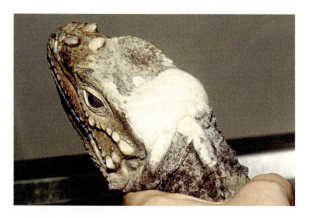

FIGURE 71-11 Healed scar on the head of a *Cyclura* sp. (heat lamp burn).

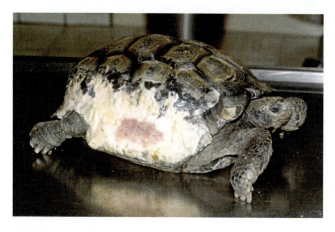

FIGURE 71-13 Healed carapace burn (heat lamp) in a Desert Tortoise *(Gopherus agassizii)*.

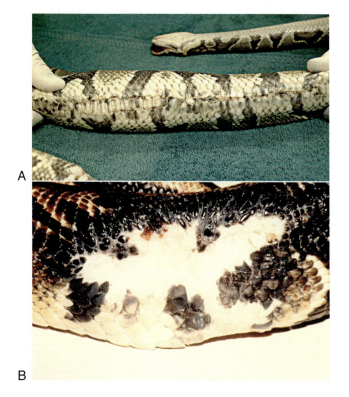

FIGURE 71-12 **A,** Resolved burn on the belly of a python. Note the side-to-side stricturing from the scar tissue (this patient is anesthestized). **B,** Healed burn wound, that left a massive scar, from a heat-lamp burn in a boa. *(Photograph courtesy S. Barten.)*

Although not discussed, many patients exposed to heat may not actually be burned but may have smoke or other toxic fume inhalation. Many melted glues and plastics produce noxious fumes and smoke that can damage delicate lung tissue. Although initially these patients may appear to be uninjured, they may have a fatal fluid build-up develop within their lungs and could potentially die if not treated properly in a timely fashion.

A complete blood count and chemistry analysis should be performed on all severely burned patients. Radiographs help assess the progression of pulmonary edema commonly seen after exposure to smoke inhalation.

SUMMARY

Understanding why reptiles are so prone to burn injury remains a mystery. But understanding the causes of burns and the mechanics of tissue injury helps us prevent such occurrences and, in the unfortunate event that they do happen, better manage their care.

Reptiles have a remarkable ability to heal. One must pay attention to aseptic technique and pain management in treatment of burn patients. Even with what appears to be severe tissue damage, the animals recover, albeit with some severe scarring (Figures 71-11 to 71-13; see also Figure 15-19).

The most important point to remember in treatment of burns in reptile patients is to be diligent, be clean, and, above all, be patient!

72

UPPER ALIMENTARY TRACT DISEASE

STEPHEN J. MEHLER and
R. AVERY BENNETT

Upper alimentary tract disease (UATD) is a general classification that refers to any disorder, disease, or condition that involves the oral cavity, the pharynx, or the esophagus. Common clinical signs of UATD include anorexia, ptyalism, tongue damage or paralysis, gingivitis, ecchymosis and petechiation, and the loss of teeth.

The oral cavity of reptiles is a complex system that relies on the coordination of many structures for proper function. The dysfunction of any part of the intricate system may be caused by or predispose to clinical inappetence; suppressed immunity; infections from bacteria, viruses, and fungi; and neoplastic disease and trauma. Presentation for disorders and diseases of the oral cavity in reptiles is a common occurrence in the clinical setting.

DISORDERS OF THE ORAL CAVITY, TEETH, AND BEAK

Congenital Disorders

Documented congenital disorders of the oral cavity of reptiles include mandibular brachygnathism, maxillary brachygnathism, and cleft palate (Figure 72-1).[1] These conditions may be the result of genetic defects, improper incubation conditions, or gravid females exposed to inappropriate temperatures or chemicals during internal incubation.[1]

Oral or Rostral Trauma

One of the most common oral conditions, which is considered iatrogenic and occurs in all species of reptiles brought into captive environments, is rostral trauma and secondary wound infection. This condition occurs as a sequela to rubbing the face on cage walls and covers (Figure 72-2). No matter how large the enclosure or with what material it is made, reptiles can have ulcerations, lacerations, calluses, and other traumatic lesions develop that are prone to bacterial or fungal infection.

Other husbandry-related injuries of the oral cavity in reptiles include thermal burns to extraoral tissues from exposed light and heat sources, intraoral burns from overheating prey items, and damage to the oral cavity during restraint, examination, and assist-feeding. Reptiles that roam freely in the presence of dogs and cats may fall prey to bite wounds (Figure 72-3).

Damage to the teeth, gingiva, and other structures of the oral cavity sometimes occurs during aggressive encounters with cage mates. Ingestion of inappropriate foreign material, loss of teeth during killing of prey, and wounds inflicted by prey during feeding can cause oral trauma (Figure 72-4). The authors have seen animals with hair or string tightly wrapped around the tongue causing constriction, swelling, and necrosis.

In chelonians, abnormalities or damage to the beak can result in anorexia (Figure 72-5). Overgrowth, softening, or damage of the rhamphotheca and rhinotheca can occur in association with congenital abnormalities, infection, nutritional secondary hyperparathyroidism (NSHP), hypovitaminosis A, trauma, and malocclusion. Some species of captive and wild tortoises are prone to rhamphotheca chips and fractures from prehending rocks (personal observation by author).

Periodontal Disease

Periodontal disease is a significant cause of morbidity in captive lizards and occurs primarily in agamids and chameleons.[2] Mastication of a natural diet provides the required texture to keep plaque from developing. When a buildup of plaque forms on the teeth, bacteria begin to colonize and cause a reversible inflammatory response in the marginal gingiva.[2] Gingivitis can become severe enough that it involves the periodontal ligament and causes irreversible damage, primarily loss of the connective tissue attachment and surrounding bone. When the disease becomes this severe, it is termed periodontitis.

In reptiles with excessive plaque buildup, a gram-positive aerobic cocci population predominates. As plaque matures, an anaerobic environment is created, and anaerobic

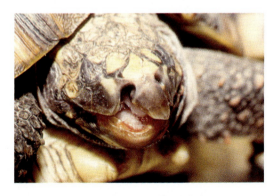

FIGURE 72-1 This Yellow-Headed Red-Foot Tortoise (*Geochelone carbonaria*) was born with a congenital defect. The animal had a cleft palate and apparent bilateral anophthalmia. (*Photograph courtesy D. Mader.*)

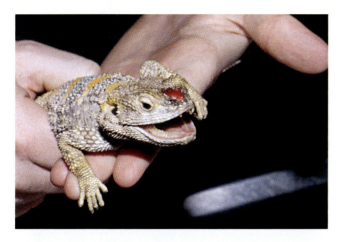

FIGURE 72-2 A Bearded Dragon *(Pogona vitticeps)* with rostral abrasions, gingival bruising, and callus formation of the rostrum, maxilla, and upper labia from chronic face rubbing on the walls of its enclosure. *(Photograph courtesy D. Mader.)*

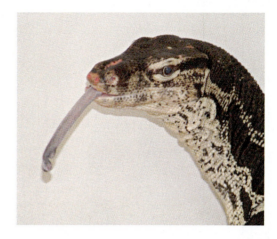

FIGURE 72-4 A Water Monitor *(Varanus salvator)* with loss of the distal tongue from trauma by live prey. This may greatly impede the lizard's ability to present molecules to the vomeronasal organ. *(Photograph courtesy S. Barten.)*

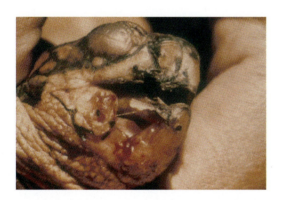

FIGURE 72-3 This Box Turtle *(Terrapene carolina)* had severe head trauma as a result of a dog bite. *(Photograph courtesy D. Mader.)*

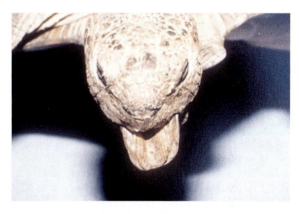

FIGURE 72-5 This California Desert Tortoise *(Gopherus agassizii)* had an overgrown lower beak. As a result, it was unable to prehend food or eat. *(Photograph courtesy D. Mader.)*

flora, including gram-negative bacteria and spirochetes, develops.[2] This change in bacterial populations occurs in both mammals and reptiles with periodontitis.

Clinical signs include gingival erythema, gingival swelling, accumulation of dental calculus, periodontal pockets, gingival recession or hyperplasia, and loosening and loss of teeth.[2] Periodontitis is often an insidious disease, and the first signs an owner observes may be a result of systemic illness. Gingivitis appears to cause some discomfort for reptiles, but many continue to eat. The early stages of the disease are usually only recognized during an oral examination. An important note is that periodontitis is commonly mistaken for stomatitis.[3]

In lizards with periodontal disease, visible calculus and marginal gingival erythema are seen on the lingual and buccal aspects of the oral cavity. As the disease progresses, more calculus builds, the gingiva becomes swollen, and the gingival margins begin to recede, exposing the underlying mandibular and maxillary bone.[2] In advanced disease, the gingiva becomes hyperplastic, and gingival pockets form.

Suppurative gingivitis and subcutaneous abscessation ensue. Areas of focal or multifocal osteomyelitis of the mandible or maxilla can develop.[2] Chameleons with oral osteomyelitis carry a grave prognosis. In the most severe cases of periodontal disease, pathologic fractures and fatal systemic infections occur.[2]

Inappropriate diet appears to be the major cause of periodontal disease in lizards. Radiographic changes associated with severe periodontal disease include bone lysis, pathologic fractures, the presence of sequestra, and adjacent areas of periosteal proliferation (Figure 72-6). Collections of samples of affected areas for culture and sensitivity and histopathology are helpful in choosing an appropriate treatment regimen.

Treatment of periodontal disease in lizards should begin with a thorough oral examination with general anesthesia. After the calculus is removed and the gingival sulci are cleaned, the mouth is irrigated with a 0.05% chlorhexadine solution.[2,4] To prevent further disease, dental prophylaxis is performed with anesthesia every 6 to 12 months. In most

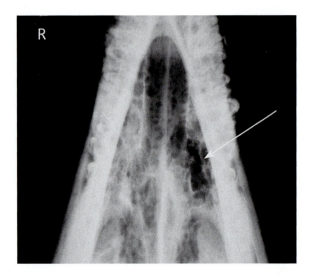

FIGURE 72-6 This crocodile was seen for anorexia. An oral examination revealed a cracked tooth. An abscess developed in the maxillary bone *(arrow)* as is evidenced by the lysis. *(Photograph courtesy D. Mader.)*

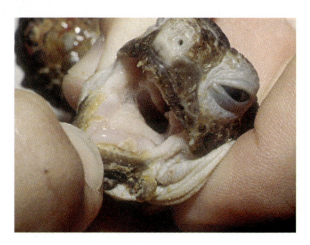

FIGURE 72-7 This Desert Tortoise *(Gopherus agassizii)* was seen for "mouth rot." It had several problems, most notably a severe oral infection that included chelitis, glossitis, and palatitis. The bacterial lesions were secondary to a herpesvirus infection. *(Photograph courtesy D. Mader.)*

cases, treatment with an appropriate systemic antibiotic is indicated. The diet must be changed to provide a varied supply of adequate textures and consistencies. Poor husbandry is addressed, and the owner is advised to make any changes necessary to help prevent further disease.

Stomatitis

Stomatitis (the hallmark of UATD) is common in reptiles and is characterized by infection of the oral mucosa and surrounding tissues. This condition may include gingivitis, glossitis, palatitis, and cheilitis.[5] Bacterial (including mycobacterial), fungal, and viral infections are known to cause stomatitis (Figure 72-7). In lay terms, this condition is commonly referred to as "mouth rot."

Common clinical signs of stomatitis include anorexia or dysphagia, ptyalism, tongue paralysis, gingivitis, ecchymosis and petechiation, and the loss of teeth. Exudates are the result of inflammation of the respiratory tract, the gastrointestinal tract, or the oral cavity. Tongue sheath abscesses are occasionally observed in chameleons, monitor lizards, and snakes (see Figure 39-9). Mucosal hemorrhages can be caused by trauma and coagulation disorders. Oral ulcers can be associated with stomatitis in most reptiles but are rare in crocodilians. Stomatitis can progress to involve the eyes, ascending the nasolacrimal duct, and respiratory tract, descending the trachea. In severe cases, it can cause septicemia and death.

The diagnostic work-up for patients with stomatitis consists of a thorough history and physical examination, appropriate cultures of affected tissues, complete blood count, and serum biochemistry analysis. Some reptiles with renal failure and secondary visceral gout have diffuse whitish plaques and nodules develop in the gingival mucosa (Figure 72-8). Imaging techniques and biopsy are performed if indicated.

Infectious stomatitis is the most common clinical form of UATD. Stomatitis may be categorized as hemorrhagic, necrotizing, proliferative, or a combination of these. Stomatitis often occurs secondary to other conditions, including

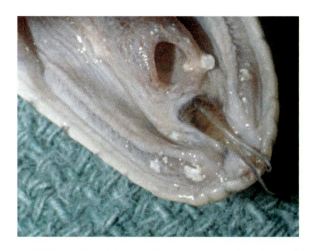

FIGURE 72-8 This colubrid had been treated for "mouth rot" with an aminoglycoside. However, supplemental fluids were not simultaneously administered, and the patient subsequently had visceral gout (white tophi) develop. *(Photograph courtesy D. Mader.)*

improper environmental husbandry, nutritional deficiencies (e.g., chronic malnutrition, vitamin/mineral imbalances), infestation with mites, oral trauma, and neoplasia. Uncomplicated stomatitis, left untreated, often progresses to other diseases such as pneumonia and chronic proliferative lesions that involve the underlying mandible or maxilla leading to osteomyelitis.

Bacterial Stomatitis

Gram-negative bacteria are predominant in the oral cavity of ill reptiles, whereas gram-positive bacteria are more prevalent in the oral cavity of healthy reptiles.[6,7] Gram-negative bacteria are reported to cause the highest morbidity and mortality rates in reptiles and commonly cause septicemia and abscesses.[8] *Pseudomonas* sp. are thought to cause both primary and secondary ulcerative stomatitis that can lead to osteomyelitis or aspiration of necrotic debris and cause pneumonia and septicemia. *Aeromonas* spp. are opportunistic bacteria commonly isolated from lizards with stomatitis. This genus can cause more severe clinical disease and septicemia, but infection generally occurs in immune-compromised individuals. *Salmonella* sp. and *Morganella* sp. have also been cultured from the oral cavity of both healthy and ill lizard species.[8]

Aeromonas hydrophilia, Escherichia coli, Pseudomonas sp. and *Salmonella* sp., *Providencia* sp., *Klebsiella* sp., and *Proteus* sp. are routinely cultured from the oral cavity of healthy snakes and from snakes with clinical stomatitis, and *Aeromonas hydrophilia, Escherichia coli, Pseudomonas* sp., and *Proteus* sp. are commonly cultured from the water source of snakes in captivity and in their natural environment.[8,9] A difficult interpretation is whether snakes contaminate their environment with these organisms and then become infected when they are immunocompromised or whether they become primarily infected and then seed their environment.

Anaerobic bacteria are a part of the normal flora of reptiles and can be found in the oral cavity, skin, conjunctiva, nasal cavity, gastrointestinal tract, and feces.[10] Species of *Bacteroides, Clostridium, Fusobacterium,* and *Peptostreptococcus* have been incriminated in diseases ranging from abscesses in the mouth and tissue necrosis to severe systemic disease. In one report, 54% of positive bacterial cultures from abscesses in reptiles contained anaerobes, with the most common isolate being *Bacteroides* sp.[10]

Mycobacterium sp. can cause chronic granulomatous or nongranulomatous lesions in the oral cavity of reptiles.[8,11] These may develop into hemorrhagic lesions and can progress to osteomyelitis. Some reptiles with mycobacterial stomatitis also have subcutaneous granulomas. *M. marinum, M. chelonei,* and *M. thamnopeos* are common mycobacterial isolates.[12] Treatment of mycobacteriosis involves a combination of enrofloxacin, rifampin, and clarithromycin (see appendix for doses). No reports have been found of successful treatment of mycobacteriosis in reptiles. Because of the apparent lack of treatment success, the chronic debilitating nature of the disease, and the zoonotic potential of the infection, euthanasia should be considered.

Treatment for bacterial stomatitis involves long-term use of appropriate antimicrobial medications and correction of any husbandry problems.[12] Prevention is best and is accomplished with appropriate husbandry combined with a low stress environment to maintain good oral health.[12] A definitive diagnosis and treatment plan are obtained from appropriate culture and sensitivity testing. If necessary, a stab incision culture protocol should be used.[12] Radiographs are made to determine bone involvement. Surgical debridement of infected oral tissue and bone is a necessary part of treatment. Abscesses that involve the structures of the head are vascular and bleed extensively during surgical debridement. **Abscesses that do not resolve with this treatment should be evaluated histologically for neoplasia, mycobacteriosis, or fungal disease.**

Antibiotic selection is best based on culture and sensitivity testing. Pending results, antibiotics such as fluoroquinolones and aminoglycosides are commonly selected because many isolates are gram-negative. Ceftazidime, carbenicillin, and chloramphenicol have also been used successfully in treatment of bacterial stomatitis in reptiles. Because of the high incidence rate of anaerobic infection, treatment should also include penicillin, cephalosporin, clindamycin, tetracycline, metronidazole, or chloramphenicol.[13]

Bacteroides spp. are frequently resistant to penicillins and tetracyclines. Because of its good activity against most gram-negative bacteria and many anaerobic bacteria, ceftazidime is often a good single antibiotic choice. Topical treatment consists of periodic debridement, irrigation with a dilute (0.05%) chlorhexidine solution, and application of a water-soluble antibiotic medication such as silver sulfadiazine cream (Figure 72-9). In mammals and humans, stomatitis is considered a painful disease process, and analgesia (see appendix for dosages) should be administered as needed (Figure 72-10).

Viral Stomatitis

Many reports are found of viral infections that cause primary and secondary pathology of the oral cavity in reptiles.[14-20] Treatment of viral diseases generally involves supportive care. The nutritional and hydration statuses of the patient

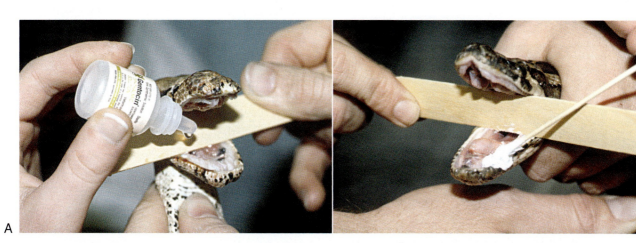

FIGURE 72-9 Mild cases of infectious stomatitis can be treated topically. In these photographs, topical aminoglycoside ophthalmic drops **(A)** and sulfadiazine cream **(B)** are applied directly to the lesions. *(Photograph courtesy D. Mader.)*

are monitored and maintained. Appropriate antibiotics or antifungals (topical and systemic) are administered for secondary infections of the oral cavity. The application of 5% acyclovir ointment and systemic acyclovir at a dose of 80 mg/kg/day orally has been described and appears to be effective in some patients with herpes viral stomatitis.[14,17] Acyclovir has efficacy only against herpesviruses.

Fungal Stomatitis

Although some investigators consider fungal infections in reptiles to be uncommon, others report that fungal diseases are common but underdiagnosed.[4,12,21,22] As in other animals, fungal infections are thought to be associated with immune compromise. *Candida albicans* is an opportunistic secondary invader that commonly infects the upper alimentary tract of reptiles, especially lizards.[12] Environmental factors including high humidity, low ambient temperature, malnutrition, overcrowding, and the buildup of contaminated debris in the animal's environment contribute to the development of fungal infections.[4,12]

Diagnosis of fungal stomatitis is with culture or histopathology. Bacterial culture and sensitivity testing are also performed because secondary bacterial infections are common. Radiographs of the affected area should be made to evaluate for secondary fungal osteomyelitis. Itraconazole has good tissue distribution, including a preferential deposition in exudates. Therapeutic protocols suggest a dose of 23.5 mg/kg orally every 24 hours for at least 4 to 6 weeks.[4,21,23-25] Treatment should include a broad-spectrum antibiotic to treat any secondary bacterial infection. Many fungal infections are systemic and potentially fatal.

Parasitic Stomatitis

Only a few parasites may be associated with the oral cavity, and even fewer may cause disease of the oral cavity (Figure 72-11).[26-28] The relationship that most parasites of reptiles have with the oral cavity appears to be transient as the parasites are delivered with food sources to the lower gastrointestinal tract or are inhaled into the respiratory tract, where the remainder of their life cycle is carried out (see Figure 21-38).

Neoplastic Diseases of the Oral Cavity

Proliferative disorders from a wide range of neoplasms are well recognized in reptiles, many of which occur as primary masses in the oral cavity.[29-32] Diagnostic evaluation for proliferative oral masses should include a biopsy of the lesion, radiographs, ultrasound examination, computed tomography (CT), and magnetic resonance imaging (MRI) as indicated. Therapies used in treatment of cancer in reptiles are similar to those used in mammals and include surgical excision, chemotherapy, cryosurgery and electrosurgery, photodynamic therapy, and radiation therapy. Chemotherapy has not been used much in reptiles because establishment of venous access is difficult. Doses for chemotherapeutic agents have been based solely on mammalian doses and should not necessarily be accepted as safe for reptiles (see Chapter 19).

Nutritional Diseases

Many of the conditions associated with the oral cavity are directly or indirectly related to inappropriate dietary husbandry. Of all the reptile groups, lizards show the greatest diversity of feeding strategies and can be classified as herbivores, insectivores, omnivores, and carnivores. Sound clinical judgments and dietary recommendations can be based on the anatomic structures found in the mouth, even if one is unfamiliar with a given species. Few, if any, truly monophagous lizards exist in the world.

The most common clinical sign of nutritional disease associated with the oral cavity in lizards is anorexia, which is commonly secondary to another disease state and may be systemically mediated in severe disease or may be from an inability to eat from damage to the oral cavity. Anorexia can be managed clinically with treatment of the primary problem and supplementation of food and fluids parenterally. Supplemental nutrition can be provided with assist-feeding, tube feeding, or placement of an esophagostomy tube (see Chapters 18 and 36). Carnivorous reptiles rarely have nutritional deficiencies develop because their diets consist of meat, organs, and bone. This combination provides balanced

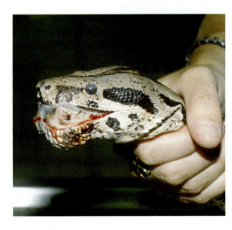

FIGURE 72-10 Boa constrictor (*Constrictor constrictor*) with severe and chronic infectious stomatitis. (*Photograph courtesy D. Mader.*)

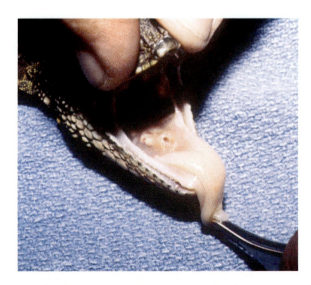

FIGURE 72-11 A tapeworm larva is encysted in the tongue muscle of this Water Dragon. (*Photograph courtesy D. Mader.*)

nutrition and allows for adequate intake of vitamin D_3, vitamin A, B vitamins, protein, and a proper calcium:phosphorus ratio.[33,34]

Nutritional Secondary Hyperparathyroidism

Nutritional secondary hyperparathyroidism (NSHP) is a common disorder seen in the herbivorous and sometimes omnivorous lizards.[33] Crocodilians, carnivorous chelonians, and carnivorous lizards fed a diet of strictly muscle or organ meat have deficiencies develop. This diet has a severely deranged calcium:phosphorus ratio. NSHP can affect the mandible and maxilla and the skeletal system, endocrine system, kidneys, gastrointestinal tract, and bone marrow. Misshapen facial bones often lead to malocclusions in the adult patient and result in chronic stomatitis from constant gingival and mucosal exposure (see Figure 61-13).

Hypovitaminosis C (Ascorbic Acid Deficiency)

Because snakes typically eat whole prey, they receive all of their required nutrients even in captivity. Few reports document the effects of hypovitaminosis C (ascorbic acid deficiency) in boas and pythons[35,36]; however, studies do suggest that Gartersnakes (*Thamnophis* spp.) are able to produce sufficient amounts of vitamin C in the kidneys, which thus is not required in the diet. Speculation exists that scorbutic animals may have spontaneous gingival bleeding and disruptions of the basement membrane of the dermis and epidermis develop.

This condition is suspected to occur because vitamin C is necessary for the hydroxylation of proline, which is involved in collagen production and function. The authors have observed a condition similar to that described for vitamin C deficiency only in severely malnourished boas in which an acute disruption of the epidermal and dermal layers of the skin developed. No gingival bleeding was observed. Vitamin C levels were not determined. Surgical repair of the skin lesion and administration of vitamin C at 10 to 20 mg/kg/day have been recommended.[36] The authors have added a broad-spectrum antibiotic to this regimen, but this condition appears to carry a grave prognosis.

Hypovitaminosis A

Hypovitaminosis A has been suggested to be more common in aquatic chelonians than in tortoises.[35] Other clinical signs commonly seen with hypovitaminosis A are lethargy, anorexia, and blepharedema from blocked nasolacrimal ducts. Treatment consists of vitamin A injectable supplementation at doses[36,37,38] and correction of the dietary husbandry problems. The diseased rhamphotheca should also be correctively trimmed because their overgrowth commonly leads to an inability to prehend food. Corrective trimming may take several months to show results, and the beak may never grow correctly (see Chapter 59).

CONCLUSION

Each species of reptile has evolved unique characteristics associated with the oral cavity, dentition, tongue, glands, and methods of mastication. These developments have provided each with an opportunity to interact with their surroundings. In captivity, the developmental relationship is often severed by the introduction of artificial surroundings and inappropriate husbandry. These changes predispose to many stresses and disorders. Disorders of the oral cavity are often a representation of what occurs systemically. Bacterial, viral, fungal, parasitic, neoplastic, and nutritional causes of disorders of the oral cavity in reptilian species are probably underestimated and likely cause a higher incidence rate of morbidity and mortality than has been reported. The misinformation that clients receive regarding husbandry may directly correlate with the frequency of oral diseases seen in a clinical setting. Prevention of disease of the oral cavity is primarily with appropriate environmental conditions and diet.

REFERENCES

1. Mader DR: Perinatology of pet reptiles. In Mader DR, editor: *Reptile medicine and surgery*, Philadelphia, 1996, WB Saunders.
2. McCracken HE: Periodontal disease in lizards. In Fowler ME, Miller RE, editors: *Zoo and wild animal medicine*, ed 4, Philadelphia, 1999, WB Saunders.
3. Mader DR: Specific diseases and conditions: upper alimentary tract disease. In Mader DR, editor: *Reptile medicine and surgery*, Philadelphia, 1996, WB Saunders.
4. Heatley JJ, Mitchell MA, Williams J, Smith JA, Tully TN: Fungal periodontal osteomyelitis in a Chameleon, *Furcifer pardalis*, *J Herp Med Surg* 11(4):7-12, 2001.
5. Mader DR: Specific diseases and conditions: upper alimentary tract disease. In Mader DR, editor: *Reptile medicine and surgery*, Philadelphia, 1996, WB Saunders.
6. Stewart JS: Anaerobic bacterial infections in reptiles, *J Zoo Wildl Med* 21(2):180-184, 1990.
7. McNamara TS, Gardiner C, Harris RK, Hadfield TL, Behler JL: Streptococcal bacteremia in two Singapore house geckos (*Gekko monarchus*), *J Zoo Wildl Med* 25(1):161-166, 1994.
8. Plowman CA, Montali RJ, Phillips LG, Schlater LK, Lowenstine LJ: Septicemia and chronic abscesses in iguanas (*Cyclura cornuta* and *Iguana iguana*) associated with a *Neisseria* species, *J Zoo Anim Med* 18(2-3):86-93, 1987.
9. Hilf M, Wagner RA, Yu VL: A prospective study of upper airway flora in healthy boid snakes and snakes with pneumonia, *J Zoo Wildl Med* 21(3):318-325, 1990.
10. Stewart JS: Anaerobic bacterial infections in reptiles, *J Zoo Wildl Med* 21(2):180-184, 1990.
11. Quesenberry KE, Jacobson ER, Allen JL, Cooley AJ: Ulcerative stomatitis and subcutaneous granulomas caused by *Mycobacterium chelonei* in a boa constrictor, *J Am Vet Med Assoc* 189(9):1131-1132, 1986.
12. Rosenthal KL, Mader DR: Special topics: microbiology. In Mader DR, editor: *Reptile medicine and surgery*, Philadelphia, 1996, WB Saunders.
13. Jacobson ER: Antimicrobial therapy in reptiles. *The Bayer proceedings, The North Atlantic Veterinary Conference*, Orlando, Fla, 33-46, 1999.
14. Schumacher J: Viral diseases. In Mader DR, editor: *Reptile medicine and surgery*, Philadelphia, 1996, WB Saunders.
15. Murray MJ: Specific diseases and conditions: pneumonia and normal respiratory function. In Mader DR, editor: *Reptile medicine and surgery*, Philadelphia, 1996, WB Saunders.
16. Schumacher J, Jacobson ER, Homer BL, Gaskin JM: Inclusion body disease in boid snakes, *J Zoo Wildl Med* 25(4):511-524, 1994.
17. Muro J, Ramis A, Pastor J, Velarde R, Tarres J, Lavin S: Chronic rhinitis associated with herpesviral infection in captive spur-thighed tortoises from Spain, *J Wildl Dis* 34(3): 487-495, 1998.

18. Une Y, Uemura K, Nakano Y, Kamiie J, Ishibashi T, Nomura Y: Herpesvirus infection in tortoises (*Malacochersus tornieri* and *Testudo horsfieldii*), *J Vet Path* 36:624-627, 1999.
19. Herbst LH, Greiner EC, Ehrhart LM, Bagley DA, Klein PA: Serological association between spirorchidiasis, herpesvirus infection, and fibropapillomatosis in green turtles from Florida, *J Wild Dis* 34(3):496-507, 1998.
20. Westhouse RA, Jacobson ER, Harris RK, Winter KR, Homer BL: Respiratory and pharyngo-esophageal iridovirus infection in a gopher tortoise (*Gopherus polyphemus*), *J Wild Dis* 32(4):682-686, 1996.
21. Pare JA, Sigler L, Hunter B, Summerbell C, Smith DA, Machin KL: Cutaneous mycoses in Chameleons caused by the *Chrysosporium* anamorph of *Nannizziopsis vriesii currah*, *J Zoo Wildl Med* 28(4):443-453, 1997.
22. Cheatwood JL, Jacobson ER, May PG, Farrell TM: An outbreak of fungal dermatitis and stomatitis in a wild population of pigmy rattlesnakes, *Sistrurus miliarius barbouri*, in Volusia County, Florida, *Proc Assoc Rept Amphib Vet* 19-20, 1999.
23. Carpenter JW, Mashima TY, Rupiper DJ: *Exotic animal formulary*, Philadelphia, 2001, WB Saunders.
24. Maxwell LK, Jacobson ER: Preliminary single-dose pharmacokinetics of enrofloxacin after oral and intramuscular administration in green iguanas (*Iguana iguana*), *Ann Proc Am Assoc Zoo Vet*, Houston, 25, 1997.
25. Gamble KC, Alvarado TP, Bennett CL: Itraconazole plasma and tissue concentrations in the spiny lizard (*Sceloporus* sp.) following once-daily dosing, *J Zoo Wildl Med* 28:89-93, 1997.
26. Page CD, Mautino M, Derendorf H, et al: Multiple dose pharmacokinetics of ketaconazole administered orally to gopher tortoises (*Gopherus polyphemus*), *J Zoo Wildl Med* 22:191-198, 1991.
27. Lane TJ, Mader DR: Special topics: parasitology. In Mader DR, editor: *Reptile medicine and surgery*, Philadelphia, 1996, WB Saunders.
28. Griffiths DA, Jones HI, Christian KA: Effect of season on oral and gastric nematodes in the frillneck lizard from Australia, *J Wild Dis* 34(2):381-385, 1998.
29. Bowman DD, Lynn RC: Arthropods. In Bowmann DD: *Georgi's parasitology for veterinarians*, ed 7, Philadelphia, 1999, WB Saunders.
30. Romagnano A, Jacobson ER, Boon GD, Broeder A, Ivan L, Homer BL: Lymphosarcoma in a green iguana (*Iguana iguana*), *J Zoo Wildl Med* 27(1):83-89, 1996.
31. Ramsay EC, Munson L, Lowenstine L, Fowler ME: A retrospective study of neoplasia in a collection of captive snakes, *J Zoo Wildl Med* 27(1):28-34, 1996.
32. Janert B: A fibrosarcoma in a Siamese crocodile (*Crocodylus siamensis*), *J Zoo Wildl Med* 29(1):72-77, 1998.
33. Abou-Madi N, Jacobson ER, Buergelt CD, Schumacher J, Williams BH: Disseminated undifferentiated sarcoma in an Indian rock python (*Python molurus molurus*), *J Zoo Wildl Med* 25(1):143-149, 1994.
34. Boyer TH: Metabolic bone disease. In Mader DR, editor: *Reptile medicine and surgery*, Philadelphia, 1996, WB Saunders.
35. Donoghue S, Langenberg J: Special topics: nutrition. In Mader DR, editor: *Reptile medicine and surgery*, Philadelphia, 1996, WB Saunders.
36. Frye F: *Biomedical and surgical aspects of captive reptile husbandry*, ed 2, vols I and II, Malabar, Fla, 1991, Krieger Publishing.
37. Rossi JV: Special topics: dermatology. In Mader DR, editor: *Reptile medicine and surgery*, Philadelphia, 1996, WB Saunders.
38. Jacobson ER: Reptile dermatology. In Kirk RW, Bonagura JD, editors: *Kirk's current veterinary therapy XI; small animal practice*, Philadelphia, 1992, WB Saunders.

73
UPPER RESPIRATORY TRACT DISEASE (MYCOPLASMOSIS) IN TORTOISES

LORI D. WENDLAND, DANIEL R. BROWN, PAUL A. KLEIN, and MARY B. BROWN

Upper respiratory tract disease (URTD) refers to a clinical syndrome that occurs in tortoises and is characterized alone or in concert by a nasal discharge, conjunctivitis, ocular discharge, and palpebral edema. Isolation of *Mycoplasma agassizii* from clinically ill tortoises and subsequent transmission studies confirmed this bacterium to be a cause of URTD.[1-3] *M. agassizii* and a second species, *M. testudineum*, are presently the only confirmed independent etiologic agents of URTD in wild North American tortoises.[1,2,4] Although other microorganisms, including *Pasteurella testudinis*, iridovirus, herpesvirus, and several fungal organisms, have been isolated from tortoises with overlapping clinical signs,[5-10] experimental transmission studies resulting in URTD have been performed only for *M. agassizii* in Desert Tortoises (*Gopherus agassizii*) and Gopher Tortoises (*Gopherus polyphemus*),[1,2] *M. testudineum* in Gopher Tortoises,[4] and a herpesvirus in Greek Tortoises (*Testudo graeca*).[11] Infection with *P. testudinis* alone failed to cause clinical disease in Desert Tortoises.[2] URTD is complicated by the fact that mycoplasmal strains and species can vary in terms of virulence and clinical disease expression.[4] Furthermore, environmental stressors and concurrent infections with other bacterial and viral organisms may also be involved in the pathogenesis of this disease, as has been observed in mycoplasmal diseases that affect other host species.[12-15]

Extensive research has been conducted to determine the causative agents of URTD, to investigate the pathogenesis of disease, to develop diagnostic tools, and to determine the distribution of mycoplasmosis in wild tortoises. The organism was originally isolated from free-ranging Desert Tortoises at the Desert Tortoise Natural Area in California and may have been a contributing factor in major tortoise population declines there during the late 1980s and early 1990s.[3,16] Subsequent population surveys in Gopher Tortoises have shown that animals exposed to and infected with *M. agassizii* occur almost throughout that geographic range of that species.[17,18]

Mycoplasmosis has also been widely documented in captive chelonians with culture and polymerase chain reaction (PCR) assays (Table 73-1). Specific antibody to *M. agassizii* has been detected in at least 24 distinct turtle and tortoise species (L. Wendland, unpublished data); however, the serologic assay has only been validated for Desert and Gopher Tortoises, and serologic results from other species must be interpreted cautiously. Despite the fact that this disease is probably one of the most extensively researched infectious diseases of chelonians, few studies have been done to establish appropriate treatment protocols and no published accounts exist that evaluate the long-term effectiveness of such regimen.

TRANSMISSION

Experimental studies suggest that the primary route of transmission for mycoplasmas in both wild and captive tortoises is through direct contact, particularly when an animal has a nasal discharge.[1,2,4] Vertical, or transovarial, transmission was not documented in early experimental infection studies involving a limited number of animals.[4] This route of transmission has been documented to occur at a very low rate in mycoplasmal infections of poultry, however.[23,24] If vertical transmission does occur in tortoises, it is likely to be influenced by the time of infection in the female tortoise, the stage of oogenesis when the animal is clinically ill, and the virulence of the organism. Additional studies with a large

Table 73-1 Tortoise Species with Confirmed Mycoplasmal Infections

Common Name	Species	Reference
Desert Tortoise	*Gopherus agassizii*	2, 3
Texas Tortoise	*Gopherus berlanderi*	19
Gopher Tortoise	*Gopherus polyphemus*	1, 4
Chaco Tortoise	*Geochelone chilensis*	20
Leopard Tortoise	*Geochelone pardalis*	3, 19-22
Indian Star Tortoise	*Geochelone elegans*	3, 20, 21
Radiated Tortoise	*Geochelone radiata*	3, 20
African Spurred Tortoise	*Geochelone sulcata*	20, 21
Travancore Tortoise	*Indotestudo travancorica*	20
Spider Tortoise	*Pyxis arachnoides*	20, 21
Flat-tailed Tortoise	*Pyxis planicauda*	20
Spur-thighed Tortoise	*Testudo graeca*	3, 20, 21
Marginated Tortoise	*Testudo marginata*	21
Egyptian Tortoise	*Testudo kleinmanni*	21
Eastern Box Turtle	*Terrapene carolina*	20
Red-footed Tortoise	*Geochelone carbonaria*	3, 21
Forsten's Tortoise	*Indotestudo forstenii*	21
Afghan Tortoise	*Testudo horsfieldi*	22
Hermann's Tortoise	*Testudo hermanni*	1, 20

number of tortoises infected at different times during the reproductive cycle are required to completely rule out vertical transmission in tortoises. Environmental transmission is unlikely in wild populations because mycoplasmas lack a cell wall and are highly susceptible to desiccation in natural environments. In captive conditions, however, increased tortoise densities and higher loads of organic material could facilitate the persistence of the organism outside the host. Fomite transmission has been documented for other mycoplasmal infections, especially in food and fiber animals.[23] Fomite transmission, particularly if equipment is contaminated with nasal exudates, should be considered possible in tortoises as well. Routine disinfection of all equipment between tortoises with a 3% to 5% bleach solution or other appropriate commercial disinfectant minimizes the chance of cross-contamination.

CLINICAL DISEASE

Mycoplasmosis is characterized by rhinitis and conjunctivitis. Clinical signs, including nasal discharge, ocular discharge, palpebral and periocular edema, and conjunctival hyperemia and edema, may develop as early as 2 weeks after infection (Figure 73-1).[1,2,4] An important note is that clinical signs may appear alone or in concert with other signs. Experimental infection studies in Gopher and Desert Tortoises suggest the following course of disease: (1) primary colonization of the upper respiratory tract with *Mycoplasma*; (2) host immune response to infection resulting in a reduction of *Mycoplasma* numbers and the development of clinical disease; and (3) progression to a chronic disease state where clinical signs and shedding of *Mycoplasma* occur intermittently. In chronically infected tortoises, clinical signs typically intensify and then abate cyclically.[2] Grooves that extend ventrally from the nares, eroded nares, and depigmentation around the nares can be observed in tortoises that have repeatedly exhibited clinical signs (Figure 73-2). Subclinical infections have also been documented, where the animal has a detectable serologic response, histopathologic lesions are present, and mycoplasmas can sometimes be recovered on culture, but the tortoise does not exhibit overt disease.[25-27] Such tortoises could serve as a source of infection for naive animals within the population or collection.

Clearance of infection may occur in a minority of tortoises, and anecdotal reports exist that claim possible clearance of the organism after treatment.[20] Clearance is difficult to document, primarily because of the nature of mycoplasmal infections in general but also because of limitations of the diagnostic assays and sampling techniques. Chronically infected animals may remain asymptomatic for years before clinical signs recur. Further, antibody titers may decrease and cultures may be negative because *Mycoplasma* numbers may be below the detectable limits of the assay or in such low numbers that they are difficult to recover with nasal flushing techniques. Which factors trigger the recrudescence of clinical signs in asymptomatic tortoises is not certain; however, environmental stressors have been shown to play a major role in mycoplasmal infections of other hosts.[28] Anthropogenic factors, such as habitat degradation, habitat destruction, and tortoise relocation, and climatic factors, including drought or excessive rainfall, have all been suggested as potential

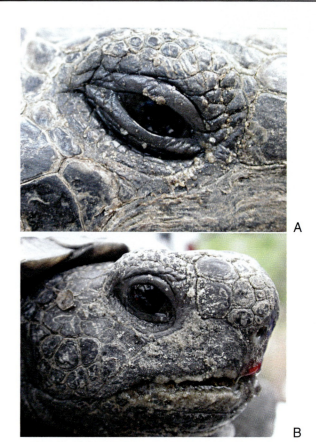

FIGURE 73-1 A, Gopher Tortoise (*Gopherus polyphemus*) with conjunctivitis, ocular discharge, and severe palpebral edema from mycoplasmosis. **B,** Epistaxis, nasal and ocular discharge, and conjunctival hyperemia are seen in this Gopher Tortoise. These signs may develop as early as 2 weeks after infection.

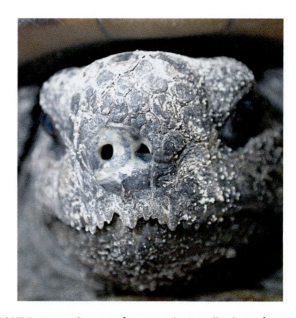

FIGURE 73-2 Grooves that extend ventrally from the nares, eroded nares, and depigmentation around the nares can be observed in tortoises that have repeatedly exhibited clinical signs. *Mycoplasma agassizii* was cultured from this individual.

influences that may result in increased morbidity and mortality rates in wild tortoises.[3,26] Increased tortoise densities, inappropriate temperature, and poor nutrition may all exacerbate mycoplasmosis in captive tortoises.

Aberrant behavior and decreased appetite have been observed in tortoises with mycoplasmosis. Decreased activity, irregular basking and burrowing behaviors, and reduced foraging have been documented in experimentally infected Gopher and Desert Tortoises and in a limited number of wild Gopher Tortoises (J. Berish, personal communication).[2,4] The impact of such behavioral changes on disease transmission and tortoise health and survival remains to be determined.

A specific antimycoplasmal antibody response develops and can be detected by 6 to 8 weeks after infection.[27] The immune response generated may not be protective, however, and may in fact exacerbate the disease. In experimental studies, infected Gopher Tortoises that were challenged a second time with *M. agassizii* had more severe clinical signs develop, and had a more intense antibody response, than from the initial infection.[4] This is consistent with the immunopathology associated with most mycoplasmal infections, where the host immune response is a key contributor to disease severity.[28] Although this evidence is limited to Gopher Tortoises, a similar response is likely in other tortoise species infected with mycoplasmas. Studies that evaluate the role of the immune response in the pathogenesis of this disease are difficult because little is known about reptilian immunology and the reagents needed for such investigations have not yet been developed.

PATHOLOGY

Mycoplasma agassizii adheres to the ciliated mucosal epithelium of the tortoise upper respiratory tract and causes severe disruption of the normal tissue architecture and function.[1-3,6,26] Gross examination of infected animals may reveal no apparent clinical signs or a serous to mucopurulent nasal and ocular discharge, edematous and erythemic conjunctiva, and periocular and palpebral edema. Severely affected tortoises may have one or both nasal cavities completely obstructed with a thick caseous discharge and varying degrees of nasal cavity erosion. Such animals may also have reduced coelomic fat or cachexia, thymus atrophy, hepatic hemosiderosis, and lymphocytic inflammation in the splenic sinusoids.[3,26] Histopathologic lesions in the nasal cavity can also vary dramatically in severity and may include multifocal to focally extensive subepithelial lymphoid aggregates; a mixed inflammatory cell infiltrate consisting of heterophils, lymphocytes, plasma cells, and macrophages; basal cell hyperplasia; mucous and olfactory epithelial metaplasia; and erosion of the ciliated epithelium.[3,6,26] In a study of 24 Gopher Tortoises, animals with URTD were more likely to have gram-negative bacteria isolated from their nasal cavity than tortoises without URTD, which strongly suggests that mycoplasmosis increases susceptibility to secondary infections.[26] This is consistent with other well-established mycoplasmal infections in mammalian and avian hosts.[28] Moribund tortoises with mycoplasmosis are often cachectic and have multisystemic disease, and death may be associated with secondary infectious, metabolic, or nutritional factors.[3,6,26]

DIAGNOSIS

The following three diagnostic tests exist for the identification of tortoises infected with or exposed to *Mycoplasma*: (1) direct mycoplasmal culture; (2) detection of mycoplasmal chromosomal DNA with PCR; and (3) detection of antimycoplasma antibodies in tortoise plasma with enzyme-linked immunosorbent assay (ELISA). These assays have been widely used for epidemiologic surveys and for captive tortoise management; however, certain features of mycoplasmal infections in tortoises and other species create a diagnostic dilemma. Representative diagnostic specimens are often difficult to obtain and mycoplasmas are notoriously difficult to culture. Further, the available serologic assay detects exposure to *M. agassizii* but has limited, if any, cross reactions with other mycoplasmas, some of which may be pathogenic. Therefore, diagnostic results must be interpreted cautiously and in the context of the clinical picture for each patient.

Mycoplasma Serology

Specific antibodies to *M. agassizii* in tortoise plasma are detected with an ELISA.[27] A positive ELISA result has been positively correlated with the presence of histologic lesions and the presence of clinical signs, especially a nasal discharge.[25,27,29] The ELISA was originally developed and validated for Gopher and Desert Tortoises, but evidence exists that the monoclonal antibodies used in the assay do recognize immunoglobulins from numerous other tortoise species (L. Wendland, unpublished data). Six to 8 weeks after infection is required for antibodies to reach a level that can be accurately detected with the assay.[27] As with other serologic assays, the ELISA can be performed on plasma or serum, and results are now reported as a titer. A single positive result indicates that the animal has been exposed to *M. agassizii*, but it does not confirm that the animal was infected at the time of sampling.

Passive transfer of maternal antibodies to hatchlings has been documented in the Desert Tortoise[30] and is likely to occur in other tortoise species. Passively acquired antibodies may persist for up to 1 year; therefore, paired titers should be performed, 6 to 8 weeks apart, to differentiate passive antibodies from acquired antibodies associated with active infection. Antibody levels are expected to increase if an active infection is present.

The current ELISA uses *M. agassizii* whole-cell lysate antigens in the analysis. The specificity of the assay is based on the affinity and avidity of antibodies produced by the tortoise in response to infection by *M. agassizii*. Other *Mycoplasma* species have been documented to share immunogenic antigens, however.[31] Experimental studies with *M. testudineum* in Gopher Tortoises revealed that this species not only caused URTD but also induced an antibody response that cross-reacted with the current ELISA and produced similar Western immunoblot results.[29,32] This *Mycoplasma* species has since been found in two wild Gopher Tortoise populations, and unlike earlier studies, serologic cross reactivity in these two populations has been limited.[17,33] The current ELISA was specifically designed to detect exposure only to *M. agassizii*, with minimal cross-reactions. Thus, the assay may miss infections by other mycoplasmal species, which demonstrates the importance of interpreting diagnostic results in the context of the individual patient. If a tortoise with clinical signs consistent with mycoplasmosis has a negative ELISA result, infection with an undescribed mycoplasmal species that does not cross-react with the current ELISA must be considered. Viral etiologies, such as herpesvirus and iridovirus, and fungal organisms are other potential differential diagnoses. The *Mycoplasma* culture and PCR tests discussed subsequently may help to clarify the clinical picture in such an animal. Additionally, an ELISA to detect exposure to *M. testudineum* is presently under development.

Mycoplasma Culture

Tortoise mycoplasmas are extremely fastidious and require specific media and growth conditions. Therefore, use of a laboratory with experience culturing this organism and established quality control procedures is essential for successful isolation. Tortoise mycoplasmas grow slowly, requiring up to 6 weeks for primary isolation in many cases.[34] SP4 medium is used for culture and can be obtained from the laboratories that provide this service or large-scale manufacturers (Remel Laboratories, Lenexa, Kan).

Numerous sampling techniques can be used to collect specimens for culture, including swabs or aspirates of a nasal discharge and flushes of the nasal cavity. Unless the animal has a significant nasal discharge, swabbing of the nasal cavity probably will be uninformative. Mycoplasmas preferentially colonize the ventrolateral depression of the tortoise nasal cavity, and this area is inaccessible in a live animal.[26] Nasal flushes can be performed with 0.5 to 5 mL of sterile saline solution or sterile phosphate-buffered saline solution (PBS) or with 0.5 to 1 mL of sterile SP4 broth. If saline solution or PBS is used for the nasal flush, enrichment of the flush sample with 10% sterile bovine serum albumin, horse or fetal calf serum, SP4 medium, or glycerol before shipping is recommended.

Mycoplasma Polymerase Chain Reaction

Polymerase chain reaction can be used to detect DNA specific to *Mycoplasma* in a nasal flush or culture sample.[32] The current assay is genus specific and therefore detects the presence of any *Mycoplasma* in the sample. *Mycoplasma* isolates are differentiated and identified on the basis of a 16S ribosomal RNA (rRNA) gene restriction fragment length polymorphism (RFLP) analysis. Five distinct patterns have been detected thus far in tortoise *Mycoplasma* isolates. Three of the variants have been established as different species.

M. testudinis was originally isolated from the cloaca of a Mediterranean Tortoise *(T. graeca)* and has not been shown to cause URTD.[35] One published report exists of *M. testudinis* recovered on a conjunctival swab from an Afghan Tortoise with rhinitis.[22] This animal was part of a breeding group of 24 tortoises, many of which were infected with *M. agassizii*, and it is possible that the tortoise may have had a dual infection. *Mycoplasma agassizii*[20,32] and *M. testudineum*[36] are recognized as distinct species, both of which have been documented to cause URTD experimentally.[1,2] The pathogenic capabilities, serologic cross reactivity with the current ELISA, and species status of the other isolates have not yet been determined.

The PCR analysis has high specificity, but the sensitivity of the assay is lower than that of the ELISA test,[37] likely because of the fastidious nature of mycoplasmas and the difficulty in obtaining representative nasal flush samples. Although contamination of samples by other organisms does not generally interfere with the PCR test, swabs containing calcium alginate may inhibit the reaction and thus should not be used.

TREATMENT

Few studies have been done to establish appropriate treatment protocols for tortoises with mycoplasmosis, and no published accounts exist that evaluate the long-term effectiveness of such regimen. Treatment recommendations are largely empirically derived or based on information extrapolated from what is known about mycoplasmal infections in other species. Further, all of the listed treatment protocols are considered extralabel use because none of these chemotherapeutic agents have been specifically labeled for chelonians.

Anecdotal reports of *Mycoplasma* clearance after treatment with various protocols exist; however, differentiation between clearance and subclinical infections can be exceedingly difficult. In other hosts, the adage "once infected always infected" is often used, particularly when making management decisions. Although treatment of free-ranging tortoises is usually impractical, captive tortoises should be isolated and treated with appropriate supportive care and antimicrobials to alleviate clinical signs and decrease the risk of disease transmission.

Mycoplasmas lack a cell wall; therefore, antibiotics that target cell wall development are ineffective. Antibacterial classes typically used to treat mycoplasmal infections in numerous hosts include tetracyclines, fluoroquinolones, lincosamides, macrolides, and certain aminoglycosides.[38-40] Detailed pharmacokinetic studies have only been performed for enrofloxacin in Gopher, Indian Star, and Hermann's Tortoises[41-43] and for clarithromycin in Desert Tortoises.[44] Further, minimum inhibitory concentrations are available for mycoplasmas that originate from other species with these antibiotics.[38,45] Consequently, enrofloxacin and clarithromycin are presently the mainstay in therapy for this disease. Given the immunopathology associated with URTD, topical antibiotic-corticosteroid combinations are often used in conjunction with oral or parenteral antibiotics to minimize the local inflammatory response.[20,46-48] Provision of necessary supportive care in terms of hydration and nutritional support and maintenance of the tortoise in the upper ranges of the preferred optimal temperature zone (POTZ) for that species improve the animal's response to treatment.

Table 73-2 lists the various treatment regimens that have been reported for mycoplasmosis in tortoises. With minor clinical disease, oral medications are generally used initially and topical therapies are added as necessary. Animals with severe disease may have reduced enteric absorption of drugs and should be administered parenteral medications. Topical ophthalmic drops or ointments that contain antibiotics such as tetracycline, oxytetracycline, gentamicin, or ciprofloxacin applied to the eyes may minimize ocular signs and provide more rapid relief for the tortoise. Therapeutic nasal

Table 73-2 Drugs Commonly Used to Treat Mycoplasmosis in Tortoises

Drug Class	Dosage	Notes
Aminoglycosides		
Gentamicin	10-20 mg/15 mL saline solution: nebulize for 30 min q12h[49]	
	40 mg/1 mL DMSO/8 mL saline solution: use for nebulization[47]	
Gentamicin/betamethasone ophthalmic drops	1-2 drops to eyes, q12-24h[46]	
	Reverse nasal flush q48-72h[46]	Drops applied to choanae and flushed-out nares as described in text
	Drops applied to external nares q12-24h[46]	
Fluoroquinolones		
Enrofloxacin	5 mg/kg IM q24-48h[41,42,50]	Most species, Gopher Tortoises, and Star Tortoises
	10 mg/kg IM q24h[43]	Hermann's Tortoises
	50 mg per 250 mL sterile water: use 1-3 mL for nasal flush per nostril q24-48h[48]	Use with oral or parenteral antibiotics until no nasal discharge
Macrolides		
Clarithromycin	15 mg/kg PO q48-72h[44,46]	Desert Tortoises
Tylosin	5 mg/kg IM q24h for 10-60 d[51]	
Tetracyclines		
Oxytetracycline	5-10 mg/kg IM q24h[46,51]	Tortoises
Doxycycline	10 mg/kg PO q24h[47]	Tortoises
	50 mg/kg IM, then 25 mg/kg q72h[43]	Hermann's Tortoises

DMSO, Dimethyl sulfoxide; *IM*, intramuscularly; *PO*, orally; *q*, every.

flushes with gentamicin/betamethasone, gentamicin/dimethyl sulfoxide (DMSO)/saline solution, and enrofloxacin/saline solution combinations or nebulization with an enrofloxacin/saline solution have all been described.[20,46-48]

A retrograde flush technique has been reported that involves placing the tortoise on its carapace, stabilizing the head, opening the beak with continuous pressure to the chin, and flooding the choanae with the gentamicin/betamethasone solution.[20,46] The tongue is then used to expel the fluid with digital pressure to the intermandibular area, forcing the tongue against the choanae. Chemical restraint may or may not be needed to perform this technique. Alternatively, the solution can be applied directly into the external nares. Some clinicians anecdotally report that the corticosteroid-antibiotic nasal flushes performed every 48 to 72 hours seem to result in a significantly lower recurrence rate of clinical disease.[20]

PROGNOSIS

Three potential outcomes exist for a tortoise with mycoplasmosis. Acute mortality has been reported but is exceedingly rare and was more commonly observed in hatchlings during the initial transmission studies.[4] Some tortoises may actually clear the infection, although this is not believed to occur very often.[2] Mycoplasmal infections that involve other hosts usually are not cleared; however, numbers of mycoplasmas may be significantly reduced during chronic phases of infection when clinical signs are not exhibited.[28] Most tortoises likely have chronic disease develop, with intermittent expression of clinical signs. The bacteria persist in the nasal cavity and damage the mucosal tissue of the upper respiratory tract, resulting in increased susceptibility to secondary infections.[6,26] In tortoises with chronic mycoplasmosis, mortality is presumed to be the result of severe debilitation and multisystemic disease.[3,6,26] Although not definitive, current data strongly suggest that the long-term effects of this disease may play a role in tortoise die-offs in selected populations, may shorten the longevity of individual tortoises, and may lower the reproductive potential of female tortoises, particularly if animals are sick during the reproductive season.[16,52,53] This could result in profound impacts to the long-term survival of rare species.

The species or strain of mycoplasma present in an individual or population is an important consideration when attempting to assess prognosis and develop appropriate management strategies. Mycoplasmas in other hosts are known to vary in virulence, and preliminary evidence suggests that this occurs in tortoises as well.[1,54,55] Early transmission studies showed that different strains of *M. agassizii* differed in terms of the number of organisms necessary to colonize and cause disease.[1] Unfortunately, knowledge of the virulence potential is available for only a limited number of isolates. Therefore, development of strategies to minimize risk from mycoplasmas in general is probably the safest approach. Actions taken depend on the ultimate disposition of the animals and the risk to cohorts.

Management Issues for Individuals, Colonies, and Wild Tortoises

Once a tortoise has been diagnosed with mycoplasmosis, it is safest to consider that animal as persistently infected and a potential source of infection for other tortoises in the collection or population. In the case of individual captive tortoises, animals with confirmed mycoplasmosis should be housed independently from other turtle and tortoise species and efforts should be made to minimize the chance of cross contamination with appropriate disinfection and sanitation protocols. Intermittent clinical disease can be treated periodically as discussed previously. Although the impact of this disease on overall longevity is unknown, many infected tortoises have continued to live and thrive for more than a decade since the original exposure. However, the full impact of chronic disease in a long-lived species may take decades to become apparent.

If a captive group of tortoises is infected, the animals can be maintained together in a single enclosure. Efforts should be made to separate eggs and hatchlings because the hatchlings may be more likely to have acute fulminant disease develop. Further, keeping hatchlings separate may result in a noninfected group of animals. Management of a large group of infected tortoises is significantly more challenging as the presence of clinically ill tortoises within the same enclosure may exacerbate disease in the nonclinical animals because tortoises with a nasal discharge are more likely to transmit the organism. Empiric experience in the management of URTD outbreaks in group-housed tortoises, and standard infection control practices for other infectious diseases, suggests that the most effective management strategy is to separate the clinically ill tortoises for treatment. Isolation of ill tortoises for more intensive monitoring and treatment may help to contain the flare-ups. Ensuring adequate husbandry practices to minimize stress within the colony may also help to decrease the frequency of clinical disease expression.

Determination of the disposition of seropositive or culture/ PCR-positive wild tortoises, particularly those that end up in rehabilitation centers, is problematic. Presently, inadequate scientific data exist to provide definitive guidelines for such tortoises. In some cases, state and federal guidelines exist that specify protocols for rehabilitation and repatriation of these animals. Often tortoises in rehabilitation facilities are exposed to other chelonians either directly with combined housing or indirectly with common grazing areas. Such practices could potentially expose tortoises to a myriad of pathogens and parasites that these animals do not normally encounter in the wild. Although mycoplasmas usually do not survive long outside the host unless protected in organic material, numerous other pathogens, viruses in particular, persist for extended periods in the environment. Rehabilitated animals that are exposed to such circumstances pose a serious threat to wild populations of tortoises when they are released.

Potential options that have been considered for the repatriation of tortoises with mycoplasmosis include the release of tortoises back to the exact site of origin, relocation to recipient populations with a high prevalence rate of infection and with resident tortoises that already express clinical signs of URTD, admission into captive breeding programs, adoption as pets, or euthanasia.[37] Each of these options has inherent problems, and no single solution is applicable for every situation. The unique circumstances of each population should be considered. The ultimate disposition of the animal depends on the rarity of the species, the value of that animal to the population, the potential risk that the animal poses to the population, and any existing regulations pertaining to that species. Certainly, decision making for such tortoises should be flexible and change as new scientific information becomes available.

Ongoing Research in Wild Tortoises

Mycoplasmal URTD is one of the most extensively characterized infectious diseases in free-ranging reptiles. Although a great deal of progress has been made to establish the etiology and distribution of the disease, and to develop diagnostic assays, information is currently lacking with regards to the long-term effects of this disease within tortoise populations. Nearly catastrophic declines in Desert Tortoise populations located in and around Kern County, California, that occurred in the late 1980s may have been associated with mycoplasmosis.[3,16] These declines led to the federal listing of Desert Tortoises north and west of the Colorado River as threatened.[56] Similar declines were observed in a Gopher Tortoise population with clinical disease consistent with mycoplasmosis on Sanibel Island, Florida.[53]

Significant Gopher Tortoise mortality events, in many cases involving hundreds of tortoises, continue to be reported (B. Blihovde, personal communication; M. Barnwell, personal communication).[57,58] The extent to which mycoplasmosis is a contributing factor in these die-offs is presently unknown; however, many of these populations are the focus of extensive investigations to determine the cause of increased tortoise mortality. Additional research that evaluates mycoplasmal disease dynamics, mycoplasmal influences on population demographics and individual tortoise survival, and anthropogenic influences on disease are presently ongoing in the southeastern and southwestern United States. Such long-term studies are critical for the development of sound, scientifically based management recommendations for free-ranging tortoises.

REFERENCES

1. Brown MB, McLaughlin GS, Klein PA, Crenshaw BC, Schumacher IM, Brown DR, et al: Upper respiratory tract disease in the Gopher tortoise is caused by *Mycoplasma agassizii*, *J Clin Microbiol* 37(7):2262-2269, 1999.
2. Brown MB, Schumacher IM, Klein PA, Harris K, Correll T, Jacobson ER: *Mycoplasma agassizii* causes upper respiratory tract disease in the desert tortoise, *Infect Immun* 62(10): 4580-4586, 1994.
3. Jacobson ER, Gaskin JM, Brown MB, Harris RK, Gardiner CH, Lapointe JL, et al: Chronic upper respiratory-tract disease of free-ranging Desert Tortoises (*Xerobates agassizii*), *J Wildl Dis* 27(2):296-316, 1991.
4. McLaughlin GS: *Upper respiratory tract disease in Gopher Tortoises, Gopherus polyphemus: pathology, immune responses, transmission, and implications for conservation and management,* Gainesville, 1997, University of Florida.
5. Harper PAW, Hammond DC, Heuschele WP: A herpesvirus-like agent associated with a pharyngeal abscess in a desert tortoise, *J Wildl Dis* 18:491-494, 1982.
6. Homer BL, Berry KH, Brown MB, Ellis G, Jacobson ER: Pathology of diseases in wild Desert Tortoises from California, *J Wildl Dis* 34(3):508-523, 1998.
7. Muller M, Sachsse W, Zangger N: Herpesvirus-Epidemie beider griechischen (*Testudo hermanni*) und der maurischen Landschildkrote (*Testudo graeca*) in der Schweiz, *Schweiz Arch Tierhelk* 132:199-203, 1990.
8. Pettan-Brewer KCB, Drew ML, Ramsay E, Mohr FC, Lowenstine LJ: Herpesvirus particles associated with oral and

respiratory lesions in a California desert tortoise *(Gopherus agassizii), J Wildl Dis* 32:521-526, 1996.
9. Snipes KP, Biberstein BL, Fowler ME: A *Pasteurella* sp, associated with respiratory disease in captive Desert Tortoises, *JAVMA* 177:804-807, 1980.
10. Westhouse RA, Jacobson ER, Harris RK, Winter KR, Homer BL: Respiratory and pharyngo-esophageal iridovirus infection in a Gopher tortoise *(Gopherus polyphemus), J Wildl Dis* 32(4):682-686, 1996.
11. Origgi FC, Romero CH, Bloom DC, Klein PA, Gaskin JM, Tucker SJ, et al: Experimental transmission of a herpesvirus in Greek tortoises *(Testudo graeca), Vet Pathol* 41:, 2004.
12. Cassel GH, Clyde WA, Davis JK: Respiratory mycoplasmosis. In Razin S, Barile MF, editors: *The mycoplasmas*, vol IV, New York, 1985, Academic Press.
13. Gourlay RN, Houghton SB: Experimental pneumonia in conventionally reared and gnotobiotic calves by dual infection with *Mycoplasma bovis* and *Pasteurella haemolytica, Res Vet Sci* 38:377-382, 1985.
14. Schoeb TR, Kervin KC, Lindsey JR: Exacerbation of murine respiratory mycoplasmosis in gnotobiotic F344/N rats by Sendai virus infection, *Vet Pathol* 22:272-282, 1985.
15. Weinack OM, Snoeyenbos GH, Smyser CF, Soerjadi-Liem AS: Influence of *Mycoplasma gallisepticum*, infectious bronchitis, and cyclophosphamide on chickens protected by native intestinal microflora against *Salmonella typhimurium* or *Escherichia coli, Avian Dis* 28(2):416-425, 1984.
16. Berry KH: *Demographic consequences of disease in two desert tortoise populations in California, USA*, 1996, Conservation, Restoration, and Management of Tortoises and Turtles: An International Conference, Purchase, NY.
17. Diemer-Berish JE, Wendland LD, Gates CA: Distribution and prevalence of upper respiratory tract disease in Gopher Tortoises in Florida, *J Herpetol* 34(1):5-12, 2000.
18. Smith RB, Seigel RA, Smith KR: Occurrence of upper respiratory tract disease in Gopher Tortoise populations in Florida and Mississippi, *J Herpetol* 32(3):426-430, 1998.
19. Willette M, Wendland LD, Cassens A, Brown MB: *Mycoplasma survey of Texas tortoises* (Gopherus berlanderi) *of the Rio Grande Valley: preliminary results*, Reno, Nev, 2002, Association of Reptilian and Amphibian Veterinarians.
20. Berry KH, Brown DR, Brown MB, Jacobson ER, Jarchow J, Johnson J, et al: Reptilian mycoplasmal infections, *J Herp Med Surg* 12:8-20, 2002.
21. Blahak S, Brown DR, Schumacher IM: *Mycoplasma agassizii in tortoises in Europe*, Berlin, 2004, The 7th International Symposium on Pathology and Medicine of Amphibians and Reptiles.
22. McArthur SDJ, Windsor HM, Bradbury JM, Yavari CA: *Isolation of* Mycoplasma agassizii *from UK captive chelonians* (Testudo horsefieldii *and* Geochelone pardalis) *with upper respiratory tract disease*, Vienna, Austria, 2002, 12th International Congress of the International Organization for Mycoplasmology.
23. Lin MY, Kleven SH: Egg transmission of two strains of *Mycoplasma gallisepticum* in chickens, *Avian Dis* 26:487-495, 1982.
24. Yoder HW: Avian mycoplasmosis. In Hofstad BWCMS, Helmboly CF, Reid WM, Yoder HW, editors: *Diseases of poultry*, Ames, 1984, Iowa State University Press.
25. Jacobson ER, Brown MB, Schumacher IM, Collins BR, Harris RK, Klein PA: Mycoplasmosis and the desert tortoise *(Gopherus agassizii)* in Las Vegas Valley, Nevada, *Chelonian Conservation Biol* 1(4):279-284, 1995.
26. McLaughlin GS, Jacobson ER, Brown DR, McKenna CE, Schumacher IM, Adams P, et al: Pathology of upper respiratory tract disease of Gopher Tortoises in Florida, *J Wildl Dis* 36(2):272-283, 2000.
27. Schumacher IM, Brown MB, Jacobson ER, Collins BR, Klein PA: Detection of antibodies to a pathogenic mycoplasma in Desert Tortoises *(Gopherus agassizii)* with upper respiratory tract disease, *J Clin Microbiol* 31(6):1454-60, 1993.
28. Simecka JW, Davis JK, Davidson MK, Ross SE, Städtlander CTKH, Cassell GH: Mycoplasmas which infect animals. In Maniloff J, McElhaney RN, Finch LR, Baseman JB, editors: *Mycoplasmas: molecular biology and pathogenesis*, Washington, DC, 1992, American Society for Microbiology.
29. Schumacher IM, Hardenbrook DB, Brown MB, Jacobson ER, Klein PA: Relationship between clinical signs of upper respiratory tract disease and antibodies to *Mycoplasma agassizii* in Desert Tortoises from Nevada, *J Wildl Dis* 33(2):261-266, 1997.
30. Schumacher IM, Rostal DC, Yates RA, Brown DR, Jacobson ER, Klein PA: Persistence of maternal antibodies against *Mycoplasma agassizii* in desert tortoise hatchlings, *Am J Vet Res* 60(7):826-831, 1999.
31. Minion FC, Brown MB, Cassell GH: Identification of cross-reactive antigens between *Mycoplasma pulmonis* and *Mycoplasma arthritidis, Infect Immun* 43:115-121, 1984.
32. Brown DR, Crenshaw BC, McLaughlin GS, Schumacher IM, McKenna CE, Klein PA, et al: Taxonomic analysis of the tortoise mycoplasmas *Mycoplasma agassizii* and *Mycoplasma testudinis* by 16S rRNA gene sequence comparison, *Int J Syst Bacteriol* 45(2):348-350, 1995.
33. Epperson DM: *Gopher tortoise* (Gopherus polyphemus) *populations: activity patterns, upper respiratory tract disease, and management on a military installation in northeast Florida*, unpublished MS thesis, Gainesville, 1997, University of Florida.
34. Brown MB, Brown DR, Klein PA, McLaughlin GS, Schumacher IM, Jacobson ER, et al: *Mycoplasma agassizii* sp. nov., isolated from the upper respiratory tract of the desert tortoise *(Gopherus agassizii)* and the Gopher tortoise *(Gopherus polyphemus), Int J Syst Evol Microbiol* 51(Pt 2): 413-418, 2001.
35. Hill AC: *Mycoplasma testudinis*, a new species isolated from a tortoise, *Int J Syst Bacteriol* 35:489-492, 1985.
36. Brown DR, Merritt JL, Jacobson ER, Klein PA, Tully JG, Brown MB: *Mycoplasma testudineum* sp. nov., from a Desert Tortoise *(Gopherus agassizii)* with upper respiratory tract disease, *Int J Syst Evol Microbiol*. In press, 2004. Published online February 27, 2004, at http://dx.doi.org/10.1099/ijs.0.02418-0.
37. Brown DR, Schumacher IM, McLaughlin GS, Wendland LD, Brown MB, Klein PA, et al: Applications of diagnostic tests for mycoplasmal infections of Desert and Gopher Tortoises, with management recommendations, *Chelonian Conservation Biol* 4:497-507, 2002.
38. Hannan PC, Windsor GD, de Jong A, Schmeer N, Stegemann M: Comparative susceptibilities of various animal-pathogenic mycoplasmas to fluoroquinolones, *Antimicrob Agents Chemother* 41:2037-2040, 1997.
39. Roberts MC: Antibiotic resistance. In Maniloff J, McElhaney RN, Finch LR, Baseman JB, editors: *Mycoplasmas: molecular biology and pathogenesis*, Washington, DC, 1992, American Society for Microbiology Press.
40. Taylor-Robinson D: *Mycoplasma* and *ureaplasma*. In Murray PR, Baron EJ, Pfaller MA, Tenover FC, Yolken RH, editors: *Manual of clinical microbiology*, Washington, DC, 1995, American Society for Microbiology Press.
41. Prezant RM, Isaza R, Jacobson ER: Plasma concentrations and disposition kinetics of enroploxacin in Gopher Tortoises *(Gopherus polyphemus), J Zoo Wildl Med* 25(1):82-87, 1994.
42. Raphael BL, Papich M, Cook RA: Pharmacokinetics of enrofloxacin after a single intramuscular injection in Indian Star Tortoises *(Geochelone elegans), J Zoo Wildl Med* 25(1):88-94, 1994.

43. Spörle H, Gobel T, Schildger B: *Blood levels of some anti-infectives in the Hermann's tortoise* (Testudo hermanni), Germany, 1991, 4th International Colloquium Pathol Med Rept Amph.
44. Wimsatt J, Johnson J, Mangone BA, Tothill A, Childs JM, Peloquin CA: Clarithromycin pharmacokinetics in the desert tortoise *(Gopherus agassizii)*, *J Zoo Wildl Med* 30(1):36-43, 1999.
45. Loria GR, Sammartino C, Nicholas RA, Ayling R: In vitro susceptibilities of field isolates of *Mycoplasma agalactiae* to oxytetracycline, tylosin, enrofloxacin, spiramycin and lincomycin-spectinomycin, *Res Vet Sci* 75:3-7, 2003.
46. Johnson JD, Mangone B, Jarchow JL: A review of mycoplasmosis infections in tortoises and options for treatment, *Assoc Rept Amph Vet* 1998.
47. Wright KM: Common medical problems of tortoises, *Proc North Am Vet Conf* 1997.
48. Jenkins JR: Medical management of reptile patients, *Compend Cont Educ Pract Vet* 13:980-988, 1991.
49. Allen DG, Pringle JK, Smith D: The use of chemotherapeutic agents in reptilian medicine. In Allen DG, editor: *Handbook of veterinary drugs*, Philadelphia, 1998, Lippincott-Raven Publishers.
50. Jacobson ER: Antimicrobial drug use in reptiles. In Prescott JF, Baggot JD, editors: *Antimicrobial therapy in veterinary medicine*, Ames, 2000, Iowa State University Press.
51. Gauvin J: Drug therapy in reptiles, *Semin Avian Exotic Pet Med* 2:48-59, 1993.
52. Rostal DC, Lance VA, Grumbles JS, Schumacher IM: *Effects of acute upper respiratory tract disease on reproduction in the desert tortoise*, Gopherus agassizii: *hormones, egg production and hatching success*, 1996, Conference on Health Profiles, Health Reference Ranges, and Diseases in Desert Tortoises, Soda Springs, Calif.
53. McLaughlin GS: *Ecology of Gopher Tortoises* (Gopherus polyphemus) *on Sanibel Island, Florida*, Ames, 1988, Iowa State University Press.
54. Davidson MK, Lindsey JR, Parker RF, Tully JG, Cassell GH: Difference in virulence for mice among strains of *Mycoplasma pulmonis*, *Infect Immun* 56:2156-2162, 1990.
55. Rodriguez R, Kleven SH: Pathogenicity of two strains of *Mycoplasma gallisepticum* in broilers, *Avian Dis* 24:800-807, 1980.
56. Interior Do: Endangered and threatened wildlife and plants: determination of threatened status for the Mojave population of the desert tortoise, *Fed Register* 55:12178-12191, 1990.
57. Gates CA, Allen MJ, Diemer Berish JE, Stillwaugh DM, Shattler SR: Characterization of a Gopher tortoise mortality event in west-central Florida, *FL Scientist* 65:185-197, 2002.
58. Seigel RA, Smith RB, Seigel NA: Swine flu or 1918 pandemic? Upper respiratory tract disease and the sudden mortality of Gopher Tortoises *(Gopherus polyphemus)* on a protected habitat in Florida, *J Herpetol* 37(1):137-144, 2003.

74
VOMITING AND REGURGITATION

RICHARD S. FUNK

Vomiting, or emesis, is defined as a forceful ejection of food from the stomach and anterior intestine. This physiologic process is under active neural control from the autonomic and somatic nervous systems. The integration of vomiting by a vomiting center in the floor of the fourth ventricle, which also receives vestibular input, is well documented in mammals but not understood in reptiles.

Regurgitation involves the discharge of undigested food immediately after eating to a few hours later and is generally passive. Regurgitation originates as an esophageal or pharyngeal problem but, in some cases, may be gastric, especially if the gastroesophageal sphincter is incompetent. These two phenomena are generally difficult to distinguish clinically in reptiles. In mammals, testing the pH may help differentiate the two, with vomitus the more acidic (usually around a pH of 2).

Often, the vomited or regurgitated material is found in the cage, and the history obtained from the owner is too incomplete to allow for a distinction to be made. If the temperature at which the reptile is kept is too cool and food is not digested well in the snake's stomach, the material may be vomited and appear to be relatively fresh. Turtles and tortoises rarely vomit or regurgitate; consequently, these are more serious symptoms in these animals. **Both vomiting and regurgitation are symptoms, not diseases.**

DIFFERENTIALS AND DIAGNOSIS

A thorough history and complete physical examination are helpful in evaluation of potential causes for vomiting or regurgitation. Behavioral etiologies (usually as a result of husbandry issues) are commonplace. Some snakes that are active and nervous and without a secure hiding box may vomit behaviorally if disturbed after eating a meal. Other snakes may vomit if handled 1 or 2 days after feeding. Cage stress, as in overcrowding, may lead to vomiting. In these cases, altering the husbandry may correct the problem.

Vomiting may be associated with diarrhea and is a common sign associated with a variety of both gastrointestinal and nongastrointestinal disorders. An animal with chronic vomiting may have acid-base and electrolyte imbalances and be dehydrated; these deficiencies need attention during treatment.

In most reptiles, vomiting, not regurgitation, is the process. Etiologies of vomiting in reptiles are less clearly elucidated than in small companion mammal species. Consumption of too large a meal, maintenance at temperatures not conducive to proper digestion, or ingestion of a prey item that was partly autolyzed may result in vomiting and may be accompanied by diarrhea.

Infectious causes are common. Parasites associated with vomiting in reptiles include cestodiasis and ascariasis,[1] cryptosporidiosis,[2] and amebiasis (Figure 74-1).[3] Vomiting has also been documented with inclusion body disease virus of boid snakes[4] and with *Chlamydiophyla* infection in a Gaboon Viper (*Bitis gabonica*).[5] It may also occur after ingestion of medicated food or ingestion of toads, resulting in *Bufo* poisoning.[6] Organophosphate or other pesticide intoxication can lead to vomiting. Bacterial and fungal gastroenteritis may also lead to maldigestion and vomiting. The role of inflammatory processes in other systems such as with pancreatitis, peritonitis, or pyometra, all of which may cause vomiting in dogs and cats, is as yet unknown in reptiles.

Anatomic intestinal obstructive lesions (such as strictures) may cause vomiting. A gastrointestinal foreign body, obstructive neoplasm or granuloma, or an intussusception may cause vomiting. The author has seen several neonatal captive-bred snakes, for example a Cornsnake (*Elaphe guttata*), California Kingsnake (*Lampropeltis getula californiae*), and Indian Cobra (*Naja naja*), with congenital defects involving an incomplete posterior intestinal tract; these snakes ate but eventually vomited because no posterior outflow was present. Iatrogenic vomiting can result from drug administration such as apomorphine, levamisole, xylazine, miticides, and organophosphates.

Several potential etiologies exist for regurgitation. Behavioral regurgitation must always be ruled out first. Other causes include esophageal, pharyngeal, or oral lesions such as stomatitis, esophagitis, neoplasia, esophageal laceration

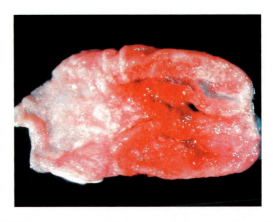

FIGURE 74-1 Cryptosporidiosis is a common cause of vomiting in snakes (see Chapter 48). This snake had a severe gastritis develop from a cryptosporidial infection. Infected animals typically vomit their meals 2 to 3 days after ingestion. An animal may commonly keep a meal down then vomit again on the next feeding, confusing the keeper into thinking that the problem has self-corrected.

or perforation, strictures, granulomas, and foreign bodies. The patient may become emaciated if it cannot keep food down. If regurgitation becomes a chronic problem, a secondary aspiration pneumonia may develop.

Diagnostic procedures that may be useful in identification of the problem include a thorough physical examination, survey and contrast radiography, bacterial and fungal cultures, fecal parasite analysis, samples for virology, laboratory analysis including a complete blood count and profile, and endoscopy of the esophagus and gastrointestinal system.

TREATMENT

Treatment is dependent on the problems identified: surgical removal of neoplasia, foreign bodies, or obstructions; administration of suitable chemotherapeutic agents[7,8]; correction of dehydration and acid-base imbalances; and correction of husbandry practices (such as handling, temperature, provision of shelters, quarantine, and hygiene). Tube-feeding or assist-feeding of a debilitated animal may be necessary once the underlying problems have been corrected (see Chapter 18). Assist-feeding or force-feeding an ill animal can do harm if the underlying pathology has not been corrected. Appropriate chemotherapeutics (antimicrobials, fluids, gastrointestinal protectants, etc.), supportive care, and dietary management are keys to a successful treatment regimen. Use of antiemetic medications such as metoclopramide, although not well-documented in reptiles, may be beneficial.

The most important point to remember is that vomiting and regurgitation are symptoms, not diseases. If the cause can be identified, the resulting symptoms can be corrected.

REFERENCES

1. Frank W: Endoparasites. In Cooper JE, Jackson OF, editors: *Diseases of the Reptilia*, San Diego, 1981, Academic Press.
2. Funk RS: *Implications of cryptosporidiosis in emerald tree boas, Corallus caninus*, Chicago, 1987, 11th International Herpetological Symposium, Captive Prop Husbandry.
3. Marcus LC: *Veterinary biology and medicine of captive amphibians and reptiles*, Philadelphia, 1981, Lea & Fibiger.
4. Jacobson ER: Viral diseases of reptiles. In Fowler ME, editor: *Zoo and wild animal medicine: current therapy* 3, Philadelphia, 1993, WB Saunders.
5. Jacobson ER, Gaskin JM, Mansell J: Chlamydial infection in puff adders (Bitis arietans), *J Zoo Wildl Med* 20(3):364, 1989.
6. Cooper JE, Jackson OF: Miscellaneous diseases. In Cooper JE, Jackson OF, editors: *Diseases of the Reptilia*, San Diego, 1981, Academic Press.
7. Funk RS: A formulary for lizards, snakes, and crocodilians, *Vet Clin North Am Exotic Anim Pract* 3(1):333-358, 2000.
8. Bonner BB: Chelonian therapeutics, *Vet Clin North Am Exotic Anim Pract* 3(1):257-332, 2000.

Section VIII
SPECIAL TOPICS

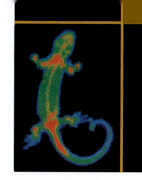

75
OVERVIEW OF AMPHIBIAN MEDICINE

KEVIN M. WRIGHT

The end of the 20th century had a surge of interest in amphibian medicine when iridoviruses and chytridiomycosis were linked with the phenomenon of global amphibian population declines. Although some advances have been seen in these particular research fields, as exemplified by the work done by the National Science Foundation's investigation of The Global Decline of Amphibians, part of the Integrated Research Challenges in Environmental Biology, amphibian medicine remains a fairly unexplored field. The amphibian immune system, critical for understanding pathogenesis of infectious disease, is poorly understood even for well-researched taxa like the Axolotl, *Ambystoma mexicanum*, and the African Clawed Frog, *Xenopus laevis*.

The veterinarian must have a thorough understanding of the biology and captive husbandry of amphibians before practicing medicine on the amphibian patient. Amphibians are a unique class of vertebrates that appear in the fossil record during the Upper Mississippian era, more than 300 million years ago. Amphibians were the first vertebrates capable of exploiting terrestrial habitats on a long-term basis, although they still relied on aquatic environments for breeding and the development of young. This class of vertebrates is named Amphibia because of the double life (*amphibios* in Greek) that is characteristic of many of its members: an aquatic larval stage followed by a terrestrial adult stage. The modern-day amphibians have been categorized in three orders: Gymnophiona, the caecilians; Urodela, the salamanders and newts; and Anura, the frogs and toads. (Throughout this chapter the word "salamander" is used to refer collectively to salamanders and newts and the word "anuran" is used to refer to frogs and toads.)

AMPHIBIAN DIVERSITY

The three orders of amphibians alive today, the Gymnophiona, the Urodela, and the Anura, are highly specialized and have greatly modified the body plan of the ancient amphibians. In fact, so many structural changes have occurred that the relationships of modern-day amphibians are in dispute.[1] Whether the group of animals termed "amphibians" represents a single ancestral amphibian lineage or three different lineages sharing similar but independently derived characters is unclear. To put this into perspective, all existing placental mammals are more closely related than the three orders of amphibians. The veterinarian must make judgment decisions in the absence of thorough medical knowledge of a given taxon and must understand that species variability may obfuscate diagnostic tests and response to treatment.

Caecilians are elongated and superficially resemble an annelid worm. Most species are fossorial, although a few are aquatic, and their anatomy is reflective of their lifestyle. The eyes are reduced or absent, and the skull is strengthened for burrowing efforts. Limbs tend to obstruct passage through burrows and are lacking in modern caecilians. Most species lack any remnant of the pectoral and pelvic girdles. Six accepted families of caecilians are found, with more than 150 species currently described. Because of their secretive nature, most species of caecilians are uncommonly found in the hands of private herpetoculturists. The most commonly encountered species are the aquatic Caecilians (*Typhlonectes* sp.), the Mexican Caecilian (*Dermophis mexicanus*), and the Sticky Caecilian (*Ichthyophis kohtaoensis*). However, interest in this group is growing as is the entire field of amphibian captive husbandry, and the clinician may begin to encounter Caecilians more frequently.

The salamanders are lizard-like in basic body plan, with an elongated body supported by four limbs and a long tail (Figure 75-1). All modern salamanders have lost one or more of the toes, and some species and families have considerably reduced limbs. Some salamanders are highly modified, such as the Lungless Salamanders (Plethodontidae) and the Eyeless Olms (Proteidae), and other species show unusual life histories. One such species with an interesting

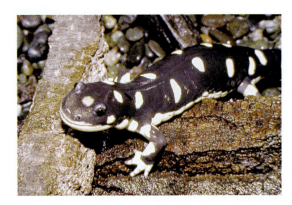

FIGURE 75-1 The California Tiger Salamander (*Ambystoma californiense*) is a species that was recently protected in California and is not available in the pet trade. *(Photograph courtesy D. Mader.)*

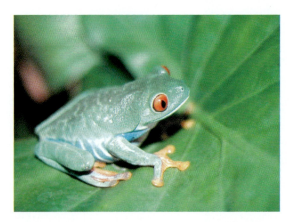

FIGURE 75-2 This Red-eyed Leaf Frog (*Agalychnis callidryas*) shows the typical body form of the anurans: four limbs and a reduced or absent tail. No external neck exists, so the head and body appear unbroken. *(Photograph courtesy D. Mader.)*

life history is the Axolotl (*Ambystoma mexicanum*). The Axolotl is a neotenic species; that is, the sexually mature adults of this species externally resemble gilled larvae. Neoteny is found among other members of the Mole Salamander family (Ambystomatidae) and is a general characteristic of the Proteidae and Sirenidae. Approximately equal numbers of aquatic and terrestrial salamanders exist within the 400 described species. These species are divided into nine commonly accepted families of salamanders. Salamanders are more popular vivarium subjects than caecilians, and some species, such as the Axolotl and European Fire Salamander (*Salamandra salamandra*), have been captive bred over many generations. Commonly encountered species include the Tiger Salamander (*Ambystoma tigrinum*), the Fire-belly Newt (*Cynops pyrrhogaster*), the Red-spotted Newt (*Notophthalmus viridescens*), and the Rough-skinned Newt (*Taricha tarosa*).

The anurans are the most speciose group of amphibians alive today, with more than 4000 species of frogs and toads described. The relationships within this order of amphibians are uncertain, but at least 20 families are generally accepted by taxonomists.

Frogs have four limbs and a reduced or absent tail. No external neck is found, so the head and body appear unbroken (Figure 75-2). The skeleton is highly modified to withstand the stresses involved in a saltatorial lifestyle, although many anurans walk more often than jump. Most frogs are terrestrial, although a few species are entirely aquatic (e.g., Surinam Toads [*Pipa* spp.] of the family Pipidae, Clawed Frogs [*Xenopus* or *Hymenochirus* spp.] of the family Xenopidae, etc.). Other than the the African Clawed Frog (*Xenopus laevis*), which is used extensively in biomedical research, the most common frogs in captivity are Hylidae (Tree Frogs), Ranidae (True Frogs), Dendrobatidae (Poison Dart Frogs), Bufonidae (True Toads), and Leptodactylidae (which includes the horned frogs, *Ceratophrys* spp.). Most of the efforts in captive husbandry and propagation of amphibians have focused on various frogs.

VIVARIUM DESIGN

The husbandry of a captive amphibian must take into account the particular microhabitat and ecological niche within which that species evolved. As a general rule, amphibians prefer cooler and moister environments than do sympatric reptiles. Many tropical amphibians do not need "sea level" tropical temperatures and are best maintained with background temperatures between 70°F and 85°F (21°C to 29°C). Many temperate amphibians do best at temperatures between 65°F and 72°F (18°C to 22°C) and may require seasonal drops of 10°F to 15°F (5°C to 8°C) or more for optimal health and breeding. A basking spot with temperatures at least 15°F (8°C) above the background temperature should be provided for all species except during brumation (hibernation). Appropriate humidity is important for normal health and activity. Even xeric-adapted amphibians need access to a humid environment daily. The relative humidity should range from 75% to 95% for most species of amphibians. A thermal and humidity mosaic should exist within the enclosure so that an amphibian can seek its preferred microenvironment.

A gradient of illumination should also exist, and a photoperiod should be maintained that is in accordance with what is found within the amphibian's natural range. Broad-spectrum illumination with small amounts of ultraviolet A and B is suggested to support vitamin D_3 synthesis and other physiologic processes. Hiding places that are appropriate to the amphibian's nature are essential to minimize the stress on a captive amphibian. A shelter that is too tall may not be perceived as shelter at all. If the preferred microenvironment is lacking, or if unpredictable major fluctuations of temperature and humidity frequently occur within the enclosure, a specimen may be severely stressed and may be more prone to health problems. Thus, a suitable stable environment is one of the most important aspects in preventive medicine for amphibians.

Caecilians can be divided into two husbandry and enclosure categories: fossorial (subterranean) and aquatic. Fossorial caecilians, such as the Sticky Caecilian (*Ichthophyis kohtaoensis*), require an enclosure provided with 1 to 4 inches (2.5 to 10 cm) of topsoil.[2-4] This author prefers to use topsoil that has been treated to eliminate unwanted arthropods (e.g., trombiculid mites, a source of vesicular skin lesions in amphibians). The topsoil can be rendered free of these arthropod parasites with baking the soil in a layer 1 inch deep (2.5 cm) for 30 to 60 minutes on a sheet in an oven heated to 200°F (95°C).

A covering of leaves and sphagnum moss should be placed on top of the soil, and cork bark or other flat pieces of bark can be added for hiding spots. As with the soil, the leaves and other decorations should be free of mites. In this case, placement of the items in the freezer for several days can eliminate the various pest arthropods. **Do not use pesticides to treat any material destined for an amphibian enclosure!**

A wet bog-like area should be provided in one corner of the cage. The bog-like area may obviate the need for a separate water source, but in the event a bog cannot be created, a shallow source of potable water is needed. Deep-water dishes should be avoided because terrestrial caecilians can become trapped and drown.

The cage should be spray-misted with chlorine-free water as needed to keep the substrate damp but not overly wet. Plants serve to increase humidity, but the roots may be damaged by the action of the caecilian inhabitants. Placing the plants within plastic pots, and burying the pot on a level with the vivarium's soil line, should adequately protect the plants. The cover for the enclosure should serve to sustain a humid environment.

Aquatic caecilians can be housed in a typical aquarium set-up with an undergravel filter and an outside canister filter.[5] Depending on the species and the preference of the herpetoculturist, the substrate can be none (bare tank bottom), sand, river mud, or pea gravel. Retreats should be provided, but care should be taken to select cage furniture with rounded edges to minimize the chance of injury to the caecilian skin. A dense mat of floating aquatic plants is desirable. A haul-out area of damp sphagnum moss is used by many specimens and should be provided. Some specimens spend a significant portion of the time buried in the moss or hiding in the aquatic plants.

The fossorial and terrestrial salamanders may be kept under similar conditions to that described for fossorial caecilians. Most salamanders are highly secretive and thrive best with a minimum of disturbance. Whereas the caecilians generally construct a tunnel system, the typical salamanders have an underground retreat and emerge from underneath the leaves and bark to forage. If conditions are correct, the salamander may be seen moving about on the surface of the cage litter.

Aquatic salamanders, both larval and adult forms, can be kept under similar conditions as described for aquatic caecilians. However, the salamanders should have easy access to haul-out places such as one provided by a smoothly sloped floor and strategically placed pieces of bark. At least part of the water area should be fairly shallow to allow the salamanders to gulp air without much struggle. Some aquatic salamanders drown if denied access to such a portion of the vivarium.

For some salamanders, such as the kinds termed "newts," generally *Cynops* sp., *Notophthalmus viridescens*, *Paramesotriton* sp., *Taricha* sp., or *Triturus* sp., the appropriate vivarium set-up depends on the stage in the life cycle of the newt. A semiaquatic set-up is recommended to encourage natural behavior and metamorphosis of the newt.

Some salamanders (e.g., Palm Salamanders of the family Bolitoglossa) are arboreal and require a more vertically oriented enclosure than as described for the terrestrial forms. Sturdy broad leaf plants should be planted in the enclosure, and tall hollow logs should also be provided for additional retreats. Heavy misting of the enclosure and an elevated water source are essential because some specimens do not descend to the ground in search of water.

The anurans have the greatest diversity in life habits and a corresponding complexity to the vivarium requirements of different species. Fossorial forms such as Spadefoot Toads (*Scaphiopus* spp.) benefit from a vivarium set-up with the appropriate soil. For some forms, topsoil is adequate, but other species may occur in sandy environments; depending on the soil type, the pH, moisture content, and other physical parameters may be very different. Thorough research is essential before the enclosure is furnished because specimens may quickly languish and die if kept in soils much different from their natural habitat. A shallow water bowl is suggested, but heavy spraying of the substrate is needed if the inhabitants are to maintain normal activity levels. Many fossorial species have brief activity periods during the year and are not accustomed to continual active life. Thus, allowing the anuran to estivate during the summer heat, or brumate (hibernate) during winter's chill, may be necessary for the long-term health of the specimen.

Aquatic anurans, such as the Clawed Frogs (*Xenopus* spp.), may be kept under conditions similar to those described for aquatic caecilians and salamanders. Terrestrial and arboreal species should be kept under conditions as have previously been described.

Although some amphibians may be kept in communal vivariums that contain different species, this is not suggested without careful planning and discussions with other experienced herpetoculturists. Many species produce skin secretions that are deadly to other species. The secretions of a pickerel frog (*Rana palustris*) incapacitate many other frogs. The feeding response of an amphibian is somewhat generalized, so the inhabitants of a communal vivarium could end up eaten by a larger cagemate. Although it has not been well documented in amphibians, the various microfauna of one species (e.g., gastrointestinal protozoa) may prove pathogenic if introduced into another species. Closely related species of salamanders may display aggressive behaviors toward each other, and the submissive salamander usually fares poorly in the closed setting of a captive enclosure. The behavioral repertoire of amphibians is far more complex than most people realize, and their social interaction may have profound effects on a successful communal vivarium.[6] Some examples of successful vivarium communities are well-planted tropical enclosures that contain green-and-black Poison Dart Frogs (*Dendrobates auratus*) and Red-eyed Tree Frogs (*Agalychnis callidrya*), and semi-aquatic temperate enclosures with Fire-bellied Toads (*Bombina orientalis*), Fire-bellied Newts (*Cynops ensicauda*), and Emperor Newts (*Tylototriton shanjing*). An attempt at a communal vivarium should be thoroughly researched before its construction and is only recommended for the advanced herpetoculturist.

More in-depth information on amphibian husbandry is readily available.[7-9]

WATER QUALITY

Water quality must be monitored in an amphibian's enclosure. Several kits are available for the measurement of water quality in tropical fish tanks, and the veterinarian should have access to a kit able to perform analysis of the following parameters: pH, dissolved oxygen, hardness, alkalinity, ammonia, nitrite, nitrate, and copper (used for medicinal purposes in tropical fish).[10] Coliform and bacterial counts of the water may need to be performed by the clinician in the evaluation of a sick amphibian, so appropriate arrangements should be made with a microbiologic laboratory or kits can be purchased for in-clinic use.

Signs of stress associated with inappropriate pH may be subtle and range from anorexia to agitation. If the ideal pH for an amphibian is unknown, a neutral or slightly acidic pH is suggested (pH, 6.8 to 7.1), to be adjusted according to the animal's response. If the amphibian is inappetent or appears irritated, a more alkaline pH may be tried (pH, 7.2 to 8). Electric eels (*Electrophorus electricus*) maintained in alkaline water (pH, 8 or higher) instead of the acidic environment of their natural habitat (pH, <6) developed in hydrocoelom, probably because hydrogren ions act as counterions to sodium in freshwater fish.[11] Maintenance in a low H+ environment (i.e., high pH) may result in accumulation of body sodium (Na^+) and subsequent fluid retention; this malady was alleviated by maintaining the eels in water with a pH of 6.5 or lower. Careful evaluation of the pH of the amphibian enclosure and knowledge of its natural habitat may reveal similar links to disease states in amphibians.

Low dissolved oxygen may cause an amphibian to frequently gulp air. This can result in listing if the air enters the gastrointestinal tract. Oxygen deprivation may also manifest as failure to feed and lethargy. Gilled amphibians may develop elaborate and elongated gill plumes in low oxygen environments. Increased aeration of the enclosure water is needed to correct this problem.

The nitrogen cycle of a stable biologic filter allows rapid conversion of nitrogenous wastes such as ammonia into less toxic forms. New filters that have not had time to build up an appropriate bacterial flora cannot cope with the wastes, and the ammonia concentration can rapidly reach dangerously high levels. Ammonia toxicity is most common in unfiltered tanks, or in tanks that have undergone stress (e.g., overpopulated tanks, heavily fed tanks, tanks that have been treated with antibiotics, tanks that have experienced power outages and subsequent underaeration).

Bacterial isolation and total and coliform bacterial counts of tank water should be performed if an epizootic of bacterial disease occurs or if the clinician suspects that husbandry has been inappropriate.

AMPHIBIAN BODY PLAN

A recent text has clinically applicable illustrations of the three basic amphibian body plans.[12] Additional detail may be found in other readily available herpetology texts.[13-15] In addition, several excellent out-of-print texts detail the anatomy and physiology of amphibians.[16-23]

Amphibians have several anatomic differences from the fish body plan, and these changes have important consequences to the veterinary clinician. The epidermis of amphibians has an external stratum corneum that provides some protection from the abrasive action of terrestrial substrates such as soil. The stratum corneum is only a few cell layers thick and is shed periodically. Some amphibians eat the shed skin. The skin of amphibians is fairly fragile when compared with the scales of a reptile, or the thick covering of skin and hair on most mammals, and can be easily damaged if an amphibian is handled improperly or in contact with inappropriate substrates. Once torn, the skin no longer proves to be an effective barrier against microorganisms. Thus, even an apparently minor abrasion can have serious consequences. The basal epithelium, the site of epidermal regeneration, lies underneath the stratum corneum and is itself only four to five layers thick and easily damaged by rough handling.

Glands within the epidermis and dermis secrete a variety of substances.[24] Mucous and waxy substances serve to reduce, but not eliminate, water loss to the atmosphere. The ability to resist cutaneous water loss varies tremendously between amphibian species, but the clinician should be aware of the need for the amphibian patient to remain in a moist setting.

The dermis is also the site of toxin-producing glands as typified by Poison-dart Frogs (Figure 75-3). Other glands are present that produce toxins (e.g., parotid gland in *Bufo* spp.; Figure 75-4), and the clinician is advised to avoid contact with an amphibian's defensive secretions because irritation and illness could result—a good reason to wear gloves when handling amphibians. Other substances have been isolated from amphibian glands, with a surprising array of bioactive properties.[24] Some of these have demonstrable antimicrobial activity and are the current subject of intensive research.

Although some amphibians may possess hard or sharp claw-like structures (e.g., African Clawed Frogs, *Xenopus laevis*), true claws and scales are lacking in amphibians. These hard protrusions are horny excrescences of modified stratum corneum and lack the vascular supply and germinal epithelium of a true nail or scale.

The respiratory system of a terrestrial amphibian has been modified so that the primary mode of respiration in the adult animal no longer requires gill structures. Gills are effective structures to extract oxygen in the water, but given the increased amount of oxygen in the atmosphere, evolution to

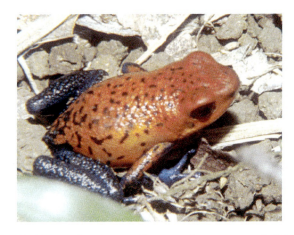

FIGURE 75-3 The skin of this Strawberry Poison-dart Frog (*Dendrobates pumilio*), as is typical of many *Dendrobates* spp. and *Phyllobates* spp., contains toxin-producing glands that can be potentially dangerous to human handlers. One should wear protective gloves when handling these animals. *(Photograph courtesy D. Mader.)*

a terrestrial environment has favored different anatomic structures for gaseous exchange.

Gaseous exchange within a living organism takes place across a moist surface. Many amphibians provide this moist surface with a simple sac-like lung or via a highly vascularized dermis. The lung or the skin is usually the primary site of respiration for terrestrial amphibians, although some respiration may occur via the lining of the oropharynx. Thus, the typical modern amphibian is able to have gaseous exchange occur by the moist surfaces of its body, both internally and externally, and no longer needs to rely on gill structures that work against the relatively low level of dissolved oxygen in an aqueous environment.

The amphibian lung lacks true alveoli. To increase the surface area of this sac-like organ, reticulate infoldings of pulmonic tissue significantly increase the sites available for gas exchange. Amphibians lack a diaphragm, so pulmonic gas exchange is accomplished with a combination of movements from the axial and appendicular muscle masses. The lung is relatively fragile and is easily ruptured if overinflated.

Amphibians that possess lungs may switch to the cutaneous form of respiration during periods of reduced oxygen availability, such as occurs during hibernation. Terrestrial amphibians that lack lungs (e.g., plethodontid and other lungless salamanders) rely primarily on cutaneous respiration, although this is not without consequences. Because the skin is somewhat less efficient a respiratory organ than lungs or gills, an amphibian that relies on cutaneous respiration must compensate for this limitation by: (1) increasing the surface area to volume ratio (e.g., plethodontid salamanders); (2) increasing the amount of skin per volume of body (e.g., the cutaneous "hairs" of the African Hairy Frog (*Trichobatrachus* spp.); or (3) possessing a metabolic rate and activity level to correspond to the limits of cutaneous gas exchange (e.g., the plethodontid salamanders).

The musculoskeletal system of an amphibian is modified to provide support for the internal organs in a terrestrial setting. Amphibians were the first vertebrates to develop a sternum, yet the ribs are poorly developed. The pectoral and pelvic girdles are attached to the vertebral column, an important anatomic characteristic that allows the limbs more efficient terrestrial locomotion of amphibians compared with fish. Dermal bone may be present in some modern amphibians and actually fuses to the skull of some frogs for additional structural support.

The amphibian circulatory system undergoes marked change during the larval metamorphosis. A larval amphibian has a single atrium and ventricle, similar to the pattern found in fish, but during metamorphosis, an intraatrial septum develops and the vascular supply to the gill arches modifies to accommodate the adult respiratory pattern (i.e., pulmonic, cutaneous, or gill respiration). Within the cardiac chamber of the adult amphibian, ridges are formed that functionally separate the blood flow to limit pulmonosystemic mixing. The fact that the heart has incomplete separation is advantageous for nonpulmonic forms of respiration and certain physiologic states such as brumation (hibernation).

Blood from the caudal portion of an amphibian drains into the hepatic portal veins, which may have some effect on the pharmacokinetics of drugs that are excreted via the hepatic route. This is in contrast to the system found in reptiles in which the renal portal system receives blood from the rear half of the body.

The excretory system of amphibians cannot concentrate its urine beyond the solute level found in its plasma. An aquatic amphibian's main nitrogenous waste product is ammonia, which is in part excreted via the gills (if present) and the skin. Urea is the main nitrogenous waste in terrestrial amphibians and may be accumulated in a primitive urinary bladder, an outpocketing of the cloacal wall. Some anurans (e.g., Waxy Tree Frog, *Phyllomedusa sauvagii*) are able to form uric acid, which makes those species less susceptible to dehydration than other amphibians. Micturition may also serve as a defensive act in some amphibians as the sudden release of urine may startle a predator and cause it to release its intended prey.

The nervous system of modern amphibians has 10 cranial nerves and lacks the accessory and hypoglossal nerves of mammals. The spinal cord is found throughout the entire vertebral column in the caecilians and salamanders, but in anurans, the caudal portion consists of a bundle of nerves known as the cauda equina. Eyes are present, except in certain cave-dwelling forms, and are keyed into movement rather than having sharp visual acuity. Amphibians were the first vertebrates to transmit sound through the air, and anurans have surprisingly well-developed ears. A dichotomy is seen in the reception of sound in many amphibian species as low frequency sounds are transmitted directly into the inner ear via the forelimbs whereas high frequency sounds are transmitted through the tympanic membrane. Many larval and aquatic adult amphibians possess a lateral line system, a series of pressure receptors that are sensitive to water movement. Smell occurs via the Jacobson's organ and appears more important in regulating behavior other than eating. Electroreceptors may be present in some species.

Despite a surprising array of reproductive strategies, the amphibian reproductive system shares many similar characteristics across orders. The gonads are paired, with associated ducts to form the gel coat of the anamniotic egg, and embryogenesis generally occurs in the environment. Fertilization is external for many amphibians, but internal fertilization is known in all three orders. An intromittent organ is present in the caecilians and in some frogs (e.g., North American

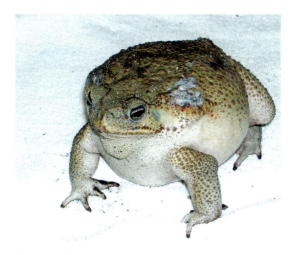

FIGURE 75-4 The *Bufo* spp. toads produce a powerful, potentially toxic secretion from the parotid glands. Gloves should always be worn when handling these species. (*Photograph courtesy S. Barten.*)

Tailed Frog, *Ascaphus truei*). Some caecilians are considered viviparous and actually secrete a substance called uterine milk for the young to feed on during development. Sexual dimorphism is present in some species of amphibians and may be permanent or seasonal. Many species show permanent dimorphism by an obvious size difference between the sexes. Seasonal dimorphism may become evident by the development of epidermal changes such as nuptial pads, dorsal crests, or altered coloration during the breeding season. The environmental cues that control reproduction are not well understood in many amphibians, and as a result, exogenous hormones often are used to induce breeding in captive amphibians.

The endocrine system of an amphibian is similar to other vertebrates (e.g., the parathyroids regulate plasma calcium levels). Some differences are found in form and function, however. The adrenal gland is homogenous in structure but has a similar role to other vertebrates. The thyroids have an additional function in amphibians not found in reptiles, birds, and mammals, in that they control morphogenesis in the metamorphosing amphibian.

All modern amphibians are primarily carnivorous as adults, and the gastrointestinal system reflects this nature. A tongue is present and may function in the capture of food by its protrusion or by assisting the jaw musculature in forming a suction to bring prey items within the oral cavity. Terrestrial species have oral glands to produce saliva and other substances needed to aid in the swallowing and predigestion of food. Cilia line the mouth and esophagus, again primarily to aid in the swallowing of food particles. Teeth are present, and many amphibians can give quite painful bites (e.g., Sirens [*Siren* spp.], Hellbender [*Cryptobranchus alleganiensis*], Horned Frogs [*Ceratophrys* spp.]). The intestine is short with minimal coiling, and feces are voided into a cloaca. The liver is usually black in color as a result of the presence of melanin within the parenchyma.

EXAMINATION AND RESTRAINT

The amphibian examination should be performed in a room that is between 70°F and 75°F (21°C to 24°C) or is in keeping with the species' preferred body temperature, if known. **Rooms suited for housing reptiles kept between 82°F and 85°F (27°C to 30°C) are unsuitably warm for most amphibians.** Unbleached paper towels wetted with chlorine-free water may be used on the examination table. A humidifier in the room may be necessary, especially if the ambient humidity is below 50%. A bottle of distilled water should be in the room to wet down the amphibian as needed. With these precautions, an amphibian may be examined without promoting dehydration.

The amphibian's skin is very sensitive to human handling. Soaps, lotions, natural oils, etc., can all irritate or damage the skin. One is wise to wear powderless vinyl or plastic gloves when handling the amphibian patients.

Clutter should be avoided in the examination room because many amphibians are fairly small and can disappear with surprising alacrity into the instruments and other accoutrements of the typical veterinary practice. For this same reason, the door to the examination room should be closed whenever the amphibian is out of its carrying case.

The physical examination of the amphibian patient should proceed in a stepwise routine manner to ensure that nothing of importance is overlooked. This initial examination should include a perusal of the animal's normal enclosure. The owner should be requested to bring in a photograph or sketch of the enclosure that should be reviewed as part of the anamnesis. A water sample from the enclosure should be provided for proper analysis. After the patient's husbandry history has been documented, the physical examination may commence. The amphibian should be observed first without handling or removal from its carrying case. Body stance, responsiveness, and general demeanor should be noted. Respiratory movements, including gular movements and pulmonary respirations, should be noted. Texture of skin and estimates of hydration status can often be assessed during this hands-off examination. The nares should be clean and free of debris, and the oropharynx should have no visible lesions. Excessive saliva or the presence of bubbles suggests respiratory complications.

The corneas should be clear, and a blink reflex should be initiated if the ocular globe is approached. Failure to blink mandates further investigation of the eye to determine whether the animal has vision. Slit lamp observation of the cornea and ocular fundus is warranted in any case.[25] Pupillary reflexes should be checked. Any cutaneous lesions should be noted. Erythema may be in response to handling or may signal a more serious underlying cause such as septicemia.

As part of the actual physical examination, coelomic (a more appropriate term for amphibians than "abdominal") palpation should be attempted, but in some species, this is not practical because many amphibians inflate themselves as a defensive maneuver. This defensive bloat appears when the amphibian is upset and should be distinguished from true bloat that remains once the animal has become calm. The stomach may be palpable in recently fed amphibians. Ingested stones and other foreign bodies may be palpated too. Oral examination is facilitated with the use of a speculum. Waterproof paper, or thin strips of firm plastic, can be used to open the mouth of the anuran. Inserting the paper at the tip of the snout works in some specimens, and inserting at the corner of the mouth works best in others. Large specimens may need a small spatula or thicker piece of plastic, such as an old credit card, to pry open the mouth. Care must be taken not to put too much torque on the mouth because the bones are thin and can easily be fractured if excess force is used. Withdrawal reflex of the limbs and righting reflex should be tested and noted. Auscultation of the pulmonic fields is rarely practical because of the small size of many amphibians.

Proper manual restraint is essential for an informative physical examination of an amphibian and for performing clinical diagnostics or administering medication. Some species produce toxic secretions, and some, such as the bicolored Poison Dart Frog (*Phyllobates bicolor*), produce toxins of a potentially lethal nature to humans. Other species (e.g., toads, *Bufo* spp.) produce toxins that irritate mucous membranes and may have lethal effects when absorbed by a human. Other amphibians defend themselves by producing mucilaginous secretions (e.g., Slimy Salamanders, *Plethodon glutinosis* complex). The clinician should wear latex gloves when handling amphibians to eliminate contact with these secretions. The gloves should be rinsed under distilled water to remove any talcum powder, which can irritate the amphibian and thereby cause the production of even more defensive secretions. Eye protection should be worn in certain cases. When pressure is applied to the parotid gland of a neotropical Giant Toad *(Bufo marinus)*, the gland's secretion may spurt several feet into the air, with unfortunate consequences to the intercepting human.

The bulk of the amphibian's body needs to be supported during manual restraint. Large anurans should be picked up by grasping behind the forelegs.[26,27] Often the anuran gives a release call, a signal to other anurans that it is either not sexually receptive or is of the wrong sex to be amplexed. The release call may sound similar to a distress call, a vocalization emitted by an anuran in response to predation, but either call may serve to startle a clinician momentarily, in which time the anuran may escape.

Many amphibians bite. Some, such as the Argentine Horned Frog *(Ceratophrys ornata)* (Figure 75-5), can inflict severe wounds on the human handler. Large anurans often kick violently when first captured, so the handler must be ready to grasp in front of the hindlegs immediately after picking up the animal behind the forelegs. Smaller anurans can be encircled with the thumb and index finger, or the hindlegs gripped in a firm fist during the examination. For a thorough physical examination, medium to small specimens may be placed inside clear plastic delicatessen cups, or small glass jars, for an unobstructed view of the entire body and ventrum.

Medium to large salamanders should be grasped behind the head and in front of the forelegs, and again immediately in front of the backlegs.[28] **Some salamanders have tail autotomy, so the handler should avoid placing any pressure on the tail.** Occasionally, despite the gentlest efforts of the handler, a specimen drops its tail anyway, so the client should be forewarned that this is a possibility. Small specimens may be examined more closely in a cup or jar as mentioned for anurans. Aquatic salamanders should not be removed from the water except for clinical diagnostics, such as collecting a skin scraping or obtaining the weight, and should be returned to the water as quickly as possible to minimize damage to the skin. Many of the larger salamanders (e.g., Hellbender, *Cryptobranchus alleganiensis*) can inflict painful bites that bleed profusely, so the handler is forewarned to maintain a firm grip when restraining these amphibians.

Caecilians and some salamanders (e.g., Amphiuma, *Amphiuma* sp.) are somewhat problematic to restrain for examination. An appropriately sized clear plastic tube, such as used for aquarium filtration equipment, or a clear glass jar or clear plastic cup is the most practical way to observe these elongated amphibians. However, to restrain the caecilian for a diagnostics such as a skin scrape, without damaging the skin on the rest of the body, can be difficult because many specimens writhe violently when pressure is applied to the body. A soft foam rubber sponge moistened with chlorine-free water can be used to pin the caecilian, and the desired portion of the body can be cautiously exposed for closer examination. Soft damp flannel may also be used. Precoating the "squeeze cage" with water-soluble gel (e.g., K-Y jelly) may be of benefit.

Anesthesia and Chemical Restraint

Physical restraint alone may not yield a thorough enough examination on certain amphibian patients or may be impractical for other reasons. Chemical restraint is often needed for a thorough evaluation of the amphibian patient. Although familiar veterinary drugs such as isoflurane and ketamine hydrochloride may be used for chemical restraint, other drugs, such as tricaine methanesulfonate and benzalkonium chloride, are the anesthetics of choice for amphibians in most cases.

Tricaine methanesulfonate is a water-soluble white powder that can be added to water with the resultant solution used to titrate to the desired anesthetic effect.[29,30] A 0.05% solution of tricaine methanesulfonate (0.5 g/L = 0.5 mg/mL) serves to anesthetize tadpoles and other amphibian larvae. A range from 0.1% to 0.2% solution (1 g/L to 2 g/L) is needed for induction of surgical level anesthesia in most frogs and salamanders, but a 0.3% solution (3 g/L) is needed for many toads (*Bufo* spp.). Because the anesthesia is titrated, the final concentration of solution does not have to be precise to be useful; a slightly more dilute or stronger concentration simply increases or decreases the time to induction of the desired plane of anesthesia.

Tricaine solution may be managed simply with premeasured amounts of drug in a container of known volume. For example, 1 gram of tricaine methanesulfonate in a 2-liter plastic soda bottle yields a 0.05% solution when 2000 mL of water is added. A 0.1% solution requires 2 g of tricaine methanesulfonate in the 2-liter soda bottle, 0.2% requires 4 g, and 0.3% requires 6 g. The concentration does not have to be exact to be effective. Precision is only necessary for a controlled study.

A clear plastic bag is an ideal induction chamber for many specimens. Large specimens need correspondingly larger chambers. Plastic sweater boxes and lock-top plastic tubs are inexpensive options. In the case of flighty anurans, the induction tub should be lined with a plastic bag. The loose fitting plastic serves to cushion the jumps during the excitatory phase of induction. Have readily available a copious supply of well-oxygenated chlorine-free water for the recovery period. If the anesthetic solution is too deep and covers the nostrils, many amphibians drown. This is less important for lungless amphibians and gilled forms that can survive total submergence for varying lengths of time. Nevertheless, use

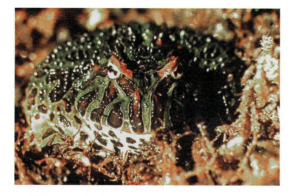

FIGURE 75-5 Many amphibians bite. Some, such as the Argentine Horned Frog *(Ceratophrys ornata)*, can inflict severe wounds on the human handler. *(Photograph courtesy D. Mader.)*

of as shallow a depth of anesthetic solution as possible is best to avoid accidents.

Tricaine methanesulfonate may be administered intracoelomically.[31] Aseptic technique must be used to prepare an injection quality solution. Intracoelomic dosages range from 50 to 300 mg/kg.

A surgical plane of anesthesia typically is induced within 20 minutes of immersion into the tricaine solution. Respiratory efforts slow down, and may stop, during tricaine anesthesia, but the cardiac rate is unaffected or even slightly increased except in very deep levels of anesthesia. Renal circulation may become reduced at high concentrations of tricaine methanesulfonate.

Erythema of the ventral skin or other light-colored skin is the first sign of anesthetic induction with tricaine methanesulfonate. The amphibian may appear agitated, and anurans often attempt escape leaps. As mentioned previously, induction of an amphibian inside a plastic bag minimizes the trauma associated with these attempts.

A light plane of anesthesia from tricaine methanesulfonate is characterized by the loss of the righting reflex and corneal reflex, but the withdrawal reflex (deep pain), spontaneous movement, gular respiration, and the cardiac impulse (visible heartbeat) are retained. A deep plane of anesthesia is the stage when only the cardiac impulse is present. The withdrawal reflex is the last reflex to go. An overdose is indicated when the cardiac impulse slows or becomes difficult to detect. Once an amphibian is in a deep plane of anesthesia, it should be placed in tricaine-free water, and the level of anesthesia can be titrated with trickling additional anesthetic solution over the amphibian's body periodically. Once the procedure is complete, anesthesia can be reversed with rinsing the body in well-oxygenated water.

Clove oil, which contains eugenol as its active anesthetic ingredient, has been used as an anesthetic in some amphibians on the basis of its anesthetic properties in fish (Whitaker, personal communication, 2000). One study used a solution of clove oil dissolved in water (final concentration of 310 to 318 mg/L) as a 15-minute bath to induce anesthesia in the Northern Leopard Frog *(Rana pipiens)*.[32,33] This anesthetic regimen achieved a deep plane of anesthesia that lasted up to 65 minutes but had a side effect of reversible gastric prolapse in 50% of the frogs treated.

Propofol has been documented as an anesthetic with intracoelomic injection[34] or intravenous injection in frogs.[33] Intracoelomic injection of 9 to 30 mg/kg resulted in deep anesthesia in White's Tree Frogs *(Pelodryas caerulea)*; a higher dosage was lethal in one specimen.[34] Intravenous injection (10 mg/kg) resulted in sedation or light sedation, but this may reflect perivascular deposition of some of the dose. Topical propofol (100 to 150 mg/kg) sedated Maroon-eyed Tree Frogs *(Agalychnis litodryas)* of less than 20 g bodyweight, with the frog rinsed in fresh water once it was sedated (Wright, unpublished data). However, topical or intracoelomic propofol is inconsistent with time of induction, depth of anesthesia, and time to recovery and offers no advantages over topical tricaine methanesulfonate.

Ketamine hydrochloride may be used to immobilize amphibians, but it is somewhat less satisfactory than tricaine methanesulfonate in that a comparatively large volume of drug may be needed, the induction time is extremely variable, the level of anesthesia achieved may vary greatly

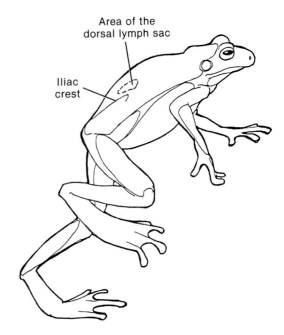

FIGURE 75-6 In some anurans, a pair of dorsal lymph sacs lies immediately lateral to the base of the sacrum.

between species (in fact, many amphibians continue to show spontaneous movement even after the withdrawal reflex is lost), and the recovery time is variable.[35,36] Ketamine may be administered intramuscularly, intravenously, lymphatically via the dorsal lymph sacs in anurans (Figure 75-6) or subcutaneously, depending on the size of the specimen and the needs of the clinician.

Dosages for ketamine are between 75 and 100 mg/kg bodyweight for most species, although some amphibians may prove extremely sensitive or resistant to ketamine and dosages must be adjusted accordingly. A minimum of 30 minutes should be allowed to pass before the anesthetic stage is evaluated. If a satisfactory level is not achieved, a supplementary dose of ketamine may be administered. If adequate anesthesia is still not achieved, one should consider delaying the effort for 24 hours and starting at a much higher initial dosage. As with tricaine methanesulfonate, anesthetic deaths are rare except in debilitated specimens or through dosage errors of several orders of magnitude.

Isoflurane is an inhalant anesthetic that may be used topically in amphibians. Several formulas may be used; a useful ratio is 1 mL isoflurane, 1 mL water, and 3 mL water-soluble gel, stirred to form a viscous liquid. This isoflurane solution is then smeared to the amphibian's ventral surface and rinsed away with fresh water once the animal is in a deep plane of anesthesia. Some amphibians, such as the Neotropical Giant Toad *(Bufo marinus)* or Argentine Horned Frog, may be anesthetized with directly dripping either halothane or isoflurane onto the skin. The problem with either topical technique using inhalant anesthetics is that the induction should be performed under a fume hood or other system for scavenging waste anesthetic gases as the agent outgases from the solution.

If inhalant anesthetics are used in an induction chamber, a saturation level of 2.5% to 3% is recommended for

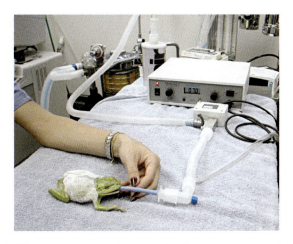

FIGURE 75-7 An uncuffed endotracheal tube is recommended to avoid damage to the tracheal tissue. This patient has been intubated and placed on a pressure-driven ventilator. No specific guidelines exist for ventilator settings. This patient was receiving six breaths per minute at 4 cm H_2O pressure, inhaling 3% to 5% isoflurane. *(Photograph courtesy D. Mader.)*

methoxyflurane,[37] halothane, and isoflurane. The amphibian should be kept in the chamber for 5 to 10 minutes after voluntary movement ceases. A deep plane of anesthesia from a chamber induction usually lasts for 10 to 30 minutes. The chamber should be moistened with fresh water for the amphibian patient's comfort. If an amphibian appears particularly irritated during the process, stop the flow of anesthetic gas and remove the animal from the chamber. Some specimens appear to not tolerate the volatile anesthetics and may suffer epidermal damage if kept in contact with halothane or isoflurane for a prolonged period of time. Large amphibians may be intubated and maintained on gaseous anesthetics, but because of alternate respiratory patterns (e.g., cutaneous, buccopharyngeal routes), maintenance of a steady level of anesthesia via this technique is difficult. An uncuffed endotracheal tube is recommended to avoid damage to the tracheal tissue (Figure 75-7).

Analagesia needs to be considered with amphibian patients. Buprenorphine injected into the dorsal lymph sac (37.6 mg/kg) may provide significant analgesia to a common laboratory test of pain and last for up to 4 hours; dexmedetomidine injected into the dorsal lymph sac (40 to 120 mg/kg) may provide analgesia up to 8 hours.[38]

Euthanasia

Two agents are noted as methods of sedation and anesthesia in many research articles that are not recommended for the amphibian patient except for euthanasia purposes: ethanol and pentobarbital. An amphibian immersed in 10% ethanol enters a deep plane of anesthesia within 15 minutes. Increasing the concentration of ethanol to 70% kills the animal. An overdose of pentobarbital (>100 mg/kg) can be administered via intracoelomic or intracardiac injection.

Decapitation as a method of euthanasia has been discussed elsewhere. Evidence exists that amphibians may still feel pain after the procedure for several minutes. If decapitation is necessary for specific reasons, the author condones this only if the animal is anesthetized.

Other methods of euthanasia have been used, such as immersing small amphibians in liquid nitrogen, but the author does not consider these to be practical in a clinical setting.

CLINICAL TECHNIQUES

Parasitologic diagnostics are similar to those reported for other orders of animals. Direct examinations and flotation concentrations are recommended for detection of most protozoal and helminth parasites. Acid-fast stains of the feces should reveal *Cryptosporidium* spp. if present.

Hematology is an underused tool in the diagnosis and treatment of disease in amphibians. Historically, part of the problem is that large volumes of blood were required to perform relatively simple tests such as hemoglobin analysis. Another problem is that most of the techniques described for blood collection in the literature were nonsurvivial techniques such as decapitation. Thus, most of the data was collected strictly for physiologic investigations, and scant attention was paid to the health or survival of the specimens.

Collection is relatively simple of blood samples adequate for white blood cell (WBC), packed cell volume (PCV), total solids (TS), and leukocyte differentials and one or two chemistries on medium-sized amphibians (40 to 80 g), and in larger specimens, one can run complete blood counts and serum or plasma chemistry panels because of the larger volume of sample that can be obtained.

Unless a blood culture is to be performed on the sample, heparinization of the syringe in venipuncture attempts is important to avoid coagulation of the sample before it is transferred to the appropriate whole blood tube. If a blood sample is to be obtained for microbial culture, no anticoagulant should be used to pretreat the syringe, needle, or capillary tube because this might affect the growth of some organisms.

Lithium heparin is the anticoagulant of choice for pretreatment of the syringe and storage of blood because it does not affect the values of plasma calcium, sodium, or ammonia. One should avoid the use of ammonium heparin when obtaining a sample that is to be analyzed for NH_3 levels or else a falsely elevated reading results. Sodium heparin should be avoided when electrolyte values are desired. Ethylenediamine tetraacetic acid (EDTA) may lyse the erythrocytes of some species of amphibians and is not recommended as an anticoagulant for amphibian blood.

Several options are available for obtaining blood from a frog. A relatively simple procedure is to bleed from the lingual venous plexus that lies immediately beneath the tongue.[39] The author has used this method on frogs as small as 25 g. Care must be taken to gently pry open the mouth to avoid breaking the thin mandibular bones. A small firm rubber spatula works well, or even a cotton minitip applicator can be used as a mouth speculum. In some animals, working from the lateral edge of the oral commissure is easier, and in other animals, insertion of the speculum into the philtrum, a small divot found just beneath the tip of the nose, is easiest. Once the mouth is opened, a cotton-tipped applicator is used to draw the tongue forward, as if the tongue were flipping out to catch a prey item (Figure 75-8). The lingual venous

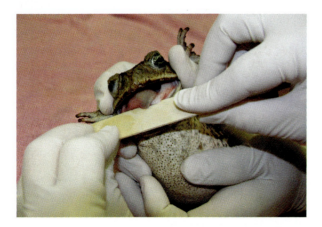

FIGURE 75-8 A soft smooth speculum can be used to open the mouth and manipulate the tongue of an anuran, such as this Neotropical Giant Toad (*Bufo marinus*). *(Photograph courtesy D. Mader.)*

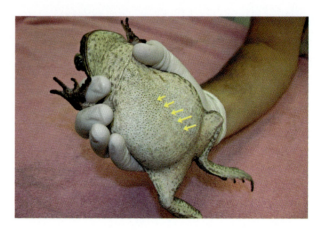

FIGURE 75-10 The midline groove on the ventrum of this Neotropical Giant Toad (*Bufo marinus*) lies immediately over the midline abdominal vein. *(Photograph courtesy D. Mader.)*

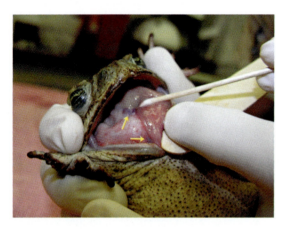

FIGURE 75-9 The lingual venous plexus is a prominent network of superficial veins that can serve as a phlebotomy site in many anurans *(yellow arrows)*. *(Photograph courtesy D. Mader.)*

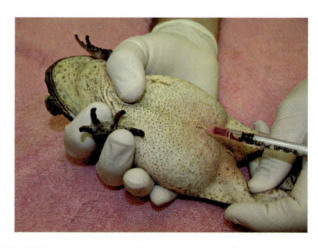

FIGURE 75-11 Obtaining a blood sample from the midline ventral vein of a Neotropical Giant Toad (*Bufo marinus*). *(Photograph courtesy D. Mader.)*

plexus is then visible on the underside of the tongue and the buccal floor. Most frogs have pale-colored tongues, so the purple to red network of veins is readily apparent (Figure 75-9). One large vein can then be punctured with a 26-gauge or 25-gauge needle, and a heparinized microhematocrit tube can be used to collect the blood that oozes from the vein. Once an adequate sample of blood is obtained, release the tongue. In most cases, this serves to put enough pressure on the vein that it stops bleeding. Occasionally, direct pressure on the venipuncture site with a cotton-tipped applicator is necessary to achieve hemostasis. The disadvantage to this technique is that the samples can be contaminated with saliva and mucus, but this can be minimalized if care is taken to swab the surface of the plexus throughly before venipuncture. In the case of a fractious animal, blood collection can be facilitated with sedating or tranquilizing the patient.

Large frogs and toads can be bled quite easily from the midline ventral vein on the ventral surface (Figures 75-10 and 75-11). A 26-gauge or 27-gauge needle can be carefully inserted in a craniodorsal direction into this vein, and gentle pressure applied to withdraw blood into the syringe. A good insertion site is the point midway between the sternum and the pelvis. Unfortunately, the passage through the bore of these small-gauge needles does tend to distort some blood cells, but a risk of lacerating the midline ventral vein is found with larger gauge needles.

Salamanders may also be bled from the anterior abdominal vein in the manner described previously, but identification of the venipuncture site in these amphibians is more difficult. An additional site for venipuncture is the ventral caudal vein, also called the tail vein, which runs immediately ventral to the vertebral bodies. In salamanders less than 80 g, a 27-gauge needle is the most practical choice for venipuncture attempts, but a 26-gauge or 25-gauge needle may be used for larger animals. Some salamanders and newts have tail autotomy, and in these species, one should not attempt this method because it could result in the loss of the specimen's tail during the venipuncture endeavor.

A final choice for the collection of hematologic samples is cardiocentesis. In the author's experience, this has worked equally well for anurans, most salamanders, and even caecilians. If the animal is difficult to restrain, it should be sedated or anesthetized to reduce the risk of pericardial, ventricular, or atrial laceration. Place the amphibian in dorsal recumbency to locate its cardiac impulse (heartbeat). The location of the heart may be quickly determined with a Doppler probe;

once located with Doppler, the cardiac impulse is easy to track visually. Once the cardiac impulse is noted, a 25-gauge, 26-gauge, or 27-gauge needle may be inserted into the central part of the impulse so as to penetrate the apex of the ventricle. Gentle pressure is applied, and the needle is slowly advanced or withdrawn until a flash of blood is visible in the hub of the syringe. If a clear yellow fluid appears instead, the needle should be withdrawn because the sample is most likely fluid from the pericardial sac. If sufficient pericardial fluid was obtained, it can be submitted for culture (if no anticoagulant was used), have cytologic specimens prepared from it, or be analyzed for biochemical parameters. Even a small quantity can be prepared for either wet mount examination or stained slides to determine whether inflammatory cells or other abnormal items are present. A new needle and syringe should be used for a second attempt, but an increased risk exists of a problem arising with each subsequent puncture of pericardial or cardiac tissue. If a blood flash is detected, pressure should be let off the syringe. A cycle of gentle pressure and release coaxes blood into the syringe with each ventricular beat. Once an adequate sample is obtained, pressure is released and the needle is withdrawn from the ventricular chamber.

Complete blood counts may be performed in the same manner as described for avian and reptilian species.[40-42] Natt-Herrick's solution allows one to make a count of WBCs and red blood cells (RBCs) from the same sample with a hemocytometer and a leukocyte Unopette (Becton, Dickinson, and Company, Rutherford, NJ). Another option is to use the eosinophil Unopette to count granulocytes and the leukocyte differential count to determine total white blood cell count. Although the eosinophil Unopette method may not work in all amphibian species, in the author's experience, it has worked well in Axolotls (*Ambystoma mexicanum*), Marine Toads, Smokey Jungle Frogs (*Leptodactylus pentadactylus*), Hellbenders (*Cryptobranchus alleganiensis*), and Sirens (*Siren intermedia*) and may be applicable to a wide variety of amphibians.

For each species encountered, the eosinophil Unopette technique is not recommended for use until it is verified for that species. This may be done by performing simultaneous WBC with the Natt-Herrick solution/Unopette method and the eosinophil Unopette method. If the counts are consistently within 5% of each other, then the eosinophil Unopette method may be used on future hematology specimens of that species. An advantage to the eosinophil Unopette method is that it is much easier to count the stained granulocytes than it is to distinguish leukocytes from erythrocytes in the Natt-Herrick solution. However, the Natt-Herrick solution allows an accurate WBC independent of the granulocyte differential count. This is important because in amphibians the granulocytes have been poorly described and may vary tremendously in staining characteristics and gross morphology between species.[43-46] Considerable expertise is needed for an accurate leukocyte differential count and interpretation.

Wright-Giemsa solution enhances the detail of the cell's internal morphology and provides consistently richer colors when compared with other commonly available stains. Important to remember is that at this point in time the granulocytes are described on the basis of their staining characteristics and that the classes of granulocytes generally are not proven to be fully homologous nor analogous to the mammalian granulocytes with similar staining characteristics.[44]

Documentation of the disease accompanying the differential leukogram is important to elucidate the role of the various leukocytes seen in amphibians. Few studies report several normal blood values for any amphibians[41] (e.g., for the American Bullfrog [*Rana catesbeiana*]; Table 75-1).

Whenever an amphibian is manually restrained, some damage occurs to the thin epidermis. For this reason, moistened latex gloves should be worn by the handler to ameliorate the cutaneous injury to the patient. Although the humoral and cell-mediated immunologic response in amphibians is poorly delineated, macrophages are responsible for phagocytic removal of cellular debris and bacteria.[44,47] Because of the presence of injured epithelial cells after handling, an amphibian's monocyte count may show a relative and absolute increase on subsequent leukocyte profiles.

Rickettsiae, parasites, and inclusions caused by viruses may be detected on appropriately stained blood smears.[48,49] Trypanosomes and microfilariare are extraerythrocytic parasites. Hemogregarine parasites are common intraerythrocytic inclusions in amphibians. The relative percentage of erythrocytes afflicted with inclusions may be important clinical prognostic indicators. Low levels are probably unimportant or may only be a minor contributing factor to the amphibian's signs. High levels of inclusions may be significant, especially if coupled with signs of anemia such as low PCV or RBC, polychromatic erythrocytes, microcytosis, or hypohemoglobinemia.

With the advent of small inexpensive dry film analyzers (e.g., Kodak Ektachem DT60 Analyzer, Eastman Kodak Co, Rochester, NY), serum or plasma chemistries on amphibians are now practical to obtain. The small volume of sample needed for analysis by these machines allows even a 0.5-mL sample to yield important results such as total protein/albumin, aspartate amino transferase (AST, also known as serum glutamic-oxaloacetic transaminase or SGOT), alanine transaminase (ALT, also known as serum glutamate pyruvate transaminase or SGPT), blood urea nitrogen (BUN), ammonia (NH_3), glucose, and electrolytes. For serum samples, the blood should be allowed to clot for a minimum of 20 minutes before centrifugation to minimize the chance of sample coagulation after separation. Plasma samples may be spun down immediately, and then the plasma may be decanted from the cellular component.

Unfortunately, given the paucity of clinicopathologic information about amphibians, even with plasma chemistry data and hematologic values it is still more of an art than a science to interpret those values in the context of the clinical picture of an amphibian. However, if a consistent systematic approach is maintained with evaluation of an amphibian as is done with evaluation of a mammal, then each practitioner has the potential to contribute to the development of this field of veterinary medicine.

Celiocentesis may be performed via the paralumbar region or just off the ventral midline. Obtained fluid should be analyzed for protein content (generally <2 g/dL), cytologic characteristics, and biochemistries and submitted for microbial cultures.

Amphibian bacteria should be cultured at 98°F (35°C) and room temperature. However, most amphibian bacterial isolates can be recovered with 98°F as the incubation temperature. Although standardized kits may yield useful information as to the identity of the bacterial isolate, more elaborate techniques are often needed to confirm the etiologic agent.

Table 75-1 Physiologic and Hematologic Values of Amphibians

Measurement	Leopard Frog (Rana pipiens) Male	Leopard Frog (Rana pipiens) Female	American Bullfrog (Rana catesbeiana)	Grass Frog (Rana temporaria)	Edible Frog (Rana esculenta)	Cuban Tree Frog (Hyla septentrionalis)	African Clawed Frog (Xenopus laevis)	Mudpuppy (Necturus maculatus)	Tiger Salamander (Ambystoma tigrinum)
BW (g)	25-42	25-46	225-306	—	—	28-35	—	—	35
Blood volume (mL/100 g BW)	—	—	3.1-3.6	—	—	7.2-7.8	—	—	—
Hematology									
PCV (%)	19-52	16-51	39-42	—	—	20-24	—	21	40
RBC ($10^3/\mu L$)	227-767	174-701	450	461	308	—	566	20	1657
Hb (g/dL)	3.8-14.6	2.7-14.0	9.3-9.7	14.34	9.7	5.6-6.8	14.9	4.6	9.4
MCV (fl)	722-916	730-916	—	—	—	—	—	10,070	—
MCH (pg)	182-221	182-238	—	—	—	—	—	2160	—
MCHC (g/dL)	22.7-26.8	19.9-27.7	21.1-25.9	—	—	25-31	—	22	—
WBC ($10^3/\mu L$)	3.1-22.2	2.8-25.9	—	14.4	6.1	—	8.2	—	4.6
Early stages (%)	—	—	—	1.5	1.0	—	0.7	—	—
Neutrophils (%)	—	—	—	6.5 ± 1.0	8.8 ± 2.1	—	8.0 ± 1.1	—	—
Lymphocytes (%)	—	—	—	68.5 ± 2.9	52.0 ± 3.3	—	65.3 ± 2.7	—	—
Monocytes (%)	—	—	—	0.8	1.3	—	0.5	—	—
Eosinophils (%)	—	—	—	14.5 ± 2.9	19.4 ± 1.3	—	?	—	—
Basophils (%)	—	—	—	24.2 ± 2.2	16.6 ± 1.3	—	8.5 ± 1.4	—	—
Plasmocytes (%)	—	—	—	0.4	1.0	—	0.2	—	—
Thrombocytes ($10^3/\mu L$)	—	—	—	20.8	16.3	—	17.1	—	—

From Carpenter JW: *Exotic animal formulary*, ed 3, St Louis, 2005, WB Saunders.
BW, Body weight; *PCV,* packed cell volume; *RBC,* red blood cell; *Hb,* hemoglobin; *MCV,* mean cell volume; *MCH,* mean corpuscular hemoglobin; *MCHC,* mean corpuscular hemoglobin count; *WBC,* white blood cell.

The laboratory used should be competent in isolating and identifying specimens from other ectotherms (i.e., reptiles and fish) because many human-oriented microbiology laboratories do not have the expertise to identify amphibian pathogens.

Cutaneous lesions should be examined with direct observation of a wet mount, stained samples, biopsy, and microbial culturing. A skin scrape of the lesion may be obtained with the blunt edge of a scalpel blade, or a dulled scalpel blade. The scraping should be viewed as a wet mount to determine the presence of fungi and protozoa. A Gram stain should be made from the scraping if fungi or bacteria are the suspected etiologic agents. A biopsy can be made of epidermal tissue with tenting the skin and removing a small oval of tissue. Tissue glue can be used to oppose the epidermal flaps. Cultures and histopathology of any samples obtained should be submitted if deemed appropriate.

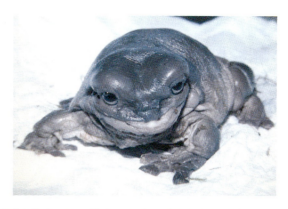

FIGURE 75-12 Mandibular, skull, and limb deformities as a result of metabolic bone disease of nutritional origin (NMBD) in a White's Tree Frog *(Pelodryas caerulea)*. *(Photograph courtesy D. Mader.)*

NUTRITIONAL DISEASES

Amphibian nutrition remains a poorly known aspect of captive husbandry. Anuran larval forms may be herbivorous, omnivorous, or carnivorous, and caecilian and salamander larvae are entirely carnivorous. Adult amphibians are entirely carnivorous, with the exception of one Tree Frog *(Hyla truncata)* that includes fruit of the coca tree in its diet.[20] The Marine Toad has been observed to consume vegetable matter in Florida, but no observations of this are reported in its natural range. As may be expected in captive insectivores, two of the major nutritional diseases are due to the fact that domestically produced insects such as crickets and mealworms do not have the levels of calcium, phosphorus, vitamin D_3, and vitamin A required by most vertebrates.

Metabolic Bone Disease of Nutritional Origin

Nutritional secondary hyperparathyroidism (NSHP) is the most common form of metabolic bone disease (MBD) in captive amphibians and is the second most commonly reported nutritional disease in a survey of captive amphibian pathology. (Starvation or emaciation is the most commonly reported nutritional disease.) An absolute or relative calcium deficiency is likely the underlying cause of most cases of NSPH in amphibians because most of the commonly fed prey items have an inverse calcium-to-phosphorus ratio and a low total calcium. At this point, no descriptions of other forms of MBD have been found in amphibians, so throughout this discussion, the simple terms NSHP and MBD will be combined to NMBD.

One of the first signs of NMBD in adult anurans is spastic tetany after strenuous movement (e.g., leaping) that subsides during rest. Coelomic distension from gastrointestinal stasis and gas buildup may be seen with or without accompanying tetany. Both of these signs are likely the result of hypocalcemia. With chronic NMBD, amphibians have spinal deformities, angulation of the long bones, and bowed mandibles (commonly called "rubber jaw" by herpetologists) develop (Figure 75-12).

High-resolution radiographs may confirm decreasing bone density in affected individuals and the presence of pathologic fractures. The lateral processes of the vertebrae become radiolucent fairly early in the course of NMBD as do the urostyles of anurans. The long bones typically become radiolucent after the "ghosting" of the lateral processes of the vertebrae and urostyle. If an apparently healthy member of the same species is available, including the healthy animal in the same exposure as the ill animal assists the clinician in evaluating skeletal structure. (Be wary in interpretation because the "healthy" animal may simply have subclinical NMBD.) The clinician may wish to retain the humerus, femur, vertebrae, and urostyle of a healthy necropsy specimen to have comparative elements for radiographic studies, in the event that a healthy specimen is not immediately available.

The author believes that different species of anurans have different calcium and vitamin needs because one species may develop signs of NMBD when fed the identical diet used to successfully maintain another species. The intake of calcium during the larval stage is especially critical for normal skeletal development and calcium homeostasis of the adult. A calcium source such as cuttlebone should be available for the tadpoles of many species; Ramsey Canyon Leopard Frog *(Rana subaquavocalis)* tadpoles that did not have access to a calcium block developed NMBD as froglets despite being fed a diet used successfully in many other ranid species.[50] Thus, any case of NMBD should elicit a thorough dietary review with an examination of the vitamin and mineral supplements administered. Consultation with others who have kept this species may provide essential tips to correct the contributing husbandry (including dietary) problems involved in NMBD.

Amphibians with NMBD require several weeks of treatment for resolution of radiographic lesions and improvement of other abnormalities. Daily baths in 2% to 5% calcium gluconate and 2 to 3 IU/mL vitamin D_3 may allow uptake of the calcium ion in many species but should be used as a supplementary aid and not the single course of corrective efforts. Injectable calcium should be given intracoelomically for amphibians in tetany[51] and may need to be administered weekly in addition to the calcium baths. Oral or injectable vitamin D_3 supplements may be required in addition to the vitamin D_3 baths.

Oral supplementation with Feline Clinical Care Liquid (Pet-Ag, Elgin, Ill) may be beneficial. The diet should be corrected so that the amounts of calcium, phosphorus, and vitamin D₃ are balanced. In some instances, the level of calcium may need to be increased over what is considered "normal" for other species—this is especially true for those amphibians that come from hard alkaline environments and those from peat bogs and other weakly acidic environments. Many amphibians are presented too late in the course of the disease to ever regain normal health. Even if calcium homeostasis and normal bone density are achieved, amphibians with deformities of the skull and hyoid bones may not be able to feed on their own. Calcitonin therapy described for reptiles[52] has not proven effective in amphibians because of the major structural differences between amphibian calcitonin and the salmon calcitonin used for the treatment of human osteoporosis.

Hypovitaminosis A

Hypovitaminosis A has been recently recognized as a significant disease in a number of captive amphibians. This nutritional disorder was first recognized in captive Wyoming Toads *(Bufo baxteri)*, an endangered species that is the subject of an intense captive propagation program to produce specimens for reintroduction to the wild. An afflicted toad sights and targets a moving cricket and then rocks forward and flicks its tongue out to capture that prey. Often the cricket walks away from this attack, seemingly missed by the tongue flick. Within the Wyoming Toad Species Survival Program (SSP), this syndrome became known as "short tongue syndrome" because it looked like the toads were undershooting their targeted prey as if their tongues were shorter than they should be. The condition appeared to be acquired with clinical signs usually occurring in subadult to adult animals and slowly worsening over time. Affected toads eventually require assist-feeding as they become completely unable to capture prey.

Pessier et al[53] determined that the underlying cause of short tongue syndrome was squamous metaplasia of the mucous glands of the tongue rather than an actual shortening of the tongue. These lingual mucous glands were not able to produce mucus. A healthy toad tongue is coated with a sticky layer of mucus that serves to "glue" a prey item to the tongue and hold the prey as the tongue is retracted into the mouth. An afflicted toad was indeed hitting a cricket with its tongue flick, but the tongue lacked the gluey coating necessary to hold the cricket. Squamous metaplasia of the mucous glands is a lesion consistent with hypovitaminosis A in other vertebrates. Since the documentation of this lesion in Wyoming toads, several other amphibians have been noted with lingual squamous metaplasia. Squamous metaplasia has also been noted in the urinary bladder and kidney and may be an underlying etiology for hydrocoelom.

Afflicted toads had mean liver retinol levels of 105 μg/g (range, 44 to 164 μg/g), whereas the toads with short tongue syndrome had a mean of 1.5 μg/g (range, undetectable to 7.3 μg/g).[53] This finding strongly supported the presumptive diagnosis of hypovitaminosis A.

Some frogs with conjunctival swellings that were nonresponsive to antibiotic treatments did have resolution after supplementation with vitamin A either orally or topically (Figure 75-13).

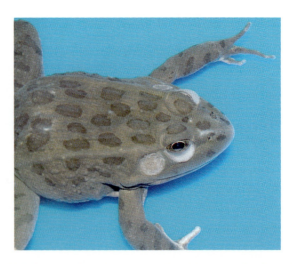

FIGURE 75-13 Bilateral conjunctival swelling typical of hypovitaminosis A.

Hypovitaminosis A is associated with an impaired immune system and secondary infections in other vertebrates. Although whether or not hypovitaminosis A impacts the secretions of glands involved in producing and maintaining the cutaneous slime layer is not yet clear, it seems likely that at least the mucus production is impaired. This may enhance colonization of the skin by various pathogens and predispose to infection by *Batrachochytrium dendrobatidis*, a fungus that feeds on keratin.

The cause of hypovitaminosis A in amphibians is unclear. Some amphibian species may have unique requirements for vitamin A or for vitamin A precursors. To date, the insects analyzed are low in vitamin A; so domestic crickets are a poor source of vitamin A, yet crickets are a mainstay of the diets for captive amphibians. One popular commercial supplement lacks vitamin A but has beta-carotene. Frogs that received only this supplement had the conjunctival lesions develop. Even multivitamin supplements with sufficient vitamin A at the time the container is opened lose their potency if the supplement is stored in areas that have high humidity, warm temperatures, or both. A multivitamin supplement should be used within 6 months of breaking the seal on the container. If the supplement is stored improperly, it should be replaced more often.

Consideration of vitamin A supplementation of any clinical ill amphibian is reasonable, particularly ones with signs similar to short tongue syndrome, swollen eyelids, evidence of infectious dermatitis, hydrocoelom, or simple failure to thrive. Commercially available vitamin A injectable solutions are too concentrated to use in all but the largest amphibians. If a sufficiently low concentration can be made at a compounding pharmacy, an intramuscular dose of 2 IU/g every 72 hours until clinical signs resolve is possible. Another possible treatment route is oral administration at a dose not to exceed 1 IU/g orally daily for 2 weeks or until clinical signs resolve. The oral vitamin A can be expressed from a human grade vitamin A supplement (liquid gel cap) and diluted with propylene glycol to an appropriate concentration. Propylene glycol may cause irritation in some amphibians, so the client should be advised of possible adverse reactions. Topical treatment with vitamin D_3 is effective in amphibians,[54] so topical administration of vitamin A likely may be absorbed too.

During a necropsy, the whole tongue should be submitted to rule out hypovitaminosis A. Because the affected glands are more prominent at the rostral tip of the tongue early on in the disease, a longitudinal section of the tongue should be examined rather than a cross section. In addition, other sensitive structures, such as the bladder, kidneys, and eyelids, should be assessed histologically for evidence of squamous metaplasia. A frozen section of the liver can be submitted for vitamin A analysis. If the levels are below 40 µg/g and histologic evidence of squamous metaplasia is seen in any of the high-risk organs, a diagnosis of hypovitaminosis A is reasonable.

Obesity

Obesity is also a common nutritional disease in captive amphibians, especially in animals that are regularly offered rodents. Some Horned Frogs (*Ceratophrys* spp.) may reach astounding proportions if fed to satiation on a regular basis. Most of an amphibian's stored fat is in the form of coelomic fat pads; thus, the obese amphibian generally has a grossly distended abdomen and normal-appearing limbs and tail (if present). Although investigations into the long-term effects of obesity in captive amphibians are lacking, obesity in amphibians undoubtedly has a major impact on health. Decreased longevity and poor reproductive performance may be associated with obesity in amphibians.

Gastric Overload or Impaction

Another common syndrome in captive amphibians is gastric overload or impaction (GOI). This potentially lethal condition is generally the result of eating a single overly large prey or consuming too many prey items in a short period of time. South American Horned Frogs and African Bullfrogs (*Pyxicephalus adspersus*) are most likely to be presented with this condition because many owners take inordinate pride in the gustatory capabilities of their animal. The owner may attempt to see how many prey items (e.g., mice) the anuran can eat in a single setting, unaware of the deleterious consequences this may have. An amphibian is often stimulated to feed when it sees movement. This may cause an amphibian to ingest a smaller cagemate, which is another cause of GOI in captive amphibians. Rocks and other foreign bodies may be ingested incidental to prey capture and swallowing, although pica has been noted in some anurans and aquatic salamanders. Some anurans retch and expel foreign bodies and large meals, but this is not often the case.

One adverse impact of swallowing an overly large meal is that the amphibian then has a decreased respiratory ability. The lung is a simple sac-like structure dorsal to the stomach, and when the stomach is distended, the tidal volume and total lung capacity are correspondingly decreased. Another complicating factor is that the digestive process may not be able to break down and assimilate the ingesta before bacterial decay sets in, leading to gastric bloat and endotoxemia. Because the prey often still moves after being swallowed, a distended stomach is prone to perforation, with subsequent contamination of the coelomic cavity with gastric contents. In the case of furred prey, the accumulated mass of undigested hair and bones may cause gastric or intestinal impaction in the course of digestion. Gastric washes with hypotonic saline solution may remove ingesta in cases of acute gastric impaction, or if gastric bloating from fermentation is noted. Endoscopic retrieval of items via the esophagus may be possible in some cases. In most cases of GOI, a gastroenterotomy to remove the items is recommended. Broad-spectrum antibiotics and appropriate fluid therapy are recommended aftercare for an amphibian with GOI. The benefit of mucosal protectants such as sucralfate is unknown. If an intestinal impaction from a trichobezoar is suspected, medical therapy (e.g., mineral oil) may be attempted.

Nutritional Support

Liquid formulas designed for the nutritional support of the domestic cat, an obligate carnivore, are generally useful for amphibians (e.g., Feline Clinical Care Liquid). A puree of cricket or mealworm abdomens, earthworms, or pinkie mice supplemented with vitamins and minerals may also serve as a tube-feeding formula, but this may need to be enzymatically digested with pancreatic enzymes to reduce its viscosity enough to flow through small-diameter tubes. Exoskeleton and skin are not digested well by pancreatic enzymes and need to be screened out of the formula to prevent clogs.

A red rubber catheter, polypropylene intravenous catheter, stainless steel gavage tube, or soft Silastic tubing may be used as a feeding tube, the choice depending on the size of the amphibian's mouth. Care should be taken to avoid injuring the esophagus or stomach with injudicious use and placement of the tube. The tube only needs to be inserted one third of the amphibian's snout-vent length to be in the stomach.

Hand-feeding (assist-feeding) may be possible for some debilitated amphibians such as the Tiger Salamander (*Ambystoma tigrinum*) or the Dumpy Tree Frog (*Pelodryas caerulea*). Even debilitated specimens often swallow a piece of food (e.g., a headless cricket) that is placed in the mouth. Removing the head of the cricket exposes the viscera of the cricket and speeds its digestion. This option is preferred to oral tubing when possible.

INFECTIOUS DISEASES

Viral Diseases

The longest studied amphibian virus is the herpesvirus that causes renal adenocarcinomas in the northern Leopard Frog (*Rana pipiens*).[55] Lucke's renal tumor is one of the better described viral-associated tumors, and its life cycle is fairly predictable. The renal tumors grow rapidly during the warm months of the year, with viral production occurring in the fall after the tumor has reached maximal size. Viral shedding occurs the following spring, during spawning, thereby ensuring the infection of the offspring and perpetuation of the disease. Affected frogs become extremely thin and generally die in the months after spawning. Hydrocoelom and hydrops may be noted in the latter stages of renal failure, and celiocentesis may yield neoplastic cells at this time. At necropsy, either or both of the kidneys may be affected, with a histopathologic diagnosis of papillary adenocarcinoma. Eosinophilic intranuclear inclusions may be detected in the kidneys of infected frogs during the winter months. In many ponds, the entire population of Leopard Frogs may be infected.

Iridoviruses have been the subject of recent intensive research efforts because of associated die-offs in wild populations of frogs and Tiger Salamanders (*Ambystoma tigrinum* spp.). Ranavirus type III is the iridovirus responsible for tadpole edema syndrome, a disease that is fatal to the tadpole, with adult anurans as asymptomatic carriers.[56,57] Infected tadpoles and metamorphosing froglets have edema and subcutaneous hemorrhage, which may be secondarily contaminated with bacteria. Grossly, the lesions appear consistent with bacterial dermatosepticemia ("red leg disease"). Histopathology reveals intranuclear inclusions within the erythrocyte; a recent finding is that basophilic intracytoplasmic inclusions may also be seen within the glandular cells of the stomach.[58] Bohle iridovirus, implicated in declines of Australian anurans, is closely related to ranavirus III.[59,60] An iridovirus has been associated with mortalities of wild populations of the European common frog (*Rana temporaria*).[61] Gross lesions include erythema, petechiae, ecchymoses, and skin ulcers. Histologically, basophilic and acidophilic intracytoplasmic inclusions may be found within hepatocytes. Secondary bacterial infections are often noted.

Other viruses have been described from amphibians (e.g., calicivirus,[62] herpesvirus[63]), as have suspected viral-induced lesions,[64] but little effort has gone into the elucidation of disease states associated with viral agents, a fact hampered by the overall paucity of information on normal histology of amphibians. In fact, "poxvirus" lesions originally described from the European Common Frog (*Rana temporaria*)[65] actually turned out to be normal melanosomes when reviewed with transmission electron microscopy.[61] Nevertheless, viral diseases seem likely to continue to be recognized as a significant source of disease and mortality in captive and wild amphibians.

Bacterial Diseases

Gram-negative bacteria such as *Aeromonas, Pseudomonas, Proteus,* and *Escherichia coli* are part of the bacterial flora that may be routinely cultured from otherwise healthy captive amphibians. Poor husbandry (as exemplified by crowding [Figure 75-14], poor water quality, inappropriate cage design [Figure 75-15], spoiled food, exposure to toxins such as pesticides, etc.) may immunosuppress an amphibian and allow any one of these organisms to cause disease. Other pathogens, such as iridovirus or *Batrachochytrium dendrobatidis*, likely may be the primary etiology of disease in many amphibians diagnosed with bacterial infections; the original pathogen may be difficult to detect by the time the amphibian shows clinical signs of illness such as ventral erythema. This clinical sign gave rise to the term *"red leg disease"* or *"red leg syndrome"* in early reports of amphibian disease. When this clinical sign is caused by a bacterial pathogen, a more appropriate term for the disease is *bacterial dermatosepticemia* (Figure 75-16).

Aeromonas is the most common genus isolated in published cases of clinical bacterial disease in amphibians. *Aeromonas*

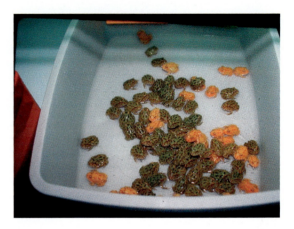

FIGURE 75-14 Many amphibians are kept under substandard conditions at wholesalers and pet stores. Crowded enclosures, such as this tub full of normal and albino Ornate Horned Frogs (*Ceratophrys ornata*), are stressful and may immunosuppress the amphibians.

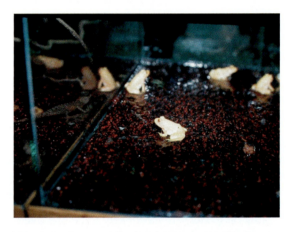

FIGURE 75-15 Improper husbandry is responsible for many of the problems seen in captive amphibians. The delicate skin of many amphibians may be injured by the stiff bristles of artificial turf carpeting. Abraded skin may be colonized more easily by pathogenic bacteria than intact skin.

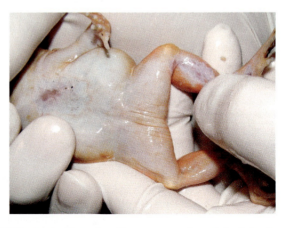

FIGURE 75-16 Ventral erythema suggestive of "red leg," more appropriately termed bacterial dermatosepticemia.

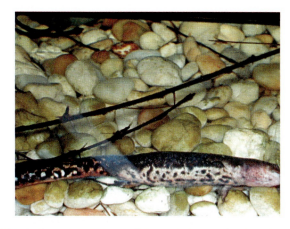

FIGURE 75-17 A Paddle-tailed Newt *(Pachytriton brevipes)* dying of bacterial dermatosepticemia. Erythema of the throat region is caused by dilatation and rupture of capillaries during this disease.

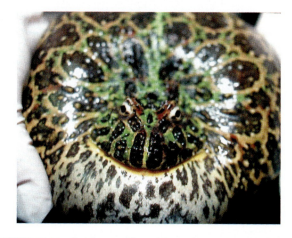

FIGURE 75-18 An Ornate Horned Frog *(Ceratophrys ornata)* with severe hydrops. Hydrops and hydrocoelom are associated frequently with septicemia but in this frog were from chronic nephritis. The weight of fluid in its coelom and subcutaneous spaces was more than the normal weight of the frog.

hydrophila has historically been associated with bacterial dermatosepticemia.[66-69] However, several other aeromonads and other gram-negative bacteria have been implicated in amphibian disease in addition to *A. hydrophila*. The following discussion is based on what is currently known about bacterial dermatosepticemia in amphibians, with the caveat that appropriate antibacterial therapy ultimately depends on the exact pathogen that has been cultured and definitively identified from the clinical case in question.

Clinical signs of bacterial dermatosepticemia may be brief and extremely rapid in chronology. Dilation of the surface capillaries and petechiation are common clinical signs and cause an erythema that is readily visible against white or pale-colored skin (Figure 75-17). This condition may progress into ecchymosis and large subcutaneous hemorrhages several hours before death; at this point, the underlying pathogenesis likely is similar to disseminated intravascular coagulation in mammals. Typically ecchymosis appears immediately before or during the agonal convulsions.

Bloating from intestinal gas, hydrocoelom (Figure 75-18), hydrops, anorexia, and lethargy may or may not be noted shortly before the onset of convulsions and sudden death. More than one animal in an enclosure is affected as a rule. Postmortem lesions are consistent with disseminated septic thrombi and may also include splenic congestion and areas of hepatic necrosis. Culture of the blood and internal organs of the dead amphibians is warranted to determine the underlying pathogen, and a blood or coelomic fluid (Figure 75-19) culture of apparently healthy amphibians within the same enclosure is suggested to determine the likelihood of further outbreaks. Some bacteria, such as *Flavobacterium* spp., have as high an epizootic potential as the classic *Aeromonas* spp.[69,70]

Because amphibians commonly have mixed infections by the time they present for clinical examination, therapy for an amphibian with signs of septicemia should target gram-negative bacteria and *Batrachochytrium dendrobatidis*. The patient should be treated immediately with aminoglycosides (5 to 10 mg/kg intramuscularly [IM] or intracoelomically [ICe] every 48 hours) or quinolones (e.g., enrofloxacin or ciprofloxacin) and then soaked for 10 minutes in 0.01% itraconazole solution or other topical imidazole solutions. Be sure to use solutions that are alcohol-free; note that many of

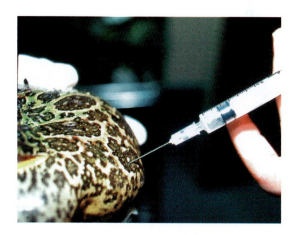

FIGURE 75-19 Fluid obtained with coeliocentesis may be subjected to cytologic, microbiologic, and biochemical analyses to help determine the underlying cause of hydrocoelom. The fluid from this ornate horned frog *(Ceratophrys ornata)* had extremely low total protein (<2 g/dL), was acellular, and did not yield any microbial isolates. The underlying etiology was severe nephritis.

the solutions do not carry this note on the bottle's label and the manufacturer must be contacted to determine whether alcohol is in the solution. If the history suggests possible exposure to sources of *Chlamydophila psittaci*, doxycycline or tetracycline therapy should also be initiated immediately. Immediate evaluation of the husbandry should be performed with the intent of eliminating contributing factors. If possible, the affected and suspect amphibians should be isolated, individually monitored, and treated on a case-by-case basis. Broad-spectrum antibiotics with anaerobic activity (e.g., metronidazole, third-generation penicillins, or cephalosporins) may be warranted as anaerobic bacteria may be isolated from ill amphibians. Even with appropriate treatment, morbidity and mortality in an outbreak are likely to be high, especially if secondary infections are noted. Soaking the patient in amphibian Ringer's solution, 0.5% to 0.6% sodium chloride, or other electrolyte solution isotonic to amphibian plasma helps combat the metabolic derangement cause by the associated skin pathology.

Chlamydophila psittaci has been reported to cause disease similar to red leg in the African Clawed Frog *(Xenopus laevis)* and the Solomon Island Eyelash Frog *(Ceratobatrachus guentheri)*.[71-74] Differentiation of this syndrome from classical bacterial dermatosepticemia relies on the absence of bacteria in the cultures obtained and detection of *Chlamydophila* inclusions in the spleen or liver. Distinguishing between chlamydial diseases and rickettsial diseases may be difficult unless antigen or polymerase chain reaction (PCR) tests are used.[75] Doxycycline is the drug of choice for chlamydophilosis, although tetracycline also may be effective.[76]

Chronic bacterial infections are uncommon. Typical presentations include cutaneous ulcers, abscesses, or an amphibian with prolonged lethargy and a poor feeding response. Skin scrapings or cultures of any lesions should be obtained to rule out mycobacterial or fungal involvement. Cutaneous ulcers and abscesses respond quite well to debridement and appropriate antibiotic therapy, both topical and parenteral. The underweight and depressed amphibian likely has internal abscesses or a granulomatous disorder. Internal abscesses are poorly responsive to treatment unless they can be surgically removed. If a granulomatous disease is confirmed, such as mycobacteriosis or chromomycosis (see subsequent), immediate euthanasia is recommended because treatment is ineffective and the diseases are likely to be zoonotic. A husbandry review is suggested to determine whether any contributing factors are present (e.g., abrasive surfaces, previous occupants that died).

Mycobacterium spp. can cause lesions in amphibians, and the species associated with amphibians are generally waterborne species or those that are soil saprophytes (e.g., *Mycobacterium marinum, M. ranae, M. xenopi*). In contrast to the more typical bacterial infections, amphibians with mycobacterial infections generally display weight loss despite a good appetite (Figure 75-20). If any cutaneous lesions are present, diagnostics should include examination of an aspirate, scraping, or biopsy to determine whether acid-fast bacteria are present. If acid-fast bacteria are detected, samples should be submitted for culture and identification. The identification of the mycobacterial species does not alter the patient's prognosis but is important because some species have a higher zoonotic potential than others. If no cutaneous lesions are found, exploratory celioscopy or celiotomy may detect internal granulomas consistent with mycobacteriosis. Finding such lesions warrants immediate euthanasia of the amphibian and counseling the client of the zoonotic potential of amphibian *Mycobacterium* spp.

Fungal and Algal Diseases

Most fungal and algal species that are involved in infectious diseases of amphibians are opportunistic invaders that invade injured or otherwise immunocompromised animals. An important exception is *Batrachochytrium dendrobatidis* (etiologic agent of chytridiomycosis) that seems to be able to cause disease in clinical healthy animals in the wild and in captivity.

Chytridiomycosis is a disease of amphibians first noted by Nichols, Smith, and Gardiner.[77] The causative agent, *Batrachochytrium dendrobatidis*, is the only known member of this family of fungi that infects vertebrates; all other known species infect invertebrates. It was first described in captive amphibians but has since been identified in free-ranging populations and has been implicated in the declines of amphibians in seemingly pristine environments.[78] (However, mounting evidence indicates that even "pristine" environments are contaminated with pollutants and pathogens originating from sites hundreds to thousands of miles away. The industrialized modern world contaminates even those wildlife preserves that have no other encroachment by humans.) Clinical signs may vary from sudden death with no obvious external signs to progressive lethargy, excessive skin shedding, ventral erythema and petechiation (Figure 75-21), deformities of the keratin beaks in tadpoles, and cutaneous lesions on the tips of the toes. Diagnosis relies on identification of the agent in skin scrapings or other tissue samples.[79] Biopsies of the drink patch or toe tips are often productive. A commercially available polymerase chain reaction (PCR) test may be used to identify chytrid DNA from skin scrapings and

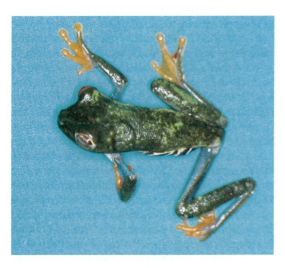

FIGURE 75-20 An emaciated Red-eyed Tree Frog *(Agalychnis callidryas)*. (Photograph courtesy D. Mader.)

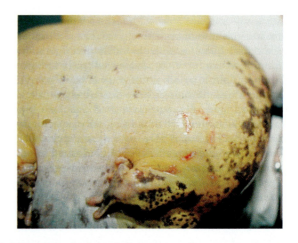

FIGURE 75-21 Epidermal ulceration on the ventrum of an Ornate Horned Frog *(Ceratophrys ornata)*. Although suggestive of an infectious etiology, these may represent abrasions that have been invaded by bacteria or fungi. A review of the enclosure should accompany the examination of the patient.

is even more sensitive than histopathology or wet mount examinations (Pisces Molecular, Boulder, CO). Fortunately, the disease seems to respond to treatment with itraconazole or miconazole baths (0.01% imidazole in 0.6% saline solution, soak for 5 minutes daily for 11 days[80]). Unfortunately, the fungus appears to persist in wild habitats and may continue to be a proximate cause of the decline of some free-ranging amphibian populations.

Other than chytridiomycosis, fungal infections are rarely encountered if an amphibian's husbandry is appropriate.[81] Many of these fungi are ubiquitous in aquatic and moist terrestrial environments. An amphibian's covering layer of mucus and other glandular secretions provides protection from invaders, but damage to the slime layer or the epidermis allows fungi to colonize. Cage furnishings may be the source of the amphibian's injury; thus, care should be taken to select decorations with nonabrasive surfaces and rounded edges.

Cagemate aggression may be the source of the traumatic injury, especially if the vivarium is overcrowded. During the breeding season, the vivarium may become functionally smaller as the inhabitants are more aware of each other and more prone to aggressive displays. In the wild, the subordinate amphibian is able to flee and avoid serious injury, but within the enclosed setting of a vivarium, little chance exists for escape. Reproductive and territorial disputes may culminate in bite wounds. Other sources of cutaneous injury are the nylon nets that are used to transfer fish and amphibians from tank to tank. Care should be taken to use soft netting or a plastic bag when capturing an amphibian to minimize the disruption afforded to the protective slime layer.

Amphibians stressed by other inappropriate husbandry techniques are especially prone to fungal infections. Proper nutrition, sanitation, and water quality are recognized as key elements in prevention of fungal disease in amphibians.

Saprolegniasis is primarily an infection of aquatic amphibians that can be caused by more than 20 different species of aquatic fungi. The characteristic sign of this fungal disease is the presence of a cotton-like material on the surface of the amphibian's skin (Figure 75-22) or in the oral cavity.[82-84] This filamentous growth covers an underlying cutaneous ulcer. The fungal mat's color can help the clinician determine the chronicity of the lesion. Acute infections are characterized by a light-colored fungal mat, and more chronic infections often turn green with algae or brown as debris is trapped in the fungal strands. If left unchecked, secondary bacterial infection may occur. A tadpole affected by saprolegniasis may starve as a result of infection of the keratin beak and ulceration of the mouth.[82] Temperature is an important factor in the progress of saprolegniasis as its incidence rate markedly decreases at water temperatures over 68°F (19°C). Wet mounts of the cottony mat reveal the characteristic fungal hyphae and confirm the lesion as saprolegniasis. Because most cases of diffuse saprolegniasis are eliminated with appropriate use of salt, itraconazole, or benzalkonium baths, it is unnecessary to speciate the etiologic agent any further. Isolated lesions respond to topical applications of miconazole, dilute benzalkonium chloride, or malachite green.

Chromomycosis is a disease of anurans that is caused by several taxa of pigmented fungi.[85,86] Cutaneous lesions are usually light-tan or gray to dark raised nodules, and the anuran may show signs of debilitation and weight loss. Presumptive diagnosis is based on finding pigmented fungi in wet mounts of scrapings from a lesion. Etiologic diagnosis requires histopathology and fungal isolation. Chromomycosis has a tendency to become systemic, unlike saprolegniasis, which is normally a cutaneous infection, and chromomycotic granulomatous lesions may spread throughout the viscera. The course of this disease may be quite slow, and therapy is usually unrewarding. Cryosurgery may be effective in eliminating individual lesions, but the commonly available antifungal agents and topical antiseptics appear to have little effect on the course of chromomycosis in amphibians. Euthanasia is recommended for infected amphibians due to the zoonotic potential of many of the fungi and the lack of viable treatment modalities to date.

Amphibian eggs often mold if kept in an inappropriate hydric environment. Dendrobatid frog eggs typically need little free water if the humidity is high and the incubation temperature is correct. Salamander eggs often mold if the water is too warm or if the dissolved oxygen of the water is low. The mold may not kill the embryo but may affect the yolk and kill the tadpole within 48 hours of hatching.

Treatment of fungal disease should be aimed at the underlying cause, so a diagnosis of fungal disease always requires a thorough husbandry review to improve the captive environment of the amphibians.

PROTOZOAL DISEASES

Amoebiasis

Entamoeba ranarum has been implicated as a cause of disease in anurans and suspected as a cause of disease in other amphibians.[87] Whether or not amphibians can recover spontaneously from this disease is questionable. Transmission is accomplished with ingestion of the cyst stage of the parasite. The direct life cycle can lead to rapid spread within a collection. Cysts are relatively durable in the environment, and once ingested, the trophozoite stage excysts to mature in the colon. Pathogenic amoebas are most likely to directly attack the colonic mucosa. Certain conditions, such as inappropriate food items, lack of ingesta, or concomitant bacterial or parasitic infections, may predispose amphibians to amoebiasis.

Renal amoebiasis has been reported in Marine Toads (*Bufo marinum*) and may have originated as an ascending infection

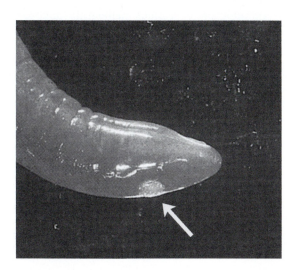

FIGURE 75-22 An aquatic caecilian with saprolegniasis.

from the cloaca. *E. ranarum* has been noted in association with hepatic abscess in a frog.

Clinical signs are limited in the early stages of amoebiasis. Anorexia, dehydration, and wasting are common signs of intestinal amoebiasis. Stools change in consistency, becoming liquid and tinged with blood. Failure to pass any stool and regurgitation may be noted at this point. Hydrocoelom and hydrops may accompany renal or hepatic disease in amphibians. Dehydration is usually associated with renal disease in terrestrial amphibians.

Antemortem diagnosis relies on a combination of clinical signs and accurate identification of the cyst or trophozoite from a fecal sample or a colonic wash. Trophozoites are typical amoeboid forms, generally with a diameter between 16 and 18 µm. Cysts are multinucleate and are between 12 and 20 µm. Direct fecal examination of feces diluted with saline solution reveals the active trophozoite. Cysts are found either with direct smears or with flotation. Detection of the cyst may be enhanced through the use of Lugol's iodine. *Entamoeba ranarum* has very similar morphologic characteristics to the familiar mammalian *E. histolytica* but generally has four to 16 nuclei. Pathogenic forms are difficult to distinguish from commensal amoebas, but a preponderance of trophozoites and cysts in the presence of clinical signs such as gastroenteritis, hydrocoelom, hydrops, or dehydration lends support to a clinical diagnosis of amoebiasis. Other stressors likely are present in most cases.

Metronidazole may be used to treat amoebiasis in amphibians, and the preferred dosage and route are 100 mg/kg orally (PO) every 14 days. Aquatic amphibians tolerate a 15-minute to 30-minute bath in metronidazole (500 mg/L), but an oral dose is preferred when practical. If severe signs of intestinal amoebiasis exist, metronidazole may be given at 50 mg/kg PO daily for 3 to 5 days. Concomitant antibiotics and fluid therapy may be necessary. If an animal displays signs of neurologic disease (e.g., listing, spasticity, lethargy), the dosage of metronidazole should be decreased. Inappropriate use of metronidazole in an herbivorous tadpole may cause an imbalance of its gut fauna. This can lead to gaseous bloat and death of the tadpole.

Ciliated Protozoa

Ciliated protozoa are reported from many families of amphibians. At present, ciliated protozoa in the gastrointestinal tract are not clearly shown to have pathogenic effects on the host.[88] Ciliated protozoa are also found in the urinary bladders of some amphibians without apparent pathogenicity.

Finding ciliated protozoa in the gastric wash, colonic wash, or feces of an amphibian is not unusual. If all other causes for an amphibian's unthriftiness have been ruled out but a high density of ciliated protozoa is voided in the feces or urine, treatment with metronidazole, tetracyclines, or paromomycin may be warranted. Gastric wash, colonic wash, and fecal parasite examinations usually reveal ciliated protozoa during the direct observation of a sample. Cysts may be found on direct examination and after concentration with flotation. Ciliated protozoa often are found in the lumen of the gastrointestinal tract at necropsy. Absence of signs of an inflammatory process such as heterophilic infiltrates supports the supposition that the ciliated protozoa are commensals. With signs of inflammation, care must be taken to rule out other etiologic agents such as amoebas, coccidia, and bacteria.

Cloudy patches of skin, ulcers, and reddened gills may be related to ciliated protozoal infections in aquatic amphibians. It is most likely to be a problem if water filtration and sanitation are poor and lead to high concentrations of organic debris. Skin scraping and direct observation with a wet-mounted sample usually reveal ciliated protozoa causing cutaneous lesions.

Oral tetracyclines and paromomycin sulfate may be warranted in an ill amphibian (with or without overt gastrointestinal disease) that has a high density of ciliated protozoa in its feces or gastric wash. Dosage is empirical, but a starting level of 50 mg/kg PO once daily (SID) for metronidazole, 50 mg/kg PO twice daily (BID) for tetracycline, or 50 to 75 mg/kg PO SID for paromomycin is suggested.

Frequent water changes and improved sanitation and filtration usually eliminate ciliated protozoa in aquatic amphibians. Baths with acriflavin, salt (10 to 25 g/L), or benzalkonium chloride may be useful in some cases.

Miscellaneous Protozoa

A variety of hemoparasites are found in amphibians, and the description and nomenclature of this group of parasites are beyond the scope of this article. A common finding in amphibian blood films is the presence of trypanosomes. Many trypanosome infections are subclinical and apparently have little affect on the captive amphibian. However, quinidine therapy may be warranted for an amphibian with signs of anemia or debilitation and concomitant trypanosomes. A suggested regimen for quinidine may begin with the method recommended for tropical fish, a 1-hour bath of quinine sulfate (30 mg/L).[89]

Sudden death may occur in amphibians with trypanosome infections. Splenomegaly is a common postmortem finding in these amphibians, and the trypanosome may often be seen in impression smears made of the spleen. Malarial parasites have been found to exert an influence on the performance and reproductive success of certain lizards, and a similar situation likely occurs with amphibians and their trypanosomes.

The introduction of various pathogenic protozoa can occur via feeder fish and via other live aquatic foods (e.g., *Tubifex* worms) or live aquatic plants placed within a vivarium. A protocol of the screening of live foods and decorative plants is suggested to minimize the accidental introduction of pathogens into a collection. Dipping the food items and live plant in a hypertonic salt bath (<5 minutes), and following that with chlorinated tap water (<30 minutes) or an acriflavin bath (1 to 2 hours), helps reduce the possibility of introducing unwanted organisms into the amphibian's enclosure.

Nematodes

Amphibians are host to a staggering variety of nematodes, only a few of which have received intensive study.[90] *Rhabdias* spp. are the best known lungworms in anurans. Infective larvae penetrate the skin and migrate, with the final

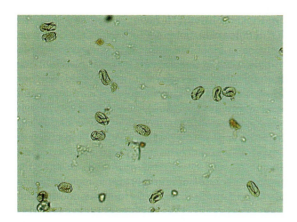

FIGURE 75-23 Embryonated nematode ova found in the feces of a White's Tree Frog *(Pelodryas caerulea)*. The type of nematode is difficult to determine based solely on the morphology of the ova. *(Photograph courtesy S. Skeba.)*

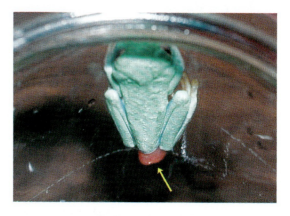

FIGURE 75-24 Cloacal prolapse in a Red-eyed Tree Frog *(Agalychnis callidryas)*. Intestinal prolapse is common with nematodiasis, gastroenteritis, or toxicoses. Prolapses of the bladder or other tissues are less common but are more typical of septicemia or toxicoses.

molt occurring in the lungs. Little damage may be noted on histopathologic examination of the lungs of an anuran with one or two adult *Rhabdias* present, but heavy infections can result in damage to the pulmonary tissue with associated inflammation and secondary infections. Diagnosis is through fecal parasite or oropharyngeal mucus examination, and the characteristic rhabditiform larvae may be seen. Embryonated ova may be detected in the feces too (Figure 75-23). Some frogs (e.g., glass frogs [*Centrolenella* spp.]) can be transilluminated and thereby reveal large adult worms in the lungs, but this is generally a postmortem finding. Because of the direct life cycle, infected amphibians should be isolated and strict hygiene practiced to prevent spread to other amphibians or superinfection of the original animal. Baths with ivermectin (10 mg/L) or levamisole (100 to 300 mg/L) weekly for 12 weeks or more may be needed to reduce or eliminate *Rhabdias* spp.

Strongyloides sp. also have a direct life cycle and may cause severe intestinal lesions (Figure 75-24). Severe strongyloidiasis may be very debilitating and contribute to protein-losing enteropathy and generalized malnutrition.[91] Treatment with anthelmintics may need to be prolonged to eliminate *Strongyloides* sp., as with *Rhabias* infections, and scrupulous attention to cage sanitation is required.

Filarid nematodes are frequently found free within the coelomic cavity or vasculature or encysted within the various organs of amphibians.[92] Microfilaria may be noted in some infections, and the presence of microfilaria in the blood of debilitated amphibians does suggest a causal relationship. Treatment with ivermectin may be attempted, but the inflammation associated with the death of the nematode could severely compromise the amphibian patient.

Some nematodes may cause signs of cutaneous hemorrhage and exfoliation. *Pseudocapillaroides xenopi* has been the causative agent of these signs in the aquatic African Clawed Frog *(Xenopus laevis)*.[93,94] The nematodes and ova can be found in both the mucus and skin scrapings from the lesions. Thiabendazole (50 to 100 mg/kg PO) and levamisole (5 mg/kg subcutaneously [SQ] followed by 10 mg/kg SQ at day 10 and day 20) was reported as efficacious in eliminating the parasite. Ivermectin baths (10 mg/L) or levamisole baths (100 to 300 mg/L) for 1 hour weekly are also effective in eliminating cutaneous nematodes.

Signs of gastrointestinal distress may accompany intestinal nematodiasis. Demonstration of parasite ova in the affected amphibian warrants anthelmintic treatment. Fenbendazole (100 mg/kg PO) or ivermectin (0.2 to 0.4 mg/kg PO) is a recommended choice for intestinal nematodiasis. Multiple weekly treatments may be needed to reduce or eliminate some nematodes.

Trematodes and Cestodes

Amphibians may be host to a variety of both trematodes and cestodes, and this situation is further complicated in that the amphibian may serve as the parasite's primary, secondary, or tertiary host or even as a paratenic host.

Larval forms are often found within an amphibian's body with a minimum of associated pathologic effects once encysted. However, significant pathology may be associated with migration of the larval forms.[95] Adult trematodes are commonly found in the lung, urinary bladder, kidney, and gastrointestinal tract and on the skin. One trematode *Ribeiroia ondatrae* has been linked with development of supernumerary limbs in a bufonid *Bufo boreas* and other limb abnormalities.[96]

Antemortem detection is rare unless the trematode is visible, as may be the case for cutaneous infections, or if the trematode is shedding ova in a way that can be detected with routine parasite examinations (e.g., gastrointestinal or urinary tract trematodes). The same may be said for cestodes. The adult cestodes may occasionally reach high enough numbers to cause wasting and anorexia by themselves or in part from obstruction of the gastrointestinal lumen.

Therapeutics of trematodiasis and cestodiasis are relatively unexplored. Praziquantel has been used in a number of species of amphibians without ill effect and with some efficacy in eliminating adult and larval trematodes and cestodes.

Other Metazoan Parasites

Microsporidial septicemia with ulcerative dermatitis has been described in the Giant Tree Frog (*Phyllomedusa bicolor*).[97] Microsporidial spores were detected in impression smears from the cutaneous ulcers. Chloramphenicol sodium succinate (5 to 10 mg/kg ICe) in combination with topical oxytetracycline hydrochloride and polymyxin B sulfate appeared an effective treatment.

Fatal renal myxosporean infection in Asian Horned Frogs (*Megophrys nasuta*) has been reported.[98] Chloramphenicol (70 mg/kg IM every 24 hours) and trimethoprim sulfadiazine (30 mg/kg IM every 24 hours) were not effective. Medicated feed containing 0.1% fumagillin DCH has been helpful in managing *Myxobolus cerebralis* infection in fish.[99]

Acanthocephalans are common gastrointestinal parasites. The ova may be detected on fecal parasite examination. Infection is usually without overt clinical signs, but if the acanthocephalan penetrates the intestinal wall, coelomitis may occur with rapid deterioration of the amphibian's condition. Acanthocephalans require an arthropod host, so the infection is self-limiting within the collection unless the arthropod food supply is contaminated or the amphibian's enclosure is contaminated with ova and suitable arthropods are introduced as prey species for the amphibian and can thereby acquire the parasite before consumption. Treatment is generally unrewarding, although high-dose ivermectin (>0.4 mg/kg ICe) may kill the acanthocephalan.

Leeches are rarely a problem of the established amphibian but may sometimes be seen in freshly imported or otherwise wild-caught specimens. Most leeches are ectoparasites, but one species actually resides within the lymphatic system of anurans. Ectoparasitic leeches are more commonly a problem of aquatic amphibians but have been noted in many nonaquatic species as well. Direct removal is necessary and may be faciliated with exposing the leech to a hypertonic salt bath.

Copepods are occasionally noted on the epidermis of aquatic amphibians. The arthropod can be diagnosed when placed in a wet mount and examined with light microscopy. Antiparasitic hypertonic salt baths as recommended for tropical fish are the suggested therapy for copepod infestation (10 to 25 g NaCl/L for 5 to 30 minutes), although ivermectin baths (10 mg/L for 60 minutes) also seem to be effective.

Trombiculid mites are an occasionally encountered parasite of terrestrial anurans and salamanders.[100] The suggestive clinical sign is the presence of erythematous vesicles in the amphibian's skin. Scrapings or biopsies of the lesions show the presence of the mites. Topical ivermectin is a suggested therapy in these cases, but hypertonic salt baths may have some effect. Antibiotic therapy may be required in amphibians with extensive cutaneous involvement. Prevention of this disease in a captive collection is established by heat-treating the soil and leaf litter used in an enclosure before its use.

An uncommonly seen but devastating parasite of terrestrial anurans is the toad fly (*Bufolucilia* spp.). The larvae infest the nasal passage of the anuran and literally eat the host until it can no longer function. Levamisole or ivermectin flushes of the nares and oropharynx may have some efficacy in killing small larvae, and brief exposure (<1 hour) to organophosphates (e.g., no-pest strips) may have some merit. More typical cutaneous and superficial bots may be manually removed.[101] Allergic reactions accompanying the removal of the bot are rare in amphibians. Flushing the wound with an antibiotic solution (e.g., gentamicin in saline solution) and concurrent administration of parenteral antibiotics is recommended.

TOXICITIES

Amphibians are exquisitely sensitive to many toxins at levels that are tolerated without ill effects by reptiles, birds, and mammals. In part, this is the result of the permeable nature of the amphibian skin, the associated vascular network in those amphibians that rely heavily on it as a respiratory organ, and the high surface area to volume ratio of small animals, all of which enhance the cutaneous absorption and assimilation of many compounds. Clinical signs of toxicosis may be quite vague, and a considerable bit of detective sleuthing is in order to uncover the underlying offending agent (e.g., polyvinyl glues used in plumbing systems).[102] In some cases, the toxin may be detected with tissue assays of dead amphibians, but the small body size of many amphibians precludes exhaustive analysis in a toxicology laboratory—simply not enough tissue is available for analysis. Environmental samples (e.g., water, soil, food sources) should be obtained for analysis in addition to the samples taken from the amphibian.

A general recommendation for the veterinary clinic is to have a supply of well-aerated chlorine-free water and several clean glass or plastic containers for the treatment of intoxicated amphibians. Avoid use of plastic containers that have held anything other than water to minimize the chance that toxic compounds are present (see subsequent iodine toxicity discussion). Rinsing the amphibian with clean water often helps remove some of the more common toxins (e.g., ammonia).

Clinical signs of toxicosis include erythema, petechia, increased mucus production, irritability, agitation, lethargy, dyspnea, convulsions, flaccid paralysis, regurgitation, and diarrhea. Many of the common disinfectants are toxic to amphibians: povidone iodine, chlorhexidine, quaternary ammonium compounds, chlorine, and ammonia. Iodine-based compounds and disinfectants that contain colorizers or perfumes are not recommended for cleaning amphibian enclosures because the plastic and organic material within the enclosure may retain these compounds and serve as a leach source that subsequently contaminates the captive environment. Treatment for disinfectant-associated toxicities is aimed at removing the source of the toxin and providing support to the amphibian patient. Rinsing with clean water, parenteral fluids, and nutritional support is indicated. If detected early, most amphibians recover from mild exposure. However, the long-term effects of the exposure may include immunosuppression and resultant secondary infections and other physiologic impairments.

High levels of chlorine and ammonia are commonly implicated in the death of amphibians. If chloramines are present in a community's tap water, an appropriate dechlorinator needs to be selected that splits the chlorine-ammonia bond and also neutralizes the resulting ammonia. The chloraminated water is recommended to be adequately aerated for

24 to 48 hours before use even if a dechlorinizer has been used to allow exhaust of the free chlorine in solution.

Sudden death, gaping, reddened skin, excess mucus, bright-red gills, disorientation, seizures, failure to gain weight, and dull colors are signs of ammonia toxicity. Diagnosis is difficult, but ammonia intoxication should be suspected if the amphibian has been kept in a vivarium with biologic filtration of the water and the system has been restarted or otherwise manipulated (e.g., major water change has occurred within past 2 weeks, antibiotics have been added to tank water). A level above 0.2 parts per million is suspicious for a diagnosis of ammonia toxicosis, and a level above 1 part per million should be considered verification of ammonia as one etiology for the clinical signs. A complete water change is the best therapy for ammonia intoxication. Sodium formaldehyde bisulfate (e.g., Amquel, Reximco International, Closter, NJ) may be used to temporarily bind the ammonia if a water change is not immediately practical. In the event this agent is used, a water change should be done at the earliest opportunity. Running the water through clay kitty litter has been suggested as another possible method of ammonia removal if a water change is impractical.

Chlorine intoxication is likely if a major water change has occurred within the past 24 hours. Test the source water to determine whether chlorine is at a dangerous level (i.e., 0.5 parts per million or higher). The affected amphibian should be placed in clean oxygenated water. A bath of 100 mg/mL sodium thiosulfate can be used to manage confirmed chlorine toxicosis. Sodium thiosulfate neutralizes the free chlorine by eliminating its oxidizing properties. After at least 30 minutes in the sodium thiosulfate solution, the amphibian should be placed in well-oxygenated chlorine-free water.

Heavy metal is an overlooked undetected killer of many captive amphibians. Plumbing generally contains copper, lead, or zinc; if tap water is used, the faucet should be allowed to run several minutes before the water is collected. Heavy metal toxicoses are far more difficult to diagnose than chlorine or ammonia toxicity. An amphibian with a heavy metal toxicosis is often beyond the point of effective therapy. The use of chelating agents (calcium versenate, calcium disodium EDTA, dimercaprol) has not been documented but may be of use in managing metallotoxicoses in amphibians.

Iodine intoxication of Poison Dart Frogs resulted in agitation and abnormal posturing before death.[103] In one reported incident, the plastic enclosure of the frogs had been treated with an iodine-containing disinfectant. Toxic levels of iodine diffused out of the plastic despite prior rinsing of the enclosure.

Salt toxicosis is rare and is generally associated with a marine aquarium near the amphibian enclosure. Amphibian enclosures should be kept well away from a marine tank, and water containers for the marine aquarium should be distinctly labeled to avoid confusion. If the possibility exists within the home, a hydrometer should be used to check the salinity of the enclosure water. Increasing the salinity of the aquarium water has been recommended to prevent ammonia build-up in unfiltered tanks. If significant evaporation occurs, the salinity may reach inappropriately high levels. Therapy for salt intoxication includes the use of hypotonic intracoelomic fluids (see dehydration) and rinsing in freshwater baths.

Pesticides are ubiquitous. The amphibian is exposed to these compounds in the wild and within the home. The effects of these compounds in amphibians include immunosuppression, reproductive failure, hepatic disorders, renal disorders, neurologic disorders, and developmental abnormalities of larvae. Even a small exposure can have long-term effects in an amphibian—just remember the devastating ecologic effects of the "safe" pesticide, dichloro-diphenyl-trichloroethane (DDT)—and pesticides do not have to be evaluated with regard to their effects on amphibians to be declared safe for the environment. Do not use pesticides around amphibians. If pesticides are used, insect growth regulators are preferred over toxicants.

Second-hand tobacco smoke appears to be irritating to amphibians. Amphibia vivaria should be kept in smoke-free rooms.

ENVIRONMENTAL CONDITIONS

Dehydration

Dehydration can quickly progress to desiccation for an amphibian without access to standing water in the absence of appropriately high humidity. Some species (e.g., *Bufo* spp.) are much more tolerant of low humidity than the average amphibian because of their decreased reliance on ammonia as an excretory product. Other amphibians (e.g., *Hyla* spp.) are able to tolerate low humidity by altering body posture to reduce surface area or by excreting protective substances on the epidermal surface. Nevertheless, all species of amphibians are susceptible to dehydration. When water loss exceeds a certain percentage of body weight (dependent on the species, as some species can tolerate over a 30% water loss without lasting ill effect), the excretory system may be damaged beyond chance of recovery. Thus, the amphibian may initially respond to therapy, but hydrocoelom and edema develop within days to weeks as the renal clearance shuts down.

The severely dehydrated amphibian often has sunken eye sockets and wrinkled and discolored skin and feels extremely tacky to the touch. Excessive tackiness of the slime coat of an amphibian may be the only sign of mild dehydration.

Rehydration is typically accomplished with placing the dehydrated amphibian in a shallow layer of well-oxygenated chlorine-free water that is at the preferred body temperature of the affected amphibian. Intracoelomic fluids may be necessary and should be slightly hypotonic. Two solutions useful for rehydrating amphibians may be made from intravenous fluids commonly available to the clinician. One solution, which has the benefit of providing some carbohydrates to the patient, consists of one part saline (0.9% NaCl) to two parts 5% dextrose. The second solution consists of seven parts saline to one part sterile water. Do not exceed 25 mL/kg body weight for an initial dose. Avoid use of potassium-containing fluids in the initial therapy. Supplemental doses may be empirically derived based on response to the freshwater baths.

Abrasions

Abrasions are an important route of invasion for secondary pathogens. The environment should be free of coarse-grained woods, sharp rocks, or any other cage furniture that is rough and likely to cause injury to an amphibian's delicate epidermis. Harsh nylon fishnets are a potential source of injury for aquatic species, so the softer fine-weave nets are preferred. Human hands can be abrasive to some amphibians, so latex gloves rinsed with aged water should be used when handling smooth-skinned amphibians. Abrasions may require treatment with topicals (e.g., benzalkonium chloride, gentamicin ophthalmic solution) if the wounds appear to be increasing in size, become erythematous, or have an opaque or serosanguineous discharge.

Water Quality

Certain parameters of water quality can cause problems if not within a narrow range: dissolved oxygen, nitrite/nitrate, ammonia, pH, hardness, and turbidity/bacterial blooms. Other parameters, such as tannin concentration, may be important to the animal but difficult to analyze. A sample of the amphibian's tank water should accompany any physical examination for illness, especially if the amphibian is entirely aquatic. Appropriate diagnostic tests should be administered to a sample of the tank water to determine whether any parameters could be contributing to the clinical signs seen. Therapy is aimed at correcting the underlying problem and restoring the tank water to appropriate parameters.

Ammonia and chlorine toxicity can be treated with sodium thiosulfate baths followed with well-oxygenated fresh water, whereas nitrite/nitrate intoxication may respond to treatment with methylene blue baths. Amphibians that have been exposed to a bacterial bloom are at risk of ocular and epidermal infections and other signs of systemic disease.

Trauma

Cagemate aggression is responsible for many of the traumatic injuries in captive amphibians. Some anurans have tusks and sharp dental projections that may be used in territorial battles and may inflict severe lacerations in a fight. Amphibians that lack such armament may still cause injury by badgering the less dominant animals and holding them at bay from food, water, and appropriate niches within the vivarium.

Dendrobatid frogs may drown if maneuvered into deep water by cagemates. Amphibians may try to ingest one another, especially if the group experiences a "feeding frenzy" as has been noted in some anurans and salamanders. This can prove fatal to both animals involved, as frequently the ingested animal is too large (see gastrointestinal overload and impaction). Some larvae are carnivorous and may eat other tankmates. If cagemate trauma is the suspected source of any injuries, animals may need to be isolated or set up in a new vivarium with more space and hiding spots. Injuries may necessitate treatment with topical or parenteral antibiotics. Corticosteroids and fluid therapy may be needed to treat shock in severely injured amphibians.

Clear-sided enclosures are another source of traumatic injury, especially to the rostrum, for many amphibians (Figure 75-25). This is especially true in active saltatorial anurans that do not recognize the glass as a barrier and

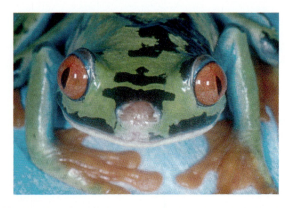

FIGURE 75-25 Rostral abrasion in a Red-eyed Tree Frog (*Agalychnis callidryas*). (Photograph courtesy S. Barten.)

may crash into the glass when startled. The clear sides may be covered with an opaque material until an amphibian has grown accustomed to its vivarium. Sudden movements and loud noises startle many amphibians, so a vivarium with these species should be kept in a quiet room with little human or pet traffic.

In addition to acting as a source of heavy metal contamination, metal screen tops can be a source of traumatic injury in anurans and should not be used. Plastic screening or drilled plastic is a preferred ventilation option for the amphibian enclosure.

Hyperthermia

Aquatic amphibians are especially susceptible to hyperthermia. Temperatures should not exceed 80°F to 85°F (26°C to 30°C). A common scenario for hyperthermia is when household heat is first turned on in a house in the fall and the vivarium that was placed on the radiator was forgotten. Hyperthermia may also be noted in the summer unless the vivarium is kept in an air-conditioned room. Broken thermostats on the enclosure's heater are another source of hyperthermia, as is the possibility that a vivarium may receive more sunlight at certain times of the year as the sun shifts in the sky with the seasons.

Signs of hyperthermia include frenzied swimming, uncoordinated jumping or walking, lethargy, and death. Autolysis is extremely rapid. If the autolysis is not far advanced, histopathology reveals congestion of the cutaneous and gill vasculature. Confirmation of hyperthermia requires skilled anamnesis in the absence of observed temperatures within the enclosure. Therapy is aimed at returning the amphibian's body temperature to normal levels rapidly and can be accomplished with bathing in freshwater ice baths and administering cool intracoelomic fluid therapy. Corticosteroid therapy is suggested in most cases. If scalding has occurred, parenteral and topical antibiotics are recommended. Unfortunately, amphibians with even minor burns have a poor prognosis because of the importance of the skin in maintaining water and electrolyte homeostasis. The amphibian may be placed into a continuous bath of full-strength amphibian Ringer's solution to combat fluid and electrolyte imbalances.

Hypothermia

Hypothermia is rarely life threatening in amphibians unless a rapid temperature drop of greater than 15°F (10°C) occurs or the absolute temperature drops below 45°F (5°C). The main clinical sign is lethargy or immobility, although regurgitation of recently eaten food or abdominal bloating may be noted. The hypothermic patient should be returned to its preferred body over the course of 12 to 24 hours. Some amphibians are immunosuppressed after hypothermia, so the affected animal should be closely monitored for signs of infection over the next 4 to 6 weeks. Antibiotics are warranted if the animal displays unusual behavior or other signs of illness.

SYNDROMES OF UNCERTAIN ETIOLOGY

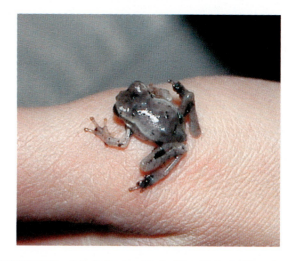

FIGURE 75-26 Spindly leg in a Masked Tree Frog (*Smilisca phaeota*). Note the poor muscling of all four limbs.

Spindly Leg

Spindly leg refers to a group of limb deformities that are associated with metamorphosing tadpoles. The classical sign is a tadpole that starts to develop hindlegs normally but the hindlegs do not complete development and are noticeably thin and may show varus or valgus deformation at the time the forelegs emerge (Figure 75-26). The deformities are not correctable, and the affected animal generally dies. Euthanasia of affected individuals is recommended. This condition has been attributed to various influences: genetic or hereditary, malnutrition, water quality, and enclosure temperature, among others.

Some dendrobatid frog enthusiasts have attributed the disease to improper nutrition of either the mother frog or the tadpoles and have recommended various dietary supplements for the parents and the tadpoles. Iodine solution has been recommended as an addition to the water to prevent development of this syndrome but has been refuted by other hobbyists. The use of water conditioners designed for tropical freshwater fish has been advocated by some. B-vitamin deficiencies and calcium deficiencies have been associated with causing abnormal metamorphosis of amphibian larvae. Several factors likely can be involved in the clinical condition called spindly leg. Careful histopathologic analysis of the affected tadpoles and concomitant standardization of the husbandry of the tadpoles and adults may well help elucidate the etiology and pathogenesis of spindly leg and indeed may recategorize this broad syndrome into a number of different diseases.

Corneal Lipidosis

Some anurans have white corneal opacities develop (Figure 75-27). In many cases, histopathologic analysis of the corneal tissue suggests the presence of cholesterol clefts; this condition is referred to as corneal lipidosis or lipid keratopathy.[2,8,104] The actual site of development of the lipid deposits may vary somewhat. It may originate from the scleral margins and advance toward the central cornea, or it may be present as a vertical line across the cornea. The opacities may remain flat or may develop into raised irregular lesions. Most affected anurans have a demonstrable

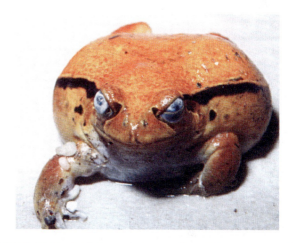

FIGURE 75-27 A Madagascan Tomato Frog (*Dyscophus antongilii*) with corneal lipidosis. (*Photograph courtesy D. Mader.*)

hypercholesterolemia. Typically, the disease is systemic, with cholesterol clefts and inflammation detected in multiple tissues besides the corneas at the time of death.

The diets offered to captive anurans typically consist of domesticated animals, such as pinkie mice and domestic crickets, which have different fatty acid profiles than their wild prey. Treatment of corneal lipidosis is generally unrewarding and consists of debulking the lesions and dietary manipulation. Unfortunately, debulking may actually exacerbate the lesion. Dietary management is aimed at the use of wild-caught insects instead of the commonly available domestic crickets and feeding small amphibians or reptiles in place of mice. Alternatively, sparingly feed high-protein low-fat foods (e.g., lean chicken heart dusted with vitamins and minerals, earthworms, domestic crickets that have not fed for 24 hours). The interested clinician may wish to investigate the potential therapeutic use of cholesterol-blocking agents in affected anurans.

Many of the species commonly reported with corneal lipidosis, such as the White's Tree Frog (*Pelodryas caerulea*), often bask and elevate their temperatures well above 100°F (39°C) in the wild. The opportunity to have this regular high body temperature is not offered to many captive specimens. These peak body temperatures may be important for normal fat metabolism. Basking spots should be offered to any amphibian with corneal lipidosis and should be considered an important aspect of husbandry in many amphibian species.

Gout

Gout has been reported in some anurans.[105] Precipitating causes in amphibians are unknown but probably include dehydration, renal failure, inappropriate diet, and toxicities. Gout is most likely to occur in those amphibians that commonly excrete a portion of their nitrogenous wastes as uric acid. Waxy Tree Frogs (*Phyllomedusa sauvagii*) are a commonly kept species that have gout and develop cystic calculi composed of uric acid.

Gastric Prolapse

Many anurans may evert their stomach and wipe its mucosa clean with their hands. This may help rid the stomach of undigestible or otherwise unpalatable materials. It has also been seen as a sign of toxicosis, anesthesia with clove oil, hypocalcemia, and various other metabolic disorders. It is a nonspecific sign in anurans and may be benign and self-correcting. It usually indicates a serious disorder when noted in salamanders.

NEOPLASTIC DISEASES

Neoplasia is commonly associated with hydrocoelom and hydrops in amphibians. Renal, integumentary, hepatic, and gonadal neoplasms are among the most commonly reported tumors of amphibians. Celiocentesis may yield cells with mytotic figures, high nucleus to cytoplasm ratios, and other histopathologic indications of neoplasia. Metastasis appears to be uncommon. Diagnosis of any of these tumors carries a grave prognosis, although some cases may be amenable to surgery (Figure 75-28).

Fibromas and papillomas are common types of benign tumors encountered. Management attempts may include surgical excision or debulking.

A comprehensive review of the literature on amphibian neoplasia that included cases filed in the Registry of Tumors in Lower Animals was recently published.[106]

Surgery

Surgery of pet amphibians has been poorly documented in the veterinary literature, although recent reviews of the subject have been found[107,108] (Figure 75-29).

Some of the larger carnivorous frogs, such as the popular Argentine Horned Frog (*Ceratophrys ornata*), are well known for pica, or eating abnormal objects, especially rocks. An occasional rock can be manually extracted with long curved Kelly forceps if it is still located in the stomach. However, foreign bodies that have passed the pylorus and entered the small intestine require an enterotomy. Many of the same techniques

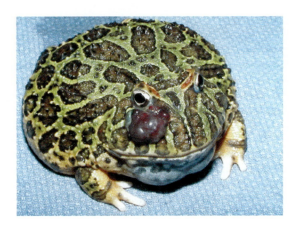

FIGURE 75-28 A purple mass on the face of an Ornate Horned Frog (*Ceratophrys ornata*). The mass, which was removed with a CO_2 laser and a local anesthetic, was described as a hemangioma. (*Photograph courtesy D. Mader.*)

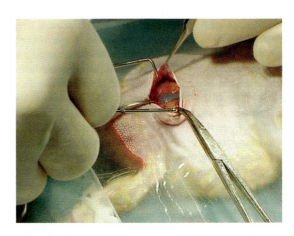

FIGURE 75-29 Ventral midline celiotomy in a frog. Surgical techniques are poorly described in amphibians but should follow closely those described for reptiles (see Chapter 35). (*Photograph courtesy D. Mader.*)

used for reptile patients work well for amphibians (see Chapter 35).

Toe Clip

Toe clipping is a standard method of permanent identification of anurans. Although some field biologists routinely perform digitectomies without sedation of the anuran, the author cannot justify this in the veterinary hospital. Reports show that complications arising from toe clipping (e.g., inflammation) can have an impact on the field population under study.[109] Small anurans can have the toe clipped with iris scissors, and direct pressure is applied to the site until bleeding stops. Larger anurans can be toe clipped with stainless steel liga-clips, and the digit distal to the clamp is removed. The clip falls off in 7 to 28 days. Many salamanders in all probability regenerate an amputated digit or limb, limiting the effectiveness of toe clipping as a permanent means of identification in this order.[110] Although the regenerated tissue is slightly different in appearance than the original tissue, this can vary and is not dependable.

Implantation of Transponder

A highly successful method of permanent identification of amphibians is the implantation of a transponder chip within the amphibian's body.[111] Some debate exists about the preferred site of implantation. A subcutaneous site (e.g., underneath the parotid gland of a toad) has been advocated by some instead of an intracoelomic site. The subcutaneous site avoids the chance of abdominal adhesions forming and associated clinical problems arising from migration of the coelomic implant. A subcutaneously placed transponder may be visible and therefore unacceptable for display animals. The intracoelomic implant avoids this problem. The intracoelomic implant may be administered via the paralumbar region or ventrally, lateral to the midline. Long-term studies comparing the advantages and disadvantages of the two site choices are lacking in amphibians, and choice is a matter of clinician preference at this point in time. Anecdotal reports are found of amphibians shedding their transponders several months after implantation. The transponder possibly migrates and is expelled through the bladder, the intestine, or even transcutaneously. Implantation of a second transponder and regular checking that both transponders are present and working are recommended for specimens that must have permanent identification.

Prolapse of Tissues out of the Cloaca

Prolapse of any tissue out of the cloaca is a life-threatening disorder of amphibians (see Figure 75-24). Rectal tissue and bladder tissue are among the most commonly seen organ prolapses. Predisposing conditions include metabolic abnormalities such as dehydration, hypocalcemia, hypoglycemia, and malnutrition, gastrointestinal foreign bodies, cystic calculi, gastroenteritis, hyperthermia, trauma, and parasitism. Radiographs to rule out gastrointestinal foreign bodies and cystic calculi are suggested. If the prolapse is detected while the mucosa is viable, the prolapse can be gently replaced. Glycerine gel may be applied to the rectal mucosa to moisten and shrink the tissue before placement. If the prolapse appears devitalized, excision of the dead intestine and anastomosis of the healthy tissue may be attempted. An antibiotic pessary may be warranted in some cases, as may parenteral antibiotics. A nylon purse-string suture should be used to close the cloaca for 2 to 3 days, and the amphibian should not be fed until after the suture has been removed. Any predisposing conditions should be corrected. Prognosis is guarded, but many anurans respond favorably.

Celioscopy

Celioscopy has proved useful in sexing nondimorphic species such as the Giant Salamanders (*Andrias* spp.) and Goliath Frogs (*Conrauagoliath*)[112,113] and as a diagnostic tool for many diseases. Incisions can be made in the paralumbar region or just lateral to the midline depending on the purpose of the celioscopy. Identification of anything other than egg mass in an ovulating female is difficult. Lateral recumbency may allow the internal organs to fall away from the hypaxial musculature and allow visualization of the testicle and kidneys. A paramedial midline incision allows best access to the liver, and care should be taken to avoid damaging the midline ventral vein. Tissue glue can be used to close the incision afterward. Large incisions may be closed with 3-0 or 4-0 nylon sutures.

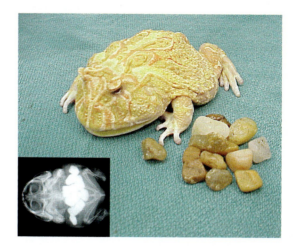

FIGURE 75-30 Postsurgical photograph of an Ornate Horned Frog (*Ceratophrys ornata*). Gastrotomy/enterotomy is a common procedure in amphibians. Note the radiograph of the patient showing the multiple ingested rocks (*inset*). (*Photograph courtesy D. Mader.*)

Celiotomy

Exploratory celiotomy is a useful diagnostic tool and can be used to confirm celioscopic diagnoses or obtain tissue samples or for therapeutic procedures such as gastrotomy (Figure 75-30). In experimental embryology laboratories, ova are routinely harvested from African Clawed Frogs (*Xenopus laevis*) with exteriorizing a portion of the egg mass through a 3-mm to 5-mm paramedial incision and excising a sample. Closure of a celiotomy site may be problematic as the cutaneous sutures are prone to dehisce. The suture line should be under as little tension as possible. A 3-0 or 4-0 nylon in an everting pattern is suggested, with further strength provided with a layer of tissue glue or with internal placement of absorbable sponge material. The patient should be confined in a small space and managed with a minimum of handling for at least 10 days after surgery. Removal of cystic calculi is a common surgery for many phyllomedusine frogs[108,114] because of the number of species that produce uric acid as a nitrogenous waste (see Figure 49-1).

FORMULARY

At present time, few studies support the extra-label use of drugs in amphibian species. This formulary consists of a variety of drugs that the author has used without ill effect in a variety of amphibian species. No claim can be made to the actual efficacy of a drug for the treatment of a given set of clinical conditions. This formulary is intended solely as a guideline for the clinician (see Figure 49-1).

Routes of Delivery

The performance of a drug in an amphibian's body is in part dependent on the route of administration. Transcutaneous administration of drugs in the form of a dip, prolonged bath, or topical application is quite effective for cutaneous diseases, such as fungal and protozoal infections. Given the extensive vascularization of the skin of amphibians, sufficient uptake of the drug may occur to achieve therapeutic levels in the blood and internal organs, and thus, antibacterial baths have been recommended in some circumstances.

Oxytetracycline baths have been advocated in the treatment of aeromoniasis in aquatic larval tanks and adult breeding tanks. Given that many aeromonads are resistant to tetracyclines, the clinician often has to use other antibiotics, and many of these antibiotics are not useful for "bath therapy." Gentamicin baths have been an option for management of septicemia, but the drug concentration must exceed 1 mg/mL solution to reach effective blood levels in *Rana pipiens*.[115,116] Ciprofloxacin 10 mg/L as a 6 to 8 hour bath has been effective in treating many bacterial infections.

Ivermectin (0.2 to 0.4 mg/kg)[117] and praziquantel (8 to 24 mg/kg) solutions have been applied topically to anurans with subsequent reduction in the numbers of parasitic ova shed via the feces. Given the small body size of many amphibians, such as Dendobatid Frogs, administration of drugs via oral or parenteral routes may be impractical. When practical, oral or parenteral routes of administration are preferred to ensure adequate uptake and distribution of any given drug.

Intracoelomic, subcutaneous, and intramuscular injections are the most common routes of drug delivery used in the treatment of amphibians of sufficient body size. Intracoelomic injections may be given in the paralumbar fossa or just off the ventral midline. The skin over the dorsum, shoulder, or pelvis is usually loose enough to allow tenting of the skin for subcutaneous injections. The epaxial musculature is a useful site for the injection of intramuscular medications in salamanders and caecilians. The forelimbs are a preferred site for anurans. The ability of the amphibian mesonephric kidney to excrete many of the commonly used drugs and drug metabolites is not poorly documented.

Amphibians with hydrocoelom or subcutaneous edema may require baths in electrolyte solutions to reduce fluid volume and correct electrolyte abnormalities of plasma. Amphibian Ringer's solution is isotonic to typical amphibian plasma (~230 milliosmoles) and can be created with dissolving 6.6 g NaCl, 0.15 g KCl, 0.15 g CaCl$_2$, and 0.2 g NaHCO$_3$ in 1.0 liter of distilled water.[118] A continuous bath in amphibian Ringer's solution is a suggested supplemental therapy for any amphibian with a bacterial or fungal infection. If amphibian Ringer's solution is not available, 0.5% to 0.6% saline solution is an alternative choice but is lacking in critical electrolytes. Hypertonic solutions may be needed when the amphibian patient has inordinate fluid overload and appears grossly distended or edematous. Simple hypertonic solutions are 0.8% to 0.9% saline or the compounds for amphibian Ringer's solution dissolved in 900 mL or less of distilled water. Dextrose (5% or higher concentration) and hetastarch solutions may also be used as short-term hypertonic baths. Monitor the amphibian while it is in the hypertonic solution and remove it if it appears distressed or when it is within 25% of its normal weight. If the amphibian starts to regain fluid when returned to normal water, it should be returned to isotonic or hypertonic solutions for additional therapy. Some amphibians may need to be maintained in isotonic solutions for several days to weeks after recovery from a severe infection.

The intravenous route is largely unused in amphibians, although euthanasia solution may be administered via cardiocentesis.

The oral route is historically how tetracycline has been administered during *Aeromonas* outbreaks. Anthelmintics and nutritional support may be given via this route. An appropriately sized over-the-cuff intravenous catheter is a useful tube-feeding apparatus for small amphibians. Waterproof paper or a thin wedge of plastic can function as a mouth speculum. Stainless steel rodent feeding tubes work well with larger amphibians.

SOURCES OF MATERIALS MENTIONED IN THE TEXT

Tetra Blackwater Conditioner, Tetra Sales, Blacksburg, Va.
Tricaine methanesulfonate (ethyl m-aminobenzoate, MS-222), Finquel, Argent Chemical Laboratories, Redmond, Wash.

REFERENCES

1. Heatwole H, Carroll RL, editors: *Amphibian biology, volume 4, paleontology, the evolutionary history of amphibians*, Chipping Norton, New South Wales, 2001, Surrey Beatty & Sons.
2. Arnheiter CJ: Husbandry of captive caecilians, *Proc 14th Int Herp Symp Captive Propagation Husbandry* 71-73, 1990.
3. Mylniczenko ND: Caecilians: husbandry and medical management, *Proc Assoc Reptilian Amphibian Vet Annual Conf* 291-297, 2001.
4. Wright KM: An Asian caecilian: *Ichthyophis kohtaoensis*, *Reptile Amphibian Mag* Sept/Oct:22-23, 1992a.
5. Wright KM: The aquatic caecilians, *Reptile Amphibian Mag* Sept/Oct:18-25, 1992b.
6. Heatwole H, Sullivan BK, editors: *Amphibian biology, volume 2, social behavior*, Chipping Norton, New South Wales, 1995, Surrey Beatty & Sons.
7. Barnett SL, Cover JF, Wright KM: Amphibian husbandry and housing. In Wright KM, Whitaker BR, editors: *Amphibian medicine and captive husbandry*, Malabar, Fla, 2001, Krieger Publishing.
8. Mattison C: *The care of reptiles and amphibians in captivity*, New York, 1992, Facts on File Publications.
9. Mattison C: *The care and breeding of amphibians*, New York, 1993, Facts on File Publications.
10. Tucker CS: Water analysis. In Stoskopf M: *Fish medicine*, Philadelphia, 1993, WB Saunders.
11. Marselas GA, Stoskopf MK, Brown MJ, Kane AS, Reimschuessel R: Abdominal ascites in electric eels (*Electrophorus electricusi*) associated with hepatic hemosiderosis and evelated water pH, *J Zoo Wildl Med* 29(4):413-418, 1998.
12. Wright KM: Anatomy for the clinician. In Wright KM, Whitaker BR, editors: *Amphibian medicine and captive husbandry*, Malabar, Fla, 2001, Krieger Publishing.
13. McDiarmid RW, Altig R, editors: *Tadpoles: the biology of anuran larvae*, Chicago, 1999, The University of Chicago Press.
14. Pough FH, Andrews RM, Cadle JE, Crump ML, Savitzky AH, Wells KD: *Herpetology*, Upper Saddle River, NJ, 1998, Prentice Hall.
15. Zug GR, Vitt LJ, Caldwell JP: *Herpetology: an introductory biology of amphibians and reptiles*, San Diego, 2001, Academic Press.
16. Dickerson MC: *The frog book*, New York, 1969, Dover Publications.
17. Duellman WE, Trueb L: *Biology of amphibians*, New York, 1986 McGraw-Hill.
18. Ecker A: *The anatomy of the frog*, Amsterdam, (reprint of original 1889 book) 1971, A. Asher.

19. Francis ETB: *The anatomy of the salamander*, London, 1934, Oxford at the Clarendon Press.
20. Mattison C: *Frogs and toads of the world*, New York, 1987, Facts on File Publications.
21. Noble GK: *The biology of the amphibia*, New York, 1955 (1931), Dover Publications.
22. Porte, KR: *Herpetology*, Philadelphia, 1972, WB Saunders Co.
23. Wells TAG: *The frog*, New York, 1964, Dover Publications.
24. Heatwole H, Barthalmus GT, editors: *Amphibian biology, volume 1, the integument*, Chipping Norton, New South Wales, 1994, Surrey Beatty & Sons.
25. Williams DL, Whitaker BR: The amphibian eye: a clinical review, *J Zoo Wildl Med* 25(1):18-28, 1994.
26. Conant R, Collins JT: *Field guide to amphibians and reptiles of Eastern and Central North America*, New York, 1991, Houghton-Mifflin.
27. Fowler ME: Amphibians and fish. In *Restraint and handling of wild and domestic animals*, Ames, 1978, Iowa State University Press.
28. Diezyck J: Lipid keratopathy of frogs, *Proc 3rd Int Colloq Path Reptiles Amphibians* 95-96, 1989.
29. Anonymous: *Argent Finquel® Package Insert*, NDC 051212-0001-1, revised October 1987.
30. Downes H: Tricaine anesthesia in Amphibia: a review, *Bull Assoc Reptilian Amphibian Vet* 5(2):11-16, 1995.
31. Letcher JL: Intracoelomic use of tricaine methane sulfonate for anesthesia of bullfrogs (*Rana catesbeiana*) and leopard frogs (*Rana pipiens*), *Zoo Biol* 11:243-251, 1992.
32. Lafortune M, Mitchell M, Smith JA: Evaluation of clinical and cardiopulmonary effects of clove oil (eugenol) on leopard frogs, *Rana pipiens*, *Proc Assoc Reptilian Amphibian Vet Annual Conf* 51-53, 2000.
33. Lafortune M, Mitchell M, Smith JA: Evaluation of medetomidine, clove oil and propofol for anesthesia of Leopard Frogs, *Rana pipiens*, *J Herpetol Med* 11(4):13-18, 2001.
34. Von Esse FV, Wright KM: Effect of intracoelomic propofol in White's tree frogs, *Pelodryas caerulea*, *Bull Assoc Reptilian Amphibian Vet* 9(3):7-8, 1999.
35. Vogelnest L: Transponder implants for frog identification, *Bull Assoc Reptile Amphibian Vet* 4(1):4, 1994.
36. Wright KM: Amputation of the tail of a two-toed amphiuma, *Amphiuma means*, *Bull Assoc Reptile Amphibian Vet* 4(1):5, 1994.
37. Wass JA, Kaplan HM: Methoxyflurane anesthesia for *Rana pipiens*, *Lab Anim Sci* 24(4):669-671, 1974.
38. Machin KL: Amphibian pain and analgesia, *J Zoo Wildl Med* 30(1):2-10, 1999.
39. Baranowski-Smith LL, Smith CJV: A simple method for obtaining blood samples from mature frogs, *Lab Anim Sci* 338-339, 1983.
40. Campbell TW: *Avian hematology and cytology*, Ames, 1988, Iowa State University Press.
41. Cathers T, Lewbart GA, Correa M, Stevens JB: Serum chemistry and hematology values for anesthetized American bullfrogs (*Rana catesbeiana*), *J Zoo Wildl Med* 28(2):171-174, 1997.
42. Wright KM: Amphibian hematology. In Wright KM, Whitaker BR, editors: *Amphibian medicine and captive husbandry*, Malabar, Fla, 2001, Krieger Publishing.
43. Hadji-Azimi I, Coosemans V, Canicatti C: Atlas of adult *Xenopus laevis laevis* hematology, *Develop Comp Immunol* 11(4):807-874, 1987.
44. Hawkey CM, Dennett TB: *Color atlas of caomparative veterinary hematology*, London, 1989, Wolfe Medical Publications, Ltd.
45. Jerret DP, Mays CE: Comparative hematology of the hellbender (*Cryptobranchus alleganiensis*) in Missouri, *Copeia* 2(22):331-337, 1973.
46. Pfeiffer CJ, Pyle H, Assashima M: Blood cell morphology and counts in the Japanese newt (*Cynops pyrrhogaster*), *J Zoo Wildl Med* 21(1):54-56, 1990.
47. Kollias GV: Immunologic aspects of infectious disease. In Hoff GL, Frye FL, Jacobson ER: *Diseases of amphibians and reptiles*, New York, 1984, Plenum Press.
48. Marcus LC: *Veterinary biology and medicine of captive amphibians and reptiles*, Philadelphia, 1981, Lea & Febiger.
49. Reichenbach-Klinke H, Elkan E: *Diseases of amphibians*, Neptune City, NJ, 1965, TFH Publications.
50. Wright KM: Nutritional secondary hyperparathyroidism in the Ramsey Canyon leopard frog, *Rana subaquavocalis*, *Proc Assoc Reptilian Amphibian Vet Annual Conf* 41-42, 2001.
51. Divers SJ: The diagnosis of nutritional metabolic bone disease and the treatment of hypocalcemic tetany in an Argentine horned frog (*Ceratophrys ornata*), *Proc Assoc Reptilian Amphibian Vet Annual Conf* 7-9, 1996.
52. Mader DR: Use of calcitonin in green iguanas, *Iguana iguana*, with metabolic bone disease, *Bull Assoc Amphibian Reptile Vet* 3(1):5, 1993.
53. Pessier AP, Roberts DR, Linn M, et al: "Short tongue syndrome," lingual squamous metaplasia and suspected hypovitaminosis A in captive Wyoming toads, *Proc Assoc Reptilian Amphibian Vet* 151-153, 2002.
54. Wright KM: Nutritional secondary hyperparathyroidism in the Ramsey Canyon leopard frog (*Rana subaquavocalis*), *Proc Am Assoc Zoo Vet, Am Assoc Wildl Vet, Assoc Reptilian Amphibian Vet, Nat Assoc Zoo Wildl Vet Joint Conf* 34-45, 2001.
55. McKinnell RG: Lucke tumor of frogs. In Hoff GL, Frye FL, Jacobson ER: *Diseases of amphibians and reptiles*, New York, 1984, Plenum Press.
56. Gruia-Gray J, Desser SS: Ultrastructural, biochemical and biophysical properties of an erythrocytic virus of frogs from Ontario, Canada, *J Wildl Dis* 25(4):487-507, 1989.
57. Gruia-Gray J, Desser SS: Cytopathologic observations and epizootiology of frog erythrocytic virus in bullfrogs (*Rana catesbeiana*), *J Wildl Dis* 28(1):34-41, 1992.
58. Green DE: Pathology of amphibia. In Wright KM, Whitaker BR, editors: *Amphibian medicine and captive husbandry*, Malabar, Fla, 2001, Krieger Publishing.
59. Hengstberger SG, Hyatt AD, Speare R, Coupar BEH: Comparison of epizootic haematopoietic necrosis and Bohle iridoviruses, recently isolated Australian iridoviruses, *Dis Aquatic Organisms* 15:93-107, 1993.
60. Speare R, Smith JR: An iridovirus-like agent isolated from the ornate burrowing frog *Limnodynastes ornatus* in northern Australia, *Dis Aquatic Organisms* 14:51-57, 1992.
61. Cunningham AA, Langton TES, Bennett PM, Lewin JF, Drury SEN, Gough RE, et al: Pathological and microbiological findings from incidents of unusual mortality of the common frog (*Rana temporaria*), *Philosoph Transact R Soc London (Biol Sci)* 351B:1539-1557, 1996.
62. Smith AW, Anderson MP, Skilling DE, Barlough JE, Ensley PK: First isolation of calicivirus from reptiles and amphibians, *Am J Vet Res* 47(8):1718-1721, 1986.
63. Garner M: Fatal systemic herpesvirus infection in three Mexican giant treefrogs, *Pachymedusa dacnicolor*, *Proc Assoc Reptilian Amphibian Vet Annual Conf* 7, 2000.
64. McNamara TS, Charles PC, Kress Y, Weidenheim K, Holmstrom W: Crystalline inclusions associated with vomeronasal organ pathology in red-eyed tree frogs (*Agalychnis callidryas*), *Proc Am Assoc Zoo Vet Annual Conf* 27-29, 1999.
65. Cunningham AA, Langton TES, Bennett PM, Drury SEN, Gough RE, Kirkwood JK: Unusual mortality associated with poxvirus-like particles in frogs (*Rana temporaria*), *Vet Rec* 133:141-142, 1993.
66. Frye FL: An unusual epizootic of anuran aeromoniasis, *JAVMA* 187(11):1223-1224, 1985.
67. Nyman S: Mass mortality in larval *Rana sylvatica* attributable to the bacterium *Aeromonas hydrophila*, *J Herpetol* 20(2):196-201, 1986.

68. Shotts EB: *Aeromonas*. In Hoff GL, Frye FL, Jacobson ER, editors: *Diseases of amphibians and reptiles*, New York, 1984, Plenum Press.
69. Taylor SK, Green DE, Wright KM, Whitaker BR: Bacterial diseases. In Wright KM, Whitaker BR, editors: *Amphibian medicine and captive husbandry*, Malabar, Fla, 2001, Krieger Publishing.
70. Olson ME, Gard S, Brown M, Hampton R, Morck DW: *Flavobacterium indologenes* infection in leopard frogs, *JAVMA* 201(11):1766-1770, 1992.
71. Honeyman VL, Mehren KG, Barker IK, Crawshaw GJ: *Bordetella* septicemia and chlamydiosis in eyelash leaf frogs, *Proc Joint Conf Am Assoc Zoo Vet and Am Assoc Wildl Vet* 68, 1992.
72. Howerth EW: Pathology of naturally occurring chlamydiosis in African clawed frogs, *Xenopus laevis*, *Vet Pathol* 21:28-32, 1984.
73. Howerth EW, Pletcher JM: Diagnostic exercise: death of African clawed frogs, *Lab Anim Sci* 36(3):286-287, 1986.
74. Newcomer CE, Anver MR, Simmons JL, Wilcke BW, Nace GW: Spontaneous and experimental infections of *Xenopus laevis* with *Chlamydia psittaci*, *Lab Anim Sci* 32(6):680-686, 1982.
75. Garner MM, Raymond J, Joslin J, Collins D, Reichard T, Nordhausen R: Three cases of a chlamydia-like or rickettsia-like infection in frogs, *Proc Assoc Reptilian Amphibian Vet Annual Conf* 171-173, 2001.
76. Wright KM: Chlamydial infections of amphibians, *Bull Assoc Reptilian Amphibian Vet* 6(4):8-9, 1996.
77. Nichols DK, Smith AJ, Gardiner CH: Dermatitis of anurans caused by fungal-like protists, *Proc Am Assoc Zoo Vet Annual Conf* 220-222, 1996.
78. Daszak P, Berger L, Cunningham AA, Hyatt AD, Green DE, Speare R: Emerging infectious diseases and amphibian population declines, *Emerg Infect Dis* 5(6):23, 1999; http://www.cdc.gov/ncidod/eid/vol5no6/daszak.htm.
79. Pessier AP, Nichols DK, Longcore JE, Fuller MS: Cutaneous chytridiomycosis in poison dart frogs (*Dendrobates* spp.) and White's treefrogs (*Litoria caerulea*), *J Vet Diagn Invest* 11:194-199, 1999.
80. Nichols DK, Laramide EW: Treatment of cutaneous chytridiomycosis in blue-and-yellow poison dart frogs (*Dendrobates tinctorius*) [poster], *Getting the Jump! on Amphibian Dis Conf* 2000.
81. Mitchell MA, Render JA, Glaze MB, Hamilton H, Spence D, Bercier C, et al: Fungal keratitis in a group of imported helmeted water toads (*Caudiverba caudiverba*), *Proc Am Assoc Zoo Vet Annual Conf* 8-9, 1997.
82. Berger L, Speare R, Thomas A, Hyatt A: Mucocutaneous fungal disease in tadpoles of *Bufo marinus* in Australia, *J Herpetol* 35(2):330-335, 2001.
83. Frye FL, Gillespie D: Saprolegniasis in a zoo collection of aquatic amphibians, *Proc 3rd Int Colloq Path Reptiles Amphibians* 43, 1989.
84. Wright KM: Saprolegniasis in aquatic amphibians, *Reptile Amphibian Mag* 58-60, 1992.
85. Ackermann J, Miller E: Chromomycosis in an African bullfrog *Pyxicephalus adspersus*, *Bull Assoc Reptile Amphibian Vet* 2(2):8-9, 1992.
86. Schmidt RE: Amphibian chromomycosis. In Hoff GL, Frye FL, Jacobson ER, editors: *Diseases of amphibians and reptiles*, New York, 1984, Plenum Press.
87. Valentine BA, Stoskopf MK: Amebiasis in a neotropical giant toad, *JAVMA* 185(1):1418-1419, 1984.
88. Poynton SL, Whitaker BR: Protozoa in poison dart frogs (Dendrobatidae): clinical assessment and identification, *J Zoo Wildl Med* 25(1):29-39, 1994.
89. Stoskopf MK: Fish chemotherapeutics, *Vet Clin North Am Small Anim Pract* 18(2):331-348, 1988.
90. Muzzall PM: Helminth infracommunities of the frogs *Rana catesbeiana* and *Rana clamitans* from Turkey Marsh, Michigan, *J Parasitol* 77(3):366-371, 1991.
91. Patterson-Kane JC, Eckerline RP, Lyons ET, Jewell MA: Strongyloidiasis in a Cope's grey tree frog (*Hyla chrysoscelis*), *J Zoo Wildl Med* 32(1):106-110, 2001.
92. Colwell GJ, Watkins KA: An incidence of fatal subcutaneous parasite load in an imported Indonesian White's tree frog, *Bull Chicago Herp Soc* 28(8):164, 1993.
93. Cosgrove GE, Jared DW: Treatment of skin-invading capillarid nematodes in a colony of South African clawed frogs, *Lab Anim Sci* 27(4):526-527, 1977.
94. Cunningham AA, Sainsbury AW, Cooper JE: Diagnosis and treatment of a parasitic dermatitis in a laboratory colony of African Clawed Frogs (*Xenopus laevis*), *Vet Rec* 138:640-642, 1996.
95. Shields JD: Pathology and mortality of the lung fluke *Haematoloechus longiplexus* (Trematoda) in *Rana catesbeiana*, *J Parasit* 73(5):1005-1013, 1987.
96. Johnson PTJ, Lunde KB, Haight RW, Bowerman J, Blaustein AR: *Ribeiroia ondatrae* (Trematoda: Diegnea) infection induces severe limb malformations in western toads (*Bufo boreas*), *Can J Zoo* 79:370-379, 2001.
97. Graczyk TK, Cranfield MR, Bicknese EJ, Wisnieski AP: Progressive ulcerative dermatitits in a captive, wild-caught, South American giant tree frog (*Phyllomedusa bicolor*) with microsporidial septicemia, *J Zoo Wildl Med* 27(4):522-527, 1996.
98. Duncan AE, Garner M, Reichard T, Bartholomew J, Nordhausen R: Renal myxosporidia in Asian horned frogs, *Megophrys nasuta*, *Proc Assoc Reptilian Amphibian Vet Annual Conf* 23-25, 2000.
99. El-Matbouli M, Hoffman RW: Prevention of experimentally-induced whirling disease in rainbow trout *Oncorrhynchus mytuss* by fumagillin, *Dis Aquatic Organisms* 2:109-113, 1991.
100. Sladky KK, Norton TM, Loomis MR: Trombiculid mites (*Hannemanias* sp.) in Canyon Tree Frogs (*Hyla arenicolor*), *J Zoo Wildl Med* 31(4):570-575, 2000.
101. Vogelnest L: Myiasis in a green tree frog (*Litoria caeulea*), *Bull Assoc Reptile Amphibian Vet* 4(1):4, 1994b.
102. Whitaker BR: The use of polyvinyl chloride glues and their potential toxicity to amphibians, *Proc Am Assoc Zoo Vet* 16-18, 1993.
103. Stoskopf MK, Wisnieski A, Piper L: Iodine toxicity in poison arrow frogs, *Proc Am Assoc Zoo Vet* 86-88, 1985.
104. Carpenter JL, Bachtrach A Jr, Albert DM, Vainisi SJ, Goldstein MA: Xanthomatous keratitis, disseminated xanthomatosis, and atherosclerosis in Cuban tree frogs, *Vet Path* 23:337-339, 1986.
105. Frye FL: Periarticular gout in a pixie frog (*Pyxicephalus delalandii*), *Proc 3rd Int Colloq Path Reptiles Amphibians* 108, 1989.
106. Green DE, Harshbarger J: Spontaneous neoplasia in amphibians. In Wright KM, Whitaker BR, editors: *Amphibian medicine and captive husbandry*, Malabar, Fla, 2001, Krieger Publishing.
107. Wright KM: Surgery of the amphibians, *Vet Clin North Am Exotic Anim Pract* 3(3):753-758, 2000.
108. Wright KM: Surgical techniques. In Wright KM, Whitaker BR, editors: *Amphibian medicine and captive husbandry*, Malabar, Fla, 2001, Krieger Publishing.
109. Golay N, Durrer H: Inflammation due to toe-clipping in natterjack toads (*Bufo calamita*), *Amphibia-Reptilia* 15:81-96, 1994.

110. Davis TM, Ovaska K: Individual recognition of amphibians: effects of toe clipping and fluorescent tagging on the salamander *Plethodon vehiculum, J Herpetol* 35(2):217-225, 2001.
111. Corn PS: Laboratory and field evaluation of effects of PIT tags, *Froglog* 4:2, 1992.
112. Gillespie D, Dresser BL, Maruska ER: Sexing goliath frogs *(Gigantorana = Conrauagoliath)* by laparoscopy, *Proc Joint Conf Am Assoc Zoo Vet and Am Assoc Wildl Vet* 62, 1988.
113. Kramer L, Dresser BL, Maruska EJ: Sexing aquatic salamanders by laparoscopy, *Proc Am Assoc Zoo Vet* 192-194, 1983.
114. Greek TJ: Cystic calculi in the frog, *Phyllomedusa sauvagei, Proc Assoc Reptilian Amphibian Vet* 3-6, 2000.
115. Riviere JE, Shapiro DP, Coppoc GL: Percutaneous absorption of gentamicin by leopard frog *(Rana pipiens), J Vet Pharmacol Ther* 2:235-239, 1979.
116. Teare JA, Wallace RS: Pharmacology of gentamicin in the leopard frog *(Rana pipiens), Proc Am Assoc Zoo Vet* 128-131, 1991.
117. Letcher JL, Glade MG: Efficacy of ivermectin as an anthelmintic in leopard frogs, *JAVMA* 200(4):527-538, 1992.
118. Wright KM, Whitaker BR: Pharmacotherapeutics. In Wright KM, Whitaker BR, editors: *Amphibian medicine and captive husbandry*, Malabar, Fla, 2001, Krieger Publishing.

76
MEDICAL CARE OF SEATURTLES

JEANETTE WYNEKEN, DOUGLAS R. MADER,
E. SCOTT WEBER III, and CONSTANCE MERIGO

SPECIES IDENTIFICATION AND BIOLOGY

Jeanette Wyneken

Seven species of seaturtles are found worldwide. Of these, the following five are considered endangered in the continental United States as defined by the International Union for the Conservation of Nature and Natural Resources (IUCN) red list of threatened species (http://www.iucnredlist.org). Leatherback (*Dermochelys coriacea*), Kemp's and Olive Ridley (*Lepidochelys kempii* and *L. olivacea*), Hawksbill (*Eretmochelys imbricata*), and Green (*Chelonia mydas*). Two species are vulnerable: Flatback (*Natator depressa*) and Loggerhead (*Caretta caretta*) (Table 76-1).

Pressures from interactions with humans (industry and recreation), poaching, predation, habitat encroachment and degradation, and disease together contribute to the worldwide decline in populations (Figures 76-1 and 76-2). Veterinarians who work along coastal regions likely will be presented with opportunities to provide veterinary care to these animals. Because of the legal implications of working with endangered and threatened species, which vary greatly from location to location, veterinarians must check with federal and local authorities regarding medical intervention with these animals. Treatment of endangered species, even under the auspices of a "Good Samaritan," can lead to fines and adjudications against licensure within certain government agencies.

This chapter is intended to give the veterinarian a working protocol for understanding basic seaturtle biology and species identification, assessing medical problems, and providing treatment. Those interested in working with these species are encouraged to pursue more advanced studies and training.

Many websites are available for gathering information on seaturtles (Table 76-2). Interested individuals are encouraged to explore these sites as a plethora of valuable information and useful contacts are accessible online. In addition, an excellent seaturtle LISTSERV, called CTURTLE, provides online support for issues ranging from conservation to rehabilitation to medicine.

Seaturtle Species and Identification

Seaturtles are taxonomically separated into the leathery-shelled (dermochelyid) and the hard-shelled (cheloniid) species. The key characteristics include the presence or absence of complete longitudinal ridges along the **carapace** versus a hard keratinous shell (Dermochelyidae versus Cheloniidae, respectively). The family Dermochelyidae is represented by just one extant species. Within the Cheloniidae, the six species can be distinguished by the number and patterns of particular scales on the head, the form of the jaws, the number of claws, and the numbers and patterns of the plates or **scutes** on the shell. The numbers and patterns of carapacial scutes are key characteristics. The **plastron** also has distinct scute patterns, but these are used most often as landmarks for internal structures rather than for species identification. **Inframarginal** (bridge) scutes are found between the carapace and plastron.[1] Inframarginal counts usually range from three to four but can be highly variable and hence are of limited use as diagnostic characters.

Scutes of the carapace are the **marginals**, **laterals (costals)**, and **vertebral (centrals)**. The first marginal behind the neck is the **nuchal**. The most posterior marginal scutes on each side are termed **supracaudals** (postcentrals). The paired scutes of the plastron (anterior to posterior) are the **gular**, **humeral**, **pectoral**, **abdominal**, **femoral**, and **anal**; unpaired **intergular** and **internal** scutes are not always present (Figure 76-3).

Table 76-1 Status and Geographic Location of Seaturtles Worldwide			
Common Name	**Scientific Name**	**Distribution**	**Status**
Green Turtle	*Chelonia mydas*	Tropical and subtropical Atlantic, Pacific, Indian Oceans	Endangered
Hawksbill	*Eretmochelys imbricata*	Tropical Atlantic, Pacific, Indian Oceans; Black Sea	Endangered
Kemp's Ridley	*Lepidochelys kempii*	Western Atlantic, Nova Scotia south to Mexico	Endangered
Olive Ridley	*Lepidochelys olivacea*	Tropical and subtropical Atlantic, Pacific, and Indian Oceans	Endangered
Leatherback	*Dermochelys coriacea*	Atlantic, Pacific, and Indian Oceans; north to Alaska and south to Australia; Mediterranean Sea; Great Britain to South Africa	Endangered
Flatback	*Natator depressa*	Tropical and subtropical Australian waters	Vulnerable
Loggerhead	*Caretta caretta*	Tropical and subtropical Atlantic, Pacific, and Indian Oceans, and Mediterranean Sea	Vulnerable

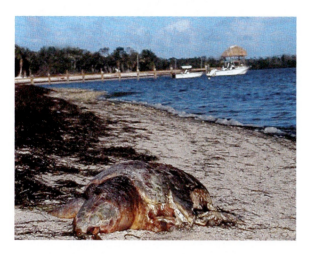

FIGURE 76-1 Seaturtles are losing the battle against man and nature. Here, a Loggerhead *(Caretta caretta)* carcass washed ashore after the turtle was struck by a boat. *(Photograph courtesy D. Mader.)*

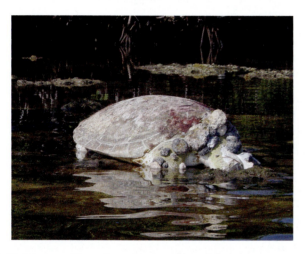

FIGURE 76-2 Natural predators, such as sharks, and natural disease also add to the decline in seaturtle populations worldwide. This adult Green Turtle *(Chelonia mydas)* was found dead in the shallows, overwhelmed with fibropapillomas. *(Photograph courtesy L. Pace.)*

Historically, far more species of seaturtles existed than we find today. Many of the various "experiments" by multiple turtle lineages invading the marine environment went extinct. Just seven species persist today: *Dermochelys coriacea* (Leatherback), *Caretta caretta* (Loggerhead), *Chelonia mydas* (Green), *Eretmochelys imbricata* (Hawksbill), *Lepidochelys kempii* (Kemp's Ridley), *Lepidochelys olivacea* (Olive Ridley), and *Natator depressa* (Flatback).

Leatherbacks lack distinct head scales as adults, have no claws, and have a thin keratin covering on the jaws. The cheloniid seaturtles are characterized and distinguished from one another by the scales on the head, carapace shape and pattern, and inframarginal scute characteristics, and the numbers of claws on the flippers. Most species have two claws associated with digits I and II. Claw I is on digit I and is usually larger than claw II; in adult males, claw I is enlarged and strongly curved ventrally. The number of claws on the front and hind limbs is the same. Figure 76-4 compares the distinguishing features of all seven species.

Table 76-2	Useful Seaturtle Websites

Archie Carr Center for Seaturtle Research Bibliography Site
http://webluis.fcla.edu/cgi-bin/cgiwrap/fclwlv3/wlv3/DGref/DBST/CM02/P1basic

A Bibliography of the Loggerhead Sea Turtle *Caretta caretta* (Linnaeus 1758)
http://www.flmnh.ufl.edu/natsci/herpetology/caretta/Caretta.htm

Marine Turtle Newsletter
http://www.seaturtle.org/mtn/PDF/MTN91.pdf

Hematocrit and Plasma Biochemical Data for Sea Turtles in Florida
http://accstr.ufl.edu/blood_chem.htm

UF Sea Turtle Necropsy Protocol
http://www.vetmed.ufl.edu/sacs/wildlife/seaturtletechniques/

UF Necropsy Report Form
http://www.vetmed.ufl.edu/sacs/wildlife/seaturtletechniques/necropsyreport2.htm

Florida Sea Turtle Grants Program administered through the Caribbean Conservation Corporation
http://www.helpingseaturtles.org

CTURTLE: An E-Mail Information Network for Sea Turtle Biology and Conservation

The Archie Carr Center for Sea Turtle Research at the University of Florida has established CTURTLE, a LISTSERV-managed e-mail network on the Internet.

This LISTSERV provides a format for rapid information exchange. Subscribers can post messages/information to the CTURTLE e-mail system that instantly send electronic message/information to all other CTURTLE subscribers. CTURTLE provides the opportunity to respond to conservation/rehabilitation issues when time is a critical factor. When an ecologic crisis involving seaturtles or their habitat occurs, the worldwide community can be informed instantly. CTURTLE is a forum for ideas, an avenue to announce job opportunities and volunteer programs, and a vehicle for discussion of research and conservation ideas or problems. The possibilities are limited only by the imagination of the participants. CTURTLE also abstracts lists and information from other LISTSERVs that are of interest to subscribers to CTURTLE. The success of CTURTLE depends on its members and their participation. The more people who subscribe, the greater the database of information.

1. To subscribe from an Internet address, send an e-mail message to LISTSERV@lists.ufl.edu with this one-line message: SUBSCRIBE CTURTLE (your first name) (your last name)
2. To post information to all subscribers on the list, send an e-mail message to CTURTLE@lists.ufl.edu.

   Because submissions to CTURTLE are restricted to subscribers only, all submissions by subscribers must be made from the e-mail address from which they subscribed.
3. For general information on LISTSERV commands, send an e-mail message to LISTSERV@lists.ufl.edu with the one-line message: GET LISTSERV REFCARD

   Note that you send only commands (e.g., SUBSCRIBE) to the LISTSERV@lists.ufl.edu address and that you send messages to be distributed to all subscribers to the CTURTLE@lists.ufl.edu address.

The hard-shelled seaturtles have keratinous scales on the dorsal and lateral head that are used in identification of species. The **prefrontal** scales are a key characteristic. They occur in pairs on the snout (Figure 76-5). *Chelonia mydas* and *N. depressa* have one pair of prefrontal scales. The other species

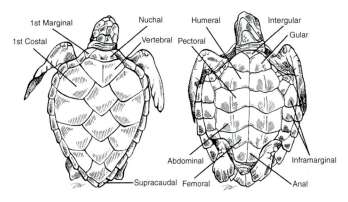

FIGURE 76-3 The scutes of the carapace and plastron are keratinous. Their pattern and number can be diagnostic in determination of species. Scutes in different parts of the carapace, bridge, or plastron are named here. *(With permission, J. Wyneken, 2001, Guide to the anatomy of sea turtles, NMFS Tech. Publication NOAA Tech., Memo NMFS-SEFSC-470.)*

all have two pairs and may have one or more **supernumerary** scales along the midline that separate the pairs. Other head scales (**supraocular, postocular, frontal, frontoparietal, parietal, interparietal, temporal,** and **tympanic scales**) may vary slightly in form but not in position relative to one another.

The form of the keratinous cover of the jaw (rhamphotheca) may be used for species identification. Most species have sharp cutting edges on crushing plates. However, in *C. mydas,* the upper rhamphotheca has a finely serrated edge; the lower rhamphotheca is serrated with spike-like projections along its edges (Figure 76-6).

Just one dermochelyid species exists: the Leatherback, *D. coriacea* (Figure 76-7). It is black with white speckling. Five dorsal ridges run the length of the carapace, two ridges form the margins, and ventral ridges are seen in hatchlings but are usually not obvious in adults. A notch occurs in each side of the upper jaw; the flippers and hind feet lack claws.

The six cheloniid species can be distinguished geographically in some cases (see Table 76-1).[2] The Flatback (*N. depressa*) is endemic to Australia; *L. kempii* (both described subsequently) is restricted to the North Atlantic. All can be distinguished from one another with external characteristics, starting with the prefrontal scales on top of the snout and the scutes on the carapace. The Green Turtle and the Flatback each have one pair of prefrontal scales (see Figure 76-5).

The Green Turtle has a smooth carapace that lacks keels and four pairs of lateral scutes (Figure 76-8). Carapace color changes with age. It is black in hatchlings and then turns brown and tan in juveniles; and in adults it is olive or gray-green, sometimes with speckles of yellow and brown. The plastron is white in hatchlings. It turns creamy yellow, sometimes temporarily pink or gray depending on the population. Adult *C. mydas* have a creamy yellow plastron except in more melanistic Pacific Green Turtles (referred to as Black Turtles) that have a gray plastron. Usually four inframarginal scutes are on each side. The Green Turtle has one claw on each limb.

The Flatback is distinct from other cheloniid species (Figure 76-9). Flatback hatchlings are light gray, and each carapacial scute is rimmed with dark gray. The marginal scutes caudal to the flippers form a serrated edge in silhouette. As Flatbacks grow, the carapace becomes solid or mottled gray; the carapacial scutes appear softer than in other cheloniids and feel waxy. The body is not as tall as in other cheloniids; however, the carapace is not flat as the name implies. The lateral margins of carapace are flat or curl slightly upward. The plastron is white or pale yellow. The flippers and hind feet typically have one claw.

The remaining cheloniid species each have two pairs of prefrontal scales, and, as young, they have keels (ridges) on their shells. The Loggerhead (Figure 76-10, *A*) has a large head and brown carapace with five, or sometimes four, lateral scutes. The nuchal scute (the marginal just dorsal to the neck) is in contact with the first lateral scute. In hatchlings, the carapace is brown with various shades of dark gray (Figure 76-10, *B*). The plastron of hatchlings is light tan to brown. In juveniles and adults, it is creamy and tan. The carapaces of juveniles often develop streaks of yellow and tan, and sometimes the scutes slightly overlap at their margins. In adults, no overlap of scutes is seen. The carapace is primarily brown, with occasional individuals retaining some tans or even black. The shells of juvenile and adult Loggerheads often host large epibiont communities. Loggerheads have two claws on each limb.

The Hawksbill has a medium to dark brown carapace and the plastron as a hatchling. The head of the Hawksbill soon elongates so that, even in turtles as small as 15 cm, the head is nearly twice as long as it is wide, and the rhamphothecae form a long narrow distinctive beak (Figure 76-11). The carapaces of juveniles and adults have distinctive patterns of yellow, black, tan and brown radiating through scutes that overlap at their margins (Figure 76-12). This color persists though adulthood. The nuchal scute does not articulate with the first lateral scute in Hawksbills. The plastron is light tan. Each plastral scute may retain a spot of dark color in very young turtles. Hawksbills have two claws on each foot.

The last two species of seaturtles that occur in United States waters are both members of the genus *Lepidochelys* (Figure 76-13). Both are primarily gray in color. The Kemp's Ridley occurs in the Gulf of Mexico and East Coast waters. The Olive Ridley occurs in Pacific and South Atlantic waters (but occasionally strays into North Atlantic regions). The hatchlings of both species are gray-brown. The carapace grows more rapidly in width than length for some periods so that both species are nearly round in silhouette. Much of this growth is in the marginal scutes, which become wide.

Olive Ridley Turtles typically have more than six normally aligned lateral scutes, six or more normally aligned vertebral scutes, and on the head, many supraoccular scales. Kemp's Ridleys, in contrast, have four or five lateral scutes and just five vertebrals. In both species, often four (sometimes three) inframarginal scutes characteristically each have a pore (Figure 76-14). Ridleys have two claws on each flipper and foot.

Natural History

Seaturtles tend to be long-lived and late maturing. In most species, longevity records are limited and often are "best guesses." Perhaps the life span is in the range of 50 to 75 years, somewhat less than the antiquity that marks other giant species such as the Galapagos and Aldabra Tortoises.

The genders can be differentiated from one another by external characteristics only after puberty, which, depending on species, ranges in age from 15 to 20 years. Mature males

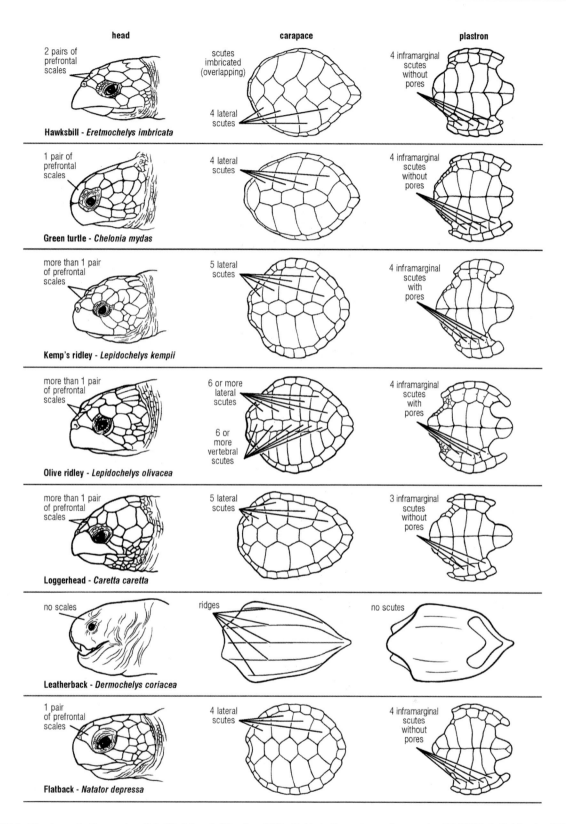

FIGURE 76-4 Key to seaturtle species. *(Modified from J. Wyneken, 2001, Guide to the anatomy of sea turtles, NMFS Tech. Publication NOAA Tech., Memo NMFS-SEFSC-470.)*

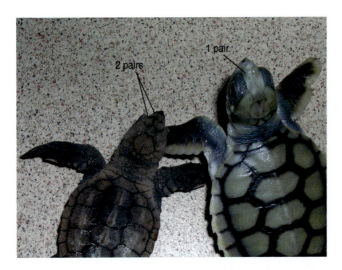

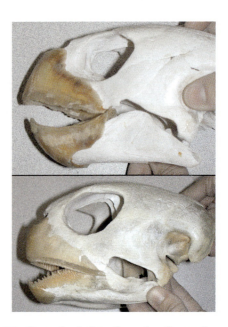

FIGURE 76-5 Prefrontal scales are a characteristic that separates the cheloniid seaturtles into two major groups. The presence of two pairs of prefrontal scales *(left)* is diagnostic for *C. caretta* (shown), *E. imbricata, L. kempii* and *L. olivacea*. One pair of prefrontal scales *(right)* is diagnostic for *C. mydas* and *N. depressa* (shown). *(Photograph courtesy J. Wyneken.)*

FIGURE 76-6 Seaturtles lack teeth, as do other turtle species. The upper and lower jaws are covered by keratinous rhamphothecae. Most species have sharp cutting edges on crushing plates *(top)*; however, the herbivorous Green Turtles *(C. mydas)* *(bottom)* have serrated edges on the rhamphothecae. *(Photographs courtesy J. Wyneken.)*

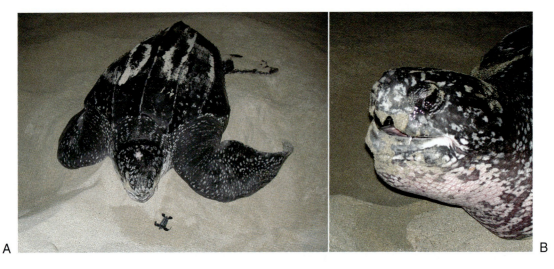

FIGURE 76-7 A, The Leatherback *(D. coriacea)* is the largest of all the seaturtles and is black with white stripes (young) or white spots (juveniles and adults). The hatchlings have scales that are lost in the juveniles. The carapace has five longitudinal ridges running its length. **B,** The jaws have little keratin, and a characteristic notch is seen in each side. *(Photographs courtesy J. Wyneken.)*

have long, prehensile tails that extend well beyond the carapace margins (Figure 76-15) and the cloacal opening is closer to the tail tip than the most caudal part of the plastron. The tails of mature females (and immature turtles) are short and seldom extend beyond the carapace except in adult Leatherbacks. The cloacal opening is close to the plastron in females.

The age to maturity is becoming better understood in several species, although several years of variability probably exist. The same species may differ in age to maturity with the ocean basin in which it lives. Maturity in cheloniid species have estimates of roughly 25 to 40 to 50 years, with the younger estimates primarily coming from Atlantic populations and the older estimates from Pacific populations.[3,4] Interestingly, the largest and the smallest species, the Leatherback and the Kemp's Ridley turtles, appear to mature at much younger ages; estimates of around 10 to 12 years are well supported.[5,6]

Adult body weights vary with species and between species from different locations. Table 76-3 lists approximate adult size and weights.

For centuries, seaturtles have been exploited. Meat, oils, leather, and jewelry were the incentive for capture and slaughter. Green Turtles and Hawksbills, with their beautiful shells, were killed for vanity purposes. The seaturtle industry has been banned in the United States and other countries. In many places, possession or trade in seaturtle artifacts is illegal.

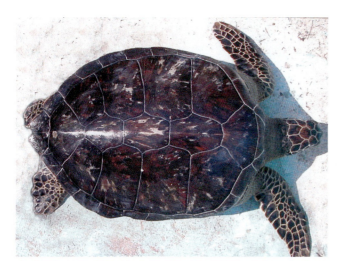

FIGURE 76-8 The Green Turtle *(C. mydas)* lacks keels on its smooth shell. This species changes colors dramatically from hatchling (black carapace with white ventral surfaces) to adult (brown, tan, or olive gray). *(Photograph courtesy D. Mader.)*

Harvest is still a problem in many countries. Members of the genus *Lepidochelys* exhibit a coordinated nesting event known as an "arribada." *L. kempii* and some smaller populations of *L. olivacea* will mass nest for several months of the year. This occurs mainly at night for *L. olivacea* and during the night and day for *L. kempii*. The synchronous emergence of 100 to 10,000 females to oviposit occurs over a 1- to 3-day period, and repeats approximately every 30 days for the season.[7] Decades of egg and turtle harvesting during these events combined with heavy incidental mortality in fisheries have taken a toll on the Atlantic Ridley population.

Current threats to seaturtles include accidental capture by fishing nets and long lines and entanglement in fishing lines and lobster or crab trap lines (Figure 76-16). Trauma from boats, personal watercraft, and dredging equipment accounts for many of the calls to rehabilitation facilities.

Environmental (chemical, agricultural run-off) may debilitate and in-water (plastic bags, other trash) pollution kills many animals before they are found. Habitat destruction, loss of nesting beaches, disorientations from artificial lighting, predation (nestlings to carnivores and adults to sharks), and natural disease are taking their toll on these remaining giant marine reptiles.

MEDICINE AND SURGERY

Douglas R. Mader

Many coastal locales have "rescue" networks or rehabilitation facilities that are capable of responding to strandings or aquatic emergencies. Once identified and located, the animals should be taken to a permitted health care facility immediately. Animals should be transported in ventral recumbency on a padded surface and be kept moistened with wet towels, misters, or some sort of irrigation.

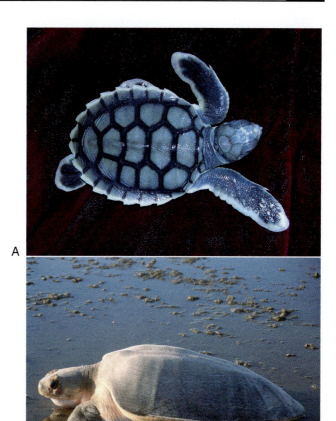

FIGURE 76-9 Flatback Seaturtles *(N. depressa)* are endemic to Australia. **A,** This species has dark pigment around each scute in hatchlings. **B,** As a juvenile or an adult, it is primarily gray or gray and tan dorsally and white or light tan ventrally. The carapace of the adult Flatback has upturned lateral edges. This species has thin keratinous scutes and scales, so the skin is pliable and the carapacial scute pattern is not easily discerned. The flippers retain more flexibility in the digits than many other cheloniids. The Flatback has powerful jaws and can have a contrary disposition. *(Photographs courtesy J. Wyneken [A] and K. Pendoley [B].)*

Extreme caution should be taken when handling any seaturtle because even ill, injured, or otherwise weakened animals may inflict a severe bite or flipper slap to unsuspecting or inexperienced handlers.

Before medical intervention is initiated, appropriate agencies should be notified and stranding reports competed. Federal and local ordinance dictates the necessary notification and documentation. Table 76-2 lists several websites with valuable information. In particular, the website for the **University of Florida Necropsy Report Form** includes an excellent "printer-friendly" **Stranding Report** that can be readily downloaded.

On arrival, a standard protocol should be used for all animals. "Lack of funds" should not be an excuse to cut medical corners when working with endangered species.

The initial diagnostic evaluation should include a complete history (as much as possible). Knowledge of how and where the animal was recovered often gives clues as to the medical problems.

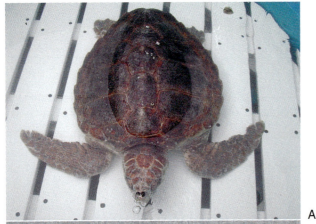

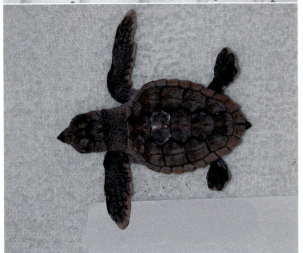

FIGURE 76-10 **A,** The Loggerhead (*Caretta caretta*) is a brown turtle with an obviously proportionately larger head than the other cheloniid species. It has two pairs of prefrontal scales and two claws on its limbs. **B,** Hatchlings, juveniles, and adults are mostly brown with gray and tan coloration. (*Photographs courtesy D. Mader [A] and J. Wyneken [B].*)

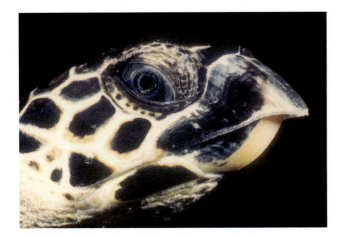

FIGURE 76-11 The head of the Hawksbill (*E. imbricata*) is elongated so that, even in turtles as small juveniles, the head is nearly twice as long as it is wide and the rhamphothecae form a long narrow distinctive beak. (*Photograph courtesy D. Mader.*)

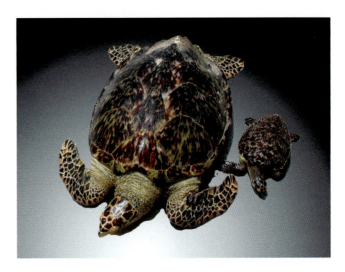

FIGURE 76-12 Hawksbills (*E. imbricata*) have overlapping scutes at most life stages. The beautiful epidermal scutes on the carapace and plastron are the source of "Tortoiseshell" used in jewelry. These colors differ little between juvenile and adult stages. (*Photograph courtesy J. Wyneken.*)

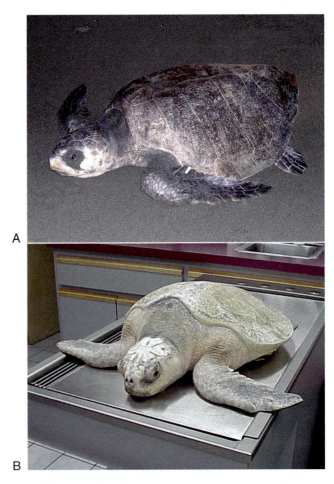

FIGURE 76-13 Both species of the Ridleys are primarily gray in color, and the carapace is nearly round in outline. **A,** The Olive Ridley (*Lepidochelys olivacea*) has many more vertebral and lateral scutes than the Kemp's Ridley (*L. kempii*). **B,** Kemp's Ridleys (*L. kempii*) have four or five lateral scutes and just five vertebrals. (*Photographs courtesy of J. Wyneken [A] and D. Mader [B].*)

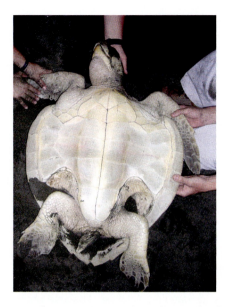

FIGURE 76-14 This ventral view of an Olive Ridley (*Lepidochelys olivacea*) shows the almost round outline of the shell, the wide marginal scutes, and the pores in the inframarginal scutes that are characteristic of this genus. (*Photographs courtesy of J. Wyneken.*)

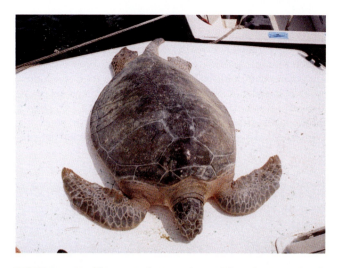

FIGURE 76-15 This ventral view of an adult male Green Turtle (*Chelonia mydas*) shows the white ventral surfaces and the long tail with the subterminally located cloacal opening. (*Photograph courtesy J. Watters*).

Table 76-3 Size, Weight, and Diet of Seaturtles

Species	SCL Hatchling	SCL Adult	Weight Range*	Natural Diets
Green Turtle (*Chelonia mydas*)	45-57 mm	59-117 cm	96-186 kg	Hatchlings omnivorous. Juveniles and adults herbivorous. Sponges, jellyfish, algae and sea grass.
Hawksbill (*Eretmochelys imbricata*)	39-50 mm	63-94 cm	78-91 kg	Hatchlings omnivorous. Adults omnivorous or spongivorous.
Kemp's Ridley (*Lepidochelys kempii*)	38-46 mm	58-75 cm	32-49 kg	Omnivorous. Vegetation, crustaceans and mollusks
Olive Ridley (*Lepidochelys olivacea*)	40-50 mm	56-78 cm	35-45 kg	Omnivorous. Vegetation, crustaceans, tunicates, and jellyfish.
Leatherback (*Dermochelys coriacea*)	56-63 mm	114-176 cm CCL	200-916 kg	Gelatinivorous. Jellyfish, cnidarians, and tunicates.
Flatback (*Natator depressa*)	56-66 mm	81-97 cm	80-90 kg	Omnivorous. Echinoderms, crustaceans, and sea grass
Loggerhead (*Caretta caretta*)	38-55 mm	70-125 cm	170-182 kg	Omnivorous-carnivorous. Mollusks, crustaceans, algae and sea grass

*Adult female.
From Bjordal KA: Foraging ecology and nutrition of sea turtles. In: Lutz PL, Musick JA (eds): *The biology of sea turtles* Boca Raton, Fla, 1997, CRC Press, p199-231; Dodd K: A Bibliography of Sea Turtles (website listed in Table 76-2); Ernst CH, Barbour RW: *Turtles of the world*, Washington, DC, 1989, Smithsonian Institute Press; Hirth H: Depart. of the Interior, Biol. Report 97(1), 120 pp 1997; Witzell WN: FAO Fisheries Synopsis No. 137, 82 pp, 1983.
CCL, Curved carapace length; *SCL*, straight carapace length.

Physical Examination

The physical assessment should be performed following a prescribed routine each time to ensure that nothing is missed. Chapter 30 describes, in detail, proper physical examination techniques for reptiles. These procedures are easily applied to seaturtles.

Saving the obvious problem(s) for last (e.g., fish hook, fractured carapace) is often recommended so that other abnormalities are not overlooked.

All animals should be weighed and the core body temperature recorded (measured from the cloaca). In addition, measurements such as straight and curved carapace lengths (SCL, CCL), straight and curved carapace widths (SCW, CCW) and straight plastron length (SPL) should be collected.[1] These data provide a proxy for estimating of maturity and a baseline for future assessment and progress.

A minimal database of complete laboratory analysis (complete blood count, plasma chemistries), whole body radiographs, and when necessary, microbiologic cultures should be collected. In some situations (such as investigation of a disease outbreak), blood and serum should be banked.

Neurologic Examination

A comprehensive neurologic examination should be performed on all patients with any neurologic abnormalities or spinal or head trauma.

The seaturtle nervous system is similar enough in form and function to mammals that a general neurologic examination, including a cranial nerve (CN) evaluation, should be effective in determining location of neurologic damage or disease.[9] Chrisman et al[9] published a complete neurologic assessment protocol based on their work with five normal and six neurologically abnormal animals. The illustration on page 8 shows a Seaturtle Neurological Assessment worksheet that Chrisman and her colleagues developed to evaluate patients.

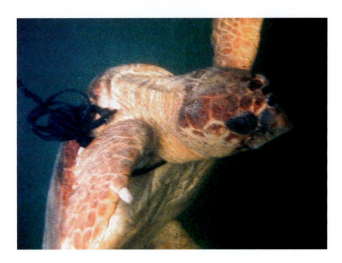

FIGURE 76-16 Entanglements in fishing lines, trap lines, and nets are a common hazard for seaturtles, such as this Loggerhead *(C. caretta)*. *(Photograph courtesy Marathon Sea Turtle Hospital.)*

Examinations should start with a quiet observation of the animal free swimming in the water (if possible). Once observations have been made, both an "Aquatic" and "Terrestrial" assessment should be performed. By following the protocol, even novice clinicians should be able to reasonably locate the site of the lesion.

Lesion identification serves two purposes. First, knowledge of the neurologic damage allows the clinician to formulate an educated prognosis, thus providing valuable information regarding potential expenditure of effort and resources (e.g., triage). Second, regular assessments provide information regarding response to treatments and likelihood of future recovery.[9]

Blood Collection

Published normal hematologic and biochemical values for seaturtles are few. Most of the available data are from private collections or small populations. The University of Florida has an ongoing database available on their website (http://accstr.ufl.edu/blood_chem.htm) for Florida seaturtles. Table 76-4 lists some normal values reported in recent literature.[8,10,11] Gicking et al[12] reported plasma protein electrophoresis values of the Atlantic Loggerhead Seaturtle (Table 76-5).[12]

Blood is best collected from either the supravertebral (dorsal occipital or cervical) sinus or the external jugular vein, or the dorsal tail vein in large turtles. Whitaker and Krum[8] also discuss blood sample collection from the metatarsal vein. The best results are obtained with a non-anticoagulated coated syringe. Fresh whole blood smears should be made immediately on collection of the sample.

Seaturtle Neurologic Assessment Form

From Chrisman CL, Walsh M, Meeks JC et al: Neurologic examination of sea turtles, *Am J Vet Med Assoc* 211(8):1043-1047, 1997.

Table 76-4	Selected Hematology, Plasma, and Serum Chemistry Values from Seaturtles[8,10]		
Parameter	A	B	C
Hematology			
Hematocrit (Hct; %)	30.1 ± 3.0	22 ± 5.33	NA
Red blood cells ($10^6/\mu L$)	NA	0.39 ± 0.08	NA
White blood cells ($10^3/\mu L$)*	NA	14.67 ± 5.8	
Chemistries			
Alanine aminotransferase (ALT; IU/L)	NA	NA	10-30
Alkaline phosphatse (ALK; IU/L)	465.3 ± 306.4	73.9 ± 36.9	10-60
Aspartate aminotransferase (AST; IU/L)	160.7 ± 42.6	122.5 ± 37.8	100-350
Bilirubin (mg/dL)	NA	NA	<0.1
Blood urea nitrogen (BUN; mg/dL)	161.7 ± 28	101.7 ± 17.8	20-80
Calcium (mg/dL)	6.3 ± 1.3	7.1 ± 0.8	6-11
Carbon dioxide (mEq/L)	NA	NA	16-29
Cholesterol (mg/dL)	NA	NA	41-160
Creatine kinase (CK; IU/L)	2832 ± 1698.6	1614.5 ± 1677	NA
Creatinine (mg/dL)	NA	NA	<0.3
Glucose (mg/dL)	118.7 ± 16.7	131.4 ± 10.2	60-120
Iron ($\mu g/dL$)	NA	NA	20-45
Lactate dehydrogenase (LDH; IU/L)	6297.7 ± 5284.8	108.8 ± 63.5	50-350
Magnesium (mg/dL)	NA	2.42 ± 0.8	NA
Phosphorus (mg/dL)	9 ± 1.8	5.3 ± 3.5	6-11
Triglycerides (mg/dL)	NA	NA	<285
Uric acid (UA; mg/dL)	NA	NA	<2
Total protein (TP; g/dL)	3.2 ± 0.6	2 ± 0.8	3-5
Albumin (g/dL)	1.6 ± 0.3	1 ± 0.26	NA
Globulin (g/dL)	1.6 ± 0.4	0.95 ± 0.65	NA
Electrolytes			
Sodium (mEq/L)	150 ± 4	157.0 ± 1	155-165
Potassium (mEq/L)	4.1 ± 0.8	4.6 ± 0.4	3-5
Chloride (mEq/L)	115.5 ± 3.9	121.0 ± 9.8	114-123

A, Rehabilitated Kemp's Ridleys (*Lepidochelys kempi*) before release from the New England Aquarium. Chemistry values from serum.[8]
B, Loggerhead Seaturtles (*Caretta caretta*) <2 kg housed at the New England Aquarium. Chemistry values from plasma.[8]
C, Mature *C. mydas, C. caretta, E. Imbricata*, and *L. Kempi*. Chemistry values from serum.[10]
*Natt and Herrick's solution.

Table 76-5	Plasma Protein Fractions Identified in 29 Loggerhead Seaturtles (*Caretta caretta*)
Parameter	Value (± SD)
Total protein	4.3 ± 0.72
Albumin	1.0 ± 0.17
Alpha	0.48 ± 0.10
Beta	0.80 ± 0.20
Gamma	1.94 ± 0.62
A:G[†]	0.33 ± 0.10

Modified from Gicking JC, Foley AM, Harr KE, Raskin RE, Jacobson ER: Plasma protein electrophoresis of the Atlantic Loggerhead Sea Turtle, *Caretta caretta, J Herp Med Surg* 14(3):13-18, 2004.
[†]Alpha globulin:Gamma globulin ratio.
SD, Standard deviation.

Hematocrit tubes should be filled, and then the balance of the sample should be transferred to a lithium heparin collection vial. Ethylenediamine tetraacetic acid (EDTA) tends to lyse turtle blood and should not be used.[13]

The supravertebral sinus is generally the most commonly used site. Blood is collected from both adults and hatchlings with this approach. For access to the supravertebral sinus, the head should be extended and slightly ventroflexed (Figure 76-17). Needle size varies with patient size, but generally 20 to 22 gauge, 1 to 1.5-inches long, for adults, and 25 to 27 gauge for hatchlings. The needle is placed to either side of the nuchal crest, 2 to 4 cm caudal to the skull, and directed axially toward the dorsal midline of the vertebra. The sinus is immediately to either side of the midline. Gentle negative pressure is applied to the syringe as soon as it enters the skin, and then the needle is advanced until it encounters bone. Generally, the tip enters the vein at this point. If no blood is aspirated, then the needle should be gently redirected cranially, caudally, medially, or laterally in small increments.

If necessary, an ultrasound probe can be used to help identify the location of the sinus. This is especially useful in large patients.

Collection of blood from extremely large patients may be difficult. Long spinal needles may be needed to reach the supravertebral vein, and sedation may be needed to prevent injury to the handlers if the animal is too strong or aggressive. In addition, accidental aspiration of lymph into the sample is not uncommon and essentially invalidates most parameters (see Chapter 28).

An alternative approach is the external jugular vein. Similarly sized needles are used as in the previous technique. Again, with the head extended and slightly ventroflexed, the vein is located paravertebrally in either the 11 o'clock or 1 o'clock position of the neck (with 12 o'clock being dorsal and 6 o'clock being ventral) (Figure 76-18). There are no obvious bony borders; however these veins lie between the paired

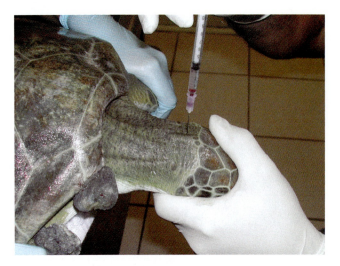

FIGURE 76-17 For access to the supravertebral sinus, the head should be extended and slightly ventroflexed. The needle (size varies with patient size, but generally 20 to 22 gauge, 1 to 1.5 inch long for adults, and 25 to 27 gauge for hatchlings) is placed to either side of the superoccipital (nuchal) crest, 2 to 4 cm caudal to the skull, and directed axially toward the dorsal midline of the vertebra. *(Photograph courtesy D. Mader.)*

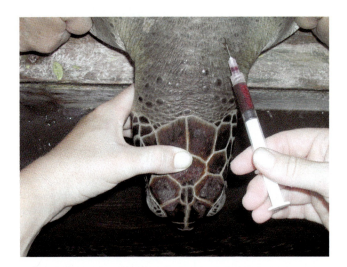

FIGURE 76-18 For a sample from the external jugular vein, the head is extended and slightly ventroflexed. The vein is located paravertebrally in either the 11 o'clock or 1 o'clock position of the neck (with 12 o'clock being dorsal and 6 o'clock being ventral). *(Photograph courtesy D. Mader.)*

suspensory muscles of the neck. Tilting the animal slightly head-down fills this vein so it is easier to access. A big advantage is that lymph contamination is not likely.

Some handlers advocate hanging the patient upside down for collection of blood samples. The theory is that the head-down position enhances blood flow to the veins and sinuses, thus making sample collection easier. Although this may be true, intraocular pressure has been shown to increase three to four times over ventral and dorsal recumbency, respectively.[14] Although no evidence exists that this practice causes problems, patient stress is likely heightened and the pressure changes may prove to be detrimental at a later date.

Either of these sites can be used for intravenous (IV) catheter placement. This author prefers a simple cutdown

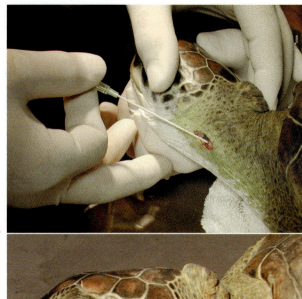

FIGURE 76-19 **A,** A simple cutdown approach exposes the external jugular vein. **B,** A standard small mammal jugular catheter is used. *(Photograph courtesy D. Mader.)*

approach with the external jugular (Figure 76-19). A standard small mammal jugular catheter is used. IV fluids, medications, and if needed, parenteral nutrition can all be administered via the IV catheter.

Cytology

Cytologic analysis is another valuable tool for diagnosis of various problems. Fecal analysis, via flotation, sedimentation, and direct saline smears, should be performed on all new patients and on hospitalized and resident seaturtles on a regular basis. Chapter 21 discusses fecal parasite analysis in great detail.

Coelomocentesis can be a useful diagnostic aid for assessment of general health. Healthy seaturtles, not uncommonly, may have some clear coelomic fluid present (incidental finding during coelioscopy). With renal, hepatic, or cardiovascular disease or inflammatory conditions (gastrointestinal foreign bodies, coelomitis), fluid may accumulate (Figure 76-20).

With the patient in ventral recumbency and one rear prefemoral fossa exposed out over the edge of a table, the area just cranial to the thigh is aseptically prepared while an assistant extends the limb. A long (6+ cm) IV catheter is inserted mid fossa, directed dorsally toward the midline at

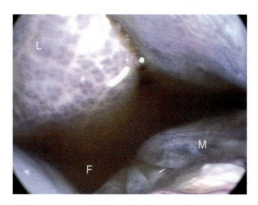

FIGURE 76-20 Coelomic fluid is not uncommon, even in normal turtles. However, in this endoscopy, the fluid is discolored and should be sampled for both cytology and microbiologic testing. L, Lung; F, fluid; M, mesentery. *(Photograph courtesy D. Mader.)*

a 45-degree angle. The needle tip passes through the skin, the subcutaneous (SQ) adipose tissue, and then the coelomic membrane, which is penetrated with an obvious "pop." Accumulated fluid readily flows into the catheter. If large amounts of fluid need to be drained, the stylet should be removed and the catheter left in place, assuming aseptic techniques are followed.

Fluid should be analyzed for cytology, protein content, and culture and sensitivity. This is a simple, rapid, and valuable aid in determination of internal damage after fish-hook ingestion (to rule out perforation).

Cerebrospinal fluid analysis (CSF) is another valuable tool for turtles with neurologic disease. The animal should be sedated to prevent movement, and the head extended and ventroflexed (as in blood sampling). The area immediately caudal to the superoccipital crest is aseptically prepared.

Standard small mammal spinal needles are used, with size based on the size of the patient. The needle is directed cranioventrally, aimed at the point of the mandible. Insertion takes the needle tip through the skin, the connective tissue, and a tough fibrous ligament dorsal to the foramen magnum. Gentle but firm pressure allows the tip to penetrate this tissue, where it is then carefully advanced to allow fluid collection. If the needle is misdirected, the sample is contaminated with blood as the vertebral sinuses are located immediately lateral to the midline on either side. In general, 1 to 3 mL of CSF can be safely collected from most adult turtles.

No normal values are listed for CSF analysis in seaturtles. However, this author uses mammal normals and clinical judgment. A cell count should be performed, with a differential analysis of a smear and total protein and glucose concentration. Blood glucose should also be measured for comparison purposes. Culture and sensitivity should be performed on the sample if meningitis is suspected.

Impression or aspiration cytology can also be performed for indications used in any other nonreptilian patient. Chapter 28 discusses techniques in detail.

Diagnostic Imaging

Radiology, ultrasound, special imaging such as computed tomography (CT) or magnetic resonance imaging (MRI), and nuclear scintigraphy are all valuable tools for diagnosis of ill

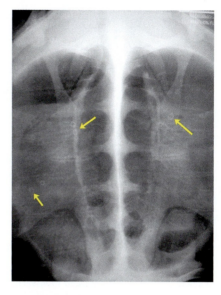

FIGURE 76-21 Barnacles and other epibiotes can appear to be lesions on radiographs *(yellow arrows)* and should be removed before imaging. *(Photograph courtesy D. Mader.)*

and injured seaturtles.[15] Techniques are covered in great detail in Chapters 29, 37, and 86.

Two challenges face the seaturtle radiographer. First, the size of many of these patients makes diagnostic radiographs difficult to obtain; not to mention the mere logistics of manipulating such large animals is significant. Portable radiology equipment like the type used for large animal medicine may be easier to maneuver in the field than trying to move a large seaturtle onto a radiology table in a hospital.

Second, before radiographs are performed, the exterior surfaces should be cleaned of barnacles because these radio-dense structures can impair detail or produce artifacts that could easily be confused as pathology (Figures 76-21). With soaking the patient in freshwater or, alternately, using a flat-edge paint scraper or plastic plaster spatula, the barnacles are usually readily removed (Figure 76-22).

Endoscopy

The principles of endoscopy are covered in Chapter 32. Both rigid and flexible endoscopy are used extensively at the Marathon Sea Turtle Hospital (MSTH). ALL patients with Green Turtle Fibropapilloma (GTFP) are endoscoped (discussed subsequently). In addition, flexible endoscopy is used for gastrointestinal (foreign bodies, obstructions) and respiratory cases.

Coelioscopy is part of the standard database analysis for all patients with GTFP. Many of these patients are debilitated, so general anesthesia is not necessary. At most, light sedation with a local analgesic at the site of insertion is all that is used (see later in chapter). Two to 4 mL of 2% lidocaine is infused in the midprefemoral fossa bilaterally. Although access to both sides of the coelomic cavity from one entry point is possible, bilateral visualization, and the addition of a second entry site, makes triangulation and use of adjuctive endosurgical devices more efficient.

The patient is held on its side. The prefemoral area is prepared, and a local is administered. A #11 scalpel blade is used to make a small stab incision, just large enough to pass the

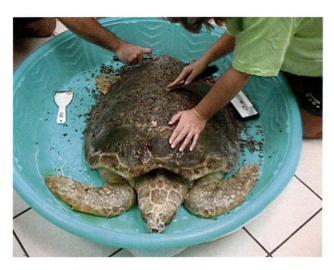

FIGURE 76-22 Soaking the seaturtle in freshwater helps loosen barnacles and other epibiotes. A dull-edged tool, such as a plaster spatula, works well to remove the barnacles. *(Photograph courtesy D. Mader.)*

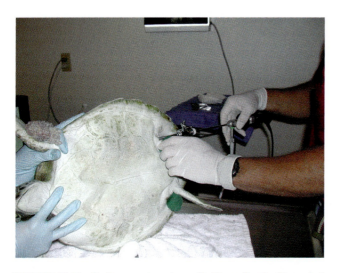

FIGURE 76-23 Endoscopy in a juvenile Green Turtle (*C. mydas*). The approach is made from either prefemoral fossa and can be performed with a combination of sedation and local analgesia. *(Photograph courtesy D. Mader.)*

trocar. The trocar is held parallel to the tabletop and aimed parallel to the inner surface of the plastron. The combination of the seaturtle's position and gravity displace the viscera in the dependent portion of the coelomic cavity. By staying parallel to the inner plastron, the lung is also avoided. After the trocar has been placed, the telescope can then be inserted into the guide for the examination (Figure 76-23).

Gently rolling the patient on its plastron permits complete visualization of the ventral surface of the lung and a partial view of the dorsal surface. The normal lung is attached along its dorsal surface to the inner (ventral) carapace along the spinal column. The lung normally folds ventrally near the cranial margin (Figure 76-24, *A*). From this same position, visualization is also possible of the inner carapace, the gonads, the kidneys, and the dorsal surface of the intestines (Figure 76-24, *B-E*).

When the patient is placed in dorsal recumbency, the viscera shift, allowing visualization of the ventral surfaces of the intestinal tract, the liver, the bladder, and the plastron (Figure 76-25, *A-C*). With a blunt probe and a separate entry point, viscera can be manipulated, allowing access to the pancreas, spleen, stomach, and gall bladder.

Biopsies and laboratory sampling can be collected from either position. Biopsies should be collected from any questionable areas. Confirmation of irreversible pathology is mandatory in a case of possible euthanasia.

Retrieval of foreign bodies, biopsies, and lung washes for cytology and microbiologic sampling are all easily accomplished with flexible endoscopy. The procedure can usually be accomplished with the patient heavily sedated. An oral speculum (a PVC coupler ring can work well in some species) is inserted and taped into the mouth to protect the endoscope for both gastrointestinal and pulmonary bronchoscopy.

The glottis is at the base of the tongue. Intubation may be necessary in some patients but is definitely recommended whenever microbiologic sampling is intended (Figure 76-26).

Seaturtles have a simple respiratory anatomy, with complete rings in the trachea, which divides internally into two primary bronchi (Figure 76-27). From there, the bronchi open into a sponge-like network of falveoli (Figure 76-28). With gentle technique and a quality small-diameter bronchoscope, maneuvering to the outer margins of the lungs is possible, thereby permitting evaluation of almost the entire lungfield.

As with other species of reptiles, endoscopy in seaturtles can be used for many indications.[16] Endoscopy allows a minimally invasive approach to various body areas that are not readily attainable with conventional means. In endangered species, this benefit alone justifies the expense of the equipment.

Common Medical Problems

Seaturtles are susceptible to any and all forms of disease and pestilence, as are any other living organisms. Surveys from various geographic locations around the world report similar conditions and problems.[17] In addition to natural disease, the seaturtles also have to deal with various forms of human impact.[18] The following discussion covers several of the more common conditions encountered when working with wild populations of seaturtles.

Trauma

Trauma comes in many forms (see Figure 76-1, Figure 76-16, and Figures 76-29 to 76-32). Boat strikes, entrapment (entanglements), and shark bites are the most common causes for morbidity and mortality in the seaturtles seen at the MSTH.

Principles of emergency medicine should be applied (see Chapter 31). Proper physical assessment should be performed as should a minimum standard database including blood analysis and radiographs.

A sequela of trauma, one that is often overlooked, is suffocation (drowning). Seaturtles are air breathers and can generally stay submerged, during rest, for 2 to 4 hours. However, if injured or struggling, time of submergence is drastically reduced. If the animal is caught below water in a trap line or other gear, or experience trauma that results in forced

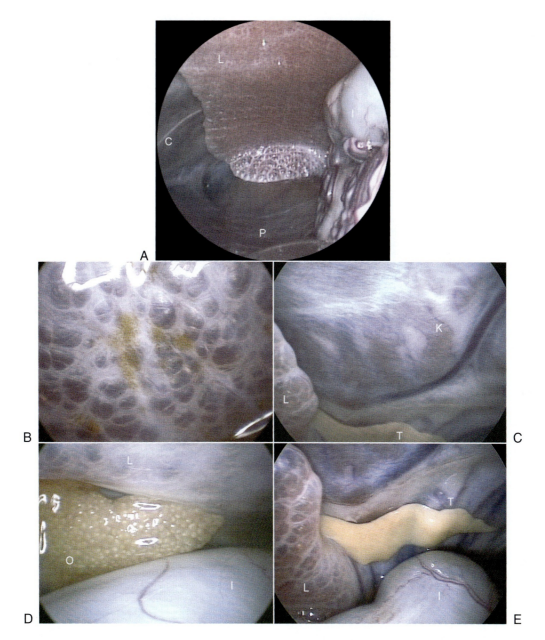

FIGURE 76-24 **A,** The cranial lung normally folds ventrally near the cranial margin. From this same entry position, visualization of the inner carapace, the gonads, the kidneys, and the dorsal surface of the intestines is also possible. *C,* Carapace; *L,* lung; *P,* plastron; *I,* intestine; *K,* kidney; *T,* testicle; *O,* ovary. **B,** Melanin pigments commonly seen during endoscopy. Heavily parasitized debilitated animals have aggregations of trematode eggs that have a similar appearance. **C, D,** and **E,** Standard views that show the kidney, testicle, and ovary. *(Photographs courtesy D. Mader.)*

submergence, these animals can aspirate or suffocate and die. Turtles with carapace punctures that penetrate the pulmonary membrane have saltwater infiltrate the lungs.

Saltwater drowning is a serious condition. Even if the patient is resuscitated, the residual seawater in the lungs induces a secondary drowning as body water follows the osmotic gradient, leaving the pulmonary tissue and entering the lungs. Treatment is difficult, and the prognosis is grave. Antibiotics, fluids, positional drainage (inclined with head down), suction, and oxygen supplementation may be necessary.

Obvious trauma needs to be treated as in any other species. Often dry-dock trauma or postoperative treatment for patients during convalescence is necessary (discussed subsequently). Severe trauma patients have been dry-docked for up to 6 weeks with no ill effects.

Open wounds are best treated as such. Rarely do seaturtles present with fresh trauma (an exception being boat strikes where the animal may be rescued immediately). As a result, debriding, packing (with sugar or honey when dry-docked), systemic antibiotics, analgesics, and fluid support are appropriate.

Depression fractures of the shell and skull should be gently elevated (generally with sedation or anesthesia). Loose pieces can be discarded because they usually do not reattach. Large fresh fractures of the carapace, plastron, or skull can be wired or plated. After fixation, the animal should be

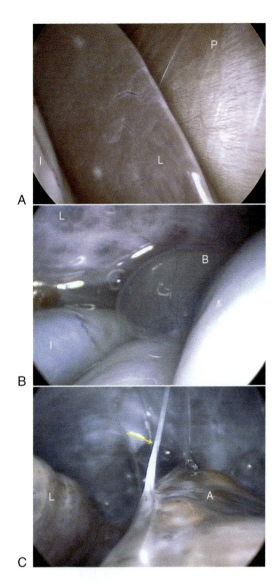

FIGURE 76-25 **A,** Endoscopic view with ventral look (left side down). *L,* Liver; *P,* plastron; *B,* bladder; *L,* lung; *I,* intestine; *A,* abscess. **B,** View of normal bladder. **C,** Adhesion and abscess inside the carapace from an infected boat strike. Wounds may appear healed on the outside, but large granulomas may be found within the coelomic cavity. *(Photographs courtesy D. Mader.)*

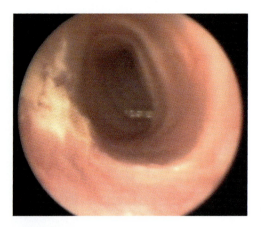

FIGURE 76-26 Flexible bronchoscopic view of the trachea. A large fibrinous plaque is seen at the 9 o'clock position. Flexible bronchoscopy allows for excellent visualization of the airways and most of the pulmonary parynchema, and provides access for cytologic and microbiologic sampling. *(Photograph courtesy D. Mader.)*

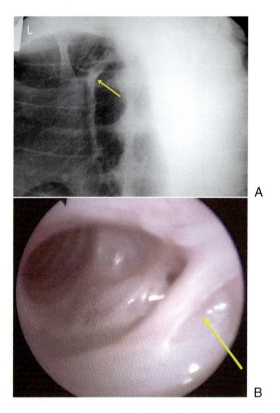

FIGURE 76-27 **A,** Dorsoventral radiograph of seaturtle with unilateral pneumonia. The *yellow arrow* points to the left primary bronchus. **B,** Endoscopic view of an occluded right primary bronchus *(yellow arrow)*. *(Photographs courtesy D. Mader.)*

dry-docked for several days to allow a surface healing before placement back in the water.

If the wounds are old, the best method is to leave them as is (other than proper cleaning and debriding) as many self-heal with secondary intention. This is evidenced by the many wild seaturtles seen with significant wounds that have healed without any veterinary intervention (Figure 76-33).

Many polytrauma cases need months of care and rehabilitation. Cost can be great, and the labor investment massive. Seaturtles have an amazing ability to heal. Patience and attention to basic principles of wound management, antibiosis, and supportive care are essential.

Fibropapillomatosis

Common to seaturtles in tropical waters worldwide is a proliferative disease known as Green Turtle Fibropapilloma (GTFP). First described in 1938 in the Green Turtle, the disease, which is caused by a herpesvirus,[19] is now found in all species of seaturtles except for the Leatherback. The reason that the disease has crossed species and has become more prevalent is not known; however, the suspicion is that human-induced environmental factors (ocean warming, algal blooms, pollution, etc.) may be co-factors.[20] Chapter 24 discusses the etiology of GTFP and other viral diseases of seaturtles in detail.

Treatment of GTFP accounts for approximately 50% of the cases at the MSTH. This debilitating disease is characterized

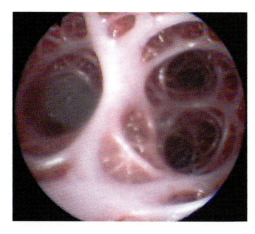

FIGURE 76-28 Deep flexible endoscopic view of the pulmonary parynchema of a seaturtle. Note that the outer pulmonary membrane can be seen at the 10 o'clock position. *(Photograph courtesy D. Mader.)*

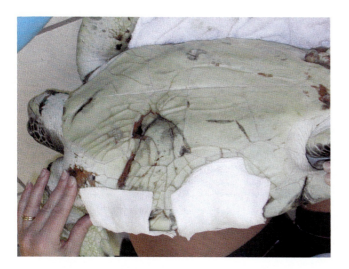

FIGURE 76-29 Shark bite in a juvenile Green Turtle *(C. mydas)*. *(Photograph courtesy D. Mader.)*

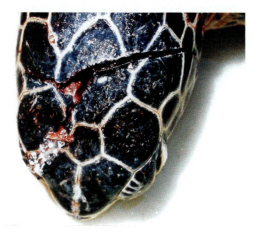

FIGURE 76-30 Boat strike on the skull of a Green Turtle *(C. mydas)*. These animals have an incredible ability to heal, and injuries that appear outwardly significant still warrant thorough diagnosis and treatment. *(Photograph courtesy D. Mader.)*

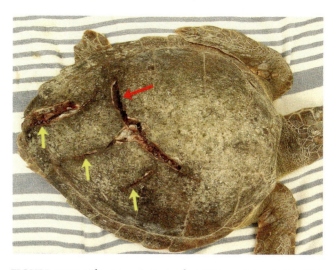

FIGURE 76-31 This juvenile Loggerhead *(C. caretta)* was struck by two separate boat propellers. The *yellow arrows* point to the row of cuts from a smaller boat. The larger *red arrow* points to a deep cut from a larger propeller. *(Photograph courtesy D. Mader.)*

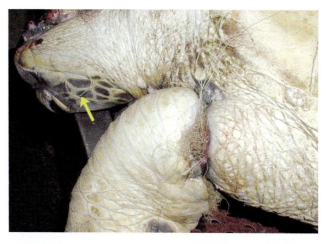

FIGURE 76-32 Loggerhead *(C. caretta)* with nylon fishing line entangling and strangling the flipper. The *yellow arrow* points to the line dangling from the mouth—an ominous sign. *(Photograph courtesy D. Mader.)*

by the proliferation of cutaneous and visceral fibropapillomas (Figure 76-34). The fibropapillomas (FP) themselves are benign, but *en masse,* these lesions debilitate the animals, causing anemia, immunosuppression, and increased susceptibility to other disease.[21-23] Fact in point, many of the GTFP cases that are brought to the MSTH have only minor lesions but arrive as a result of some other injury (e.g., trauma from boats, sharks).

If FP occurs on the eyes, it can lead to blindness, which results in the inability to find food, and ultimately starvation. Likewise, small lesions on the flippers, skin, or carapace generally do not cause problems for the patient; however, if the FP grows to a large size, or massive numbers, it affects the hydrodynamics, the ability to swim, and poses an increased risk of entanglement. Debilitation is the key to eventual mortality.

On the basis of experience and hundreds of cases presented to the MSTH, the FP appears to start externally,

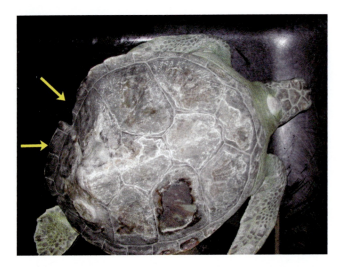

FIGURE 76-33 This animal was found alive with evidence of an old traumatic amputation of the left rear flipper *(yellow arrows)*. This was likely the result of a shark attack. Animals in the wild have an amazing ability to heal, even from significant wounds, without the benefit of veterinary intervention. *(Photograph courtesy D. Mader.)*

then over time, internal FP develops (Figure 76-35). All animals presented to the MSTH are radiographed to check for evidence of internal tumors (Figure 76-36). MRI has been shown to be superior and more sensitive at identification of internal FP,[24] which are most commonly found in the lung tissue. The liver, gallbladder, intestinal tract (both mesentery and mural), the kidneys, and the shell are other locations where FP has been seen. In our experience, if internal FP exists, the patient's prognosis is grave and the animal is immediately euthanized and necropsied. As a result, every effort is made to make the correct diagnosis (see Figure 29-43).

Magnetic resonance imaging is an excellent tool for diagnosis of FP. However, it is expensive and not readily available in some regions. At the MSTH, all FP cases are endoscopically examined. Endoscopic examinations are readily performed, even on the most debilitated animals.

In experienced hands, endoscopy is effective in locating even FP lesions that are too small to show up on radiographs (Figure 76-37). Limitations to endoscopic examination include FP lesions on the dorsal side of the lungs (between the attachment of the lung to the internal carapace) and intraparynchemal lesions.

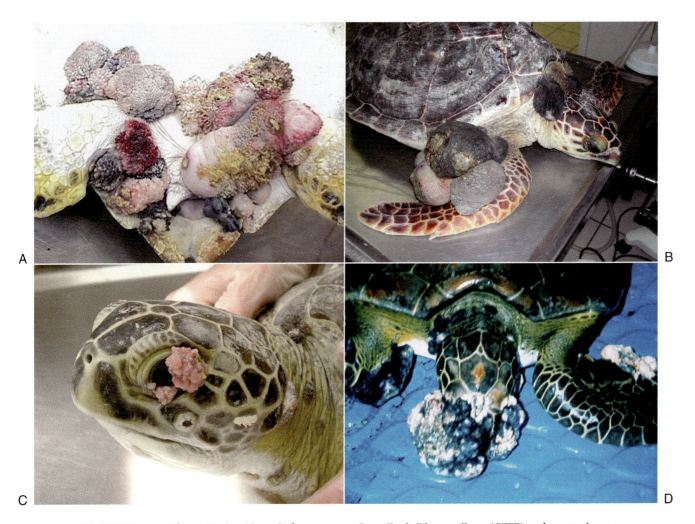

FIGURE 76-34 **A,** The multicolored large fleshy masses are Green Turtle Fibropapilloma (GTFP) on the ventral rear quarters of a juvenile Green Turtle *(C. mydas)*. **B,** Large external fibropapilloma (FP) on the flippers and neck of this Hawksbill-Loggerhead hybrid. **C,** FP on the sclera and nictitating membrane of a juvenile Green Turtle. **D,** Severe, multiple, debilitating FP lesions of the head, face, eyes, and flippers of this Green Turtle. *(Photographs courtesy D. Mader [A, B], W. Mader [C], and The Marathon Sea Turtle Hospital [D].)*

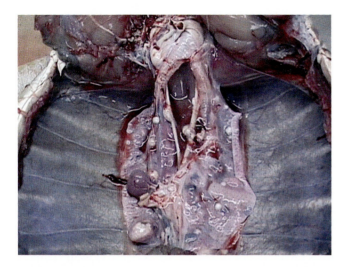

FIGURE 76-35 Prosection shows multiple ivory-colored nodules (fibropapilloma [FP]) in the lungs of a turtle. *(Photograph courtesy D. Mader.)*

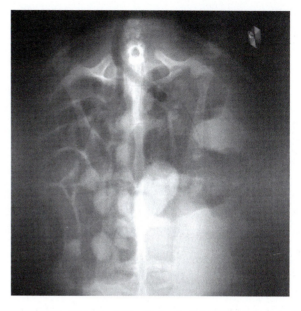

FIGURE 76-36 Dorsoventral radiograph of the lungs in a seaturtle. Note the multiple radiodense nodules throughout the pulmonary region. These are fibropapillomas (FP). *(Photograph courtesy D. Mader.)*

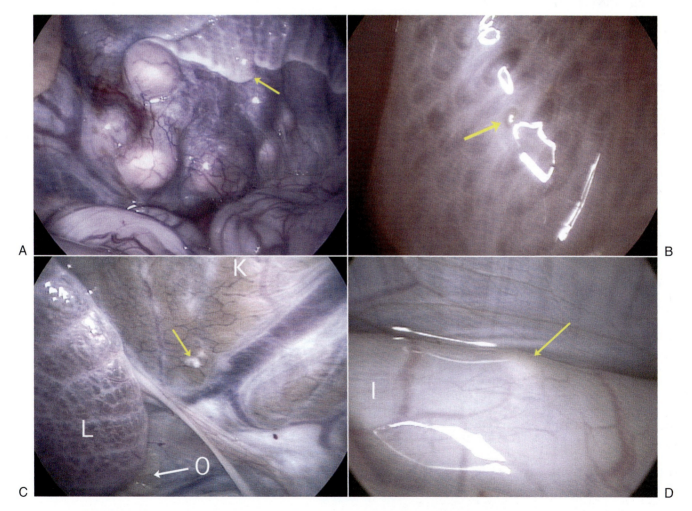

FIGURE 76-37 **A,** Endoscopic view of multiple pulmonary fibropapilloma (FP). **B,** Endoscopic view of a trematode granuloma in the lung. This should not be mistaken for FP. If any doubt exists, the lesion should be biopsied. **C,** FP lesion in the kidney. *L,* Lung; *K,* kidney; *O,* ovary. **D,** FP lesion in the wall of the intestine *(yellow arrow). I,* Intestine. *(Photograph courtesy D. Mader.)*

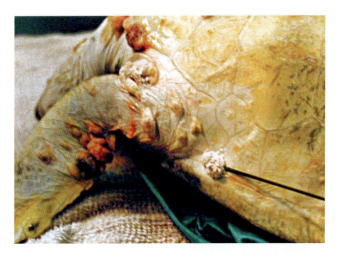

FIGURE 76-38 Cryosurgery used to remove fibropapilloma (FP) lesions in a Green turtle *(C. mydas). (Photograph courtesy D. Mader.)*

No formal study has been conducted that identifies one best method of treatment. Discussions of vaccines and antivirals have occurred, but technology has not materialized.

To date, the most effective method of controlling GTFP appears to be surgical removal. At the MSTH, we have seen the evolution of FP removal starting with cold-steel (scalpel) to radioscalpel to cryosurgery (Figure 76-38) to the CO_2 laser. These masses can hemorrhage extensively when surgical resection is attempted with the scalpel, which, in debilitated animals, can be significant.

In early treatment regimes, sliding skin grafts were attempted to cover sometimes large deficits in the skin. However, the sutures would pull out and the grafts would dehisce. Regardless, the wounds would progress to healing via secondary intention even though they were not closed.

The CO_2 laser has revolutionized removal of the masses. Minimal hemorrhage occurs, even in the larger lesions. After removal, the laser can be used to shrink and seal the site so that no sutures are necessary (Figure 76-39). The patients are started on antibiotics and analgesics after surgery, held out of the water for 24 hours, then placed back in their tanks.

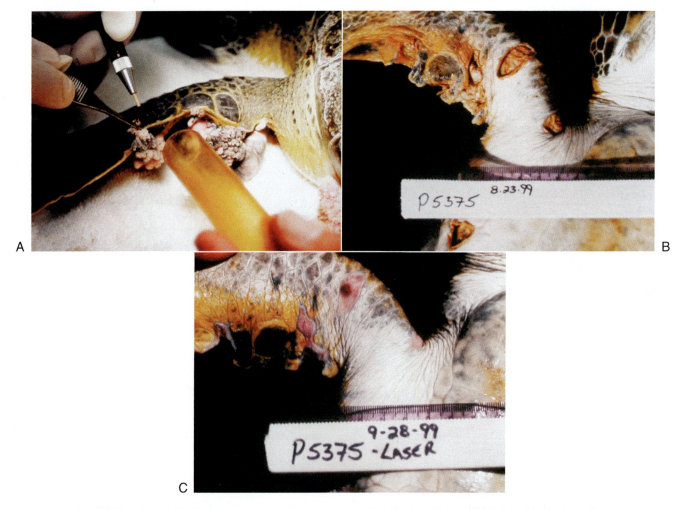

FIGURE 76-39 A, CO_2 laser surgery is used to remove multiple fibropapilloma (FP) lesions. **B,** Postoperative appearance of the skin after CO_2 laser removal of several FP lesions. **C,** Same animal less than 5 weeks later. The large defects have completely filled in with new epithelial tissue. *(Photographs courtesy D. Mader.)*

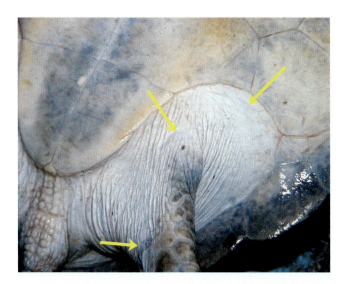

FIGURE 76-40 This patient had multiple fibropapillomas (FPs) removed with the CO_2 laser approximately 8 weeks previously. The wounds (*yellow arrows*) were allowed to heal with secondary intention. (*Photograph courtesy D. Mader.*)

Evidence of the surgery is difficult to find in as little as 12 weeks after surgery (Figure 76-40).

No formal studies have been conducted to determine the amount of time FP animals need to be held after mass removal before being released back to the wild. Empirically, at the MSTH, patients are kept for 1 year. If no regrowth occurs in that time, the animals are released. If FP returns, the procedure/time clock starts over.

Mass removal is prioritized on the basis of location and overall medical condition of the patient. Eyes (palpebra, conjunctiva, and cornea) are always done first. Even in marginally stable patients, the first procedure attempted is to laser cut the FP from the eyes. This is generally a fairly simple procedure as the masses are almost always conjunctival. The laser scalpel readily "peels" the mass from the globe without damaging the underlying tissue. If the globe is infiltrated or the cornea is effaced, the eye must be enucleated (discussed in the surgery section).

In patients with multiple FP, generally only half the animal is cleared at a time. Usually a 4-week to 6-week waiting period is needed, and then the remaining FP are removed.

Much remains to be learned about this disease. The debilitating disease is not seen in adults, which suggests that an immunity may develop. We have seen some lesions develop and then regress, but that is the exception. Seaturtles with untreated GTFP have a grave prognosis.

At present, surgical removal of lesions and careful postoperative monitoring seems to offer the best hope for these animals. At the MSTH, we have several "lifers," seaturtles that for various reasons cannot be released and that have gone more than 10 years in captivity with no regrowth of FP.

Fish Hooks and Gastrointestinal Injury

The gastrointestinal tract, in some fashion, is commonly involved with seaturtle morbidity. Ingestion of fish hooks, fishing line, plastic bags, garbage, and more can contribute to both fast and slow deaths in these animals (Figures 76-41 and 76-42).[25,26]

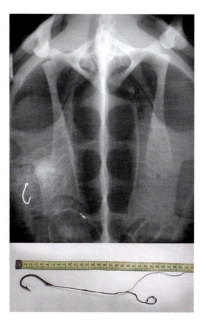

FIGURE 76-41 Dorsoventral radiograph shows a hook and leader. Sinkers, which are made of lead, are toxic. Whenever this combination is seen, one must remember that line always connects the two parts. The *bottom image* shows the typical relationship between the hook, line, and sinker. (*Photograph courtesy D. Mader.*)

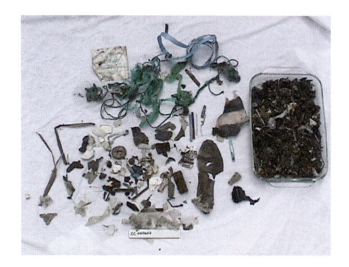

FIGURE 76-42 All of this trash was removed from the intestinal tract (during necropsy) of a single patient. Garbage and cast-off fishing products are lethal to seaturtles. (*Photograph courtesy the Marathon Sea Turtle Hospital.*)

Fish hooks may be readily apparent in the oral cavity if swallowed, with the line trailing from the mouth or cloaca. They may be occult and incidental findings on survey radiographs. Most hooks are designed to rust and eventually be eliminated by the animal. However, if they become lodged, or if the line is pulled, the hook may perforate the intestinal tract, causing a potentially life-threatening coelomitis.

Additional problems with hooks and lines include strangulation one or both flippers with trailing line, erosions to the lateral commissures of the mouth from the line (see Figure 76-32), and lead intoxication from the ingested sinkers. In general, whenever there is a hook, there is usually a line. If a hook and a sinker/swivel are seen on the radiograph, a line

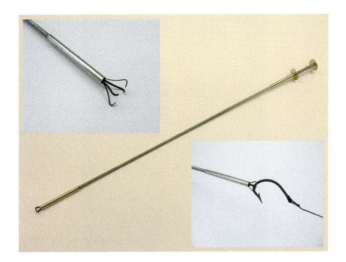

FIGURE 76-43 This automotive tool is used for retrieval of fish hooks in the esophagus of seaturtles at the Marathon Sea Turtle Hospital. The *inset (upper left)* shows the four strong jaws that can grasp, dislodge, and hold onto hooks *(inset: bottom right). (Photograph courtesy D. Mader.)*

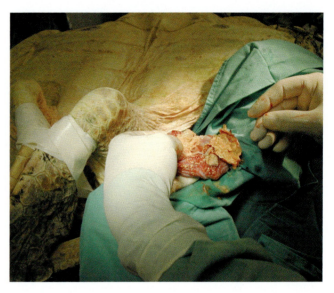

FIGURE 76-44 Surgical access to most of the intestinal tract, including the greater curvature of the stomach, can be accomplished through either of the prefemoral fossae in larger seaturtles. *(Photograph courtesy the Marathon Sea Turtle Hospital.)*

is likely between the two. This line acts like a typical linear foreign body and can cause perforations and strangulation to the intestines. These findings must be corrected via either endoscopic extraction or surgery.

Approach to fish hook removal is similar to that in dogs and cats. If the line is still attached, it can be passed through a hard plastic hose or tube and then, the tube can be used to gently dislodge the hook. Commercial dehooking devises are now relatively common and are recommended for certain kinds of dehookings by some facilities. If not retrievable by standard visual means, an endoscope can be used to follow the line down to the hook and retrieve it.

At the MSTH, we use an automotive tool designed to reach into small spaces and retrieve nuts and bolts. This is a rigid, sturdy instrument, approximately 40 cm (16 in) long. It has a syringe-like plunger on one end and a four-pronged grasper on the opposite (Figure 76-43). If the line is present, it can be threaded through the grasper and then followed directly to the hook if it is within reach. If not, an endoscope can be used to locate the hook; then, the grasper can follow the scope to the hook.

If the hook cannot be reached with a scope or the grasper and examination suggests perforation or a lead sinker is present, every attempt should be made to retrieve it surgically. Several approaches have been described.[27-29] If the hook cannot be accessed via the oral or supraplastron approach nearly the entire intestinal tract can be reached through either prefemoral fossa (Figure 76-44).

Entanglements

Entanglements are common with fish hooks, nets, and trap lines. The offending fibers need to be carefully removed, and the tissue tested for viability. Strangulation injuries, not uncommonly, occur, devitalizing limbs. Amputation is generally the only option in these cases (discussed subsequently).

Intestinal impactions are likewise potentially lethal. These impactions can lead to buoyancy problems, pressure necrosis, and intestinal perforations.

Seaturtles with intestinal impactions often present in marked states of emaciation. Ingestion of floating plastic (apparently appears to look or taste like jellyfish, a natural diet of many seaturtles) and garbage (see Figure 76-42) eventually kills the animal if it does not pass or is not removed. In addition, seaturtles are commonly seen with mollusk shell impactions in the transverse and distal colon.

Mineral oil gavages (0.25% body weight), lactulose (15 to 60 mL total dose per day), and psyllium (1 to 3 g per turtle per day) have been used with success at the MSTH. Avoid docusate (stool softener) because it has been shown to be toxic in reptiles.[30]

Hydration is extremely important in these patients. Oral (PO) fluid administration seems to be the most practical and useful; however, intracoelomic (ICe) administration is also beneficial in dehydrated patients. Antimicrobials should be used as needed. Breakup and passage of the impaction can take days to weeks. Every attempt to treat conservatively should be made before an invasive enterotomy is performed.

Flotation (Buoyancy) Abnormalities

Several potential causes exist for "floater" seaturtles that are unable to maintain proper buoyancy or have difficulty in diving. Trauma, which causes small or large tears in the lung, causes air to leak from the lung where it then gets trapped in the coelom. The lung tears act as "one-way" valves, and the air cannot return back into the lung. As a result, a pneumocoelom develops and the animal floats and bobs at the surface like a cork.

Any gas-producing coelomic infection can result with the seaturtle floating.

Intestinal impactions, where ileus is a consequence of the blockage, frequently manifest with buoyancy problems.

Animals with neurologic damage, such as spinal trauma, may not be able to dive properly and appear to have buoyancy problems.

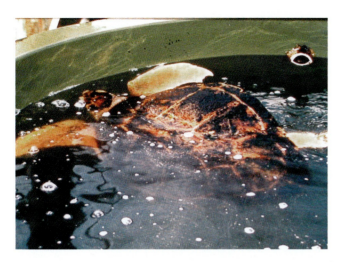

FIGURE 76-45 An adult Loggerhead (*C. caretta*) with buoyancy abnormalities is housed in a small observation tank. These turtles are called "floaters." (*Photograph courtesy D. Mader.*)

Cold-stunned animals, simply from weakness, may not be able to dive and, as a result, are found floating on the surface.

Likely many other causes have yet to be elucidated.

Floaters can present with total body floating, but it is rare. Most commonly, they are either floating high on one side or the rear quarters are elevated (Figure 76-45).

Aside from the inciting problem (which can be life threatening in itself), these animals become exhausted in their attempts to dive and search for food. Large calluses develop across the dorsal cervical region in the animals float with a strong elevation of the hindquarters; the carapace rubbing the back of the neck causes thickening of the skin to develop.

Grimm and Mader[31] performed a study with 33 healthy *C. mydas*, evaluating their coelomic pressure during the respiratory cycle. Mean resting coelomic pressures were 0 mm Hg. Peak inspiratory pressure was –3 mm Hg. Although not definitive, this study suggests that measurement of coelomic pressures may aid in diagnosis.

Treatment and correction of floating problems centers on identifying and reversing the cause. In general, if the problem can be found (e.g., lung injury, intestinal impaction), the floating can be corrected. Unfortunately, the cause cannot always be found.

Removal of excessive air in the coelom has been attempted and found to be successful in some cases. In general, coelomic air is removed until the coelomic pressure is as close to 0 mm Hg as possible. Some of these animals remain neutrally buoyant; however, more often than not, the floating problem returns in a few days if the underlying problem has not been corrected.

Placement of the animal in freshwater helps because the specific gravity is lower than that of seawater. The animals are naturally not as buoyant in freshwater, and in some cases, the floating problem self-corrects. Note, however, that these animals should not be left unattended because swimming in fresh water takes more effort and the animals may become exhausted and drown.

At the MSTH, the general "floater" protocol involves collection of the minimal database, including vertical and horizontal beam radiographs. MRI or CT imaging where available is helpful in locating the source of the trapped gas.

If the source is not readily apparent, the animal is started on four-quadrant antimicrobial therapy, such as amikacin and penicillin. These animals may be left on this for weeks to months, with their blood values monitored on a regular (weekly) basis. The animals are fed or assist fed, and fluid therapy is administered as needed. Not uncommonly, these cases slowly resolve over weeks to months, eventually returning to normal, even though the cause was never determined.

Contamination with Oil, Fuel, and Other Toxins

Fossil fuels, heavy metals, and environmental toxins are a problem for seaturtles worldwide.[32-36] Oil and the byproducts can be problematic through both ingestion and surface contamination. Heavy metals and toxins are ingested through water and food contamination. Not unexpectedly, high levels of toxicants are seen in areas of greater human populations.

Lutcavage et al[32] reported that oiled turtles had up to a four-fold increase in white blood cell counts, a 50% reduction in red blood cell counts, and red blood cell polychromasia. Most serum blood chemistries (e.g., blood urea nitrogen [BUN], protein) were within normal ranges, although glucose returned more slowly to baseline values than in the controls.[32]

Gross and histologic changes were present in the skin and mucosal surfaces of oiled turtles, including acute inflammatory cell infiltrates, dysplasia of epidermal epithelium, and a loss of cellular architectural organization of the layers of the skin. The cellular changes in the epidermis may increase susceptibility to infection. Lutcavage et al[32] observed that the physiologic insults resolved with a 21-day recovery period but pointed out that the long-term biologic effects of oil on seaturtles remain completely unknown.

External oil can be removed with animal-safe detergent baths (such as Dawn dishwashing liquid, Procter and Gamble, www.pg.com), vegetable oil, or mayonnaise. After the turtle is covered with the mayonnaise, it is rinsed off. If the mouth is affected, start with the head and mouth (congealed petroleum often occludes the mouth, gluing to the jaws and partially occluding the airways.) The process is repeated until the patient is clean. Human handlers should wear protective gear when handling oiled animals.

Internal contamination can be countered with activated charcoal, 2 to 8 g/kg per day. Patients should have their blood counts and chemistries monitored every few days.

Parasites

All wild seaturtles have a natural burden of both endoparasites and ectoparasites.[37-40] In a healthy seaturtle host, these rarely cause problems. However, when stressed with disease, trauma, or environmental imbalances, these parasites can cause pathology. Parasites are covered in detail in Chapter 21.

Helminths such as trematodes and nematodes are a part of the normal flora. Monogenetic and digenetic trematodes are found in many species of seaturtles. The monogenetic trematode *Lophotaspis vallei* resides mainly in the stomach and upper small intestine of Loggerhead. They are not known to cause damage to their hosts.

Most digenetic trematodes have evolved to a level of mutual coexistence, and little or no pathology is inflicted. These live in nearly every soft tissue organ in the body of their reptilian hosts, although most reside in the gastrointestinal tract.

Spirorchiidae, a group of digenetic flukes whose adults live in blood vessels and the heart, are pathogenic. Sometimes the adults may be numerous enough to block smaller vessels (capillaries), causing ischemia and damage to the tissue not being fed or oxygenated. The fluke eggs can accumulate, causing the same problem, and some of those eggs that leave the gut are trapped by the host, forming granulomas.

Raidal et al[40] evaluated causes of morbidity and mortality in juvenile *C. mydas* off the coast of western Australia. Histopathologic examination showed severe multifocal to diffuse granulomatous vasculitis, aggregations of spirorchid fluke eggs, and microabscesses throughout various tissues including intestines, kidney, liver, lung, and brain.

Adnyana, Ladds, and Blair[41] evaluated praziquantel in six spontaneously infected *C. mydas*. After treatment, the animals were necropsied and evaluated. The absence of flukes in treated, but not control, turtles indicated that a 1-day course of treatment at a dose rate of 3×50 mg/kg body weight, administered orally, was effective. Jacobson et al,[42] in a pharmacokinetic study in *C. caretta*, found that oral administration of 25 mg of praziquantel/kg 3 times at 3-hour intervals may be appropriate for treatment of Loggerhead Seaturtles with spirorchidiasis.

Sulcascaris sulcata is a nematode of the stomach of Loggerheads; it uses oysters as its intermediate host. Although no pharmacokinetic studies have been done with fenbendazole in seaturtles, at the MSTH, all patients are routinely treated with 25 mg/kg, repeated in 2 weeks.

Caryospora cheloniae, a coccidial pathogen, was implicated in the deaths of 70 wild Green Turtles in southeast Queensland, Australia, over 6 weeks in spring 1991. On the basis of the necropsy of 24 turtles, a severe enteritis or encephalitis was found.[39] Before this report, *C. cheloniae* had only been reported in farm-raised *C. mydas*.

Eimeria caretta, also a coccidial parasite, has been found in Loggerheads but has not been associated with pathology.[43]

Marine leeches (*Ozobranchus margoi*) are found in large numbers on Green Turtles, Atlantic Hawksbills, Loggerheads, and Atlantic Ridleys. High populations of this leech usually are seen on severely emaciated turtles (Figure 76-46). Fresh-water baths usually suffice to rid the turtles of the leeches.

Infectious Diseases

Seaturtles are susceptible to a myriad of infectious diseases. Bacterial, fungal, and viral diseases are commonplace, especially in animals that have been immunocompromised from reasons already discussed.[17,22,40,44-50] Chapters 16 and 24 discuss these various pathogens in detail. Signs vary with pathogen and condition, but generalized debilitation is common to most.

A thorough physical examination needs to be performed on all patients. The standard minimum database should be performed on all patients. Microbial cultures and sensitivities, cytology, and biopsy should be performed as needed. Treatment should be directed at the specific findings.

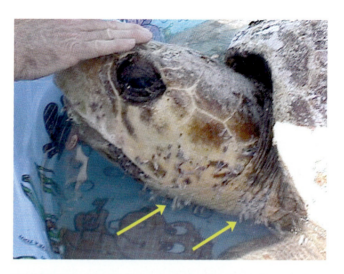

FIGURE 76-46 Debilitated seaturtles not uncommonly present covered with marine leeches (*Ozobranchus margoi*). A short soak in a freshwater bath usually kills and removes the ectoparasites. *(Photograph courtesy D. Mader.)*

Neoplasia

Neoplasia has been documented in wild seaturtles (see Figure 19-6).[51,52] Other than that discussed with the GTFP, treatment of neoplasia in seaturtles has not been reported.

Certainly, considering the endangered status of most seaturtles, if neoplasia is encountered, attempts at proper diagnosis and treatment should be considered (see Chapter 19 for approach to neoplasia in reptiles).

Anorexia

Anorexia is a symptom, not a disease. Chapter 44 discusses the general approach to anorexia in reptiles.

Seaturtle anorexia can be caused by anything from maladaptation to captivity to disease. Recent captives may not recognize captive diets as food and may refuse to eat. A complete physical examination with minimal standard database must be performed on all patients with anorexia. In general, when the underlying problems are identified and corrected, the animal resumes or starts eating.

Table 76-6 lists a recipe for a gel diet that can be used for captive seaturtles. In addition, medications can easily be added to this diet and facilitate treatment of ill animals.

Ill and debilitated animals do need alimentation. Parenteral nutritional support has not been described, but this should not discourage clinicians from attempting such, with standard techniques. This necessitates placement of a jugular catheter (previously discussed).

At the MSTH, weak or anorectic animals are routinely assist (tube) fed. The ingredients in the gruel diet are based on the species supplemented. The patients are strapped to a restraint board or rack and tipped head-up (Figure 76-47). This helps gravity to assist flow of the gruel readily into the stomach.

A semirigid plastic tube with a smooth end (like an equine gastric tube) is lubricated and gently passed into the stomach as described in Chapter 36 for other turtle species. Gruel is administered at 0.5% to 3% of the body weight, generally

Table 76-6	Gelatin Diet for Seaturtles	
Ingredient	Weight (g)	Percent of Diet
Staple Diet		
Trout chow	425	8
Fish, various species	565	10.6
Squid (viscera removed)	282	5.3
Peeled shrimp	282	5.3
Carrots (fresh, washed)	142	2.7
Spinach (fresh or frozen)	142	2.7
Gelatin (unflavored)	450	8.5
Water	2800 mL	53
Supplements		
Sea Tabs (Pacific Research Labs, Inc, El Cajon, Calif) #4	500 mg tabs	0.04
Amino Acid Complex 1000 #4	500 mg tabs	0.04
Spirolina (Lightforce, Santa Cruz, Calif)	50 mL powder (28 g)	0.5
Rep-Cal (Rep-Cal Research Labs, Los Gatos, Calif)	200 mL powder (180 g)	3.4

Modified from Stamper MA, Whitaker BR: *Medical observations and implications on "healthy" sea turtles prior to release into the wild*, Pittsburgh, Pa, 1994, Proc AAZV.

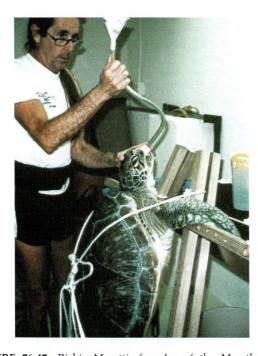

FIGURE 76-47 Richie Moretti, founder of the Marathon Sea Turtle Hospital, tube feeds a debilitated Green Turtle (*C. mydas*). Positioning the patient on an inclined rack facilitates passing the stomach tube and also helps prevent regurgitation after feeding. The patient is left inclined for approximately 30 minutes after feeding. (*Photograph courtesy the Marathon Sea Turtle Hospital.*)

once or twice daily. In emaciated animals where the stomach has atrophied, smaller, more frequent meals may be needed at first. General principles of nutritional support for debilitated reptiles, as outlined in Chapter 18, should be followed.

Anecdotal reports of the use of pharyngostomy tubes in seaturtles have been described. For animals that need prolonged enteral supplementation, a feeding tube is a consideration. Chapters 36 and 18 both describe pharyngostomy tube placement in turtles. However, this is a difficult procedure and the benefits should outweigh the risks.

Weak, Lethargic, and Moribund

Many reasons exist for a seaturtle to present in a weak, lethargic, or moribund condition. These animals may wash up on the shore or be found floating in the ocean. Systemic disease, heavy parasite burdens, toxins, trauma, or blood loss from trauma and starvation or combinations of these conditions, and others, can all be contributing factors.

Cold-stunned animals present obtunded or moribund. A complete discussion of cold stunning follows at the end of this chapter.

For an occasional animal to present in such a fashion is not uncommon. However, finding multiple animals in a similar condition within a short period of time is a cause for alarm. Two recent epizootics involving Loggerheads have been reported.[54,55]

Dubbed "Lethargic Syndrome" and "Debilitated Loggerhead Syndrome," these episodes occurred in the fall-winter 2000-2001 and 2003 in Florida and along the southeast Atlantic cost of the United States, respectively. Many similarities were seen in both events. In general, the strandings were emaciated subadult Loggerheads in various stages of ill health or were dead. Many of the seaturtles were covered with small barnacles on both their shells and skin (Figure 76-48). Epibiota (barnacles, bryozoans, and other encrusting organisms) are not uncommonly found on a seaturtle's shell; however, they are not usually found on the skin of healthy animals.

Health assessment revealed that the Florida seaturtles were suffering from a wide variety of ailments, including bacterial and parasitic infections. Clinically, live animals presented weak and dehydrated and with varying degrees of paralysis. The palpebral (blink), menace, and corneal reflexes were absent in many animals, and several had developed corneal ulcers (Figure 76-49). Swallowing and gag reflexes were also absent in the more severely affected animals. Deep pain appeared to be absent in the distal extremities. Three of the patients were bradycardic (heart rate, <10 beats per minute, with normal being 30 to 40 beats per minute).

Most of the animals had a tenacious mucoid respiratory/oral discharge. Bronchoscopy revealed hyperemia, mucoid fluid accumulation, and plaques in the trachea and bronchi (see Figure 76-26). In severe cases, brownish caseous material was found occluding both the upper and the lower airways.

Hematologic and plasma biochemical findings included leukocytosis (primarily a heterophilia), hyperglycemia, and hypermagnesemia. The leukocytosis and hyperglycemia were presumed to be a stress response. The hypermagnesemia was thought to be the result of the fact that many of the animals were so weak they could not effectively hold their heads out of the water and were aspirating seawater into their lungs.

Investigation of the former epizootic involved many institutions. Extensive testing was performed, including neurologic evaluation of live animals, laboratory analysis, toxicology, and more. No definitive conclusions were made as to the cause of the epizootic; however, several observations were documented.

Neurologic and electrophysiologic examinations and pathologic changes within peripheral nerve specimens

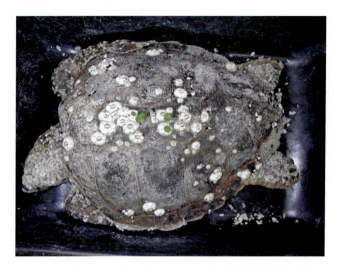

FIGURE 76-48 A debilitated Loggerhead Seaturtle (*C. caretta*) is covered with epibiotes. Barnacles are not uncommonly found on the shell, but finding them on the skin is usually a sign of a severely ill animal. *(Photograph courtesy D. Mader.)*

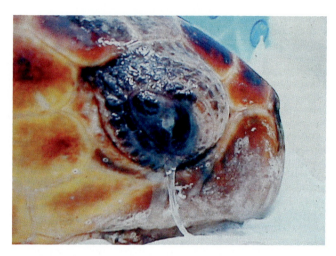

FIGURE 76-49 The "Lethargic Loggerheads" presented with varying degrees of paralysis. Most had no menace, palpebral, or corneal reflexes. As a result, many presented with corneal ulcers. The viscous tears are normal. *(Photograph courtesy D. Mader.)*

supported a diagnosis of either demyelinating polyneuropathy or neuromuscular junction transmission block.[54] Eighteen Loggerheads were necropsied, and histopathology indicated generalized and neurologic spirorchiidiasis (*Neospirorchis* sp.).

Evaluation for heavy metals, organophosphates, and environmental toxins showed some minor perturbations from the normal in some of the affected animals, but none were considered high enough to be the sole cause of the outbreak. The authors concluded that the clinical signs and pathologic changes seen in the affected Loggerheads resulted from combined heavy spirorchiid parasitism and possible chronic exposure to a novel toxin present in the diet of the Loggerheads.[54]

Whenever any moribund animal presents, assessment and treatment should follow standard medical protocols. A thorough physical examination, minimal database, and supportive care should be administered until laboratory results dictate otherwise. Any abnormal presentation or unusual series of events should always be brought to the attention of authorities. Documentation of the event is paramount as it provides clues to cause and helps with future treatment.

THERAPEUTICS

Therapeutics are covered in depth in Chapter 36. Principles of treatment for seaturtles should follow standard guidelines. More efforts are being made to establish seaturtle specific drug dosages.[56-59] Chapter 89 lists drugs that have been used successfully in reptile patients in general. Obviously, any drug used should be selected on the basis of patient assessment, laboratory data, and microbiologic analysis.

After initial diagnostics and establishment of a treatment plan, the seaturtles should be housed in isolation pools. If patients are too weak to raise their heads out of the water to breathe, they can be placed in shower pools (Figure 76-50) or covered with petrolatum jelly and moist towels to prevent dehydration. In addition, they should also be placed on foam padding to protect their plastron because their weight is not supported by the water column. Animals with slightly more energy can be placed in shallow tanks, and those with normal activity should be housed in deep pools to promote swimming and exercise.

Dehydrated and parasite-covered seaturtles should receive a soaking in a freshwater pool. The freshwater assists in the correction of the dehydration and also helps rid the animal of the ectoparasites.

Normal seawater should be used in the rehabilitation and hospitalization tanks. The salinity should be approximately 35 parts per thousand (ppt). Chlorine can be added to the salt water (0.5 mg/L to achieve a level of 0.5 parts per million [ppm]) to reduce bacterial and algal growth. The water should be tested because chlorine levels greater than 1 ppm can be irritating to the turtle's eyes.[10]

The water temperature at subtropical facilities generally does not need to be regulated; however, at more tropical or more temperate locations the water temperature may need regulation. Indoor pools should be kept between 25°C and 30°C (77°F to 86°F). Water that is too cold can be immunosuppressive, depress appetite, and delay healing, and water that is too warm can cause hyperthermia and also have other metabolic consequences.[10] Partial shade is required in outdoor tanks.

Medications are generally administered either orally, intramuscularly (IM), intracoelomically (ICe), or intravenously (IV). The general adage "if the mouth works, use it," does apply to seaturtles. However, in animals that are debilitated, have gastrointestinal stasis, or are large and dangerous, the oral route may not be practical.

Intramuscular injections can be administered in the pectoral or pelvic limbs. ICe medications and fluids are best administered in the prefemoral fossa cranial to each thigh. Placement of an ICe catheter is possible for ease of treatment (Figure 76-51).[60] IV medications can be given in any of the veins discussed for venipuncture, or a jugular catheter can be placed. Although intraosseous (IO) catheters have been discussed in seaturtles, this author (DRM) does not like to use them as they are commonly associated with complications such as clogging, slow operation, infection (cellulitis and osteomyelitis), and pain.

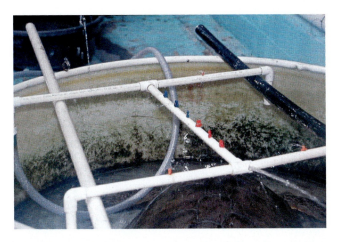

FIGURE 76-50 Animals too weak to be housed in pools can be kept in shower tanks to prevent dehydration. *(Photograph courtesy D. Mader.)*

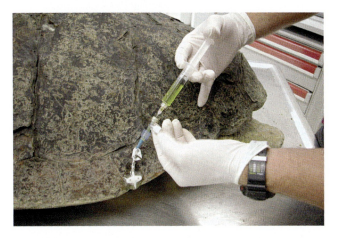

FIGURE 76-51 Medication is administered via an intracoelomically implanted catheter. This facilitates administration of fluids and medications that cannot be given either subcutaneously (SQ) or intramuscularly (IM). *(Photograph courtesy D. Mader.)*

Much controversy exists regarding the best fluid to give reptile patients. Excellent discussions are found in both Chapters 31 and 36. The important point to remember is that no single best fluid exists for all reptile patients. Fluid choice should be based on patient assessment and blood results.

Hypoglycemic patients can be started on either an IV or ICe dextrose solution. Once the condition is normoglycemic, this author routinely chooses either 0.9% NaCl or Normosol-R as a maintenance crystalloid, unless laboratory values dictate otherwise.

Anorectic patients are supported nutritionally as previously described. Hatchling seaturtles are tube fed an oral glucose-electrolyte solution approximately 5% to 7% of their body weight until strong enough to self-feed. Chopped fish, shrimp parts, floating chow, and gelatin diets can all be offered to convalescing turtles. Daily weights should be recorded on all hospitalized patients, labor permitting.

Treatments should be continued for several days to weeks after clinical response. At the MSTH, all convalescing patients must be able to demonstrate an ability to compete for and catch their own food before being considered for release.

Anesthesia

As with any patient, a thorough preoperative assessment and anesthetic plan should be developed before induction. Ideally, animals should be properly warmed and hydrated before anesthesia.

Seaturtles present a unique challenge as anesthetic patients. These animals are capable of shunting their pulmonary circulation (dive response) and holding their breath for several hours.

Seaturtles can be premedicated before induction. For potentially painful procedures, administration of analgesics before the event is recommended.

Moon and Stabenau[61] discuss unpremedicated direct orotracheal intubation and isoflurane induction in *L. kempii*. An isoflurane concentration of $3.4 \pm 0.3\%$ provided anesthetic induction in 7 ± 1 minutes. The mean duration of the recovery was 241 ± 31 minutes. The duration of the recovery phase was not affected by the duration of anesthesia, type of carrier gas, method of ventilatory weaning, or use of selected pharmacologic agents. The recovery phase was characterized by hypoxemia, progressive acidemia, hypercapnia, and lactic acidosis. Awakening in the turtles was preceded by a characteristic tachycardia and tachypnea. All seaturtles recovered from isoflurane anesthesia without apparent adverse effects within 24 hours.

Chittick et al[62] used premedications in their study on 13 Loggerhead Seaturtles. Anesthesia was induced with a premedication cocktail of medetomidine (50 mcg/kg, IV) and ketamine (5 mg/kg, IV); the patient was intubated and then maintained with sevoflurane (0.5% to 2.5%) in oxygen. Sevoflurane was delivered with a pressure-limited intermittent-flow ventilator. Administration of sevoflurane was discontinued 30 to 60 minutes before the end of the surgical procedure. Atipamezole (0.25 mg/kg, IV) was administered at the end of surgery.

Median induction time was 11 minutes (range, 2 to 40 minutes; n = 11). Median delivered sevoflurane concentrations 15, 30, 60, and 120 minutes after intubation were 2.5 (n = 12), 1.5 (n = 12), 1.25 (n = 12), and 0.5 (n = 8), respectively. Heart rate decreased during surgery to a median value of 15 beats/minute (n = 11). End-tidal partial pressure of CO_2 ranged from 2 to 16 mm Hg (n = 8); median blood gas values were within reference limits. Median time from atipamezole administration to extubation was 14 minutes (range, 2 to 84 minutes; n = 7). The authors concluded that a combination of medetomidine and ketamine for induction and sevoflurane for maintenance provides safe, effective, controllable anesthesia in injured Loggerhead Seaturtles.

At the MSTH, various anesthetic protocols have been tried. Telazol (Fort Dodge Animal Health, Overland Park, Kan) at 3 mg/kg, IV or IM, has proven an effective sedative for large or overly aggressive animals. At that dose, the patient is not anesthetized and intubation is not necessary. However, they are generally relaxed enough to undergo intubation if needed or to tolerate endoscopy with the addition of local analgesia at the coelomic insertion site. When Telazol is used with isoflurane, recovery times may be prolonged (several hours).

Propofol (Abbott, Abbott Park, Ill, *www.abott.com*) at 3 mg/kg IV provides rapid induction and good sedation for minor procedures. The patient should be intubated and started on positive pressure ventilation for prolonged or painful surgeries.

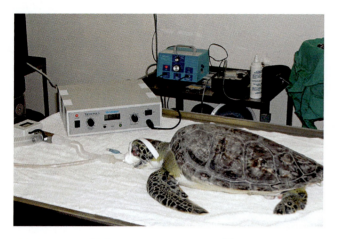

FIGURE 76-52 With a surgical plane of anesthesia, seaturtles must be placed on a ventilator. This Green Turtle (*C. mydas*) is ventilated with a Vetronics pressure-driven unit. *(Photograph courtesy D. Mader.)*

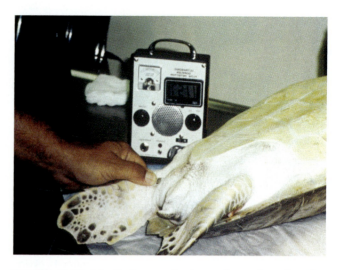

FIGURE 76-53 Monitoring anesthesia can be performed with a combination of patient reflexes, pulse oximetry, ultrasonography, and other techniques. This animal is monitored with a Doppler flow detector. *(Photograph courtesy D. Mader.)*

At surgical planes of anesthesia, some form of mechanical ventilation is necessary (Figure 76-52). The tidal volume can be estimated to be approximately 50 mL/kg. Ventilatory pressure should not exceed 15 cm H_2O, and the rate should be approximately 2 to 8 breaths per minute.[8] The anesthetic carrier gas should be either 100% oxygen or a 50:50 mixture of oxygen and nitrous oxide. If nitrous oxide is used, it should be discontinued at least 5 minutes before the end of surgery.

The patient should be placed on a warm surgical table or provided with supplemental heat. Ideally, the animal should be on a warm fluid drip, but this is not always practical or possible.

Anesthetic monitoring is discussed in detail in Chapter 27. In general, reflexes such as jaw tone, palpebral reflex, and flipper pinch can be a crude estimate of anesthetic depth. Heart/pulse rate may be monitored with an ultrasound, a pulse oximeter, or Doppler flow detector (Figure 76-53). None of these techniques offer information regarding the physiologic status of the animal during anesthesia, but they do provide a means to monitor heart rate and trends. An electrocardiogram (ECG) can be used; however, because the reptilian heart can beat even after death, the tracing may prove to be of little value.

Postanesthetic recovery may take from minutes to hours, depending on the preanesthetic and anesthetic used, the length of the procedure, the patient's body temperature, and individual variation. An intubated patient should never be left unattended. Before recovery, generally an increase is seen in both spontaneous respirations and heart rate.[61]

An important word of caution here is that the endotracheal tube should *not* be removed on initial evidence of recovery. Seaturtles commonly go through several episodes of apparent recovery before consciousness is actually completely regained. Patients extubated too early may become apneic and die.

Finally, at the MSTH, patients are kept out of the water and not returned to their tanks for at least 24 hours after anesthetic recovery.

Pain Management

Pain management is a serious concern in all patients, and sea turtles are no exception. However, to date, no pharmacodynamic or pharmacokinetic studies are available for analgesics in seaturtles. Hence, anything that is recommended is strictly anecdotal or trial and error.

Caution should be taken with any novel medication in these animals. Earlier on, in an attempt to provide analgesia to two Green Turtles that had just undergone extensive FP removal surgery, this author administered flunixin meglumine at 1 mg/kg IM, after surgery. Within 12 hours, both animals developed hemorrhagic enteritis. One animal survived, but the second died within the next 24 hours.

Currently, the analgesia protocol at the MSTH is to administer torbugesic at 0.5 mg/kg, IM twice daily (bid) for 2 days after surgery. Obviously, this protocol is open for discussion, and much more research needs to be done to identify effective pain control protocols.

Surgery

Surgical techniques are similar to those used in other chelonian species (see Chapter 35). Just as in other water turtles, return of seaturtles to the aquatic environment is based on procedure, anesthesia, and risk assessment.

Shell repair is also similar to that in land turtles (see Chapter 67).[63,64] An exception here is that the marine environment tends to favor healing for small or open wounds. At the MSTH, small cracks and shell deficits are routinely left open to allow healing with secondary intention.

Seaturtles do have an amazing ability to heal, provided supportive care and attention to sepsis prevention are addressed. An example is that of a Green Turtle with a plastron wound that opened to the coelomic cavity.[55] Over the course of 4 weeks and an abundance of nursing care, the turtle was returned to a pool. Evaluation 1 year later showed that the patient made a complete recovery (Figures 76-54).

Of interest to note is the effect of the marine environment on skin sutures. Govett et al[66] evaluated tissue response to

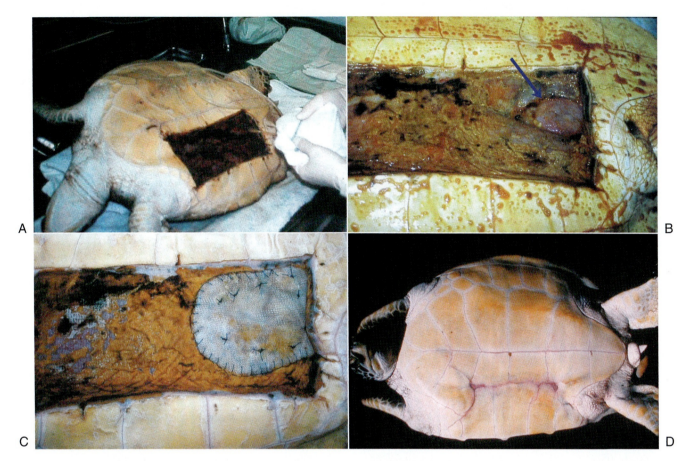

FIGURE 76-54 **A,** An attempt at a plastronotomy to remove an intestinal foreign body failed, and the plastron wedge devitalized. **B,** The animal presented to the Marathon Sea Turtle Hospital with an open coelomic fistula *(blue arrow* points to the intestines). **C,** A polytetrafluoroethylene patch was placed over the fistula, and the animal was dry-docked for approximately 4 weeks to promote healing. **D,** The same patient, just before release, 1 year later. *(Photographs courtesy D. Mader.)*

four different absorbable skin sutures. Chromic gut, polyglyconate, polyglactin 910, and poliglecaprone 25 were used in 258 turtles to close a wound produced at the time of laparoscopic sex determination. Gross and histologic tissue reactions to the different suture types were analyzed. Histologically, polyglactin 910 produced a greater tissue reaction than any other suture type. Poliglecaprone 25 and polyglyconate caused the least tissue reaction of the four suture types examined in seaturtle skin.

At the MSTH, only nonabsorbable monofilament sutures are used for skin closure. In general, skin sutures need to be left in place for a minimum of 4 to 6 weeks. In our experience, the absorbable sutures tend to break down before adequate healing has a chance to occur.

All skin closures are performed with a horizontal everting pattern. In areas where tension, motion, or dehiscence is a concern, plastic stints (made from IV line tubing) are added for additional strength. The stints are removed after 3 to 4 weeks, with the skin sutures removed 2 or more weeks later.

Several seaturtle-specific surgeries have been described in the literature.[27-29,67] In general, surgical approaches are similar to those for any other chelonian. The coelomic cavity can be approached from either prefemoral fossa. In small animals, endoscope-assisted visualization of internal organs or endosurgery may be the techniques of choice.

At the MSTH, FP removal is the most common surgical procedure performed. Second to FP, amputation of flippers for various reasons is the next most common surgery.

Amputations are generally performed at either the shoulder or hip joints, although distal amputations are possible. Seaturtles cope with amputations well. After surgery, the animals are placed in large pools to provide rehabilitation and exercise. The animals do not take long to learn to swim and steer, regardless of whether the amputation was front or rear.

We have had a number of seaturtles with dual ipsilateral or contralateral amputations (Figure 76-55). Amazingly, these animals have done well, although we have not released any dual amputees. Single amputees are routinely released. Verbal reports have documented single amputee animals nesting in subsequent seasons.

Enucleations are another common surgical procedure. Be it from trauma or FP, on occasion an eye must be removed. Because of the lack of distensible skin and a paucity of subcutaneous fat, a closed enucleation is nearly impossible to perform. Enucleations were initially attempted using standard procedures, such as the eyelid splitting technique. Regardless of the technique used, the majority of the incisions dehisced. After noting that these open lesions healed by granulation, future enucleations were performed by simply removing the globe and palpebra, in toto. The optic vessels are ligated with

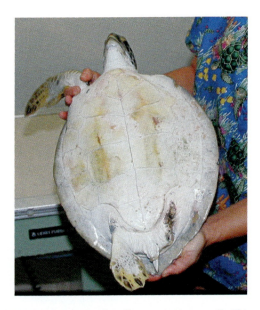

FIGURE 76-55 Seaturtles handle amputations well. This animal was able to swim and collect food even after ipsilateral flippers were amputated. The turtle presented to the Marathon Sea Turtle Hospital missing the left forelimb (probably a traumatic amputation; e.g., shark bite). The left rear flipper had been entangled in fishing line and also had to be amputated. *(Photograph courtesy D. Mader.)*

nonabsorbable suture, and the open lesion is then allowed to heal by granulation (Figure 76-56). As with other surface wounds, the saltwater seems to facilitate healing. Antibiotics and analgesics are provided after surgery. The patient is allowed back in its pool 24 hours post-operatively. Healing via secondary intention and granulation takes approximately 3 months.

Necropsy

Because of the intrinsic value of these animals, all seaturtles that die or are euthanized must be necropsied. In some regions, performing a complete post mortem examination, documenting the findings, and reporting them to the appropriate authorities is a legal requirement.

Chelonian necropsy technique is described in detail in Chapter 34. A comprehensive **seaturtle-specific necropsy protocol** is available via the Internet at the University of Florida's website http://www.vetmed.ufl.edu/sacs/wildlife/seaturtletechniques/, and a downloadable printable necropsy form can be found at http://www.vetmed.ufl.edu/sacs/wildlife/seaturtletechniques/necropsyreport2.htm. A more generic reptilian necropsy form is available in Chapter 34.

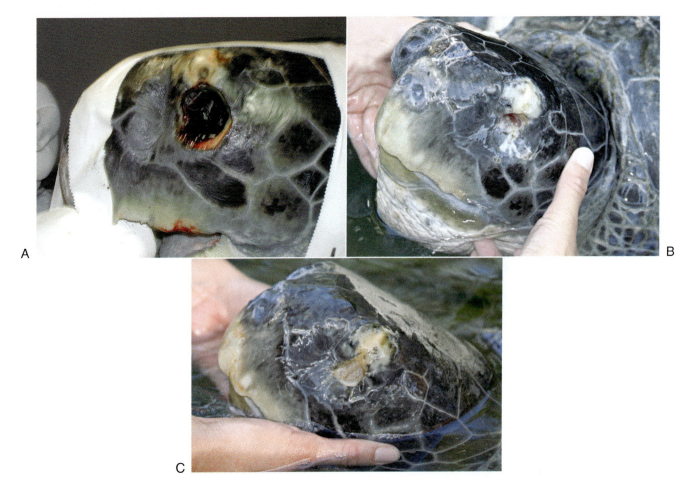

FIGURE 76-56 **A,** Traumatic enucleation in an adult Green Turtle *(C. mydas)*. The palpebra are removed during the enucleation, and the orbit is left open to heal through secondary intention. **B,** Three months after surgery. **C,** One year after surgery. *(Photographs courtesy Theater of the Sea.)*

MEDICAL MANAGEMENT OF COLD-STUNNED SEATURTLES

E. Scott Weber III and Constance Merigo

"Cold-stunning" of seaturtles in the northeastern United States and Europe has been reported for many years.[68-76] Juvenile seaturtles frequent these areas during the summer months but normally migrate to warmer waters before winter.[77,78] Those animals that do not leave the northern waters are susceptible to severe hypothermia in autumn as water temperatures rapidly drop. Although the reasons for these cold-stun events are not completely understood, geographic, oceanographic, and meteorologic conditions are thought to be involved.[72] The peak period of strandings is late November to late December when water temperature drops below 12°C (54°F).[68-72] In North America, most strandings occur when water temperature is below 10°C (50°F).[72,74] Unfortunately, 35% to 85% of cold-stunned turtles are already dead when they are found on the beach.[69,71,79]

In Massachusetts, the average number of cold-stunned seaturtle strandings has steadily increased in the past 30 years. A total of 1381 cold-stunned turtles were found in Massachusetts between 1979 and 2003. On average, less than 30 turtles per year were stranded in the 1980s, increasing to an average of 144 turtle strandings per year from 1999 to 2003.[74]

At the New England Aquarium (NEAQ) between 1994 and 2004, 529 live cold-stunned cases have been presented. Eighty-three percent of these animals were Kemp's Ridleys, 13% were Loggerheads, 3% were Green turtles, and 1% were hybrids. Of 290 cold-stunned animals found between 1982 and 1997 in New York, 66% were Kemp's Ridleys, 29% were Loggerheads, and 6% were Green turtles.[69]

A classification system for cold-stunned seaturtles from New York was suggested by Sadove, Pisciotta, and DiGiovanni[80] in 1998. This system uses four classes of assessment, with class I being fairly strong alert animals and class IV being moribund animals. New England cold-stunned turtles are mainly class III and class IV animals. Despite this, NEAQ achieves a high rate of survival with a standard treatment regime. For the years 1999 to 2004, NEAQ had an overall survival rate of 69%. Gerle, DiGiovanni, and Pisciotta[69] in 1998 reported a survival rate of 56.8% for 95 cold-stunned seaturtles in New York between 1982 and 1997.[69] Excluding turtles that die within the first 3 days of presentation, NEAQ had an 88% success rate between 1999 and 2004. Many of the animals that die within the first 3 days show no indication of being alive other than weak cardiac contraction seen with echocardiography. One could argue that some of these animals are clinically dead and thus should not necessarily be considered treatment failures. The authors do not classify an animal as dead until no cardiac activity is visible with echocardiography.

In Massachusetts, the Massachusetts Audubon Society patrols beaches for stranded seaturtles in November and December during predicted stranding conditions. They coordinate transport of all live animals from these beaches to NEAQ for medical care. In transport, the animals are secured in padded boxes, and efforts are made to keep the animals at ambient temperature to avoid rapid warming. Experience has shown that immediate rapid warming results in higher mortality rates than does controlled gradual warming as discussed subsequently.

Assessment and Treatment of Cold-Stunned Seaturtles

Table 76-7 provides a step-by-step initial assessment protocol for all potential cold-stunned seaturtles. An admission data sheet (Figure 76-57), which includes standard measurements (Figure 76-58), should be completed for each animal.

Cold-stunned turtles should initially be kept within 2°C to 3°C (3°F to 5°F) of their core body temperature. Animals are placed on towels or padding in a modified intensive care unit incubator (ICU) that increases the core temperature to 13°C (55°F) over the first 24 hours. The ICU unit is effective in maintaining temperature, providing 100% oxygen and proper humidity. Before a turtle is placed in the ICU, the carapace is covered with water-soluble lubricant gel and ophthalmic lubricant ointment is applied to the eyes. Temperature maintenance can also be achieved with various heaters and heat lamps, with care taken to protect animals from rapid heating, overheating, and thermal burns.

Table 76-7 Initial Evaluation of Cold-Stunned Seaturtles

1. Perform a complete physical examination.
2. Measure core body temperature via cloacal probe.*
3. Subjectively assess mentation, activity, and attitude; most seaturtles are quiet and partially responsive.
4. Evaluate heart rate with Doppler. If no cardiac sounds are detected with Doppler, use echocardiography. Bradycardia is common, with heart rate at admission generally 1 to 12 bpm.
5. Evaluate respiratory rate. Apnea or severe bradypnea is common, with respiratory rate at admission between one breath per minute and one breath per 15 to 20 minutes.
6. Complete admission data sheet (Figure 76-57), including standard measurements (Figure 76-58).
7. Weigh the animal.
8. Perform oral examination and cleaning of the oral cavity.
9. Use fluorescent corneal stain to detect corneal damage or ulceration. Corneal damage from desiccation and predation is common.[79]
10. Assess and photograph the carapace and plastron, flippers, tail, and head, noting any lesions. Traumatic wounds and fractures are common.
11. Assess hydration status both subjectively and objectively.
12. Subjectively assess nutritional status and body condition.
13. Immediately assess hematocrit, electrolytes, blood glucose, and blood gas status with a point-of-care analyzer.
14. Submit blood for a complete blood count and plasma chemistry profile.
15. Obtain a cloacal lavage, fecal sample, or cloacal swab for parasitology, cytology, and microbiology.
16. Consider euthanasia in cases of severe brain or spinal trauma; severe, bilateral ocular trauma; or if multiple flippers are amputated. Be conservative with euthanasia decisions; turtles can often heal from severe injuries. Discuss any seaturtle euthanasia plan with federal authorities in advance.
17. Develop a treatment plan on the basis of physical examination, blood glucose, electrolyte, and blood gas status.

*Admission temperatures at New England Aquarium (NEAQ) are generally 4°C to 13°C (39°F to 55°F).

Intake Transport Form

Arrival Measurements: Date_______ Initials_____ **Transport Measurements:** Date______ Initials____

Straight Length	**Curved Length**	**Straight Length**	**Curved Length**
Notch to Notch (cm):__________	Notch to Notch (cm):__________	Notch to Notch (cm):________	Notch to Notch (cm):________
Notch to Tip (cm):__________	Notch to Tip (cm):__________	Notch to Tip (cm):__________	Notch to Tip (cm):__________
Straight Width (cm):________	**Curved Width (cm):** __________	**Straight Width (cm):**______	**Curved Width (cm):** _______

Photos: Carapace_____ Plastron_____ Head_____ Wounds_______ **Photos:** Carapace_____ Plastron____ Head____ Wounds___

FIGURE 76-57 Admission data sheet used for cold-stunned seaturtles at the New England Aquarium (NEAQ).

COLD-STUNNED TURTLE HEALTH ASSESSMENT

MH No:_______ **BAND COLOR**_______ **DATE OF EXAM:**______ **ST No.**_______

PHYSICAL EXAMINIATION:

Heart Rate: ____________Quality: absent weak irregular strong other:_____________

Respiration: ___________Character: rapid labored shallow normal other:______________

Temperature:___________ F/C **Weight :**_______________(kg)

Nares: R: Occluded: Yes/No; Discharge: Yes/No Color:___________ Other:_______________

L: Occluded: Yes/No; Discharge: Yes/No Color:___________ Other:_______________

Eyes: R: Clear: Yes/No; Tearing: Yes/No; Discharge: Yes/No; Stain: Pos/Neg Other:________

L: Clear: Yes/No; Tearing: Yes/No; Discharge: Yes/No; Stain: Pos/Neg Other:_________

Mouth/Beak: Lesions/Wounds Description: Color:________ Other:_____________________

Hydration: Normal Slight dehyd. Mod. dehyd. Severe dehyd. Other:______________

Urine: None Clear Cloudy Color:_______ **Feces:** None Formed Diarrhea Color:__________

Behavior: Normal Aggressive Depressed Lethargic **Attitude:** Bright Alert Responsive Quiet

State of Nutrition: Normal Fat Underweight Very underweight

Plastron: Normal Sunken Bruising **Skin:** Normal Cracking Bleeding Moist Other:________

External Wounds: Mark on diagram below: **Comment:** On reverse side

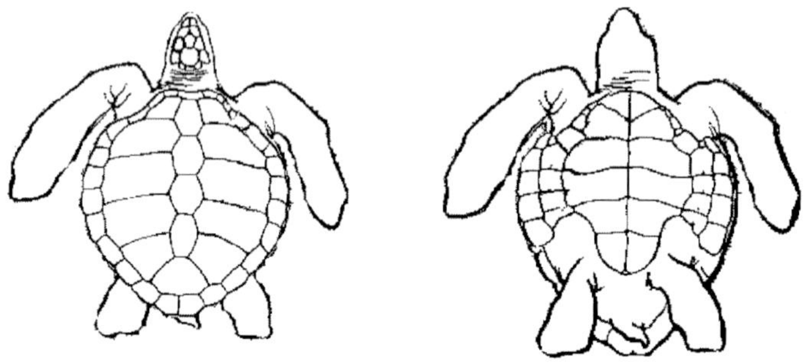

FIGURE 76-58 Standard seaturtle measurement sheet used for cold-stunned seaturtles at the New England Aquarium (NEAQ).

Most animals are given hypotonic balanced electrolyte and glucose solution (1 part lactated Ringer's solution, 2 parts 2.5% dextrose/0.45% saline solution) at 1% to 2% of body weight SQ on the basis of hydration status. This is often divided between a morning and afternoon dose. Fluid temperatures are kept at 10°C to 13°C (50°F to 55°F) initially to prevent rapid warming. Subsequent fluid doses are adjusted to the patient's current core body temperature. In the authors' experience, intracoelomic fluids offer no benefit over SQ fluids in cold-stunned seaturtles and may cause iatrogenic coelomitis. Oral fluids may also be used, and some individuals drink voluntarily when bathed. Gavage tube administration of fluids at 1% to 2% of body weight daily is useful, but SQ fluids are generally more efficient when large numbers of turtles strand simultaneously.

In animals with poor cardiac contractility and severe bradycardia, the authors have had some success with IV fluids, atropine (0.05 to 0.2 mg/kg IV), and 10% calcium gluconate (0.5 to 1.5 mL/kg IV). Other authors have reported the use of dopamine (5 mg/kg/min IV) and dexamethasone (0.15 to 5 mg/kg IV) in addition to the drugs mentioned previously.[79,81] The choice of crystalloid products for IV use in seaturtles is largely empirical but should be based on the current metabolic and hydration status of the patient. For example, some cold-stunned turtles are severely hyperkalemic and likely benefit from administration of 0.9% sodium chloride, rather than potassium-containing fluids. In other cases, hypokalemia or hypoglycemia may warrant supplementation of fluids with potassium and dextrose, respectively. One should note that most drugs and fluid protocols have not been evaluated by controlled study in seaturtles, and their use as discussed here is based on clinical experience.

Hypoglycemic patients (glucose, <80 mg/dL) may benefit from IV 50% dextrose (1 mL/5 kg).[79] The authors prefer to dilute dextrose to a strength of 10% with 0.9% saline solution before infusion.

For apneic animals, doxapram (5 mg/kg) may be administered intravenously with variable success. Endotracheal intubation and positive pressure ventilation may be required. NEAQ uses an "ambubag" to provide room air, rather than 100% oxygen to intubated cold-stunned patients.

All turtles get a supervised shallow freshwater bath adjusted to their core body temperature within the first 24 hours. Freshwater helps to clean the carapace of algae, marine parasites, and debris. Some individuals drink voluntarily when freshwater is offered, and this may help to correct dehydration and hypernatremia. Each animal is evaluated for its ability to move and swim voluntarily. Stronger turtles may be given access to shallow seawater within 24 to 48 hours, and weaker turtles continue with shallow freshwater bathing until their hydration is improved.

After the first day of care, patient temperature is raised 3°C (5°F) per day until the temperature reaches 25°C (78°F).

Start broad-spectrum antibiotic and antifungal coverage when the turtle is at least 21°C (70°F; e.g., Ceftazidime [22 mg/kg IM every 72 hours] and Fluconazole [21 mg/kg SQ loading dose, then 10 mg/kg SQ every 5 days]).[59,82]

Hematology and Plasma Biochemical Abnormalities of Cold-Stunned Seaturtles

Clinical laboratory findings generally indicate metabolic disturbances, dehydration, and organ failure.

Common plasma biochemical abnormalities include hypoglycemia, hyperglycemia, hypernatremia, hyperchloremia, hypophosphatemia, hyperphosphatemia, hypocalcemia, hypoproteinemia, hypokalemia, hyperkalemia, hypermagnesemia, reduced BUN, and elevated tissue enzymes including lactate dehydrogenase (LDH), aspartate aminotransferase (AST), and creatine kinase (CK).[78,80,82] Lactate levels may also be elevated from hypoventilation, poor perfusion, and anaerobic metabolism.

Complete blood cell counts often reveal heterophilic leucocytosis.[79,81,83,84]

Blood gas evaluation generally reveals metabolic and respiratory acidosis.

For future study, bank serum at -56°C (-70°F) for all animals on arrival, two weeks after arrival, and before release.

Convalescent Care and Monitoring of Cold-Stunned Seaturtles

All turtles should have dorsoventral, horizontal beam craniocaudal, and horizontal beam lateral whole body radiographs and flipper radiographs taken as soon as possible, after the animal's core temperature has been stabilized at 25°C (78°F) and they have started antibiotics.

Monitor hematocrit, electrolytes, blood glucose, and blood gas values every other day for the first 10 days of convalescence. Acid-base and electrolyte abnormalities often resolve with general supportive care.

Resolution of hyperkalemia with fluid therapy appears to be a favorable prognostic sign. Be cautious to monitor for rebound hypokalemia as diuresis begins. Persistence and exacerbation of hyperkalemia, despite fluid therapy, appears to be a negative prognostic sign.

Perform complete blood count and plasma biochemical profiles weekly for 2 weeks and then monthly for duration of rehabilitation, unless otherwise required. Common signs of improvement include resolution of anemia, resolution of leukocytosis, increasing BUN, and resolution of elevated tissue enzyme levels.[79,84]

A blood culture for aerobic bacteria and fungal pathogens should be performed when the core body temperature is over 21°C (70°F), before antibiotics and antifungal therapy are started, and repeated in 2 weeks.

Each turtle receives a "swim plan" according to its activity level, attitude, and overall physical condition. Supervised swims are permitted in shallow pools until the animals are strong enough for deep-water activity.

Cold-stunned seaturtles are generally not fed until they are able to swim on their own and their hydration and electrolytes have returned to within normal limits. These patients often present with functional ileus. In some cases, premature feeding may cause additional complications. Body condition, attitude, and activity level should be carefully evaluated before assist-feeding is instituted. In many cases, turtles begin feeding in several weeks voluntarily. Anorexic turtles receive an injection of vitamin B complex 0.1 mL/kg IM at least once and repeated in a week if anorexia persists. Initially, only small amounts of filleted fish are offered. Once regular defecation is observed, larger meals may be offered. Diets are prepared after review of several factors such as species, body condition, activity level, and appetite. Kemp's Ridleys are generally offered a variety of shrimp, herring, squid, capelin, mackerel, and live crabs. Live crustaceans should not be fed at the onset of rehabilitation because they may cause impaction.

Because cold-stunned turtles in Massachusetts are almost exclusively juveniles, nutritional requirements are calculated by factoring growth, healing, and current body condition. Generally food intake is gradually increased to between 3% and 7% of body weight daily depending on body condition, injuries, age, attitude, and activity level.

Injectable vitamin A, D, and E (vitamin A 100,000 IU/mL, vitamin D 10,000 IU/mL, vitamin E 20 IU/mL) 0.15 mL/kg is given IM once a month.

Oral vitamin B_1 (25 mg/kg of fish) is given on a daily basis to prevent thiamine deficiency for animals that eat previously frozen fish.

If the turtle has two negative blood cultures and a normal CBC and is clinically stable, discontinue antibiotics and antifungals after 3 weeks.

Common pathologic conditions that have been documented during rehabilitation of cold-stunned seaturtles at NEAQ include: bacterial and fungal pneumonia; systemic bacterial and fungal infection; buoyancy disorders; osteomyelitis; coelomitis; hepatic necrosis; diffuse inflammation of spleen, pancreas, fat, and digestive tract; renal tubular dilation with red blood cell casts; and bone marrow hypoplasia.[79,85]

Diagnostic testing, including needle aspiration, biopsy, tracheal wash, microbiology culture, ultrasound, endoscopy, magnetic resonance imaging, computed tomography, and nuclear scintigraphy, may be used to thoroughly evaluate the patient during rehabilitation.[15]

Transport for Cold-Stunned Seaturtles to Outside Facilities

The cold-stun stranding season in Massachusetts is short and finite. Live strandings generally begin in early November and finish by late December. During years of excessive numbers of turtle strandings, transportation of turtles to other rehabilitation centers for care may be necessary. In 1999, a total of 144 critical seaturtles were admitted to NEAQ within a 51-day period; therefore, some had to be transported to other facilities for care. Because of space and resource constraints, following the criteria outlined herein may not always be possible; however, these criteria should be followed as closely as possible. In general, each transport or release candidate should meet the criteria outlined in Table 76-8.

Summary

Rescue, rehabilitation, and research on seaturtles is a necessary and rewarding endeavor. Successful rehabilitation and release help to maintain the reproductive potential of the individual and may contribute to the overall gene pools of the populations. As veterinarians and biologists continue to gather data and share experiences, the survival rate for seaturtles is hoped to increase.

The location of release is usually determined by governing authorities with assistance from biologists and veterinarians. Release is generally attempted in geographic areas where or near the animal was found or normally occurs. All released animals must be permanently tagged with flipper tags, living tags, or pit tags (Figure 76-59). These tags are registered with appropriate government agencies for future tracking purposes.

Successful release of a rehabilitated seaturtle is a momentous event. Very few people get the chance to help perpetuate an endangered species. The work done well today may well pay off several times over for the next century.

ACKNOWLEDGMENTS

Many individuals have contributed to the development of these cold-stunned seaturtle protocols. We are grateful to the staff and volunteers of the Rescue and Rehabilitation and the Animal Health Departments at the New England Aquarium, staff and volunteers of the Wellfleet Bay Wildlife Sanctuary, and NOAA Fisheries. Special thanks go to Dr Charles Innis for his role in coordinating this document and keeping the authors to a strict deadline. We also acknowledge past veterinarians at the New England Aquarium for their efforts in establishing the basis for cold-stun response, which provided a foundation for these protocols.

REFERENCES

1. Wyneken J: *Guide to the anatomy of sea turtles*, 2001, NMFS Tech Publication, NOAA Tech, Memo NMFS-SEFSC-470 Miami, Fla US Department of Commerce.
2. Ernst CH, Barbour RW: *Turtles of the world*, Washington, DC, 1989, Smithsonian Institute Press.
3. Bjorndal KA: Conservation of hawksbill sea turtles: perceptions and realities, *Chelonian Conserv Biol* 3(2):174-176, 1999.
4. Chaloupka M, Limpus C, Miller J: Green turtle somatic growth dynamics in a spatially disjunct Great Barrier Reef metapopulation, *Coral Reefs* 23(3):325-335, 2004.
5. Zug G, Parham J: Age and growth in leatherback turtles, Dermochelys coriacea (Testudines: Dermochelydae): a skeletochronological analysis, Chelonian Conserv Biol 2:173-183, 1996.

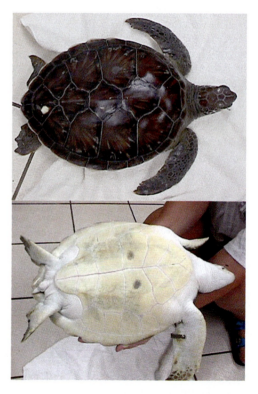

FIGURE 76-59 All released seaturtles must be tagged for future identification and tracking. Pit tags, living tags (shown here on carapace and plastron), and flipper tags (*bottom image*, front flipper) can all be used, although the flipper tags run the risk of infection and being lost. (*Photographs courtesy D. Mader.*)

Table 76-8	Criteria for Transport and Release

Pretransport for Cold-Stunned Seaturtles
- Warmed to temperature of 25°C (78°F)
- Well hydrated
- Electrolytes normalized
- Complete blood count within normal range
- Consuming food voluntarily on a regular basis
- No radiographic signs of pneumonia
- Fractures healed or stabilized
- Attitude robust and strong

Prerelease Criteria for Cold-Stunned Seaturtles
- Hematology and chemistry results must be within normal limits
- All previous medical conditions resolved
- *Off antibiotics for minimum of 1 month*
- Activity and attitude strong
- Body weight restored to normal status
- External wounds healed
- Ability to forage on own

6. Shaver DJ, Caillouet CW Jr: More Kemp's Ridley turtles return to south Texas to nest, *Marine Turtle Newsletter* 82:2-5, 1998.
7. Hamman M, Limpus CJ, Owens DW: Reproductive cycles of males and females. In Lutz PL, Musick JA, Wyneken J: *The biology of sea turtles*, VII, Boca Raton, Fla, 2003, CRC Press.
8. Whitaker B, Krum H: Medical management of sea turtles in aquaria. In Fowler M, Miller RE, editors: *Zoo and wild animal medicine: current therapy*, ed 4, New York, 1999, WB Saunders.
9. Chrisman CL, Walsh M, Meeks JC, Zurawka H, LaRock R, Herbst L, et al: Neurologic examination of sea turtles, *J Am Vet Med Assoc* 211(8):1043-1047, 1997.
10. Campbell TW: Sea turtle rehabilitation. In Mader DR, editor: *Reptile medicine and surgery*, Philadelphia, 1996, WB Saunders.
11. Bradley TA, Norton TM, Latimer KS: Hemogram values, morphological characteristics of blood cells and morphometric study of Loggerhead sea turtles, *Caretta caretta*, in the first year of life, *Assoc Reptilian Amphibian Vet* 8(3):8-16, 1998.
12. Gicking JC, Foley AM, Harr KE, Raskin RE, Jacobson ER: Plasma protein electrophoresis of the Atlantic Loggerhead sea turtle, *Caretta caretta*, *J Herp Med Surg* 14(3):13-18, 2004.
13. Bolten AB, Jacobson ER, Bjorndal KA: Effects of anticoagulant and autoanalyzer on blood biochemical values of loggerhead sea turtles *(Caretta caretta)*, *Am J Vet Res* 53(12):2224-2227, 1992.
14. Chittick B, Harms C: Intraocular pressure of juvenile loggerhead sea turtles *(Caretta caretta)* held in different positions, *Vet Rec* 149(19):587-589, 2001.
15. Smith CR, Turnbull BS, Osborn AL, Dube K, Johnson KL, Solano M: Bone scintigraphy and computed tomography: advanced diagnostic imaging techniques in endangered sea turtles, *Proc AAZV/IAAAM* 217-221, 2000.
16. Pressler BM, Goodman RA, Harms CA, Hawkins EC, Lewbart GA: Endoscopic evaluation of the esophagus and stomach in three loggerhead sea turtles *(Caretta caretta)* and a Malaysian giant turtle *(Orlitia borneensis)*, *J Zoo Wildl Med* 34(1):88-92, 2003.
17. Oros J, Torrent A, Calabuig P, Deniz S: Diseases and causes of mortality among sea turtles stranded in the Canary Islands, Spain (1998-2001), *Dis Aquat Organ* 63(1):13-24, 2005.
18. Samuel Y, Morreale SJ, Clark CW, Greene CH, Richmond ME: Underwater, low-frequency noise in a coastal sea turtle habitat, *J Acoust Soc Am* 117(3 Pt 1):1465-1472, 2005.
19. Lackovich JK, Brown DR, Homer BL, Garber RL, Mader DR, Moretti RH, et al: Association of herpesvirus with fibropapillomatosis of the green turtle *Chelonia mydas* and the loggerhead turtle *Caretta caretta* in Florida, *Dis Aquat Organ* 37(2):89-97, 1999.
20. Jones AG: Sea turtles: old viruses and new tricks, *Curr Biol* 14(19):R842-R843, 2004.
21. Swimmer JY: Biochemical responses to fibropapilloma and captivity in the green turtle, *J Wildl Dis* 36(1):102-110, 2000.
22. Work TM, Balazs GH, Wolcott M, Morris R: Bacteraemia in free-ranging Hawaiian green turtles *Chelonia mydas* with fibropapillomatosis, *Dis Aquat Organ* 53(1):41-46, 2003.
23. Adnyana W, Ladds PW, Blair D: Observations of fibropapillomatosis in green turtles *(Chelonia mydas)* in Indonesia, *Aust Vet J* 75(10):736-742, 1997.
24. Croft LA, Graham JP, Schaf SA, Jacobson ER: Evaluation of magnetic resonance imaging for detection of internal tumors in green turtles with cutaneous fibropapillomatosis, *J Am Vet Med Assoc* 225(9):1428-1435, 2004.
25. Tomas J, Guitart R, Mateo R, Raga JA: Marine debris ingestion in loggerhead sea turtles, *Caretta caretta*, from the Western Mediterranean, *Mar Pollut Bull* 44(3):211-216, 2002.
26. Bugoni L, Krause L, Petry MV: Marine debris and human impacts on sea turtles in southern Brazil, *Mar Pollut Bull* 42(12):1330-1334, 2001.
27. Jaegger GH, Wosar MA, Harms CA, Lewbart GA: Use of a supraplastron approach to the coelomic cavity for repair of an esophageal tear in a Loggerhead Sea Turtle, *J Am Vet Med Assoc* 223(3):353-355, 2003.
28. Miller SM, Koike B, Lobue C: Treatment of an esophageal foreign body in a Kemp's Ridley sea turtle, *Lepidochelys kempii*, *Assoc Reptilian Amphibian Vet* 7(1):6-9, 1997.
29. Moraes-Neto M, D'Amato AF, Dos Santos AS, Godfrey MH: Retrieval of an esophageal foreign body (fish hook) using esophagostomy in an Olive Ridley turtle, *Lepidochelys olivacea*, *J Herpe Med Surg* 13(3):26-28, 2003.
30. Paul-Murphy J, et al: *Necrosis of esophageal and gastric mucosa in snakes given oral dioctyl sodium succinate*, Hawaii, 1987, Proceedings of the 1st International Conference of Zoological and Avian Medicine.
31. Grimm K, Mader D: *Measuring intracoelomic pressure in Green Sea Turtles, Chelonia mydas*, Orlando, Fla, 2001, Proc Assoc Rept Amphib Vet.
32. Lutcavage ME, Lutz PL, Bossart GD, Hudson DM: Physiologic and clinicopathologic effects of crude oil on loggerhead sea turtles, *Arch Environ Contam Toxicol* 28(4):417-422, 1995.
33. Day RD, Christopher SJ, Becker PR, Whitaker DW: Monitoring mercury in the loggerhead sea turtle, *Caretta caretta*, *Environ Sci Technol* 39(2):437-446, 2005.
34. Keller JM, Kucklick JR, Stamper MA, Harms CA, McClellan-Green PD: Associations between organochlorine contaminant concentrations and clinical health parameters in loggerhead sea turtles from North Carolina, USA, *Environ Health Perspect* 112(10):1074-1079, 2004.
35. Gardner SC, Pier MD, Wesselman R, Juarez JA: Organochlorine contaminants in sea turtles from the Eastern Pacific, *Mar Pollut Bull* 46(9):1082-1089, 2003.
36. Franzellitti S, Locatelli C, Gerosa G, Vallini C, Fabbri E: Heavy metals in tissues of loggerhead turtles *(Caretta caretta)* from the northwestern Adriatic Sea, *Comp Biochem Physiol C Toxicol Pharmacol* 138(2):187-194, 2004.
37. Manfredi MT, Piccolo G, Prato F, Loria GR: Parasites in Italian sea turtles. I. The leatherback turtle *Dermochelys coriacea* (Linnaeus, 1766), *Parassitologia* 38(3):581-583, 1996.
38. Manfredi MT, Piccolo G, Meotti C: Parasites of Italian sea turtles. II. Loggerhead turtles *(Caretta caretta* [Linnaeus, 1758])*, Parassitologia* 40(3):305-308, 1998.
39. Gordon AN, Kelly WR, Lester RJ: Epizootic mortality of free-living green turtles, *Chelonia mydas*, due to coccidiosis, *J Wildl Dis* 29(3):490-494, 1993.
40. Raidal SR, Ohara M, Hobbs RP, Prince RI: Gram-negative bacterial infections and cardiovascular parasitism in green sea turtles *(Chelonia mydas)*, *Aust Vet J* 76(6):415-417, 1998.
41. Adnyana W, Ladds PW, Blair D: Efficacy of praziquantel in the treatment of green sea turtles with spontaneous infection of cardiovascular flukes, *Aust Vet J* 75(6):405-407, 1997.
42. Jacobson ER, Harman GR, Maxwell LK, Laille EJ: Plasma concentrations of praziquantel after oral administration of single and multiple doses in loggerhead sea turtles *(Caretta caretta)*, *Am J Vet Res* 64(3):304-309, 2003.
43. Upton SJ, Odell DK, Walsh MT: *Eimeria caretta* from the loggerhead sea turtle, *Can J Zool* 68:1268, 1990.
44. Greer LL, Strandberg JD, Whitaker BR: Mycobacterium chelonae osteoarthritis in a Kemp's ridley sea turtle *(Lepidochelys kempii)*, *J Wildl Dis* 39(3):736-741, 2003.
45. Oros J, Delgado C, Fernandez L, Jensen HE: Pulmonary hyalohyphomycosis caused by *Fusarium* spp in a Kemp's Ridley Sea Turtle *(Lepidochelys kempi)*: an immunohistochemical study, *N Z Vet J* 52(3):150-152, 2004.

46. Cabanes FJ, Alonso JM, Castella G, Alegre F, Domingo M, Pont S: Cutaneous hyalohyphomycosis caused by *Fusarium solani* in a loggerhead sea turtle *(Caretta caretta* L.), *J Clin Microbiol* 35(12):3343-3345, 1997.
47. Oros J, Arencibia A, Fernandez L, Jensen HE: Intestinal candidiasis in a loggerhead sea turtle *(Caretta caretta)*: an immunohistochemical study, *Vet J* 167(2):202-207, 2004.
48. Manire CA, Rhinehart HL, Sutton DA, Thompson EH, Rinaldi MG, Buck JD, et al: Disseminated mycotic infection caused by *Colletotrichum acutatum* in a Kemp's ridley sea turtle *(Lepidochelys kempi)*, *J Clin Microbiol* 40(11):4273-4280, 2002.
49. Torrent A, Deniz S, Ruiz A, Calabuig P, Sicilia J, Oros J: Esophageal diverticulum associated with *Aerococcus viridans* infection in a loggerhead sea turtle *(Caretta caretta)*, *J Wildl Dis* 38(1):221-223, 2002.
50. Harms CA, Lewbart GA, Beasley J: Medical management of mixed nocardial and unidentified fungal osteomyelitis in a Kemp's ridley sea turtle, *Lepidochelys kempii*, *J Herp Med Surg* 12(3):21-26, 2002.
51. Oros J, Tucker S, Fernandez L, Jacobson ER: Metastatic squamous cell carcinoma in two loggerhead sea turtles *Caretta caretta*, *Dis Aquat Organ* 58(2-3):245-250, 2004.
52. Oros J, Torrent A, Espinosa de los Monteros A, Calabuig P, Deniz S, Tucker S, et al: Multicentric lymphoblastic lymphoma in a loggerhead sea turtle *(Caretta caretta)*, *Vet Pathol* 38(4):464-467, 2001.
53. Stamper MA, Whitaker BR: *Medical observations and implications on "healthy" sea turtles prior to release into the wild*, Pittsburgh, Pa, 1994, Proc AAZV.
54. Jacobson ER, Homer BL, Stacy BA, et al: Epizootic of neurological disease in wild loggerhead sea turtles *(Caretta caretta)*, *Dis Aquatic Organ*, In press.
55. Norton T, et al. *Debilitated Loggerhead Turtle (Caretta caretta) syndrome along the southeastern US coast: incidence, pathogenesis and monitoring*, Proc AAZV, AAWV, WDA Joint Conference, San Diego, Calif, 2004.
56. Rhinehart HL, Manire CA, Byrd L, Garner MM: Use of human granulocyte colony-stimulating factor in a green sea turtle, *Chelonia mydas*, *J Herp Med Surg* 13(3):10-14, 2003.
57. Manire CA, Rhinehart HL, Pennick GJ, Sutton DA, Hunter RP, Rinaldi MG: Steady-state plasma concentrations of itraconazole after oral administration in Kemp's ridley sea turtles, *Lepidochelys kempi*, *J Zoo Wildl Med* 34(2):171-178, 2003.
58. Stamper MA, Papich MG, Lewbart GA, May SB, Plummer DD, Stoskopf MK: Pharmacokinetics of florfenicol in loggerhead sea turtles *(Caretta caretta)* after single intravenous and intramuscular injections, *J Zoo Wildl Med* 34(1):3-8, 2003.
59. Stamper MA, Papich MG, Lewbart GA, May SB, Plummer DD, Stoskopf MK: Pharmacokinetics of ceftazidime in loggerhead sea turtles *(Caretta caretta)* after single intravenous and intramuscular injections, *J Zoo Wildl Med* 30(1):32-35, 1999.
60. Mader DR, Schaff S, Moretti R, Rose C: *Intracoelomic catheters in sea turtles*, Reno, Nev, 2002, Proc ARAV.
61. Moon PF, Stabenau EK: Anesthetic and postanesthetic management of sea turtles, *J Am Vet Med Assoc* 208(5):720-726, 1996.
62. Chittick EJ, Stamper MA, Beasley JE, Lewbart GA, Horne WA: Medetomidine, ketamine, and sevoflurane for anesthesia of injured Loggerhead Sea Turtles: 13 cases (1996-2000), *J Am Vet Med Assoc* 221(7):1019-1025, 2002.
63. Naganobu K, Ogawa H, Oyadomari N, Sugimoto M: Surgical repair of a depressed fracture in a green sea turtle, *Chelonia mydas*, *J Vet Med Sci* 62(1):103-104, 2000.
64. Neiffer DL, Marks SK, Klein EC, Brady NJ: Shell lesion management in two loggerhead turtles, *Caretta caretta*, with employment of PC-7 epoxy paste, *Assoc Reptilian Amphibian Vet* 8(4):12-17, 1998.
65. Mader DR: *The use of a Gortex mesh to repair a traumatic coelomic fistula in a juvenile Green Sea Turtle, Chelonia mydas*, Kansas City, Mo, 1998, Proc ARAV.
66. Govett PD, Harms CA, Linder KE, Marsh JC, Wyneken J: Effect of four different suture materials on the surgical wound healing of loggerhead sea turtles, *Caretta caretta*, *J Herpe Med Surg* 14(4):6-11, 2004.
67. Nutter FB, Lee DD, Stamper MA, Lewbart GA, Stoskopf MK: Hemiovariosalpingectomy in a loggerhead sea turtle *(Caretta caretta)*, *Vet Rec* 146(3):78-80, 2000.
68. Morreale SJ, Meylan A, Sadove SS, Standora EA: Annual occurrence and winter mortality of marine turtles in New York waters, *J Herp* 26(3):301-308, 1992.
69. Gerle E, DiGiovanni R, Pisciotta RP: A fifteen year review of cold-stunned sea turtles in New York waters. In Abreu-Grobois FA, Briseño-Dueñas R, Márquez R, Sarti L, compilers: 1998, 2000, Proceedings of the Eighteenth International Sea Turtle Symposium. US Dept Comm NOAA Tech Memo NMFS-SEFSC-436, 293.
70. Burke VJ, Standora EA, Morreale: Factors affecting strandings of cold-stunned juvenile Kemp's ridley and loggerhead sea turtles in Long Island, NY, *Copeia* 4:1136-1138, 1991.
71. Bentivegnal F, Paolo Breber P, Hochscheid S: Cold stunned loggerhead turtles in the south Adriatic Sea, *Marine Turtle Newsletter* 97:1-3, 2000.
72. Still BM, Griffin CR, Prescott R: Climatic and oceanographic factors affecting daily patterns of juvenile sea turtle cold-stunning in Cape Cod Bay, Massachusetts, *Chel Cons Biol* 4(4):883-890, 2005.
73. Still B, Tuxbury K, Prescott R, Ryder C, Murley D, Merigo C, et al: A record cold stun season in Cape Cod Bay, Massachusetts, USA. In Mosier A, Foley A, Brost B, compilers: 2000, 2002, Proceedings of the Twentieth Annual Symposium on Sea Turtle Biology and Conservation, NOAA Tech Memo NMFS-SEFSC-477, 369.
74. Dodge KD, Prescott R, Lewis D, Murle D, Merigo C: A review of cold-stun strandings on Cape Cod Massachusetts from 1979-2003. In Proceedings of the Twenty Fourth Annual Symposium on Sea Turtle Biology and Conservation, NOAA Technical Memorandum. In press.
75. Witherington WB, Ehrhart L: Hypothermic stunning and mortality of marine turtles in the Indian River lagoon system, Florida, *Copeia* 696-703, 1989.
76. Schwartz F: Behavioral and tolerance responses to cold water temperatures by three species of sea turtles (Reptilia, Cheloniidae) in North Carolina, *Florida Mar Res Publ* 33: 16-18, 1978.
77. Lazell JD: New England waters: critical habitat for marine turtles, *Copeia* 2:290-295, 1980.
78. Morreale SJ, Standora EA: Western North Atlantic waters: crucial developmental habitat for Kemp's ridley and loggerhead sea turtles, *Chel Cons Biol* 4(4):872-882, 2005.
79. Turnbull BS, Smith CR, Stamper MA: Medical implications of hypothermia in threatened loggerhead *(Caretta caretta)* and endangered Kemp's ridley *(Lepidochelys kempi)* and Green *(Chelonia mydas)* sea turtles, *Proc AAZV/IAAAM* 31-35, 2000.
80. Sadove SS, Pisciotta R, DiGiovanni R: Assessment and initial treatment of cold-stunned sea turtles, *Chel Cons Biol* 3(1): 84-87, 1998.
81. Pisciotta RP, Durham K, DiGiovanni R, Sadove SS, Gerle E: A case study of invasive medical techniques employed in the treatment of a severely hypothermic Kemp's ridley sea turtle. In Keinath JA, Barnard DE, Musick JA, Bell BA, compilers: 1995, Proceedings of the Fifteenth Annual Symposium on Sea Turtle Biology and Conservation, NOAA Technical Memorandum NMFS-SEFSC-387, 355.

82. Mallo KM, Harms CA, Lewbart GA, Papich MB: Pharmacokinetics of fluconazole in loggerhead sea turtles *(Caretta caretta)* and single intravenous and subcutaneous injections, and multiple subcutaneous injections, *J Zoo Wild Med* 33(1):29-35, 2002.
83. Carminati C, Gerle E, Kiehn LL, Pisciotta RP: Blood chemistry comparison of healthy vs. hypothermic juvenile Kemp's ridley sea turtles *(Lepidochelys kempi)* in the New York bight. In Bjordnal KA, Bolten AB, Johnson DA, Eliazar PJ, compilers: 1994, Proceedings of the Fourteenth Annual Symposium on Sea Turtle Biology and Conservation, NOAA Technical Memorandum NMFS-SEFSC-351, 323.
84. Smith CR, Hancock AL, Turnbull BS: Comparison of white blood cell counts in cold-stunned and subsequently rehabilitated loggerhead sea turtles *(Caretta caretta), Proc AAZV/IAAAM* 50-53, 2000.
85. Matassa K, Early G, Wyman B, Prescott R, Ketton D, Krum H: A retrospective study of Kemp's ridley *(Lepidochelys kempi)* and loggerhead *(Caretta caretta)* in the area of the Northeast stranding network and associated clinical and postmortem pathologies. In Bjordnal KA, Bolten AB, Johnson DA, Eliazar PJ, compilers: 1994, Proceedings of the Fourteenth Annual Symposium on Sea Turtle Biology and Conservation, NOAA Technical Memorandum NMFS-SEFSC-351, 323.

77

BIOLOGY, CAPTIVE MANAGEMENT, AND MEDICAL CARE OF TUATARA

WAYNE BOARDMAN and BARBARA BLANCHARD

BIOLOGY

The three currently recognized Tuatara taxa are the only extant representatives of the suborder Sphenodontia[2] (meaning "wedge toothed"). These include *Sphenodon punctatus punctatus*, the Northern Tuatara (total population circa 10,000 on 28 islands), an unnamed subspecies of *S. punctatus* or Cook Strait Tuatara (total population circa 45,000 on four islands), and *S. guntheri*, Brothers Island Tuatara (total population circa 400 on three islands). They are slow-growing reptiles that take between 9 and 13 years to reach sexual maturity. Life expectancy is thought to be 60 to 100 years.[4]

Subfossil evidence now indicates they were previously found throughout New Zealand until about 2000 years ago[11] when the arrival of rats associated with humans significantly reduced numbers. Tuatara are now currently found on 35 offshore islands that range from 0.4 to 3100 hectares. In suitable habitat, as found on Takapourewa (Stephens Island), Tuatara stocking density can be as high as 2000 per hectare. *Sphenodon guntheri* is considered vulnerable and has been translocated to other islands as a precaution. Captive breeding of remnant populations of Northern Tuatara has been successful, and after head starting, juvenile Tuatara have been released back onto these islands with weights of more than 80 g and snout-vent lengths of 120 mm. All three taxa are listed as CITES Appendix 1.

With superficial resemblance to lizards, Tuatara differ anatomically from them in several respects including the absence of an external auditory meatus and external copulatory organ.[9] Other interesting features include a functioning nictitating membrane, a small median parietal eye or "third eye," uncinate processes on the ribs, and a gastralia.[8] Anatomic features of the skull distinguish them most significantly from lizards. They have a diapsid skull with a fixed quadrate bone. Teeth in the upper jaw are arranged in two rows, the lower jaw has only one row, and they do not have sockets. Adult males tend to be larger and have greater crest development than females. Males weigh 400 to 850 g, females weigh 200 to 550 g, and hatchlings weigh 3 to 6 g[14] (Figure 77-1).

Physiologically, Tuatara are adapted to cool temperatures. They differ from other reptiles because of a significantly lower preferred body temperature range. Tuatara are most active at temperatures between 11°C and 17°C and continue to show activity at temperatures as low as 6°C.[6] Temperatures in excess of 29°C result in death, and sustained temperature over 25°C can be detrimental. In contrast to the male annual reproductive cycle, females lay eggs on average once every 4 years because of slow vitellogenesis and egg shelling, which takes 6 to 8 months. Natural incubation takes approximately 15 months. In winter, they go through a period of brumation (hibernation) but often bask on sunny days.

CAPTIVE MANAGEMENT

Diet

Tuatara are carnivorous. In the wild, they take predominantly moving prey such as darkling beetles (*Mimopeus* sp.), wetas (*Stenopelmatidae* and *Deinacridae*), spiders, isopods, lizards, young Tuatara, and, during summer, eggs and hatchling sea birds (e.g., Fairy prions [*Pachyptila turtur*]).[6]

In captivity, Tuatara can be offered a range of invertebrates including larval *Tenebrio molitor*, galleria moth larvae, and occasionally larval huhu (*Prionoplus* sp.), but the most important items are adult crickets. Adults are fed three crickets sprinkled with calcium powder once weekly (four for females in summer), and juveniles are fed one to two once weekly all year round. Fortnightly monitoring of weights can reveal trends, which can be used to determine the feeding frequency

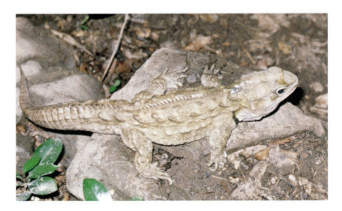

FIGURE 77-1 An obese male Tuatara that weighs about 950 g. (*Photograph courtesy A. Cree.*)

and quantities. Females increase noticeably in weight before egg laying, which should not be confused with obesity.

Housing

Rostral abrasions should be avoided with provision of nonabrasive linings from ground level to 20 cm high in all enclosures. To prevent predation, off-display adult enclosures should have a wire mesh roof and sides, the spacing of which should be 6 to 10 mm. Concrete footings prevent escape by Tuatara and access by rodents. A minimum of 1.5 m² of floor space is allowed per animal.[12]

A friable, well-drained earth floor should be contoured (mounds should be approximately 0.3 m high). Logs and rocks can also act as visual barriers. Substrate should be changed with fresh leaf mold every 6 weeks. Moving-water features or shallow dishes should allow adults to submerge.

An artificial burrow is provided for each animal and comprises a timber box (30 × 30 × 30 cm) that is partially buried in the substrate. Extra artificial burrows should be provided for refuges. The burrow should contain dry leaf mold and have two lids, with the upper one insulated to maintain suitable conditions. Shading should be provided for the boxes. For escape and ventilation, two 100-mm internal diameter corrugated plastic pipes, with drain holes 600 mm long, lead from the base of the boxes through the substrate to the surface. Burrow occupancy can vary; often animals of both genders occupy a single burrow. Natural excavation of burrows should be discouraged.

Young should be reared separately from the adults for several years to prevent predation. For the first 6 months, hatchling Tuatara can be housed together indoors in spacious vivaria. Logs and stones are provided for cover, and the substrate comprises a deep layer of leaf litter. A shallow dish of water is provided. Artificial ultraviolet lighting (e.g., Trulite tubes, Durolite International, Fairlawn, NJ) should be provided 75 cm above the substrate for several hours each day, and small pieces of cuttlebone can be offered in a bowl. A 40-watt incandescent bulb can also be used to provide additional localized heat for basking. These enclosures allow for close observation and environmental control during the hatchlings' early stages of development. From 6 months, hatchlings can be territorial, so separation of incompatible individuals, which become sedentary and lose weight, is important. From 12 months, they are transferred to outside rearing units that have the same features as the adult holding areas except they can be much smaller. Partly buried terracotta plant pots can act as juvenile dens.

Air temperature should stay within the range of 4°C to 15°C (39°F to 59°F) in winter and 10°C to 25°C (50°F to 77°F) in summer. Ventilation should be adequate, with positive ventilation being best. In regions where the summer temperature can exceed 30°C, an overhead sprinkler system can cool the environment rapidly.

Temperature, humidity, and photoperiod should vary seasonally if the animals are held in indoor enclosures. Regular misting provides humidity. Double-glazing of windows can be important for exhibits to reduce vibration and noise.

Reproduction

Male Tuatara have an annual reproductive cycle and can potentially mate each year. Males are territorial during the breeding season, and access to females resident within their territories should be controlled. Aggressive encounters between males include displays with crest erection and throat inflation, chases, and fights. Biting during fights may inflict physical injury (e.g., tail loss), although only one death from fighting has been recorded.[3] Mating occurs in late summer and can last for 2 hours.

Females lay eggs in spring in a group situation.[15] Oviposition occurs in spring. Females lay only once every 4 years on average, although 2 years has been known in captivity. On average, 11 eggs are laid[7] in an excavated hollow or burrow, and the next few nights are spent backfilling the entrance with soil. Incubation may last up to 16 months depending on the temperature of the soil at the nest site.[6]

Intracoelomic injection of 1 IU/100 g of body weight of oxytocin into a normal gravid Tuatara (diagnosed radiologically) in spring induces laying within 3 hours (but may continue for up to 24 hours). With too-early induction, however, substandard eggs can be produced. These and eggs laid in enclosures should be removed for artificial incubation. Successful incubation can be achieved with vermiculite and water (96 mL of water to 120 g of vermiculite) and temperatures between 15°C and 25°C.[13] Hatchlings usually take 7 to 9 months to appear. Incubation temperatures of 18°C are thought to produce females and 23°C males.[8] Mean weight at hatching is 5.2 g, and at 12 months is 20.8 g.[3]

MEDICAL CARE

Handling, Signs of Health, and Sampling

Tuatara are relatively slow reptiles, and capture poses few problems. Adults, however, have sharp teeth and strong jaws that can inflict a painful bite. Physical examination can be achieved with grasping the animal from behind the jaws around the neck while holding the tail and lower body extended. Holding the Tuatara with their feet on a forearm makes them feel less insecure, and they can be calmed with stoking their abdomen firmly from chest to pelvis with one finger. Handling must be kept to a minimum to reduce stress. Tuatara emit croaking noises when agitated. Hatchlings are generally more active than adults and need additional care because rough handling may result in tail loss.

Healthy Tuatara should have elastic glossy skin that is free from injuries, pressure marks, or old skin. Moulting usually takes 1 month. Gradual weight loss, dehydration, refusal to eat for more than 1 week, and prolonged reduced activity can be indicators of ill health.

Tuataras, like other captive reptiles, are susceptible to metabolic disorders such as nutritional secondary hyperparathyroidism (NSHP) (Figure 77-2).

Blood sampling is best performed by a single operator.[3] The animal is held upright and a 23-gauge × 1-inch needle attached to a 2-mm preheparinized syringe, directed craniodorsally at 10 to 20 degrees, is inserted into ventral midline tail, seven to eight scales caudal to the cloaca. Normally only 1% of the body weight should be removed. Colonic lavage with saline solution may be useful to collect a stool sample.

Tuatara have the largest red blood cells of any known reptile, with a surface area of 252 μm.[2,10]

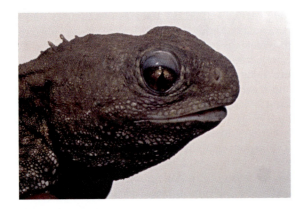

FIGURE 77-2 A juvenile female Tuatara kept indoors that shows nutritional secondary hyperparathyroidism (fibrous osteodystrophy of the mandible and exophthalmia). *(Photograph courtesy A. Cree.)*

Table 77-1 Reference Range for Hematologic and Serum Biochemistry Parameters		
Parameters	Mean	Range (n = 25)
PCV (%)	34.2	22-53
Hemoglobin (g/L)	64.6	45-91
MCHC (g/L)	18.9	14.3-26.4
Estimated total WBC	7.5	1.2-21
Total protein (g/L)	41.1	18.7-58.4
Calcium (mmol/L)	2.9	1.6-5.8
Phosphorus (mmol/L)	1.9	1-3.4
ALT (U/L)	1.8	0-9
AST (U/L)	27	4-112
Creatinine (µmol/L)	40.8	30-63
Urea (mmol/L)	2.8	1.3-7.2
Uric acid (µmol/L)	0.17	0.01-0.5
Glucose (mmol/L)	6.7	4.6-13.9

Results from Batchelar Animal Health Laboratory, Palmerston North, New Zealand.
PCV, Packed cell volume; *MCHC*, mean corpuscular hemoglobin count; *WBC*, white blood cell count; *ALT*, alanine aminotransferase; *AST*, aspartate aminotransferase.

Table 77-1 shows limited reference ranges of hematologic and biochemistry parameters.

Identification

Microchip implants can be inserted in the left inguinal region. Toe clipping is still used, usually in juveniles, for fieldwork. Insertion of a wire containing colored beads into the crest of males has been used. Juveniles can be identified with dots of white marking fluid along the dorsum until they are old enough to be implanted. Repeated marking is necessary.

Surgery and Anesthesia

Few operations have been performed on Tuatara. Cloacal gland amputation and eye enucleation have been performed with general anesthesia.[3] Sutures should be retained for at least 12 to 16 weeks because of their slow metabolic rate. Tissue adhesive is not recommended. Laparoscopy in the Tuatara has been used to assess the stage of vitellogenesis and thus assess the female Tuatara reproductive status[5] (Figure 77-3).

In addition, this technique has been used to diagnose disease of the coelomic cavity and for liver biopsies. After swabbing the lateral body wall with 70% ethanol, 0.1 to 0.2 mL of local anesthetic is injected and a 0.6-mm incision site (through which an endoscope can be introduced) is made halfway between the pectoral and pelvic girdles midway up the left lateral body wall.

Isoflurane inhalation anesthesia with masking and then intubating has been used to good effect.[3] Ketamine has been used unsuccessfully; it may take too long to be eliminated from the organs because of the low metabolic rate of the Tuatara. Intermittent positive-pressure ventilation (IPPV) should be used at a rate of three times per minute. Tuatara can be masked down with 5% isoflurane (Forane, Abbott Laboratories Ltd, Queensborough, Kent, United Kingdom) and a 1-L oxygen flow rate. Occasional pressure on the chest helps to induce inhalation of the anesthetic. Pedal reflexes in both fore and hind limbs can be used to assess the depth of anesthesia. After approximately 10 minutes, the mask can be removed and a 2.5-mm endotracheal tube inserted and secured to the forelimbs with string. An Ayres T piece can be attached and can be used at the rate of three times per minute with an isoflurane concentration of 2% to 3%. The pedal reflex disappears during deep anesthesia, and assessment of the heart rate is difficult at any stage of the procedure. When finishing, IPPV can be continued with oxygen only at the rate of two to three times per minute until spontaneous breathing occurs, usually after 30 minutes.

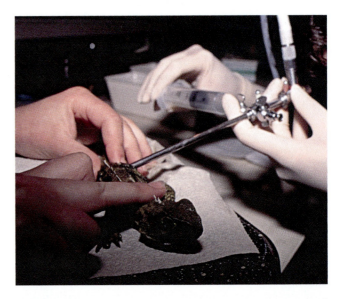

FIGURE 77-3 A wild Tuatara reproductive examination with laparoscopy. *(Photograph courtesy A. Cree.)*

DISEASES

A list of infectious diseases in captive Tuatara includes bacteremia associated with a pure growth of *Achromobacter xylosoxidans*[3] and disseminated granuloma formation, bacteremia associated with *Proteus rettgeri*, necrotizing ulcerative fungal and bacterial dermatitides (either primary or secondary), necrotic stomatitis associated with *Pseudomonas maltophilia* and

Table 77-2 Selected Noninfectious Diseases of Tuatara

Disease	Etiology/Suspected Associations	Prevalence/Signs	Management
Nutritional myopathy	Vitamin E/selenium deficiency High fat diet (i.e., galleria)	Uncommon Hind limb paralysis, weight loss	Supplementation with vitamin E/selenium in diet
Nutritional secondary hyperparathyroidism	Vitamin D deficiency Calcium/phosphorus imbalance in diet Associated with overcrowding in juveniles; smallest prevented from basking and eating	Common in juveniles Cessation of growth Rubber jaw, hind limb paralysis Generalized radiolucency of long bones	Full-spectrum lighting; calcium in diet Reduce overcrowding and isolate the smallest Increase space and visual barriers for basking and eating
Heat stress	High ambient temperatures	Common outside New Zealand Found in extremis or dead	Control temperature environment Provide sprinklers
Egg peritonitis	Unknown Suspect calcium imbalance and limited access to nesting sites	Seen several times Females perioviposition and postoviposition Weight loss, inappetence, lethargy	Radiograph all females Supportive therapy and laparotomy
Rostral abrasions	Trauma to rostral maxilla Overcrowding; too many males in enclosure	Common in males Loss of rostral skin with ulceration and osteomyelitis	Soft nonabrasive lining to enclosure to prevent damage Separation to heal with treatment for skin wounds and osteomyelitis Reduce overcrowding
Acute spontaneous periovarian hemorrhage	Unknown Artificial indoor environment and photoperiod and increased nutritional status	Noted in ovulating females Sudden-onset lethargy, anemia, death from hypovolemic shock	Vitamin K and C therapy; colloidal blood expander; attempt blood transfusion
Squamous cell carcinoma	Unknown Excessive exposure to ultraviolet light	Uncommon Slow-growing cloacal mass	Reduce exposure to ultraviolet light
Systemic gout	Unknown Suspect high protein levels in diet, excess calcium and vitamin D_3, and dehydration	Uncommon; possibly associated with male dominance (i.e., eating most food) Associated with ventral dermatitis Lethargy, weakness, and death	Provide optimal conditions Reduce protein in diet and increase access to water
Cloacal gland impaction	Unknown	Uncommon; seen in males Enlarged gland; may become infected	Manual correction and topical antibiotic ointments

Klebsiella sp., osteomyelitis after trauma, granulocytic pneumonia, body wall abscesses after trauma, skin fold dermatitis associated with moist conditions, and myositis from *Plistophora* sp.[13]

No work has been done on antibiotic therapy in Tuatara. Dose rates used are standard lizard dose rates found in the literature. However, because of the low metabolic rate, decreasing the dose rate and increasing the dose interval should be considered while at the same time maintaining the environmental temperature around 20°C. No drugs so far have been found to be toxic at standard reptile dose rates.

Haemogregarina tuatarae has been found on blood smears.[1] No pathology has been associated with the infection. A trematode *Dolichosaccus leiolopismae* and a nematode *Hatterianema hollandiae* have also been recorded from Tuatara. Ticks *Aponomma sphendonti* and *Neotrombicula sphendonti*[1] are believed to be host specific and have been commonly recorded infesting Tuatara without causing illness.

A list of noninfectious diseases (Table 77-2) includes nutritional myopathy,[16] systemic gout, hyperthermia, rostral abrasions, acute spontaneous periovarian hemorrhage, metabolic bone disease, cloacal gland impaction, trauma from fighting, egg peritonitis, and squamous cell carcinoma.

ACKNOWLEDGMENTS

Particular thanks to Richard Jakob-Hoff, Mike Goold, and Paul Prosée for help with records.

REFERENCES

Ainsworth R: *Parasites of New Zealand reptiles,* Adelaide, 1994, Proceedings of the Second World Congress of Herpetology.

Benton MJ: Classification and phylogeny of the diapsid reptiles, *Zoo J Linnean Soc* 84:97-164, 1985.

Boardman WSJ, Sibley MD: *The captive management, diseases and veterinary care of tuatara,* Calgary, 1991, Proceedings of the American Association of Zoo Veterinarians.

Castenet J, Newman DG, Saint Girons H: Skeletochronological data on the growth, age and population structure of the tuatara, *Sphenodon punctatus*, on Stephens and Lady Alice Islands, New Zealand, *Herpetologica* 44:25-37, 1988.

Cree A, Cockrem JF, Brown MA, Watson PR, Guilette LJ Jr, Newman DG, et al: Laparoscopy, radiography, and blood analyses as techniques for identifying the reproductive condition of female tuatara, *Herpetologica* 47:238-249, 1991.

Cree A, Daugherty CH: Tuatara sheds its fossil image, *New Scientist* 1739:22-26, 1990.

Cree A, Daugherty CH, Schafer SF, Brown D: Nesting and clutch size of tuatara on North Brothers Island, Cook Strait, *Tuatara* 31:8-16, 1991.

Cree A, Thompson MB: Tuatara sex determination, *Nature* 375(6532):543, 1995.

Evans HE: *Zoo and wild animal medicine,* ed 2, Philadelphia, 1986, WB Saunders.

Frye FL: *Biomedical and surgical aspects of captive reptile husbandry,* Edwardsville, 1981, Veterinary Medicine.

Holdaway RN: A spatio-temporal model for the invasion of the New Zealand archipelago by the Pacific Rat, *Rattus exulans, J Roy Soc N Z* 29:91-105, 1999.

Newman DG, Crook IG, Moran LR: Some recommendations on the captive maintenance of tuataras *Sphenodon punctatus* based on observations in the field, *Int Zoo Yearbook* 19:68-74, 1979.

Si-Kwang Liu, King FW: Microsporidiosis in the tuatara, *JAVMA* 159(11):1578-1582, 1971.

Thompson MB, Cree A, Daugherty CH: *Tuatara husbandry: guidelines for maintenance and breeding,* Victoria, 1988, University of Wellington.

Thompson MB: Incubation of eggs of tuatara, *Sphenodon punctatus, J Zoo Lond* 222:303-318, 1990.

Tintinger V: Breeding the tuatara, *Sphenodon punctatus*, at Auckland Zoo, *Int Zoo Yearbook* 26:183-186, 1987.

78

LARGE COLLECTIONS: SPECIAL CONSIDERATIONS

DONALD SCOTT GILLESPIE

Management of large reptile collections can be both a rewarding and a frustrating clinical experience for veterinarians who work with these types of facilities. Facility design, personnel expertise, and rate of turnover of specimens kept in the facility vary among zoos, large private breeder operations, and pet shops or dealers that sell to the general public. Thus, the types of medical problems encountered and management solutions vary. Quarantine protocols and disease screening should generally be easier to maintain in the zoologic and large breeder operations, with fewer specimens generally entering and leaving the collection. Nevertheless, in many instances, the level of cooperation and interest of personnel actually managing the collection to follow good medical care or quarantine procedures determines the effective level of medical care more so than any other factors, including facility design.

ZOOLOGIC PARKS

Quarantine

Zoologic parks vary in size from less than 50 animals to collections with many rare and large reptiles in numbers approaching 1000. Staff expertise also varies widely from part-time keepers of the reptile area to staff herpetologists of world-class knowledge. Even with this wide variety of facilities and expertise present in zoos, quarantine principles should be followed whenever possible.

A quarantine room physically separated from the main collection area should be established. If possible, sections within this area can be physically segregated between species and especially between shipments of animals. Hospital keepers may care for the animals during the quarantine period. Reptile staff often service the area in smaller collections but must always work in the section only after working in the regular collection. After servicing the quarantine area, keepers should not return to the main collection until the next workday. This is in part to meet minimum American Zoo and Aquarium Association (AZA) standards regarding quarantine standards. Written procedures should be established for all personnel. Footbaths should be maintained at all room entrances and cleaned as often as needed. Footbath disinfectant may be chlorhexidine, quaternary ammonium agents, or synthetic phenols. Instrument-cleaning or cage-cleaning tools should also have their own dedicated disinfectant bath per room or section of the reptile house. In some cases, ammonia products may be used if *Cryptosporidium* problems have been encountered, but this use is often relegated to cleaning tools or instruments.

Quarantine procedures should include as a minimum two fecal examinations, including both a fecal direct and flotation. Physical examination should be performed including the oral cavity, palpation, reference weight, and other procedures such as ultrasound or radiography as needed. Handling of venomous reptiles for such procedures may necessarily be limited for safety reasons depending on the individual case and staff expertise with a particular species. Blood should be drawn on specimens that exceed 100 g body weight, and often a basic reptile complete blood count and serum chemistry panel can be drawn on specimens down to as little as 50 g in weight. A reference cloacal culture is considered valuable to include *Salmonella* and *Campylobacter* species. Paramyxovirus titers on viper and other susceptible species should be done at the beginning and, if possible, at the end of the quarantine period.

The quarantine period should be a minimum of 30 days in length. Animals suspected of long-term problems such as paramyxovirus may be quarantined as long as 90 days to be observed for normal appetite, activity, and shedding. Quarantine is also a period for the new arrival to adjust to the stress of shipping, often a new environment if recently wild caught, and perhaps a new diet. Keepers and veterinary staff must recognize these adjustments during the quarantine. All efforts should be made to ensure that the basic and any special needs of the species are met during this time. This may include delaying certain handling procedures or examinations until the new arrival is sufficiently acclimated.

Accurate records are a vital part of assessment of specimens during the quarantine period. Cage cards of various types are used to denote shedding, food amounts that are offered and actually eaten, defecations, fecals obtained for examination, and other significant behavior or husbandry items. Information should be recorded on daily reports, both veterinary and keeper sections, to ensure accurate inclusion in the specimen's Animal Record Keeping System (ARKS) and Medical Records Keeping System (MEDARKS).

Preventive Husbandry and Health

Facility design may limit ideal procedures for separation of feeding and cleaning functions. In these cases, deliberate efforts to structure the daily routine are mandatory such that the kitchen area is not used for food preparation and cage or exhibit furniture cleaning in the same time periods. Food preparation should always occur first in these situations. Hand washing after food preparation, good footbath maintenance, handwashing between servicing each exhibit or handling specimens, and soaking of cage-cleaning tools in appropriate disinfectants for sufficient time periods are all parts of a good daily routine. These procedures should also be in written form and included in formal training sessions by managers for staff. Failure or success to emphasize and maintain these basic procedures is the single most important factor for prevention of the spread of many common disease problems in a reptile facility.

Climate control is essential for proper temperature gradients for specimens and proper ventilation. Airflow systems should ideally produce 12 to 15 air changes per hour in all sections of exhibits and in the service areas to help prevent the spread of airborne diseases and growth of mold or other fungi, especially in exhibit substrate, and to assist in odor control. Specific rooms may vary in ambient temperature or humidity depending on the species kept, which may require added humidifiers, dehumidifiers, or air conditioning according to the season and whether or not the specimens are brumated (hibernated) or maintained at cooler temperatures for part of the year. Temperature gradients within individual cages in dedicated rooms can be adjusted with use of heating tape, heating pads, heat lamps, or ceramic heaters. Use of infrared temperature guns and ultraviolet (UV) light intensity meters aid in maintaining desired ambient conditions. Timers for heaters and lights help in energy conservation, variance of light, UV intensity, and heat through a daily cycle as needed.

Water quality should not be neglected in assessment of quality environmental control. If aquatic reptiles are maintained in mixed exhibits with fish or invertebrates, water quality parameters must first be maintained to support the wholly aquatic animals. If reptiles are the sole occupants of an aquatic display, attention should be directed to maintaining salinity and pH in the same range as animals encounter in their native environment, which appears to be necessary for normal skin and eye health of reptiles from brackish environments.

Arthropod pests may be a common problem in moderate to large collections. Snake mites (*Ophionyssus natricis*) have been implicated in the spread of gram-negative septicemia and may play a role in viral transmission as well. Vigilant detection of infested reptiles during quarantine may represent the best opportunity for timely elimination of this serious pest.

Flies, roaches, and ants represent other pest problems either as disease vectors, odor or sanitation problems, or physical dangers to reptiles maintained outdoors in many parts of the southern United States. Care must be taken to use nontoxic insecticide remedies around the actual holding areas and in the service area of the facility because of possible ingestion of insects and secondary poisoning effects. Pest control companies should not be allowed to place bait in service and holding areas; this should be done, if at all, directly by the reptile staff. In the author's experience, pest control technicians do not seem to fully appreciate the danger of placing insecticides in close proximity to zoo animal exhibits. Even then, in one zoologic operation, an assistant curator chose to spray large amounts of chlorpyrifos for a harmless species of ant in a poorly ventilated enclosure. In this mixed pit viper and watersnake exhibit, species differences were seen in symptoms, but many individuals had seizures and died in spite of appropriate treatment. Efforts to ventilate the exhibit probably resulted in the spread of the insecticide levels to other parts of the small building and service area. Infertility, infertile eggs, and an increase in accompanying dystocias were seen in pit vipers and elapid species in other exhibits for a number of years afterwards. Whether or not this represented a true delayed organophosphate toxicity syndrome was never proved. Safe alternatives for insect control include baited fly water traps, boric acid in strategic locations, UV bug "zappers," and peanut butter mixed with ivermectin compounds. Finally, fire ants can be an actual physical hazard to smaller reptiles housed outdoors much of the year in many parts of the southern United States. Control measures include vigilance to recognize colonies or other fire ant activity, removal of reptiles if problems are seen, and appropriate insecticide use around the actual colonies of fire ants in the immediate area.

Safety

Keeper and veterinary staff should establish standard methods of restraint for all dangerous or venomous reptiles. It can make for an unpleasant day if everyone involved with restraint of a large snake or aquatic turtle is not on the same page, so to speak. Review of the procedures and expected actions from each team member is always a sound procedure even if the working group is familiar with one another. This review becomes crucial with venomous snake procedures, and a carefully written policy is necessary for accredited zoos under the AZA. Snakebite procedures should be reviewed periodically, and alarm systems tested at least quarterly. Generally, a good reptile curator should handle the logistics of space and personnel involved to accomplish the designated medical procedure. Rarely may modification of the plan be necessary if the veterinarian feels uncomfortable with the safety level involved. Remember, it is better to be "safe than sorry." Your own safety and liability are often on the line also. NEVER try to accomplish venomous animal procedures when you feel sick, are stressed to complete the procedure quickly, or have a low level of safety that may be regretted later. Specific snakebite emergency procedures are covered later in this section.

PRIVATE BREEDER COLLECTIONS

General

The same general principles discussed for zoologic operations should be used in the large private breeder collection. That is, food preparation should not be mixed with cage-cleaning activities and should take place first if done in the same area. Normal specimens should be serviced first, then any sick reptiles, and finally new arrivals undergoing quarantine. If absolutely no dedicated room exists in which to place new arrivals, placement of the cage area should be done next to unrelated species and preferably no closer than 10 feet from the closest related species to reduce chances of airborne disease spread. Because many of these operations are often in conjunction with the owner's house, a portion of an infrequently used room of the house often suffices as a temporary quarantine room. If this is done, security measures must be taken to ensure that other household animals cannot contact the new arrivals or that children cannot gain access to the room in the case of large or dangerous reptiles. If quarantine is done in an outside facility, the owner must also take steps to safeguard against predation from wild animals or, in parts of the southern continental United States, fire ants.

Preventive Health

Careful initial examination by the contract veterinarian of new arrivals may be the optimum time in these situations to treat initial problems or eliminate arthropod infestations such as mites. Examination may be conveniently scheduled at the veterinarian's clinic before placement in the new holding cages or shortly after arrival. Wild-caught specimens may be treated at this time with various anthelmintics or metronidazole at the appropriate dosages while in hand for examination.

Records should be kept as in the zoo situation but may vary according to owner expertise and preference. Again, major behavior and feeding or defecation should be recorded and easily deciphered from whatever system is used.

Routine cleaning schedules and use of disinfectants should be discussed with the facility manager or owner. Spot cleaning between regular cleaning times should be encouraged to prevent pathogen and odor buildup. Disinfectants may be dispensed from the clinic. One routine schedule might be chlorhexidine or quaternary ammonium compounds several times weekly and then use of sodium hypochlorite (i.e., bleach) at a 1:32 or 1:100 dilution after complete cage stripping or at more extensive cage cleaning times. If sodium hypochlorite is used, emphasis must be placed on control of fumes for personnel and the specimens during use and until after the chlorine is dissipated, which includes adequate ventilation, setting objects out in the sun and wind to help eliminate chlorine, or flushing with copious amounts of water after sufficient contact time. In any event, specimens should not be returned to the disinfected environment until the chemical has been eliminated. Use of all disinfectants must occur after organic matter is removed from the surface. This appears to be one of the hardest principles of cleaning for both experienced herpetologists and professional zoo staff to accept, perhaps because it often doubles the cleaning time involved. Personnel in private facilities should be encouraged to practice extensive hand washing and other personal hygiene steps such as not eating, drinking, or smoking while cleaning reptile areas or handling specimens. See Chapter 85 for a detailed discussion of cleaning and disinfection.

A set of basic medical emergency supplies should be maintained, such as fecal cups, culture swabs, hemostatic powder, bandaging material, and emergency veterinarian or hospital telephone numbers. Instructions for use of each of these items are required. Experienced clients can often be easily trained on proper specimen submission to help keep routine fees lower.

Safety

If large reptiles are kept in the collection, especially venomous reptiles, thought should be given to potential liability situations that may arise. Veterinarians should also assess their true capabilities with such animals and be ready to refer extremely dangerous reptiles to an experienced reptile veterinarian.

Keeping the appropriate antivenin may be impractical or impossible for the many varieties of cobras, vipers, and other venomous snakes kept in many collections. A call to the local zoo or human hospital to see what antivenins are kept and to determine the expertise of local doctors in snakebite treatment is a wise precaution if procedures are planned on venomous species. In many cases, lack of appropriate antivenin or treatment expertise may make such procedures highly inadvisable from a safety standpoint.

Fees

In many parts of the country, experienced reptile breeders and many pet shops tend to try to do their own medical treatments or do not treat their specimens in any significant manner. This practice often has been because of lack of qualified reptile veterinarians in the area or the tendency of many individuals to not regard reptiles as an animal or pet worth the expense of typical veterinary fees. These people have often managed to acquire common antibiotics, parasiticides, or other drugs from a variety of sources and learned how to administer these in one fashion or another. Although this practice may not be ideal, it is nevertheless the mindset of many (but not all) in the reptile breeder and pet shop industry today. Thus, charging full fees for all work, especially on a contract basis, probably results in a very low caseload if you are a veterinarian interested in working with these types of operations. A basic approach that may be successful involves the following considerations:

- Set the basic contract fees for routine visits and fecal examinations on a minimum basis. Set the effective number of visits for the facility and fees involved clearly in writing for all parties involved. For some pet shops, initial physical examinations and follow-up client animal examinations are negotiated as free procedures.
- Set prices for routine parasiticides and other drugs at cost or a reasonable amount above.
- Charge full fees for actual medical cases presented from the facility.

This type of arrangement becomes profitable primarily on the basis of referrals from the breeder facility or new owners of animals from a pet shop becoming steady clients. If the veterinarian begins a relationship with a good facility or pet shop, the word-of-mouth referrals for reptile patients can be significant. Knowledge gained from working with a good private breeder in approaching many common husbandry problems or special problems with a particular species represents another solid benefit to these types of relationships.

PET SHOPS

Although good pet shops do exist in the industry, all too commonly reptiles are kept in such businesses as a third-tier or fourth-tier product in sales and importance with staff that know little or nothing about their care. Education about basic husbandry, disinfectant use, proper diet, and lighting assumes more importance with veterinary work in these facilities than with zoos or private breeders. Unless the veterinarian works with all the animals in the business, it may be hard to justify the time and expense involved in working with the reptiles kept in these types of pet shops. More specialized pet shops that carry a number of reptiles along with primarily aquatic animals may present a better long-term choice for building a good referral base of clients that justifies the time and expense involved.

Summary

Areas of emphasis in building a good animal health program are similar to considerations for zoos and private breeders and include:

- Proper lighting and temperature gradients for common species kept in the pet store.
- Proper cage orientation and cage furniture for the species involved (e.g., no arboreal reptiles in 10-gal or 20-gal horizontal aquariums with no perches).
- Proper diet and supplements for common species kept.
- Parasite detection and treatment for both internal and external parasites.
- Training of staff of good cleaning, disinfectant use, and hand washing between cages or specimens.
- Encouragement of the pet shop owner to not acquire reptiles with special or high maintenance requirements. Even better, encourage sale only of captive-raised reptiles.

Because pet shops are not dedicated reptile facilities run by herpetologists, realistic expectations in working with these types of animal business are needed. Fees may be set along the general lines discussed under the section for private breeders, but remember that profit margins are fairly slim for many pet shop operations. In some cases, humane euthanasia of critically ill reptiles may be a viable alternative because of financial considerations.

79
REPTILE ZOONOSES AND THREATS TO PUBLIC HEALTH

CATHY A. JOHNSON-DELANEY

Most veterinary practitioners are familiar with canine and feline zoonoses and are well-versed at educating their clients regarding the importance of prevention. Reliable diagnostic tests and treatments are available, and client educational materials are widely distributed. Physicians are less familiar with reptile zoonoses and are not familiar with veterinary technology, diagnostics, and treatments that minimize the risks of zoonoses. The physician rarely seeks consultation with the patient's veterinarian about potential or diagnosed problems. Frequently, the only information the veterinarian receives from the client is that "x family member has been diagnosed with (blank) disease and they have been instructed to get rid of the animal." Veterinarians must be able to counsel their clients about responsible pet care and also be able to educate physicians regarding alternatives to "getting rid of the pet."

Veterinarians who see reptiles are often asked by reptile owners what diseases their pet can carry that could be a danger to them, which species are more likely to carry the disease organism, and what can be done to either prevent transmission or rid the pet of the organism (Figure 79-1). Veterinarians and their staff should be knowledgeable about potential zoonotic pathogens of reptiles. Client educational handouts that cover prevention of zoonotic disease from reptiles are helpful, but the information can be emphasized by the technician or veterinarian discussing its significance with the owner.

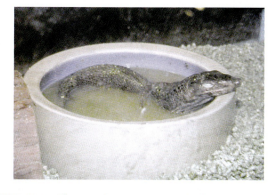

FIGURE 79-1 The number one cause of disease transmission between reptiles and humans is poor hygiene, usually resulting in fecal (reptile)–oral (human) transmission. Captive herps must be kept in properly sanitized environments and provided with fresh food and water, and excreta must be removed on a regular basis. In addition, herp handlers must practice proper hygiene when working around or handling any animal. (*Photograph courtesy D. Mader.*)

Humans that are particularly at risk for most zoonoses include immunosuppressed or immunocompromised individuals: infants and children under the age of 5 years, the elderly, and those with chronic disease that compromises the immune system. Patients on immunosuppressive therapy are at a greater risk.[1-6]

The importance of the human-animal bond and its positive effects are well known, and the healing effects provided by the pet during illness or incapacitation are well documented (see Chapter 3).[7] A teamwork approach to the situation by the veterinarian, the physician, and the owner/patient provides the best possible living arrangement for the pet-owning household.

Reptiles have been documented to carry many potential pathogens that can cause infections in humans under the right circumstances; however, the recovery of such an organism from the reptile does not mandate that the pathogen will be passed to the human and cause disease.[8-10] Evaluation of the risk potential includes identification of any possible pathogenic organisms, the amount of contact the owner has with the reptile, sources of infection or reinfection by the reptile (i.e., food sources, sanitation measures, housing and husbandry practices), original source of the reptile (e.g., wild caught, domestically bred, exposure to other reptiles), and sources of infection to the reptile during transport and sale (e.g., shipping conditions, pet store housing).

Herpetologists and hobbyists may be at greater risk through exposure to more reptiles and species than an owner of a single pet. On the other hand, the reptile hobbyist may be more aware of enzootics and potential pathogens and practice better husbandry and sanitation. Zoo personnel are usually well trained in biosafety measures for themselves and protective measures for the public; however, they may be exposed to wild-caught reptiles and those considered dangerous, including venomous or aggressive species.[1,11] Veterinary clinic staff need to be aware of potential hazards for their own protection and the protection and education of the client.[6]

Domestically bred reptiles may be infected with fewer pathogens if the breeders have been careful about screening their wild-caught breeding stock and are meticulous about sanitation. In reality, although some parasitic organisms have been eliminated from the domestically bred reptile, largely because of lack of appropriate intermediate host or other determinant in the life cycle, bacterial organisms are still found in abundance.[12] These bacterial pathogens, such as *Salmonella* spp., *Edwardsiella* spp., *Klebsiella* spp.,

Campylobacter spp., and *Proteus* spp., can originate from contaminated food sources. Risk of transmission may be greater from a live food, such as a chick or mouse, than from processed food containing poultry or beef products.[10,13,14]

The veterinarian is in an excellent position to train staff, pet owners, reptile handlers, caretakers, and herpetologists on how to minimize the risk of zoonotic infections.[6] Proper handling and restraint of the different species should be stressed to minimize bites and scratches. Bites or scratches from nonvenomous reptiles should be treated as contaminated injuries.[15,16] Wounds should be promptly scrubbed with soap and plenty of water. Topical or systemic antimicrobial therapy may be necessary. Serious wounds should be attended by a physician. A tetanus booster may be recommended, particularly after a puncture wound.[16] Appropriate soaps for wound treatment include Hibiclens (Stuart Pharmaceuticals, Wilmington, Del), Betadyne Skin Cleanser or Surgical Scrub (Purdue Frederick Co, Norwalk, Conn), Nolvasan Scrub (Fort Dodge Laboratories, Fort Dodge, Iowa), and even household hand soaps.[6,16]

Reptiles should not be housed in the kitchen or other area where food is prepared or eaten. The most important thing to decrease the chance of zoonoses from the reptile is to always thoroughly wash hands after handling the reptile, its dishes, water, or cage.[6] Young children should not handle or kiss reptiles. If they do, it should only be under close supervision to minimize the risks of transmission. Children are notorious for putting their hands and other objects, including small reptiles, in their mouths. Protective gloves should be worn while cleaning the reptile habitat. This is particularly important when removing fecal material or during changing of the reptile's bathing or soaking water. Water and fecal materials should be drained into the toilet rather than dumped in the sink or bathtub. The reptile should have its own pool rather than the use of the owner's sink or bathtub.[6,16,17] The soaking pool can be cleaned after each use with an appropriate disinfectant, such as Roccal-D (Winthrop, New York, NY), Nolvasan (Fort Dodge Laboratories), or One-Stroke Environ (Ceva, Overland Park, Kan), or 1:10 dilution of chlorine bleach and water, then rinsed thoroughly and dried (see Chapter 85, Disinfectants for the Vivarium). A splash-guard face shield is recommended to minimize inhalation of potential aerosols or water-borne pathogens coming in contact with mucous membranes during the cleaning process.[10,12]

Habitats should be designed with sanitation in mind: nonporous surfaces whenever possible, ease of changing substrates or water pools, and good ventilation and humidity control. They should also permit easy and safe capture and handling of the reptile. Other pets in the household, such as dogs and cats, should not have contact with the reptile or its cage, water pool, fecal material, or foods. In particular, other pets should not be allowed to drink out of the reptile's water or come in contact with caging materials or substrates that may contain fecal material. Likewise, letting other pets lick or play with the reptile is not advisable. Not only could the reptile be injured, but at the same time, it could potentially transmit a bacterial organism such as *Salmonella* spp. or *Campylobacter* spp. to the pet.[18] The risk of transmission can also be minimized by screening the reptile for pathogens as part of a regular preventive health maintenance program (Table 79-1).[10,12]

Table 79-1 Prevention of Reptilian Zoonoses

Pet reptiles may carry a number of bacterial, fungal, protozoal, or parasitic organisms that can potentially cause disease in people. Children, elderly, and immunosuppressed individuals, such as patients on chemotherapy or those with AIDS, are most at risk.

To protect yourself and your family, follow these simple rules:

Do's

Do wash your hands with hot soapy water after handling any reptile, cage, or cage accessories.
Do wear gloves and face protection while cleaning the reptile cage or during changing of the reptile's water tub, pond, or soaking pool.
Do disinfect reptile caging and cage accessories frequently.
Do supervise children handling reptiles. Minimize their contact with reptiles.
Do house reptiles away from the kitchen, dining room, and eating or food preparation areas.
Do keep other pets away from the reptile, its caging, and its water tub/pond/pool.
Do have your reptile examined by a veterinarian frequently and have laboratory testing done to screen for potentially harmful disease organisms.

Do Not's

Do not use your bathtub, sink, or shower as a tub, pond, or soaking pool for your reptile.
Do not kiss your reptile.
Do not eat, drink, or smoke while handling your reptile or while cleaning its housing or water tub, pond, or pool.
Do not clean the cage or dump the water in an area where food is prepared, where dishes are washed (the kitchen sink), or where faces are washed and teeth are brushed (bathroom sink).
Do not ignore bites or scratches received from your pet; wash them with plenty of hot soapy water, stop bleeding, consult your physician. Reptile-induced wounds can become infected easily.
Do not keep venomous reptiles as pets.
For additional information and client education materials, consult the website for the Association of Reptilian and Amphibian Veterinarians: www.arav.org.

BACTERIAL ZOONOSES

Salmonellosis

The most recognized reptilian zoonosis is salmonellosis. *Salmonella* spp. are gram-negative straight rods, usually flagellated, and facultative anaerobes.[19,20] More than 2400 serotypes exist. The classification system has recently changed. See Chapter 68 for current nomenclature. Salmonellae are pathogenic to a variety of animals, and although some serotypes are host specific (e.g., *S. java* and *S. urbana* of turtles), all serotypes within *S. enteritidis* should be considered as potential pathogens for animals and humans (Table 79-2).[21]

The zoonotic significance of salmonellosis was first reported in 1963 when a 7-month-old infant acquired the disease from a pet turtle, although the potential had been recognized since 1946 when *Salmonella* spp. were originally isolated from turtles.[22] In this initial case, none of the other family members were ill, although the agent *S. hartford* was isolated from a

Table 79-2	*Salmonella* Serotypes Implicated in Cases of Reptile Zoonoses[8,9,25,26,32,46,47,49,54-56]

S. abaetetuba	S. lome
S. agona	S. marina
S. anatum	S. miami
S. arizonae*	S. monschaui
S. berta	S. montevideo
S. blockley	S. muenchen
S. braenderup	S. muenster
S. brandenburg	S. newport
S. cerro	S. oranienburg
S. chameleon	S. overschie
S. chester	S. panama
S. ealing	S. paratyphi-B
S. enteritidis	S. phoenix
S. florida	S. poana
S. fluntern	S. pomona
S. give	S. poona
S. hartford	S. rubislaw
S. heidelberg	S. saint-paul
S. houten	S. san-diego
S. infantis	S. schwarzengrund
S. jangwani	S. stanley
S. java†	S. thompson
S. javiana	S. typhimurium
S. kralendyk	S. urbana†
S. litchfield†	S. wassenaar

*In older literature, *S. arizonae* may be classified as *Arizona hinshawii*, *A. arizonee*, or *Paracolobactrum arizonae*.
†*S. urbana*, *S. litchfield*, and *S. java* are at least four times more specifically associated with turtle-to-man transmission than other serotypes.

3-year-old sibling. *S. hartford* and two other *Salmonella* serotypes were isolated from the pet turtle, but the family dog cultured negative. Twenty-five turtles, obtained from the same source, all cultured positive for *S. hartford*.

In 1968, in response to information about the association of human salmonellosis and pet turtles, the State of Washington issued a regulation requiring that turtles sold in the state be certified as *Salmonella*-free.[9,23] Because positive conclusion that a turtle was free of *Salmonella* spp. was virtually impossible, in large part because of variability in excretion of the organism, this regulation effectively stopped the sale of pet turtles in Washington. Subsequently, other state public health departments conducted detailed surveys of the incidence of turtle-associated salmonellosis.

In New Jersey, in 124 families with children between the ages of 1 and 10 years diagnosed with salmonellosis, 22.6% were found to own pet turtles versus only 5.7% of control families. The most frequently isolated serotype was *S. java*. Ownership of pet turtles was found to be four times more common in families with overt disease from *Salmonella* infection than in other families in their neighborhoods.[23]

Data from 1965 to 1968 from the Seattle-King County area of Washington were evaluated to see whether the state regulation had any effect in the incidence rate of salmonellosis. Children under the age of 10 years were most at risk, and a significant decrease (30.3% to 31.6%) was found in turtle-associated salmonellosis cases from 1968 to 1969 after enactment of the regulation.[22,24,25] Other epidemiologic studies show that 14% or approximately 280,000 of the estimated 2 million cases of salmonellosis in the United States seen yearly were turtle associated.[22,24,25] This was based on a calculation derived from an estimated 15 million turtles sold annually in the United States in 1971, average life span in captivity of 2 months, and 60 million households with 4.2% owning turtles. On the basis of the estimated 15 million turtles sold annually, the risk of becoming infected with *Salmonella* organisms from a pet turtle was approximately 2%.[22]

Although this sounds like a small degree of risk to the general public, children and immunosuppressed individuals are likely to be at a greater risk. Even at this predicted low level of incidence, one survey suggested that at least 22% of cases required hospitalization, which denotes a serious health hazard. A great number of cases probably occur that go unreported because signs may be nonspecific and self-limiting.[26] Symptoms in humans include abdominal pain, cramps, diarrhea, dysentery, nausea, vomiting, and fever.[24,26] Serious complications, such as meningitis or brain abscesses, have occurred in cases of salmonellosis in young children.[24]

In 1972, the Department of Health, Education, and Welfare, United States Food and Drug Administration (FDA), banned the importation of turtles and turtle eggs and interstate shipment of turtles not certified free of *Salmonella* spp. or *Arizona hinshawii* (now classified as *S. arizonae*) by the state of origin.[19,27] Certification was done by submitting 60 turtles from each lot to be shipped to domestic markets for testing by a state health authority. Detection of *Salmonella* excretion was done with bacteriologic assay of the water the turtles had been kept in for 72 hours.[28,29] This method proved to be variable in effectiveness: many turtles were certified *Salmonella*-free but later shown to harbor *Salmonella* spp. An epidemiologic study in 1971 evaluated copper sulfate treatments to breeding and holding ponds of commercial turtle farms in Louisiana.[22,44] High levels of bacterial contamination were found in the water of the breeding ponds and in adjacent swamp and bayou waters. Similar serotypes were isolated from all locations, including turtle nests in the pond banks. *Salmonella* spp. were not isolated from the feed. Eggs were gathered daily and hatched in boxes containing sterile sawdust. Transovarian transmission, although postulated, was not shown. Infection of the neonates appeared to result from *Salmonella* spp. in the pond penetrating newly laid eggs. A trial was made to add 2 to 5 parts per million of copper sulfate to a test pond to see if that could control the *Salmonella* contamination. Although this level had proven germicidal in the laboratory, it failed to eliminate the organisms from the pond environment or from the intestinal tract of the adult breeder turtles. Decontaminating turtle ponds was complicated by the fact that the ponds have dirt banks for egg laying and a dirt bottom, which was necessary for breeding stock to hibernate during the winter. The ponds also held stagnant water that was rich in organic material and turtle feces. Copper sulfate was deemed unusable as a decontaminant for turtle ponds.

In another study, latent *Salmonella* infections were "activated" by simply dehydrating the turtles for 10 to 14 days.[30] The authors of the study suggested that many human infections that resulted from turtles certified to be free of *Salmonella* organisms actually were acquired from animals who had latent infections exacerbated by the stress of shipping and new and unnatural environments, such as pet stores, holding facilities, and diet alterations. In June 1975, the FDA ruled it illegal in the United States to sell viable turtle eggs or live turtles with a carapace length less than 10.2 cm (4 inches), with exceptions made for educational or scientific institutions and marine turtles (families Dermochelidae and Chelonidae). Marine turtles had not been shown to be a reservoir of *Salmonella* spp. and are used to restock coastal waters through United States conservation programs. Also exempt are turtles sold or held for sale and distribution, turtle eggs not used in connection with a business, and turtles and turtle eggs destined for export only.[31]

Carapace length (<4 inches [10.2 cm]) was used as a measure of potential to transmit *Salmonella*. The assumption was that larger turtles were less likely to be purchased or handled by children under the age of 10 years, the age group most at risk.[22,23,31,32] Baby turtles (*Pseudemys* [*Trachemys*, *Chrysemys*] *scripta elegans*, Red-eared Slider Turtle) have also been documented to perhaps have a *Salmonella* excretion rate ranging from 0 to 66.7% over a 3-year period and shed intermittently or continuously for more than a year after hatching.[24]

After enactment, a 77% decrease in turtle-associated salmonellosis was recorded in a study covering years 1970 to 1976.[25,33] Under the law, violators are given a written demand to destroy lots of turtles cultured positive under the supervision of the FDA within 10 working days. Any person who violates any provision of the law, including any person who sells or offers for any type of commercial or public distribution viable eggs or live turtles (carapace length <4 inches [10.2 cm]) or who refuses to destroy the turtles may be subject to a fine of not more than $1000 or imprisonment of not more than a year or both for each violation. Despite regulations, *Salmonella* colonization of pet turtles continues and cases of human infection from pet turtles continue, although infections from lizards have increased.[34,35]

Although more than 2000 recognized serotypes (serovars) of *Salmonella* exist, close to 1000 different serotypes have been isolated from reptiles, many of which have been associated with zoonotic disease in humans.[20] Virulence factors within serotypes may dictate infectivity and severity, although all serotypes are considered potentially pathogenic for humans.[9,18-20] As many as five serotypes can be isolated from a single reptile and are usually different from those commonly associated with human disease.[22,28] The variability in excretion of *Salmonella* from reptiles has contributed to the difficulties in isolating the organisms and identifying carriers.[3,36] Turtles cultured negative with routine cloacal swabbing and water examination for periods up to 6 months have then actively excreted the organism.[30] The latent phase of excretion may be interrupted by stress. The organism may be cultured from the feces or cloaca one day and not the next.[3,9,36]

Salmonella organisms can remain virulent for 89 days in tap water, 115 days in pond water, 120 days in pasture soil, 280 days in garden soil, 28 months in avian feces, and 30 months in bovine manure.[37] Reptiles may become carriers in a number of ways. Turtles kept in large breeding ponds are often overcrowded, are exposed to offal, and refuse feeding that may be contaminated with enteric pathogens. Reptile eggs buried in moist soil or sand may pick up organisms in that substrate. Eggs may become exposed during passage through the cloaca as well. *Salmonella* readily penetrates turtle eggs with contamination of the internal contents within 1 hour of exposure.[38]

Estimates of reptiles harboring *Salmonella* spp. have been reported to be as high as 83.6% to 93.7%, depending on the method of testing. Turtles may be infected at a rate of 12.1% to 85%, snakes 16% to 92%,[9] and lizards 36% to 77%.[9,39,40] One survey in Canada between 1979 and 1983 tested 150 pet reptiles submitted for necropsy: 51% of the snakes, 48% of the lizards, and 7% of the turtles cultured positive for *Salmonella* spp., with 31 different serotypes identified.[14] *S. arizonae* is more prevalent in snakes, estimated at 78.8% harboring the organism. A recent study with polymerase chain reaction (PCR) to detect prevalence of *Salmonella* in hatchling Green Iguanas (*Iguana iguana*) showed a 67% infection rate in one population and a 94% rate in the second population.[41] In 1996, the Centers for Disease Control (CDC) estimated that of the 2 to 6 million human salmonellosis cases per year in the United States, approximately 3% to 5% may be reptile associated, on the basis of the estimated pet reptile population.[2,3,41] Increasingly reported are human cases associated with iguanas.[2,3,6,36,42-47]

Although the rate of infection is quite high, reptiles usually do not show signs of disease from *Salmonella* infection and the relationship may indeed be a saprophytic one.[8] Table 79-3 lists serotypes cultured from apparently healthy reptiles and ponds. Experimental infections in snakes, tortoises, and lizards with oral inoculation resulted in fecal shedding without observable disease in the host or formation of agglutinins, indicating some sort of immune response. Infection via subcutaneous, intracardial, or intraperitoneal routes resulted in the formation of specific agglutinins without lesion development. Some strains of *Salmonella* have been implicated as the etiologic agent in spontaneous disease in reptiles that may manifest as septicemia, pneumonia,

Table 79-3	Potentially Zoonotic *Salmonella* Serotypes Cultured from Apparently Healthy Turtles, Lizards, Snakes, and Turtle Ponds[13,14,24,30,33,57,46,47]
S. adelaide	*S. luciana*
S. agiobo	*S. madelia*
S. alachua	*S. manhattan*
S. anatum	*S. marina*
S. arizonae	*S. montevideo*
S. bareilly	*S. morbificans*
S. bovis	*S. mowanjum*
S. bredeney	*S. muenchen*
S. carrau	*S. new-brunswick*
S. chameleon	*S. newport*
S. durham	*S. ohio*
S. gaminara	*S. oslo*
S. give	*S. panama*
S. harmelen	*S. poona*
S. heidelberg	*S. saint-paul*
S. houten	*S. subgenus II, IV*
S. infantis	*S. typhi phage type F*
S. jangwani	*S. typhimurium*
S. kralendyk	*S. urbana*
S. krefeld	*S. weltevreden*

coelomitis, abscess, granuloma, hypovolemic shock, and death (Table 79-4).[14,48] However, highly virulent strains occur in clinically healthy reptiles.[9] Isolation of the organism from the reptile does not really elucidate its role in causing disease in the reptile or potential for zoonotic transmission.

Reptiles, including lizards and snakes, have been implicated as sources of human salmonellosis and the cause of infection in livestock and poultry.[9,39,49] A well-documented outbreak of human salmonellosis in Otago, New Zealand, traced the source of *S. saint-paul* to the wild lizard, *Leiolopisma zelandica* (Common Skink), and Gecko (*Hoplodactylus pacificus*), which frequently were found in the kitchens and play areas of the affected humans. Another source was traced to goose meat; the goose had been observed feeding on lizards.[39] Another risk previously undocumented was from indirect contact from reptiles in a zoologic exhibit to children. The children were determined to have become infected from touching the wooden barrier that the reptiles (Komodo Dragons, *Varanus komodoensis*) had contaminated.[3,50]

Although the public is generally aware of the relationship between turtles and *Salmonella*, they are not as well informed about the connection between other species of reptiles, particularly iguanas and *Salmonella*. In 1990, in Indiana, two cases in infants (3 months old and 2 weeks old) were linked to pet iguanas. The iguanas had come from different pet stores supplied by the same distributor who in turn was supplied by one importer. The 3-month-old infant had diarrhea and fever develop and was hospitalized for 6 days. Diarrhea persisted for 20 days. Household contacts and household well water were negative for *Salmonella*; however, a stool culture from the only indoor pet, an iguana, yielded *S. marina*. The iguana was housed in a wooden cage, and the infant's father fed the pet and cleaned the cage. The mother and infant had no known direct contact with the Iguana or its environment.[49] The second case involved a low–birth weight newborn who had watery diarrhea develop 5 days after discharge from the hospital (at 12 days old). A stool culture from the infant yielded *S. marina*. The diarrhea resolved within 10 days on antibiotic therapy; however, stool cultures remained positive for 7 months. No *Salmonella* illness was found in other neonates or hospital staff on the ward where the infant had been. Household contacts and well water were also negative. The only indoor pet was an iguana housed in a glass aquarium. A stool culture from the iguana was negative; however, two of nine cultures taken from the aquarium's surface yielded *S. marina*. The infant's mother reported that she washed her hands after feeding the iguana and cleaning its cage. Direct contact with the reptile does not appear to be necessary for transmission.[49]

Since these reports, cases from iguanas have greatly increased as the popularity of iguanas as pets has increased.[1-3,5,6,34,41,43-47] Other lizards, including chameleons, have also been implicated as sources of *Salmonella* infection in humans.[47]

Unfortunately, because iguanas from different countries are often shipped together in a single lot and are not tagged during the shipping process, trace-backs are not possible. The exporting country issues a certificate of health for each lot of Iguanas shipped, but no quarantine or health inspections are required for entry into the United States. Infection with *Salmonella* may occur in the country of origin or after contact with other iguanas during shipping or subsequent housing in pet stores.

The public sale of reptiles is a major enterprise in the United States. Reptiles and their surrounding environment may become contaminated with *Salmonella*, causing a public health hazard to household members and zoologic curators. Owners should be made aware of the potential health hazards, especially when children, the elderly, or the immunosuppressed are involved. Knowledge of potential health hazards with proper sanitation is usually sufficient. Repeated fecal, cloacal, and water samples taken from pet or exhibit reptiles are useful but not conclusive in identifying carriers because shedding is intermittent and many negative results may be false negative.[3,36] Veterinarians may be asked to "screen" an individual reptile or group of reptiles for carriage of *Salmonella*. Requests may come from physicians or public health departments in cases of potential zoonotic exposure or from breeders, zoos, or pet store owners seeking to certify their animals as "*Salmonella*-free."[3,36] This may be impossible to do in reality. A succession of three cultures, at 2-week intervals, has been considered the most reliable screening protocol, but this does not guarantee the animal is *Salmonella*-free because of intermittent shedding.[3,36] Most infections occur within the first month of exposure to the reptile. Treatment of asymptomatic carriers with antibiotics is probably ineffective because clearing positive animals or accurately identifying that the animal is truly clear may be difficult.[9,41]

Treatment aimed at eliminating the organism from the reptile is often difficult because antibiotics may merely suppress the excretion of detectable organisms without their complete elimination. *Salmonella* is unlikely to be eliminated from the intestinal tract of reptiles.[51] Treatment failure may promote the development of drug-resistant strains.[41] A recent study of in vitro inhibition of *Salmonella* organisms isolated from reptiles concluded that antibiotics should not be used to eliminate *Salmonella* organisms from reptiles because of the development of antibiotic resistance.[52] Excretion of the organisms after antibiotic treatment may not take place for periods up to 8 weeks.[28,41,48,53] Because of the intermittent excretion, determination of whether treatment is effective and has eliminated the carrier state may also be difficult. Reptiles that do not display clinical signs associated with salmonellosis are recommended to be left untreated. These animals should not be used in a zoologic exhibit or area frequented by children.[41]

The only regulations in effect to deal with the *Salmonella* problem are the regulations concerning small pet turtles. Although these are efficient vehicles for *Salmonella* transmission because they seem like a relatively harmless pet (they are small; easy to raise, ship, and distribute worldwide; inexpensive; attractive; quiet; and tame), all turtles whatever their

Table 79-4	*Salmonella* Serotypes Implicated in Reptilian Deaths[14,48]
S. agioboo	S. muenchen
S. anatum	S. oslo
S. carrau	S. pomona
S. chameleon	S. thompson
S. durham	S. typhimurium
S. infantis	S. saint-paul
S. krefeld	S. subgenus II
S. montevideo	S. subgenus IV

size can be *Salmonella* carriers. The *Salmonella* public health precautions should be extended to cover all reptiles, and the veterinarian has responsibility for educating the reptile owner.[1,6] (See Figure 68-1 for information on obtaining *Salmonella* client brochures.)

Aeromonas

Aeromonas spp. are gram-negative, fermentative, and oxidase-positive bacteria that have been associated with diseases in fish, frogs, and reptiles. They are also opportunistic pathogens and have been frequently cultured from clinically healthy reptiles.[58] In one survey of turtles (*T. scripta elegans*) purchased from 27 different suppliers, *Aeromonas* spp. were isolated from 63%.

Aeromonas spp. are common bacteria in lakes, ponds, and water housing reptiles, amphibians, or fishes. Potential infection may occur from contact with the water in open wounds or injuries or from bites or scratches inflicted by reptiles living in water environments. Two cases of *A. hydrophilia* infection after alligator attacks have been documented. In one case, the man was actually in the water after a boating accident; in the other case, the man was on the bank of a ditch in his backyard and did not come in contact with the water. *Aeromonas* spp. are considered part of the normal mouth flora of alligators.[59] In addition to the *Aeromonas* infections, *Pseudomonas* spp. and *Serratia* spp., and *Enterobacter* spp., respectively, were also isolated from the alligator-bite wounds.

Campylobacter

Campylobacter spp. (*C. jejuni*, *C. fetus*, etc.) are enteric bacteria that can cause diarrhea and acute gastroenteritis in humans. *Campylobacter* is frequently linked as a zoonotic pathogen in cases of diarrhea in children with the source being the family dog.[60] During the course of a *Salmonella* investigation involving a family in California in 1984, *C. fetus* was isolated from ill humans (a 9-month-old, a 2-year-old, and the father) and a pet Taylor-Baur's Box Turtle (*Terrapene bauri*), which had been purchased 2 months before the illness began. No *Salmonella* was cultured from any of the humans or the turtle. The symptoms of diarrhea, nausea, vomiting, abdominal cramps, and fever exhibited in the humans are consistent with a *Campylobacter* infection. The turtle appeared clinically healthy but, in subsequent cultures several months later, continued to excrete *C. fetus*. The turtle had met the *Salmonella* requirement of carapace length greater than 10.2 cm (4 inches) and was apparently free of *Salmonella* spp. The investigators concluded that pet turtles may also be reservoirs for *Campylobacter* spp. infections.[56]

OTHER ENTERIC BACTERIA

Many other species of potentially pathogenic bacteria can be isolated from both clinically healthy (asymptomatic) and diseased reptiles. *Aeromonas* spp., *Citrobacter* spp., *Enterobacter* spp., *Klebsiella* spp., *Proteus* spp., and *Serratia* spp. were isolated in one study of bacterial flora in pet turtles (*P. scripta elegans*).[58] These bacteria have also been implicated in enterocolitis and diarrhea in children and infants. *Enterobacter cloacae* and *Klebsiella pneumoniae* are frequently diagnosed as causes of genitourinary infections in humans, and the possible public health significance of having a pet reptile shedding these organisms in the home environment should be considered.[58] The authors recommend caution, particularly concerning children and their contact with the reptiles or the water used by the reptile for soaking or swimming.[58]

Clinically asymptomatic lizards and snakes are also known to carry *Klebsiella* spp., *Proteus* spp., and a variety of gram-negative enteric bacteria.[8,61,62] *Proteus* spp. may cause diarrhea in humans. It is transmitted from the reptile to the human via direct contact. Many wild or wild-caught reptiles may carry potentially pathogenic bacteria because of contamination of their environment.

Erysipelothrix rhusiopathiae has been isolated from American Alligators (*Alligator mississippiensis*) and American Crocodiles (*Crocodilus* spp.). Human erysipeloid is usually an occupational disease of handlers of infected animals, meats, fish, and seafood products, with swine and poultry being the primary sources. However, keepers of crocodilians, particularly those fed infected meat or fowl, could potentially be exposed to the bacteria and contract the disease. In humans, erysipeloid is primarily a cutaneous infection, causing pain, a burning sensation, pruritus, arthritis if the joints are involved, and rarely a generalized septicemic form that may lead to endocarditis and death.[63] Humans are infected through wounds or skin abrasions. Veterinarians have been infected through needle-stick injuries after injection of an infected swine or during the vaccination process with the combination virulent vaccine and hyperimmune serum.[63]

Yersinia enterocolitica can cause a variety of illnesses in humans, including a severe gastroenteritis with abdominal pain that mimics appendicitis. It is common in many species of animals and the environment. The reservoir and mode of transmission of virulent strains are not clearly delineated, but outbreaks generally are associated with environmental sources. *Y. enterocolitica* and the closely related *Y. intermedia* have been isolated from a number of wildlife species, including Snapping Turtles (*Chelydra serpentina*), in a survey done in New York State.[64] *Y. pseudotuberculosis* has also been isolated from reptiles.[63] Although no epidemiologic evidence points to the reptile as a source for human infection, the rodents that some reptiles consume may be a source, particularly if the rodents are wild caught or exposed to infected rodent stock. Epizootic outbreaks have occurred in guinea pigs, hares, cats, rats, sheep, wild birds, turkeys, ducks, pigeons, and canaries. The disease primarily affects children, adolescents, and young adults, with the most common clinical signs including mesenteric adenitis, acute abdominal pain mimicking appendicitis, and vomiting; some cases progress to more systemic forms including arthritis, nephritis, erythema nodosum, and iritis. Septicemia is more likely to develop in the elderly or immunocompromised.[63]

Pseudomonas spp., gram-negative rods, have been cultured from both clinically healthy and diseased reptiles.[48,61,65] *P. aeruginosa* O serovars have been isolated from hospital-linked purulent infections in humans. *Pseudomonas* spp. are common bacteria in oral lesions in snakes.[65] Humans contract infection through direct contact with the organism after scratches or bite wounds, inhalation, or ingestion.[61]

Table 79-5	Potential Zoonotic Pathogens Isolated from Diseased Reptiles[12,48,57,65,66]
Actinobacillus sp.	*Leptospira* sp.
Bacteroides sp.	*Mycobacterium* sp.
Citrobacter sp.	*Neisseria* sp.
Clostridium sp.	*Pasteurella* sp.
Corynebacterium sp.	*Staphylococcus* sp.
Edwardsiella tarda	*Streptococcus* sp.
Escherichia coli	

Many potential zoonotic pathogens have been isolated from diseased reptiles (Table 79-5). Although most probably are not considered health risks to healthy human adults, they could pose potential disease risks for the immunocompromised, infants and young children, and the elderly.

Mycobacterium

Mycobacterium spp. are acid-fast bacilli. Several species known to cause infection in humans have been isolated from reptiles including *M. marinum*, *M. avium*, and *M. tuberculosis*.[48,66,67] *M. marinum* has been implicated in cutaneous and subcutaneous nodular disease in humans.[66] Direct contact with the organism through scratches in the skin, during handling the animal, or while cleaning its habitat resulted in the human infection.[68] *Mycobacterium* spp. cause a wide variety of pathologic lesions in reptiles, usually chronic, including both granulomatous and nongranulomatous lesions, involving the lungs, liver, spleen, skin, subcutaneous tissue, oral mucosa, gonads, bone, and central nervous system.[48,67,69] Potential routes of transmission of *Mycobacterium* spp. organisms to humans from infected pet reptiles include direct contact through defects, scratches, or bites in the skin or with inhalation and contact with oral or respiratory mucosa. The veterinarian, technicians, and staff who handle reptiles with chronic, purulent, or granulomatous lesions should protect themselves by wearing appropriate gloves, mask, face/eye shield (particularly when cleaning caging, tanks), and other garments. Treatment of infected reptiles is not recommended because of the zoonotic potential. The owner should be instructed in proper methods of sanitizing the reptile's environment to minimize exposure and eliminate the organisms.

Q Fever—*Coxiella burnetii*

In 1978, a cluster of human cases of Q fever caused by the rickettsia *Coxiella burnetii* was diagnosed in employees of an exotic bird and reptile importing company in New York State. These employees had been involved in unpacking and deticking a shipment of Ball Pythons *(Python reguis)* imported from Ghana. Three types of ticks were identified, including *Amblyomma nuttalli*, the vector of Q fever. Although two types of rickettsial organisms were isolated from the hemolymph of five ticks but not characterized further, direct isolation of the organism from samples of Python blood, spleen, and liver and from 15 live ticks and five frozen ticks was negative. Speculation was that the employees had been infected by inhaling aerosolized particles containing *C. burnetii* during the handling of the Pythons or ticks or excreta of the ticks or Pythons.[70] *C. burnetii* is a gram-positive rod-shaped organism that can assume spherical or diplococcoid forms. It has been identified in snakes, lizards, and turtles during serologic surveillance of wildlife, and speculation exists that reptiles may serve as reservoir hosts for the transmission of *C. burnetii* by infected ticks to mammals.[48,71]

FUNGAL INFECTIONS

Zygomycosis

Zygomycosis, also known as phycomycosis, mucormycosis, or entomophthoromycosis, refers to a group of diseases in man caused by several genera and species of fungi belonging to the class Zygomycetes, orders Entomophthorales and Mucorales.[63] Zygomycetes are ubiquitous saprophytes that produce a large number of spores. These fungi are opportunistic pathogens because they invade tissues of patients weakened by other diseases, on long-term antibiotic therapy, or immunosuppressed. Humans contract the infection through inhalation, ingestion, inoculation, or contamination of the skin with the spores.[63] They are common inhabitants of the gastrointestinal tract of reptiles and amphibians and are considered common fungi of decomposing organic material. Organisms from the order Entomorphthoales have been isolated from gastroenteric mycoses in reptiles.[48] Entomophthorales contains members of *Basidiobolus ranarum (B. haptosporus)*, which has been documented to cause a granulomatous disease in man primarily in the subcutaneous tissues. Cases have occurred in Africa, Southeast Asia, Latin America, and the United States. Disease from *Conidiobolus* spp. produces lesions in the nasal concha, subcutaneous facial tissues, paranasal sinuses, pericardium, mediastinum, and lungs. *Conidiobolus* cases have occurred primarily in the tropics.

Order Mucorales contains the genera *Absidia*, *Mucor*, *Rhizopus*, *Cunninghamella*, and *Rhizomucor*. *Mucor* spp. and *Rhizopus arrhizus* have been isolated from various reptile species with pneumonia.[48] Infections in humans usually begin in the nasal mucosa and paranasal sinuses and then spread to the eye, meninges, and brain. Other routes of dissemination include the pulmonary system, the gastrointestinal system, and subcutaneous tissue if the infection was a consequence of deep burns, injections, or contaminated bandages over wounds. The rhinocerebral form has been diagnosed mainly in patients with diabetes mellitus. Immunosuppressed patients, whether from immunosuppressive disease or from prolonged treatments with immunosuppressant medications, have been seen with the pulmonary or disseminated mucormycoses form.[15,63] Although no documentation of transmission of these fungal agents from the diseased reptile directly to the human can be found, the potential for infection exists.

To minimize potential inhalation, ingestion, or contamination of the skin with fungal agents from reptiles, the veterinarian and staff should wear gloves, masks, and face shields when handling the animal, its feces, and contaminated housing, and during necropsy procedures. Owners should be educated in the proper handling of fecal materials and sanitation of the caging.

Deep and Superficial Mycoses

Many different mycotic agents have been isolated from diseased reptiles that could also cause infection in humans. *Aspergillus* spp. have been isolated from skin, pulmonary, and systemic lesions in chelonians, crocodilians, lizards, and snakes. *Candida* spp. have been cultured from pulmonary and hepatic lesions. *Trichosporon* spp. and *Trichophyton* spp. have also been isolated from reptiles. Zoonotic transmission of fungal agents, although possible, has not been documented.[48]

VIRAL AGENTS

Reptiles may act as reservoir hosts to western equine encephalitis (WEE; genus: *Alphavirus;* family: Togaviridae). The exact mechanism for the maintenance of the virus over the winter and the insertion into the transmission cycle is unclear. In one study in Utah, the virus was isolated from the blood of 37 of 84 snakes of three genera (*Thamnophis, Coluber,* and *Pituophis*), captured, and examined in the early spring. The viremia in the snakes is cyclic with changes in the ambient temperature. A rise in ambient temperature is accompanied by the reappearance of the viremia. The viremia in the snakes was sufficiently high to infect a large percentage of the vector, *Culex tarsalis*, that were allowed to feed on the snakes. Viremia was also found in the progeny of infected snakes.

In a Canadian survey of wild reptiles and amphibians, snakes of the genus *Thamnophis* and frogs (*Rana pipiens*) were found to be viremic. Wild-caught reptiles from endemic areas may be infected. Reptiles should not be housed outdoors during an epizootic outbreak in horses in an area.[48] Public health notifications usually discuss precautions for humans, horses, and birds but do not mention reptilian or amphibian collections that may be housed outdoors (Figure 79-2).

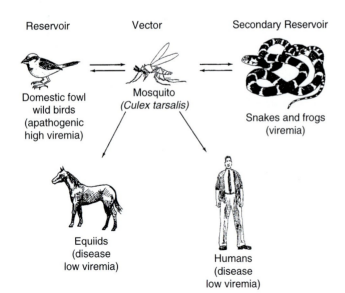

FIGURE 79-2 Life cycle of western equine encephalitis.

Veterinarians may need to contact reptile owners about the possible role of the reptile in the disease and to encourage owners to house reptiles indoors during epizootic outbreaks. WEE affects humans and horses.

West Nile virus (WNV) is a mosquito-borne flavivirus that is transmitted by various species of adult *Culex* mosquitoes (see Chapters 17, 24, and 41 for additional information on the virus and disease). WNV is known to have zoonotic potential as a result of infectivity in a wide variety of mammals and birds.[72] Although flaviviruses and arboviruses have been reported to affect ectotherms and in some cases serve as reservoirs, reptiles and amphibians were not initially considered as primary species at risk.[73] The virus emerged in North America in 1999 when it infected and caused deaths in humans, horses, and birds.[72] By the year 2001, WNV had spread into the southeastern United States, including Georgia and Florida. During the fall of 2001 and 2002, two epizootics occurred in captive alligators (*A. mississippiensis*) housed on an alligator farm in Georgia.[73] The disease was also reported in three wild alligators from central Florida and in one captive Crocodile Monitor (*Varanus salvadori*) with neurologic signs from the District of Columbia and Maryland area.[74] The disease had previously been reported in farmed Nile Crocodiles (*Crocodylus niloticus*) in Israel.[72,74] In 2004, WNV also was reported in alligator farms in Louisiana and at an alligator farm in Idaho that received young alligators from Florida.[72] Serologic surveys of reptiles in Israel in 1965 to 1966 had found hemagglutination-inhibiting antibodies in one turtle (*Clemmys caspica*).[74] Experimentally, a Russian strain of WNV resulted in a high level of viremia in Lake Frogs (*Rana ridibunda*).[75] At publication, North American species that may serve as reservoirs, or that may be affected by the virus, are under study. The potential role of reptiles and amphibians in the life cycle and epidemiology of WNV is not known.[74] If wild and captive species are susceptible, then the range of WNV and zoonotic potential will increase if North American and captive nonnative herpetologic species can serve as reservoirs for the virus.[76]

PROTOZOA

Despite the high numbers of protozoal organisms found in reptiles, most are ectotherm specific, that is, reptile specific. Many varieties are not associated with known disease in the reptile, and their significance as zoonotic pathogens is also unknown. Many may be opportunistic pathogens of the reptile and opportunistic zoonotic pathogens to susceptible humans, with infants and the elderly, the immunocompromised, or debilitated most at risk.

Cryptosporidia

Cryptosporidium is a coccidian protozoan in the family Cryptosporidiidae, suborder Eimeriina. The parasite is not species specific and can easily be transmitted from one mammalian species to another or from animal to man. It has been isolated in many different hosts including mammals, birds, and reptiles.[77] No documented evidence has shown that reptilian cryptosporidiosis is zoonotic. Cattle and poultry have served as primary reservoirs of infection.[63]

PENTASTOMIASIS (ARMILLIFERIASIS)

The pentastomes are currently classified in a separate phylum, Pentastomida, because they exhibit characteristics of both the phyla Arthropoda and Annelida.[63,78,79] They have also been called linguatulids or tongue worms because of their distinct tongue-shaped appearance. Infection by pentastomids may be referred to as pentastomiasis, linguatuliasis or linguatulosis, porocephalosis, or porocephaliasis.[79] Pentastomes are almost exclusively parasites of reptiles, with the exception of species of *Linguatula* with carnivorous mammals as definitive hosts and *Reighardia sternae* with seagulls and terns as definitive hosts.[78,79]

Nine genera have been identified in snakes, three in lizards, four in crocodiles, and two in turtles. *Armillifer* spp. are the most common genera identified from pythonids and viperids, *Kiricephalus* spp. from colubrids, and *Porocephalus* spp. from boids and crotalids.[79] A variety of herbivorous vertebrates may serve as intermediate hosts, including rodents and artiodactylids. Carnivores, nonhuman primates, and humans may serve as incidental hosts.[78,79] Figure 79-3 shows a typical presentation of the adult parasites in the lung tissue from a primate. Figure 21-1 depicts the characteristic life cycle of a pentastomid.

The larval stage of the pentastome bores through the intestinal wall of the intermediate host and passes into the blood, then migrates to the mesenteric lymph nodes, liver, lungs, omentum, or other organs where it becomes encysted. The larva becomes quiescent and metamorphoses into the vermiform nymphal stage that may pass through a series of molts. After this series of molts, a third-stage larva may break out of the cyst and migrate through the peritoneal cavity of the intermediate host. The reptilian definitive host is infected by ingestion of the intermediate host with the encysted nymphal forms or migrating third-stage larvae. The infective larvae penetrate the host's intestine and migrate to the respiratory system. They develop to sexually mature adult parasites in the lungs, trachea, or nasal passages of the reptile. Female pentastomids may produce several million fully embryonated eggs, each containing a single larva. Eggs are coughed up by the host, swallowed, and passed to the environment in the feces.[80] The life cycle of the pentastomid is considered an oddity in that the intermediate host (rodent, mammal) is higher in the phylogenic scheme than the definitive host (snake, reptile), an uncommon occurrence among parasites.[78,79]

Man, an aberrant host, contracts the infection by consuming water or foods contaminated with eggs eliminated in the saliva or feces of snakes, by consuming raw or undercooked snake meat, or by handling infected reptiles and then placing contaminated hands in the mouth. Other intermediate hosts are infected through ingestion of contaminated water, plants, or the snakes themselves.[63]

In the aberrant host, such as man, dogs, or cats, pentastomes may cause minimal to moderate inflammatory responses. The larvae are eventually surrounded by scar tissue with minimal mononuclear infiltrate. Eosinophilic response is generally absent. Despite the host response, the pentastomes can excyst and migrate. Whether the larvae eventually die of their own accord or are killed by the host immune response is unclear. Most larvae are thought to die and calcify within 2 years of infection.[78] Usually, the incidental host is asymptomatic with the larval invasion, and migration nymphs or larvae are often found at necropsy or during radiographic examination. The organisms may show up as radiopaque C-shaped or serpiginous objects on radiographs (see Figure 21-61). A case has been published of fatal pentastomiasis from *Armillifer armillatus*, although the parasite infestation was not definitively established as the cause of death.[16,81] The fact that humans can serve as incidental hosts for reptilian pentastomes should alert veterinarians to recognize the zoonotic potential of these parasites.

At present, no successful therapy exists against the larval forms in the incidental hosts. In cases of limited infection in humans, surgical removal of free or encysted larvae has been tried. Experimental trials with oral mebendazole and antihistamines in dogs infected with larval *P. crotali* proved ineffective in controlling the organisms. Severe allergic responses in the incidental host may be triggered by the death of numerous larval pentastomes, which may be an unwanted consequence of treatment with some of the newer anthelmintics. Surgical removal may be difficult because of the extensive tissue distribution of the larvae and cysts.[78,79]

Treatment of infected reptiles may be attempted, but anthelminthic drugs may not be effective because of the extraintestinal location of the adult parasites. Levamisole hydrochloride (Ripercol, American Cyanamid, Wayne, NJ) given intracoelomically in snakes at a rate of 5 mg/kg along with antibiotics to treat associated pneumonia or secondary bacterial infections has been tried.[10,63] Supportive fluids, vitamins, diuretics, and oxygen supplementation should also be provided as necessary.[10] See Chapter 21 for a more thorough discussion of treatment options, including endoscopic retrieval of adult worms, in reptile patients.

Veterinarians need to educate pet owners about the zoonotic potential of pentastomiasis. Newly acquired reptiles, whether purchased at pet stores or captured from the wild, should be examined. Only "clean" laboratory/commercially bred and reared rodents should be fed to pet or captive reptiles to minimize the chances for infection. Ideally at least two successive fecal specimens from the reptile should

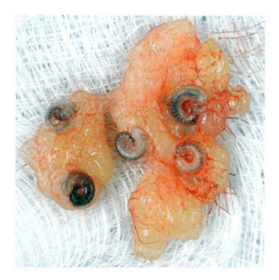

FIGURE 79-3 Pentastomid parasite from the lung tissue of a primate. See Figure 21-1 for the life cycle and transmission of this common zoonotic parasite.

be examined to reduce the possibility of false-negative results. The need for prompt removal of feces from the reptile's habitat should be stressed. The owner should be instructed in the proper disposal of snake feces (i.e., flush down the toilet versus the family garbage can) and to wear gloves while doing so. Reptile food sources (such as live rodents) should not be allowed to come in contact with the reptile's feces.

HELMINTHS

Reptiles act as the second intermediate hosts for cestodes in the genera *Spirometra* and *Diphyllobothrium*. *Spirometra mansoni, S. mansonoides, S. erinaceieuropaei (D. erinacei), S. theileri,* and *S. proliferum* have been associated with sparganosis in humans (i.e., infection with the second-stage larvae called the sparganum or plerocercoid). The definitive hosts are mainly domestic and wild canids and felids. Amphibians and reptiles become infected after ingesting the first intermediate host, a copepod *Cyclops* found in water environments worldwide, or by ingesting other animals that harbor sparga. Man is generally infected through ingestion of raw or undercooked infected amphibian, reptile, bird, or wild mammal meat or through direct contact with infected amphibian meat used as a poultice for antiphlogistic effects in some Southeast Asian cultures. Use of the poultice has been linked to an ocular form of sparganosis. The assumption is that man can also be infected via drinking water containing infected copepods (first-stage larvae). Man is an accidental host and usually does not play a role in the life cycle of the parasite.[63]

Because of the life cycle and environmental conditions needed along with the fact that most pet reptiles are not going to be a food source, risk of sparganosis from captive and pet reptiles is low. Freshwater sources devoid of the copepod negate the possibility of maintaining the life cycle (Figure 79-4).

Mesocestoidiasis is a rare infection in man caused by *Mesocestoides lineatus* or *M. variabilis*. The definitive hosts are dogs, cats, and several species of wild carnivores. The first intermediate host appears to be an arthropod, and many vertebrates can harbor the tetrathyridium larval form including reptiles, amphibians, birds, and mammals. Man has been infected through the ingestion of raw meat of the intermediate host. In Japan, several cases have been connected to the consumption of raw snake liver.[63] Pet and captive reptiles not used as food sources pose no zoonotic risk.

ARTHROPODA

Arthropods that affect reptiles do not pose a direct zoonotic threat. Instead, their importance may be as vectors for viral or bacterial diseases, with the reptile serving as a reservoir. The arthropods may cross species, biting reptiles, birds, and mammals, including humans. *Aedes* and *Culex* genera of mosquitoes may feed on reptiles, serving as possible reservoirs for western equine encephalitis virus.[63,82]

Ornithodoros turicata, also known as the relapsing fever tick, is native to the United States and Mexico and can occasionally be found on reptiles. Heavy infestations have been found on the Box Turtle (*Terrapene* spp.), on the Gopher

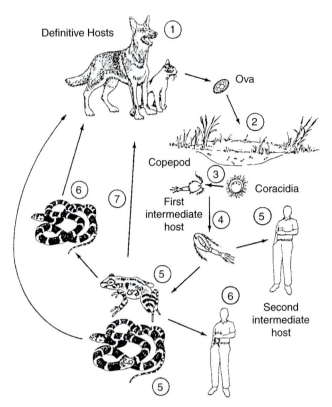

FIGURE 79-4 Transmission cycle in sparganosis. *1*, Definitive host (canids, felids). Plerocercoid attaches to intestinal mucosa, matures in 10 to 30 days, produces eggs. *2*, Eggs passed in feces, end up in water containing copepods of the genus *Cyclops*. In the water, eggs become free ciliated embryos called coracidia. *3*, Coracidia ingested by first intermediate host (*Cyclops*). *4*, Develop into first-stage larvae, "procercoid," in the tissues of *Cyclops*. *5*, Ingestion of procercoids in infected *Cyclops* via water by second intermediate host (vertebrates: reptiles, amphibians, birds, small mammals [rodents, insectivores], swine, nonhuman primates, man). *6*, Develops into a "plerocercoid" or "sparganum" in the tissues of the vertebrate host. Plerocercoids in an ingested infected vertebrate can encyst in new vertebrate host. Man can be infected with ingestion of either a procercoid or a plerocercoid. *7*, Infected vertebrate host with plerocercoids ingested.

Tortoise (*Gopherus polyphemus*), and on rattlesnakes (*Crotalus* spp.). It transmits relapsing fever (also known as tick-borne relapsing fever, borreliosis, or spirochetosis) in man. The tick may also be a vector of *Leptospira pomona*. All stages readily attack man.[82]

Immature stages of *Haemaphysalis punctata* have been found on lizards in Europe, northwestern Africa, and southwestern Asia and on the European Viper (*Vipera berus*). This tick may transmit the agent of Siberian tick typhus (*Rickettsia siberica/Dermacentroxenus sibericus*). Immature stages of another tick, *H. concinna*, have been found on various reptiles in Europe and northern Asia. This tick transmits the agents of Russian spring-summer encephalitis (a flavivirus) and Siberian tick typhus.[82]

The immature stages of *Ixodes pacificus* are found on Gartersnakes (*Thamnophis* spp.) and lizards (*Sceloporus* spp.) in the Pacific coastal region of North America. It is also called the California black-legged tick and is quite common. The bite itself causes irritation and trauma in man and has been implicated in the transmission of tularemia (*Francisella tularensis*). It also may transmit Lyme disease (*Borrelia burgdorferi*). In Europe, immature stages of *I. ricinus* rarely occur on lizards. However, this tick's bite also causes severe irritation and paralysis in man and may transmit central European tick-borne encephalitis, Lyme disease, and agents of Boutonneuse fever (*R. conorii/D. conorii*).[82]

Larvae of trombiculid mites have been found on reptiles caught in the wild or maintained in outdoor habitats in endemic areas. The most common species in North America is *Eutrombicula alfreddugesi* (also called *Trombicula irritans*), the common chigger. It has been found throughout the Western Hemisphere on Box Turtles (*Terrapene* spp.), various snakes including racers (*Masticophis* spp.), Hog-nosed Snakes (*Heterodon* spp.), Kingsnakes (*Lampropeltis* spp.), Gartersnakes (*Thamnophis* spp.), and various lizards. *E. splendens*, common in the southeastern United States, has been found on snakes and lizards. In Europe, *Neotrombicula autumnalis*, the common harvest mite, has been found on lizards and snakes. Only the larvae of these genera are parasitic. The adults are free-living. Control of the reptile includes topical insecticides and cleansing of the environment. All of these mites have been reported to cause dermatitis in man.[82]

Ophionyssus natricis, a dermanyssid mite of snakes and occasionally lizards, may bite humans. The mite is worldwide in distribution, and heavy infestations can lead to severe anemia, anorexia, lethargy, and death of the host snake. *O. natricis* is known to transmit *Aeromonas hydrophilus*, which has caused fatal hemorrhagic septicemia in snakes. A documented case in humans involved an infested pet python. The family had pruritic papular lesions that had black central dots from skin puncture and bleeding. Some of the lesions appeared vesicular or bullous. They had noticed what they called "small insects" fixed on their skin and large numbers of the same on the snake and in the chair the snake usually occupied. The snake, its cage, and the chair were liberally dusted with a pyrethrum powder. No further bites were noted.[83]

HAZARDS OF KEEPING VENOMOUS REPTILES

Although, by definition, bites from venomous reptiles do not constitute a zoonotic disease, the potential for human injury is real. The topic warrants discussion. See also Chapter 81, Working with Venomous Species, for more information and emergency protocols.

Venomous snakes or lizards are not recommended to be kept as pets or as part of private collections. If owners cannot be dissuaded from owning these animals, precautionary measures such as lining up sources of antivenin for the species owned and contacting local emergency facilities that can handle such bites should be made. Too often a bite occurs and the victim reports to an emergency facility. The staff then tries to locate a veterinarian or contact the veterinary or reptile departments of the local zoo to find the necessary antivenin. Most zoos stock antivenin to deal with the species housed. Their keepers and staff have been drilled in emergency procedures and have worked out a protocol with a local hospital. Although they may try to help in an emergency, they cannot always be counted on to have the necessary antivenin or to be immediately accessible.

Table 79-6　Venomous Snakes in the United States

Pit Vipers (*Crotalidae*)
　Cottonmouths and Copperheads (*Agkistrodon*)
　Rattlesnakes (*Crotalus*)
　　Eastern Diamondback (*C. adamanteus*)
　　Sidewinder (*C. cerastes*)
　　Rock (*C. lepidus*)
　　Black-tailed (*C. molossus*)
　　Red Diamond (*C. ruber*)
　　Tiger (*C. tigris*)
　　Ridge-nosed (*C. willardi*)
　　Western Diamondback (*C. atrox*)
　　Timber (*C. horridus*)
　　Speckled (*C. mitchelli*)
　　Twin-spotted (*C. pricei*)
　　Mojave (*C. scutulatus*)
　　Western (*C. viridis*, 5 subspecies)
Massauga and Pigmy Rattlesnakes (*Sistrurus*)
　Massauga (*S. catenatus*)
　Pigmy (*S. miliarius*)
Coralsnakes (*Elapidae*)
　Sonoran Coralsnake (*Micruroides euryxanthus*)
　Eastern Coralsnake (*Micrurus fulvius*)

Clinicians who see venomous reptiles need to have a well-trained staff not only in handling the animals but in first aid and emergency protocols. Only highly trained individuals, such as the veterinarian, should handle the reptile, and it should be transported in a locking carry box. A snake hook or long-handled tongs is useful. An acrylic tube that is sealed at one end and can be used for restraint and for gas anesthesia is a necessary piece of equipment.

Most cases of venomous snake or lizard bites in the United States occur outdoors in the environment of the wild reptile.[84] However, a number occur when people try to capture or keep the wild-caught reptile as a pet. Only two lizards in North America, the Gila Monster (*Heloderma suspectum*) and the Beaded Lizard (*H. horridum*), are known to be venomous.[15] Their venom contains hyaluronidase, phospholipase A, and one or more salivary kallikreins.[84] Signs, symptoms, and clinical course are similar to those of a mild to moderate case of Western Diamondback Rattlesnake (*Crotalus atrox*) bite. Localized pain, swelling and edema, ecchymosis, lymphangitis, and lymphadenopathy are the most common manifestations. Systemic involvement may develop with moderate to severe poisoning that includes weakness, sweating, thirst, headache, tinnitus, and rarely cardiovascular collapse.

In the United States, about 20 species of venomous snakes are found (Table 79-6). Most are Pit Vipers (*Crotalidae*), although a few are Coralsnakes (*Elapidae*). Rattlesnakes (*Crotalus* spp.) account for about 70% of venomous snake bites and for almost all deaths. Coralsnakes inflict less than 1% of all bites. Other reported snake bites are from Copperheads and Cottonmouths, both in the genus *Agkistrodon*. Estimates are that more than 45,000 people are bitten by snakes per year in the United States, with less than 8000 cases of venom poisoning reported. Fewer than 15 fatalities per year occur, and these are reported to be mostly in children or the elderly, in untreated or undertreated cases, or in handlers of venomous nonindigenous snakes. Imported snakes found in zoos, schools, snake

Table 79-7	Antivenins

Antivenin (Crotalidae) Polyvalent (U.S.P)

Crotalidae Polyvalent Antivenin Equine Origin, BIO. 210

Veterinary product: Fort Dodge Laboratories, Inc, 800 Fifth Street, Fort Dodge, IA 50501.

- For use in the neutralization of venom from most Pit Vipers worldwide.
- Venoms used in preparation: Eastern Diamondback Rattlesnake (*C. adamanteus*), Western Diamondback Rattlesnake (*C. atrox*), Cascabel (*C. durissus terrificus*), Barba Amarilla (*Bothrops atrox*).
- Vials contain ammonium sulfate, concentrated lyophilized globulins, equine origin (reconstituted: 10 mL/vial).

Antivenin (Crotalidae) Polyvalent Immune Fab (OVINE)-CroFab

Protherics Inc, Nashville, TN Phone: 6153271027 Fax: 6153201212

- Indication for use: Treatment of minimal and moderate North American Crotalidae envenomation
- CroFab [Crotalidae Polyvalent Immune Fab (Ovine)] is a sterile, nonpyrogenic, purified, lyophilized preparation of ovine Fab (monovalent) immunoglobulin fragments obtained from the blood of healthy sheep flocks immunized with one of the following North American snake venoms: *Crotalus atrox* (Western Diamondback Rattlesnake), *Crotalus adamanteus* (Eastern Diamondback Rattlesnake), *Crotalus scutulatus* (Mojave Rattlesnake), and *Agkistrodon piscivorus* (Cottonmouth or Water Moccasin).
- The dose is 4-6 vials per patient, best used if administered within 6 hours of the envenomation. Each vial of CroFab should be reconstituted with 10 mL of sterile water, then further diluted in 250 mL of 0.9% sodium chloride USP. The reconstituted and diluted product should be used within 4 hours.

Antivenin (Micrurus Fulvus; Coral Snake; U.S.P)

North American Coral Snake Antivenin: Wyeth-Ayerst Laboratories, Division of American Home Products Corp, PO Box 8299, Philadelphia, PA 19101. Medical emergencies: day: (800) 934-5556; night (610) 688-4400.

- Prepared from the venom of the Eastern Coral Snake *M. fulvus*.
- Concentrated lyophilized horse serum antivenin, reconstituted to 10 mL/vial.
- Each vial neutralizes approximately 2.5 mg of *M. fulvus* venom and *M. nigrocinctus* (Black-banded Coral Snake).

Ineffective against: *M. mipartitus* (Black-ringed Coral Snake), *Micruroides euryxanthus* (Arizona Coral Snake).

Antivenins are available in most countries for use in the treatment of indigenous venomous snake poisoning.[81] Consult the country's public health department or ministry for information on manufacturer and availability of a specific antivenin.

Table 79-8	First Aid for Venomous Snakebite in Animals[82-84]

General Considerations:

Treatment must be started immediately. Treatment aims:

- A. Prevent or control shock.
- B. Neutralize venom.
- C. Minimize necrosis.
- D. Prevent secondary infections and toxicities.

For Dogs, Cats, and Other Companion Animals:

1. Keep the animal quiet.
2. Identify the snake if possible to differentiate between *Crotalid* and *Elapid* for antivenin choice.
3. Start intravenous isotonic fluids to combat hypotension and hypovolemic shock. Lactated Ringer's solution, 9% sodium chloride, or colloids.
4. Administer appropriate antivenin intravenously (IV) via slow injection. All animals should be skin tested before antivenin administration, although false-positive or false-negative reactions may occur. Follow the skin-test directions in the package insert. Diphenhydramine (Benadryl, Parke-Davis, Morris Plains, NJ), 10 to 25 mg/animal IV before administration of the antivenin, may help to calm the animal and pretreat against allergic reactions to the antivenin. Monitor the inner pinna for hyperemia as an indicator of a systemic reaction. Epinephrine should be available for acute anaphylaxis. If the patient has a reaction, discontinue the antivenin and administer diphenhydramine IV. Waiting a few minutes is advisable before starting antivenin administration more slowly under close observation. If a reaction recurs, stop the injection and seek consultation. If the initial skin test is positive, antivenin administration should still be tried with very close monitoring of the patient. Antivenin treatment is most effective when given early, and repeated administration may be needed, depending on clinical signs and laboratory results.
5. Obtain baseline laboratory data on presentation of the patient. Data should include: complete blood cell count (CBC), platelet count, coagulation profile, serum electrolytes, blood urea nitrogen (BUN), creatinine, creatine phosphokinase (CPK), and glucose. Electrocardiographic monitoring and respiratory support may be needed.
6. Administer broad-spectrum antibiotics. Tetanus antitoxin and toxoid administration may be indicated as for any puncture wound.

farms, and private and professional collections account for about 15 reported bites per year.[84] Although snakebite should always be treated as a medical emergency, important to remember is that envenomation may not occur in all bites. For example, 20% to 30% of Crotalid bites contain no venom.[84] If no envenomation has occurred, then the bite wound should be treated like other bite and puncture wounds. If envenomation has occurred, signs, symptoms, and clinical course may vary considerably depending on the site of the bite, species of snake, degree of envenomation, time elapsed, depth of the bite, and size of the victim.

Most references try to categorize snake venoms as neurotoxins, hemotoxins, cardiotoxins, and others, but in fact, most snake venoms are complex mixtures of toxins with many systemic effects. Venoms contain many pharmacologically active substances including phospholipase A, phosphodiesterase (exonuclease), L-amino acid oxidase, proteolytic enzymes (peptide hydrolases), hyaluronidase, and other enzymes.[85] Many have actions at the intracellular/intranuclear level, and the action is complicated by the release of serotonin and histamine from the host's damaged tissues.[84]

Although North American Elapid venom can cause major changes in neuromuscular transmission and have central nervous system effects, because of the small size of the snake relative to the victim, the small amount of venom injected, and the nonaggressive nature of these snakes, few Elapid bites are recorded or reported to cause major complications. Elapid venom can cause local tissue damage, necrosis, systemic hematologic changes, and respiratory and renal complications, but these have been reported largely from Elapids in Australia, Asia, and Africa.[85,86]

Identification of the snake is important for treatment; however, great care must be exercised in capturing a wild snake that has inflicted a bite. Usually the snake is assumed to be a native Crotalid: the commercial antivenin (Antivenin [Crotalidae] Polyvalent, Wyeth-Ayerst Laboratories, Philadelphia, Pa) is multivalent for Cottonmouths, Copperheads, and Rattlesnakes (Table 79-7). With captive snakes, identification is usually not a problem; even so, the severity of the bite and envenomation may be difficult to tell.

Signs and symptoms of a Crotalid venomous snakebite may include local progressive edema, muscle fasciculations, hypotension, arrhythmias, increased salivation, or enlarged painful regional lymph nodes. Elapid bites may be locally painful, but minimal local swelling occurs. Clinical signs of respiratory distress or collapse may not occur for several hours, but once signs develop, they are rapidly progressive. To clip the hair and thoroughly scrub the bite site is prudent with any suspected snakebite because local secondary infection is possible. Treatment guidelines are outlined in Table 79-8.

REFERENCES

1. Glynn MK, Mermin JH, Durso LM, et al: Knowledge and practices of California veterinarians concerning the human health threat of reptile-associated salmonellosis (1996), *J Herp Med Surg* 11(2):9-13, 2001.
2. Anonymous (Centers for Disease Control and Prevention): Reptile-associated salmonellosis: selected states, 1996-1998, *MMWR* 48:1009-1013, 1999.
3. Cambre RC, McGuill MW: *Salmonella* in reptiles. In Bonagura JD, editor: *Current veterinary therapy XIII*, Philadelphia, 2000, WB Saunders.
4. Glaser CA, Angulo FJ, Rooney JA: Animal-associated opportunistic infections among persons infected with the human immunodeficiency virus, *Clin Infect Dis* 18:14-24, 1994.
5. Chomel B: Zoonoses of house pets other than dogs, cats, and birds, *Pediatr Infect Dis J* 11:479-487, 1992.
6. Bradley T, Angula F, Mitchell M: Public health education on *Salmonella* spp and reptiles, *JAVMA* 219(60):754-755, 2001.
7. Wood L: A compelling case for compassionate management, *Vet Econ* 34(8):38, 1993.
8. Anonymous: Reptilian salmonellosis, *Lancet* 2(8238):130, 1981.
9. Chiodini RJ, Sundberg JP: Salmonellosis in reptiles: a review, *Am J Epidemiol* 113:494, 1981.
10. Frye FL: *Biomedical and surgical aspects of captive reptile husbandry*, Edwardsville, Kan, 1981, Veterinary Medicine Publishing.
11. Miller RE: *AZA guidelines for animal contact with the general public*, Wheeling, WV, 1997, American Zoo and Aquarium Association policy.
12. Barten SL: The medical care of iguanas and other common pet lizards, *Vet Clin North Am Small Anim Pract* 23(6):1213, 1993.
13. Jephcott AE, Martin DR, Stalker R: *Salmonella* excretion by pet terrapins, *J Hyg Cambridge* 67:505, 1969.
14. Onderka DK, Finlayson MC: *Salmonellae* and salmonellosis in captive reptiles, *Can J Comp Med* 49(3):268, 1985.
15. Bisseru B: Reptiles and amphibians. In *Diseases of man acquired from his pets*, London, 1967, William Heinemann Medical Books.
16. Marcus LC: Common reptilian zoonoses, *Proc North Am Vet Conf Small Anim Exotics* 16:822-823, 2002.
17. Stair GM, Tacal JV Jr, Lawrence W, et al: Association of *Salmonella typhimurium* infection with a household iguana, *Calif Morbidity* 42:1989.
18. Pelzer KD: Salmonellosis, *JAVMA* 195(4):456, 1989.
19. Krieg NR, Holt JG, editors: *Bergey's manual of systematic bacteriology*, vol I, Baltimore, 1984, Williams & Wilkins.
20. McWhorter-Murlin AC, Hickman-Brenner FW: *Identification and serotyping of Salmonella and an update of the Kauffmann-White Scheme*, Atlanta, 1994, Centers for Disease Control and Prevention.
21. Fox JG: *Campylobacter* infections and salmonellosis, *Semin Vet Med Surg Small Anim* 6(3):212, 1991.
22. Lamm SH, Taylor A, Gangarosa EJ, et al: Turtle-associated salmonellosis: I: an estimation of the magnitude of the problem in the United States, 1970-1971, *Am J Epidemiol* 95(6):511, 1972.
23. Altman R, Gorman JC, Bernhardt LL, et al: Turtle-associated salmonellosis: II: the relationship of pet turtles to salmonellosis in children in New Jersey, *Am J Epidemiol* 95(6):518, 1972.
24. Kaufmann AF, Fox MD, Morris GK, et al: Turtle-associated salmonellosis: III: the effects of environmental salmonellae in commercial turtle breeding ponds, *Am J Epidemiol* 95(6):521, 1972.
25. Cohen ML, Potter M, Pollard R, et al: Turtle-associated salmonellosis in the United States: effect of public health action, 1970-1976, *JAVMA* 243(12):1247, 1980.
26. D'Aoust JY, Lior H: Pet turtle regulations and abatement of human salmonellosis, *Can J Public Health* 69:107, 1978.
27. Anonymous: *Fed Reg* 37:224, 1972.
28. Siebeling RJ, Neal PM, Granberry WD: Evaluation of methods for the isolation of *Salmonella* and *Arizona* organisms from pet turtles treated with antimicrobial agents, *Appl Microbiol* 29:240, 1975.
29. Wells JG, Clark GM, Morris GK: Evaluation of methods for isolating *Salmonella* and *Arizona* organisms from pet turtles, *Appl Microbiol* 27:8, 1974.
30. Duponte MW, Nakamura RM, Change EML: Activation of latent *Salmonella* and *Arizona* organisms by dehydration in red-eared turtles, *Pseudemys scripta elegans*, *Am J Vet Res* 39(3):529, 1978.
31. Anonymous: Part 1250-control of communicable disease: ban on sale and distribution of small turtles, *Fed Reg* 40:22543, 1975.
32. Fujita K, Murono K, Yoshioka H: Pet-linked salmonellosis, *Lancet* 2(8245):525, 1981.
33. Anonymous: Turtle-associated salmonellosis: Ohio, *MMWR* 35(47):733, 1986.
34. Shane SM, Gilbert R, Harrington KS: *Salmonella* colonization in commercial pet turtles (*Pseudemys scripta elegans*), *Epidemiol Infect* 105:307-315, 1990.
35. D'Aoust JY, Daley E, Crozier M, Sewell AM: Pet turtles: a continuing international threat to public health, *Am J Epidemiol* 32(2):233-238, 1990.
36. Burnham BR, Atchley MS, DeFusco RP, et al: Prevalence of fecal shedding of *Salmonella* organisms among captive green iguanas and potential public health implications, *JAVMA* 2113(1):48-50, 1998.
37. Morse EV, Duncan MA: Salmonellosis—an environmental health problem, *JAVMA* 165:1015, 1974.
38. Feeley JC, Treger MD: Penetration of turtle eggs by *Salmonella braenderup*, *Public Health Rep* 84:156, 1969.

39. DeHamel FA, McInnes HM: Lizards as vectors of human salmonellosis, *J Hyg Cambridge* 60:247, 1971.
40. Cambre RC, Green DE, Smith EE, et al: Salmonellosis and arizonosis in the reptile collection at the National Zoological Park, *JAVMA* 9:800, 1980.
41. Mitchell MA, Shane S: *Salmonella* in reptiles, *Sem Avian Exotic Pet Med* 10(1):25-35, 2001.
42. Anonymous (Centers for Disease Control and Prevention): Reptile-associated salmonellosis-selected states, 1994-1995, *MMWR* 44:347-350, 1995.
43. Ackerman DM, Drabkin P, Birdhead G, et al: Reptile-associated salmonellosis in New York State, *Pediatr Infect Dis J* 14:955-959, 1995.
44. Mermin J, Hoar B, Angula FJ: Iguanas and *Salmonella marina* infection in children: a reflection of the increasing incidence of reptile-associated salmonellosis in the United States, *Pediatrics* 99:299-402, 1997.
45. Dalton C, Hoffman R, Pape C: Iguana-associated salmonellosis in children, *Pediatr Infect Dis J* 14:319-320, 1995.
46. Sanya D, Douglas T, Roberts R: *Salmonella* infection acquired from reptilian pets, *Arch Dis Child* 77:345-346, 1997.
47. Woodward DL, Khakhria R, Johnson WM: Human salmonellosis associated with exotic pets, *J Clin Microbiol* 35(11):2786-2790, 1997.
48. Frye FL: Infectious diseases: fungal actinomycete, bacterial, rickettsial, and viral diseases. In *Biomedical and surgical aspects of captive reptile husbandry*, Melbourne, Fla, 1991, Krieger Publishing.
49. Anonymous: Iguana-associated salmonellosis: Indiana, *MMWR* 41(3):38, 1990.
50. Friedman CR, Torigian C, Shilam P, et al: An outbreak of salmonellosis among children attending a reptile exhibit at a zoo, *J Pediatr* 132:802-807, 1997.
51. Bradley T, Angulo FJ, Raiti P: Association of Reptilian and Amphibian Veterinarians guidelines for reducing risk of transmission of *Salmonella* spp. from reptiles to humans, *J Am Vet Med Assoc* 213(1):51-52, 1998.
52. Wooley RE, Ritchie BW, Currin MFP, et al: In vitro inhibition of *Salmonella* organisms isolated from reptiles by an inactivated culture of microcin-producing *Escherichia coli*, *AJVR* 62(9):1399-1401, 2001.
53. Marcus LC: Salmonellosis in reptiles. In Kirk RW, editor: *Current veterinary therapy 6*, Philadelphia, 1977, WB Saunders.
54. Anonymous: Lizard-associated salmonellosis: Utah, *MMWR* 41(33):610, 1992.
55. Anonymous: *Salmonella wassenar*: Canada, *MMWR* 25(41):332, 1976.
56. Harvey S, Greenwood JR: Isolation of *Campylobacter* fetus from a pet turtle, *J Clin Microbiol* 21(2):260, 1985.
57. Otis VS, Behler JL: The occurrence of salmonellae and *Edwardsiella* in the turtles of the New York Zoological Park, *J Wildl Dis* 9:4, 1973.
58. McCoy RH, Seidler RJ: Potential pathogens in the environment: isolation, enumeration, and identification of seven genera of intestinal bacteria associated with small green pet turtles, *Appl Microbiol* 25(4):534, 1973.
59. Raynor AC, Bingham HG, Caffee HH, et al: Alligator bites and related infections, *J Fla Med Assoc* 70(2):107, 1983.
60. Saeed AM, Harris NV, DiGiacomo RF: The role of exposure to animals in the etiology of *Campylobacter jejuni/coli* enteritis, *Am J Epidemiol* 137(1):108, 1993.
61. Clark B: *Zoonotic diseases*, ed 2, Topeka, Kan, 1990, American Association of Zoo Keepers.
62. Timm KI, Sonn RJ, Hultgren BD: Coccidioidomycosis in a Sonoran Gopher snake, *Pituophis melanoleucus affinis*, *J Med Vet Mycol* 26(2):101, 1988.
63. Acha PN, Szyfres B: *Zoonoses and communicable diseases common to man and animals*, ed 2, Washington, DC, 1987, Pan American Health Organization, World Health Organization.
64. Shayegani M, Stone WB, DeForge I, et al: *Yersinia enterocolitica* and related species isolated from wildlife in New York State, *Appl Environ Microbiol* 52(3):420, 1986.
65. Jacobsen ER: Snakes, *Vet Clin North Am Small Anim Pract* 23(6):1179, 1993.
66. Marcus LC: Specific diseases of herpetofauna. In Marcus LC: *Veterinary biology and medicine of captive amphibians and reptiles*, Philadelphia, 1981, Lea & Febiger.
67. Brownstein DG: Mycobacteriosis. In Hoff GL, Frye FL, Jacobson ER, editors: *Diseases of amphibians and reptiles*, New York, 1984, Plenum Press.
68. Cannon CA: Personal communication, 1993.
69. Quesenberry KE, et al: Ulcerative stomatatitis and subcutaneous granulomas caused by *Mycobacterium chelonei* in a boa constrictor, *JAVMA* 189(99):1131, 1986.
70. Anonymous: Q fever: New York, *MMWR* 27:321, 1978.
71. Yadav MD, Sethi MS: Poikilotherms as reservoirs of Q fever (*Coxiella burnetii*) in Uttar Pradesh, *J Wildl Dis* 15:15, 1979.
72. Jacobson ER: West Nile virus infection in crocodilians, *Proc Assoc Reptilian Amphib Vet* 85-86, 2004.
73. Miller DL, Manuel MJ, Baldwin C, et al: West Nile Virus in farmed alligators, *Emerg Infect Dis* 9(7):794-799, 2003 (on-line serial).
74. Steinman A, Banet-Noach C, Shlomit T, et al: West Nile Virus infection in crocodiles, *Emerg Infect Dis* 9(7):887-889, 2003 (on-line serial).
75. Kostiukov MA, Cordeeva ZSE, Bulychev VP, et al: The lake frog (*Rana ridibunda*)—one of the food hosts of blood-sucking mosquitoes in Tadzhikistan—a reservoir of the West Nile fever virus, *Med Parazitol (Mosk)* 3:49-50, 1985.
76. Kierney B: *Federal scientists refocus on West Nile Virus impacts on wildlife [news release]*, Reston, Va, 2003, US Geological Survey, www.usgs.gov/public/press/public_affairs/press_releases/pr1720m.html.
77. Schantz PM: Emergence of newly recognized parasitic zoonoses, *Compend Cont Ed Pract Vet* 5(3):163, 1983.
78. Drabick JJ: Pentastomiasis, *Rev Inf Dis* 9(6):1087, 1987.
79. Hendrix CM, Blagburn BL: Reptilian pentastomiasis: a possible emerging zoonosis, *Compend Cont Ed Pract Vet* 10(1):46, 1988.
80. Barnard SM: Color atlas of reptilian parasites: part III: miscellaneous endoparasites and ectoparasites, *Compend Cont Ed Pract Vet* 8(5):287, 1986.
81. Lavarde F, Fornes P: Lethal infection due to *Armillifer armillatus* (Porocephalida): a snake-related parasitic disease, *Clin Infect Dis* 29:1346-1347, 1999.
82. Flynn RJ: Arthropods. In *Parasites of laboratory animals*, Ames, 1973, Iowa State University Press.
83. Schultz H: Human infestation by *Ophionyssus natricis* snake mite, *Br J Dermatol* 93:695, 1975.
84. Berkow R, editor: *The Merck manual of diagnosis and therapy*, ed 15, Rahway, NJ, 1987, Merck.
85. Minton S: Snake bite. In Steele JH, editor: *CRC Handbook series in zoonoses: section C: parasitic zoonoses*, vol III, Boca Raton, Fla, 1982, CRC Press.
86. US Department of Navy: *Poisonous snakes of the world*, U.S. Department of the Navy, Bureau of Medicine and Surgery, Mineola, NY, 1991, Dover Publications.

80
LAWS AND REGULATIONS: EUROPEAN AND AMERICAN

MARGARET E. COOPER, GREGORY A. LEWBART, and DANIEL T. LEWBART

INTRODUCTION

The hobby of captive herpetology is gaining momentum, and more people and herptile (amphibians and reptiles) species are becoming a part of this expanding industry. Although captive breeding is much more popular and successful than it has been in decades past, many wild-caught specimens still find their way into captivity (some illegally) (Figure 80-1). In some cases, maintenance of cultivated herptiles may also be against certain laws (Figure 80-2). This chapter focuses on the international, federal, national, state, and local laws regarding herptiles and the authorities that enforce these regulations. Several examples of specific regulation enforcement are also included and discussed.

THE CONVENTION ON INTERNATIONAL TRADE IN ENDANGERED SPECIES OF WILD FAUNA AND FLORA (CITES)

Most readers are familiar with the acronym "CITES." This multinational agreement was originally written in 1973, was entered into force in 1975, and is meant to protect vulnerable and endangered plants and animals throughout the world. The 1973 draft was based on a prior document written by the International Union for the Conservation of Nature (IUCN). CITES is strictly a political agreement among the participating countries, and enforcement of the CITES regulations is up to the individual country (so regulation of CITES is far from consistent). To date, 167 countries have ratified the CITES agreement. The following countries have signed but have not ratified the agreement: Ireland, Kuwait, and Losotho. For details about CITES, see the informative web site at www.cites.org.

Listed CITES animals fall into one of three categories (Appendix I, II, or III), with Appendix I the most protective. However, even Appendix I species can be commercially exploited through a loophole called a "Reservation," which allows participating countries to make exemptions for certain species (e.g., Japan's taking of seaturtles). CITES regulations only apply to the international import and export of listed species, which means legally imported CITES species can be transported, traded, or sold within a given country. The following paragraphs summarize the separate CITES appendices.

Appendix I

These organisms are currently threatened with extinction and may be further threatened by international trade. Listed species can only be imported or exported with special permits and not for commercial trade (Figure 80-3, *A*). Some CITES Appendix I herptiles include the Giant Chinese/Japanese Salamander (*Andrias* sp.), Golden Toad (*Bufo periglens*), most crocodilians (some are listed in more than one appendix because of farming and ranching), Tomato Frog (*Dyscophus antongilii*), Bog Turtle (*Clemmys muhlenbergi*), Galapagos Tortoise (*Geochelone elephantopus*), Tuatara (*Sphenodon punctatus*), all seaturtles, Fiji Island Iguana (*Brachylophus* sp.), and Hawksbill Seaturtle (*Eretmochelys imbricata*) (Figure 80-3, *B*).

Appendix II

These organisms are not currently threatened with extinction, and commercial trade is legal with special

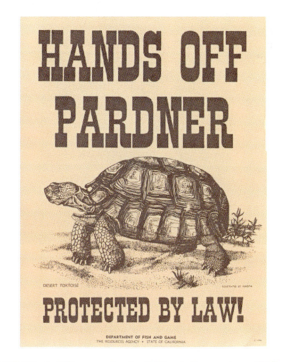

FIGURE 80-1 This poster by the California Department of Fish and Game clearly shows the status of the California Desert Tortoise (*Gopherus agassizii*).

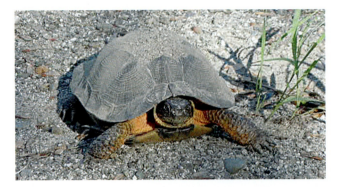

FIGURE 80-2 This female Wood Turtle *(Clemmys insculpta)* had probably just finished a nest on the shoulder of a Maine road (note sand on the carapace). This species is not protected in Maine (although a permit may be required to keep one) but is considered threatened in Virginia. Conversely, the Eastern Box Turtle *(Terrapene carolina)* is protected in Maine but not in Virginia. *(Photograph courtesy G. Lewbart.)*

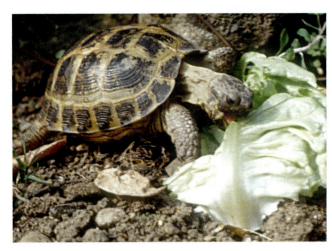

FIGURE 80-4 This Horsfield or Russian Tortoise *(Testudo horsfieldi)*, like all tortoises, is listed as CITES II. A permit is required to import this tortoise from overseas. Certain states may require permits for possession of this species and other exotic herpetofauna. *(Photograph courtesy G. Lewbart.)*

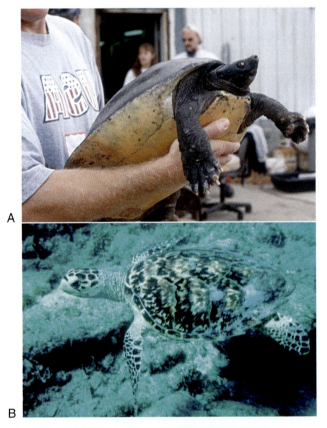

FIGURE 80-3 A, This River Terrapin *(Batagur baskar)* was one of approximately 7500 turtles seized on December 11, 2001, by authorities in Hong Kong. The illegal shipment of Southeast Asian turtles was destined for use as food and traditional medicine. Many of the surviving turtles were shipped to the United States and Europe for medical treatment and rehabilitation. *Batagur baskar*, native to Sumatra, Thailand, and the Malay Peninsula, is considered critically endangered and is listed as CITES I. **B,** This Wild Hawksbill Turtle *(Eretmochelys imbricata)* was photographed in the U.S. Virgin Islands. Like all seaturtles, it is listed as CITES I and cannot be used in commercial trade. *(Photographs courtesy G. Lewbart.)*

permits (Figure 80-4). Some CITES Appendix II herptiles include the Eastern Box Turtle *(Terrapene carolina)*, Wood Turtle *(Clemmys insculpta)*, land tortoises *(Geochelone* spp.), Gopher Tortoises *(Gopherus* sp.), Axolotl *(Ambystoma mexicanum)*, Poison Dart Frogs *(Dendrobates* sp.), and Boa Constrictor *(Boa constrictor)*.

Appendix III

These organisms are subject to trade regulations within certain individual nations and require multinational cooperation to regulate international trade. Permits are required from the country that listed the species. Some CITES Appendix III herptiles include the Atlantic Coral Snake *(Micrurus diastema)* in Honduras and Russell's Viper *(Vipera russellii)* in India.

All CITES and US required permits are available through the U.S. Fish & Wildlife Service Office of Management Authority, 4401 Fairfax Drive, Room 432, Arlington, VA 22203. Visit their web site at www.fws.gov.

EUROPEAN LEGISLATION REGARDING REPTILES

Margaret E. Cooper

INTRODUCTION

General

The geographic area of Europe extends from the west of Iceland to the east of Russia and from Norway in the Barents Sea above the Arctic Circle to Crete in the Mediterranean Sea and comprises many countries that are diverse in their geography, ecology, history, culture, legal systems, and attitudes towards animals.

Not surprisingly, considerable variation exists in the legislation relating to animals, including reptiles, from one country to another not only as to content, form, and stage of development but also in effectiveness and enforcement.

Sources of Information on Legislation

One can usually obtain printed copies of national legislation from the official government printer, and in some countries (e.g., France and Germany), publishers produce bound volumes of codes of legislation that are to be found in the larger bookshops. International and regional, and in some countries, national, legislation is available on the Internet. The laws of individual countries normally are produced in the national language; however, in countries where the language is not widely spoken (such as the Scandinavian counties, the Netherlands, or the new members of the European Union [EU; Table 80-1]), a translation may be available in, for example, English or French. The EU web site provides links to legal sources of member countries. Collections of useful EU links are provided at http://www.hse.gov.uk/aboutus/europe/links.htm. The legislation is available via EUR-Lex at http://europa.eu.int/eur-lex/en/index.html, a comprehensive web site on EU law. The ECOLEX web site provides access to a wide range of environmental laws at http://www.ecolex.org/ecolex/index.php.

Specialist bodies, such as the herpetological societies or wildlife or animal welfare organizations, may have copies of translations of legislation and may also have information or expertise on the application or enforcement of laws relevant to their fields of operation. The newsletter and web site of the Federation of European Veterinarians (http://www.fve.org/news/pdf/newsletters/2004_2_Newsletter.pdf) is a valuable source of information on recent or forthcoming changes in laws relevant to the veterinary profession.

Levels of Legislation

As mentioned at the beginning of this chapter, legislation can be found at several levels, ranging from global conventions to city bylaws. These are described in Table 80-2, and examples of the legislation relevant to reptiles that has been produced at these levels are shown in Table 80-1. Where global or regional legislation on a particular field of law exists, countries that are parties are likely to have some similarity in the content of their relevant national laws.

Implementation and Enforcement of Legislation

Differences also exist in the legal systems between individual nations. For instance, many have codified legislation (e.g., France) and written constitutions (most nations), whereas Britain has neither of these. Countries may also have fundamentally different judicial systems. For this reason, the implementation (i.e., legal obligations put into effect) usually with legislation and enforcement (i.e., that the legislation is obeyed) of global and regional legislation is the responsibility of individual countries.

European Regional Legislation

The two regional European law-making bodies are the European Community (EC; the major part of the EU) and the Council of Europe (COE). Table 80-3 provides some information that may help to clarify their status and the effect of their legislation on reptiles.

REPTILES IN THE WILD

General

The legal protection of reptiles in the wild includes both species protection and habitat protection. Thus, a country's law may specifically afford protection for particular species of reptile, but in addition, reptiles also derive benefit from protection of the habitat in which they can be found.

Substantial wildlife conservation legislation is relevant to reptiles at all levels. This legislation is set out in Table 80-1. Most countries have national species and habitat legislation, which is usually a combination of their implementation of global and regional legislation and national provisions. The legislation specifies species and habitats to be protected, methods of protection, offences, penalties, and enforcement powers.

Protected Species

Free-living reptiles have the benefit of protective legislation at a regional and national level. The species covered vary from country to country and relate primarily to the species that occur naturally in that country. Table 80-4 shows the listings of protected reptiles for the COE, EU, and by way of an example of national law, English conservation legislation.

Typical Prohibited or Controlled Activities Relating to Reptiles in the Wild

Core offences likely to be included in a country's species protection legislation are:

- Deliberate killing, taking, or injuring of a protected reptile or its young or eggs.
- Deliberate disturbance of a protected reptile.
- Deliberate disturbance of its breeding or resting place.
- Use of prohibited or nonselective methods (e.g., poison, nets, traps, lights, vehicles) of capture or killing of protected reptiles that may deplete or disturb local populations or are inhumane.

Table 80-1 Levels of Wildlife Conservation Legislation Relevant to Reptiles

International: (Lyster, 1985)	Convention on Wetlands of International Importance, Especially as Waterfowl Habitat 1971 (Ramsar Convention) Convention concerning the Protection of the World Cultural and Natural Heritage 1972 (World Heritage Convention) Convention on Trade in Endangered Species of Wild Fauna and Flora 1973 (CITES) (Washington Convention) Convention on the Conservation of Migratory Species of Wild Animals 1979 (Bonn Convention) Convention on Biological Diversity 1992 (Biodiversity Convention)
Regional: EU	Council Directive 92/43/EEC of May 21, 1992, on the conservation of natural habitats and wild fauna and flora (Habitats Directive) Council Regulation (EC) No. 338/97/EC of December 9, 1996, on the protection of species of fauna and flora and regulating trade therein Commission Regulation (EC) No. 1808/2001 of August 30, 2001, laying down rules concerning the implementation of Council Regulation (EC) No. 338/97 on the protection of species of wild fauna and flora by regulating trade therein Commission Regulation (EC) No. 349/2003 of February 25, 2003, suspending the introduction into the Community of specimens of certain species of wild fauna and flora Commission Regulation (EC) No. 1497/2003 of August 18, 2003, amending Council Regulation (EC) No. 338/97 on the protection of species of wild fauna and flora by regulating trade therein
Regional: COE	Convention on the Conservation of European Wildlife and Natural Habitats 1979 (Berne Convention)
National (and state)	Each country has its own wildlife conservation legislation that is likely to include protection for specified reptiles. England, Scotland, and Wales share most of this legislation. Northern Ireland has its own very similar laws. EC Regulations on CITES (see previous) have direct application. Control of Trade in Endangered Species (Enforcement) Regulations 1997 (SI 1997/1372) (COTES) Wildlife and Countryside Act 1981 (as amended) (WCA) Countryside and Rights of Way Act 2000 (CROW) Conservation (Natural Habitats, etc.) Regulations 1994 (SI 1994/2716; Habitats Regulations)
Useful web sites:	
General	http://www.biodiv.org/convention/partners-websites.asp http://www.jncc.gov.uk/legislation/default.htm http://www.eu-wildlifetrade.org/pdf/en/2_national_legislation_en.pdf
COE	http://www.coe.int/t/e/Cultural_Co-operation/Environment/Nature_and_biological_diversity/Nature_protection/default.asp#TopOfPage
CITES Convention	http://www.cites.org/
EC CITES	http://www.cites.org/eng/news/sundry/new_append.shtml http://www.europa.eu.int/comm/environment/cites/legislation_en.htm http://www.wcmc.org.uk/species/trade/eu/
EC CITES Regulations	http://www.eu-wildlifetrade.org/html/en/wildlife_trade_regulations.asp http://www.ukcites.gov.uk/intro/cites_species.htm#EC%20Regulation%20Annexes http://www.ukcites.gov.uk/pdf_files/1497-2003%20EN.pdf http://www.jncc.gov.uk/
British CITES	http://www.wcmc.org.uk/species/trade/eu/tradereg.html#species http://www.ukcites.gov.uk/intro/leg_frame.htm http://www.ukcites.gov.uk/default.asp

EC, European Community; *COE*, Council of Europe.

Table 80-2 Levels of Legislation Relating to Reptiles

Level	Description	Type of Legislation	Subjects Relevant to Reptiles
International (or global)	Treaties that all countries may join and that give rise to legal obligations.	International treaties, conventions, agreements.	International conservation conventions.
Regional	Multilateral legislation in which countries of a certain region are eligible to participate.	European Community Regulations and Directives. Council of Europe Conventions.	Legislation on conservation, animal health, animal transport, veterinary profession, veterinary medicines, health, and safety.
National (or federal)	Legislation of individual countries. Note: In the United Kingdom, much of the older legislation applies to England, Wales, and Scotland, but since devolution (July 1, 1999), the three countries make some laws separately through the English and Scottish Parliaments and the Welsh Assembly, causing divergence of content. Northern Ireland always has its separate legislation.	Primary laws passed by national parliament. Secondary legislation: orders or regulations made under primary legislation.	Laws on conservation, zoos, research, animal welfare, import/export, veterinary profession, medicinal products, health, and safety.
State	In countries with a federal constitution, each constituent state (e.g., a land in Germany and a canton in Switzerland) may have its own laws (as in the states of the United States or Australia and the provinces of Canada).	Laws produced by individual constituent states and effective only within that state.	As for national (see previous), depending on scope given to state by national (federal) law or constitution.
Local	Laws made by local government authorities. Sometimes they also implement national laws.	Laws or bylaws made or implemented by local government authorities under national or state legislation.	Laws on keeping animals for specified purposes (e.g., exhibition). Bylaws regulating, for example, the keeping of animals.

Table 80-3 European Institutions That Make Regional Wildlife Conservation Legislation

Institution	Membership	Legislation	Legislation Relevant to Reptiles	Implementation
EC (part of EU) Primary aims of EC: economic, political, and legislative EU aims: also foreign policy and crime prevention	25 member states: Austria, Belgium, Denmark, Finland, Germany, Greece, Ireland, Italy, Luxembourg, Portugal, Spain, Sweden, The Netherlands, United Kingdom together with (joined May 1, 2004) Cyprus, Czech Republic, Estonia, Hungary, Latvia, Lithuania, Malta, Poland, Slovenia, Slovakia.	Regulations have direct application in EU member countries. Directives have to be transposed by each EU country into its national law. Enforcement is responsibility of each EU country. Member countries can be required by the European Court of Justice to implement Directives, backed by financial penalty.	*Habitats Directive Transport Directive Scientific Research Directive *CITES Regulations (full titles in text) Professional Directives Medicines Directives	Should be implemented by all member countries.
COE Primary aims: social and cultural, especially democracy, rule of law, and human rights	COE has 46 members and 5 observer countries (including Canada, the Holy See, Japan, Mexico, United States). Nonmembers of COE can join its conventions. 350 NGOs have consultative status.	Conventions must be implemented by member countries that have ratified or acceded to them. Other countries can accede. No specific means to make a country implement a convention.	Relevant Conventions: Wildlife conservation (Berne) Welfare of animals during transport 1968 Revised 2003 Scientific research Pets	Ratified by: 45 members, 6 other countries and EC 24 countries and Russia 3 countries 17 countries and EC 18 countries

*See Table 80-1 for the full titles of these laws.
EC, European Community; *EU*, European Union; *COE*, Council of Europe; *NGO*, nongovernmental organization.

Table 80-4 Comparative Table of Protected Reptiles in Europe

Council of Europe Convention applies to 51 countries **Berne Convention**	European Union Directive applies to 25 countries	An example of national legislation England	
Appendix II	**EC Habitats Directive Annex IV (a)**	**WCA**	**Habitats Regulations**
Specially protected species	Animal and plant species of community interest in need of strict protection	Fully or partially protected species listed in WCA	"European protected species" (i.e., those species listed on Annex IV of the Habitats Directive whose natural range includes any area in Britain)
Reptiles			
Testudines			
Testudinidae			
Testudo graeca	Testudo graeca		
Testudo hermanni	Testudo hermanni		
Testudo marginata	Testudo marginata		
Emydidae			
Emys orbicularis	Emys orbicularis		
Mauremys caspica	Mauremyscas pica		
Mauremys leprosa	Mauremys leprosa		
(Mauremys caspica leprosa)			
Dermochelyidae			
Dermochelys coriacea	Dermochelys coriacea	Dermochelys coriacea	Dermochelys coriacea
Chelonidae			
Caretta caretta	Caretta caretta	Caretta caretta*	Caretta caretta
Chelonia mydas	Chelonia mydas	Chelonia mydas*	Chelonia mydas
Eretmochelys imbricata	Eretmochelys imbricata	Lepidochelys kempii*	Lepidochelys kempii
Lepidochelys kempii	Lepidochelys kempii	Eretmochelys imbricata*	Eretmochelys imbricata
Trionychidae			
Rafetus euphraticus			
Trionyx triunguis			
Sauria			
Gekkonidae			
Cyrtodactylus kotschyi	Cyrtopodion kotschyi		
Tarentola angustimentalis	Tarentola angustimentalis		
Tarentola boettgeri	Tarentola boettgeri		
Tarentola delalandii	Tarentola delalandii		
Tarentola gomerensis	Tarentola gomerensis		
Phyllodactylus europaeus	Phyllodactylus europaeus		
Agamidae			
Stellio stellio	Stellio stellio		
(Agama stellio)			
Chamaeleontidae			
Chamaeleo chamaeleon	Chamaeleo chamaeleon		

Continued

Table 80-4 Comparative Table of Protected Reptiles in Europe—Cont'd

Lacertidae

Algyroides fitzingeri	Algyroides fitzingeri		
Algyroides marchi	Algyroides marchi		
Algyroides moreoticus	Algyroides moreoticus		
Algyroides nigropunctatus	Algyroides nigropunctatus		
Archaeolacerta bedriaga (Lacerta bedriagae)			
Archaeolacerta monticola (Lacerta monticola)			
Gallotia galloti	Gallotia atlantica		
	Gallotia galloti		
	Gallotia galloti insulanagae		
Gallotia simonyi (Lacerta simonyi)	Gallotia simonyi		
Gallotia stehlini	Gallotia stehlini		
Lacerta agilis	Lacerta agilis	*Lacerta agilis*	Lacerta agilis
Lacerta clarkorum			
Lacerta dugesii	Lacerta bedriagae		
Lacerta graeca	Lacerta danfordi		
Lacerta horvathi	Lacerta dugesii		
Lacerta lepida	Lacerta graeca		
Lacerta parva	Lacerta horvathi		
Lacerta princeps			
Lacerta schreiberi	Lacerta monticola		
Lacerta trilineata	Lacerta schreiberi		
Lacerta viridis	Lacerta trilineata		
	Lacerta viridis		
	Lacerta vivipara pannonica	Lacerta vivipara†	
Ophisops elegans	Ophisops elegans		
Podarcis erhardii	Podarcis erhardii		
Podarcis filfolensis	Podarcis filfolensis		
	Podarcis hispanica atrata		
Podarcis lilfordi	Podarcis lilfordi		
Podarcis melisellensis	Podarcis melisellensis		
Podarcis milensis	Podarcis milensis		
Podarcis muralis	Podarcis muralis		
Podarcis peloponnesiaca	Podarcis peloponnes iaca		
Podarcis pityusensis	Podarcis pityusensis		
Podarcis sicula	Podarcis s icula		
Podarcis taurica	Podarcis taurica		
Podarcis tiliguerta	Podarcis tiliguerta		
Podarcis waglerianus	Podarcis wagleriana		

Anguidae

Ophisaurus apodus	Ophisaurus apodus	Anguis fragilis†	

Scincidae

Ablepharus kitaibelli	Ablepharus kitaibelli
Chalcides bedriagai	Chalcides bedriagai
Chalcides occidentalis	Chalcides occidentalis

Chalcides ocellatus	Chalcides ocellatus	
Chalcides sexlineatus	Chalcides sexlineatus	
Chalcides simonyi (Chalcides occidentalis)		
Chalcides viridianus	Chalcides viridianus	
Ophiomorus punctatissimus	Ophiomorus punctatissimus	
Ophidia		
Colubridae		
Coluber cypriensis		
Coluber gemonensis		
Coluber hippocrepis	Coluber hippocrepis	
Coluber jugularis	Coluber jugularis	
Coluber caspius (Coluber jugularis caspius)	Coluber caspius	
	Coluber laurenti	
Coluber najadum	Coluber najadum	
Coluber rubriceps (Coluber najadum rubriceps)		
	Coluber nummifer	
Coluber viridiflavus	Coluber viridiflavus	
Coronella austriaca	Coronella austriaca	Coronella austriaca*
	Eirenis modesta	
Elaphe longissima	Elaphe longissima	
Elaphe quatuorlineata	Elaphe quatuorlineata	
Elaphe situla	Elaphe situla	
Natrix megalocephala		
	Natrix natrix cetti	Natrix natrix†
	Natrix natrix corsa	
Natrix tessellata	Natrix tessellata	
Telescopus fallax	Telescopus fallax	
Viperidae		
Vipera albizona		
Vipera ammodytes	Vipera ammodytes	
Vipera barani		
Vipera kaznakovi		
Vipera latasti		
Vipera lebetina		
Vipera schweizeri (Vipera lebetina schweizeri)	Vipera schweizeri	
	Vipera seoanni (except Spanish populations)	
Vipera pontica		
Vipera ursinii	Vipera ursinii	
Vipera wagneri		
Vipera xanthina	Vipera xanthina	
		Vipera berus†
Boidae		
	Eryx jaculus	

EC, European Community; WCA, Wildlife and Countryside Act.
*Full protection.
†Partial protection (killing, injuring, sale).

- Trade (e.g., sale, exchange, barter, transport, or display for sale) in live animals, dead specimens, or derivatives thereof.
- Release of alien (nonnative) species.

Many of these activities can be authorized by licence for specified purposes (e.g., conservation, research, education, exhibition, captive breeding, trade in captive-bred specimens, public health, or crop or property protection).

Variation in National Laws

National laws that incorporate some or all of the previous laws may also vary in quantity, quality, and effectiveness, but some uniformity of content does exist within the EU or COE (because the national laws must reflect the regional laws) and among countries that have implemented the global Conventions (see Table 80-4 and relevant Convention web sites). However, the level of protection of a particular species can also vary because its conservation status can differ from one country to another. This may be so in spite of the listed status of a species at the regional level because a country may derogate from the main legislation when a species is not at risk, not present, or a country is not willing to protect it; conversely, a country may impose a higher status or stricter regulation than that required by the regional legislation. Likewise, the quality of enforcement is variable, for example because of the extent of the powers provided or the different degrees of political will or financial resources.

Fieldwork That Involves Reptiles

In addition to the foregoing legislation, those who carry out scientific research in the field using free-living reptiles may need to obtain research authorization, licences to comply with the species protection laws, or permission to enter the area where the reptiles are studied. If the work involves population management, one should have regard to the IUCN Guidelines on reintroductions, translocation, and other topics (IUCN, various) and, in the case of health monitoring, Woodford (2001).

REPTILES IN CAPTIVITY

General

The keeping of animals, including reptiles, is mainly regulated by national or state legislation, although day-to-day control may be the responsibility of local government authorities. The sort of control is likely to depend on the nature of the species and the purpose for which they are kept. Regulation may include provisions for licensing and inspection and require compliance with standards or guidelines.

Reptiles Kept as Pet, Companion, or Hobby

The private keeping of reptiles is often controlled, usually at local government authority level, especially if the species (e.g., the large or poisonous reptiles) represent a risk to the public. Some countries may regulate the keeping of any species of reptile. Others may be selective, as in Britain where the keeping of specified species is subject to licensing and inspection under the Dangerous Wild Animals Act 1976 (as amended). The animals must be kept in secure and appropriate accommodations, and the keeper must be insured. Reptiles subject to the Act include alligators, caimans, crocodiles, some Colubridae, elaphid snakes, the front-fanged venomous vipers, and the Helodermatidae, although the list is under review. See http://www.defra.gov.uk/wildlife-countryside/gwd/wildact.htm.

The COE European Convention for the Protection of Pet Animals 1987 has broad provisions for the responsible keeping of pets, defined as "any animal kept or intended to be kept by man in particular in his household for private enjoyment and companionship." It requires the keeper of a pet animal to adhere to basic principles of animal welfare (see subsequently), and Article 4 provides that a pet should not be caused unnecessary pain, suffering, or distress nor be abandoned. The keeper of a pet must be responsible for its health and welfare and provide accommodations, care, and attention that take account of the ethologic needs of the animal in accordance with its species and breed. In particular, keepers must give it suitable and sufficient food and water and adequate opportunities for exercise and take reasonable measures to prevent its escape.

Keeping of Protected Species

Restrictions may exist under national wildlife laws (see previous) on the possession of reptiles, particularly wild-caught ones. A licence may be necessary to keep, breed, or trade in native or specified wild-caught or captive-bred reptiles.

Exhibition, Display, and Entertainment

Reptiles are used or displayed for purposes such as zoos, circuses, cabarets, or education; such activities are likely to be subject to controls, usually through licensing by a local government authority. Great variation exists in the legislation, enforcement, and actual quality of care provided for exhibited animals in different countries. Countries are required to implement several supranational laws, which are mentioned subsequently.

The COE Pets Convention applies general welfare provisions (see previous) to pets, including reptiles, that are used in exhibitions, entertainment, and competitions and requires that these activities must not interfere with their health and well being.

The Council Directive 1999/22/EC relating to the keeping of wild animals in zoos applies to collections open to the public and requires EU countries to regulate zoos as briefly summarized:

- The directive applies to collections of "wild species" that are exhibited to the public on 7 or more days in a year.
- Zoos must be licensed and inspected.
- Accommodation for animals must take into account their biological and conservation needs and provide enrichment; zoos must provide good husbandry, veterinary care, and nutrition.

- Records must be kept; measures must be taken to prevent escapes of animals or the access of pests and to provide for dispersal of animals in the event of closure.
- Zoos must also make a contribution to conservation (e.g., by way of research, training, exchange of information, captive breeding, reintroduction) and to public education relating to their animals and their habitats.
- The Directive was modelled on the British Zoo Licensing Act 1981 (although the latter has been amended to comply with the Directive).
- British zoos must also comply with the Secretary of State's Standards of Modern Zoo Practice. See http://www.defra.gov.uk/wildlife-countryside/gwd/zooprac/index.htm.

The EC CITES Regulations (see Table 80-1), in addition to regulating international trade in CITES species (see subsequent), also requires that any use of species listed on Annex A of the Regulation for commercial purposes must be authorized by an Article 10 or, for zoos, Article 30 certificate. This applies not only to the usual aspects of trade but also to display, which is interpreted to include any exhibit with a commercial element such as zoos, cabarets, and trade shows. Annex A includes all CITES Convention Appendix I animals together with a number of other species that have been upgraded to that status within the EU (http://www.ukcites.gov.uk/pdf_files/1497-2003%20EN.pdf).

Scientific Research

Regional Legislation

The COE European Convention for the Protection of Vertebrate Animals used for Experimental and other Scientific Purposes was formed in 1987.

The EC Council Directive 86/609/EEC of November 24, 1986, on the approximation of laws, regulations, and administrative provisions of the Member States concerned the protection of animals used for experimental and other scientific purposes.

This legislation relates to experimental or other scientific use of an animal that may cause pain, suffering, distress, or lasting harm and applies to all nonhuman vertebrates, including reptiles, both captive and free-living. Some countries also have detailed regulations or guidance that supplements the main legislation. The controls can include (as in Britain) licensing, inspection, and ethical review; pain controls; veterinary supervision; and the training of researchers. Other countries may or may not have controls of varying content.

Trade

International: CITES Convention

For the titles of the legislation see Table 80-1.

Worldwide trade of species listed on Appendices I, II, and III of CITES is controlled via CITES (http://www.cites.org/eng/append/appendices.shtml) import and export permits (see subsequent).

The essential principles of trade under CITES are:

- Certain species of reptile are listed on Appendices I, II and III of the Convention.
- Any international trade (as defined subsequently) of such CITES listed species must be authorized by a CITES import and export permit.
- Trade means international (cross-frontier) movement, whether commercial or not and for whatever purpose.
- In the case of Appendix I species, a permit may be given only for movement that is not of a primarily commercial nature.
- Permits may be provided for the commercial movement of Appendix II and captive-bred specimens of Appendix I species.
- Special certificates may also be given for the movement of captive-bred animals that are pets or in a travelling exhibition.
- Specific criteria exist for the issue of permits.

The detailed provisions of CITES are complex, and further information can be obtained from the CITES Convention web site at http://www.cites.org/ and at national sites such as the UK Government CITES web site at http://www.ukcites.gov.uk/.

Derivatives of CITES Specimens

The CITES provisions apply not only to live specimens but also to carcases, parts, and other derivatives. Originally envisaged to include material such as ivory, traditional medicines, plumage, and the like, the provisions also apply to biological and veterinary diagnostic specimens and samples. The agreement at the 12th Conference of the Parties (CoP) to CITES, held in Santiago, Chile, in November 2002, was that a simplified permit procedure (similar to that in place for museum specimens) should apply to the movement of specified types of non-commercial time-sensitive biological and veterinary samples (Cooper, 2000). This may not yet be in place in many countries but is included in a draft EC Regulation that will replace Regulation (EC) No1808/2001. A proposal exists for the 13th CoP that DNA samples should be designated as not subject to CITES.

For a detailed study of the functioning of CITES, see Wijnsteker (2000).

Regional

The EC CITES Regulations are listed in Table 80-1.

The essential provisions of EU legislation have been summarized as the EC CITES Regulations that operate directly in the member countries. Other countries in Europe operate CITES by implementing the global Convention on an individual basis.

- The Regulations implement CITES directly in all EU member countries; they do not have national legislation on CITES.
- Exception: enforcement is the responsibility of individual EU countries (e.g., in Britain by the Control of Trade in Endangered Species [Enforcement] Regulations 1997).
- Many species (in addition to those on the CITES Appendices) are included in Annexes A to D of the Regulation. The species listed and the status accorded to them may be stricter than the requirements of the CITES Convention. For example, some CITES Convention Appendix II species such as the Mediterranean Tortoises have been upgraded to

Annex A (equivalent to CITES Convention Appendix I status) and others, not listed on the Convention, have been put onto Annex B (Appendix II status).
- Once legally in the EC, CITES specimens can be moved freely around the EU.
- The importation into the EU of certain Annex B species (including many reptiles) has been suspended (see lists in Commission Regulation [EC] No 349/2003).

For current lists of CITES Convention and EC CITES species, see Wildlife Conservation Monitoring Centre (WCMC) (2001) and the list of web sites in Table 80-1.

National Laws: In-Country Trade in CITES Species

Within the EU area and within individual EU countries, the trade of Annex A (which includes, *inter alia*, all CITES Appendix I species) is additionally controlled under the CITES Regulations as follows:

- Annex A species may not be used for primarily commercial purposes.
- Annex A species that have been captive-bred from captive-bred parents may be used for commercial purposes if authorized by an Article 10 certificate (or Article 30 for zoos).
- To obtain a certificate, one must produce evidence to show that the animal was legally imported or captive-bred.
- Annex A species in commercial use must be permanently marked with a microchip transponder that conforms to ISO Standards 11784:1996 (E) and 11785:1996 (E) (where this is not physically possible, then with another permanent form of identification). Note: In Britain, while hatchling tortoises are less than 10 centimeters long, they do need not to be marked.
- A CITES animal that has been legally imported or for which an Article 10 certificate has been issued can be traded (in accordance with the terms of the certificate) freely within the EU.
- For an example of these provisions at a national level, see the Guidance Notes issued by the Britain's Department for Environment, Food and Rural Affairs, (DEFRA) (DEFRA, various) also available at http://www.ukcites.gov.uk/.

Other national provisions:

- A thriving trade exists in captive-bred reptiles as pets, among hobbyists, or for other purposes.
- Licensing controls are often seen in the case of indigenous (and possibly other) reptiles under national wildlife legislation and in conformity with the Habitats Directive and the Berne Convention.
- Local authority controls may relate to pet traders and their premises.
- Law enforcement measures are important to deal with illegal trade.

Animal Health Controls

Animal health laws also apply cross-frontier controls, but they operate entirely separately from the CITES provisions described previously.

European Community Directives on Import and Export

Animal health legislation often requires authorization (usually issued by the ministry responsible for agriculture) to import many species of mammal and bird. This legislation also involves veterinary health certification and quarantine for live animals. For such controls to apply to reptiles is unusual. However, permission may be necessary to import pathogenic reptile material, for example, blood or tissues, particularly when the samples are not fixed. Authorization may include conditions relating to packaging, storage, and disposal of the material.

National Wildlife Legislation: The Export of Indigenous Species

Some countries forbid the export of indigenous species or derivatives thereof except under licence. In addition, national controls may be found on the export and exploitation of genetic materials under legislation implementing the Biodiversity Convention. This might apply to material derived from reptiles and intended to be screened for potential value in developing modern medicines.

Customs and Excise

Animals imported normally are subject to a country's taxes such as customs duty and value added (sales) tax.

Reptiles and Veterinary Practice

Veterinary Professional Law

Veterinary practice in most European countries is regulated according to the usual provisions that relate to the registration of veterinarians and control of the profession, together with restrictions on the practice of veterinary medicine by lay persons.

Because the legislation is at national level, the precise provisions and levels of enforcement vary from country to country. To verify whether a reptile must be treated by a veterinarian, one must inquire as to whether reptiles are included in the range of species that must be treated by a registered veterinarian and whether the procedure is one that must be carried out by a veterinarian.

European Union nationals with EU veterinary qualifications are entitled to practice in any EU country. They must register in the given country. Directives 78/1026/EEC and 78/1027/EEC concern the recognition of qualifications and freedom of movement. The nationals may also have to provide a certificate of good standing from the EU country in which they were first or previously registered.

Britain also gives recognition to some (British) Commonwealth degrees from Australia, Canada, New Zealand, and South Africa and also American Veterinary Medical Association (AVMA)–recognized veterinary degrees from the United States. (See http://www.rcvs.org.uk/.)

Veterinary Medicinal Products

Directive 2004/28/EC of March 31, 2004, amends Directive 2001/82/EC on the community code relating to veterinary medicinal products.

The pharmaceutical legislation that controls the sale, supply, prescription, and administration of veterinary drugs varies from very strict in some European countries (with prosecutions and professional conduct [malpractice] proceedings in respect of breaches of the law or for the abuse or mishandling of substances) to lax in other countries.

The sale, supply, and administration of veterinary medicinal products are controlled by national legislation and, in the EU, in accordance with *(inter alia)* the Directives previously mentioned.

Prescription-only medicines for use in animals should normally be prescribed by a veterinarian. In light of the relatively few drugs that are approved for use in reptiles, the veterinarian may have to resort to "off-label" prescribing. In the EU, this must be done with the client's consent and the drugs chosen in accordance with the "cascade" principles (British Veterinary Association, 2000; http://www.vmd.gov.uk/lu/amelia/amelia8r.pdf).

If any patient is eventually to be used for food, then strict withdrawal periods must be observed. The EC provisions regarding "off-label" prescribing are under review; for further information see http://www.fve.org/news/pdf/newsletters/2004_2_Newsletter.pdf.

Occupational Health and Safety

Occupational health and safety legislation is strong in some countries, particularly in the EU where many directives exist on the subject. In countries in which the legislation is strictly enforced, the management of health and safety is all-pervasive and requires employers use the principles of risk assessment. Thus, in the case of reptiles kept in a zoo or veterinary practice, a risk assessment must be made of the hazards involved, the risks they pose, and the persons affected. Measures to remove or reduce the risk, written records, and provision for monitoring and reviewing the procedures must be put in place. Legislation may also exist for specific health and safety situations, such as radiographs and dangerous substances, fire, and first aid. Information on the EC legislation is available at the web site of the European Agency for Safety and Health at Work at http://europe.osha.eu.int/legislation/.

In other countries, little development may be seen of health and safety so far, and any measures that the veterinarian takes are on a voluntary basis and reduce the risk of compensation claims (on the basis of negligence or employers' liability) that arise from accidents.

Welfare

Regional Legislation

No international welfare laws relate to cruelty of animals, but at the regional level, some broad provisions exist in the COE European Convention for the Protection of Pet Animals 1987 (ratified by 13 countries). It covers "any animal kept or intended to be kept by man in particular in his household for private enjoyment and companionship" and therefore includes reptiles kept as pets.

Article 3: Basic principles for animal welfare includes:

1. Nobody shall cause a pet animal unnecessary pain, suffering, or distress.
2. Nobody shall abandon a pet animal.

The article also contains provisions for responsible pet keeping (see previous).

National Legislation

Most countries have national legislation against cruelty to animals, and some may have extensive welfare law. The species covered by animal protection laws vary greatly, so examination of a country's legislation in detail is necessary to find whether it extends to reptiles, captive or free-living.

The provisions vary a great deal, but the forms of animal use or abuse that are addressed may include:

- Specific acts of cruelty.
- A general category: causing unnecessary suffering.
- The responsibility of the keeper of an animal to provide food, water, and suitable environment.
- Poisoning, trapping, and cruel sports.
- Mutilations (e.g., tying of venom ducts in snakes).
- Use of anesthesia (and analgesics) during surgery.
- Specific uses such as research and zoos if separate legislation is not provided.
- Transportation (see subsequent).

Some laws include most of the foregoing topics under one law; others have separate provisions, for example, for animals used in scientific research. The English legislation is currently under revision, and a new Animal Welfare Act is expected in 2005 or 2006 (see http://www.defra.gov.uk/animalh/welfare/bill/index.htm).

Welfare During Transportation

Regional legislation exists on the humane transportation of animals, and this should have been transposed into national legislation. For example, in the English law there are provisions both general and specific that apply to reptiles.

Under the European Convention for the Protection of Animals during International Transport 1968, revised 2003, COE member countries must make provision for the welfare of vertebrate animals (including reptiles) during international transport. The requirements for noncommercial transportation are basic (i.e., that the animal should be fit to travel and that its health and welfare should be safeguarded during the journey). The stipulations for commercial transport are more stringent.

The EC Council Directive 91/628/EEC of November 19, 1991, on the protection of animals during transport (as amended) lays down requirements for the conditions of transport of vertebrate animals within, to, and from the Member States of the EU. Those most relevant to reptiles are:

- "No animal shall be transported unless it is fit for the intended journey and unless suitable provisions have been made for its care during the journey and on arrival at the place of destination. Animals that are ill or injured shall not be considered fit for transport. However, this provision shall not apply to:
  - animals that are slightly injured or ill whose transport would not cause unnecessary suffering;
  - animals that fall ill or are injured during transport shall receive first-aid treatment as soon as possible; they shall be given appropriate veterinary treatment and if necessary undergo emergency slaughter in a way which does not cause them any unnecessary suffering." Chapter II, Article 3 (1).
- "Cold-blooded animals shall be transported in such containers, under such conditions, in particular with

regard to space, ventilation and temperature, and with such supply of water and oxygen as are considered appropriate for the species. They shall be transported to their destination as soon as possible." Chapter V, Article 46.

In England, the Welfare of Animals (Transport) Order 1997 SI No. 1480 (as amended) (WATO) implements the European legislation and therefore has requirements that are applicable to reptiles.
- Animals of any sort, including invertebrates, must not be transported in any way that causes or is likely to cause them injury or unnecessary suffering.
- In the case of commercial or other nonprivate transportation of animals, additional requirements apply to the provision of suitable containers and vehicles, food, water, ventilation, temperature, and attendance.
- "Other vertebrate animals and cold-blooded animals shall be transported in such receptacles or means of transport, under such conditions (in particular with regard to space, ventilation, temperature and security) and with such supply of liquid and oxygen as are appropriate for the species concerned." Schedule 6 & Article 4(7).
- Animals that are CITES-listed species must be transported in accordance with the CITES "Guidelines for transport and preparation for shipment of live wild animals and plants" (CITES, 1980). In the case of air transport, they must be transported at least in accordance with the most recent airline rules governing the transport of live animals (IATA, annual).

For further information on the legislation see http://www.defra.gov.uk/animalh/welfare/farmed/transport/legislation.htm.

Additional, miscellaneous provisions on transport are:
- Public road and rail carriers may also have their own requirements.
- IATA Regulations, although not law, are applied by most airlines to all animals transported via air (IATA, annual).
- CITES Guidelines (not law) apply to any form of transport provided for CITES species (CITES, 1980).
- The WATO (see previous) makes it a legal requirement to comply with the IATA Regulations and CITES.
- Other guidelines where they are applicable.
- International and national postal regulations may forbid the transport by mail of living reptiles. Very precise requirements also exist for the mailing of animal carcasses and pathogens, including special packaging and labeling.

Case studies

There are various sources of reports of law enforcement. CITES infringements and associated prosecutions in many countries are reported in the TRAFFIC Bulletin (http://www.traffic.org/publications/index.html#bulletin). The Royal Society for the Protection of Birds (based in UK) provides case reports of enforcement of CITES, wild bird and other legislation that may also be relevant to reptiles (http://www.rspb.org.uk/policy/wildbirdslaw/rspb_publications.asp). Herpetological societies will often note significant cases that have implications for their members.

CONCLUSION

A wide variety of legislation relates to reptiles either specifically or by way of general application. Although an extensive body of national legislation cannot be detailed here, this chapter attempts to bring together as many as possible of the relevant principles that may be found in the law of the many countries of Europe. It is also intended to guide the reader towards appropriate sources of further and more specific information on the subject of reptile law.

SUGGESTED READING

British Veterinary Association: *BVA code of practice on medicines*, London, 2000, British Veterinary Asociation.
CITES: *Guidelines for transport and preparation for shipment of live animals and plants*, Geneva, 1980, Secretariat of the Convention on International Trade in Endangered Species of Wild Fauna and Flora.
Cooper ME: Legal considerations in the international movement of diagnostic and research samples from raptors: a conference resolution. In Lumeij JT, Remple JD, Redig PT, Liertz M, Cooper JE, editors: *Raptor biomedicine III*, Lake Worth, 2000, Zoological Education Network.
DEFRA: *Guidance notes (on aspects of the CITES regulations)*, Bristol, various, Department of the Environment, Transport and the Regions.
Lyster S: *International wildlife law*, Cambridge, 1985, Grotius.
IATA: *Live animals regulations*, Montreal and Geneva, annual, International Air Transport Association.
IUCN: http://www.iucn.org/themes/ssc/pubs/policy/index.htm.
IUCN: *Guidelines for the prevention of biodiversity loss caused by alien invasive species*, 2000, SSC Invasive Species Specialist group (adopted by IUCN Council).
IUCN/SSC: *Guidelines for re-introductions*, 1995, Re-introductions specialist group (adopted by IUCN council).
IUCN: *Guidelines for the placement of confiscated animals*, 2000, (adopted by IUCN council).
IUCN: *Policy statement on state gift of animals*, 1987 (adopted by IUCN council).
IUCN: *Position statement on translations of living organisms: introductions, re-introductions and re-stocking*, 1987 (adopted by IUCN Council).
IUCN: *Policy statement on captive breeding*, 1987, Captive breeding Specialist Group (adopted by IUCN Council).
WCMC: *Checklist of herpetofauna listed in the CITES appendices and in EC Regulation 338/97*, ed 8, 2001, http://www.wcmc.org.uk.
Woodford MH: *Quarantine and health screening protocols for wildlife prior to translocation and release into the wild*, Paris, 2001, Veterinary Specialist Group/Species Survival Commission of the World Conservation Union (IUCN), Gland, Care for the Wild International, Rusper and the European Office International des Epizooties.
Wijnstekers W: *The evolution of CITES*, ed 7, 1995, Secretariat of the Convention on International, http://www.cites.org/eng/resources/publications.shtml.

UNITED STATES FEDERAL REGULATIONS

Gregory A. Lewbart and
Daniel T. Lewbart

The US Endangered Species Act (ESA) is a federal act that was established in 1973 to protect rare animals and plants, both native and nonnative (Figure 80-5). The ESA has also been a model for state endangered species programs and serves as the state regulatory plan in those states without their own legislation. All species of included animals and plants are listed as either threatened or endangered. It also implements CITES in the United States (http://endangered.fws.gov/pubs/esa_basics.pdf). The details of the ESA can be found in title 50, part 17, of the Code of Federal Regulations (ref: 50 CFR 17). Special permits are required for just about any activity involving a listed species (currently about 125 species of herptiles are listed). Some endangered herptiles are Wyoming Toad (*Bufo baxteri*), Shenandoah Salamander (*Plethodon shenandoah*), American Crocodile (*Crocodylus acutus*), Leatherback Seaturtle (*Dermochelys coriacea*), Jamaican Iguana (*Cyclura collei*), and Puerto Rican Boa (*Epicrates inornata*). Some threatened herptiles are Goliath Frog (*Conraua goliath*), Loggerhead Seaturtle (*Caretta caretta*), Turks and Caicos Iguana (*Cyclura carinata carinata*), and Giant Gartersnake (*Thamnophis gigas*).

Some "special rules" apply to certain situations involving threatened (not endangered) species. These rules eliminate the normal ESA permit requirements. Examples of these special rules include the American Alligator (state laws apply) and by-catch (accidental capture) Loggerhead, Olive Ridley, and Green Seaturtles.

NATIONAL MARINE FISHERIES SERVICE REGULATIONS

The ESA regulations are enforced by both the United States Fish and Wildlife Service (USFWS) and the National Marine Fisheries Service (NMFS); USFWS has jurisdiction only when seaturtles are ashore. Incidental capture permits are required by fishermen who are likely to accidentally take seaturtles. Detailed requirements exist for handling both living and dead-by-catch seaturtles (50 CFR 222.50 and 227.72).

The ESA permits for endangered species are only granted for the following reasons: legitimate scientific research, propagation, species survival, and incidental take. Permits for threatened species may be granted for zoologic exhibition, educational purposes, and those listed previously for threatened species. ESA and CITES permits are required for species subject to both documents (in the United States, a single ESA permit fulfills CITES requirements). The ESA only regulates transactions at the interstate level (intrastate commercial activities involving legally obtained species are not regulated by the ESA). Individual states may restrict commercial activity of threatened and endangered species.

DESIGNATED UNITED STATES PORTS OF ENTRY

All wildlife entering the United States must do so via one of the following ports of entry unless specified otherwise (50 CFR 14.11 and 14.12): Atlanta, Baltimore, Boston, Chicago, Dallas/Fort Worth, Honolulu, Los Angeles, Miami, Newark, New Orleans, New York, Portland (Ore), San Francisco, or Seattle. All wildlife shipments are subject to inspection by both the USFWS and the US Customs Service. Specific ports of entry exceptions exist for wildlife (not requiring special permits) originating in Canada and Mexico.

SPECIAL TURTLE REGULATIONS

The U.S. Food and Drug Administration (FDA) and Public Health Service (PHS) regulate the import of any turtle under 4 inches carapace length or turtle eggs. Restrictions on foreign imports can be found in the PHS regulations (42 CFR 71). Six or fewer turtles and eggs can be imported without a PHS permit for noncommercial purposes. Seven or more turtles/eggs may be authorized with a permit if used for legitimate scientific, educational, or exhibition purposes. Interstate and intrastate transport is governed by the FDA (21 CFR 1240). No turtles less than 4 inches carapace length or turtle eggs may be sold as pets in the United States. Exceptions include legitimate scientific, educational, or exhibition purposes. Confiscated turtles and eggs in violation are subject to humane destruction by the FDA. For more information, go to www.fda.gov.

STATE LAWS

Most U.S. states have their own laws governing the taking and keeping of native reptile species. Some states also regulate the sale and captivity of exotic amphibian and reptile species. See Table 80-5 for a complete listing of state regulatory agencies. Current web sites have been included because laws relating to herptiles are dynamic and the web sites allow the interested reader to browse various pertinent web pages.

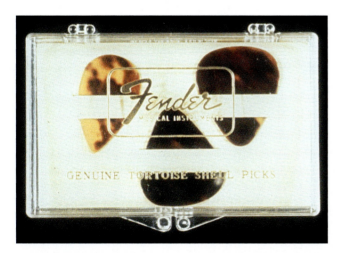

FIGURE 80-5 Several Hawksbill Seaturtle guitar picks are shown. Although popular with some musicians, possession of such materials made after 1973 (the year the Endangered Species Act was instituted) is illegal. (*Photograph courtesy NCSU-CVM Biomedical Communications.*)

Table 80-5 U.S. State Agencies That Regulate Herptiles

Alabama Department of Conservation and Natural Resources
Game and Fish Division
Law Enforcement Section
64 North Union Street
Montgomery, AL 36130
www.dcnr.state.al.us

Alaska Department of Fish and Game
PO Box 25526
Juneau, AK 99802-5526
www.adfg.state.ak.us

Arizona Game and Fish Department
Permits Coordinator
2221 West Greenway Road
Phoenix, AZ 85023
www.gf.state.az.us

Arkansas Game and Fish Commission
2 Natural Resources Drive
Little Rock, AR 72205
www.agfc.state.ar.us

California Department of Fish and Game
1416 Ninth Street
Sacramento, CA 95814
www.dfg.ca.gov

Colorado Division of Wildlife
6060 Broadway
Denver, CO, 80216
www.wildlife.state.co.us

Connecticut Department of Environmental Protection
Wildlife Division
79 Elm Street
Hartford, CT 06102
www.dep.state.ct.us

Delaware Department of Natural Resources and Environmental Control
Division of Fish and Wildlife
89 Kings Highway
Dover, DE 19901
www.dnrec.state.de.us/fw/index.htm

Florida Fish and Wildlife Conservation Commission
Bureau of Protected Species Management
620 South Meridian Street OES-BPS
Tallahassee, FL 32399
www.floridaconservation.org/psm

Georgia Department of Natural Resources
Wildlife Resources Division
Law Enforcement Section
2070 US Highway 278, Southeast
Social Circle, GA 30025
www.dnr.state.ga.us/dnr/wild

Hawaii Department of Land and Natural Resources
Division of Forestry and Wildlife
1151 Punchbowl Street, Room 325
Honolulu, HI 96813
www.dofaw.net

Idaho Department of Fish and Game
600 South Walnut Street
PO Box 25
Boise, ID 83707
www.fishandgame.idaho.gov

Illinois Department of Natural Resources
Endangered Species Protection Board
524 South Second Street
Springfield, IL 62701
www.dnr.state.il.us/espb/index.htm

Indiana Department of Natural Resources
Division of Fish and Wildlife
402 West Washington, Room W273
Indianapolis, IN 46204
www.in.gov/dnr/fishwild

Iowa Department of Natural Resources
Fish and Wildlife Division
Law Enforcement Bureau
Henry A. Wallace Building,
502 East 9th Street
Des Moines, IA 50319-0034
www.iowadnr.com

Kansas Department of Wildlife and Parks
Law Enforcement
512 Southeast 25th Avenue
Pratt, KS 67124-8174
www.kdwp.state.ks.us

Kentucky Department of Fish and Wildlife Resources
1 Game Farm Road
Frankfort, KY 40601
www.kdfwr.state.ky.us

Laws and Regulations 1047

Louisiana Department of Wildlife and Fisheries
2000 Quail Drive
Baton Rouge, LA 70808
www.wlf.state.la.us

Maine Department of Inland Fisheries and Wildlife
284 State Street
41 State House Station
Augusta, ME 04333-0041
www.state.me.us/ifw

Maryland Department of Natural Resources
Wildlife and Heritage Service
Tawes State Office Building
580 Taylor Avenue, E-1
Annapolis, MD 21401
www.dnr.state.md.us/wildlife

Massachusetts Division of Fisheries and Wildlife
251 Causeway Street, Suite 400
Boston, MA 02114-2152
www.state.ma.us/dfwele/dfw

Michigan Department of Natural Resources
Mason Building
PO Box 30028
Lansing, MI 48909
www.dnr.state.mi.us

Minnesota Department of Natural Resources
500 Lafayette Road
St. Paul, MN 55155-4040
www.dnr.state.mn.us

Mississippi Department of Wildlife, Fisheries and Parks
1505 Eastover Drive
Jackson, MS 39211-6374
www.mdwfp.com

Missouri Department of Conservation
2901 West Truman Boulevard
PO Box 180
Jefferson City, MO 65102
www.conservation.state.mo.us

Montana Department of Fish, Wildlife, and Parks
Law Enforcement Division
1420 East Sixth Avenue
PO Box 200701
Helena, MT 59620-0701
www.fwp.state.mt.us

Nebraska Game and Parks Commission
2200 North 33rd Street
Lincoln, NE 68503
www.ngpc.state.ne.us

Nevada Department of Wildlife
1100 Valley Road
Reno, NV 89512
www.ndow.org

New Hampshire Fish and Game Department
2 Hazen Drive
Concord, NH 03301
www.wildlife.state.nh.us

New Jersey Department of Environmental Protection
Division of Fish and Wildlife
PO Box 400
Trenton, NJ 08625-0400
www.state.nj.us/dep/fgw

New Mexico Department of Game and Fish
1 Wildlife Way
Santa Fe, NM 87507
www.wildlife.state.nm.us

New York State Department of Environmental Conservation
Division of Fish, Wildlife, and Marine Resources
625 Broadway
Albany, NY 12233-4750
www.dec.state.ny.us/website/dfwmr

North Carolina Wildlife Resources Commission
Division of Wildlife Management
512 North Salisbury Street
Raleigh, NC 27604-1188
www.ncwildlife.org

North Dakota Game and Fish Department
100 North Bismark Expressway
Bismark, ND 58501-5095
www.state.nd.us/gnf

Continued

Table 80-5 U.S. State Agencies That Regulate Herptiles—Cont'd

Ohio Department of Natural Resources
Division of Wildlife
2045 Morse Road
Bldg.G
Columbus, OH 43229-6693
www.dnr.state.oh.us/wildlife

Oklahoma Department of Wildlife Conservation
1801 North Lincoln Boulevard
Oklahoma City, OK 73105
www.wildlifedepartment.com

Oregon Department of Fish and Wildlife
3406 Cherry Avenue N.E.
Salem, OR 97303
www.dfw.state.or.us

Pennsylvania Department of Conservation and Natural Resources
7th Floor Rachel Carson State Office Building
PO Box 8767
400 Market Street
Harrisburg, PA 17105-8767
www.dcnr.state.pa.us

Rhode Island Department of Environmental Management
Division of Fish and Wildlife
4808 Tower Hill Road
Wakefield, RI 02879
www.dem.ri.gov

South Carolina Department of Natural Resources
Rembert C. Dennis Building
1000 Assembly Street
Columbia, SC 29201
www.dnr.sc.us

South Dakota Department of Game, Fish and Parks
523 East Capitol Avenue
Pierre, SD 57501
www.sdgfp.info

Tennessee Wildlife Resources Agency
Ellington Agricultural Center
PO Box 40747
Nashville, TN 37204
www.state.tn.us/twra

Texas Parks and Wildlife Department
4200 Smith School Road
Austin, TX 78744
www.tpwd.state.tx.us

Utah Department of Natural Resources
Utah Division of Wildlife Resources
1594 West North Temple
Salt Lake City, UT 84116
www.wildlife.utah.gov

Vermont Fish and Wildlife Department
Law Enforcement Division
103 South Main Street
Waterbury, VT 05671-0501
www.vtfishandwildlife.com

Virginia Department of Game and Inland Fisheries
4010 West Broad Street
Richmond, VA 23230
www.dgif.state.va.us

Washington Department of Fish and Wildlife
600 Capitol Way North
Olympia, WA 98501-1091
www.wdfw.wa.gov

West Virginia Division of Natural Resources
Capitol Complex, Building 3, Room 663
1900 Kanawaha Boulevard, East
Charleston, WV 25305-0660
www.wvdnr.gov

Wisconsin Department of Natural Resources
101 South Webster Street
PO Box 7921
Madison, WI 53707-7921
www.dnr.state.wi.us

Wyoming Game and Fish Department
5400 Bishop Boulevard
Cheyenne, WY 82006
http://gf.state.wy.us/index.asp

Note: The United States Fish and Wildlife Service maintains a web database of state, territorial, and tribal organizations: http://offices.fws.gov/statelinks.html

THE LACEY ACT

(Text from the USFWS web site.) Passed in 1900, the Lacey Act prohibits import, export, transportation, sale, receipt, acquisition, or purchase of fish, wildlife, or plants that are taken, possessed, transported, or sold in violation of any federal, state, tribal, or foreign law. The 1981 amendments to the Act were designed to strengthen federal laws and improve federal assistance to states and foreign governments in enforcement of fish and wildlife laws. The Act has become a vital tool in efforts to control smuggling and trade in illegally taken fish and wildlife. Another aspect of the Lacey Act regulates the transportation of live wildlife, requiring that animals be transported into the United States under humane and healthful conditions. The Act also allows the Interior Secretary to designate those wildlife species considered injurious to humans and prohibit their importation into the country.

Individuals convicted of violating the Lacey Act may be fined up to $100,000 and sentenced up to 1 year in jail for misdemeanors and up to $250,000 and 5 years of imprisonment for felony violations. Fines for organizations in violation of the Act are up to $250,000 and $500,000 for misdemeanor and felony violations, respectively. In addition, vehicles, aircraft, and equipment used in the violation and illegal fish, wildlife, and plants may be subject to forfeiture.

Persons who provide information on violations of the Lacey Act may be eligible for cash rewards.

CASE EXAMPLES

Case I

Facts
Federal and Pennsylvania Fish and Boat Commission agents raided a Pennsylvania man's home in June 1999. The man was charged with illegal possession and sale of reptiles and amphibians, which included rattlesnakes and an American Alligator. The sting was part of a coordinated interstate crackdown, which resulted in simultaneous arrests in 12 other states.

Laws Violated
CITES
ESA
Pennsylvania Wildlife Laws

Outcome
The man was charged with violating state and federal wildlife laws, pled guilty, and was fined $5,000 and sentenced to 1½ years' probation.

Case II

Facts
A foreign national was charged with numerous violations of the Lacey Act and the Federal Anti-Smuggling Statute, 18 USC § 545, for illegally importing reptiles. The perpetrator was charged with smuggling approximately 60 Pig-nose or Fly River Turtles (*Carettochelys insculpta*) and 113 Irian Jaya Snake-neck Turtles (*Chelodina siebenrocki*). On another occasion, the perpetrator flew from Japan to San Francisco, carrying six Red Mountain Racer Snakes and two Mandarin Ratsnakes in his luggage. A grand jury returned a five-count indictment against the perpetrator.

Laws Violated
Federal Anti-Smuggling Statute
ESA
CITES

Outcome
The defendant was sentenced to 5 years of probation (unsupervised provided that he would leave the United States), a fine of $5,000, and a special assessment of $200.

Case III

Facts
The defendant, a notorious international wildlife dealer, was charged with illegally importing exotic reptiles by concealing them in express delivery packages, airline baggage, and large commercial shipments of legally declared animals. A number of species were involved in the smuggling activity, including Komodo Dragons, Plowshare Tortoises, Fiji Banded Iguanas, Bengal Monitor Lizards, and Indian Soft-shelled Turtles. The defendant's smuggling activities violated CITES.

Laws Violated
CITES
ESA

Outcome
The defendant was sentenced to 71 months in federal prison and was ordered to pay a $60,000 fine.

Case IV

Facts
A 31-year-old man was charged with conspiracy to smuggle wildlife into the United States and trade of protected species in interstate commerce. The perpetrator was a reptile dealer known for the breeding of small lizards. U.S. Fish and Wildlife inspectors discovered a mail parcel from Spain addressed to the perpetrator, and when opened, the package contained 13 Lilford's Wall Lizards, which are small blue lizards that inhabit the Balcatic Islands off the coast of Spain. The lizards are protected under CITES, and both the United States and Spain are signatories of the CITES treaty. A federal search warrant was issued, and additional species were discovered, including European Ladder Ratsnakes, Box Turtles, venomous Massasauga Rattlesnakes, a Timber Rattlesnake, Great Plains Ratsnakes, and two Desert Tortoises. The perpetrator was charged with violating the US ESA and CITES. The Lacey Act was also violated because some of the species were protected by the Illinois state law, including the Dangerous Animals Act, which prohibits the possession of dangerous wildlife, including venomous snakes. The case was prosecuted by the U.S. Attorney for the Southern District of Illinois and the U.S. Department of Justice, Wildlife and Marine Resources Section, Washington, DC.

Laws Violated
CITES
ESA
United States Postal Laws
Illinois State Wildlife Laws

Outcome
The perpetrator pled guilty and faced 5 years of incarceration or $250,000 fine or both.

Case V

Facts
A U.S. reptile dealer was charged with wildlife smuggling, conspiracy, and money laundering. The dealer was apprehended in Orlando, Florida, in August 1998 after expulsion from Belize in Central America. The perpetrator trafficked protected reptiles from Australia, Indonesia, South America, and the Caribbean. A multicount indictment was levied against the perpetrator, his wife, and two former employees for the black market reptile trade. Reptiles were smuggled and concealed in suitcases and transported on commercial flights to the United States. The reptiles included Madagascar Tree and Ground Boas, Radiated Tortoises, and Spider Tortoises. Smuggling of these reptiles violated CITES and the Lacey Act. Defendants faced sentences of up to 20 years in prison and penalties as high as $500,000 per count.

Laws Violated
CITES
ESA
Lacey Act

Outcome
In January 1999, the Florida businessman pled guilty to seven felony counts of conspiracy, smuggling, and violating the Lacey Act and CITES. In April 1999, he was sentenced to 30 months in prison. The conviction of the smuggler was made possible by Operation Chameleon, a sting operation run by the U.S. Fish and Wildlife Service with cooperation from authorities in Florida, Virginia, Canada, Germany, Mexico, The Netherlands, South Africa, Belize, and Japan.

SUGGESTED READING

Allen WB: *State lists of endangered and threatened species of reptiles and amphibians and laws and regulations covering collecting of reptiles and amphibians in each state,* ed 3, Pittsburgh, 1988, privately printed, Pittsburgh Zoo.

Levell JP: *A field guide to reptiles and the law,* ed 2, Malabar, Fla, 1997, Serpents Tail Publications, Krieger Publishing.

81
WORKING WITH VENOMOUS SPECIES: EMERGENCY PROTOCOLS

BRENT R. WHITAKER and
BARRY S. GOLD

Approximately 450 species of venomous snakes and two species of venomous lizards (Table 81-1) exist, many of which are kept in captivity (Figures 81-1 and 81-2). Of approximately 8000 venomous bites a year in the United States, fewer than six typically result in death. Of those bitten, about half are young intoxicated males who are handling or antagonizing the animal. Most bites occur on the extremities (Figure 81-3). Only about 100 bites are from exotic species kept by zoos, aquariums, or hobbyists.[1] Of these, the cobra bite is the most common.

Reptile venoms are complex substances, comprised mainly of protein with enzymatic activity, that bind to receptor sites and cause physiologic changes in the victim. Although venoms have been previously classified as "neurotoxins," "hemotoxins," "myotoxins," and "cardiotoxins," each victim may have a unique clinical picture because of the wide range of effects produced by the various venom components. The enzymes of pit viper venom, for example, can produce serious physiologic effects, but mortality may be caused by the smaller low-molecular-weight polypeptides.

Venomous reptiles are kept at most zoos, at a few aquariums, and by some hobbyists. Although bites are rare, the development and then the following of appropriate emergency protocols minimize the likelihood of mortality or permanent disability from an accidental envenomation. Emergency protocols for alerting support staff of a venomous animal bite, for the recapture of a venomous animal, for the administration of first aid, and for the transport of an injured person to a medical facility where proper medical care can be given are needed before working with venomous animals. This chapter provides the information needed to develop site-specific emergency protocols for handling venomous reptiles. Additional procedures and general considerations for the attending physician are also provided.

DEVELOPMENT OF EMERGENCY PROTOCOLS FOR THE MANAGEMENT OF VENOMOUS ANIMAL BITES

Emergency protocols for handling venomous reptiles should be developed and implemented before the acquisition of a venomous animal. These protocols include:

A venomous animal escape/recovery plan
A venomous animal bite plan
First-aid procedures for a venomous animal bite
A medical treatment plan

Sources of information that may be useful in the development of these protocols include the American Association of Zoos and Aquariums Resource Center (www.aza.org), where emergency plans developed by several zoos have been published, and direct contact with other zoos or aquariums. In addition, the *Antivenin Index*, published and updated periodically by the American Zoo and Aquarium Association and the American Association of Poison Control Centers, lists the amount and location of available antivenoms for most venomous species. Information obtained on the Internet must be interpreted with caution unless it has been peer reviewed or published by a reliable source. Additional literature that may be useful is listed under "Suggested Reading" at the end of this chapter.

Table 81-1 Examples of Venomous Code 1 and Code 2 Reptiles

Family	Code 1	Code 2
Viperidae (Crotalinae: Pit Vipers)	Rattlesnake, Cottonmouth, Copperhead, Lance-headed Pit Viper, Fer-de-lance, Bushmaster, and Asiatic Pit Viper	
Viperidae (Viperinae: True Vipers)	African, European, and Middle Eastern Vipers	
Elapidae	Cobras, Mambas, Kraits, Coral Snakes, and all venomous snakes of Australia	
Hydrophiidae	True Sea Snakes	
Colubridae	Boomslang, Bird or Twig Snake, and Red-necked Keelback	Brown Vine Snake, Amazonian Vine Snake, and Cat-eyed Snake
Laticaudidae	Sea Kraits	
Atractaspididae	African and Middle East Mole Vipers	
Helodermatidae	Gila Monster and Mexican Beaded Lizard	

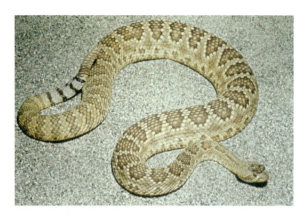

FIGURE 81-1 The venom of the Mojave Rattlesnake, *Crotalus scutulatus scutulatus*, is primarily neurotoxic and causes a paucity of local symptoms or signs unlike other pit vipers, which are capable of causing pain, edema, erythema, ecchymoses, fasciculations, paresthesias, nausea, vomiting, diaphoresis, generalized weakness, hypotension, shock, and spontaneous bleeding from mucous membranes. Deaths from Mojave Rattlesnake envenomations are generally the result of respiratory depression. *(Photograph courtesy B. Gold.)*

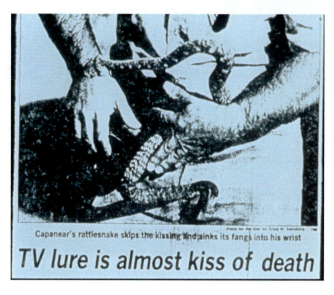

FIGURE 81-3 Most venomous reptile bites occur when proper handling precautions are ignored. This handler survived after hospitalization and administration of antivenom. *(Photograph courtesy B. Gold.)*

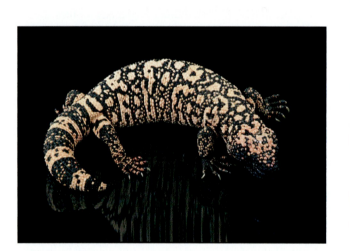

FIGURE 81-2 The venom of Beaded Lizards such as this animal, *Heloderma horridum*, is delivered through grooves on the surface of the animal's canines as the animal grasps and chews its prey. If bitten, one should place the animal on the floor to encourage it to release its grip. These lizards tend to keep their jaws clamped when held suspended in the air. If this does not work, other options include immersing the animal in water, placing a flame under the animal's jaw, or spraying ammonia into its mouth. Pain, tachycardia, generalized weakness, edema, lymphadenopathy, lymphangitis, erythema, nausea, vomiting, and leukocytosis may be associated with a bite from this animal. *(Photograph courtesy G. Grall, National Aquarium, Baltimore.)*

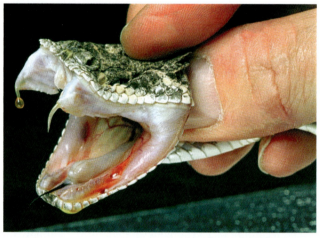

FIGURE 81-4 Emergency protocols must be prepared and appropriate antivenoms acquired in advance of receiving venomous reptiles. *(Photograph courtesy G. Grall, National Aquarium, Baltimore.)*

In development of emergency protocols for venomous animal bites, differentiation between venomous animals capable of inflicting life-threatening injury and less dangerous species may be helpful. For example, we classify our venomous reptiles as code 1 and code 2 animals. The venom of a code 1 animal is capable of causing death, long-term illness, or permanent disability, and the venom of a code 2 animal is unlikely to have severe or long-lasting effects. The protocols developed must be specific for the type and number of venomous reptiles in the collection (Figure 81-4). Maintenance of antivenom, for example, that is expired or inappropriate for the bite received can be life threatening. For each protocol, contact information for responsible staff and outside consultants must be readily available (Table 81-2). We recommend that a physician knowledgeable in the treatment of venomous reptile bites be consulted in the development of protocols for venomous animal bites. Once developed, these protocols should be given to authorities at the medical facility that will be responsible for treating an envenomation. In addition, we recommend that a medical toxicologist or physician with experience treating venomous animal bites be identified in advance of an actual emergency.

Venomous Animal Bite Plan

Prompt, appropriate first aid minimizes the risk of death or long-term debilitation after a venomous reptile bite. For this

Table 81-2	Example of a Table for Emergency Numbers

	Title or Facility	Contact Number
HOSPITALS		
LOCAL CONSULTANTS		
OUT-OF-STATE CONSULTANTS		
STAFF		

Table 81-3	Protocols for Code 1 Venomous Animal Bites

Victim

Leave area
Secure area to prevent animal escape
Activate emergency bite alarm
Notify others in area of the bite, type of animal, and whether the animal is secured
Remain calm; remove all jewelry to prevent further injury from swelling

First Assistant

Call 911; report that a venomous animal bite has occurred and give address
Call for further assistance
Ensure jewelry has been removed, and keep victim calm
Administer first aid
When help arrives, ensure that the antivenom, *Antivenin Index*, and other reference documents accompany victim to hospital

Second Assistant

Enlist trained staff to recapture venomous animal, if necessary
Gather antivenom, *AZA Antivenin Index*, and other documents needed to accompany victim to hospital

Table 81-4	Protocols for Code 2 Venomous Animal Bites

Victim

Recapture and secure animal if easily done
Leave area and close door
Request assistance from staff
Remove all jewelry to prevent swelling-associated injuries
Begin first aid

Assistant

Treat as a code 1 venomous animal bite if victim is in severe pain or shows signs of shock or other systemic effects
If available, request an emergency medical technician; otherwise, take victim directly to a medical facility for treatment
Notify appropriate staff of injury

---

reason, an emergency bite alarm, which can be easily activated by the victim and identifies the victim's location, is recommended in facilities that maintain code 1 animals.

Example protocols are provided for the response to code 1 (Table 81-3) and 2 (Table 81-4) venomous animal bites. We recommend that at least two *trained* people be present with handling of code 1 venomous reptiles. Alternatively, a second trained person should be close enough to respond to an emergency in less than 1 minute. If possible, both the victim and the uninjured person should leave the area and secure it. If not, the noninjured person should assume responsibility for containing the animal until additional help arrives. In the event that a second trained person is not present, the injured person should sound the alarm, secure the area, and seek assistance from nearby staff to monitor the location of the venomous animal until trained personnel arrive. Attending staff should begin first aid as soon as possible.

Routine emergency drills are important to ensure that personnel are prepared and alarms are working properly. Appropriate antivenoms, if available, must be acquired, properly stored, and replaced when expired.

Venomous Animal Escape Plan

Every facility that holds venomous reptiles must have a plan for recapturing escaped animals. A well-developed plan is critical for management of a situation in which an envenomation has occurred but emergency assistance has not yet arrived. The plan must include procedures for managing an escape into both public and contained areas and a course of action if the animal cannot be located (Table 81-5). The plan must also include a contact list of staff who are authorized to respond to an escape, with descriptions of their predetermined roles. All equipment necessary for the capture and handling must be readily available. Two trained staff are needed to recapture a code 1 venomous reptile.

First-Aid Procedures for a Venomous Animal Bite

First aid for bites by a code 1 animal (Table 81-6) should be administered immediately after activating the venom alarm and calling 911 (see Venomous Animal Bite Plan). Do not activate the venom alarm or call 911 for code 2 animal bites (Table 81-7) unless the victim is in severe pain or shock. Staff should be trained in the use and location of the venom emergency first-aid kits, which must contain everything needed to provide first aid for the bite of any venomous reptile kept on the premises (Table 81-8). One staff person must be responsible for replenishing the kit after each use and inspecting it monthly to ensure all materials are present.

A Sawyer Extractor (Sawyer Products, Safety Harbor, Fla; Figure 81-5) may aid in the extraction of venom from viperid and crotalid bites if applied to the bite site within 5 minutes of the injury and left in place for up to 60 minutes. Although the effectiveness of this device has not been proven, it does not cause harm and may be of some benefit. The technique of lancing bites and sucking out venom is ineffective and may result in greater tissue damage and possible infection. The use of a tourniquet or an ice pack is contraindicated. Pressure bandages are not recommended if the venom has proteolytic

Table 81-5	Example Protocols for the Recapture of Venomous Animals

Contained Escape (i.e., in a secured area)

Alert appropriate staff of the escape, including the type of animal and its location, via radio, pager, or telephone

Alert any personnel in the immediate vicinity of an animal escape

For code 1 animals, secure the area and wait until a minimum of two trained staff members arrive before recapture is attempted

Code 2 animals may be recaptured by one trained staff person

If alone or untrained in the capture of venomous reptiles, secure the area and monitor the animal from a distance until trained staff arrives

Recapture and secure animal

Report incident to appropriate staff

Public Area Escape

Report escape to appropriate staff, including the type of animal and its location, via radio, pager, or telephone

If members of the public are present, evacuate them from area

Secure area. This may include:
    Closing doors, windows, or other escape routes
    Shutting off escalators and elevators

Recapture and secure animal

Maintain communication with appropriate staff, such as the head of Visitor Services, Security, and other departments that need to ensure public and staff safety

Missing Venomous Animal

Report to appropriate staff that an animal is missing; include the type of animal and location of escape

Once the animal has been confirmed missing, appropriate actions are determined by:
    The species of animal
    The area involved
    The potential risk to visitors or staff

Table 81-6	Code 1 Venomous Animal Bite First Aid

Do:

Activate venom alarm and call 911

Have victim lie down or sit

Keep victim as calm as possible

Remove all jewelry

Maintain an airway at all times

Identify bite site

Apply Sawyer Extractor within 5 minutes of the bites of Vipers and Pit Vipers; leave in place for up to 60 minutes

Apply pressure wrap to the bites of Sea Snakes and Sea Kraits and some species of Cobras whose venom is not associated with tissue necrosis

If Bite is on Extremity:

Begin at bite site and wrap firmly toward trunk

If Bite is on Trunk:

Apply continuous pressure with a hand-held pad until arrival of medical support staff

Immobilize bitten limb with a splint and crepe bandage to prevent motion of limb; rest bitten limb at or below the level of the heart

Do Not:

Apply a pressure wrap to the bites of vipers and pit vipers

Leave victim unattended

Apply ice or heat to the bite site

Lance wound or attempt to suck out venom

Administer products containing stimulants (e.g., caffeinated beverages, caffeinated analgesics)

Administer aspirin to victims of crotalid or viperid bites

Table 81-7	Code 2 Venomous Animal Bite First Aid

Do:

Victim:

Secure animal

Seek immediate assistance of nearby staff

Remove jewelry in case of swelling

Assistant:

If severe pain, treat as a code 1 emergency

Seek medical attention or identify another person to transport victim and caregiver to a medical facility

Cleanse bite site

Apply suction over fang punctures with a Sawyer Extractor; leave extractor in place

Do Not:

Activate venom alarm

Call 911 unless victim is in severe pain or going into shock

Apply pressure wrap

Apply heat or cold to bite site

Incise the wound

properties, which cause tissue necrosis (e.g., vipers; Figure 81-6). A pressure wrap is recommended for bites by sea snakes, sea kraits, or other animals whose venom has primarily cardiotoxic or neurotoxic effects (Figure 81-7).

Many types of venom can cause respiratory failure. Therefore, maintenance of an airway at all times is important.

Medical Treatment Plan

Table 81-9 provides a summary of signs, symptoms, and medical treatments for code 1 envenomations. In the event of a venomous snakebite (see Table 81-9 for treatment of lizard bites), the physician should perform the following procedures without delay:

- If a crepe bandage has been applied as a first-aid measure to retard the absorption of venom, **do not remove** the bandage until the patient is receiving antivenom or it has been determined that an envenomation did not occur. If a tourniquet has been applied, place a constriction band above the tourniquet before removing the tourniquet. Leave the constriction band in place until either the patient is receiving antivenom or it has been determined that an envenomation did not occur.
- Establish control of Airway, Breathing, and Circulation.
- The patient should be continuously monitored in the Emergency Department/Intensive Care Unit. Detailed history with respect to the bite (i.e., time of bite, circumstances, first-aid measures used) should be obtained along with any significant medical history, medications, and allergies.
- Start a peripheral intravenous line (18-gauge catheter) with 0.9% normal saline solution or lactated Ringer's

Table 81-8 Venomous Bite Emergency First Aid Kit

Antiseptic isopropyl swabs and Betadine swabs
Self-adherent sterile bandages; Coban self-adherent wrap
Sawyer Extractor
Extremity splints
Sling
Nonsterile hypoallergenic gloves
Ring cutter for the removal of jewelry
A copy of the Venom Emergency First-Aid Procedures
    (to be transported to hospital with victim)
A copy of the current *AZA Antivenom Index*

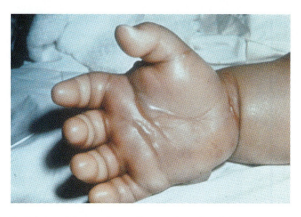

FIGURE 81-6 The swollen and edematous hand of a victim bitten by an Eastern Diamondback, *Crotalus adamanteus*, emphasizes the need to remove all jewelry soon after a bite from a venomous animal. Pressure bandages should not be applied to bites from venomous animals such as vipers that cause tissue necrosis. (*Photograph courtesy B. Gold.*)

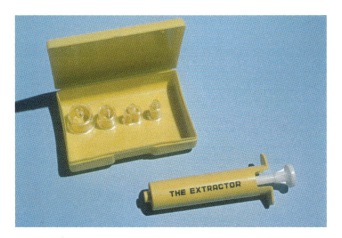

FIGURE 81-5 The Sawyer Extractor creates a negative pressure over the bite wound and may aid in venom removal. Although the effectiveness of this device is not proven, it is easily used and may provide some benefit if applied within the first 5 minutes of the envenomation. (*Photograph courtesy B. Gold.*)

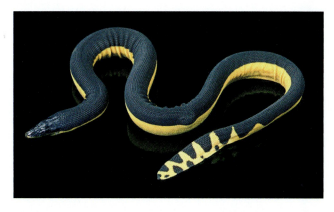

FIGURE 81-7 A pressure wrap should be applied to the bite of venomous reptiles, such as this Yellow-bellied Sea Snake, *Pelamis platurus*, whose venom has primarily cardiotoxic or neurotoxic effects. (*Photograph courtesy G. Grall, National Aquarium, Baltimore.*)

solution at a rate of 200 mL/hr in the unaffected upper extremity
- Draw blood from the contralateral arm, and obtain urine for the following STAT laboratory studies:
    1. Complete blood count (CBC) with differential and platelet count
    2. Coagulation profile to include prothrombin time (INR), activated partial thromboplastin time (APTT), fibrinogen level, fibrin degradation products
    3. Serum electrolytes, blood urea nitrogen (BUN)/creatinine, calcium, phosphorus
    4. Lactate dehydrogenase
    5. Type and cross match for two units of packed red blood cells
    6. Creatinine kinase (CK)
    7. Urinalysis (macroscopic and microscopic)
- Electrocardiogram
- Continuous urine output monitoring (insert indwelling Foley catheter if necessary)
- On the basis of the type of snake, some of the previous laboratory studies should be repeated every 4 hours or after each course of antivenom, whichever is sooner.
- Observe patient closely for signs/symptoms of envenomation including laboratory abnormalities, which may manifest within minutes to hours after the bite, depending on the type of snake

If any signs/symptoms of crotaline (pit viper) envenomation become apparent, institute antivenom therapy as follows:
An intradermal skin test for hypersensitivity should be performed on a contralateral extremity with Wyeth Crotalidae Polyvalent Antivenin. A control of 0.02 mL of 0.9% normal saline solution should be performed on the other extremity. This should be read after 30 minutes. **A skin test should never be performed until the need for antivenom has been determined.** If no evidence exists of erythema or a vesicular response, the test should be considered negative. A positive skin test is not a contraindication to treatment with antivenom. **A negative skin test does not preclude the occurrence of a hypersensitivity reaction.** In the presence of a positive skin test, the risk/benefit ratio should be assessed and, if necessary, antivenom can be administered after pretreatment

Table 81-9 Code 1 Envenomations: Signs, Symptoms, and Medical Treatment

Family	Distribution/Examples	Principal Action of Venom	Serious Risks	Symptoms of Envenomation	Treatment Recommendations	Other Considerations
Viperidae Subfamily: Viperinae (True Vipers)	Africa, Europe, Middle East: *Bitis arietans* (Puff Adder), *B. gabonica* (Gaboon Viper), *B. nasicornus* (Rhinoceros Horned Viper), *Echis* sp. (Saw-scaled Viper), *Cerastes* sp. (Horned or Desert Vipers), *Vipera* sp. (Vipers) Indian subcontinent and southeast Asia: *Daboia russelii* (Russell's Viper)	Hemostatic and cardiovascular effects, local tissue necrosis	Alterations in clotting mechanisms, hypovolemic shock, myocardial toxicity	Swelling and pain at site of bite; hypotension/shock; cardiac arrhythmias; spontaneous bleeding from mucous membranes, orifices, bite site (incoagulable blood)	Evidence of local envenomation by species known to cause local necrosis (e.g., *Bitis*, *Echis*, *Vipera* sp.; digit bites, rapid progressive swelling, swelling involving more than half of the bitten extremity) Evidence of systemic envenomation (spontaneous systemic bleeding, incoagulable blood, hypotension, shock, arrhythmia, abnormal ECG, impaired consciousness, neurotoxicity) Antivenom: Monospecific is preferred over polyspecific if available Dosage is based on severity of envenomation	Antivenom is indicated in all cases of systemic and severe local envenomation Supportive care: Administer appropriate tetanus toxoid Administer antibiotics based on culture/sensitivity testing
Viperidae Subfamily: Crotalinae (Pit Vipers)	North, South, Central America; Asia: *Crotalus* sp. (Rattlesnakes), *Agkistrodon* sp. (Copperhead and Cottonmouth), *Bothrops* sp. (Lance-headed Pit Vipers), *Lachesis muta* (Bushmaster), *Trimeresurus* sp. (Asiatic Pit Vipers)	Local tissue damage, vascular defects, hemolysis, defibrination, neuromuscular dysfunction	Cardiovascular collapse, coagulopathies, respiratory failure	Pain (e.g., Mojave Rattlesnake), erythema, ecchymoses, edema, fasciculations, paresthesias, unusual tastes (Rattlesnakes), hypotension, shock, spontaneous bleeding from mucous membranes, nausea, vomiting, diaphoresis, generalized weakness, respiratory depression, altered mental status	Antivenom administration is recommended for moderate to severe envenomations Two types of antivenom: Equine-derived (Wyeth) and ovine-derived (Tab) Envenomations are graded on the basis of the most severe clinical sign, symptom, or laboratory abnormality at any given time (e.g., local swelling	Grades of envenomation: *Mild*: Local swelling only, normal laboratory results *Moderate*: Local swelling, non-life threatening signs of systemic envenomation, moderate laboratory abnormalities *Severe*: Rapidly progressing local effects, severe systemic effects, markedly abnormal laboratory results Skin testing must be performed before treatment with equine-derived

				antivenom; however, a positive skin test does not preclude treatment with antivenom, nor does a negative skin test eliminate the possibility of hypersensitivity reaction Immediate hypersensitivity reactions are seen in as many as 50% or more of patients after administration of equine-derived antivenom Serum sickness (type III hypersensitivity reaction) is often seen with administration of >5 vials of equine-derived antivenom and occurs 1 to 2 weeks after antivenom administration; treat with a tapering course of steroids
			with markedly abnormal laboratory results is graded as a severe envenomation)	
Hydrophiidae Subfamily: Laticaudinae (Sea Kraits) Subfamily: Hydrophiinae (True Sea Snakes)	East coast of Africa to the West coast of the Americas	Neurotoxic, myotoxic	Rhabdomyolysis, flaccid paralysis, respiratory failure, muscle necrosis with renal failure	Myalgias, dizziness, dry throat, nausea, vomiting, generalized weakness, pseudotrismus, headache, diaphoresis, swelling of tongue, myoglobinuria, flaccid paralysis progressing to respiratory paralysis	Antivenom is indicated in the presence of paralysis or laboratory evidence of myolysis (i.e., myoglobinuria and elevated CK) Antivenom is most effective if given within 8 hr of bite but may still be effective 24 to 36 hr after bite In the presence of myoglobinuria, good hydration is essential and requires aggressive IV fluid therapy Renal function may be impaired from rhabdomyolysis; consequently BUN/creatine and K should be monitored ECG may be helpful in detection of hyperkalemia	Muscle weakness and movement pain are the classic indicators of systemic Sea Snake envenomation Muscle pain is severe; reluctance to move may be misinterpreted as paralysis Bite is often painless with usually little or no local reaction Up to 80% of bites cause little or no systemic effect Systemic effects typically appear within 30 min to 3.5 hr; cases of severe envenomation generally manifest within 2 hr If no evidence exists of myoglobinuria or envenomation within 4 hr of bite, serious effects are unlikely Myoglobinuria may be evident in 3 to 6 hr; monitor CBC for leukocytosis, CK, and liver enzymes (AST primarily)

Continued

Table 81-9 Code 1 Envenomations: Signs, Symptoms, and Medical Treatment—Cont'd

Family	Distribution/ Examples	Principal Action of Venom	Serious Risks	Symptoms of Envenomation	Treatment Recommendations	Other Considerations
Elapidae	Tropical and warm temperate zones: *Naja* sp. (Cobras), *Dendroaspis* sp. (Mambas), *Bungarus* sp. (Kraits), *Micrurus*, *Calliophis*, and *Maticora* sp. (Coralsnakes), and most venomous snakes of Australia	Neurotoxic (with exception of Spitting Cobras), tissue necrosis	Cranial nerve palsies, respiratory paralysis	African Spitting Cobras (*Naja katiensis*, *N. mossambica*, *N. nigricollis*, *N. pallida*, *Hemachatus haemachatus*): Bite: Intense local pain and rapidly developing swelling with blistering "Spat" venom: Intense ocular pain with blepharospasm, palpebral edema, leukorrhea, corneal erosions, secondary infection (panophthalmitis) Other Cobras (*Naja* sp.) and Mambas (*Dendroaspis* sp.): Headache, dizziness, paresthesias, cranial nerve palsies, heaviness of eyelids, blurred vision, tingling of tongue and lips, vomiting, salivation, sweating, diarrhea, slurred speech, abdominal pain, paralysis	Evidence of systemic or several local envenomation calls for treatment Antivenom: Monospecific is preferred over polyspecific if available SAIMR polyspecific antivenom effectively neutralizes most Cobra venoms Dosage is based on severity of envenomation	Spitting Cobra bites: Venom in the eyes causes blepharospasm, palpebral edema, and corneal erosions; hypopyon and anterior uveitis also occur; secondary infection of corneal ulcers may lead to panophthalmitis and corneal opacities Mambas, Egyptian and Cape Cobra: Bites cause severe neurotoxic effects Shield-nose and Coral Snakes: Rarely are envenomations fatal to adults; venoms of many Cobras and Mambas are neurotoxic; the venom of the African Spitting Cobra is not neurotoxic to humans; neurotoxicity is progressive, and effects are reversible with administration of antivenom or prolonged supportive care (1 to 7 d)
Colubridae	Africa: *Dispholidus typus* (Boomslang), *Thelotornis* sp. (Bird Snake) Includes rear-fanged snakes Asia: *Rhabdophis tigrinus* (Yamakagashi), *R. subminiatus* (Red-necked Keelback)	Hemotoxic with incoagulable blood, defibrination, elevated fibrin(ogen) and fibrin degradation products, severe thrombocytopenia and anemia	Persistent bleeding from fang marks (earliest symptom), nausea, vomiting, colicky abdominal pain, headache, bleeding from old and recent wounds, diffuse spontaneous bleeding, intravascular hemolysis, renal failure	Nausea, vomiting, abdominal pain, headache, bleeding from gums and wounds (old and new)	Specific antivenom is not available except for the Boomslang, for which a monospecific antivenom (SAIMR boomslang antivenom) is made by South African Vaccine Producers, Johannesburg, South Africa	Site of bite may show some swelling Symptoms develop quickly or may be delayed up to 24 hr Investigations may reveal incoagulable blood, defibrinogenation, elevated fibrin and fibrinogen degradation products, severe thrombocytopenia, and anemia Consultation with Poison Center is strongly recommended for suggestions regarding cross reactivity of other antivenoms

Atractaspididae	Africa, Middle East: *Atractaspis* sp. (Burrowing Asp), *Macrelaps microlepidotus* (Natal Black Snake)	Proteolytic activity, enzymatic activity, hemotoxic activity, cardiotoxic activity	Acute respiratory failure, AV conduction disturbances, myocardial ischemia, prolonged INR, elevated alkaline phosphatase and AST, abnormal liver histology	Local: Pain, swelling, blistering, local necrosis at the bite site, painful lymphadenopathy Systemic: Fever, nausea, headache, faintness, generalized weakness	No specific antivenom No specific evidence of cross reactivity to other antivenoms Treatment is supportive	Bites are extremely rare
Helodermatidae	Southwestern United States, Mexico, Guatemala: *Heloderma* sp. (Gila Monster, Beaded Lizard)	Vasodilatory activity, hyaluronidase activity	Hypotension	Pain, tachycardia, generalized weakness, edema, lymphadenopathy, lymphangitis, erythema, nausea, vomiting, leukocytosis	No antivenom available Treatment is supportive on basis of degree of envenomation Vasopressor agents are rarely necessary Hypotension and tachycardia usually respond to fluid administration At least 6 hr of observation is recommended Wound must be explored for foreign bodies (e.g., teeth); radiographs are of limited value in finding these foreign bodies High incidence rate of secondary infection Tetanus prophylaxis as necessary	Degree of envenomation based on: Size of the animal Duration and depth of bite (tends to bite and maintain bite on victim with venom flow augmented by chewing motion); rapid removal of the animal should be attempted to decrease severity of envenomation; removal may be attempted with application of a flame under the animal's lower jaw for 3 to 5 sec or with spraying ammonia into the animal's mouth The teeth involved: Venom delivery is predominantly through the base of the canines Location of bite: Obstruction between lizard and victim (e.g., glove, fabric) Animal disposition before bite (e.g., feeding-response bite)

AV, Atrioventricular; *BUN*, blood urea nitrogen; *CBC*, complete blood count; *CK*, creatinine kinase; *ECG*, electrocardiography; *INR*, prothrombin time; *IV*, intravenous.

with antihistamine. While awaiting skin test results, dilute the contents of the antivenom to prepare for administration. **If using the Crotalidae Polyvalent Immune Fab (CroFab; Ovine), skin testing is not necessary.**

- Dilute and administer antivenom per package insert directions. The amount of antivenom required varies on the basis of the species of snake and the severity of the envenomation. Regional Poison Centers **(National Hotline, 800-222-1222)** maintain a roster of experts available to assist in the treatment of envenomations, if needed. The rate of administration should be adjusted accordingly to avoid fluid overload; however, a brisk urine output should be a treatment goal. If a reaction occurs during antivenom administration, the infusion should be stopped immediately and subcutaneous epinephrine, and H_1 and H_2 receptor blockers should be administered to control the acute reaction. The need for continued antivenom treatment should be reassessed on the basis of the risk/benefit ratio and progression of local, systemic, and coagulopathic effects.
- The patient should remain under direct observation for at least 30 minutes after the infusion of antivenom.
- The patient's clinical status must be constantly reassessed. If the patient's condition does not improve or worsens, additional antivenom should be administered until marked regression or reversal of the venom effects is seen.
- Monitor suspected victims of snakebites containing neurotoxic venom components (i.e., elapids) in the hospital for a minimum of 12 hours because venom effects may be delayed or develop suddenly hours after the bite and are not easily reversed. Frequent monitoring of O_2 saturation along with peak flow and vital capacity is essential because of the potent neurotoxic venom component. Ventilatory support may be necessary.

GENERAL CONSIDERATIONS

The patient should remain in the intensive care unit until free of symptoms or signs for at least 24 hours and should remain under observation in the general hospital for at least 24 hours after all symptoms have abated.

Skin testing is not innocuous and should only be performed after the decision has been made to treat with antivenom. Although no predictive value to skin testing exists, it must be performed with the Wyeth Crotalidae Polyvalent Antivenin for medical-legal purposes.

Pertinent medical history must be obtained with particular attention to prior exposure to equine-derived products, atopic history, and underlying medical problems.

Hypersensitivity, pyrogenic, and serum sickness–type reactions can occur with **any** foreign protein (i.e., antivenoms).

Antivenom should **never** be injected directly into fingers or toes.

Antibiotics are rarely indicated and should not be given prophylactically.

For snakes with neurotoxic venom, narcotic analgesics along with sedative/hypnotics should be avoided in the early stages of observation/treatment because they may mask life-threatening, early neurologic manifestations.

Antiplatelet drugs (e.g., aspirin) should be avoided in viperid and crotalid bites.

In cases of hypovolemic shock unresponsive to antivenom therapy and intravenous fluid administration, plasma volume expanders or vasopressors may be administered.

In a consumptive coagulopathy, blood products (e.g., fresh frozen plasma, platelets) are not advisable in the presence of unneutralized venom because they are consumed and increase levels of fibrin degradation products, which are also anticoagulants.

The appropriate tetanus prophylaxis should be administered.

The bitten extremity should be immobilized in a functional position at or below the level of the heart. Early attention should be given to maintaining limb function.

Delayed hypersensitivity reactions (serum sickness) may occur 7 to 21 days after the administration of equine-derived or ovine-derived antivenom. It manifests as pruritus, urticaria, fever, lymphadenopathy, and arthralgias. Mild cases may be managed with diphenhydramine. More severe cases respond to a tapering course of prednisone over 7 to 10 days.

Surgical intervention should be avoided unless objective evidence of compartment pressure syndrome is manifested by compartment pressure measurements that exceed 30 mm of mercury for greater than 1 hour. Visual evidence of swelling is not a reliable indicator of compartment pressures.

All individuals with neurotoxicity from elapid bites (e.g., Asiatic Cobra species) should be given a test dose of the short-acting cholinesterase inhibitor edrophonium chloride (10 mg intravenously [IV]). If this dose is successful in reversing neurotoxic effects, administer neostigmine sulfate (0.5 mg IV or subcutaneously [SC] every 20 minutes). Pretreatment with atropine sulfate (0.6 mg IV) is required before the dose of edrophonium chloride and each dose of neostigmine sulfate to prevent the unpleasant muscarinic effects of acetylcholine.

The use of heparin or steroids is not indicated in the treatment of an acute envenomation.

ACKNOWLEDGMENTS

We extend our sincere appreciation to Reva Arnoff, RN, for her valuable contribution to this manuscript. Her attention to detail and dedication to the completion of this manuscript are greatly appreciated. In addition, we thank Valerie Lounsbury and Jack Cover, who assembled the National Aquarium in Baltimore's *Venom Emergency Procedures Manual*, which was used in the development of this manuscript.

REFERENCES

1. Gold B: Venomous snakes. In Beers H, Berkow R, editors: *Merck manual*, ed 17, Whitehouse Station, NJ, 1999, Merck.

2. Hooker K, Caravati E: Gila monster envenomation, *Ann Emerg Med* 24(4):731, 1994.

SUGGESTED READING

Campbell J, Lamar W: *The venomous reptiles of Latin America*, New York, 1989, Cornell University Press.

Dart R, Russell F: Animal poisoning. In Hall B, Schmidt G, Wood L, editors: *Principles of critical care*, New York, 1992, McGraw-Hill.

Gold B: Snake venom poisoning. In Rakel, R, editor: *Conn's current therapy*, New York, 2000, Saunders.

Gold B: Neostigmine for the treatment of neurotoxicity following envenomation by the Asiatic cobra, *Ann Emerg Med* 28(1):87, 1996.

Gold B, Wingert W: Snake venom poisoning in the United States: a review of therapeutic practice, *S Med J* 87(6):579, 1994.

Gold BS, Dart RC, Barish RA: Current concepts: bites of venomous snakes, *NEJM* 347(5):347, 2002.

Gold BS, Barish RA, Dart RC: North American snake envenomation: diagnosis, treatment, and management, *Emerg Med Clin N Am* 22:423-443, 2004.

Johnson-Delaney C: Reptile zoonoses and threats to public health. In Mader D, editor: *Reptile medicine and surgery*, Philadelphia, 1996, WB Saunders.

Jurkovich G, Luterman A, McCullar K, Ramenofsky M, Curreri P: Complications of Crotalidae antivenom therapy, *J Trauma* 28(7):1032, 1988.

Klauber L: *Rattlesnakes*, Los Angeles, 1982, University of California Press.

Meier J, White J: *Clinical toxicology of animal venoms and poisons*, New York, 1995, CRC Press.

Russell F: Snake venom poisoning, Great Neck, NY, 1983, Scholium International.

Spawls S, Branch B: *The dangerous snakes of Africa*, Sanibel Island, Fla, 1995, Ralph Curtis Books.

82
UNDERSTANDING DIAGNOSTIC TESTING

JIM WELLEHAN

In testing for infectious agents, one should first determine what information is sought. Are you looking for a pathogen, such as a virus or bacterium, or are you looking for a reaction to a pathogen, such as an antibody response?

Some tests, such as pathogen isolation or polymerase chain reaction (PCR), give information regarding the presence of pathogen. These tests require pathogen to be present in the sample submitted. Choice of sample for these tests is highly important. For example, in a patient with a viral infection that is not viremic at the time of sample collection, test results on blood are negative. This does not mean that virus does not exist elsewhere in the patient. For pathogen isolation, the pathogen needs to be viable, so the sample needs to be collected and stored in a manner so that the pathogen is not inactivated.

Other tests measure immune response to a pathogen. Immunologic testing gives evidence that an animal has had an immune response to a pathogen but does not give information on whether the pathogen is currently present. A look at changes in immune response over time is typically needed to determine the current relevance of an immune response; this requires assay of immune response at more than one time point.

Also important is consideration of whether the patient has had time to develop an immune response to a pathogen. This may take several weeks in reptiles.[1] In acute infections, a specific immune response may not be present. Large seasonal and temperature effects and species differences are seen on the immune response of reptiles.[2-4] Other factors, including reproductive status and exogenous corticosteroid administration, may also affect development of a measurable immune response.[5,6]

In testing immune response, consideration of what aspect of the immune system is being measured is also important. A humoral immune response primarily produces antibodies to fight pathogens extracellularly, whereas a cellular immune response primarily uses cytotoxic T cells to trigger self-destruction of host cells infected with pathogens. Cellular and humoral immune responses are often found together, but not always. An animal may have a cellular immune response without a significant humoral immune response, and vice versa. Most common assays measure humoral immunity. A cellular immune response is typically most protective for intracellular pathogens such as viruses.

Neither the presence of an infectious agent nor the presence of an immune response to an infectious agent necessarily indicates disease. The clinician needs to correlate this information with other appropriate diagnostic information, such as histopathology, to diagnose disease.

The following describes the most common laboratory tests used to diagnose reptilian disease. One must understand the limitations and peculiarities of each test to maximize the diagnostic value and avoid misinterpretations.

A test result that is positive from a patient that is actually negative is defined as a false-positive result. A test result that is negative from a patient that is actually positive is defined as a false-negative result.

PATHOGEN ISOLATION

Culture of a pathogen from a diseased animal is considered the gold standard for identification of infectious agents whenever possible. For some bacterial pathogens such as coliforms and pseudomonads, isolation and identification is fairly straightforward. For other pathogens such as some viruses, pathogen isolation is difficult and has a high false-negative rate even with skilled personnel. Culture specimens should be collected before antimicrobial therapy is begun. All specimens should be transported in labeled, tightly sealed, leak-proof containers that are not externally contaminated.

Many infectious agents that affect reptiles grow best at temperatures lower than those that affect mammalian hosts. Samples should be incubated at a variety of temperatures. Microbial identification kits for diagnostic laboratories are developed around organisms likely to be found in mammals or birds. If an identification appears unusual, questioning the result with a microbiologist is appropriate.

Both aerobic and anaerobic bacterial pathogens are found in reptiles. They may also be part of normal fauna of the gastrointestinal and upper respiratory tracts and the skin. Consequently, a sample culture alone is insufficient to make a causal association. Samples commonly submitted for bacterial culture include swabs from body orifices, cavity washes, tissue aspirates, blood cultures, and biopsies.

Selection of appropriate transport media is essential for useful bacterial culture results. Less fastidious organisms, such as pseudomonad and coliform bacteria, are relatively hardy and can be reasonably expected to survive overnight transport at room temperature on a standard collection swab such as Stuart's or Amies transport media. For noncoliform bacteria, Amies is preferable. Anaerobic samples should be placed immediately into anaerobic transport media such as thioglycollate agar. More fastidious bacteria such as *Mycoplasma* spp., *Chlamydia* spp., and many others require specific transport media.

Samples for *Mycoplasma* spp. should immediately be placed into a mycoplasma culture broth such as SP4 or Frey's. Because *Mycoplasma* spp. lack cell walls, they are highly susceptible to desiccation. If the sample is taken with a swab, chances for successful culture are greatly improved with premoistening swabs in sterile mycoplasma broth. Many *Mycoplasma* spp. are slow growing, and culture results may take up to several weeks. Concurrent serology or PCR are recommended if mycoplasmal disease is suspected (see Chapter 73).

Mycobacterial or actinomycete cultures are often most successful when taken from tissue samples. Biopsies should be sent directly to the laboratory in a sterile sealed container. *Mycobacterium* spp. are slow growing, and culture results may take weeks to months. Concurrent histology with acid-fast staining is recommended if mycobacterial or nocardial disease is suspected.

Chlamydophila spp. and *Chlamydia* spp. cultures also require specialized chlamydia transport media. As with *Mycoplasma* spp., if the sample is taken with a premoistened swab, chances for successful culture are greatly improved. Concurrent PCR testing is recommended if disease associated with *Chlamydophila* spp. is suspected. For identification of unusual bacteria, PCR amplification of 16S ribosomal DNA (rDNA) and sequencing is helpful for identification.

Fungal cultures are best collected directly from biopsy tissue samples. Biopsies should be sent directly to the laboratory in a sterile sealed container. In cases in which fungal pneumonia is suspected and bronchoscopic biopsy specimens are not available, fungal culture of a pulmonary wash can be used. When fungal skin infection is suspected, the skin is cleaned with alcohol and allowed to dry and the biopsy is collected and then imbedded into culture media. Reptiles are often infected with unusual fungal species not commonly encountered in many diagnostic laboratories, so finding a laboratory with expertise in this area is important (see Chapter 16).

Concurrent histology with special staining is recommended if fungal disease is suspected. For identification of unusual fungi, PCR amplification of 18S rDNA and sequencing is helpful for identification.

Some viruses, including herpesviruses, paramyxoviruses, and flaviviruses, are not tolerant of multiple freeze-thaw cycles. For isolation of these viruses, biopsy samples should be shipped refrigerated in viral transport media as soon as possible. Other viruses, including reoviruses, adenoviruses, poxviruses, and iridoviruses, are tolerant of freezing. For isolation of these viruses, biopsy samples should be shipped frozen. In spite of research, successful culture (virus isolation) methods for a number of reptile viruses have not been found.

POLYMERASE CHAIN REACTION

Polymerase chain reaction directly tests for the presence of nucleic acid from an infectious agent (pathogen). Like other pathogen isolation techniques, this requires that the clinician submit an appropriate sample that contains the actual pathogen. A negative test does not mean that the pathogen is not present elsewhere in the patient. Unlike pathogen isolation, with PCR the suspected agent does not need to be viable.

DNA is composed of two complementary strands oriented in opposite directions (Figure 82-1, *A*). Primers (short single-stranded segments of DNA) are designed to match the sequence of the two strands of pathogen DNA in a manner such that they face one another. The DNA is heated so that

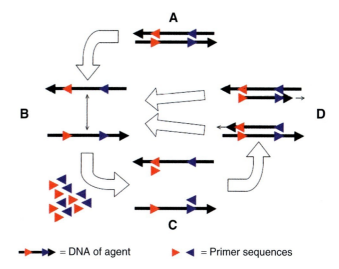

FIGURE 82-1 Polymerase chain reaction (PCR).

the two strands separate (Figure 82-1, *B*). The temperature is then decreased to an appropriate temperature for the primers to anneal (bind) with the DNA (Figure 82-1, *C*). If the primers do not match with the DNA sequence, they do not anneal and no product is formed.

The temperature is then increased to an appropriate temperature for thermostable DNA polymerase to extend the primer, making a matching strand for the DNA (Figure 82-1, *D*). The amount of DNA between the primers present is thus doubled. The cycle starts over again as the DNA is reheated to separate the strands. The cycle is repeated many times, and the amount of DNA increases geometrically.

The PCR product must then be validated, meaning that it must be determined to be the appropriate product and not an accidental binding of the primers to an unexpected site on a different DNA template. The most definitive way to determine the identity of the PCR product is to sequence it. Alternatively, a labeled piece of DNA containing part of the target sequence may be used to probe the PCR product. The probe must be designed to a sequence unique to the pathogen found within the PCR product. When done in the appropriate conditions, binding of the probe to the PCR product indicates that the PCR product is correct. Some protocols, such as TaqMan, have the probe incorporated in the PCR routine.

Another method of determination of the identity of the PCR product is restriction enzyme digestion. A restriction enzyme recognizes a short sequence of DNA, typically four to six base pairs, and cuts at the site. The sizes of the pieces generated are then typically measured with electrophoresis on a gel. When the DNA product is cut into pieces of the expected size, this suggests that the appropriate product has been generated. This is known as restriction fragment length polymorphism (RFLP), which is less specific than sequencing or probing but indicates that the PCR product was of the appropriate size and that restriction enzyme digestion sites were spaced to result in the expected fragment sizes.

A fourth method of checking the identity of the PCR product is to measure the size of the product, typically with electrophoresis on a gel. This is the least rigorous method of product identification.

Before primers can be designed, the nucleic acid sequence must be known. Some nucleic acid sequences are specific to a pathogen, and a PCR with unique primer sequences done at appropriate conditions that results in appropriate sized products is unlikely. This should be verified with extensive testing before diagnostic testing.

Other nucleic acid sequences have stayed the same through evolution and are found in many organisms. These are known as consensus sequences. Genes that are conserved throughout evolution are typically essential for function of the organism, such as ribosomal RNAs (rRNAs) or viral polymerases. In reptile medicine, many pathogens remain to be identified. If primers designed to conserved sequences are used in a PCR, the PCR amplifies all organisms that contain the conserved sequence. Although consensus sequence PCR is useful for amplification of sequence from novel pathogens, it should be accompanied by sequencing of the PCR product.

Polymerase chain reaction is a highly sensitive technique, and the potential for false-positive results from slight contamination anywhere from collection to laboratory is high. As such, measures must be taken to avoid contamination during sample collection and transport and appropriate controls must be run.

IMMUNOHISTOCHEMISTRY AND DNA IN SITU HYBRIDIZATION

Immunohistochemistry and DNA in situ hybridization directly test for the presence of an infectious agent. Like pathogen isolation, this requires the clinician to submit an appropriate sample that contains the pathogen, and a negative test result does not mean that pathogen does not exist elsewhere in the patient. Unlike pathogen isolation, the pathogen does not need to be viable. Samples for both tests should first be screened with standard histology. This provides the opportunity to find histologic lesions caused by the pathogen, indicating that disease is also present with the infection. The pathogen may be detected either with an antibody or with a labeled DNA probe.

With immunohistochemistry, the pathogen is detected with a labeled antibody to the pathogen (Figure 82-2, *A*). Immunohistochemistry requires an antibody to an infectious agent for detection. To make an antibody for an infectious agent, the infectious agent must be cultivated and injected into an animal to make antibodies. Not all currently known infectious agents of reptiles have been cultivated, meaning that antibodies may not be available for testing purposes.

With DNA in situ hybridization, the pathogen is detected by a labeled piece of DNA that matches a known target sequence from the pathogen's genome (Figure 82-2, *B*). DNA in situ hybridization requires knowledge of at least partial nucleotide sequence of an infectious agent.

The specificity of both antibody and the DNA probe varies according to the specificity of antibody or DNA probe design and the binding conditions. An assay of low stringency may require further diagnostic investigation for more specific identification of the pathogen.

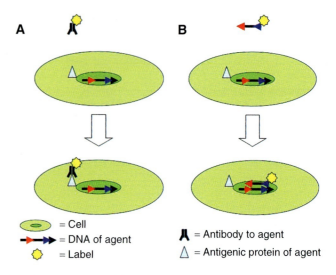

FIGURE 82-2 Immunohistochemistry and DNA in situ hybridization.

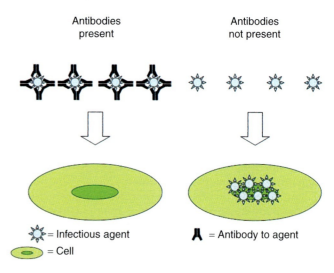

FIGURE 82-3 Serum neutralization.

SERUM NEUTRALIZATION

Serum neutralization (SN) tests for the presence of a humoral immune response to an infectious agent. It is typically considered the gold standard serologic test for viruses. The pathogen is grown in cell culture, and serum from the patient is added to the culture. If antibodies are present in the serum, they bind to the pathogen and prevent invasion of the cells (Figure 82-3). Cytopathic effects (changes in the cells from infection) are only seen if the cells are infected. This requires cell culture, which is labor intensive and slow (days to weeks) and requires skills at virus cultivation. As a result, fewer laboratories are equipped to perform this gold standard test.

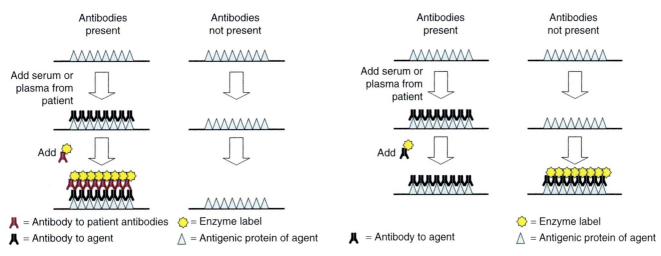

FIGURE 82-4 Enzyme-linked immunosorbent assay (ELISA).

FIGURE 82-5 Competitive enzyme-linked immunosorbent assay (ELISA).

ENZYME-LINKED IMMUNOSORBENT ASSAY

Enzyme-linked immunosorbent assay (ELISA) usually tests for the presence of a humoral immune response to an infectious agent. A sample plate is coated with antigen from the infectious agent. Serum or plasma from the patient is added to the plate, and if antibodies to the infectious agent are present, they bind to the antigen. Bound antibodies are then detected with an enzyme-labeled secondary antibody against the constant (Fc) portion of the patient's antibody (Figure 82-4). Enzymatic activity indicates the presence of bound antibody. This test is rapid and relatively easy to run. The test is designed to look at specific antibody classes, and thus, an early immunoglobulin M (IgM) response is detected separately from a later immunoglobulin G (IgG) response. Several reagents are required to run this test. First, the infectious agent must be cultivated to coat the plate with antigen. Second, a secondary antibody specific to the Fc portion of the patient's antibody must be made. This means that an ELISA is host species specific. Secondary antibodies are not available for many reptile species, and all available secondary antibodies for reptiles to date are IgG specific. Secondary antibody must be validated for every new species to be tested.

A variation on this test is the competitive ELISA. This test may be done without secondary antibodies specific to the host antibodies. In this test, a plate is coated with antigen from the infectious agent. Serum or plasma from the patient is added to the plate, and if antibodies to the infectious agent are present, they bind to the antigen. Enzyme-labeled antibody against the antigen is added. If the antigen is already covered with antibodies from the patient, the enzyme-labeled antibody does not have sites on the antigen to bind (Figure 82-5). The competitive ELISA does not require a secondary antibody specific to the Fc portion of the patient's antibody. Antibody to the infectious agent is needed instead.

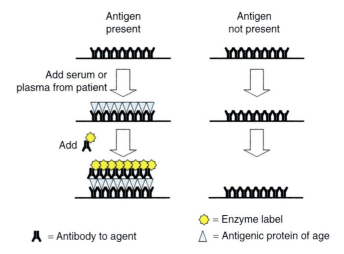

FIGURE 82-6 Antigen capture enzyme-linked immunosorbent assay (ELISA).

Thus, new reagents are not necessary for each host species, although the test does need to be validated for each species. Potential drawbacks to this method include the possibility that the host antibody and the reagent antibody bind to different sites on the antigen. If this occurs, the patient antibodies do not block the binding of the reagent antibody and a false-negative result occurs. Competitive ELISAs generally tend to be less sensitive than a traditional ELISA.

An ELISA to directly detect infectious agent can be designed. A plate is coated with antibody to an infectious agent. Serum or plasma from the patient is then added, and if infectious agent is present in the serum or plasma, it binds to the antibodies on the plate. A labeled antibody to the infectious agent is then added to detect bound antigen. Like any test for the presence of infectious agent, this test is only useful if the agent is present in the sample, in this case serum or plasma (Figure 82-6).

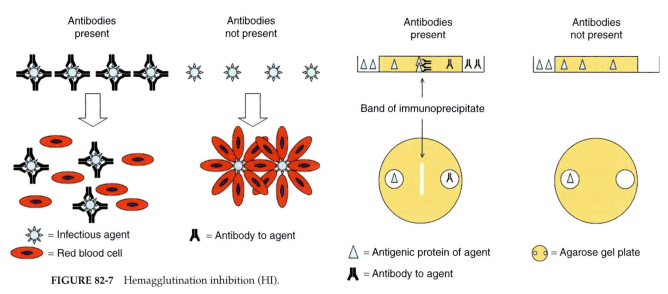

FIGURE 82-7 Hemagglutination inhibition (HI).

FIGURE 82-8 Agarose gel immunodiffusion (AGID).

HEMAGGLUTINATION INHIBITION

Hemagglutination tests for the presence of a humoral immune response to an infectious agent. Some infectious agents, such as paramyxoviruses, hemagglutinate erythrocytes. Serum is added to the infectious agent, and then erythrocytes are added. If antibodies are bound to the infectious agent, they block the ability of the infectious agent to hemagglutinate the erythrocytes (Figure 82-7). This test is relatively rapid and easy to perform. The test does not require host-specific secondary antibodies as reagents. Limitations of this test include the requirement that the infectious agent hemagglutinate erythrocytes; most do not. The infectious agent must also be able to be cultured.

AGAROSE GEL IMMUNODIFFUSION

Agarose gel immunodiffusion (AGID) tests for the presence of a humoral immune response to an infectious agent. When antibody and antigen are combined at equal proportions, a precipitate forms. Serum or plasma from the patient is put into a well in an agarose gel plate, and antigen from the infectious agent is put in a separate well. Antigen diffuses out from the antigen well, with the highest concentration near the well. If antibody is present, it diffuses out from the serum or plasma well, and where antigen and antibody are in equal concentration, a band of immunoprecipitate becomes visible (Figure 82-8). This test typically requires 48 to 72 hours for the antigen and antibody to diffuse. The infectious agent must also be able to be cultured to provide antigen.

INDIRECT FLUORESCENT ANTIBODY

Indirect fluorescent antibody (IFA) assays involve detection of an antibody with a second fluorescently labeled antibody. Depending on how they are used, they are either a variation on immunohistochemistry (detecting infectious agent) or similar to ELISA (detecting humoral immune response). If used in immunohistochemistry, a second fluorescent dye-labeled antibody detects bound antibody to the infectious agent. If used in a manner similar to ELISA, a fluorescent dye-labeled secondary antibody is used rather than an enzyme-labeled secondary antibody. IFA tests for humoral immune response generally tend to be less sensitive than ELISAs and are being replaced in many laboratories by ELISAs. The clinician should consult with the laboratory to determine specifically what type of test is being run.

T CELL PROLIFERATION ASSAYS

T cell proliferation assays test for the presence of a cellular immune response to an infectious agent. A cellular immune response is typically the protective response for an intracellular pathogen. In a cellular immune response, the T cell receptor (TCR), rather than the antibody, is the pathogen-adapted molecule. Unlike antibodies, which recognize shapes of whole antigens, TCRs recognize only antigenic proteins that have been broken down into shorter peptides and are presented on a major histocompatibility complex (MHC) by an antigen-presenting cell. In a T cell proliferation assay, antigen-presenting cells and T lymphocytes of the patient are cultured with antigen from the infectious agent. In a host that has had a previous cellular immune response to the infectious agent, T cells with antigen specific TCRs are present and the T cells proliferate rapidly (Figure 82-9). This proliferation is measured with a metabolic marker, such as uptake of tritiated thymidine.

T cell proliferation assays require viable white blood cells from the patient to be run. They also require infectious agent to be cultivated to produce antigen. Most importantly, they require lymphocyte purification and culture, which is labor intensive and slow (days to weeks) and requires specialized skills. T cell proliferation assays for reptiles are

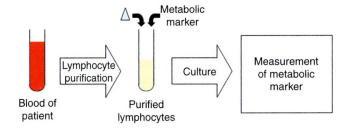

△ = Antigenic protein of agent

FIGURE 82-9 Lymphocyte proliferation assay.

currently not available, and no good methods of assaying cellular immune responses are available to clinicians at this time. This method is mentioned because advances in diagnostic testing are rapidly progressing, and it may be available in the future.

REFERENCES

1. Lock BA, Green LG, Jacobson ER, Klein PA: Use of an ELISA for detection of antibody responses in Argentine boa constrictors (Boa constrictor occidentalis), Am J Vet Res 64:388-395, 2003.
2. Zapata AG, Varas A, Torroba M: Seasonal variations in the immune system of lower vertebrates, Immunol Today 13: 142-147, 1992.
3. el Masri M, Saad AH, Mansour MH, Badir N: Seasonal distribution and hormonal modulation of reptilian T cells, Immunobiology 193:15-41, 1995.
4. Munoz FJ, De la Fuente M: The immune response of thymic cells from the turtle Mauremys caspica, J Comp Physiol [B] 171:195-200, 2001.
5. Saad AH, el Deeb S: Immunological changes during pregnancy in the viviparous lizard, Chalcides ocellatus, Vet Immunol Immunopathol 25:279-286, 1990.
6. Mondal S, Rai U: Dose and time-related in vitro effects of glucocorticoid on phagocytosis and nitrite release by splenic macrophages of wall lizard Hemidactylus flaviviridis, Comp Biochem Physiol C Toxicol Pharmacol 132:461-470, 2002.

83
REPORTED TOXICITIES IN REPTILES

KEVIN T. FITZGERALD and REBECCA VERA

INTRODUCTION

Dosage differentiates the poison from the remedy.
Paracelsus

An ever-expanding array of substances has been shown to be toxic to lizards, snakes, and turtles. Intoxication in reptiles, once merely an anecdotal domain, has grown tremendously in the last few years thanks to more detailed published accounts of poisoning and some in-depth pharmacologic studies. Certainly, thousands of different molecules have the capacity to poison living reptiles. Unfortunately, less than 5% of all potential toxins have antidotes or effective physiologic antagonists. This index of poisons, although by no means complete, focuses on the most common poisonings of reptiles, their mechanisms of action, and their potential treatments.

IVERMECTIN

Ivermectin is an antiparasitic from a family of chemicals called avermectins. These are marocylic lactones made from fermentation broth of the fungus *Streptomyces avermitilis*.[1] The macrolide ivermectin is available as an injectable, a spray, and an oral formulation. It has activity against a variety of parasites, including nematodes, arthropods, and arachnids.

Mechanism of Action

Avermectins work by potentiating the effects of the inhibitory neurotransmitter gamma-aminobutyric acid (GABA).[1] They stimulate release of GABA by presynaptic sites and increase GABA binding to postsynaptic receptors, which causes neuromuscular blockage. Avermectins also open chloride channels in membranes of the nervous system and further depress neuronal function. These actions cause paralysis and death of susceptible parasites. Ivermectin is absorbed systemically by host tissues. When parasites bite the host, they then absorb the ivermectin. Ivermectin is active against intestinal parasites, mites, microfilariae, and developing larvae.[1] Concurrent treatment with diazepam, which also works through GABA potentiation, may heighten deleterious effects.

Clinical Signs

Ivermectin can cause depression, paralysis, coma, and death in chelonians.[2] Species susceptible to ivermectin toxicosis may have a blood-brain barrier more permeable than in nonsensitive species. This greater permeability may be the result of p-glycoprotein mutation in membranes of the central nervous system (CNS). Another, separate theory postulates the existence of a specific protein receptor only present in the brains of ivermectin-sensitive species. This has not yet been demonstrated. Ivermectin toxicity has also been reported in several species of lizards and snakes.[3] Ball Pythons *(Python regius)* in particular may show mild neurologic signs when treated.[3]

Treatment

No known antidote or physiologic antagonist exists for ivermectin. Treatment is supportive and should include decontamination of any topical sprays with soap and water, fluid therapy, nutritional support, monitoring of electrolytes, and respiratory (ventilator) support. Recovery may take days to weeks. One debilitated tortoise recovered fully after 6 weeks. We have seen two box turtles *(Terrapene* sp.) completely recover in 4 weeks.

Summary

Ivermectin should **never** be given to chelonians, pregnant animals, or neonatal individuals. Also, for particularly tiny species, other therapies should be investigated. If any question exists, it should be used only as a topical or until an alternative is found.

ORGANOPHOSPHATES AND CARBAMATES

Organophosphates are the most commonly used insecticides worldwide. In the United States alone, 250 million pounds of organophosphates are used annually at a cost of $2.4 billion to produce.[4] They are found in agriculture, in the home, and on or around various domestic animals. Some organophosphates are meant to stay on surfaces to which they are applied, and others are absorbed and become systemic in animals. They are the active ingredient in a long list of products. For animal use as insecticides, they are formulated as dips, sprays, topical medications, systemic parasitic agents, and flea collars. This group of insecticides includes: chlorpyrifos (Dursban), dichlorvos, diazinon, cythioate (Proban), fenthion (ProSpot), malathion, ronnel, parathion, trichlorfon, and vaponna. Their cousins the carbamates include carbaryl (Sevin), bendiocarb, methiocarb, propoxur, and carbofuran. As newer, safer insecticides are marketed, this group is involved in fewer accidental poisonings but still accounts for a large number of intoxications.

Mechanism of Action

Organophosphates and carbamates interfere with metabolism and breakdown of acetylcholine at synaptic junctions.[5] Acetylcholinesterase is the enzyme responsible for breaking down the neurotransmitter at these sites. Acetylcholinesterase is inhibited by organophosphates and carbamates at these cholinergic sites. As a result, acetylcholine accumulates at the synapses, which at first excites and then paralyzes transmission in these synapses, giving it the characteristic "nerve gas" signs associated with organophosphate toxicity. This inhibition of the synapse is irreversible with organophosphates and reversible with carbamates. Organophosphates are readily absorbed by all routes—dermal, respiratory, gastrointestinal, and conjunctival. Overdose with organophosphates may happen more readily if given together with imidothiazoles such as levamisole.

Clinical Signs

Clinical signs seen in reptiles include salivation, ataxia, muscle fasciculations, inability to right themselves, coma, and respiratory arrest.[6] Death results from massive respiratory secretions, bronchiolar constriction, and effects on respiratory centers in the medulla, leading to the cessation of breathing.

Treatment

Animals with dermal exposure should be washed with a mild dishwashing detergent and copious amounts of water. Animals should be dried after rinsing to prevent further uptake of the insecticide. The need for fluid therapy to counter dehydration and electrolyte imbalances should be considered. The specific physiologic antidote, the muscarinic antagonist atropine, should be given (0.4 mg/kg intramuscularly [IM]). This should help with salivation, bronchospasm, and dyspnea. Diazepam may be given as needed for seizures. Use of antihistamines to cover insecticide poisonings is controversial and most likely not that effective. Prognosis is dependent on dosage, duration of exposure, and size of the animal.

Summary

Therapies both more effective and safer than organophosphates exist for treatment of parasites in captive reptiles. These therapy regimens are outlined in detail elsewhere in this volume.

VITAMIN A TOXICITY

Vitamin A is necessary for normal skin and periocular tissue health, particularly in chelonians. Turtles with hypovitaminosis A typically show ocular discharge, palpebral edema, blindness, hyperkeratosis of skin and mouthparts, and aural abscesses. Patients can improve with vitamin A supplementation (2000 IU/kg every 7 days) and better diets.[7]

Unfortunately, excessive iatrogenic administration of vitamin A can cause its own set of problems (see Chapter 59). This can cause inappetence, full-thickness skin sloughing, secondary bacterial infection, discoloration of the skin, and extreme lethargy. These results usually happen at dosages of 10,000 IU/kg or higher given IM as a single injection.[8] Treatment involves ceasing vitamin A administration, antibiotics, fluid therapy, and nutritional support. The skin lesions may heal slowly, but animals managed supportively can completely recover. Prognosis varies depending on the severity of the lesions.

VITAMIN D TOXICITY

For water-soluble vitamins, in which excesses can be excreted into the urine, the margin of safety is very large. For fat-soluble vitamins like A and D, this is not the case. Owners, breeders, and veterinarians often oversupplement captive reptiles with disastrous results. Dosages of 50 to 1000 times the minimum daily requirement are often given for weeks to months. This can be insidious, particularly when the minimum daily requirement of most mammalian vertebrates for vitamin D is only 10 to 20 IU/kg body weight.[9] Minimum daily requirements have not been established for reptiles.

The mechanism of action of the toxicity of vitamin D is related to the hypercalcemia it induces. This prolonged hypercalcemia causes dystrophic calcification of the gastrointestinal tissues, the kidneys, lungs, blood vessels, and joints. Complete removal of vitamin D–containing supplements and cortisone may help control hypercalcemia, but resolution of soft-tissue calcification may not be successful.

In light of the inherent calcium problems of captive reptiles, veterinarians must counsel clients about proper husbandry, nutrition, and dietary requirements and ensure that *no* supplements are given to animals without veterinary approval. Veterinarians must provide up-to-date advice to reptile caretakers concerning every aspect of the health of the animals.

See also the discussion on cholecalciferol.

ZINC TOXICOSIS

Zinc is an essential trace element. It is necessary for the synthesis of more than 200 enzymes required for cell division, growth, and gene expression.[10] Chronic zinc deficiency from improper diet is more commonly seen than acute zinc poisoning from excessive zinc intake. Zinc toxicosis may result from overzealous administration of supplements, ingestion of galvanized metal objects, zinc oxide ointment, or ingestion of pennies. Before 1982, pennies were more than 90% copper; since that time, they are 97% zinc. We have seen two iguanas and one snake with gastrointestinal tracts full of pennies that showed signs of zinc toxicity.

Mechanism of Action

The precise mechanism of action of zinc toxicosis is not known. However, the red blood cells, kidney, and liver are most affected. Intravascular hemolysis is the most consistent abnormality seen. Zinc is thought to cause oxidative mechanisms that lyse the red blood cell membrane, leading to anemia.[10]

Clinical Signs

Clinical signs of zinc toxicosis depend on the amount and form of the zinc ingested. Signs are delayed if coins are the source of the zinc. As few as one or two pennies can cause a toxicity. First, the animal may be anorectic and lethargic, and the zinc ingestion may mimic a gastrointestinal enteritis. This is followed by intravascular hemolysis, hemoglobinemia, yellow discoloration of the skin and mucous membranes, and weight loss. Palpation may be positive for coins, but in larger animals, radiographs may be necessary to reveal the pennies.

Treatment

Treatment consists of removal of the zinc-containing foreign object. Endoscopy or surgery may be necessary to remove the coins. Additional supportive therapy involves fluid treatment to maintain hydration, possible blood transfusion to control anemia, and in severe cases, use of a zinc chelator. However, chelators such as D-penicillamine and calcium-EDTA have been shown to be of questionable value once the source of the exposure has been removed.

Summary

Successful treatment of zinc toxicity involves removal of the zinc-containing objects through surgery or endoscopy and supportive care. Prognosis depends on the amount of zinc ingested, the duration of the toxic exposure, and the severity of the resulting anemia. Reptiles must be kept in environments free of potential sources of zinc ingestion.

CHLORHEXIDINE TOXICITY

Soaking living animals in any solution can be potentially life threatening. Recently, turtles soaked for 1 hour in chlorhexidine scrub have been shown to become intoxicated.[11] Cutaneous absorption of the solution and possible oral ingestion of these soaks has been postulated as the cause of the problem. Before any substances are used as a soak, the literature should be checked for preferred usage, dosage, and duration of the soak. Affected animals should be removed from the soak, rinsed, and supported with warmth and fluids. Remember to *never* leave any reptile unattended in a bath. Animals can drown much faster than anticipated.

FIREFLY TOXICOSIS

Reptile caretakers often supplement the diet of captive animals with freshly caught insects. Fireflies of the genus *Photinus* have been shown to contain steroidal pyrones (lucibufagins) that are poisonous.[12] These pyrones are structurally similar to cardenolides of plants and bufodienolides of toads, both of which are well-studied toxins.[4,13] These two compounds cause nausea and vomiting at low concentrations and can be potentially cardiotoxic at higher dosages. If extrapolations from mammals are correct, less than one half of a firefly could be lethal to a 100-g lizard.

Bearded Dragons (*Pogona vitticeps*) have shown fatal intoxication after ingestion of fireflies.[14] In both cases documented, the lizards showed signs 30 to 60 minutes after ingestion. Clinical signs included pronounced oral gaping, intense color change in the neck area, and dyspnea. Both animals died within 90 minutes of eating the fireflies. At present, no effective therapy is known.

Lucibufagins protect fireflies from predators. Spiders, birds, and several species of lizard have been shown to avoid fireflies.[15-18] Like many lizards, Bearded Dragons show indiscriminate eating strategies and may ingest toxic substances. Furthermore, the Bearded Dragon, an Australian native, has no natural contact with *Photinus* species of fireflies and thus may exhibit no self-protective avoidance behavior.

Other lizard species have been shown to eat fireflies without lethal results. In one study, both Fence Lizards (*Scleroporus undulates*) and Skinks (*Eumeces laticeps*) were fed fireflies.[18] Both species readily attacked and ate the insects but immediately spit them out, wiping their mouths and rubbing their faces on the ground. When offered fireflies a second time (even days later), they refused to eat them and exhibited the same mouth wiping that they displayed after tasting the insects. Next, the authors stuffed five to seven fireflies into live crickets. Both types of lizards ate the crickets but subsequently regurgitated all the crickets they had eaten. No lizards of either species died after eating fireflies. This study concluded that fireflies were distasteful and could cause regurgitation and vomiting. The conclusion was that the ingestion of fireflies was not always lethal to all lizard species.

Keepers must be advised to feed only safe food items. Any questions should be referred to a veterinarian. Fireflies should not be fed to reptiles, nor any insects that sequester cardenolides such as monarch butterflies (*Donaeus plexxipus*), queen butterflies (*Donaeus gillipus*), and lygaeid bugs (*Oncopeltus fasciatus*).[14] Other lizard species and other captive reptiles may be susceptible to intoxication after firefly ingestion, and they should not be offered as food.

FENBENDAZOLE

Fenbendazole is a benzimidazole type of antiparasitic drug.[19] It is safe and effective for treatment of many helminth parasites in animals. Fenbendazole inhibits glucose uptake in the parasites.[19] Because of its wide range of activity, its high degree of efficacy, and its broad margin of safety, this anthelminthic is frequently prescribed by veterinarians. Fenbendazole has a good margin of safety and has been reported to be well tolerated even at six times the recommended dosage and three times the recommended duration.[19] It has been extensively used as an anthelminthic therapy in reptiles at a dosage of 50 to 100 mg/kg orally (PO) once (repeated in 2 weeks) or 50 mg/kg PO every 24 hours for 3 to 5 days.[20-22]

Toxic effects have been reported in birds, rats, cats, and dogs.[23-27] Recently, evidence of fenbendazole overdose has been reported in individuals of a small snake species given an exceedingly large dose of the drug.[20] Four adult Fea's Vipers (*Azemiops feae*) died after administration of single dosages of fenbendazole ranging from 428 mg/kg to 1064 mg/kg. Necropsy findings were suggestive of intestinal changes consistent with fenbendazole toxicity. Fenbendazole is regarded as a safe anthelminthic drug; this study documents adverse effects that can appear if the medication is used at more than the recommended dosages.

Fenbendazole and mebendazole have been shown to cause agranulocytosis in mammals in extremely high dosages and also have been implicated in liver toxicities.[24,26,27]

No antidote exists for this poisoning, and treatment is supportive and symptomatic.

METRONIDAZOLE

Metronidazole is used as an antibacterial, an antiprotozoal, and an appetite stimulant in reptiles. It is formulated as a suspension, as an injectable, and as a tablet. Strict attention must be paid to the dosage, the frequency, and the size of the animal.

Mechanism of Action

The activity of metronidazole is specific for anaerobic bacteria and protozoa.[28] It is specific particularly for *Giardia* organisms. Metronidazole disrupts DNA in target microbes through reaction with intracellular metabolites.

Clinical Signs

The most severe side effect of metronidazole is dose-related CNS toxicity. High dosages can cause ataxia, inability to walk, nystagmus, opisthotonos, tremors of the lumbar muscles and hind limbs, seizures, and death.[29,30]

Treatment

Treatment is symptomatic and supportive and involves administration of fluids and both warmth and respiratory support. With supportive care, most patients recover. In severe cases, the patient may need to be placed on a ventilator. Recovery time is dependent on the extent of the toxicity, taking anywhere from 1 to several days.

Summary

Metronidazole has been recommended for a variety of conditions in reptiles. Particular care must be taken when this drug is used regarding dosage, duration, and size of the animal.

PYRETHRINS AND PYRETHROIDS

Pyrethrin is the oldest used botanic insecticide. It is made from the dried and ground flowers of *Chrysanthemum cinerifolium*.[31] Pyrethroids are synthetic derivatives of pyrethrin and are widely available. Pyrethroid insecticides have enhanced stability, potency, and half-life compared with the parent molecule. A variety of dilute pyrethrin-containing and pyrethroid-containing sprays have been recommended for reptiles.

Mechanism of Action

The mechanism of action of both pyrethrins and pyrethroids is the same. These molecules affect parasites by altering the activity of the sodium ion channels of nerves. These poisons prolong the period of sodium conductance and increase the length of the depolarizing action potential.[31] This results in repetitive nerve firing and death. With the right conditions or at higher dosages, these compounds can intoxicate host animals. Because of the potential for transcutaneous absorption, pyrethrin and pyrethroid sprays must be thoroughly rinsed from the animal immediately after application. Rinsing with lukewarm water is usually sufficient.

Like ivermectin, organophosphates, and carbamates, pyrethrins and pyrethroids should never be given concurrently with other cholinesterase-inhibiting compounds.

Clinical Signs

Clinical signs have been reported for pyrethrins and pyrethroids particularly if sprays used also contain insect growth regulators (like methoprene). Animals can have signs develop within 15 minutes of application. Signs include salivation, ataxia, inability to right themselves, and muscle fasciculations.[32] Idiosyncratic reactions to pyrethrins can happen at much lower doses than expected. A small percentage of animals appear to be extremely sensitive to pyrethrins and pyrethroids.

Treatment

No known antidote exists for these molecules. If caught early enough, treatment for pyrethrin/pyrethroid toxicity involves dermal decontamination, isotonic fluids, atropine, and diazepam for seizures. Care must be taken to keep pyrethrin/pyrethroid sprays away from the reptile's eyes and mouth to prevent intoxication. Prognosis depends on the strength of the agent used, the duration of the exposure, and the size of the animal involved. Animals that are treated do best. Pyrethrins and pyrethroids should be used in the smallest amounts that are effective. For instance, permethrin is used as a spray diluted to 0.002% to 0.007%. Pyrethrin levels in mite sprays for birds is as low as 0.03%, whereas those levels in dog and cat flea sprays can be in the 0.3% range. Extreme caution must be used with these molecules, and labels must be read before these products are used.

Summary

A variety of pyrethrins and pyrethroids have been recommended for use against the parasites of reptiles. If used prudently, they are both safe and effective. Animals are saturated with the spray. As soon as the parasiticide is applied, it should be rinsed off. This brief exposure is enough to kill the parasites. Pyrethrin/pyrethroid sprays should not be left on to prevent absorption and systemic toxicity in host animals. In smaller animals that have larger surface-to-volume ratios, most sprays should be diluted to the smallest effective dosage to prevent accidental intoxication from transcutaneous absorption.

BLEACH

Various hypochlorite bleach solutions can be found in most households. Typically, these are 3% to 6% hypochlorite solutions in water.[33] Bleaches are moderately irritating. If contact with skin is prolonged, the damage is worsened. Bleaches can be effective in treatment of cage parasites of reptiles but should **never** be applied to live animals. Bleach can cause alkali-type burns if splashed in the eyes of lizards and turtles. Immediate irrigation of the eye with copious amounts of water minimizes the damage done by the bleach. Skin exposed to bleach should be washed with a mild soap and lukewarm water. Animals should be kept out of recently bleached cages a minimum of 24 hours to prevent respiratory tract irritation. Cages should be allowed to air out at least this long. In addition, residual disinfectant can be removed by wiping with a clean cloth or towel and exposing the area to direct sunlight for a few hours.

ANTIFUNGAL TOXICITY

A variety of fungal infections have been documented in reptiles. Ranging from dermatophytes to systemic mycotic infections, these conditions are treated with a variety of antifungal medications. Because of the often small size of the reptilian patient, the mechanism of action of these drugs, and idiosyncrasies of reptilian physiology, improper treatment with antifungals can lead to serious intoxications.

Amphotericin B

Amphotericin B is a macrolide class of antibiotic unrelated to erythromycin. This antifungal inhibits ergosterol synthesis. Ergosterol is a component of the cell membrane unique to fungal organisms. Amphotericin is a potent nephrotoxin. It produces signs of renal toxicity in 80% of patients that receive it.[34] Its action causes renal vasoconstriction, reduces glomerular filtration rate, and has direct toxic affects on the membranes of the renal tubule cells.[35] Through these mechanisms, amphotericin B causes acute tubular necrosis. Almost 35% of human patients treated with amphotericin have hypokalemia develop sufficient to warrant potassium supplementation.[34]

Clinical signs mimic acute renal failure, anorexia, lethargy, weight loss, etc. Elevated blood urea nitrogen (BUN) and creatinine levels, with decreased potassium and sodium levels, are commonly seen in mammals but may not be relevant in reptiles.

Treatment includes discontinuation of the drug, aggressive fluid therapy to prevent further kidney damage, and diminishment of renal effects with sodium chloride–containing fluids. Treatment with mannitol may help increase the elimination of amphotericin B.[36]

Prognosis after amphotericin B toxicity depends on the severity of the renal damage. Amphotericin B is still listed as a treatment for aspergillosis in reptiles (1 mg/kg intracoelomically once daily for 2 to 4 weeks).[37] Safer drugs may be available. A less toxic, new formulation of amphotercin B is available for humans and may soon be available for veterinary use. Amphotericin B should not be used in animals that already have renal disease.

Griseofulvin

This antifungal works by inhibiting fungal spindle activity and leads to distorted weakened fungal hyphae. It has also been shown to cause bone marrow suppression in mammals, although the mechanism of this action is unknown.[38]

Anorexia, lethargy, diarrhea, and anemia have been reported in intoxicated animals. In reptiles, the recommended dosage for fungal dermatitis is 20 to 40 mg/kg PO every third day for five treatments.[39] It is available as a tablet and a topical ointment.

Treatment includes discontinuation of the drug and symptomatic support. No specific antidote exists. Griseofulvin has been shown to be teratogenic in pregnant animals of many species.[40] Topical treatments can be removed with tepid water and gentle hand soap. Antifungal overdoses can be best avoided with prevention of fungal infection through good husbandry.

Imidazoles (Ketoconazole) and Triazoles (Fluconazole and Itraconazole)

These antifungal drugs inhibit fungal replication by interfering with ergosterol synthesis. Ketoconazole also has direct effects on the fungal membrane.[40] These fungistatic drugs are metabolized by the liver. Itraconazole is more potent than ketoconazole and is better tolerated.

Clinical signs of intoxication include anorexia, lethargy, weight loss, and diarrhea. Elevated liver enzymes may be present in intoxicated animals. Dosages recommended for reptiles include 2 to 5 mg/kg PO daily for 5 days for fluconazole, 25 mg/kg PO daily for 3 weeks for ketoconazole, and 23.5 mg/kg PO once daily for itraconazole.[39] Little problem seems to exist with miconazole preparation applied topically.

No specific antidote exists for toxicity by these antifungals. Treatment involves stopping the drug, decontaminating any topicals, and supportive therapy (fluids, warmth). For ketoconazole, treatment includes countering the hepatotoxicity. Mild intoxications usually improve with simple cessation of the drug.

The safest, most effective drugs must be selected for use in fungal infections in reptiles, and they must reflect the severity of the infection, the size of the animal, and the condition of the animal before treatment. Dosages must be meticulously checked, particularly for topicals and dips to be used on reptiles. Many treatments are best administered by veterinarians and not clients. Finally, reptiles must **never** be left alone in any bath or medicated dip.

RODENTICIDES

Each year, rodents destroy crops in the field, eat food in storage, serve as vectors for human diseases, bite people, and cause material damage by gnawing. As a result, a variety of rodenticides are ubiquitously used in an attempt to control populations of these animals. These substances prove to be nearly as dangerous to humans and nontarget species as they are to rodents. Rodenticide intoxication has been documented in a variety of species, including reptiles. The original container housing the poison is beneficial if brought in with the animal so that active ingredients can be positively identified and appropriate treatment can be initiated.

Anticoagulants

The long-acting anticoagulants are responsible for 80% of rodenticide poisoning in humans and animals in the United States.[41] These long-acting agents have the same action as warfarin. However, they are more potent, and their half-life is longer. They are effective in single or very limited feedings when compared with older rodenticides. They act by decreasing the activity of the vitamin K–dependent blood-clotting factors (II, VII, IX, X). When clotting factors are sufficiently reduced, bleeding occurs. The most common and most toxic second-generation anticoagulants in use are brodifacoum and bromadilone.

Clinical signs depend on the site and extent of hemorrhage. Most intoxicated animals show anorexia, weakness, and lethargy. The number one clinical sign is dyspnea.[42] Typically, animals bleed into body cavities, abdomen, thorax, joints, etc. Most of these poisons are packaged as molasses-soaked grain laced with the anticoagulants. These various plant materials can attract herbivorous or omnivorous reptiles. Newer formulation of these baits are dyed turquoise.

The authors have seen one Green Iguana (*Iguana iguana*) and one box turtle intoxicated by anticoagulant bait ingestion. Baseline determinations of one-stage prothrombin time (PT) are helpful in animals suspected of consuming anticoagulant poisons in mammals. Comparison PT can be measured in known healthy animals for reptiles. The antidote for anticoagulant poisoning, vitamin K_1, should be administered in animals if the PT is increased. Daily dosage recommendations in mammals for vitamin K_1 are 2.5 mg/kg.[42] Therapy with this antidote must be maintained until toxic amounts of the poison are no longer present in the animal. Length of treatment depends on the dose and type of anticoagulant ingested but may be as long as 3 to 4 weeks. A PT test should be run 48 hours after cessation of vitamin K_1 treatment. If clotting time is normal, therapy is discontinued. If the clotting time is increased, therapy is continued for another week. Vitamin K_1 treatment can be given with subcutaneous injection or orally. Intravenous injections have a high incidence rate of anaphylactic reaction in mammals.[42] This has not been reported in reptiles. Treatment includes vitamin K_1 and possible oxygen support and plasma transfusions.

Bromethalin

Bromethalin is one of the newer rodenticides that has not been reported to cause poisonings in reptiles, but because of increasing popularity, the possibility for intoxication exists. It is formulated in baits of pelleted grain and dyed green or turquoise. Bromethalin is a neurotoxin, but because of its name, it can be confused with the long-acting anticoagulants bromadilone and brodifacoum. Again, one should encourage clients to bring in original containers to obtain valuable label information concerning ingredients.

The mechanism of action of bromethalin is to uncouple oxidative phosphorylation. The brain is the primary target for bromethalin because of its unique dependence on oxidative phosphorylation. The drug causes brain electrolyte disturbances and results in the development of cerebral edema.[41]

Clinical signs include hind limb paralysis, abnormal postures, fine muscle tremors, and seizures. Severely poisoned animals are comatose. Clinical signs are usually seen within 24 hours of ingestion.[43]

Bromethalin is a nonselective vertebrate poison. No antidote exists, and treatment is initially directed at reducing gastrointestinal absorption and providing symptomatic and supportive care. Treatment must also aim at control of cerebral edema seen in severe poisonings. Administration of dexamethasone and mannitol have been recommended to control bromethalin-induced cerebral edema in mammals.[43] Unfortunately, the efficacy of these diuretic agents in controlling bromethalin-poisoned animals is not very successful. Animals with severe signs such as seizures, paralysis, or coma generally have a grave prognosis.

Cholecalciferol

Cholecalciferol (vitamin D_3), a newer rodenticide, exploits the fact that rodents are extremely sensitive to small percentage changes in the calcium balance in their blood. Cholecalciferol causes hypercalcemia through mobilization of the body stores of calcium predominantly found in bone. This dystrophic hypercalcemia results in calcification of blood vessels, organs, and soft tissues. It leads to nerve and muscle dysfunction and cardiac arrythmias.[41]

The rodenticide is formulated in pelleted baits of grain or seed. Accidental ingestion of human medication with vitamin D_3 or its analogs by animals is also possible. Iatrogenic oversupplementation of vitamin D_3 to reptiles is likewise possible.[44]

Clinical signs include depression, weakness, and anorexia. Eventually, signs of renal disease become evident as glomerular filtration rate decreases.[41]

Treatment usually involves corticosteroid and diuretic therapy. Corticosteroids suppress bone resorption and intestinal calcium absorption and promote calciuresis. Prednisone (6 mg/kg) and furosemide (1 to 4 mg/kg) have been recommended in intoxicated mammals.[44] Supportive fluids are essential. Calcitonin therapy has been recommended, but its efficacy is questionable. Pamidronate disodium (Aredia), a biphosphonate, has been recommended in dogs, with 1 to 2 mg/kg given slowly over 2 hours.[45]

Prognosis is poor in animals in which dystrophic mineralization has already occurred.

METALDEHYDE

Metaldehyde is the active ingredient in most slug and snail baits.[46] It is formulated in granules, powder, pellets, and liquid. Protein-rich material such as bran or grain is usually added to the bait to make it more attractive to snails. Unfortunately, other animals find it more palatable as a result. Metaldehyde poisoning has been reported in a wide range of species ranging from dogs to livestock. This is not a common intoxication for reptiles; however, the authors did see one captive tortoise fatality after the poison was encountered in a household backyard garden.

The mechanism of action of metaldehyde poisoning was once thought to be a result of the degradation of the compound to acetaldehyde. Recent studies suggest metaldehyde itself may be the agent that affects the CNS.[47] GABA levels are decreased by metaldehyde, and this decrease can lead to depression, seizures, and coma.

Clinical signs include ataxia, incoordination and locomotor signs, muscle spasms, abnormal postures, and convulsions.[46] The tortoise involved was comatose and nonresponsive and had the head and legs rigidly extended. Clinical signs develop within a few hours of ingestion.

No specific antidote exists for metaldehyde poisoning. Instead, animals are treated supportively. Fluids should be given and oxygen administered to counter respiratory depression. Mammals display the "shake and bake" syndrome and are treated with diazepam or other appropriate anticonvulsant, and steps are taken to counter the hyperthermia. Prognosis is generally better if the animal survives the first 36 hours.[46] The public is strangely unaware of the hazards of this potent poison.

ANTIMICROBIAL TOXICITY

Selection of antibiotics should be made judiciously. Selection depends on experience of the clinician, empirical considerations, the type of infection present based on culture and sensitivity and Gram stains, and last but not least, the size, age, species, and condition of the reptilian patient. No antibiotic can be relied on to be effective for all situations. In addition, antibiotics are no substitute for good wound management, nursing care, nutrition, or husbandry.

Gentamicin

Gentamicin is an aminoglycoside antibiotic. Other aminoglycosides include amikacin, tobramycin, neomycin, streptomycin, and kanamycin. Gentamicin is bacteriocidal and is broad spectrum except for streptococci and anerobic bacteria.[48] Its mechanism of action inhibits bacterial protein synthesis by binding to 30S ribosomes. Historically, gentamicin has been used for acute serious infections, such as those caused by gram-negative bacteria. Amikacin has a greater antimicrobial range, is less toxic and, for the most part, has replaced gentamicin as the drug of choice for severe gram-negative sepsis in reptile patients.

Nephrotoxicity of gentamicin in reptiles is well documented.[49] Patients must have adequate fluid and electrolyte balance during therapy. Ototoxicity in reptiles has also been reported.[50] Recommended dosage for gentamicin varies from 1.5 to 2.5 mg/kg given no sooner than every third day.[51]

Amikacin

Amikacin is also an aminoglycoside, is bactericidal, is broad spectrum in activity, and operates on bacteria through the same mechanism of action as gentamicin.[48] It is indicated particularly against gram-negative organisms, where it may have greater activity than gentamicin.[48,52]

Like gentamycin, nephrotoxicity is the most dose-limiting toxicity of amikacin. Patients must be maintained in fluid and electrolyte balance during therapy. Ototoxicity has also been reported. If used together with anesthetic agents, aminoglycosides may show neuromuscular blockade in mammals.[48] Dosages for amikacin vary. See Chapter 89 for drug dosages.[51]

Chloramphenicol

Chloramphenicol is an antibacterial with a broad spectrum of activity against gram-positive bacteria, gram-negative bacteria, and *Rickettsia*. Its mechanism of action is by inhibition of bacterial protein synthesis by binding with ribosomes.[48]

The major toxicity of chloramphenicol is hematologic.[53] In all vertebrates studied, it produces direct, dose-dependent bone marrow depression that results in reductions in red blood cells, white blood cells, and platelets in mammals.[53] This manifestation is aggravated by inappropriate dosages, extended treatments, and repeated use of the drug. Treatment of chloramphenicol intoxication is supportive and may require blood transfusions. The drug has also been reported to be appetite-suppressive. Like gentamycin, chloramphenicol is used less frequently as safer antibiotics appear. The recommended dosage for chloramphenicol is 50 mg/kg administered once daily or every other day.[51]

Enrofloxacin

Enrofloxacin is a fluoroquinolone antibacterial drug. It is bactericidal with a broad spectrum of activity. Its mechanism of action inhibits DNA gyrase, thus inhibiting both DNA and RNA synthesis. Sensitive bacteria include *Staphylococcus*, *Escherichia coli*, *Proteus*, *Klebsiella*, and *Pasteurella*.[48] *Pseudomonas* is moderately susceptible but requires higher dosages. In some species, enrofloxacin is partially metabolized to ciprofloxacin.

Damage to cartilage has been seen in growing mammals treated with fluoroquinolones. This has not been reported in reptiles, but caution is advised for very young herps. Dosages of enrofloxacin range from 2.5 to 5 mg/kg.[51] Enrofloxacin can cause severe muscle necrosis if administered IM (see Figure 36-17).

VENOMOUS AND POISONOUS ANIMALS

Snake Evenomations

Snake venoms are complex mixtures of enzymatic and nonenzymatic proteins.[54,55] Derived from modified salivary glands, snake venoms immobilize prey and begin to predigest their tissues (Table 83-1). Hyaluronidase is present in most snake venom and works by catalyzing the cleavage of internal glycoside bonds and mucopolysaccharides.[55] This action potentiates the activity of many of the other toxic agents. Phospholipase A_2, which causes hydrolytic breakdown of membrane phospholipids, is common to many snake venoms. This molecule displays cytotoxic, anticoagulant (prevents activation of clotting factors), and neurotoxic activities.[54,55] Collagenase is also found in snake venom and leads to the digestion of collagen and breaking down of connective tissue.

Table 83-1	Some Typical Enzymes Found in Pit Viper Venom
Phospholipase A	Protease
Phospholipase B	Arginine ester hydrolase
Acetycholinesterase	Collagenase
Phosphodiesterase	Biogenic amines
Hyaluronidase	RNAase, DNAase

Snake venoms are incredibly complex diverse combinations of toxins and may vary even between closely related species.[54-56] Many of the toxic principals in snake venom have yet to be precisely identified. Snake venom toxins are usually named either after the snake venom they were first identified in or after their primary pharmacologic effect on the victim.

Snake venoms are approximately 90% water and, in addition to enzymatic and nonenzymatic proteins, can contain lipids, carbohydrates, and biogenic amines.[54] The actual toxins that compose the "killing fraction" are referred to as *venins*. The entire mixture is called *venom*. Not only does much variability exist in venom composition among snake species, tremendous variability is also seen in susceptibility to different snake venoms by potential prey species.

Since ancient times, venomous snakes have been proposed to be more resistant or even immune to their own venom. Venomous snakes do appear to be relatively more resistant to their own venom.[54] Neutralizing antibodies have been documented in the serum of many snakes to the toxins of their own venom.[57] However, the authors have seen fatalities in venomous snakes bitten by conspecifics. The severity of the response appears to be dependent on the location of the bite, the volume of venom injected, and the size of the bite recipient. We have also seen bites between conspecifics and self-inflicted bites that were nonfatal.

Certain nonvenomous snake species that prey on other snakes (including venomous ones), such as the Kingsnake *Lampropeltus getulus*, also appear to have some resistance to venom.[58] Other species such as pigs have been reported to be resistant to snake venom. However, their alleged resistance has been shown to be provided by their thick skin and large layers of subcutaneous fat that retard venom absorption into the bloodstream. Pigs have been shown to be sensitive to both intramuscular and intravenous injections of venom. Humans repeatedly bitten by venomous snakes have claimed immunity to their bite. Satisfactory serologic evidence for these claims has not been established. Effective antivenins exist for many venomous snakebites. A vaccine against rattlesnake bites (Rattlesnake vaccine, Red Rock Biologics, www.redrockbiologics.com) has recently been marketed for dogs. However, its overall effectiveness has not been determined.

Poisonous Lizards

Of the approximately 3000 species of lizards, only two known poisonous species exist.[59] The Gila Monster, *Heloderma suspectum* (with two subspecies), and the Mexican Beaded Lizard, *H. horridum* (with three subspecies), comprise the venomous lizards and are found only in the Americas. Their venom is only used in defense.[59]

The venom of these lizards is antigenically unrelated to snake venom.[60] The venom glands are in the lower jaw, and the venom is delivered to the gums at the base of the teeth. Delivery of the venom is dependent on intense chewing action.

Heloderma venom consists of multiple enzymatic proteins including hyaluronidase, phospholipase, arginine hydrolase, and kallikrein-like enzymes.[59] Other proteins have been identified in this venom, including gilatoxin and helothermine.

Hyaluronidase acts as a spreading factor, decreases the viscosity of connective tissue, and catalyzes the cleavage of acid mucoglycosides.[59] Arginine hydrolase causes hydrolysis of peptide linkages, and the kallikrein-like enzymes cause vasodilation, increase capillary permeability, lead to edema, and affect the contraction or relaxation of extravascular smooth muscle.

Phospholipase has been documented in many venoms and contributes by releasing other enzymes, leading to membrane destruction. It also stimulates histamine, kinin, and serotonin release. Gilatoxin is a neurotoxic protein.[61] Helothermine has been shown to depress the body temperature in mice subjected to this poison.[62] Bites of these lizards on people have been reported as very painful. Currently, no specific antivenin is available for venomous lizard bites, and treatment is supportive. Gila Monsters appear to be relatively resistant to the effects of their own venom. The evolution of the venom in these lizards and their primitive delivery system appears to be for defense, for it is not used in the apprehension of prey. This sets it apart from snake and spider venoms, which are used in defense but are primarily designed for immobilization and predigestion of prey.

Amphibian Toxins

Certain amphibians are poisonous and can cause intoxications. In the United States, two toad species (genus *Bufo*) are the source of most toad poisonings.

The Cane or Marine Toad (*Bufo marinus*) and the Colorado River Toad (*B. alvarius*) are the two species most implicated.[63]

All *Bufo* species of toads have parotid glands that release toxic substances when the animals are threatened. These are biologically active compounds such as dopamine, norepinepherine, epinepherine, serotonin, bufotenine, bufagenin, bufotoxins, and indolealkylamines.[64] Severe toxicosis has been seen in small animals that bite, masticate, or hold these toads in their mouths. The active compounds secreted from the toad parotid gland are rapidly absorbed by the mucous membranes of the predator and enter the systemic circulation.

Once these compounds have entered the circulation, the greatest effects are seen on the peripheral vascular system, the CNS, and the heart. Bufotenine has pressor effects on blood vessels but may act as a hallucinogen as well.[64] Bufagenin has digitalis-like effects.[65] It causes alterations in heart rate and rhythm. Bufotoxins are vasoconstrictors and add to pressor effects.[65] Indolealkylamines have activity similar to the hallucinogen lysergic acid diethylamide.[64]

Dogs are the animals most commonly affected by amphibian parotid toxins. However, adverse reactions have also been reported in cats and ferrets. Exposure in reptiles has not been documented but anecdotal reports of poisonings do exist. Collectors have reported that Poison Arrow Frogs fed to pet snakes have killed the snakes. Therefore, the assumption is logical that predatory reptiles that include amphibians in their diet might encounter and ingest poisonous toads. No specific antidote is available, and treatment is supportive. Therapy includes thorough flushing of the oral cavity with running water. Severely affected animals may need seizure intervention and medications to stabilize heart rhythms. Supportive care involving fluids may be necessary in badly debilitated animals. Many other toxicoses and conditions can lead to neuropathies, and cardiac arrhythmias can present with signs similar to those of toad poisonings. Differential diagnosis must always be considered and explored.

Fire Ants

In the early 1900s, the imported fire ant reached the United States from South America. The black fire ant *Solenopsis richteri* has remained in a small area of central Alabama and Mississippi. The red imported fire ant *Solenopsis invicta* has now reached 13 southern states from Texas to North Carolina.[66] The highly adaptive insects both supplant and interbreed with local species. New hybrids display a greater tolerance for cold and drought, which enables their spread much further into the continental United States.[67] In some areas, as many as 60% of local humans report being stung at least once annually.[66] For humans, 1% of those stung display hypersensitivity reactions.[66]

The fire ants and hybrids are small and similar in appearance to native house and garden ants. These fire ants bite *and* sting. First, the ant uses powerful mandibles to bite and anchor itself to the skin of the victim, then it uses its abdominal stinger to inject venom in a series of stings rotating in a circle around the head. Unlike the venom of most stinging insects, ant venom is composed primarily of alkaloids, particularly piperadine. Ant venoms have local necrotic and hemolytic effects.[66,67]

The authors have seen several small reptiles victimized by these predatory ants in Louisiana and Florida. Neonatal reptiles are especially vulnerable to these aggressive insects. In Florida, we saw several small snakes fall prey to them.

No antidote therapy exists; however, the use of antihistamines, topical steroid ointments (1% hydrocortisone), topical alcohol, and warm water baths may provide symptomatic relief.

Fire ants generally build mounds in warm sunny areas, places similar to where reptiles typically bask. We can expect more reptile species to fall victim to the bites of these ants as these predatory insects continue to expand their range. Efforts to control the spread of these ants so far have not been effective.

PLANT POISONINGS

Some plants produce very powerful poisons. For many years, veterinary toxicology largely dealt with livestock suffering from plant poisonings. The last 20 years have seen tremendous growth in our understanding of small animal intoxications.

Because many reptiles are either partially or entirely herbivorous, the potential for the accidental ingestion of toxic plants is real (Table 83-2). Although consideration of all plants potentially toxic to reptiles is beyond our present discussion, this section examines more frequently encountered plant poisonings and those commonly reported in the literature.

Table 83-2	Factors That Affect the Potential Toxicity of Poisonous Plants

Geographic and Seasonal Variables

Plants known to be poisonous in one part of the world may not be as toxic in other areas.
Season may also affect toxicity of plants.

Plant Part Ingested

Not all parts of poisonous plants are always toxic.

    Example: Tomato:
        Very edible fruit
        Stems and leaves contain toxic alkaloids
    Example: Apples, peaches, apricots:
        Have cyanide-containing seeds
        Fruit is edible

Absorbability of Toxins

Apples, peaches, apricots: cyanide not released unless seeds are broken
Castor bean: poison (ricin) not released unless seeds are chewed

Species That Ingest the Plant

Much of poisonous plant intoxication depends directly on which species has done the ingesting.

Heaths

The heath family plants (azaleas, laurel, rhodendrons) are commonly planted in the United States as ornamental shrubbery. These plants contain grayanotoxins (diterpenoids) that interfere with membrane-based sodium channels.[68] The toxin is found in the stem, leaves, flowers, and nectar.[69] Dogs and people may be seen with bradycardia. Ingestion of small amounts can lead to gastrointestinal signs; larger amounts can cause depression, ataxia, and convulsions.[69] No antidote exists; treatment is supportive. We have seen two iguanas stricken after eating azalea plants, one of which died. Both lizards were recumbent and nonresponsive a few hours after ingestion. Toxic levels in dogs begin at 7 mg/kg.[68] The one lizard died shortly after presentation.

Yews

Ground hemlock, Florida yew, English yew, Pacific yew, and Japanese yew are all members of a group that contains taxine, a cardiotoxic alkaloid.[68] This substance is a sodium channel blocker that can cause both cardiac and neurologic toxicity.[70] The bark, leaves, and seeds are poisonous but not the red fruit surrounding the seeds of these ornamental shrubs.[68] No antidote exists. Poisonings have been reported in livestock, dogs, and caged birds.[70]

Lilies

Easter lily, tiger lily, day lily, Japanese showy lily, and Asiatic lily are known to be poisonous to cats by causing renal toxicosis.[68] All parts of the plant are poisonous.[68] In addition, lily of the valley contains a potent cardiac glycoside.[71] In our experience, toxic plant ingestion by reptiles is more than possible; captivity exposes animals to all sorts of never encountered plants. We have administered activated charcoal to an iguana that ingested Easter lilies. The animal survived with supportive therapy including fluids, warmth, and oxygen.

Fruit Seeds

The seeds of apples, apricots, cherries, peaches, plums, and the jetberry bush contain cyanogenic glycosides.[68] The seeds are dangerous if the seed capsule is broken. In humans, as few as five to 25 broken seeds can cause cyanide toxicosis.[72] Cyanide disrupts the ability of cells to use oxidative phosphorylation by poisoning mitochondria. The net effect is tissue hypoxia. The onset of clinical signs may be very rapid, and death can occur suddenly. Treatment for cyanide toxicosis is often not successful but does include 100% oxygen administration, supplemental fluids, and perhaps sodium nitrate or sodium thiosulfate. Attention must be given to what captive reptiles are eating, being fed, or are able to come into contact with.

Avocado

Avocado (*Persea americana*) has been shown to be toxic to rabbits, mice, and caged birds.[68,73] All above-ground parts of the plant are toxic.[68] Persin, a compound isolated from the leaves, is believed to be the toxin responsible for avocado toxicity.[73] Intoxicated mammals display cardiac arrhythmias, necrosis of the myocardium, and acute death.[73] Caged birds show respiratory distress.[68,73]

Mader (personal communication) reports observing Green Iguanas (*Iguana iguana*) in the wild eating avocados that have fallen on the ground. However, with all the negative information available regarding ingestion of avocados, they should not be included in the diet of herbivorous captive reptiles until more is known concerning the nature of avocado poisoning.

Ricins (Castor Bean Intoxication)

Castor bean plants contain ricins, a potent toxin that stops protein synthesis. The poison is present in the whole plant but most concentrated in the seed.[68] Chewing or breaking of the seed coat is necessary before intoxication can take place. For mice, rats, rabbits, and dogs, one seed can be fatal. In dogs, clinical signs involve the gastrointestinal tract but can include kidney failure and convulsions.[74] No known antidote is available. All ingestions of castor beans should be taken seriously because of the high toxicity of ricin. However, seed coats are not always chewed or broken when animals ingest seeds. Often the seeds pass undigested, and animals show no clinical signs.

Cycad (Sago) Palms

These palms are used as houseplants and are naturally occurring in tropical and subtropical regions. All parts of the plant are toxic.[68] The nuts (seeds) are most toxic and only produced by female plants.[68] Toxins involve gastrointestinal and hepatic signs (cycasin), neurologic signs (B-methylamino-L-alanine), and an unknown toxin that causes additional neurologic signs.[69] Gastrointestinal signs generally appear within 24 hours of ingestion.[75] No antidote exists; treatment is supportive. Clients should be encouraged to bring in the chewed plant to help identify the species.

Holly, Mistletoe, and Poinsettia

During the holiday season, several potentially toxic plants are often brought into the home. Although their toxicity is exaggerated, reptiles may blunder into them. Here is an overview of the most common holiday plants.

Mistletoe (*Phoradendron* spp.) are evergreen parasitic plants that grow on trees. Human exposures usually involve the berries either eaten by small children or the berries brewed into tea.[68] Attempts to reproduce clinical signs in animals have been unsuccessful. In humans, the most common clinical signs are gastrointestinal. No antidote is available, and treatment is supportive. In human children and mammalian companion animals, this intoxication is not lethal.

Holly (*Ilex* spp.) includes English or Christmas holly, American or white holly, and winterberry. Berries contain the sapponin ilicin, which is a potent gastrointestinal irritant.[68] In humans and companion mammalian species, the most common sign is upset of the digestive tract. No antidote exists, and treatment is symptomatic. In mammalian companion animals, these types of poisonings are not lethal.

Poinsettia (*Euphorbia pulcherrima*) possesses a milky sap rich in diterpenoids.[68] These molecules are fairly irritating to the skin, mucous membranes, and gastrointestinal tract. Reports of toxicity stem from a single account.[76] Poisoning is rare, and treatment is supportive.

Plants Containing Cardiac Glycosides

Several plants contain cardiac glycosides, including oleander (*Nerium oleander*), foxglove (*Digitalis purpurea*), and lily of the valley (*Convallaria majulis*).[68] For oleander, all parts of the leaf are poisonous; a single leaf well chewed has been reported to be lethal.[77] Foxglove leaves and seeds are toxic. Lily of the valley poisoning comes from leaves, flowers, and roots. The cardiac glycosides are gastrointestinal irritants, may be responsible for a variety of cardiac arrhythmias (irregular pulse, bradycardia, rapid thready pulse, ventricular fibrillation) and can be fatal.[77] With plant ingestions, the exact amount of toxin involved is never known.

Ivy

Ivy (*Hedera* spp.) is used in greenhouses, as a houseplant, and as a ground cover. English ivy, Irish ivy, Persian ivy, Atlantic ivy, etc. are all potentially toxic.[68] These plants, particularly the berries, contain terpenoids.[68] These molecules can cause salivation, gastrointestinal irritation, and diarrhea. Most ingestions are not serious, and treatment is supportive.

Plants Containing Nicotine

Tobacco products including pipe tobacco, cigarettes, cigars, chewing tobacco, and snuff contain the alkaloid nicotine. Nicotine is a stimulant of the CNS and cardiovascular system.

It stimulates sympathetic ganglia and increases heart rate and blood pressure. High-dose exposures can cause paralysis of chest muscles and lead to respiratory compromise and cardiac arrest.[78] Cigarettes average from 15 to 25 mg of nicotine depending on the brand. Cigars have four to five times the nicotine of cigarettes. Chewing tobacco is even more palatable to animals because of flavors added (e.g., honey, sugar, molasses, cinnamon, licorice, and various syrups). Aids to stop smoking can also be a source of accidental nicotine ingestion. Nicotine patches usually contain between 7 and 25 mg, and nicotine gum contains 2 to 4 mg per piece. Some garden spray insecticides contain 40% nicotine (Black Leaf 40).

Captive reptiles may ingest cigar and cigarette butts, pipe tobacco, chewing tobacco, or nicotine patches and gums. We have seen death in one tortoise and one Green Iguana after eating several cigarette butts. Clinical signs of high-dose nicotine intoxication include excitement followed by depression, diarrhea, seizures, coma, and respiratory or cardiac arrest.[79] No known antidote exists. Treatment includes frequent monitoring of heart rate, and animals may benefit from fluid therapy and oxygen administration. Prognosis is poor for high-dose intoxications. As few as two cigarettes have been shown to cause lethal poisonings in puppies. No data exists for secondary smoke intoxication, but an association between chronic respiratory conditions in captive reptiles and households with one or more smokers have long been suspected by the authors (personal observation).

Oak Poisoning

Oak trees are found almost worldwide. Acorns, buds, twigs, and leaves have been implicated, but most incidents of intoxication involve either immature leaves in the spring or freshly fallen acorns in the spring.[80]

Toxicosis from oak is produced by high concentrations of tannic acid and its metabolites, gallic acid and pyrogallol. Ingestion of toxic amounts of oak have been shown to cause ulcerative lesions in the upper and lower gastrointestinal tract, liver lesions, and necrosis of proximal renal tubular epithelial cells.

A fatal episode of oak intoxication has been reported in a tortoise.[81] An African Spurred Tortoise (*Geochelone sulcata*) was found dead in an outdoor enclosure where numerous oak trees hung over and into the area. On necropsy, the stomach of the tortoise was markedly distended with partially digested oak leaves. Extensive necrosis was found in the oral cavity, esophagus, stomach, and kidneys. The proximal renal tubules showed 45% necrosis.

Reports of this type show the importance for both caretakers and veterinarians to be aware of the potential for toxicity of any plant material ingested either in browsing or as an intentional part of the captive diet. Nutrition of captive reptiles must be carefully considered and continually monitored.

Marijuana

Marijuana continues to be by far the most used illicit drug in the United States.[82] *Cannabis sativa* has been used for centuries for its hemp fiber, as rope, and for its psychoactive resins. Totally or partially herbivorous captive reptiles may encounter growing marijuana plants or ingest dried stems, leaves, and flowers.

The main active ingredient of marijuana is tetrahydrocannibinol (THC). The highest concentration of this psychoactive constituent is found in the leaves and the flowering tops of plants.[83] Hashish is the dried resin of flower tops. The precise mechanism of action of THC is unknown, but the psychoactive effects of this drug are thought to stem from a number of sites within the CNS, including cholinergic dopaminergic, serotonergic, noradrenergic, and GABA receptors. Ingested marijuana shows effects much more slowly than the results of the inhaled smoke; however, the effects of ingested THC last much longer.

Clinical signs after ingestion of marijuana include mydriasis, weakness, ataxia, bradycardia, hypothermia, and stupor. The extent of clinical signs after marijuana ingestion is almost totally dose related.

Treatment for marijuana ingestion is primarily supportive and symptomatic. Marijuana toxications are rarely fatal because of the wide margin of safety of THC. Activated charcoal administration is recommended to decrease enterohepatic recirculation. Despite its relative safety margin, recovery after ingestion may be prolonged and take up to 3 to 4 days. Fluids and monitoring of body temperature may be beneficial.

We have seen two reptiles ingest fairly large amounts of marijuana. A 10-pound Sulcata Tortoise showed no effects after eating four marijuana cigarettes. However, a 6-pound male Green Iguana was stuporous after eating into a "baggie" of marijuana and needed support. Both animals recovered completely.

Undoubtedly other "under-the-counter" drugs have been blundered across by reptiles. Various "over-the-counter" drugs kept on nightstands, kitchen counters, or bathroom shelves may be encountered by captive reptiles given free range in the house. For their own safety, captive animals should be confined and **all** medications kept in their original containers in child-proof and animal-proof cabinets.

DIOCTYL SODIUM SULFOSUCCINATE

Dioctyl sodium sulfosuccinate (DSS) is an anionic surfactant substance that traditionally has been recommended as a laxative and stool softener for a variety of vertebrates ranging from humans to rodents. Likewise, DSS has been advocated for the same use in reptiles.

It is generally regarded as a relatively safe pharmaceutical agent with a low toxicity. However, reports of toxic effects exist in the literature for horses, dogs, monkeys, rats, rabbits, guinea pigs, and mice after both oral and topical administration.[84-90] Furthermore, fatalities in reptiles after oral use of DSS have been reported.[91] One study documents severe changes in gastric and esophageal mucosa in Gophersnakes (*Pituophis melanoleucus*) given oral DSS at a dosage of 250 mg/kg.

A specific dose of DSS has not been established for reptiles, but dosages for other species range from 15 to 40 mg/kg for dogs and cats to 200 mg/kg for horses.[89,92] Concentrations (dilutions) of 1:30 have been recommended for reptiles.[93]

The study in the gophersnakes and the several reports in various other species indicate that DSS may not be as innocuous as once popularly believed. These studies demonstrate that DSS can have adverse effects, and in reptiles, levels greater than 250 mg/kg can cause caustic changes to epithelial surfaces. In addition, the potential for overzealous administration of DSS leading to aspiration pneumonia clearly exists in captive reptiles. Extreme care must be employed if DSS is to be used, and other laxatives, stool softeners, and enhancers of gastric motility should be explored.

ACKNOWLEDGMENTS

The authors thank Dr Douglas Mader for his encouragement and support in contributing to this project. Also, we thank Dr Alvin C. Bronstein for his tireless enthusiasm for toxicology and for his unselfish aid of poisoned small animal patients. Finally, we thank Dr Robert A. Taylor and the entire staff at Alameda East Veterinary Hospital for providing such a wonderful place to treat, study, and help sick reptiles. We hope that there are always wild reptiles on our planet.

REFERENCES

1. Papich MG: Ivermectin. In Papich MG, editor: *Handbook of veterinary drugs*, London and New York, 2002, WB Saunders.
2. Teare JD, Bush M: Toxicity and efficacy of ivermectin in chelonians, *J Am Vet Med Assoc* 183(11):1195, 1983.
3. Wosniak EJ, et al: Ectoparasites, *J Herp Med Surg* 10(3):15-21, 2000.
4. Carlton FB, Simpson WM, Haddad LM: The organophosphates and other insecticides. In Haddad LM, Shannon MW, Winchester JF, editors: *Clinical management of poisoning and drug overdose*, Philadelphia, 1998, WB Saunders.
5. Blodgett DJ: Organophosphate and carbamate insecticides. In Peterson ME, Talcott PA, editors: *Small animal toxicology*, Philadelphia, 2001, WB Saunders.
6. Jamal GA: Neurological syndromes of organophosphorus compounds, *Adv Drug React Toxicol Rev* 16(3):133-170, 1997.
7. Rossi JV: Dermatology. In Mader DR, editor: *Reptile medicine and surgery*, Philadelphia, 1996, WB Saunders.
8. Frye FL: *Biomedical and surgical aspects of captive reptile husbandry*, ed 2, vol 2, Malabar, Fla, 1991, Krieger Publishing.
9. Lewis LD, Morris ML Jr, Hand MS: *Small animal clinical nutrition*, Topeka, Kan, 1987, Mark Morris.
10. Talcott PA: Zinc poisoning. In Peterson ME, Talcott PA, editors: *Small animal toxicology*, Philadelphia, 2001, WB Saunders.
11. Lloyd ML: Chlorhexidine toxicosis in a pair of red-bellied short-necked turtles, *Emydura subglosa*, *Bull Assoc Rept Amph Vet* 6(4):6-7, 1996.
12. Eisner T, et al: Lucibufagins: defensive steroids from the fireflies *Photinus ignitus* and *Photinus marginellus* (Coleoptera: Lampyridae), *Proc Natl Acad Sci* 75:905-908, 1978.
13. Fieser LF, Fieser M: *National products related to phenanthrene*, Reinhold, NY, 1999.
14. Glor R, et al: Two cases of firefly toxicosis in Bearded Dragons, *Pogona vitticeps*, *Proc Assoc Rept Amph Vet* 27-30, 1999.
15. Eisner T, et al: Firefly "femme fatales" acquire defensive steroids (lucibufagins) from their firefly prey, *Proc Natl Acad Sci* 94:9723-9728, 1997.
16. Sexton OJ: Differential predation by the lizard *Anolis carolinensis* on unicoloured and polycoloured insects after an interval of no contact, *Anim Behav* 12:101-110, 1964.
17. Lloyd JE: Firefly parasites and predators, *Coleopt Bull* 27:91-106, 1998.
18. Sydow SL, Lloyd JE: Distasteful fireflies sometimes emetic, but not lethal, *Entomol* 58:312, 1998.
19. Papich M: *Handbook of veterinary drugs*, London and New York, 2002, WB Saunders.
20. Alvarado TP, et al: Fenbendazole overdose in four Fea's vipers (*Azemiops feae*), *Proc Assoc Rept Amph Vet* 35-36, 1997.
21. Stein G: Reptile and amphibian formulary. In Mader DR, editor: *Reptile medicine and surgery*, Philidelphia, 1996, WB Saunders.
22. Carpenter JW, Mashima TY, Rupiper DJ: *Exotic animal formulary*, Philadelphia, 2001, WB Saunders.
23. Dalvi RR: Comparative studies on the effect of fenbendazole on the liver and liver enzymes of goats, quail, and rats, *Vet Res Commun* 13:135-139, 1989.
24. Howard LL, et al: Benzimidazole toxicity in birds, *Proc Annu Conf Am Assoc Zoo Vet* 36, 1999.
25. Papendick RI, et al: Suspected fenbendazole toxicity in birds, *Proc Annu Conf Am Assoc Zoo Vet* 144-146, 1998.
26. Shoda T, et al: Liver tumor promoting effects of fenbendazole in rats, *Toxicol Pathol* 27:553-562, 1999.
27. Stokol T, et al: Development of bone marrow toxicosis after albendazole administration in a dog and a cat, *J Am Vet Med Assoc* 210:1753-1756, 1997.
28. Papich MG: Metronidazole. Papich MG: *Handbook of veterinary drugs*, London and New York, 2002, WB Saunders.
29. Bennett RA: Neurology. In Mader DR, editor: *Reptile medicine and surgery*, Philadelphia, 1996 WB Saunders.
30. Lawton MPC: Neurological disease. In Benyon PH, editor: *Manual of reptiles*, Ames, 1992, Iowa State Universty Press.
31. Hansen SR: Pyrethrins and pyrethroids. In Peterson ME, Talcott PA, editors: *Small animal toxicology*, Philadelphia, 2001, WB Saunders.
32. Denardo D, Wozniak EJ: Understanding the snake mite and current therapies for control, *Proc Assoc Rept Amph Vet* 137-147, 1997.
33. Mcguigan MA: Bleach, soaps, detergents, and other corrosives. In Haddad EM, Shannon MW, Winchester JF, editors: *Clinical management of poisoning and drug overdose*, ed 3, Philadelphia, 1998, WB Saunders.
34. Haddad LM, Herman SM: Antibiotics and anthelminthics. In Haddad LM, Shannon MW, Winchester JF, editors: *Clinical management of poisoning and drug overdose*, Philadelphia, 1998, WB Saunders.
35. Hoitsma AJ, et al: Drug-induced nephrotoxicity aetiology, clinical features, and management, *Drug Safety* 6(2):131, 1991.
36. Plumb DC: *Veterinary drug handbook*, ed 3, Ames, 1999, Iowa State University Press.
37. Bonner BB: Chelonian therapeutics, *Vet Clin North Am Exotic Pract* 3(1):257-232, 2000.
38. Roder JD: Antimicrobials. In Plumlee KH, editor: *Clinical veterinary toxicology*, St Louis, 2004, Mosby.
39. Funk RS: A formulary for lizards, snakes, and crocodilians, *Vet Clin North Am Exotic Pract* 3(1):333-358, 2000.
40. Scott FW, et al: Teratogenesis in cats associated with griseofulvin therapy, *Teratology* 11:79, 1975.
41. Metts BC, Stewart NJ: Rodenticides. In Haddad LM, Shannon MW, Winchester JF, editors: *Clinical management of poisoning and drug overdose*, Philadelphia, 1998, WB Saunders.
42. Murphy JM, Talcott PA: Anticoagulant rodenticides. In Peterson ME, Talcott PA: *Small animal toxicology*, Philadelphia, 2001, WB Saunders.
43. Dorman DL: Bromethalin. In Peterson ME, Talcott PA: *Small animal toxicology*, Philadelphia, 2001, WB Saunders.

44. Rumbeiha WK: Cholecalciferol. In Peterson ME, Talcott PA: *Small animal toxicology,* Philadelphia, 2001, WB Saunders.
45. Morrow CK, Volmer PA: Cholecalciferol. In Plumlee KH, editor: *Clinical veterinary toxicology,* St Louis, 2004, Mosby.
46. Puschner B: Metaldehyde. In Peterson ME, Talcott PA, editors: *Small animal toxicology,* Philadelphia, 2001, WB Saunders.
47. Gfeller RW, Messonnier SP: Metaldehyde. In Gfeller RW, Messonnier SP: *Handbook of small animal toxicology and poisonings,* St Louis, 2004, Mosby.
48. Papich MG: *Handbook of veterinary drugs,* Philadelphia, 2002, WB Saunders.
49. Montali RJ, Bush M, Smeller JM: The pathology of nephrotoxicity of gentamycin in snakes, *Vet Pathol* 16:108-115, 1979.
50. Bagger-Sjoback D, Wesall J: Toxic effects of gentamycin on the basillar papilla in the lizard *Calotes versicolor, Acta Otolaryngol* 81:57, 1976.
51. Funk RS: A formulary for lizards, snakes, and crocodilians, *Vet Clin North Am Exotic Pract* 3(1):333-358, 2000.
52. Klingenberg RJ: Therapeutics. In Mader DR, editor: *Reptile medicine and surgery,* Philadelphia, 1996, WB Saunders.
53. Holt D, Harvey J, Hurley R: Chloramphenicol toxicity, *Adverse Drug Reactions Toxicol Rev* 12:83-95, 1993.
54. Fowler ME: *Veterinary zootoxicology,* Boca Raton, Fla, 1993, CRC Press.
55. Peterson ME, Talcott PA: *Small animal toxicology,* Philadelphia, 2001, WB Saunders.
56. Walter FG, Fernandez MC, Haddad LM: North American venomas snakebites. In Haddad LM, Shannon MW, Winchester LF, editors: *Clinical management of poisoning and drug overdose,* 1998, WB Saunders.
57. Ovadia M, Kochua E: Neutralization of Viperidae and Elapidae snake venoms by sera of different animals, *Toxicon* 15:541, 1977.
58. Philpot VB, Smith RG: Neutralization of pit viper venom by king snake serum, *Proc Soc Exp. Biol Med* 74:521, 1950.
59. Peterson ME: Poisonous lizards. In Peterson ME, Talcott PA: *Small animal toxicology,* Philadelphia, 2001, WB Saunders.
60. Fowler ME: Venomous lizards. In Fowler ME: *Veterinary zootoxicology,* Boca Raton, Fla, 1993, CRC Press.
61. Heradon RA, Tu AT: Biochemical characterization of the lizard toxin gilatoxin, *Biochemistry* 20:3517-3522, 1981.
62. Mocha-Morales J, Martin BM, Possani LD: Isolation and characterization of helothermine, a novel toxin from *Heloderma horridum horridum* (Mexican beaded lizard) venom, *Toxicon* 28:299-309, 1990.
63. Peterson ME: Toad venom toxicity. In Tilley LP, Smith WK, editors: *The five-minute veterinary consult,* Philadelphia, 1997, Williams & Wilkins.
64. Peterson ME: Amphibian toxins. In Peterson ME, Talcott PA: *Small animal toxicology,* Philadelphia, 2001, WB Saunders.
65. Butler VP, et al: Heterogeneity and liability of endogenous digitalis-like substances in the plasma of the toad *Bufo marinus, Am J Physiol* 271:R325-R332, 1996.
66. Tunney FX: Stinging insects. In Haddad LM, Shannon MW, Winchester JF, editors: *Clinical management of poisoning and drug overdose,* Philadelphia, 1998, WB Saunders.
67. Tracy J, et al: The natural history of exposure to the imported fire ant *(Solenopsis invicta), J Allergy Clin Immunol* 95:824, 1995.
68. Plumlee KH: Plant hazards, *Toxicol Vet Clin North Am Small Anim Prac.* 32(2):383-395, 2002.
69. Puschner B: Grayanotoxins. In Plumlee KH, editor: *Clinical veterinary toxicology,* St Louis, 2003, Mosby.
70. Casteel S: Taxine alkaloids. In Plumlee KH, editor: *Clinical veterinary toxicology,* St Louis, 2004, Mosby.
71. Hall J: Lily. In Plumlee KH, editor: *Clinical veterinary toxicology,* St Louis, 2004, Mosby.
72. Fitzgerald KT: Cyanide. In Peterson ME, Talcott PA: *Small animal toxicology,* Philadephia, 2001, WB Saunders.
73. Pickerell JA, Oehme F, Mannala SA: Avocado. In Plumlee KH, editor: *Clinical veterinary toxicology,* St Louis, 2004, Mosby.
74. Albretsen JC: Evaluation of castor bean toxicosis in dogs: 98 cases, *J Am Anim Hosp Assoc* 36:229-233, 2000.
75. Albretson JC: Cycasin. In Plumlee KH, editor: *Clinical veterinary toxicology,* St Louis, 2004, Mosby.
76. Kunkel DB, Brailberg G: Poisonous plants. In Haddad LM, Shannon MW, Winchester JF, editors: *Clinical management of poisoning and drug overdose,* Philadelphia, 1998, WB Saunders.
77. Galey FD: Cardiac glycosides. In Plumlee KH, editor: *Clinical veterinary toxicology,* St Louis, 2004, Mosby.
78. Plumlee KH: Nicotene. In Peterson ME, Talcott PA: *Small animal toxicology,* Philadephia, 2001, WB Saunders.
79. Haddad LM: Nicotene. In Haddad LM, Shannon MW, Winchester JF, editors: *Clinical management of poisoning and drug overdose,* Philadelphia, 1998, WB Saunders.
80. Plumlee KH: Tannic acid. In Plumlee KH, editor: *Clinical veterinary toxicology,* 2004, St Louis, Mosby.
81. Rotstein DS, et al: Suspected oak Quercus, toxicity in an African Spurred Tortoise, *Geochelone sulcata, J Herp Med Surg* 13(3):20-21, 2003.
82. Martin B, Szara S: Marijuana. In Haddad LM, Shannon MW, Winchester JF, editors: *Clinical management of poisoning and drug overdose,* Philadelphia, 1998, WB Saunders.
83. Volmer PA: Drugs of abuse. In Peterson ME, Talcott PA: *Small animal toxicology,* Philadephia, 2001, WB Saunders.
84. Case MT, et al: Acute mouse and chronic dog toxicity studies of danthron, dioctyl sodium sulfosuccinate, poloxalkol and combinations, *Drug Chemical Tox* 1(1):89-101, 1977-1978.
85. Donowitz M, Binder HJ: Effect of dioctyl sodium sulfosuccinate on colonic fluid and electrolyte movement, *Gastroenterology* 69:941-950, 1975.
86. Fox DA, et al: Surfactants selectively ablate enteric neurons of the rat jejunum, *J Pharm Exp Ther* 277(2):538-544, 1983.
87. Karlin DA, et al: Effect on dioctyl sodium sulfosuccinate feeding on rat colorectal 1,2-dimethylhydrazinc carcinogenesis, *JNCL* 64:791-793, 1980.
88. Lish PM: Some pharmacological effects of dioctyl sodium sulfosuccinate on the gastrointestinal tract of the rat, *Toxicol Appl Pharmacol* 41(6):580-584, 1961.
89. Moffatt RE, et al: Studies on dioctyl sodium sulfosuccinate toxicity: clinical, gross and microscopic pathology in the horse and guinea pig, *Can J Comp Med* 39:434-441, 1975.
90. Saunders DR, et al: Effect of dioctyl sodium succinate on structure and function of human and rodent intestine, *Gastroenterology* 69(2):380-386, 1975.
91. Paul-Murphy J, et al: *Necrosis of esophageal and gastric mucosa in snakes given oral dioctyl sodium succinate,* Proceedings of the 1st International Conference of Zoological and Avian Medicine, Hawaii, 1987.
92. Kirk RW: *Current veterinary therapy in small animal practice,* Philadelphia, 1976, WB Saunders.
93. Frye FL: Biomedical and surgical aspects of captive reptile husbandry, Edwardsville, Ky, 1981, Veterinary Medical Publishing.

84
ARTIFICIAL LIGHTING
WILLIAM H. GEHRMANN

A variety of factors can influence the selection of one or more lamp types for use in herpetoculture. Some of these factors are enclosure size and design, species to be illuminated, lamp cost, and light characteristics. Lamps can be described by the kinds of radiation emitted. For example, most lamps are designed to radiate visible light, but various amounts of infrared (heat) and ultraviolet (UV) radiation are also produced (Table 84-1). Additional features of light output from a lamp are the intensity (total power output as illuminance or irradiance) and quality. Light quality can refer to the (1) color temperature of emitted light (e.g., reddish, bluish, whitish light), (2) color-rendering index (the appearance of colors of reptiles that are illuminated), and (3) spectral power distribution (the power at different wavelengths or within color bands).[1] These features of lamps are available from the manufacturer.

Photoperiod is a feature of the light environment that is external to the lamp. A variety of timers are available that automatically turn lamps on and off at preset times. The period length of the photophase may be kept constant or varied to correspond to the photoperiod observed at a selected latitude. Twelve hours of light per day is often used and corresponds to the year-round daylength at the equator. The time of lights on/off may likewise be set to parallel the phasing at a given latitude. Photoperiod effects have been systematically studied in relatively few species. Photoperiod has been shown to influence a variety of physiologic rhythms, including thermoregulation and reproduction, in some species. Irrespective of the details, a light-dark cycle of some sort is indicated for reptiles in captivity.

The principal consideration in evaluation of the photoenvironment of captive reptiles involves analysis of the thermal conditions. Temperature is important in facilitating normal behavioral and physiologic processes. A variety of symptoms are presented by reptiles maintained in an inappropriate thermal environment.[2] The primary heat source for a vivarium may be an incandescent lamp. Reflector lamps serve a dual purpose in establishing a thermal gradient with a basking area and supplying visible light. The magnitude of the gradient can be selected with use of a lamp of the appropriate wattage or by changing the distance between the lamp and the substrate. Non–light-emitting heat sources, such as hot rocks (within-enclosure and under-enclosure types), heating pads, or ceramic bulbs may be used separately or in conjunction with a light source. Preferred thermal environments vary among species. Conditions recommended for selected species are described in Chapter 4.

In the last decade, a proliferation of manufacturers and distributors has marketed lamps presumably designed for reptiles. Interestingly, virtually no hard experimental data exist underpinning various claims of benefit to reptiles.[3]

The assumption is often made that the lamp that emits light most similar to natural light is the most suitable for herpetocultural purposes. A major problem with this assertion is that natural light and lamp light are fundamentally different in several ways. In general, natural light is variable, whereas lamp light is comparatively constant. The intensity and quality of natural light change daily and are seasonally related to movement of the earth, cloud cover, type of habitat, and other factors. To reconcile these differences, the further assumption is made that natural light at a color temperature of about 5000°K, at which color balance is optimal (at least to human eyes) and which occurs at about midday, is "best" for the overall health and well-being of reptiles in captivity.

These ideas were formalized more than 25 years ago by Duro-Test Corporation in the phrase "full spectrum," which was used to describe the light quality from the Vita-Lite lamp (note: Duo-Test Corporation has been out of business since 2000). By definition, full-spectrum light has a color temperature

Table 84-1	Representative Light Sources and Principal Types of Radiation
Source	**Principal Radiation**
Sun	UVB (290-320 nm)
	UVA (320-400 nm)
	Visible (400-700 nm)
	Infrared (>700 nm)
Incandescent	Visible, infrared
Frosted bulbs	
Reflector	
Flood	
Spot	
Halogen Lamps	Visible, infrared
Fluorescent	Visible; wide variety of visible band emitters available; cool white and warm white lamps are common examples
Plant lamps	Emphasize blue and red
Blacklights	High UVA, some UVB
Sun lamps	UVB, some UVA
Reptile full-spectrum lamps	Visible, UVA, UVB
High-intensity Discharge	
Metal halide	Visible, infrared; UVA and UVB, usually shielded
Mercury vapor	Visible, infrared, UVA, UVB (includes Westron Active UVHeat)

UVA, ultraviolet A; *UVB*, Ultraviolet B.

Table 84-2 Photometric Characteristics of Selected Lamps

Lamp	Spectronics Corp		UVP, Inc		Illuminance (lux)	Photo Product Formed (%)[†]
	UVA ($\mu W/cm^2$)	UVB ($\mu W/cm^2$)	UVA ($\mu W/cm^2$)	UVB ($\mu W/cm^2$)		
Cool White (General Electric Co)	2 (4.3)*	2 (1.8)*	3 (4.3)*	0 (1.8)*	861	0.09
Instant Sun (Verilux, Inc)	4	2	6	1	635	0.03
Reptisun 2.0 (Zoo Med Labs)	6 (9.8)*	2 (1)*	9 (9.8)*	1 (1)*	753	None detected
Reptisun 5.0 (Zoo Med Labs)	12 (36.5)*	13 (4.1)*	41 (36.5)*	47 (4.1)*	420	0.13
Super UV Daylight (ESU, Inc)	4	3	6	5	624	0.10
Desert 7% (ESU, Inc)	30	9	102	31	560	None detected
350 Blacklight (Sylvania Lighting)	53	16	209	63	<100	0.24

Measurements were made at 30 cm from the center of each lamp with Spectronics Corp and UVP, Inc, handheld ultraviolet radiometers and a General Electric Type 214 light meter. Photoproducts formed from 7-dehydrocholesterol were calculated from ampules exposed to a lamp for 1 h at 30 cm.
*Measured by Lighting Sciences Canada, Ltd, with an Ocean Optics, Inc, recording spectroradiometer.
[†]Ampules were evaluated in the laboratory of Michael F. Holick, PhD, MD, Boston University Medical Center, 715 Albany St, Bldg M 1013, Boston, MA 02118. For information regarding availability and processing of ampules, contact Dr. Holick.
UVA, Ultraviolet A; *UVB*, ultraviolet B.

of about 5500°K, a color-rendering index of 90 or above, and a spectral power distribution for UV and visible light similar to that of open-sky natural light at noon. During the ensuing years, the original concept of full spectrum has evolved to the point of being unrecognizable and almost meaningless. At best, full spectrum refers to fluorescent lamps produced by a variety of manufacturers that are reasonably close to the original criteria. These include a variety of reptile lamps (Table 84-2). At worst, the phrase is used to describe any fluorescent lamp that is not a cool white or plant lamp.

One of the most inventive uses of "full spectrum" is its reference to incandescent lamps whose glass contains the element neodymium. The quality of light from any incandescent lamp is quite different from that of natural light and is rendered even more deviant by the absorption of yellow wavelengths by the neodymium. To be sure, the light appears "whiter" to a human and the color rendering is improved, but the spectral power distribution is significantly different from that of natural light. Ultraviolet A (UVA) from these lamps is no greater than that of any incandescent lamp of an equivalent wattage, and no ultraviolet B (UVB) is radiated. The importance of UVB from these lamps for vitamin D_3 synthesis and calcium metabolism still occasionally appears, incorrectly, in advertising. The UVA irradiances are comparatively low, and assertions that the UVA contributes to the health of reptiles are unsubstantiated and misleading.

Until differences in biologic efficacy among lamps are experimentally verified, one may take comfort in the fact that a large body of anecdotal data indicates that many species, including heliophilic lizards, can successfully adapt to a wide range of light qualities.

Many lamps emit UV radiation. All visible-light fluorescent lamps emit some UVA and UVB, although at irradiances considerably less than in natural light.[4] Blacklight fluorescent lamps radiate UVA at irradiances about 15 times those found in visible-light lamps; UVB from blacklights, however, is only slightly greater. Blacklight blue (BLB) tubes are essentially blacklights from which the visible blue wavelengths are absorbed by an additional phosphor. Incandescent lamps radiate a small amount of UVA, usually less than that from fluorescent lamps, and no UVB. Variation exists in the degree of transmission of UV radiation through various materials (Table 84-3).

The importance of UV light for different species remains largely problematic at this time. Several species of lizards have been shown to possess lateral eye sensitivity to UVA. Blacklight (UVA) has been shown to stimulate agonistic and reproductive behaviors in various lizard species. Some herpetocultural facilities routinely use a blacklight in conjunction with visible-light lamps. Perhaps UVA in the photo-environment contributes in some way to the health of reptiles, but this remains to be demonstrated.

Emission of UVB is a primary consideration in evaluating lamps for use in herpetoculture. UVB has been shown to promote the cutaneous photolysis of 7-dehydrocholesterol (provitamin D_3 [proD_3]) to previtamin D_3 (preD_3) in reptiles.[5,6] PreD_3 is then thermally isomerized to vitamin D_3 (D_3), signaling the importance of thermal options available to reptiles in a vivarium. The rate of conversion from proD_3 to preD_3 is related to the amount of UVB. The amount of UV is commonly described by the irradiance, which is the power density (e.g., microwatt/cm^2). However, not all wavelengths within the UVB band (285 to 320 nanometers) are equally effective. Maximum conversion occurs at 295 nanometers, and about 60% is converted between 290 and 300 nanometers (calculated from MacLaughlin, et al[7]). Because not all wavelengths are equally effective in promoting preD_3 conversion, different types of lamps with the same irradiance recorded by a UV meter can differ significantly in their preD_3-producing ability.

The UVB irradiance from a lamp at different wavelengths can be measured with a recording spectroradiometer, an instrument that is generally not available, in part because of its expense. Photometric features of various lamps used in

Table 84-3	Transmission of Ultraviolet Radiation Through Various Materials		
		% Transmittance	
Material		UVA	UVB
Window glass, single thick		78	4
Acrylite GP acrylic, 0.635 cm (CYRO Industries)		6	0
Acrylite OP-4 acrylic, 0.318 cm (CYRO Industries)		89	79
UV-T plexiglass, 0.635 cm (Rohm and Haas Co)		89	64
Cellulose triacetate, 0.025 cm		67	30
Galvanized mesh, 0.318 cm		67	71
Galvanized mesh, 1.270 cm		82	83

UVA, Ultraviolet A; *UVB*, Ultraviolet B.

herpetoculture as measured with an International Light, Inc (Newburyport, MA) spectroradiometer were recently reported by Lindgren.[8] Approximation of total UVA or UVB irradiances can be read from less expensive handheld broadband radiometers. Such meters should have a resolution to at least 1 microwatt/cm^2 if measurements from fluorescent reptile lamps are to be evaluated. Greater resolutions, such as 10 microwatt/cm^2 increments for the Spectronics DM 300X, do not permit comparisons among these lamps. The only handheld meter in this category less than $1000 that is currently available is the Model UVX manufactured by UVP, Inc (Upland, CA, www.uvp.com). Spectronics Corporation (Westbury, NY) stopped manufacture of its DM 365N and DM 300N models several years ago, although the meters were widely distributed and some are still in use. A comparison of UV irradiances from each of these instruments for several types of reptile lamps is shown in Table 84-2. Irradiances from a given lamp are observed to generally differ depending on which meter is used. This is in part attributable to the different transmission characteristics of the sensor filter and processing software. The actual irradiances for three of the lamps, as measured with a recording spectroradiometer, are also shown in Table 84-2. Clearly, direct comparison of irradiances for a given lamp cannot be made between meter types. However, comparisons of relative irradiances among lamps of a given type (e.g., reptile lamps) with a given meter are valid. A meter may also be used to estimate transmission of UV through various materials (see Table 84-3). One should note that an erroneously high irradiance reading is recorded if high illuminances of visible light and infrared enter the sensor. These handheld meters are not designed for use outdoors in direct sunlight or close to high-intensity lamps. Several moderately priced (about $2500 and up) handheld meters are available that are more suited for use with natural light and high-intensity lamps, as well as fluorescent lamps. These are available from Gigahertz-Optik, Inc (Newburyport, MA, www.gigahertz-optik.de), International Light, Inc (Newburyport, MA, www.intl-light.com) and Solar Light Co, Inc (Philadelphia, PA, www.solar.com). Recently, an inexpensive (about $200.) handheld UVB meter has become available from Solartech, Inc (Harrison Township, MI, www.solarmeter.com). The meter has been adjusted to filter extraneous red and infrared wavelengths and can be used to estimate UVB in natural light.[9]

A realistic way to measure the actual ability of UVB from a lamp to produce preD$_3$ is to subject a known amount of proD$_3$ to radiation from the lamp. Such a system is available as a boron-silicate ampule containing a known quantity of proD$_3$ dissolved in an ethanol vehicle. After exposure to a light source, the quantity of vitamin D photoproducts, primarily preD$_3$, is measured by high performance liquid chromatography (HPLC) and is used to calculate the percent of photoproducts formed from proD$_3$. Photoproduct-forming ability of various lamps is presented in Table 84-2. Two recent studies relate photoproduct-synthesizing ability to different meters as well as different light sources.[9,10]

Considerable anecdotal data indicate that dietary D$_3$ can adequately substitute for UVB-produced D$_3$. A major problem with dietary input is assuring the correct dose; both hypervitaminosis D and hypovitaminosis D have been reported. Some herpetoculturists speculate that UVB photosynthesis of D$_3$ is less likely to lead to hypervitaminosis D, as has been shown in some mammals. It has been demonstrated that Panther Chameleons (*Furcifer pardalis*) will behaviorally adjust their exposure to UVB in a gradient depending on their D$_3$ status.[11] Further experimental studies are required in order to clarify the relative efficacy of dietary D$_3$ compared to UVB-synthesized D$_3$ for various species.

What lamps can effectively substitute for natural light? A variety of fluorescent reptile lamps are available. The UVA and UVB output is highly variable depending on the manufacturer as well as the model number, (e.g., Reptisun 2.0 versus Reptisun 5.0 [see Table 84-2]). Each type must be evaluated separately. Self-ballasted, high-intensity discharge lamps that emit UV, visible, and infrared radiation, but are designed to emit more UV than is usual for this type of lamp, are available for herpetoculture. One such, previously known as Wonderlite and Dragon Light, is currently called Active UVHeat and is manufactured by Westron Corporation (Oceanside, NY) and is officially distributed by T-REX Products, Inc (Chula Vista, CA). However, it may also be sold by other lamp vendors under a generic label such as: self-ballasted mercury vapor lamp, made in Canada, followed by wattage, voltage, width ("R" number), flood or spot UV, and base type. Zoo Med Laboratories, Inc, (San Luis Obispo, CA) has recently started marketing a self-ballasted, mercury-vapor lamp manufactured in Japan with the brand name of Powersun UV. A considerable number of anecdotal accounts support the view that this type of lamp is able to maintain various species, especially lizards, in "good health" and possibly reverse certain pathologies, for example, metabolic bone disease of nutritional origin (NMBD). It has been demonstrated that Westron lamps are comparable to a Sylvania 350 BL fluorescent blacklight and incandescent reflector lamp combination in their ability to support normal growth and bone development in juvenile Chuckwallas (*Sauromalus obesus*) maintained on a D$_3$-free diet. The Westron lamps were capable of maintaining serum 25-hydroxy D$_3$ levels comparable to those measured in wild-caught individuals.[12]

UVB-emitting sunlamps (fluorescent and high-intensity discharge types) are restricted from general distribution, although they are readily available to the medical community. By federal law, these lamps must carry an appropriate warning. Potentially, sunlamps can be used for UVB phototherapy of hypovitaminosis D, but the dose necessary for different species is unknown. Furthermore, they must be used with care because serious UVB burns can occur. They are unsuitable for general herpetocultural use.

What are the UVB requirements of various reptile species, described either as irradiance meter readings or ampule D_3 photoproduct-synthetic ability? Unfortunately, this question cannot be definitively answered for most reptiles because the range of tolerance for UVB for various physiologic and behavioral functions is unknown. Ferguson, et al.[13,14] have reported irradiances and ampule conversion values required for maturation and the subsequent production of viable eggs and hatching success in captive-raised female Panther Chameleons. Clearly, further studies of a variety of species are called for.

SUMMARY

With the recognition that infrared (heat) radiation is of paramount importance for many species, incandescent lamps can be used to maintain temperatures in enclosures above ambient. Reflector lamps are ideal for establishing a thermal gradient with basking spots. Visible light from lamps with a color temperature between 5000°K and 6500°K, a color-rendering index of 88 or above, and a spectral power distribution similar to that of natural light optimize the visual features of reptiles and their environment for the human viewer and may be beneficial for some reptiles as well. Several brands of full-spectrum fluorescent reptile lamps as well as the Westron Corp. and Zoo Med Laboratories mercury-vapor lamps appear capable of maintaining health in captive reptiles. A blacklight may facilitate behaviors, for example, reproduction, not otherwise seen in some species. UVB-emitting sunlamps may be beneficial for the short-term treatment of NMBD but must be used with great care because of the potential to cause burns. Generally, these sunlamps are not available to the herpetocultural community.

REFERENCES

1. Gehrmann WH: Spectral characteristics of lamps commonly used in herpetoculture, *Vivarium* 5(5):16-29, 1994.
2. Lillywhite HB, Gatten RE: Physiology and functional anatomy. In Warwick C, Frye FL, Murphy JB, editors: *Health and welfare of captive reptiles*, New York, 1995, Chapman and Hall.
3. Gehrmann WH: Light requirements of captive amphibians and reptiles. In Murphy JB, Collins JT, Adler K, editors: *Captive management and conservation of amphibians and reptiles*, Ithaca, NY, 1994, Society for the Study of Amphibians and Reptiles.
4. Gehrmann WH: Ultraviolet irradiances of various lamps used in animal husbandry, *Zoo Biol* 6:117-127, 1987.
5. Chen TC: Photobiology of vitamin D. In Holick MF, editor: *Vitamin D: molecular biology, physiology, and clinical applications*, Totowa, NJ, 1999, Humana Press.
6. Holick MF: Vitamin D: importance in the prevention of cancers, type 1 diabetes, heart disease, and osteoporosis, *Amer J Clin Nutrit* 79:362-371, 2004.
7. MacLaughlin JA, Anderson RR, Holick MF: Spectral character of sunlight modulates photosynthesis of pre-vitamin D_3 and its photoisomers in human skin, *Science* 216:1001-1003, 1982.
8. Lindgren J: UV-lamps for terrariums: their spectral characteristics and efficiency in promoting vitamin D_3 synthesis by UVB irradiation, *Bull Chicago Herp Soc* 40(1):1-9, 2005.
9. Gehrmann WH, Jamieson D, Ferguson GW, Horner, JD, Chen TC, Holick MF: A comparison of vitamin D-synthesizing ability of different light sources to irradiances measured with a solarmeter model 6.2 UVB meter, *Herp Review* 35(4): 361-364, 2004.
10. Gehrmann WH, Horner JD, Ferguson GW, Chen TC, Holick MF: A comparison of responses by three broadband radiometers to different ultraviolet-B sources, *Zoo Biol* 23: 355-363, 2004.
11. Ferguson GW, Gehrmann WH, Karsten KB, Hammack SH, McRae M, Chen TC, Lung NP, Holick MF: Do panther chameleons bask to regulate endogenous vitamin D_3 production? *Physiol Biochem Zool* 76:52-59, 2003.
12. Aucone BM, Gehrmann WH, Ferguson GW, Chen TC, Holick MF: Comparison of two artificial ultraviolet light sources used for chuckwalla *Sauromalus obesus*, husbandry, *J Herp Med Surgery* 13(2):14-17, 2003.
13. Ferguson GW, Jones JR, Gehrmann WH, Hammack SH, Talent LG, Hudson RD, et al: Indoor husbandry of the panther chameleon *Chamaelo [Furcifer] pardalis*: effects of dietary vitamins A and D and ultraviolet irradiation on pathology and life-history traits, *Zoo Biol* 15:279-299, 1996.
14. Ferguson GW, Gehrmann WH, Chen TC, Dierenfeld ES, Holick MF: Effects of artificial ultraviolet light exposure on reproductive success of the female panther chameleon (*Furcifer pardalis*) in captivity, *Zoo Biol* 21:525-537, 2002.

85
DISINFECTANTS FOR THE VIVARIUM
EILEEN SLOMKA-McFARLAND

Although often used interchangeably, cleaning, disinfecting and sterilizing are not the same. Cleaning refers to the physical act of removing organic matter and solid debris. Dirt, grease, blood, body fluids, and the like need to be removed from any item that is to be disinfected or sterilized. Although thorough cleaning removes this material, it does little to reduce pathogens such as bacteria, fungi, or viruses.

Disinfection of hard nonporous surfaces reduces the pathogen load but does not eliminate it. A properly disinfected cage or food preparation area still harbors a low level of bacteria, fungi, and viruses, but the pathogen level is usually so low that it does not cause problems for otherwise healthy inhabitants.

Sterilization, as opposed to simple cleaning or disinfecting, kills all life—bacteria, fungi, and viruses. Exposure to steam at high pressures and certain chemicals such as ethylene oxide gas and formalin are options. These methods require special equipment and safety considerations.

Disinfection techniques differ depending on specific needs. Maintenance of hygiene in a single private home cage versus a large breeding colony versus a dynamic pet store or quarantine facility can vary dramatically. Veterinarians must properly advise clients with specific instructions for specific needs.

Many disinfectants are on the market, and choosing the right one can be confusing. One must take the time to read labels to choose the right disinfectant. Labels are full of important information and make the decision much easier, and more importantly, maximize the disease control program.

In choosing a disinfectant, one should keep in mind that it should have a broad spectrum of activity, be easy to use and fast acting, and have predictable risk to animals in the vivarium.

Good housekeeping is the best ally against disease. Cleaning and disinfecting on a scheduled basis prevent the spread of disease. Few disinfectants work in the presence of organic debris (blood, feces, and urine).

Thorough cleaning before disinfection ensures that the disinfectant works properly. Wash all cages, bowls, and accessories in hot water with a mild detergent. Dish soaps work well because they are easily rinsed and generally effective against grease. After washing, items must be rinsed thoroughly in hot water.

Disinfectants should be mixed following the manufacturer's directions. Too dilute a concentration is ineffective, and too strong may be toxic, hard to rinse, and expensive.

Avoid mixing chemicals without prior knowledge of their compatibility. Ammonia and bleach can produce toxic, potentially lethal fumes.

Plastics and rubber may retain chemicals. Disinfectants used on these materials, if not thoroughly rinsed and soaked, can leech out back into an animal's environment, water, or substrate with potentially toxic effects.

Ammonia and bleach are both excellent, inexpensive, and readily available disinfectants. Ammonia can be used undiluted (full strength), and bleach should be diluted to a working concentration of 5% (50 mL of household bleach to 1 L of water; 0.125-oz cup of bleach added to 1 gal of water). Either of these solutions is adequate to kill most common pathogens.

Contact time is the key to effectiveness. Soak items for a minimum of 5 to 30 minutes. Placement of disinfectants in spray bottles is an excellent way to disperse the material (one should wear proper personal protective devices such as eye protection and a face mask when using aerosolized chemicals). Rinse well, and allow to air dry.

Ammonia can be rinsed with water. Chlorine bleach can be neutralized with the addition of a dechlorinator to the rinse water, or with placement of the items in direct sunlight for a few hours (sunlight deactivates the chlorine).

Extra bowls and cages allow rotation of items through this cleaning process with minimal stress to caged herps. Substrates (such as dirt, paper, corn cob, crushed walnut, etc.) should be changed or discarded when soiled.

In choosing a disinfectant, determination of what organisms or pathogens are targeted is necessary. More than one disinfectant may be needed to prevent the spread of disease.

Five basic categories of disinfectants exist. Each has a different spectrum of activity, advantages, and disadvantages, and each is used for a variety of applications. See Table 85-1 for an overview of each category.

In addition to choosing and using disinfectants properly, use of extra caution and protection is also wise, such as gloves, aprons, and disposable cleaning items (towels, brushes, mops, etc.).

One must also remember that proper disinfection of porous items such as wood or other permeable items is impossible. Whenever possible, if contaminated, these items are best thrown away.

Nothing replaces elbow grease; it is absolutely essential that items are cleaned, thoroughly and with vigor, before any efforts toward disinfection. If not, any attempts at pathogen control will fail.

Table 85-1 Characteristics of Common Disinfectants

Types	Examples	Dilutions	Spectrum of Activity	Advantages/Disadvantages	Common Uses	Contact Time
Halogen and halogen-containing compounds Iodophore solutions	Betadine Povidine-iodine	10%-100% solution	Effective antimicrobial; limited activity against bacterial spores. Good activity against enveloped and nonenveloped viruses; good activity against TB organisms and mycoplasma.	Inactivated by organic debris and alcohol. Stains skin and porous material.	Wound antiseptic, preoperative scrubs.	1-5 min depending on concentration.
Chlorine	Sodium hypochlorite solutions (bleach)	2%-10% solution	Good germicidal activity on nonenveloped and enveloped against viruses; bactericidal; good activity against TB organisms and mycoplasma.	Corrosive, irritant, strong fumes, germicidal activity decreases in high water pH. Inactivated by some soaps. Must be rinsed well.	Hard surfaces.	10 min.
Biguanides, chlorhexidine Gluconates	Nolvasan Chlorhexiderm Virosan	90 mL/gal	Bactericidal on most gram-positive, few gram-negative. Does not destroy spores. Fair viricidal activity against enveloped viruses; low to moderate fungicidal activity. Good activity against TB organisms and mycoplasma.	Not inhibited by organic matter or alcohol. May be affected by alkaline pH.	Disinfect instruments and cages. All hard surfaces. Preoperative scrub.	10 min.

Quaternary ammonium compounds	Roccal-D Parvosol Disintegrator		Good bactericidal activity; moderate fungicidal activity. Poor activity on nonenveloped viruses. Fair activity on enveloped viruses. Good activity against TB organisms. Fair activity against mycoplasma.	Inhibited by organic matter. Poor activity in hard water. Inactivated by soaps.	Disinfect rubber equipment and instruments and all hard surfaces.	10 min.
Alcohols	Ethyl alcohol Isopropyl alcohol	Full strength	Strong bactericidal; some viricidal activity; slight fungicidal activity. Does not destroy bacterial spores.	Good skin antiseptic. Inactivated by organic matter, fumes may be irritating.	Disinfect instruments and skin.	20 min.
Phenol-based compounds	Lysol SynPhenol-3	Full strength	Bactericidal; more effective against gram-positive than gram-negative species. Fungicidal and viruses.	Not inactivated by organic material. Toxic to cats and reptiles. Must be rinsed well. Irritating and corrosive to skin.	Hard surfaces, floors. Laundry rinse.	10 min.
Aldehydes	Glutaraldehyde	Full strength	Inactivate many microbial agents such as bacteria (including mycobacteria), viruses, and *Chlamydia*.	Work in the presence of organic debris. Corrosive, toxic, and irritating to the eyes, skin, and respiratory tract.	Used for sterilization of endoscopic equipment and also as a fixative for electron micropsy.	20 min.

TB, Tuberculosis.

86

COMPUTED TOMOGRAPHY AND MAGNETIC RESONANCE IMAGING ANATOMY OF REPTILES

JEANETTE WYNEKEN

The need for good anatomic information extends from the veterinary community to a diversity of basic research areas. Although detailed dissection of carcasses is useful, suitable dissection material is not always available. Up until the present, radiographic and ultrasonographic methods have been the primary noninvasive ways to get anatomic information. The dissection of fresh dead animals can provide a wealth of information, including some landmarks, organ structure, and the overall arrangement of organ systems. However, the normal relative positions and sizes of living organs in vivo and their functions, particularly of very dynamic organ systems, and most vasculature cannot easily be seen in dead animals, or even in "flat film" radiographs.

Recent advances in three-dimensional imaging and the availability of high-resolution diagnostic imaging tools make the understanding of anatomy, in even the most unusual species, possible. The following provides descriptions of magnetic resonance imaging (MRI) and computed tomography (CT) with basics for understanding the images. Examples demonstrate their use while providing baseline reptile anatomy in several taxa.

COMPUTED TOMOGRAPHY

Computer-assisted radial tomography (CT) is a three-dimensional radiographic procedure that uses thousands of fast projections taken with a radiograph tube that spins around the subject.[1] Computer software is used to reconstruct the images in two or three dimensions. **CT provides two-dimensional or three-dimensional images of all or part of the animal and is particularly good for supplying detail of hard structures (bones, eggs), or airways.** Because the images are collected serially along the axis specified by the clinician, CT scans can provide flat section images or the images may be put together in three-dimensional reconstructions[2] (Figure 86-1). CT image collection is fast, and the CT data can be reviewed in serial sections (Figure 86-2) or reconstructed in a variety of ways to allow for the retention of three-dimensional landmarks (see Figure 86-1). Virtual endoscopy is possible with appropriate software. Vasculature may be visualized with a radiopaque contrast injection medium; however, the solution is fairly viscous and is not suitable for small subjects.

Data are collected in series, and sequential data series are put together with software to form the three-dimensional image. If the animal moves during the exposure, the sequential data may not be in register with one another. The chameleon's tail in Figure 86-3 shows this artifact.

MAGNETIC RESONANCE IMAGING

High-resolution MRI and the proliferation of MRI facilities have made machines accessible (and financially realistic)

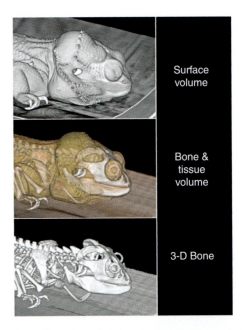

FIGURE 86-1 These lateral views of a Bearded Dragon's head and torso show the versatility of computed tomography (CT) data. They may be reconstructed in three dimensions to emphasize different structure densities and to allow understanding of external landmarks and the internal structures (skeleton in this case). The same dataset from a single CT scan shows the results of three reprocessing modes. Different threshold settings allow the same dataset to be reconstructed as a surface image, showing the whole volume of the animal *(Surface volume)*, a translucent tissue image of the whole volume with the skeleton detected *(Bone + tissue volume)*, and a three-dimensional image of the skeleton alone. Bony sutures are not seen in this image because their small size was below the level of sampling resolution. Cartilage cannot be seen when reprocessing for the bone but is included with other reconstruction settings that include the denser soft tissues. *Pogona vitticeps*, snout-vent length = 22.5 cm.

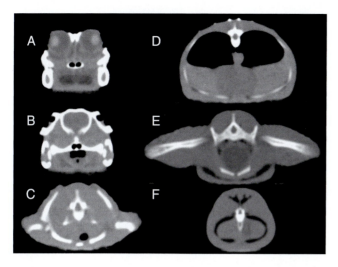

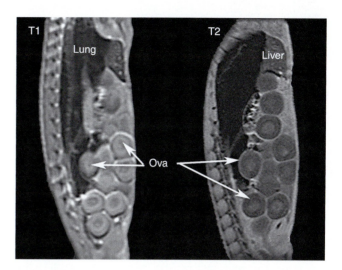

FIGURE 86-2　Two-dimensional axial images along the body of an alligator. At the level of the eyes (A), the jaws form the most bony parts of the skull. Teeth can be seen extending from the lower jaw upward. The bony palate ventral to the choanae resides between spaces that are the palatal vacuities. The vitreous and the tongue are dark. The scleral ossicles appear light. (B), Posterior to the orbits, the palate is complete and the internal choanae can be seen joining the glottis. Dorsally is the oval braincase with posterior temporal bars extending ventrally and laterally. At the level of the shoulders (C), the vertebrae are mostly surrounded by the scapulae and procoracoids. The single element ventral to the trachea is the interclavical. (D), Posterior to the forelimbs, the body wall is supported by dorsal ribs and ventral ribs. The sternum is not detected. The dark heart can be seen ventral to the paired lungs. Two osteoderms are visible dorsal to the trunk vertebra. (E), The hindlimbs are supported by robust ilia articulating with sacral vertebrae. The anterior aspect of the paired pubic bones can be seen ventrally. (F), The tail vertebra and ventral Y-shaped chevron bone are surrounded by muscle (*gray*) and tendon (*black*). *Alligator mississippiensis*, snout-vent length = 22 cm.

FIGURE 86-4　Two sagittal images of a female iguana torso taken at roughly the same position. Cranial is toward the top of the image. In the T1 image, fat is bright, air is black, fluid (blood, edema, cerebrospinal fluid [CSF], or yolk) is dark, and cortical bone is dark. Parts of the spinal nerves can be seen as the white dots running along the spine on the left side of the image. In T2 images, fluids are bright; fats are gray, and bone is dark. The posterior trunk vertebrae and muscles are easy to identify. This T2 section caught little blood flow (seen immediately to the left of the more anterior ova). The more liquid centers of the yolked ova are clear in both images.

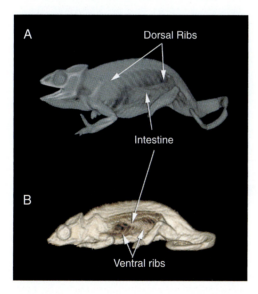

FIGURE 86-3　Chameleons have thin bones and large sac-like lungs. The ribs are jointed at the articulations of the dorsal ribs, spine, and ventral ribs (Gastralia) from the belly. Chameleon ribs extend along the length of the trunk. These computed tomography (CT) scans show the large areas of low density lungs and the large numbers of ribs. In *A*, the data were reconstructed from 0.6-mm serial images and reprocessed so that both skeletal and airway data could be seen. Postprocessing of the image data with false color (*B*) shows the lung field and intestine after a virtual cut to remove the overlying skin image. *Furcifur pardalis*, snout-vent length = 12.6 cm.

for scanning almost real-time images of live animals in a non-invasive fashion. **MRI is particularly good for visualization of soft tissues and fluids**. Often in diagnostics, one is looking for fluid, gas, changes in the brain or nerve cord, or circulatory anomalies.[1] MRI is good for understanding the forms and positions of these soft tissues. The pictures provide detailed information and landmarks and can provide an understanding of normal positions of soft tissues, such as the gastrointestinal tract, liver, and lung. Functional MRI (fMRI) is used to assess organ function, cardiopulmonary performance, blood flow patterns, or sites of fluid accumulation. Two-dimensional and three-dimensional pictures taken with fMRI can be used to show soft tissue functional anatomy with landmarks.

Magnetic resonance imaging is a set of techniques that uses the different biochemical and biophysical properties of the tissues in response to the magnetic pulses to produce images. An MRI machine focuses a magnetic field that rapidly spins around the subject. Protons in tissues or liquids temporarily respond in tissue-specific ways to generate an image. Images are composed of a series of two-dimensional images or slices that may be viewed alone or in three dimensions. The image data are reconstructed with computer software to create "serial sections" or three-dimensional images.

The images can be exposed in many different ways. For basic needs, two major categories of images can be used: T1-weighted and T2-weighted images (Figure 86-4). The terms refer to the biophysical properties of protons in tissues in response to magnetic fields and differ in what is seen. Many special techniques for specific application are based on these two main types of images. In T1 images, fat is bright, fluid (blood, edema, cerebrospinal fluid [CSF]) is dark, and

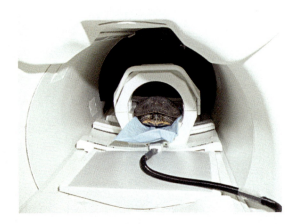

FIGURE 86-5 The closed magnetic resonance imaging (MRI) machine has a donut-shaped magnet as its largest component. It produces and sends and can receive signals. For small-bodied animals like this turtle, a smaller receiver coil mounted inside the gantry provide better images.

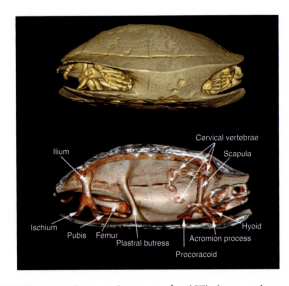

FIGURE 86-6 Computed tomography (CT) data can be reconstructed to show three-dimensional skeletal anatomy. Postprocessing software allows for the reconstructed images as whole skeletons that then can be cut virtually to show internal anatomy. *Trachemys scripta*, straight-line carapace length unknown, adult.

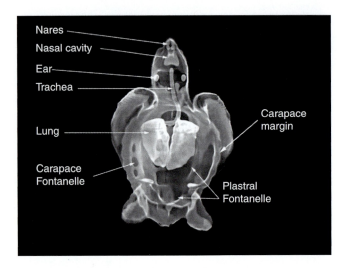

FIGURE 86-7 This computed tomography (CT) scan of a small juvenile seaturtle was reconstructed applying threshold values to the data to make the bones and airways translucent and the surfaces and margins appear as outlines. The partial secondary palate of seaturtles allows the nares to be seen clearly and separately from the trachea, which opens in the tongue. The lungs attach to the carapace and along the vertebral column. Unossified fontanelles are in the margin carapace and make up the center of the plastron. The otic chamber *(labeled ear)* is air filled. Other areas of trapped air appear in the neck and inguinal pockets. *Caretta caretta*, straight-line carapace length = 6.3 cm.

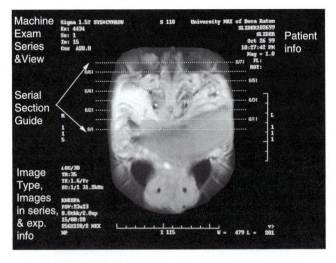

FIGURE 86-8 Both computed tomography (CT) and magnetic resonance images (MRI) are set up with a short exposure "scout image" on which a map of slices or section, their thickness, and extent are set. This image is often termed a "localizer" and is useful to include with the films or files. In addition to patient information, the scan type, and number of sections in the examination, the localizer provides the key to identifying where in the body the two-dimensional images were taken. In this case, a frontal image of a slider from an MRI is used to map out an examination of transverse or axial images. Because most commercially available MRI and CT machines have software specifically for human patients, one must carefully explain to the technician what planes of view are needed from the nonhuman patient. The images are often presented as if the animal were on its back so that its right is on the left side of the image. This MRI was used to map image collection for the cranial half of the turtle in a series of 80 slices. This localizer maps them out in groups of 10, starting at mid body and progressing toward the head.

cortical bone is dark. T1 techniques are good for imaging brain and spinal cord because of the high levels of fat in the spinal cord and brain. In T2 images, fluids are bright, fats are gray, and bone is dark. Bone marrow, because of the fat within, appears bright. T2 is good for visualizing circulation.[1]

Magnetic resonance imaging may also be used to assess function. This is particularly true in assessment of circulation or lack of circulation. Gas and blood can be distinguished in some modalities. Pooling of blood or hematomas may be detected with or without intravenous contrast media. In the author's experience, Gadolinium-positive contrast solution (at 1 to 2 mL/kg) gave sufficient contrast to detail the circulation in several species of turtles, pythons, and agamid lizards with no detectable adverse effects. This dose is similar to that which produces good results in dogs.[3]

The MRI machine consists of a magnet that produces the signals and a receiver. Closed MRI machines give better

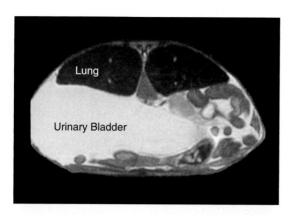

FIGURE 86-9   This T2-weighted magnetic resonance image (MRI) is a transverse or axial section from the slider midbody, designated by the line labeled 6/1 in the localizer image (Figure 86-8). The turtle was oriented with the plastron down; left and right are not reversed in the image. At this level, the large fluid-filled urinary bladder extends anteriorly and occupies most of the left half of the image. Bone is barely visible as a thin dark outline. Dorsally are the black spaces occupied by the lungs; their paired pulmonary artery and vein can be seen as white dots. To the right are the grey intestines; fat, intracoelomic fluid, and mesenteric blood are bright. The darker gray caudal tip of the liver is ventral. The left side of the turtle was outside of the scanned area. This image was magnified slightly in processing the data. *Trachemys scripta*, adult. Straight-line carapace length unknown.

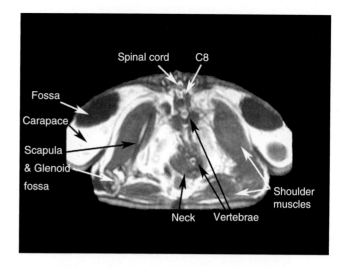

FIGURE 86-11   This section is 30 slices more cranial than section 21 (designated 6/51) in the localizer (Figure 86-8). At this level, the carapace bone appears thick because the "cut" traverses its curvature. The black spaces dorsolaterally are fossae where the fore limbs may retract. Medullary bone is bright. Muscle is dark gray. Both sets of shoulder muscles and the left scapula are in this plane. In the middle of the body is the retracted neck at the level where the vertebrae form an s-curve. As a result, parts of vertebrae C8, C7 or C6, and C3 are seen from dorsal to ventral. Fat and fluid are bright.

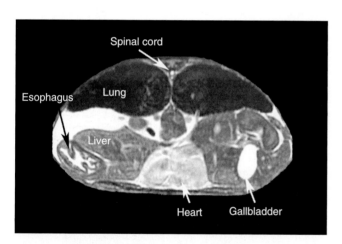

FIGURE 86-10   This section is 20 slices more cranial than section 1 (designated 6/21) in the localizer (Figure 86-8). At this level, the esophagus can be seen to the left. The liver has two large lobes that fill much of the ventral half of the body and one small one dorsal to the heart. The heart is light gray and is found midventrally. The dark lungs are dorsal and abut the vertebrae. The spinal cord can be seen as a white dot between the medial and dorsal parts of the lungs. Blood is bright, as is fat.

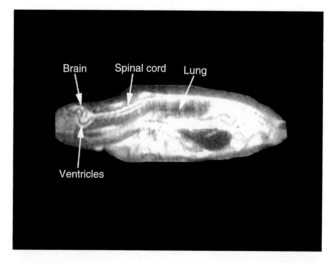

FIGURE 86-12   This T1-weighted image of a posthatchling Leatherback Turtle is a nearly midsagittal view. The brain and spinal cord are bright. The cerebrospinal fluid (CSF) in the ventricles and the spinal canal appear dark gray. This species has a great deal of lipid in its shell and the residual yolk; hence, much of the body is bright. Gas appears black. *Dermochelys coriacea*, straight-line carapace length = 5.7 cm.

resolution than open MRI machines. The images presented here were all collected with a closed MRI. For large-bodied animals, the donut-shaped magnet and a receiver are housed together. For smaller animals or parts of the animal, smaller receivers, termed coils, may be used to provide clearer images by increasing the signal to noise ratio (Figure 86-5), reducing artifacts. In the author's experience, head, knee, or wrist coils provide good quality images where the length of the animal or the region of interest is not great. Some animals that move little when handled may need little or no restraint. Others may be briefly anesthetized with a nonvolatile anesthetic. No metal can be on or in the animal because it may heat up during imaging and can cause discomfort or burns or may leave large artifacts in the image, obscuring the site of interest.

Basic reptile skeletal, landmark, and soft tissue anatomy are illustrated in the following series of CT and MRI pictures (Figures 86-6 to 86-27). Data were processed to maximize the

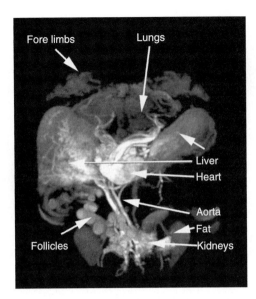

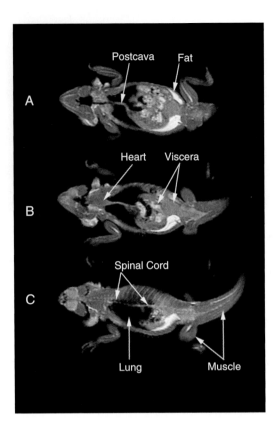

FIGURE 86-13 Soft tissue anatomy of a slider turtle in ventral view is outlined in this T2-weighted functional magnetic resonance image (fMRI) with the vasculature highlighted by gadolinium contrast medium. The heart plus the highly vascular liver, pulmonary arteries and veins, and kidneys are clearly outlined. Forelimbs are outlined less densely. The two systemic aortas join in the midbody as the single dorsal aorta. The larger vessel paralleling the dorsal aorta is the post caval vein. Follicles and fat pads are shown caudally. *Trachemys scripta,* straight-line carapace length unknown.

FIGURE 86-15 These three images are of an adult male Bearded Dragon viewed serially from ventral to dorsal in frontal sections. The exposures are T1 weighted so fat is bright. Medullary bone tends to be bright as well. Fluid and nonfatty tissues appear gray. Air appears black. The most ventral section (A) passes dorsal to the tongue and through the trachea, lungs, postcava, liver, viscera, and through the proximal tail. Long bones and muscles of the limbs can be seen. More dorsally, (B) the lungs, heart, aorta, liver, viscera, and fat pads are clear. In the most dorsal view, (C) the air-filled nasal passages, the eyes, left lung, parts of the spinal cord (light), abdominal fat pads, and tail muscles and tendons can be discriminated. *Pogona vitticeps,* snout-vent length = 17.6 cm.

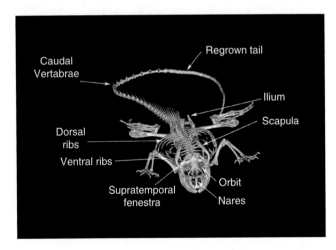

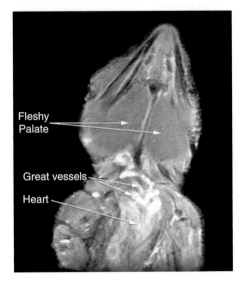

FIGURE 86-14 This three-dimensional reconstruction of an adult iguana skeleton shows normal anatomy, including the multiple fenestrae in the skull, arrangement of the vertebral spinous processes, and the dorsal girdle elements and a few common artifacts found in computed tomography (CT) images. First, rib elements appear to be missing laterally. The thinnest rib ends and cartilaginous parts between the dorsal and ventral ribs are not detected in this kind of reconstruction. The thin nasal bones just behind the nares also appear to be missing. Their data fall outside of the threshold used by the software to make this kind of reconstruction. The striping, most apparent on the skeleton, is from reconstruction of sequential two-dimensional images. *Iguana iguana,* snout-vent length = 41.8 cm.

FIGURE 86-16 This two-dimensional frontal section functional magnetic resonance image (fMRI) was at the level of a Bearded Dragon's fleshy palate. Contrast medium shows that the great vessels are in the same plane. This is a T1-weighted image after gadolinium contrast medium was injected. *Pogona vitticeps,* snout-vent length = 22.5 cm.

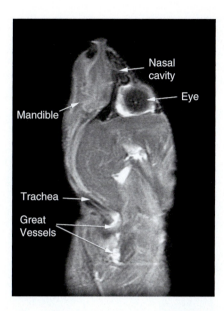

FIGURE 86-17 This two-dimensional parasagittal section of a Bearded Dragon is a functional magnetic resonance image (fMRI). It shows muscle, the medial edge of the lower jaw, and the nasal cavity. The jaw joint and part of the adjacent circulation (external jugular vein) appear white. This is a T1-weighted image with gadolinium contrast medium in the vessels. Parts of the great vessels are caught in this plane of section, as is a small section of the trachea. *Pogona vitticeps*, snout-vent length = 22.5 cm.

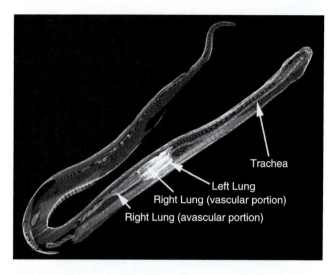

FIGURE 86-19 Python computed tomography (CT) reconstructed for airway resolution. The truncated left lung just has a vascular portion (more dense tissue). The full-sized right lung has a vascular portion connecting to an avascular air sac, which extends posteriorly. *Python regius*, adult. Snout-vent length unknown.

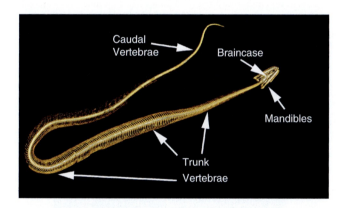

FIGURE 86-18 Ventral view of a Python skeleton. The separate mandibles are easily seen. Snakes lack a secondary palate, so the roof of the mouth is also the floor of the braincase. Cervical vertebrae are limited to the anterior two and cannot be distinguished in this computed tomography (CT) reconstruction. Trunk vertebrae have ribs and extend most of the length of the snake. Snakes lack ventral ribs. Caudal vertebrae lack ribs. The slight shift in registration of the reconstructed sections in the midbody are associated with one breath taken by the snake during scanning. *Python regius*, adult. Snout-vent length unknown.

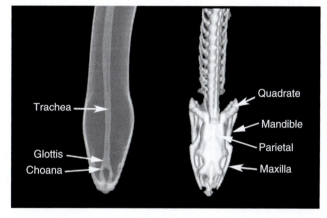

FIGURE 86-20 This close-up computed tomography (CT) scan of the head structure shows the relationship of the airways in a Cornsnake to its skull and neck. Although snakes lack a secondary palate, the airways through the choanae and to the glottis are clear. Snake skulls are highly kinetic. Joints between the parietals, quadrate, and mandibles contribute to the snake's large gape. Highly mobile maxillae assist in prey capture and manipulation for swallowing. No rigid joint is found between the two mandibles or the maxillae. *Elaphe guttata*, adult. Snout-vent length unknown.

landmark information with several different post-processing modalities. The different processing options are presented, not only to enhance the reader's appreciation of reptilian anatomy but also to provide an introduction to the versatility of CT and MRI technologies.

ACKNOWLEDGMENTS

The author thanks Fred Steinberg, MD, Medical Director, University MRI, Boca Raton, for providing access to his high-resolution CT and fMRI equipment and software.

Section VIII SPECIAL TOPICS

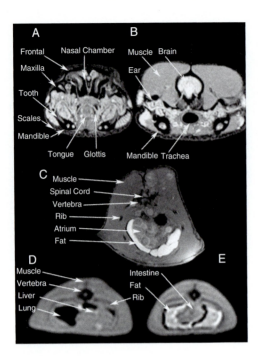

FIGURE 86-21 Python magnetic resonance image (MRI) axial composite. MRI of whole snakes is difficult because of the tubular geometry of the animals. Often the snake must be examined in a series of sequential parts to avoid losing image quality (A to C). Snake images taken without the aid of a small imaging coil or in an open MRI may be of limited value because they tend to be noisy (D and E). For an MRI machine to have sufficient range to scan a whole snake, or even part of a large snake, the distance between the snake and receiver needs to be maximized. However, this large distance leads to images with a great deal of noise and hence, low image quality. Alternatively, one can scan snakes in small segments and use a small coil, but the entire animal (and sometimes the entire organ) cannot be examined in one scan. These T1-weighted axial scans show nasal passages and mouth (A), more caudally on the head, the brain is white, and muscles are various shades of gray (B). Sections through the trunk show the vertebrae and ribs as dark patches seen in part by the plane of view; the spinal cord is light. Fat and fluids also appear light (B, C, and E). Bone and air appear dark in T1 images. *Python molurus*, adult male. Total length = 2.9 m.

Gina Boykin, Andrew Kaufman, and Steve Rubel collected the images at UMRI Boca Raton. Dale Wilke at OMI of Jupiter taught the author much of what she knows about the techniques and procedures; he collected most of the turtle images presented here. The author is grateful to these talented individuals for fine assistance and willingness to work with reptiles.

REFERENCES

1. Lee SH, Rao KCVG, Zimmerman RA: *Cranial and spinal MRI and CT*, ed 4, Kingsport, 1999, McGraw-Hill Professional.
2. Wu YT: *From CT image to 3D model*, 2001, Advanced Imaging.
3. Jordin D, Green MS, Reed A, Omary MS, Finn JP, Chung Y-C, et al: Two- and three-dimensional MR coronary angiography with intraarterial injections of contrast agent in dogs: a feasibility study, *Radiology* 226:272-277, 2003.

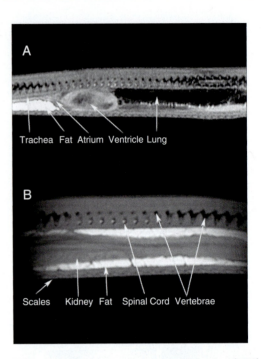

FIGURE 86-22 Python magnetic resonance imaging (MRI) trunk composite. This composite of images taken in the sagittal or parasagittal planes shows major structures of the anterior (A) and posterior trunk (B). The head is to the left in both images. These T1 images show the heart and lungs in less detail than the lobular kidney. Because the image was not timed to the heart beat, some movement artifacts are seen in the anterior body. The thyroid and parathyroid glands could not be distinguished from the fat with this imaging mode. *Python molurus*, adult male. Total length = 2.9 m.

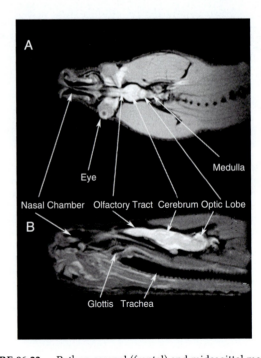

FIGURE 86-23 Python coronal (frontal) and midsagittal magnetic resonance images (MRI). This pair of images shows the major brain anatomy and some of the landmarks associated with the mouth. The two images show the muscle masses surrounding the brain and braincase (A) and the close proximity of the brain to the primary palate bones (B). *Python molurus*, adult male. Total length = 2.9 m.

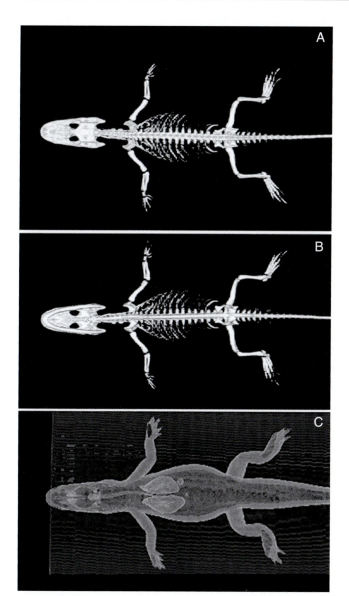

FIGURE 86-24 The skeleton of a small juvenile alligator from a CT scan. The diapsid skull architecture, in dorsal view (A), includes paired superior and lateral fenestrae located posterior to the large orbits. The ventral view (B) shows the large secondary palate separating air and food passages. Paired palatal fenestrae (palatal vacuities) occur ventral to the orbits. The internal choanae, posterior to these openings, appear unpaired along the midline because of the resolution of this scan. The glottis in this lung volume reconstruction (C) aligns with the internal choanae. Crocodilians have cervical ribs (B), dorsal ribs that attach to a sternum and extensive ventral ribs; the latter are not detected in this construction. The pectoral girdle of crocodilians is simple, with paired scapulae dorsally (A) and procoracoids ventrally (B); primitively it retains an unpaired interclavical. The pelvis is attached to the axial skeleton by robust sacral vertebrae (A). The more proximal caudal vertebrae have prominent lateral processes; these are absent near the end of the tail (A and B). The alligator's lungs occupy a relatively small volume in the body (C). *Alligator mississippiensis*, snout-vent length = 22 cm.

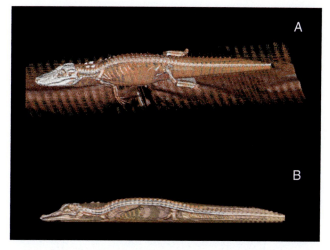

FIGURE 86-25 Here the computed tomography (CT) data are reconstructed in three dimensions. The bone and tissue together provide landmarks. The reconstruction is cut virtually (B), showing the skull's internal architecture, spine, lungs, and pelvis. In both views, the terminal tail vertebrae were beyond the scanned field. *Alligator mississippiensis*, snout-vent length = 22 cm.

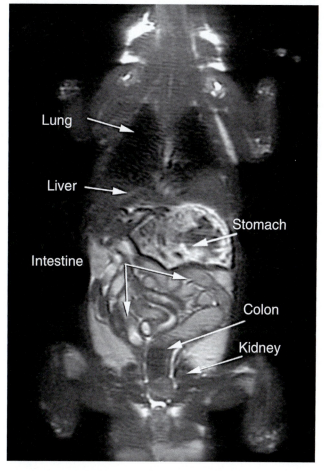

FIGURE 86-26 This T2-weighted magnetic resonance image (MRI) of a juvenile alligator torso is a two-dimensional image. The plane of view is a frontal section of the ventral one third of the animal. The gastrointestinal tract and its contents are clearly visible as shades of gray. Fluids in the coelomic cavity and throat are bright. Fat is dark gray, and air is black. Portions of the kidneys are visible adjacent to the colon. *Alligator mississippiensis*, snout-vent length = 29 cm.

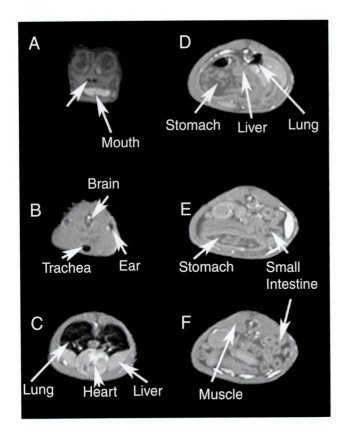

FIGURE 86-27 These MRI axial sections of a small alligator provide a survey of different parts of the animal from the head to the lower abdomen. The eyes appear as light gray ovals with dark gray centers (the vitreous); air in the nares, trachea, and ear cavities is black; and the brain is white with gray surrounding bone *(A and B)*. At the level of the heart *(C)*, great vessels and the pulmonary circulation appear bright; the lungs are black; muscles and liver appear gray; and the spinal cord and cerebrospinal fluid (CSF) appear white. At the midbody, the lung sections are small. The stomach and liver are large, and major vessels including the abdominal veins and aortae can be seen *(D)*. More posteriorly, the remainder of the gastrointestinal tract can be seen, and gray back muscles occupy much of the dorsal body *(E to F)*. Compare this composite with Figure 86-2 to see the differences in the two imaging modes. *Alligator mississippiensis*, snout-vent length = 22 cm.

RECOMMENDED READING

Kardong KV: *Vertebrates: comparative anatomy, function, evolution*, ed 3, New York, 2002, McGraw-Hill.

Romer AS: *The vertebrate body*, Philadelphia, 1970, WB Saunders.

Witherington D, Wyneken J: Chelonian anatomy, *Exotic DVM* 4(6):35-41, 2003.

Witherington D, Wyneken J: Snake anatomy, *Exotic DVM* 5(5): 38-42, 2003.

Wyneken J: The external morphology, musculoskeletal system, and neuroanatomy of sea turtles. In Lutz P, Musick J, Wyneken J, editors: *The biology of sea turtles*, vol II, Boca Raton, Fla, 2003, CRC Press.

Wyneken J: Respiratory anatomy: form and function in reptiles, *Exotic DVM* 3(2):17-22, 2001.

Wyneken J: *Guide to the anatomy of sea turtles*, 2001, NMFS Tech Publication NOAA Tech, Memo NMFS-SEFSC-470.

87
RADIOGRAPHIC ANATOMY

DOUGLAS R. MADER

After the challenge of taking a diagnostic-quality radiograph has been mastered, the task of interpreting the images comes. A thorough knowledge of the internal anatomy helps the clinician evaluate radiographs. An impossible task is to have normals for all 7000-plus species of reptiles. However, this chapter presents some of the common body forms and a general layout of the various reptilian body parts. The reader is referred to Chapter 29, Diagnostic Imaging, for radiographic techniques and Chapters 5 to 8, Biology Section, for more information on species anatomy.

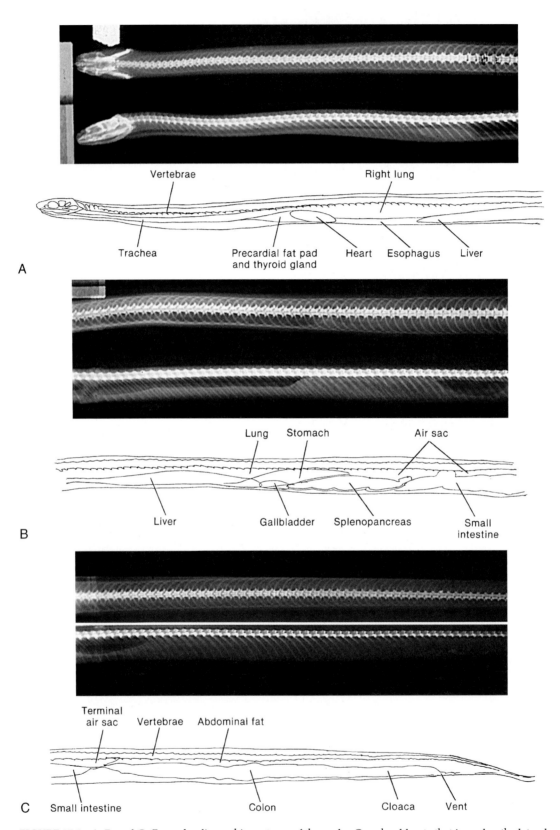

FIGURE 87-1 **A, B,** and **C,** General radiographic anatomy of the snake. One should note that in snakes the lateral view provides the most diagnostic view.

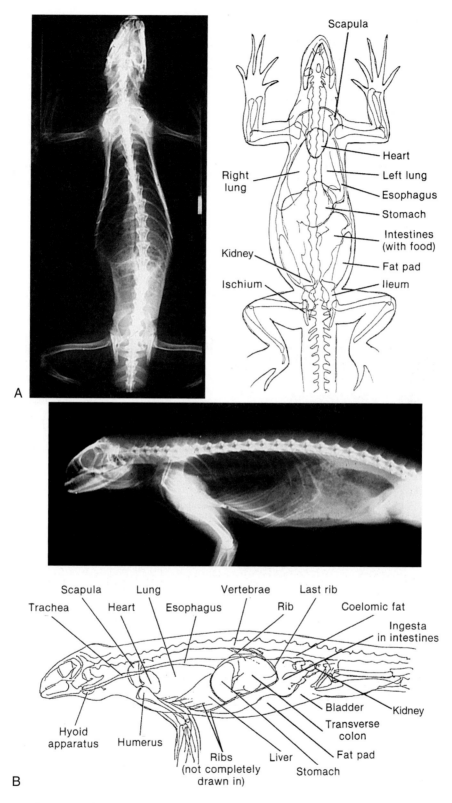

FIGURE 87-2 Dorsoventral (**A**) and lateral (**B**) views of the common Green Iguana *(Iguana iguana).* Of particular interest is the position of the heart within the pectoral girdle. The healthy reptilian kidney is located within the pelvic girdle and is not normally seen on either a dorsoventral or a lateral image.

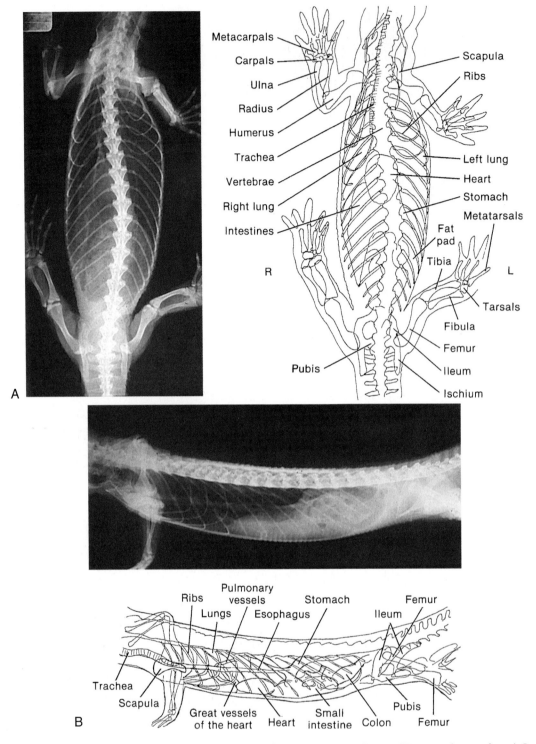

FIGURE 87-3 Dorsoventral **(A)** and lateral **(B)** views of an Asian Water Monitor *(Varanus salvator salvator)*. In comparison with the Green Iguana *(Iguana iguana)*, the heart of the monitor lizard is located almost in the midbody region. Unlike the iguana, the kidneys in the monitor are midcoelomic and cannot normally be seen.

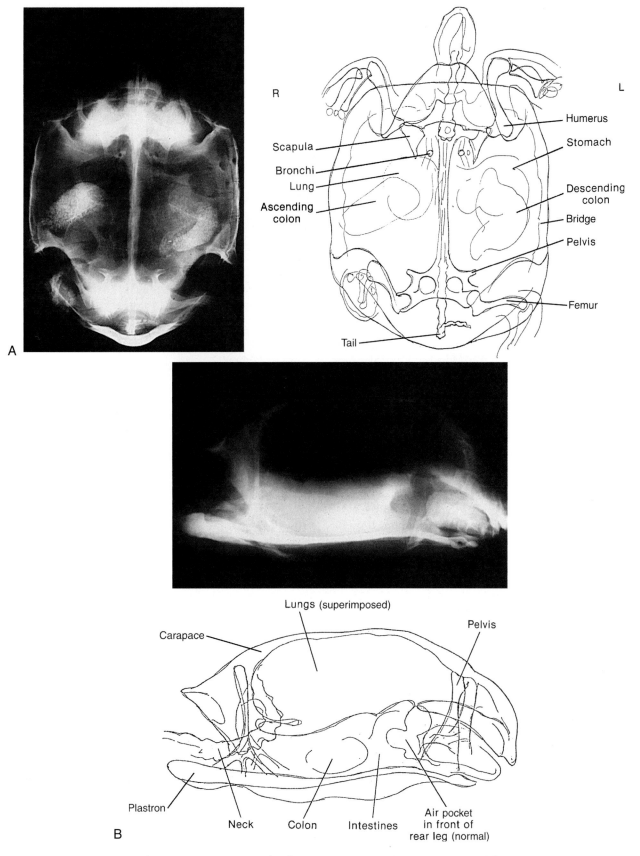

FIGURE 87-4 A. The dorsoventral view in the chelonians is most useful for evaluation of the gastrointestinal and urinary systems. The lateral (B) and craniocaudal (C) views are beneficial in evaluation of lung fields. The craniocaudal view is the only projection that allows distinction between the left and right lung fields.

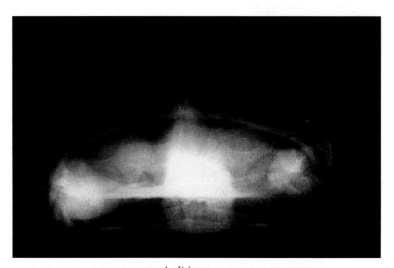
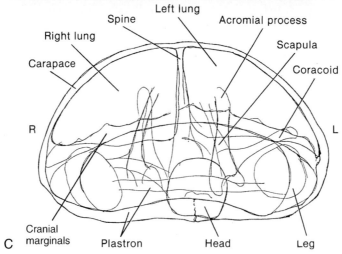

FIGURE 87-4, cont'd

88
HEMATOLOGIC AND BLOOD CHEMISTRY VALUES IN REPTILES

GERALDINE DIETHELM and GEOFF STEIN

Hematologic and Serum Biochemical Values of Reptiles

Measurements	Boa Constrictor (*Boa Constrictor*)[3,26,ISIS]	Rainbow Boa (*Epicrates cenchiria*)[ISIS]	Emerald Tree Boa (*Corallus caninus*)[ISIS]
Hematology			
PCV (%)	24-40	28 (11-40)	23 (6-57)
RBC (10^6/mL)	1.0-2.5	0.34-1.74	0.05-5.05
Hgb (g/dL)	3.3-15.3	6.5-13.1	9.6 (6.1-18.7)
MCV (fL)	159-625	174-534	–
MCH (pg)	85-208	83-160	113-149
MCHC (g/dL)	21-42	21-40	30-60
WBC (10^3/mL)	4-10	9.2 (1.5-35)	5 (0.5-5)
Heterophils (%)	20-65[b]	–	–
Lymphocytes (%)	10-60	–	–
Azurophils (%)	1.5(0-5.8)	–	–
Monocytes (%)	0-3	–	–
Eosinophils (%)	0-3	–	–
Basophils (%)	0-20	–	–
Chemistries			
AP (IU/L)	421 (242-652)	85 (14-593)	109 (14-323)
ALT (IU/L)	6 (0-20)	11 (1-31)	5 (1-11)
AST (IU/L)	5-35	41 (8-136)	34 (5-115)
Bilirubin, total (mg/dL)	0.3 (0.2-0.4)	0.4 (0-0.8)	0.2 (0.1-0.3)
BUN (mg/dL)	<1-10	1-3	0-4
Calcium (mg/dL)	10-22	13.7 (11.3-18.9)	12.8 (8.9-17.4)
Chloride (mEq/L)	16.8 (14.1-23.7)	119 (94-141)	130 (106-150)
Cholesterol (mg/dL)	118 (107-124)	225 (140-394)	289 (101-539)
Creatine kinase (IU/L)	87 (53-138)	–	–
Creatinine (mg/dL)	<0.1-0.3	0.4 (0.1-0.7)	0-1.1
Glucose (mg/dL)	10-60	28 (2-67)	28 (10-56)
LDH (IU/L)	30-300	309 (102-661)	495 (76-1680)
Magnesium (mEq/L)	–	–	–
Phosphorus (mg/dL)	3.6 (2.6-4.9)	5.2 (3.4-7.7)	4.5 (1.8-11.2)
Potassium (mEq/L)	3.0-5.7	3.6 (1.2-5.7)	4.9 (1.8-8.7)
Protein, total (g/dL)	4.6-8.0	6.5 (3.7-8.4)	42.3-8.3
Albumin (g/dL)	3.1 (1.9-5.3)	2.9 (1.8-4.8)	2.7 (1.2-4)
Globulin (g/dL)	4 (2.2-6.9)	3.9 (2.8-5.8)	2.8 (1-3.8)
A:G (ratio)	–	–	–
Sodium (mEq/L)	130-152	157 (137-170)	148-175
Thyroxine (mg/dL)	–	–	–
Uric acid (mg/dL)	1.2-5.8	6 (1.3-27.5)	5.6 (1.2-19.8)

Continued

Hematologic and Serum Biochemical Values of Reptiles—cont'd

Measurements	Diamond-backed Water Snake (*Nerodia* sp.)[21]	Ball Python (*Python regius*)[16,ISIS]	Pythons (*Python* spp.)[a,26]
Hematology			
PCV (%)	–	18 (16-21)	25-40
RBC (10^6/mL)	–	0.8 (0.3-1.3)	1.0-2.5
Hgb (g/dL)	–	6.7 (5.5-7.9)	–
MCV (fL)	–	211-540	–
MCH (pg)	–	82-139	–
MCHC (g/dL)	–	25-40	–
WBC (10^3/mL)	–	12.2 (7.9-16.4)	6-12
Heterophils (%)	–	62 (56-67)	20-80[b]
Lymphocytes (%)	–	14 (7-21)	10-60
Azurophils (%)	–	17 (12-22)	-
Monocytes (%)	–	1 (0-1)	0-3
Eosinophils (%)	–	–	0-3
Basophils (%)	–	1 (0-2)	0-10
Chemistries			
AP (IU/L)	69 (27-157)	106 (96-116)	–
ALT (IU/L)	–	14 (12-16)	–
AST (IU/L)	–	33 (15-51)	5-30
Bilirubin, total (mg/dL)	0.6 (0.3-1.0)	0.3 (0-2.1)	–
BUN (mg/dL)	1 (0-3)	0-3	<1-10
Calcium (mg/dL)	7 (6-8)	14 (13-14)	10-22
Chloride (mEq/L)	127 (117-131)	120 (109-130)	–
Cholesterol (mg/dL)	–	124 (23-302)	–
Creatine kinase (IU/L)	262 (92-572)	–	–
Creatinine (mg/dL)	0.7 (0.3-1.8)	0-0.5	<0.1-0.3
Glucose (mg/dL)	33 (4-97)	29 (28-30)	10-60
LDH (IU/L)	191 (69-538)	209 (77-782)	40-300
Magnesium (mEq/L)	1.2 (0.9-1.5)	–	–
Phosphorus (mg/dL)	31.4 (0.7-2.5)	3 (2.7-3.4)	–
Potassium (mEq/L)	4.6 (2.8-6.4)	–	3.0-5.7
Protein, total (g/dL)	5.8 (4.3-7.6)	5.2 (5.0-5.6)	5-8
Albumin (g/dL)	–	2.2 (1-3.7)	–
Globulin (g/dL)	–	4.6 (2.1-9)	–
A:G (ratio)	–	–	–
Sodium (mEq/L)	166 (154-175)	138-173	130-152
Thyroxine (mg/dL)	–	–	–
Uric acid (mg/dL)	–	3.6 (3.2-4.1)	1.2-5.6

Hematologic and Serum Biochemical Values of Reptiles—cont'd

Measurements	Jungle Carpet Python (Morelia spilota cheynei)[2,ISIS]	Green Tree Python (Morelia [Chondropython] viridis)[ISIS]	Reticulated Python (Python reticulatus)[ISIS]
Hematology			
HCT (%)	30 (23-37)	8-38	25 (17-45)
RBC (10^6/mL)	0.89 (0.54-1.3)	0.4-1.3	0.41-1.33
Hgb (g/dL)	8.6 (4-15.5)	4-8.3	10 (5.2-30)
MCV (fL)	282 (178-414)	207-250	331 (176-428)
MCH (pg)	113.5 (66.7-159)	100	78-86
MCHC (g/dL)	40 (23.5-53.2)	33.2-40	29-45
WBC (10^3/mL)	8.5 (5.7-11.3)	3.5-22.1	8 (1.8-17.7)
WBC (Natt Herrick)	7.3 (4.5-10.2)	–	–
Heterophils (%)	53 (38-68)	–	–
Lymphocytes (%)	43 (35-51)	–	–
Monocytes (%)	0 (0-1)	–	–
Azurophils (%)	2 (0-5)	–	–
Eosinophils (%)	0 (0-1)	–	–
Basophils (%)	1 (0-3)	–	–
Chemistries			
AP (IU/L)	36 (13-60)	4.6-6	84 (4-183)
ALT (IU/L)	19 (6-38)	43 (8-132)	27 (5-96)
AST (IU/L)	25 (2-120)	29 (8-79)	24 (2-105)
Bilirubin, total (mg/dL)	0.5	0.2	0.3 (0.1-0.6)
BUN (mg/dL)	2 (1-3)	2 (0-2)	3 (0-6)
Calcium (mg/dL)	25.6 (12.4-100)	14 (10.3-18.5)	18.8 (8.6-48)
Chloride (mEq/L)	112 (102-123)	128 (119-138)	122 (107-141)
Cholesterol (mg/dL)	333 (199-594)	204 (116-360)	263 (81-371)
Creatine kinase (IU/L)	479 (27-1537)	524 (198-992)	1086
Creatinine (mg/dL)	1.1 (0.3-3.7)	0.2 (0-0.5)	0.3 (0.1-0.5)
Glucose (mg/dL)	31 (16-71)	67 (5-223)	36 (12-81)
LDH (IU/L)	306 (48-547)	206	–
Magnesium (mEq/L)	–	–	–
Phosphorus (mg/dL)	8.7 (2.1-37)	6.7 (2.8-26.3)	7.2 (2.5-15.4)
Potassium (mEq/L)	5.4 (3.7-9)	5.3 (2.8-6.4)	5.5 (3.4-10.2)
Protein, total (g/dL)	8.3 (4.7-14)	5.7 (3.9-6.9)	7.5 (5.5-10.1)
Albumin (g/dL)	3 (1.9-6.2)	2 (1.4-2.8)	2.9 (1.3-7.2)
Globulin (g/dL)	5.5 (2.7-8)	4.4 (3.2-5.4)	4.7 (2.6-8.3)
A:G (ratio)	–	–	–
Sodium (mEq/L)	149 (135-158)	160 (157-163)	160 (142-176)
Thyroxine (mg/dL)	–	–	–
Uric acid (mg/dL)	7 (1.9-25.4)	5.8 (1-20.4)	8.6 (3-34.2)

Continued

Hematologic and Serum Biochemical Values of Reptiles—cont'd

Measurements	Gopher Snake (*Pituophis melanoleucus*)[9,19,ISIS]	Red Rat Snake (*Elaphe guttata*)[ISIS]	Yellow Rat Snake (*Elaphe obsoleta quadrivitatta*)[24]
Hematology			
PCV (%)	25 (15-38)	31 (21-52)	25 (9-46)
RBC (10^6/mL)	1.09	1.16 (0.62-1.86)	0.21-1.56
Hgb (g/dL)	10 (6.9-12.7)	11.5 (9.7-13.5)	9 (2.8-15.2)
MCV (fL)	189-568	291 (170-403)	384 (179-961)
MCH (pg)	123-160	127 (110-143)	137 (90-217)
MCHC (g/dL)	27-37	32-40	34 (26-54)
WBC (10^3/mL)	6.2 (1.7-20)	9.2 (1.02-31.4)	9 (0.4-32)
Heterophils (%)	—	—	—
Lymphocytes (%)	—	—	—
Monocytes (%)	—	—	—
Azurophils (%)	—	—	—
Eosinophils (%)	—	—	—
Basophils (%)	—	—	—
Chemistries			
AP (IU/L)	60 (9-133)	64 (18-297)	92 (55-130)
ALT (IU/L)	22 (11-65)	34 (2-64)	18 (7-29)
AST (IU/L)	53 (16-127)	42 (9-224)	59 (15-103)
Bilirubin, total (mg/dL)	0.2 (0.1-0.4)	0.6 (0.1-1)	0.3 (0.1-0.8)
BUN (mg/dL)	2 (1-5)	2 (0-6)	4 (0-20)
Calcium (mg/dL)	14.4 (13.0-15.7)	15.8 (12-19.6)	17.7 (11.3-73.2)
Chloride (mEq/L)	137 (109-148)	122 (108-137)	119 (68-140)
Cholesterol (mg/dL)	327 (138-702)	314-572	371 (101-745)
Creatine kinase (IU/L)	78-1918	433 (77-2460)	716 (200-1231)
Creatinine (mg/dL)	0.3 (0.1-0.6)	0.6 (0.2-2)	0.5 (0.3-1.3)
Glucose (mg/dL)	88 (24-129)	54 (31-88)	62 (26-117)
LDH (IU/L)	97 (6-313)	173 (48-444)	203 (86-320)
Magnesium (mEq/L)	—	—	2.5
Phosphorus (mg/dL)	4.1 (2.5-5.7)	3.8 (1.9-6)	4.4 (1.7-14.7)
Potassium (mEq/L)	6.6 (3.6-10.0)	6.8 (1.9-13.2)	5 (1.6-8.5)
Protein, total (g/dL)	4.3 (2.8-7.3)	6.6 (4.6-8.4)	6.6 (3.3-10.6)
Albumin (g/dL)	1.9 (1.6-2.1)	2.6 (1.8-3.4)	2.4 (1.6-4.4)
Globulin (g/dL)	3.2 (1.9-5.4)	4.4 (3.3-5.7)	4.3 (2.6-8.3)
A:G (ratio)	—	—	—
Sodium (mEq/L)	171 (161-180)	164 (147-183)	162 (151-177)
Thyroxine (mg/dL)	—	—	—
Uric acid (mg/dL)	6.7 (2-17.6)	7 (1.3-19.9)	6.6 (1.6-32.1)

Hematologic and Serum Biochemical Values of Reptiles—cont'd

Measurements	Common Kingsnake (Lampropeltis getulus)[ISIS]	Milksnake (Lampropeltis triangulum)[ISIS]	Indigo Snake (Drymarchon corais)[8]
Hematology			
PCV (%)	30 (12-45)	27 (8-48)	–
RBC (10^6/mL)	2.65 (0.35-14)	0.9 (0.5-2)	–
Hgb (g/dL)	–	10 (6.9-11.9)	–
MCV (fL)	318 (28-500)	369 (135-615)	–
MCH (pg)	–	119 (89-164)	–
MCHC (g/dL)	–	34 (29-45)	–
WBC (10^3/mL)	12 (1-42)	10 (1.2-39)	–
Heterophils (%)	–	–	–
Lymphocytes (%)	–	–	–
Monocytes (%)	–	–	–
Azurophils (%)	–	–	–
Eosinophils (%)	–	–	–
Basophils (%)	–	–	–
Chemistries			
AP (IU/L)	90 (17-478)	105 (70-168)	123 (80-161)
ALT (IU/L)	23 (8-40)	7 (0-17)	–
AST (IU/L)	40 (0-124)	29 (0-102)	46 (6-163)
Bilirubin, total (mg/dL)	0-0.1	0.5 (0.1-0.9)	–
BUN (mg/dL)	2 (0-4)	4 (2-14)	–
Calcium (mg/dL)	20 (6.8-60)	15 (12-18)	159 (30-337)
Chloride (mEq/L)	114 (88-136)	125 (109-137)	119 (100-129)
Cholesterol (mg/dL)	294 (55-1083)	390 (154-822)	–
Creatine kinase (IU/L)	514 (82-1634)	202 (92-332)	644 (68-1923)
Creatinine (mg/dL)	0.4 (0-1.6)	0.5 (0.2-1.1)	–
Glucose (mg/dL)	42 (7-90)	56 (15-124)	46 (28-89)
LDH (IU/L)	179 (24-488)	816 (18-2807)	313 (13-1055)
Magnesium (mEq/L)	–	–	–
Phosphorus (mg/dL)	6.2 (0.7-24.6)	7.3 (2.9-25)	35 (8-69)
Potassium (mEq/L)	4.9 (2.1-9.2)	5.3 (2.2-9.7)	8.1 (4.3-14.3)
Protein, total (g/dL)	7.1 (3.6-12)	6.6 (3.8-11.6)	8.9 (5.9-12.3)
Albumin (g/dL)	2.3 (1.1-6.8)	2.2 (1.2-3)	2.5 (1.7-4.6)
Globulin (g/dL)	4.6 (1.8-7.9)	–	–
A:G (ratio)	–	–	–
Sodium (mEq/L)	161 (132-184)	166 (157-178)	157 (143-170)
Thyroxine (mg/dL)	–	–	–
Uric acid (mg/dL)	7.1 (1.9-28)	7.4 (2.1-35.6)	8.6 (2.2-17.2)

Continued

Hematologic and Serum Biochemical Values of Reptiles—cont'd

Measurements	Tokay Gecko (*Gekko gecko*)[ISIS]	Egyptian Spiny-tailed Lizard (*Uromastyx aegyptius*)[ISIS]	Blue Tongued Skink (*Tiliqua scincoides*)[ISIS]
Hematology			
PCV (%)	30 (25-34)	27 (18-40)	10 (6-13)
RBC (10^6/mL)	0.67 (0.63-0.74)	0.73 (0.46-0.99)	1.05 (0.73-1.36)
Hgb (g/dL)	–	5.8 (3.6-8.2)	10.4 (6-13)
MCV (fL)	467 (432-492)	308 (242-391)	299 (266-354)
MCH (pg)	–	87 (78-95)	98 (44-173)
MCHC (g/dL)	–	28 (20-36)	33 (16-57)
WBC (10^3/mL)	10 (4-20)	11 (4-32)	7 (2-20)
Heterophils (%)	–	–	–
Lymphocytes (%)	–	–	–
Monocytes (%)	–	–	–
Azurophils (%)	–	–	–
Eosinophils (%)	–	–	–
Basophils (%)	–	–	–
Chemistries			
AP (IU/L)	54	98 (53-164)	82 (39-162)
ALT (IU/L)	5	3	13 (2-34)
AST (IU/L)	61 (9-146)	37 (14-81)	45 (7-106)
Bilirubin, total (mg/dL)	0.5	0.3 (0.1-0.7)	–
BUN (mg/dL)	–	3 (1-4)	1 (0-2)
Calcium (mg/dL)	17-18	11.3 (8.6-14.1)	13.2 (8.2-20.6)
Chloride (mEq/L)	119	126 (111-135)	113 (111-115)
Cholesterol (mg/dL)	–	317 (306-328)	192 (72-429)
Creatine kinase (IU/L)	117	2003 (556-3454)	2099 (73-5832)
Creatinine (mg/dL)	–	0.3 (0.2-0.4)	0.3 (0.1-0.6)
Glucose (mg/dL)	141 (105-173)	184 (102-248)	130 (63-176)
LDH (IU/L)	189	639 (197-1235)	735 (364-1106)
Magnesium (mEq/L)	–	–	–
Phosphorus (mg/dL)	5.6 (2.8-7.7)	4.5 (1.3-10)	5.3 (2.8-7.7)
Potassium (mEq/L)	–	3.7 (3-4.6)	5.6 (4.3-8.6)
Protein, total (g/dL)	–	5.2 (3.1-8)	6 (4.4-7.6)
Albumin (g/dL)	2.7	1.6 (0.9-2.4)	2 (1.2-2.9)
Globulin (g/dL)	–	2.6 (2.2-4.6)	3.8 (3.2-5.2)
A:G (ratio)	–	–	–
Sodium (mEq/L)	158	173	148 (142-158)
Thyroxine (mg/dL)	–	–	–
Uric acid (mg/dL)	5.9 (1.4-12.2)	3.8 (2.6-5.6)	3.3 (0.7-8.5)

Hematologic and Serum Biochemical Values of Reptiles—cont'd			
Measurements	Bearded Dragon (*Pogona vitticeps*)[4]	Iguanid Lizard (*Dipsosaurus dorsalis*)[17]	Green Iguana (*Iguana iguana*)[7,10,12,13,ISIS]
Hematology			
PCV (%)	24 (17-28)	–	25-38
RBC (10^6/mL)	1.1 (0.8-1.8)	–	1-1.9
Hgb (g/dL)	–	–	6-10
MCV (fL)	–	–	165-305
MCH (pg)	–	–	48-78
MCHC (g/dL)	–	–	20-38
WBC (10^3/mL)	9.4 (5.9-14.3)	–	3-10
Heterophils (%)	–	–	0.35-5.2[c]
Lymphocytes (%)	64 (54-76)	–	0.5-5.5[c]
Monocytes (%)	–	–	0-0.1[c]
Azurophils (%)	3 (0-8)	–	0-1.7[c]
Eosinophils (%)	–	–	0-0.3[c]
Basophils (%)	–	–	0-0.5[c]
Chemistries			
AP (IU/L)	151 (15-447)	14 (4-30)	50-290
ALT (IU/L)	11 (4-20)	13 (3-38)	5-68[d]
AST (IU/L)	27 (0-92)	179 (34-400)	5-52[d]
Bilirubin, total (mg/dL)	0.5 (0-3.7)	0.2 (0.1-0.5)	0.3 (0-4.9)
BUN (mg/dL)	3 (3-4)	2 (1-5)	2 (0-11)
Calcium (mg/dL)	10 (8-13)	11 (8-30)	8.8-14.0
Chloride (mEq/L)	126 (107-163)	120 (12-155)	117-122
Cholesterol (mg/dL)	425 (160-900)	243 (100-399)	107-333
Creatine kinase (IU/L)	1211 (59-7000)	4500 (700-14,240)	272 (73-666)
Creatinine (mg/dL)	0.2 (0-0.6)	0.5 (0.2-1.8)	0.5 (0.1-1.3)[d]
Glucose (mg/dL)	232 (211-261)	355 (255-575)	169-288
LDH (IU/L)	296 (35-628)	789 (145-2915)	443 (36-3861)
Magnesium (mEq/L)	–	–	3.2 (2.4-4)[d]
Phosphorus (mg/dL)	5.6 (2.7-15.1)	5.5 (2.8-10.0)	4-6[18]
Potassium (mEq/L)	3.8 (1.3-6.3)	2.6 (0.4-7.0)	1.3-3.0[d]
Protein, total (g/dL)	2.2 (2.0-2.7)	3.8 (2.4-5.4)	5.0-7.8
Albumin (g/dL)	2.6 (1.3-4.6)	2.3 (1.6-3.0)	2.1-2.8[d]
Globulin (g/dL)	2.3 (1-4.4)	1.5 (0.8-2.4)	2.5-4.3
A:G (ratio)	–	1.7 (1.0-2.3)	–
Sodium (mEq/L)	156 (137-186)	164 (137-245)	158-183[d]
Thyroxine (mg/dL)	–	–	3.81 (2.97-4.65)
Triglycerides (mg/dL)	310 (93-459)	–	53-691
Uric acid (mg/dL)	4.5 (2.9-10.0)	5.6 (2.4-13.3)	1.2-2.4[d]

Continued

Hematologic and Serum Biochemical Values of Reptiles—cont'd

Measurements (all iguanas kept in natural environment, outdoors)[12]	Green Iguana, male (*Iguana iguana*)[12]	Green Iguana, Female gravid (*Iguana Iguana*)[12]	Green Iguana, female (*Iguana iguana*)[12]	Green Iguana, juvenile (*Iguana iguana*)[12]
Hematology				
PCV (%)	34 (29.2-38.5)	–	38 (33-44)	38 (30-47)
RBC (10^6/mL)	1.3 (1.0-1.7)	–	1.4 (1.2-1.8)	1.4 (1.3-1.6)
Hgb (g/dL)	8.6 (6.7-10.2)	–	10.6 (9.1-12.2)	9.6 (9.2-10.1)
MCV (fL)	266 (228-303)	–	270 (235-331)	–
MCHC (g/dL)	25.1 (22.7-28)	–	27.9 (24.9-31)	–
Fibrinogen	100 (100-200)	–	100 (100-300)	100 (100-300)
WBC (10^3/mL)	15.1 (11.1-24.6)	–	14.8 (8.2-25.2)	16.3 (8.0-22.0)
Heterophils (10^3/mL)	3.6 (1.0-5.4)	–	3.2 (0.6-6.4)	2.2 (1.0-3.8)
Lymphocytes (10^3/mL)	9.7 (5.0-16.5)	–	9.9 (5.2-14.4)	12.9 (6.2-17.2)
Monocytes (10^3/mL)	1.3 (0.2-2.7)	–	1.2 (0.4-2.3)	0.4 (0.3-0.6)
Azurophils (10^3/mL)	–	–	–	–
Eosinophils (10^3/mL)	0.1 (0.0-0.3)	–	0.1 (0.0-0.2)	0.3 (0.0-0.4)
Basophils (10^3/mL)	0.4 (0.1-1.0)	–	0.5 (0.2-2.1)	0.5 (0.1-0.7)
Chemistries				
AP (IU/L)	39 (14-65)	37.5 (34-41)	59 (22-90)	–
ALT (IU/L)	32 (4-76)	7.6 (5.3-10)	45 (5-96)	–
AST (IU/L)	33 (19-65)	21 (12-29)	40 (7-102)	41 (13-72)
Bilirubin, total (mg/dL)	0.8 (0.1-1.4)	0.9 (0.2-2.1)	1.5 (0.3-3.1)	–
BUN (mg/dL)	–	–	–	–
Calcium (mg/dL)	11.3 (8.6-14.1)	32.5 (22.5-47.5)	12.5 (10.8-14.0)	14.3 (12.1-23.2)
Ionized Calcium[6]	0.37 (0.34-0.4)[6]	0.37 (0.34-0.4)[6]	0.37 (0.34-0.4)[6]	0.37 (0.34-0.4)[6]
Chloride (mEq/L)	119 (115-124)	121.3 (117-124)	121 (113-129)	–
Cholesterol (mg/dL)	161 (82-214)	339 (253-453)	255 (204-347)	–
CO_2 (mEq/L)	19.9 (15.2-24.7)	19.3 (15.1-21.7)	19.1 (16-23.2)	–
Anion gap (mEq/L)	21.8 (12.1-29.5)	25.8 (19.7-36.8)	29 (18.8-41)	–
Glucose (mg/dL)	166 (70-244)	140 (126-153)	170 (105-258)	273 (131-335)
LDH (IU/L)	–	–	–	–
Magnesium (mEq/L)	–	–	–	–
Phosphorus (mg/dL)	5.3 (3.2-7.6)	12 (8.4-17.5)	6.3 (2.8-9.3)	7.7 (4.3-9.0)
Potassium (mEq/L)	4 (2.8-6.1)	3.9 (3.2-5.0)	3.6 (2.0-5.8)	–
Protein, total (g/dL)	5.4 (4.4-6.5)	7.5 (7.0-8.2)	6.1 (4.9-7.6)	5 (4.2-6.1)
Albumin (g/dL)	2 (1.3-3.0)	2 (1.5-2.5)	2.4 (1.5-3.0)	2.3 (92.0-2.8)
Globulin (g/dL)	3.5 (2.5-4.4)	5.5 (4.9-6.7)	3.8 (2.8-5.2)	2.7 (2.2-3.0)
A:G (ratio)	0.6 (0.4-0.9)	0.4 (0.2-0.5)	0.7 (0.3-1.0)	0.8 (0.7-0.9)
Sodium (mEq/L)	157 (152-162)	162.5 (161-164)	163 (156-172)	–
Thyroxine (mg/dL)	–	–	–	–
Uric acid (mg/dL)	2.7 (1.5-5.8)	3.3 (2.2-4.9)	3.6 (0.9-6.7)	3.3 (0.7-5.7)

Hematologic and Serum Biochemical Values of Reptiles—cont'd

Measurements	Prehensile-tailed Skink (*Corucia* sp.)[30]	Tegu Lizard (*Tupinambus teguixin*)[ISIS]	Green Crested Basilisk (*Basiliscus plumifrons*)[ISIS]
Hematology			
PCV (%)	35 (24-60)	37 (23-55)	34 (27-41)
RBC (10^6/mL)	1.5 (0.8-1.4)	0.8 (0.4-1.1)	–
Hgb (g/dL)	9.6 (7.4-11.6)	9.1 (8.8-9.3)	8.9 (8.6-9.1)
MCV (fL)	263 (152-600)	425 (299-677)	–
MCH (pg)	69 (42-111)	185 (130-239)	–
MCHC (g/dL)	28 (17-56)	39	26 (22-29)
WBC (10^3/mL)	12.4 (3.9-22.4)[e]	17.4 (3.9-47.1)	12 (3.3-31)
Heterophils (%)	37 (16-58)	–	–
Lymphocytes (%)	22 (2-40)	–	–
Monocytes (%)	0.6 (0-6)	–	–
Azurophils (%)	–	–	–
Eosinophils (%)	4 (0-18)	–	–
Basophils (%)	15 (4-26)	–	–
Chemistries			
AP (IU/L)	–	160 (38-358)	137 (77-230)
ALT (IU/L)	–	33 (11-65)	13 (5-21)
AST (IU/L)	19 (<4-76)	18 (5-52)	60 (14-136)
Bilirubin, total (mg/dL)	–	0.3 (0.1-0.5)	0.6 (0.5-0.8)
BUN (mg/dL)	–	1 (0-1)	5 (1-20)
Calcium (mg/dL)	13 (11-21)	12.2 (11.1-14.1)	10 (7-13)
Chloride (mEq/L)	124 (123-129)	121 (113-138)	127 (125-129)
Cholesterol (mg/dL)	144 (11-252)	206 (137-290)	845 (550-1237)
Creatine kinase (IU/L)	210 (27-940)	641 (50-1904)	5355 (2691-9436)
Creatinine (mg/dL)	–	0.3 (0.2-0.4)	0.4 (0.2-0.8)
Glucose (mg/dL)	100 (70-122)	128 (98-205)	283 (60-280)
LDH (IU/L)	–	540 (33-1234)	–
Magnesium (mEq/L)	–	–	–
Phosphorus (mg/dL)	3.7 (2.8-6.7)	5.6 (3.5-11.4)	0.5 (6.2-11.6)
Potassium (mEq/L)	3.6 (1.4-5.0)	3.4 (0.7-3.6)	3 (2.4-3.5)
Protein, total (g/dL)	6.5 (5-8)	6.6 (3.5-8.5)	5.7 (4.0-8.3)
Albumin (g/dL)	–	3.6 (2.2-4.6)	3.1 (2.6-3.5)
Globulin (g/dL)	–	2.9 (0.7-4.5)	2.9 (2.1-4.9)
A:G (ratio)	–	–	–
Sodium (mEq/L)	158 (145-167)	159 (156-166)	1663 (145-172)
Thyroxine (mg/dL)	–	–	–
Uric acid (mg/dL)	1.6 (<0.3-3.1)	3.2 (0.5-6.2)	10.9 (1-96.6)

Continued

Hematologic and Serum Biochemical Values of Reptiles—cont'd

Measurements	Savannah Monitor (*Varanus exanthematicus*)[ISIS]	Nile Monitor (*Varanus niloticus*)[ISIS]	American Alligator (*Alligator mississippiensis*)[5,10,15]
Hematology			
PCV (%)	32 (21-51)	33 (21-40)	25 (12-40)
RBC (10^6/mL)	1.22 (0.63-1.58)	0.6	0.6 (0.23-1.29)
Hgb (g/dL)	10.4 (6.2-13.2)	–	7.8 (3.7-11.6)
MCV (fL)	291 (229-392)	667	445 (230-1174)
MCH (pg)	94 (89-99)	–	139 (58-370)
MCHC (g/dL)	32 (26-39)	-	32 (18-65)
WBC (10^3/mL)	4.8 (1.2-11.3)	8.2 (2.6-24)	0 (1.8-29)
Heterophils (%)	–	–	–
Lymphocytes (%)	–	–	–
Monocytes (%)	–	–	–
Azurophils (%)	–	–	–
Eosinophils (%)	–	–	–
Basophils (%)	–	–	–
Chemistries			
AP (IU/L)	77 (5-675)	79 (24-141)	39 (0-109)
ALT (IU/L)	58 (5-374)	75 (3-255)	39 (0-154)
AST (IU/L)	30 (1-170)	24 (8-50)	289 (0-700)
Bilirubin, total (mg/dL)	0.2 (0-0.6)	–	0.3 (0-5.1)
BUN (mg/dL)	2 (0-6)	2 (1-4)	2 (0-13)
Calcium (mg/dL)	14 (11-18)	12.8 (10.7-14.8)	11 (0-15.6)
Chloride (mEq/L)	115 (105-129)	111 (103-117)	110 (0-130)
Cholesterol (mg/dL)	117 (46-231)	57 (45-65)	94 (0-245)
Creatine kinase (IU/L)	1540 (150-9080)	1324 (436-2001)	2022 (0-8620)
Creatinine (mg/dL)	0.4 (0-0.8)	0.3 (0.1-0.6)	0.4 (0-1.3)
Glucose (mg/dL)	109 (40-159)	137 (93-206)	91 (0-198)
LDH (IU/L)	596 (29-3699)	375 (127-584)	485 (0-2000)
Magnesium (mEq/L)	3.1	2.9	0
Phosphorus (mg/dL)	4.9 (1.6-14.3)	6.5 (4.5-10)	4.4 (0-9.4)
Potassium (mEq/L)	4.6 (2.7-10.8)	4.9 (2.9-7)	3.8 (0-6)
Protein, total (g/dL)	6.9 (4.2-10.5)	6.4 (4.3-7.8)	5.3 (2.5-9.4)
Albumin (g/dL)	2.1 (1.2-3.5)	2.1 (1.6-2.9)	1.6 (0.8-2.3)
Globulin (g/dL)	4.9 (3.4-6.6)	5 (2.7-6)	3.5 (1.6-6)
A:G (ratio)	–	–	–
Sodium (mEq/L)	155 (146-166)	164 (157-176)	146 (0-165)
Thyroxine (mg/dL)	–	–	–
Uric acid (mg/dL)	7 (1.2-18)	8.6 (2.4-19.5)	1.6 (0-5.7)

Hematologic and Serum Biochemical Values of Reptiles—cont'd

Measurements	Dwarf Caiman (Paleosuchus palpebrosus)[ISIS]	Common Box Turtle (Terrapene carolina)[10,22,28,ISIS]	Ornate Box Turtle (Terrapene ornata)[ISIS]
Hematology			
PCV (%)	22 (16-29)	22 (7-35)	25 (17-37)
RBC (10^6/mL)	0.64 (0.43-0.89)	0.5 (0.09-1)	0.6 (0.5-0.8)
Hgb (g/dL)	7.3 (5.3-8.8)	5.1	7.2 (6-9)
MCV (fL)	382 (180-540)	420 (229-1000)	408 (350-463)
MCH (pg)	119 (98-140)	102	122 (108-136)
MCHC (g/dL)	31 (23-38)	28 (26-29)	33 (31-33)
WBC (10^3/mL)	5.7 (2.5-10.6)	7 (1.7-16)	8.9 (2-24)
Heterophils (%)	–	11	–
Lymphocytes (%)	–	56	–
Monocytes (%)	–	9.4	–
Azurophils (%)	–	–	–
Eosinophils (%)	–	–	–
Basophils (%)	–	8	–
Chemistries			
AP (IU/L)	13 (6-29)	62 (29-102)	664 (300-1267)
ALT (IU/L)	52 (24-93)	7 (2-14)	30 (9-47)
AST (IU/L)	111 (42-221)	124 (2-620)	156 (33-517)
Bilirubin, total (mg/dL)	0.3 (0-1)	0.5 (0.1-1)	0.1
BUN (mg/dL)	2 (1-4)	49 (20-102)	38 (4-64)
Calcium (mg/dL)	11.3 (0.7-14.4)	13.6 (6.5-26.4)	10.4 (8-13.6)
Chloride (mEq/L)	119 (99-137)	106 (101-112)	105 (96-112)
Cholesterol (mg/dL)	127 (66-344)	240 (65-496)	167 (107-276)
Creatine kinase (IU/L)	2350 (37-9890)	463 (37-898)	1550 (88-4155)
Creatinine (mg/dL)	0.2 (0-0.5)	0.4	1.2 (0.2-2.4)
Glucose (mg/dL)	77 (29-187)	84 (33-153)	67 (8-110)
LDH (IU/L)	1986 (80-6615)	206 (111-313)	664 (300-1267)
Magnesium (mEq/L)	–	3.5	–
Phosphorus (mg/dL)	5.3 (2.6-13.6)	4 (1.6-8.2)	3.8 (2.9-4.8)
Potassium (mEq/L)	4.6 (3.3-7.9)	5.6 (3-9.7)	6.6 (4-8.8)
Protein, total (g/dL)	5.5 (3.6-7.4)	5.6 (2.7-7.5)	4.4 (2.7-6)
Albumin (g/dL)	1.6 (0.9-2.7)	2.2 (1.2-3.2)	2.1 (1.6-2.4)
Globulin (g/dL)	4.1 (3-5.4)	3.4 (2.5-4.7)	2.5 (1.2-3.6)
A:G (ratio)	–	–	–
Sodium (mEq/L)	150 (140-162)	144 (138-149)	147 (132-183)
Thyroxine (mg/dL)	–	–	–
Uric acid (mg/dL)	2.2 (0.7-4.5)	1.6 (0.5-3.1)	2 (0.6-5.6)

Continued

Hematologic and Serum Biochemical Values of Reptiles—cont'd

Measurements	Radiated Tortoise (T. radiata)[20,ISIS]	Red-footed Tortoise (Geochelone carbonaria)[ISIS]	Star Tortoise (Geochelone elegans)[ISIS]
Hematology			
PCV (%)	22 (9-40)	27 (15-47)	22 (12-34)
RBC (10^6/mL)	0.5 (0.2-0.7)	2 (0.5-6.3)	0.5 (0.3-0.7)
Hgb (g/dL)	6.1 (4-8)	7-7.9	7.6 (6-8.5)
MCV (fL)	481 (319-700)	347 (71-468)	409 (354-475)
MCH (pg)	125 (82-174)	136 (123-149)	135 (122-163)
MCHC (g/dL)	28 (24-33)	31 (29-32)	31 (26-35)
WBC (10^3/mL)	4.3 (0.7-18)	7.8 (1.1-15)	12 (0.8-61)
Heterophils (%)	2 (0.7-3.4)[e]	–	–
Lymphocytes (%)	1.6 (0.4-3.4)[e]	–	–
Monocytes (%)	0.15 (0.03-0.47)[e]	–	–
Azurophils (%)	0.18 (0.03-0.53)[e]	–	–
Eosinophils (%)	0.34 (0.10-0.94)[e]	–	–
Basophils (%)	–	–	–
Chemistries			
AP (IU/L)	200 (83-392)	73 (23-162)	173 (38-379)
ALT (IU/L)	9 (0-48)	9 (2-18)	13 (0-30)
AST (IU/L)	139 (25-383)	214 (87-616)	96 (12-296)
Bilirubin, total (mg/dL)	0.2 (0-1.8)	0.1	0.2 (0-0.4)
BUN (mg/dL)	16 (2-90)	12 (1-22)	4 (0-11)
Calcium (mg/dL)	10.5 (6.1-18)	12.6 (9.1-15.8)	11.6 (5.4-22)
Chloride (mEq/L)	99 (70-114)	98 (89-105)	105 (90-118)
Cholesterol (mg/dL)	105 (60-154)	144 (47-284)	127 (77-252)
Creatine kinase (IU/L)	723 (170-1892)	754 (56-1798)	1099 (144-8518)
Creatinine (mg/dL)	0.3 (0.1-1.6)	0.3 (0.2-0.4)	0.3 (0.2-0.5)
Glucose (mg/dL)	60 (46-93)	01 (17-171)	115 (39-212)
LDH (IU/L)	691 (222-2227)	428 (118-880)	667 (402-1512)
Magnesium (mEq/L)	–	–	–
Phosphorus (mg/dL)	4.4 (2.1-8.4)	3.6 (1.8-5.8)	3.8 (2.2-5.7)
Potassium (mEq/L)	5.5 (3.9-8.2)	5.3 (4.2-6.8)	5.2 (3.9-6.1)
Protein, total (g/dL)	4.0 (3.2-5.0)	4.5 (2.9-7.2)	4.6 (3-6)
Albumin (g/dL)	1.1 (0.8-1.3)	1.7 (1-2.8)	1.5 (0.2-3.1)
Globulin (g/dL)	2.3 (1.3-3.7)	3 (1.7-5.3)	3.1 (2.3-4.2)
A:G (ratio)	0.38	–	–
Sodium (mEq/L)	127 (121-147)	128 (116-133)	131 (122-150)
Thyroxine (mg/dL)	–	–	–
Uric acid (mg/dL)	0.8 (0-1.8)	0.8 (0.2-1.3)	3 (1-8.1)

Hematologic and Serum Biochemical Values of Reptiles—cont'd			
Measurements	Desert Tortoise (*Gopherus agassizii*)[11,25,ISIS]	Gopher Tortoise (*Gopherus polyphemus*)[29]	Mediterranean Tortoises (*Testudo* spp.)[10,14,15]
Hematology			
PCV (%)	23-37	23 (15-30)	28-34
RBC (10^6/mL)	1.2-3.0	0.54 (0.24-0.91)	0.7-1.0
Hgb (g/dL)	6.9-7.7	6.4 (4.2-8.6)	9.1-11.3
MCV (fL)	377-607[f]	–	384-944[f]
MCH (pg)	113-126[f]	–	125-314[f]
MCHC (g/dL)	19-34[f]	–	27-40[f]
WBC (10^3/mL)	6.6-8.9	15.7 (10-22)	–
Heterophils (%)	35-60[g]	30 (10-57)	–
Lymphocytes (%)	25-50[g]	57 (32-79)	–
Monocytes (%)	0-4[g]	7 (3-13)	–
Eosinophils (%)	0-4[g]	–	–
Basophils (%)	2-15[g]	6 (2-11)	–
Chemistries			
AP (IU/L)	32 (29-35)	39 (11-71)	–
ALT (IU/L)	6.1 (3.8-8.3)	15 (2-57)	–
AST (IU/L)	59 (47-70)	136 (57-392)	–
Bilirubin, total (mg/dL)	0.1 0-0.2)	0.02 (0-0.1)	–
BUN (mg/dL)	46 (30-62)	30 (1-130)	–
Calcium (mg/dL)	10 (9.6-10.3)	12 (10-14)	2.3-4.0
Chloride (mEq/L)	110 (109-112)	102 (35-128)	95-100
Cholesterol (mg/dL)	74 (60-89)	76 (19-150)	–
Creatine kinase (IU/L)	2079 (52-6945)	160 (32-628)	–
Creatinine (mg/dL)	0.13 (0.12-0.14)	0.3 (0.1-0.4)	–
Glucose (mg/dL)	75 (69-82)	75 (55-128)	78
LDH (IU/L)	25-250	273 (18-909)	–
Magnesium (mEq/L)	2.1 (1.8-2.4)	4.1 (3.3-4.8)	–
Phosphorus (mg/dL)	4.2 (1.2-13.5)	2.1 (1.0-3.1)	–
Potassium (mEq/L)	4.7 (2.2-6.6)	5 (2.9-7.0)	4.4-7.8
Protein, total (g/dL)	3.7 (1.2-7.7)	3.1 (1.3-4.6)	6.6
Albumin (g/dL)	1.1 (0.4-3)	1.5 (0.5-2.6)	–
Globulin (g/dL)	2.2 (1.2-4.7)	–	–
A:G (ratio)	–	–	–
Sodium (mEq/L)	130-157	138 (127-148)	127
Thyroxine (mg/dL)	–	–	–
Uric acid (mg/dL)	2.2-9.2	3.5 (0.9-8.5)	–

Continued

Hematologic and Serum Biochemical Values of Reptiles—cont'd

Measurements	African Spurred Tortoise (*Geochelone sulcata*)[ISIS]	Leopard Tortoise (*Geochelone pardalis*)[ISIS]	Aldabra Tortoise (*Geochelone sp.*)[27,ISIS]
Hematology			
PCV (%)	28 (13-48)	22.5 (7-60)	17 (11-27)
RBC (10^6/mL)	0.9 (0.4-1.3)	5.1 (0.4-27)	0.4 (0.25-0.65)
Hgb (g/dL)	10.9 (6.4-17)	10.4 (4.3-28)	5.4 (3.2-8.0)
MCV (fL)	384 (201-575)	364 (179-542)	452 (375-537)
MCH (pg)	133 (91-165)	83	146 (118-185)
MCHC (g/dL)	36 (27-62)	33 (25-46)	33 (28-40)
WBC (10^3/mL)	7.2 (0.6-27)	8.8 (1.3-23)	3.4 (1.0-8.3)
Heterophils (%)	–	–	71 (32-79)
Lymphocytes (%)	–	–	22 (2-40)
Monocytes (%)	–	–	2 (0-8)
Eosinophils (%)	–	–	0.5 (0-7)
Basophils (%)	–	–	2 (0-4)
Chemistries			
AP (IU/L)	38 (12-63)	148 (54-272)	111 (29-182)
ALT (IU/L)	9 (0-47)	3 (1-8)	7 (0-26)
AST (IU/L)	114 (34-401)	79 (35-344)	57 (5-138)
Bilirubin, total (mg/dL)	0.4 (0-2.6)	0.2 (0.1-0.2)	0.2 (0-0.3)
BUN (mg/dL)	2 (0-6)	24 (1-100)	33 (21-57)
Calcium (mg/dL)	11.8 (6.6-19.2)	13.6 (9.1-22.1)	12 (6-20)
Chloride (mEq/L)	108 (93-121)	106 (75-137)	93 (87-107)
Cholesterol (mg/dL)	147 (58-394)	117 (36-237)	275 (52-631)
Creatine kinase (IU/L)	1228 (103-6205)	413 (32-3397)	303 (12-4210)
Creatinine (mg/dL)	0.3 (0.1-0.5)	0.4 0.3-0.6)	0.1 (0.1-0.2)
Glucose (mg/dL)	139 (54-277)	85 (15-207)	50 (22-113)
LDH (IU/L)	1114 (258-1980)	324 (78-546)	532 (127-2484)
Magnesium (mEq/L)	–	–	5.1 (4.8-5.5)
Phosphorus (mg/dL)	3.9 (1.5-7.8)	3.4 (1.7-6.6)	4.3 (1.6-12.1)
Potassium (mEq/L)	5.5 (3.6-10.2)	6 (4.9-7.5)	4.7 (3.2-6.1)
Protein, total (g/dL)	4 (2.3-7)	3.2 (1.6-6.4)	4.1 (0.6-6.2)
Albumin (g/dL)	1.6 (1.3-2)	1.6 (0.5-2.6)	1.5 (0.3-2.6)
Globulin (g/dL)	2.1 (1.4-2.9)	2.2 (1.1-4.1)	2.6 (0.3-3.6)
A:G (ratio)	–	–	–
Sodium (mEq/L)	139 (121-155)	135 (125-154)	133 (129-136)
Thyroxine (mg/dL)	–	–	–
Uric acid (mg/dL)	5.1 (2.1-10.5)	3.1 (0.5-15.3)	1.6 (0-4.9)

Hematologic and Serum Biochemical Values of Reptiles—cont'd

Measurements	Red-eared Slider (Trachemys scripta)[5,10,15,ISIS]	Painted Turtle (Chrysemys picta)[ISIS]
Hematology		
PCV (%)	29 (16-47)	22 (2-40)
RBC (10^6/mL)	0.8 (0.3-2.2)	0.6 (0.4-0.7)
Hgb (g/dL)	8.0	5.6
MCV (fL)	179-1000[f]	271 (183-365)
MCH (pg)	95-308[f]	–
MCHC (g/dL)	31[f]	28
WBC (10^3/mL)	13 (3.5-25.5)	5.5 (0.4-13)
Heterophils (%)	–	–
Lymphocytes (%)	–	–
Monocytes (%)	–	–
Eosinophils (%)	–	–
Basophils (%)	–	–
Chemistries		
AP (IU/L)	212 (81-677)	208
ALT (IU/L)	16 (1-66)	–
AST (IU/L)	230 (0-522)	137 (62-280)
Bilirubin, total (mg/dL)	0.3 (0.1-1)	0.1
BUN (mg/dL)	23 (4-54)	20
Calcium (mg/dL)	12.8 (8.3-18)	11.4 (5.5-19)
Chloride (mEq/L)	102 (97-107)	95 (88-99)
Cholesterol (mg/dL)	167 (106-227)	–
Creatine kinase (IU/L)	1952 (108-4856)	168 (35-355)
Creatinine (mg/dL)	0.3 (0.2-0.5)	1
Glucose (mg/dL)	67 (20-138)	98 (68-175)
LDH (IU/L)	1702 (371-5763)	724 (412-1035)
Magnesium (mEq/L)	2.2	–
Phosphorus (mg/dL)	4.8 (2.7-7.7)	4.8 (1.7-17)
Potassium (mEq/L)	4.9 (3.5-9.1)	2.9 (2.6-3.2)
Protein, total (g/dL)	4.5 (2.8-6.6)	3.2 (1.9-6.5)
Albumin (g/dL)	1.8 (0.8-2.5)	1.2
Globulin (g/dL)	2.6 (1.2-3.7)	1.2
A:G (ratio)	–	–
Sodium (mEq/L)	137 (124-144)	131 (126-137)
Thyroxine (mg/dL)	–	–
Uric acid (mg/dL)	1.2 (0.3-3.2)	1 (0.2-2.2)

[a]Includes Burmese *(Python molurus)*, Ball *(P. regius)*, and Reticulated *(P. reticulatis)* Pythons.
[b]Heterophils and neutrophils.
[c]Absolute values ($10^3/\mu L$).
[d]Elevated in gravid females; vitamin D_3 higher in female Green Iguanas *(Iguana iguana)*.[23]
[e]Includes 22% (8% to 42%) azurophils.
[f]Calculated from data.
[g]Greatly differing percentages have also been reported: heterophils, 33% ± 15%; lymphocytes, 23% ± 7%; monocytes, 11% ± 7%; azurophilic monocytes, 2% ± 2%; eosinophils, 1% ± 0.5%; and basophils, 30% ± 11%.[1]

PCV, Packed cell volume; *RBC*, red blood cell; *Hgb*, hemoglobin; *MCV*, mean cell volume; *MCH*, mean corpuscular hemoglobin; *MCHC*, mean corpuscular hemoglobin concentration; *WBC*, white blood cell; *AP*, alkaline phosphatase; *ALT*, alanine aminotransferase; *AST*, aspartate aminotransferase; *BUN*, blood urea nitrogen; *LDH*, lactate dehydrogenase; *A:G*, albumin:globulin.

REFERENCES

1. Alleman AR, Jacobson ER, Raskin RE: Morphologic and cytochemical characteristics of blood cells from the desert tortoise (Gopherus agassizii), Proc Assoc Amph Rept Vet 51-55, 1996.
2. Centini R, Klaphake E: Hematologic values and cytology in a population of captive jungle carpet pythons, Morelia spilota cheqnei, Proc Assoc Rept Amph Vet 107-111, 2002.
3. Chiodini RJ, Sundberg JP: Blood chemical values of the common boa constrictor (Constrictor constrictor), Am J Vet Res 43:1701-1702, 1982.
4. Cranfield M, Graczyk T, Lodwick L: Adenovirus in the bearded dragon, Pogona vitticeps, Proc Assoc Amph Rept Vet 131-132, 1996.
5. Crawshaw GJ: Comparison of plasma biochemical values in blood and blood-lymph mixtures from red-eared sliders, Trachemys scripta elegans, Bull Assoc Rept Amph Vet 6:7-9, 1996.
6. Dennis PM, Bennet Ra, Harr KE, et al: Plasma concentration of ionized calcium in healthy iguanas, J Am Vet Med Assoc 219:326-328, 2001.
7. Divers SJ, Redmayne G, Aves EK: Haematological and biochemical values of 10 green iguanas (Iguana iguana), Vet Rec 138:203-205, 1996.
8. Drew ML: Hypercalcemia and hyperphosphatemia in indigo snakes (Drymarchon corais) and serum biochemical reference values, J Zoo Wildl Med 25:48-52, 1994.
9. Fleming GJ: Capture and chemical immobilization of the Nile crocodile (Crocodylus niloticus) in South Africa, Proc Assoc Amph Rept Vet 63-66, 1996.
10. Frye FL: Reptile clinician's handbook, Malabar, Fla, 1994, Krieger Publishing.
11. Gottdenker NL, Jacobson ER: Effect of venipuncture sites on hematologic and clinical biochemical values in desert tortoises (Gopherus agassizii), Am J Vet Res 56:19-21, 1995.
12. Harr KE, Alleman AR, Dennis PM, et al: Morphologic and cytochemical characteristics of blood cells and hematologic and plasma biochemical reference ranges in green iguanas, J Am Vet Med Assoc 218:915-921, 2001.
13. Hernandez-Divers SJ, MacDonald J: Diagnosis and surgical treatment of thyroid adenoma-induced hyperthyroidism in a green iguana (Iguana iguana), J Zoo Wildl Med 32:465-475, 2001.
14. Jackson OF: Chelonians. In Beynon PH, Cooper JE, editors: Manual of exotic pets, Gloucestershire, Great Britain, 1991, British Small Animal Veterinary Association.
15. Jacobson ER: Evaluation of the reptile patient. In Jacobson ER, Kollias GV Jr, editors: Exotic animals, New York, 1988, Churchill Livingstone.
16. Johnson JH, Benson PA: Laboratory reference values for a group of captive ball pythons (Python regius), Am J Vet Res 57:1304-1307, 1996.
17. Kopplin RP, Tarr RS, Iverson CNM: Serum profile of the iguanid lizard (Dipsosaurus dorsalis), J Zoo Anim Med 14:30-32, 1983.
18. Mader DR: Personal communication, 2003.
19. Mader DR, Horvath CC, Paul-Murphy J: The hematocrit and serum profile of the gopher snake (Pituophis melanoleucas catenifer), J Zoo Anim Med 16:139-140, 1985.
20. Marks SK, Citino SB: Hematology and serum chemistry of the radiated tortoise (Testudo radiata), J Zoo Wildl Med 21:342-344, 1990.
21. McDaniel RC, Grunow WA, Daly JJ, et al: Serum chemistry of the diamond-backed water snake (Nerodia rhombifera rhombifera) in Arkansas, J Wildl Dis 20:44-46, 1984.
22. Mitruka BM, Rawnsley HM: Clinical, biochemical, and hematological reference values in normal experimental animals and normal humans, ed 2, New York, 1981, Masson.
23. Nevarez J, Mitchell M, LeBlanc C, Graham P: Determination of plasma biochemistries, ionized calcium, vitamin D3, and hematocrit values in captive green iguanas (Iguana iguana) from El Salvador, Proc Assoc Rept Amph Vet 87-91, 2002.
24. Ramsey EC, Dotson TK: Tissue and serum enzyme activities in the yellow rat snake (Elaphe obsoleta quadrivittata), Am J Vet Res 56:423-428, 1995.
25. Rosskopf WJ Jr: Normal hemogram and blood chemistry values for California desert tortoises, Vet Med Small Anim Clin 85-87, 1982.
26. Rosskopf WJ Jr, Woerpel RW, Yanoff SR: Normal hemogram and blood chemistry values for boa constrictors and pythons, Vet Med Small Anim Clin 822-823, 1982.
27. Samour JH, Hawkey CM, Pugsley S, et al: Clinical and pathological findings related to malnutrition and husbandry in captive giant tortoises (Geochelone species), Vet Rec 299-302, 1986.
28. Stein G: Hematologic and blood chemistry values in reptiles. In Mader DR, editor: Reptile medicine and surgery, Philadelphia, 1996, WB Saunders.
29. Taylor RW Jr, Jacobson ER: Hematology and serum chemistry of the gopher tortoise, Gopherus polyphemus, Comp Biochem Physiol 72A:425-428, 1982.
30. Wright KM, Skeba S: Hematology and plasma chemistries of captive prehensile-tailed skinks (Corucia zebrata), J Zoo Wildl Med 23:429-432, 1992.

WEBSITE LISTINGS

ISIS International Species Information System: file://D:/USAPages/74051018.html

89
REPTILE FORMULARY

RICHARD S. FUNK and
GERALDINE DIETHELM

The dosages in this formulary have been compiled from several sources over several years. The authors have not attempted to verify all of the dosages, as many of the reported dosages have been derived empirically by reptilian practitioners with many years of experience. The most recent reference for each dose has been cited should the reader have an interest in exploring the original use of any of these drugs.

In addition, it is important to mention that there are no drugs currently approved by the FDA for use in reptiles and amphibians. Although most of the following dosages have been taken from "reliable" published reports, many of these drugs have not withstood the rigors of research and safety testing, and some of the original authors actually give warnings regarding their use (when warnings were made, they have been included in this formulary). Substantial additional experience is needed with many of these pharmaceuticals. All practitioners should be cognizant of the legal implications when using extra- and off-label drugs and are encouraged to discuss these eventualities with their clients prior to using each medication.

In some cases, certain drugs may have markedly different dosages listed for treatment options. It is not uncommon to find one source citing a drug with a dose that differs from a second source by a factor of 10 or greater. In these cases, instead of hybridizing and creating an artificially wide range, the authors have included all dosages that appear in print. The reader must decide on an appropriate dose based on the clinical situation. If two authors report similar dosages, the common value is listed and both sources are cited.

Drug dosages that have been pharmacokinetically derived based on actual research are designated "PD." Bear in mind, however, that many of these reports are based on a single species, and, in some case, only a single administration of the medication. Recommended dosages are extrapolations of these single-dose trials. Readers interested in original research involving reptile therapeutics are referred to Chapter 36.

All of the dosages supplied are to be used as a "place to start." In clinical veterinary medicine, it is not practical for practitioners faced with therapeutic challenges to perform proper clinical trials every time they have an ill patient. The drugs listed have been used with limited success and fulfill the requirement of "acceptable standards of practice."

Please use the information contained herein with care and thought. The authors encourage all reptile practitioners to keep accurate records of drug usage and report any relevant information in the appropriate literature. It will be through such efforts that our understanding of these unique patients will further be defined.

Table 89-1 Antimicrobial Agents Used in Reptiles*

Agent	Dosage	Species/Comments
Amikacin	—	Potentially nephrotoxic; maintain hydration; frequently used with penicillin or cephalosporin
	5 mg/kg IM, then 2.5 mg/kg q 72 h[138]	Snakes/PD (Gophersnakes); house at high end of optimum temperature range during treatment; use 1 mg/kg for Blood Pythons and 2 mg/kg for Black-headed and Rock Pythons[148]
	3 mg/kg q 72 h SC, IM[107]	Pythons/PD (Ball Pythons)
	5 mg/kg IM, then 2.5 mg/kg q 72 h[7,60]	Lizards
	5 mg/kg IM q 24 h[7]	Lizards
	5 mg/kg IM q 48 h[34]	Chelonians/PD (Gopher Tortoises)
	5 mg/kg IM, then 2.5 mg/kg q 72 h[143]	Chelonians
	2.5-3.0 mg/kg IM q 72 h × 5 treatments[200]	Seaturtles
	2.25 mg/kg IM q 72 h[98]	Crocodilians/PD (alligators)
	50 mg/10 mL saline solution × 30 min nebulization q 12 h[153]	Most species/pneumonia
	50-75 mg/10 mL saline solution × 30 min nebulization q 12 h[125]	Aminophylline at 25 mg/9 mL of sterile saline solution in nebulizer before antibiotics for bronchodilation[169]; addition of hyaluronidase to nebulization solution (100-150 U/100 mL) aids in breakdown of proteinaceous debris[125]
	2.5 mg/7.5 mL DMSO q 12-24 h topical × 3-4 wk[189]	For deep local penetration; abscesses involving bone

Continued

Table 89-1 Antimicrobial Agents Used in Reptiles*—cont'd

Agent	Dosage	Species/Comments
Amoxicillin	22 mg/kg PO q 12-24 h[66]	Use with aminoglycoside
	10 mg/kg IM q 24 h[195]	Use with aminoglycoside
Ampicillin	—	May be used with aminoglycoside
	3-6 mg/kg PO, SC, IM q 12-24 h[64,66]	Most species
	10 mg/kg SC, IM q 12 h[104] or 20 mg/kg SC, IM q 24 h[19,189]	Most species, including chameleons
	20 mg/kg IM q 24 h[143,161]	Chelonians
	6 mg/kg IM q 12 h[100]	Chelonians/ulcerative shell disease
	50 mg/kg IM q 12 h[93,188]	Tortoises/preliminary study
Azithromycin	10 mg/kg PO q 2-7 d[42]	Ball Pythons; only single-dose study done; may cause nonregenerative anemia; *Mycoplasma, Cryptosporidium, Giardia,* and other susceptible organisms; location dictates dosage frequency: skin q 3 d, respiratory tract q 5 d, liver/kidneys q 7 d
Carbenicillin	400 mg/kg IM q 24 h[121]	Snakes/PD
	200 mg/kg IM q 24 h[88]	Carpet Pythons
	400 mg/kg SC, IM q 24 h[7]	Lizards/may be used with an aminoglycoside (administer at different time of day)
	400 mg/kg IM q 48 h[122]	Chelonians/PD (*Testudo* spp.)
	200-400 mg/kg IM q 48 h[143,161]	Chelonians/may be used with aminoglycoside; may cause skin sloughing in Desert Tortoises
Cefotaxime	20-40 mg/kg IM q 24 h[66,161]	May be used with aminoglycoside
	100 mg/10 mL saline solution × 30 min nebulization q 12 h[153]	Most species/pneumonia; addition of hyalurondiase (Wydase) to nebulization solution (100-150 U/100 mL) aids in breakdown of proteinaceous debris[125]
Ceftazidime	20 mg/kg SC, IM, IV q 72 h[7,96,120]	Most species/PD (snakes); especially effective against gram − (i.e., *Pseudomonas*); q 24-48 h in chameleons[190]
	20 mg/kg IM, IV q 72 h[194]	Seaturtles
Ceftiofur	2.2 mg/kg IM q 48 h[195]	Snakes
	2.2 mg/kg IM q 24 h[195]	Turtles
	4 mg/kg IM q 24 h[66]	Tortoises/respiratory infection
	5 mg/kg SC, IM q 24 h[18]	Lizards (*Iguana iguana*)
Cefuroxime	50 mg/kg IM q 48 h[2]	Most species
	100 mg/kg IM q 24 h[53,66]	Most species, including snakes/may be used with an aminoglycoside
Cephalexin	20-40 mg/kg PO q 12 h[195]	Most species
Cephaloridine	10 mg/kg SC, IM q 12 h[64]	Most species
Cephalothin	20-40 mg/kg IM q 12 h[66]	Most species
Cephazolin	20 mg/kg SC, IM q 24 h[137]	Most species/burns
Cefoperazone	100 mg/kg IM q 96 h[186]	Snakes/PD (Ground Snakes)
	125 mg/kg IM q 24 h[186]	Lizards/PD (Tegus)
Chloramphenicol	—	Most species/public health concern; may result in permanent pigmentation change in chameleons given IM; may cause bone marrow suppression in watersnakes;[93] because it is bacteriostatic, it has limited usefulness in reptiles
	40 mg/kg PO, SC, IM q 24 h, or 20 mg/kg PO, SC, IM q 12 h[93,100,102,146,161]	Most species/20 mg/kg may be given q 24 h in larger crocodilians
	40 mg/kg SC q 24 h[32]	Snakes/PD (Gophersnakes)
	50 mg/kg SC q 12-72 h[39,94,97]	Snakes/PD; q 12 h in Indigo Snakes, Ratsnakes, Kingsnakes; q 24 h in boids, Moccasin Snakes; q 48 h in Rattlenakes; q 72 h in Red-bellied Watersnakes
	Topical ophthalmic ointment[100]	Most species
Chlorhexidine	Topical 0.05% aqueous solution or ointment[8,35]	All species/topical disinfection; infectious stomatitis
	1:30 aqueous solution[24]	Most species/topical disinfection; infectious stomatitis; middle ear infection flush in Box Turtles
	1:10 aqueous solution, irrigation q 24 h[146]	Lizards/periodontal disease (irrigation of gingival pockets)
	1:10 dilution, soak 1 h q 12 h[100]	Lizards, snakes/in conjunction with antibiotic therapy; soak at 27°C-30°C (81°F-86°F)
Chlortetracycline	200 mg/kg PO q 24 h[2]	Most species
Ciprofloxacin	10 mg/kg PO q 48 h[53]	Most species
	11 mg/kg PO q 48-72 h[113]	Pythons/PD (Reticulated Pythons)
Clarithromycin	15 mg/kg PO q 48-72 h[105,203] (mycoplasmosis)	Tortoises/PD (Desert Tortoises); upper respiratory tract disease

Table 89-1 Antimicrobial Agents Used in Reptiles*—cont'd

Agent	Dosage	Species/Comments
Clindamycin	2.5-5.0 mg/kg PO q 12 h[64]	Most species/gram + and anaerobes
	5 mg/kg PO q 24 h[195]	Most species
Dihydrostreptomycin	5 mg/kg IM q 12-24 h[66,195]	Most species/maintain hydration
Doxycycline	5-10 mg/kg PO q 24 h × 10-45 d[2,66,102]	Most species/respiratory infection (i.e., mycoplasmosis); may use nystatin concurrently to prevent secondary yeast infections[148]
	10 mg/kg PO q 24 h[206]	Tortoises
	50 mg/kg IM, then 25 mg/kg q 72 h[93,107]	Tortoises
Enrofloxacin	5-10 mg/kg q 24 h PO, SC, IM, ICe[2]	Most species/IM administration is painful and may result in tissue necrosis and sterile abscesses; may cause skin discoloration or tissue necrosis if given SC
	5 mg/kg PO, IM q 24 h[144]	Lizards/PD (Green Iguanas); marked pharmacokinetic variability with PO administration may make IM more suitable in critically ill animals
	10 mg/kg IM q 5 d[89]	Monitors/PD (Savannah Monitors); preliminary data
	6.6 mg/kg IM q 24 h, or 11 mg/kg IM q 48 h[113]	Pythons/PD (Reticulated Pythons); *Pseudomonas*
	10 mg/kg IM q 48 h[208]	Snakes/PD (Burmese Pythons); *Pseudomonas*
	10 mg/kg IM, then 5 mg/kg q 48 h[208]	Snakes/PD (Burmese Pythons)
	5 mg/kg IM q 24-48 h[19,166]	Chelonians and most other reptiles/PD (Gopher Tortoises); hyperexcitation, incoordination, diarrhea reported in Galapagos Tortoise[37]
	5 mg/kg IM q 12-24 h[172]	Chelonians/PD (Star Tortoises); q 12 h for *Pseudomonas* and *Citrobacter*; q 24 h for other bacteria
	5 mg/kg IM q 48 h[200]	Seaturtles
	10 mg/kg IM q 24 h[188]	Chelonians/PD (Hermann's Tortoises)
	5 mg/kg IV q 36 h[81]	Crocodilians/PD (alligators); mycoplasmosis; neurologic symptoms reported in American Alligator
	1-3 mL (50 mg/250 mL sterile water) nasal flush/nostril q 24-48 h[102]	Upper respiratory infection; use until no discharge; use concurrently with parenteral antibiotics
	11.4 mg/7.5 mL DMSO topical q 12-24 h × 3-4 wk[189]	For deep local penetration; abscesses involving bone
Gentamicin	—	Nephrotoxicity has been reported, especially in snakes; maintain hydration; commonly used with penicillin or cephalosporin
	2.5 mg/kg IM q 72 h[32,33]	Snakes/PD (Gopher Snakes)
	2.5-3.0 mg/kg IM, then 1.5 mg/kg q 96 h[85]	Snakes/PD (Blood Pythons)
	3 mg/kg IM q >96 h[9]	Turtles/PD (Eastern Box Turtles); lower dose may be more appropriate
	5 mg/kg IM q 72 h[143,161]	Chelonians
	6 mg/kg IM q 72-96 h[171]	Turtles/PD (Red-eared Sliders)
	2-4 mg/kg IM q 72 h[100]	Tortoises
	1.75-2.25 mg/kg IM q 72-96 h[93,98]	Crocodilians/PD (alligators); respiratory infection
	10-20 mg/15 mL saline solution × 30 min nebulization q 12 h[73,125]	Most species/pneumonia; addition of hyalurondiase (Wydase) to nebulization solution (100-150 U/100 mL) aids in breakdown of proteinaceous debris
	50 mg/9 mL saline × 30 min nebulization q 12 h[169]	Most species; aminophylline at 25 mg/9 mL of sterile saline solution in nebulizer before antibiotics for bronchodilation
	40 mg/1 mL DMSO/8 mL saline solution, nebulization[206]	Tortoises
	Topical ophthalmic ointment[100] or drops	Most species/superficial ocular infection; lesions in oral cavity[134]
Gentamicin/ betamethasone ophthalmic drops	1-2 drops to eye q 12-24 h[105]	Tortoises/upper respiratory infections; may also be given as a reverse nasal flush q 48-72 h or intranasal q 12-24 h
Kanamycin	10-15 mg/kg IM, IV q 24 h (or in divided doses)[64]	Most species/avoid in cases of dehydration or renal or hepatic dysfunction; maintain hydration
Lincomycin	5 mg/kg IM q 12-24 h[53]	Most species/wound infection; potentially nephrotoxic; maintain hydration
	10 mg/kg PO q 24 h[53]	
Marbofloxacin	10 mg/kg PO q 48 h[43]	Ball Python

Continued

Table 89-1 Antimicrobial Agents Used in Reptiles*—cont'd

Agent	Dosage	Species/Comments
Metronidazole	20 mg/kg PO q 24 h × ≥7 d[95]	Most species/anaerobes; dose range 12.5-40 mg/kg[64]
	20 mg/kg PO q 24-48 h[119]	Iguanas/PD; use q 24 h for resistant anaerobes
	20 mg/kg PO q 48 h[118]	Snakes/PD (Yellow Ratsnakes)
	50 mg/kg PO q 48 h[21]	Cornsnake
	50 mg/kg PO q 24 h × 7-14 d[113]	Most species/may be administered concurrently with amikacin for broader spectrum; because of potential side effects at this dose, a lower dose may be prudent[113]
Neomycin	10 mg/kg PO q 24 h[53]	Most species
Oxytetracycline	6-10 mg/kg PO, IM, IV q 24 h[53,64]	Most species/may produce local inflammation at injection site
	5-10 mg/kg IM q 24 h[105]	Tortoises/upper respiratory tract infection (mycoplasmosis)
	10 mg/kg PO q 24 h[164]	Alligators
	10 mg/kg IM, IV q 5 d[82]	Crocodilians/PD (alligators); mycoplasmosis
	41 mg/kg IM, then 21 mg/kg IM q 72 h -or-	Loggerhead Seaturtle
	82 mg/kg IM, then 42 mg/kg IM q 72 h[70]	For minimum plasma concentration of 1 μg/mL or 2 μg/mL, respectively
Penicillin, benzathine	10,000 units/kg IM q 48-96 h[64]	Most species/frequency dependent on temperature; may be used with aminoglycoside
Penicillin G	10,000-20,000 IU/kg SC, IM, IV, ICe q 8-12 h[64]	Most species/infrequently used
Piperacillin	50-100 mg/kg IM q 24 h[64]	Most species/broad-spectrum bactericidal agent; maintain hydration; may use with aminoglycoside
	100-200 mg/kg IM q 24-48 h[104,189]	Most species (including chameleons)/can be administered SC in most species
	50 mg/kg IM, then 25 mg/kg q 24 h[195]	Snakes
	100 mg/kg IM q 48 h[86]	Snakes/PD (Blood Pythons)
	100 mg/10 mL saline solution × 30 min nebulization q 12 h[153,125]	Most species/pneumonia; addition of hyalurondiase (Wydase) to nebulization solution (100-150 U/100 mL) aids in breakdown of proteinaceous debris
Polymyxin B, neomycin, bacitracin cream	Topical[164]	All species
Povidone-iodine solution (0.05%) or ointment	Topical[164]	All species/can soak in 0.005% aqueous solution ≤ 1 h q 12-24 h
Silver sulfadiazine cream	Topical q 24-72 h[134,164]	All species/broad-spectrum antibacterial for skin (i.e., wounds, burns) or oral cavity; dressing is generally not necessary
Streptomycin	10 mg/kg IM q 12-24 h[64]	Potentially nephrotoxic; maintain hydration; avoid in cases of dehydration or renal or hepatic dysfunction
Sulfadiazine	25 mg/kg PO q 24 h[195]	Maintain hydration
Sulfadimethoxine	90 mg/kg IM, then 45 mg/kg q 24 h[64]	Potentially nephrotoxic; maintain hydration
Tetracycline	10 mg/kg PO q 24 h[100]	Most species/seldom used
Ticarcillin	50-100 mg/kg IM q 24 h[64]	Most species/maintain hydration
	50 mg/kg IM, IV q 24 h × 7-10 d or 100 mg/hk IM q 48 h for 5 tx[142]	Loggerhead Seaturtles (n = 3), may cause vomiting; combination with aminoglycoside or β-lactamase inhibitior recommended
Tobramycin	—	Potentially nephrotoxic; maintain hydration; potentiated by β-lactams
	2.5 mg/kg IM q 24-72 h[2,66]	Most species
	2.5 mg/kg IM q 72 h[190]	Chameleons/more frequent administrations have been reported[104]
	10 mg/kg IM q 24 h[53]	Chelonians/can be given q 48 h in tortoises
Trimethoprim/sulfadiazine	—	Maintain hydration; parenteral form must be compounded
	15-25 mg/kg PO q 24 h[195]	Most species
	20-30 mg/kg PO, SC, IM q 24-48 h[113]	Most species
	30 mg/kg IM q 24 h × 2 d, then q 48 h[6,94,143]	Most species; also administered PO or SC
Trimethoprim/sulfamethoxazole	10-30 mg/kg PO q 24 h[64]	Most species/maintain hydration
Tylosin	5 mg/kg IM q 24 h × 10-60 d[66,100]	Most species/mycoplasmosis

*Because reptiles are ectothermic, pharmacokinetics of drugs are influenced by ambient temperature. Antimicrobial therapy should be conducted at the upper end of the patient's preferred optimum temperature zone.
IM, Intramuscularly; *q*, every; *PD*, Pharmacokinetically derived; *SC*, subcutaneously; *DMSO*, dimethyl sulfoxide; *PO*, orally; *IV*, intravenously; *ICe*, intracoelemically.

Table 89-2 Antiviral Agents Used in Reptiles

Agent	Dosage	Species/Comments
Acyclovir	80 mg/kg PO q 24 h × 10 d[113]	Tortoises/antiviral (i.e., herpes virus dermatitis); nebulization may help[158]
	Topical (5% ointment) q 12 h[175]	Tortoises/antiviral (i.e., herpes virus dermatitis)

PO, Orally; q, every.

Table 89-3 Antifungal Agents Used in Reptiles

Agent	Dosage	Species/Comments
Amphotericin-B	0.5-1 mg/kg IV, ICe q 24-72 h × 14-28 d[53]	Most species/aspergillosis
	1 mg/kg IT q 24 h × 2-4 wk[101]	Most species/respiratory infection; dilute with water or saline solution
	0.5 mg/kg IV q 48-72 h[64]	Most species/nephrotoxic; can use in combination with ketoconazole; administer slowly
	0.1 mg/kg intrapulmonary q 24 h × 4 wk[83]	*Testudo Graeca*/pneumonia
	5 mg/150 mL saline solution × 1 h nebulization q 12 h × 7 d[92]	Most species/pneumonia
Chlorhexidine	20 mL/gal water bath[204]	Lizards/dermatophytosis
Clotrimazole	Topical[175]	Most species/dermatitis; may bathe q 12 h with dilute organic iodine before use
Fluconazole	5 mg/kg PO q 24 h[204]	Lizards/dermatophytosis
	21 mg/kg SC once, then 10 mg/kg SC 5 d later[69,140]	Loggerhead Seaturtle (*Caretta caretta*)
Griseofulvin	20-40 mg/kg PO q 72 h × 5 treatments[175]	Most species/dermatitis; limited success
Itraconazole	23.5 mg/kg PO q 24 h[65]	Lizards/PD (Spiny Lizards); after 3-d treatment, therapeutic plasma concentration persists for 6 d beyond peak concentration; treatment interval was not determined
	5 mg/kg PO q 24 h[78]	Panther Chameleon
	5 mg/kg PO q 24 h or 15 mg/kg PO q 72 h[141]	Kemp's Ridley Seaturtles
Ketoconazole	—	May use antibiotics concomitantly to prevent bacterial overgrowth; may use concurrently with thiabendazole
	15-30 mg/kg PO q 24 h × 2-4 wk[66]	Most species
	25 mg/kg PO q 24 h × 3 wk[93]	Snakes, turtles
	15-30 mg/kg PO q 24 h × 2-4 wk[143,162]	Chelonians/PD (Gopher Tortoises); systemic infection
	50 mg/kg PO q 24 h × 2-4 wk[195]	Crocodilians
Malachite green	0.15 mg/L water × 1 h bath × 14 d[53]	Dermatitis
Miconazole	Topical[175]	Most species/dermatitis; may bathe q 12 h with dilute organic iodine before use
Nystatin	100,000 IU/kg PO q 24 h × 10 d[92]	Most species/enteric yeast infections; limited success
Thiabendazole	50 mg/kg PO q 24 h × 2 wk[100]	Chelonians/pneumonia; dermatitis; may use concurrently with ketoconazole
Tolnaftate 1% cream	Topical q 12 h prn[2]	Most species/dermatitis; may bathe q 12 h with dilute organic iodine before use

IV, Intravenously; *ICe*, intracoelemically; *q*, every; *IT*, intratracheal; *PO*, orally; *SC*, subcutaneously; *PD*, Pharmacokinetically derived; *prn*, as required.

Table 89-4 Antiparasitic Agents Used in Reptiles

Agent	Dosage	Species/Comments
Albendazole	50 mg/kg PO[195]	Most species/ascarids
Carbaryl powder (5%)	Topical q 7 d prn[7]	Most species, primarily snakes/mites; apply sparingly; may rinse after 1-5 min; must treat environment concurrently; alternatively, dust empty cage lightly, place animal in cage for 24 h, then bathe animal and wash cage
Chloroquine	125 mg/kg PO q 48 h × 3 treatments[195]	Tortoises/hemoprotozoa
Dimetridazole	100 mg/kg PO, repeat in 2 wk,[94] or 40 mg/kg PO q 24 h × 5-8 d[147]	Snakes (except Milksnakes and Indigo Snakes)/amoebae, flagellates; not available in United States
	40 mg/kg PO, repeat in 2 wk[94]	Milksnakes and Indigo Snakes/amoebae, flagellates
Emetine	0.5 mg/kg SC, IM q 24 h × 10 d[2]	Most species/amoebae, trematodes; higher doses (2.5-5 mg/kg) have been reported[114]; avoid use in debilitated animals
Fenbendazole	—	Drug of choice for nematodes; may have an antiprotozoan effect[111]; can be given percloacally or use powdered form on food in tortoises[90]
	25 mg/kg PO q 7 d for up to 4 treatments[112]	All species
	50-100 mg/kg PO, repeat q 14 d prn[7,92,94,143]	All species/use 25 mg/kg in Ball Pythons
	50 mg/kg PO q 24 h × 3-5 d[67]	All species; in chameleons for flagellates, nematodes, and giardia[116]
	50 mg/kg PO q 24 h × 3 d q 7-10 d[116]	Chameleons, nematodes
	50 mg/kg PO q 24 h × 3 d or 100 mg/kg PO q 14-21 d[206]	Tortoises
	100 mg/kg PO q 48 h × 3 treatments; repeat 3 treatments in 3 wk[24,148]	Turtles/lower dose (25 mg/kg) has also been recommended[109]
Fipronil	Spray or wipe over q 7-10 d[55]	Most species/mites, ticks; beware of reactions to alcohol carrier; use with caution; use in reptiles needs further evaluation[35]
Ivermectin	—	Do not use in chelonians (may be toxic),[198] crocodilians,[111] Indigo Snakes, and skinks[29]
	0.2 mg/kg PO, SC, IM, repeat in 2 wk[7,61,93,202]	Snakes (except Indigos), lizards (except skinks)[29]/nematodes, mites; caution: colored animals may have skin discoloration at injection site; rarely, adverse effects have been observed in chameleons, possibly associated with breakdown of parasites[7]; do not use within 10 d of diazepam and tiletamine/zolazepam; can dilute with propylene glycol; narrower range of safety than fenbendazole; rare deaths and occasional nervous system signs, lethargy, or inappetence have been reported (especially in lizards);[111] used for Pentastomids in Monitor Lizards (used with dexamethasone 0.2 mg/kg q 2 d)[61]; surgical removal may still be necessary[58]
	5[2,112]-10 mg[112]/L water topical q 4-5 d up to 4 wk[112]	Snakes, lizards/mites; spray on skin and in cage; some wash cage out 15 min later, others let cage dry before replacing reptile; some recommend ivermectin spray for the animal and pyrethroid or larval inhibitor for environment[110]
Levamisole	5-10 mg/kg SC, ICe, repeat in 2 wk[113] (5 mg/kg in chelonians[143]; 10 mg/kg in lizards,[7] snakes[92])	Most species/nematodes (including lungworms); very narrow range of safety; main advantage is that it can be administered parenterally; avoid concurrent use with chloramphenicol; avoid use in debilitated animals; low dose may stimulate depressed immune system; can be used IM, but less effective
	10-20 mg/kg SC, IM, ICe[101]	Most species, including turtles
Mebendazole	20-100 mg/kg PO, repeat in 14 d[55]	Most species/strongyles, ascarids
Metronidazole	—	Protozoan (i.e., flagellates, amoebae) overgrowth; may stimulate appetite; may cause seizures if overdosed[93]; for small patients, injectable form can be administered PO; oral liquid is not available in United States, but can be compounded

Table 89-4 Antiparasitic Agents Used in Reptiles—cont'd

Agent	Dosage	Species/Comments
	25-40 mg/kg PO on days 1, 3 or q 24 h for up to 1 wk[112]	Most species
	50 mg/kg PO q 48 h[21]	Cornsnake
	40-125 mg/kg PO, repeat in 10-14 d[111,113]	Most species/q 72 h × 5-7 treatments for amoebae
	100 mg/kg PO q 3 d × 2-3 wk[8]	Most species
	100 mg/kg PO, repeat in 2 wk[7,93-95]	Most species (except Uracoan Rattlesnakes, Milksnakes, Tricolor Kingsnakes, and Indigo Snakes)
	125-250 mg/kg PO, repeat in 2 wk[64,161]	Most species/recommend using lower end of dose range
	40 mg/kg PO, repeat in 2 wk[94]	Uracoan Rattlesnake, Milksnake, Tricolor Kingsnake, and Indigo Snakes
	40-60 mg/kg PO q 7-14 d × 2-3 treatments[190]	Chameleons
	50 mg/kg PO q 24 h × 2-5 d[116]	Chameleons, when accompanied by increased GI symptoms
	40-200 mg/kg PO, repeat in 2 wk[150]	Geckos/ocular lesions (40 mg/kg) and subcutaneous lesions (200 mg/kg) caused by *Trichomonas*
	50 mg/kg PO q 24 h × 3-5 d or 100 mg/kg PO q 14-21 d[206]	Chelonians (tortoises)/use lower dosage for severe cases
Milbemycin	0.25-0.50 mg/kg SC[20] prn	Chelonians/nematodes; parenteral form is not commercially available in United States; fenbendazole preferred
	0.5-1 mg/kg PO[20] prn	Chelonians/nematodes; fenbendazole preferred
Nitrofurazone	25.5 mg/kg PO[201]	Most species/coccidia; seldom used
Olive oil	Coat q 7 d[7]	Most species, especially small, delicate lizards/mites; wash animal with mild soap (and rinse well) the next day; messy to use; environment must be treated
Oxfendazole	68 mg/kg PO, repeat in 14-28 d prn[55]	Most species/nematodes
Paromomycin	35-100 mg/kg PO q 24 h × ≤4 wk[64,92,202]	Most species/amoebae
	300-360 mg/kg PO q 48 h × 14 d[163]	Lizards (Gila Monsters)/cryptosporidia
	300-800 mg/kg PO q 24 h[41] prn	Geckos/cryptosporidia; reduced clinical signs; does not eliminate organism
	100 mg/kg PO q 24 h × 7 d, then 2 ×/wk × 3 mo[46]	Snakes/cryptosporidia; reduced clinical signs and oocyte shedding; does not eliminate organism
Permethrin	Topical, repeat in 10 d[22]	Most species/mites; pyrethroid; safer than pyrethrins; use with care; dilute to 1% solution and apply lightly via spray bottle in well-ventilated enclosure (with water bowl removed for 24 h); blot off excess; administer in conjunction with environmental control; Proventamite topically on tortoises, treatment of substrate in lizards and snakes after removal from environment[31]
Piperazine	40-60 mg/kg PO, repeat in 2 wk[2]	Most species/nematodes
	50 mg/kg PO, repeat in 2 wk[100]	Crocodilians
Praziquantel (Droncit, Mobay)	8 mg/kg PO, SC, IM, repeat in 2 wk[7,94,104]	Most species/cestodes, trematodes; doses >8 mg/kg have shown potential for treating pentastomids[114]; higher dosages have been administered PO[3,19]
	5-10 mg/kg PO q 14 d[116]	Chameleons; flukes may best be left untreated if not causing a problem[116]
	25 mg/kg PO q 3 h × 3 treatments[99]	Seaturtles/PD Loggerhead Seaturtles
Pyrantel pamoate	5 mg/kg PO, repeat in 2 wk[64]	Most species/nematodes
Pyrethrin spray (0.09%)	Topical q 7 d × 2-3 treatments	Most species/use water-based sprays labeled for kittens and puppies; apply with cloth; can also spray cage, wash out after 30 min; use sparingly and with caution; pyrethroids are safer (see permethrin, resmethrin)
Quinacrine	19-100 mg/kg PO q 48 h × 2-3 wk[201]	Most species/some hematozoa
Quinine sulfate	75 mg/kg PO q 48 h × 2-3 wk[201]	Most species/some hematozoa; toxic at >100 mg/kg q 24 h; ineffective against exoerythrocytic forms

Continued

Table 89-4 Antiparasitic Agents Used in Reptiles—cont'd

Agent	Dosage	Species/Comments
Resmethrin spray or shampoo	Topical[139], repeat prn q ≥10 d	Most species/mites; pyrethroid; safer than pyrethrins; use with care; spray (0.35%) or shampoo entire animal, then rinse off immediately in running, tepid water; protect eyes (other than snakes) with 1 drop of mineral oil; lightly spray environment, wipe off in 5-10 min
Spiramycin	160 mg/kg PO q 24 h × 10 d[45,46]	Snakes/cryptosporidia; may reduce clinical signs and oocyte shedding; does not eliminate organism
Sulfadiazine, sulfamerazine	25 mg/kg PO q 24 h × 3 wk[7,100,201]	Snakes, lizards/coccidia; avoid in cases of dehydration or renal dysfunction
	50 mg/kg PO q 24 h × 3 d, off 3 d, on 3 d[107]	Most species/avoid in cases of dehydration or renal dysfunction
	75 mg/kg PO, then 45 mg/kg q 24 h × 5 d[64,201,116]	Most species/coccidia
Sulfadimethoxine (Albon, Roche)	—	Coccidia; avoid in cases of dehydration or renal dysfunction
	50 mg/kg PO q 24 h × 3-5 d, then q 2 d prn[107,115]	Most species
	90 mg/kg PO, IM, IV, then 45 mg/kg q 24 h × 5-7 d[66,92,201]	Most species
Sulfadimidine (33% solution)	1 oz/gal drinking water × 10 d[201]	Most species/coccidia
	0.3-0.6 mL/kg PO q 24 h × 10 d[201]	Most species/coccidia; alternatively, 0.3-0.6 mg/kg, then 0.15-0.30 mg/kg q 24 h × 2-10 d
Sulfamethazine	75 mg/kg PO, IM, IV, then 40 mg/kg q 24 h × 5-7 d[2,66,92]	Most species/coccidia
	50 mg/kg PO q 24 h × 3 d, off 3 d, on 3 d[107]	Most species/coccidia
	25 mg/kg PO, IM q 24 h × 7-21 d[2,201]	Snakes/coccidia
Sulfamethoxydiazine	80 mg/kg SC, IM, then 40 mg/kg q 24 h × 4 d[201]	Most species/coccidia
Sulfaquinoxaline	75 mg/kg PO, then 40 mg/kg q 24 h × 5-7 d[92]	Most species/coccidia
Thiabendazole	50-100 mg/kg PO, repeat in 2 wk[64,94]	Most species/nematodes; fenbendazole preferred
Trimethoprim/sulfa	30 mg/kg IM q 24 h × 2 d, then 15 mg/kg q 48 h × 5-14 d[201]	Most species/coccidia; may be administered SC[148]
	30 mg/kg PO q 24 h × 7 d, or 15 mg/kg PO q 12 h × 7 d[102]	Most species/coccidia
	30 mg/kg PO q 24 h × 2 d, then q 48 h × 3 wk[7,201]	Most species/coccidia
	30-60 mg/kg PO q 24 h × 2 mo[2]	Snakes/use in treatment of cryptosporidia is of questionable value; may be toxic at this dosage
Vapona No-Pest Strip	6-mm strip/10 ft^3 × 3-5 d; 2.5 cm^2 in perforated plastic film container × 2-5 d[64,66]	Most species/mites; use with caution; prevent contact with animals (i.e., place strip above cage); avoid in cases of renal or hepatic dysfunction; remove water container; some recommend not to use continuously (expose 2-3 h, 2-3×/wk for 3-4 wk)[107] because of its toxicity and availability of safer alternatives, use is discouraged
Water	Bath × 30 min[133]	Snakes, lizards/mites; use lukewarm water; safe, but not very effective; does not kill mites on head

PO, Orally; *q*, every; *prn*, as required; *SC*, subcutaneously; *IM*, intramuscularly; *ICe*, intracoelemically; *GI*, gastrointestinal; *IV*, intravenously.

Table 89-5 Chemical Restraint/Anesthetic/Analgesic Agents Used in Reptiles

Agent	Dosage	Species/Comments
Acepromazine	0.05-0.25 mg/kg IM[102]	Most species/can be used as preanesthetic with ketamine
	0.1-0.5 mg/kg IM[151,160]	Most species/preanesthetic; reduce by 50% if used with barbiturate
Alphaxalone/alphadalone	6-9 mg/kg IV, or 9-15 mg/kg IM[123]	Most species/good muscle relaxation; variable results; drug requires more evaluation; may have violent recovery;[11] don't use within 10 days of DMSO treatment; not available in United States
	9 mg/kg IV, intracardiac[151]	Snakes/induction 5 min; good muscle relaxation; variable results; minimal effect if administered IM
	15 mg/kg IM[151]	Lizards, chelonians/induction 35-40 min; duration 15-35 min; good muscle relaxation; variable results
	24 mg/kg ICe[68]	Chelonians (Red-eared Sliders)/surgical anesthesia with good relaxation
Atipamezole	5× medetomidine dose IM, IV[62,185,183]	Medetomidine reversal; causes severe hypotension in Gopher Tortoises when given IV[48]
Atropine	0.01-0.04 mg/kg SC, IM,[23] IV,[64] ICe[180]	Most species/preanesthetic; bradycardia; rarely indicated; generally use only in profound or prolonged bradycardia[153]; does not work at this dose in Green Iguana[159]
Buprenorphine	0.005-0.02 mg/kg IM q 24-48 h[74]	Analgesia
	mg/kg IM[16]	Analgesia
	0.01 mg/kg IM[124]	Analgesia
Butorphanol	—	Butorphanol combination follows; see ketamine for combinations
	0.4-1.0 mg/kg SC, IM[180]	Analgesia; sedation; preanesthetic; 0.2 mg/kg IM used experimentally in tortoises[74]
	0.05 mg/kg IM q 24 h × 2-3 d[132]	Lizards (iguanas)
	1.0-1.5 mg/kg SC, IM[180]	Lizards/administer 30 min before isoflurane for smooth, shorter induction
	1-2 mg/kg IM[16]	Snakes, analgesia
	0.5-2 mg/kg IM or 0.2-0.5 mg/kg IV, IO[16]	Preanesthetic
Butorphanol (B)/midazolam (M)	(B) 0.4 mg/kg/(M) 2 mg/kg IM[15]	Preanesthetic; administer 20 min before induction
Carprofen	1-4 mg/kg PO, SC, IM, IV q 24 h,[124] follow with ½ dose q 24-72 h[145]	Analgesia; nonsteroidal antiinflammatory
Chlorpromazine	0.1-0.5 mg/kg IM[64]	Most species/preanesthetic; not commonly used
	10 mg/kg IM[11]	Chelonians/preanesthetic
Diazepam	—	Diazepam combination follows; see ketamine for combinations
	—	Muscle relaxation; give 20 min before anesthesia; potentially reversible with flumazenil
	2.5 mg/kg IM, IV[176]	Most species/seizures
	0.2-0.8 mg/kg IM[180]	Snakes/used in conjunction with ketamine for anesthesia with muscle relaxation
	2.5 mg/kg PO[177]	Iguanas/reduce anxiety, which often leads to aggression
	0.2-1.0 mg/kg IM[180]	Chelonians/used in conjunction with ketamine for anesthesia with muscle relaxation
Diazepam (D)/ succinylcholine (S)	(D) 0.2-0.6 mg/kg IM, followed in 20 min (S) 0.14-0.37 mg/kg IM[187]	Alligators
Disoprofol	5-15 mg/kg IV to effect[28]	All species/anesthesia; similar characteristics to propofol; not available in United States
Doxapram	5 mg/kg IM, IV[15] q 10 min prn	Respiratory stimulant; reduces recovery time; reported to partially "reverse" effects of dissociatives[127]
	4-12 mg/kg IM, IV[180]	Respiratory stimulant
Etorphine	0.3-2.75 mg/kg IM[123]	Crocodilians, chelonians/very potent narcotic; crocodilians: induction, 5-30 min; duration, 30-180 min; chelonians: induction, 10-20 min; duration, 40-120 min; not very effective in reptiles other than the alligator[160]; poor relaxation; adequate for immobilization and minor procedures; requires antagonist; limited use because of expense and legal restrictions
	0.3-0.5 mg/kg IM[151]	
Flumazenil	1 mg/20 mg of zolazepam,[127] IM, IV[170]	Crocodilians, chelonians/reversal of zolazepam
Flunixin meglumine	0.1-0.5 mg/kg IM q 12-24 h[124]	Analgesia; use for maximum of 3 d
	1-2 mg/kg IM q 2 4h × 2 treatments[28,191]	Lizards/postsurgical analgesia; see Table 89-7

Continued

Table 89-5: Chemical Restraint/Anesthetic/Analgesic Agents Used in Reptiles—cont'd

Agent	Dosage	Species/Comments
Gallamine	0.4-1.25 mg/kg IM[13]	Crocodiles/results in flaccid paralysis, but no analgesia; larger animals require lower dosage; reverse with neostigmine; use in alligators questionable; unsafe in alligators at ≥1.0 mg/kg[160]
	0.6-4 mg/kg IM[128]	
	0.7 mg/kg IM[152]	
	1.2-2 mg/kg IM[62]	
Glycopyrrolate	0.01 mg/kg SC,[23] IM, IV[15]	Most species/preanesthetic; for excess oral or respiratory mucus; rarely indicated; generally use only in profound or prolonged bradycardia; may be preferable to atropine[64]; does not work at this dose in Green Iguana[159]
Halothane	3%-4% induction, 1.5%-2.0% maintenance[23,64]	Most species/isoflurane preferred; in lizards, in particular, use lowest concentration needed
Hyaluronidase	25 IU/dose SC[127]	Crocodilians/combine with premedication, anesthetic, or reversal drugs to accelerate SC absorption
Isoflurane	3%-5% induction,[101] 1.0%-3.0% maintenance[1,29]	Most species/inhalation anesthetic of choice in reptiles; induction, 6-20 min; recovery, 30-60 min; not as smooth in reptiles as compared with other animals; intubation and intermittent positive pressure ventilation advisable; may preanesthetize with low dose of propofol, ketamine, etc
Ketamine	—	Ketamine combinations follow
	—	Muscle relaxation and analgesia may be marginal; prolonged recovery with higher doses; larger reptiles require lower dose than smaller reptiles; painful at injection site; safety is questionable in debilitated patients; avoid use in cases with renal dysfunction; snakes may be permanently aggressive after ketamine anesthesia[11]; generally recommended to be used only as a preanesthetic before isoflurane for surgical anesthesia
	22-44 mg/kg SC, IM[11-13]	Most species/sedation
	55-88 mg/kg SC, IM[12,13]	Most species/surgical anesthesia; induction, 10-30 min; recovery, 24-96 h
	10 mg/kg SC, IM q 30 min[23]	Most species/maintenance of anesthesia; recovery, 3-4 h
	20-60 mg/kg IM, or 5-15 mg/kg IV[102]	Most species/muscle relaxation improved with diazepam 2-5 mg/kg[44]
	20-60 mg/kg SC, IM[23,106]	Snakes/sedation; induction, 30 min, recovery, 2-48 h
	60-80 mg/kg IM[29]	Snakes/light anesthesia; intermittent positive pressure ventilation may be needed at high dose
	5-10 mg/kg IM[180]	Lizards/decreases incidence of breath-holding during chamber induction
	20-30 mg/kg IM[60]	Lizards/sedation (i.e., facilitates endotracheal intubation); preanesthetic; requires lower dose than other reptiles
	30-50 mg/kg SC, IM[23,106]	Lizards/sedation; variable results
	20-60 mg/kg IM[87,106,160]	Chelonians/sedation; induction 30 min; recovery ≥24 h; potentially dangerous in dehydrated and debilitated tortoises
	25 mg/kg IM, IV[200]	Seaturtles/sedation; used at higher doses (50-70 mg/kg), recovery times may be excessively long and unpredictable; combination of ketamine and acepromazine gives more rapid induction and recovery
	38-71 mg/kg ICe[205]	Green Seaturtles/anesthesia; induction, 2-10 min; duration, 2-10 min; recovery, <30 min
	60-90 mg/kg IM[106,151]	Chelonians/light anesthesia; induction, <30 min; recovery h to d; requires higher doses than most other reptiles
	20-40 mg/kg SC, IM, ICe (sedation), to 40-80 mg/kg (anesthesia)[127]	Crocodilians/induction, <30-60 min; recovery, h to d; in larger animals, 12-15 mg/kg may permit tracheal intubation[180]
Ketamine (K)/butorphanol (B)	(K) 10-30 mg/kg, (B) 0.5-1.5 mg/kg IM[180]	Chelonians/minor surgical procedures (i.e., shell repair)
	See (K) dosages, (B) ≤1.5 mg/kg IM[180]	Snakes/anesthesia with improved muscle relaxation
Ketamine (K)/diazepam (D)	(K) 60-80 mg/kg,[151] (D) 0.2-1.0 mg/kg IM[180]	Chelonians/anesthesia; muscle relaxation
	See (K) dosages, (D) 0.2-0.8 mg/kg IM[180]	Snakes/anesthesia with improved muscle relaxation
Ketamine (K)/medetomidine (M)	—	Reverse medetomidine with atipamezole
	(K) 10 mg/kg, (M) 0.1-0.3 mg/kg IM[54]	Most species

Table 89-5 Chemical Restraint/Anesthetic/Analgesic Agents Used in Reptiles—cont'd

Agent	Dosage	Species/Comments
	(K) 5-10 mg/kg IM, (M) 0.10-0.15 mg/kg IM, IV[76]	Lizards (iguanas)
	(K) 3-8 mg/kg, (M) 0.025-0.080 mg/kg IV[129]	Giant Tortoises (Aldabra)
	(K) 5 mg/kg, (M) 0.05 mg/kg IM[156]	Tortoises (Gopher)/light anesthesia; tracheal intubation; inconsistent results
	(K) 5-10 mg/kg IM, (M) 0.10-0.15 mg/kg IM, IV[76]	Tortoises (small-medium)
	(K) 7.5 mg/kg, (M) 0.075 mg/kg IM[156]	Tortoises (Gopher)/anesthesia; tracheal intubation
	(K) 10-15 mg/kg, (M) 0.15-0.25 mg/kg IM juveniles[79]	American Alligator/juveniles
	(K) 5-10 mg/kg, (M) 0.1-0.15 mg/kg IM adult[79]	Alligators/adults
	(K) 4 mg/kg, (M) 0.04 mg/kg IM[80]	Green Seaturtle
	(K) 5 mg/kg, (M) 0.05 mg/kg IV[38]	Loggerhead Seaturtle, induction of anesthesia for intubation
	(K) 10-20 mg/kg IM, (M) 0.15-0.30 mg/kg IM, IV[76]	Turtles (freshwater)
Ketamine (K)/ midazolam (M)	(K) 20-40 mg/kg, (M) ≤2 mg/kg IM[19]	Chelonians/sedation; muscle relaxation
	(K) 60-80 mg/kg,[151] (M) ≤2 mg/kg IM[180]	Chelonians/anesthesia; muscle relaxation
Ketamine (K)/propofol (P)	(K) 25-30 mg/kg IM, (P) 7 mg/kg IV[167]	Chelonians/administer propofol ≈70-80 min after ketamine; see propofol
Ketoprofen	2 mg/kg SC, IM q 24 h[124]	Analgesia
Lidocaine (0.5%-2.0%)	Local or topical[180]	Local analgesia; infiltrate to effect (i.e., 0.01 mL 2% lidocaine used for local block for IO catheter placement in iguanas)[13]; often used in conjunction with chemical immobilization
Medetomidine	—	See ketamine for combination injectables
	—	Produces poor to no immobilization alone; reversible with atipamezole
	0.10-0.15 mg/kg IM[15]	Most species
	0.15 mg/kg IM[183,185]	Crocodilians, Desert Tortoises (Gopherus agassizii)/sedation; incomplete immobilization; bradycardia, bradypnea
Meloxicam	0.1-0.2 mg/kg PO q 24 h[124]	Analgesia (orthopedic pain); not available in United States
Meperidine	5-10 mg/kg IM q 12-24 h[74]	Analgesia; no noticeable effect in snakes, even at 200 mg/kg[11]
	2-4 mg/kg ICe[2]	Nile Crocodiles/analgesia
Methohexital	5-20 mg/kg SC,[13] IV[64]	Most species/induction, 5-30 min; recovery, 1-5 h; use at 0.125%-0.5% concentration; much species variability; decrease dose 20%-30% for young animals; avoid use in debilitated animals
	9-10 mg/kg SC,[154] ICe	Colubrids/induction, ≥22 min; recovery, 2-5 h; does not produce soft tissue irritation seen with other barbiturates; may need to adjust dosage in obese snakes
Methoxyflurane	3%-4% induction, 1.5%-2.0% maintenance[64]	Not commonly used
Metomidate	10 mg/kg IM[55,178]	Snakes/profound sedation; not available in United States
Midazolam	—	See butorphanol, ketamine for combinations; potentially reversible by flumazenil
	2 mg/kg IM[11,13]	Most species/preanesthetic; increases efficacy of ketamine; effective in Snapping Turtles, not in Painted Turtles[13]
	1.5 mg/kg IM[157]	Turtles (Red-eared Sliders)/ sedation; onset, 5.5 min; duration, 82 min; recovery, 40 min; much individual variability
Morphine	0.5-4 ICe[185]	Crocodilians/analgesia
Neostigmine	0.063 mg/kg IV[128]	Crocodiles/gallamine reversal; may cause emesis and lacrimation; fast 24-48 h before use; effects enhanced if combined with 75 mg hyaluronidase per dose when administered SC, IM
	0.03-0.25 mg/kg IM[128]	
	0.07-0.14 mg/kg IM[152]	
Oxymorphone	0.025-0.10 mg/kg IV[64]	Some species/analgesia; avoid in cases with hepatic or renal dysfunction; no noticeable effect in snakes, even at 1.5 mg/kg[11]

Continued

Table 89-5	Chemical Restraint/Anesthetic/Analgesic Agents Used in Reptiles—cont'd	
Agent	**Dosage**	**Species/Comments**
Oxymorphone—cont'd	0.5-1.5 mg/kg IM[64]	Some species/analgesia
	0.05-0.2 mg/kg SC, IM q 12-48 h[74]	
Pentazocine	2-5 mg/kg IM q 6-24 h[74]	Analgesia
Pentobarbital	15-30 mg/kg ICe[151]	Snakes/induction, 30-60 min; duration, ≥2 h; prolonged recovery (risk of occasional fatalities); venomous snakes require twice as much as nonvenomous snakes[11]; avoid use in lizards
	10-18 mg/kg ICe[151]	Chelonians
	7.5-15 mg/kg ICe, or 8 mg/kg IM[11,151]	Crocodilians
Pethidine	20 mg/kg IM q 12-24 h[124]	Analgesia; not available in United States
Prednisolone	2-5 mg/kg PO, IM[124]	Analgesia (chronic pain)
Proparacaine	Topical to eye[136]	Desensitizes surface of eye; ineffective in animals with spectacles
Propofol	—	See ketamine for combination
	—	Anesthesia; rapid, smooth induction; may give 15-25 min anesthesia and restraint in most species; rapid, excitement-free recovery; must be administered (slowly) IV (no inflammation if goes perivascularly); may be administered IO; dosages may be reduced by as much as 50% in premedicated (i.e., ketamine) animals; may get apnea and bradycardia; intubation and assisted ventilation generally required; considered by many to be the parenteral agent of choice for inducing anesthesia
	5-10 mg/kg IV, intracardiac[5,178]	Snakes
	3-5 mg/kg IV, IO[75,76]	Lizards (i.e., iguanas)/intubation and minor diagnostic procedures; may need to give an additional increment in 3-5 min; less cardiopulmonary depression than occurs with higher doses
	5-10 mg/kg IO,[17] IV	Iguanas/higher dose is recommended for induction for short-duration procedures or intubation
	10 mg/kg IV, IO[17,55]	Lizards, snakes/0.25 mg/kg/min may be given for maintenance[10]
	2 mg/kg IV[15]	Giant Tortoises
	12-15 mg/kg IV[51]	Chelonians/lower dosages (5-10 mg/kg IV[180]) may be used; 1 mg/kg/min may be given for maintenance[180]
	10-15 mg/kg IV[127]	Crocodilians/duration, 0.5-1.5 h; maintain on gas anesthetics; experimental IM with hyaluronidase[135]
Sevoflurane	prn[75,173]	Most species/anesthesia; rapid induction and recovery when intubated
Rocuronium	0.25-0.5 mg/kg IM	Neuromuscular blocking agent; no analgesia; for intubation only and small, nonpainful procedures[108]
Succinylcholine	—	No analgesia; narrow margin of safety; intermittent positive pressure ventilation generally required; paralysis occurs in 5-30 min; avoid if exposed to organophosphate parasiticides within last 30 d; administer minimal amount required to perform procedure
	0.25-1 mg/kg IM[101]	Most species
	0.75-1 mg/kg IM[23]	Large lizards
	0.1-1 mg/kg IM[104]	Chameleons
	0.5-1 mg/kg IM[29]	Box Turtles/induction, 20-30 min
	0.25-1.5 mg/kg IM[160,161]	Chelonians/induction, 15-30 min; recovery, 45-90 min; facilitates intubation
	0.4-1 mg/kg IM[160]	Alligators/rapid onset; 3-5 mg/kg in smaller animals has been used[13]
	0.5-2 mg/kg IM[13,106]	Crocodilians/variable induction and recovery periods
Thiopental	19-31 mg/kg IV[205]	Green Seaturtles/anesthesia; induction 5-10 min; recovery <6 h; erratic anesthesia
Tiletamine/zolazepam	—	Sedation, anesthesia; severe respiratory depression possible (may need to ventilate)[29]; variable results; may have prolonged recovery; use lower end of dose range in heavier species; good for muscle relaxation before intubation[63,170]
	4-5 mg/kg SC, IM[13]	Most species/sedation; induction, 9-15 min; recovery, 1-12 h; adequate for most noninvasive procedures

Table 89-5 Chemical Restraint/Anesthetic/Analgesic Agents Used in Reptiles—cont'd

Agent	Dosage	Species/Comments
	5-10 mg/kg IM[15]	Most species
	3 mg/kg IM[76]	Snakes/facilitates handling and intubation of large snakes; induction, 30-45 min; prolongs recovery
	10-30 mg/kg IM,[151] to 20-40 mg/kg IM[101,179]	Snakes, lizards/induction, 8-20 min; recovery, 2-10 h; variable results; longer sedation and recovery times at 22°C than at 30°C[196]; good sedation in Boa Constrictors at 25 mg/kg IM[196]; generally need to supplement with inhalation agents for surgical anesthesia; some snakes died at 55 mg/kg
	3.5-14 mg/kg IM[151] (generally, 4-8 mg/kg)	Chelonians/sedation; induction, 8-20 min; does not produce satisfactory anesthesia even at 88 mg/kg[160]
	5-10 mg/kg IM, IV[180]	Large tortoises/facilitates intubation; if light, mask with isoflurane rather than redosing
	2-10 mg/kg IM[180]	Large crocodilians/may permit intubation
	5-10 mg/kg SC, IM, ICe (sedation), 10-40 mg/kg (anesthesia)[127]	Crocodilians
	15 mg/kg IM[40]	Alligators/induction, >20 min; adequate for minor procedures
Xylazine	—	Infrequently used; variable effects; potentially reversible with yohimbine; preanesthetic for ketamine
	0.10-1.25 mg/kg IM, IV[64]	Most species
	1-2 mg/kg IM[127,160]	Nile Crocodiles
Yohimbine	0.1 mg/kg IM[127]	Xylazine reversal

IM, Intramuscularly; *IV*, intravenously; *DMSO*, dimethyl sulfoxide; *ICe*, intracoelemically; *SC*, subcutaneously; *q*, every; *IO*, intraosseously; *PO*, orally, *prn*, as required.

Table 89-6 Hormones and Steroids Used in Reptiles

Agent	Dosage	Species/Comments
Arginine vasotocin	0.01-1 μg/kg IV (preferred), ICe[126] q 12-24 h × several treatments	Most species/dystocias; administer 30-60 min after Ca lactate/Ca glycerophosphate; more effective in reptiles than oxytocin but not commercially available for use in animals; higher doses have been reported; 0.5 μg/kg commonly recommended
Calcitonin	1.5 IU/kg SC q 8 h × 2-3 wk prn[64]	Most species (i.e., iguanas) severe nutritional secondary hyperparathyroidism; administer after Ca supplementation; do not give if hypocalcemic
	50 IU/kg IM, repeat in 2 wk[14,195]	
Dexamethasone	0.60-1.25 mg/kg IM, IV[64]	Shock (septic/traumatic)
	2-4 mg/kg IM, IV q 24 h × 3 d[181]	Inflammatory, noninfectious respiratory disease
Dexamethasone NaPO4	0.10-0.25 mg/kg SC, IM, IV[66]	Shock (septic/traumatic)
Levothyroxine	0.02 mg/kg PO q 48 h[155]	Tortoises/hypothyroidism; stimulates feeding in debilitated tortoises
Nandrolone	1 mg/kg IM q 7-28 d[52]	Anabolic steroid; reduces protein catabolism; may stimulate erythropoiesis
Oxytocin	—	Dystocias; results are variable; works well in chelonians, less so in snakes and lizards; generally administer 1 h after Ca administration; use multiple doses with caution
	1-10 IU/kg IM[60,102]	Most species/higher end of range is commonly used; may be repeated up to 3 × at 90 min. intervals with increasing dosage[91]
	2 IU/kg IM q 4-6 h × 1-3 treatments[8]	Most species
	1-5 IU/kg IM,[50] repeat in 1 h	Lizards/alternatively, 5 IU/kg by slow IV or IO over 4-8 h[50]
	1-2,[25] 2-20,[66,143] or 10-20[24] IU/kg IM	Chelonians
Prednisolone	2-5 mg/kg PO, IM[124]	Analgesia (chronic pain)
Prednisolone Na succinate	5-10 mg/kg IM, IV,[64] IO[52]	Shock; brain swelling from hyperthermia; may help reduce nephrocalcinosis
Stanozolol	5 mg/kg IM q 7 d prn[66]	Most species/anabolic steroid; management of catabolic disease states

IV, Intravenously; *ICe*, intracoelemically; *q*, every; *SC*, subcutaneously; *prn*, as required; *IM*, intramuscularly; *IO*, intraosseously; *PO*, orally.

Table 89-7 Nutritional/Mineral/Fluid Support Used in Reptiles

Agent	Dosage	Species/Comments
Calcium	PO prn	Sources include crushed cuttlebone, oyster shell, Ca lactate, or other commercially available products[114]
Ca carbonate	PO prn	Most species/Ca supplement
Ca gluconate	10-50 mg/kg IM[101]	Most species/hypocalcemia; dystocia
	100 mg/kg SC, IM, ICe[8,195] q 8 h[14]	Most species/nutritional secondary hyperparathyroidism; hypocalcemic muscle tremors; seizures or flaccid paresis in lizards; when patient is stable, switch to oral Ca
	100-200 mg/kg SC, IM[182]	Most species/nutritional secondary hyperparathyroidism; hypocalcemia; dystocia
Ca gluconate/Borogluconate	10-50 mg/kg IM[2]	Most species/hypocalcemia; hypocalcemic dystocia
Ca glubionate	10 mg/kg PO q 12-24 h[2] prn	Most species/nutritional secondary hyperparathyroidism; hypocalcemia; dystocia
Ca lactate/Ca glycerophosphate	1-5 mg/kg SC, IM[2]	Most species/hypocalcemia; hypocalcemic dystocia
	10-25 mg/kg SC, IM[66]	Most species/hypocalcemia; dystocia
	10 mg/kg SC, IM, ICe q 24 h × 1-7 d[7,14]	Lizards (iguanas)/nutritional secondary hyperparathyroidism
Clinicare—feline and canine	After 48-96 h of water or electrolyte solution PO, start on nutritional supplementation[207]	Omnivorous/herbivorous species: canine formula; carnivorous species: feline formula; initially dilute with water 1:1 and gradually increase to full strength over 48 h
Critical Care for Herbivores	20 mL/kg PO[35]	Herbivorous species; nutritional support; anorexia; debility; prepare product according to directions
Crystalloid (nonlactated) solutions	PO, SC, IV, ICe, EpiCe, IO prn[28]	Fluid therapy; can mix with equal parts 5% dextrose[165] (if patient is hypoglycemic) or 0.45% NaCl for initial rehydration[28]
Dextrose (2.5%, 5.0%)	PO, SC, IV, ICe, EpiCe, IO prn[35]	Fluid therapy; can mix with crystalloid solutions
Electrolyte solutions	20-30 mL/kg PO q 24 h[49]	Oral fluid therapy; anorexia
Emeraid Critical Care	20 mL/kg PO[35]	Most species (especially herbivores); nutritional support, prepare according to directions
Iodine	2-4 mg/kg PO q 24 h × 2-3 wk, then q 7 d[66]	Herbivorous species/iodine deficiency (i.e., goiter); use in species maintained on goitrogenic diet; alternatively, can use balanced vitamin-mineral mixture or iodized salt (0.5% of feed)[114]
Iron dextran	12 mg/kg IM 1-2×/wk × 45 d[197]	Crocodilians/iron deficiency; also used in other species, but dose not established
Lactated Ringer's solution (LRS)	10-25 mL/kg IV,[130] SC, ICe q 24 h[35]	Fluid therapy; to prevent nephrotoxicity from aminoglycosides; use extracoelomically in chelonians; use in reptiles is controversial and other fluids may be preferable
Metronidazole	—	May stimulate appetite by affecting bacterial flora or protozoa levels
	12.5-50 mg/kg PO[64]	Most species
	50-100 mg/kg PO[103]	Chameleons
Ringer's solution for reptiles	—	Fluid therapy; 1 part LRS, 2 parts 2.5% dextrose/0.45% saline solution; or 1 part LRS, 1 part 5% dextrose, 1 part 0.9% saline solution[201]; to prevent nephrotoxicity from aminoglycosides; can use epicoelomically in chelonians
	15 (large reptiles) to 25 (small reptiles) mL/kg q 24 h or divided q 12 h for maintenance[8]	All species
	10-25 mL/kg ICe q 24 h[66]	All species
	20 mL/kg q 12 h[8]	All species/severe dehydration
Selenium	0.028 mg/kg IM[2]	Lizards/deficiency; myopathy
Sodium chloride (0.45%)	PO, SC, IV, ICe, EpiCe, IO prn[35]	Fluid therapy; can mix with crystalloid solutions
Vionate (ARC)	500 mg (¼ tsp)/kg PO q 24 h[182]	Most species/vitamin, mineral supplement
Vitamin A	—	Hypovitaminosis A; may have value in infectious stomatitis; overdose may cause epidermal sloughing; for less severe cases (especially in chelonians); oral vitamin A can be supplied via cod liver oil (2 drops 2×/wk) or commercial reptile vitamin products[114]
	2000 IU/kg PO, SC, IM q 7-14 d × 2-4 treatments[8,24,29,190]	Most species
	1000-5000 IU/kg IM q 7-10 d × 4 treatments[3,66]	Most species

Table 89-7. Nutritional/Mineral/Fluid Support Used in Reptiles—cont'd

Agent	Dosage	Species/Comments
	2000 IU/30 g PO once, repeat in 7 d[71,77]	Chameleons
	200 IU/kg[56] SC, IM	Turtles/hypovitaminosis A; give in conjunction with PO vitamin A (2000-10,000 IU/kg feed DM)
Vitamins A, D_3, E	0.15 mL/kg IM, repeat in 3 wk[102]	Most species/hypovitaminosis A, D_3, or E; product contains alcohol and may sting when administered; product without alcohol can be compounded commercially
	0.3 mL/kg PO, then 0.06 mL/kg q 7 d × 3-4 treatments[24]	Box Turtles/hypovitaminosis A; parenteral use may result in hypervitaminosis A and D; given PO may enhance Ca uptake
Vitamin B complex	5-10 mg/kg SC, IM	Most species/appetite stimulant; hypovitaminosis B
	25 mg thiamine/kg PO q 24 h × 3-7 d[8]	Most species/appetite stimulant; hypovitaminosis B
Vitamin B_1 (thiamine)	25 mg/kg PO q 24 h prn[176] or × 3-7 d[176]	Thiamine deficiency (i.e., in piscivorous species)
	30 g/kg feed fish PO[66]	Crocodilians/treat or prevent deficiency
Vitamin B_{12} (cyanocobalamin)	0.05 mg/kg SC, IM[66]	Lizards, snakes/appetite stimulant
Vitamin C	10-20 mg/kg SC, IM q 24 h[67,182]	All species/hypovitaminosis C; supportive therapy for bacterial infections; higher doses (i.e., 100 mg/kg) may be used for severe burns[148]
	100-250 mg/kg PO q 24 h[67]	Most species/infectious stomatitis
Vitamin D_3	—	Nutritional secondary hyperparathyroidism; hypocalcemia; herbivores are sensitive to excess; excessive supplementation may result in soft-tissue calcification
	200 IU/kg IM q 4 wk[114]	Most species
	1000 IU/kg IM, repeat in 1 wk[26,27,29]	Most species
	200 IU/kg PO, IM q 7 d[7,14]	Lizards (i.e., iguanas)/PO may be safer than IM, but absorption may be poor
Vitamin E	1 IU/kg[57]	Most species/hypovitaminosis E
	25 mg/kg IM[59]	Lizards/hypovitaminosis E (see vitamins A,D_3,E)
Vitamin K_1	0.25-0.50 mg/kg IM[102]	Most species/hypovitaminosis K_1; coagulopathies

PO, Orally; *prn*, as required; *IM*, intramuscularly; *SC*, subcutaneously; *ICe*, intracoelemically; *q*, every; *IV*, intravenously; *EpiCe*, epicoelomic; *IO*, intraosseously; *DM*, dry matter.

Table 89-8. Miscellaneous Agents Used in Reptiles

Agent	Dosage	Species/Comments
Allopurinol	10[143]-20[52,168] mg/kg PO q 24 h	Most species/gout; decreases production of uric acid[131]; long-term therapy; tortoises may respond best
	50 mg/kg PO q 24 h × 1 mo, then q 72 h[117]	Chelonians
Aluminum hydroxide	100 mg/kg PO q 12-24 h[130]	Hyperphosphatemia (associated with renal disease); decreases intestinal absorption of P; use cautiously in patients with gastric outlet obstruction
Amidotrizoate	7.5 mL/kg PO[149]	Tortoises/gastrointestinal contrast agent; give via gavage; mean transit times: 2.6 h at 30.6°C; 6.6 h at 21.5°C
Aminophylline	2-4 mg/kg IM[64]	Bronchodilator
Atropine	0.01-0.04 mg/kg IM, IV q 8-24 h[148]	Dry up excess mucous secretions with infectious stomatitis
	0.1-0.2 mg/kg IM[102]	Organophosphate toxicity prn
	0.2 mg/kg SC, IM[176]	Respiratory distress associated with excessive secretions
Barium sulfate	5-20 mL/kg PO[36]	Gastrointestinal contrast studies
Cyanoacrylate	Topical[102]	Hemostasis of bleeding toenails
Cyanoacrylate	Topical[184]	May protect burns, noninfected lesions, surgical sites
Cimetidine	4 mg/kg PO, IM q 8-12 h[66]	Gastric and duodenal ulceration; esophagitis; gastroesophageal reflux
Cisapride	0.5-2.0 mg/kg PO q 24 h[195]	Motility modifier; gastrointestinal stasis; not commercially available in United States, may be compounded; proven ineffective in Desert Tortoises at 1 mg/kg[199]

Continued

Table 89-8 Miscellaneous Agents Used in Reptiles—cont'd

Agent	Dosage	Species/Comments
Dioctyl Na sulfosuccinate	1-5 mg/kg PO[67]	Most species/constipation; use 1:20 dilution
Doxorubicin	1 mg/kg IV q 7 d × 2 treatments, then q 14 d × 2 treatments, then q 21 d × 2 treatments[174]	Snakes/chemotherapy for sarcoma (also lymphoma, carcinoma, etc); treatment periods variable
Ferric subsulfate powder	Topical[102]	Hemostasis (i.e., cut toenails)
Flunixin meglumine	0.1-0.5 mg/kg IM, IV q 12-24 h × 1-2 d[66,143]	Nonsteroidal antiinflammatory; antipyretic
	0.5-1.0 mg/kg IM, IV q 24-72 h[74]	Nonsteroidal antiinflammatory
	2 mg/kg IM q 24 h × 2 treatments[191]	Iguanas/analgesia (after surgery)
	—	Do not use in Sea Turtles because of potential for gastric ulcers[130]
Furosemide	5 mg/kg PO, IM, IV q 12-24 h[66,102]	Diuretic for edema and pulmonary congestion
Hydrochlorothiazide	1 mg/kg q 24-72 h[52]	Promotes diuresis; monitor hydration status
Insulin	1-5 IU/kg IM, IC q 24-72 h[193]	Snakes/chelonians; doses are empirical, must be adjusted on basis of response to therapy and serial blood glucose
	5-10 IU/kg IM, IC q 24-72 h[193]	Lizards/crocodilians; see previous
Iodine compound	500 mg/kg IV, IO[52]	Lizards/intravenous urography; take radiographs 0, 5, 15, 30, and 60 min after injection
Iohexol (240 mg I/mL)	5-20 mL/kg[35]	Gastrointestinal contrast studies; nonionic, organic iodine solution; good alternative to barium[36]; faster transit time than barium; can be diluted 1:1 with water
K-Y Jelly	1-3 mL of 50% K-Y Jelly and 50% warm water/100 g[4]	Enema
Lactulose	0.5 mL/kg PO q 24 h[192]	Lizards/fatty liver disease
Liquid paraffin (medicinal)	20-30 mL (50:50 with electrolyte solution)/kg PO q 24 h[49]	Constipation; administer via gavage; use cautiously because of risk of regurgitation and aspiration; seldom indicated[35]
Methimazole	2 mg/kg q 24 h × 30 d[71,72]	Snakes; for excessive shedding from hyperthyroidism, limited success
Metoclopramide	0.06 mg/kg PO q 24 h × 7 d[49,195]	Stimulates gastric motility
	1-10 mg/kg PO q 24 h[206]	Tortoises/stimulates gastric motility; proven ineffective in Desert Tortoise at 1 mg/kg[199]
Mineral oil	PO prn	Constipation; use cautiously because of risk of regurgitation and aspiration; seldom indicated[35]
New Skin (Medtech)	Topical[176]	Spray-on bandage
Oral cleansing gel	Topical[190]	Stomatitis; periodontitis
Pentobarbital	60[1,30]-100[30] mg/kg IV, ICe	Euthanasia
Polyurethane barrier	Topical[184]	Encourages healing of cutaneous wounds
Potassium chloride	2 mEq/kg IV, ICe[14]	Euthanasia; cardioplegic; administer after euthanasia solution
Probenecid	Not established[131]	Gout; increases uric acid excretion
Silver nitrate	Topical[102]	Hemostasis (i.e., cut toenails)
Silver sulfadiazine cream	Topical q 24-72 h[131,164]	Broad-spectrum antibacterial for skin or oral cavity; dressing is generally not necessary
Simethicone	PO prn	Gastrointestinal disturbance (gas)
Sodium bicarbonate	0.5-1 mg/kg IV[195]	Hypoxic acidosis after anesthesia
Sodium hypochlorite (3%)	Disinfectant	Disinfectant for cages, water bowls, etc; rinse well after use
Sodium pentosan polysulfate	0.83 mg/kg q 22 d × 4 treatments[84]	Arthritis; anecdotal
Sucralfate	500-1000 mg/kg PO q 6-8 h[64]	Oral, esophageal, gastric, and duodenal ulcers
Sulfinpyrazone	Not established[131]	Gout; increases uric acid excretion
Tamoxifen 60d time release pellets	Pellets containing 5 mg tamoxifen implants ICe[47]	Leopard Gecko; inhibition of follicular development for 60 d if implanted before vitellogenesis
Tegaderm	Topical[35]	Wound dressing

PO, Orally; *q*, every; *IM*, intramuscularly; *IV*, intravenously; *prn*, as required; *SC*, subcutaneously; *IO*, intraosseously; *ICe*, intracoelemically.

REFERENCES

1. Report of the AVMA panel on euthanasia, *J Am Vet Med Assoc* 202:243-249, 1993.
2. Allen DG, Pringle JK, Smith D: *Handbook of veterinary drugs*, Philadelphia, 1993, JB Lippincott.
3. Anderson NL: Diseases of *Iguana iguana*, *Compend Cont Educ Pract Vet* 14:1335-1343, 1992.
4. Anderson NL, Wack RF: Basic husbandry and medicine of pet reptiles. In Birchard SJ, Sherding RG, editors: *Saunders Manual of Small Animal Practice*, ed 2, Philadelphia, 2000, WB Saunders.
5. Anderson NL, Wack RF, Calloway L: Cardiopulmonary effects and efficacy of propofol as an anesthetic agent in brown tree snakes, *Boiga irregularis*. *Bull Assoc Rept Amph Vet* 9:9-15, 1999.
6. Barrie MT: Chameleon medicine. In: Fowler ME, Miller RE, editors: *Zoo & wild animal medicine: current therapy 4*, Philadelphia, 1999, WB Saunders.
7. Barten SL: The medical care of iguanas and other common pet lizards, *Vet Clin North Am Small Anim Pract* 23:1213-1249, 1993.
8. Bauck L, Boyer TH, Brown SA, et al: *Exotic animal formulary*, Lakewood, Colo, 1995, American Animal Hospital Association.
9. Beck K, Loomis M, Lewbart G, et al: Preliminary comparison of plasma concentrations of gentamicin injected into the cranial and caudal limb musculature of the eastern box turtle (*Terrapene carolina carolina*), *J Zoo Wildl Med* 26:265-268, 1995.
10. Bennett RA: *Personal communication*, 1999.
11. Bennett RA: A review of anesthesia and chemical restraint in reptiles, *J Zoo Wildl Med* 22:282-303, 1991.
12. Bennett RA: Current techniques in reptile anesthesia and surgery, *Proc Assoc Rept Amph Vet Am Assoc Zoo Vet* 36-44, 1994.
13. Bennett RA: Anesthesia. In Mader DR, editor: *Reptile medicine and surgery*, Philadelphia, 1996, WB Saunders.
14. Bennett RA: Management of common reptile emergencies, *Proc Assoc Rept Amph Vet* 67-72, 1998.
15. Bennett RA: Reptile anesthesia, *Semin Avian Exotic Pet Med* 7:30-40, 1998.
16. Bennett RA, Divers SJ, Schumacher J, et al: Anesthesia, *Bull Assoc Rept Amph Vet* 9:20-27, 1999.
17. Bennett RA, Schumacher J, Hedjazi-Haring K, Newell SM: Cardiopulmonary and anesthetic effects of propofol administered intraosseously to green iguanas, *J Am Vet Med Assoc* 212:93-98, 1998.
18. Benson KG, Tell LA, Young LA, et al: Pharmacokinetics of ceftiofur sodium following intramuscular and subcutaneous injection in the common green iguana (*Iguana iguana*), *Am J Vet Res* 64:1278-1282, 2003.
19. Bienzle D, Boyd CJ: Sedative effects of ketamine and midazolam in snapping turtles, *J Zoo Anim Med* 23:201-204, 1992.
20. Bodri MS, Hruba SJ: Safety of milbemycin (A_3-A_4 oxime) in chelonians, *Proc Joint Meeting Am Assoc Zoo Vet Am Assoc Wildl Vet* 156-157, 1992.
21. Bodri MS, Rambo TM, Wagner RA, et al: Pharmacokinteics of metronidazole administered as a single oral bolus to corn snakes, *Elaphe guttata*, *Assoc Rept Amph Vet* 121-122, 2001.
22. Boyer DM: IME: snake mite (*Ophionyssus natricis*) eradication utilizing permectrin spray, *Bull Assoc Rept Amph Vet* 5:4-5, 1995.
23. Boyer TH: Clinical anesthesia of reptiles, *Bull Assoc Rept Amph Vet* 2:10-13, 1992.
24. Boyer TH: Common problems of box turtles (*Terrapene* spp) in captivity, *Bull Assoc Rept Amph Vet* 2:9-14, 1992.
25. Boyer TH: Emergency care of reptiles, *Semin Avian Exotic Pet Med* 3:210-216, 1994.
26. Boyer TH: Metabolic bone disease. In Mader DR, editor: *Reptile medicine and surgery*, Philadelphia, 1996, WB Saunders.
27. Boyer TH: Diseases of the green iguana, *Proc North Am Vet Conf* 718-722, 1997.
28. Boyer TH: Emergency care of reptiles, *Vet Clin North Am Exotic Anim Pract* 1:191-206, 1998.
29. Boyer TH: *Essentials of reptiles: a guide for practitioners*, Lakewood, Colo, 1998, AAHA Press.
30. Burns RB, McMahan W: Euthanasia methods for ectothermic vertebrates. In Bonagura JD, editor: *Kirk's current veterinary therapy XII: small animal practice*, Philadelphia, 1995, WB Saunders.
31. Burridge MJ, Simmons L-A: Control and eradication of exotic tick infestations on reptiles, *Proc Assoc Rept Amph Vet* 21-23, 2001.
32. Bush M, Smeller JM, Charache PN, et al: Preliminary study of antibiotics in snakes, *Proc Am Assoc Zoo Vet* 50-54, 1976.
33. Bush M, Smeller JM, Charache P, et al: Biological half-life of gentamicin in gopher snakes, *Am J Vet Res* 39:171-173, 1978.
34. Caligiuri R, Kollias GV, Jacobson E, et al: The effects of ambient temperature on amikacin pharmacokinetics in gopher tortoises, *J Vet Pharmacol Therapeut* 13:287-291, 1990.
35. Carpenter JW: *Personal communication*, 2003.
36. Carpenter JW: Radiographic imaging of reptiles, *Proc North Am Vet Conf* 873-875, 1998.
37. Casares M, Enders F: Enrofloxacin side effects in a Galapagos tortoise (*Geochelone elephantopus nigra*), *Proc Am Assoc Zoo Vet* 446-448, 1996.
38. Chittick EJ, Stamper MA, Beasley JF, et al: Medetomidine, ketamine, and sevoflurane for anesthesia of injured loggerhead sea turtles: 13 cases (1996-200), *J Am Vet Med Assoc* 221:1019-1025, 2002.
39. Clark CH, Rogers ED, Milton JT: Plasma concentrations of chloramphenicol in snakes, *Am J Vet Res* 46:2654-2657, 1985.
40. Clyde VC, Cardeilhac P, Jacobson E: Chemical restraint of American alligators (*Alligator mississippiensis*) with atracurium or tiletamine-zolazepam, *J Zoo Wildl Med* 25:525-530, 1994.
41. Coke RL, Tristan TE: *Cryptosporidium* infection in a colony of leopard geckos, *Eublepharis macularius*, *Proc Assoc Rept Amph Vet* 157-163, 1998.
42. Coke RL, Hunter RP, Isaza R, et al: Pharmacokinetics and tissue concentrations of azithromycin in ball pythons (*Python regius*), *Am J Vet Res* 64:225-228, 2003.
43. Coke RL, Isaza R, Koch DE, et al: Pharmacokinetics of marbofloxacin in ball pythons (*Python regius*), *Proc Assoc Rept Amph Vet* 116, 2004.
44. Cooper JE: Anaesthesia of exotic animals, *Anim Technol* 35:13-20, 1984.
45. Cranfield MR, Graczyk TK: An update on ophidian cryptosporidiosis, *Proc Am Assoc Zoo Vet* 225-230, 1995.
46. Cranfield MR, Graczyk TK: Cryptosporidiosis. In Mader DR, editor: *Reptile medicine and surgery*, Philadelphia, 1996, WB Saunders.
47. DeNardo DF, Helminski G: Birth control in lizards? Therapeutic inhibition of reproduction, *Proc Assoc Rept Amph Vet* 65-66, 2000.
48. Dennis PM, Heard DJ: Cardiopulmonary effects of a medetomidine-ketamine combination administered intravenously in gopher tortoises, *J Am Vet Med Assoc* 220:1516-1519, 2002.
49. Divers SJ: Constipation in snakes with particular reference to surgical correction in a Burmese python (*Python molurus bivittatus*), *Proc Assoc Amph Rept Vet* 67-69, 1996.
50. Divers SJ: Medical and surgical treatment of pre-ovulatory ova stasis and post-ovulatory egg stasis in oviparous lizards, *Proc Assoc Amph Rept Vet* 119-123, 1996.

51. Divers SJ: The use of propofol in reptile anesthesia, *Proc Assoc Amph Rept Vet* 57-59, 1996.
52. Divers SJ: Clinician's approach to renal disease in lizards, *Proc Assoc Rept Amph Vet* 5-11, 1997.
53. Divers SJ: Empirical doses of antimicrobial drugs commonly used in reptiles, *Exotic DVM* 23, 1998.
54. Divers SJ: Anesthetics in reptiles, *Exotic DVM* 7-8, 1999.
55. Divers SJ: Clinical evaluation of reptiles, *Vet Clin North Am Exotic Anim Pract* 2:291-331, 1999.
56. Donoghue S: Nutritional problems of reptiles, *Proc North Am Vet Conf* 762-764, 1999.
57. Donoghue S, McKeown S: Nutrition of captive reptiles, *Vet Clin N Am Exotic Anim Pract* 2:69-91, 1999.
58. Driggers T: Respiratory diseases, diagnostics, and therapy in snakes, *Vet Clin North Am Exotic Anim Pract* 3:519-530, 2000.
59. Farnsworth RJ, Brannian RE, Fletcher KC, Klassen S: A vitamin E-selenium responsive condition in a green iguana, *J Zoo Anim Med* 17:42-45, 1986.
60. Faulkner JE, Archambault A: Anesthesia and surgery in the green iguana, *Semin Avian Exotic Pet Med* 2:103-108, 1993.
61. Flach EJ, Riley J, Mutlow AG, McCandlish IAP: Pentastomiasis in Bosc's Monitor Lizards *(Varanus exanthemicus)* caused by an undescribed *Sambonia* species, *J Zoo Wildl Med* 31:91-95, 2000.
62. Fleming GJ: Capture and chemical immobilization of the Nile crocodile *(Crocodylus niloticus)* in South Africa, *Proc Assoc Amph Rept Vet* 63-66, 1996.
63. Fleming GJ: Crocodilian anesthesia, *Vet Clin North Am Exotic Anim Pract* 4:119-145, 2001.
64. Frye FL: *Reptile clinician's handbook*, Malabar, Fla, 1994, Krieger Publishing.
65. Gamble KC, Alvarado TP, Bennett CL: Itraconazole plasma and tissue concentrations in the spiny lizard *(Sceloporus* sp.) following once-daily dosing, *J Zoo Wildl Med* 28:89-93, 1997.
66. Gauvin J: Drug therapy in reptiles, *Semin Avian Exotic Pet Med* 2:48-59, 1993.
67. Gillespie D: Reptiles. In Birchard SJ, Sherding RG, editors: *Saunders manual of small animal practice*, Philadelphia, 1994, WB Saunders.
68. Hackenbroich C, Failing K, Axt-Findt U, Bonath KH: Alphaxalone-alphadolone-anaesthesia in *Trachemys scripta elegans* and its influence on respiration, circulation and metabolism, *Proc 2nd Conf Europ Assoc Zoo Wildl Vet* 431-436, 1998.
69. Harms CA, Lewbart GA, Beasley J: Medical management of mixed nocardial and unidentified fungal osteomyelitis in a Kemp's Ridley sea turtle, *Lepidochelys kempii, J Herp Med Surg* 12:3,21-26, 2001.
70. Harms CA, Papich MG, Stamper MA, et al: Pharmacokinetics of oxytetracycline in loggerhead sea turtles *(Caretta caretta)* after single intravenous and intramuscular injections, *J Zoo Wildl Med* 35:477-488, 2004.
71. Harkewicz KA: Dermatology of reptiles: a clinical approach to diagnosis and treatment, *Vet Clin North Am Exotic Anim Pract* 4:411-461, 2001.
72. Harkewicz KA: Dermatologic problems of reptiles, *Semin Avian Exotic Pet Med* 11:151-161, 2002.
73. Hawk CT, Leary SL: *Formulary for laboratory animals*, Ames, 1995, Iowa State University Press.
74. Heard DJ: Principles and techniques of anesthesia and analgesia for exotic practice, *Vet Clin North Am Small Anim Pract* 23:1301-1327, 1993.
75. Heard DJ: Advanced reptile anesthesia and medicine, *Proc Avian Specialty Advanced Prog/Small Mam Rept Prog (Annu Conf Assoc Avian Vet)* 113-119, 1998.
76. Heard DJ: Advances in reptile anesthesia, *Proc N Am Vet Conf* 770, 1999.
77. Heard D, Fleming G, Lock B, et al: Lizards. In Meredith A, Redrobe S., editors: *BSAVA manual of exotic pets*, ed 4, Gloucester, England, 2002, British Small Animal Veterinary Association.
78. Heatley J, Mitchell M, Williams J, et al: Fungal periodontal osteomyelitis in a Chameleon, *Fucifer pardalis, J Herp Med and Surg* 11:7-12, 2001.
79. Heaton-Jones TG, Ko J, Heaton-Jones DL: Evaluation of medetomidine-ketamine anesthesia with atipamezole reversal in American Alligators *(Alligator mississippiensis)*, *J Zoo Wildl Med* 33:36-44, 2002.
80. Helmick KE, Bennett A, Ginn P, et al: Intestinal volvulus and stricture associated with a leiomyoma in a green turtle *(Chelonia mydas)*, *J Zoo Wildl Med* 31:221-227, 2000.
81. Helmick KE, Papich MG, Vliet KA, et.al: Pharmacokinetics of enroflaxacin after single-dose oral and intavenous administration in the American Alligator *(Alligator mississippiensis)*, *J Zoo Wildl Med* 35:333-340, 2004.
82. Helmick KE, Papich MG, Vliet KA, et al: Pharmacokinetic disposition of a long-acting oxytetracycline formulation after single-dose intravenous and intramuscular administrations in the American alligator *(Alligator mississippiensis)*, *J Zoo Wildl Med* 35:341-346, 2004.
83. Hernandez-Divers SJ: Pulmonary candidiasis caused by *Cadida albicans* in a Greek tortoise *(Testudo graeca)* and treatment with intrapulmonary amphotericin B, *J Zoo Wildl Med* 32:352-359, 2001.
84. Hernandez-Divers SJ: Diagnosis and surgical repair of stifle luxation in a spur-thighed tortoise *(Testudo graeca), J Zoo Wildl Med* 33:125-130, 2002.
85. Hilf M, Swanson D, Wagner R, et al: A new dosing schedule for gentamicin in blood pythons *(Python curtus)*: a pharmacokinetic study, *Res Vet Sci* 50:127-130, 1991.
86. Hilf M, Swanson D, Wagner R, et al: Pharmacokinetics of piperacillin in blood pythons *(Python curtus)* and in vitro evaluation of efficacy against aerobic gram-negative bacteria, *J Zoo Wildl Med* 22:199-203, 1991.
87. Holz P, Holz RM: Evaluation of ketamine, ketamine/xylazine, and ketamine/midazolam anesthesia in red-eared sliders *(Trachemys scripta elegans), J Zoo Wild Med* 25:531-537, 1994.
88. Holz PH, Burger JP, Pasloske K, Baker R, et al: Effect of injection site on carbenicillin pharmacokinetics in the carpet python, *Morelia spilota, J Herp Med Surg* 12:12-16, 2002.
89. Hungerford C, Spelman L, Papich M: Pharmacokinetics of enrofloxacin after oral and intramuscular administration in savanna monitors *(Varanus exanthematicus), Proc Am Assoc Zoo Vet*: 89-92, 1997.
90. Innis C: IME: per-cloacal worming of tortoises, *Bull Assoc Rept Amph Vet* 5:4, 1995.
91. Innis CJ, Boyer TH: Chelonian reproductive disorders, *Vet Clin Exotic Anim Pract* 5:555-578, 2002.
92. Jacobson ER: Use of chemotherapeutics in reptile medicine. In Jacobson ER, Kollias GV Jr, editors: *Exotic animals*, New York, 1988, Churchill Livingstone.
93. Jacobson ER: Antimicrobial drug use in reptiles. In Prescott JF, Baggot JD, editors: *Antimicrobial therapy in veterinary medicine*, Ames, 1993, Iowa State University Press.
94. Jacobson ER: Snakes, *Vet Clin North Am Small Anim Pract* 23:1179-1212, 1993.
95. Jacobson ER: Use of antimicrobial therapy in reptiles. In *Antimicrobial therapy in caged birds and exotic pets*, Trenton, NJ, 1995, Veterinary Learning Systems.
96. Jacobson ER: Bacterial infections and antimicrobial treatment in reptiles, *Proc North Am Vet Conf* 771-774, 1999.
97. Jacobson ER: Use of antimicrobial drugs in reptiles. In Fowler ME, Miller RE, editors: *Zoo & wild animal medicine: current therapy 4*, Philadelphia, 1999, WB Saunders.

98. Jacobson ER, Brown MP, Chung M, et al: Serum concentration and disposition kinetics of gentamicin and amikacin in juvenile American alligators, *J Zoo Anim Med* 19:188-194, 1988.
99. Jacobson E, Harman G, Laille E, Maxwell L: Plasma concentrations of praziquantel in loggerhead sea turtles, *Caretta caretta*, following oral administration of single and multiple doses, *Assoc Rept Amph Vet Proc* 37-39, 2002.
100. Jacobson E, Kollias GV Jr, Peters LJ: Dosages for antibiotics and parasiticides used in exotic animals, *Compend Cont Educ Pract Vet* 5:315-324, 1983.
101. Jenkins JR: *A formulary for reptile and amphibian medicine*, University of California, Davis, 1991, Proc Fourth Annu Avian/Exotic Anim Med Symp.
102. Jenkins JR: Medical management of reptile patients, *Compend Cont Educ Pract Vet* 13:980-988, 1991.
103. Jenkins JR: Diagnostic and clinical techniques. In Mader DR, editor: *Reptile medicine and surgery*, Philadelphia, 1996, WB Saunders.
104. Jenkins JR: Husbandry and diseases of Old World chameleons, *J Small Exotic Anim Med* 1:145-192, 1992.
105. Johnson JD, Mangone B, Jarchow JL: A review of mycoplasmosis infections in tortoises and options for treatment, *Proc Assoc Rept Amph Vet* 89-92, 1998.
106. Johnson JH: Anesthesia, analgesia and euthanasia of reptiles and amphibians, *Proc Am Assoc Zoo Vet* 132-138, 1991.
107. Johnson JH: *Clinical pharmacology of reptiles*, Texas A&M University, College Station, 1995, Symp Rept Med.
108. Kaufman GE, Seymour RE, Bonner BB, et al: Use of rocuronium for endotracheal intubation of North American Gulf Coast box turtles, *J Am Vet Med Assoc* 222:1111-1115, 2003.
109. Klingenberg RJ: The box turtle: a practitioner's approach, *Proc Assoc Amph Rept Vet* 37-39, 1996.
110. Klingenberg RJ: Management of the anorectic ball python, *Proc North Am Vet Conf* 830, 1996.
111. Klingenberg RJ: New perspectives on reptile anthelmintics, insecticides and parasiticides, *Proc North Am Vet Conf* 831-832, 1996.
112. Klingenberg RJ: Parasitology for the practitioner, *Proc North Am Vet Conf* 826-827, 1996.
113. Klingenberg RJ: Therapeutics. In Mader DR, editor: *Reptile medicine and surgery*, Philadelphia, 1996, WB Saunders.
114. Klingenberg RJ: Reptiles. In Aiello SE, editor: *The Merck veterinary manual*, ed 8, Whitehouse Station, NJ, 1998, Merck & Co.
115. Klingenberg RJ: Treating coccidia in reptiles, *Proc North Am Vet Conf* 779, 1999.
116. Klingenberg RJ: Diagnosing parasites of Old World chameleons, *Exotics DVM* 1.6:17-21, 2000.
117. Koelle P: Efficacy of allopurinol in European tortoises with hyperuricemia, *Proc Assoc Rept Amph Vet* 185-186, 2001.
118. Kolmstetter CM, Frazier D, Cox S, Ramsey EC: Pharmacokinetics of metronidazole in the yellow rat snake, *Elaphe obsoleta quadrivitatta*, *J Herp Med Surg* 11:4-8, 2001.
119. Kolmstetter CM, Frazier D, Cox S, Ramsey EC: Pharmacokinetics of metronidazole in the green iguana, *Iguana iguana*, *Bull Assoc Rept Amph Vet* 8:4-7, 1998.
120. Lawrence K, Muggleton PW, Needham JR: Preliminary study on the use of ceftazidime, a broad spectrum cephalosporin antibiotic, in snakes, *Res Vet Sci* 36:16-20, 1984.
121. Lawrence K, Needham JR, Palmer GH, et al: A preliminary study on the use of carbenicillin in snakes, *J Vet Pharmacol Therapeut* 7:119-124, 1984.
122. Lawrence K, Palmer GH, Needham JR: Use of carbenicillin in 2 species of tortoise (*Testudo graeca* and *T. hermanni*), *Res Vet Sci* 40:413-415, 1986.
123. Lawton MPC: Anaesthesia. In Beynon PH, Lawton MPC, Cooper JE, editors: *Manual of reptiles*, Ames, 1992, Iowa State University Press.
124. Lawton MPC: Pain management after surgery, *Proc North Am Vet Conf* 782, 1999.
125. Lightfoot T: Nebulization therapy in tortoise pneumonia, *Exotic DVM* 2.6, 2001.
126. Lloyd ML: Reptilian dystocias review: causes, prevention, management and comments on the synthetic hormone vasotocin, *Proc Am Assoc Zoo Vet* 290-296, 1990.
127. Lloyd ML: Crocodilian anesthesia. In Fowler ME, Miller RE, editors: *Zoo & wild animal medicine: current therapy 4*, Philadelphia, 1999, WB Saunders.
128. Lloyd ML, Reichard T, Odum RA: Gallamine reversal in Cuban crocodiles (*Crocodilus rhombifer*) using neostigmine alone versus neostigmine with hyaluronidase, *Proc Assoc Rept Amph Vet/Am Assoc Zoo Vet* 117-120, 1994.
129. Lock BA, Heard DJ, Dennis P: Preliminary evaluation of medetomidine/ketamine combinations for immobilization and reversal with atipamezole in three tortoise species, *Bull Assoc Rept Amph Vet* 8:6-9, 1998.
130. Mader DR: Personal communication, 2003.
131. Mader DR: Gout. In Mader DR, editor: *Reptile medicine and surgery*, Philadelphia, 1996, WB Saunders.
132. Mader DR: Reproductive surgery in the green iguana, *Semin Avian Exotic Pet Med* 5:214-221, 1996.
133. Mader DR: Specific diseases and conditions. In Mader DR, editor: *Reptile medicine and surgery*, Philadelphia, 1996, WB Saunders.
134. Mader DR: Antibiotic therapy in reptiles, *Proc North Am Vet Conf* 791-792, 1998.
135. Mader DR: Common bacterial disease and antibiotic therapy in reptiles, *Suppl Compend Contin Educ Pract Vet* 20:23-33, 1998.
136. Mader DR: Understanding local analgesics: practical use in the green iguana, *Iguana iguana*, *Proc Assoc Rept Amph Vet* 7-10, 1998.
137. Mader DR: Understanding thermal burns in reptile patients, *Proc Assoc Rept Amph Vet* 143-147, 1998.
138. Mader DR, Conzelman GM, Baggot JD: Effects of ambient temperature on the half-life and dosage regimen of amikacin in the gopher snake, *J Am Vet Med Assoc* 187:1134-1136, 1985.
139. Mader DR, Palazzolo C: Common reptile parasites not always easy to treat, *Vet Prod News* 32-33, 1995.
140. Mallo DKM, Harms CA, Lewbart GA, Papich MS: Pharmacokinetics of fluconazole in loggerhead sea turtles (*Caretta caretta*) after single intravenous and subcutaneous injections, and multiple subcutaneous injections, *J Zoo Wildl Med* 33:29-35, 2002.
141. Manire CA, Rhinehart HL, Pennick GJ, et al: Steady-state plasma concentrations of itraconazole after oral administration in Kemp's Ridley sea turtles, *Lepidochelys kempi*, *J Zoo Wild Med* 34:171-178, 2003.
142. Manire CA, Hunter, RP, Koch DE, et al: Pharmacokinetics of Ticarcillin in the loggerhead sea turtle (*Caretta caretta*) after single intravenous and intramuscular injections, *J Zoo Wildl Med* 36:44-53, 2005.
143. Mautino M, Page CD: Biology and medicine of turtles and tortoises, *Vet Clin North Am Small Anim Pract* 23:1251-1270, 1993.
144. Maxwell LK, Jacobson ER: Preliminary single-dose pharmacokinetics of enrofloxacin after oral and intramuscular administration in green iguanas (*Iguana iguana*), *Proc Am Assoc Zoo Vet* 25, 1997.
145. McArthur SD, Wilkinson RJ, Barrows MG: In Meredith A, Redrobe S, editors: *BSAVA manual of exotic pets*, ed 4, Gloucester, England, 2002, British Small Animal Veterinary Association.
146. McCracken HE: Periodontal disease in lizards. In Fowler ME, Miller RE, editors: *Zoo & wild animal medicine: current therapy 4*, Philadelphia, 1999, WB Saunders.

147. McFarlen J: Commonly occurring reptilian intestinal parasites, *Proc Am Assoc Zoo Vet* 120-127, 1991.
148. Messonnier S: Formulary for exotic pets, *Vet Forum* 46-49, 1996.
149. Meyer J: Gastrographin® as a gastrointestinal contrast agent in the Greek tortoise *(Testudo hermanni)*, *J Zoo Wildl Med* 29:183-189, 1998.
150. Miller HA, Brandt PJ, Frye FL, et al: *Trichomonas* associated with ocular and subcutaneous lesions in geckos, *Proc Assoc Rept Amph Vet/Am Assoc Zoo Vet* 102-107, 1994.
151. Millichamp NJ: Surgical techniques in reptiles. In Jacobson ER, Kollias GV Jr, editors: *Exotic animals*, New York, 1988, Churchill Livingstone.
152. Morgan-Davies AM: Immobilization of the Nile crocodile *(Crocodilus niloticus)* with gallamine triethiodide, *J Zoo Anim Med* 11:85-87, 1980.
153. Murray MJ: Pneumonia and normal respiratory function. In Mader DR, editor: *Reptile medicine and surgery*, Philadelphia, 1996, WB Saunders.
154. Nichols DK, Lamirande EW: Use of methohexital sodium as an anesthetic in two species of colubrid snakes, *Proc Assoc Rept Amph Vet/Am Assoc of Zoo Vet* 161-162, 1994.
155. Norton TM, Jacobson ER, Caligiuri R, et al: Medical management of a Galapagos tortoise *(Geochelone elephantopus)* with hypothyroidism, *J Zoo Wildl Med* 20:212-216, 1989.
156. Norton TM, Spratt J, Behler J, Hernandez K: Medetomidine and ketamine anesthesia with atipamezole reversal in private free-ranging gopher tortoises, *Gopherus polyphemus*, *Proc Assoc Rept Amph Vet* 25-27, 1998.
157. Oppenheim YC, Moon PF: Sedative effects of midazolam in red-eared slider turtles *(Trachemys scripta elegans)*, *J Zoo Wildl Med* 26:409-413, 1995.
158. Origgi FC, Jacobson ER: Diseases of the respiratory tract of chelonians, *Vet Clin North Am Exot Anim Pract* 3:537-549, 2000.
159. Pace L, Mader D: Atropine and glycopyrrolate, route of administration and response in the Green Iguana *(Iguana iguana)*, *Proc Assoc Rept Amph Vet* 79-84, 2002.
160. Page CD: Current reptilian anesthesia procedures. In Fowler ME, editor: *Zoo & wild animal medicine: current therapy 3*, Philadelphia, 1993, WB Saunders.
161. Page CD, Mautino M: Clinical management of tortoises, *Compend Cont Educ Pract Vet* 12:79-85, 1990.
162. Page CD, Mautino M, Derendorf H, et al: Multiple-dose pharmacokinetics of ketoconazole administered orally to gopher tortoises *(Gopherus polyphemus)*, *J Zoo Wildl Med* 22:191-198, 1991.
163. Paré JA, Crawshaw GJ, Barta JR: Treatment of cryptosporidiosis in gila monsters *(Heloderma suspectum)* with paromycin, *Proc Assoc Rept Amph Vet* 23, 1997.
164. Pokras MA, Sedgwick CJ, Kaufman GE: Therapeutics. In Beynon PH, Lawton MPC, Cooper JE, editors: *Manual of reptiles*, Ames, 1992, Iowa State University Press.
165. Prezant RM, Jarchow JL: Lactated fluid use in reptiles: is there a better solution? *Proc Assoc Rept Amph Vet*, 83-87, 1997.
166. Prezant RM, Isaza R, Jacobson ER: Plasma concentrations and disposition kinetics of enrofloxacin in gopher tortoises *(Gopherus polyphemus)*, *J Zoo Wildl Med* 25:82-87, 1994.
167. Pye GW, Carpenter JW: Ketamine sedation followed by propofol anesthesia in a slider, *Trachemys scripta*, to facilitate removal of an esophageal foreign body, *Bull Assoc Amph Rept Vet* 8:16-17, 1998.
168. Raiti P: Veterinary care of the common kingsnake, *Lampropeltis getula*, *Bull Assoc Rept Amph Vet* 5:11-18, 1995.
169. Raiti P: Administration of aerosolized antibiotics to reptiles, *Exotic DVM* 4.3:87-90, 2002.
170. Raphael BL: Chelonians (Turtles, tortoises). In Fowler ME, Miller RE, editors: *Zoo & wild animal medicine*, ed 5, Philadelphia, 2003, WB Saunders.
171. Raphael B, Clark CH, Hudson R Jr: Plasma concentrations of gentamicin in turtles, *J Zoo Anim Med* 16:136-139, 1985.
172. Raphael BL, Papich M, Cook RA: Pharmacokinetics of enrofloxacin after a single intramuscular injection in Indian star tortoises *(Geochelone elegans)*, *J Zoo Wildl Med* 25: 88-94, 1994.
173. Rooney MB, Levine G, Gaynor J, et al: Sevoflurane anesthesia in desert toroises *(Gopherus agassizii)*, *J Zoo Wild Med* 30: 64-69, 1999.
174. Rosenthal K: Chemotherapeutic treatment of a sarcoma in a corn snake, *Proc Assoc Rept Amph Vet/Am Assoc Zoo Vet* 46, 1994.
175. Rossi J: Practical reptile dermatology, *Proc North Am Vet Conf* 648-649, 1995.
176. Rossi JV: Emergency medicine of reptiles, *Proc North Am Vet Conf* 799-801, 1998.
177. Rossi JV: Practical iguana psychology, *Proc North Am Vet Conf* 798-799, 1998.
178. Schaeffer DO: Anesthesia and analgesia in nontraditional laboratory animal species. In Kohn DF, Wixson SK, White WJ, Benson GJ, editors: *Anesthesia and analgesia in laboratory animals*, New York, 1997, Academic Press.
179. Schobert E: Telazol® use in wild and exotic animals, *Vet Med* 82:1080-1088, 1987.
180. Schumacher J: Reptiles and amphibians. In Thurman JC, Tranquilli WJ, Benson GJ, editors: *Lumb and Jones' veterinary anesthesia*, ed 3, Baltimore, 1996, Williams & Wilkins.
181. Schumacher J: Respiratory diseases of reptiles, *Semin Avian Exotic Pet Med* 6:209-215, 1997.
182. Scott BW: Nutritional diseases. In Beynon PH, Lawton MPC, Cooper JE, editors: *Manual of reptiles*, Ames, 1992, Iowa State University Press.
183. Sleeman JM, Gaynor J: Sedative and cardiopulmonary effects of medetomidine and reversal with atipamezole in desert tortoises (Gopherus agassizii), *J Zoo Wildl Med* 31: 28-35, 2000.
184. Smith DA, Barker IK, Allen OB: The effect of certain topical medications on healing of cutaneous wounds in the common garter snake *(Thamnophis sirtalis)*, *Can J Vet Res* 52: 129-133, 1988.
185. Smith JA, McGuire NC, Mitchell MA: Cardiopulmonary physiology and anesthesia in crocodilians, *Proc Assoc Rept Amph Vet* 17-21, 1998.
186. Speroni JA, Giambeluca L, Errecalde EO: *Farmacocinetica de cefoperazona tras su administracion intramuscular a Tupinambis teguixin (Sauria, Teidae)*, Buenos Aires, Argentina, 1989, AHA Comm Meeting.
187. Spiegel RA, Lane TJ, Larsen RE, et al: Diazepam and succinylcholine chloride for restraint of the American alligator, *J Am Vet Med Assoc* 185:1335-1336, 1984.
188. Spörle H, Gobel T, Schildger B: *Blood-levels of some anti-infectives in the Hermann's tortoise (Testudo hermanni)*, Germany, 1991, 4th Internat Colloquium Path Med Rept Amph.
189. Stahl SJ: Osteomyelitis in lizards and snakes, *Proc North Am Vet Conf* 759-760, 1997.
190. Stahl SJ: Common medical problems of old world chameleons, *Proc North Am Vet Conf* 814-817, 1998.
191. Stahl SJ: Reproductive disorders of the green iguana, *Proc North Am Vet Conf* 810-813, 1998.
192. Stahl SJ: Medical management of bearded dragons, *Proc North Am Vet Conf* 789-792, 1999.
193. Stahl SJ: Diseases of the reptile pancreas, *Vet Clin Exotic Anim Pract* 6:191-212, 2003.
194. Stamper MA, Papich MG, Lewbart GA, et al: Pharmacokinetics of ceftazidime in loggerhead sea turtles *(Caretta caretta)* after single intravenous and intramuscular injections, *J Zoo Wildl Med* 30:32-35, 1999.

195. Stein G: Reptile and amphibian formulary. In Mader DR, editor: *Reptile medicine and surgery*, Philadelphia, 1996, WB Saunders.
196. Stirl R, Krug P, Bonath KH: Tiletamine/zolazepam sedation in boa constrictors and it's influence on respiration, circulation and metabolism, *Proc Europ Assoc Zoo Wildl Vet* 115-119, 1996.
197. Suedmeyer WK: Iron deficiency in a group of American alligators: diagnosis and treatment, *J Small Exotic Anim Med* 1:69-72, 1991.
198. Teare JA, Bush M: Toxicity and efficacy of ivermectin in chelonians, *J Am Vet Med Assoc* 183:1195-1197, 1603.
199. Tothill A, Branvold H, Paul C, et al: Effect of cisapride, erythromycin, and metoclopramide on gastrointestinal transit time in the desert tortoise, *Gopherus agassizii*, *J Herp Med Surg* 10:16, 2000.
200. Whitaker BR, Krum H: Medical management of sea turtles in aquaria. In Fowler ME, Miller RE, editors: *Zoo & wild animal medicine: current therapy 4*, Philadelphia, 1999, WB Saunders Co.
201. Willette-Frahm M, Wright KM, Thode BC: Select protozoal diseases in amphibians and reptiles: a report for the Infectious Diseases Committee, American Association of Zoo Veterinarians, *Bull Assoc Rept Amph Vet* 5:19-29, 1995.
202. Wilson SC, Carpenter JW: Endoparasitic diseases of reptiles, *Semin Avian Exotic Pet Med* 5:64-74, 1996.
203. Wimsatt J, Johnson J, Mangone BA, et al: Clarithromycin pharmacokinetics in the desert tortoise *(Gopherus agassizii)*, *J Zoo Wildl Med* 30:36-43, 1999.
204. Wissman MA, Parsons B: Dermatophytosis of green iguanas *(Iguana iguana)*, *J Small Exotic Anim Med* 2:133-136, 1993.
205. Wood FE, Critchley KH, Wood JR: Anesthesia in the green sea turtle, *Chelonia mydas*, *Am J Vet Res* 43:1882, 1602.
206. Wright KM: Common medical problems of tortoises, *Proc North Am Vet Conf* 769-771, 1997.
207. Wright K: Omphalectomy of reptiles, *Exotic DVM* 3.1:11-15, 2001.
208. Young LA, Schumacher J, Jacobson ER, et al: Pharmacokinetics of enrofloxacin in juvenile Burmese pythons *(Python molurus bivittatus)*, *Proc Assoc Rept Amph Vet/ Am Assoc Zoo Vet* 97, 1994.

WEBSITE LISTINGS

ISIS *International Species Information System*, file://D:/USAPages/74051018.htm.

90
AMPHIBIAN FORMULARY
KEVIN M. WRIGHT

Table 90-1 Antimicrobial Agents Used in Amphibians*,†

Agent	Dosage	Species/Comments
Amikacin	5 mg/kg SC, IM, ICe q 24-48 h[47]	Most species; may be used in combination with piperacillin[47]
	5 mg/kg IM q 36 h[17]	Bullfrogs/PD
Carbenicillin	100 mg/kg SC, IM q 72 h[5]	
	200 mg/kg SC, IM, ICe q 24 h[25]	
Chloramphenicol	50 mg/kg SC, IM, ICe q 12-24 h[25]	
	20 mg/L bath[25]	Change daily
Ciprofloxacin	10 mg/kg PO q 24 h[47]	
	500-750 mg/75 L as 6-8 h bath q 24 h[47]	May be used for large numbers of animals
Doxycycline	10-50 mg/kg PO q 24 h[29]	African Clawed Frogs/chlamydiosis
	5-10 mg/kg PO, q 24 h[44]	Chlamydiosis
Enrofloxacin	5-10 mg/kg PO, SC, IM q 24 h[17, 47]	Most/PD (Bullfrogs)[17]; ICe and topical routes also used but not documented with PD[47]
Gentamicin	2-4 mg/kg IM q 72 h × 4 treatments[12]	
	2.5 mg/kg IM q 72 h[32]	Coldwater salamanders (e.g., *Necturus*)/PD; more frequent dosing may be needed if temperature >4°C (39.2°F)
	3 mg/kg IM q 24 h @ 22.2°C (72°F)[33]	Leopard Frogs/PD[33]; at higher temperatures, serum concentration is lower
	1.3 mg/L × 1 h bath q 24 h × 7 d[12]	Bacterial dermatoses; can be toxic
	Topical to eyes[42]	All/ocular infections; dilute to 2 mg/mL
Isoniazid	12.5 mg/L bath[29]	Mycobacteriosis
Metronidazole	10 mg/kg PO q 24 h × 5-10 d[24]	For chronic diarrhea[24]
	12 mg/kg topically q 24 h × 5-10 d[47]	For chronic diarrhea[47]
	50 mg/kg PO q 24 h × 3 d[47]	Anaerobic infections
	60 mg/kg topically q 24 h × 3 d[47]	Anaerobic infections
	10 mg/kg IV q 24 h × 2 d[47]	Anaerobic infections
	50 mg/L × 24 h bath[47]	Anaerobic infections
Neomycin, polymixin	Apply to wound topically q 24 h[10]	Microsporidian infections[10]
Nifurpirinol	250 mg/38 L × 1 h bath q 24 h[12]	
Nitrofurazone	10-20 mg/L × 24 h bath[5]	Change daily
Oxytetracycline	25 mg/kg SC, IM q 24 h[25]	Most species
	50 mg/kg PO q 12-24 h[25]	Most species
	50-100 mg/kg IM q 48 h[17]	Bullfrogs/PD[17]; especially useful in cases of chlamydiosis (use up to 30 d)[47]
	100 mg/L × 1 h bath[47]	Most species
	1 g/kg feed × 7 d[25]	
Piperacillin	100 mg/kg SC, IM q 24 h[47]	Anaerobes; may be used in combination with amikacin[47]
Rifampin	25 mg/L × 24 h bath[9]	Potentially effective for mycobacteriosis
Silver sulfadiazine 1%	Topical q 24 h[45]	Antibiotic cream
Sulfadiazine	132 mg/kg PO q 24 h[25]	
Sulfamethazine	1 g/L bath to effect[25]	Change daily
Tetracycline	50 mg/kg PO q 12 h[5]	
	150 mg/kg PO q 24 h × 5-7 d[40]	
	167 mg/kg (5 mg/30 g) PO q 12 h × 7 d[12]	
Trimethoprim/ sulfadiazine	15-20 mg/kg IM q 48 h[19]	

Continued

Table 90-1	Antimicrobial Agents Used in Amphibians*,†—cont'd	
Agent	**Dosage**	**Species/Comments**
Trimethoprim/ sulfamethoxazole	15 mg/kg PO q 24 h[47]	Chronic diarrhea
	20 μg/mL and 80 μg/mL in 0.5% or 0.15% salt solution × 24 h bath	Bacterial dermatosepticemia; make fresh bath daily[20]
Trimethoprim/sulfa	3 mg/kg PO, SC, IM q 24 h[5]	Unspecified sulfa

*Water baths containing antibiotics or topical applications may not provide as consistent distribution as parenteral administration.
†SC can be administered in dorsal lymph sac of anurans.[6]
SC, Subcutaneously; *IM*, intramuscularly; *ICe*, Intracoelomically, *q*, every; *PO*, orally; *IV*, intravenously; *PD*, .

Table 90-2	Antifungal Agents Used in Amphibians	
Agent	**Dosage**	**Species/Comments**
Amphotericin-B	1 mg/kg ICe q 24 h[47]	Internal mycoses
Benzalkonium chloride	2 mg/L × 1 h bath q 24 h[25]	Saprolegniasis
	1:4,000,000 bath[25]	Saprolegniasis; change water 3×/wk
	0.25 mg/L × 72 h bath[5]	
Fluconazole	60 mg/kg PO q 24 h[47]	
Itraconazole	0.01% in 0.6% salt solution as 5 min bath q 24 h × 11 d[23]	Topical route best choice to treat chytridiomycosis[23]
	10 mg/kg PO q 24 h[47]	
Ketoconazole	10 mg/kg PO q 24 h[25]	
	10-20 mg/kg PO q 24 h[47]	
	Topical cream[7]	Topical route best choice to treat chytridiomycosis[46]
Malachite green	0.15-0.2 mg/L × 1 h bath q 24 h[12]	Cutaneous mycoses; caution: mutagenic, teratogenic; potentially toxic
Mercurochrome	4 mg/L × 1 h bath q 24 h[41]	Saprolegniasis
Methylene blue	2-4 mg/L bath to effect[5]	Tadpoles/reduces mortality in newly hatched tadpoles
	4 mg/L × 1 h bath q 24 h[41]	Saprolegniasis
Miconazole	5 mg/kg ICe q 24 h × 14-28 d[43]	Systemic mycoses
	Topical cream[47]	Topical route best choice for chytridiomycosis; solutions containing alcohol may cause irritation
Nystatin 1% cream	Topical[46]	Cutaneous mycoses[46]
Potassium permanganate	1:5000 water × 5 min bath q 24 h[3]	Cutaneous mycoses
Sodium chlorite (NaOCl$_2$)	20 mg/L as 6-8 h bath[45]	Cutaneous mycoses
Tolnaftate 1%	Topical[12]	Cutaneous mycoses

ICe, Intracoelomically; *q*, every; *PO*, orally.

Table 90-3 Antiparasitic Agents Used in Amphibians*

Agent	Dosage	Species/Comments
Acriflavin	0.025% bath × 5 d[25]	Protozoa
	500 mg/L × 30 min bath[39]	Protozoa
Benzalkonium chloride	2 mg/L × 1 h bath q 24 h to effect[39]	Protozoa
Copper sulphate	0.1 mg/L as continuous bath to effect[47]	Some protozoa; copper may be toxic to some amphibians
	500 mg/L × 2 min bath q 24 h to effect[25]	Protozoa
Distilled water	3 h bath[25]	Fenbendazole combinations follow
Fenbendazole	—	
	30-50 mg/kg PO[6]	Gastrointestinal nematodes
	50 mg/kg PO q 24 h × 3-5 d, repeat in 14-21 d[47]	Resistant nematode infections
	50-100 mg/kg PO,[24] repeat in 2-3 wk prn	Most species/gastrointestinal nematodes
	100 mg/kg PO,[36] repeat in 14 d	Gastrointestinal nematodes
Fenbendazole (F)/ invermectin (I)	(F) 100 mg/kg PO on d 1, then (I) 0.2 mg/kg PO on d 2, 11[36]	Gastrointestinal nematodes
Fenbendazole (F)/ metronidazole (M)	(F) 100 mg/kg PO, repeat in 10-14 d + (M) 10 mg/kg PO q 24 h for 5 d[36]	Concurrent gastrointestinal nematodes and protozoa
Formalin (10%)	—	Do not use if skin is ulcerated
	1.5 ml/L × 10 min bath q 48 h to effect[7]	Protozoans; may be toxic in some species
	0.5% × 10 min bath once[25]	Monogenic trematodes; may be toxic to some amphibian species
Ivermectin	0.2-0.4 mg/kg PO, SC, repeat q 14 d prn[6]	Nematodes, including lungworms, mites
	2 mg/kg topically, repeat in 2-3 wk[16]	Especially useful for small specimens[47] and *Rana* spp.[16]
	10 mg/L as 60 min bath, repeat in q 14 d prn[47]	Best route for treating mites[47]
Levamisole	—	May cause paralysis in some species at suggested dosages[47]
	10 mg/kg topically,[47] IM,[5] ICe,[45] repeat in 2 wk	Nematodes, including lungworms
	12 mg/L bath × 4 d[11]	African Clawed Frogs/cutaneous nematodes; use ≥4.2 L of tank water/frog
	100-300 mg/L × 24 h bath, repeat in 1-2 wk[47]	Nematodes, including subcutaneous nematodes in aquatic amphibians; water-soluble form is available through aquaculture supply companies
	100 mg/L × ≥72 h bath[47]	Resistant nematodes
Malachite green	0.15 mg/L × 1 h bath q 24 h to effect[25]	Protozoa; caution: mutagenic, teratogenic; potentially toxic
Metronidazole	—	See fenbendazole combinations
	10 mg/kg PO q 24 h × 5-10 d[36]	Protozoa; for unfamiliar or sensitive species
	50 mg/kg PO q 24 h × 3-5 d[47]	Confirmed cases of amoebiasis and flagellate overload
	100 mg/kg PO q 3 d[7]	Protozoa
	100-150 mg/kg PO, repeat in 2-3 wk or prn[25]	Protozoa (e.g., *Entamoeba, Hexamita, Opalina*)
	500 mg/100 g feed × 3-4 treatments[5]	Ciliates
	0.05 mL of 1.008 mg/mL on dorsum q 24 h × 3 d[21]	Fire-bellied Toads (1.8 g/protozoa; rinse 1 h after treatment; results in absorption of 23 mg/kg BW of metronidazole)
	50 mg/L × 24 h bath[29]	Aquatic amphibians/protozoa
Moxidectin	200 μg/kg SC q 4 mo[28]	Nematodes
Oxfendazole	5 mg/kg PO[40]	Gastrointestinal nematodes
Oxtetracycline	25 mg/kg SC, IM q 24 h[39]	Protozoa
	50 mg/kg PO q 12 h[39]	Protozoa
	1 g/kg feed × 7 d[39]	Protozoa
Paromomycin	50-75 mg/kg PO q 24 h[43]	Gastrointestinal protozoa
Piperazine	50 mg/kg PO, repeat in 2 wk[12]	Gastrointestinal nematodes
Potassium permanganate	7 mg/L × 5 min bath q 24 h to effect[25]	Ectoparasitic protozoa
Praziquantel	8-24 mg/kg topically, PO, SC, ICe,[47] repeat q 14 d	Trematodes, cestodes
	10 mg/L × 3 h bath,[47] repeat q 7-21 d	Trematodes, cestodes
Salt (sodium chloride)	4-6 g/L bath[25]	Ectoparasitic protozoa
	6 g/L × 5-10 min bath q 24 h × 3-5 d[39]	Ectoparasitic protozoa
	25 g/L × ≤10 min bath[7]	Ectoparasitic protozoa
Sulfadiazine	132 mg/kg q 24 h[39]	Coccidiosis
Sulfamethazine	1 g/L bath[39]	Coccidiosis; change daily to effect
Tetracycline	50 mg/kg PO q 12 h[39]	Protozoa
Thiabendazole	50-100 mg/kg PO,[12] repeat in 2 wk prn	Gastrointestinal nematodes
	100 mg/L bath, repeat in 2 wk[41]	Verminous dermatisis
Trimethoprim/sulfa	3 mg/kg PO, SC, IM q 24 h[39]	Coccidiosis

*SC can be administered in dorsal lymph sac of anurans.[6]
q, Every; *PO*, orally; *prn*, as needed; *SC*, subcutaneously; *IM*, intramuscularly; *ICe*, intracoelomically; *BW*, body weight.

Table 90-4 Chemical Restraint, Anesthetic, and Analgesic Agents Used in Amphibians*

Agent	Dosage	Species/Comments
Atipamezole	Titrate to effect	Antagonist for dexmedetomidine[18]
Benzocaine	—	Anesthesia; not sold as fish anesthetic in United States; available from chemical supply companies; do not use topical anesthetic products marketed for mammals; prepare stock solution in ethanol (poorly soluble in water); store in dark bottle at room temperature
	50 mg/L bath to effect[6]	Larvae/dissolve in ethanol first
	200-300 mg/L bath to effect[6]	Frogs, salamanders/dissolve in ethanol first
	200-500 mg/L bath[4]	Dissolve in acetone first
Buprenorphine	38 mg/kg SC[18]	Analgesia, >4 h; ED_{50} in Leopard Frog[18]
Butorphanol	0.2-0.4 mg/kg IM[27]	Analgesia; dosage not determined but assumed to be similar to that in mammals
Clove oil (eugenol)	0.3 mL/L (~310-318 mg/L)[14]	Anesthesia; deep anesthesia after 15 min bath; caused reversible gastric prolapse in 50% of Leopard Frogs[14]
	0.45 ml/L (~473 mg/L)[21]	Anesthesia; deep anesthesia induced in 80% of Tiger Salamanders
Codeine	53 mg/kg SC[18]	Analgesia, >4 h; ED_{50} in Leopard Frog[18]
Dexmedetomidine	40-120 mg/kg SC[18]	Analgesia, >4 h; ED_{50} in Leopard Frog[18]
Diazepam	—	See ketamine combination
Fentanyl	0.5 mg/kg SC[18]	Analgesia, >4 h; ED_{50} in Leopard Frog[18]
Halothane	4%-5% to effect[6]	Terrestrial species/induction chamber
	Bubbled into water to effect[29]	Aquatic species
	5%[2]	Prolonged exposure for euthanasia
Isoflurane	—	Anesthesia; induction chamber, inhalant of choice
	3%-5% induction, 1%-2% maintenance[27]	Terrestial species
	0.28 mL/100 mL bath[30]	Induce in closed container
	Bubbled into water to effect[30]	Aquatic species
	Topical application of liquid isoflurane[30]	*Bufo* spp. (0.015 mL/g BW),[30] African Clawed Frog (0.007 mL/g BW)[30]/induce in closed container, once induced, remove excess from animal
	Topical mixture of isoflurane (3 mL), KY Jelly (3.5 mL), and water (1.5 mL)[30]	*Bufo* spp. (0.035 mL/g BW),[30] African Clawed Frog (0.025 mL/g BW)[30]/induce in closed container; once induced, remove excess from animal
	5%[2]	Terrestrial species/euthanasia; induction chamber
Ketamine	—	May have long induction and recovery times; does not provide good analgesia so may not be suited for major surgical procedures; other agents preferred; ketamine combination follows; see lidocaine
	50-150 mg/kg SC, IM[6]	Most species
Ketamine (K)/diazepam (D)	(K) 20-40 mg/kg + (D) 0.2-0.4 mg/kg IM[27]	Variable results
Lidocaine 1%-2%	Local infiltration[13]	All/local anesthesia; with or without epinephrine; 2% lidocaine in combination with ketamine has been used for minor surgeries[27]; use with caution
Meperidine	49 mg/kg SC[18]	Analegesia, >4 h; ED_{50} in Leopard Frog[18]
Methoxyflurane	0.5-1 mL in 1 L container (cotton soaked)[13]	Induction in 2 min; surgical anesthesia maintained for about 30 min; recovery within 7 h; not recommended because of potential of overdose[27]
Morphine	38-42 mg/kg SC[18]	Analgesia, >4 h
Nalorphine	122 mg/kg SC[18]	Analgesia, >4 h
Naloxone	10 mg/kg SC[18]; titrate to effect	Antagonist for butorphanol, buprenorphine, codeine, fentanyl, meperidine, morphine
Naltrexone	1 mg/kg SC[18]; titrate to effect	Antagonist for butorphanol, buprenorphine, codeine, fentanyl, meperidine, morphine
Pentobarbital sodium	40-50 mg/kg ICe[27]	Frogs, toads/seldom used, other agents preferred; can also administer in dorsal lymph sac; anesthesia and recovery are prolonged
	60 mg/kg ICe,[2] IV	Euthanasia, ICe is preferred route; can also be administered in lymph sacs in anurans
Propofol	100-140 mg/kg topically[46]	Unpublished data; Maroon-eyed Tree Frogs (*Agalychnis litodryas*); 15-20 min to maximal effect at 100 mg/kg dose, 10-15 min to maximal effect at 140 mg/kg[46]; sedation to deep anesthesia; remove and rinse when desired level achieved; recommended only for animals <50 g

Table 90-4 Chemical Restraint/Anesthetic/Analgesic Agents Used in Amphibians*—cont'd

Agent	Dosage	Species/Comments
Propofol—cont'd	10-30 mg/kg ICe[35]	Pilot study in White's Tree Frogs; use lower dosage for sedation or light anesthesia; induction within 30 min; recovery in 24 h
	60-100 mg/kg ICe[35]	Euthanasia
Tiletamine/zolazepam	10-20 mg/kg IM[27]	Results variable between species; recovery rapid; not suitable as single anesthetic agent for anurans[15]
Tricaine methanesulfonate (MS-222)	—	Anesthesia; buffer acidity by adding sodium bicarbonate to buffer solution to pH 7-7.1[8]; aerate water to prevent hypoxemia; remove from bath on induction or overdosing can easily occur; after bath, place terrestrial amphibians on moist towel or in very shallow water to recover[5]; some species can be induced at much lower concentrations than listed here[43]; in some cases, anesthesia can be maintained by dripping dilute solution of drug (100-200 mg/L) over the skin or by covering the animal with a paper towel moistened with anesthetic[43]
	1 g/L bath to effect[8]	Most gill-less adult species (unless very large)/induction
	100-200 mg/L bath to effect[38]	Larvae/induction
	200-500 mg/L bath to effect[6]	Tadpoles, newts/induction in 15-30 min
	0.5-2 g/L bath to effect[6]	Frogs, salamanders/induction in 15-30 min
	2-3 g/L bath to effect[47]	Toads/induction; takes 15-30 min
	50-200 mg/kg SC, IM, ICe[8]	Most species/may be irritating administered SC, IM (neutral solution is preferred)[8]
	100-200 mg/kg ICe[31]	Leopard Frogs
	100-400 mg/kg ICe[31]	Bullfrogs
	10 g/L bath[2]	Euthanasia; can be administered ICe or in lymph sacs
Yohimbine	Titrate to effect[18]	Antagonist to dexmedomidine

*SC can be administered in dorsal lymph sac in anurans.
SC, Subcutaneously; ED_{50}, effective dose for 50% of the population; IM, intramuscularly; BW, body weight; ICe, intracoelomically; IV, intravenously.

Table 90-5 Hormones Used in Amphibians*

Agent	Dosage	Species/Comments
Gonadotropin-releasing hormone (GnRH)	0.1 mg/kg SC, IM, repeat prn[25]	Induction of ovulation in those nonresponsive to PMSG or hCG; administer to females 8-12 h before males
	10 μg SC to female followed by additional 20 μg after 18 h; 5 μg SC to male[37]	Ovulation and spermiation in Tomato Frog (*Dyscophus guineti*)
Human chorionic gonadotropin (hCG)	50-100[6] to 300[25] IU SC, IM	For mating or release of sperm in males; follow with GnRH in 8-24 h
	250-400 IU SC, IM[6]	African Clawed Frogs, Axolotls, etc./induction of ovulation; may be used with PMSG or progesterone or both
Luteinizing hormone-releasing hormone	10 μg in 0.05 mL of 40% DMSO applied to ventral drink patch[26]	Induced spermiation in 70% of male *Bufo americanus* or *B. Valliceps*[26]
	5 μg ICe per salamander	Induced oviposition in 94% of *Desmognathus ochrophaeus*[34]
Pregnant mare serum gonadotropin (PMSG)	50-200 IU SC, IM[6]	African Clawed Frogs, Axolotls, etc./induction of ovulation; administer 600 IU hCG IM, SC 72 h later[25]
Progesterone	1-5 mg SC, IM[6]	African Clawed Frogs, Axolotls, etc./used in addition to PMSG or hCG for induction of ovulation

*SC can be administered into the dorsal lymph sac of anurans.
SC, Subcutaneously; IM, intramuscularly; prn, as needed; DMSO, dimethyl sulfoxide; ICe, intracoelomically.

Table 90-6 Miscellaneous Agents Used in Amphibians*

Agent	Dosage	Species/Comments
Amphibian Ringer's solution (ARS)	6.6 g NaCl, 0.15 g KCl, 0.15 g $CaCl_2$, and 0.2 g $NaHCO_3$ in 1 L water	For treating hydrocoelom and subcutaneous edema; place animal in shallow ARS bath until stabilized (≈24 h or more); replace with fresh solution daily; may need to wean animal off ARS by placing it in gradually more dilute solutions[47]; hypertonic solution created by using 800-950 mL water instead of 1 L and may be more effective for some cases of hydrocoelom[47]
Atropine	0.1 mg SC, IM prn	Organophosphate toxicosis[47]
Calcium glubionate	1 mL/kg PO q 24 h	Nutritional secondary hyperparathyroidism[47]
Calcium gluconate	100-200 mg/kg SC[47]	Hypocalcemic tetany[47]
	2.3% continuous bath (with 2-3 IU/mL vitamin D_3)[47]	Nutritional secondary hyperparathyroidism[47]
Cyanoacrylate surgical adhesive	Topical on wounds[7]	Produces seal for aquatic and semiaquatic species
Dexamethasone	1.5 mg/kg SC, IM[42]	Vascularizing keratitis; same dose IM or IV for shock
Dextrose 5% solution	Bath	For treating hydrocoelom and subcutaneous edema[46]; place animal in shallow bath until stabilized (≈24 h or more); replace with fresh solution daily; may need to wean animal off dextrose by placing it in gradually more dilute solutions; 7.5%-10% solutions may be more effective for some cases of hydrocoelom
Feline Clinical Care Liquid	1-2 mL/50 g PO q 24 h[46]	Dosage is approximate; may be more appropriate to offer larger volume less frequently for easily stressed animals
	3-6 mL/50 g PO q 72 h[46]	
Flunixin meglumine	1 mg/kg SC, IM q 24 h[47]	Analgesia; adjunct treatment for septicemia
Hill's Feline A/D	PO[7]	Nutritional support; mix 1:1 with water; generally gavaged
Laxative	PO[7]	Laxative, especially for intestinal foreign bodies
Methylene blue	2 mg/mL bath to effect[47]	Nitrite and nitrate toxicoses
Orabase	Topical on wounds[7]	Protective water-resistant ointment; antibiotics can be incorporated into the ointment[7]; do not use preparation containing local anesthetic such as benzocaine[46]
Oxygen	100% for up to 24 h[47]	Adjunct treatment of septicemia
Prednisolone sodium succinate	5-10 mg/kg IM, IV[47]	Shock
Sodium thiosulfate	1% solution as continuous bath to effect[47]	Halogen toxicoses
Vitamin B_1	25 mg/kg feed fish[19]	Deficiency resulting from thiaminase-containing fish
Vitamin D_3	2-3 IU/mL continuous bath (with 2.3% calcium gluconate)[47]	Nutritional secondary hyperparathyroidism
	100-400 IU/kg PO q 24 h[47]	
Vitamin E (alpha-tocopherol)	200 IU/kg feed[25]	Steatitis
	1 mg/kg IM, PO q 7 d[47]	
Waltham Feline Concentration	PO[7]	Nutritional support; mix 120 mL with 40-80 mL water, generally gavaged

*SC can be administered into the dorsal lymph sac of anurans.
SC, Subcutaneously; IM, intramuscularly; prn, as needed; PO, orally; q, every; IV, intravenously.

REFERENCES

1. Anver MR, Pond CL: Biology and disease of amphibians. In Fox JG, Cohen BJ, Loew FM, editors: *Laboratory animal medicine*, Orlando, Fla, 1984, Academic Press.
2. Burns RB, McMahan W: Euthanasia methods for ectothermic vertebrates. In Bonagura JD, editor: *Kirk's current veterinary therapy XII: small animal practice*, Philadelphia, 1995, WB Saunders.
3. Campbell TW: Amphibian husbandry and medical care. In Rosenthal KL, editor: *Practical exotic animal medicine* (Compendium Collection), Trenton, NJ, 1997, Veterinary Learning Systems.
4. Copper JE: Anesthesia of exotic animals, *Anim Technol* 35:13-20, 1984.
5. Crawshaw GJ: Amphibian medicine. In Kirk RW, Bonagura JD, editors: *Kirk's current veterinary therapy XI: small animal practice*, Philadelphia, 1992, WB Saunders.
6. Crawshaw GJ: Amphibian medicine. In Fowler ME, editor: *Zoo & wild animal medicine: current theraphy 3*, Philadelphia, 1993, WB Saunders.
7. Crawshaw GJ: Amphibian emergency and critical care, *Vet Clin North Am: Exotic Anim Pract* 1:207-231, 1998.
8. Downes H: Tricaine anesthesia in amphibia: a review, *Bull Assoc Rept Amph Vet* 5:11-16, 1995.
9. Fox WF: Treatment and dosages, *Axolotl Newsletter* 9:6, 1980.
10. Graczyk TK, Cranfield MR, Bichnese EJ, et al: Progressive ulcerative dermatitis in a captive wild-caught South American giant treefrog *(Phyllomedusa bicolor)* with microsporidial septicemia, *J Zoo Wildl Med* 27:522-527, 1996.
11. Iglauer F, Willamann F, Hilken G, et al: Anthelmintic treatment to eradicate cutaneous capillariasis in a colony of South African clawed frogs *(Xenopus laevis)*, *Lab Anim Sci* 47:477-482, 1997.
12. Jacobson E, Kollias GV, Peters LJ: Dosages for antibiotics and parasiticides used in exotic animals, *Compend Contin Educ Pract Vet* 5:315-324, 1983.
13. Johnson JH: Anesthesia, analgesia and euthanasia of reptiles and amphibians, *Proc Am Assoc Zoo Vet* 132-138, 1991.
14. Lafortune M, Mitchell MA, Smith JA: Evaluation of clinical and cardiopulmonary effects of clove oil (eugenol) on leopard frogs, *Rana pipients*, *Proc Assoc Rept Amph Vet* 51-53, 2000.
15. Letcher J: Evaluation of use of tiletamine/zolazepam for anesthesia of bullfrogs and leopard frogs, *J Am Vet Med Assoc* 207:80-82, 1995.
16. Letcher J, Glade M: Efficacy of ivermectin as an anthelmintic in leopard frogs, *J Am Vet Med Assoc* 200:537-538, 1992.
17. Letcher J, Papich M: Pharmacokinetics of intramuscular administration of three antibiotics in bullfrogs *(Rana catesbeiana)*, *Proc Assoc Rept Amph Vet/Am Assoc Zoo Vet* 79-93, 1994.
18. Machin KL: Amphibian pain and analgesia, *Zoo Wildl Med* 30:2-10, 1999.
19. Maruska EJ: Procedures for setting up and maintaining a salamander colony. In Murphy JB, Adler K, Collins JT, editors: *Captive management and conservation of amphibians and reptiles*, Ithaca, NY, 1994, Society for the Study of Amphibians and Reptiles.
20. Menard MR: External application of antibiotic to improve survival of adult laboratory frogs *(Rana pipiens)*, *Lab Anim Sci* 34:94-96, 1984.
21. Mitchell M: *Personal communication*, 2003.
22. Mombarg M, Claessen H, Lambrechts L, et al: Quantification of percutaneous absorption of metronidazole and levamisole in the fire-bellied toad *(Bombina orientalis)*, *J Vet Pharmacol Ther* 15:433-436, 1992.
23. Nichols DK, Lamirander EW, Pessier AP, et al: Experimental transmission and treatment of cutaneous chytridiomycosis in poison dart frogs, *Dendrobates auratus* and *Dendrobates tinctortius*, *Proc Am Assoc Zoo Vet/Int Assoc Aquatic Anim Med* 42-44, 2000.
24. Poynton SL, Whitaker BR: Protozoa in poison dart frogs *(Dentrobatidae)*: clinical assessment and identification, *J Zoo Wildl Med* 25:29-39, 1994.
25. Raphael BL: Amphibians, *Vet Clin N Am: Small Anim Pract* 23:1271-1286, 1993.
26. Rowson AD, Obringer AR, Roth TL: Non-invasive treatments of luteinizing hormone-releasing hormone for inducing spermiation in American *(Bufo americanus)* and Gulf Coast *(Buffo valliceps)* toads, *Zoo Biol* 20:63-74, 2001.
27. Schumacher J: Reptiles and amphibians. In Lumb WV, Jones EW, editors: *Veterinary anesthesia*, ed 2, Philadelphia, 1996, Williams & Wilkins.
28. Shilton CM, Smith DA, Craswshaw GJ, et al. Corneal lipid deposition in Cuban tree frogs *(Osteopilus septentrionalis)* and its relationship to serum lipids: an experimental study, *J Zoo Wild Med* 32:305-319, 2001.
29. Stein G: Reptile and amphibian formulary, In Mader DR, editor: *Reptile medicine and surgery*, Philadelphia, 1996, WB Saunders.
30. Stetter MD, Raphael B, Indiviglio F, et al: Isoflurane anesthesia in amphibians: comparison of five application methods, *Proc Am Assoc Zoo Vet* 255-257, 1996.
31. Stoskopf MK: Pain and analgesia in birds, reptiles, amphibians, and fish, *Invest Ophthalmol Visual Sci* 35:775-780, 1994.
32. Stoskopf MK, Arnold J, Mason M: Aminoglycoside antibiotic levels in the aquatic salamander *(Necturus necturus)*, *Zoo Anim Med* 18:81-85, 1987.
33. Teare JA, Wallace RS, Bush M: Pharmacology of gentamicin in the leopard frog *(Rana pipiens)*, *Proc Am Assoc Zoo Vet* 128-131, 1991.
34. Verrel PA: Hormonal induction in ovulation and oviposition in the salamander *Desmognathus ochrophaeus* (Plethodontidae), *Herp Rev* 20:42-43, 1989.
35. von Esse FV, Wright KM: Effect of intracoelomic propofol in White's tree frogs, *Pelodryas caerulea*, *Bull Assoc Rept Amph Vet* 9:7-8, 1999.
36. Whitaker BR: Developing an effective quarantine program for amphibians, *Proc North Am Vet Conf* 764-765, 1997.
37. Whitaker BR: Reproduction. In Wright KM, Whitaker BR, editors: *Amphibian medicine and captive husbandry*, Malabar, Fla, 2001, Krieger Publishing.
38. Whitaker BR, Wright KM, Barnett SL: Basic husbandry and clinical assessment of the amphibian patient, *Vet Clin North Am: Exotic Anim Pract* 2:265-290, 1999.
39. Willette-Frahm M, Wright KM, Thode BC: Select protozoan diseases in amphibians and reptiles, *Bull Assoc Rept Amph Vet* 5:19-29, 1995.
40. Williams DL: Amphibians. In Beynon PH, Cooper JE, editors: *Manual of exotic pets*, Gloucestershire, England, 1991, British Small Animal Veterinary Association.
41. Williams DL: Amphibian dermatology. In Bonagura JD, editor: *Kirk's current veterinary therapy XII: small animal practice*, Philadelphia, 1995, WB Saunders.
42. Williams DL, Whitaker R: The amphibian eye—a clinical review, *J Zoo Wildl Med* 25:18-28, 1994.
43. Wright KM: Amphibian husbandry and medicine. In Mader DR, editor: *Reptile medicine and surgery*, Philadelphia, 1996, WB Saunders.
44. Wright KM: Chlamydial infections of amphibians, *Bull Assoc Rept Amph Vet* 6:8-9, 1996.
45. Wright KM: Trauma. In Wright KM, Whitaker BR, editors: *Amphibian medicine and captive husbandry*, Malabar, Fla, 2001, Krieger Publishing.
46. Wright KM: *Personal communication*, 2004.
47. Wright KM, Whitaker BR: Pharmacotherapeutics. In Wright KM, Whitaker BR, editors: *Amphibian medicine and captive husbandry*, Malabar, Fla, 2001, Krieger Publishing.

APPENDIX A
REPTILE VIRAL DISEASES—SUMMARY TABLE
STEPHEN J. HERNANDEZ-DIVERS

Appendix A

Herpesviruses

General Characteristics:

Enveloped and pleomorphic; 100-200 nm.
Nuclear replication; hence, INIB.
Usually host adapted, causing little pathology but chronic latent infections.
Severe disease in non-host adapted species.
Horizontal transmission with direct contact, oculonasal and respiratory secretions, saliva, and feces.
Commonly affect the GI tract, respiratory tract, eye, and integument. Secondary bacterial or mycotic infections common.
Cell-to-cell transmission; hence, evade immune system. Survivors develop protective immunity against severe disease but do not clear virus (latency).
Diagnosis with viral neutralization (but assays generally epitope and hence, viral strain specific), ELISA, EM, histology, PCR (may be nonspecific and useful for multiple species), and virus isolation in TH-1 cells.
Treatment and control: supportive care (broad-spectrum antimicrobials, fluids, nutritional support, temperature, lesion debridement, nebulization), acyclovir, strict isolation, improvement of hygiene (sensitive to common disinfectants; e.g., sodium hypochlorite), reduction of stress (e.g., overcrowding), improvement in husbandry and nutrition.
Quarantine: 3 to 6 months, VN/ELISA, PCR at beginning and end of quarantine.
Any reptile infected with herpesvirus should be considered latently infected. May be demonstrated by persistent antibody titer. Paired titers 8 to 12 weeks apart to demonstrate active infection.

Disease	Species	Clinical Signs	Pathology	Specific Diagnosis	Comments
Herpesvirus of Freshwater Turtles	Pacific Pond Turtle (ChHV-2) Painted Turtle (ChHV-3) Map Turtle	Lethargy, anorexia, muscular weakness, edema	Ecchymotic hemorrhages on limbs, neck, plastron; limb and pulmonary edema; hepatomegaly and hepatic necrosis; splenic hypertrophy	INIB in liver, spleen, lung, kidney, and pancreas EM Virus isolation	Antimicrobials to control secondary infections Acyclovir
Herpesvirus of Tortoises	More than 50 spp., especially *Geochelone*, *Gopherus*, and *Testudo*, including Argentine Tortoise (ChHV-4) Desert Tortoise Spur-thighed Tortoise Gopher Tortoise Hermann's Tortoise Afghan Tortoise Marginated Tortoise	Oculonasal discharge, regurgitation, anorexia, lethargy, rhinitis, stomatitis, dyspnea, conjunctivitis, pharyngitis, glossitis, pneumonia, ataxia, and lymphoproliferative diseases	Ulcerative, necrotizing, hyperplastic lesions of the oropharynx, GI, and respiratory tracts; serous atrophy of fat; hepatic fatty degeneration; CNS involvement if severe	Large eosinophilic INIB in liver, spleen, lung, kidney, brain, GI tract EM ELISA VN PCR Virus isolation	Mortality up to 100% Antimicrobials to control secondary infections Acyclovir therapy Seroconversion takes 4 to 9 weeks
Herpesvirus of Seaturtles					
Gray-patch Disease (ChHV-1)	Captive-bred/reared Green Seaturtles 56 days to 1 year old	Epizootics of small circular papular skin lesions, coalesce into patches, then ulcerate	Ulcerative/necrotizing lesions	Basophilic INIB in epidermal cells EM Virus isolation	Predisposed by overcrowding and elevated temperatures Mortality 5% to 10% in severely affected individuals Acyclovir may be useful Outbreaks concentrate around January to August Disease experimentally reproduced

Lung, Eye, Trachea Disease	Green Seaturtles of more than 1 year	Harsh respiratory sounds; ulcerations/caseous debris over globe, oropharynx, and trachea; buoyancy problems; symptoms develop in 2 to 3 weeks	Keratitis, conjunctivitis, periglottal necrosis with mixed inflammatory infiltrate, necrotizing/caseous tracheitis, severe bronchopneumonia, multifocal white nodules in liver	Amorphous INIB in epithelial cells of trachea and lung EM	High mortality rate over weeks or months Disease experimentally reproduced Virus survives for up to 120 hours in sea water
Fibropapillomatosis	Free-ranging Green Seaturtles Kemp's and Olive Ridley and Loggerhead, rarely Hawksbill	Papillomatous tumors, gray to black, 2 to 20 cm; focal to multifocal; head, limbs, tail, plastron, carapace, cornea; internal papillomas affecting kidney, liver, GI tract, lung; cachexia of free-ranging turtles	Fibropapillomas: marked hyperplasia of epidermis, vacuolation of cytoplasm and ballooning degeneration of epidermal cells, proliferating fibroblasts in dermis	Eosinophilic INIB in fibropapilloma lesions EM	Wide surgical removal of external lesions (internal lesions have poor prognosis) Theorized causes are infection (herpes and reovirus) and environmental factors Disease experimentally reproduced and not directly associated with spirorchidiasis Possible transmission by Ozobranchus leech (mechanical vector)
Herpesvirus of Squamates:					
Herpesvirus of Boa Constrictors	Two neonate Boa Constrictors	Clutch of 16; 9 stillborn, 6 died in less than 1 year, 1 survived	Fatty degeneration of liver, multifocal hepatic and splenic necrosis, exudative glomerulonephritis	Amphophilic INIB in liver EM	
Venom Gland Herpesvirus Infection of Elapids and Viperids	Indian Cobra Banded Krait Siamese Cobra Mojave Rattlesnake	Thick tenacious venom, swollen venom glands	Multifocal necrosis of columnar glandular epithelium, mixed inflammatory infiltration	INIB in venom and venom gland	
Iguana Herpesvirus 1	Green Iguana	Subclinical, anorexia, lethargy, brilliant green coloration, lymphocytosis, spontaneous hemorrhage	Lymphocytosis; splenomegaly; histiocytic infiltrates of liver, spleen, myocardium, and bone marrow	INIB EM	Clinical signs of disease experimentally reproduced
Iguana Herpesvirus 2	San Esteban Chuckwallas	Fibrotic gingival hyperplasia, death	Hemorrhagic and congested lungs, pale necrotic liver, necrotic spleen, empty GI tract	INIB in liver PCR	
Herpesvirus of Agamas	Agamas	None; died within 6 months of capture	Hepatic and splenic necrosis, exudative pneumonia	INIB in liver and lung	
European Green Lizard Herpesvirus	European Green Lizards	Cutaneous papillomas associated with bites from mating	Characteristic papillomatous lesions	INIB in papillomas	Also in conjunction with papovavirus and reovirus
Gerrhosaurid Herpesviruses 1-3	Sudan Plated Lizards Black-lined Plated Lizards	Stomatitis, dyspnea	Labial and periglottal stomatitis	INIB in oral epithelium	

Continued

Appendix A

Adenoviruses

General Characteristics:

Nonenveloped; 70-90 nm.
Nuclear replication; hence, basophilic INIB.
Usually host-adapted, causing little pathology but disease in young, and in adults, asymptomatic chronic infections become clinical with concomitant disease/stress.
Commonly affect the GI tract, respiratory tract, liver, kidney, CNS, often asymptomatic.
Disease rare in animals with functional immune system. Concurrent bacterial, fungal, viral, or parasitic infections common.
Horizontal and vertical transmission generally by fecal-oral route.
Diagnosis with basophilic INIB, viral neutralization, EM, in situ hybridization with liver biopsy, PCR.
Treatment and control: supportive care (broad-spectrum antimicrobials, fluids, nutritional support, temperature), strict isolation, improvement in hygiene (removal of feces, persists in environment), treatment of underlying disease, reduction of stress (e.g., overcrowding), improvement in husbandry and nutrition.
Formalin, aldehyde, and iodophore disinfectants are effective.
Quarantine: 6 months, strict hygiene (remove feces), PCR detection.

Disease	Species	Clinical Signs	Pathology	Specific Diagnosis	Comments
Nile Crocodile Adenovirus	Nile Crocodiles	Underweight, no signs before death	Necrotizing enteritis; hepatic necrosis; congestion of lung, intestine, and kidney	Basophilic INIB in hepatocytes and crypt epithelial cells EM	Diseases occurred in two animals in Zimbabwe
Bearded Dragon and Rankin Dragon Adenoviruses	Bearded Dragons Rankin Dragons	None, to failure to thrive; anorexia; paresis; coelomic distension; depression; lethargy	Subcutaneous, coelomic, intestinal, and perirenal petechial to ecchymotic hemorrhages; enlarged yellow mottled liver with necrosis and vacuolar hepatic lipidosis; interstitial, peritubular nephritis and tubular lipidosis; pancreatitis, and lung congestion	Basophilic INIB in liver, kidney, intestine, pancreas, bile ducts EM	Concurrent coccidia and microsporidia Co-infected with dependovirus
Monitor Adenoviruses	Water Monitors Savannah Monitors	No signs, death	Hepatitis, proliferation of mucosal epithelial cells	Basophilic INIB in liver EM	Neonatal boa experimentally infected with intracoelomic injection of Savannah Monitor innoculant Died 14 days later of multifocal hepatic necrosis
Chameleon Adenoviruses	Mountain Chameleon Jackson's Chameleon Veiled Chameleon	None, to anorexia, tracheitis, esophagitis, opisthotonos, death in less than 3 days	Enteritis, tracheitis, esophagitis, mononuclear infiltrate	Basophilic INIB in epithelial cells of trachea, esophagus, enterocytes EM	Mountain Chameleon was wild-caught and strictly quarantined, so natural infections can occur
Boa Constrictor Adenovirus	Boa Constrictors	Lethargy, dehydration, anorexia, dermatitis, regurgitation, head tilt, death	Edematous small intestine containing excessive mucus, hepatomegaly with mottling and necrosis, lung congestion	Large basophilic INIB in hepatocytes only EM Viral isolation in viper heart cells	Concurrent enterohepatic amoebiasis, bacterial ulcerative enteritis, retroviral infection No bacteria isolated from liver; hence, viral hepatopathy

Disease	Clinical Signs	Pathology / Specific Diagnosis	Comments
Rosy Boa Adenovirus	Rosy Boas — No signs, death	Multifocal hemorrhages in intestinal serosa and liver	Basophilic INIB in hepatocytes, renal epithelial cells, heart EM, PCR Viral isolation in viper heart cells
Kingsnake Adenovirus	Mountain Kingsnakes — Regurgitation, dehydration, CNS disturbance, unresponsiveness, death	Gastroenteritis and necrotic enteritis with segmental mucosal necrosis and hyperplasia with villus blunting and fusion, hepatitis; gliosis in cerebrum, brainstem, and cervical spinal cord	Basophilic INIB in hepatocytes, renal epithelial cells, heart EM Adenoviral DNA by PCR	Gram-negative bacteria or *Clostridium* implicated in death Concurrent parvovirus
Mojave Rattlesnake Adenovirus	Mojave Rattlesnake — Abdominal mass detected day before death	Severe intestinal lesions with multifocal hemorrhage and ulceration	Basophilic INIB in enterocytes EM	Concurrent amoebiasis and renal carcinoma
Other Serpentine Adenoviruses	Four-lined Ratsnake, Boa Constrictor, Aesculpian Snake, Gaboon Viper, Royal Python, Palm Viper — Regurgitation, diarrhea, CNS signs, holding mouth open	Gastroenteritis, hepatitis, encephalitis, often subclinical; multifocal degeneration and necrosis of esophagus and mouth	Basophilic INIB in enterocytes and hepatocytes EM	Concurrent infections with parvovirus, picornavirus, herpesvirus, paramyxovirus

Paramyxoviruses

General Characteristics:

Enveloped, RNA viruses, pleomorphic, 150-300 nm.
Cytoplasmic replication; hence, eosinophilic ICIB, but can also produce INIB.
Multiple strains may infect different reptile species; generally low host specificity.
Commonly affect the respiratory tract, but also brain and pancreas.
Snakes, especially boas and pythons, may become chronic asymptomatic shedders for at least 10 months.
Horizontal transmission with direct contact, respiratory secretions, formites, ectoparasites (especially mites).
Seroconversion takes at least 8 weeks.
Development of HI ab does not correlate with cessation of virus shedding.
Recovered animals may be immune or persistent shedders.
Diagnosis eosinophilic ICIB in lung/pancreas, HI ab, virus isolation, PCR, FAT, in situ DNA hybridization.
Treatment and control: supportive care (broad-spectrum antimicrobials, diazepam for seizures, fluids, nutritional support, temperature), strict isolation, improvement in hygiene to reduce formite spread, reduction of stress (e.g., overcrowding), improvement in husbandry and nutrition, and different species not mixed.
Sodium hypochlorite, lysol, phenol, formalin disinfectants are effective. If organic contamination, must use detergent first.
Quarantine: 4 months, strict hygiene, test for HI ab at start and end. Serial EM or PCR on lung lavage/fecal samples. Eliminate ectoparasites (especially mites).

Disease	Species	Clinical Signs	Pathology	Specific Diagnosis	Comments
Ophidian Paramyxovirus	Mainly Viperidae (Fer-de-lance, *Crotalus*, *Vipera*, *Bothrops*, *Trimeresurus*, *Bitis*, *Ophiophagus*, *Agkistrodon*, *Hydrodynastes*) But also reported in: Elapidae	Peracute: death Acute (1-3 days): severe respiratory disease, dyspnea, brown to hemorrhagic discharge from nostrils and trachea, opisthotonos, head tremors, loss of righting reflex, convulsions, star-gazing	Lung edema, hemorrhage and hypertrophy, proliferation of type II alveolar cells Secondary bacterial infections and caseous pneumonia; hepatic necrosis, enlarged pancreas, multifocal gliosis, and perivascular cuffing in brain	Submit lung and pancreas Eosinophilic ICIB HI ab titers >1:20 suspect, >1:80 positive Single titer to document seroconversion (takes at least 8 weeks) Paired plasma HI ab titers at least 8-10 weeks apart to document active infection	Predisposed by poor husbandry, especially suboptimal temperature, old age Secondary bacterial pneumonias are common Concomitant adenovirus enteritis reported

Continued

Paramyxoviruses—cont'd

Disease	Species	Clinical Signs	Pathology	Specific Diagnosis	Comments
	Colubridae Boidae Pythonidae	Chronic (weeks to >1 year): mild respiratory disease leading to chronic pneumonia, often secondary bacterial infections, progressive neurologic disease, hypophagia, anorexia, regurgitation, emaciation		Virus isolation on VH cells PCR FAT In situ DNA hybridization	Prognosis generally grave, but Copperheads have remained asymptomatic Free-ranging, seroconverted Copperheads have been documented Incubation may be as short as 21 days, generally >90 days HI ab titers are not comparable between laboratories
Caiman Lizard Paramyxovirus	Caiman Lizard	Pneumonia	Proliferative pneumonia. ICIB in lung	EM Virus isolation in VH cells	Cross-reacted with ophidian paramyxovirus
Bearded Dragon Paramyxovirus	Bearded Dragon	Ascites		EM; paramyxovirus particles in ascitic aspirate	

Retroviruses

General Characteristics:
Nonenveloped, 95-110 nm.
Variable effects from subclinical to acute neurologic disease, and neoplasia.
Cytoplasmic replication; hence, eosinophilic ICIB.
Horizontal transmission with direct contact, aerosol, excrement, and snake mites implicated. Vertical transmission strongly suspected but unproven. Do not mix species.
Diagnostic biopsies of liver, kidney, esophageal tonsils, gastric mucosa, pancreas for eosinophilic ICIB on histopathology, EM, virus isolation on primary kidney or brain cells. PCR, serology and immunohistochemistry may become available in future.
Treatment and control: supportive care (broad-spectrum antimicrobials, fluids, nutritional support, temperature), strict isolation, excellent hygiene, reduction of stress (e.g., overcrowding), improvement in husbandry and nutrition, control of snake mites, and no mixing of different species, particularly boas and pythons.
Euthanatize confirmed cases.
Unstable outside host, so routine disinfectants effective.
Quarantine: 6 months, eliminate ectoparasites (especially mites). Use of sentinel Royal Pythons considered unreliable.

Disease	Species	Clinical Signs	Pathology	Specific Diagnosis	Comments
Inclusion Body Disease	Boidae, especially Burmese python Boa constrictor Also Vipers, Kingsnake	Pythons: acute; head tremors, opisthotonos, loss of righting reflex Boas: chronic; regurgitation, loose feces, stomatitis, dermatitis, dysecdysis, cutaneous neoplasia, leukemia, pneumonia, poor striking ability, dull mentation, anorexia, star-gazing, blindness, head tilt, disorientation	WBC (lymphs) normal or high Acute: nonsuppurative meningoencephalitis (python more than boa), hepatitis, hepatic lipidosis, ulcerative dermatitis, pneumonia Chronic: splenic/ pancreatic fibrosis, pancreatic atrophy, fat/muscle atrophy	Eosinophilic ICIB in pancreas > kidney/liver > stomach, lung, spleen, heart EM Virus isolation	More common in Burmese Pythons before the 1980s, now more common in Boas Mortality up to 100% in neonates, more protracted in adults; Boa Constrictors may be persistently infected reservoirs Do not mix Boas and Pythons

Disease	Species	Clinical Signs	Pathology	Specific Diagnosis	Comments
Other Retroviruses Identified from Snakes (with or without obvious pathology)	Jararacussu Viper Russell's Viper Cornsnake California Kingsnake Boa Constrictor Brazilian Lancehead Four-lined Chicken Snake Burmese Python	Palpable mass in 1 snake, otherwise none	Normal venom and spleen, pericardial myxofibroma, embryonal rhabdomyosarcoma, leukemia, erythroleukosis, fibrosarcoma, lymphosarcoma, transitional cell carcinoma, adenocarcinoma, renal and mesenchymal tumors	Retroviruses detected with EM	Disease has been experimentally reproduced in Burmese Pythons Incubation <2 weeks (Pythons) to many months (Boas) Secondary bacterial and protozoal diseases common Often type C retroviruses
Green Seaturtle Retrovirus	Green Seaturtle	None to fibropapillomas	None to fibropapillomas	EM retrovirus in healthy and fibropapillomatosis cases; heart, lung	Reverse transcriptase activity higher in fibropapillomatosis cases Retrovirus may be precipitating factor for fibropapillomatosis
Tuatara Retrovirus	Tuatara	None	None	EM	Endogenous retrovirus

Reoviruses

General Characteristics: Nonenveloped, RNA viruses, 70-85 nm in diameter, nearly spherical icosahedral particles.
Cytoplasmic replication; hence, eosinophilic ICIB.
Respiratory, Enteric and **Orphan**; often found without evidence of disease.
Many are nonpathogenic; few cause high morbidity and mortality depending on host age, strain virulence, route of exposure, and concurrent disease.
Horizontal transmission with direct contact or excrement. Incubation in reptiles unknown (2-9 days in birds).
Diagnosis: EM or virus isolation from tissues or feces (but may be present in normal animals).
Treatment and control: supportive care (broad-spectrum antimicrobials, fluids, nutritional support, temperature), strict isolation, good hygiene, reduction of stress (e.g., overcrowding), improvement in husbandry and nutrition.
Stable outside the host, especially in organic debris, resistant to many disinfectants. Infectivity reduced by prolonged contact with high concentrations of iodine, ethanol, or formalin.
Standard quarantine procedures.

Disease	Species	Clinical Signs	Pathology	Specific Diagnosis	Comments
Chinese Viper Reovirus	Chinese Vipers	Recently imported, no signs of disease before death	Hepatic necrosis, vacuolar degeneration of hepatocytes and enteritis	EM of intestinal cells Virus isolation in VH cells	
Rattlesnake Reovirus	Western Rattlesnake	Incoordination, propioceptive deficits, convulsions	Concurrent intestinal nematodiasis No gross or histologic lesions	EM in brain	
Spur-thighed Tortoise Reovirus	Spur-thighed Tortoise			EM of tongue, esophagus, lung, liver, kidney	
Royal Python Reovirus	Royal Python	Moribund		EM, viral isolation	Syncytium formation in chicken embryo fibroblasts, but no CPE in TH cells

Continued

Appendix A

Poxviruses

General Characteristics:
- DNA virus, large brick-shaped, enveloped virions up to 400 nm.
- Replicates in cytoplasm; hence, ICIB (Bollinger bodies).
- Very stable outside host, can remain infectious for years in organic debris.
- Horizontal transmission from environment or direct contact. Many require damage to epithelium to invade host.
- Incubation in reptiles unknown, persistent infections postulated in crocodilians.
- Diagnosis: histologic demonstration of large eosinophilic ICIB (Bollinger bodies) or EM of biopsies.
- In general, uninfected papules heal without scarring unless secondary infection.
- Treatment and control: debridement and wound cleansing, topical and if warranted systemic antimicrobials, supportive care (fluids, nutritional support, temperature), strict isolation, good hygiene, reduction of stress (e.g., overcrowding), improvement of husbandry and nutrition.
- Autogenous vaccination in crocodiles.
- Resistant to many disinfectants; KOH, steam, NaOH, phenols likely to be effective.
- Standard quarantine procedures.

Disease	Species	Clinical Signs	Pathology	Specific Diagnosis	Comments
Caiman Poxvirus	Spectacled Caiman	1-mm to 3-mm gray-white papular skin lesions over entire body but especially on head, may coalesce to form patches	Edematous dermatitis, mononuclear cellular infiltrates and large eosinophilic ICIB in hypertrophied epithelial cells	Histopathology, EM	Lesions resolved in two thirds of caiman over 1 month. Lesions progressed to patches, and third animal euthanatized
Crocodile Poxvirus	Nile Crocodiles	Yearlings only 2-mm to 8-mm yellow-brown proliferative, diffuse skin lesions, especially around eyes (can cause blindness), nostrils, mouth, ventral neck and body, limbs and tail base 2-mm to 5-mm brown blotches on gums and tongue	Multifocal hyperkeratosis, parakeratosis, large eosin ICIB	Histopathology, EM (virus not documented in oral lesions)	Reported from Africa 40% morbidity rate, 27% mortality rate. Signs usually regressed over 3-4 weeks leaving translucent scar. No disease reported in adjacent ponds. Stress and poor water quality considered predisposing factors in outbreak
Tegu Poxvirus	Golden Tegu	Brown papular dermatitis	Eosin ICIB of epithelial cells	Histopathology, EM	Spontaneously resolved in 3-4 months
Chameleon Poxvirus	Flap-necked Chameleons	None	ICIB within monocytes and macrophages in spleen and liver	Histopathology, EM	Chlamydophila inclusions also identified

Iridoviruses

General Characteristics:
- DNA virus, 120-300 nm, enveloped and icosahedral.
- Replicates in cytoplasm; hence, ICIB (but INIB also reported, especially in RBCs).
- Some reptile iridoviruses antigenetically related to frog virus 3 (*Ranavirus*); virus may cross taxonomic divides.
- Very stable outside host, can remain infectious for months in water or organic debris.
- Diagnosis: histologic demonstration of ICIB (or INIB in RBCs) or EM. PCR available for frogs and turtles.
- Treatment and control: supportive care (antimicrobials, fluids, nutritional support, temperature), strict isolation, good hygiene, reduction of stress (e.g., overcrowding), improvement in husbandry and nutrition.
- Standard quarantine procedures.

Disease	Species	Clinical Signs	Pathology	Specific Diagnosis	Comments
Hermann's Tortoise Iridovirus	Hermann's Tortoise	Either no signs before death, or stomatitis similar to herpesvirus lesions	Multiple gray spots in liver, congested spleen with small white foci on cut surface, hepatic necrosis, basophilic ICIB in hepatocytes and intestinal cells	Liver and spleen EM Virus isolation in TH cells and chicken fibroblasts PCR	
Spur-thighed Tortoise Iridovirus	Spur-thighed Tortoise	None		EM	Undetermined clinical importance
Gopher Tortoise Iridovirus	Gopher Tortoise	Upper respiratory tract disease, rhinitis, conjunctivitis, stomatitis, tracheitis	Necrotizing ulcerative tracheitis, pharyngitis, esophagitis, multifocal pneumonia Large ovoid to round basophilic ICIB	EM of trachea and lung	
Box Turtle Iridovirus	Box Turtle	Moribund		EM, virus isolation	Related to frog virus 3 (*Ranavirus*)
Soft-Shelled Turtle Iridovirus	Soft-shelled Turtle	"Red-neck disease"		EM, virus isolation	
Burmese Star Tortoise Iridovirus	Burmese Star Tortoise	Nasal discharge, stomatitis, conjunctivitis, cervical edema		PCR (related to frog virus 3)	
Variegated Dtella Iridovirus	Variegated or Tree Dtella Gecko		ICIBs, vasculitis, necrotizing splenitis, conjunctivitis, esophagogastroenteritis, glomerulonephritis, epicarditis, interstitial pneumonia	EM	Undetermined clinical importance
Chameleon Iridoviruses, Including Lizard Erythrocytic Virus	Chameleons, Geckos, Lacertids		INIBs in peripheral RBCs	EM	Undetermined clinical importance
Gryllus Bimaculatus Iridescent Virus (GbIV)	Bearded Dragon Spotted Chameleon Frilled Lizard		INIBs in peripheral RBCs	Virus isolation in VH cells EM PCR	PCR for frog virus 3 negative 100% identity with GbIV, an invertebrate iridescent virus of undetermined clinical importance in reptiles
Snake Erythrocytic Virus	Northern Watersnakes	None	None, more rounded RBCs with pyknotic nuclei	ICIB	Previously misidentified as *Toddia* sp. parasites
Green Tree Python Ranavirus	Green Tree Python	Nasal ulceration, stomatitis, edema	Ulceration, necrotizing inflammation of pharyngeal mucosa with heterophil and macrophage infiltration, edema	IHC, EM, ELISA, PCR In situ hybridization	Novel ranavirus of illegally imported snakes into Australia from Indonesia

Papillomaviruses

General Characteristics: DNA virus, 45-50 nm, nonenveloped, icosahedral.
Replicates in nucleus, producing INIB.
Papilloma viruses are generally highly host-specific and cause benign skin tumors (papillomas).
Difficult to replicate in cell culture, identification with molecular techniques (sequencing, cloning, hybridization) with nucleic acid from lesions.
Horizontal transmission, suggested routes by epidermal trauma (e.g., biting during mating).
Persist in the environment, inactivated by sodium hypochlorite, iodophores, and formaldehyde.
Diagnosis: histologic demonstration of INIB, EM.

Continued

Papillomaviruses—cont'd

Treatment and control: surgical removal but often recur, prolonged treatment with salicylic acid, supportive care (e.g., topical antimicrobials), strict isolation, good hygiene, reduction of stress (e.g., overcrowding), improvement in husbandry (i.e., reduction of skin trauma from abrasive substrates, reduction of aggression), and nutrition.
Potential for autogenous vaccines.
Standard quarantine procedures: 6 months.

Disease	Species	Clinical Signs	Pathology	Specific Diagnosis	Comments
Bolivian Side-neck Turtle Papillomavirus	Bolivian Side-neck Turtles	Pale, flat to oval skin lesions, especially on head; focal to coalescing patches; plastron lesions typically ulcerate and secondarily infected	Thickened stratum corneum, hyperplastic, acanthotic epidermis, vacuolated nuclei	INIBs in epidermal cells EM	
European Green Lizard Papillomavirus	European Green Lizards	Firm, gray to black, 2-mm to 20-mm proliferative masses, especially on neck and tail base, not on ventrum	Hyperkeratotic, hyperplastic epidermal cells	INIBs in epidermal cells EM	Herpesvirus and reovirus also found in lesions Surgical removal effective in mild cases

Parvoviruses

General Characteristics:
DNA virus, 18-26 nm, nonenveloped, icosahedral.
Replicates in nucleus, producing large basophilic INIB (Cowdry type A inclusions).
Often in association with a helper virus, adenovirus, or herpesvirus. All reptile parvoviruses have been in association with other viruses.
Replicate in rapidly growing cells; hence, predilection for intestinal tract and causing severe diarrhea.
Horizontal transmission by fecal-oral route, very stable outside host.
Inactivated by formalin or sodium hypochlorite. Parvoviruses destroyed by 0.5% formaldehyde for 15 minutes.
Diagnosis: histologic demonstration of INB (Cowdry type A inclusions) or EM.
Treatment and control: supportive care (antimicrobials, fluids, nutritional support, temperature), strict isolation, good hygiene, reduction of stress (e.g., overcrowding), improvement in husbandry and nutrition.
Standard quarantine procedures.

Disease	Species	Clinical Signs	Pathology	Specific Diagnosis	Comments
Kingsnake Parovirus	Juvenile Californian Mountain Kingsnake	Regurgitation, dehydration, death <72 hours	Gastroenteritis; pylorus and SI dilated and filled with pasty yellow ingesta; multifocal petechial hemorrhages of GI tract serosa, intestinal mucosal edema, and necrosis; crypt distension with sloughed enterocytes, hyperplasia and villus blunting	Basophilic Cowdry type A INIB in enterocytes peripheral to necrosis EM: parvovirus (15-18 nm) and adenovirus (65-70 nm)	Other snakes including adults of same species were unaffected These juveniles were fed wild-caught Fence Lizards that were proposed as a possible source of infection
Bearded Dragon Dependovirus	Neonate Bearded Dragons	Nonspecific signs, death	Enteritis	Basophilic INIBs in liver and small intestine EM: adenovirus in liver and intestine, dependovirus in liver	
Serpentine Adeno-associated Virus (SAAV), Dependovirus	Boa Constrictor Royal Python			Virus isolation in VH cells	Unknown clinical importance

Togaviruses and Flaviviruses

General Characteristics:
- RNA virus, icosahedral enveloped particles, 40-70 nm.
- Transmitted by arthropod vectors, especially mosquitoes and ticks.
- Reptiles implicated in maintenance and transmission of WEE, EEE, VEE, JE, and West Nile viruses.
- Serologic evidence of togaviruses in 25 spp. snakes, 14 spp. lizards, 12 spp. chelonia, 1 crocodilian.
- Many reptiles serve as subclinical natural reservoirs; high viremia for improved vector infection and transmission.
- Horizontal and vertical transmission.
- Serologic activity documented in free-ranging reptiles; viremia ceases after solid immune response, often subclinical.
- Disease in non-host adapted species, generally encephalitis and enteritis.
- Unstable outside the host, inactivated by common disinfectants.
- Diagnosis: serology, virus isolation, EM, PCR, immunoperoxidase staining with monoclonal antibodies.
- Treatment and control: prevent contact with vectors (i.e., control arthropods or move outdoor reptiles inside during high vector prevalence), supportive care (antimicrobials, fluids, nutritional support, temperature), reduction of stress (e.g., overcrowding), improvement in husbandry and nutrition.
- Standard quarantine procedures, remove arthropods and control mosquitoes.

Disease	Species	Clinical Signs	Pathology	Specific Diagnosis	Comments
Japanese Encephalitis Virus	Soft-shelled Turtle Skinks	None	None	Virus isolation, EM	Unknown clinical importance
Western Equine Encephalitis Virus	Gartersnakes Gophersnakes Blue Racers Texas Tortoises	None	None	Virus isolation from blood, EM Serology: HI, CF, VN	Cyclic viremia associated with temperature changes 44% of tortoises were positive 70% of infected tortoises developed neutralizing antibodies Snakes brumated (hibernated) 11 days PI developed viremia Snakes brumated (hibernated) 19 days PI did not
Eastern Equine Encephalitis Virus	Gartersnakes Spotted Turtles Cuban Iguanas	None	None	Virus isolation, EM	Viremia lasted 36 days to >6 months
West Nile Virus	American Alligators	Depression, lethargy, neurologic disease	Heterophilic lymphoplasmocytic meningoencephalomyelitis; coelomic effusion; fibronecrotic oral mucosal exudate, glossitis, necrotic stomatitis; enlarged pale liver with red mottling, hepatic lipidosis, necrotic hepatitis, splenitis; myocardial degeneration and necrosis, mild interstitial pneumonia, adrenalitis	Virus isolation, EM, PCR Immunoperoxidase staining monoclonal antibody	High viremia, potential amplification hosts, 3.3% mortality rate
	Green Iguanas Florida Gartersnakes Red-eared Sliders	None	None	Virus isolation, EM	Low but detectable viral loads in blood, oral or cloacal swabs, or organs

Continued

Caliciviruses

General Characteristics:
RNA virus, 35-40 nm, nonenveloped, icosahedral.
Replicates in cytoplasm, may find INIB and ICIB.
Transmission unknown.
Inactivated by sodium hypochlorite.
Diagnosis: histologic demonstration of inclusions, EM, PCR, virus isolation.
Treatment and control: supportive care (antimicrobials, strict isolation, good hygiene), reduction of stress (e.g., overcrowding), improvement in husbandry and nutrition.
Standard quarantine procedures.

Disease	Species	Clinical Signs	Pathology	Specific Diagnosis	Comments
Reptilian Calicivirus Crotalus Type 1	Aruba Rattlesnake, Rock Rattlesnake, Eyelash Viper	Diarrhea, lethargy, death	Enteritis, hepatitis	EM, virus isolation in vero cells from cloacal swabs	Isolated viruses not definitively associated with particular disease. Virus recovered from cloacal swabs of normal animals and SI, liver, and kidney of diseased animals at necropsy. Experimental infection in Western Rattlesnake died 61 days PI. Also recovered from pinnipeds

Adapted from Schumacher J: Viral Diseases. In Mader D: *Reptile medicine and surgery*, ed 1, Philadelphia, 1996, WB Saunders; and Ritchie B: Virology. In Mader D: *Reptile medicine and surgery*, ed 2, St Louis, 2006, Saunders. *INIB*, Intranuclear inclusion bodies; *ELISA*, enzyme-linked immunosorbent assay; *EM*, electronmicroscopy; *PCR*, polymerase chain reaction; *VN*, virus neutralization; *ChHV*, chelonid herpesvirus; *GI*, gastrointestinal; *CNS*, central nervous system; *ICIB*, intracytoplasmic inclusion bodies; *HI ab*, hemagglutination inhibition antibody; *FAT*, fluorescent antibody test; *VH*, viper heart cells; *WBC*, white blood cell; *SI*, small intestine; *CPE*, cytopathic effect; *TH*, tortoise heart cells; *KOH*, potassium hydroxide; *RBC*, red blood cell; *IHC*, immunohistochemical staining; *EEE*, Eastern equine encephalitis; *VEE*, Venezuelan equine encephalitis; *JE*, Japanese encephalitis; *SGP*, snake globulin precipitation; *CF*, complement fixation; *WEE*, Western equine encephalitis; *PI*, postinfection.

APPENDIX B
REPTILE PARASITES—SUMMARY TABLE

STEPHEN J. HERNANDEZ-DIVERS

Appendix B

Reptile Parasites

Parasite	Host	Location and Clinical Signs	Pathology	Diagnosis	Treatment
ECTOPARASITES					
Ticks					
Hard-bodied ticks: *Amblyomma*, *Aponomma*, *Ixodes*, *Hyalomma*, *Haemaphysalis*	Many species of lizards, snakes, chelonians, crocodilians	Axillae, around joints, cloaca, nostrils, eyes, between plastron and carapace	Localized skin damage and entry of secondary infections. Transmit disease (viruses, bacteria, and blood parasites; e.g., *Coxiella burnetti* of Ball Pythons, *Amblyomma marmoreum* and *A. sparsum*; transmits *Cowdria ruminantum* from African Tortoises). Anemia in large numbers, can be fatal. Transmit zoonoses: Tularemia, Siberian tick typhus, Lyme disease	Physical examination	Physical removal. Permethrin, ivermectin (not chelonia)
Soft-bodied ticks: *Argasidae*, *Ornithodoros*	Many species of lizards, carapace snakes, chelonians, crocodilians	Axillae, around joints, cloaca, nostrils, eyes, between plastron and carapace	Localized skin damage, and entry of secondary infections. Transmit disease (blood parasites, viruses, bacteria). Anemia in large numbers. *Ornithodoros* transmits the filarid, *Macdonaldius*, to snakes. Transmit zoonosis: Relapsing fever	Physical examination	Physical removal. Permethrin, ivermectin (not chelonia)
Mites					
Ophionyssus natricis	Snakes, Some lizards	Under scales, especially around eyes, nostrils, pits, cloaca	Irritation, anemia, disease transmission (*Aeromonas hydrophila* septicemia, viruses)	Physical examination, microscopy	Permethrin, ivermectin, OPs, environmental control. Use of predatory mites, *Hypoaspis*.
Hirstiella: *H. pyriformis*, *H. trombidiiformis*	Lizards	Under scales, especially around eyes, nostrils, axillae, tail base, cloaca, and skin folds	Irritation, anemia, potential disease transmission (bacteria, viruses)	Physical examination, microscopy	Permethrin, ivermectin, OPs, environmental control
Prostigmatid mites: *Ophioptidae*, *Cloacaridae*	Snakes, Snapping Turtle, Painted Turtle	Under scales. Cloacal mucosa	Minimal, mild irritation	Physical examination, microscopy	Rarely indicated; permethrin

Chiggers: *Trombiculid larvae*	Snakes Lizards	Skin folds	Unknown, probably mild irritation	Physical examination, microscopy (three-legged larval mite)	Rarely indicated; permethrin, ivermectin, OPs
Flies and Mosquitoes					
Calliphorid (blowflies)	All terrestrial reptiles	Open wounds	Maggot infestation, secondary bacterial infection, toxemia	Physical examination	Wound irrigation, maggot removal, permethrins, ivermectin (not chelonians), supportive care Vector control Protect wounds
Cuterebra (bot flies)	Box Turtles and other terrestrial reptiles	Neck and limbs, and softer skin areas Localized swellings, anorexia and debilitation if numerous	Fistulous tract leading to incubating bot larva Local inflammation, secondary infection	Physical examination	Surgical removal, vector control
Culex (mosquitoes)	All terrestrial reptiles	Usually none	Usually none, but may transmit viruses and hemoparasites; anemia if severe	Physical examination	Vector control
Leeches					
Hirundinea (leeches) *Placobdella papillifera* *Placobdella multilineata*	Aquatic reptiles, especially alligators	In and around mouth, cervical and axillary areas	Rarely cause disease, but may transmit other diseases (e.g., *Haemogregarina crocodilnorum*)	Physical examination	Salt or freshwater baths Topical vinegar or alcohol
ENDOPARASITES					
Amoebiasis					
Entamoeba invadens	Snakes (especially Watersnakes) Lizards Turtles (especially Giant Tortoises)	Gastrointestinal tract causing ulcerative gastroenteritis, colitis, dysentery Hematogenous spread to liver and kidneys	Ulcerative gastroenteritis, hematogenous spread causing abscess and necrosis Mortality ≤ 100% in snakes, 13-77 d PI Pathology in carnivores appears related to absence of plant starch, which *Entamoeba* require for completion of life cycle; if unavailable, invades intestinal cell for glycogen alternative	Fecal flotation, direct smear Lugols iodine may help Culture	Metronidazole and increase temperature Avoid mixing carriers and susceptible species Gartersnakes, Black Racers, Eastern Box Turtles, and crocodilians considered carriers Kingsnake and King Cobra considered more resistant

Continued

Reptile Parasites—cont'd

Parasite	Host	Location and Clinical Signs	Pathology	Diagnosis	Treatment
Coccidiosis					
Eimeria	Snakes, lizards, chelonia, crocodilians	Gastrointestinal and bile duct epithelium. Anorexia, dehydration, regurgitation, hemorrhagic enteritis	Protozoan causes cellular destruction. Intestinal ulcers, fibrosis, secondary septicemia	Oocysts in feces (4 sporocysts, 2 sporozoites)	Trimethoprim/sulfonamides, sulfa drugs. Hygiene and isolation
Isospora	Snakes, lizards, crocodilians	Gastrointestinal and bile duct epithelium. Anorexia, dehydration, regurgitation, hemorrhagic enteritis. Renal infection in one boa constrictor	Protozoan causes cellular destruction, may migrate from cloaca to kidneys. Intestinal ulcers, fibrosis, secondary septicemia	Oocysts in feces (2 sporocysts, 4 sporozoites)	Trimethoprim/sulfonamides, sulfa drugs. Hygiene and isolation
Caryospora	Uncommon Snakes, lizards	Gastrointestinal epithelium. Anorexia, dehydration, regurgitation, hemorrhagic enteritis	Protozoan causes cellular destruction. Intestinal ulcers, fibrosis, secondary septicemia	Oocysts in feces (1 sporocyst, 8 sporozoites)	Trimethoprim/sulfonamides, sulfa drugs. Hygiene and isolation

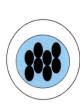

Cryptosporidiosis

Cryptosporidium serpentis	Snakes	Snakes, varanids, Frilled Lizard: Gastric causing regurgitation, weight loss, midbody swelling	Parasite inhabits parasitophorous vacuole in microvillus; sporulation within host cells immediately infectious; no need for sporulation outside host	None 100% effective; TMS, sulfa drugs, paromomycin, spiramycin
Cryptosporidium saurophilum	Lizards Leopard Gecko Frilled Lizard Varanids	Asymptomatic snakes (Rough Greensnake, Common Gartersnake) and chelonians: Died with small intestinal and proximal large intestinal lesions	Snakes: hypertrophic gastritis Lizards: hypertrophic enteritis Hyperplasia, mononuclear infiltration Loss of fat bodies and muscle mass	Oocysts (<5 μm) in feces, gastric lavage, gastric biopsy, ELISA (ab) IFA 16× better than acid-fast stain	Hyperimmune bovine serum, toltrazuril Disinfection: ammonia, formaldehyde
		Most lizards (Leopard Geckos): Intestinal causing weight loss, anorexia, diarrhea, lethargy Not considered zoonotic for immunocompetent humans			

Hemoprotozoa

Haemogregarines: Little clinical disease, occasional anemia, all require invertebrate intermediate host or vector

Adeleiina		Usually asymptomatic	Gametogony and schizogony in reptile; gametocytes in RBCs ± WBCs; may accumulate in liver, spleen, and lung	Blood smear; gametocytes	Therapeutic information lacking
Haemogregarina H. crocodilnorum	Aquatic spp. American Alligator	Transmitted usually by ingestion of arthropod or annelid vector; sporogony in invertebrate vector			
Hepatozoon Karyolyses	Terrestrial spp. Old-World lizards and treesnakes	May cause problems in young with concomitant disease/captivity stress (e.g., granulomatous hepatitis in southern water snakes)			

Continued

Reptile Parasites—cont'd

Parasite	Host	Location and Clinical Signs	Pathology	Diagnosis	Treatment
Eimeriina *Schellackia Lainsonia*	Lizards, snakes Many species worldwide	Transmitted usually by ingestion of arthropod or annelid vector; sporogony and gametogony in reptile, present in RBCs and lymphs Usually asymptomatic	Usually nonpathogenic May cause problems in young with concomitant disease/captivity stress	Blood smear	Therapeutic information lacking
Aegyptianella Babesia Sauroplasma Serpentoplasma	Chelonians, snakes, lizards Rare	Transmitted by biting insects and arthropods Small nonpigmented RBC inclusions (piroplasms) Usually asymptomatic	Usually nonpathogenic	Blood smear	Therapeutic information lacking
Plasmodium and Haemoproteus: Peripheral blood, intraerythrocytic with schizogony stages in RBCs					
Plasmodiidae Plasmodium Fallisia Saurocytozoon Haemoproteus	Snakes; *Plasmodium, Haemoproteus* only Lizards, turtles; all four genera	Arthropod transmission (e.g., Culex) Usually asymptomatic	Usually nonpathogenic, mild anemia Characteristic pigment in RBCs *Plasmodium mexicanum* fatal in juvenile lizards because of hemolytic anemia	Blood smear	Chloroquine
Trypanosomiasis: Peripheral blood, extracellular trypanomastigote					
Trypanosoma spp.	Lizards, snakes, chelonians, crocodilians Worldwide distribution	Transmitted by intermediate hosts; dipteran biting flies or leeches to crocodiles and caiman Usually asymptomatic	Usually nonpathogenic	Blood smear; extracellular	Therapeutic information lacking
Leishmaniases: Peripheral blood					
Leishmania spp.	Rare disease of some lizards	Transmitted by sand flies Intracytoplasmic in thrombocytes, lymphocytes, or monocytes Usually asymptomatic	Usually nonpathogenic	Tissue culture techniques preferred as difficult to show in blood smears (round to oval 2-4 μm)	Therapeutic information lacking
Sarcosporidia					
Myxosporidia Microsporidia	Lizards Chelonians	Small protozoan intracellular parasites Cysts may infect heart and skeletal muscle or gallbladder in aquatic chelonians Usually asymptomatic, may cause swollen muscles, anorexia, lethargy, weight loss, death	White fusiform streaks in muscles, myositis, myocarditis Hepatic necrosis in Bearded Dragons; parasites also seen in epithelial cells of kidneys, lungs, stomach, enterocytes, capillary endothelial cells, and brain	Histologic demonstration of parasites	None reported
Ciliated Protozoa					
Balantidium Nyctotheroides	Common in chelonians	Lower intestinal tract commensals, usually asymptomatic	Nonpathogenic, no evidence of disease, but numbers may increase secondary to other disease/stressor	Fecal float, direct smear	Rarely required, metronidazole

Flagellated Protozoa				
Hexamita *Trichomonas* *Giardia* *Leptomonas*	Lizards, snakes, chelonians, crocodilians	Gastrointestinal and urinary tracts Usually asymptomatic commensal, may cause anorexia, weight loss, unthriftiness	Usually nonpathogenic Probably requires concomitant primary disease/stressor to become pathogenic Hexamita: reported to be pathogenic to chelonians but not crocodilians; may cause nephritis, enteritis, colitis	Fecal float, direct smear	Rarely required, metronidazole
Trematodes				
Monogenea	Freshwater chelonians	Flukes <3 mm length in urinary bladder, nose, mouth, esophagus	Nonpathogenic, no disease reported, but possible in captivity given direct life-cycle	Adult fluke or eggs in feces/urine	None reported; try praziquantel, albendazole
Aspidogastrea	Freshwater chelonians	External and internal (gastrointestinal) No clinical signs reported	None reported, nonpathogenic Freshwater snails intermediate hosts Disease in captivity unlikely because of lack of intermediate hosts	Adult fluke or eggs in feces	None reported; try praziquantel, albendazole
Digenea				
Refifers *Renifers* *Dasymetra* *Ochetosoma* *Stomatrema* *Pneumatophilus* *Zeugorchis* *Lechriorchis*	Indigo Snakes Watersnakes Kingsnakes Hog-nosed Snakes Gartersnakes	Mouth, oral cavity, esophagus, trachea, lungs Usually asymptomatic, occasional pneumonia Amphibian (or fish) intermediate host	Nonpathogenic in oral cavity Ulcerating lesions in lungs, secondary pneumonia	Adult flukes on oral examination Eggs in feces or lung wash	Manual removal, praziquantel, albendazole
Spirorchidae *Laeredius* spp. *Spirorchis* spp.	Aquatic chelonians (and other reptiles)	Listlessness, anorexia, fluid accumulation (circulatory disturbance), floatation abnormality (secondary pneumonia), ischemic necrosis (egg granulomas), pitting ulcerations of the shell, secondary infections, especially pneumonia Prepatent period 6 wk to 4 mo Snail intermediate host (egg → miracidia → cercaria)	Cercariae penetrate mucous membranes or skin causing dermatitis Adults reside in heart and blood vessels and release eggs into circulation causing egg granulomas in various tissues or ischemic necrosis if block terminal arterioles; eggs can penetrate gastrointestinal tract to escape in feces	Adults at necropsy, ELISA Eggs; feces (sediment), or tissues	None reported; try praziquantel, albendazole Often found in association with fibropapillomas in Green Seaturtles
Styphlodoro (renal flukes)	Kingsnakes, Cottonmouth Moccassins Indigosnakes Ratsnakes Bushmasters Boa Constrictors	Renal flukes found in renal tubules, ureters, and cloaca Clinical signs rare, unless high numbers	Renal tubular damage, characteristic nodules of small calcified exudate	Adult flukes (round to oval) or eggs in urine	Praziquantel

Continued

Reptile Parasites—cont'd

Parasite	Host	Location and Clinical Signs	Pathology	Diagnosis	Treatment
Alaria marcinae	Texas Indigo Snake Red-eared Slider	Soft fluctuant masses in tail, mandibular and cervical regions	Minimal	Clinical signs, histopathology	Surgical resection, drainage

Cestodes

Proteocephalidea: All indirect with invertebrae, fish, or amphibian intermediate host; various paratenic hosts

Parasite	Host	Location and Clinical Signs	Pathology	Diagnosis	Treatment
Proteocephalus *Acanthotaenia* *Crepidobothrium* *Ophiotaenia*	Varanid lizards Varanids, snakes Snakes Snakes, aquatic chelonia	Adults located in proximal small intestine, few if any clinical signs Ophiotaenia most common in NA snakes from ingestion of infected frogs None reported in crocodilians	Nonpathogenic unless very high numbers	Eggs or segments in fecal float or direct smear	Praziquantel

Pseudophyllidea: Complex life cycles with several intermediate hosts, coracidium → procercoid (crustacean) → pleurocercoid (vertebrates)

Parasite	Host	Location and Clinical Signs	Pathology	Diagnosis	Treatment
Spirometra *Bothriocephalus*	Various snakes, especially Australia, Africa, East Asia	Snakes are intermediate hosts (felids and canids definitive hosts) Soft tissue swellings in dorsolateral body, especially posterior region; rarely secondary infection leads to rupture; heavy infestation causes lethargy, anorexia, weight loss Zoonosis	Pleurocercoids encyst in SQ muscle, called Spargana, cause soft tissue parasitic cysts	Pleurocercoid identification	Surgical removal Praziquantel
Bothridium *Duthiersia* *Scyphocephalus*	Boas and Pythons Varanids Varanids	Adults in gastrointestinal tract	Nonpathogenic unless very high numbers leading to obstruction Enteritis reported in Green Tree Pythons	ID adult cestodes (10-80 cm) or eggs in feces	Praziquantel

Mesocestoidea: All indirect with invertebrate, fish, or amphibian intermediate host; reptiles can be intermediate or definitive hosts

Parasite	Host	Location and Clinical Signs	Pathology	Diagnosis	Treatment
Nematotaeniidae	Lizards	Intestinal tract	None	Identification of adult cestodes or eggs in feces	Praziquantel
Anoplocephalidae	Lizards Chelonians Snakes	Ingestion of cysticeroids in arthropod intermediate host Medium to large cestode in intestinal tract	None	Identification of adult cestodes or eggs in feces	Praziquantel
Dilepididae	Snakes Small lizards	Adult cestode of birds and mammals Reptiles are intermediate hosts, cysticeroids in peritoneum and liver	Local parasitic cysts, minimal reaction	Identification of cysticeroid in peritoneum or tissues	None reported, surgical removal, praziquantel

Parasite	Host	Life cycle / Location	Clinical signs / Pathology	Diagnosis	Treatment
Mesocestoididae	Kingsnakes, Rattlesnakes, Iguanid lizards	Adult cestodes in mammal intestinal tract. In reptiles, second-stage tetrathyridea encyst in kidney, intestinal wall, liver, lung, coelomic cavity, and serosal surfaces of other organs. Zoonosis: eating raw snake liver	Local tetrathyridium cysts, minimal reaction	Identification of tetrathyridium cysts in reptile tissues	None reported; surgical removal, praziquantel. Tetrathyridium cysts may asexually reproduce in rattlesnakes and mice; do not feed fresh wild rodents

Nematodes

Ascarididea: Large worms with thick double-walled eggs

Parasite	Host	Life cycle / Location	Clinical signs / Pathology	Diagnosis	Treatment
Ophidascaris labiatopapillosa	Watersnakes, Kingsnakes, Hog-nosed Snakes, Black Racers	L3 larvae ingested with intermediate host (amphibians, rodents), migrate from gastrointestinal tract to lungs, adults in esophagus, stomach, small intestine	Larval migration can cause ulcerations and abscesses in lungs/trachea; Ophidascaris adults may bury into mucosa and submucosa; gastrointestinal perforations or obstructions in heavy infestations	Adults or eggs in feces (or vomit). Adults, eggs or larvae in skin biopsy, skin examination	Benzimidazoles, ivermectin (not Chelonia)
Ophidascaris moreliae Polydelphis anoura	Pythons	Regurgitation, weight loss, anorexia, death			
Sulcascaris Angusticaecum	Chelonia	Direct life cycle in herbivores	Can cause extensive damage and mortality. Necrotizing ulcerative gastritis in juveniles		
Dujardinascaris waltoni Paratrichosoma crocodilus	Crocodilians	Adults reside below skin, larvae migrate through stratum corneum causing zigzag marks	Minimal, but results in significant reduction in skin value		
Anisakiidae	Marine turtles	Cranial small intestine	Minimal, but zoonotic	Adults or eggs in feces	Benzimidazoles

Rhabdiasidea: Free living and parasitic, parthenogenetic phases; not reported in chelonians or crocodilians

Parasite	Host	Life cycle / Location	Clinical signs / Pathology	Diagnosis	Treatment
Rhabdias sp.	Snakes	L3 penetrate mucosa or skin and migrate to lungs; adult females in lungs (rarely coelom and pericardial sac)	Severe pneumonia reported in captive snakes (direct life cycle)	Eggs or larvae in feces, oral secretions, or lung wash	Benzimidazoles, Ivermectin, levamisole
Enteromelas sp.	Lizards	Larvated eggs or larvae up trachea, swallowed and passed in feces	Usually no signs, but can cause significant disease in captivity (poor temp, ventilation, humidity, hygiene); respiratory distress, open mouth breathing, anorexia, weight loss, death		
Strongyloides	Many snakes	Adults in small intestine	Diarrhea, weight loss	Larvated eggs or free larvae in feces	Benzimidazoles, Ivermectin
	Burmese Pythons	Ureters, kidneys, enteritis, aberrant location? Parthenogenetic females → eggs in feces → larvae may penetrate skin or mature as free-living adults	Rare in nature, may cause gastroenteritis in captivity		

Continued

Appendix B

Reptile Parasites—cont'd

Parasite	Host	Location and Clinical Signs	Pathology	Diagnosis	Treatment
Strongylidea: Small to medium sized worms found throughout the gastrointestinal tract; feed on host blood and tissue fluids					
Diaphanocephaloidea (hookworms) *Diaphanocephalus* *Kalicephalus* *Spineoxys*	Snakes Some lizards Freshwater turtles	Ingested or skin penetration of L3, adults in gastrointestinal tract from esophagus to large intestine Adults feed on blood Asymptomatic in nature, can cause severe disease in captivity, especially in unsanitary conditions, as result of direct life cycle Anorexia, debilitation, regurgitated worms	Gastrointestinal ulceration, obstruction, intussusception Small worms may be missed on necropsy	Adults in feces/vomit, fecal float, and direct for eggs	Improved hygiene Benzimidazoles, ivermectin (not chelonia)
Filariidae: Produce microfilaria not eggs, usually subclinical					
Oswaldofilaria spp. *Befilaria* spp. *Conofilaria* spp. *Piratuba* spp. *Piratuboides* spp. *Solafilaria* spp. *Foleyella* spp.	Crocodilians and lacertid lizards Chameleon, lacertids	Mosquito or tick vector ingest microfilaria and inject second host Adults reside in posterior vena cava or renal veins Usually subclinical but clinical signs including edema and necrosis	Usually nonpathogenic At necropsy, adults may be found in blood vessels, free in coelom, or under skin Thrombosis causes edema, aneurysms, necrosis May cause extensive dermal lesions in Asian Pythons from microfilariae in capillaries	Microfilaria in blood smear; SQ removal of adult *Foleyella*	Control vectors Treatment of a patent infection (ivermectin) may cause death from degeneration of adult worms Monthly prevention with avermectins possible (not chelonia) Surgical removal of adults (SQ or intracoelomic)
Cardianema spp. *Pseudothamugadia* spp. *Thamugadia* spp.	Chelonia, lacertids				
Saurositus spp. *Macdonaldius* spp.	Lacertids Snakes and lizards				
Oxyuridea: Small, pin-shaped worms, very common, often host specific, usually nonpathogenic; not reported from crocodilians					
Oxyurus (>100 spp.)	Lizards Chelonia Some snakes	Ingested eggs → larvae → adults in large intestine No apparent cross contamination between different species Usually asymptomatic	Usually float, or direct nonpathogenic Mortality in Red-foot Tortoises from Proatractis in caecum and colon Viviparous → autoinfection possible Report of impaction in Fiji Banded Iguana	Adults in stool, fecal for eggs, direct smear, or Baermann technique for larvae	Benzimidazoles, ivermectin (not chelonia)
Trichuridea: Hepatic worms, life cycles largely unknown, real pathologic significance yet to be determined					
Capillaria spp. *Eustrongylides* spp.	Lizards Snakes Crocodilians	Adults in intestinal tract Usually subclinical but disease more likely with involvement of liver, bile ducts, or oviducts; few clinical signs reported Snake deaths associated with migrating	Little reported; pathologic significance unknown Migrating *Eustrongylides* larvae found in skin, lungs, body cavity, and along spinal column	Eggs in fecal float or direct	Benzimidazoles Ivermectin

Capillaria recurva	American Crocodile	*Eustrongylides* larvae; snake can serve as paratenic hosts Adults in intestine but migrate to lay eggs in stratum corneum	No pathology associated with migrating adults or eggs in epidermis	Eggs in skin biopsy, adults in intestinal tract
Spiruridea:				
Dracunculoidea *Dracunculus* *Paraspirura* *Spirura*	Snakes Varanids Crocodilians Chelonians	Invertebrate intermediate host, L3 migrates to SQ sites and escapes through skin (requires water contact and macerated epidermis) Skin lesions, pustular dermatitis	Reptiles may serve as definitive, paratenic, or intermediate hosts Generally nonpathogenic, occasional intestinal, ocular, or renal pathology Enteritis and obstruction	Eggs in feces or histologic demonstration of migrating larva	Benzimidazoles Ivermectin (not chelonia)
Physaloptera	Horned lizards	Ants are intermediate hosts, enteritis			
Trichinella zimbabwaensis	Varanids, snakes crocodilians, chelonians	Encysted larvae in gastric mucosa			
Acanthocephalans: Spiny-headed worms, amphibians are normal definitive hosts					
Acanthocephala	Snakes, terrestrial chelonians	Larvae can survive in unsuitable hosts, may migrate to tissues and encyst in mesentery, viscera, and SQ tissues Clinical signs rare unless nodules formed under skin	Rare, encysted worms in skin, mesentery, and viscera	Histologic demonstration of encysted parasites Fecal centrifugation, oval eggs (larva with hooks)	Levamisole or ivermectin (not chelonia) Degenerating cysts may cause severe tissue reactions
	Aquatic chelonians	Intermediate stage ingested in aquatic snail, adults in small intestine Most infections asymptomatic	Nodular granulomas or ulceration of intestinal mucosa caused by spines of worm's protruding proboscis		
Pentastomiasis: Primitive arthropods (not helminths)					
Raillietiella sp. *Porocephalus* sp.	Lizards, snakes US Rattlesnakes, Cottonmouth Moccasin US nonvenomous snakes Vipers, African Python	Adults in lung, but can bore through to penetrate skin Usually asymptomatic with little inflammatory response, but can cause severe disease in captivity	Dependent on immune status of host, numbers of ingested parasites, concurrent disease/stressors Major pathology from local tissue damage from parasite attachment to lung	Endoscopy, fecal float or direct, eggs (larva with four legs)	Often self-limiting in captivity because of lack of intermediate hosts (dietary control) Surgical removal, ivermectin (but possible reactions to dying parasites in lungs)
Kiricephalus sp. *Armillifer* sp. *Sambonia* sp.	Monitor Lizards	Eggs with four-legged larvae swallowed → feces → ingested intermediate host (rodent), develop into nymphs → ingested → migrate to lungs			

Continued

Reptile Parasites—cont'd

Parasite	Host	Location and Clinical Signs	Pathology	Diagnosis	Treatment
Sebekia spp. *S. oxycephala* *S. mississippiensis*	Crocodilians American Alligators African Dwarf Crocodiles	Anorexia, weight loss, constipation, dehydration, respiratory distress, and secondary bacterial pneumonia, death Life cycle as previous, 95% prevalence rate in some populations Intermediate host is mosquito fish Young captives most susceptible Anorexia, weight loss, respiratory distress, and secondary bacterial pneumonia, death	Severe inflammation and damage to lung, secondary bacterial infection, pneumonia, hepatitis Often asymptomatic in many crocodilians, can be acutely fatal in hatchlings (e.g., African Dwarf Crocodiles)	Fecal float or direct, eggs (larva with four legs)	Improved hygiene, dietary control (freezing mosquito fish at −10°C for 72 hrs killed parasites) Ivermectin (but possible reactions to dying parasites in lungs)

PI, postinfection; *ELISA*, enzyme-linked immunosorbent assay; *IFA*, immunofluorescent antibody test; *TMS*, trimethoprimsulfa; *RBC*, red blood cell; *WBC*, white blood cell; *NA*, ; *SQ*, subcutaneous; *ID*, identification.

APPENDIX C
ENVIRONMENTAL, DIETARY, AND REPRODUCTIVE CHARACTERISTICS OF REPTILES

Environmental, Dietary, and Reproductive Characteristics of Reptiles[1,3-9]

Species	Temperature[a-c]	RH (%)	Diet[d]	Method of Reproduction[e]	Gestation/Incubation Period (d)[f]
Snakes					
Boa Constrictor (*Boa constrictor*)	28°C-34°C (82°F-93°F)	50-70	C	V	120-240
Sand Boa (*Eryx* sp.)	25°C-30°C (77°F-86°F)	20-30	C	V	120-180
Burmese (Indian) Python (*Python molurus*)	25°C-30°C (77°F-86°F)	70-80	C	Ov	56-65
Ball (Royal) Python (*Python regius*)	25°C-30°C (77°F-86°F)	70-80	C	Ov	90
Gartersnake (*Thamnophis sirtalis*)	20°C-35°C[2] (68°F-95°F)	60-80	C	V	90-110
Kingsnake (*Lampropeltis getulus*)	23°C-30°C (73°F-86°F)	50-70	Op/c	Ov	50-60
Chelonians					
Spur-thighed Tortoise (*Testudo graeca*)	20°C-27°C (68°F-81°F)	30-50	H/om	Ov	60
Common Box Turtle (*Terrapene carolina*)	24°C-29°C (75°F-84°F)	60-80	C/f	Ov	50-90
Desert Tortoise (*Gopherus agassizii*)	25°C-30°C (77°F-86°F)	—	H	Ov	84-120
Red-eared Slider (*Trachemys scripta elegans*)	22°C-30°C (72°F-86°F)	80-90	C	Ov	59-93
Painted Turtle (*Chrysemys picta*)	23°C-28°C (73°F-82°F)	—	H/I/o	Ov	47-99
Musk Turtle (*Sternotherus odoratus*)	20°C-25°C (68°F-77°F)	—	O/I	Ov	60-87
Lizards					
Green Iguana (*Iguana iguana*)	29.5°C-39.5°C (85.1°F-103.1°F)	60-80	H	Ov	73
Leopard Gecko (*Eublepharis macularius*)	25°C-30°C (77°F-86°F)	20-30	I	Ov	55-60
Green Anole (*Anolis carolinensis*)	23°C-29°C (73°F-84°F)	70-80	I/c	Ov	60-90
Jackson's Chameleon (*Chamaeleo jacksonii*)	21°C-27°C (70°F-80°F)	50-70	I	V	90-180
Plumed Basilisk (*Basiliscus plumifrons*)	23°C-30°C (73°F-86°F)	70-80	C/f	Ov	60-64
Water Dragon (*Physignathus lesueuri*)	25°C-34°C (77°F-93°F)	80-90	I/om	Ov	90

Continued

Environmental, Dietary, and Reproductive Characteristics of Reptiles[1,3-9]—cont'd

Species	Environmental Preference		Diet[d]	Method of Reproduction[e]	Gestation/Incubation Period (d)[f]
	Temperature[a-c]	RH (%)			
Crocodilian					
American Alligator (*Alligator mississippienis*)	30°C-35°C (86°F-95°F)	—	C/p	Ov	62-65

[a]Temperatures shown are ideal ambient daytime temperature gradients. These should be allowed to fall by approximately 5°C (9°F) during the night. "Hot-spot" temperatures should generally be 5°C (9°F) greater than the highest temperature shown.

[b]Preferred daytime temperature range for other commonly housed captive snakes are: Rosy Boa (*Lichanura trivirgata*), 27.0°C-29.5°C (80°F-85°F); Green Tree Python (*Morelia viridis*), 24°C-28°C (75°F-82°F); Carpet Python (*Morelia spilota*), 27°C-29.5°C (80°F-85°F); Cornsnake (*Elaphe guttata*), 25°C-30°C (77°F-86°F); Yellow Ratsnake (*Elaphe obsoleta*), 25°C-29°C (77°F-84°F); Gopher/Bullsnake (*Pituophis melanoleucus*), 25°C-29°C (77°F-84 °F).

[c]Preferred daytime temperature range for other commonly housed captive lizards are: Day Gecko (*Pheluma* sp.), 29.5°C (85°F); Chameleons, montane (*Chamaeleo* spp.), 21°C-27°C (70°F-80°F); Chameleons, lowland (*Chamaeleo* spp.), 27°C-29°C (80°F-84°F); Bearded Dragon (*Pogona vitticeps*), 26.7°C-29.4°C (80°F-85°F); Blue-tongued Skink (*Tiliqua* sp.), 27.0°C-29.5°C (80°F-85°F); Monitor Lizards (*Varanus* spp.), 29°C-31°C (84°F-88°F); Tegus (*Tupinambis* spp.), 27°C-30°C (80°F-86°F).

[d]*C*, Carnivorous; *F*, frugivorous; *H*, herbivorous; *I*, insectivorous; *O*, molluscavorous; *Om*, omnivorous; *Op*, ophiophagous; *P*, piscivorous. Uppercase letters denote principal dietary requirements; lowercase denotes secondary preference.

[e]*V*, Viviparous; *Ov*, oviparous.

[f]Temperature-dependent.

REFERENCES

1. Barrie MT: Chameleon medicine. In Fowler ME, Miller RE, editors: *Zoo and wild animal medicine: current therapy 4*, Philadelphia, 1999, WB Saunders.
2. Cooper JE: Physiology (reptiles). In Fowler ME, editor: *Zoo and wildlife medicine*, ed 2, Philadelphia, 1986, WB Saunders.
3. Cunningham AA, Gili C: Management in captivity. In Beynon PH, Lawton MPC, Cooper JE, editors: *Manual of reptiles*, Ames, 1992 (reprinted 1994), Iowa State University Press.
4. Divers SJ: Administering fluid therapy to reptiles, *Exotic DVM* 1:5-10, 1999.
5. Dundee HA, Rossman DA: *The amphibians and reptiles of Louisiana*, Baton Rouge, La, 1989, Louisiana State University Press.
6. Harless M, Morlock H: *Turtles: perspective and research*, New York, 1979, John Wiley & Sons.
7. Jarchow JL: Hospital care of the reptile patient. In Jacobson ER, Kollias GV Jr, editors: *Exotic animals*, New York, 1988, Churchill Livingstone.
8. McKeown S: General husbandry and management. In Mader DR, editor: *Reptile medicine and surgery*, Philadelphia, 1996, WB Saunders.
9. Stahl SJ: Reproductive disorders of the green iguana, *Proc North Am Vet Conf* 810-813, 1998.

APPENDIX D
SELECTED SOURCES OF REPTILIAN PRODUCTS

Selected Sources of Reptilian Products in the United States*

Foods and Supplements

Five Star Diets	800-747-0557
Fluker Farms	800-735-8537
Drs Foster & Smith	800-443-1160
Kaytee	800-529-8331
LM Tropical Magic	800-332-5623
Mazuri	800-227-8941
Pretty Pets	800-356-5020
Rep-Cal	408-356-4289
San Francisco Bay Brand	510-792-7200
Sticky Tongue Farms	909-672-3876
Zoo Med	888-496-6633
ZuPreem	800-345-4767

Live/Frozen Foods for Carnivores

Bayou Rodents	800-722-6102	Frozen mice, rats
Carolina Mouse Farm	864-944-6192	Frozen mice, rats
Essex Pets	800-336-6423	Frozen mice, rats
G&A Frozen Rodents	718-456-0067	Frozen mice, rats, chicks
Perfect Pets, Inc	800-366-8794	Frozen mice, rats, chicks, guinea pigs, gerbils
Pinkies & Fuzzies	903-683-5212	Frozen mice
The Gourmet Rodent, Inc	352-495-9024	Frozen mice, rats
The Mouse Factory	432-837-7100	Live and frozen mice, rats

Live Foods for Insectivores

Arbico	800-827-2847	Crickets, mealworms, waxworms, flies
Bassett's	800-634-2445	Crickets, mealworms
Drosophila	800-545-2303	Fruitflies
Fluker Farms	800-735-8537	Crickets, mealworms, fruitflies
Ghann's Cricket Farm	800-476-2248	Crickets, mealworms
Grubco	800-222-3563	Crickets, mealworms, fly larvae, waxworms, superworms
Millbrook Cricket Farm	800-654-3506	Crickets, mealworms
Rainbow Mealworms	800-777-9676	Crickets, mealworms
Russell's Cricket Farm	800-224-4668	Crickets
Sunshine Mealworms	800-322-1100	Crickets, mealworms
Top Hat Cricket	800-638-2555	Crickets, mealworms, waxworms
Topline Wholesale Dist Co	888-922-0464	Worms, roaches

Lights

Chromolux	800-788-5781	Incandescent, heat
Energy Savers Unlimited	310-851-8999	Ultraviolet coil lamp
Fluker Farms	800-735-8537	Incandescent, heat
General Electric	800-688-5826	Fluoroscent (Vita-Lite), incandescent, basking, heat
Hikari Sales USA	800-621-5619	Ultraviolet lighting
Nature's Zone	800-782-3766	Ultraviolet heat lamp
T-Rex Products	800-991-TREX	Ultraviolet heat lamp
Wild Inside	775-573-2352	Ultraviolet heat lamp
Zoo Med	888-496-6633 or 805-542-9988	Fluorescent (Reptisun, Iguana Light), heat/basking, incandescent

Heating Devices

Fluker Farms	800-735-8537	Undercage heaters
Helix Controls	619-566-8335	Thermostats, temperature controls, heating systems
The Bean Farm	425-861-7964	Heat pads
Zoo Med	888-496-6633	Temperature controls

*See Chapter 2 for more information on resources for reptilian clinicians.
Many pet stores sell live and frozen food for reptiles and many of the products listed.
Numerous sources of information were used to compile these tables.

APPENDIX E
UNITED STATES COMMERCIAL AND ANALYTICAL LABORATORIES

Commercial Analytical Laboratories in the United States

Laboratory	Test/Procedure
Antech Diagnostics 10 Executive Boulevard Farmingdale, NY 11735 (800) 745-4727 (800) 872-1001	**Reptiles:** Hematology, chemistries, microbiology, *Mycoplasma*, sexing (Green Iguanas)
Avian & Exotic Animal Clin Path Labs 2712 North Highway 68 Wilmington, OH 45177 (800) 383-3347 (800) 350-1122	**Avian:** Hematology, chemistries, bile acid, electrophoresis, histopathology, cytology, microbiology, *Chlamydia*, *Mycoplasma*, parasitology, *Giardia*, blood lead and zinc, iron assays **Reptiles:** Similar to previous; *Cryptosporidium*
Avian and Wildlife Laboratory Division of Comparative Pathology University of Miami School of Medicine PO Box 016960 (R-46) Miami, FL 33101 (305) 243-6700 (800) 596-7390	**Reptiles:** Hematology, chemistries, histopathology, microbiology
California Avian Laboratory PO Box 5647 El Dorado Hills, CA 95762 (916) 933-0898 (877) 521-6004	**Avian:** Hematology, chemistries, cytology, histopathology, necropsy, microbiology, *Chlamydia*, *Mycoplasma*, parasitology, radiology consultation **Reptiles:** Similar to previous
Clinical Virology Laboratory Room A239 College of Veterinary Medicine University of Tennessee 2407 River Drive Knoxville, TN 37996 (865) 974-5643	**Reptiles:** Ophidian paramyxovirus
Comparative Toxicology Laboratories College of Veterinary Medicine Kansas State University Manhattan, KS 66506 (785) 532-5679	General toxicologic analyses: heavy metals, pesticides, mycotoxins, other environmental contaminants
Diagnostic Laboratory College of Veterinary Medicine PO Box 5786 Ithaca, NY 14852 (670) 253-3900	**Avian:** West Nile virus
Infectious Diseases Laboratory Department of Medical Microbiology College of Veterinary Medicine 510 DW Brooks Drive University of Georgia Athens, GA 30602 (706) 542-8092	**Reptiles:** *Salmonella* spp. (DNA probe)

Continued

Commercial Analytical Laboratories in the United States—cont'd

Laboratory	Test/Procedure
Jacobson, Elliot, DVM, PhD Dept of Small Animal Clinical Sciences College of Veterinary Medicine University of Florida PO Box 100126 Gainesville, FL 32610 (352) 392-4700 (x5700)	**Reptiles:** Ophidian paramyxovirus
Mycoplasma Research Laboratory University of Florida 1600 SW Archer Road BSB 350 Gainesville, FL 32610 (352) 392-4700 (x3968)	**Reptiles:** Tortoise *Mycoplasma* testing
National Veterinary Services Laboratory APHIS USDA PO Box 844 (Send specimens to 1800 Dayton Street) Ames, IA 50010 (515) 663-7266 Note: Submission of samples requires approval by the federal veterinarian in charge of your area	**Avian:** Microbiology culture and serology (aspergillosis, avian adenovirus, herpes, influenza, paramyxovirus, Pacheco's virus, poxvirus, reovirus, *Chlamydia*, *Mycoplasma*, *Mycobacterium*, *Salmonella*, Newcastle disease, etc.), toxicology, parasitology **Reptiles:** Similar to previous
Northwest ZooPath 654 West Main Street Monroe, WA 98272 (360) 794-0630	Pathology
Quest Diagnostics APL Veterinary Laboratories 4230 S. Burnham Avenue Las Vegas, NV 89119 (702) 733-7866 (800) 433-2750	**Avian:** Hematology, chemistries, pathology, aspergillosis, AGID serology (also other fungal diseases), *Chlamydia*, *Mycoplasma* and *Mycobacterium* culture, TSH stimulation **Reptiles:** Similar to previous
Texas Veterinary Medical Diagnostic Laboratory Texas A&M University PO Drawer 3040 College Station, TX 77841-3040 (409) 845-3414 (888) 646-5623 (Send specimens to 1 Sippel Road, College Station, TX 77843)	**Avian:** *Chlamydophila*, Pacheco's virus, polyomavirus, chemistries, necropsy, histopathology, cytology, microbiology, serology, toxicology **Reptiles:** Similar to previous
Veterinary Medical Diagnostic Laboratory College of Veterinary Medicine University of Missouri PO Box 6023 Columbia, MO 65205 (573) 882-6811	General toxicologic analyses, pesticide screen, heavy metal screen, lead, mycotoxin screen
Zoo/Exotic Pathology Service 2825 KOVR Drive West Sacramento, CA 95605 (916) 725-5100 (800) 457-7981	Pathology
Zoogen, Inc 1902 East 8th Street Davis, CA 95616 (530) 750-5757 (800) 955-02473	**Reptiles:** Sex determination (Green Iguanas)

Similar services are also offered at most of these laboratories for other exotic animals.

APPENDIX F
WEIGHTS AND MEASURES CONVERSIONS

Common Weight, Liquid Measure, and Length Conversions

Weights

1 milligram (mg) = 1000 micrograms (mcg or µg)
1 grain (gr) = 64.8 mg (~65 mg)
1 gram (g) = 15.43 grains (~15 grains) = 1000 mg
1 kilogram (kg) = 1000 g
1 ounce (oz) = 28.35 g (~30 g)
1 pound (lb) = 454 g = 16 oz = 0.45 kg
2.2 pound = 1 kg

Liquid Measures

1 drop = 0.05 (1/20) milliliter (mL)
1 cubic centimeter (cc) = 1 mL
1 liter (L) = 1000 mL
1 teaspoon (tsp) = 5 mL
1 tablespoon (Tbs) = 15 mL
1 fluid ounce (fl oz) = 29.57 mL (~30 mL)
1 quart = 2 pints = 32 fl oz (~0.95 L)
1 gallon = 4 quarts = 3.785 L
1 cup = 8 fl oz = 237 mL = 16 Tbs

Linear Measures

1 millimeter (mm) = 0.039 inches (in)
1 centimeter (cm) = 0.39 in
1 meter (m) = 39.37 in
1 inch (in) = 2.54 cm
1 foot (ft) = 30.48 cm
1 yard (yd) = 91.44 cm

APPENDIX G
CELSIUS VERSUS FAHRENHEIT CONVERSIONS

Equivalents of Celsius (Centigrade) and Fahrenheit Temperature Scales

°C	°F	°C	°F	°C	°F
0	32.0	17	62.6	34	93.2
1	33.8	18	64.4	35	95.0
2	35.6	19	66.2	36	96.8
3	37.4	20	68.0	37	98.6
4	39.2	21	69.8	38	100.4
5	41.0	22	71.6	39	102.2
6	42.8	23	73.4	40	104.0
7	44.6	24	75.2	41	105.8
8	46.4	25	77.0	42	107.6
9	48.2	26	78.8	43	109.4
10	50.0	27	80.6	44	111.2
11	51.8	28	82.4	45	113.0
12	53.6	29	84.2	46	114.8
13	55.4	30	86.0	47	116.6
14	57.2	31	87.8	48	118.4
15	59.0	32	89.6	49	120.2
16	60.8	33	91.4	50	122.0

Temperature formulas: $°C = 5/9 \, (°F - 32)$; $°F = (°C \times 9/5) + 32$.

APPENDIX H
US-IU (BLOOD VALUES) CONVERSION

US and International Unit (Blood Values) Conversion

	Conventional (US) Unit	Conversion Factor	SI Unit
Hematology			
Red blood cell count	$10^6/\mu L$	1	$10^{12}/L$
Hemoglobin	g/dL	0.1	g/L
MCH	pg/cell	1	pg/cell
MCHC	g/dL	0.1	g/L
MCV	μm^3	1	fl
Platelet count	$10^3/\mu L$	1	$10^9/L$
White blood cell count	$10^3/\mu L$	1	$10^9/L$
Plasma Chemistry			
Alkaline phosphatase	u/L	1	IU/L
ALT (SGPT)	u/L	1	IU/L
Albumin	g/dL	10	g/L
Ammonia (NH_4)	$\mu g/dL$	0.5871	$\mu mol/L$
Amylase	u/L	1	IU/L
AST (SGOT)	u/L	1	IU/L
Bilirubin	mg/dL	17.1	$\mu mol/L$
Calcium	mg/dL	0.2495	mmol/L
Carbon dioxide	mEq/L	1	mmol/L
Chloride	mEq/L	1	mmol/L
Cholesterol	mg/dL	0.02586	mmol/L
Cortisol	$\mu g/dL$	27.59	nmol/L
Creatine kinase	u/L	1	IU/L
Creatinine	mg/dL	88.4	$\mu mol/L$
Fibrinogen	mg/dL	0.01	g/L
Glucose	mg/dL	0.05551	mmol/L
Iron	$\mu g/dL$	0.1791	$\mu mol/L$
Lipase			
Sigma Tietz	u/dL	280	IU/L
Cherry Crandall	u/L	1	IU/L
Lipid, total	mg/dL	0.01	g/L
Osmolality	mOsm/kg	1	mmol/kg
Phosphate (as inorganic P)	mg/dL	0.3229	mmol/L
Potassium	mEq/L	1	mmol/L
Protein, total	g/dL	10	g/L
Sodium	mEq/L	1	mmol/L
Thyroxine (T_4)	$\mu g/dL$	12.87	nmol/L
Urea nitrogen	mg/dL	0.357	mmol/L*
Uric acid	mg/dL	59.48	$\mu mol/L$

Modified from: *The Merck veterinary manual*, ed 8, Whitehouse Station, NJ, 1998, Merck and Co. as adapted from *The SI manual in health care*, Metric Commission, Canada, 1981.
*Urea.
SI, International System of Units; *MCH*, mean corpuscular hemoglobin; *MCHC*, mean corpuscular hemoglobin count; *MCV*, mean cell volume; *ALT*, alanine aminotransferase; *SGPT*, serum glutamate pyruvate transaminase; *AST*, aspartate aminotransferase; *SGOT*, serum glutamate oxaloacetate transaminase.

APPENDIX I
PHARMACOLOGY ABBREVIATIONS

Common Abbreviations Used in Prescription Writing

Abbreviation	Definition	Abbreviation	Definition
ac	before meals	mL	milliliter
ad	right ear	od	right eye
ad lib	at pleasure	os	left eye
adm	administer	ou	both eyes
aq	water	oz	ounce
as	left ear	pc	after meals
au	both ears	PO	per os
bid	twice a day	prn	as needed
c	with	q	every
cap(s)	capsule(s)	qd	every day
cc	cubic centimeter	q4h	every 4 hours, etc
disp	dispense	q24h	once a day
fl oz	fluid ounce	qid	four times a day
g (gm)	gram	qod	every other day
gr	grain	qs	a sufficient quantity
gtt(s)	drop(s)	®	trademarked name
h (hr)	hour	SC (SQ)	subcutaneously
hs	at bedtime	sig:	instructions to patient
IC	intracardiac	sol'n	solution
ICe	intracoelomic	stat	immediately
IM	intramuscularly	susp	suspension
inj	inject	tab(s)	tablet(s)
IV	intravenously	Tbs	tablespoon
kg	kilogram	tid	three times a day
lb	pound	tsp	teaspoon
mg	milligram	ut dict	as directed

GLOSSARY

LONNY B. PACE

Aberrant   Deviating from the normal form, structure, or course.
Abiotic   All nonliving components of the environment (e.g., weather and geology).
Acrodont   With teeth fused to the summit of the jawbones.
Ad Libitum   As one wishes or pleases.
Adipose   Fat.
Aerobic   Living or active only in the presence of oxygen.
Albumen   The white protein part of an egg.
Allanto-chorion   An embryonic membrane.
Allantois   A sac in the developing egg that primarily functions as a vessel for waste products.
Ambient   External or outside.
Ambient temperature   The surrounding temperature.
Amniote   A tetrapod that arises developmentally from an amniotic egg (e.g., reptiles, birds, and mammals).
Amplexus   Amplex (v.), amplectant (adj.), amplectic (adj.). The copulatory behavior of frogs in which the male sits on the female's back and grasps her with his forelimbs; amplexus can be inguinal (forefeet grasping body immediately in front of hindlimbs), axillary (immediately behind forelimbs), cephalic (on head or neck), straddled (male sits on shoulders of female while frogs are vertical and sperm flows down the female's back), or glued (male is attached to females back by adhesive substance). In amplexus, the cloacae of the male and female are adpressed, and sperm and eggs are extruded simultaneously. Amplexus is absent in some frogs.
Anamniote   A tetrapod that lacks an amniotic egg in its development (e.g., amphibians).
Anemia   Below-normal erythrocytes, hemoglobin, or hematocrit.
Anomaly   Anomalies (pl.). Abnormality or birth defect.
Anorexia   Loss of appetite.
Anterior   The front or head end of an animal.
Anthelmintic   A medicine that kills or ejects worms usually of the intestines.
Anthropomorphic   Attributing human qualities or emotions to animals.
Antibody   Any of a large number of proteins of high molecular weight that are produced normally by specialized white blood cells (B lymphocyte cells) after stimulation by an antigen and act specifically against the antigen in an immune response.
Anticoagulant   Any substance that prevents or retards the clotting of blood.
Antigen   Any substance, usually protein or carbohydrate (as a toxin or enzyme), capable of stimulating an immune response.
Antiseptic   Preventing infection; any substance that prevents the growth of microorganisms.
Antivenene   Serum produced to combat the effects of (snake) venom.
Arcade   Parts of the skull roof that separate the orbits and the temporal openings.
Aspirate   The act of sucking up, sucking in, or withdrawing fluids or gases from a body cavity (e.g., lungs, thorax, peritoneum, urinary bladder).
Atrophy   The physiologic or pathologic reduction in size of a cell, tissue, organ, or region in the body.
Auditory   meatus—The ear canal, either external or internal.
Autoinfection   Infection by an organism within the body.
Autolysis   The destruction of cells by enzymes within them that occurs after death or by some diseases.
Autotomy   The voluntary shedding of parts of the body in animals usually in defense. Autotomy of the tail is common in many lizard species.
Axilla   Axillary (adj.). At the forelimb insertion.
Bacteriophage   A virus that infects bacteria.
Bacteriostasis   Bacteriostatic (adj.). Inhibition of the growth of bacteria without destruction.
Basal   Pertaining to the most fundamental, basic, lowest, least, or deepest level.
Bifurcate   Forked; divided into, or the site of, two parts or branches.
Bilateral   Pertaining to two sides.
Biological clock   An internal biological rhythm that is responsible for periodic changes in an animal's behavior.
Biopsy   The removal and examination of tissue, cells, or fluids from the living body.
Biota   Biotic (adj.). All living components of the environment.
Bipedal   Moving on two limbs.
Brackish   Slightly salty (e.g., water in marshes near seas).
Brill   The transparent immovable spectacle that covers the eye in snakes and some lizards.
Brumation   Brumate (v.) A period of prolonged cool temperature without actual hibernation. This is the new term that is being used in reptiles. It replaces the old term, hibernation, which should only be used in mammals.
Buccal   The mouth cavity.
Calcareous   Of, like, or containing calcium.
Calculi   Any abnormal stony deposit formed in the body (e.g., bladder, kidney).
Canker   An ulcer-like sore, especially in the mouth.
Cannibalism   Eating one's own kind.
Carapace   The upper shell of a turtle (and other animals with horny protective coverings).
Carbohydrate   An organic compound that comprises the starches, sugars, celluloses, and dextrins.
Cardiovascular   Pertaining to the heart and the blood vessels as a unified body system.
Carnivore   Carnivorous (adj.). A flesh-eating organism.

Carrion Decaying flesh of a dead body that may serve as food for scavenging animals.
Caseous Cheesy; of or like cheese.
Cataract Opacity of the crystalline lens or capsule of the eye.
Cathartic Purgative; in medicine, a substance used to stimulate the evacuation of the bowels.
Catheter A rigid or flexible tube used to pass fluids into or out of a body cavity, passage, or vessel.
Caudally Towards the tail.
Cecum The cavity in which the large intestine begins and into which the ileum opens.
Cellulitis Inflammation of connective tissue.
Cervical Of the neck.
Chemotherapy The treatment or prevention of disease with the use of drugs.
Chimaera Literally, monster.
Chitin Chitinous (adj.). The structural material of some animals, mainly those in the phylum Arthropoda.
Cilia Cilium (sing.). Hairlike cytoplasmic processes of cells, comprised of microtubules, that serve in locomotion or in the movement of substances.
Clade A group of organisms that contains an ancestor and all its descendants.
Classification Node name or node-based name. This classification category name labels a clade that stems from the immediate common ancestor of two or more designated descendants.
Cloaca A common chamber for the passage of feces, urine, and reproductive material.
Coelomic cavity The cavity of most higher multicellular animals in which the visceral organs are suspended.
Conduction The transmission of heat (and electricity, etc) by the passage of energy from particle to particle.
Congenital Existing before or at birth.
Conspecifics Conspecific (adj.). Individuals or populations of the same species.
Constriction A method used by some snakes to overpower prey that uses the application of pressure from the coils to cause asphyxia.
Convection A transference of heat caused by the differences in density of air as a result of temperature; the upward movement of warm light air.
Coprophageous Eating feces.
Copulation Copulate (v.). The act of sexual intercourse; coitus.
Core temperature Temperature within the body.
Cortex The outer portion of an organ situated just beneath the capsule.
Cranial Of, toward, or pertaining to the skull.
Crepuscualar Active at dawn or dusk.
Cross feeding Transferring an uneaten food animal from one snake's cage to another.
Crotalid Any member of the rattlesnake family Crotalidae.
Crustacean An aquatic arthropod that includes the shrimp, crab, barnacle, and lobster.
Cryptic Hidden.
Culture The growth of microorganisms on artificial media.
Curettage The process of cleaning or scraping tissues from body surfaces.
Cutaneous Of, belonging to, or involving the skin.
Cyst A structural form in the life cycle of certain parasites in which they form a protective wall; a saclike structure in the body that when abnormal is filled with fluid or diseased matter.
Cytology The study of cell structure.
Debride The cutting away of tissue: the cutting away of dead or contaminated tissue from a wound to prevent infection; chemical agents may be used to achieve similar results.
Decapitation Removal of the head.
Decongestant A medication used to relieve congestion, as in nasal passages.
Definitive host A host in which sexual maturation of a parasite occurs.
Dehydrate To remove water as in the body.
Disarticulation Separation at a joint.
Disinfectant Any substance used to destroy pathogens.
Display A ritualized pattern of behavior directed at other animals for sexual, territorial, or protective motives.
Distal Toward the tip of an extremity (i.e., closest to the body).
Diuretic Any substance that increases the flow of urine.
Diurnal Active in daytime.
Dorsal Pertaining to the back part of the body.
Dorsal ventral Extending in a direction from the dorsal surface to the ventral surface.
Double clutching Producing two clutches in less than 1 year. Used for pythons and boas, although clutch refers to eggs.
Duct A small enclosed tube conducting fluid.
Durophagous Eating hard-bodied prey; often used in herpetology for snakes and lizards that prey on skinks or related lizards armored with osetoderms beneath scales.
Dysecdysis Unable to slough off outer epidermis.
Dyspnea Labored breathing.
Dystocia Slow or difficult labor.
Ecdysis Sloughing off outer epidermis.
Ectoparasite An organism that lives on another organism (host).
Ectotherm An animal that regulates its body temperature by using energy derived from external sources. This term accurately describes the thermogenic behavior of most reptiles.
Edema Excessive accumulation of fluid in cells, tissues, or cavities of the body that results in swelling.
Edentate Lacking teeth.
Encephalomyelitis Inflammation of the brain and spinal cord.
Encyst To form a cyst.
Endemic Restricted to or constantly present in a particular locality.
Endogenous Originating from within; internally.
Endothelium The epithelium lining of internal cavities of the body.
Endotherm An animal whose thermal energy is a byproduct of its own metabolism. This includes mammals, birds, and some reptiles. For example, female pythons regulate their body temperature during egg brooding cycles with shivering thermogenesis.
Enteric Intestinal.
Enzootic Affecting animals in a certain area, climate, or season.
Erythrocyte Red blood cell.
Estivate The act of becoming dormant to survive hot, dry conditions.
Ethological Relating to behavior.

Etiology Etiological (adj.). The scientific study of the causes of disease.
Euthanize Euthanasia (n.). To kill painlessly; painless death.
Excreta Waste matter eliminated (excreted) from the body, especially feces and urine.
Exogenous Coming from outside the animal.
Exostosis The condition of a bone having a rugose surface, commonly arising from the fusion of bone and dermis or osteoderms.
Exsanguinate To remove the circulating blood.
Exoskeleton Any hard external supporting structure of a body.
Extant The state of a population or species of being alive now; not extinct.
Exudate Any substance discharged through pores, incisions, etc.
Fang A large specialized tooth adapted for the injection of poison into prey.
Femoral pores A number of hollow scales arranged on the underside of the thighs in many lizards. Usually better developed in males, they can be used in some species as a means of gender identification. Their function is not understood.
Fertilization The penetration of the ova's cell membrane by the sperm and the fusion of the sperm and ovum pronuclei to reestablish a diploid state.
Fertilization External: The condition in which the sperm and ovum come in contact external to the reproductive tract or cloaca of a female.
Fertilization Internal: The condition in which the sperm and ovum come in contact within the reproductive tract or cloaca of a female.
Fibropapilloma Fibroadenoma; a benign tumor that contains both fibrous and glandular elements.
Fibrosis Abnormal increase in fibrous connective tissue.
Filarial Pertaining to parasitic nematodes in the superfamily.
Filarioidea Adults live in the vertebrate host's circulatory or lymphatic systems, the connective tissues, or serous cavities; larval forms (microfilaria) are found in the bloodstream or lymph spaces.
Flagella Flagellum (sing.). A tail-like structure on microorganisms and sperm used for propelling the organism.
Flora The entire plant life of any geographic area.
Folivore Folivorous (adj.). A foliage-eating organism.
Follicle The structure in the ovary that contains the developing ovum.
Fossorial Living underground; not all fossorial animals are burrowers, but instead they may use preexisting holes and cavities in the earth.
Frugivore Frugivorous (adj.). A fruit-eating organism.
Fungus Fungi (pl.). A parasite that feeds on living organisms or dead organic material; includes mold, mildew, rust, smut, and the mushroom.
Fuzzies Newborn rodents that have just begun to grow hair.
Gait The pattern of limb movement.
Gastroenteritis Inflammation of the stomach and intestines.
Genital pore An external opening to the male or female reproductive structures.
Gingiva Gingival (adj.). The mucous membranes and underlying soft tissue that surround a tooth and the gums.

Gnathotheca The horny covering of the lower mandible of the beak.
Goiter Enlargement of the thyroid gland.
Gonad An ovary or testis.
Gout A disease characterized by an excess of uric acid in the blood and deposits of uric salts in various tissues, especially the viscera and joints.
Grade A group of organisms that possess a similar adaptive level of organization.
Gram negative Pertaining to microorganisms that appear pink microscopically after the Gram's stain process is completed.
Granulation Formation into granules, such as new capillaries on the surface of a wound.
Granuloma Granulomatous (adj.). A mass or nodule of chronically inflamed tissue with granulations that is usually associated with an infective process.
Gravid Pregnant.
Gular Of or pertaining to the throat.
Harderian gland A gland situated a the inner junction of the eyelids (inner canthus) in vertebrates, but especially those with a well-developed nictitating membrane.
Hatchling An animal recently hatched from an egg. The duration of the hatchling state is variable, although its end in reptiles might be fixed by the disappearance of the yolk-sac scar.
Heart water A disease of ruminants caused by infection with *Cowdria ruminantium*.
Heliophilic Sun-loving.
Heliothermic Deriving heat from the sun.
Helminth Refers to worms of the platyhelminthes, nematoda, or annelida.
Hematocrit The portion of blood cells to the volume of blood.
Hematologic Referring to the blood, its nature, functions, and disease.
Hemipenes The paired sex organ of the male, typical in lizards and snakes. The singular term is "hemipenis," not "hemipene."
Hemipenis Hemipenes (pl.). Either one of the paired copulatory organs situated laterally in a cavity at the base of the tail of snakes and lizards.
Hemorrhagic Heavy bleeding or characterized by blood.
Hepatotoxic Any substance that is injurious or lethal to liver cells.
Herbivore Herbivorous (adj.). A plant-eating organism.
Herpetologist One who studies reptiles and amphibians.
Herpetology The study of amphibians and reptiles.
Herpitliary An outside enclosure used for keeping both amphibians and reptiles in near-natural conditions.
Herptile A name used to collectively describe an amphibian or reptile.
Heterodont Processing teeth of several types (e.g., tearing, cutting, crushing, grinding).
Hexacanth embryo Pertaining to the six-hooked Eucestoda larva (oncosphere) within an egg.
Hibernaculum An artificial or natural place where certain animals spend the winter in a dormant condition.
Hibernation The act of spending the cold winter months in a state of torpor. This is a mammalian term and is no longer used for reptiles.

Homeotherm An animal whose body temperature is relatively consistent (±2°C). Some reptiles can regulate their body temperature within a narrower range than this, especially during periods of activity.
Homeothermic The ability of an organism to maintain itself at a constant temperature.
Homodont Processing teeth of a single type.
Homoxenous Living within only one host during a parasite's life cycle.
Hormone Any chemical substance produced by an organ or cells of an organ that is carried by bloodstream or other body fluids to cells for a specific regulatory effect.
Hybrid The usually sterile young produced as a result of a cross mating between two different species.
Hybridization Cross-breeding.
Hydration Fluid replacement.
Hydroscopic Having the capacity to absorb or take up fluids from bodily tissue.
Hyperplasia An abnormal increase in the number of cells that compose a tissue or organ.
Hyperthermia The elevation of the body temperature via exogenous sources (e.g., the treatment of disease with inducing fever).
Hypertonic Excessive or above normal in tone or tension, especially muscles; having an osmotic pressure greater than that of physiologic salt solution or of any other solution taken as a standard.
Hypoglycemia An abnormally low concentration of sugar in the blood.
Hypotensive Abnormally low blood pressure.
Hypothermia Abnormally low body temperature.
Hypoxia Hypoxic (adj.). An abnormal condition that results from oxygen deficiency.
IM Intramuscular
Immunosuppressive The action of inactivating a specific antibody by various agents to permit the acceptance of a foreign substance by an organism.
Inanition A state of starvation.
Inbreeding Reproduction of the same or closely related genetic material.
Inclusion body A minute foreign particle within a cell (e.g., a virus).
Indigenous Naturally of, or belonging to, a region or country; innate; inherent; inborn.
Inflammation The body's reaction to injury characterized clinically by heat, swelling, redness, and pain.
Insectivore An insect-eating organism, although commonly used for an organism that eats any arthropod.
Intergrade An animal that may show the mixed characteristics of two different subspecies at the border of their respective ranges.
Intermediate host An organism that harbors the asexual or intermediate phases of a parasite.
Intracelluar Within the cell.
Intravenous Within or into the veins.
Intussusception Telescoping, slipping, prolapsing, or passage of one part of the intestine into another.
IV Intravenous.
Jacobson's organ A pair of organs situated in the anterior part of the palate that correspond with and are closely allied to the internal nares. Used to smell the contents of the mouth and may be used in conjunction with the forked tongue.

Keratitis Inflammation of the cornea.
kg Kilogram. One thousand grams (1000 g) or 2.2 pounds.
Kinesis The ability of a lizard to raise the upper part of the skull through movement of the quadrate.
Labial Pertaining to the lips.
Larva Larvae (pl.). The free-living immature form of any animal that changes structurally when it becomes an adult.
Lateral Away from the midline of the body; on the side.
Lavage The irrigation or washing out of an organ.
Lethargy Pathologic drowsiness.
Leukocyte White blood cell.
Life cycle Stages through which an organism passes, generation after generation.
Lumen The cavity or channel within a tubular structure or organ.
Malnutrition Poor nourishment that results from improper diet.
Manu Hand or forefoot.
Medial Toward the midline of the body.
Medulla The central portions of certain organs (e.g., adrenal glands).
Melanism A condition in which an animal possesses an unusually abundant amount of dark pigment in the skin such as to make it appear black. Fairly common in certain lizard and snake species.
Melena The discharge of feces colored black by altered or digested blood.
Meningoencephalitis Combined inflammation of the membranes that cover the brain (meninges) and the spinal cord.
Mesonephros The adult kidney of fishes and amphibians.
Metabolism Metabolic (adj.). The process of assimilating food into complex elements that are then dissimilated into simple ones to produce energy.
Metanephric Pertaining to the permanent kidney of reptiles, birds, and mammals that develops from an excretory organ lying behind the mensonephros in an embryo. In higher vertebrates, the mesonephros develops into the epididymis and vas deferens.
Meter A unit of length in the metric system equal to 39.37 inches.
mg An abbreviation for milligram. One one-thousandth of a gram ($1/1000$ g).
Microfilaria Microfilaria (pl.). First-stage juvenile of any filariid nematode that is viviparous and is usually found in the blood or tissue fluids of the definitive host.
Microflora Flora of a small area; in medicine, the microorganisms of the intestines
Micron (μ). One-thousandth of a millimeter ($1/1000$ mm).
Milligram (mg). One one-thousandth of a gram ($1/1000$ g).
Milliliter (mL). One one-thousandth of a liter ($1/1000$ L); is equal to one cubic centimeter (1 cc).
Minimum and maximum critical temperatures The upper and lower thermal tolerance limits, where the righting reflex is lost in 50% of animals.
mL Milliliter. One one-thousandth of a liter ($1/1000$ L); is equal to one cubic centimeter (1 cc).
Molluscivore Molluscivorous (adj.). A mollusk-eating organism.
Monogenetic Pertaining to animals without alternating asexual and sexual generations.

Monotypic   Having only one type (e.g., a genus consisting of only one species, the feeding of only one food type).

Montane   Mountain dwelling.

Morbidity   A diseased state or condition.

Morph   A particular body form or colored group of individuals. Morph is used regularly in discussion of polymorphism and variation of individuals within a population of species.

Morphology   The study of an organism's form or shape, or the shape of one or more of an organism's parts.

Mucosa   Mucosal (adj.). Mucous membrane; the membrane lining body cavities that come in contact with air.

Mycobacterial   Infection, etc, caused by rod-shaped, aerobic, gram-positive bacteria of the family Mycobacteriaceae.

Mycotic dermatitis   Inflammation of the skin from a fungus infection.

Myoglobin   The respiratory pigment of muscle fibers, differing from blood hemoglobin in that it has a higher affinity for oxygen and a lower affinity for carbon dioxide.

Myiasis   A condition that results from the invasion of tissues or organs of humans and other animals by dipterous larva.

Nanometer   (nm). A unit of length equal to one-billionth of a meter.

Nares   Nasal passages; the nostrils.

Necropsy   Examination of a dead animal; postmortem examination.

Necrosis   The death of tissue.

Necrotizing dermatitis   Inflammation of the skin that results in the death of the tissue.

Nectivore   A nectar-eating organism.

Neonate   Neonatal (adj.). A newly born infant.

Neoplasm   A tumor or aberrant new growth of abnormal cells or tissues.

Neotropic   Neotropical (adj.). Of the zoogeographic region that includes South America, the West Indies, Central America, and tropical Mexico.

Nephritis   An acute or chronic disease of the kidneys characterized by inflammation, degeneration, fibrosis, etc.

Nephrotoxic   A toxic substance that destroys the cells of the kidneys.

Neurotoxic   A toxic substance that destroys the cells of nerve tissue.

Nictitating membrane   Thin transparent conjunctival tissue in certain vertebrates (e.g., birds, reptiles) called the third eyelid that serves to protect the eyeball without obscuring vision.

Nocturnal   Active at night.

Nodule   A small node.

Nonpathogenic   Not causing disease.

Obligatory   Required; necessary.

Occlude   To prevent the passage of.

Occult   Concealed from observation. Not apparent without symptoms; hidden.

Ocular   Of or pertaining to the eye.

Olfaction   The sense of smell.

Omnivore   Omnivorous (adj.). Any animal that feeds on both plant and animal matter.

Oocyst   Cyst stage of apicomplexans containing sporozoites, resulting from sporogony.

Oogenesis   The process of egg formation.

Operculum   Opercular (adj.). A lid or covering.

Opisthotonic spasm   Describes a condition in which the head (and lower limbs of animals other than snakes) is bent backwards while the body is arched forward.

Opportunistic   Referring to any organism that is incapable of inducing disease in a healthy host but is able to produce infections in a less resistant or injured host.

Organic   Derived from or pertaining to living organisms.

Osteoderm   A bony deposit in the form of a plate or scale found in the dermal layers of the skin.

Osteoid   Bone-like; young hyaline bone matrix in which calcium salts are deposited.

Osteomalacia   A bone disease characterized by a softening as a result of a deficiency of calcium.

Osteomyelitis   Infection of the bone marrow or bone structure, usually caused by a bacterium (e.g., *Staphylococcus*).

Oviparous   Oviparously (adj.). Producing eggs that hatch after leaving the body of the female.

Oviposit   To lay eggs.

Oviposition   The act of laying or depositing eggs in specific sites.

Ovoviviparous   Having nonshelled eggs that hatch internally.

Ovulation   Release of mature eggs or ova.

Ovum   An egg, in both pythons and boas, whether fertilized or not, is an ovum; the plural is ova.

Palate   The roof of the mouth that separates oral cavity from nasal cavity.

Palpebral membrane   A transparent "eye" lid that lies beneath the true eyelids and can extend horizontally from its resting position in the inner corner of the eye to the outer corner.

Palatine   The main bone plate in the palate.

Palpate   To examine by touching.

Palpebra   Palpebral (adj.). Having to do with the eyelids.

Panophthalmitis   Inflammation of all of the tissues of the eyeball.

Paramyxovirus   Also known as OPMV, ophidian paramyxovirus infection has been isolated in a wide variety of reptilian and mammalian cell types; clinical signs of illness are variable from going unnoticed altogether to loss of appetite, muscle tone, or equilibrium; in one epizootic, a snake underwent violent convulsions.

Parasite   Any organism that lives in or on another organism (host) to obtain some advantage but contributes nothing useful in return.

Parasiticide   A substance or agent used to destroy parasites.

Paratenic host   A host in which a parasite survives without undergoing further development; a transport host.

Parenteral   Brought into the body in a way other than the digestive tract (e.g., via injection).

Parietal eye   A vestigial "third eye" situated in the center of the skull between the parietals. A sensory structure capable of light reception that may serve as a temperature detector.

Parthenogenesis   Parthenogenetic (adj.). Reproduction with the development of an unfertilized egg, seed, or spore.

Parthenogenetic   Describing a method of reproduction in which the ova develop without fertilization by the male gamete, producing offspring genetically identical to the parent.

Parturition   The act of giving birth.

Pathogen   Pathogenic (adj.). An organism producing or capable of producing disease.

Perinatal Pertaining to the period shortly before and after birth.
Periocular Surrounding the eye.
Peristalsis Rhythmic muscular contractions often associated with the gastrointestinal tract or other tubular structures.
Pes Foot, specifically the hind foot.
Petecchial Referring to the minute rounded spot(s) of hemorrhage on body surfaces, such as skin, mucous and serous membranes, or on the cross-sectioned surface of an organ.
Phenotype The external appearance of a living organism.
Pheromone A chemical signal secreted by one animal that conveys specific information to another animal, usually a conspecific, and often elicits a specific behavioral or physiologic response.
Photoperiod The number of daylight hours best suited to an organism for proper growth and maturation.
Pinkies Newborn rodents without hair.
Plastron The under or ventral shell or of a chelonian.
Pleurodont With teeth set in a cavity on the inner side of the jawbone.
Poikilotherm Poikilothermic (adj.). Ectotherm; an animal that is "cold-blooded" such as a reptile.
Poikilotherm An animal whose body temperature is variable. This is not the same as an ectotherm; indeed, many mammals, particularly those that undergo hibernation, could correctly be termed poikilothermic.
Polyphyodont With teeth that are replaced more than once.
Posterior Posteriorly (adj.). Situated behind or to the back of a part.
Post mortem After death.
Post partum The period of time after parturition.
POTZ Preferred optimum temperature zone. The range of temperatures within which a specific ectotherm functions optimally overall. It is the thermal environment within which a reptile engages in normal activities. Important to note is that all physiologic functions have a temperature at which they function optimally, but within a species, not all functions are optimized at the same temperature. The term POTZ is somewhat misleading because it implies a conscious choice. Activity temperature range (ATR) may be a better term because it is less anthropomorphic.
Prehensile Adapted for holding or grasping.
Premaxilla The teeth-bearing bone at the front of the upper jaw.
Primary host First or main host.
Primitive A character or condition that is the same as an ancestral character or condition.
Proboscis An elongated structure located at the anterior end of the organism.
Progeny Children; descendants; offspring.
Proglottid Any of the segments of a tapeworm's body; each segment has both male and female reproductive organs.
Prolapse The falling down or sinking of a part or viscous procidentia from its usual position (e.g., forceful extrusion of the cloaca associated with straining).
Prophylaxis The prevention or protection against disease.
Proteolytic The breaking down of proteins to form more simple substances.
Proteroglyphous Appertaining to snakes with canalized venom fangs at the front of the upper jaw that are usually fixed (e.g., in the Elapidac).

Protozoa Unicellular eukaryotes in the Kingdom Protista.
Pupa Pupae (pl.). An insect in the stage of development between the larval and adult forms.
Purgative A substance used to stimulate evacuation of the bowels (a cathartic).
Purse-string suture A running stitch placed in a circle and pulled together to close an opening.
Purulent Consisting of, containing, or forming pus.
Quadrate The part of the upper jaw that forms the point of articulation.
Quadrupedal Moving on four limbs.
Quarantine The act of isolating individuals, for purposes of examination, for the duration of the incubation period of most diseases from which they may have been exposed.
Radiograph Radiographically (adj.). To make a photograph on a sensitive film with projection of roentgen rays through a part of the body.
Raphe A seam or ridge.
Renal-portal system Refers to the anatomic variation of reptiles whereby blood leaving the tail and pelvic limbs of these animals passes through the kidneys before returning to the heart.
Rectilinear locomotion A mode of limbless locomotion dependent on a wavelike pattern of rib movement.
Recrudescence The reappearance or regrowth.
Regurgitation The return of food from the stomach.
Reservoir host An animal that provides a parasite with a suitable environment and while doing so, serves as a source of infection for other animals.
Reticulated Having a pattern of color that resembles a net.
Rhamphotheca The horny covering or sheath of the beak.
Rhinotheca The horny covering or sheath of the upper mandible of the beak.
Rostral Pertaining to or resembling a beak or projection.
Rupicolous Living on walls or rocks.
SC Or SQ. Subcutaneous.
Saline solution A salt solution. Physiologic saline solution contains 0.9 grams of sodium chloride to 100 mL of water.
Salmonellosis Infection of an organism in the genus salmonella (e.g., septicemia, gastroenteritis, food poisoning).
Saltatory Moving by jumping, either bipedally or quadrupedally.
Saurian Reptile in the order Sauria; lizard.
Scansorial Climbing in bushes, shrubs, and other relatively low growing vegetation; capable of climbing but not arboreal.
Scolex Head of a tapeworm.
Scute A horny, chitinous, or bony external plate or scale, as on the shell of a turtle or the underside of a snake. Also called scutum.
Selected body temperature T_s. The temperature selected by an individual when placed in an artificial thermal gradient. This varies over time because the temperature selected mirrors the optimal temperature for the physiologic function perceived as most important at that time. It is synonymous with preferred body temperature T_p. This is sometimes expressed as a range of temperatures that reflects the middle 50% to 67% of the body temperatures measured during an animal's circadian temperature fluctuation.
Self-limiting A disease that is limited by its own characteristics rather than outside influence.

Septicemia Septicemic (adj.). A disease spread throughout the body via the bloodstream by pathogenic microorganisms and their toxic products.

Sequelae A pathologic condition that results from a disease.

Serpentine A mode of limbless undulatory locomotion in which all portions of the body pass along the same path and use the same frictional surfaces for pushing the body forward.

Sexual dimorphism The condition in which the male and female of a species show obvious differences in color or structure.

Sidewinding A specialized mode of serpentine locomotion in which only two parts of the body touch the ground simultaneously.

Sister group The taxon sharing the most recent common ancestor with another taxon. A pair of taxa sharing the same common ancestor.

Somatic Pertaining to the framework of the body but not to the viscera.

Spargana Sparganum (sing.). Cestode plerocercoids of unknown identity.

Species A taxonomic group of individuals similar in morphology and physiology.

Spermatophore A mucoid pedestal to support the sperm packets of some male salamanders; it is produced in the cloaca.

Spurious Not true or genuine; false.

Sputum Salvia, mucus, etc, that is spit out of the mouth.

Steatitis Inflammation of adipose tissue.

Stem name or stem-based name This classification category name labels a clade of all taxa that are more closely related to a specified set of descendants than to any other taxa.

Stomatitis Inflammation of the oral cavity.

Stress A condition in animals in which psychologic effects reduce resistance to disease. Applies particularly to newly captured wild specimens.

Subcaudal Scales after the cloaca on the snake's ventral surface.

Subcutaneous SC, SQ. Under the skin.

Subspectacular Referring to the area just beneath the fixed transparent watchglass-like covering (spectacle; eye cap) of the eye in snakes and some lizards.

Substrate In zoology, the ground or other solid material on which an animal moves or is fastened.

SVL Snout-vent length; straight-line distance from the tip of the snout to the anterior edge of the vent.

Symbiont Symbiotic (adj.). Any organism involved in parasitic, commensalistic, or mutualistic relationship with its "host."

Symbiosis The interaction of organisms whereby one lives on, in, or with another.

Symmetrical Exhibiting corresponding characteristics on opposite sides of a plane.

Sympatric Occurring in the same geologic area.

Symphysis The joining of two bones with interlocking parts.

Syndrome A set of signs or a series of events that occur together and often point to a single disease or condition as the cause.

Taxa Taxon (sing.). A group or category, at any level, in a system for classifying plants or animals.

Taxonomy The study of the theory, rules, and procedure of classification.

Tectorial membrane A membrane in the inner ear that covers a patch of sensory hairs.

Tepid Moderately warm.

Teratogenic Tending to produce anomalies of formation or teratism. Causing birth defects.

Terrestrial Mainly ground dwelling.

Thecodont Having teeth inserted in sockets.

Therapeutic Serving to cure or to heal; a curative.

Thermoreceptor A heat-detecting organ (e.g., the "pit" in Pit Vipers).

Thermoreglate To control temperature.

Thermoregulation The process used by ectotherms to maintain their preferred body temperature by moving in and out of areas of environmental warmth.

Thiaminase An enzyme present in raw fish (and in certain bacteria) that causes the cleavage of thiamine, rendering it unavailable to the body.

Thigmotherm An animal that derives its energy by thermal conduction from items in the environment. This applies to many crepuscular reptiles.

TL Tail length or total length. For tail length, it is distance from posterior edge of the vent to the tip of the tail; and for total length, distance from tip of snout to tip of tail.

Tomia Tomium (pl.). The cutting edge of a beak.

Torpid A state of being dormant or inactive.

Tractable Tame, "handleable."

Transient Temporary.

Transport host Host in which a parasite survives without undergoing further development; also known as a paratenic host.

Tumor A swelling on some part of the body, especially a mass of new tissue growth independent of its surrounding structures, having no physiologic function.

Tympanum Tympana (pl.). Eardrum.

Ulcer Ulcerate (v.). An open sore on the skin or mucous membrane that often discharges pus.

μm Micrometer (micron). One one-thousandth of a millimeter ($1/1000$ mm).

Undulatory A group of limbless locomotion patterns in which the body moves through a series of curves.

Urate A salt of uric acid.

Uric acid A product of protein metabolism that is present in the blood and urine of animals living in arid areas.

Vent The external opening of the cloaca.

Venter Ventral (adj.). The underside or lower surface of an animal.

Ventral Pertaining to the belly.

Vermiculite Alteration of mica, producing hydrous silicate minerals that occur in tiny leafy scales that expand greatly when heated.

Vermin Verminous (adj.). Any animal regarded as objectionable by humans (e.g., flies, roaches, lice, rats).

Vertebrate An animal that possesses a spinal column.

Vertical transmission The transmission of a trait, disease, etc, from parent to offspring across the placenta.

Vestigial Referring to a remnant of something formerly present or more fully developed.

Virus A vast group of minute infectious structures that rely totally on living cells for reproduction and metabolism.

Viscous Glutinous; sticky; semifluid; having high viscosity.

Vitellogenesis Development of the yolk part of an egg in the ovary.
Viviparous Bearing live offspring.
Viviparous Livebearers; those species that give birth to offspring in an advanced state of development.
Xeric Habitat with low moisture level or water availability; adapted to dry or arid conditions.
Yeast Single-celled ascomycete.
Yolk Aspherical mass of (usually) yellow nutritive fluid enclosed by the yolk sac and supportive of the developing embryo.
Zoonoses Diseases that may be transmitted to man from animals. Very few reptilian diseases are pathogenic to man.

Index

A

Abdominal distension. *See* Snakes
Abdominal scutes, 972
Abelpharus sp. *See* Oscellated Skink
Aberrant host (AH), 343, 344f
Ablation, usefulness, 620
Abnormal skin, 776
Abrasions, 201
   impact. *See* Amphibians
Abscesses, 201-202, 715. *See also* Aural abscesses; Internal abscesses; Renal abscesses
   clinical signs, 716
   debridement, 745
   diagnosis, 716-717
   follow-up, 717
   formation, 716
   impact, 854-855
   inciting causes, 715-716
   masses, lamellar appearance, 716f
   recurrence, 715
   resolution, problems, 927
   samples, no growth yield, 379f
   in toto excision, 202
   trauma, result, 716f
   treatment, 717
Academy of Veterinary Homeopathy, 439
Acanthamebic meningoencephalitis, 248
Acanthocephala, 346t, 353-354
Acanthocephalan egg, 355f
Acanthocephalans, 299
   eggs, 353-354
Acanthocephalans, commonness, 962
Acanthosaurus crucigera. *See* Horn-headed Lizard
Acariasis, 720
   clinical signs, 723-726
   diagnosis, 726-727
   parasite natural history, 720-723
   pathogenesis, 720-723
   treatment, 373, 727-733
Acarids
   historic treatments, partial list, 727t
   therapy, proposal treatments, 728t
AccuVet CO_2 superpulse laser, 619f
Acellular low-protein coelomic transudate, 807
Acetylcholine, impact, 143
Acetylcysteine, 656
Acetylglucosamine, 265
Acid base, 462-463
Acid/base ratio, 463
Acid-fast bacilli, 1023
Acid-fast bacteria, 152
Acid-fast organisms, identification, 234

Acid-fast stain/staining, 227, 758
Acidic urine, observation, 883
Acid-loving bacteria, maintenance, 32
Acid phosphatase, 139
Acinar cells, hyperplasia, 859
Acrochordus arafurae. *See* File Snake
Acrus lipoideus corneae. *See* Mediterranean Tortoise
Acrylic, usage, 525
Acrylic positioning devices, 484f
Acrylite OP-4, 87
ACTH. *See* Adrenocorticotropic hormone
Activated partial thromboplastin time (APTT), 1055
Activated vitamin D_3, 463
Active UVHeat, 1083
Activity
   fractional decreases/increases, 253t
   reduction, case report, 283
Acupuncture, 432-434. *See also* Aquapuncture; Electroacupuncture points. *See* A-shi acupuncture points; Lizards; Turtles
Acute central/peripheral nerve trauma, treatment, 244
Acute gouty arthritis, 795
Acute hepatitis, 807
Acute pain
   analgesic agents, usage, 451t
   local anesthetic agents, usage, 451t
   management, 451
Acute proptosis, 331
Acute renal failure, mimicking, 1072
Acyclovir
   treatment, 397
   usage, 1123t
Acyl-coenzyme A (CoA), 811
Adeleorina (suborder), 801
Adeno-like virus, 153
Adenosine triphosphate (ATP), anaerobic metabolism, 543
Adenoviral DNA, detection, 399
Adenovirus, 397-401, 1150-1151. *See also* Crocodilians; Lizards; Snakes
   clinical features, 397-398
   control, 400-401
   diagnosis, 400
   epizootiology, 398
   immunity, 400
   implication, 398
   incubation, 399
   opportunistic pathogens, 399
   pathogenesis, 399
   pathology, 399-400
   recovery, 398

Adenovirus—cont'd
   transmission, 399
   treatment, 401
   vertical transmission, 399
   virus strains, relationship, 398-399
Adenovirus-associated disease, 398
Adrenal glands
   location, 53f
   necropsy examination, 576
Adrenocorticotropic hormone (ACTH), 120
Adriamycin, administration, 318
Advanced imaging, 299
Aerobic bacteria, blood culture, 1003
Aerobic bacterial pneumonias, suspicion, 875
Aerobic cultures, execution, 227f
Aerobic gram-negative bacteria, 183
Aeromonas, 202, 232-233, 956
Aeromonas hydrophila, culturing, 233f
Aeromonas sp., culture, 607f
Aeromonas spp., 1022
   isolation, 233
   transmission, 208f
Afferent renal portal veins, 127
African *geochelone*, 92
African House Snake (*Lamprophis fulginosus*), neurologic behavior, 680f
African Spurred Tortoise (*Geochelone sulcata*)
   hematologic values, 1116
   laser cystotomy, contact mode, 625f
   oral examination, metal mouth gag (usage), 509f
   popularity, 92f
   serum biochemical values, 1116
African tick (*Ambylomnia* spp.), 734
   presence, 208f. *See also* Leopard Tortoise
Agalychnis callidryas. *See* Red-eyed Leaf Frog
Agamidae, 59
Agamids, teeth, 63
Agarose gel immunodiffusion (AGID), 1066
   illustration, 1066f
Agents, usage, 1133t-1134t. *See also* Amphibians; Analgesic agents; Anesthetic agents; Antifungal agents; Antimicrobial agents; Antiparasitic agents; Antiviral agents; Chemical restraint
Aggression. *See* Defensive aggression; Offensive aggression
AGID. *See* Agarose gel immunodiffusion
Agkistrodon c. contortrix. *See* Copperhead; Southern Copperhead
Agkistrodon contortrix. *See* Venomous Copperhead
Aglyphous teeth, 48

Page numbers followed by f indicate figures: t, tables.

Agrionemys horsfieldi. See Russian Tortoise
AH. *See* Aberrant host
AIDS inpatients, 760
Airborne disease spread, chances, 1014
Air-dried smears, 520
Airway markings, distinction, 484
Airway resolution, CT reconstruction. *See* Pythons
Alabama, herpetological societies, 6t
Alanine aminotransferase (ALT), 653, 807
   activity, 462, 464
Aldabran Tortoise (*Dipsochelys elephantina*), dorsal coccygeal vein (blood collection), 515f
Aldabran Giant Tortoise, species, 92
Aldabra Tortoise (*Geochelone* sp.)
   hematologic values, 1116
   serum biochemical values, 1116
Aldehydes, treatment, 401
Alethinophidia (infraorder), 45-46
Aleuris sp., posterior end, 359f
Alfalfa flakes, supplementation, 371
Alimentary tract, necropsy examination, 577-578
Alkaline phosphatase (AP/ALP), 652, 807
   activity, 462
Alleles, 678
Alligatorinae (subfamily), life span, 102-103
Alligator mississippiensis. See American Alligator
Alligators
   anorexia, radiography, 158f
   behavioral fever, 114
   body, two-dimensional axial images, 1089f
   bronchi, caseous material, 710f
   climatic conditions, impact, 111f
   crocodilians, distinctions, 103f
   CT data, reconstruction, 1094f
   ECG results. *See* American Alligator
   enteritis, 712f
   enterocolitis, 710f
   follicle groups, hierarchy (development), 109
   intestinal mucosa, fibrotic membrane, 712f
   kidneys, position, 142f
   length, 116
   lesions, healing, 712
   lymphohistiocytic proliferative syndrome (PIX disease), 709
      gross lesions, 709f
   mandibular lesions, 708f
   MRI axial sections, 1095f
   nest preparation. *See* Female alligators
   oral cavity, 147f
   pathogenic mycoplasmosis, emergence, 650-651
   rear limb lesion, 711f
   renal anatomy, 143f
   scleral ossicles, appearance, 1089f
   skeleton, CT scan, 1094f
   skin pigmentation, 709f
   temperature-dependent sex determination, 111f
   tissue necrosis, 711f
   torso, T2-weighted MRI (two-dimensional image), 1094f
   vascular anatomy, 143f
Alligator Snapping Turtle (*Macrochelys temminckii*), 81f

Alligator Snapping Turtle —cont'd
   hind foot, plantar surface (fibroid mass), 315f
Allometric scaling, 419
   aM^b, formula, 419
   formulary, 424t-425t
   usefulness, 421
   worksheet, 426t
Allometry. *See* Chelonians
   controversies, 420-423
Allopurinol
   dosages, reports, 799t
   impact. *See* Uric acid
   usage, 798
ALP. *See* Alkaline phosphatase
Alpha$_2$-agonists, usage, 444, 445
Alpha-globulin fraction, increase, 817
Alpha-keratin, synthesis, 778
ALSV. *See* Avian leukosis/sarcoma viruses
ALT. *See* Alanine aminotransferase
Alternaria sp., 209
   isolation, 220f
Alternative veterinary therapies, 428
   natural history, considerations, 428-429
Althea officinalis. See Marsh mallow root
Ambient temperature, impact, 198
Amblyomma dissimile. See Ticks
Amblyrhynchus cristatus. See Marine Iguana
Ambu bag, usage, 547f
Ambubag, usage. *See* New England Aquarium
Ambystoma californiense. See California TigerSsalamander
Ameba, 347f
Amelanistic Green Iguana (*Iguana iguana*), 59f
American Academy of Veterinary Acupuncture, 439
American Alligator (*Alligator mississippiensis*)
   bacteria, isolation, 707t-708t
   carpal wound, infection, 513f
   cartilaginous crura, 109f
   congenital abnormality, 711f
   copulatory organ, ventral groove, 109f
   death, 361
   Dujardinascaris sp., 357f
   ECG results, 188t
   head tilt, 710f
   hematologic values, 1112
   investigation, 109
   mandibular fracture, 711f
   raising, circular building, 705f
   respiratory rate, 106
   serum biochemical values, 1112
   treatment, case study, 432
   ultrasound examination, 667f
   vasovagal response, induction, 513f
   WNV, 710f
American Association of Poison Control Centers, 1051
American Association of Zoos and Aquariums Resource Center, 1051
American Association of Zoo Veterinarians, conferences, 13
American Holistic Veterinary Medical Association, 439
American laws/regulations, 1031

American Society of Ichthyologists and Herpetologists (ASIH), 9
American Veterinarians and Chiropractors Association, 440
American Veterinary Medical Association (AVMA), 12, 1042
   reptile recognition, 14f
American Zoo and Aquarium Association (AZA), 1013
   written policy, 1014
Amikacin
   comparison. *See* Gentamicin
   impact, 1074
   ineffectiveness, 717
   pharmacokinetics
      determination, 646
      environmental temperature, impact, 647
   usage, 1119t
Amino acids, 139
   usage. *See* Intravenous amino acids
Aminoglycosides, 934
   gold standard, 645
   half-lives, 645
   usage, 645-647
Aminophylline, 656
Aminosuberic arginine vasotocin, activity, 790
Amitriptylline, disadvantages, 431
Ammonia
   end product, 793
   excretion, 141
   levels, 962-963
Amoebiasis, 959-960, 1161
   antemortem diagnosis, 960
   clinical signs, 960
   signs, 347
Amphibian-Reptilia, 10
Amphibians
   abrasions, impact, 963-964
   agents, usage, 1155t
   algal diseases, 958-959
   analgesia, consideration, 949
   analgesic agents, usage, 1143t-1144t
   anesthesia, 947-949
   anesthetic agents, usage, 1143t-1144t
   antimicrobial agents, usage, 1140t-1141t
   antifungal agents, usage, 1141t
   antiparasitic agents, usage, 1142t
   bacteria, culturing, 951
   bacterial diseases, 956-958
   behaviors, 164t
   body
      bulk, 947
      plan, 944-946
   catalepsy, 175-178
   celioscopy, usage, 967
   celiotomy, usage, 967
   chemical restraint, 947-949
      agents, usage, 1143t-1144t
   circulatory system, 945
   clinical techniques, 949-953
   cloacal tissue, prolapse, 967
   corneal lipidosis, 965-966
   death feigning, 175-178
   defensive behaviors, 175-176
   dehydration, impact, 963
   diversity, 941-942
   eggs, 959
   enclosure, water quality, 943-944

Amphibians—cont'd
  endocrine system, 946
  environmental conditions, 963-965
  euthanasia, 949
  examination, 946-949
  excretory system, 945
  existence. See Communal vivariums
  formulary, 967-968, 1140
    delivery routes, 967-968
  fungal diseases, 958-959
  gastric prolapse, 966
  GOI, 955
  gout, 966
  hematologic values, 952t
  hormones, usage, 1144t
  hyperthermia, 964
  hypothermia, 965f
  hypovitaminosis A, 954-955
  improper husbandry, 956f
  infections, 957-958
  infectious diseases, 955-959
  lung, alveoli (absence), 945
  MBD, nutritional origin, 953-954
  medicine, overview, 941
  moisture conservation, 176
  morphologic adaptations, 164t, 177-178
  musculoskeletal system, 945
  neoplastic diseases, 966-967
  nervous system, 945
  NHSP, 953
  NMBD, 842f, 953
  nonrespiratory gas exchange, capability, 133f
  nutritional diseases, 953-955
  nutritional support, 955
  obesity, 955
  pedal luring, 176
  physical examination, 946
  physiologic values, 952t
  protozoal diseases, 959-962
  reproductive behavior, 176-177
  restraint, 946-949
  shed skin, consumption, 177
  skin, sample-taking, 200f
  spindly leg, 965
  substandard conditions, 956f
  sudden death, occurrence, 960
  surgery, 966
  syndromes, etiology, 965-966
  toe clip, 966
  tonic immobility, 175-178
  toxicities, 962-963
  toxins, 1075-1706
  trauma, impact, 964
  unken reflex, 175-178
  viral diseases, 955-956
  water quality, 964
Amphigonia retardata (sperm storage), 365
Amphophilic inclusions. See Bearded Dragon
Amphophilic intranuclear inclusion bodies, herpesvirus (presence), 396
Amphotericin B, impact, 1072
Ample gel, application, 666f
Amputation. See Limb amputation; Tails
  appropriateness. See End-stage limb disease
  considerations, 610f. See also Chelonians

Anabolic steroids, usage. See Hepatic lipidosis
Anaconda (*Eunectes* sp.)
  oviduct, incision, 627f
  prolapsed colon, 752f
Anaerobic agents, culturing, 783
Anaerobic bacteria, 235
Anaerobic cultures
  collection, 652
  execution, 227f
Anaerobic metabolism, 133
Analgesia, 442, 450-451.
    See also Intraoperative analgesia; Postoperative analgesia
  drug administration, routes, 445
  maintenance/monitoring, 448-449
  premedication, 443-444
  recovery/postoperative care, 449-450
Analgesic agents, usage, 1127t-1131t.
    See also Acute pain; Amphibians; Chronic pain
Analgesic regimens, 450-451
Anal glands. See Cloacal scent glands
Analog endovideo cameras, 553
Anal scutes, 972
Anamnesis, 880
Anatomic strictures, 788f
Ancillary diagnostic techniques, 484-489
Andrews, RM, 12
Anemia
  etiologies, 454
  prognosis, 460
Anesthesia, 442
  agents, usage, 444t
  cardiac monitoring, usage, 193
  drug administration, routes, 445
  impact. See Endoscopy
  induction, 446-447
  light plane, 948
  maintenance/monitoring, 448-449.
    See also Green Iguana
  necessity, 897
  postoperative care, 449-450
  premedication, 443-444
  recovery, 449-450, 586
  surgical plane, 948, 998
Anesthetic agent, IM administration, 445
Anesthetic agents. See Injectable anesthetic agents; Local anesthetic agents
  usage, 1127t-1131t. See also Amphibians
Anesthetic gas, usage, 600f
Anger. See Loss
Aniliidae, 45
Animal Record Keeping System (ARKS), 1013
Animals. See Poisonous animals; Venomous animals
  bad news, delivery, 20
  biology, understanding, 2
  body, handling, 19
  bonds. See Humans
  curator/caretaker bonds, 16f
  deceased, examination, 19
  health controls, 1042-1043
  loss
    clinician/client concerns, 20-22
    replacement, clinician concerns, 22
  needs, understanding, 2
  restraint, 666

Ankylosis, spreading, 908f
Annular pad. See Equatorial annular pad
Anolis carolinensis. See Green Anoles
Anomalepididae, 44
Anomochilidae, 45
Anophthalmia, 333
Anorexia, 156, 739. See also Complete anorexia; Crocodilians; Partial anorexia; Seaturtles; Snakes
  death, 352
  diagnosis, 740-741
  environmental causes, 688
  husbandry, relation, 739f, 740f
  medical causes, 688
  social/reproductive factors, impact, 740
  symptom, 739-740
  temperatures, impact, 739
  treatment, 741
Antarchoglossa, 59-60
Antebrachium, splint usage, 603f
Antegrade double contrast digestive tract examination, 481
Antennas, 614-615
  implantation, 616, 617f. See also Snakes
Anterior chamber, 338-339
  anatomy, 338
Anterior lung, biopsy, 520
Anteromedial Harderian gland, 831
Anthelminthic therapy, 1070
Antibacterials
  preparations, usage, 584f
  usage, 645-649
Antibiotics
  impact, 247
  therapy, 920
  usage, 213
    concerns, 645
Antibodies, concentrations, 400
Anticoagulants, impact, 1073
Anti-*Cryptosporidium* immunoglobulins, action, 759
Antifungal agents, usage, 1123t
Antifungal coverage, 1003
Antifungal drugs, pharmacokinetics, 875
Antifungal medication, transcarapacial intraluminal instillation, 226
Antifungals, usage, 654-655
Antifungal toxicity, 1072
Antigen capture ELISA, 1065f
  comparison, 902
Antihyperuricemic drugs, usage, 796, 798
Antimicrobial agents, usage, 1119t-1122t.
    See also Amphibians
Antimicrobials, 644-645
  administration, techniques (usage), 655-657
  beads, 657
  nebulization, 656
  recommendation, 232t
  selection, 644
Antimicrobial toxicity, 1074
Antimycotics, 213
Antineoplastic drugs, systemic administration, 317
Antiparasitic agents, usage, 1124t-1126t.
    See also Amphibians
Anti-tortoise herpesvirus antibodies, detection, 817
Antivenins, 1028t

Antiviral agents, usage, 1123t
Antivirals
 usage, 654
 in vivo use, 654
Anurans
 dorsal lymph sacs, location, 948f
 flight, 947
 hind leg, fourth segment, 177
 speciose group, 942
Anura (order), 941
Aorta, calcification, 187f
Aortic arch, aneurysm. See Green Iguana
Aortic bodies, necropsy examination, 576
Aortic stenosis, 187f
AP. See Alkaline phosphatase
Apalone spinifera. See Spiny Softshell Turtle
Apalone spp. See Softshell Turtle
Apalone (Triomyx) s. spiniferus. See Eastern Spiny Softshell Turtle
Apnea, 127
Appendicular osteomyelitis, 478
Appendicular skeletal frames, 477
Appetite, decrease, 933
APTT. See Activated partial thromboplastin time
Aquapuncture, 437
 advantage. See Lizards
Aquaria, size. See Box Turtles
Aquatic anurans, 943
Aquatic assessment, 980
Aquatic caecilian, saprolegniasis (presence), 959f
Aquatic carnivores, thiamin deficiency (susceptibility), 289
Aquatic salamanders, 943
Aquatic turtles, 95-98
 diet, 97t
 feeding, 97-98
 haul out area, 97
 head, middle ear abscess (MRI), 243f
 housing, 95-96
 infection, 874
 mice/pinkies, consumption, 98
 neonatal care, 98
 nesting areas, 97
 taxonomy, 95
 temperature, 97
 water quality, 96-97
ARAV. See Association of Reptilian and Amphibian Veterinarians
Arboreal reptiles
 plastic container, usage, 31f
 screen mesh, hazard, 774f
Archosauria, classification, 43
Arcus lipoides corneae, 691
Argasidae. See Soft ticks
Argentine Horned Frog (Ceratophrys ornata)
 bite wounds, 748f
 bladder stone, 763f
 humans, wounds, 947
 laser coeliotomy/enterotomy, 627f
 NMBD, 842f
Arginine vasotocin, 790
 activity. See Aminosuberic arginine vasotocin
Argos system, usage, 615
Arizona, herpetological societies, 6t
Arkansas, herpetological societies, 6t

ARKS. See Animal Record Keeping System
Armillifer armillatus, indirect life cycle, 344f
Armilliferiasis. See Pentastomiasis
Arm waving. See Circumduction
Arterial blood, supply, 135, 137
Arterial oxygen saturation (SpO_2)
 monitoring, 193f. See also Green Iguana
 trends, 449
Arterial PCO_2 values, correlation, 449
Arthrodesis, 607-608
Arthropoda, 1026-1027
Arthrotomy. See Green Iguana
 performing, 608
Artifacts (pseudoparasites), 805
Artificial lighting, usage, 1081
Artificial turf, usage, 31, 775
Ascaphis truei. See North American Tailed Frog
Ascarida (order), 356
Ascarididae, 155
Ascarid nematode, lips, 357f
Ascarids, families, 154
Ascites, 181f, 506f, 699. See also Coelomic transudate
 impact, 693
Ascorbic acid deficiency. See Hypovitaminosis C
Asepsis, importance, 529-530
Asexual reproduction, 377
A-shi acupuncture points, 433f
Ashley, LM, 10
Asian Box Turtle (Cuora flavomarginata)
 popularity, 96f
 radiograph, 174f
Asian Pond Turtle (Mauremys mutica)
 calcified egg, ultrasound image, 672f
 ovary, ultrasound image, 672f
 ultrasound examination, 668f
Asian Water Dragons (Physignathus concincinus)
 closed eyes, cotton wool/tape (wrapping), 502f
 heart, Doppler ultrasound assessment, 508f
 rostral abrasions, 506f
 underwater rest/sleep, 171f
Asian Water Monitor (Varanus salvator salvator)
 dorsoventral view, 1100f
 lateral view, 1100f
ASIH. See American Society of Ichthyologists and Herpetologists
Aspartate aminotransferase (AST), 461, 807
 activity, 464
 increase, 817
 levels, increase, 651
 parameters, 881
Aspergillus spp., 154, 218-219
Aspicularis tetraptera, 345f
Aspidobothrid trematodes, 351
Aspirate, collection, 870f
Aspiration cytology, 983
Assist feeding, 278f, 535, 536f, 856
 need, 536f
 risks, 280
 usage, 955
Association of Food and Drug officials, impact, 420

Association of Reptilian and Amphibian Veterinarians (ARAV), 903f
 conferences, 13
Associations, 9-10
AST. See Aspartate aminotransferase
Asymptomatic hyperuricemia, 795
Ataxia. See Lizards; Terrapins; Tortoises; Turtles
At-home euthanasia, 19
Atipamezole, administration, 444
ATP. See Adenosine triphosphate
Atractaspidae, 46
Atrial systole, 126
Atropine, usage, 876
Atypical bacteria, 872
Aural abscesses, 742
 ancillary diagnostic testing, 744
 diagnostic plan, 744
 etiopathogenesis, 742-744
 hematogenous/traumatic etiologies, 743-744
 inflammatory response, 744
 semifirm swellings, 744
 systemic evaluation, 744
 therapeutic plan, 744-746
 unilateral/bilateral firm swellings, 744
Auroscope, usage, 323
Auscultation, 495. See also Green Iguana; Heart; Lungs
 enhancement, gauze sponge (usage), 182f
Autoanalyzers, usage, 533
Autogenous bacterins, usage, 658
Autogenous vaccines, usage, 412
Autoimmune diseases. See Humans
Autolysis, 683
Autolytic artifact, 570
Autotomy. See Surgical autotomy; Tails
Aviadenoviral nucleic acid probe, usage, 399
Avian leukosis/sarcoma viruses (ALSV), 404
Avian leukosis viruses, subgroup division, 405-406
Avian medicine, growth, 549
Avian orthoreoviruses, serotypes, 407
Avian radiographic positioning, 474
AVMA. See American Veterinary Medical Association
AVM Instrument Company, 615
Avocado, impact, 1077
Axial alignment, 604f
Axolotol, examination, 666f
Axoplasmic aberration, 436
Ayurvedic medicine, 429
AZA. See American Zoo and Aquarium Association
Azole derivatives, 154
Azurophils, 458f

B

Baby chameleons, plastic containers (usage), 31f
Baby mice (pinkies), 371
Bacteria, potential role, 244
Bacterial colonies, detection, 908
Bacterial dermatosepticemia. See Red leg
Bacterial dermatosepticemia, clinical signs, 957

Bacterial diseases, 152-153, 217, 227
  diagnosis, 223-225
  diagnostic techniques, 227-230
  therapy, 225-226
Bacterial DNA gyrase, fluoroquinolones (impact), 649
Bacterial enteritis, 753
Bacterial growth, 228f
Bacterial infections, 248, 329, 577. See also Chronic bacterial infections
  etiology, 782-783
  reoccurrence, 839
Bacterial isolates, recommendation, 232t
Bacterial isolation, 944
Bacterial keratitis. See Mediterranean Tortoise
Bacterial organisms, isolation, 872
Bacterial phagocytosis, 466f
Bacterial pneumonia, 872
Bacterial stomatitis, 926-927
Bacterial zoonoses, 1018-1022
Bacteroides spp., 235f, 927
Balantidium, 350f
Balling behavior, 169
Ball Python (*Python regius*)
  anorexia, 739
  bite wounds, 748f
  blood sample collection, cardiocentesis (usage), 194
  dyspnea, 500f
  endoscopic view, 521f
  gaping response, 679f
  granulomatous pneumonia, 521f
  hematologic values, 1104
  intestine, *Bothridium* sp., 353f
  lesion, radiograph, 907f
  longevity record, 56
  mycotic dermatitis, 498f
  open-mouth breathing, 500f, 866f
  oral cavity, opening, 635f
  pancreas/spleen/gallbladder triad, 823f
  prey bite, 235f
  rat bite, 907f
  retained spectacle, 499f
  sentinels, usage, 407
  serum biochemical values, 1104
  trachea chondroma, 679f
  wrinkled spectacle, 791f
Baltimore Zoo study, 756
Bandage, reinforcement, 601-602
Bandy Bandy (*Vermicillia anulata*), 164
Barbour, RW, 11
Bargaining. See Loss
Barium studies, 757, 759
Bark chips. See Reptiles
Barthalmus, GT, 11
Bartlett, PP, 10
Bartlett, RD, 10
Basidobolus, 209
Basiliscus plumifrons. See Green Crested Basilisk; Plumed Basilisk
Basilisk (*Basilicus plumifrons*), housing, 69f
Basking
  areas, absence, 696
  spots, 966
Basophilic inclusions, presence, 454
Basophilic intranuclear inclusion bodies, 399
  detection, 400

Basophils, 456f
  size, 456
Batagur baskar. See River Terrapin
Beaded Lizard (*Heloderma* sp.)
  coelomic musculature, bipolar incision, 627f
  venom, delivery/characteristic, 1052f
Beak
  congenital disorders, 924
  deformities, 202
  disorders, 924-929
  oral/rostral trauma, 924
Bearded Dragon (*Pogona vitticeps*)
  amphophilic inclusions, 400f
  bicephalic condition, 374f
  blepharospasm, 506f
  bone volume, 1088f
  captive breeding, 293
  cardiac silhouette, enlargement, 487f
  carpus, deformity, 286f
  cohabitation, 74f
  conjoined twins, 684f
  conjunctivitis, 506f
  cricket, consumption, 266f
  CT data, usefulness, 1088f
  dorsal ventral radiograph, 487f
  dorsal view, 1092f
  dorsolateral cervical region, mass, 686f
  Eimeria sp., 348f
  epidermal necrosis, 225f
  feces, components, 257f
  feeding trial, 259f
  fMRI, two-dimensional parasagittal section, 1093f
  gingival bruising, 925f
  hematologic values, 1108
  hemopericardium, 184f
  hepatocytes, lipidosis, 252f
  hyperkeratosis, 225f
  idiopathic head tilt, 692f
  intranuclear basophilic inclusions, 400f
  isoflurane, administration, 299f
  Isopora amphiboluri, 348f
  lateral views, 1088f
  lesions, cleansing, 225f
  lip, mucocutaneous junction (mass), 319f
  liver
    hepatic lobes, swelling, 400f
    hepatocytes, number, 400f
    hexagonal viral particles, intranuclear paracrystalline array, 398f
  lung lavage catheter, placement, 520f
  nerve-sheath tumor, 319f
  nutritional secondary hyperparathyroidism, 286f
  obesity, 284f
  oral cavity, flashing, 168f
  Oxyurid spp., 155f
  pancreas, necropsy specimen, 823f
  parasite elimination, 35f
  parenchyma, appearance, 400f
  pericardial fluid, presence, 487f
  pressure-driven mechanical ventilator, usage, 449f
  pressure-driven ventilator, usage, 545f
  radiograph, 520f
  rostral abrasions, 925f

Bearded Dragon—cont'd
  rostrum/maxilla/upper labia, callus formation, 925f
  scoliosis, 286f
  serum biochemical values, 1108
  siblings, dominance, 508f
  Snake mite (*Ophionyssus natricis*) infestation, 685f
  surface volume, 1088f
  surgical debridement, 225f
  systemic itraconazole, usage, 226f
  threat display, 168f
  throat region, inflation, 168f
  tissue volume, 1088f
  topical silver sulphadiazine, usage, 226f
  two-dimensional frontal section fMRI, usage, 1092f
  ventral view, 1092f
  whole blood transfusion, receiving, 545f
Bedding. See Herbivores
Behavioral adaptations, 163
Behavioral fevers, 253
Belly-hugging, case report, 288
Bending stability, 604f
Benzalkonium chloride, 947
  usage, 964
Benzocaine hydrochloride, usage, 566
Benzodiazepines, usage, 246, 444
Berber Skink (*Eumeces schneider*), bite wound (infection), 504f
Berlander's Tortoise (*Gopherus berlandieri*), dorsoventral radiograph, 894f
Berries, consumption, 267
Betadine
  usage, 584f
  water combination, usage, 782
Betadyne Skin Cleanser, 1018
Beta-lactamase-producing pseudomonal species, 652
Bian Que, 438
Bicornuate reproductive system, 753
Big-headed Turtle (*Platysternon megacephalum*), 81f
Bilary ductal epithelium, 406
Bilateral calcium phosphate ureteroliths. See Red-eared Slider
Bilateral cut-down procedures, 887
Bilateral microphthalmia, 333
Bile, storage, 148
Bile acids, assessment usefulness, 807
Bile ducts, necrosis, 402
Biliary ductal epithelium, 406
Bilirubin, analysis, 884
Biliverdin, 807
Binocular magnification loupes, adequacy, 583f
Bioactive substrates, 27
  usage, 34. See also Captive reptiles
Bioactive substrate systems (BSS), usage, 36-37
Biochemical parameters. See Green Iguana
Biochemistry. See Pneumonia
  parameters, usage. See Livers
Biological shut down, 631
Biological tissue, laser (effects), 619f
Biologic data, remote monitoring, 614
Biology, basics, 25-27
Biology of the Reptilia, 10

Biopsies, 570-572
  forceps, 552
    types, 552f
  impact. See Endoscopy
  precision, 561-562
  preparation/submission. See Small
      biopsies
  prognosis, relationship, 676f
  sample, procurement, 569-578
  specimens
    collection, usefulness, 838
    handling, 572t
  techniques, 809f
    overview, 569
  usage, 523
Biosynthetic absorbent wound dressing,
    748-749
Biotelemetry, 613
  complications, 615
  power sources, 614
  units, suppliers, 614t
Biotin deficiency, 243-244, 680
  clinical signs, 243-244
Bipolar coagulation, 623f
Bipolar forceps, 623f
Birds, virus activity (documentation), 391t
Bites. See Prey bites
  wounds, prevention, 747
Black and White Tegu (Tupinambus
    teguixin), HO/lesions, 849f
Blacklight blue (BLB) tubes, 1082
Black Racer (Coluber constrictor)
  copulatory bursa, 356f
  dietary requirements, 740f
  Kalicephalus sp., 355f
Black spot disease, 220
Bladder. See Slider; Tortoises
  biopsy, 527
  calculi, ventral midline, 769f
  catheterization, 888
    (blind-stick), 882
  distention. See Green Iguana
  endoscopic biopsy, 527
  excisional biopsy, 527
  prefemoral soft-tissue approach,
      usage, 770f
  prolapse, 961f. See also Frogs
  stones
    increase, 769f
    weight/size, radiograph, 766f
Blanding's Turtle (Emydoidea blandingi)
  carapace, fracture, 897f
Blanding's Turtle (Emydoidea blandingi),
    tongue (excised mass), 468f
Blastomyces dermatitidis, 223
BLB. See Blacklight blue
Bleach
  impact, 1072
  necessity, 34
  solutions, dilution, 731
Blepharedema, 326, 832f
Blepharitis, 326
Blepharospasm, 326, 335, 691
Blind diverticula, similarity.
    See Hemipenes
Blindness, 404. See also Terrapins; Tortoises;
    Turtles
  differential diagnosis, inclusion, 854

Blind Snakes (Rhamphotyphlops braminus),
    44-45, 49f
  parthenogenesis, 49
Blind-stick. See Bladder
Blister disease, 202-203, 219. See also Florida
    KingSnake
  dampness, impact, 497f
Bloating, 842. See Terrapins; Tortoises;
    Turtles
  intestinal gas, 957
Blood
  agar plates, usefulness, 230f
  analysis, 883. See also Pneumonia
  biochemical tests, 461
  biochemistry, influences, 825
  chemistry values, 1103-1117
  chloride concentration, 462
  CO_2 levels, increase, 129
  collection, 513-516, 533-534, 981.
      See also Heparin
  cultures, 227
    performing, 949
    underutilization, 227f
  data, 513
  definition, 429t
  film. See Burmese Python; Desert
      Tortoise; Green Iguana; Slider
    examination, 562
  flow evaluation, radioisotope scans
      (usage), 191f
  gas evaluation, 1003
  glucose
    factors, 823-825
    sampling, 825
    values, 825
  insulin levels, usefulness, 825-826
  oxygen, affinity, 128
  parasites, 349, 802t
    transmission, 208f
  positive dipstick reaction, 883
  sample collection, 461
  smear, value, 533
  system, analysis, 513-517
  transfusion. See Whole blood transfusion
  vessels, noncontact laser treatment, 626f
  volumes, percentages. See Total body
      water
Blood-borne infection, 205
Blood-borne viral pathogens,
    transmission, 726
Blood creatinine concentration, 462
Blood-feeding mites, mouthparts, 722
Blood Python (Python curtis)
  ovary
    echolucent previtellogenic follicles,
        386f, 387f
    ultrasound image, 671f
  oviduct, echogenic egg, 387f
Blood-sucking parasites, 454
Blood urea nitrogen (BUN), 993
  reduction, 1003
  values, 461-462
Blossoms, consumption, 267
Blue-eye, 779
Blue-staining granules, 456f
Blue-tailed Monitor (Varanus doreanus)
  nematode egg, 355f
  visceral gout, 27f

Blue-tongued Skink (Tiliqua scincoides)
  dorsal recumbency, 636f
  hematologic values, 1108
  serum biochemical values, 1108
Bluff, displays, 167-168
Blunt dissection, usage, 557
Boa constrictor. See Red-tailed Boa
Boa Constrictor (Boa constrictor)
  bacterial dermatitis, 498f
  bacterial stomatitis, 499f
  bite wounds, 749f
  boid IBD, 496f
  bone phase, nuclear scan, 910f
  brain, nonsuppurative
      encephalitis/demyelination, 837f
  buccal erythema, 499f
  burn, healing, 204f
  Capillaria sp. egg, 359f
  coeliotomy, 527f
  distal esophagus, esophageal tonsils
      (endoscopic examination), 839f
  docility, 43f
  dorsal spinous process, biopsy, 911f
  dysecdysis, 497f
  echolucent germinal disc, echogenic
      yolk, 387f
  eosinophilic intracytoplamic inclusions,
      presence, 836f
  fetus, caudal end (ultrasound image), 387f
  fibrosis/scarring, 204f
  gastric mucosal cells, cytoplasm, 836f
  hematologic values, 1103
  hemorrhages, 499f
  IBD, 839f
  infectious stomatitis, 928f
  kidney
    cell culture (cytoplasm), vacuoles (viral
        particles), 837f
    cranial pole, close-up, 886f
  lateral horizontal radiograph, 886f
  liver, IBD, 836f
  neurons, degeneration, 837
  one-piece shedding, 779f
  osteomyelitis, 478f
  radiograph, 472f
  renal biopsy, 527f
  renal carcinoma, 299
  renal gout, 886f
  restraint, 496f
  rib, proximal portion (distortion), 478f
  rodent bite wounds, 748f
  secondary mineralization, 886f
  SEM, 204f
  serum biochemical values, 1103
  single bite wound, 747f
  skin necrosis, 498f
  spinal ankylosis, 245f
  spinal osteopathy, 245f, 910f
  stomach, IBD, 836f
  tapeworm egg, 354f
  wet-to-dry bandages, change, 749f
Boa Constrictor (Constrictor constrictor),
    blister disease/retained slough, 203f
Boaedon fuliginosus. See Brown House Snake
Body
  cavity (mesentery), tumors, 311t-312t
  positioning, 586
  surfaces, sampling, 227-228

Body—cont'd
  systems, stress (effects), 120-121
  temperatures
    evaluation, 535f
    range, 631
  wall, opening, 573
  water distribution, 540
  work, 438
Body weight (BW), 252
  carapace length, relationship, 276f
  conversion table, 422t
  graph, 279f
Boidae, 46
  electromagnetic radiation imaging systems, 340
  longevity, 56t
Boids, 42f
  coiling, 169
  conspecific aggression levels, increase, 172
  gestation, 172-173
  IBD, 248-249
  incubation behavior, 172-173
  Snakes, spurs (location), 380
  stargazing, 170-171
  vestigial pelvic appendages, 51f
Boinae, 46
Bollinger's bodies, 408
  visibility, 709
Boltzman factor, 420
Boluses, administration, 277
Bolyeriidae, 46
Bombyx mori. See Silkworm larva
Bone marrow. See Gelatinous bone marrow; Trabecular bone marrow
  aspiration. See Yemen Chameleon
  distribution, 578f
  hematologic evaluation, 516-517
  necropsy examination, 578
Bones
  angular deformities, 476
  bacterial infection, fluid/cellular debris, 697f
  biopsy, 523, 525
    bacterial cultures, 910
    challenge, 571-572
  bulbous distortion, 476
  calcium, depletion, 389
  culture, 910
  curettes, 894
  destruction, 906
  elevation, 590f
  fractures. See Facial bone fractures; Long bone fractures
    response, 477
  grafts, 605-606
  loss, orthopedic abnormalities, 601
  matrix, deposition. See Organic bone matrix
  pathology treatment, calcium (usage justification), 846
  plates, removal, 605
  plating, treatment, 605f
  radiopacity, evaluation, 476
  remodeling, 601f
  rongeur, usage, 578
  roungers, 894
  scan. See Green Seaturtle
  stimulator, usage, 606

Bony bridge, cranial/caudal limits, 637
Borrel bodies, 408
  visibility, 709
Bothridium sp. See Ball Python
Bothrochilus boa. See Ringed Python
Bothrops sp., 356f
Bovine serum albumin, 934
Bowel, exteriorization, 598
Box Turtles (*Terrepene* sp.), 89-91. See also Asian Box Turtle; Eastern Box Turtle
  acclimatization, 90-91
  aquaria, size, 90
  aural abscess, 742f
  automobile accident, rhinotheca fracture, 541f
  beak, overgrowth, 509f
  carapace, bony plates, necrosis, 896f
  chronic nutritional problems, 90
  diet, 91t
  epidermal sloughing, 834f
  feeding, 90
    tubes, advantage, 541f
  fly larva infestation, 209f
  head, jaw removal, 743f
  hypervitaminosis A, effect, 834f
  indoor housing, 90
  inspissated aural abscess, 745f
  intromission, 173
  isoflurane, administration, 299f
  lateral carapace, fractures, 899f
  nutritional secondary hyperparathyroidism, 286f
  outdoor housing, 90
  pharyngostomy tube, advantage, 541
  pseudoshell, formation, 896f
  reproduction, 90
  temperature, control, 90
  toes, lacerations, 776f
  volume-driven mechanical ventilator, usage, 448f
  water, supply, 90
Boyer, TH, 11
Bradycardia, occurrence, 128
Brain
  destruction, entry point, 567f
  neuroendocrine response, 120
  paramyxovirus infection, 860f
  viral cultures, 710
Brazos WaterSnake (*Nerodia harteri*), characteristics, 25f
Breathing difficulty, 816
Breath sounds, abnormality. See Terrapins; Tortoises; Turtles
Breeding. See Captive breeding
  soundness, evaluation, 559
  stock, 384
Bridging spondylosis, 914f
Brille, 327
Broad-headed Skink (*Eumeces laticeps*), jowls/head coloration, 175f
Broad-spectrum antibiotics, 656, 957
  initiation, 1003
Broad-spectrum lighting, usage, 880
Bromethalin, impact, 1073
Bronx Zoo (New York Zoological Garden), 36
Brown House Snake (*Boaedon fuliginosus*), tick (presence), 207f

Brown spot disease. See Crocodilians
Browse, consumption, 267
Brumation. See Snakes
BSS. See Bioactive substrate systems
Buccal cavity, 519
Buccopharyngeal membranes, 133
Bufagenin, 1075
Bufodienolides, 1070
Bufo marinus. See Neotropical Giant Toad
Bufo spp. toads, parotid glands (toxic secretion), 945f
Bufotoxins, 1075
Bufo viridis. See Green Toad
Bullous diseases, 202-203
Bullous spectaculopathy, 331
Bumps, 681
BUN. See Blood urea nitrogen
Buoyancy
  abnormalities, 394
  problems, 992
Bupivacaine, administration, 445
Buprenorphine, usage, 451, 616
Burmese Brown Tortoise (*Manouria emys*), species, 93
Burmese Mountain Tortoise (*Manouria emys emys*)
  gallbladder, ultrasound image, 670f
  inguinal region, subcutaneous space (usage), 636f
  tomia, manipulation, 640f
Burmese Python (*Python molurus bivittatus*), 42f
  anorexia/weight loss/coelomic mass, 316
  bilateral anophthalmia, 374f
  blood film, 456f-459f
  body mass, 421f
  cardiomegaly, 187f
  chronic constipation, lateral radiograph, 316f
  cloaca, metastatic lesion, 316f
  coelomic fat bodies, 316f
  core contents, aspiration, 716f
  corneal injury, 784f
  death, pneumonia/chronic paramyxovirus infection, 860f
  disorientation, 837f
  egg hatching, 366f
  feeding trial, 260f
  heart, ultrasound image, 668f
  heat lamp, coiling, 918f
  immature erythrocytes, 454f
  kinks, 907f
  lesions, enrofloxacin administration (impact), 643f
  liver, ultrasound image, 669f
  lung, resected portion, 860f
  lymphosarcoma, 500f
  mandibles, radiograph, 175f
  mandibular swelling, 500f
  microphthalmia, 374f
  neurologic signs, acute onset, 837f
  OPMV infection, signs, 858f
  proliferative segmented spondylosis/proliferative spinal osteopathy, 907f
  renal adenocarcinoma, 316f
  righting reflex, 837f
  Strongyloides infection, 355

Burmese Python—cont'd
  submandibular bacterial cellulitis, 500f
  subspectacular abscess, 499f
  tracheal/lung wash cytology, 466f
Burn-damaged keratin, 896
Burns, 203-204. *See also* Chemical burns; First-degree burns; Fourth-degree burns; Second-degree burns; Thermal burns; Third-degree burns
  commonness, 917f
  debridement, 203
  treatment, 919-923, 920t
  types, 918-919
Burrowing Python (*Calavaria reinhardtii*), 166f
  defensive balled position, 169f
Bursalis muscles, 327
Buspirone HCL, disadvantages, 431
Butcher's paper, usage, 31
Butorphanol, administration, 451. *See also* Green Iguana
BW. *See* Body weight

C

Cable tie shell repair, 899
Cachectic reptile, urine, 883f
Cachexia (poverty lines), 281-282, 816
  indication, 497
Cachexic snake, skin ridges, 498f
Cadle, JE, 12
Caecilians, elongation, 941
Caenophidia (infraorder), 46
Cages
  accessory, 33
    change, impact, 39
  changing, impact, 39
  furniture, 780
  hiding ability, 33
  mates
    aggression, 959, 964
    confrontations, avoidance, 36f
  shapes, 32-33
  size/construction. *See* Captive reptiles
  substrate, 675
Caging, requirements (minimum). *See* Snakes
Caicos Rock Iguana (*Cyclura carinata*), ontogenetic change, 71
Caiman (*Caiman*)
  chemical burns, 204f
  eversion, digital palpation (usage). *See* Male caiman
  genera, 103
  length, 116
  snouts, narrowness, 103f
  temperature-dependent sex determination, 111f
Caiman (*Caiman* sp.), pox viral infection, 708f
Caiman (*Dracaena* sp.), transparent third eyelid, 325f
Caiman Lizard (*Dracaena guianensis*), cheek teeth, 64f
Calavaria reinhardtii. *See* Burrowing Python
Calcitonin (CT)
  impact, 845
  mediation, 463
Calcitrol, formation, 848

Calcium
  calcitonin/parathyroid hormone, physiologic interrelationship, 843f
  deficiencies, 285-289, 389, 965
    signs, 286
    treatment, 286-289
  deficits, 842
  importance. *See* Gastrointestinal peristalsis
  metabolism, 463
    aberration, 879
  supplements, 273
    commercial availability, 272t
  tolerances, 291
Calcium-deficient diets, 464
Calcium-EDTA, 1070
Calculi. *See* Urinary calculi
  signs, 765
Caledonian Lizard (*Rhacodactylus* sp.), autotomy, 502f
Caliciviruses, 411, 1158
California, herpetological societies, 6t
California Department of Fish and Game, poster, 1031f
California Desert Tortoise (*Gopherus agassizii*)
  aural abscess, 745f
  beak, overgrowth, 925f
  coelomic cavity, impaction, 853f
  egg shape, abnormality, 787f
  head tilt, 854f
  herpesvirus, 815f
  measurements, 89f
  NMBD, 842f
  pseudo calculi, 765f
  rear leg usage, inability, 853f
  status, poster, 1031f
  twins, 374f
  urinary calculi, presentations, 768f
  uroliths, 771f
  vagosympathetic trunk damage, pharyngostomy feeding tube misplacement, 854f
California Giant Red-sided Gartersnake (*Thamnophis sirtalis*), live birth, 366f
California Kingsnake (*Lampropeltis getulus getulus*)
  bicephalic condition, 374f
  bone lysis, radiograph, 245f
  intestinal adenocarcinoma, 318f
  metastatic lesions, 318f
  neoplastic lesion, 318f
  swelling, 245f
  vertebral osteomyelitis, 245f
California Tiger Salamander (*Ambystoma californiense*), protection, 942f
California Turtle and Tortoise Club, 9
Callus formation, 201
Calorie sources, 253-256
  factors, 256
  genetics, impact, 256
  ontogenic shifts, 256
  seasonal variations, 256
  species variations, 256
Campylobacter spp., 1022
Candida, 209
Candida albicans bacteria, 920f
Canine acupoints, transposition, 433f
Cannibalism, 294

Cannibal mites, 732
CANV. *See Chrysosporium* anamorph of *Nannizziopsis vriesii*
Capillaria sp. *See* Green Tree Python egg. *See* Boa Constrictor
Capillary refill time (CRT), 182
Capnometry, uses, 449
Captive amphibian, husbandry, 942
Captive-bolt stun gun, usage, 567f
Captive breeding, 384-389
Captive Green Iguana, diet (recommendation), 72t
Captive iguana diet, description, 71
Captive propagation, genetic mutations. *See* Snakes
Captive reptiles, 1040-1044
  bioactive substrates, usage, 36-37
  cage size, 32-33
    minimums, 32t
  closed collections, disease transmission (control), 35
  construction, 32-33
  death, 120f
  disinfection, 34
  examinations, 34
  feeding, 38-39
  heat sources, 29f
  hospitalization, 33
  humidity, 30-31
  lighting, 37
  light quality, 30
  long-term hospitalization, 28
  multiindividual/multispecies enclosures, 35-36
  natural light, usage, 30f
  nutrition, impact, 38
  parasite control, 34-35
  photoperiod, 30
  POTR, 26t
  quarantine, 33-34
  seasonal cooling period, 384
  staff training, 28
  stress, 39, 119
    measurement, 39f
  substrate, usage, 31-32
  temperature, 29-30
    ranges, preference, 26t
  water, availability, 37-38
Captive snake, shed skin (examination), 213f
Captive tortoises, reproductive data, 95t
Captivity
  impact. *See* Parasitism
  stress, 120f, 121-122
Carapaces
  bones, 893
  coccygeal vertebrae, disarticulation, 575f
  fractures, presence, 475f
  length, 1020
  removal, 574f, 575f
  scutes, nomenclature, 84f
Carbamates, 1068-1069
  action, mechanism, 1069
  clinical signs, 1069
  intoxication, 246
  treatment, 1069
Carbenicillin, 652, 927
  pharmacokinetics, 643-644
Carbohydrates, fermentation, 292

Carbon dioxide (CO$_2$)
  elimination, 442
  incubation, 900
  levels. See Blood
  movement, 133
  superpulse laser. See AccuVet CO$_2$
    superpulse laser
Carbon dioxide (CO$_2$) lasers
  beam, focusing, 620
  contact/noncontact modes,
    diagrammatic comparison, 621f
  diode lasers, comparison, 620t
  equipment, 620
  popularity, 619
  power density, 620
  spot size, 620
  tips, usage, 621f
  usage, 583, 612, 621f. See also Seaturtle;
    Tortoises
Carbonization area, 623
Carbonized-tip technique, 621-622
Carcass
  disposition, 566-568
  sternal recumbency, 575
Carcinomas, 404
Cardiac contractility, difference, 487
Cardiac diseases, 185. See also Clinical
    cardiac disease
Cardiac evaluation, practicality, 487
Cardiac glycosides
  impact, 1077
  usage, care, 185
Cardiac monitoring, usage. See Anesthesia
Cardiac shunting, 128
Cardiac silhouette, confusion, 191f
Cardiac size, estimation, 182f
Cardiac ultrasonography. See Honduran
    Milksnake
Cardiac ultrasound. See Echocardiography
Cardiocentesis, 194, 515
  achievement, 516
Cardiology, 181
  diagnostic techniques, 186-194
Cardiomegaly, 677. See also Burmese
    Python; Monitor Lizards
Cardiomyopathy, diagnosis, 184f
Cardiopulmonary anatomy, 124
Cardiopulmonary physiology, 124
Cardiopulmonary systems, radiographic
    interpretation, 482-484
Cardiotoxins, 1051
Cardiovascular anatomy, 124
Cardiovascular function, assessment, 517
Cardiovascular performance, 448
Cardiovascular physiology, 127-129
Cardiovascular system
  necropsy examination, 578
  tumors, 313t-314t
Caretakers, bonds. See Animals
Caretta caretta. See Loggerhead Seaturtle;
    Loggerhead Turtle
Carettochelys insculpta. See Fly River Turtle;
    Pig-nosed Turtle
Carnitine, impact. See Hepatic lipidosis
Carnivores
  calorie sources, 254
  feeding trials, 279
  fuel sources, 255f

Carnivores—cont'd
  pellets, consumption, 270
  pet foods, supply, 271
  tube feeding diets, 273
Carnivorous neonatal reptiles, foods
    (usage), 373t
Carotene-rich foods, usage, 833
Carotid bodies, necropsy examination, 576
Carpal walking, 843
Carpenter, JW, 11
Carpet Python (*Morelia spilotus
    variegatus*), 44f
  heart, swelling (radiograph), 185f
  midbrain
    gliosis, 413f
    region, glial cells, 413f
    myenteric ganglion, 413f
    perivascular lymphoid cuff, 413f
Cartilaginous granuloma, 599f
Caruncle, presence. See Oviparous
    species
Caryospora cheloniae, implication, 994
Caseated keratitis, 394
Caseous conjunctivitis, 335
Caseous pneumonia, commonness, 402
Castor bean intoxication, 1077
Cast padding, usage, 601
Castration, 172
Castroviejo needle holders, 583
Casts, observation, 885
Catalepsy, 163-165. See also Amphibians
Cataracts, 339f. See also Mediterranean
    Tortoise
  rarity, 681
  surgery, 339
Catecholamines, 706
Catheterization, 525
Catheters
  flash, evidence, 538
  insertion, 636
  site, closure, 657
Cats, reptile replacement, 15f
Caudal coelomic cavity, 577
Caudal luring, 167
Caudal pole, kidneys (fusion), 138f
Caudal trachea, 520
Caudal vascular anatomy, contrast
    angiography. See Green Iguana
Caudal vena cava, blood flow, 589f
Cava, communication, 60
CAVM. See Complementary and alternative
    veterinary medicine
CBC. See Complete blood count
CCD. See Charge coupled device
CCL. See Curved carapace length
CCW. See Curved carapace widths
CE. See Competitive exclusion
Cecal anaerobes, CF3, 659
Cedar shavings, 70
Cefoperazone
  evaluation, 648
  pharmacokinetics, 648
Ceftazidime, 920
  discontinuation, 921f
  pharmacokinetics, 647
Celiocentesis, performing, 951
Celioscopy. See Exploratory celioscopy
  usage. See Amphibians

Celiotomy, 586-595
  incision. See Snakes
  usage. See Amphibians
Cell culture, usage, 391
Cell-mediated components, 632
Cell-mediated responses, 213
Cell membrane, osmotic forces, 541f
Cellular compartment, contraction, 542f
Cellular debris, accumulation, 529
Cellulitis, 685. See also Pythons
  suppurative infection, 716f
Cell wall synthesis, 652
Centers for Disease Control and
    Prevention, 658
Central nervous system (CNS)
  cephalosporins, entry, 647
  damage, 248, 852f
  disease, 815-816
    pathogenic mechanism, 816
  fluoroquinolones, adverse effects, 649
  impact, 401
  inclusions, presence, 818
  membranes, 1068
  tumors, 680
Centrals, 972
Centrolenidae. See Glass Frog
Cephalic flexure, 239
Cephalic vein
  exposure, 537f
  location. See Lizards
  usage, 638-639
Cephalosporins, 927
  usage, 647-648
Ceratophrys ornata. See Argentine Horned
    Frog; Ornate Horned Frog
Cerclage, 601f. See also Hemicerclage
Cerebrospinal fluid (CSF), 242f
  analysis, 239, 242-243
  blood contamination, 530
  collection, 529
  sampling, 529-530
  tap, positioning. See Green Iguana
  tool, 983
Cestodes, 346t, 1166-1167
  antemortem detection, 961
  eggs. See Pythons
  impact, 961
  orders, 155
CF3. See Continuous flow culture
Chaetomium sp., isolation, 220f
Chamaeleo calyptratus. See Veiled Chameleon
Chamaeleo deremensis
  nutritional secondary
    hyperparathyroidism, 287f
  radius/ulna, fracture, 287f
Chamaeleo dilepis. See Flap-necked
    Chameleon
Chamaeleonidae, 59
Chamaeleo calyptratus. See Yemen
    Chameleon
Chamaeleo jacksoni. See Jackson's Chameleon
Chameleon Information Network, The, 10
Chameleons (*Chamaeleo* sp.)
  bones, characteristics, 1089f
  cloacal region, ventral view, 684f
  eyelids, papilloma, 326f
  fruit flies, consumption, 372f
  heart, pectoral girdle location, 191f

Chameleons—cont'd
  iatrogenic hypovitaminosis A, 683
  IO catheter, placement, 540f
  kidney anatomy, normal separation, 138f
  Klebsiella pneumonia, 234f
  lateral midsagittal view, 62f
  lateral recumbency positioning, 585f
  lowland species, growth rates, 253f
  lungs
    characteristics, 1089f
    lobe, nematode (presence), 875f
  paper tape splint, 602f
  partial sloughing. See Flap-necked
      Chameleon
  ribs, characteristics, 1089f
  seminal plugs, removal, 684f
  subcutaneous tissue, *Foleyella furcata*
      removal, 360f
  vitamin A, need, 289
  water, delivery (consistency), 258f
Chameleons (*Chamaeleo verrucosus*),
      emaciation, 693
Chamaeleo parsoni. See Parson's Chameleon
Chamaeleo verrucosus. See Chameleons
Chapiniella sp. egg. See Ornate Box Turtle
Charge coupled device (CCD), 550
  imaging, 552
Charges, estimates, 3
Cheese-like plugs, 715
Chelonia, 78, 173-175
  hind leg fold, midcranial portion
      (incision site), 556f
  lens capsule, thinness, 339
  ultrasonography, 192
Chelonia mydas. See Green Seaturtle; Green
      Turtle
Chelonians
  abnormality, 702f
  allometry, 276f
  amputation, considerations, 610f
  anatomy, 871
  anesthesia, induction, 446-447
  aquatic signs, 852-853
  body systems, tumors, 300t-301t
  brumation, 88
  carnivore-omnivore gel diets, usage.
      See Zoological Society of San Diego
  celiotomy, 588-593
  circling, 853
  claw length, 86
  coelomic cavities, schematic
      representation, 554f
  craniocaudal view, 1101f-1102f
  dietary intake, essential nutrients, 274
  difference, 86
  digestive tract, contents, 480
  dorsoventral view, usefulness, 1101f
  dystocia
    diagnosis, 789
    surgery, 791
  egg laying, location, 388
  exoskeletons, injuries, 478
  fan-shaped mesovaria, 596f
  fractured humerus/femur, 603f
  gait, abnormality, 853
  girdles, 84
  gonads, pairing, 86
  gravid females, 95

Chelonians—cont'd
  head
    positions, abnormality, 854
    tilt, 854
  heart
    CT scans, 189-190
    imaging, CT scan, 190f
    MRI imaging, 189-190
    visualization, 190f
  hemipenes, 528-529
  herbivore gel diets, usage. See Zoological
      Society of San Diego
  herpesvirus, pathology, 395-396
  hindlimb-frontlimb paresis/paralysis,
      853-854
  intestinal walls, visualization, 190f
  lateral view, 1101f-1102f
  liver, coelioscopic view, 809f
  lungs
    field, evaluation, 1101f-1102f
    pairing, 131f
  males, plastron shape, 380
  maturity, length, 376
  movement, reluctance, 853
  nasal discharge, abnormality, 701f
  neurologic disorders, 852-854
  nontraditional therapeutic methods, 658
  nutritional secondary
      hyperparathyroidism, 286f
  open-mouthed breathing, 702f
  oral cavity access, difficulty, 640f
  organs, mobility, 667f
  outdoor enclosures, planning, 93
  palpebral reflex, 448
  penile prolapse, 701f
  phallus, 528-529
    location, 137
  plastron, cutting, 592f
  positioning, 473-474
  POTZ, 87
  pulmonary evaluation,
      craniocaudal/lateral projections
      (usage), 483
  radiographic survey films, 189f
  renal portal systems, 87
  reproduction/courtship, 173
  respiration, difficulty, 84
  respiratory tract, anatomy, 129
  restraint, 473-474
    radiograph beam, lateral/craniocaudal
        views, 473f
  sac-like lungs, 129
  scutes
    loss, 204
    sloughing, abnormality, 204
  sexual dimorphism, 87
  shell
    damage, 204
    hinges, 81
    removal, 573-575
  spirorchid flukes, presence, 184
  survey radiographs, 482
  tails, enlargement, 381
  teeth, absence, 85
  towel clamps, ineffectiveness, 586f
  ulcerative shell disease, 213
  urinary bladder, 597
  vaccination, 658

Chelonians—cont'd
  water, access, 90f
  whole body twitching/tremors, 853
Cheloniid species, 974
Chelus fimbriatus. See Mata Mata
Chelydra serpentis. See Snapping Turtle
Chelydridae, 79-80
Chemical burns, 203, 677
  impact, 697
Chemical restraint. See Amphibians
  agents, usage, 1127t-1131t
Chemosensory detection. See Foods
Chemosensory system, inclusion, 240-241
Chemotherapeutic agents, 317
Chemotherapeutics, 639
Chemotherapy, 317-318, 320. See also
    Intralesional chemotherapy
  agents, toxicity (potential), 318
  drugs/dosages/administration
      routes, 317t
  usage, 159-160
Cherry-head Red-foot Tortoise (*Geochelone
    carbonaria*)
  lateral recumbency, 636f
  red-rubber feeding tube,
      premeasurement, 640f
Chicago Herpetological Society, 9
Chicken ESP, analysis, 272
Chiggers, infestation. See Collared Lizard
Chi Institute, 440
Chinese medical terms, definitions, 429t
Chinese Water Dragon (*Physignathus
    cocincinus*)
  endangerment, 103
  lateral horizontal execretory urogram, 886f
  scoliosis/hydrocephalus, 374f
  tibia
    nonunion fracture, radiograph, 606f
    osteomyelitis, 607f
Chiropractic, 434-438. See also Snakes
  manipulations, 437-438
Chitin, 257
  structure, 265-266
Chitinases, activities, 257t
Chitobiases, activities, 257t
Chitra indica. See Narrowhead Softshell
    Turtle
Chlamydia, 234
Chlamydial LPS antigens, 234
Chlamydia sp., recovery, 184
Chlamydiophila psittaci, reports, 958
Chlamydophila, 534
Chlamydosaurus kingii. See Frilled Dragon
Chloramphenicol, 717
  impact, 1074
  pharmacokinetic studies, 648
  plasma concentrations, 648
  usage, 642, 648
Chlorhexadine, 246
  solution, 927
Chlorhexidine
  soaks, usage, 781
  toxicity, 1070
  usage, 584f, 749
Chloride, absorption/transportation, 462
Chlorine
  intoxication, 963
  levels, 962-963

Chlorine-free water, 962
Choana, 229f
Cholecalciferol, impact, 1073
Cholecystocentesis, performing, 488
Cholesterol-blocking agents, 965
Cholesterol crystals, infiltration.
  See Peripheral cornea
Choline, usage. See Hepatic lipidosis
Chorioallantoic placenta, 377
Chromatophores, 67, 197
Chromic gut suture, avoidance, 590
Chromomycosis, 959
Chronic bacterial infections, 958
Chronic coxofemoral luxation, 608
Chronic glomerulonephritis, 826
Chronic pain
  analgesic agents, usage, 451t
  local anesthetic agents, usage, 451t
  management, 451
Chronic poor doer, 858
Chronic renal failure, physical
    presentation, 879f
Chronic respiratory tract disease, 690
Chronic weight loss, 839
Chrysemys picta. See Painted Turtle
Chrysemys picta dorsalis. See Southern
    Painted Turtle
Chrysosporium anamorph of *Nannizziopsis vriesii* (CANV), 217-218
  attention, 221
  infection, 224f
  isolation, 220, 225
Chuckwalla (*Sauromalus* sp.)
  chronic dermatitis (mite infestation), 197f
  skin, depigmentation, 197f
  skin, red mites (*Ophionyssus acertinus*), 720f
Chytrid DNA, identification, 958
Cicatrization, 207
Cilate trophozoite. See Star Tortoise
Ciliated protozoa, 350, 1164
  impact, 960
Ciprofloxacin
  plasma half-life, 650
  usage, 335, 337
Circular saw blades, availability, 584f
Circulatory disturbances, 245
Circumduction (arm waving), 171
Cirrhosis, 812
CITES. See Convention on International
    Trade in Endangered Species of Wild
    Fauna and Flora
CK. See Creatine kinase
Claw
  deformities, 202
  overgrowth, 202
Cleaning schedules, 1015
Clear-sided enclosures, 964
Clemmys guttata. See Spotted Turtle
Clemmys insculpta. See Wood Turtle
Clemmys marmorata, *Hexamita*, 350f
Client
  education, 19
  services. See Reptile practice
  support, 19-20
Climate control, 1014
Clindamycin, 927
Clinical cardiac disease, 181-182

Clinical chemistries, 460-465
  sample collection/handling, 461
Clinical hypocalcemia, 843
Clinically healthy animals, paramyxovirus, 858-859
Clinical pathology, 453
Clinical reproductive anatomy, 376
Cloaca
  anatomy. See Female lizard; Male turtle
  catheter, insertion, 522
  derivation, 135
  digital palpation, 383
  evacuation, 481
  fecal staining, absence, 504
  foreign body, presence (lateral
      projection), 480f
  GI tract terminus, 148
  hemorrhage, 165
  irrigation, 481
  mass, protrusion, 700-702
  probing, 381
  problems, 913
  purse-string suture, 389
  sterile swab, placement, 228, 228f
  stimulation, 525
  temperature, measurement, 495
  urates, impaction, 701
Cloacal glands, 529
Cloacal organ prolapse, 751-755
Cloacal prolapse, 389, 598-599, 701f, 751.
      See also Lizards
  anatomy, 751
  sign. See Nutritional metabolic bone
      disease
Cloacal scent glands (anal glands), 52f
Cloacal soft tissue masses, evaluation
      difficulty, 482
Cloacal vent, bleeding, 701
Cloacocolonic biopsy, 527
Cloacocolonic lavage, 522
Cloacoscopy, 559
Closed MRI machine, usage, 1090f
Clot formation, prevention, 637
Cloudy eyes, 681
Clove oil, usage, 948
Clutch
  dynamics, 378
  size
    trade-off. See Offspring size
    variation, 378
CNS. See Central nervous system
CNs. See Cranial nerves
CO_2. See Carbon dioxide
CoA. See Acyl-coenzyme A
Coagulase-positive infection, development.
      See Pythons
Coagulase-positive staphylococci,
      pathogenic quality, 231
Coaptation. See External coaptation;
      Postcoaptation
Coccidia, 155
  direct life cycle, 344
  prevention, 34
Coccidian oocysts, 348
Coccidiasis, 348
Coccidiosis, 347-349, 1162
Coccygeal vertebrae, disarticulation.
      See Carapaces

Coddidioides immitis, 223
Code 1 envenomations,
    signs/symptoms/medical treatment,
    1056t-1059t
Code 1 venomous animal bites
  first aid, 1054t
  protocols, 1053t
Code 2 venomous animal bites
  first aid, 1054t
  protocols, 1053t
Coelioscopy, 554-556
Coeliotomy, 131f
  alternate approach, 593f
  biopsy, 526-527, 886. See also Pneumonia
  techniques, 525
Coelom
  distention, 693
  insufflation, 549
  mass, 703
  soft-tissue approach, 769
Coelomic cavity
  entrance, 593
  sterility, 575f
Coelomic fluid
  estimation, 473
  presence, 473f
Coelomic masses, 500, 788f
Coelomic membranes, incisions, 553
Coelomic musculature, bipolar incision.
      See Beaded Lizard
Coelomic transudate (ascites), 671-672
Coelomic wall, removal, 576f
Coelomitis, threat, 991
Coelomocentesis, 982-983
COE Pets Convention, 1040
Coiled tail display. See Ring-necked
    Snake
Coiling
  behavior, 169
  syndrome, 246
Cold-blooded animals, transportation,
    1043-1044
Cold-blooded reptiles, 251
Cold-stunned animals, 992
Cold-stunned Seaturtles
  admission data sheet. See New England
      Aquarium
  assessment/treatment, 1001-1003
  convalescent care, 1003-1004
  evaluation, 1001t
  hematology abnormalities, 1003
  medical management, 1001-1004
  monitoring, 1003-1004
  plasma biochemical abnormalities, 1003
  release criteria, 1004t
  transport, 1004
    criteria, 1004t
Collapsed eggs, dehydration, 368f
Collards, usage, 266
Collared Lizard (*Crotaphytes collaris*)
  gastrointestinal impaction
      (radiograph), 70f
  lesions, enrofloxacin administration
      (impact), 643f
  trombiculid mites (chiggers),
      infestation, 725f
Colletotrichum acutatum, isolation, 222
Collins, JT, 11

Colloid oncotic pressure (COP), 543-544.
    See also Intravascular COP
  increase, 545
  transcapillary forces, 541f
Colloids, characteristics, 545.
    See also Synthetic colloids
Colon
  examination, 501
  prolapse, 753-755
  suturing, 598f
Colopexy technique, 598f
Coloration, sexual dimorphism (rarity), 50f
Color change, 168. See also Green Iguana
Colorectal atresia, performing, 597
Coluber constrictor. See Black Racer
Colubridae, 46
  classification, 42
  longevity, 56t-57t
  mouth rot, 926f
Colubrids, 42f, 44f
  nervousness, 500
Colubrid snake, splenopancreas
    (appearance), 823f
Colubroidea, 46
Coma. See Lizards; Terrapins; Tortoises;
    Turtles
Commercial animals, 15
Commercial diets, 270-271
Commercial lightbulbs, UV A/B
    emission, 272f
Common Box Turtle (*Terrapene carolina*)
  hematologic values, 1113
  serum biochemical values, 1113
Common Kingsnake (*Lampropeltis getulus*)
  hematologic values, 1107
  serum biochemical values, 1107
Common Musk Turtle (*Sternotherus
    odoratus*)
  carapace/bridge, fractures, 898f
  fractures, stabilization, 898f
Communal vivariums, amphibians
    (existence), 943
Competitive ELISA, 1065f
Competitive exclusion (CE) cultures, 659
Competitive exclusion (CE) products,
    658-659. See also Nontraditional
    therapeutic methods
Complementary and alternative veterinary
    medicine (CAVM), 428
  plan, 433
  practitioners, 429
Complementary veterinary therapies, 428
  natural history, considerations, 428-429
Complete anorexia, 386
Complete blood count (CBC), 717,
    results, 157
  usage, 740f
Compressive myelopathy, 436
Computed tomography (CT), 484-486, 1088
  data, reconstruction, 1090f. See also
    Alligators
  localizer image, 1090f
  reconstruction. See Pythons
  scan. See Alligators
    close-up. See Cornsnake
    inclusion, 151
    reconstruction. See Seaturtle
  scout image, 1090f

Computed tomography—cont'd
  settings, manipulation. See Desert
      Tortoise
  significance, 158
  studies, 478, 485
  usefulness, 241
Conant, R, 11
Concertina locomotion, 51
Concurrent histology, 1063
Conduction, 916
Conductive heat, 917
Cone-rich retina, 340
Conference of the Parties (CoP), 1041
Conferences, 13
Congenital abnormalities. See Globes
Congenital cardiovascular anomalies, 185
Congenital neuropathies, 246
Congenital spinal abnormalities, 856
Conical scutes, growth. See Star Tortoise;
    Tortoises
Conjunctiva, 334-336
Conjunctival fornix, foreign bodies
    (presence), 334-335
Conjunctivitis, 335, 394
  sign, 815
Constipation. See Lizards; Terrapins;
    Tortoises; Turtles
  report, 751
Constrictor constrictor. See Boa Constrictor
Contact dermatitis, 206
Contact duration, 918
Contia tenius. See Sharp-tailed Snake
Continuous flow culture (CF3), 659.
    See also Cecal anaerobes
Contrast media, injection, 190f
Conus papillaris, function (problems), 340
Convection, involvement, 916
Convective heat, 917
Convention on International Trade in
    Endangered Species of Wild Fauna
    and Flora (CITES), 78, 1031-1032,
    1041-1042
  appendix I, 1031
  appendix II, 1031-1032
  appendix III, 1032
  convention. See International trade;
      Regional trade
  parameters, establishment, 100
  specimens, derivatives, 1041
Convulsions. See Lizards
  occurrence, 680
Cooper, JE, 11
Cooter (*Pseudemys* sp.). See Florida Cooter
  radiograph, 473f
COP. See Colloid oncotic pressure
CoP. See Conference of the Parties
Copepods, observation, 962
Copperhead (*Agkistrodon c. contortrix*), 45f
  anesthetization. See Venomous
      Copperhead
Copulation, 385
  injuries, 385
Copulatory organ prolapse, 751-752
Coracidia, ingestion, 1026f
Corallus caninus. See Emerald Tree Boas
Coralsnakes
  antivenin, 1028t
  defensive behaviors, 166f

Core biopsies, 571
Core body temperature, monitoring, 193f
Corneal cholesterol dystrophy.
    See Red-eared Slider
  occurrence, 336
Corneas, 336-338
  abnormalities. See Lizards
  anatomy, 336
  clarity, 946
  keratitis, 337-338
  lesions, 393
  lipidosis. See Amphibians; Madagascan
      Tomato Frog
  refraction, loss, 336
  ulceration, 336
  viral infection, 338f
Cornsnake (*Elaphe guttata guttata*)
  cloacal mass, 159f
  fecal specimens, 758f
  fibrosarcoma, 210f
    histological presentation, 210f
  gastric mucosa, mass (origination), 677f
  granulosa cell tumor, bipolar
      coagulation/dissection, 627f
  head structure, CT scan (close-up), 1093f
  lipomas/liposarcomas, 319f
  midbody swelling, 158f
  multilobular cysts, 316f
  prosection, 679f
  pseudoparasite, 346f
  subcutaneous mass, 316f
  ventral coccygeal vein, propofol
      administration, 445f
Coronavirus, 706
Cortical bone biopsy instruments,
    usage, 523
Corticocancellous grafts, harvesting, 606f
Corticosteroid therapy, 964
Corticosterone, role (complication),
    120-121
Corucia zebrata. See Prehensile-tailed Skink
Costals, 972
Costovertebral joints, 908
Council Directive 86/609/EEC, 1041
Council Directive 91/628/EEC, 1043
Council Directive 1999/22/EC, 1040
Courtship injuries, 385
Cowdria ruminantium, transmission, 207
Coxiella burnetii, 1023
CPK. See Creatinine phosphokinase
Cranial caudal projection, usefulness, 484
Cranial coeliotomy, 520
Cranial edge, trapezoidal incision, 590f
Cranial kinesis, 606
Cranial nerves (CNs), 239-240
  damage, 852f
  evaluation, 979-980
  involvement, 241, 246
Cranial tail cut-down biopsy, 526.
    See also Pneumonia
  techniques, 525
Cranial trachea, sampling, 519-520
Craniocaudal view, horizontal beam
    projections, 867
Cranium, lateral aspects, 495
Creatine kinase (CK), 461
  muscle-specific enzyme, 464
Creatine values, 881

Creatinine, 462
  values, 881
Creatinine phosphokinase (CPK), 652
  parameters, 881
Crickets, food, 71-73, 263
Critical care. *See* Emergency/critical care
Critical reptile patient
  assessment, 545
  dose administration, 545
  fluid selection, 539-546
  nutritional support, 534-535
  therapeutics, 534-535
  treatment response, monitoring, 545
Crocodile Monitor (*Varanus salvadorii*),
    glossitis/tongue sheath
    infection, 687f
Crocodilians, 100, 175
  adenovirus, 398
  anatomic fold, 105f
  anesthesia, induction, 447
  anorexia, 706, 926f
  basking, 115f
  behaviors, 113-114
  bellowing, 110f
  birth defects, 111-112
  bite block, placement, 116f
  blood collection, 516f
  body systems, tumors, 302t
  captive husbandry, 705
  cardiopulmonary anatomy/physiology,
      126-127
  carnivores, 38-39
  celiotomy, 587-588
  characteristics, 101f
  circulation, 106
  circulatory system, 106
  classification, 100-102, 100t
  climatic conditions, impact, 111f
  coelomic cavities, schematic
      representation, 555f
  coelomic design, complexity, 555
  conical teeth, 102f
  death, 706
  dermatophilosis (brown spot disease), 708
  developmental malformations, 111
  diagnostic techniques, 512-513
  diet, variation, 115f
  differential diagnosis, 705
  digestive system, 107-108
  distinctions. *See* Alligators
  ears, 107
  eggs
    laying, 110
    rigid shell, 377f
  endangerment, 101-102
  environmental temperature, 115
  evolution, 100-102, 145
  external auditory meatus, 107
  eyes, 106-107
  farming, 102f
  feeding, 115-116
  food conversion ratio, 116
  gallop, 112
  gastrointestinal disease, 712-713
  gender determination, 110-111
  glottis, 132
    location, 130f
  gular fold, 105f

Crocodilians—cont'd
  hatchlings, 115
  head
    restraint, 116f
    slapping, 110f
    tags, 113f
  heart
    dorsal view, 127f
    images, 190
    lungs/coelomic viscera, separation, 132f
    ventral view, 127f
  hemipenes, 528-529
  hemodynamics, 106
  homing instinct, 107
  identification, 112-113
    methods, 113f
  immunosuppression, 705-706
  incoordination, 854
  incubation range, 111f
  integumentary disease, 706-709
  integumentary system, 108
  jaws, taping, 105f, 116f
  lethargy, 706
  life span, 102-105, 102t
  locomotion, 112
    difficulties, 854
  longevity, 102t
  mating, 110
    season, 110f
  microchips, implantation, 113f
  muscle twitching, 854
  muscular weakness, 854
  musculoskeletal disease, 711-712
  mycobacteriosis, 711
  mycoplasmosis, 710-711
  nervous system, 106-107
  nesting, 110
  neurologic disease, 709-711
  neurologic disorders, 854
  nonspecific clinical signs, 706
  nontraditional therapeutic methods,
      657-658
  nutrition, 115-116
  oral cavity, anatomy, 642
  osmoregulation, 114-115
  osteodermal armor, 101f
  penile groove, 109
  pox virus, 708-709
  renal portal system, 126-127
  reproduction, behavior, 110
  reproductive activity, 109-112
  reproductive system, 108-109. *See also*
      Female crocodiles; Male crocodiles
  respiratory disease, 710
  respiratory system, 105-106
  respiratory tract, anatomy, 132-133
  restraint, 116-117
  saltwater, tolerance, 115
  scleral ossicles, absence, 333
  shunt, 126
  skeletal system, 105
  skin, 197
  skull, 105
  small intestine, 108
  smell, sense, 107
  species/subspecies, 101t
  stomach, division, 108
  stress, 705-706

Crocodilians—cont'd
  systemic mycosis, 220-221
  tags, usage, 112
  tail-notching method, 113f
  teeth, 107
    oral examination, 926f
    sockets, location, 145
  thermoregulation, 114
  throat flap, 105f
  toe tags, 113f
  transponders, usage, 112-113
  transportation, 116-117
  valve-like flaps, 105
  VAV, 587-588
  velum palati, location, 130f
  water, periodic submergence, 115
  WNV, 709-710, 854
Crocodilia (order), 138
Crocodylia, order, 100
Crocodylinae (subfamily), life span, 103-104
Crocodylus intermedius. *See* Orenoco
    Crocodile
Crocodylus porosus. *See* Indopacific
    Crocodile; Saltwater Crocodile
Crocodylus siamensis. *See* Siamese Crocodile
Crocoydlus niloticus. *See* Nile Crocodile
CroFab. *See* Crotalidae Polyvalent
    Immune Fab
Cross-contamination, chance
    (minimization), 932
Cross-transmission studies.
    See Cryptosporidiosis
Crotalidae
  antivenin, 1028t
  polyvalent antivenin equine origin, 1028t
Crotalidae Polyvalent Immune Fab
    (CroFab), 1060
Crotalinae
  electromagnetic radiation imaging
      systems, 340
  longevity, 56t
Crotalus adamanteus. *See* Eastern
    Diamondback Rattlesnake
Crotalus cerastes laterorepens. *See* Sidewinder
Crotalus s. scutulatus. *See* Mojave
    Rattlesnake
Crotaphytes collaris. *See* Collared Lizard
Crouching, case report, 288
Crowding, 778
CRT. *See* Capillary refill time
Crus, splint usage, 603f
Cryosurgery, 990
Crypsis, 168
Cryptodira (suborder), 78, 79f
Cryptosporidia, 1024
Cryptosporidiosis, 349, 756, 1163
  carrier state, 757
  clinical manifestation, 757
  clinical signs, 757
  control, 761
  cross-transmission studies, 757t
  diagnostics, 758-760
  gross pathology, 757
  histology, 757-758
  impact, 676. *See also* Vomiting
  life cycle, 756
  species specificity, 756-757
  subclinical manifestation, 757

Cryptosporidiosis—cont'd
  transmission, 756
    studies, 756-757
  treatment, 760
  zoonotic implications, 756-757
Cryptosporidium, presence (proof), 349
Cryptosporidium muris, 346f
Cryptosporidium sp., infection, 760f
Cryptosporidium sperpentis
  direct wet smear preparation,
    759f, 7575f
  modified acid-fast stain, usage, 758f
Cryptosporidium spp., 156
Crystal growth, 764
Crystalloids, proportion, 541-545
Crytosporidia, prevention, 34
CSF. See Cerebrospinal fluid
C-shaped trachea, 599
CT. See Calcitonin; Computed tomography;
    Computerized tomography
Ctenosaura pectinata. See Spiny-tailed Iguana
CTURTLE, seaturtle biology/conservation
    (e-mail information network), 973t
C-type oncornavirus, 299
Cuban Boa (Epicrates angulifer), focal
    wound, 498f
Cuff overinflation, minimization, 447
Cultivars, 53f
Culture
  data, 230-231
  media, selection, 230
  results, interpretation, 230-231
Culturing, 228f
Cuora flavomarginata. See Asian Box Turtle
Curators, bonds. See Animals
Current Veterinary Therapy, 10
Curved carapace length (CCL), 979
Curved carapace widths (CCW), 979
Customs/excise. See Reptiles
Cutaneous lesions
  biopsy, 224
  examination, 953
  lasers, usage, 615
Cutaneous mycoses, 219-221. See also
    Subcutaneous mycoses
Cutaneous sutures, dehiscence, 967
Cut-down procedures. See Bilateral
    cut-down procedures
Cutting scissors, 553
Cyanoacrylate ester, usage, 897
Cyanosis, 181f
Cyanotic mucous membranes, 867
Cycad palms (sago palms), impact, 1077
Cycloheximide, 224
Cyclura carinata. See Caicos Rock Iguana
Cyclura cornuta. See Rhinocerous Iguana
Cyclura sp., head scar (healing), 923f
Cyclura spp. See Ground Iguanas
Cyfluthrin, 733
Cylindrophidae, 45
Cylindrophis maculates. See Sri Lankan Pipe
    Snake
Cyst, resting stage, 347
Cystacanth larvae, 353
Cystic calculi, 281, 504, 788f.
    See also Uromastyx
  development, 966
  presence, 595

Cystic calculi—cont'd
  removal, 770
  sizes/shapes, 771f
Cystic dilatation, 859
Cystic perforation, 527
Cystic urinary calculus, 751
Cystine stones, 766
Cystocentesis, 525. See also Pneumonia
Cystotomy, 597
Cytologic interpretation
  imprint technique, usage, 571f
  smear technique, usage, 571f
  swab technique, usage, 571f
Cytologic sample, evaluation, 465-468
Cytology, 569. See also Seaturtle
  treatment, 329-330
Cytoplasm, inclusions. See Erythrocytes

D

D'Albert's Python (Liasis albertisii),
    shedding problems, 780f
Dangerous Wild Animals Act (1976), 491
Data
  collection, 278
  extrapolation, 875
  quality, 418
  range, limitations, 418-420
  transmission systems, usage, 613
Dawley, EM, 11
Daylight film emulsions, 551
Daytime air temperatures, guideline, 29
DDT. See Dichlorodiphenyltrichloroethane
Death. See Crocodilians
  feigning, 163-165, 175. See also
    Amphibians
  Salmonella serotypes, implication, 1021t
Debilitated Loggerhead Syndrome, 995
Decapitation, acceptability, 566f
Decision levels, 461
Deep friction massage, response.
    See Traumatic fibrosis
Deep mycoses, 226, 1024
Deep shell abscesses, 894, 896
Defensive aggression, 171-172
Defensive behaviors. See Amphibians;
    Coralsnake; Reptiles; Snakes
Defensive posture, 176
Definitive host (DH), 343, 344f
  genera. See Reptiles
Dehooking devices, 992
Dehydration, 280
  commonness, 258-259
  degree, 448
  impact. See Amphibians
  occurrence, 632-633
  tolerance, 546
Delaware, herpetological societies, 6t
Delayed secondary enrichment (DSE), 901
Dendrobates pumilio. See Strawberry
    Poison-dart Frog
Dendrobatid frogs, drowning, 964
Dennett, TB, 11
Dental calculus, accumulation, 925
Dental picks, 894
Deoxygenated blood, 126
Depo-Provera, disadvantages, 431
Depression, 292. See also Loss
Dermal fistulas, 699

Dermatemydidae, 79
Dermatitis, 205-206. See also Contact
    dermatitis; Foreign body dermatitis;
    Foreign-body dermatitis
  mite infestation. See Chuckwalla
Dermatologic diagnosis, laboratory
    investigations, 200
Dermatology, 196
  clinical signs, 201
  clinical techniques,
    observation/examination, 199
  collection samples, 199-200
  developmental abnormalities, 206
  discoloration, 206
  diseases, 201-213
  environment, role, 199
  genetic abnormalities, 206
  necrosis, 210
  neoplasms, 210-211
  nutritional disorder, 211-212
  patches, 212
  treatment, 213-214
  viral diseases, 213
Dermatomycoses, treatment, 225-226
Dermatomycosis
  cases, documentation, 220-221
  documentation, rarity, 221
  lesions, diagnosis, 223-225
Dermatophagy, 294
Dermatophilosis (brown spot disease), 206.
    See also Crocodilians
  reports, 685
Dermochelyidae, 79
Dermochelyid species, existence, 974
Dermochelys coriacea, straight-line carapace
    length, 1091f
Desert enclosure setup. See Snakes
Desert Iguana (Disposaurus dorsalis),
    pathological spinal fracture, 600f
Desert Monitor (Varanus griseus), ovary
    (ultrasound image), 670f
Desert Tortoise (Gopherus agassizii), 81f.
    See also California Desert Tortoise
  automobile accident, 534f
  bladder, 560f
  blood film, 455f, 456f, 459f
  carapace burn, healing, 923f
  CT series, 869f
  CT settings, manipulation, 486f
  cystocentesis, 882f
  eggs
    calcified shells, 483f
    radiograph, 386f
  emaciation, pancreas, 824f
  foreign bodies, evidence (dorsoventral
    view), 474f
  hematologic values, 1115
  intestinal obstruction, 474f
  jugular vein, location, 538f
  large colon, Oxyurid larva
    (impaction), 358f
  lateral view pulmonary examination, 484f
  lesions, enrofloxacin administration
    (impact), 643f
  maxilla, lysis (radiograph), 235f
  mouth rot, 926f
  MRI, 486f
Mycobacterium chelonei osteomyelitis, 235f

Desert Tortoise—cont'd
  mycoplasmosis, 740
  nares, erosion, 702f
  nebulization chamber, 656f
  proctodeum, 560f
  prolapsed colon, 752f, 753f
  prolapsed oviducts, 753f
  pulmonary abscess, 869f
  radial paralysis, 609f
  radiopaque urinary bladder calculus, presence, 482f
  sand impaction, 480f
  scutes
    seams, erythema, 698f
    sloughing, 698f
  serum biochemical values, 1115
  short clipping, 776f
  skin, removal, 538f
  thyroid hormones, measurement, 290
  ultrasound examination, 669f
  urinary bladder
    calculus, 483f
    trauma, 753f
  urinary calculus, 482f
  ventral coeliotomy, 753f
Desiccation retardation, 778
Deutonymphs, activity, 721
Devcon 5 Minute Epoxy, usage, 898
Developmental abnormalities, 374f.
  See also Dermatology
De Vosjoli, P, 11
Dewlaps, 68
  extension, 171
  pressure, 277
Dextran-40, concentration, 545
Dextrose molecules, impact, 542f
DH. *See* Definitive host
DHCC. *See* Dihydroxycholecalciferol
Diabetes mellitus
  contrast. *See* Hyperglycemia
  suggestion, 464
Diadophis sp. *See* Ring-necked Snake
Diagnostic Center for Population and Animal Health (Michigan State University), iohexol assays/GFR calculation, 528
Diagnostic decision making, 550
Diagnostic images, 158
Diagnostic imaging, 471, 534.
  See also Seaturtle
Diagnostic sample collection, 513-519
Diagnostic techniques, 490. *See also* Ancillary diagnostic techniques
  considerations, 490-495
  legislation, 491
Diagnostic testing, 151-152
  understanding, 1062
Diamond-backed Water Snake (*Nerodia* sp.)
  hematologic values, 1104
  serum biochemical values, 1104
Diarrhea, 772. *See also* Lizards; Snakes
  diagnosis, 773
  parasites, impact, 773f
  treatment, 773
Diarthrodial joints, movement, 906
Diazepam, usage, 246, 444, 1069
Dichlorodiphenyltrichloroethane (DDT), 732

Dichlorvos strips
  advocacy, 731
  usage. *See* Mite infestation
Diet
  evaluation, 288
  offering, 965
  repetition, problems, 739
Dietary deficiency/intoxication, signs, 273
Dietary supplements, 659
Differential diagnoses, symptom categorization, 492t-495t
Diff-Quik stain, 465f, 468f, 838
  usage, 453
Diffuse spongiosis, 406
Digenetic flukes, 994
Digenetic spirorchid flukes, encounter, 184
Digenetic trematodes, 351, 994
Digestible sand, impact, 69f
Digestion, venom (impact), 148
Digestive system
  body temperature, impact, 384
  radiographic interpretation, 478-481
Digestive tract, 479
  mucosal pattern, 481
  necropsy examination, 577-578
  radiographic contrast procedures, 480
  tissue opacity, 485
Digital thermometers, usage, 535f
Digits. *See* Iatrogenic digits
  abnormalities, 774
    history, 774
    physical examination, 774
  fractures, 604, 775-776
    ball bandage, usage, 604f
  treatment, 776-777
Dihydroxycholecalciferol (DHCC), 841
Diiodithyronine (DIT), 290
Dimethyl sulfoxide (DMSO)
  acid-fast fecal technique, 759t
  usage, 935
Dimorphic fungi, 223
Dioctyl sodium sulfosuccindate (DSS), impact, 1078-1079
Diode lasers
  advantages, 619
  comparison. *See* Carbon dioxide lasers
  equipment, 620-622
  noncontact mode, 622
  open surgery usage, 622
  power settings, 622
  usage, 583
Diomed lasers, 620
Diphtheritic necrotizing gastritis, 152
Diploglossa, 60
Dipsosaurus dorsalis. See Desert Iguana; Iguanid lizard
Dipstick specific gravity assays, correlation, 884
Direct arterial blood pressure measurements, 448
Direct life cycle, 343
Discoloration. *See* Dermatology
Disepithelization, presence, 817
Disinfectant-associated toxicities, 962
Disinfectants
  characteristics, 1086t-1087t
  usage. *See* Vivarium
Disorientation, 404, 873, 963

Dissociative agents, 445
Distal esophagus, feeding tube placement, 277, 635f
Distal femur, splint usage, 603f
Distal humerus, 603
  splint usage, 603f
Distal lens designs, 552
Distal lens offsets
  comparisons, 551f
  consideration, 551
Distal tubule, 139-140
Distal ureters, concretions, 763f
DIT. *See* Diiodithyronine
Diuretics, 185, 1025
Diurnal animals
  sunshine, relationship, 842, 844f
  UV radiation, exposure, 841
Diurnal cage temperatures, range, 70-71
Diurnal temperature gradients, 70
DMSO. *See* Dimethyl sulfoxide
DNA in situ hybridization, 1064
  relationship. *See* Immunohistochemistry
DNA probes, 391
Documentation devices, 553
Docusate, usage, 992
Dodd, Jr., CK, 11
Dogs, reptile replacement, 15f
Doppler flow detector, usage, 448.
  See also Peripheral pulses
Doppler flow probe, placement. *See* Green Iguana
Doppler ultrasonic flow detector monitoring, 193-194
Doppler ultrasound assessment. *See* Asian water Dragons
Dormitor, usage, 639
Dorsolateral articular facets, 908
Dosing syringe, insertion, 641f
Double contrast upper GI radiographic contrast procedures, 480-481
Double layered closure, 597
Dove, usage, 920
Doxycycline, 957
  therapeutic regimen, 653
D-Penicillamine, 1070
Dracaena guianensis. See Caiman Lizard
Dracaena sp. *See* Caiman
Dragon Light, 1083
Dremel tools, 894
Dri-Die, 732
Drowning fatality, 690
Drugs
  administration
    routes. *See* Analgesia; Anesthesia
    technique, 875
  distribution, 644
  metabolic/excretory pathways, 644
  overdose, 491
  pharmacokinetics, 644
Dry docking, recommendation, 894
Dry-dock trauma treatment, 986
Dry eye. *See* Keratoconjunctivitis sicca
Dry film analyzers, 951
Drymarchon corais. See Indigo Snake
Drymarchon couperi. See Eastern Indigo Snake; Indigo Snake
DSE. *See* Delayed secondary enrichment
DSS. *See* Dioctyl sodium sulfosuccindate

D-tubocurarine, 324
Dual-binding protein, detection, 289
Duellman, WE, 11
Dujardinascaris sp. *See* American Alligator
Dursban, usage, 1068
Dusting, 265
Dwarf Boa *(Tropidophis canus curtus)*, 44f
Dwarf Caiman *(Paleosuchus palpebrosus)*
   hematologic values, 1113
   serum biochemical values, 1113
Dyscophus antongilii. *See* Madagascan Tomato Frog
Dysecdysis, 206-207, 778, 914f.
   See also Lizards; Snakes
   association, 685
   clinical signs, 779-781
   ectoparasites, impact, 780f
   factors, 782t
   histologic examination, 206f
   localization, 201
   pearls of practice, 785
   prevention, 784-785
   problems, 780
   prognosis, 785
   treatment, 206-207, 781-783
Dysecdysis-retained spectacles, 783-784
Dyspnea, 679. *See also* Lizards; Terrapins; Tortoises; Turtles
   occurrence, 222
   presence, 866
Dystocia, 389, 787. *See also* Lizards; Nonobstructive dystocias; Obstructive dystocias
   causes, 787-788
   complications, 789
   diagnosis, 788-789
   etiology, 787-788
   hormonal stimulation, 789-790
   obstructive causes, 689
   physical manipulation, 789
   recurrence, 792
   reports, 787
   reproduction, 791
      prevention, 792
   result, 681
   surgery, 790-791
   treatment, 789-792

E

Ears
   anatomy, 742
   sampling, 531
Eastern Box Turtle *(Terrapene carolina carolina)*
   carapace, fracture (healing), 897f
   carapacial bone, lytic lesion, 854f
   commonness, 89f
   iris color, 86f
   rear legs, paralysis, 854f
   shell growth, abnormality, 699f
   ultrasound examination, 667f, 668f
Eastern Diamondback Rattlesnake *(Crotalus adamanteus)*
   venomoid surgery, 612f
   victim's hand, swelling, 1055f
Eastern equine encephalomyelitis (EEE), 410-411

Eastern Hog-nosed Snake *(Heterodon platirhinos)*
   death feigning, 165f
   dorsal recumbency, position, 165f
   threat removal, 165f
Eastern Indigo Snake *(Drymarchon couperi)*, bilateral wounds, 172f
Eastern Kingsnake *(Lampropeltis getulus getulus)*, pancreas (necropsy specimen), 823f
Eastern Painted Turtle, testicle, 559f
Eastern Spiny Softshell Turtle *(Apalone (Triomyx) s. spiniferus)*, cutaneous lesions, 222f
Eastern tent caterpillar *(Mallacosoma americanus)*, safety, 266
EC. *See* Extracellular
Ecchymoses, 181f
Ecdysis, 52, 198-199. *See also* Monitor Lizards
   completion, difficulty, 239
   frequency, problems, 781
   hormonal regulation, 784-785
   occurrence, 582
   regeneration/healing, forms, 198-199
ECF. *See* Extracellular fluid
ECG. *See* Electrocardiograms
Echocardiography (cardiac ultrasound), 192-193
Ectoparasite-infected skin, 723
Ectoparasites, 343, 346-347, 518, 1160-1161
   diagnosis, 735
   impact, 781. *See also* Dysecdysis
   presence, 677
   treatment, 207
   visibility, 201
Ectotherms, 251
   fasts, withstanding, 281
Edema, 207, 699. *See also* Peripheral edema; Pleural edema
   control, 863
Edematous conjunctiva, 933
EDTA. *See* Ethylenediaminetetraacetic acid
EEE. *See* Eastern equine encephalomyelitis
Eggs
   artificial incubation, substrates (usage), 367f
   artificial pipping, necessity, 370f
   binding, 546, 857. *See also* Postovulatory egg binding; Preovulatory egg binding
   collection, 367
   contents, removal, 790
   death. *See* Slider Turtle
      causes, 369t
      signs, 368f
   dehydration. *See* Collapsed eggs
   development, 376-377
   embryo, removal, 371f
   free-living stages, 732
   harvesting, 370f
   hatching, 90
      time, 389
   incubation, 50, 388-389
      substrates, usage. *See* Reptiles
      times, 369
   laying, failure, 702-703
   malformation/breakage, 787f

Eggs—cont'd
   management, 367-370
   manual extraction, impossibility, 790f
   milking, 593f, 790-791, 791f
      danger, 593
   misting, 368
   monitoring, 369
   mottling/discoloration, 368f
   movement, wax pencil mark (usage), 368f
   pipping, neonate placement, 371f
   placement. *See* Prewarmed incubator
   radiographic exposure, effects, 386
   retention, 857. *See also* Milksnake; Snakes
   slugs, passage, 368f
   treatment, 642-643
   triangular wedge, cutting, 370f
   viability, checking, 368f, 369f. *See also* Snakes
Eggshell powder (ESP), 272
   presence. *See* Herbivores
   safety, 272
Eggs or fetuses, viability. *See* Retained eggs or fetuses
Egg yolk coelomitis, reports, 789
Egyptian Spiny-tailed Lizard *(Uromastyx aegyptius)*
   hematologic values, 1108
   serum biochemical values, 1108
Egyptian Tortoise *(Testudo kleinmanni)*
   hepatic membrane, incision, 809f
   liver, biopsy forceps (insertion), 809f
Eimeria sp. *See* Bearded Dragon
Eimeria tokayae. *See* Tokay Gecko
Eimeriorina (suborder), 802
Ektachem DT60 Analyzer, 951
Elaphe guttata. *See* Ratsnake; Red Ratsnake
Elaphe guttata guttata. *See* Cornsnake
Elaphe obsoleta quadrivittata. *See* Yellow Ratsnake
Elaphe sp. *See* Ratsnake
Elaphe vulpina. *See* Foxsnakes; Western Foxsnakes
Elapidae, 46
   longevity, 57t
Electric timers, usage, 30
Electroacupuncture, usage, 437f
Electrocardiograms (ECG)
   appearance, 193
   interpretation, 188
   usage, 189, 998. *See also* Mammals
Electrocardiographic leads
   attachment, 193
   placement. *See* Green Iguana
Electrocardiographic monitoring, 193
Electrocardiographic normal readings, 187f
Electrocardiographic results, evaluation. *See* Reptiles
Electrocardiographic tracing, 187f
Electrocardiography, 186-189
Electrocardiography (ECG), 448
Electrodiagnostic techniques, 241-243
Electrolytes, 462-463
   homeostasis, 964
Electromagnetic memory, 432
Electromyography, usage, 241
Electron microscopy, 153
   impact, 454
   usage, 391. *See also* Virions

Electron Microscopy Laboratory
(University of Georgia), 396
Electroretinographic (ERG) studies, 325
Elephant foot appearance, 477
ELISA. *See* Enzyme-linked immunosorbent
assays
Elliptical cup forceps, 552f
Embryo
nutrition, 260
necessity, 366
removal. *See* Eggs
Embryonic development, 365-366
Emerald Tree Boas (*Corallus caninus*)
blood film
erythrocytic cytoplasmic *Sauroplasma*
(*Serpentoplasma*), 803f
Hepatozoon, 803f
trypanosome, 804f
chronic abdominal distention, 481f
emaciation, muscling loss, 275f
fetuses, ultrasound image, 672f
hematologic values, 1103
plastic containers, usage, 31f
serum biochemical values, 1103
Emergencies, common cases, 546-547
Emergency/critical care, 533
Emergency diagnostics, 533-534
Emergency numbers table, example.
See Venomous reptiles
Emerging Diseases Research Group
(University of Georgia), 403
Emesis. *See* Snakes; Terrapins; Tortoises;
Turtles
Emydidae (family), 79, 80f
Emydoidea blandingi. See Blanding's Turtle
Enclosures
setups. *See* Snakes
usage. *See* Naturalistic enclosures;
Outdoor enclosures
Endocrine disorders, laboratory
evaluation, 465
Endocrine pancreas, 822-823
Endocrine system, tumors, 300t
Endocrine tissues, necropsy examination,
575-576
Endoparasites, 343, 347-349, 1161-1170
Endoscopes, 552
2.7mm, recommendation, 552
protectors, placement. *See* Plastic
endoscope protectors
Endoscopic biopsy, 521. *See also* Bladder;
Pneumonia
Endoscopic examination, 809f
documentation, 551
indications, 555, 556t
Endoscopic gender determination, 559
Endoscopic orchidectomy, monopolar
radiosurgery (usage). *See* Green
Iguana
Endoscopic telescope, introduction, 868-869
Endoscopy, 549. *See also* Pneumonia;
Seaturtle
anesthesia, impact, 554
biopsy, impact, 559-561
contraindications, 562
hand instrumentation, 552-553
indications, 562
instrument care, 553-554

Endoscopy—cont'd
light guide cables, requirement, 551-552
light sources, requirement, 551
special techniques, 556-562
sterilization, usage, 553-554
technique, evolution, 549-550
tools, requirement, 551-553
Endothelial cells, detection, 399
Endotherms, infection/trauma, 274
Endotracheal intubation, 447
Endovideo cameras, quality, 560
End-stage limb disease, amputation
(appropriateness), 610f
End tidal CO_2, monitoring, 193f
End-tidal PCO_2 monitoring, usage, 449
Energy
disorders, 281-285
intakes. *See* Standard metabolic rate
maintenance, 251-253
requirements, 252
sources. *See* Omnivores
Enodiotrema sp. *See* Loggerhead Seaturtle
Enophthalmia, 704
Enrichment broths, efficacy, 901
Enrofloxacin
evaluation, 649-650
impact, 1074
ineffectiveness, 717
injections, impact, 609f
negative side effects, 651
usage, 642, 650
Entamoeba invadens, danger, 855
Entamoeba ranarum, implication, 959
Enterals, feeding appropriateness, 273
Enteric bacteria, 1022-1023
Enteritis, 152-153, 757. *See also* Alligators
Enterocolitis. *See* Alligators
Enterotomy. *See* Argentine Horned Frog
Entomoeba invadens trophozoite, 347f
Enucleation. *See* Globes
requirement, 338
Environment
pristine condition, 958
role. *See* Dermatology
Environmental heat, provision, 631
Environmental humidity, impact, 633
Environmental temperature
impact, 581
inadequacy, 696
Enzyme-linked immunosorbent assays
(ELISA), 153, 900-902. *See also* Antigen
capture ELISA; Competitive ELISA
development, 873
illustration, 1065f
performing, 933
sensitivity, 396
test
representation, 759
sensitivity/specificity, estimation,
902-903
usage, 1065
deficiencies, 349
extensiveness, 901-902
Eosin methylene blue agar, 900
Eosinophilic inflammation, 466
Eosinophilic intranuclear inclusion
bodies, 395
Eosinophils, 455f, 456f

Epaxial muscles, 616f
Epicrates angulifer. See Cuban Boa
Epicrates cenchria. See Rainbow Boa
Epistaxis, occurrence, 690
Epithelioid cells, presence, 466
Epizootiology. *See* Adenovirus;
Herpesvirus; Paramyxoviridae;
Retroviridae
Epoxy
glue, usage, 898
resin, usage, 590
usage, 525
Epoxy-fiberglass-epoxy sandwich, 590
Equatorial annular pad, 339
Eretmochelys imbricata. See Hawksbill Turtle
ERG studies. *See* Electroretinographic
studies
Ernst, CH, 11
Ernst, EM, 11
Erycinae, 46
Erysipelothrix rhusiopathiae, isolation, 1022
Erythema, 290f. *See also* Tortoises
Erythemic conjunctiva, 933
Erythroblastosis, 404
Erythrocytes. *See* Reptiles
counts, obtaining, 460
cytoplasm
inclusions, 455f, 457f
vacuoles, artifacts, 457f, 459f
immature cells. *See* Burmese Python
nucleation, 453
responses, 454
Erythromycin, resistance, 643
Erythron, status, 453
Erythrophagocytosis. *See* Monocytes
Erythroplastids, 454
ESA. *See* U.S. Endangered Species Act
Escherichia coli, 234
ESF. *See* External skeleton fixation
Esophageal mucosal cells, 406
Esophagitis, 505, 510
Esophagostomy tube, placement, 639-640
Esophagus. *See* Snakes
anatomic/physiologic features, 147
conical papilla, endoscopic view.
See Seaturtle
function, 146-147
ESP. *See* Eggshell powder
Ethylenediaminetetraacetic acid (EDTA)
impact, 453, 533
lysing tendency, 981
usage, 949
Ethylene oxide, option, 554
Etiopathogenesis. *See* Aural abscesses
Etorphine HCl, investigation, 447
Eublepharines, 170
Eublepharis macularius. See Leopard Gecko
Eugenol, usage, 948
Eukaryotic organisms, 218
Eumeces fasciatus. See Five-lined Skink
Eumeces laticeps. See Male Broad-headed
Skink
Eumeces schneider. See Berber Skink
Eunectes sp. *See* Anaconda
Euparadistomum sp. *See* Green-eyed
Gecko
European conservation legislation (levels),
relevance, 1034t

European laws/regulations, 1031, 1033, 1040-1044
  case studies, 1044
  implementation/enforcement, 1033
  information, sources, 1033
  levels, 1033, 1034t
  national laws, variation, 1040
European Lizard (*Lacerta* sp.), papillomata, 326f
European protection, comparative table, 1037t-1039t
European regional legislation, 1033, 1041
European regional wildlife conservation legislation, European institutions (involvement), 1036t
European Tortoise, renal gout (renal ultrasound), 798f
European Union (EU), 1033
Eustachian tube
  connection, 743f
  openings, 146
  presence, 742
Euthanasia, 16-17, 564. *See also* At-home euthanasia
  guidelines, 19-20
  longevity, impact, 16
  methods, 565-566
  permission, 567
  physical means, acceptability, 566f
  protocols, 564-565
  questions, 20-22
  solution
    administration, 566
    pithing/injection, 566f
    sterility, 565
  techniques, 565-566
    recommendation, 565t
  therapeutic option, 659-660
Excisional biopsy. *See* Bladder
Exocrine tissues, secretion, 148-149
Exophthalmia, 704
Exophthalmos, 334
Exoskeleton injuries, evaluation, 474
Exotic DVM, 10
Exploratory celioscopy, 958
Exposure factors, 472-474
Exposure gingivitis, 676
External coaptation, 599-604
  application, 601
External fibropapillomas, 393
  response, 397
External fixation, complications, 606
External incubation, viability. *See* Ova
External morphology, sexual dimorphism (rarity), 50f
External skeleton fixation (ESF), 604
External structures, endoscopic examination, 556
Extracellular (EC) compartment, proportion, 541f
Extracellular (EC) distribution volumes, impact, 543f
Extracellular (EC) matrix, usage, 749
Extracellular fluid (ECF)
  osmolality, 258
Extracellular fluid (ECF), proportion, 541f
Extracoelomic masses, 500
Extraosseous calcium storage, 287

Extremities, fractures, 244
Exudates. *See* Inspissated exudates; Lizards
  cellular content, 468
Eyecap, 327
Eyelids, 325-327
  anatomy, 325
  cellular debris, 833
  papilloma. *See* Chameleons
  retractors, 583
  swelling, 704
  trauma, 326
Eyes. *See* Blue-eye; Snakes
  abrasions, 328
  caps, removal. *See* Retained eye cap
  debridement, 328
  hemorrhage, 165
  intraocular pressure, 333
  sampling, 530
  sunkenness, 704
Eye scale, 327

F
Facial bone fractures, 606-607
Facial ganglioneuritis, 412
Facial nerve, 240
Facial scars, 612
Facilitation hypothesis, 436
False Gharials (*Tomistominae schlegelii*), 104-105
False-positive fecal examination, 345
False spitting cobras, 163
Farancia abacura reinwardti. *See* Mud Snake
Farm-raised crocodiles, vitamin A deficiency, 832-833
Fasting, 260-261
Fatal renal myxosporean infection, 962
Fat bodies, 673
Fat frail, 261
Fat pads, tophi deposition, 796f
Fat presence, 810
Fatty acid oxidation, 812
Fatty change, 810
Fatty liver, diagnosis, 806
FBD. *See* Foreign-body dermatitis
FDA. *See* U.S. Food and Drug Administration
Feces
  characteristics, 344
  components, 257f
  examination, 34, 758, 874. *See also* False-positive fecal examination
    technique, 344-345
  fixing, PVA (usage), 344
  laboratory investigation, 490f
  PCR-based screening, 403
Feeding. *See* Assist-feeding; Slap feeding
  ecology, 149
  fractional decreases/increases, 253t
  management, 273-280
  needles (ball-tipped stainless steel), 277f
  schedules, 278-279. *See also* Snakes
Feeding tubes
  insertion, 640
  passage, ease, 277f
  placement, 539. *See also* Distal esophagus; Stomach
  premeasurement, 635f
  withdrawal, 641f

Feet
  infection. *See* Shingle-backed Skink
  withdrawal/response, 241
Feline Clinical Care Liquid, 955
  oral supplementation, 953-954
Female alligators, nest preparation, 111f
Female crocodiles, reproductive system, 108-109
Female injury, 385
Female isolation, 791
Female reproductive anatomy, 376
Femoral scutes, 972
Femur fractures, 602
Fenbendazole
  impact, 1070-1071
  usage, 1070
Fertilization
  time, 365
  timing, 385
Fetal development, 365-366
Fetal monsters, abnormalities, 373
Fetal slugs, milking, 593f
  danger, 593
Fetuses, milking, 790-791
Fiber
  consideration, 293
  foods, 283
  level, maintenance, 267
  sources. *See* Long-stem fiber sources
  usage, 255-256
Fiber disorders, 292-293
Fibriscesses, 201
Fibropapilloma-associated herpesvirus, 814
Fibropapilloma (FP), 986-991. *See also* External fibropapillomas; Green Turtle fibropapilloma; Internal fibropapillomas; Seaturtle
  cause, 299
  lesions, cryosurgery (usage). *See* Green Turtle
Fibropapillomatosis. *See* Green Turtle; Seaturtle
Fibrosis, 207
Fieldwork. *See* Reptiles
Filarid genera, 184
Filarid nematodes, presence, 961
Filarioidea, genera, 360t
Filarioidea (order), 359-360
File Snake (*Acrochordus arafurae*), parthogenesis, 49
Fipronil, usage. *See* Mite infestation
Fire ants, impact, 1706
Firearm, usage, 567f
Firefly ingestion, impact, 247
Firefly toxicosis (toxicity), 247, 266, 1070
First-degree burns, 918-919, 919f
First-time-in-man (FTIM) dose selection, 420
Fish hooks, hazard. *See* Seaturtle
Fistulas, exploration, 606
Five-lined Skink (*Eumeces fasciatus*), tail autotomy, 67f
Fixation, 436. *See also* Internal fixation
  complications. *See* External fixation; Internal fixation
Flaccid paresis, 703
Flagellated protozoa, 1165

Flap-necked Chameleon *(Chamaeleo dilepis)*
  partial sloughing, 198f
  spleen
    histiocytes/erythrocytes,
      intracytoplasmic eosinophilic
      inclusions, 409f
    splenic sinusoid, macrophage, 409f
Flatback Turtles *(N. depressa)*
  Australia location, 977f
  carapace, characteristics, 977f
Flatworms, 352-353
Flaviviruses, 410-411, 1157
  transmission, 1024
Flexible endoscopy. *See* Snakes
  contrast. *See* Rigid endoscopy
Flexor carpi ulnaris muscles, 639
Floater protocol, 993
Floating, unevenness, 702
  dorsal plane, 702f
Florfenicol
  serum half-lives, 549
  thiamphenicol, relationship, 648
  usage, 648-649
Florida, herpetological societies, 6t
Florida Cooter *(Pseudemys floridana)*
  cranial-to-caudal radiograph
    projections, 485f
  pneumonia, 485f
Florida Kingsnake *(Lampropeltis getulus floridana)*
  blister disease, vesicular dermatitis, 233f
  cutaneous lesion, fine needle
    aspiration, 518f
Flowers, consumption, 38
Fluconazole
  impact, 1072
  triazole compounds, 655
Fluid
  balance, 633-634
  base, variations (tolerance), 633
  compositions, characteristics, 544t
  pharmacology, 541
  rates, empiric recommendations, 634
  selection. *See* Critical reptile patient;
    Replacement fluid
  supplementation, 634
  support. *See* Hepatic lipidosis
  usage, 1132t-1133t
Fluid administration. *See* Hypotonic fluid
    administration
  intracoelomic route, 642
  intramuscular/intravenous routes, 642
  parenteral route, 642
  routes, 634-639
  subcutaneous route, 642
Fluid-filled blisters, 685
Fluid light cable, 552
Fluid therapy, 535-536.
    See also Therapeutics
  indication, 586
  initiation, 443
  principles, 540
  requirements, 542f
Fluke egg *(Lophotaspis vallei)*, 351f
Fluke infestation, diagnosis, 184
Fluorescein dye, usage, 329.
    See also Lacrimal system
Fluorescent bulbs, usage, 37

Fluoridated water, components, 259
Fluoroquinolones
  adverse effects. *See* Central nervous
    system
  impact. *See* Bacterial DNA gyrase
  resistance, selection, 649
  usage, 649-654
Fly larva infestation. *See* Box Turtles
Fly River Turtle *(Carettochelys insculpta)*, 80f
Fly strike. *See* Myiasis
fMRI. *See* Functional MRI
Foleyella furcata, removal. *See* Chameleons
Foleyella genera, 184
Follicles, development, 376-377
Follicle-stimulating hormone (FSH), 109
Foods, 261-273
  acquisition, visual detection, 149
  calorie/nutrient content. *See* Herbivores
  chemosensory detection, 149
  commercial suppliers, 261t
  conversion ratio. *See* Crocodilians
  FDA definition, 438
  items. *See* Regurgitated food items
  offering. *See* Reptiles
  prehension
    impairment, 275f
    inability, 203f
  scenting, 371-372
  warming, 372
Foot. *See* Feet
Forages, usage, 271
Foraging strategy, understanding, 149
Forceps. *See* Biopsies; Grasping forceps;
    Retrieval forceps
  5-French elliptical, 561
  usage, 329
Foreign bodies, 716
  conjunctival hyperplasia. *See*
    Mediterranean Tortoise
  dermatitis, 206
  impact, 294, 334-335
  removal, 597
Foreign-body dermatitis (FBD), 205, 206
Forked tails, development, 914f
Formalin, treatment, 401
Formalin-preserved specimens, 569
Formulary. *See* Allometric scaling;
    Amphibians; Reptiles
Fossorial salamanders, 943
Four-quadrant antimicrobial therapy, 993
Fourth-degree burns, 919
Fovea, presence, 340
Fowler, Me, 11
Foxsnakes *(Elaphe vulpina)*, outdoor
    enclosures, 36
FP. *See* Fibropapilloma
Fractures. *See* Skull
  advanced treatment, 605-606
  forces, 600f
    exertion, 599
  healing, 603
  management, 604, 607f
  repair, 599
  stabilization difficulty. *See* Pathologic
    fractures
  treatment, 603f, 607f
    failure, 606
Free-living reptiles, 199-200

Free-ranging egg-eating reptiles, 243
Free-ranging Green Iguanas *(Iguana iguana)*,
    plant selection, 293
Free-ranging reptiles, 401-402
Free-ranging tortoises, 346
  BW/allometric relationships, 275-276
Free-roaming prey, offering, 266
Freeze damage, 246, 853
Freeze-dried insects, impact, 633
Freshwater terrapin
  edema, 207f
  foot, skin injury, 212f
  shell, ulcerated lesions, 207f
Freshwater Turtles *(Pseudomys scripta)*
  anuria, occurrence, 143
  hyperglycemia, 824
Freshwater Turtles *(Trachemys scripta elegans)*
  blood film, hemogregarine, 803f
  carapacial lesions, 212f
  shell injury, epoxy resin repair, 204f
  Spiroxis sp., mouth parts, 357f
Frilled Dragon *(Chlamydosaurus kingii)*,
    vertical branches (need), 69f
Frogs
  prolapsed bladder, 752f
  ventral midline celiotomy, 966f
Frontal scales, 974
Frontlimb paresis/paralysis. *See* Chelonians
Frontoparietal scales, 974
Fruit
  additives, 269f
  consumption, 267
  nutritional value, limitation, 39
  seeds, impact, 1077
Fruit-flavored medications, usage, 639
Fruit flies
  consumption. *See* Chameleons
  nutritive value, augmentation, 372f
Frye, FL, 11, 12
FSH. *See* Follicle-stimulating hormone
FTIM. *See* First-time-in-man
Fudge, AM, 11
Fulgurating current, 623
Full-thickness burn, 920
Fully rectified waveform, 622
Functional MRI (fMRI), 1089
  two-dimensional parasagittal section.
    See Bearded Dragon
  usage. *See* Bearded Dragon; Slider Turtle
Fundoscopy, achievement, 323-324
Fungal cystitis, 223
Fungal diseases, 153-154, 217, 329
  diagnosis, 223-225
  therapy, 225-226
Fungal etiologic agents, 154
Fungal growth, support, 873
Fungal infections, 210, 1023-1024. *See also*
    Retained skin
  presence, 329
Fungal isolates, identification, 225
Fungal keratitis, causes, 338
Fungal pneumonia, 222, 873-874
  diagnosis, 873-874
Fungal stomatitis, 928
Fungus, isolation, 224
Fungus-reptile interaction, 218-219
Furcifer minor. *See* Lesser Chameleon
Furcifer pardalis. *See* Panther Chameleon

Fusarium, 209
Fusarium oxysporum, 223
Fusarium semitectum, impact, 222f
Fusarium solani, 223
Fusiform testes. *See* Snakes
    recrudescence, 50f
Fusobacter spp., 235f

G

GABA. *See* Gamma-aminobutyric acid
Galapagos Tortoise (*Geochelone* sp.), 92f
Gallamine triethiodide, usage, 117
Gallbladder. *See* Snakes
    liver, contiguity, 148
    necropsy examination, 577
Gamma-aminobutyric acid (GABA), 246, 1068
    agonist, 730
    GABA-regulated chloride channels, 730
Gamma-glutamyltransferase (GGT), 807
Gaping, 963
Gartersnake (*Thamnophis sirtalis*)
    neurologic function, quality, 497f
    retained spectacle, 330f
    righting inability, 856f
    thiamine deficiency, 497f
Gaseous exchange, 945
Gas exchange, 133
Gas-fluid interface level, 473f
Gas-producing coelomic infection, 992
Gastric biopsy, 759
    preparation, 757f
Gastric lavage, 522-523
    test sensitivity, 758
    usage, 349
Gastric mucosa
    histologic section, 760f
    impact, 757
Gastric overload or impaction (GOI), 955. *See also* Amphibians
Gastric prolapse. *See* Amphibians
Gastric rugae, endoscopic view, 758f
Gastritis, 152. *See also* Diphtheritic necrotizing gastritis
Gastroenteritis, cause, 740
Gastrointestinal (GI) anatomy/physiology, 145
Gastrointestinal (GI) diseases, 152-160
    diagnostic testing, 151-152
Gastrointestinal (GI) foreign bodies, 157-158, 740
Gastrointestinal (GI) impactions, 740
Gastrointestinal (GI) injury. *See* Seaturtle
Gastrointestinal (GI) microflora, 149-150
Gastrointestinal (GI) motility, 148
Gastrointestinal (GI) neoplasia, 158-160
Gastrointestinal (GI) parasites, 429
Gastrointestinal (GI) parasitism, 675
Gastrointestinal (GI) peristalsis, calcium (importance), 844f
Gastrointestinal (GI) procedures, 597-598
Gastrointestinal (GI) signs. *See* Lizards
Gastrointestinal (GI) system
    diagnostic techniques, 521-523
    neoplasms, 158
    tumors, 301t, 302t-304t, 306t-309t

Gastrointestinal (GI) tract
    culturing, 228
    disease
        diagnostics, 150-151
        history, 150-151
        physical examination, 150-151
    endoscopic examination, 558-559
    foreign bodies, presence, 157
Gastrointestinal (GI) transit time, 85
Gastroscopy, 523f
Gavialinae (subfamily), life span, 104
Gavialis gangeticus. See Indian Gharial; True Gharial
Geckos
    eggs, rigid shells, 377f
    elbows/carpus/phalanges, tophi (periarticular accumulation), 795f
    Hemidactylus sp., mite cluster, 197f
    joints, radiograph, 795f
    periarticular gout, 795f
    scales, cleaning, 171f
    skin fragility, 168-169
    spectacle cleaning, 170
    tongue, usage, 171f
    thermoregulation, 169f
    treatment, case study, 429
Gekko gecko. See Tokay Gecko
Gekkonidae, 59
Gekkonids, parietal eye (absence), 325
Gekko smithii. See Green-eyed Gecko
Gelatinous bone marrow, 578
Gel stand-off pad, usage. *See* Lizards
Gender determination. *See* Endoscopic gender determination
Genetic abnormalities. *See* Dermatology
Genetics, impact. *See* Calorie sources
Genitourary system, radiographic interpretation, 481-482
Genotyping, 384
Gentamicin
    accumulation, 646
    Amikacin, comparison, 645
    dehydration, 680
    disposition kinetics, 645-646
    glomerular filtration, excretion process, 646
    iatrogenic overdosage, 680
    impact, 1074
    ophthalmic solution, 964
    pharmacokinetics, 186
        determination, 646
        differences, 646
    resistance, 643
    treatment, 642-643
Geochelone carbonara. See Yellow-headed Red-Footed Tortoise
Geochelone carbonaria. See Cherry-head Red-Foot Tortoise
Geochelone denticulata. See Yellow-footed Tortoise
Geochelone elegans. See Indian Star Tortoise; Star Tortoise
Geochelone pardalis. See Leopard Tortoise
Geochelone sp. *See* Aldabra Tortoise; Galapagos Tortoise
Geochelone sulcata. See Spurred Tortoise; Sulcata Tortoise; African Spurred Tortoise

Geographic positioning systems (GPS)
    unit, integration, 615
    usage, 614
Geophagy, 294
Georgia, herpetological societies, 6t
Geotrichum, 209, 219
Geriatric snakes, susceptibility, 401
Gerrhosauridae, 60
Gestation, 387-388
GFR. *See* Glomerular filtration rate
GGT. *See* Gamma-glutamyltransferase
Ghara, 175
Giant Snakes, 57
Giant Tortoise, goiter (case report), 291
Giardia lamblia, 350f
Gibbs-Donnan effect, 541
Giemsa stain, 453
Gila Monster (*Heloderma suspectum*)
    handling, 28f
    venemoid surgery, 613
    venom gland, location, 613f
Gilatoxin, 1075
Gingival erythema, 925
Gingival recession, 925
Gingival swelling, 925
Gingivitis, 924-926. *See also* Exposure gingivitis
Girling, S, 11
Glass fiber optic cable, 552
Glass Frog (*Centrolenidae*), ventrum transparency, 177f
Glial cells, amphophilic inclusions (usage), 412
Gliosis, identification, 248
Globes, 333-334
    anatomy, 333
    bacterial infection, 334
    congenital abnormalities, 333
    enucleation, 334
    fungal infection, 334
Glomerular filtration, reduction, 643
Glomerular filtration rate (GFR), 528, 878. *See also* Nephron GFR
    determination, 888
    reports, 889
Glomerular mesangial cells, 406
Glomeruli
    blood flow, 186
    development, 139, 143f
    necrosis, 879
Glottis
    location, 146
    opening, 229f
    sampling, 519-520
Glucocorticoids, 706
    impact, 292
Gluconeogenesis, 120
Glucose, 706
    analysis, 883
    metabolism, laboratory evaluation, 464
Glucosuria, 825
Glutaraldehyde
    soak tray, 553f
    usage, 554
Glycoprotein, 139
Glycosides, impact. *See* Cardiac glycosides

Goggle, 327
GOI. *See* Gastric overload or impaction
Goiter, case report. *See* Giant Tortoise
Goitrogens, 290
Gonads, 529
Gophersnake *(Pituophis catenifer)*, albinism, 53f
Gophersnake *(Pituophis melanoleucas)*
  hematologic values, 1106
  radiolucent foreign body, intestinal obstruction, 480f
  serum biochemical values, 1106
Gopher Tortoise *(Gopherus polyphemus)*
  conjunctivitis, 932f
  food, transit times, 293
  hematologic values, 1115
  mycoplasmosis, impact, 932f
  nares, grooves, 932f
  ocular discharge, 932f
  palpebral edema, 932f
  SCEP, 242f
    cytoplasm, artifact (Wright stain), 805f
  serum biochemical values, 1115
Gopherus agassizii. See California Desert Tortoise; Desert Tortoise
Gopherus berlandieri. See Berlandier's Tortoise; Texas Tortoise
Gopherus polyphemus. See Gopher Tortoise
Gout, 281, 793, 879. *See also* Pseudogout
  causes, 793-795
  diagnosis, 796
  impact, 259
  occurrence, 712
  treatment, 281, 796, 798
    medications, usage. *See* Mammals
  types, 795
GPS. *See* Geographic positioning systems
Gram-negative bacteria, 230f
  development, 925
  impact, 1074
  infections, 227
  relationship. *See* Resident flora
Gram-negative facultative anaerobes, 900
Gram-negative isolates, 232-235
Gram-negative straight rods, 1018
Gram-positive isolates, 231
Gram-positive organisms, 230
Gram stain, usage, 227
Granulation, impact, 749
Granulocytic leukocytes, presence, 248
Granulomas, formation. *See* Lungs
Graspers, 552-553
Grasping forceps, 552-553
Grassland tortoises, feces, 292ff
Grass Snake *(Natrix natrix)*, mycotic infection (histologic section), 209f
Grey-patch disease, 393-395, 814
  ChHV-1, 395
  reproduction, 395
Gray's Monitor Lizard *(Varanus olivaceous)*, ontogenetic change, 71
Graze, consumption, 267
Greek Tortoise *(Testudo graeca)*
  conjunctivitis, 815f
  jaw, oral discharge, 816f
  jugular vein, blood collection, 515f

Greek Tortoise—cont'd
  liver
    coelioscopic view, 809f
    histologic section, 810f
    melanomacrophage aggregation, multifocal pigmentated areas, 524f
    nuclei, paucity, 810f
  oral cavity, diphteritic plaques, 815f
  oral examination, 509f
  oral mucosa, hemorrhagic inflammation, 815f
  pinworms, presence, 358f
  secondary nutritional hyperparathyroidism, 511f
  shell, deformation, 511f
Green Anoles *(Anolis carolinensis)*, hypovitaminosis A, 289
Green Crested Basilisk *(Basiliscus plumifrons)*
  hematologic values, 1111
  serum biochemical values, 1111
Greene, HW, 11
Green-eyed Gecko *(Gekko smithii)*, *Euparadistomum* sp., 351f
Green Iguana *(Iguana iguana)*. *See* Amelanistic Green Iguana
  abscess, 202f
    surgical debulking, 777f
  acute bilateral humeral fractures, occurrence, 477f
  alertness, 503f
  anesthesia, maintenance/monitoring, 449f
  antebrachium, swelling, 507f
  aortic arch, aneurysm, 183f
  arterial oxygen saturation (SpO_2), monitoring, 449f
  ascending avascular necrosis, 914f
  assist feeding, 741f
  automobile accident, 534f
  bilateral fibroma/osteoma, intraoral appearance, 506f
  bilateral ovariosalpingectomy, 791f
  bilateral submandibular swelling, 505f
  bilateral thyroid adenomas, 319f
  biopsy site, hemorrhage, 809f
  bladder, distention, 139f
  blood film, 455f-457f, 459f
    erythrocyte, cytoplasm, 804f
  body fat/muscling, loss, 282f
  bone opacity
    normal quality, 477f
    poor quality, 476f
  bone production, 479f
  bumps, 685f
  burns, 921f
    wound, healing, 922f
  calcium deficiency, 286f
  carpal walking, 845f
  carpus/first digit, bilobed abscess, 777f
  caseous plug, exposure, 718f
  cat food diet, impact, 793f
  caudal edge liver biopsy, 5-French biopsy forceps (usage), 809f
  caudal vascular anatomy, contrast angiography, 139f
  cecum, zinc intoxication (radiograph), 247f
  choanal slits, 557f

Green Iguana—cont'd
  chronic bilateral draining carpal wounds, presence, 479f
  chronic nutritional metabolic bone disease, 476f
  chronic renal disease, 507f
  cloacal prolapse, 508f
  coeliotomy, 888f
    Tru-Cut renal biopsy, 526f
  coelomic distension, 506f
  coin ingestion, radiograph, 688f
  coins, removal, 247f
  color, change, 170f
  coloration, 175f
  combat, 173f
  coprodeum, 560f
  corneal ulceration, flourescein dye (usage), 337f
  cortical bone biopsy, 524f
  cortical remodeling, 476f
  cortical thinning, 476f
  cranial pleuroperitoneal cavity, view, 555f
  crests, development, 508f
  CSF tap, positioning, 530f
  cystocentesis, 882f
  demineralization, 476f
  depression, 503f
  dewlap
    development, 508f
    movement, oral cavity examination, 505f
    surface area-to-volume ratio, increase, 252f
  diet, recommendation. *See* Captive Green Iguana
  distal humeral epiphysis, osteolysis (presence), 479f
  distended colon, oxyurids, 359f
  Doppler flow probe, placement, 299f
  dorsal surfaces, burns, 504f
  dorsoventral survey radiograph, 637f
  dorsoventral view, 1099f
  dystocia, commonness, 791f
  elbow
    joint, arthrotomy, 609f
    osseous union/arthrodesis, 609f
    osteomyelitis, 608f
    postsurgery radiographs, 609f
  electrocardiographic (ECG) lead placement, 188f
  emaciation, 507f
  endoscopic orchidectomy, monopolar radiosurgery (usage), 628
  eustachian tube, 558f
  expansile lytic region, periosteal reaction, 479f
  eye, gross distension, 506f
  femoral fracture, healing, 476f
  femoral pores, 65f, 379f
    thigh location, ventral aspect, 65f
  femur, bulbous distortion, 476f
  fibrous osteodystrophy, 844f, 845f
  fungal blepharitis, 220f
  glomerulonephrosis, 879f
  glottis, 443f
    inspiration, 557f
  granulomatous nephromegaly, 64f
  gravid iguana, 472f

Green Iguana—cont'd
  gravid ova, 483f
  growth
    diet, relationship, 257f
    dietary protein, impact, 270f
  gular region, lesions, 849f
  hatchlings, 71
    soil consumption, 150
  head
    coloration, 175f
    conformations, abnormality, 505f
    trauma, 503f
  heart
    auscultation, 518f
    long axis view, 192f
    radiograph, 183f
  hematologic values, 1109-1110
  hemipenal plug, removal, 529f
  hemipenis
    necrosis, amputation, 863f
    penile prolapse, 863f
    prolapse, 389f, 863f
  hemorrhage, occurrence, 611f
  herbivores, 71, 150
  hindlimb, swelling, 507f
  HO, 849f
  idiopathic stenosis, 690f
  incubator recovery, 450f
  induction, propofol (usage), 446f
  inspissated impacted plugs,
      infection/pain, 914f
  intestinal obstruction, signs, 480f
  intramuscular butorphanol,
      premedication, 446f
  intrapelvic kidneys, coelioscopic
      examination (endoscopic
      technique), 887f
  iohexol excretion curve, 889f
  iris dilation, intracameral injection, 324f
  jowls
    coloration, 175f
    development, 508f
  jugular vein, location, 638f
  kidneys, 137f
    caudal pole exposure, cranial tail cut-
      down procedure, 526f
    endoscopic view, 529f
    enlargement, 507f, 797f
    evaluation, ultrasound probe
      position, 672f
    ultrasonogram, 887f
  large vessels, radiograph, 183f
  lateral horizontal beam radiograph, 886f
  lateral radiograph, 671f, 867f
  lateral view, 1099f
  limb
    fracture, 287f
    superimposition, 867f
  liver (evaluation), transducer position, 669f
  lumbar spine, osteosarcoma, 909f
  lumbosacral CSF tap, 530f
  lumps, 685f
  lung fields
    horizontal beam lateral view, 868f
    superimposition, 867f
  mandible, 63f
    abscess, 718f-719f
    misshape, 286f

Green Iguana—cont'd
  mask induction, sevoflurane
      (administration), 446f
  masturbation, 914f
  maxilla, softening/compressibility, 505f
  MBD, 841f
  menace reflex, 240f
  metabolic derangement, 503f
  mineralization, 477f
  mite infestation, 725f, 781f
  monitoring, multimodal monitor
      (usage), 193f
  necropsy specimen, 63f
  neurologic disease, 852f
  NMBD, 476f, 847f
    early stages, 845f
    radiograph, 844f
  nostril, chronic sinusitis, 67f
  NSHP, 841f
  nutritional secondary
      hyperparathyroidism, 286f, 287f,
      505f, 534f
  oral abnormalities, 506f
  osteolysis, identification, 478f
  ovarian teratoma, 30f
  ovary, 559f
  overriding, 476f
  oviductal blood vessels, coagulation, 626f
  oviposition, problem, 847f
  Ozolaimus sp., 358f
  pancreas, endoscopic evaluation, 826f
  paramedian celiotomy incision, 63f
  pectoral girdle, heart position, 1099f
  periocular dermatomycosis, 220f
  periosteal reaction, 476f
  pharyngeal edema, chronic renal disease
      (impact), 506f
  postural abnormalities, 855f
  preanal/femoral pores,
      reduction/absence, 508f
  prolapsed colon, 754f
  propioceptive placement deficit, 503f
  pulse oximeter, usage validation, 194f
  pulse rate, monitoring, 449f
  radiolucent fat bodies, calcification, 477f
  radiopaque gravel fragments, 471f
  reflectance pulse oximeter probe,
      placement, 299f
  renal abscesses, 764f
  renal damage disease, biochemical
      parameters, 881t
  renomegaly (gout), 797f
  resected aorta, 183f
  right-sided head tilt, 503f
  RMBD, 849f
  rostrum, trauma, 275f
  Salmonella spp. dermatitis, 232f
  scapula, verticality, 845f
  scoliosis, 847f,
  SCT, NSHP treatment protocol, 846t
  secondary pyoderma, 781f
  sepsis, 503f
  septic arthritis, 479f
  serum biochemical values, 1109-1110
  soft tissue
    callus, presence, 476f
    opacities, 472f
    swelling, 479f

Green Iguana—cont'd
  spinal fracture, 507f, 534f, 844f
  spinal lesions, 855f
  spleen, endoscopic view, 517f
  stifle, osteomyelitis, 540f
  stomach, ultrasound image, 670f
  stomatitis, 152f
  tail
    amputation, 611f
    base, enlargement, 379f
    fracture, 914f
    rigidity/enlargement, 478f
    vertebrae, ankylosis, 909f
  thermoregulation, 170f, 917f
  tibia, intraosseus catheter placement, 637f
  tissue contrast, 471f
  TMJ, 558f
  toes, mass (presence), 775f
  tonometry, 324
  treatment, case study, 434
  tubulonephrosis, 879f
  unicameral lung, collapse, 557f
  urinary bladder
    calculus, lamellar pattern, 482f
    ultrasound image, 673f
  urinary papilla, saline solution infusion
      technique, 560f
  urine, urate crystals (presence), 884f
  ventral abdominal vein, intravenous
      catheter (placement), 446f
  ventral burns, 203f
  ventral midline incision, CO_2 laser
      (usage), 625f
  ventral view, 60f, 380f
  ventrum, burns, 504f
  vitellogenic ova, highlight, 671f
  vitellogenic postovulatory ova, 672f
  wet-to-dry sterile bandages,
      application, 921f
Green Lizard (Lacerta viridis)
  epithelial proliferation, 211f
  papilloma, histologic appearance, 211f
Green phase Burmese Python (Python
      molurus bivatattus), 53f
Greens
  consumption, 267
  proportion, 267
Green Seaturtle (Chelonia mydas), 79, 80f
  bone scan, 488f
  carapacial bone, papilloma
      growth, 488f
  Learedius learedi, 352f
  pappillomas, presence, 394f
  shells, keels (absence), 977f
Green Toad (Bufo viridis), dorsoventral
      radiograph, 178f
Green Tree Python (Morelia viridis)
  Capillaria sp., 359f
  cloacocolonic prolapse, 500f
  head tilts, 856f
  hematologic values, 1105
  motor function, loss, 838f
  musculature, paralysis, 838f
  neurologic disorders, 856f
  serum biochemical values, 1105
  star gazing, 856f
Green Tree Python (Morelia viridis),
    tapeworm egg, 354f

Green Turtle (*Chelonia mydas*)
  death, fibropapillomas, 973f
  endoscopy approach, 984f
  FP lesions (removal), cryosurgery (usage), 991f
  palpebra, removal, 1000f
  shark bite, 986f
  skull, boat strike, 986f
  traumatic enucleation, 1000f
  tube feeding. *See* Marathon Sea Turtle Hospital
  ventral view, 979f
Green Turtle fibropapilloma (GTFP), 393, 983, 987, 988f
  database analysis, 983
  description, 986
Griseofulvin
  impact, 1072
  improvement, failure, 226
Griswold, B, 10
Gross anatomy, 135-138
Gross hepatomegaly, 808
Gross pathology. *See* Cryptosporidiosis
  comparison, usefulness. *See* Ultrasound images
Gross photography, 579-580. *See also* Lizards
  quality, absence, 579f, 580f
Ground Iguanas (*Cyclura* spp.), herbivores, 71
Growth-associated problems, 282
Growth hormone, release, 432
Grzimek, HCB, 11
GTFP. *See* Green Turtle fibropapilloma
Guilt. *See* Loss; Pets
Gular, 972
  pumping, 702
Gurley, R, 11
Gut-inhabiting flagellated protozoa, 349-350
Gut-loading. *See* Invertebrate prey
Gymnophiona (order), 941

H

Habitat design, 1018
Haemaphysalis punctata, immature stages, 1026
Haemogregarina tuatarae, 1011
Haemogregarinids. *See* Hemogregarines
Halofuginone, usage, 760
Halothane, 949
Hand feeding, 955
Hand instrumentation. *See* Endoscopy
Hapalotrema loossi. *See* Loggerhead Seaturtle
Harder, Johan, 332
Harderian gland, secretion, 332
Hard-shelled insect prey, 689
Hard-shelled seaturtle, 973-974
Hard-shelled ticks, 726f
Hard structures, detail, 1088
Hard ticks (Ixodidae), 346
Hard water, components, 259
Hatch failure. *See* Lizards
Hatching success, humidity (impact), 722
Hatchlings
  manual removal, requirement, 370
  pip location, 369
  reptiles, aggressiveness. *See* Reptiles
  rigid shells. *See* Tortoises

Hawkey, CM, 11
Hawksbill Turtle (*Eretmochelys imbricata*)
  commercial trade, nonusage, 1032f
  guitar picks, possession (illegality), 1045f
  head (characteristic), 978f
  scutes, overlap, 978f
Hay, consumption, 267
Hay-based pellets, 271
H&E. *See* Hematoxylin and eosin
Head
  abnormalities, 852
  bobbing, 171
  examination, 504
  hiding behavior, 166f
  muscles, tophi deposition, 796f
  tremors, 401, 404
Head tilts, 404. *See also* Lizards
  association, 852
  IBD, impact, 680
  rarity, 680
Healing
  forms, 198-199
  time, reduction, 776
Healing Oasis Wellness Center, 440
Hearing, development, 240
Heart
  auscultation, 504
  caudal placement. *See* Monitor Lizards
  landmark orientation, 667
  placement, 47-48
  position, radiographic view, 190f
  rate
    decrease, 127-128
    variations, 127
  swelling, 181f
  visualization, 482
    clarity, 189
    nonselective angiography, 190f
Heartwater disease, 734
Heat
  conductance, 918
  injury, 917-918
  regulation, 778
  sources, 70, 367. *See also* Captive reptiles
    temperature, 918
  supplementation, requirement, 535f
  transfer, 916
Heaths, impact, 1706
Heating cages, availability, 535f
Heating pads, usage, 29f
Heatwole, HF, 11
Heavy-bodied juvenile snakes, hemipene eversion (impossibility), 381
Heavy metal
  impact, 963
  intoxication, 247
Helminths, 1026
  fixatives, 346t
Heloderma horridum. *See* Mexican Beaded Lizard
Heloderma sp. *See* Beaded Lizard
Heloderma suspectum. *See* Gila Monster
Hemagglutination inhibition (HI), 859, 1066
  antibodies, development, 402
  illustration, 1066f
  test, 872
  usage. *See* Ophidian paramyxovirus

Hemagglutinin-neuraminidase, comparison, 402
Hemangiomas, 404
Hematologic parameters, usage. *See* Livers
Hematologic samples, collection, 950-951
Hematologic values, 1103-1117
Hematology, 453-460
  usage, 949. *See also* Pneumonia
  usefulness, 460
Hematopoietic system, tumors, 300t, 302t, 303t, 310t-311t
Hematopoietic tissues, necropsy examination, 578
Hematoxylin and eosin (H&E) stain, 760f, 836
  usage, 347
Hemicerclage, 601f
Hemipenal plug forms, 529
Hemipenes. *See* Chelonians; Crocodilians
  blind diverticula, similarity, 383
  eversion, 167
    popping technique. *See* Snakes
    saline solution injection technique, 382f
  hydrostatic eversion, 381-383
  manual eversion, 381
  mineralized hemibacula, presence. *See* Monitors, heart (caudal placement)
  pairing. *See* Lizards
Hemipenile prolapse, 389
Hemipenis
  base, double ligation, 389
  uselessness, 382f
Hemiphractinae subfamily, 177
Hemocrit, evaluation, 536t
Hemoglobin, absorption coefficient, 619f
Hemogram
  evaluation, 453
  interpretation, considerations, 460
Hemogregarines (haemogregarinids), 801
  Hepatozoon. *See* Snakes
  life cycle, 801
Hemoparasites, 349, 801
  presence, 960
Hemopericardium. *See* Bearded Dragon; Python
Hemopoietic system, analysis, 513-517
Hemoprotozoa, 1163-1164
Hemoptysis, occurrence, 690
Hemorrhage, minimization, 613
Hemostasis, 459-460
  laboratory evaluation, 460
  morphology, 459
  response, 460
Hemostat
  introduction, 641f
  usage, 640
Hemotoxins, 1051
Hepatic abscess, ultrasound imagery, 665f
Hepatic aspirates (obtaining), ultrasound (usage), 487-488
Hepatic disease, 632
  classification, 807
Hepatic encephalopathy, 680
Hepatic hemosiderosis, 933
Hepatic lipidosis, 283-284, 406, 806
  anabolic steroids, usage, 812
  anamnesis (history), 806-807

Hepatic lipidosis—cont'd
  carnitine, impact, 811-812
  choline, usage, 812
  diagnosis, 806-810
  diagnostic imaging, 808, 810
  examination, 284
  fluid support, 811
  histopathologic features, 810-811
  laboratory investigations, 807
  methionine, usage, 812
  nutritional support, 811
  pathologic features, 810-811
  physical examination, 806-807
  postmortem features, 810
  recommendations, 812
  thyroxine, usage, 812
  treatment, 811-812
Hepatic necrosis, 402
Hepatic piston, 133
Hepatic-portal circulation system, 317
Hepatic vein, 125
Hepatobiliary disease, 464
Hepatocytes, lipidosis. See Bearded Dragon
Hepatozoon. See Emerald Tree Boas; Snakes
Herbal energetics, 281
Herbal medicine
  dosage calculation, 431
  usage, 429-431
Herbivores
  bedding, 271
  caloric requirements. See Mammals
  calorie sources, 255-256
  dependence, 149
  diets, low-level antibiotics (presence), 271
  foods, calorie/nutrient content, 268t
  fuel sources, 255f
  pellets, consumption, 270
  poisonous plants, access (restriction), 269
  protein
    relationship, 256-257
    requirements, 267
Herbs
  active constituents/actions, 430
  usage, 430-431
Hermann's Tortoise (*Testudo hermanni*)
  adhesion separation, laser usage (contact mode), 625f
  gender determination, tail size (usage), 512f
  liver, paleness, 524f
  nictitating membrane, protrusion, 509f
  water intake, 271f
Heparin, blood collection, 460
Herpes-like virus
  recovery, 394
  reports. See Upper respiratory disease
Herpesviral DNA, reports, 816
Herpesvirus, 392-397, 1148-1149.
    See also Marine Turtles; Pond turles;
    Tortoises
  clinical features, 393
  control/prevention, 396-397
  epizootiology, 394-395
  global distribution, 394
  immunity/diagnosis, 396
  impact. See Nasal discharge
  infections
    documentation, 393
    seasonality, impact, 819

Herpesvirus—cont'd
  instability, 397
  outbreaks, 397
  pathology, 395-396. See also Chelonians;
    Reptiles
  presence. See Amphophilic intranuclear
    inclusion bodies
  transmission, 395
  treatment/vaccination, 397
Herpesvirus, suspicion, 211
Herpesvirus-association lesions,
    commonness, 395
Herpesvirus-like particles, 814
Herpetofauna, radiotelemetry
    (practicality), 613
Herpetological journals, 10
Herpetological Natural History, 10
Herpetological societies, 6t-7t
Herpetologic surgery
  lasers, usage, 624-625
  radiofrequency, 626
Herpetologists League, 9
Herpetology
  online sources, 12-13
  websites, 12-13
Herptiles, US state agency regulation,
    1046t-1048t
HES. See Hydroxyethyl starches
Heterodon nasicus. See Rear-fanged
    Hog-nosed Snake
Heterodon platirhinos. See Eastern
    Hog-nosed Snake
Heterodon simus. See Hog-nosed Snakes
Heterophilic inflammation, 465f
Heterophilic rhinitis, cytodiagnosis, 465f
Heterophilic tracheitis, cytodiagnosis,
    465f, 466f
Heterophils, 455f, 458f. See also
    Nondegenerate heterophils; Toxic
    heterophils
  abnormality, 458
  cytoplasmic granules, 455
  degeneration, 467f
  granules, 465
  macrophages, mixture, 466f
Hexamita. See *Clemmys marmorata*
Hexamitiasis, 349
HI. See Hemagglutination inhibition
Hibernaculum. See Indoor hibernaculum
Hibernation (brumation)
  option, 91
  temperatures, 29-30
  need. See Montane reptiles
Hibiclens, 1018
Hidden-neck Turtle, example. See Leopard
    Tortoise
High-fat diet, 291
High-humidity retreat, provision, 28f
High-protein diets, impact, 879-880
High tail amputation, suture, 612f
Hilaire's Side-neck Turtle (*Phrynops*
    genus), 79f
Hindlimb paralysis. See Chelonians
Hindlimb paresis, 703. See also Chelonians
Hinge-backed Tortoises (*Kinixys* sp.),
    bilateral hinges, 174f
Hirstiella mites, presence. See Iguanas
Hirstiella trombidiiformis. See Lizard mites

Histopathologic analysis, 776
Histoplasma capsulatum, 223
History form, 491t
HO. See Hypertrophic osteopathy
Hog-nosed Snakes (*Heterodon simus*), 163
  outdoor enclosures, 36
  righting, 164
Holly, impact, 1077
Homeopathy, 431-432
Honduran Milksnake (*Lampropeltis
    triangulum hondurensis*)
  cardiac ultrasonography, 668f
  ultrasound examination, 667f
Hopkins telescope, usage, 810
Horizontal beam projections.
    See Craniocaudal view
Hormonal changes, inclusion, 432
Hormones, usage, 1131t. See also
    Amphibians
Horned Lizards (*Phrynosoma cornutum*),
    blood (squirting), 66, 165
Horner's syndrome. See Mediterranean
    Tortoise
Horn-headed Lizard (*Acanthosaurus
    crucigera*)
  coleom, distension, 693f
  thigh swelling (femur osteomyelitis), 683f
Hosemys spinosa. See Spiny Turtle
Hospitalization, 33
Hospitals
  cages, necessities, 28f
  reptile caging, requirement, 2f
Host-parasite relations, 197-198
Host-specific retroviruses, 404
Hot rocks, 916
  danger, 918f
  problems, 70
  shorting out, 917
  usage, 29
Housing, considerations, 33-34
HPA. See Hypothalamic-pituitary-adrenal
Human-reptile relationship
  printed material, 23
  resources/information, 23
Human-reptile relationship,
    understanding, 14
Humans
  animals, bond, 14
  autoimmune diseases, 404
  calculi analysis, 768
  salmonellosis, outbreak, 1021
Humeral scutes, 972
Humerus fractures, 602
  stabilization, 604f
Humidifiers, usage, 31
Humidity. See Captive reptiles
  box
    characteristics, 31f
    construction, 783t
  impact. See Shedding
Humpback. See Kyphosis
Husbandry. See Captive amphibian
  impact, 784, 787
  management, 25
  optimization, 896
  requirements, 27-39
Hyaline fungal hyphae, 220f
Hyalohyphomycosis, 154

Hyaluronidase administration, 546
Hydration. *See* Interstitial hydration; Intracellular hydration
  importance, 992
  status, 946
Hydrocoelom, 957
Hydrops, 955
Hydroregulation, 27
Hydrosaurus amboinensis. See Soa-soa Sailfin Lizard
Hydrosaurus pustulatus. See Sailfin Lizard
Hydrostatic pressure, transcapillary forces, 541f
Hydroxyethyl starches (HES), 545
Hymenolepis diminuta, 345f
Hymenolepis nana, 345f
Hypercapnia, 134
  impact, 443
Hypercholesterolemia, 246
Hyperchromia. *See* Keratin
Hyperechoic outer line, 670
Hyperglycemia, 822. *See also* Stress-associated hyperglycemia
  approach, 825-826
  cases, reports, 827t
  diabetes mellitus, contrast, 822
  histopathology, 826
  induction, 824
  management, 826, 828
  necropsy, 826
  physical examination, 825
Hyperimmune bovine colostrum, results, 760
Hyperimmune bovine colostrum treatment, results, 761t
Hyperkeratosis, 201
Hyperkeratosis, focal area, 408
Hyperlactatemia, 543
Hypermetabolic patients, feeding frequency, 277
Hypermetabolism, role, 274
Hypermetric gait. *See* Terrapins; Tortoises; Turtles
Hyperopia, 336
Hyperparathyroidism. *See* Nutritional secondary hyperparathyroidism; Renal secondary hyperparathyroidism
Hyperphosphatemia, 504
Hyperpigmentation, 206
Hyperplasia, 925
Hyperproteinemia, 464
Hypersensitivity reaction, occurrence, 1055
Hyperthermia. *See* Amphibians
  signs, 964
Hypertonic fluids, characteristics, 542
Hypertonic saline solution injection, impact, 542f
Hypertrophic cardiomyopathy, mistake, 668f
Hypertrophic osteopathy (HO), 683, 848
  differentials, 848
Hyperuracemia, 246
Hyperuricemia, 462
Hypervitaminosis A, 292, 697, 831. *See also* Iatrogenic hypervitaminosis A
  impact. *See* Terrestrial chelonians
Hypervitaminosis D, 292
Hyphema. *See* Red-eared Slider

Hyphema, presence, 338
Hypoalbuminemia, 807
Hypocalcemia, 244, 504, 689. *See also* Prolonged hypocalcemia
Hypocalcemic tetany, 546, 845f, 855
Hypochloremia, 462
Hypoechoic center line, 670
Hypoglycemia, 245
  causes, 464
Hypohydration, 280
Hypokalemia, 462
Hypomineralization, 605
Hypoproteinemia, 632
Hypopyon, presence, 338
Hypothalamic-pituitary-adrenal (HPA) axis, 120
Hypothermia. *See* Amphibians
Hypothiaminosis (leukoencephalopathy), 243
Hypothyroidism, association. *See* Selenium
Hypotonic fluid administration, 542
Hypovitaminosis, 831
Hypovitaminosis A, 831-833. *See also* Amphibians
  bilateral conjunctival swelling, 954f
  clinical signs, 831
  commonness, 929
  diagnosis, 831-833
    basis, 832
  imbalance, 865
  pathogenesis, 831
  role, 211
  treatment, 833
Hypovitaminosis C (ascorbic acid deficiency), commonness, 929
Hypoxia, impact, 443

I

IATA Regulations, 1044
Iatrogenic digits, 776
Iatrogenic hypervitaminosis A, 833-834
  clinical signs, 834
  pathogenesis, 834
  treatment, 834
Iatrogenic hyponatremia, 462
Iatrogenic mandibular fractures, 607f
Iatrogenic tail swelling/infection, 913
IBD. *See* Inclusion body disease
IC. *See* Intracardiac
ICe. *See* Intracoelomic
Icterus, 687
Idaho, herpetological societies, 6t
IEGL. *See* Inner epidermal generation layer
IFA. *See* Immunofluorescence antibody; Indirect fluorescent antibody
IgG. *See* Immunoglobulin G
IgM. *See* Immunoglobulin M
Iguana: Conservation, Natural History and Husbandry of Reptiles, 10
Iguana iguana. See Amelanistic Green Iguana; Green Iguana; Wild Green Iguanas
Iguanas
  basking space, quest, 121f
  biopsy forceps, insertion, 528
  caudal kidney, exposure (surgical technique), 887f
  diet. *See* Captive iguana diet
  egg impaction, 788

Iguanas—cont'd
  egg-yolk coelomitis, death, 789f
  endoscopic scissors, insertion, 528
  glomerulonephrosis, histology, 879f
  head bobs, 171
  heart, pectoral girdle location, 191f
  Hirstiella mites, presence, 503f
  kidneys
    caudal pelvic window, image, 672f
    endoscopic evaluation/biopsy, 528, 888f
    histology, 879f
    location, bony pelvis, 880f
    ultrasonography, 887f
  lettuce, unsuitability, 267
  renal mineralization, histology, 879f
  renal portal system, behavior, 643
  rust color, 170
  tail, craniolateral aspect, 887f
  torso, sagittal images, 1089f
  treatment, case study, 431, 432
  tubulonephrosis, histology, 879f
Iguania, groups, 59
Iguanid Lizard (*Dipsosaurus dorsalis*)
  hematologic values, 1109
  serum biochemical values, 1109
IH. *See* Intermediate host
Illinois, herpetological societies, 6t
Image detail, decrease, 484f
Image generation, tissue-specific ways, 1089
Imaging techniques, 241-243
Imidazoles, impact, 1072
Immobilization, agents (usage), 444t
Immune-mediated condition, 906
Immune response. *See* Therapeutics
Immune system
  efficiency, 218-219
  humoral component, 632
  innate component, 632
Immunofluorescence antibody (IFA), 156
  usage, 758
Immunofluorescence staining, usage, 860
Immunoglobulin G (IgG), 1065
Immunoglobulin M (IgM), 1065
Immunoglobulin production, 213
Immunohistochemistry, 1064
  DNA in situ hybridization, relationship, 1064f
Immunoperoxidase staining, 860
Immunosuppression, presence, 880
Implantation sites, 616f
Import/export, European Community directives, 1042
Impressed Tortoise (*Manouria impressa*), mortality rate/food refusal, 256f
Impression cytology, 983
Impression smears, 519
Imprint technique, usage. *See* Cytologic interpretation
Incised skin, inversion tendency, 582f
Incising scissors, 553
Inclusion body disease (IBD), 406f. *See also* Boids
  acute stage, 837-838
  clinical changes, 404
  etiologic agent, 836
  impact. *See* Head
  incidence rate, 405

Inclusion body disease—cont'd
  index, 407
  outbreak, 405
  remission, 838
  retrovirus
    association, 404-405
    impact, 153
  supportive care, 839
  vertical transmission, 406
  virus, 836
    antemortem diagnosis, 838
    clinical management/treatment, 839
    clinical signs, 837-838
    diagnosis, 838-839
    pathology, 836-837
    postmortem diagnosis, 838-839
    prevention/control, 839-840
Inclusions, appearance, 837
Incubation media, fungal contamination, 689
Incubators
  availability, 535f
  egg, placement. See Prewarmed incubator
  neonates, placement, 372f
  temperature, 367
Indented spectacle. See Royal Python
Indiana, herpetological societies, 6t
Indian Gharial (Gavialis gangeticus), characteristics, 104f
Indian Python (Python molurus)
  edema, 203f
  epidermis, raising, 203f
  granulocytic infiltration, 203f
Indian Star Tortoise (Geochelone elegans), 92, 93f
Indigenous species, export, 1042
Indigo Snake (Drymarchon couperi) (Drymarchon corais)
  hematologic values, 1107
  hypercalcemia, 464
  lungs
    pentastomid, inflammatory response, 362f
    pentastomid, removal, 362f
    radiodense serpiginous pattern, 360f
  radiograph, 360f
  Salmonella spp. dermatitis, 232f
  serum biochemical values, 1107
Indirect fluorescent antibody (IFA) assays, 1066
Indirect life cycle, 343. See also Armillifer armillatus
Indirect ophthalmoscopy, usage, 323. See also Mediterranean Tortoise
Indolealkylamines, 1075
Indoor hibernaculum, 88
Indopacific Crocodile (Crocodylus porosus), 103
Induction chamber, 947
Indwelling catheter placement, 535. See also Jugular vein
Indwelling gastrostomy tubes, indication, 277
Indwelling pharyngostomy tubes
  indication, 277
  usefulness, 278f
Infection clearance, 932
Infection-damaged keratin, 896

Infectious arthritis, 478
Infectious diseases, 152-156, 183-184. See also Noninfectious diseases
  classification, 196
Infectious neuropathies, 248-249
Infectious stomatitis, 152, 676f, 926
  mild cases, 927f
Influenza C virus, 706
Inframarginal scutes, 972
Ingesta, identification, 479
Inhalational agents, 445-446
Injectable anesthetic agents, 444-445
Injuries, multiple projections, 475f
Inner epidermal generation layer (IEGL), 198f
Insect-based diets, 263
Insecticides, impact, 246
Insectivorous reptiles, feeding, 156
Insect prey. See Hard-shelled insect prey
Insects, food, 98
In Situ Hybridization Laboratory (University of Georgia), 400
Inspiration, time limit, 449
Inspiratory radiograph, 472f
Inspissated exudates, 499
Insufflation
  achievement, 549
  gas filter, 550f
Insulin resistance, 823-824
Integument. See Lizards; Snakes
  biologic samples, collection, 517-519
  examination, 496-497, 502, 504
Integumentary sense organs (ISO), 107
Integumentary system, tumors, 300t, 302t, 304t, 309t-310t
Intensive care unit (ICU) incubator, usage, 1001
Interendothelial pore size, 541f
Interfragmentary wires, 601f
Intergular scutes, 972
Intermediate host (IH), 343
  requirement, 362
Intermittent positive pressure ventilation (IPPV), 448
  negative effects, 449
  usage, 1010
Internal abscesses, 716, 717f
  diagnosis, radiographs, 717f
Internal anatomy, differences, 487
Internal fibropapillomas, 393
Internal fixation, 604-605
  complications, 606
Internal scutes, 972
Internal space-occupying masses, 675
International Association for Veterinary Homeopathy, 440
International Commission on Zoological Nomenclature, 100
International Conference on Exotics, 13
International Herpetological Symposium, 13
International Species Information System (ISIS), 12
International trade, CITES convention, 1041
International Veterinary Acupuncture Society, 440
Internet, usage, 12-13. See also Reptile practice
Interparietal scales, 974

Interstitial compartment, contraction, 542f
Interstitial fibrosis, 402
Interstitial fluid replacement, 546
Interstitial hydration, 546
Interstitial integrity, water (impact), 539
Interstitial nephritis, 826, 879
Interstitial pneumonia, 406
Interstitium, overhydration, 545
Intestinal cramping, 842
Intestinal flagellates, examination, 349
Intestinal impactions, 992
Intestinal mucosa, calcium/phosphorus absorption, 464
Intestinal parasites, 692
Intestinal tract, viewpoint, 668
Intestines. See Snakes
  digestion process, 148
  evaluation, 481
  walls/tears, 598f
Intracardiac (IC) catheters, 537
  advantage, 539f
  usage. See Snakes
Intracellular compartment, proportion, 541f
Intracellular hydration, 546
Intracameral injection. See Neuromuscular blocking agents
Intracoelomic (ICe) fluid
  replacement route, 634
  therapy, 964
Intracoelomic (ICe) implant, 967
Intracoelomic (ICe) pressure, regulation, 549
Intracoelomic (ICe) route, fluid administration, 635-636
Intracytoplasmic eosinophilic inclusions, 409f
Intralesional chemotherapy, 299
Intralesional fungal elements, 222f
Intramuscular (IM) administration, 403
Intramuscular (IM) butorphanol, administration, 443. See also Green Iguana
Intramuscular (IM) injections, avoidance, 642
Intranuclear basophilic inclusions. See Bearded Dragon
Intranuclear coccidia, 874
Intranuclear inclusion bodies, presence, 399-400
Intraoperative analgesia, 443
Intraoperative blood loss, 686
Intraosseous (IO) catheters
  difficulty, 636-637
  placement, 62
    effort, 443
    radiographic confirmation, 540f
    routes, usage, 540f
  usage. See Snakes
Intraosseous (IO) fluids
  administration, 636
  replacement route, 634
Intrapelvic kidneys, coelomic approaches, 526
Intrapulmonic administration, 656-657
Intravascular compartment, volume expansion, 542f
Intravascular COP, 543, 545
Intravascular volume, 546
Intravascular volume depletion, 546
  fluid plan, 543

Intravenous (IV) amino acids, usage, 280
Intravenous (IV) catheters
  advantages, 537f
  placement, 47, 62, 535-536
    effort, 443
Intravenous (IV) cut-down techniques, 536-539
Intravenous (IV) fluids
  replacement route, 634
  therapy, 637
Intravenous (IV) urography, usage, 885
Intussusception, 577
Invertebrate prey, 263-266
  calorie/nutrient content, 263
  diet characteristics, 266t
  dust, collection, 265
  feeding. See Reptiles
  gut-loading, 264-265
  mineral concentrations (dry matter basis), 264t
  nutrient composition, 264t
  nutritional composition, factors, 264
  protein quality, 263-264
  risks, 265-266
  supplementation, 265
  supplements, sticking (failure), 265f
Invertebrates
  endoskeleton, absence, 263
  size, guideline, 266
IO. See Intraosseous
Iodine
  binding, 267
  deficiency, 290-291
  intoxication, 963
Iodophors, treatment, 401
Iohexol
  assays, 889
  clearance studies, 888
  excretion curve. See Green Iguana
Ion concentration, difference, 541
Ionized calcium concentration, 464
Iowa, herpetological societies, 6t
IPPV. See Intermittent positive pressure ventilation
Iridoviruses, 409-410, 1154-1155
Iridovirus-like particles, detection, 409-410
Iridovirus nucleic acid (detection), PCR-based assay, 410
Iris, composition, 240
Iris forceps, 583
Iris hooks, 583
Iris scissors, 583
Iron deficiency, 454
Isenbugel, E, 12
ISIS. See International Species Information System
ISO. See Integumentary sense organs
Isoflurane, 949
  administration. See Bearded Dragon; Box Turtles
  anesthetic usage, 75
  induction, 997
  inhalant anesthetic, 948
  inhalation anesthesia, 1010
  MAC, 446
Isolates, retrieval, 150
Isopora amphiboluri. See Bearded Dragon
Isospora amphiboluri, 155-156

ISO standards, 1042
Isotonic replacement crystalloid (LRS)
  administration, 543f
Itraconazole
  evaluation, 655
  impact, 1072
  selection, 226
  triazole compounds, 655
IUCN Guidelines, 1040
Ivermectin, 1068
  absorption, 1068
  action, mechanism, 1068
  clinical signs, 1068
  flushing usage, 330
  impact, 246-247
  intoxication, signs, 247
  safety margin, 732
  treatment, 1068
  usage, 968. See also Mite infestation; Ticks
Ivermectin-induced hepatic lipidosis, 807
Ivory, usage, 920
Ivy, impact, 1077
Ixodes pacificus, 1026-1027
Ixodidae. See Hard ticks

J
Jackson, OF, 11
Jackson's Chameleon (*Chamaeleo jacksonii*)
  bullous lesions, 220f
  chelitis, 833f
  dehydration, 281f
  dermatomycotic lesions, 220f
  egg yolk formation/embryo nutrition, 260f
  esophagitis/tracheitis, 400
  exfoliative lesions, 220f
  hyperkeratosis, 833f
  lung lobe accessory, 131f
  ocular turret, involvement, 691f
  temporal gland dorsolateral, abscessation, 687f
  ulcerative lesions, 220f
Jacobson, ER, 11-12
Jamshidi, 523
JAVMA. See Journal of the American Veterinary Medical Association
Jaws. See Rubber jaw
  shape, problems, 847
Jeweler's forceps, 583
Joints
  capsule, destabilization, 906
  surgery, 607-609
  swelling, 703
Journal of the American Veterinary Medical Association (JAVMA), 10
Journals, 10. See Herpetological journals; Veterinary journals
Jugular catheters
  placement, 638
  usage, 638. See also Snakes
Jugular vein
  bulge, 536
  exposure, 537
  indwelling catheter placement, 537
  location, 637
  visibility, 513

Jungle Carpet Python (*Morelia spilota cheynei*)
  hematologic values, 1105
  serum biochemical values, 1105

K
Kale, usage, 267
Kalicephalus sp. See Black racer
  anterior end, 356f
  impact, 207
  larva. See Snakes
Kansas, herpetological societies, 6t
Kaplan, M, 12
Karl Storz Veterinary Endoscopy, 549, 886
Kemp's Ridley (*Lepidochelys kempii*), scutes/vertebrals characteristics, 978f
Keratectomy. See Superficial keratectomy
Keratin. See Burn-damaged keratin; Infection-damaged keratin
  infection, focus, 206f
  layers, 778
  pitting/hyperchromia, 205f
Keratitis. See Caseated keratitis; Corneas
Keratoconjunctivitis sicca (dry eye), 332-333. See also Mediterranean Tortoise
Keratolysis, 222f
Ketaconazole, usage. See Oral ketoconazole
Ketamine
  administration, 444, 446
  combination, 447, 639
  dosage, 447, 948
Ketamine hydrochloride, usage, 117, 444, 948
Ketoconazole, 654
  impact, 1072
Ketones, analysis, 883
Ketosis, 826
Kidneys. See Green Iguana; Water Monitor
  anatomy. See Snakes
    normal separation. See Chameleon
  caudolateral aspect, 526
  digital palpation, 880f
  endoscopic technique, 561-562
  fusion. See Caudal pole
  laboratory evaluation, 461-462
  location. See Turtles
  mucoid substances, secretion, 141
  ovaries/oviducts/urethra, relationship, 141f
  position. See Alligator
  stones, 763
  tophic deposition, 796f
Kingsnake (*Lampropeltis* sp.)
  intracoelomic mass, 500f
  subcutaneous nematode, 207f
  ventrum, thermal burn, 497f
Kinixys sp. See Hinge-backed Tortoises
Kinosternidae (family), 80f
Klebsiella, 234
Klebsiella pneumonia. See Chameleons
  association, 338
  pure culture, presence, 872f
Klebsiella sp., 927
  hypopyon. See Snakes
KOH. See Potassium hydroxide
Kollias, GV, 11-12
Komodo Dragon (*Varanus komodoensis*)
  circulating vitamin D_3 levels, 287
  pulse oximeter, usage, 194f

Kübler-Ross, Elisabeth, 17
Kupffer cells, 400
   detection, 399
Kyphosis (humpback), 907f, 910

L

Laboratory samples, inoculation, 229-230
Lacerta agilis, body temperature, 631
Lacerta lepida. *See* Lizards
Lacerta sp. See European Lizard
Lacerta viridis. *See* Green Lizard
Lacerta vivipara. *See* Lizards
Lacertids, 324
Lacey Act, 1049
Lacrimal system, 332-333
   anatomy, 332
   fluorescein dye, usage, 332
   patency, testing, 332
Lactalbumin, 263
Lactate dehydrogenase (LD/LDH), 461, 652, 807
   parameters, 881
Lactated Ringer's solution (LRS), usage, 543, 616, 633
Lactulose, usage, 992
Lameness, effect, 389
Lampropeltis getulus. *See* Common Kingsnake
Lampropeltis getulus floridana. *See* Florida Kingsnake
Lampropeltis getulus getulus. *See* California Kingsnake; Eastern Kingsnake
Lampropeltis sp. See Kingsnake
Lampropeltis triangulum campbelli. *See* Pueblan Milksnake
Lampropeltis triangulum elapsoides. *See* Scarlet Kingsnake
Lampropeltis triangulum hondurensis. *See* Honduran Milksnake
Lampropeltis triangulum sp. See Milksnake
Lampropeltis triangulum syspila. *See* Red Milksnake
Lamprophis fulginosus. *See* African House Snake
Lamps, photometric characteristics, 1082t
Land turtles, plasma sodium concentration, 543
Langaha sp. See Leaf-nosed snakes
Large collections. *See* Reptiles; Zoologic parks
   concerns, 16
   considerations, 1012
Larval dracunculids, 299
Lasers
   coagulation usage, 625
   coeliotomy. *See* Argentine Horned Frog
   cystotomy, contact mode. *See* African Spurred Tortoise
   effects. *See* Biological tissue
   light, 618
   physics, 618-620
   production, diagrammatic representation, 618f
   radiofrequency safety, 624
   surgery, 617-618
      appropriateness, 315
      performing. *See* Rats

Lasers—cont'd
   tissue penetrations, diagrammatic representation. *See* Nonpigmented tissue; Pigmented tissue
   usage. *See* Herpetologic surgery
Laser stone ablation, 770
Lateral incisions, 590f
Laterals, 972
Lateral undulation, 51
Lavage. *See* Gastric lavage
   posttreatment, 745
Law of similars, 432
Lay-box. *See* Ovipositorium
LD. *See* Lactate dehydrogenase
LDH. *See* Lactate dehydrogenase
Lead citrate, 398f, 409f
Lead-shot nutria, 706
Leaf-nosed Snakes (*Langaha sp.*), dimorphism, 50f
League of Florida Herpetological Societies, 9
Learedius learedi. *See* Green Seaturtle
Leatherback Seaturtle (*D. coriacea*), size, 976f
Leatherback Turtle, T1-weighted image. *See* Posthatchling Leatherback Turtle
Leaves, consumption, 267
Leeches, 346-347
   discovery, 208
   presence, 208f
   problem, 962
Leiolopisma telfairii. *See* Rare Skink; Skink
Length, examination, 491
Lenses, 339
   anatomy, 339
Leopard Gecko (*Eublepharis macularius*)
   gastrointestinal impaction, 69f
      radiograph, 69f
   one-piece shedding, 779f
   pseudomonas infection, 337f
Leopard Tortoise (*Geochelone pardalis*)
   advantage, 92f
   African tick, presence, 208f
   carapace, bilateral abrasions, 201f
   carapacial damage, 205f
   cloacalith, 764f
   feces, production, 772f
   fiber supplementation, absence, 292f
   focal bacterial hepatitis, 524f
   hematologic values, 1116
   hidden-neck turtle example, 79f
   liver, paleness, 524f
   nasal discharge, cytology, 465f
   precocious birth, 365f
   pyramidal shell growth, 700f
   red rubber feeding tube, usage, 278f
   serum biochemical values, 1116
   shell defect, East African materials (usage), 205f
   species, 92
   tracheal/lung wash cytology, 465f
   tube feeding, esophagostomy tube (usage), 811f
Lepidochelys kempii. *See* Kemp's Ridley
Lepidochelys olivacea. *See* Olive Ridley
Lepidosauria, classification, 43
Leptin, 283
Leptotyphlopidae, 44-45

Lesions
   bisection, 202f
   contents, coagulation, 685-686
   repair, 204
Lesser Chameleon (*Furcifer minor*), disseminated mycosis, 223f
LET. *See* Lung-eye-trachea
LETD. *See* Lung eye and trachea disease
Lethargic Syndrome, 995
Lethargy, 957. *See also* Crocodilians
Lettuce, unsuitability. *See* Iguanas; Tortoises
Leukemias, 404
   reports, 459
Leukocytes. *See* Reptiles
   analysis, 884
   counts, obtaining, 460
   differentials, 949
   response, 458-459
Leukoencephalopathy. *See* Hypothiaminosis
Levamisole, usage, 1025
LIA. *See* Lysine iron agar
Liasis albertisii. *See* D'Albert's Python
Liasis papuanus. *See* Papuan Python
Lichanura trivirgata. *See* Rosy Boa
Lidocaine, usage, 519
Light
   amount, impact, 30
   quality. *See* Captive reptiles
   sources
      representation, 1081t
      requirement. *See* Endoscopy
Lightbulbs, UV A/B emission. *See* Commercial lightbulbs
Light-carrying bundles, volume (selection), 550
Lighting, usage. *See* Artificial lighting
Lilies, impact, 1706-1077
Limbal conjunctiva, needle (advancement), 324
Limbs
   amputation, 609-610
   electrodes, usage, 188
   extension. *See* Withdrawn limbs
Lingual lesion, 233f
Lipid, holes (appearance), 810
Lipidosis, 400f, 632
Lipopolysaccharid structure, variations, 232
Liquid diets, continuous feeding (recommendation), 278
Liquid light cable, 552
Lissencephalic reptiles, 239
Lithium heparin, 949
Lithophagy, 294
Lithotripsy, usage, 770
Live-bearing reptiles, 377
Live prey food, usage, 38
Livers, 806
   anatomy, 806
   biopsy, 523, 810
   disease, assessment
      biochemistry parameters, usage, 808t
      hematologic parameters, usage, 808t
   endoscopic technique, 561
   histopathologic changes, 826
   laboratory evaluation, 464
   necropsy examination, 577-578
   originates, 806

Livers—cont'd
  physiology, 806
  removal, 577f
  samples, ultrasound guidance, 523
  tissue opacity, 485
  tophi deposition, 796f
  ventral acoustic window, usage, 487
Living reptiles, clades, 59
Lizard mites (*Hirstiella trombidiiformis*)
  presence, 724f
  problems, 35
Lizards, 59. *See also* Poisonous lizards
  abrasions, 684
  activity, 69f
  acupuncture points, 435f
  adenovirus, 398
  adrenal glands, 68
  aggression, 75, 692
  anatomy, 60-68
  anesthesia, induction, 447
  anorexia, 688
  aquapuncture, advantage, 437f
  arboreal species, 68
  ataxia, 691-692
  behavior, 75
    changes, 692
  bite trauma, 233f
  blisters, 685-686
  blood collection, 514f
  body systems, tumors, 303t-305t
  breeding seasons, 64
  cages, 74
  caging, 68
  captive reptile husbandry, 68
  carcass, gross photograph, 579f
  cardiovascular system, 60-62
  carnivore classification, 73
  caudal tail/vein, blood collection, 514f
  cecum, 64
  celiotomy, 587-588
  cephalic vein, location, 639f
  chamber wall thickness, measurement, 192
  classification, 42
  claws, 68
  cloaca, 64
  cloacal anatomy, 136f
  cloacal opening, circumferential purse-string sutures (problems), 863f
  cloacal prolapse, 689
  coelom
    distension, 692-693
    pigmentation, 573f
  color/color change, abnormalities, 686
  coma, 691-692
  communal housing/handling, 74
  constipation, 689
  convulsions, 691-692
  cornea, abnormalities, 691
  crusts, 684-685
  deformities, 683-684
  dental disease, 688
  dermatitis, 684
  diagnostic techniques, 501-504
  diarrhea, 689
  dietary intake, essential nutrients, 274
  differential diagnosis, 683
  digestive system, 63-64
  disinfection, 74

Lizards—cont'd
  dysecdysis, 684-685
  dyspnea, 690
  dystocia, 689-690
    diagnosis, 788-789
    surgery, 791
  ears, 65
  endocrine system, 68
  environmental captivity
    philosophy, 68
    requirements, 68-75
  exudates, 686-687
  eyes, 65-66, 691
  feeding, 71, 73
  feet, caseated abscess, 233f
  femoral pores, 65
  firefly consumption, 1070
  flaccid paralysis, 855
  flakes, 684-685
  flavored medications, preference, 641
  gastrointestinal signs, 688-689
  gender identification, 65
  glottis, location, 130f
  gonads, ultrasonic evaluation, 65
  hatch failure, 689
  head tilts, 691-692, 854-855
  heart
    caudal placement, 191f
    dorsal view, 125f
    ventral view, 125f
  hemipenes, pairing, 140f
  herbivore classification, 71
  hormone fluctuations, 74
  hyperkeratotic epidermis, proliferation, 211f
  imagery, gel stand-off pad (usage), 666f
  infertility, 689
  insectivore classification, 71, 73
  integument, 67-68, 684-686
  internal fertilization, 64-65
  intravenous cut-down techniques, 536
  jugular vein, location, 638f
  keepers, 74
  Lacerta lepida, head (scale size/appearance), 196
  Lacerta vivipara, hypovitaminosis A, 211f
  lameness, 683
  lenses, abnormalities, 691
  lethargy, 694
  lips, 63
  longevity, 75-76
    records, 75t
  lungs, 130
    pairing, 131f
    respiratory surfaces, location, 132f
    symmetry, 131f
  lysis, radiograph, 381f
  meridian points, 433f
  mesenteric interstitium, melanophore accumulation, 573f
  mucous membrane color, 687
  muscle weakness/twitching, 855
  musculoskeletal signs, 683-684
  nasal discharge, 690
  nasal salt glands, 66
  nervous system, 65
    behaviors, 691-692
  neurologic disorders, 854-855

Lizards—cont'd
  nitrogenous waste, excretion, 64
  nodules, 685-686
  nontraditional therapeutic methods, 658
  nutrition, 71, 73
  one-piece shedding, 779f
  open sores, 684
  oral cavity, 686-688
  oral discharge, 687
  oral multicellular mucous glands, 145
  osmoregulation, 71
  palpebral abnormalities, 691
  parakeratotic epidermis, proliferation, 211f
  paralysis/paresis, 692
  parental care, 366
  petechiae, 686
  pharyngeal edema, 687
  physical restraint, 501f
  pleuroperitoneal cavity, 555
    schematic representation, 554f
  polydipsia/polyuria, 694
  positioning, 472, 474-475
  precloacal pores, 65
  protection, 75
  PSO, presence, 909f
  ptyalism, 687
  quarantine, 74
  regurgitation, 688-689
  renal anatomy, 139f
  reproduction, 692
  reproductive signs, 689-690
  reproductive system, 64-65
  respiratory signs, 690-691
  respiratory system, 66-67
  respiratory tract
    anatomy, 129-128
    evaluation, lateral views, 484
  restraint, 75, 474-475
    towel wrap technique, 502f
  ribs, 67
  scabs, 684-685
  scars, 686
  sexual characteristics, 508f
  single-handed restraint, 502f
  skeletal abnormalities, 683
  skeletal system, 67
  skin, 67
  special senses, 65-66
  spectacle abnormalities, 691
  spinal abnormalities, 683
  squamate reproduction/courtship, 171-173
  stillbirths, 689
  stomach, 64
    black pigmentation, gross photograph, 573f
    tubing, 811
  stomatitis, 686-687
  substrate, usage, 68-70
  sudden death, 694
  swellings, 685-686
  systemic signs, 692-694
  tails, 683
    autotomy, 914f
    dropping, fear (impact), 275f
    regrowth, 167
  teeth, 688
  thermoregulation, 70-71

Lizards—cont'd
　thin-walled bladder, 64
　tongue, 64
　　characteristics, 687-688
　treatment, case study. See Uromastix
　　Lizards
　twitching, 691-692
　ulcerations, 684, 686-687
　ultraviolet (UV) light requirements, 73
　uric acid excretion, 256
　urinary system, 64-65
　vascular anatomy, 139f
　VAV, 515, 587-588
　venomous species, 63
　visual security, 74
　vocalizations, abnormality, 690-691
　vomition, 688-689
　weight loss, 692
Lizard *(Scleroporus magister)*, middle/inner
　　ear relations, 743f
Local anesthetic agents, 445
　usage, 451. See also Acute pain; Chronic
　　pain
Localizer. See Slider
　image. See Computed tomography;
　　Magnetic resonance imaging
Locomotion. See Concertina locomotion;
　　Rectilinear locomotion; Snakes
　abnormality, 389
Loggerhead Seaturtle *(Caretta caretta)*
　buoyancy abnormalities, 993f
　carapace length, 1090f
　carcass, 973f
　debilitation, 996f
　dorsal cervical sinus, blood
　　collection, 516f
　Enodiotrema sp., 352f
　entanglements, hazard, 980f
　Hapalotrema loossi, 352f
　head, proportionate size, 978f
　lethargy, 996f
　Neospirorchis sp., 352f
　nylon fishing line, entanglement, 986f
　Orchidasma amphiorchis, 351f
　Pachypsolus irroratus, 352f
　plasma protein fractions,
　　identification, 981t
　Sulcascaris sulcata, 356, 357f
Loggerhead Turtle *(Caretta caretta)*
　duplicate flipper, 374f
　erythrocytes, cytoplasm (artifacts), 805f
　histiosarcoma, 318f
Longitudinal folds, presence, 148
Long-stem fiber sources, appearance, 292
Long-term feeding, nutritional
　　problems, 263
Long-term hospitalization. See Captive
　　reptiles
Lophotaspis vallei. See Fluke egg
Loreal pits, impaction, 724
Loss
　anger, 18, 20
　　helping process, 18
　clinician/client concerns. See Animals
　concentration, reduction, 17
　crying, acceptability, 22
　depression, 19
　　helping process, 19

Loss—cont'd
　guilt/bargaining, 18
　　helping process, 18
　guilty feelings, 21
　pessimism, 17
　reactions, 17-19
　replacement, clinician concerns, 22
　shock/denial, 17-18, 20
　　helping process, 17-18
　support groups/web sites, 23
Louisiana, herpetological societies, 6t
Lovich, JE, 11
Lower-phosphorus diets, 273
Low-grade infections, fulmination, 387
Low Skin Resistant (LSR) points, 433
Loxocemes bicolor. See Neotropical Sunbeam
　　Snake
Loxocemidae, longevity, 46, 56t
LRS. See Isotonic replacement crystalloid;
　　Lactated Ringer's solution
LSR. See Low Skin Resistant
Lucke's renal tumor. See Renal
　　adenocarcinomas
Lumbosacral CSF tap. See Green Iguana
Lumps, 681
Lung eye and trachea disease (LETD), 335
　association, 396
　investigation, 814
　lesions. See Ulcerative LETD lesions
Lung-eye-trachea (LET) disease, 338
Lungs
　auscultation, 504
　biopsy, 520-521
　culturing, 576f
　endoscopic entry, 521
　evaluation, 473
　falveolar lining, 558f
　fields, visualization, 190
　granulomas, formation, 871f
　lavage, 520
　nonrespiratory portion, caudal view, 558f
　paramyxovirus infection, 860f
　Pseudomonas aeruginosa pneumonia, 233f
　sac-like appearance, 484
　sterility, 575f
　structure, difference, 483-484
　tissue, edematous appearance, 233f
　tophi deposition, 796f
　visualization, 482
　wash, 520
　　cytology. See Burmese Python; Leopard
　　　Tortoise; Red-tailed Boa
　　fluid retrieval, 229f
Lungworms, impact, 874
Luteinizing hormone, 432
Lymph contamination, complication, 516
Lymph infiltration, 778
Lymphocyte proliferation assay, 1067f
Lymphocytes, 456f, 457f
　concentration, 458
　function, 459
　influx, 466
　production, impact, 632
　resemblance, 457
Lymphocytes, mobilization, 213
Lymphocytic inflammation, 933
Lymphocytic myocarditis, 412
Lymphocytosis, occurrence, 459

Lymphohistiocytic proliferative syndrome
　　(PIX disease). See Alligators
Lymphoid tissues, necropsy
　　examination, 578
Lymphomas, 404
Lypolysis, 120
Lysine iron agar (LIA), usage, 900-901
Lysis, radiograph. See Lizards
Lytic proliferative spinal osteopathy, 244

M

Mab. See Monoclonal antibody
MAC. See Minimum alveolar concentration
MacConkey agar, 900
Macdonaldius genera, 184
Macrochelys temminckii. See Alligator
　　Snapping Turtle
Macrolides
　pharmacokinetics, determination, 651
　usage, 651
Macroparasites, 207-209
　visibility, 201
Macrophages
　influx, 466
　production, 219
Macrophagic inflammation, 467
Madagascan Tomato Frog *(Dyscophus
　　antongilii)*, corneal lipidosis, 965f
Madagascar Leaf-tailed Gecko *(Uroplatus
　　fimbriatus)*, serrated vertical
　　pupil, 66f
Magnetic resonance imaging (MRI).
　　See Aquatic Turtles; Desert Tortoise;
　　Savannah Monitor Lizard
　axial composite. See Pythons
　axial sections. See Alligators
　inclusion, 151
　localizer image, 1090f
　machine, usage. See Closed MRI machine
　pulsating external magnetic field,
　　usage, 242
　scout image, 1090f
　significance, 158
　trunk composite. See Pythons
　usage, 1088-1093
Magnetic resonance (MR), 486-487
Maine, herpetological societies, 6t
Major histocompatibility complex
　　(MHC), 1066
Maladaptation syndrome, 120f
Malaria-causing parasites, 803-804
Malathion, usage, 1067
Male caiman (penis), eversion (digital
　　palpation, usage), 383f
Male crocodiles, reproductive system, 109
Male reproductive anatomy, 376
Male snakes
　sexual segment, 49f
　urodeum, ureteral papilla, 137f
Male tortoise, penis, 142f
　extension, 86f
Malignant neoplasia, 465, 467
　diagnosis, cytologic criteria, 467
Mallacosoma americanus. See Eastern tent
　　caterpillar
Malocclusion, 924
Malochochersus tornieri. See Pancake
　　Tortoise

Mammalian insulin
    radioimmunoassays, 825
Mammals
  ECG usage, 193
  gout (treatment), medications
      (usage), 799t
  herbivores, caloric requirements, 150
  metabolic bone diseases, types
      (examples), 841t
  synthetic salmon calcitonin, effects, 846t
Mandibles
  deformation, 389
  malleability, 601
  pressure, 505
Mandibular deformities, NMBD
    (impact), 847f
Mandibular fibrous osteodystrophy, 847
Mandibular osteomyelitis, lytic process, 478
Man-made toxins, impact, 158-159
Manouria emys. See Burmese Brown Tortoise
Manouria emys emys. See Burmese Mountain
    Tortoise
Manouria impressa. See Impressed Tortoise
Manual veterinary therapies, 432-438
Manus, fractures (ball bandage usage), 604f
Marathon Sea Turtle Hospital (MSTH),
    983, 984
  animal presentation, open coelomic
      fistula, 999f
  assist feeding, 994
  fish hook retrieval, 992f
  Green Turtle, tube feeding, 995f
  lifers, 991
  patients, convalescence, 997
  turtle presentation, forelimb
      (absence), 1000f
Marathon Veterinary Hospital, logo, 5
Marcus, LC, 12
Marginals, 972
Marijuana, impact, 1078
Marine Iguana *(Amblyrhynchus cristatus)*,
    serrated teeth, 145, 146f
Marine leeches *(Ozobranchus margoi)*,
    coverage, 994. *See also* Seaturtle
Marine turtles, herpesvirus, 393-394
Marrow space, limitation, 539
Marsh mallow root *(Althea officinalis)*,
    prescription, 430
Maryland, herpetological societies, 6t
Marzec, G, 12
Masked Tree Frog *(Smilisca phaeota)*,
    spindly leg, 965f
Masking tape, usage, 585f
Massachusetts, herpetological societies, 6t
Massage, 438
Mass lesions, 716
Mata Mata *(Chelus fimbriatus)*
  side-neck turtle member, 79f
  underside, 697f
Material safety data sheets (MSDS), 12
Maternal care, 379
Mating, time, 365
Mattison, C, 12
Mauremys mutica. See Asian Pond Turtle
Maxilla, pressure, 505
Maxillary osteomyelitis, lytic process, 478
MBD. *See* Metabolic bone diseases
McArthur, S, 12

MCHC. *See* Mean cellular hemoglobin
    concentration
MCV. *See* Mean cellular volume
ME. *See* Metabolized energy
Mean cellular hemoglobin concentration
    (MCHC), 453-454
Mean cellular volume (MCV), 453
Mean inhibitory concentration (MIC),
    230-231
Meat-based dietary component, retention,
    254-255
MEDARKS. *See* Medical Records Keeping
    System
Medetomidine
  combination, 447, 639
  usage, 444
Media plate, specimen inoculation, 229
Medical emergency supplies, set, 1015
Medical Records Keeping System
    (MEDARKS), 1012
Medical treatment plan. *See* Venomous
    reptiles
Mediterranean Tortoise *(Testudo graeca)*
  acrus lipoideus corneae, 336f
  bacterial keratitis, 337f
  cataracts, 339f
  cornea, postinflammatory
      pigmentation, 338f
  dry eye, 332f
  ear abscess, 335f
  eyelid flap, corneal ulceration, 337f
  eyes, pus, 335f
  foreign body (sand substrate),
      conjunctival hyperplasia, 334f
  grass seed foreign body, 334f
  hematologic values, 1115
  Horner's syndrome, 323f
  indirect ophthalmoscopy, usage, 324
  microphthalmos, 333f
  orbital cellulitis, 335f
  serum biochemical values, 1115
Melanin, absorption coefficient, 619f
Membrana vasculosa retinae, 340
Menac reflex. *See* Green Iguana
Meninges, location, 239
Mentation, alteration, 546
Merck Veterinary Manual, The, 10
Meriflour *Cryptosporidium/Giardia* Mab
    combination reagent, 759f
Mesenchymal cell neoplasms, 467
Mesentery. *See* Body
Mesocestoidiasis, 1026
Mesocestoididea, 155
Mesophilic saprophytic fungi, 225
Mesorchium, 576
Mesovarium, 576
  Mesovasorum, variation, 587
Metabolic bone diseases (MBD), 475, 841.
    See also Renal metabolic bone
    disease
  facial deformities. *See* Postnutritional
      MBD facial deformities
  femurs, radiographic comparison, 850f
  forms, 601
  impact, 683, 686, 913
  non-nutritional origin, 847-850
  nutritional origin. *See* Amphibians
  types, examples. *See* Mammals

Metabolic bone diseases of nutritional
    origin (NMBD), 30
Metabolic derangements, 246
Metabolic neuropathies, 245-246
Metabolic states, 259-261
Metabolized energy (ME), 251
  percentage, 254, 263
Metaldehyde, impact, 1073-1074
Metallic markers, 475f
Metanephric reptiles, 633
Metastatic disease/rate, 317
Metastatic mineralization, 690
Metatarsal-phalangeal joints, gout
    (presence), 774-775
Metazoan parasites, detection, 885
Methionine, usage. *See* Hepatic lipidosis
Methoxyflurane, 949
Methylene blue, usage, 454
Methylmethacrylate beads,
    implantation, 606
Methylprednisolone acetate, usage, 748
Metronidazole, 927
  action, mechanism, 1071
  clinical signs, 1071
  impact, 247
  toxicity, 651
  treatment, 1071
  usage, 651-652, 960
Mexican Beaded Lizard *(Heloderma
    horridum)*, yolk sac (fungal hyphae
    proliferation), 223f
Meyer, J, 12
MHC. *See* Major histocompatibility
    complex
MIC. *See* Mean inhibitory concentration;
    Minimum inhibitory concentration
Mice
  food, usage, 39
  purchase/thawing. *See* Prekilled
      pinkie/adult mice
Michigan, herpetological societies, 7t
Microbiologic culture, 151
  test sensitivity/specificity, estimation,
      902-903
Microbiologic isolation methods.
    See Salmonella
Microbiologic sampling, 534
Microbiology, 217
Microfilaria, 804-805
Microflora. *See* Gastrointestinal microflora
Microhepatica, 808
Micromark, 584
Micromosquito hemostats, 583
Micronutrient imbalances, 439
Microorganisms, 231-235
Microscopic evaluation, usage, 391
Microsporidiosis, 350
Micurus fulvus, antivenin, 1028t
Midazolam, usage, 444
Midcoelomic region, catheter passage, 522
Middle ear cavity, swelling, 696
Midline incision, importance, 587-588
Migration nymphs, 1025
Milbemycin, usage, 247
Milksnake *(Lampropeltis triangulum* sp.)
  egg retention, 789f
  hematologic values, 1107
  serum biochemical values, 1107

Mineralization process, 601f
Mineral oil gavages, 992
Minerals
　deficiencies, 291
　　traces, 267
　intoxication, 292-293
　supplements, need, 39
　support, usage, 1132t-1133t
Minimum alveolar concentration (MAC), 446. *See also* Isoflurane
Minimum inhibitory concentration (MIC), requirement, 643, 652
Minnesota, herpetological societies, 7t
Missing toes. *See* Toes
Missouri, herpetological societies, 7t
Mistletoe, impact, 1077
MIT. *See* Monoiodothyronine
Mite infestation, 727f. *See also* Snakes
　clinical signs, 727
　impact, 686
　prevention
　　alternate methods, 731-732
　　dichlorvos strips, usage, 730-731
　　fipronil, usage, 730
　　ivermectin, usage, 730
　　organophosphates, usage, 729-730
　　pyrethrins/pyrethroids, usage, 729
Mite-infested animals, appearance, 723
Mite-related anemia, 730
Mites, 346
　biologic control, 732
　control, 35
　growth regulators, 732
　isolation/quarantine, 728
　life cycle-directed control strategies, 732-733
　pockets, 197
　prevention program, 735
　prognosis, 735-736
　sanitation/cleaning, 728-729
　treatment protocols, 727-728
　zoonotic potential, 733-735
Mixed-cell inflammation, 466f
Mixed greens, usage, 267
Modified transudates, 468
Moisture conservation. *See* Amphibians
Moisture-containing substrates, usage, 31, 37
Mojave Rattlesnake (*Crotalus s. scutulatus*)
　shed skin, fungal growth, 218f
　venom, characteristic, 1052f
Molecular diagnostics, 153
Monclonal antibody (Mab), 759f
　combination reagent. *See* Meriflour *Cryptosporidium/Giardia* Mab combination reagent
Monitor Lizards (*Varanus* spp.)
　cardiomegaly, 181f
　caudal/tail vein, lateral approach (blood collection), 515f
　dorsoventral/lateral views, 873f
　ecdysis, 66f
　glottis, location, 130f
　heart, caudal placement, 191f
　hemipenes, mineralized hemibacula (presence), 383t
　orthogonal views, 873f

Monitor Lizards—cont'd
　ultrasound examination, manual restraint, 667f
　unilateral bacterial pneumonia, 872f
Monoclonal antibodies, 234
Monocytes, 455f, 457f, 458f
　erythrophagocytosis, 458f
　occurrence, 459
　resemblance, 457
Monofilament absorbable suture, 597
Monogenetic trematodes, 351
Monoiodothyronine (MIT), 290
Mononuclear cell infiltrates, 249
Monophagous lizards, existence, 928
Monopolar/bipolar applications, 622
Montane reptiles, brumation temperatures (need), 29
Montane species, temperature/feeding, 282
Morbidity, catastrophic outbreaks, 392
Morelia spilotus cheynei. *See* Jungle Carpet Python
Morelia spilotus variegatus. *See* Carpet Python
Morelia viridis. *See* Green Tree Python
Morphologic adaptations, 163, 173-175. *See also* Amphibians; Reptiles
Morphology, 145-149
Morus nigra. *See* Mulberry larva
Mosquito forceps, usage, 535
Motor function, progressive loss, 873
MOTT. *See* Mycobacteria tuberculosis complex
Mouth
　rot, 676f
MR. *See* Magnetic resonance
MRI. *See* Magnetic resonance imaging
MSDS. *See* Material safety data sheets
MSTH. *See* Marathon Sea Turtle Hospital
Mu, definition, 429t
Mucolytic agents, usage, 875-876
Mucoprotein, 139
Mucorales (order), 1023
Mucormycosis, 154
Mucor sp., isolation, 220
Mucous membranes. *See* Pale tongue/mucous membranes
Mucus
　examination, 758
　excess, 963
Mucus-secreting cells, gastric hyperplasia. *See* Snakes
　wet mount preparation, sheared light illumination, 758f
Mud Snake (*Farancia abacura reinwardti*), parental care, 45f
Mulberry larva (*Morus nigra*), nutrient/energy composition, 265t
Muller-Kauffmann tetrathionate, usage, 901
Multifocal hyperkeratotic fungal dermatitis, 222f
Multinucleated giant cells, production, 219
Multinucleated mesenchymal cells, 468f
Murphy, JB, 12
Muscles
　atrophy. *See* Temporal muscle atrophy
　biopsy, 525f
　fasciculations, 843

Muscles—cont'd
　injury, laboratory detection, 464-465
　tremors, 710
Muscular contraction, series, 127
Muscular ridge, 127
Muscular tone, evaluation, 299
Muscular ventricle, presence, 668f
Musculature, palpation, 34
Musculoskeletal deformities, 678
Musculoskeletal disorders, 711-712
Musculoskeletal signs. *See* Snakes
Musculoskeletal system
　diagnostic techniques, 523-525
　necropsy examination, 578
　tumors, 301t, 302t, 305t, 313t
Musk glands, 529
Musk Turtles (*Sternotherus* sp.)
　morphologic appearance, 80f
　prolapsed/ruptured globe, 334f
Mycelia, 338
Mycobacteria, 534
Mycobacteria tuberculosis complex (MOTT), 234
Mycobacteriosis. *See* Crocodilians
Mycobacterium, 234, 1023
Mycobacterium chelonei osteomyelitis. *See* Desert Tortoise
Mycobacterium sp., 202
Mycoplasma, 534
　clearance, 934
　culture, 934
　PCR, 934
Mycoplasma, 234
Mycoplasmal infections, confirmation. *See* Tortoises
Mycoplasma serology, 933-934
Mycoplasmosis. *See* Crocodilians
　drug treatment. *See* Tortoises
　emergence, 653
　impact. *See* Gopher Tortoise
　management issues. *See* Wild tortoises
Mycoses. *See* Cutaneous mycoses; Deep mycoses; Subcutaneous mycoses; Superficial mycoses; Systemic mycoses
Mycotic fungal diseases, 209-210
Mycotic pneumonia, 853
Myelin degeneration, 249
Myeloblastosis, 404
Myeloid leukosis, 404
Myenteric ganglia, 406
Myiasis (fly strike), 208-209, 209f, 346
　diagnosis, 209
　impact, 684
Myotoxins, 1051

N

N. depressa. *See* Flatback Turtles
Nails, short clipping, 776
Naja naja. *See* Spectacled Cobra
Naloxone, impact, 432
Nares
　depigmentation, 701
　erosion, 701. *See also* Desert Tortoise
　occlusion, 675
　sampling, 519-520
　tissue, distortion, 702

Narrowhead Softshell Turtle *(Chitra indica)*, pentastome, 361f
Nasal discharge, 816, 933
　herpesvirus, impact, 701
　lower respiratory pathology, 866f
Nasolacrimal duct, patency (investigation), 331
Nasolacrimal system, blockage, 331
National Institutes of Health (NIH)
　research, 850
　web site, 428
National laws. *See* Reptiles
National Marine Fisheries Service regulations, 1045
National Pet Week, poster, 14f
National wildlife legislation, 1042
Natricine, 44f
Natrix natrix. See Grass Snake
Natt-Herrick solution, 951
Natural environment toxins, impact, 158-159
Naturalistic enclosures, usage, 35-36
Natural killer (NK) cells, 218
Natural light, usage. *See* Captive reptiles
NEAQ. *See* New England Aquarium
Nebraska, herpetological societies, 7t
Nebulization, 656
　antibiotics, usage, 876t
　chamber, 656. *See also* Desert Tortoise
Necropsy, 572-578
　equipment, purchase, 572
　instruments, usage, 572f
　sample procurement, 569-578
　specimens
　　handling, 572t
　　tissue collection protocol, 573t
　submission form, 570f
　techniques, overview, 569
　usage, 564-565
Necrosis. *See* Dermatology
Necrotic material (soup), 722
Necrotic stomatitis, 675
Needle driver, usage, 535
Negative energy balance, 632
Neguvon, usage, 729
Nematodes, 346t, 354-360, 1167-1169
　eggs. *See* Blue-tailed Monitor; Red Ratsnake
　encountering, 154
　impact, 960-961
　lips. *See* Ascarid nematode
　search, 345
　signs, impact, 961
　treatment, 155
Nematophila sp. *See* Yellow-footed Tortoise
Neodymium-yttrium aluminum garnet (YAG) lasers, 620
　effects, 623
Neonatal colubrid snakes, sexual determination, 381
Neonatal lizards/snakes, aggression, 371
Neonatal prey, mineral/fat-soluble vitamin contents, 262
Neonates
　conditions, impact, 372-373
　feeding, 371-372
　housing, 370-371
　morbidity/mortality, 373-375

Neonates—cont'd
　placement. *See* Incubators
　quarantine/hygiene, 375
　treatments, 373
Neoplasia, 158, 326-327, 506f. *See also* Gastrointestinal neoplasia; Malignant neoplasia; Seaturtle
　impact, 854-855
　indication, 479f
　reports, 775
Neoplasms. *See* Dermatology
Neoplastic diseases. *See* Amphibians
Neospirorchis sp. *See* Loggerhead Seaturtle
Neostigmine methysulfate, usage, 117
Neotropical Giant Toad *(Bufo marinus)*
　lingual venous plexus, phlebotomy site, 950f
　midline ventral vein, blood sample (obtaining), 950f
　mouth, opening (speculum usage), 950f
　ventrum, midline groove (location), 950f
Neotropical Sunbeam Snake *(Loxocemes bicolor)*, 43f
Nephrocalcinosis, 577
Nephron, 140
　blood supply, 140
Nephron GFR, 878
Nephrosclerosis, 826
Nephrotoxic antibiotics, misuse, 795
Nephrotoxins, exposure, 880
Nerodia erythrogaster flavigaster.
　See Yellow-bellied Water Snake
Nerodia harteri. See Brazos Watersnake
Nerodia harteri harteri. See Watersnakes
Nerodia sp. *See* Diamond-backed Water Snake
Nerve gas, characteristic, 1069
Nerves
　compression, 436
　depolarization, 842
　receptors, heat sensation, 918
Nervous system
　diagnostic techniques, 529-531
　necropsy examination, 578
　signs. *See* Snakes
　tumors, 305t
Nests
　guarding, 379
　side, benefit, 388
Network Of Animal Health (NOAH), 12
Neuroanatomy, 239
Neurodystrophic hypothesis, 436
Neurologic disorders, 852
Neurologic dysfunction, report, 751
Neurologic examination, 239-241
Neurologic function, improvement, 242f
Neurology, 239
Neuromuscular blocking agents, intracameral agents, 324
Neuronal degeneration, 406
Neuron degeneration, 249
Neuropathies. *See* Congenital neuropathies; Infectious neuropathies; Metabolic neuropathies; Toxic neuropathies; Trauma-induced neuropathies
Neurotransmitters, response, 293
Nevada, herpetological societies, 7t
Newcastle disease virus, 402

New England Aquarium (NEAQ), 1001
　admittance, 1004
　ambubag, usage, 1003
New England Aquarium (NEAQ), cold-stunned seaturtles
　admission data sheet, 1002f
　measurement sheet, 1002f
New Guinea Blue-tongued Skink *(Tiliqua gigas)*, lung lavage, 520f
New Hampshire, herpetological societies, 7t
New Jersey, herpetological societies, 7t
New Mexico Chinese Herbal Veterinary Medicine Course, 440
Newspapers
　shredded, usage, 31
　substrate, usage, 28f
　usage. *See* Reptile practice
Newts, 943
New World Python, renaming, 43f
New York, herpetological societies, 7t
New York Herpetological Society, 7t, 9
New York Zoological Garden. *See* Bronx Zoo
Nicotine, impact, 1077-1078
NIH. *See* National Institutes of Health
Nile Crocodile *(Crocoydlus niloticus)*
　bite, 212f
　predation, reports, 102
Nile Monitor *(Varanus nioloticus)*
　aggressiveness, 75f
　hematologic values, 1112
　serum biochemical values, 1112
Nitrites, analysis, 884
Nitrogen
　excretion, 765
　concerns, 257
　sources, 256-257
Nitrous oxide, usage, 998
NK. *See* Natural killer
NMBD. *See* Nutritional metabolic bone disease
NMBO. *See* Metabolic bone diseases of nutritional origin
NOAH. *See* Network Of Animal Health
No growth sample results, interpretation, 231
Nolvasan Scrub, 1018
Noncontact temperature measurement, 87
Noncrocodilian reptiles
　cardiopulmonary anatomy/physiology, 124-126
　circulation, 126f
Nonculture diagnostic methods. *See* Salmonella
Nondegenerate heterophils, 465f
Noninfectious diseases, 156-160
　classification, 196
Noninflammatory osteoarthritis, 906
Non-light-emitting heat sources, 1081
Nonmetastatic tumors, surgery (preference), 299, 315
Non-native tortoise herpesvirus PCR, usage, 817
Nonobstructive dystocias, 787-788
Nonpigmented tissue, penetrations (diagrammatic representation), 622f

Nonprotein nitrogen (NPN)
    amount, 257
    source, 281
Nonspecific clinical signs, differentials (list), 706
Non-steroidal antiinflammatory drug (NSAID)
    treatment, 433
    usage, 451
Nonsupportive interstitial pneumonia, 412
Nonsuppurative encephalitis, 249
Nontraditional therapeutic methods, 657-659
    CE products, 658-659
Nonunion fracture, 605
    radiograph. See Chinese Water Dragon
Nonvenomous snakes, nervousness, 496f
Nonvestibular lesions, occurrence, 854
Normosol, usage, 633
Normosol-R, 543
North American Tailed Frog (Ascaphis truei), 177f
North American Veterinary Conference, 13
Northern California Herpetological Society, 10
Northern Ohio Association of Herpetologists, 10
Nose-to-tail physical examination, 774
Nostrils, hemorrhage, 165
Novafil, usage, 616
NPN. See Nonprotein nitrogen
NSAID. See Non-steroidal antiinflammatory drug
NSHP. See Nutritional secondary hyperparathyroidism
Nuchal, 972
Nuclear medicine, 488-489
Nucleic acid
    breakdown, 793f
    degradation, 793
Nucleotide formation, 793f
Nutraceuticals, usage, 438-439
Nutrients
    disorders, 284
    trial dosages. See Reptiles
Nutrition, 251. See also Embryo
    assessment, 274-276
    diseases, 182-183, 280-294. See also Amphibians
    disorder. See Dermatology
    metabolism, relationship, 251-261
    neuropathies, 243-244
    requirements, 38
    support, 273-280. See also Hepatic lipidosis; Parenteral nutrition support
        commercial liquid products, 279t
        techniques, 276-277
        usage, 1132t-1133t
Nutritional deficiencies, 680
Nutritional metabolic bone disease (NMBD), 475f, 476f, 601, 600f. See also Green Iguana
    cloacal prolapse, sign, 844f
    impact. See Mandibular deformities
    mouth, opening, 607f
    prelude, 845f

Nutritional secondary hyperparathyroidism (NSHP), 286f, 287f, 601, 841-847
    commonness, 929
    consequence, 847
    lesions
        association, 211
        deformities, 929f
    physiologic response, 842-843
    problem, 285
    sequelae, 692
    signs, 286
    treatment, 843-847
        goals, 845
Nycotherus (merthiolate stain), 350f
Nyctisaura, 59
Nyctotherus, 350f
Nylon
    pursestring suture, usage, 967
    usage, 581
Nystagmus, 852
Nystatin, usage, 210

O

Oak poisoning, 1078
Obesity, 282-283
Obstructive dystocias, 787. See also Nonobstructive dystocias
Occupational health/safety legislation, 1043
Occupational Safety and Health Administration (OSHA), 12
Ocular discharge, 704, 816, 933
Ocular system, tumors, 314t
OEGL. See Outer epidermal generation layer
Offensive aggression, 172
Offspring size, clutch size (trade-off), 378
Ohio, herpetological societies, 7t
Oil-emulsion vaccine, 658
Oklahoma, herpetological societies, 7t
Oldham, JC, 12
Old World Chameleons, exception, 130
Olfaction, 240
Olive Ridley (Lepidochelys olivacea)
    color/carapace characteristics, 978f
    ventral view, 979f
Omnivores
    calorie sources, 254-255
    energy sources, 255f
    pellets, consumption, 270
Oncology, 299
    local therapy, 299, 315, 317
    principles/diagnostics/staging, 299
    treatment options, 299, 315-320
One-Stroke Environ, 1018
Ontogenetic stage, 128
Ontogenic shifts. See Calorie sources
Oochoristica. See Tokay Gecko
Oocysts, 348
    morphology, 348t
    shedding, 757
    transmission agents, 756
OP. See Osteoporosis
Opheodrys aestivus. See Rough Greensnakes
Ophidian paramyxovirus (OPMV), 403, 858
    diagnosis, 872
    laboratory tests, HI usage, 859t
Ophionyssus acertinus. See Red mites
Ophionyssus natricis. See Snake mite

Ophiophagous snake, proximity, 56
Ophioptid mites, 724
Ophisthotonos, 404
Ophthalmic examination, 323-324
Ophthalmic instruments, advantages, 583
Ophthalmology, 323
Opioid agents
    investigation, 447
    usage, 444, 445, 451
Opisthoglyphous teeth, 48
OPMV. See Ophidian paramyxovirus
Opportunistic bacterial infections, 156
Optic nerve, role, 240
Oral cavity. See Alligator; Snakes
    characteristics, 145-146
    ciliated mucous epithelium, lining, 145
    congenital disorders, 924
    disorders, 924-929
    examination, 151, 499
    flashing. See Bearded Dragon
    flora, 228
    neoplastic diseases, 928
    nutritional diseases, 928-929
    oral/rostral trauma, 924
Oral exudates, 687
Oral gavage, 539
Oral ketoconazole, usage, 210
Oral membranes, edema, 676
Oral neoplasma, 687
Oral trauma. See Beak; Oral cavity; Teeth
Orchidasma amphiorchis. See Loggerhead Seaturtle
Orchidectomy, 595-597
Orenoco Crocodile (Crocodylus intermedius), distribution, 103
Organ hypertrophy, 500
Organic bone matrix, deposition, 601f
Organomegaly, 506f
Organophosphates, 1068-1069
    action, mechanism, 1069
    clinical signs, 1069
    intoxication, 246
        insidious chronic form, 731
    neurotoxic action, 730
    treatment, 1069
    usage. See Mite infestation
Ornate Box Turtle (Terrapene ornata)
    botfly pores, visibility, 696f
    carapaces, whitish areas, 698f
    Chapiniella sp. egg, 356f
    hematologic values, 1113
    scutes, missing, 698f
    serum biochemical values, 1113
Ornate Horned Frog (Ceratophrys ornata)
    acellular fluid, protein level, 957f
    chronic nephritis, 957f
    face, hemangioma, 966f
    hydrops, 957f
    postsurgical photograph, 967f
    substandard conditions, 956f
    ventrum, epidermal ulceration, 958f
Ornithodoros talaje. See Ticks
Ornithodoros turicata, 1026
Orogastric tube, insertion, 85f
Oropharynx, discharges, 690
ORO stain, 810
Orthomolecular medicine, usage, 438-439
Orthopedics, 581, 599

Orthoplast, 602
Oscellated Skink (*Abelpharus* sp.), spectacles, 66
OSHA. *See* Occupational Safety and Health Administration
Osmoregulation, 462
Osmoregulatory function, assessment, 527
Osmosis, principles, 540
Osseous metaplasia, 908
Ossifying spondylosis, 683
Osteitis deformans, 856, 908
Osteodermal armor. *See* Crocodilians
Osteoderms, 67-68
Osteolaemus tetraspis. *See* West African Dwarf Crocodile
Osteolysis, 857-858
Osteomyelitis, 856-857
   radiographic signs, 909
Osteopetrosis, 404
Osteoporosis (OP), 848-849
   differentials, 849
Osteotomy, 590f
   necessity, 871
   performing. *See* Three-sided osteotomy
Oswaldofilaria, 184
Outdoor enclosures. *See* Reptiles; Snakes
   planning. *See* Chelonians
   usage, 36
Outer epidermal generation layer (OEGL), 198f
Ova, external incubation (viability), 482
Ovarian follicles, development, 594f
Ovarian teratoma. *See* Green Iguana
Ovarian vessels, ligation, 598f
Ovariectomy, 595f
   performing, 595
Ovaries
   identification, 669
   removal, 594
Ovariosalpingectomy, 593-595
Ovary
   elevation, 595f
   vena cava, proximity, 595f
Overfeeding, concerns, 284
Overgrown rhamphotheca, 698, 699f
Oversupplementation, intoxications, 292
Oviduct
   characteristics, 753f
   prolapse, 752-753
Oviductal blood vessel, pinpoint coagulation, 627f
Oviductal epithelial cells, 406
Oviductal openings, avoidance, 527
Oviductal prolapse, 389
Oviductal scarring/stricture, 791
Oviducts, 529
   characteristics, 791f
Oviparous species, caruncle (presence), 369f
Oviposition, 367, 387-388
   history, 788
   occurrence, 1009
Ovipositorium (lay-box), 388
Ovocentesis. *See* Percutaneous ovocentesis
Owner present euthanasia, 565
Oxygen
   affinity, 128
   chamber, usage, 134
   dissociation curves, 128

Oxygen—cont'd
   dissolution, 944
   movement, 133
   saturation, 128
   supplement, need, 450
   supplemental therapy, 876
Oxygen-rich circuits, oxygen-poor circuits (contrast), 47
Oxytetracycline, usage, 642
Oxytocin, administration, 388, 789-790
Oxyurida (pinworms). *See* Green Iguana
   genera, 358t
   larva, impaction. *See* Desert Tortoise
   order, 357-358
Oxyurid spp. *See* Bearded Dragon
Ozolaimus sp. *See* Green Iguana
   posterior end, 358f

P

Pachypsolus irroratus. *See* Loggerhead Seaturtle
Pachytritoni brevipes. *See* Paddle-tailed Newt
Packed cell volume (PCV), 546, 949
   assessment, 533
   decrease, 652
   determination, 453
   values, 632
Paddle-tailed Newt (*Pachytritoni brevipes*)
   bacterial dermatosepticemia, 957f
   throat, erythema, 957f
Paecilomyces lilacinus, isolation, 222f
Paecilomyces pneumonia, isolation, 222-223
Paget's disease (PD), 850, 908
Paget's syndrome, 678
PAH. *See* Para-amino-hippurate
Pain control, studies, 776
Painted Turtle (*Chrysemys picta*)
   hematologic values, 1117
   serum biochemical values, 1117
Palatine-pterygoid veins, visualization, 514
Paleosuchus palpebrosus. *See* Dwarf Caiman
Pale tongue/mucous membranes, 700
Palmaris longus muscles, 639
Palpebral edema, 933
Palpebrum, caseous exudate (presence), 832f
Pamidronate, usage, 292
Pancake Tortoise (*Malochochersus tornieri*)
   fontanels, presence, 174f
   shell, flattening, 84f
Pancreas. *See* Endocrine pancreas
   biopsy, 826
   function, 148-149
   necropsy examination, 576
   paramyxovirus infection, 860f
Pancreatic acinar cells, 406
Pancreatic ducts, hyperplasia, 859
Pancreatic polypeptide (PP) cells, 822
Panizza, foramen, 106
Panniculus reflex, 241
Panophthalmoscope, usage, 323
Panther Chameleon (*Furcifer pardalis*)
   abscess, 715f
   balance problems, 855f
   belly-hugging crouching stance, 287f
   carotid artery, occlusion, 855f
   growth, 252f

Panther Chameleon—cont'd
   head tilt, 855f
   nutritional secondary hyperparathyroidism, 287f
Paper medical tape, usage, 585f
Paper towels, substrate, 370
Papillomatosis, 201
Papillomatous lesions, characteristics, 412
Papillomavirus-associated skin lesions, documentation, 412
Papillomaviruses, 1155-1156
Papovaviridae, 411-412
   clinical features, 412
   control/treatment, 412
   immunity/diagnosis, 412
   pathology, 412
   transmission, 412
Papuan Python (*Liasis papuanus*), incoordination/disorientation (signs), 838f
Para-amino-hippurate (PAH), variation, 878
Paracoccidioides brasiliensis, 223
Parakeratosis, focal area, 408
Paramedian incision, disadvantage, 588
Paramyxo-like virus, 248
Paramyxoviridae, 401-404
   clinical features. *See* Snakes
   clinical progression, 401
   control, 403-404
   diagnosis, 403
   epizootiology, 401-402
   immunity, 403
   pathology, 402-403
   transmission, 402
   treatment, 403-404
   vaccination, 404
Paramyxovirus-associated lesions, 402
Paramyxoviruses, 858, 1151-1153. *See also* Clinically healthy animals
   acute signs, 858
   clinical signs, 857-858
   diagnosis, 859-860
   documentation, 401
   global distributions, 401
   identification, 706, 872
   infection
      impact, 402
      snake tissues, 860f
   isolates, recovery, 402
   peracute signs, 858
   prevention/control, 860-861
   risk, 33
   stability, 403-404
   titers, 1012
Parasite-covered seaturtles, 996
Parasites, 1160-1170
   control. *See* Captive reptiles
   dead end, 343
   diagnosis, 344-346
   elimination. *See* Bearded Dragon
   treatment, 362-363
Parasitic diseases, 154-156, 184-185
Parasitic enteritis, 753
Parasiticides, usage, 213
Parasitic infections, 248, 577
Parasitic pneumonia, 874
Parasitic stomatitis, 928

Parasitism
  captivity, impact, 720
  diagnosis, 35
Parasitology, 343
Paratenic host, 343
Parathion, usage, 1067
Parathormone (PTH) mediation, 463
Parathyroid gland
  necropsy examination, 576
  negative feedback, 845
Parathyroid hormone (PTH)
  physiologic interrelationship.
    See Calcium
  release, 842
Paratrichosoma, impact, 207
Paravertebral muscles, IM injections, 445
Parenchyma, appearance. See Bearded
    Dragon
Parental care, 366
Parenteral nutrition support, 280
Parenteral vitamin A, high doses (impact).
    See Tortoises
Paresis. See Flaccid paresis; Hindlimb
    paresis
Parietal eye, 324-325
  anatomy, 324-325
  physiology, 325
Parietal scales, 974
Paromomycin, usage, 760
Parotid gland, development, 176
Parson's Chameleon (*Chamaeleo parsoni*)
  dental radiographs, 479f
    mandibular rami, osteolysis (rostral
      portions), 479f
Parthenogenesis, 377
Partial anorexia, 386
Partially rectified waveform, 622
Partial nucleic acid sequences,
    comparison, 402
Parturition date, prediction, 383
Parviridae, 410
  clinical features, 410
Parvoviruses, 1156
PAS. See Periodic acid-Schiff
Passive range-of-motion exercises, 612
Pasture, usage. See Sulcata Tortoise
Patches. See Dermatology
Patency, testing. See Lacrimal system
Pathogenic flora, distinction, 228f
Pathogenicity, recommendation, 232t
Pathogenic mycoplasmosis, emergence.
    See Alligators
Pathogenic protozoa, introduction, 960
Pathogen isolation, 1062-1063
Pathologic fractures, 605
  NSHP, impact, 775
  stabilization, difficulty, 601f
Pathologic spinal fractures, occurrence, 244
Patients
  assessment. See Critical reptile patient
  examination, 666-673
  positioning, 585, 666
  restraint/positioning, 472-474
PBS. See Phosphate buffer saline
PCR. See Polymerase chain reaction
PCV. See Packed cell volume
PD. See Paget's disease
PDT. See Photodynamic therapy

Pectoral girdle, 554
Pectoral scutes, 972
Pedal luring. See Amphibians
Pellets
  consumption. See Carnivores;
    Herbivores; Omnivores
  soaking, 271f
Pelodryas caerulea. See White's Tree Frog
Pelomedusa sp. See Side-necked Turtle
Pelvic bones, injury (avoidance), 590f
Penicillin, 927
  usage. See Semisynthetic penicillins
Penicillium sp., isolation, 220f
Penile prolapse, 389, 862-864. See also
    Terrapins; Tortoises; Turtles
Pen light, usage, 323
Pennsylvania, herpetological societies, 7t
Pentastomiasis (armilliferiasis), 1025-1026
Pentastomids (pentastomes), 360-362, 874.
    See also Narrowhead Softshell Turtle;
    Pythons
  eggs, 361f
  hosts/genera, 360t
  inflammatory response. See Indigo Snake
  life cycle, 360
  parasite, 1025
Peppermint, dosage, 431
Peptostreptococcus spp., 235f
Peracetic acid solution, usage, 554
Percutaneous ovocentesis, 790
Performance pet foods, 286
Perfusion, 545
  evaluation. See Renal perfusion
Periarticular bony proliferation, 908
Pericardial sac
  evidence, 576f
  tophi deposition, 796f
Perinatology, 365
Periocular edema, 933
Periocular lesions, 393
Periodic acid-Schiff (PAS) staining, 227, 458
  positive/negative values, 459
Periodontal disease, 924-926
  treatment, 925-926
Periodontal pockets, 925
Perioperative antibiotics, usage, 613
Peripheral blood, necropsy examination, 578
Peripheral cornea, cholesterol crystals
    (infiltration), 336
Peripheral edema, 181f
Peripheral insulin resistance, 274
Peripheral nerves
  biopsy, 531
  composition, 239
Peripheral pulses, doppler flow detector
    (usage), 182f
Perivascular cuffing, identification, 248
Permectrin II, usage, 729
Permethrin, 733
Per os (PO) fluid replacement route, 634
Pes, fractures (ball bandage usage), 604f
Pesticides
  avoidance, 943
  exposure, 956
  ubiquity, 963
Pest problems, 1014
Petechiae, 511. See also Lizards; Terrapins;
    Tortoises; Turtles

Pets
  caring, concerns, 21
  death, guilt, 21
  foods. See Performance pet foods
    supply, 270-271. See also Carnivores
  loss
    discussion, 21
    support groups/web sites, 23
  memorialization, 21
  remains
    disposal questions, 21
    retrieval, 567
  reptiles, 14-15, 1040
    sedation, 490
  stores, interaction. See Reptile practice
Pet shops, 1015-1016
Phagocitized microorganisms,
    destruction, 455
Phallus. See Chelonians; Crocodilians
Pharmacognosy, 430
Pharyngeal edema. See Lizards
Pharyngostomy feeding tube,
    premeasurement, 640f
Pharynx, visualization, 558
Phelsuma guentheri. See Round Island Gecko
Phelsuma standingii. See Standings Day
    Gecko
Phialophera, 209
Philtrum, visualization, 558
Phobosuchus, species, 100
Phosphate buffer saline (PBS), 815
Phospholipids, 139
Phosphorus, metabolism, 463
Photodynamic therapy (PDT), 299
  morbidity, chance, 315
Photometric characteristics. See Lamps
Photoperiod. See Captive reptiles
  impact, 30
  inhospitability, 784
Phrynops genus. See Hilaire's Side-neck
    Turtle
Phrynosoma cornutum. See Horned Lizards
Phthisis bulbi, 334
Physical examination, 533
Physical restraint/examination, 490
Physical therapy (PT), 612
Physignathus cocincinus. See Chinese Water
    Dragon; Water Dragon
Physignathus concincinus. See Asian Water
    Dragons
Physignathus sp. See Water Dragon
Physiologic behavior, 169-171
Physiology, 145-149
Pianka, ER, 12
Pica, 955
Pigmented tissue, penetrations
    (diagrammatic representation), 622f.
    See also Nonpigmented tissue
Pig-nosed Turtle (*Carettochelys insculpta*), 80f
Pineal gland, necropsy examination, 575-576
Pinesnake (*Pituophis melanoleucus mugitus*),
    shed skin (fungal growth), 218
Pinkies. See Baby mice
  exclusive diet, 842
Pin purchase, maximization, 605f
Pinworms
  genera. See Oxyurida
  presence. See Greek Tortoise

Piperacillin, 656
Pirhemocyton, 804
Piroplasms, 802
Pituitary gland, necropsy examination, 575-576
Pituophis catenifer. See Gophersnake
Pituophis melanoleucas. See Gophersnake
Pituophis melanoleucus mugitus. *See* Pinesnake
Pit viper venom, enzymes (presence), 1075t
PIX disease. *See* Alligators
Plantar/palmar flap, usage, 609
Plant-based pellets, characteristics, 270
Plants, 266-270
　constituents/actions, 430t
　feeding. *See* Reptiles
　nutritional contents, 267
　poisonings, 1706-1078
　risks, 267-269
　toxicity, factors. *See* Poisonous plants
Plaques
　location, 894
　presence, 335
Plasma
　biochemical abnormalities, 1003
　biochemistries, indication, 838
　increase, 883
　laboratory evaluation, 464
Plasma cell cholinesterase activity, 731
Plasma chemistry profile, 652
Plasma CK activity, 464
Plasmalyte-A, 543
Plasma phosphorus concentrations, 464
Plasma potassium concentrations, 462
Plasma retinol, measurement, 832
Plasma uric acid, 462
Plasmodium, species, 803-804
Plastic boxes, environmental enrichment (absence), 55f
Plastic drapes, usage, 585, 586f
Plastic endoscope protectors, placement, 553f
Plastron
　bones, 893
　distraction, 592f
　hinges, 173
　nomenclature, 84f
　pattern, 972
　removal, 575f
　　pelvic bones, damage (avoidance), 590f
Plastronotomy
　flap, seal, 591f
　healing, 591f
　incisions, 592f
　performing, 770
　usage, 769f
Platysternidae, 80-81
Platysternon megacephalum. See Big-headed Turtle
Plerocercoids, 299
Pleroceroid
　attachment, 1026f
　development, 1026f
Pleural edema, 181f
Pleural membranes, incision, 553
Pleurodirans, 78
Pleurodira (suborder), 79f
Pluck, removal, 573

Plumed Basilisk *(Basiliscus plumifrons)*, facial abscess, 519f
PMMA. *See* Polymethylmethacrylate
Pneumonia, 865. *See also* Bacterial pneumonia; Fungal pneumonia; Parasitic pneumonia; Viral pneumonia
　biochemistry, 880-881
　blood analysis, 880-881
　clinical investigation, 880-882
　clinical signs, 865
　coeliotomy biopsy, 887-888
　commonness. *See* Caseous pneumonia
　cranial tail cut-down biopsy, 887
　cystocentesis, 882
　cytodiagnosis, 467f
　diagnostic plan, 865-872
　differential diagnosis, 872-874
　endoscopic biopsy, 888
　endoscopic catheterization, 882
　endoscopy, 868, 871, 886
　hematology, usage, 880
　history, 865
　noninfectious causes, 874-875
　physical examination, 865-867, 880
　radiography, usage, 867, 885-886
　renal biopsy, 886-888
　scintigraphy, 886
　suggestions, 466f
　systemic evaluation, 872
　transtracheal wash, usage, 867-868
　treatment, 875-876
　ultrasonography, 886
　ultrasound-guided biopsy, 888
　urinalysis, 881-882
　urine
　　diagnostic imaging, 885-886
　　dipstick evaluation, 882-883
　voided urine, examination, 881-882
PO. *See* Per os
Pogona vitticeps. See Bearded Dragon
Poikilothermic reptiles, 133-134, 251
Poinsettia, impact, 1077
Poisonous animals, 1074-1706
Poisonous lizards, 1075
Poisonous plants
　tolerance, 269
　toxicity, factors, 1706t
Poliglecaprone, recommendation, 864
Polychromasia, 454
Polydelphis sp. *See* Reticulated Python
Polydipsia, 292. *See also* Lizards
Polyene macrolide antibiotics, 154
Polyene macrolide derivatives, 154
Polyglyconate, recommendation, 864
Polymerase chain reaction (PCR), 153. *See also* Mycoplasma; Reverse transcriptase PCR
　amplification, 224
　assay, 156, 931
　　false negative results, 902
　　test sensitivity/specificity, estimation, 902-903
　illustration, 1063f
　PCR-based assay, 400-401
　　usage, 407. *See also* Iridovirus nucleic acid; Viral nucleic acid

Polymerase chain reaction—cont'd
　PCR-based screening. *See* Feces; Tracheal washes
　PCR-based testing. *See* Secretions
　benefit, 396
　sensitivity, estimation, 903
　technique, 900, 902
　usage, 234, 1063-1064
Polymerase genes, comparison, 402
Polymethylmethacrylate (PMMA), 657
　beads, 657
Polypropylene, usage, 581
Polypropylene IV catheter, 955
Polysaccharide, 257
Polytetrafluoroethylene patch, placement, 999f
Polytrauma cases, 986
Polyurea. *See* Lizards
Polyuria, 292
Polyvinyl alcohol (PVA), 344
　usage. *See* Feces
Polyvinyl chloride (PVC)
　coupler ring, 984
　tube, usage, 642
Pond turtles, herpesvirus, 393
Poor doer. *See* Chronic poor doer
Poor doing, 839
　history, 284
Porcine reproductive and respiratory syndrome virus (PRRSV), 816
Pore reflection coefficient, 541f
Postcaval vein, 125
Postcoaptation, 602f
Postcooling period, 385
Posterolateral lacrimal gland, 831
Posthatchling Leatherback Turtle, T1-weighted image, 1091f
Postmortem diagnosis, 403
Postmortem examinations, 759-760
Postmortem specimens, electrocardiogram analysis, 565
Postnutritional MBD facial deformities, 848f
Postocular scales, 974
Postoperative analgesia, 443
Postoperative treatment, 986
Postovulatory conditions, 594f,
Postovulatory egg binding, 594
Postprandial handling, 675
Postprandial hyperuricemia, 462
Postpulmonary septum, location, 554
Potassium, absorption/transportation, 462-463
Potassium hydroxide (KOH), treatment, 209
Potentiated sulfas, usage, 653-654
POTR. *See* Preferred optimum temperature range
POTZ. *See* Preferred optimum temperature zone
Pough, FH, 12
Poverty lines. *See* Cachexia
Povidone-iodine, usage, 749
Power sources. *See* Biotelemetry; Telemetry
Pox-like viruses, identification, 708
Poxviruses (pox viruses), 1154. *See* Crocodilians
　evidence, 326
　lesions, 956

Poxviruses—cont'd
  outbreak, 408
  pathogen, 657-658
Poxviridae, 408-409
  clinical features, 408
  control, 409
  diagnosis, 408
  transmission, 408
  treatment, 409
PP. *See* Pancreatic polypeptide
Praziquantel, usage, 968
Preanesthetic evaluation, 443
Precaval veins, 125
Precooling period, 385
Prefemoral fossae, 511
Preferred optimum temperature range
    (POTR), 26-27. *See also* Captive
    reptiles; Species-species POTR
  environmental temperature,
    increase, 450
  maintenance, 29, 448
Preferred optimum temperature zone
    (POTZ), 87, 127, 193.
    See also Chelonians
  maintenance, 533, 865
  top level, 213
  upper ranges, 934
Prefrontal scales, 974
Pregnancy
  determination, 385-387
  identification, 482
  latter stages, 377
Prehensile-tailed Skink (*Corucia zebrata*)
  hematologic values, 1111
  serum biochemical values, 1111
  technicium scan, 488f
Prekilled pinkie/adult mice,
    purchase/thawing, 262f
Premedication. *See* Analgesia; Anesthesia
Preovulatory condition, 594f, 595f
Preovulatory egg binding, 594
Preplaced nonabsorbable sutures, 598f
Pressure-driven mechanical ventilator,
    usage. *See* Bearded Dragon
Prewarmed incubator, egg placement, 368f
Prey bites, 747
  treatment, 747-749
Prey food, usage. *See* Live prey food
Prey odors, absence, 263
Prey presentation, 282
Print pages, usage. *See* Reptile practice
Private breeders/collections, 1014-1015
  fees, 1015
  preventative health, 1015
  safety, 1015
Proban, usage, 1068
Procercoid
  development, 1026f
  ingestion, 1026f
Productive osteolysis, 159f
Prolapse. *See* Cloaca; Green Iguana;
    Hemipenile prolapse; Oviductal
    prolapse; Penile prolapse
  sedation, necessity, 863
Proliferative spinal osteopathy (PSO), 906
  bacterial involvement, 907-908
  clinical signs, 909-910, 910t
  etiologies. *See* Vertebrates

Proliferative spinal osteopathy—cont'd
  presence, 909. *See also* Lizards
  radiographic evidence, 910
Prolonged hypocalcemia, 601f
Propofol
  administration, 447. *See also* Cornsnake;
    Green Iguana
  anesthetic use, documentation, 948
  induction agent, 445
  premedication, 446
  usage, 997
Proprioception
  absence, 856
  assessment, 496
Prosthesis, providing, 610f
Protected species, keeping. *See* Reptiles
Protective glasses/facemasks, 624f
Protein
  analysis, 883
  deficiency, 284
  electrophoresis, 461
  metabolism, end product, 141, 143f
  quality, 254
    examination, 285
  relationship. *See* Herbivores
  synthesis, inhibition, 648
Protein-bound calcium, increase, 464
Protein-losing nephropathy, 882
Proteocephalidae, 155
Proteroglyphous teeth, 48
Prothrombin time (PT), 1073.
    See also One-stage PT
Protonymphs, 721, 732
Protozoa, 960, 1024. *See also* Ciliated
    protozoa; Flagellated protozoa;
    Gut-inhabiting flagellated protozoa
  diseases. *See* Amphibians
  impact, 347
  infestation, 155
Protozoan parasites, detection, 885
Providencia, 233
PRRSV. *See* Porcine reproductive and
    respiratory syndrome virus
Psammophis sp. *See* Sand Snake
Pseudemys floridana. *See* Florida Cooter
Pseudemys sp. *See* Cooter
Pseudoabscess, formation, 335
Pseudoaneurysm, cases, 685
Pseudoarthrosis formation, 477
Pseudobuphthalmos, 331-332
Pseudo calculi. *See* California Desert
    Tortoise
Pseudodiaphragm, 520
Pseudogout, 794
Pseudomonal resistance, 652
Pseudomonas, 202, 232
  infection. *See* Leopard Gecko
Pseudomonas aeruginosa
  bacteria, 920f
  pneumonia. *See* Lungs
Pseudomonas sp. dermatitis, 518
Pseudomonas spp., 1022
  bacteria, growth, 71
Pseudomys scripta. *See* Freshwater Turtles
Pseudoparasites, 344, 345f.
    See also Artifacts; Cornsnake
Pseudophyllidae, 155
Pseudotumors, 201

PSO. *See* Proliferative spinal osteopathy
Psyllium, usage, 992
PT. *See* Physical therapy; Prothrombin time
PTH. *See* Parathormone; Parathyroid
    hormone
Ptyalism, 499. *See also* Lizards
Pubis/umbilical scar, surgical stab, 588f
Public health, threats, 1017
Pueblan Milksnake (*Lampropeltis triangulum
    campbelli*)
  body, kinks, 678f
  fungal dermatitis, 220
Pulmonary disease, squash preparation, 184
Pulmonary lymphofollicular
    hyperplasia, 412
Pulmonary mycoses, 226
Pulmonary vascular resistance, increase, 134
Pulmonary veins, 125
Pulse oximeter, usage. *See* Komodo Dragon
  validation. *See* Green Iguana
Pulse oximetry, 194
  usage. *See* Seaturtle
Pure filtered wave form, 622
Purine metabolism, end product, 793
Purines, degradation, 794f
Purse-string suture. *See* Cloaca
  removal, 863
Push-ups, 171
PVA. *See* Polyvinyl alcohol
PVC. *See* Polyvinyl chloride
P wave, 186
Pylorus, negotiation, 523
Pyogranulomatous hepatitis, 402
Pyramidal shell growth, 699
Pyramiding, 284
Pyrethrins/pyrethroids, 1071-1072
  action, mechanism, 1071
  clinical signs, 1071
  treatment, 1071
  usage. *See* Mite infestation
Pyrimidines, catabolism, 793
Python curtis. *See* Blood Python
Pythoninae, 46
Python molurus bivatattus. *See* Green phase
    Burmese Python
Python molurus bivitattus. *See* Burmese
    Python
Python regius. *See* Ball Python; Royal
    Python
Python reticulatus. *See* Reticulated Python
Python sebae. *See* Rock Python
Pythons (*Python* sp.)
  airway resolution,
    CT reconstruction, 1093f
  blood collection, cardiocentesis
    (impact), 514f
  burns, resolution, 923
  cellulitis, 29f
  cestodes
    eggs, 353f
    larva, 354f
  cloacocolonic internal examination, 501f
  coagulase-positive infection,
    development, 232f
  coronal frontal MRI, 1094f
  eggs
    brooding, 173
    coiling, 379f

Pythons—cont'd
　hematologic values, 1104
　hemopericardium, 184
　labial pits, snake mites (Ophionyssus
　　　natricis), 720f
　midsagittal MRI, 1094f
　mouth rot, aminoglycoside
　　　treatment, 797f
　MRI
　　axial composite, 1094f
　　trunk composite, 1094f
　pentastomid parasite, close-up, 361f
　radiograph, 185f
　serum biochemical values, 1104
　shivering, 173
　skeleton, ventral view, 1093f
　slough, dorsal head section, 498f
　spectacle, wedge resection, 530f
　submandibular skin laceration, 497f
　subspectacular exudates,
　　　drainage/collection, 530f
　tapeworm egg, 355f
　tophi depositions, 797f
　traumatic wound, suturing, 232f

Q

Q fever, 1023
Qi
　concept, 433
　definition, 429t
QRS, widening, 187f
QRS complex, 186
Q-T intervals, 182
Quarantine, usefulness, 728
Queen Snakes (Regina septemvittata),
　　outdoor enclosures, 36
Quick-core disposable biopsy needle,
　　usage, 810

R

Radiant heat, 916, 917
Radiant lamps, availability, 535f
Radiated Tortoise (T. radiata)
　hematologic values, 1114
　serum biochemical values, 1114
Radiation
　therapy, 299
　types, 1081t
Radio, usage. See Reptile practice
Radiodense urolith. See Tortoises
Radiofrequency. See Herpetologic
　　surgery
　safety. See Lasers
Radiographic anatomy, 1097
Radiographic exposures,
　　recommendations, 472t
Radiographic findings, abnormalities, 562
Radiographic interpretation, 475-484
Radiographic plates, multiple
　　exposures, 475f
Radiographs, characteristics, 471
Radiography, 189-191
　usage, 383
Radioisotope scans, usage, 191f.
　　See also Blood flow evaluation; Renal
　　perfusion
Radiology, 472-484
Radiopacity, increase, 484f

Radiosurgery, 617-618
　equipment, 622-623
　waveforms, surgical uses, 623f
Radiotelemetry, transmission distances, 615
Railietiella frenatus. See Tokay Gecko
Raillietiella spp., occurrence, 360
Rainbow Boa (Epicrates cenchria)
　hematologic values, 1103
　serum biochemical values, 1103
　spectacle, hole, 748f
Rainbow uromastyx (Uromastyx benti),
　　muscle loss, 275f
Raiti, P, 1116
Rappaport-Vassiliadis broth, 900
Rare Skink (Leiolopisma telfairii), squamous
　　cell carcinomas, 211f
Rats
　buccal mucosa, laser surgery, 623
　food, usage, 39
　obesity, 806
Ratsnake (Elaphe guttata). See Red Ratsnake
　caudal tail/vein, blood collection, 514f
　oral swab cytology, 466f
Ratsnake (Elaphe sp.), pulmonary
　　parasitism, 485f
Raytek Ranger ST, 87
RBC. See Red blood cell
rDNA. See Ribosomal DNA
Rear-fanged Hog-nosed Snake (Heterodon
　　nasicus), 146f
Receivers, 615
Rectilinear locomotion, 51
Rectum, sterile swab placement, 228f
Red blood cell (RBC)
　cholinesterase activity, 731
　usage, 951
Red-eared Slider (Trachemys scripta elegans)
　aural abscess, 744f
　bilateral calcium phosphate
　　　ureteroliths, 763f
　blepharedema, 833f
　carapace
　　deep shell abscessation, 895f
　　superficial erosions, 894f
　corneal cholesterol dystrophy, 336f
　cutaneous ulceration, 509f
　hematologic values, 1117
　hyphema, 338f
　keratin scute material, exposure, 894f
　lung inflation, granulomatous
　　　inflammation, 561f
　mycotic dermatitis, 509f
　penile prolapse, 862f
　Salmonella, occurrence, 643
　serum biochemical values, 1117
　Siamese twins, 374f
　subcarapacial site venous sinus, blood
　　　collection, 516f
　valve control, 186
Red-eyed Leaf Frog (Agalychnis callidryas)
　body form, 942f
　cloacal prolapse, 961f
　emaciation, 958f
　rostral abrasion, 964f
Red-footed Tortoise (Geochelone
　　carbonaria)
　gender determination, plastron shape
　　　(usage), 512f

Red-footed Tortoise—cont'd
　hematologic values, 1114
　serum biochemical values, 1114
Red leg (bacterial dermatosepticemia),
　　ventral erythema (relationship), 956f
Red Milksnake (Lampropeltis triangulum
　　syspila)
　eggs, characteristics, 388f
　ovipositoria placement, 388f
Red mites (Ophionyssus acertinus), 720f.
　　See also Chuckwalla
Red Ratsnake (Elaphe guttata)
　hematologic values, 1106
　nematode egg (Rhabdias sp.), 355f
　serum biochemical values, 1106
Red-tailed Boa (Boa constrictor)
　cerebrum, 406f
　　glial cells/neuron cell bodies,
　　　cytoplasm (inclusions), 406f
　chondrosarcoma, 319f
　chronic infectious stomatitis, 315f
　esophagram, mucosal folds, 481f
　granulomatous tissue, 315f
　lungs, visualization (dorsal ventral
　　　projection), 483f
　ribs, mass (attachment), 319f
　tracheal/lung wash cytology, 466f, 467f
Refeeding syndrome, 282
Reference
　intervals, obtaining (difficulty), 461
　sources, 10-12. See also Reptile clinicians
Reflectance pulse oximeter probe,
　　placement. See Green Iguana
Reflexes, evaluation, 448
Regeneration, forms, 198-199
Regina septemvittata. See Queen Snakes
Regional trade, CITES convention, 1041-1042
Regurgitated food items, 758
Regurgitation, 939. See also Lizards; Snakes;
　　Terrapins; Tortoises; Turtles
　differentials/diagnosis, 939-940
　treatment, 940
Rehydration, completion, 963
Reinsemination, 379
Renal abscesses, 764f
Renal adenocarcinomas (Lucke's renal
　　tumor), 394
Renal amoebiasis, 959-960
Renal anatomy, 135
Renal biopsy, 525-527. See also Pneumonia
　endoscopic biopsy, 527
　ultrasound-guided biopsy, 527
Renal calculi, occurrence, 795
Renal cysts, 879
Renal damage disease, biochemical
　　parameters. See Green Iguana
Renal disease, 879-880
　diagnosis/clinical management, 878
　dietary changes, 281
Renal edema, 879
Renal failure, 280, 394, 692
　physical presentation. See Chronic renal
　　　failure
　syndrome, 694
Renal function
　assessment, 888-889
　evaluation, 527-528, 889
Renal metabolic bone disease (RMBD), 841

Renal neoplasms, 404
Renal parynchema, homogenous appearance, 798f
Renal perfusion evaluation, radioisotope scans (usage), 191f
Renal physiology, 135, 140-144, 878-879. See also Reptiles
Renal-portal circulation system, 317
Renal portal system, 185-186, 643-644. See also Chelonians; Crocodilians
Renal portal veins, 138
Renal secondary hyperparathyroidism (RSHP), 847-848
Renal tubular disease, 462
Renin-angiotensin system, 462
Renoliths, reports, 764f
Reoviridae, 407-408
   clinical features, 407
   control, 408
   diagnosis, 407-408
   transmission, 407
Reoviruses, 1153
Replacement fluid, selection, 633-634
Reproduction
   stimuli, 378, 385
   timing/frequency. See Reptiles
Reproductive anatomy. See Clinical reproductive anatomy; Female reproductive anatomy; Male reproductive anatomy
Reproductive behavior, 171-173
Reproductive biology, 376
Reproductive cycles. See Reptiles
Reproductive disorders, 389
Reproductive system
   diagnostic techniques, 528-529
   tumors, 301t, 302t, 305t, 312t
Reproductive tract
   necropsy examination, 576-577
   visualization, 669
   yolks, release, 596f
Reptile-associated salmonellosis, 658
Reptile-origin *Salmonella*, implication, 906
Reptile practice, 1042-1043
   building, 1
   client
      diagnosis, 4
      services, 2-4
   community member, establishment, 5
   equipment, 1-2
      list, recommendation, 547t
   facilities, 1-2
   identity, establishment, 4
   integrated practice, 1
   Internet, usage, 5
   marketing, 4-8
   pet stores, interaction, 5
   print/yellow pages, usage, 4-5
   promotional items, 5, 8
   revenue generation, 8
   staff, 2
   television/radio/newspapers, usage, 5
   value, establishment, 2-3
Reptiles. See Pets
   aggressiveness. See Hatchling reptiles
   anatomy, 442-443
   bad news, delivery, 20
   bark chips, 69

Reptiles—cont'd
   behaviors, 163t
   caging, requirement. See Hospitals
   clinicians, reference sources, 9
   companion, 1040
   customs/excise, 1939
   defensive behaviors, 163-169
   DH, genera, 360t
   diagnostics, 535f
   dietary intake, essential nutrients, 273f
   display, 1040-1041
   dog/cat cages, modification/usage, 33f
   ECG
      results, evaluation, 188t
      value, 193f
   ectothermic quality, 26
   egg incubation, substrates (usage), 367t
   entertainment, 1040-1041
   erythrocytes, 453-454
   escape artists, 68
   exhibition, 1040-1041
   fieldwork, 1040
   food
      offering, 263
      usage. See Carnivorous neonatal reptiles
   formulary, 1119
   functional diaphragm, absence, 132f
   hatchlings, aggressiveness, 372f
   hazards. See Venomous reptiles
   herpesvirus, pathology, 248
   hobby, 1040
   hosts, 353t
      genera, 358t
   incubator, design, 367f
   invertebrate prey, feeding, 266
   large collections, 15-16
      emotion/finance, 15f
   leukocytes, 454-459
   medicine, stress (importance), 122
   microscopic anatomy, 138-140
   morphologic adaptations, 164t
   national laws, 1042
   nonrespiratory gas exchange, capability, 133f
   nutrients/supplements, trial dosages, 439t
   outdoor enclosures, 36f
   owners, groups/types, 4
   patient, therapeutics. See Critical reptile patient
   personalities/affection, reports, 15f
   physiology, 442-443
   plants, feeding, 269-270
   plastic container, usage. See Arboreal reptiles
   protected species, keeping, 1040
   protection. See Wild reptiles
   pulmonary disease, placement, 134f
   questions, 20-22
   racks, usage/construction, 28f
   replacement. See Cats; Dogs
   reproduction
      frequency, 378-379
      timing, 378
   reproductive condition, ultrasonography (usage), 383
   reproductive cycles, 376-379
   reproductive mode, 378t

Reptiles—cont'd
   retroviridae, 405
   scientific research, 1041
   sexual determination, 379-384
      probing method, 382f
      technique, preference, 380t
   skin, 196-198
      sample-taking, 200t
      shedding cycle, 198f
   species, global movement, 391
   surgery pack, 582
   temperature ranges, preference. See Captive reptiles
   trade, 1041-1042
   virus activity, documentation, 391t
Reptiles, 10
Reptisun lights (ZooMed), 37
Resection-anastomosis, 597
Resident flora, gram-negative bacteria (relationship), 230
Respiration, control, 443
Respiratory anatomy, 129-133, 442-443
Respiratory distress, coalescing lesions (impact), 393
Respiratory epithelium, degeneration, 466f
Respiratory infections, caseous component, 866f
Respiratory performance, 448-449
Respiratory physiology, 129, 133-134, 442-443
Respiratory signs. See Snakes
Respiratory system
   diagnostic techniques, 519-521
   histologic lesions, 859
   modification, 944-945
   tumors, 300t-301t, 314t
Respiratory tract
   anatomy, 129-133
   endoscopic examination, 556-558
   necropsy examination, 578
   neoplasms, 690
   sampling, 228
Retained eggs or fetuses, viability, 791-792
Retained eye cap, removal, 784f
Retained eye shields. See True retained eye shields
   elevation, 783-784
Retained ocular spectacle tissue, 780
Retained skin
   fungal infections, 783
   removal, 780f
Retained spectacle, 330-331. See also Gartersnake
   diagnosis, 330-331
   treatment, 331
Reticulated Python *(Python reticulatus)*
   hematologic values, 1105
   Polydelphis sp., 357f
      jugular vein, example, 638f
   serum biochemical values, 1105
Retinal forceps, 583
Retinas, 340-341
   anatomy, 340
   disease, 341
   visual tracts, 340
Retinol-binding protein, 834
Retractor bulbi muscles, 327
Retrieval forceps, 552-553

Retroviridae, 404-408. *See also* Reptiles
  clinical features, 404
  clinical presentations, 405
  control, 407
  diagnosis, 406-407
  epizootiology, 405-406
  immunity, 406-407
  pathogenesis, 406-407
  pathology, 406
  transmission, 406
  vaccination, 407
Retroviruses
  association. *See* Inclusion body disease
  detection. *See* Type-C retrovirus
Reverse transcriptase PCR (RT-PCR), 153, 710, 817
Rhabdias sp. *See* Red Ratsnake
Rhabditoidea (order), 354-355
Rhacodactylus Gecko
  hemipenal prolapse, 508f
  spectacled eye, 506f
Rhacodactylus sp. *See* Caledonian Lizard
Rhamphotheca. *See* Overgrown rhamphotheca
  moisture/dried mucus, 700
Rhamphotyphlops braminus. *See* Blind Snakes
Rheumatoid arthritis, 906
Rheumatoid immune mediated-type arthritis, 906
Rhinitis (runny nose), 815
  diagnosis, 817
Rhinocerous Iguana (*Cyclura cornuta*)
  abdomen, swelling, 319f
  caudal coelom, radiograph, 319f
  ovarian carcinoma, 319f
  tapeworm egg, 354f
Rhode Island, herpetological societies, 7t
Rhynchocephalia (order), 137
Ribbonsnakes (*Thamnophis proximus*), outdoor enclosures, 36
Ribosomal DNA (rDNA), PCR amplification, 1063
Ribosomal RNA (rRNA), 934, 1064
Ribosome inhibition, 651
Ricins, impact, 1077
Rickettsia, 951
Righting reflexes, loss, 401, 404, 496f
Rigid endoscopes, handling, 553
Rigid endoscopy, flexible endoscopy (contrast), 550-551, 550t
Ringed Python (*Bothrochilus boa*), 44f
Ringer's solution, 964, 968
  usage. *See* Lactated Ringer's solution
Ring-necked Snake (*Diadophis* sp.), coiled tail display, 166f
River terrapin (*Batagur baskar*), seizure (illegal shipment), 1032f
RMBD. *See* Renal metabolic bone disease
RNA activity, increase, 467
Roccal D, 729
Roccal-D, usage, 34, 1018
Rock Python (*Python sebae*)
  skin damage, 199f
  wound, adhesive drape (usage), 204f
Rocuronium, 422
  investigation, 447
Rodenticides, 1072-1073

Rodents
  bite trauma, 677-678
  colony, maintenance, 735
  prey, average weight/length, 262t
Romanowsky stains, 455
Ronnel, usage, 1068
Rose Bengal dye, usage, 329
Ross, RA, 12
Rossi, JV, 12
Rossi, R, 12
Rostral trauma. *See* Beak; Oral cavity; Teeth
Rosy Boa (*Lichanura trivirgata*), 44f
Rotary power tools, 894
Rough Greensnakes (*Opheodrys aestivus*), outdoor enclosures, 36
Round Island Gecko (*Phelsuma guentheri*), liver TEM, 802f
Rous sarcoma virus, 299
Royal Python (*Python regius*)
  abraded spectacle, 328f
  dyspnea, 500f
  endoscopic view, 521f
  granulomatous pneumonia, 521f
  indented spectacle, 331f
  mycotic dermatitis, 498f
  open-mouth breathing, 500f
  retained spectacle, 499f
rRNA. *See* Ribosomal RNA
RSHP. *See* Renal secondary hyperparathyroidism
RT-PCR. *See* Reverse transcriptase PCR
Rubber Boa (*Charina bottae*), tail behavior, 166f
Rubber jaw, 953
Rubel, GA, 12
Russian Tortoise (*Agrionemys horsfieldii*), oral examination, 151f

S

Sago palms. *See* Cycad palms
Sailfin Lizard (*Hydrosaurus pustulatus*), dermatitis (inflammation/ulceration/crusts), 685f
Salads, bite-sized portions, 270
Salamanders
  bleeding, 950
  digits, regeneration, 966
  tail autotomy, 947
Salicylic acid treatment, 412
Saline solution, infusion, 558
Salivary gland, paramyxovirus infection, 860f
Salmon calcitonin (SCT)
  dosage, 846
  effects. *See* Mammals
  protocol treatment. *See* Green Iguana (*Iguana iguana*)
  side effects, 846
Salmonella, 232, 900
  diagnostic methods, 900
  elimination, enrofloxacin (usage), 650
  infection rate, 1020
  isolation, microbiologic culture techniques, 901
  microbiologic isolation methods, 900-901
  nomenclature, 900
  nonculture diagnostic methods, 901-902
  occurrence. *See* Red-eared Slider

Salmonella—cont'd
  serotypes, 902
  cultures, 1020t
  implication. *See* Death; Zoonoses
  test results, interpretation, 904
Salmonella spp.
  dermatitis. *See* Green Iguana; Indigo Snake
  growth, selective medium, 230
Salmonellosis, 1018-1022
  zoonotic significance, 1018
Salpingotomy, 790
Salt glands, function, 169
Salt glands, usage, 259
Salt-secreting cells, 332
Salt toxicosis, 963
Saltwater Crocodile (*Crocodylus porosus*), salt glands, 169
Saltwater drowning, 985
Salvadora grahamiae. *See* Texas Patch-nosed Snake
Sample collection. *See* Blood; Clinical chemistries; Diagnostic sample collection
  holding, 534
Sample handling, 229-230. *See also* Clinical chemistries
Sampling devices, variety, 521
Sampling techniques, 227
Sand impaction. *See* Desert Tortoise
Sand Snake (*Psammophis* sp.), sloughing, 199f
Saprolegnia, 209
Saprolegniasis, 959
  presence. *See* Aquatic caecilian
Saprophytic molds, 218
Sarcomas, 404
Sarcosporidia, 1164
Sarocystis sp. *See* Viper
Sauria (suborder), 135
Saurocytozoon, identification, 804
Sauromalus sp. *See* Chuckwalla
Savannah Monitor Lizard (*Varanus exanthematicus*)
  anorexia/lethargy, 317f
  colon, ultrasound image, 673f
  cortices, 849f
  free coelomic fluid, ultrasound image, 673f
  gallbladder, ultrasound image, 670f
  gastric adenoma, confirmation, 523f
  gastroscopy, 523f
  hematologic values, 1112
  hepatomegaly, radiograph, 693f
  kidney, ultrasound image, 673f
  liver
    ultrasound image, 670f
    vasculature, 673f
  lymphoma, 317
  medullary cavities, 849f
  necropsy, 574f, 693f
  nuclear scan, 243f
  obesity, 284f, 807f
  OP, 849f
  oral cavity, mucous membranes, 687f
  oral discharge, 865f
  pluck, removal, 574f
  serum biochemical values, 1112

Savannah Monitor Lizard—cont'd
  spinal cord trauma, MRI, 242f
  thoracic spine, inflammation
    (hot spot), 243f
  ticks, presence, 503f
  ultrasound examination, 527f
  ventral view, 61f
  WBC, 317f
Sawyer Extractor, usage, 1055f
SC. See Subcutaneous
Scales
  abnormalities, 373
  biopsies, 519
  ventrolateral incision, 790-791
Scaling
  pharmacologic application, 421-423
    derivation, 422-423
    model, selection, 422
    technique, review, 421-422
  physiologic application, 421
Scanning electron microscopy (SEM).
    See Boa Constrictor; Skink;
    Snake mite
Scapulae, rotation, 843
Scarlet Kingsnake (*Lampropeltis triangulum elapsoides*), 42f
Scenting. See Foods
SCEP. See Spinal cord evoked potential
Schellackia, 802-803
Schizogony, occurrence, 803
Scintigraphy. See Pneumonia
Scissors. See Cutting scissors; Incising scissors
SCL. See Straight carapace length
Scleral ossicles, absence. See Crocodilians
Scolecophidia (infraorder), 44-45
Scout image. See Magnetic resonance
    imaging: Computed tomography
Scout studies, 486f
Scrapings, culture, 223
Screen mesh, hazard. See Arboreal reptiles
SCT. See Salmon calcitonin
SCUD. See Septicemic cutaneous ulcerative
    disease
Scutes
  abnormalities, 373
  loss. See Chelonians
  nomenclature. See Carapaces
  pattern, 972
  terminology, 81
SCW. See Straight carapace widths
Sea level tropical temperatures, 942
Seasonal cooling, 384-385
  period. See Captive reptiles
Seattle-King County, data, 1019
Seaturtle
  age to maturity, 976
  amputations, 1000f
  anesthesia, 997-998
    monitoring, 998f
    surgical plane, 998f
  anorexia, 994-995
  barnacles/epibiotes, lesion appearance
    (radiographs), 983f
  biology/conservation, e-mail information
    network. See CTURTLE
  blood collection, 980-982
  bronchi, dorsoventral view, 868f

Seaturtle—cont'd
  buoyancy abnormalities, 992-993
  carapace
    adhesion/abscess, infected boat
      strike, 986f
    scutes, 974f
  coelomic fluid, commonness, 983f
  cranial lung, fold, 985f
  CT scan, reconstruction, 1090f
  cutdown approach, 982f
  cytology, 982-983
  debilitation, 994f
  dehydration, 996
  diagnostic imaging, 983
  diet, 979t
  dorsal cervical sinuses, usage, 516
  dystrophic mineralization, 190f
  endoscopic view, 986f
  endoscopy, 983-984
  entanglements, 992
    hazard, 980f
  enucleations, 999-1000
  esophagus
    conical papilla, endoscopic view, 147f
    fish hooks, retrieval, 992f
  external jugular vein
    exposure, 982f
    sample, 982f
  fibropapillomatosis, 986, 990
  fish hooks, hazard, 991-992
  flipper tags, usage, 1004
  flotation abnormalities, 992-993
  FP removal, CO_2 laser surgery
    (usage), 990f
  fresh water soaking, 984f
  gastrointestinal injury, 991-992
  gelatin diet, 995t
  geographic location, 972t
  hematology, values, 981t
  hook/sinker, dorsoventral
    radiograph, 991f
  infectious diseases, 994
  intestinal tract, surgical access, 992f
  lethargy, 995-996
  LISTSERV, 972
  lungs
    dorsoventral radiograph, 989f
    evaluation, prefemoral approach, 871f
    trematode granuloma, endoscopic
      view, 989f
  marine leeches (*Ozobranchus margoi*),
    coverage, 994f
  median induction time, 997
  medical care, 972
  medical management. See Cold-stunned
    Seaturtles
  medical problems, 984
  medication administration,
    intracoelomically implanted catheter
    (usage), 997f
  medicine/surgery, 977-1000
  melanin pigments, 985f
  moribund behavior, 995-996
  natural history, 97-977
  necropsy, 1000
    intestinal tract, trash removal, 991f
  neoplasia, 994
  neurological assessment, 980f

Seaturtle—cont'd
  neurologic examination, 979-980
  oil/fuel/toxins, contamination, 993
  otic chamber, 1090f
  pain management, 998
  parasites, 993-994
  physical examination, 979
  pit tags, usage, 1004
  plasma values, 981t
  plastron, scutes, 974f
  plastronomy, attempt, 999f
  pneumonia, dorsoventral radiograph, 986f
  populations, decline, 973
  prefrontal scales, differentiating
    characteristic, 976f
  pulmonary FP, endoscopic view, 989f
  pulmonary parynchema, endoscopic
    view, 986f
  pulse oximetry, usage, 998f
  rear flipper, traumatic amputation, 988f
  recovery, episodes, 998
  serum chemistry values, 981t
  shower, housing, 997f
  size, 979t
  species, 972-974
    biology, 972-977
    identification, 972-974
    key, 975f
  specific necropsy protocol, 1000
  status, 972t
  supravertebral sinus, access, 982f
  surgery, 998-1000
  swim plan, 1003
  tagging, 1004f
  teeth, absence, 976f
  therapeutics, 996-1000
  trachea
    bronchoscopic view, 986f
    dorsoventral view, 868f
  trauma, 984-986
  trematode eggs, presence, 985f
  ultrasonography, usage, 998f
  ventilator, usage, 998f
  water temperature, 996
  weakness, 995-996
  websites, 973t
  weight, 979t
Sebaceous cysts, reports, 685
Sebekia sp. See Softshell Turtle
  infestation, 361-362
Secondary bacterial infections, 836
  prevention, 776
Secondary gram-negative bacterial
  infection, 394
Secondary nutritional
  hyperparathyroidism, 504
Secondary sexual characteristics, 379-381
Second-degree burns, 919, 919f
Secretions, PCR-based testing, 403
Sedimentation, usage, 344-345
Seizures, 963
  occurrence, 680
Selenite broth, 900
Selenium
  deficiency, 692
    hypothyroidism, association, 290
  intoxication, 291
Self-adhesive bandages, usage, 896

Sellotape, usage, 329
SEM. *See* Scanning electron microscopy
Seminal plugs, formation, 862
Semisynthetic penicillins, usage, 652-653
Senescence, 261
Sensitivity data, 230-231
    support, 233
Sensory pits, 240
Sepsis, 546
    attention, 921f
Septic arthritis. *See* Green Iguana
Septicemia, 467f
    evaluation, blood culture
        (recommendation), 245
    production, 183
Septicemic cutaneous ulcerative disease
    (SCUD), 213, 896
    impact, 698
Septic inflammation, 467f
    term, usage, 466f
Septic tracheitis, cytodiagnosis, 467f
Septum horizontale, 129
Serial blood sampling, 888
Serpentes (suborder), 135-137
Serratia, 233
Serratia marcescens, growth, 233f
Serum antibody titers, 758-759
Serum neutralization (SN), 1064
    illustration, 1064f
    test, 817
Serum proteins, laboratory evaluation, 464
Serum sodium values, increase, 546
Services, commercial suppliers, 261t
Sevoflurane
    administration. *See* Green Iguana
    anesthetic usage, 75
Sevoflurone, usage, 616
Sexing probes, 382f
    usage, 501f
Sexual characteristics. *See* Secondary sexual
    characteristics
Sexual determination. *See* Reptiles; Surgical
    sexual determination; Temperature-
    dependent sexual determination
    accuracy, 379
Sexual dimorphism, 338. *See also* Chelonians;
    Coloration; External morphology;
    Leaf-nosed Snakes
Sexual maturity, onset, 376
Sexual production, temperature
    (determination), 383
SG. *See* Stratum germinativum
Shake-and-bake technique, 265
Sharp-tailed Snake *(Contia tenius)*, body
    mass, 421f
Shed cilia, 466f
Shedding. *See* Snakes
    age, impact, 781
    complex, 778
    cycle. *See* Reptiles
    humidity, impact, 780-781
    problems, 914f. *See also* D'Albert's Python
        scars, 779f
    skin, assistance, 782
Shells. *See* Soft shells
    abnormalities, 373
    abscesses. *See* Deep shell abscesses;
        Superficial shells

Shells—cont'd
    algae growth, 697
    anatomy, 893
    biopsy, 523, 525
    bridge (incision), striker saw (usage), 574f
    damage, 204-205, 893
    defect, 898
    dermal bone, exposure, 896
    distortion, 699
    dorsal midline, vertebrae fusion, 897
    erosions. *See* Superficial shells
    fractures, 698, 896-897
        treatment, 897
    glands, 753f
    growth. *See* Pyramidal shell growth
    hemorrhage/infection. *See* Tortoises
    injury. *See* Turtles
    modifications, 81
    repair, 998. *See also* Cable tie shell repair
    rot, 697-698
    sloughing, 697
    therapeutic endpoint, 896
    treatment, 897-898
    ulceration, 697-698
    whitish areas, 697
Shine, R, 12
Shingle-backed Skink *(Trachydosaurus
    rugosas)*, foot (infection), 775f
Shock/denial. *See* Loss
Shu, definition, 429t
Shudder bob, 171
Siamese Crocodile *(Crocodylus siamensis)*, 104
Siamese twins. *See* Red-eared Slider
Sick room, 397
Side-necked Turtle *(Pelomedusa sp.)*, urea
    production, 27f
Side-neck Turtle
    example. *See* Mata Mata
    Phrynops genus. *See* Hilaire's Side-neck
        Turtle
Sidewinder *(Crotalus cerastes laterorepens)*, 45f
    metabolic changes, 279
Sidewinding, 51
Silica gel powder, abrasion, 732
Silkworm larva *(Bombyx mori)*,
    nutrient/energy composition, 265t
Silver sulfadiazine burn cream, application.
    See Snakes
Single-cusped atrioventricular valves, 125
Site-specific emergency protocols, 1051
Skeletal system, radiographic
    interpretation, 475-478
Skin. *See* Abnormal skin
    algorithm, 200f
    biopsies, 519
    blueing, 778
    closure, everting suture pattern
        (usage), 582f
    eversion, 583f
    heating, 127
    inflammation, 205
    inversion tendency. *See* Incised skin
    lesions, scraping, 519f
    necropsy examination, 572-573
    pigmentation, 624
    punch biopsy, 519
    reddening, 963
    rehydration, 782f

Skin—cont'd
    removal. *See* Retained skin
    retained ringlets, 774f
    sample-taking. *See* Amphibians; Reptiles
    scrapes, 519
    shedding, 198-199, 219
    sloughing, 290f, 697, 779f, 784f
    staples, characteristics, 582f
    surfaces, 227-228
    surgery preparation, difficulty, 584f
    test, 1055
    whitish growth, 697f
    wounds, 212
Skink *(Leiolopisma telfairii)*
    burns, recovery, 922f
    hot-rock burn, penetration, 922f
    jowls/head coloration. *See* Broad-headed
        Skink
    mandibular symphysis separation, 608f
    SEM, 196f
    suboptimal bone health, 608f
Skink *(Tiliqua sp.)*
    epithelium, keratinization, 196f
    external barrier, 196f
Skin surfaces, sampling, 227-228
Skull
    fractures, 607-608
    shape, 146
Slap feeding, 372
Slide containers, 569
Slider
    bladder, 141f
    bone, visibility, 1091f
    fluid-filled urinary bladder, 1091f
    localizer, 1091f
    midbody, T2-weighted MRI, 1091f
    MRI
        frontal image, 1090f
        section, 1091f
Slider *(Trachemys scripta elegans)*, blood
    film, 456f
Slider Turtle *(Trachemys sp.)*
    soft tissue anatomy, ventral view, 1092f
    T2-weighted fMRI image, 1092f
Slider Turtle *(Trachemys sp.)*, egg death, 374f
Sliming, 371
Sloughing, 198-199
Slow Worms, 324
Slurries, administration, 277
Small biopsies, preparation/submission,
    562-563
Small-toothed forceps, usage, 535
Smear samples, performing, 569
Smear technique, usage. *See* Cytologic
    interpretation
SMEC. *See* Specific minimum energy cost
Smilisca phaeota. *See* Masked Tree Frog
Smith, HM, 12
SMR. *See* Standard metabolic rate
SN. *See* Serum neutralization
Snake mite *(Ophionyssus natricis)*, 208f,
    1027. *See also* Pythons
    activity/behavior, 722
    color, 724f
    commonness, 346
    eggs, 721
    hematophagous characteristic, 373
    importance, 207-208

Snake mite—cont'd
- infestation, 728. *See also* Bearded Dragon
- life cycle, 721
  - duration, 723t
- presence, 723f
- problems, 35
- recovery, 518f
- removal, 330
- SEM, 208f
- species specificity, 735
- teardrop appearance, 724f

Snakes, 42. *See also* Blind Snakes; Giant Snakes
- abdominal distension, 677
- adenovirus, 398
- aggression, restraint, 495-496
- air sacs, 133f
- anatomy, 46-53
- anesthesia, induction, 447
- anorexia, 599f, 675
- ataxia, 855-856
- basic enclosure setup, 55
- behavior, 55-56
  - changes, 681
- bites, first aid. *See* Venomous snakes
- bladders, absence, 763f
- blood film, *Hepatozoon*, 803f
- blue color, 678
- body
  - position/movement, abnormality, 856-857
  - systems, tumors, 306t-314t
- brumation, 56
- bumps, 681
- caging, requirements (minimum), 54-55, 55t
- captive propagation, genetic mutations, 53f
- captivity, longevity, 56t-57t
- cardiovascular system, 46-48
- carnivorous quality, 53-54
- celiotomy, 586-587, 600f
  - incision, 587f
- chiropractic, manual spinal manipulation, 437f
- classification, 42, 43t
- cloacal opening, circumferential pursestring sutures (problems), 863f
- coelomic cavity abnormalities, palpation, 151
- C-shaped trachea, 132f
- defensive behaviors, 165-167
- dentition, 48-49
- depression, 599f, 680
- desert enclosure setup, 55
- diagnostic view, 1098f
- diarrhea, 676
- dietary intake, essential nutrients, 274
- diets, suggestions, 54t
- differential diagnoses, 675
- digestive system, 48
- dorsal recumbency, 241f
- dysecdysis, 52
- dystocia
  - diagnosis, 788
  - surgery, 790-791
- early scale lesion, 205f
- ears, 50

Snakes—cont'd
- ectothermic quality, 53
- eggs
  - retention, 790f
  - viability checking, ultrasound transducer (usage), 369f
- emesis, 675-676
- endocrine system, 52
- envenomations, 1074-1075
- environmental captivity requirements, 54-55
- environment/maintenance, 53-54
- esophageal tear, endoscopic view, 147f
- esophagus, 48, 676
- excisional lung biopsy, 521
- eyes, 50-51, 680-681
  - format, 333
- fat reserves, 500
- feeding, 53-54, 739
  - comparisons, 279
  - schedules, 278-279
- flexible endoscopy, 557f
- fusiform testes, 50
- gallbladder, 828f
- gastric mucosa, 760f
- gastritis, 939f
- gastrointestinal tract, signs, 675-677
- gender determination, 366, 501f
- glass, striking, 607f
- glottis, 48, 130, 132
  - location, 442, 447
- gross anatomy, ventral view, 47f
- hatchling
  - hemipene, eversion (popping technique), 381f
  - pliable egg, 377f
- head tilt, 857
- heart
  - dorsal view, 122f
  - enlargement, midbody swelling, 677f
  - rate, determination, 193
  - transverse echocardiographic view, 192f
  - ventral view, 122f
- hematocrit, level, 48
- hemipenes, presence, 50
- hyperemia, 205f
- IBD, 153
- incoordination, 855-856
- infection, 205f
  - signs, 498f
- infrared-sensitive sensory structures, 149
- integument, 51-52
- integumentary signs, 677-678
- intestines, 676-677
- intracardiac catheters, usage, 537-538
- intraosseous catheters, usage, 538-539
- intravenous cut-down techniques, 537-539
- iris, characteristic, 338
- jugular catheters
  - anesthesia/analgesia, requirement, 538f
  - usage, 537f
- jugular vein, location, 638f
- kidneys
  - anatomy, 140f
  - ultrasound appearance, 673f
- *Klebsiella* sp. hypopyon, 234f

Snakes—cont'd
- lateral body wall, subcutaneous space, 635f
- lead placement, challenge, 188f
- locomotion, 51
- longevity, 56-57
- longitudinal rugae, exaggeration, 760f
- lumps, 681
- lungs, 132
  - characteristic, 471
  - size, 484f
  - tube shape, 133f
- meals
  - frequency, 54
  - sizes, 278-279
- meridian points, difficulty, 433f
- mite infestation, 518f
- mucosal thickening, 760f
- mucus-secreting cells, gastric hyperplasia, 757
- muscle twitching, 855-856
- muscularis obliquus, 132
- musculoskeletal signs, 678
- musculoskeletal system, 51
- natural setups, 55
- nervous system, 50-51
  - signs, 679-680
- neurologic disorders, 855-857
- nontraditional therapeutic methods, 658
- nutrition, 53-54
- open-mouth breathing, 599f
  - abnormality, 679f
- opisthotonos, 857
- oral cavity, 676
  - access, 641f
  - *Kalicephalus* sp. larva, 356f
- oral multicellular mucous glands, 145
- outdoor enclosures, 55
- ovaries/oviducts, length, 593f
- palpation, 386
- paralysis, 856
- paramyxoviridae, clinical features, 401
- parthenogenesis, 377
- positioning, 474
- prey strike, inability, 856-857
- radiographic anatomy, 1098f
- regurgitation, 675-676
- renal anatomy, 140f
- reproductive signs, 681
- reproductive system, 49-50
- respiratory cycle, 132
- respiratory disease, 866f
- respiratory signs, 679
- respiratory sounds, 679
- respiratory system, 48
- respiratory tract
  - anatomy, 130-132
  - lateral views, 484
- restraint, 474, 495-496
- righting reflex, loss, 856-857
- rodents/chicks, food, 274
- scales, 51-52
- scoliosis, 908f
- sexual segment. *See* Male snakes
  - histologic appearance, 143f
- shedding, 52f, 779
- shed skin, examination. *See* Captive snake

Snakes—cont'd
  silver sulfadiazine burn cream, application, 920f
  skin, fragility, 212
  soaking, attention, 782f
  spinal osteopathy, 908f
  splenopancreas, 828f
  squamate reproduction/courtship, 171-173
  star gazing, 857
  stomach, 48, 676
    tubing, 811
  strapping, 585f
  stress, 55f
  surgery, 612-613
  swamp tea setup, 55
  taxonomy, 42-46
  teeth, 48
  thermoregulation, 53
  three-layer enclosure setup, 55
  thyroid glands, 52
  tissue destruction, 205f
  tongue, 48
  toxemia, sign, 498f
  trachea, 48
  transmitters/antennas, implantation, 616f
  uric acid excretion, 256
  urinary system, 49-50
  vascular anatomy, 140f
  venom, 48-49
    categorization, 1028
    enzymes, presence, 49
    glands, 49
  vomiting, 675-676
  weight loss, 681-682
  wet/dry enclosure setup, 55
Snapping Turtle (Chelydra serpentis)
  caseous debris, removal, 895f
  inspiration, 85
  liver
    hepatic lipidosis, 561f
    melanomacrophages, 561f
  lung collapse, 561f
  necrotic tissue/bone, removal, 895f
  scutes, peeling, 895f
  seasonally active ductus deferens, 559f
Snout-vent length (SVL), 495
  percentage, 499-500, 517, 520
Soaking cycle, completion, 554
Soa-soa Sailfin Lizard (Hydrosaurus amboinensis), teeth, 63f
Societies, 9-10
Society for the Study of Amphibians and Reptiles (SSAR), 9
Sodium, absorption/transportation, 462
Sodium hypochlorite, usage, 1015
Sodium nitrate, usage, 344
Sodium pump number, 421
Soft bone, collapse, 601f
Soft-shelled ticks, 726f
Soft shells, 698
Softshell Turtle (Apalone spp.). See also Spiny Softshell Turtle
  exoskeleton, dorsal ventral projection, 474f
  integumentary/buccopharyngeal gas exchange, 133f

Softshell Turtle—cont'd
  pentastome. See Narrowhead Softshell Turtle
  Sebekia sp., 361f
Soft ticks (Argasidae), 346
Soft tissue
  anatomy, ventral view. See Slider Turtle
  biopsy specimens, 571
  calcification, 287, 477, 1069
  prefemoral incision, 592, 593f
Soft tissue surgery, 581
  instrumentation, 582-584
  postoperative care, 586
  preoperative care, 584-586
  preparation, 584-586
Solar radiation, provision, 631
Solenoglyphous teeth, 48
Solomon Island Skink (Corucia zebrata), gastric lavage, 522f
Solute-free water, distribution, 542f
Somatoautonomic dysfunction, 436
Southern copperhead (Agkistrodon c. contortrix), tails (caudal luring), 167f
Southern Painted Turtle (Chrysemys picta dorsalis), 80f
  advantage, 96f
SP4 medium, 934
Space-occupying lesions, 875
Sparganosis, transmission cycle, 1026f
Sparganum, development, 1026f
Spark-gap tissue destruction, 623
Special senses, diagnostic techniques, 529-531
Species-species adenovirus, infection, 399
Species-species POTR, 442
Specific minimum energy cost (SMEC), 422
Spectacled Cobra (Naja naja), hood expansion, 45f
Spectacles, 327-332. See also Retained spectacle; Ulcerated spectacle
  abrasions, 327-328. See also Royal Python
  anatomy, 327
  appearance, 329
  cleaning. See Geckos
  composition, 327
  dermal fungal infection, 329f
  diagram. See Tertiary spectacle
  indenting. See Royal Python
  loss, 328-329
    desiccated eye, 329f
  retaining. See Gartersnake
  sulcus, 330
  surgical wedge resection, 530
  trauma, 327-328
  ulcers, 327-328
  vascularization, 327
Speculum
  necessity, 640
  usage, 634, 639
Sperm storage. See Amphigonia retardata
Sphagnum moss
  misting, 368
  usage, 367
Sphenodontia (suborder), 1008
Spinal ankylosis. See Boa Constrictor
Spinal cord
  fractures, 853
  injury, 245

Spinal cord evoked potential (SCEP), 241, 242f. See also Gopher Tortoise
Spinal fracture, occurrence, 847
Spinal osteopathy, 244-245, 906. See also Boa Constrictor
  clinical signs, 909-910
  diagnosis, 910
  pathogenesis, 906-909
  prognosis, 911
  treatment, 910-911
Spindly leg. See Amphibians
Spine
  ankylosis, 244-245
  biomechanics, 437f
  kyphosis, 684
  scoliosis, 684
Spiny-tailed Iguana (Ctenosaura pectinata), fibrous osteodystrophy, 844f
Spiny Softshell Turtle (Apalone spinifera), 80f
  intraosseous femoral catheter, placement, 637f
  uncomplicated penile prolapse, 862f
Spiny-tailed Lizard (Uromastyx aegyptius), dorsoventral radiograph, 886f
Spiny Turtle (Hosemys spinosa), importation, 96f
Spiramycin, usage, 760
Spirochetes, 925
Spirochid blood fluke eggs, 696
Spirometra, larval tapeworms, 353
Spirorchid infections, treatment, 184-185
Spirorchiidae, 352
Spiroxis sp., mouth parts. See Freshwater Turtles
Spirurida (group), 356
Spiruridea, 1169-1170
Spiruroids, 299
SPL. See Straight plastron length
Spleen
  biopsies/aspirates, 517
  necropsy examination, 578
Splenic fibrosis, 406
Splenic lymphocytes, depletion, 406
Splenic macrophages, 400
Splenopancreas. See Snakes
  organ, location, 517
Splinting, variety, 601
SpO_2. See Arterial oxygen saturation
Sporocysts, 348
Sporogony, 802
  occurrence, 803
Sporozoites, 348
Spotted Turtle (Clemmys guttata), aural abscess, 509f
Spring-handled scissors, 583
Spring water, usage, 367f
Sprouts, addition, 267
Spurred Tortoise (Geochelone sulcata), pyramidal shell growth, 700f
Spurs, relationship. See Vestigial pelvis
Spur-thighed Tortoise, pinworm, 358f
SQ. See Subcutaneous
Squamata (order), 135-137
Squamate groups, relationships, 59
Squamate reproduction/courtship. See Lizards; Snakes
Squamates, 175
  medication ease, 640

Squamous metaplasia, 326
Sri Lankan Pipe Snake (*Cylindrophis maculates*), automimicry (exhibition), 43f
Sri Lankan Shield-tailed Snake (*Uropeltis phillipsi*), 43f
SSAR. *See* Society for the Study of Amphibians and Reptiles
Stab incisions, 617f
Staining methods, 227
Stainless steel liga-clips, 966
Standard metabolic rate (SMR)
    calculations, 252
    energy intakes, 254f
    estimates, 253t
Standings Day Gecko (*Phelsuma standingii*), emaciation, 275f
Stargazing, 404
Stargazing (star gazing). *See also* Boids
Starling's forces, principles, 540
Starling's Law, 541f
Star Tortoise (*Geochelone elegans*)
    cilate trophozoite, 347f
    conical scutes, growth, 285f
Stat stains, 465
Stebbins, RC, 12
Steel suture, necessity, 581
Steep-sided water containers, 37
Steinmann pins usage, 604f
Sterile field, necessity, 586f
Sterile nonbacteriostatic saline solution, usage, 870f
Sterile swab, placement. *See* Cloaca
Sterilization, usage. *See* Endoscopy
Sternotherus odoratus. *See* Common Musk Turtle; Stinkpot
Sternotherus sp. *See* Musk Turtles
Sternum, xiphoid process, 520
Steroids, usage, 1131t
Stillbirths. *See* Lizards
Still photography, usage, 553
Stinkpot (*Sternotherus odoratus*), 80f
    carapace/bridge, fractures, 898f
    fractures, stabilization, 898f
S-T intervals, 182
Stomach. *See* Snakes
    components, 147-148
    feeding tube placement, 635f
    functions, 147-148
Stomatitis, 153, 926-928. *See also* Bacterial stomatitis; Fungal stomatitis; Green Iguana; Lizards; Parasitic stomatitis; Viral stomatitis
    diagnosis, 817
    term, reference, 814-815
Storz Avian Sheath system, 549f
    instrumentation, visualization, 550f
    top instrument port, advantage, 549f
Storz diagnostic sheath system, 559
Storz Model 600 Flash Generator, TTL flash measurement, 551f
Storz sheath, closeup, 550f
Strabismus, sign, 852f
Straight carapace length (SCL), 979
Straight carapace widths (SCW), 979
Straight plastron length (SPL), 979
Stranding Report, 977
Stratum germinativum (SG), 198f

Strawberry Poison-dart Frog (*Dendrobates pumilio*), skin (toxin-producing glands), 944f
Streptococci spp., identification, 378f
Stress. *See* Captive reptiles; Lizards; Snakes
    definition, 119
    disorders, 293-294
    effects. *See* Body systems
    handling, 121
    importance. *See* Reptiles
    nutritional management, 293
    signs, 944
Stress-associated hyperglycemia, 823-824
Stress response, 490
    nonadaptivity, timing, 121
    reason, 120
    regulation, 120
Striker saw, usage, 578. *See also* Shells
Strongyloides sp., life cycle, 961
Stump, trauma, 610f
Subacute myocarditis, 406
Subacute periportal hepatitis, 406
Subclinical viral infection, 391
Subcutaneous (SC/SQ) adipose tissue, 983
Subcutaneous (SC/SQ) fat, dissection, 592
Subcutaneous (SC/SQ) fluids
    replacement route, 634
    usage, 635
Subcutaneous (SC/SQ) hemorrhages, 498f
Subcutaneous (SC/SQ) injections, administration, 635
Subcutaneous (SC/SQ) mycoses, 219-221
Subcutaneous (SC/SQ) tissue
    closure, subcuticular pattern, 617f
    tophi deposition, 796f
    tumors, 309t-310t
Subdermal mites, skin scraping, 725f
Subluxations, 434
    pathophysiology, 436
Submerging, inability, 702
Subspectacular abscess, 329-330, 335
    lancing, 330f
Subspectacular fluid, drainage, 497
Subspectacular space
    distention, 691
    flushing, 328f, 329-330
    increase, 331f
Subspectacular swelling, 497-499
Substrate
    changing, impact, 39
    selection, 33
    usage. *See* Captive reptiles; Eggs; Lizards
Succinylchlorine chloride, usage, 117
Sudden death, 963
    occurrence. *See* Amphibians
Sulcascaris sulcata. *See* Loggerhead Seaturtle
Sulcata Tortoise (*Geochelone sulcata*)
    calcium deficiency, 286f
    carapace, deformity, 286f
    hatchling nourishment, 256f
    pasture, usage, 269f
    pyramiding, 284f
    vitamin D_3 deficiency, 286f
Sulfadiazine cream, usage, 927f
Sulfa drugs, bacteriostatic characteristic, 653
Sullivan, BK, 11
Summer estivation, 256
Superficial keratectomy, 337

Superficial mycoses, 1024
Superficial shells, abscesses/erosions, 893-894
Superficial tissues, sampling, 376f
Superglue, usage, 897
Supernumerary scales, 974
Supersaturated solution, seeding, 764
Superworms (*Zophobas mori*), food, 263f
Supplements. *See* Dietary supplements
    trial dosages. *See* Reptiles
    usage, 271-273
Supplies, commercial suppliers, 261t
Suppurative gingivitis, 925
Supracaudals, 972
Supraocular scales, 974
Supravertebral sinus, usage, 981
Surface electrodes, placement, 186
Surface mites, visibility, 725f
Surgery. *See* Joints; Lasers; Mammals; Radiosurgery; Soft tissue surgery
Surgical autotomy, 611
Surgical implantations, 615-617
Surgical lasers, usage, 583
Surgical Scrub, 1018
Surgical sexual determination, 383
Surgitron
    unit, 623f
    usage, 583, 622
Sutures. *See* Preplaced nonabsorbable sutures
    materials, 581-582
    removal
        delay, 581f
        skin, sticking, 582f
    tightening, 598f
SVL. *See* Snout-vent length
SV wave, 186
Swab technique, usage. *See* Cytologic interpretation
Swamp tea setup. *See* Snakes
Swim plan. *See* Seaturtle
Sympatholytics, 185
Synovial fluid, crystallization, 794
Synthetic colloids
    characteristics, 545
    disadvantages, 545
Synthetic salmon calcitonin, effects. *See* Mammals
Syphacia muris, 345f
Systemic analgesic agents, 445
Systemic antibiotics, usage, 749
Systemic antifungal chemotherapeutics, 154
Systemic deep mycoses, diagnosis, 873
Systemic disease, 692
Systemic drugs, selection, 226
Systemic itraconazole, usage. *See* Bearded Dragon
Systemic lesions, biopsy, 224
Systemic mycoses, 221-223
Systole, 126. *See also* Atrial systole

T

T. radiata. *See* Radiated Tortoise
T1-weighted image. *See* Posthatchling Leatherback Turtle
T2-weighted fMRI image. *See* Slider Turtle
T2-weighted MRI. *See* Slider
    two-dimensional image. *See* Alligators

Tachypnea, 499, 710
  occurrence, 222
Tags, usage. *See* Crocodilians; Seaturtle
Tails
  amputation, 610-611
    suture. *See* High tail amputation
  avascular necrosis, 683
  avulsion, 914f
  behavior. *See* Rubber Boa
  damage, 913-915
  development. *See* Forked tails
  displays, 165-167. *See also* Ring-necked Snake
    ventrum, 166f
  hydrostatic pressure, 382
  ischemic necrosis, 879
  lashing, 171
  loss (autotomy), 167. *See also* Five-lined Skink; Lizards
  masses, 913
  partial damage, 914f
  regrowth, 914f. *See also* Lizards
  skin, damage, 913
  swellings, 913
  tips, 678-679
    avascular necrosis, 679
  vascular integrity, 611
  vein, blood (course), 589f
  vertebrae, disarticulation, 574-575
Tantalum powder, infusion, 485f
Tapeworms, 352-353
  competition, 353
  eggs. *See* Boa Constrictor; Green Tree Python; Pythons; Rhinoceros IIguana
  genera, 353t
  presence. *See* Water Dragon
Tapotement, 438
Tap water, adequacy, 71
Tarsal plate, development, 325
Taxonomic uncertainty, 419
Taylor, J, 11
TBW. *See* Total body water
T-cell lymphocytes, usage, 632
T cell proliferation assays, 1066-1067
T cell receptor (TCR), 1066
TCID. *See* Tissue culture infectious dose
TCR. *See* T cell receptor
TCVM. *See* Traditional Chinese veterinary medicine
TDSD. *See* Temperature-dependent sexual determination
Tear-secreting ophthalmic glands, 831
Technicians, training, 28f
Technicium scan. *See* Prehensile-tailed Skink
  vascular phase, 488f
Teeth
  congenital disorders, 924
  disorders, 924-929
  oral/rostral trauma, 924
  visualization, 558
Teflon catheter, length, 538f
Teflon guide, 553
Tegaderm, usage, 894
Tegu Lizard (*Tupinambis teguixin*)
  electrocardiography, 518f
  hematologic values, 1111
  serum biochemical values, 1111
Tegu (*Tupinambis* sp.), infection, 382f

Telazol, usage, 444, 565, 638, 997
Telemetry. *See* Biotelemetry
  complications, 615
  power sources, 614
  units
    attachment, 614t
    suppliers. *See* Biotelemetry
Telescope, diameter (selection), 550
Television, usage. *See* Reptile practice
Telezol, usage, 616
TEM. *See* Transmission electron micrograph
Temperature-dependent sexual determination (TDSD), 110, 111f, 383-384
Temperature gradients, providing (failure), 251
Temporal muscle atrophy, 703
Temporal scales, 974
Temporomandibular joint (TMJ). *See* Green Iguana
  visualization, 558
Tenesmus, cause, 755
Tennessee, herpetological societies, 7t
Terrapene carolina. *See* Common Box Turtle
Terrapene carolina carolina. *See* Eastern Box Turtle
Terrapene carolina triunguis. *See* Three-toed Box Turtle
Terrapene spp. *See* American Box Turtle
Terrapins, 78
  ataxia, 703
  behavioral thermoregulation, 87
  blindness, 703-704
  bloating, 700
  blood collection, 515-516
  breath sounds, abnormality, 702
  brumation, 88-89
  captive care, 87-98
    considerations, 87-89
  circling, 703
  circulatory system, 87
  clinical anatomy/physiology, 81-87
  coma, 703
  constipation, 700
  cutaneous signs, 696-699
  cutaneous swelling, 696
  diagnostic techniques, 504-512
  diarrhea, 700
  differential diagnosis, 696
  dyspnea, 702
  emaciation, 700
  emesis, 700
  erythema foul odor, 696
  gastrointestinal signs, 699-701
  gastrointestinal system, 85
  genitourinary system, 85-86
  hypermetric gait, 703
  integumentary system, 84
  lameness, 703
  lighting, 87
  musculoskeletal signs, 703
  musculoskeletal system, 81-84
  nasal discharge, 701
  neurologic signs, 703
  ophthalmologic signs, 703-704
  paralysis, 703
  penile prolapse, 702
  penis, extension, 86f
  petechia, 696

Terrapins—cont'd
  predators, impact, 87
  regurgitation, 700
  reproductive signs, 702-703
  respiratory signs, 701-702
  respiratory system, 84-85
  sexual dimorphism, 86-87
  shell, 696
  skin, 696
    wound, povidone iodine preparation treatment, 212f
  subcarapacial site, availability, 515
  taxonomy, 78-81
Terrepen sp. *See* Box Turtles
Terrestrial assessment, 980
Terrestrial chelonians, hypervitaminosis A (impact), 212
Terrestrial salamanders, 943
Terrestrial tortoises, uric acid excretion, 256
Tertiary spectacle, diagram, 327f
Testes, recognition, 669
Testicle
  elevation, 597f
  vascular supply, 596f
Testudinata, 78
Testudines (order), 78, 137-138
Testudinidae, 80, 91
  scales, thickness, 84
Testudo genus, 91
Testudo graeca. *See* Greek Tortoise; Mediterranean Tortoise
Testudo hermanni. *See* Hermann's Tortoise; Tortoises
Testudo kleinmanni. *See* Egyptian Tortoise
Testudo Tortoise
  carapace, full-thickness shell biopsy, 524f
  cloaca, prolapse, 512f
  cloacocolonic lavage, 522f
  corneal lesion, 530f
  forelimb, enlargement, 510f
  growth, excessiveness, 511f
  oviduct, prolapse, 512f
  penile prolapse, 512f
  scapulohumeral joint aspiration, 525f
Tetany, 843, 844. *See also* Hypocalcemic tetany
Tetracycline, 927
  resistance, 643
  therapy, 957
  usage, 653
Tetrahydorcannibinol (THC), 1078
Tetrathionate broth, 900
Tevcocin, plasma concentrations, 648
Texas, herpetological societies, 7t
Texas Patch-nosed Snake (*Salvadora grahamiae*), characteristics, 27f
Texas State Diagnostic Laboratory
  serologic testing, 403
  testing, 859
Texas Tortoise (*Gopherus berlandieri*)
  carapacial scutes, progressive infection, 222f
  necrotizing scute disease, 222f
  radiograph, 157f
TH-1 cells
  cytopathic effect, absence, 407
  irido-like virus, recovery, 408-409
  virus isolation, 396

Thamnophis proximus. See Ribbonsnakes
Thamnophis sirtalis. See California Giant Red-sided Gartersnake; Gartersnake
THC. *See* Tetrahydorcannibinol
Therapeutic plan
   development, 631-660
   environmental considerations, 631-632
Therapeutics, 230-231, 631. *See also* Chemotherapeutics; Seaturtle; Trial-and-error therapeutics
   administration, 639-642
   fluid therapy, 632-639
   immune response, 632
   methods. *See* Nontraditional therapeutic methods
   nutritional status, 632
   option. *See* Euthanasia
Thermal burns, 203, 677, 916, 918
   impact, 697
   thermodynamics, 916-917
Thermal energy, transfer, 917f
Thermal gradients, providing, 70
Thermal insulation, 806
Thermal neutral zone (TNZ), 53
Thermoregulation, 70-71. *See also* Geckos; Green Iguana; Lizards; Snakes
   function, 169-170
   necessity, 27f
Thermoregulatory functions, absence, 631
Thermotolerance, 225
Thiaminase, levels, 853
Thiamin deficiencies, 289-290, 709
Thiamine deficiencies, 243, 680
Thiamphenicol, relationship. *See* Florfenicol
Thigmothermy, 169
Third-degree burns, 919, 919f
Third-stage larva, 1025
Threat, displays, 167-168. *See also* Bearded Dragon
Three-layer enclosure setup. *See* Snakes
Three-sided osteotomy, performing, 589
Three-toed Box Turtle (*Terrapene carolina triunguis*)
   blepharedema, 832f
   carapace, fracture (healing), 897f
   mucopurulent ocular discharge, 832f
   rhamphothecal, distortion, 700f
   seam growth, 700f
Thrombocytes, 459-460. *See also* Toxic thrombocytes
   appearance, 459
   laboratory evaluation, 460
   morphology, 459
   response, 460
   Wright's stain, usage, 456f, 459f, 460f
Thrombocytopenia, 696
Thrombosis, 205
Through-the-lens (TTL) flash metering, 551
Thymus, necropsy examination, 578
Thymus atrophy, 933
Thyroglobulin, 290
Thyroid follicular cells, 406
Thyroid gland
   evidence, 576f
   necropsy examination, 576
   single/paired, 53f
Thyroid hormones, 432
Thyroid size, 576

Thyronine (amino acid), 290
Thyroxine, usage. *See* Hepatic lipidosis
Tick-infested tortoise premises, 733
Ticks (*Haemaphysalis punctata*), immature stages, 734
Ticks (*Ornithodoros talaje*) (*Amblyomma dissimile*), 184, 346. *See also* Hard-shelled ticks; Soft-shelled ticks
   anatomic surgery, 723
   attacks, variety, 734
   genera, 721
   identification, 727
   location. *See* Tortoises
   mouthparts, 722
   parasitization capability, 734f
   presence, 726f. *See also* Savannah Monitor Lizard
   prevention program, 735
   prognosis, 735-736
   removal, 733
      forceps, usage, 733f
      ivermectin, usage, 733
   zoonotic potential, 733-735
Tiletamine
   administration, 447
   usage, 444
Tiliqua gigas. See New Guinea Blue-tongued Skink
Tiliqua scincoides. See Blue-tongued Skink
Tilt. *See* Head tilts
Timber Rattlesnake (*Crotalus horridus*)
   restraint, 496f
   ulcerative dermatitis, 222f
Tissue
   amputation, 752
   appearance, assessment, 560-561
   coagulation, 621
   damage, 752
   devitalization, 755
   effects/healing, 623-624
   imprints, 569
   injury, 917-918
   laser welding, 624
   preservation, optimization, 572
Tissue culture infectious dose (TCID), 816
Titer level, 858
TMS. *See* Tricaine methane sulfonate
TNZ. *See* Thermal neutral zone
Toenails
   absence, 774-775
   asymmetric wear, 703
   overgrowth, 698
Toes. *See* Twitching toes
   absence, 774-775
   clip. *See* Amphibians
Togaviruses, 410-411, 1157
   recovery, 411
Tokay Gecko (*Gekko gecko*)
   Eimeria tokayae, 348f
   hematologic values, 1108
   Oochoristica, 354f
   Railietiella frenatus, 361f
   serum biochemical values, 1108
   tear drainage (failure), 331f
Tomistominae schlegelii. See False Gharials
Tomistominae (subfamily), life span, 104-105

Tongues
   glottis, 984
   membranes. *See* Pale tongue/mucous membranes
   variation, 146
   visualization, 558
Tonic immobility, 163-165, 175. *See also* Amphibians
Tonometry. *See* Green Iguana
Tophaceous gout, 795
Tophi
   deposition, common sites, 796f
   presence, 775
Topical aminogylcoside opthalmic drops, usage, 927f
Topical antibiotics, usage, 749
Topical antiseptics, variety, 654
Topical silver sulphadiazine, usage. *See* Bearded Dragon
Topical wound management, 655-656
Torpor, 260-261
Torso electrodes, usage, 188
Tortoises, 78, 91-95
   ataxia, 703
   beak lesions, 203f
   behavioral thermoregulation, 87
   bladder, 141f
      stone, 788f
   blindness, 703-704
   bloating, 700
   blood
      collection, 515-516
      erythrocytic inclusion, 803f
   bone destruction, uric acid crystals (impact), 797f
   breath sounds, abnormality, 702
   brumation, 88-89
   BW, 275-276
   captive care, 87-98
      considerations, 87-89
   carapace
      bilateral abrasions. *See* Leopard Tortoise
      fracture, dog attack, 511f
   carapacial bones, burns, 511f
   circling, 703
   circulatory system, 87
   clinical anatomy/physiology, 81-87
   clitoris. *See* Female tortoise
   coma, 703
   conical scutes, growth, 285f
   constipation, 700
   cutaneous signs, 696-699
   cutaneous swelling, 696
   diagnostic techniques, 504-512
   diarrhea, 700
   diet, 94t
   differential diagnosis, 696
   digestibility, diet (impact), 292
   digital ballotment, 766f
   dorsoventral radiograph, 870f
   dyspnea, 510f, 702
   eggs, rigid shell, 377f
   emaciation, 700
   emesis, 700
   enlarged prolapsed penis, 752f
   erythema, 510f
      foul odor, 696

Index

Tortoises—cont'd
  feces. *See* Grassland Tortoises
  feeding, 94
  fontanels, presence. *See* Pancake Tortoise
  forelimb, osteoderms (radiograph), 197f
  gastrointestinal signs, 699-701
  gastrointestinal system, 85
  genitourinary system, 85-86
  glottis, location, 130f
  gross anatomy
    midsagittal view, 83f
    ventral view, 82f, 83f
  hatchlings
    rigid shell, 377f
    water supply, 258f
  heart, cranial transverse view, 192f
  herbivores, 38
  herpesvirus, 393, 814
    clinical diagnosis, 816
    clinical signs, 814-816
    conservation, 819-820
    diagnosis, 816-818
    histology, 817-818
    laboratory diagnosis, 816-817
    postmortem diagnosis, 817
    serologic testing, diagnostic laboratories (list), 818t
    therapy/prevention/management, 818-819
  horizontal beam cranial-caudal view, 870f
  hospitalization/water soaking, 37f
  hypermetric gait, 703
  iatrogenic hypervitaminosis A, 510f
  indoor housing, 93
  integumentary system, 84
  intestinal tract, length/attachment, 591f
  intravenous infusion pump, connection, 538f
  keratin scutes, sloughing, 511f
  lameness, 703
  lettuce, unsuitability, 267
  lighting, 87
  limbs
    skin punch biopsy, 519f
    trauma, fox attack, 510f
  longevity, 78
  lungs
    biopsy, 521f
    parynchema, transcarapacial approach, 871f
    Tru-Cut biopsy, 521f
  males/females, distinctions, 87f
  musculoskeletal signs, 703
  musculoskeletal system, 81-84
  mycoplasmosis, drug treatment, 935t
  nasal discharge, 701
  neonatal care, 95
  neurologic signs, 703
  NMBD, 842f
  open-mouth breathing, 510f
  ophthalmologic signs, 703-704
  osteomyelitis, plastron infection, 512f
  outdoor hazards, 93
  outdoor housing, 93
  ovarian vessels (photo-coagulation), CO_2 laser usage, 626f
  oviducts, vascular mesosalpinx support, 596f

Tortoises—cont'd
  paralysis, 703
  parenteral vitamin A, high doses (impact), 290f
  penile prolapse, 702
  penis. *See* Male tortoise
  petechia, 696
  predators, impact, 87
  prolapsed bladder, 752f
  radiodense urolith, 767f
  regurgitation, 700
  reproduction, 94
  reproductive data. *See* Captive tortoises
  reproductive signs, 702-703
  respiratory signs, 701-702
  respiratory system, 84-85
  right-sided head tilt, 797f
  scutes, hemorrhage/infection, 511f
  sexual dimorphism, 86-87
  shell, 696
    hemorrhage/infection, 511f
  skin, 696
    sloughing, 510f
  species, mycoplasmal infections (confirmation), 931t
  splints, 603
  stomach, *Chapiniella* infestation, 355-356
  subcarapacial site, availability, 515
  substrates, 93-94
  taxonomy, 78-81
  testicles, attachment, 83f
  Testudo hermanni, shell lesion, 210f
    histologic section, 210f
  tethering, 93
  ticks, location, 727f
  unilateral pneumonia, development, 870f
  urine, amoeba (presence), 885f
  voluntary eating, 278f
  water
    bowls, 94
    supply, 94
Tortoiseshell, origin, 978f
Total body water (TBW)
  blood volumes, percentages, 373
  distribution, 540, 541f, 542f
Total plasma calcium, association, 464
Total protein (TP) values, 632
Total red blood count (TRBC), 453
Total solids (TS), 949
  parameters, 546
Towel clamps, 585
  ineffectiveness. *See* Chelonians
Toxic heterophils, 459f
Toxicities, reports, 1068
Toxic neuropathies, 246-247
Toxic reactions, treatment, 856
Toxic thrombocytes, 459f
Toxin-producing glands, 944
Toxins
  exposure, 956
  impact, 156-157, 247
  secreting glands, distribution, 176
Toxoplasmosis, 248
TP. *See* Total protein
Trabecular bone marrow, 578

Trachea
  lateral skin incision, 600f
  monofilament absorbable suture, usage, 600f
  visualization, 868
Tracheal cartilage, impact, 599f
Tracheal catheter, usage, 485f
Tracheal resection, 599
Tracheal tissue (damage avoidance), uncuffed endotracheal tube (recommendation), 949f
Tracheal washes
  PCR-based screening, 403
  performing, 228
Tracheitis, 222
Trachemys scripta
  optokinetic studies, 340
  straight-line carapace length, 1090f
Trachemys scripta elegan. See Red-eared Slider
Trachemys scripta elegans. See Freshwater Turtles; Slider
  optics/ocular physiology, studies, 340
Trachemys sp. *See* Slider Turtle
Trachydosaurus rugosas. See Shingle-backed Skink
Traditional Chinese veterinary medicine (TCVM), 428
  framework, 432
  philosophy, 432
Transcapillary forces. *See* Colloid oncotic pressure; Hydrostatic pressure
Transcarapacial intraluminal instillation. *See* Antifungal medication
Transducer frequency, impact. *See* Ultrasound images
Transendoscopic radiosurgery, usage, 517
Transillumination, 495
Transmission electron micrograph (TEM), 810-811. *See also* Round Island Gecko
Transmitters, 614
  implantation. *See* Snakes
Transport host, 343
Transport media
  bacteria, addition, 231f
  buffered fluid/semisolid media, 229f
  specialization, 229-230
Transtracheal wash, 874
  usage. *See* Pneumonia
Transudates. *See* Modified transudates
Transverse echocardiographic view. *See* Snakes
Transverse hinge, presence, 893
Trauma
  impact, 854-855
  nature, impact, 610
  rib periosteal response, 477
Trauma-induced neuropathies, 244-245
Traumatic fibrosis, deep friction massage response, 438
TRBC. *See* Total red blood count
Trematodes, 346t, 351-352, 874, 1165-1166. *See also* Digenetic trematodes; Monogenetic trematodes
  antemortem detection, 961
  eggs, presence. *See* Seaturtle
  impact, 961
Trematodiasis, therapeutics, 961

Trial-and-error therapeutics, 373
Triamcinolone acetonide, usage, 748
Triangulation, requirement, 615
Triazoles
　impact, 1072
　investigation, 655
Tricaine methanesulfonate, 947
Tricaine methane sulfonate (TMS), 566
Trichlorfon, usage, 729, 1068
Trichophyton. See Unspeciated Trichophyton
Trichosporon, 219
Trichuroidea (genera), 358-359
Triiodothyronine (T_3), 290
Trimethoprim sulfadimethoxine, usage, 653-654
Trimethoprin sulfa, usage, 760
Trionychidae, 79
Triple sulfa, resistance, 643
Trombiculids (chiggers), 720
　infestation. See Collared Lizard
　larvae, 722
Trophozoite
　direct smear, presence, 350
　immune status, 347
　stage, 347
Tropidophiidae, 46
Tropidophis canus curtus. See Dwarf Boa
Tru-cut biopsies (Tru-Cut biopsies), 526-527, 887
Trueb, L, 11
True Gharial (Gavialis gangeticus), characteristics, 104f
True retained eye shields, 783
Trypanosomatids, 804
Trypanosomes, blood-sucking invertebrate host requirement, 804
TS. See Total solids
TTL. See Through-the-lens
Tuatara
　air temperature, 1009
　anesthesia, 1010
　artificial burrow, provision, 1009
　biology, 1008
　blood sampling, 1009
　captive management, 1008-1009
　classification, 43
　diet, 1008-1009
　difference, 1008
　diseases, 1010-1011
　handling, 1009-1010
　health, signs, 1009-1010
　hematologic parameters, reference range, 1010t
　housing, 1009
　identification, 1010
　kidneys, 137
　mandible/exophthalmia, fibrous osteodystrophy, 1010f
　medical care, 1008-1010
　noninfectious diseases, 1011t
　obesity, example, 1008f
　reproduction, 1009
　reproductive examination, laparoscopy (usage), 1010f
　sampling, 1009-1010
　serum biochemistry parameters, reference range, 1010t
　surgery, 1010

Tubular traction splints, usage, 603, 603f
Tubules, necrosis, 879
Tufts University. See Wildlife Rehabilitation Database
Tui Na, 438
Tumors, treatment, 211
Tunica media, calcification, 183
Tupinambis sp. See Tegu
Tupinambis teguixin. See Tegu Lizard
Tupinambus teguixin. See Black and White Tegu
Turtle-associated salmonellosis, 1019
　decrease, 1020
Turtles, 78. See also Aquatic turtles
　acupuncture points, 436f
　ataxia, 703
　beak lesions, 203f
　behavioral thermoregulation, 87
　bladder, meridians (inaccessibility), 434f
　blindness, 703-704
　bloating, 700
　blood collection, 515-516
　breath sounds, abnormality, 702
　brumation, 88-89
　　survival, 88
　cage, scrubbing/rinsing, 96-97
　calcium requirements, 287
　captive care, 87-98
　　considerations, 87-89
　carapacial lesions. See Freshwater Turtles
　circling, 703
　circulatory system, 87
　clinical anatomy/physiology, 81-87
　cloacal anatomy, 136f
　coma, 703
　constipation, 700
　cranial peritoneal cavity, 556f
　craniocaudal pulmonary examination, 484f
　cutaneous signs, 696-699
　cutaneous swelling, 696
　diagnostic techniques, 504-512
　diarrhea, 700
　differential diagnosis, 696
　dog-gnawing trauma, 88f
　dyspnea, 702
　emaciation, 700
　emesis, 700
　erythema foul odor, 696
　gallbladder, meridians (inaccessibility), 434f
　gastrointestinal signs, 699-701
　gastrointestinal system, 85
　genitourinary system, 85-86
　glottis, location, 130f
　heart
　　dorsal view, 125f
　　ventral view, 125f
　herbivores, 38
　hypermetric gait, 703
　integumentary system, 84
　intravenous cut-down techniques, 536-537
　intromission. See Male Box Turtles
　IO catheter placement, 539
　kidneys
　　location, 140f
　　meridians, inaccessibility, 434f
　lameness, 703

Turtles—cont'd
　lighting, 87
　liver
　　lobe, 562f
　　meridians, inaccessibility, 434f
　lungs, FP, 989f
　males/females, distinctions, 87f
　meridians
　　difficulty, 433f
　　inaccessibility, 434f
　movement, degree, 173-174
　musculoskeletal signs, 703
　musculoskeletal system, 81-84
　nasal discharge, 701
　neurologic signs, 703
　ophthalmologic signs, 703-704
　paralysis, 703
　penile prolapse, 702
　penis, extension, 86f
　petechia, 696
　predators, impact, 87
　regulations, 1045
　regurgitation, 700
　reproductive signs, 702-703
　respiratory signs, 701-702
　respiratory system, 84-85
　sexual dimorphism, 86-87
　shell, 696
　　injury, epoxy resin repair. See Freshwater Turtles
　skin, 696
　species interactions, 98
　stomach meridians, inaccessibility, 434f
　subcarapacial site, availability, 515
　substrate preference, 31-32
　table characteristics, 30f
　taxonomy, 78-81
　trachea, bifurcation, 131f
　vascular anatomy, 142f
　water
　　change, 96
　　impact, 96
Turtle Survival Alliance, 78
T wave, 186
Twitching. See Lizards
Twitching toes, 776
Two-dimensional frontal section fMRI, usage. See Bearded Dragon
Two-wavelength spectrophotometer, usage, 194
Tympanic abscess, verification, 505
Tympanic cavity, variability, 742
Tympanic membranes, swelling, 696
　middle ear abscess, sign, 697f
Tympanic scales, 974
Type-C retrovirus, detection, 405
Type II topoisomerase, 649
Typhlopidae, 44

U

UATD. See Upper alimentary tract disease
Ulcerated spectacle, 328f
Ulcerations. See Lizards
Ulcerative dermatitis, 406. See also Timber Rattlesnake
Ulcerative diphtheroid-necrotizing stomatitis/glossitis, 395
Ulcerative gastritis, development, 347

Index

Ulcerative lesions, 213
Ulcerative LETD lesions, 393
Ultimobranchial body, necropsy examination, 576
Ultrasonography, 487-488, 665. *See also* Pneumonia
 significance, 158
 usage. *See* Reptiles; Seaturtle
Ultrasound equipment, 665-666
Ultrasound examination. *See* American Alligator; Asian Pond Turtle; Desert Tortoise; Eastern Box Turtle; Honduran Milksnake
 manual restraint. *See* Monitor Lizards
Ultrasound-guided biopsy. *See* Pneumonia; Renal biopsy
Ultrasound images. *See* Burmese Python
 advantages, 488
 gross pathology, comparison (usefulness), 665f
 interpretation, 665f
 obtaining, methods, 487
 transducer frequency, impact, 666f
Ultrasound transducer, usage. *See* Snakes
Ultrasound waves, transmission, 665
Ultraviolet A (UVA) light, 30
 emission, 1082
Ultraviolet B (UVB) light, 30
 emission, 1082
 exposure, 285
 meter, 1083
 radiation, 288
 sources, 73
Ultraviolet-excimer lasers, 618
Ultraviolet (UV) light
 necessity, 30
 providing, 95
 reflection, 175
Ultraviolet (UV) meters, 87
Ultraviolet (UV) radiation
 exposure. *See* Diurnal animals
 transmission, 1083t
Ultraviolet (UV) wavelengths, importance, 73
Umbilical stalk, severing/ligation, 371f
Uneven floating. *See* Floating
Unicameral lung, 556
Unilateral microphthalmia, 333
Unilateral pathology, 868
United States
 case examples, 1049-1050
 federal regulations, 1045-1050
 ports, designated entry, 1045
 state agency regulation. *See* Herptiles
 state laws, 1045
University of Florida
 laboratory testing, 859
 Necropsy Report Form, 977
 serologic testing, 403
University of Tennessee, serologic testing, 403
Unken relfex, 176. *See also* Amphibians
Unopette, usage, 951
Unpremedicated direct orotracheal intubation, 997
Unspeciated *Trichophyton*, 221
Up-and-down bob, 171

Upper alimentary tract disease (UATD), 924
 clinical signs, 925
Upper eyelids, anatomy, 325
Upper respiratory disease, herpes-like virus (reports), 393
Upper respiratory tract disease (URTD), 816, 866f, 931
 clinical disease, 932-933
 diagnosis, 933-934
 pathology, 933
 prognosis, 935-936
 transmission, 931-932
 treatment, 934-935
Uranyl acetate, 398f, 409f
Urates
 evaluation, 881-882
 laboratory investigation, 490f
 salt types, 767f
Urate stones, 766
Urea cycle, defects, 812
Ureter, connection, 137
Urethral catheter, endoscope-guided placement, 882
Uric acid, 143f, 462, 652
 derivation, 794
 presence, 794
 production (decrease), allopurinal (impact), 798f
 secretion, 141
Uricemia, 259
Uricotelic reptiles, 765
Urinalysis, 525, 1055. *See also* Pneumonia
 technique, 882
Urinary bladders. *See* Chelonians
 existence, 135t, 137
 neck, entrance, 137
 presence, 671-672
 prolapse, 753
 portion, 753
 visualization, 671
Urinary calculi, 763
 constituents, 769t
 detection, gold standard, 765-766
 diagnosis, 765-769
 effects, 765
 presentations. *See* California Desert Tortoise
 treatment, 769-770
Urinary formation, etiology, 763-765
Urinary stasis, 259
Urinary system
 diagnostic techniques, 525-528
 dysfunction, 586
 tumors, 301t, 305t, 313t
Urinary tract
 necropsy examination, 577
 ultrasound evaluation, 488
Urine. *See* Cachectic reptile
 beta-hydroxybutyrate, increase, 883
 diagnostic imaging. *See* Pneumonia
 dipstick evaluation. *See* Pneumonia
 dipstick ketone assays, 883
 evaluation, 881-882
 examination. *See* Voided urine
 flora, qualitative/quantitative data, 885
 gross evaluation, 882
 laboratory investigation, 490f
 microbiology, 525

Urine—cont'd
 microscopic examination, 767
 observation. *See* Acidic urine
 pH, 882-883
 sediment evaluation, 884-889
 specific gravity, 884
Urine-filled bladder, impression, 751
Urobilinogen, analysis, 884
Urodela (order), 941
Urodeum, ureteral papilla. *See* Male snakes
Urogenital papillae, avoidance, 537
Urogenital tract, viewpoint, 668
Urolithiasis (stones), 577
Uroliths
 lamellar onion-like construction, 764f
 presence/reports, 763f
 radiographic appearance, 764f
 space-occupying lesion, 766f
Uromastix Lizards
 cloacocolonic lavage, 522f
 treatment, case report, 437
Uromastyx aegyptius. *See* Egyptian Spiny-tailed Lizard; Spiny-tailed Lizard
Uromastyx benti. *See* Rainbow Uromastyx
Uromastyx spp.
 biting plates, 145
 stomach/intestine radiopacity, 157f
Uromastyx (*Uromastyx* sp.), cystic calculi, 770f
Uropeltidae, 43f, 45
Uropeltis phillipsi. *See* Sri Lankan Shield-tailed Snake
Uroplatus fimbriatus. *See* Madagascar Leaf-tailed Gecko
URTD. *See* Upper respiratory tract disease
U.S. Endangered Species Act (ESA) (1973), 1045f
U.S. Fish and Wildlife Service (USFWS), 1049
U.S. Food and Drug Administration (FDA), 1019, 1045
 ban, implementation, 642
 definition. *See* Foods
USFWS. *See* U.S. Fish and Wildlife Service
Utah, herpetological societies, 7t
UV. *See* Ultraviolet
Uveal tract, 338-339
 anatomy, 338
Uveitis, 338-339

V

Vaccines, usage, 657
Vacuum-assisted closure, 899
Vagal-vagal response, 241
Valgus deformation, 965
Value establishment, method, 3
Vaponna, usage, 1068
Vaporizers, usage, 31
Varanids, heart (caudal placement), 191f
Varanus doreanus. *See* Blue-tailed Monitor
Varanus exanthematicus. *See* Savannah Monitor Lizard
Varanus griseus. *See* Desert Monitor
Varanus komodoensis. *See* Komodo Dragon
Varanus nioloticus. *See* Nile Monitor
Varanus olivaceous. *See* Gray's Monitor Lizard
Varanus salvadorii. *See* Crocodile Monitor

Varanus salvator. See Water Monitor
Varanus salvator salvator. See Asian Water Monitor
Varanus spp. See Monitor Lizard
Varus deformation, 965
Vascular clips
 availability, 583f
 insertion, 597f
Vascular necrosis, 210
Vas deferens, 529
Vasodilators, 185
Vasovagal response, 502
VAV. See Ventral abdominal vein
VEE. See Venezuelan equine encephalomyelitis
Vegetables
 consumption, 267
 cooking, 38
 mixture, 371
Veiled Chameleon *(Chamaeleo calyptratus)*
 basking light, closeness, 251f
 carpal joints, nodules (presence), 794f
 casque, surface area-to-volume ratio (increase), 251f
 chronic renal failure, 477f
 crouching/belly-hugging, case report, 288
 dehydration, 281f
 digits, difficulty, 794f
 dystrophic mineralization, 477f
 epidermis/superficial dermis, fungal proliferation, 224f
 gout, 281f
 gravid ova, 483f
 growth, 252f
 protein deficiency, 285f
 radiograph projections, 483f
 sepsis, development, 281f
 shedding, multiple pieces, 779f
 splenic imprint, 467f
 stress coloration, 252f
Vena cava, gonad attachment, 596
Venemoid surgery, 612-613
 completion, 613f
Venezuelan equine encephalomyelitis (VEE), 410-411
Venipuncture, 513-516
 attempts, 949
 sites, 514
  cotton-tipped applicator, usage, 950
  usage, 61-62
Venom, impact. See Digestion
Venom duct, double ligation, 612
Venomous animal bites
 first aid. See Code 1 venomous animal bites; Code 2 venomous animal bites
 procedures, 1053-1054
 management, emergency protocols (development), 1051-1060
 plan, 1052-1053
 protocols. See Code 1 venomous animal bites, protocols; Code 2 venomous animal bites, protocols
Venomous animals, 1074-1706
 differentiation, 1052
 escape plan, 1053
 recapture, protocols (example), 1053t
Venomous bite emergency first aid kit, 1055t

Venomous Code 1 and 2 reptiles, examples, 1051t
Venomous copperhead *(Agkistrodon contortrix)*, anesthetization, 496f
Venomous reptiles
 antivenoms, acquisition, 1052f
 bites
  improper handling, 1052f
  pressure wrap, application, 1055f
 emergency numbers table, example, 1053t
 hazards, 1027-1028
 medical treatment plan, 1054-1055, 1060
Venomous snakes, 1027t
 bites, first aid, 1028t
Venomous species
 considerations, 1060
 emergency protocols, 1051
Venous sinuses, identification, 590f
Ventilation, disadvantages, 917
Ventilators, usage, 547f
Ventral abdominal vein (VAV). See Crocodilians; Lizards
 avoidance, 588f
 bilateral pelvic veins, confluence, 587f
 blood flow, 589f
 confluence, 587
 mesovasorum support, 588f
 venous access sites, 447
Ventral coccygeal vein, venous access sites, 447
Ventral coelomic membrane, incision/manipulation, 591f
Ventral erythema, relationship. See Red leg
Ventral midline
 abdominal vein, presence, 587
 usage, 587
Ventral scutes, movements (observation), 182f
Ventricle, division, 125
Ventricular enlargement, 187f
Ventricular hypertrophy, 187f
Vermicillia anulata. See Bandy Bandy
Vermiculite, usage, 367f
Vertebrae, fusion, 893
Vertebral column
 exotoses, 856
 stiffness, 910
Vertebral scutes, 972
Vertebrate prey, 262-263
 nutrient composition, 262t
 nutritional composition, factors, 262
 risks, 262-263
 scenting, 263
Vertebrates, proliferative spinal osteopathy (etiologies), 908t
Vertebrobasilar arterial insufficiency, 436
Vesicular dermatitis. See Florida Kingsnake
Vesicular diseases, 202-203
Vestigial pelvis, spurs (relationship), 51f
Veterinary cutable plates, usage, 604
Veterinary Information Network (VIN), 12
Veterinary journals, 10
Veterinary medicinal products, 1042-1043
Veterinary practice, 1042-1043
Veterinary professional law, 1042

Veterinary therapies. See Alternative veterinary therapies; Complementary veterinary therapies; Manual veterinary therapies
Vetronics Small Animal Ventilator, 448
Vet thermoplastic, 602f
Vi-Drape Adhesive, 585
VIN. See Veterinary Information Network
Vincristine, administration, 318
Viper, *Sarocystis* sp., 348f
Viperidae, 46
 longevity, 56t
Viperinae, longevity, 56t
Viral agents, 1024
Viral cultures. See Brain
 obtaining, 572
Viral diseases, 153, 1147. See also Dermatology
Viral etiology, disease, 412
Viral-induced disease, 391
Viral infections, 248-249, 335-336. See also Corneas; Subclinical viral infection
Viral isolation, 153
Viral nucleic acid (discovery), PCR-based assay (usage), 411
Viral pneumonia, 872-873
Viral stomatitis, 927-928
Viral transmission, routes, 399
Virginia, herpetological societies, 7t
Virio damsela, recovery, 184
Virions
 presence, electron microscopy (usage), 859-860
 spread, 396
Virology, 391
Virus-damaged epithelial tissues, 394
Viruses
 activity, documentation. See Birds; Reptiles
 isolation. See TH-1 cells
 strains, relationship. See Adenovirus
 susceptibility, 392
Virus-neutralizing antibodies, 411
Viscera
 dorsal view, 577f
 ventral view, 576f, 577f
Visceral bacterial cultures, obtaining, 572
Visual tracts. See Retinas
Vitamin A
 deficiency, 289, 475f, 831
 dietary source, 289
 dosages (injectable/oral), 289t
 high doses, impact. See Tortoises
 injections, 326
 supplementation, 954-955
 toxicity, 1069
Vitamin B deficiencies, 965
Vitamin C deficiency, 273
Vitamin D
 deficiency, 475f
 toxicity, 287, 1069
Vitamin D_3
 balance, 954
 deficiency, 285-289
  signs, 286
  necessity, 30

Vitamin E
  deficiencies, 111, 289-290, 692
  dosages, 290
  supplement, 277
Vitamin K
  deficiency, 562
  intoxication, 292
Vitamin K_1, administration, 562
Vitamins
  deficiencies, 291
  intoxication, 291-292
  supplements
    mixture, 705
    need, 39
Vitellogenesis, 260
Vitt, LJ, 12
Vivarium
  design, 942-943
  disinfectants, usage, 1085
  sunlight, receiving, 964
Viviparity, 377
  documentation, 365
Viviparous species
  maternal care, 379
  ultrasonographic appearance, 386-387
Voided urine, examination, 525. *See also* Pneumonia
Volume depletion, cause, 543-544
Volume-driven mechanical ventilator, usage. *See* Box Turtles
Vomiting, 939. *See also* Snakes
  cryptosporidiosis, impact, 939f
  differentials/diagnosis, 939-940
  treatment, 940
Voriconazole, 226
V trough, balance/usage, 585

W

Walking position, 602f
Warwick, C, 12
Wasting, 347
Watchglass, 327
Water
  absorption coefficient, 619f
  adequacy. *See* Tap water
  balance, 462
  coliform bacteria, absence (requirement), 259
  conservation, 142-143
  containers. *See* Steep-sided water containers
  disorders, 280-281
  homeostasis, 964
  impact. *See* Interstitial integrity
  importance/access, 258-259
  loading, 878
  misting, advantage, 782
  movement, 540-541
  providing, process, 37
  quality. *See* Amphibians
  regulation, 27
  shift, 542f, 543f
  soaks, 833
  substance, metals/contaminants (upper limits), 259t
  substrate preference, 32

Water Dragon (*Physignathus cocincinus*)
  chronic ileus, 488f
  oviduct, shelled eggs, 594f
  tongue muscle, tapeworm larva (presence), 928f
Water Dragon (*Physignathus* sp.)
  rostral damage, 201f
  tarsal plate, 325f
Water Monitor (*Varanus salvator*)
  distal tongue, loss, 925f
  kidneys, 138f
Watersnakes (*Nerodia harteri harteri*), outdoor enclosures, 36
Water-soluble vitamin A, impact, 834
Water Wizard, usage, 96
WATO. *See* Welfare of Animals Transport Order
Waxworms
  food, 285f
  obesity, 806
WBC. *See* White blood cell
WEE. *See* Western equine encephalomyelitis
Weight
  accuracy, importance, 507f
  examination, 491
  loss, 156, 292, 816. *See also* Chronic weight loss; Lizards; Snakes
    case report, 283
  reduction programs, 282-283
Welfare laws, 1043-1044
  national legislation, 1043
  regional legislation, 1043
  transportation, concerns, 1043-1044
Welfare of Animals Transport Order (WATO), 1044
West African Dwarf Crocodile (*Osteolaemus tetraspis*)
  restraint, 513f
  venipuncture sites, 516f
Western equine encephalitis, life cycle, 1024
Western equine encephalomyelitis (WEE), 410-411
Western Foxsnakes (*Elaphe vulpina*), male combat, 172f
Western Veterinary Conference, 13
West Nile Virus (WNV), 410, 709-710. *See also* American Alligator; Crocodilians
  reports, 1024
Wet/dry enclosure setup. *See* Snakes
Wet-to-dry bandages, usage, 897
Wet-to-dry sterile bandages, application. *See* Green Iguana
Wheezing, occurrence, 222
White blood cell (WBC) count, 373, 949. *See* Savannah Monitor Lizard
  usage, 951
White muscle disease, 182
White rubber sealing bonnet, 550
White's Tree Frog (*Pelodryas caerulea*), embryonated nematode ova (feces location), 961f
Whole blood transfusion, 545
Whole blood twitching. *See* Chelonians
Wild-caught breeding stock, 1017
Wild-caught reptiles, exposure, 1017
Wild Green Iguanas (*Iguana iguana*), folivores, 71

Wildlife Rehabilitation Database (Tufts University), 12
Wild reptiles
  prohibited/controlled activities, relationship, 1033, 1040
  protected species, 1033
  protection, 1033, 1040
Wild tortoises
  mycoplasmosis, management issues, 935-936
  research, 936
Wilkinson, R, 12
Winter cool-down, 256
Wire retrieval basket, 553
Wisconsin, herpetological societies, 7t
Withdrawal reflex, 917
Withdrawn limbs, extension, 510
WNV. *See* West Nile Virus
Wolvekamp, P, 12
Wonderlite, 1083
Wood-base substrates, complications, 633
Wood Turtle (*Clemmys insculpta*), protection (Maine), 1032f
World Chelonian Trust Newsletter, 10
Wounds
  bandages, 748-749
  cleansing, 920
  healing, 581
  management. *See* Topical wound management
Wright, KM, 12
Wright's Giemsa, 838
Wright's stain, usage, 454f-459f, 465, 466f-467f
Wyoming, herpetological societies, 7t

X

Xanthomatosis, 245-246
Xantusia vigilis. *See* Yucca Night Lizard
Xenopeltidae, 45-46
  longevity, 56t
Xenophidiidae, 46
Xenosauridae, 60
Xiphoid process. *See* Sternum
XLD. *See* Xylose-lysine-desoxycholate
XLT-4. *See* Xylose-lysine-tergitol 4
Xylose-lysine-desoxycholate (XLD) agar, usage, 900
Xylose-lysine-tergitol 4 (XLT-4), usage, 900, 903

Y

YAG. *See* Neodymium-yttrium aluminum garnet
Yang, definition, 429t
Yeasts, 218
Yellow-bellied Water Snake (*Nerodia erythrogaster flavigaster*), 44f
  venom, characteristic, 1055f
Yellow-foot Tortoise (*Geochelone denticulata*)
  eating refusal (stomatitis), 278f
  feeding trial, 260f
  Nematophila sp., 351f
  pharyngostomy tube, placement, 278f
Yellow fungus disease, 220
Yellow-headed Red-footed Tortoise (*Geochelone carbonara*)
  bilateral anophthalmia, 924f
  cleft palate, 924f

Yellow-headed Red-footed Tortoise—cont'd
  congenital defect, 924f
  prolapse oviduct, 751f
Yellow pages, usage. *See* Reptile
  practice
Yellow Ratsnake *(Elaphe obsoleta
  quadrivitatta)*
  hematologic values, 1106
  serum biochemical values, 1106
Yemen Chameleon *(Chamaeleo calyptraptus)*
  retrobulbar venous plexus,
   trauma/engorgement, 506f
  tibia, bone marrow aspiration, 517f
Yews, impact, 1706
Yin, definition, 429t
Yolk coelomitis, 596f
  result, 595
Yucca Night Lizard *(Xantusia vigilis),*
  parental care, 366

Z

Ziehl-Neelsen (ZN) stain, usage, 234
Zigzag lesions, 708
Zinc toxicosis, 247, 1069-1070
  action, mechanism, 1069-1070
  clinical signs, 1070
  treatment, 1070
ZN. *See* Ziehl-Neelsen
Zolazapem
  administration, 447
  usage, 444
Zoological Society of San Diego, chelonian
  herbivore/carnivore-omnivore gel
  diets (usage), 91t
  nutrient analysis, 92t
Zoologic parks
  large collections, 1013-1014
  preventative husbandry/health,
   1013-1014

Zoologic parks—cont'd
  quarantine procedures, 1013
  safety, 1014
ZooMed. *See* Reptisun lights
Zoo Med Laboratories, 1083
Zoonoses, 1017. *See also* Bacterial zoonoses
  prevention, 1018t
  Salmonella serotype, implication, 1019t
  source, 490-491
Zoonotic pathogens, isolation, 1023t
Zophobas mori. See Superworms
Zug, GR, 12
Zygomycetous fungi, 224
Zygomycosis, 1023-1024